THE DEFENSE POLICIES
OF NATIONS

THE DEFENSE POLICIES OF NATIONS

A Comparative Study

SECOND EDITION

Edited by

Douglas J. Murray and Paul R. Viotti

THE JOHNS HOPKINS UNIVERSITY PRESS
Baltimore and London

The Johns Hopkins University Press
701 West 40th Street
Baltimore, Maryland 21211
The Johns Hopkins Press Ltd., London

The views and conclusions expressed by military and other government personnel in material contained in this volume are those of the authors and not necessarily those of the U.S. Air Force Academy, the Department of Defense, any particular service thereof, or any other government agency.

The paper used in this publication meets the minimum requirements of American National Standard for Information Sciences—Permanence of Paper for Printed Library Materials, ANSI Z39.48-1984.

Library of Congress Cataloging-in-Publication Data

The Defense policies of nations: a comparative study/edited by Douglas
J. Murray and Paul R. Viotti.—2nd ed.
    p.   cm.
  Bibliography: p.
  Includes index.
  ISBN 0-8018-3599-2.—ISBN 0-8018-3600-X (pbk.)
  1. Military policy—Case studies. 2. Armed Forces—Case studies.
I. Murray, Douglas J. II. Viotti, Paul R.
UA11.D387 1989
355′.0335—dc20   89-7947
                                                              CIP

To Richard F. Rosser and the late Fred Sondermann,
whose contributions to international relations and
security studies have given impetus to the development
of the comparative study of defense policy

Contents

Acknowledgments

As would be expected in an enterprise of this magnitude, our debts are many. Not only do we thank all of our contributors for their efforts, but also we wish to acknowledge the collaboration of Harold Maynard during the early and very important conceptualization phase of the first edition that was published in 1982. In soliciting manuscripts for both editions of this volume, we have quite consciously sought both a mix of civilian and military authors and a similar blend of American and foreign contributors. Not only was such a balance our own preference, but it was also the consensus that emerged from a survey of over 400 academics and policy makers.

For both editions we have relied on many others for help. We appreciate the efforts of our research assistants on this edition—Greg Giletti, Monte Kleman, Greg Mang, Miten Merchant, Paul Rendessy, Tim Robinson, Brian Ruhm, and Chad Sevigny. We are indebted to our colleagues who so willingly gave of their time to read and comment on manuscripts and engage in the laborious task of proofreading: Bill Barry, Ed Boring, Barrett Clay, Chuck Costanzo, Phil Davis, Ginny Dietvorst, Nelson Drew, Tom Drohan, Steve Else, Pete Hays, Gwen Hall, Lynn Hollerbach, Pete Jordan, Bob Stephan, Jeff Larsen, Ken Rogers, Brenda Vallance, and Al Van Tassel. We acknowledge Bruce Doyle's support, the substantive contributions of our copy editor, Peter Dreyer, and the editorial assistance of Henry Tom and his assistant, Denise Dankert, both of the Johns Hopkins University Press.

Secretarial support was also invaluable. In particular, we would like to acknowledge the efforts of Deborah Kurrle, Kay McGrew, Charlotte Bond, Kay Schneider, and Wendie Sumrell. We would also like to thank Beverlee Carlisle, Barbara Feduska, Gertrude Pollok, and Chris Skully. Illustrations were prepared in the first edition by Richard Mohr and in this edition by Mickiko Goodman and John Wendt, with typesetting by Teresa Linn.

Finally, but certainly one of the most important considerations that has made this effort possible, was financial backing for copyright permissions and clerical support from the Johns Hopkins University Press and the Air Force Academy's Academic Support Fund. In addition, a contribution in 1979 by the National Security Education Program at New York University, directed at the time by the late Frank Trager, enabled us to convene a meeting of our authors prior to the first edition. The National Defense University provided a convenient location and excellent facilities for a similar conference in 1986.

Contributors

The Editors

DOUGLAS J. MURRAY, permanent professor and head of the Department of Political Science at the U.S. Air Force Academy, is the author and editor of articles and studies on U.S.-Canadian relations and other defense issues. His most recent work is *We Stand On Guard for Thee: The Theory and Practice of Canadian Defense Policy*. Murray has a Ph.D. from the University of Texas at Austin.

PAUL R. VIOTTI, professor and deputy head of the Political Science Department at the U.S. Air Force Academy, is the author and editor of articles and studies on national security and international relations, including *International Relations Theory: Realism, Pluralism, Globalism* and *Conflict and Arms Control*. Viotti has a Ph.D. from the University of California, Berkeley.

Country Studies

WILLIAM E. BERRY, JR., currently director of Field Studies Programs and assistant director of National Security Policy at the National War College in Washington, D.C., previously taught in the Department of Political Science at the U.S. Air Force Academy and has had extensive experience in Asia with assignments in Vietnam, the Philippines, and the Republic of Korea. Berry has been selected to be air attaché in Malaysia. A Cornell Ph.D., Berry has written many journal articles and chapters in edited books on U.S. security interests in Asia and other Asian-related topics. Westview Press is publishing his book on the Philippine base negotiations.

MICHAEL J. DZIEDZIC earned a Ph.D. from the University of Texas at Austin. A tenured faculty member at the U.S. Air Force Academy, he recently served, while on sabbatical, as a research fellow at the International Institute for Strategic Studies in London. He has particular expertise in Latin American politics and has done extensive field research in the region leading to a number of publications.

JERROLD F. ELKIN holds a J.D. from Columbia University and a Ph.D. from the University of Pennsylvania. Formerly an analyst with the Defense Intelligence Agency and subsequently a member of the Air Force Academy's Department of Political Science. Elkin has contributed extensively to the literature on Indian and South Asian defense policy.

JOHN E. ENDICOTT, former deputy head of the U.S. Air Force Academy's Department of Political Science, is director of research at the National Defense University in Washington.

The author of *Japan's Nuclear Option*, coauthor of *The Politics of East Asia*, and coeditor of the fourth edition of *American Defense Policy*, he earned a Ph.D. from the Fletcher School of Law and Diplomacy at Tufts University.

DAVID GREENWOOD is the director of the Centre for Defence Studies at the University of Aberdeen, Scotland. He is an economist with degrees from the University of Liverpool. A former member of the Royal Air Force, he has served as economic adviser to the Ministry of Defence, as visiting fellow at the International Institute for Strategic Studies, and in several governmental advisory posts concerned with national security and arms control. The author of numerous publications in these fields, Greenwood is particularly noted for his work on defense budgeting.

ROBERT H. GROMOLL, coauthor of the article on American defense policy, currently is scholar in residence at the U.S. Arms Control and Disarmament Agency. He has written articles about the strategic defense initiative (SDI), arms control verification, and Middle Eastern politics. He has also served as a professor at the University of Pittsburgh. Gromoll earned a Ph.D. from the School of International Service at American University.

WILLIAM R. HEATON, JR., holds a Ph.D. in political science from the University of California, Berkeley. Formerly a faculty member at the U.S. Air Force Academy and the National War College, Heaton is currently a senior analyst with the Central Intelligence Agency. He is the author of numerous articles and books, including *The Politics of East Asia* and *Insurgency in the Modern World*. Heaton has travelled extensively in China and has lived in Hong Kong.

MARK VEBLEN KAUPPI completed the chapter on South African defense policy while he was a professor at the University of Colorado, Colorado Springs. He is currently a political scientist on the faculty of the Defense Intelligence College in Washington, D.C. Kauppi

holds a Ph.D. from the University of Colorado, Boulder. He is an editor of and contributor to *International Relations Theory: Realism, Pluralism, Globalism*. Kauppi has also contributed to the literature on ethnicity and on the Soviet role in Africa and the Middle East.

CATHERINE MCARDLE KELLEHER directs the Center for International Security Studies at the University of Maryland. Kelleher's governmental experience includes a position on the National Security Council staff during the Carter Administration and a series of consulting assignments in the office of the assistant secretary of defense for international affairs, the Arms Control and Disarmament Agency, and the Department of the Army. She has also been on the faculties of the University of Denver and the National War College. Kelleher earned a Ph.D. in Political Science at the Massachusetts Institute of Technology.

LAWRENCE J. KORB, former assistant secretary of defense for manpower, reserve affairs and logistics, and former dean of the Graduate School of Public and International Affairs at the University of Pittsburgh, is now director of the Center for Public Policy Education at the Brookings Institution. He has also been a faculty member at the Naval War College and director of Defense Policy Studies at the American Enterprise Institute for Public Policy Research (AEI) in Washington, D.C. Prior to assuming this position, he also served as coeditor of the AEI *Foreign Policy and Defense Review*. Among his many contributions to the national security field are: *The Joint Chiefs of Staff*, *The Price of Preparedness*, *The System for Educating Military Officers*, and *The Fall and Rise of the Pentagon: American Defense Policies in the 1970s*. Korb holds a Ph.D. from the State University of New York at Albany.

BARD E. O'NEILL is the director of Middle East Studies at the National War College and an adjunct professor in the Department of Politics at Catholic University. He is the author or editor of several books and numerous articles including *Armed Struggle in Palestine* and *Insurgency in the Modern World*. O'Neill earned a Ph.D. from the Graduate School of International Studies, University of Denver, and is currently working on a manuscript analyzing the nature of insurgency.

JOSEPH C. RALLO is currently associate professor of political science at Michigan Technological University. He is the author of *The Technological Politics of Alliance Relations* and *Defending Europe in the 1990s*, as well as a number of articles on West European politics. Rallo was a NATO-Fulbright recipient in 1987. He holds a Ph.D. from Syracuse University.

ANDREW RITEZEL, coauthor of the article on Indian defense policy, is a U.S. Army officer with particular expertise on southern Asia. In addition to his army assignments, he also has served as an analyst with the Defense Intelligence Agency.

ALAN NED SABROSKY, director of studies at the Strategic Studies Institute and holder of the General of the Army Douglas MacArthur Chair of Research at the U.S. Army War College, also teaches at Georgetown University and the Johns Hopkins School of Advanced International Studies. An adjunct senior fellow of political-military studies at the Center for Strategic and International Studies, he also has served on the faculty at the U.S. Military Academy at West Point. Sabrosky earned a Ph.D. from the University of Michigan.

PETER N. SCHMITZ, formerly a branch chief in NATO's international military staff's Plans and Policy Division, is currently commander of a Pershing I missile wing in the Federal Republic of Germany. He has served in various assignments in the German Air Force and in the Ministry of Defense, and was an international research fellow at the National Defense University, Washington, D.C. He graduated from the Federal Armed Forces Command and Staff College in Hamburg and from the NATO Defense College in Rome.

EDWARD L. WARNER III, now a senior defense analyst for the RAND Corporation, holds a Ph.D. from Princeton University. Formerly a faculty member in the Department of Political Science at the U.S. Air Force Academy and later an assistant air attaché in Moscow, he also headed the staff group that assists the air force chief of staff in Washington. Warner currently conducts studies on U.S. and Soviet defense and arms control policies. Among his many publications is *The Military in Contemporary Soviet Politics: An Institutional Analysis*.

Bibliographic Essays

HAROLD COLSON is currently a public services and collection development librarian at the University of California at San Diego. Colson's other positions have included social science reference librarian at Auburn University's Ralph Brown Draughon Library, government documents librarian at Stetson University's duPont-Ball Library, and instructor and staff officer at the U.S. Army Ordnance Center and School, Aberdeen Proving Ground, Maryland. Colson earned his M.A. in Latin American Studies from Indiana University.

THOMAS A. DROHAN, a specialist in East Asian politics, is an assistant professor in the Air Force Academy's Department of Political Science. He has an M.A. from the University of Hawaii's East-West Center and is currently working on a doctorate in political science at Princeton University.

CHRIS L. JEFFERIES is currently assigned to the Military Airlift Command headquarters as director of administration. He has had assignments as a staff group member in the office of the secretary of the air force, as a defense policy analyst and planner with the U.S. Mission to NATO, and as a faculty member in the Political Science Department at the U.S. Air Force Academy. He has a master's degree from the University of Pittsburgh and frequently contributes articles on public administration to professional journals. Jefferies also has expertise in the politics of the defense budgetary process.

JEFFREY A. LARSEN, formerly an assistant professor of political science at the U.S. Air Force Academy, is currently pursuing a Ph.D. in political science at Princeton University. He earned an M.A. in national security affairs and West European area studies from the Naval Postgraduate School in Monterey, California. Larsen has written articles on Spanish politics, Danish security policy, and U.S. environmental policy as it relates to military deployments in West Germany.

RICHARD J. LATHAM is a career officer in the U.S. Air Force who is a specialist in East Asian, particularly Chinese, politics and regional foreign and defense policies. He has a Ph.D. from the University of Washington. Latham has served as air attaché in Hong Kong and as a member of the political science faculty at the U.S. Air Force Academy.

JAY L. LORENZEN, an assistant professor of political science at the U.S. Air Force Academy, is currently pursuing a doctorate at Denver University's Graduate School of International Studies. Lorenzen also studied as an Olmsted Scholar at the University of Tübingen in West Germany. Lorenzen has done environmental policy studies in Europe. He earned his M.A. in international affairs from the Fletcher School of Law and Diplomacy at Tufts University.

JEROME V. MARTIN is a faculty member in the Department of Military Studies at the U.S. Air Force Academy and has particular expertise in Soviet defense policy. He has served as an intelligence analyst in the Federal Republic of Germany and in Thailand. He is completing his doctorate at the University of Indiana.

MARY PAYROW-OLIA holds a master's degree in political science. Formerly a faculty member at the Air Force Academy, she has particular expertise on the politics of Middle Eastern countries. Also an air force intelligence officer, Payrow-Olia is currently an analyst at the U.S. Central Command.

KENNETH A. ROGERS is an associate professor and director of comparative and area studies in the Political Science Department at the U.S. Air Force Academy. He is a Soviet and East European area specialist and has served as a post-doctoral fellow at the University of Edinburgh, Scotland. Rogers travels to the Soviet Union where he conducts arms control inspections as a U.S. team chief. He earned a Ph.D. from the American University in Washington, D.C.

FRANK L. ROSA is currently an associate professor of political science at the U.S. Air Force Academy. He also has served as a senior teaching fellow at the University of Notre Dame, where he holds a Ph.D. in International Relations. He has taught courses in Latin American politics, American defense policy, and political violence. Rosa has particular expertise in the defense planning process, strategic defense policy, and arms control issues.

MARION DAVID TUNSTALL is presently assigned as an intelligence officer with the Tactical Air Command in Norfolk, Virginia. He has served as a faculty member in the Department of Political Science at the U.S. Air Force Academy and has also taught as an adjunct member of faculties at Florida State University and the University of Colorado, Colorado Springs. Tunstall has particular expertise in Latin American politics and has served with the U.S. Southern Command in Panama. He holds a Ph.D. from the University of Virginia.

Part One

DEFENSE POLICY
The International Environment

Introduction

DEFENSE POLICY IN COMPARATIVE PERSPECTIVE

Douglas J. Murray and Paul R. Viotti

In the introduction to the first edition of this work in 1982 we wrote that the field of comparative defense or national security policy[1] was relatively new. In the years since the first edition, growth of the field has continued and interest in the subject matter has increased steadily.

To our knowledge, the first study that introduced this field in America was a volume based on contributions to a 1973 conference and edited by our colleagues Barry Horton, Edward L. Warner, and Anthony Rogerson.[2] Subsequently, there has been substantial evidence of growing interest in this field. In 1975, for example, John Baylis and several of his colleagues published a volume of comparative essays (which they updated in a 1987 revised edition) that examined the defense policies of the United States, the Soviet Union, China, the United Kingdom, and France.[3] In 1978, another effort to advance this growing field was made by a well-attended conference of the International Studies Association's section on military studies, the entire proceedings of which were devoted to comparative defense policy.[4]

Our own effort, of which this is the second edition, was published by Johns Hopkins University Press in 1982. Host in 1986 for a preliminary conference of our contributors to this edition was the National Defense University, which has also encouraged scholarly work on the comparative study of defense policy. There has also been some work in the field on Europe and other regions. A noteworthy example is a volume on European defense policies edited by Catherine Kelleher and Gale Mattox.[5]

A related enterprise has been the study of comparative military-political sociology, led by Morris Janowitz, Charles Moskos, Sam Sarkesian, Catherine Kelleher, and others. A useful product from that endeavor was a 1974 volume edited by Kelleher on "political-military" systems. Another volume, published in 1988 and edited by Moskos and Frank R. Wood, takes a cross-national cut at the military profession and civil-military relations in Great Britain, West Germany, France, Australia, the Netherlands, Greece, Switzerland, and Israel.[6] The semiannual *Journal of Political and Military Sociology* and the Inter-University Seminar's quarterly, *Armed Forces and Society*, have been primary vehicles for promoting further research in this area. Other scholarly journals dealing with comparative defense studies include *International Security, Defence Analysis,* and *Comparative Strategy.* Finally, credit must be given to works produced primarily in the 1950s and 1960s which examine military elites, particularly in the Third World, where they are often seen as agents of modernization and political development.[7]

This work is built upon the foundation laid by these earlier studies. At the same time, it attempts to expand this emerging field further by applying to additional countries the same framework for analysis used in the first edition. Our attempt is to develop (1) the conceptualization or paradigm that organizes knowledge in this field, and (2) the methodology to study it. What follows, then, is not theory, but, we hope, the prelude to it. It is the basis upon which hypotheses for comparative study can be constructed and tested.

Approaches to the Comparative Study of Defense Policy

In the period since 1973, several approaches to comparative defense studies have appeared. One such approach is to select such recurring issues as military doctrine, force posture, the decision-making process, and weapons acquisition and then to compare and contrast how different countries deal with these issues. This, in essence, was the organizational device used in the 1973 edition of *Comparative Defense Policy*.

An alternative approach, used by Aaron Wildavsky and others, is to focus upon the budget.[8] Two of the contributors to this volume—Lawrence Korb and David Greenwood—have a demonstrated preference for

such a methodology. Greenwood has even asserted that expenditure is policy. To the extent that policy involves the allocation of scarce resources expressed in monetary terms, the budget is a handy device for comparative description. Understanding how the budget comes to be, furthermore, engages one in the politics of the budgetary process—a relevant focus for the theoretical task of developing defense policy explanation.

Of course, a substantial limitation associated with any budget-oriented methodology is data availability. Intentionally or unintentionally, some countries conceal defense expenditures in other budget categories; others do not publish such data at all. Indeed, much of what we say we know of Soviet budget allocations is inferred from observed force posture, weapons acquisition, and research and development programs. Needless to say, numerous assumptions are made in estimating the Soviet budget. As a result, conclusions are almost always subject to considerable dispute.

The approach that we have adopted in this volume is a "country study" one that uses a common framework for analysis. This framework is founded upon our perception of defense policy as a dynamic process that can best be understood by studying it from several different dimensions. Samuel Huntington writes that defense policy is Janus-like—existing in the worlds of both international and domestic politics.[9] At the same time, it involves a threat frequently generated in the international politico-economic environment and responded to in the domestic or national one. Glenn Snyder adds a further dimension by arguing that national security policy involves two concepts— deterrence and defense. He writes:

Essentially, deterrence means discouraging the enemy from taking military action by posing for him a prospect of cost and risk which outweighs his prospective gain. Defense means reducing our own prospective costs and risks in the event that deterrence fails. Deterrence works on the enemy's intentions; the deterrent value of military forces is their effect in reducing the likelihood of enemy military moves.

Defense reduces the enemy's capability to damage or deprive us; the defense value of military forces is their effect in mitigating the adverse consequences for us of possible enemy moves, whether such consequences are counted as losses of territory or war damage. . . .

Perhaps the crucial difference between deterrence and defense is that deterrence is primarily a peacetime objective while defense is a wartime value. Deterrence value and defense value are directly employed in different time periods.[10]

Given these views of national security policy concerns, we constructed a four-part framework that we asked our contributors to use to describe the defense policy of an individual state. The four parts are: (1) the international environment as it is perceived by the state; (2) the particular national objectives, strategy, and military force employment doctrine of that state; (3) the state's defense policy-making process; and (4) various recurring issues—force posture, the use of force, weapons acquisition, arms control, and civil-military relations. The framework is discussed in greater detail in the next section.

As editors, we are quite pleased that the contributors have been willing to follow this framework as closely as they have. We make no claim to have developed a comprehensive theory of comparative defense or national security policy any more than this has been achieved in other fields of inquiry in political science. Nevertheless, after almost a decade of using the framework in classrooms and in research at a number of institutions, we believe we have identified at least some of the important variables or factors that would likely be part of such a theory.

A Framework for Analysis

The security dilemma in which all states find themselves (and with which all governments must cope) arises from the absence of any authority over states—no guarantor of order among states. The defense policy of any state, then, is closely tied to its position within what we refer to as an international system of interacting states. This international environment can be understood as both the source of "opportunities" the state may wish to pursue and the source of "threats" to its security. Certainly, it is our view that the study of a country's defense policy should begin with an assessment of the country's position within the international system.

The second part of our organizational outline or framework conforms fairly closely to a rational actor model of national security policy decision making. Given national objectives, possessing certain capabilities, and facing various constraints, decision makers acting for the state establish national strategy and military force employment doctrine. We do not claim that national strategy, force posture, military doctrine, or other elements of national security policy necessarily conform to this logical pattern. We asked our contributors to examine objectives, strategies, and doctrines in the various countries they chose to study with an eye toward identification of both consistencies and contradictions. It may be, for example, that national strategy, force employment doctrine, and the range of feasible national objectives they serve are determined by capabilities provided by the existing force posture. In short, do strategy and doctrine give rise to a given force posture, or does the latter determine the former? Or, under what circumstances do these different relations obtain? Whatever may be the case, we asked our contributors to provide an exposition of these factors as they saw them in the separate empirical realms they chose to examine.

In the third part of the framework, we address many of the questions raised by the first and second parts. How does the defense policy process actually work? How important are organizational processes or bureaucratic politics among agencies (or bureaucrats representing these agencies)? What is the relative importance of domestic and international factors in determining defense policy outcomes?

Finally, we address what we call the recurring defense policy issues (civil-military relations, weapons acquisition, force posture, arms control, and the use of force), treating them in the context of the conceptual discussion in the first three parts of the framework for analysis. These recurring issues are the substance of defense policy outputs—the decisions and actions made by government officials. Rather than discuss them at the end, some of our contributors exercised the option of incorporating these recurring issues in the main body of the chapter. Often these issues are used as empirical illustrations of conceptual arguments related to the first three parts of the framework. To facilitate any comparative analysis in which our readers might wish to engage, we are including the framework or outline used by our contributors as an appendix to this introduction.

The organization in this book reflects a view strongly held by the editors that any defense or national security study must begin with some consideration of factors external to the state. Thus, we begin our effort with the chapter entitled "Defense Policy: The International Environment." Chapters 2 and 3 are an examination of the American and Soviet superpowers. Following that are country chapters on countries throughout the world. Indeed, we have added a number of countries to this edition to include representative Third World examples that were not included in the first edition. We conclude with a comparative essay that represents our effort to summarize some of the findings in this collective effort. In this regard, we have been assisted by the written work of our contributors, as well as by their comments during conferences held in 1979 and 1986.

One of our aims in this book is to provide readers with bibliographic sources, a choice of methodological tools, and empirical data on various countries in order to facilitate any comparative analysis in which they may wish to engage. In addition to this aim of providing a stimulus to further work in the field of comparative defense policy, we hope that this book will be of use to both policy makers and academics concerned with such matters. The policy maker who wishes a broad overview of a given country's defense policy will find that what he or she wants is in this volume. Those engaged in national security and defense studies should also find this book to be a useful source even if their efforts are concentrated solely on American national security issues, since a cursory knowledge of the defense policies and processes of other states is important in understanding those of the United States.

The student of foreign policy or comparative and international politics should also find use for this volume. Security, though by no means the only important issue, is clearly a core concern in any country's foreign policy. Those interested in political institutions and processes will find considerable resource material in this book for European, East Asian, and Third World studies.

Appendix: Organizational Outline

I. International Environment
   A. Relative Position in the International System
      1. Power and status
      2. Relative capabilities
   B. Threats
      1. Internal and external threats
      2. Nature of the threat (military, political, cultural, economic, etc.)
      3. Source of the threat
      4. Perceptions of the threat by decision makers
      5. Vulnerabilities of the state
   C. Self-perceived Role and Opportunities for the State within the International System (World View)
      1. Role in the past
      2. Changes in the role since World War II
      3. Changes in the role in the next five to ten years
   D. Linkages and Interdependencies
      1. Alliances
      2. Dependencies and interdependencies

II. National Objectives, National Strategy, and Military Doctrine
   A. National Security Objectives
      1. Changes in objectives over time
      2. Degree of consensus or dissensus
         a. Voicing of dissent
         b. Effectiveness of dissent
      3. Direction of objectives
         a. Internal (domestic affairs)
         b. External (state's actions in international system)
         c. Relative importance of internal versus external objectives
   B. Determining National Objectives
      1. Relative importance of ideology, culture, and capabilities

2. The effect of national experiences and "lessons" learned

C. Capabilities for Accomplishing National Security Objectives
   1. Military capabilities
   2. Economic capabilities
   3. Technological capabilities
   4. Political capabilities
   5. Psychosocial capabilities

D. National Strategy for Achieving National Security Objectives
   1. Formally (and publicly) stated versus implicit (must be inferred from observation of actual practice)
   2. Degree of consensus or dissensus among individuals, factions, and bureacratic agencies

E. Domestic Determinants of National Strategy
   1. Political system type
   2. Economic system type
   3. Geography
   4. Public opinion
   5. National "will"
   6. Level of political and economic development
   7. Technology
   8. Population size and educational level
   9. Other factors

F. Military Doctrine (Force Employment Doctrine)
   1. Conventional forces
   2. Nuclear forces
   3. Relation between doctrine and national strategy
   4. Relation between doctrine and national security objectives
   5. Formally (and publicly) stated versus implicit military doctrine (must be inferred from observation of actual practice)
   6. Degree of consensus or dissensus on military doctrine among individuals, factions, and bureaucratic agencies

III. The Defense Decision-Making Process
   A. The Nature of the Process
   B. Degree of Concentration or Fragmentation of Power Domestically
      1. Effect of concentration or fragmentation on comprehensiveness and responsiveness of policy outputs
      2. The important actors in the process
   C. Relative Importance of Bureaucratic Politics in the Process
      1. Domestic and external influences on policy choices
      2. Relative importance of different bureaucratic actors
      3. Resolution of disputes among bureaucratic actors
   D. Relative Importance of Personality in the Process; Other Idiosyncratic Factors
   E. Constraints on Defense Decision Makers
      1. Opposition from other states
      2. Economic and budgetary limitations
      3. Technological insufficiencies
      4. Manpower
         a. Number, age, sex
         b. Conscripted or "volunteer" forces
         c. Reserves
         d. Capability for mobilization of reserves
      5. Military hardware
         a. Weapons systems
         b. Spare parts
         c. Fuel
         d. Logistical capabilities
         e. Defense industry capability
         f. Foreign dependencies
      6. Implementation difficulties (bureaucratic opposition and delaying tactics)
      7. Public opinion, interest groups, and political parties as sources of opposition
      8. Ideological and cultural orientations
      9. Past lessons "learned"
      10. Law and ethical norms

IV. Recurring Issues: Defense Policy Outputs
   A. Civil-Military Relations
      1. Domestic role of the military

2. Alienation or integration of the military and society
3. Recruitment and social groups
4. Social status of the military
B. Weapons Acquisition
  1. Domestic industry production
  2. Technology level (degree of domestic autonomy or foreign dependency)
  3. Foreign supply
    a. Dependency on foreign supply
    b. Reliability of foreign supply
  4. Cooperative production projects
  5. Percentage of GNP spent on weapons acquisition
C. Force Posture
  1. Weapons systems and military units maintained
  2. Deployment
  3. Effectiveness of the recruitment program
  4. Effectiveness of force employment
  5. Responsiveness of force posture to national objectives, strategy, and military doctrine (does doctrine determine force posture or vice versa?)
D. Arms Control
  1. Feasibility
    a. Quantitative restrictions
    b. Qualitative restrictions
  2. Threat perceptions
  3. Existing agreements
  4. Future prospects
E. The Use of Force
  1. Type and extent of employment
    a. Passive role (deterrent)
    b. Active role (fighting)
  2. Objectives sought through use of the military instrument
  3. Constraints on the use of force posed by other countries
  4. Technological developments and the use of force
  5. Domestic constraints on the use of force
F. Other Issues

Notes

1. In this volume we use the terms national security policy and defense policy interchangeably. Some would disagree, arguing that national security policy is the broader term, covering a wide range of political, social, economic, and military issues, whereas the term defense policy refers primarily to military-political concerns. Although a case can be made for such differentiation, we prefer to regard the terms as synonyms. Indeed, preference for this usage was also the consensus at a conference of our country study contributors.
2. See Frank B. Horton III, Anthony C. Rogerson, and Edward L. Warner III, eds., *Comparative Defense Policy* (Baltimore: Johns Hopkins University Press, 1974).
3. See John Baylis et al., *Contemporary Strategy: Theories and Policies* (New York: Holmes & Meier, 1975). The revised and enlarged second edition is in two volumes, the second of which deals with the defense policies of the nuclear powers. Contributors include Baylis, Ken Booth, John Garnett, and Phil Williams. See Baylis et al., *Contemporary Strategy* 2 vols. (New York: Holmes and Meier, 1987).
4. Many of the papers presented at that conference were published in a volume edited by James Roherty. See James Roherty, ed., *Defense Policy Formation: Towards Comparative Analysis* (Durham, N.C.: Carolina Academic Press, 1979).
5. See Catherine M. Kelleher and Gale A. Mattox, eds., *Evolving European Defense Policies* (Lexington, Mass.: D.C. Heath/Lexington Books, 1987). Another example of regionally focused comparative defense studies is James W. Morley, ed., *Security Interdependence in the Asia Pacific Region* (Lexington, Mass.: D.C. Heath/Lexington Books, 1986).
6. See Catherine M. Kelleher, ed., *Political Military Systems: Comparative Perspectives* (Beverly Hills, Calif.: Sage Publications, 1974) and Charles C. Moskos and Frank R. Wood, eds., *The Military: More Than Just a Job?* (Washington, D.C.: Pergamon-Brassey's, 1988).
7. For example, see Lucian Pye, "Armies in the Process of Political Modernization," *Archives Européennes de Sociologie* 2 (1961); John J. Johnson, ed., *The Role of the Military In Underdeveloped Countries* (Princeton: Princeton University Press, 1962); idem, *The Military and Society in Latin America* (Stanford: Stanford University Press, 1964); Samuel E. Finer, *The Man on Horseback: The Role of the Military in Politics* (New York: Penguin, 1962); Morris Janowitz, *The Military in the Political Development of New Nations* (Chicago: University of Chicago Press, 1964); Robert J. Alexander, "The Army in Politics," in *Government and Politics in Latin America*, ed. Harold Eugene Davis (New York: Ronald, 1958); Edwin Lieuwen, *Arms and Politics in Latin America* (New York: Praeger, 1964); J.C. Hurewitz, *Middle East Politics: The Military Dimension* (New York: Praeger, 1969); and Amos Perlmutter, "The Praetorian State and the Praetorian Army," *Comparative Politics* I (April 1969): 382-404. For a critique

of the military elite as modernizer, see Eric A. Nordlinger, "Soldiers in Mufti: The Impact of Military Rule upon Economic and Social Change in the Non-Western States," *American Political Science Review* 64 (December 1970): 1131-48. See also an anthology edited by Sheldon Simon, *The Military and Security in the Third World: Domestic and International Impacts* (Boulder, Colo.: Westview Press, 1978). Certainly, if one is to explain defense policy outcomes or the defense policy process in various countries, one cannot ignore the military as an institutional actor and the entire range of civil-military issues; however, our focus on comparative defense policy in this volume is broader in scope than the concerns of comparative military-political sociology, although these concerns do form a vital part of our effort.

8. See Aaron Wildavsky, *Budgeting: A Comparative Theory of Budgetary Process* (Boston: Little, Brown, 1975), and his earlier *Politics of the Budgetary Process* (1964; reprinted, Boston: Little, Brown, 1979).

9. See Samuel Huntington, *The Common Defense* (New York: Columbia University Press, 1961).

10. See Glenn H. Snyder, *Deterrence and Defense: Toward a Theory of National Security* (Princeton: Princeton University Press, 1961) as excerpted and reprinted in various editions of *American Defense Policy*. For example, see the 4th edition edited by John E. Endicott and Roy W. Stafford, Jr. (Baltimore: Johns Hopkins University Press, 1977), pp. 39-40 and the 5th edition edited by John F. Reichart and Steven R. Sturm (Baltimore: Johns Hopkins University Press, 1982), pp. 154-55.

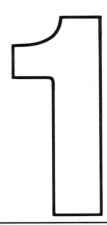

INTERNATIONAL RELATIONS AND THE DEFENSE POLICIES OF NATIONS: INTERNATIONAL ANARCHY AND THE COMMON PROBLEM OF SECURITY

Paul R. Viotti

The comparative study of defense policy begins with examination of the international political environment. Indeed, the study of the national security or defense policy of any given state must originate by observing the international context within which the state, its bureaucratic agencies, and its decision makers are immersed. The absence of any superordinate authority or world government that would maintain order among states gives rise to a security problem with which all states must cope. Although survival is by no means the only objective states seek, this concern with national security is common to all. Indeed, it is the underlying condition of anarchy—the absence of any central authority over states—that gives rise to the defense policies of nations or states.[1] In a world of states that claim to be sovereign

entities, there is no global authority that would provide security. Accordingly, given national security objectives, states formulate their own defense policies, attempting to develop the necessary strategies, forces, and force-employment doctrines.

In its broadest formulation, the term *security* goes well beyond military considerations. Security can be understood not only as *defense* against external (or internal) threats, but also as the overall socioeconomic well-being of a society and the individuals who compose it. In fact, in the defense and security policy literature, they often are used interchangeably, as they are in this volume. When they are used interchangeably, it is the narrower, or military, meaning of security that is intended as being synonymous with defense. Although there are exceptions, to reduce confusion and to underscore their primary focus, the country studies in this volume usually refer to the *defense* policies of nations.

Specifying this distinction between *security*, the more inclusive term, and *defense*, a component of security, is more than semantics. Defense spending, for example, may contribute to security by deterring or dissuading would-be adversaries—making attacks by them less likely. Economic benefits from defense spending would include increased employment of domestic labor forces and the development of new, nonmilitary industries based on commercial "spin-offs" from emergent defense technologies. On the other hand, large allocations of a society's resources to defense may be at the cost of social or other programs that the state otherwise would be in a position to finance. Beyond these "opportunity costs," defense expenditures that are excessive or wasteful of societal resources may even weaken the economy and reduce the economic and social well-being of the citizenry (or portions of it). Not all measures taken in the name of defense necessarily make a contribution to overall security.

They may not even enhance security in the narrower, defense-related meaning of the term. As John Herz and others have pointed out, states may still find themselves in a security "dilemma."[2] Allocating more resources to defense may induce other states to do likewise, in effect giving impetus to an arms race. Instead of enhancing security, such arms competition may set into motion a train of actions and reactions that undermines security for all parties concerned.

Security in an anarchic world of sovereign states is, in the final analysis, the responsibility of individual states. Kenneth Waltz refers to it as a "self-help" system. States are on their own to provide for their defense in a potentially hostile world. To bolster their security in response to threats, they can take actions both *internally* (such as raising armies and strengthening their economies) or *externally* (for example, engaging in diplomacy or forming alliances).[3]

If security in the narrow, defense-related sense is the minimum objective common to *all* states, then *strategy* refers to the way in which a state mobilizes and coordinates the use of its resources or capabilities in the attainment of this and other objectives. Formulation of strategy as a means of providing for the common defense is the state's response to the security problem it faces in an anarchic world.

Realism, Security, and the Emergence of a World System of Sovereign States

Realism is the school of thought most concerned with problems of security for states in an anarchic world system. The roots of realism in Western thought extend at least as far back as Thucydides (471–400 B.C.), who wrote about the Peloponnesian War among ancient Greek city-states. Growth in the power of Athens and the fear this caused in Sparta were seen by Thucydides as the underlying cause of the war. Power and the balance of power among city-states were key concepts for Thucydides, much as contemporary realists use the same concepts to describe relations among states in the present-day world.

The contemporary international, or state, system emerged formally from events that occurred in Europe during the sixteenth and seventeenth centuries. The idea of a temporal unity in Europe, always more myth than reality, even in medieval Europe, lost whatever credibility it had with the onset of the Reformation and the resultant fracturing of "Christendom." Conflict between Catholic and Protestant princes would be settled ultimately by granting to the sovereign the right to determine the religion of the inhabitants in a given realm (*Cujus regio ejus religio*).

Although the issue ostensibly was religion, a very important principle was established that went well beyond religion. Indeed, if the prince had the *right* to establish the religion of his subjects, his temporal authority in secular matters must also be quite substantial. Although this idea was also part of the earlier Peace of Augsburg in 1555, it was the Peace of Westphalia in 1648 that not only ended the Thirty Years War, but also provided formal ground for the emergence of the concept of sovereignty. Indeed, the ideas of sovereign state and a system of sovereign states persist to the present day.

States or, more specifically, their sovereigns, came to have both the "internal" *right* to exercise complete jurisdiction within their own territories and the "external" *right* to be independent or autonomous in their relations with other states or sovereigns. The Peace of Westphalia constituted formal recognition of a system and organizing principle (decentralization of authority to states or to their kings, dukes, or princes) that had evolved over time. Princes would not need to turn to emperors, popes, or other central authorities for the source of their own authority.

For a brief time, Napoleon upset this European state system by imposing French imperial rule; however, immediately after his final military defeat, the state system was restored by the diplomats who gathered at the Congress of Vienna in 1815. Indeed, that international politics should be organized as a system of sovereign states gained additional legitimacy by this formal reimposition in the nineteenth century of ideas that were part of the seventeenth-century Westphalia settlement.

Sovereign authority, then, was to be held only by states, whether exercised by their monarchs or by their legislatures. Among others, the sixteenth- and seventeenth-century writings of Bodin, Machiavelli, and Hobbes reflect this understanding of sovereignty. Although states varied considerably in relative power— the resources or capabilities at their disposal— each would be equal in terms of sovereign authority. Some states would use their power to coerce other states, but none would have the *right* to do so.

Be that as it may, the absence of central authority or world government with the power to prevent or stop aggression by some states against the sovereign prerogatives of others produces a security problem for all states. Hobbes stated the problem most starkly in chapter 13 of *Leviathan*: "Kings and persons of sovereign authority, because of their independency, are in continual jealousies and in the state and posture of gladiators, having their weapons pointing and their eyes fixed on one another; that is, their forts, garrisons and guns

upon the frontiers of their kingdoms, and continual spies upon their neighbors, which is a posture of war."

Although the formal origins of the sovereign state were in Europe, this Western idea was, in effect, imposed upon the rest of the world during the colonial and imperial periods. National independence movements in the eighteenth and nineteenth centuries and decolonialization in the twentieth century, particularly after World War II, established a truly global system of states, each state claiming to be sovereign.

Universal membership in the United Nations (UN), an international organization that explicitly recognizes the sovereignty and independence of its members, amounts to a further grant of legitimacy to this system of states. There is considerable variation in types of political, economic, and social structures of states in the contemporary international system. Nevertheless, regardless of type, *all* states continue to claim both internal and external dimensions of sovereignty.

Maintaining National and International Security in an Anarchic World

Maintaining a balance of power among states or alliances of states is a prescription offered by many realists. On the other hand, balance-of-power politics arguably have been as much the cause of, as the obstacle to, war. Indeed, a classic formulation of the balance of power saw the use of force in small wars as part of balance-of-power maintenance. Correctly or not, formation of balance-of-power alliances was blamed by many as having caused World War I. At least partly as a result of this thinking, alliances were to be avoided in the interwar period. Secret alliances and secret defense agreements among states were particularly onerous among those who shared the Wilsonian preference for open covenants openly arrived at.

The concept of *collective security* in the League of Nations was to replace alliance formation and balance-of-power thinking. Aggression and the use of force were outlawed. The enforcement mechanism rested with law-abiding states that were to band together to stop law-breaking, aggressor states. Notwithstanding what may have been the best of intentions, not only did collective security fail, but also the absence of alliances in the interwar period posed no obstacle to a Nazi Germany determined to expand beyond its borders.

Following World War II, collective security was restored within the United Nations organization, but it would again prove to be of limited utility, although UN peace-keeping efforts (including the deployment of international military forces under the UN flag) would meet with some success, whether providing buffers between adversaries or maintaining peace in areas torn by civil strife. Nevertheless, the experiences of both the United Nations and the earlier League of Nations have not built much confidence in collective security as a principal source of international order. Alliances and counteralliances would be formed, exercising a claimed right of collective defense recognized under Article 51 of the UN Charter.

Although the terms *collective security* and *collective defense* are often used interchangeably in common parlance as if they were synonymous, it is useful to underscore that alliances or collective defense arrangements are part and parcel of realist thought on the balance of power, whereas the collective security approach has attempted, however unsuccessfully, to establish a peace based on legal principles with collective enforcement of them. Collective security—concerted action by "law abiding" states against aggressors—was intended to be a substitute for, not the equivalent of, alliance or "balance-of-power" politics. For their part, world federalists, taking a different approach, propose to transform international relations by creating a world government, thus ending the condition of international anarchy. However desirable or undesirable world government may seem, few consider this outcome very likely.[4]

While realist advocates of a balance of power may turn to the writings of Thucydides, Machiavelli, and Hobbes for inspiration, those who advocate world order through rules or law also owe an intellectual debt to the thinking of Hugo Grotius (1583–1645). Aside from forma-

tion of alliances, security also may be addressed by the establishment of *regimes*—sets of formal, or tacitly understood, norms or rules to govern the international relations of states in a wide variety of issue areas. Some of these rules may have the formal, binding quality of law even if there is no central enforcing authority. Regimes also may have formal institutions associated with them, but such formal institutionalization is not prerequisite for a regime to exist. Although constructing regimes and establishing routines of international behavior are different from the power and countervailing power notions so central to much of realist thought, this "Grotian" approach is also compatible with realism. Indeed, the late Hedley Bull, a realist, observed how much international order depends on both "Hobbesean" (balance-of-power) and "Grotian" (rule-oriented) approaches.[5]

Given the security problem that confronts states in an anarchic international environment, there is at least some incentive for them to attempt reduction of uncertainties in their relations by creating rules to make the behavior of states somewhat more predictable. The construction of regimes dealing with trade, the exchange of currencies, investment, navigation, fishery rights, technology transfer, air and water pollution and other environmental concerns, health, communications, and other socioeconomic and scientific issues has been the subject of numerous studies, but there has been much less conceptual and empirical work done on the construction of international *security* regimes. As shown in table 1, international security regimes tend to deal with armaments numbers and types, geographic limits on arms and their uses, and functional issues including communications between or among adversaries at peace and in crises. Policy makers may seek to construct and maintain such regimes. Indeed, established or agreed rules and norms that comprise the regimes to which states adhere undoubtedly will influence their defense policy choices as well.

Arms control or, more specifically, the building of arms control regimes, is an effort to manage arms races, even if armaments cannot be reduced or eliminated. A related approach

Table 1. International Security Regimes:
Conflict and Arms Control

Geographic
  Antarctica
  Space
  Nuclear Free Zones
  Seabed
  European Security (CSCE)
  Tacit Spheres of Influence

Instrumental Means
  Communications
    Hot Line
    Nuclear Accidents
    Risk Reduction Centers
  Other Confidence-Building Meaures

Armaments
  Strategic Arms Reductions/Limitations
  Conventional Force Reductions
  Nuclear Nonproliferation
  Nuclear Test Bans
  Chemical Weapons Prohibitions
  Biological Weapons Prohibitions
  Conventional Arms Transfers

is establishing rules for managing conflicts, if not totally eliminating them. The strength of regimes or regime rules comes from the degree to which they are accepted *voluntarily* by sovereign states as being in their collective or enlightened self-interest. They are by no means perfect, but do represent a method by which sovereign states have met with at least some success in reducing some uncertainty and some feelings of insecurity—in effect establishing at least some degree of control over the international anarchy that surrounds states.

In themselves, these regimes do not alter in any way the underlying condition of international anarchy. States remain sovereign; there is still no central authority over them. By constraining and routinizing the international behavior of states, however, regimes to some degree reduce the unpredictability and uncertainty that otherwise would inhere in these relations. That is how regimes contribute to international security.

The conflicting parties to regimes that include adversaries (as have been established among the superpowers and other states in the arms control field) do have a logical purpose in common with parties to nonsecurity regimes. This common element—reduction of uncertainty—is a dominant motive for constructing all types of regimes. In fact, the uncertainty-reduction purpose would appear to be as in-

tense (and probably even more intense) in the process that results in the construction of regimes between adversaries as it is in the construction of other categories or types of international regimes. For example, the stakes are rather high in relations between the superpowers: the parties are driven to reduce uncertainty in what are inherently conflictual relations. The seeming contradiction in the idea of collaboration between or among adversaries can thus be accommodated by introducing the common purpose of uncertainty reduction. Parties to arms and conflict control negotiations may express their purposes as lessening the likelihood of war, reducing damage or devastation should war occur, and lowering costs—the defense expenditures that would result from continuing an arms race. These purposes are clearly attempts to reduce the uncertainty associated with adversarial relations.

That the parties may also be seeking advantage over other states is a further example of an attempt to control environmental uncertainty. In short, conflict remains central to adversary regimes, but the construction of such regimes can be understood as a routinization of conflict relations. When policy makers agree upon rules (and even procedures) that make mutual behavior somewhat more predictable, they are obviously reducing uncertainty. More to the point, they are attempting to gain some control over an unpredictable external environment by agreeing to define the limits or constraints within which conflict will continue to take place.[6]

The International Environment: Structural Considerations

An important question is the extent to which the external environment determines (or constrains) the policy choices made by the decision makers of states. Certainly, international-level considerations cannot be ignored. The relations between the superpowers, for example, affect the security calculations of the other states. Kenneth Waltz refers to this condition as the bipolar structure of the contemporary international system.[7] If by structure we mean the distribution (concentration or dispersion) of capabilities or power within the global system, then a strong case can be made for bipolarity. In this regard, Waltz is quick to note that to say the world is bipolar is not to say that the superpowers necessarily *control* the policies of other states; it is only to say that, given their relative power positions, the United States and the Soviet Union pursue policies that have pervasive *influence*. These policies cannot be ignored. The impact of their actions can be felt globally, something that really cannot be said about any other country. Moreover, their superpower status does not depend on nuclear weapons. Even if neither side possessed these weapons of mass destruction, residual military and economic capabilities still would confer superpower status upon them.

Stanley Hoffmann, by contrast, argues that the world is asymmetrically multipolar.[8] Central to his thesis is the view that power calculations vary from issue to issue. Thus, in such nondefense issues as international trade and monetary relations, he sees the world as decidedly multipolar. But even Hoffmann agrees with Waltz that in security or "strategic" relations the bipolar description applies. Although both would appear to agree on this point, Waltz rejects attempts by Hoffmann and others to disaggregate the concept of power. The classic view, expressed most clearly by E. H. Carr,[9] is that power is an integrity: it cannot be divided. Given linkages among issues, the attempt to separate the military, econonmic, and other components of power is artificial at best. Indeed, those who hold this view that power is an integrity observe, for example, that relations within the European Economic Community (EEC) cannot be separated from the fact that these relations occur under the security umbrella of one of the superpowers. Similarly, seen from this perspective, the attempt to view the economic relations of East European countries as separate from the security relations these countries have with the other superpower is misleading.

The distribution of capabilities among states is uneven. Not only is there asymmetry in the distribution of capabilities *among* states, but also the composition of a given state's capabilities may differ substantially from other states. For example, Japanese military capabilities are relatively small compared to other states of its rank, but Japan has assumed the role of a major power due primarily to its growth in *economic* capacity. For their part, Western European states have substantial economic and military capabilities, but they do not act as a unity and, as such, their separate capabilities are not additive. So long as this is true, Europe cannot do more than aspire to superpower status on a par with the United States and the Soviet Union. Some progress has been (and continues to be) made in coordination of social and economic policies among EEC members, but a greater degree of unity is required on these, security, and other issues if Europe is to be considered a great power (or superpower) in its own right.

In any event, few would disagree with the contention that policies pursued by the superpowers and relations between them affect the defense policy choices of other states; their impact is far greater than that of most lesser powers that have regional rather than global scope. Accordingly, given their relative importance, the defense policies of the United States and the Soviet Union are the first two country studies in this volume. As a reading of the Korb and Warner chapters makes clear, the policies of the other superpower are a principal concern of both the United States and the Soviet Union. This is not an exclusive focus, of course. Both countries are also concerned with alliance management and threats posed by other countries. For example, the Soviet Union keeps a close eye on China, the European states (especially West Germany), and the countries of the Middle East and South Asia on the periphery of the USSR.

Some writers, however, object to bipolar and most multipolar conceptions of structure as oversimplifications that ignore the effect of such factors as the resource dependency of Northern Hemisphere countries upon those of the "South"—the less industrially developed states of the Southern Hemisphere or the "Third World." They point out, for example, that, when acting in concert (as they did in the 1970s), states belonging to the Organization of

Petroleum Exporting Countries (OPEC) can assert considerable leverage over states dependent on them as a source of oil and natural gas. Resource availability is not just an economic issue. Indeed, national security depends upon maintenance of either domestic or external sources of petroleum and other mineral resources. Moreover, massive debts incurred in the late 1970s and the 1980s by Third World countries to banks and other financial institutions in the advanced, industrial countries of the "North" have important security implications for both lenders and debtors. The viability of private banks and the global financial system depends upon continued servicing of Third World debts. Although creative approaches have been used to reduce these burdens somewhat, massive defaults—completely writing these debts off—would be a disaster both for private banks and the world financial system. At the same time, if they are to service their debts, debtor countries are forced to make sacrifices that affect negatively their economies and the well-being of their populations.

From this perspective, then, the Third World is more than just an arena or stage upon which superpower and other great power relations are played out; structural images must certainly capture the systemic role played by Third World countries. Because bipolar and multipolar images as they are now represented tend to have an East-West focus, critics argue that structural images used by students of international relations should be made more sensitive to North-South considerations.

Power: Interdependence and Perceptions as Moderating Factors

Having noted the importance of power and its distribution as factors that affect defense policy choices, one must also acknowledge the limits of power as an explanatory variable. Neither superpower has the power to impose its designs on the other. But even in their relations with other states, the superpowers moderate their relative positions by their degree of dependence or interdependence.[10] For example,

given the superpower status of the United States, one would expect American-Canadian relations to be dominated by the United States. In fact, Canada exercises considerable autonomy in its international relations concerning both security and nonsecurity questions. That Canada is not totally dependent on the United States in these issues contributes to the country's policy independence. Even in security matters, Canada is able to pursue a more independent path than one would otherwise suppose. In North American air defense, for example, Ottawa can be sure that the United States will provide for air defense, even if Canada chooses not to participate in the arrangement.[11]

Washington can be expected to make expenditures for North American air defense with or without Canadian contributions. Given this situation, it is the United States that becomes somewhat dependent on Canada for its continuing contribution to the common effort—a contribution measured not only in dollar expenditures, but also in terms of radar sites and associated communications nets that Canada's geographic location offers. In short, dependency by one party equates to some degree of leverage for the other party quite apart from "objective" power calculations.

Assuming that states are the principal actors, "sensitivity" interdependence addresses the external effects on other states of actions taken by a given state or group of states. Beyond mere sensitivity is the degree of vulnerability of various states to the actions of other states. One criticism of this state-centric approach to defining interdependence is that it does not take direct account of such transnational actors as multinational banks and corporations that operate across the boundaries of individual states. The same criticisms, of course, can be directed against this volume, given the country-study approach followed here.

In any event, there is no consensus among scholars as to whether global interdependence (however defined) is increasing, decreasing, or remaining substantially the same.[12] Even more contentious is the question of whether increasing interdependence is conducive to peace.

That rising interdependence is associated with peace is certainly the common wisdom deeply set in the Western liberal tradition, but this causal relation has been challenged. Indeed, closer association of states may result in a higher probability of conflicts that could lead to war; from this perspective isolation from other states—an autarkic position—is the best posture for avoiding conflicts that lead to war.[13] On the other hand, those who believe that interdependence promotes peace argue that ties of mutual dependency make these relations too costly to break and thus make war less likely. Indeed, there are opportunity costs associated with breaking relations.

The power of states (defined by some as the capabilities that give a state the capacity to influence) would also seem to be moderated by such factors as national will. Indeed, some scholars have considered power to be a multiplicative function such that power is the product of perceived will (or credibility) and capability. For example, as either credibility or capability decline, the overall power of the state is similarly reduced. From this perspective, the subjective dimension of perceptions is at least as important as "objective" calculations of capability.[14] Furthermore, it is argued that even the capabilities factor is moderated by perceptions.

Although a common focus in security policy studies is on threats and threat perceptions, note should also be taken of the obverse side of the same security coin: perceived opportunities the state may wish to pursue.[15] Indeed, policy makers may see little or nothing within the international environment that would obstruct or otherwise impede the attainment of certain goals. To the contrary, other actors may be supportive of these purposes and be willing to collaborate in a common effort to achieve collective goals.

Decision makers hold certain images of the role their states should play internationally. A substantial change in power position relative to other states inevitably alters these perceptions; however, there is sometimes a considerable lag between changes in the "objective" situation and "subjective" realization (and acceptance) of a new role.

Strategy and the Formation of Alliances: State Responses to Insecurity

Recognizing the lack of any central, directive authority in international relations has led realists and others to observe that an inherently conflictual international environment is necessarily a consequence. Politics in this view amount to a zero-sum game, with one side's gains equating to the other side's losses. Strategies of states in such a world are competitive.[16]

Because the world may be described as anarchic does not mean that international politics are necessarily conflictual. If, instead of a zero-sum game, the parties see it as "variable sum," with the possibility of all parties gaining (a "positive sum" outcome), then competitive strategies can yield to cooperative ones—not just among allies, but among adversaries as well. Achieving such outcomes is the stuff of arms control and other security and nonsecurity negotiations. The best diplomatic (or business) deal, it can be said, is one in which all parties register some gain and thus feel good about agreements reached. Collaboration, even among adversaries, becomes possible. Again, competitive strategies, following this logic, yield to cooperative ones.

Kenneth Waltz deals with this issue in *Man, the State and War*.[17] Considering states as if they were the hunters in Rousseau's allegorical tale, Waltz relates how hunters in a mythical state of "nature" (an imaginary world without central authority or, for that matter, any other social structure) come to deal with their own security problem. If all the hunters are needed to capture the stag that will provide for their collective sustenance, would it be rational for any one of them to defect from the group in pursuit of a hare that will serve the needs of only one hunter (especially if he thinks any of the other hunters may do so first)? Waltz answers that going for the hare may be perfectly rational, an optimal choice clearly preferable to waiting around to join the others in the joint hunting of a deer for their common use. Waltz sees serving the short-run self-interest (going for the hare) as most likely. Others, such as Stanley Hoffmann and Ernst Haas, have disagreed. According to Haas, an "upgrading" of the "common interest" is at least as possible as serving narrow, individual, short-term interests.[18] Constructing and maintaining international regimes are the kinds of collaborative activities that result from pursuing cooperative strategies. Upgrading the common, longer-term interest is achieved in negotiations that limit or reduce armaments and set parameters for conflicts when and if they occur.

Strategy is a *voluntarist* formulation by which states (i.e., their statesmen) try to maximize their positions, achieving at least an adequate degree of security or defense capability in a potentially hostile world. Statesmen exercise their will (this is the meaning of "voluntarist") as they try to influence international outcomes. How much is a matter of volition and how much is determined—beyond the control of statesmen, regardless of what they try to effect? It is the age-old problem of effective free will (voluntarism) versus determinism. How much freedom of action do statesmen have or, put another way, how much is determined by the structure of power relations within the international environment or by other actors with which the state must interact? Formulation of a strategy amounts to an assertion that statesmen *can* make a difference—that they can affect the course of events even though, at the same time, they face both internal factors (within their states and themselves) and external factors (within the international environment) that constrain their behavior to some degree.

The effective policy space—the area within which statesmen can have some effect—is not always a function of power. The observation reported by Thucydides that the strong do what they will and the weak do what they must[19] does not always hold. True, some issues are almost the exclusive domain of the superpowers and other major powers. On the other hand, small states can act independently in many areas and can even have decisive impact (particularly when they are acting in concert) on other defense and security matters.

In a particularly insightful article that relies heavily on the writings of Clausewitz, Michael Howard identifies four "dimensions" of strategy applicable to the use of military forces: the operational, the logistical, the social, and the technological.[20] It is not enough to focus only on operational capabilities—tactical considerations on the battlefield. The effectiveness of military forces is also influenced by their technological and logistical capabilities. The nature of society itself—the morale, social cohesion, and capabilities of the people in both civil and military pursuits—is also part of the strategic calculation. Although the relative importance of each of these factors is arguable, ignoring any one of them can have devastating consequences. In particular, Howard warns that the West appears "to be depending on the technological dimension of strategy to the detriment of its operational requirements, while [ignoring] its societal implications altogether."[21]

Operational capability on the battlefield depends on the social dimension directly, as well as on the logistical and technological dimensions, which are related to each other and, in turn, to the social dimension underlying them. The important point, however, is that Howard effectively combines socioeconomic considerations (viz., the social, logistical, and technological) with the purely military or operational elements of national strategy.

Some states choose to go it alone, opting for nonalignment or neutrality. Others seek to augment their power (or countervailing power) against adversaries by forming alliances. The literature on alliances is extensive and offers a variety of approaches to the subject.[22] Certainly, understanding the politics both *within* and *between* alliances is central also to understanding the defense policies of most of the countries in this volume. Particular attention is directed, of course, toward both the Warsaw Pact and North Atlantic Treaty organizations as competing alliances.

The military "balance" (or, to use Soviet terminology, the "correlation of forces") in Europe favors Soviet and Warsaw Pact forces in numbers of personnel and most categories of armaments deployed there. The United States and its NATO allies rely on such factors as advanced technology, flexibility in combat, and the morale and fighting spirit of their forces to offset the Warsaw Pact's quantitative advantage.[23] Moreover, the presence of nuclear weapons and a commitment to use them first, if necessary, to stop Warsaw Pact aggression are central to the Western military position.

Both sides also depend heavily on the integrity of their alliances and on effective command, control, and communications functions when engaged in combat operations. In addition to these social and operational dimensions, both face major logistical problems in any war efforts, particularly if escalation to the use of nuclear weapons occurs. It is in this context that Howard's treatment of the dimensions of national strategy seems particularly relevant. Indeed, evaluating the military balance in Europe and elsewhere in the world depends heavily upon the relative importance one places on each of the factors Howard identifies. In turn, the evaluation that each party makes of the military capabilities of the other is key to maintaining stability in the deterrence relations between them.

Diverse Approaches to Security, Peace, and the Comparative Study of Defense Policy

Political *realism*, a school of thought often said to be preoccupied with questions of security (relegating far less attention to socioeconomic and other "welfare" issues), typically uses as its starting point the state-as-actor, focusing on its relations with other states in an anarchic world. Critics argue that this perspective loads the dice, leading those who think about strategy to competitive (rather than cooperative) approaches to achieving national objectives. One finds competitive (and "countervailing") strategies offered by policy-oriented realists.

Realists often address the power of given states and the balance of power among states. The competition can be zero-sum or variable sum, depending in part upon the predisposition of the actors and the established pattern of their relations. By contrast, most "peace theorists" adopt a different point of departure. They are prone to reject international anarchy and the balance of power to the extent that

these are metaphors that predispose one to thinking in competitive, particularly zero-sum, terms.

Peace theorists are by no means of one mind (any more than realists are). In fact, peace studies are an interdisciplinary blend, drawing from psychology, social psychology, anthropology, political science, and other fields in the social sciences and the humanities. Peace studies were developed after World War II in academic communities in nonaligned and in smaller allied countries, particularly in Scandinavia. This new academic focus on *peace* (rather than *war*, *defense*, or *security*) studies spread to other countries to include the United States, especially in the aftermath of the Vietnam War.

Some peace theorists consider the legitimacy of using force as a value that has been learned and that pacific or accommodative modes of dealing with conflicts should be promoted instead. The realist notion that peace rests fundamentally on military preparedness (*si vis pacem, para bellum*: if you desire peace, then prepare for war) is alien to this more irenic mode of thought. New peace-oriented modes of thought and action *can* be learned.

Often relying heavily upon insights drawn from psychology and social psychology, peace theorists look toward building confidence among individuals and among states that otherwise might be adversaries. Structuring military forces so that they are not provocative— advocacy of a "defensive defense" posture—is one approach to confidence building.[24] The exchange of observers and advance notification of military exercises agreed upon within the CSCE (Conference on Security and Cooperation in Europe) process are measures designed to make these military activities less threatening. Improving communications, particularly the capacity for rational communications in crises, is an important area to some peace researchers, as it is to many realists as well.

Indeed, the research agendas of realists and peace researchers do overlap. There is interest by scholars in both groups in negotiation and conflict resolution or, if conflicts cannot be resolved, at least to management of them, thus precluding the outbreak of war. It is the peace researcher, however, who is less prone to accept the status quo, realist assumptions about the nature of international politics and the present world order. Some look to the rational construction of new world orders, advancing justice and other global values.[25] To the extent that the absence of central authority is acknowledged by peace theorists as a cause of war, they may be committed to world federalism or some other form of world government.

There is also overlapping between peace theorists and realists, especially as both may look to Grotian modes of thought. Moreover, both may have an interest in dealing with transnational actors and such transnational phenomena as terrorism. But their points of departure and the degree of attention they focus on alternative *means* of maintaining peace or security diverge significantly.

Another school of thought, which can be labeled pluralist,[26] does not see the state as a unitary actor, but instead looks within it to find the actions and interactions of individuals, groups, and bureaucracies as key to understanding policy outcomes. Some peace theorists are also pluralists, but many other pluralists have tended to avoid security or peace issues as such, studying instead the wide range of socioeconomic or "welfare" issues often overlooked by realists. To pluralists, states are not the only important actors. The wide range of nonstate actors are also worth studying— such diverse units as multinational corporations, banks, churches, and terrorist groups. Although state membership is the defining characteristic of such *international organizations* as the European Communities (EC), the UN, the World Bank, and the International Monetary Fund, these organizations achieve a degree of independence, enabling them to perform roles and engage in activities that go well beyond the charter of any given state.[27] Regional integration efforts such as have occurred in Europe have been carried out by elites in the different countries seeking to achieve near-term socioeconomic goals that, if carried to their logical conclusion, would transform the political economy of the region and its relations to the rest of the world.[28]

Operating separately from pluralists, real-ists, and peace theorists are scholars directly (or indirectly) influenced by the thinking of Karl Marx, who see world politics and security matters affected by class or dependency relations, not just within a given state, but also on a global scale. Such ideas may have an influence in defense policy formulation in the Soviet Union, China, East Germany, and other Marxist-Leninist states (although some would argue that realist analyses apply at least equally well in these countries). A Marxist analysis of international security, however, would go beyond merely recognizing the influences of domestic or international classes and class conflict on defense policy formulated in a given state. Instead, it would itself be an alternative way of conceptualizing the comparative study of defense policy. One would see the world, and security relations within it, through class analytical lenses.

While acknowledging the insights offered by these alternative approaches to international security questions and the defense policies of nations, the editors and contributors to this volume have drawn upon both state-centric and pluralist approaches. The first two parts of the framework for analysis that examine the international environment and the state's objectives, strategy, and force-employment doctrine within that environment conform to a rational and state-centric, realist view. The third part of the framework is a pluralist approach used to discover the actors and bureaucratic processes associated with defense decision making. In short, because we recognize that understanding a country's defense policy requires consideration of diverse factors at international, national, and subnational levels, our effort explicitly combines realist and pluralist analyses, albeit in separate parts of our framework for the analysis of the defense policies of nations.

Notes

1. The relation between international conflict and international anarchy is developed in Kenneth N. Waltz, *Man, the State and War* (New York: Columbia University Press, 1954, 1959), especially chapters 6, 7,

and 8. Cf. his later work in *Theory of International Politics* (Reading, Mass.: Addison-Wesley, 1979). The late Hedley Bull dealt at length with anarchy as an underlying condition of international relations in his *The Anarchical Society: A Study of Order in World Politics* (New York: Columbia University Press, 1977).

2. A classic article on the "security dilemma" for states produced by international anarchy is John H. Herz, "Idealist Internationalism and the Security Dilemma," *World Politics* 5, no. 2 (January 1950): 157–80.

3. See Kenneth N. Waltz, "Theory of International Relations" in Fred I. Greenstein and Nelson W. Polsby, eds., *Handbook of Political Science*, vol. 8 (Reading, Mass.: Addison-Wesley, 1975), pp. 36–37.

4. For a classic treatment of balance of power, collective security, and world government as alternative approaches to world order, see Inis L. Claude, Jr., *Power and International Relations* (New York: Random House, 1962).

5. See Bull, *Anarchical Society*, pp. 24–27 and 65–71.

6. I develop this idea further in a case study on management of conflict relations in Berlin. See Paul R. Viotti, "Berlin and Conflict Management with the USSR," *Orbis* 28, no. 3 (Fall 1984): 575–91.

7. Although it has been repeated in subsequent works by Waltz cited in nn. 1 and 3 above, an earlier statement of his contention that the structure of international politics is bipolar is his "International Structure, National Force, and the Balance of Power," *Journal of International Affairs* 21 (1967): 215–31. The article is reprinted in James N. Rosenau, ed., *International Politics and Foreign Policy*, rev. ed. (New York: Free Press, 1969), pp. 304–14.

8. The term *asymmetric multipolarity* is used in Stanley Hoffmann, "Choices," *Foreign Policy* 7 (Summer 1972): 4. Hoffmann's position is developed further in his *Primacy or World Order* (New York: McGraw-Hill, 1978). Cf. his earlier *Gulliver's Troubles* (New York: McGraw-Hill, 1968), esp. pp. 54–71, and "Weighing the Balance of Power," *Foreign Affairs* 50, no. 4 (July 1972): 618–44.

9. See E. H. Carr, *Twenty Years' Crisis, 1919–1939* (1939; New York: Harper and Row, 1964), especially chap. 8. Carr states: "Power, which is an element of all political action, is one and indivisible" (p. 132).

10. For a well-developed discussion, see Robert Keohane and Joseph Nye, *Power and Interdependence* (Boston: Little, Brown, 1976).

11. For a good example of this, see the case study on the Canadian purchase of a new long-range patrol aircraft in Douglas J. Murray, *We Stand on Guard for Thee: The Theory and Practice of Canadian Defense Policy* (Washington, D.C.: NDU Press, 1989).

12. For an empirical analysis that challenges the "conventional wisdom" of a continuing trend toward rising interdependence, see Richard Rosecrance, "Whither Interdependence?" *International Organization* (Summer 1977).

13. For a development of this argument, see Kenneth N. Waltz, "Conflict in World Politics," in *Conflict in World Politics*, ed. Steven L. Spiegel and Kenneth N. Waltz (Cambridge, Mass.: Winthrop Publishers, 1971), pp. 454–74.

14. For one of the better treatments of perceptual factors and their impact on international politics, see Robert Jervis, *Perception and Misperception in International Politics* (Princeton: Princeton University Press, 1976).

15. See, for example, the discussion in Waltz, *Man, the State and War*, p. 204.

16. Indeed, the idea of "competitive strategies" has been advanced within the U.S. Department of Defense. For example, see the annual *Report of the Secretary of Defense Caspar W. Weinberger to the Congress on the FY 1988/FY 1989 Budget and FY 1988–92 Defense Programs* (Washington, D.C.: U.S. Government Printing Office, 1987), pp. 65–69. The zero-sum nature of a competitive strategy is clear: "aligning enduring American strengths against enduring Soviet weaknesses" and "even within their strengths we should seek weaknesses—chinks in their armor—that we exploit, thereby rendering Soviet military power less potent over time" (p. 66).

17. See Waltz, *Man, the State and War*, pp. 167–71. For an alternative view, see Stanley Hoffmann, "Rousseau on War and Peace," *American Political Science Review* 57, no. 2 (June 1963): 317–33. Cf. Jean Jacques Rousseau, "A Discussion on the Origins of Inequality," in *The Social Contract and Discourses*, trans. G. D. H. Cole (New York: E. P. Dutton, 1950), pp. 235–38.

18. See Ernst B. Haas, *Beyond the Nation-State* (Stanford: Stanford University Press, 1964), pp. 69–71.

19. See "The Melian Dialogue" in Thucydides, *History of the Peloponnesian War*, trans. Rex Warner (New York: Penguin Books, 1982), pp. 400–408.

20. See Michael E. Howard, "The Forgotten Dimensions of Strategy," *Foreign Affairs* 57, no. 5 (Summer 1979): 975–86.

21. Ibid.

22. A representative sample of this literature, but by no means an exhaustive list, would include Francis A. Beer, ed., *Alliances: Latent War Communities in the Contemporary World* (New York: Holt, Rinehart and Winston, 1970); George F. Liska, *Nations in Alliance: The Limits of Interdependence* (Baltimore: Johns Hopkins University Press, 1962); William H. Riker, *The Theory of Political Coalitions* (New Haven: Yale University Press, 1962); and Julian Friedman, Christopher Bladen, and Steven Rosen, eds., *Alliances in International Politics* (Boston: Allyn and Bacon, 1970).

23. For further elaboration of these offsetting factors, see Jonathan Dean, *Watershed in Europe* (Lexington, Mass.: D.C. Heath/Lexington Books, 1987), pp. 38–58 and F. W. von Mellenthin and R. H. S. Stolfi with E. Sobik, *NATO under Attack: Why the Western Alliance Can Fight Outnumbered and Win in Central Europe without Nuclear Weapons* (Durham, N.C.: Duke University Press, 1984).

24. See, for example, Johan Galtung, "Transarmament: From Offensive to Defensive Defense," *Journal of Peace Research* 21, no. 2 (1984): 127–39.

25. See Richard A. Falk, *A Study of Future Worlds* (New York: Macmillan/Free Press, 1975).

26. For elaboration, see Paul R. Viotti and Mark V. Kauppi, eds., *International Relations Theory: Realism, Pluralism, Globalism* (New York: Macmillan, 1987), pp. 7–9 and 192–216.

27. For a classic study of this issue, see Haas, *Beyond the Nation-State*.

28. For an explanation of why European integration

has not moved as quickly as originally anticipated, see Ernst B. Haas, "Turbulent Fields and the Theory of Regional Integration," *International Organization* 30, no. 2 (Spring 1976): 173–212. A more detailed treatment is in Haas, *The Obsolescence of Regional Integration Theory* (Berkeley, Calif.: University of California Institute of International Studies, 1975). For a summary of the argument, see Viotti and Kauppi, pp. 206–09.

Part Two

THE SUPERPOWERS

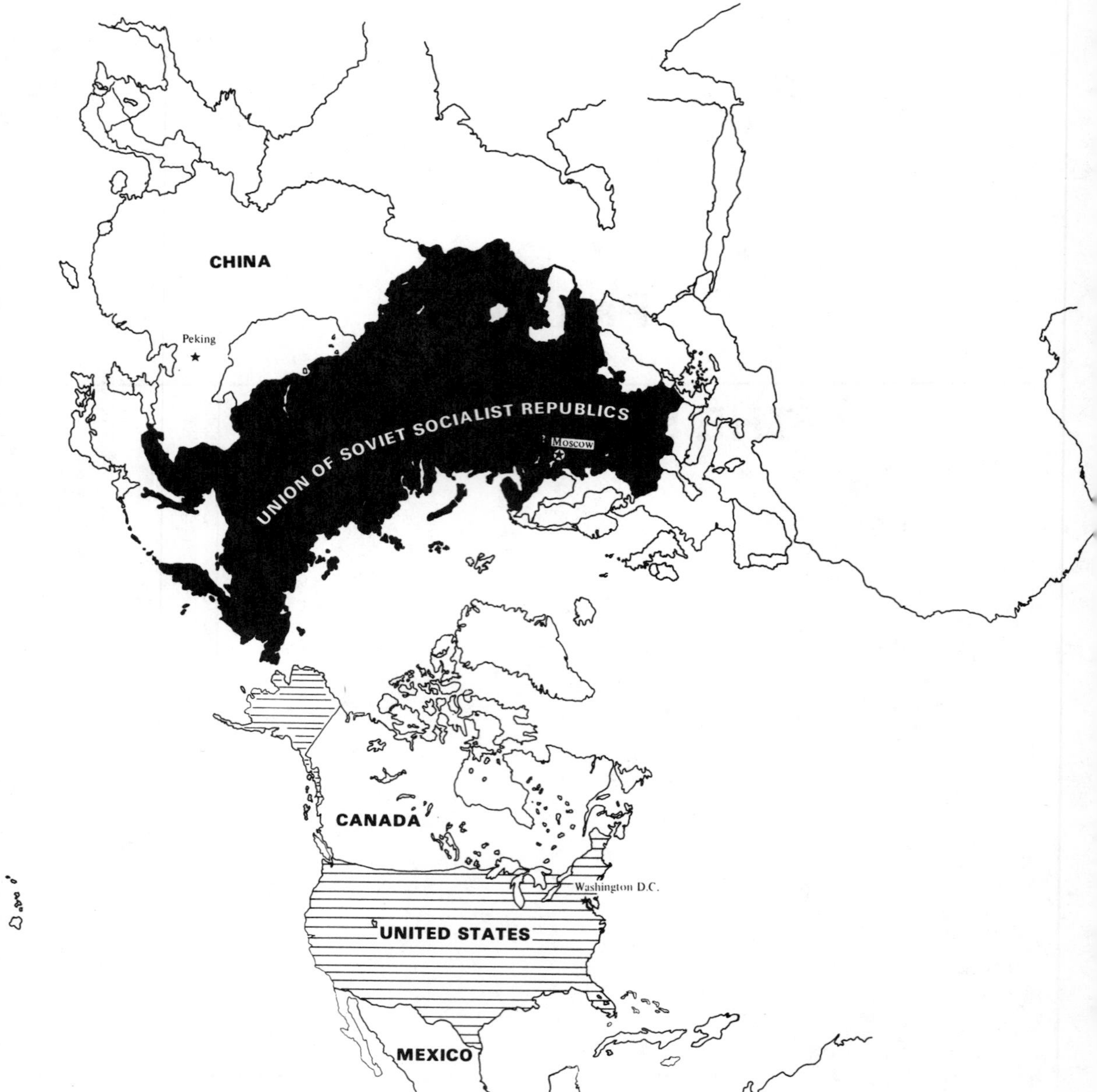

CHINA
Peking
UNION OF SOVIET SOCIALIST REPUBLICS
Moscow
CANADA
Washington D.C.
UNITED STATES
MEXICO
Mexico City

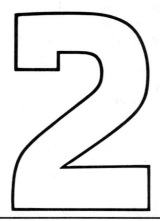

THE UNITED STATES

Lawrence J. Korb and Robert H. Gromoll

American defense policy is an abiding interest among virtually all who study and practice international affairs. In combined military and economic terms, the United States is the most powerful nation in the international system. No nation, therefore, can avoid being influenced by the American defense establishment. That influence may be direct—for example, through the employment of U.S. military power, maintenance of alliances, and arms transfers, or by the stationing of American military personnel and dependents abroad—or less direct, through the attitudes of American leaders concerning the use of military force or the impact U.S. defense spending has on national and international economies. No nation, however, stands unaffected by the Pentagon.

What, then, are the elements of U.S. defense policy? In considering that question, this chapter identifies and examines the context, processes, and substance of the American defense establishment by focusing on the international environment that shapes—and is shaped

by—U.S. defense programs; U.S. national objectives, strategy, and military doctrine; the defense decision-making process; and defense policy outputs.

International Environment

The United States emerged from World War II as the world's preeminent power; no other nation on earth could rival it economically or militarily. Pre–World War II centers of power were virtually destroyed by the war and the defeated Axis powers literally lay in ruins. The victorious British and Russians were not in much better shape. The six long years of war had bankrupted the British Empire, and the Soviet Union had suffered almost twenty million casualties and severe damage to its industrial base. Throughout the next two decades, the United States remained the world's preeminent economic and military power; however, Western Europe and Japan made great strides economically, as did the Soviet Union—although its greatest accomplishments were in military capability.

During the 1970s, the Russians increased defense spending by about 5 percent annually in real terms. They invested substantially in their military and improved the efficiency, quality, and capacity of their weapons and equipment. During this period they managed to surpass the United States in most quantitative indicators of military power. There were a number of reasons for this. All considered, the Vietnam War cost about half a trillion 1985 dollars—expenditures that otherwise could have gone into U.S. defense investment. The war ultimately cost the United States about six to eight years of defense modernization, while, as figure 1 indicates, the Soviet Union forged ahead in defense investment expenditures.[1] United States spending was also constrained

by antimilitary sentiments generated by the Vietnam War and President Carter's preference for a moderate, nonconfrontational tone vis-à-vis the USSR, as well as by high U.S. inflation rates and unanticipated cost overruns in the development of new weapons.

The United States nevertheless managed to retain qualitative advantages in many nuclear and conventional military technologies, so the superpowers coexisted throughout the 1970s in a state of rough equivalence. Many military analysts, however, decried what they perceived to be a "decade of neglect" during this period and doubted that the United States could cling to military parity with the USSR if it did not soon undertake a major military modernization effort.[2] Indeed, presidential candidate Ronald Reagan campaigned on the charge that his predecessors had allowed the Soviet

Figure 1. A Comparison of U.S. Defense Investment Expenditures with the Estimated Dollar Cost of Soviet Investment Expenditures

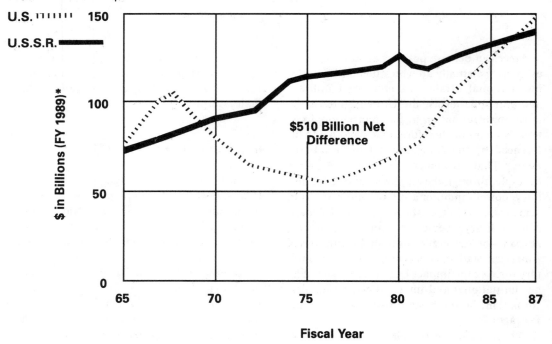

* Includes RDT&E, Procurement and Military Construction, and Non-DOD-Funded Programs.

Source: U.S. Department of Defense Annual Report to Congress, FY 1989.

Union to gain a "margin of superiority" over the United States.

When President Reagan entered office in 1981, the United States remained an economic and military superpower, but its preeminence was gone. It still had the world's largest gross national product (GNP), but it no longer dominated world trade. It exported over $150 billion in manufactured and agricultural goods annually, but it had run a negative trade balance since 1971. It was also more heavily dependent upon imported raw materials that were critical for national security. And inflation in the United States had risen to as high as 7 percent or more per year, reaching double digits in some years, with real growth in the economy falling from 5 percent to below 2 percent.

The Reagan administration brought the rate of inflation down to as little as 3 percent by the mid 1980s, but it did little to increase productivity or to reduce the size of the federal budget deficit. Real growth in the economy that averaged 5 percent in the 1960s averaged about 2 percent in the first half of the 1980s. Federal budget deficits averaged nearly $200 billion per year in the Reagan years, more than doubling the size of the national debt, and making interest on national debt the fastest growing item in the federal budget. That figure grew from less than $50 billion per year at the beginning of the Reagan presidency to over $200 billion by the end of Reagan's first term.

President Reagan also made a firm commitment to arrest the serious deterioration in U.S. military capabilities that had occurred during the 1970s.[3] His administration was also inclined to reassess fundamental strategic concepts that had guided U.S. defense policy since the end of World War II with the idea that many of these no longer applied in such vastly changed strategic and political environments.[4] It initiated a long-term modernization program by immediately submitting amendments to increase real growth in the outgoing Carter administration's defense spending program by 12 percent. Obligational authority was immediately increased by $32.6 billion and defense outlays by $5.8 billion. Over the period of Carter's proposed five-year program, defense spending jumped in real terms by an amazing $195 billion.[5] During fiscal year 1982 through fiscal year 1985, the Reagan administration spent $1.1 trillion on national defense, about 36 percent more in real terms than what was spent in the previous four years.[6]

Despite this unparalleled peacetime defense effort, the Pentagon reported in 1986 that Moscow had achieved parity in every category of land force technology, that a decline was also occurring in "virtually every major category where the United States enjoyed a lead in deployed air and naval technology," and that Soviet quantitative and qualitative advances in offensive and defensive systems had "significantly altered the strategic balance."[7] A year later, however, under domestic pressure to show that the administration's military buildup over the previous five years had been productive, Secretary of Defense Caspar Weinberger reported that the negative trends of earlier years had begun to reverse.[8]

As early as FY 1984, however, concerns about the $185 billion federal deficit and mounting charges that the administration was overspending on high technology and underspending on mundane, but essential, components of readiness and sustainability caused public and congressional enthusiasm for higher defense spending to wane.[9] The high rate of growth in defense expenditures consequently diminished, and congressional action in the FY 1986 budget gave the Reagan administration its first experience with negative growth in the defense budget, a development Weinberger warned would "undermine" U.S. security against growing Soviet threats.[10] Questions persisted, however, concerning the prudence of the administration's penchant for "big ticket" items, like acquiring technically troubled B-1B bombers and building up to fifteen aircraft carrier task groups for a controversial offensive maritime strategy.[11]

No matter how one assesses it, though, U.S. military power at the end of the 1980s was truly formidable. U.S. strategic forces in FY 1987 had some 7,834 nuclear warheads deployed on 1,992 strategic offensive missiles, including ten new MX/Peacekeeper intercontinental ballistic missiles (ICBMs) that could deliver as many as ten nuclear warheads apiece.[12] Some 327 U.S. strategic bombers were deployed, including the new B-1B and around 100 B-52Gs, newly fitted with air-launched cruise missiles (ALCMs) to enhance penetration capabilities against the USSR's unmatched air defense system.[13] And to add to the U.S. nuclear reserve, nuclear sea-launched cruise missiles (SLCMs) were deployed aboard attack submarines and surface vessels, thus extending strategic nuclear roles to weapons platforms that had previously performed tactical missions only.[14] In addition to strategic nuclear forces, the United States had 5,800 forwardly deployed tactical nuclear weapons, 567 ships, 14 carrier air wings, 37 air force tactical fighter wings, and 21 active and 11 reserve divisions.[15]

Thus, whereas much was made of declining American power relative to the Soviet Union at the outset of the 1980s, the Defense Department claimed toward the end of the decade that American military strength had been "reconstituted." However, it was quick to add, in light of Congress' revived inclination to cut defense spending, that Moscow still enjoyed significant advantages, and that U.S. modernization efforts had to be sustained because the Soviet threat was growing.[16]

Another important aspect of the military environment—as evidenced by the guerrilla wars in Afghanistan, Central America, the Philippines, Kampuchea, and Africa—was that Third World conflicts continued to be numerous and, for the most part, of "low-intensity" varieties. These conflicts posed special problems for the United States because visible American military intervention in them would readily mobilize local nationalistic sentiments against American involvement. And because these conflicts derived from the sociopolitical fabric of the countries they afflicted, they were more likely to be unresponsive to the conventional strategies and tactics to which American military forces continued to be wed.[17]

Also, because by the end of the decade the population of weapons manufacturers and suppliers was increasingly diversified, larger amounts of military equipment and advanced technology were available globally. This contributed to high-intensity conflicts like the Falklands and Iran-Iraq wars, which produced staggering casualty rates by anyone's standard.[18] This development had grave implications for U.S. defense policy because it made projecting U.S. military power riskier.

U.S. economic power also declined—a disturbing trend considering that political influence derives in the long run more from a "highly productive, competitive economy" than from military power.[19] The United States remained the most productive nation in the world, of course, and its gross national product continued to grow: in 1974 the GNP was $2,729 billion, and by 1986 it had risen to $3,702 billion (both figures expressed in 1982 dollars). American economic growth was slower than expected, only a little more than 2 percent in 1986, for example, but this was still greater than that experienced by America's trading partners in Western Europe and much of the Third World. In previous years, from 1982 to 1985, real GNP in Europe grew at an annual rate of only 2.2 percent, roughly one-half that of the United States, Canada, and Japan.[20]

This uneven economic recovery, combined with other factors like an overvalued U.S. currency, declining interest rates, lower levels of savings and investment, and a fall in labor productivity and technological advance, contributed to a serious decline in U.S. ability to compete successfully in international markets, and consequently to unprecedented trade imbalances.[21] Significant, too, was the fact that many technological advances upon which U.S. political, military, and economic power were based continued to diffuse globally, enabling South Korea and Taiwan, along with reemergent Japan and Western Europe, to enjoy lower production costs, greater competitiveness, and rising rates of return on investments.[22]

The last overall American trade surplus occurred in 1980. In that year the surplus was $57 billion, but by 1984 the trade deficit was $83.6 billion. By 1985 the imbalance was $132 billion, and in 1986 it reached the unexpected high of $166.3 billion, which slowed overall economic growth and contributed to recessions in key industries.[23] From 1982 to 1986 the imbalance in merchandise trade worsened in nine of ten major product groups, and U.S. bilateral trade balances worsened against all top U.S. trading partners, as well as against nineteen of the top twenty.[24] With Japan alone, the deficit rose from $18.3 billion in 1981 to $58.6 billion in 1986, amounting to more than 35 percent of the total U.S. trade deficit with the world.[25] Compounding this were slow economic growth and a heavy burden of external debt among developing countries, which prompted greater economic austerity on their part and reduced demand for U.S. exports. In 1981 developing countries purchased 41 percent of all U.S. merchandise exports, but by 1985 that figure was only 34 percent. Beyond its negative impact on trade, the unsettling level of Third World debt—over $800 billion in 1987—also suggested that some key U.S. financial institutions were dangerously overextended, and this cast doubt on the stability of world financial markets.[26]

These unfavorable developments for U.S. international trade generated increasing economic nationalism in the United States, charges of unfair trading practices against friends and allies, and mounting protectionist sentiments. The Reagan administration, while maintaining that trade problems were attributable mostly to uneven economic recovery between the United States and its major trading partners, was nevertheless pressured by domestic interests to protect U.S. manufacturers against Japanese imports. And many of the administration's Democratic opponents concluded that a stronger protectionist stance on their part would work to their advantage in the 1988 elections. Indeed, polls in the late 1980s reported that Japanese and Americans were increasingly characterizing relations between their two countries as "unfriendly."[27] From the standpoint of national defense, these responses to the trade problem raised concerns about the long-term impact on political relations between the United States and its major trading partners, most of whom were mainstays of the Western alliance system.

The international political environment in which American defense policy was conducted had several notable characteristics. Foremost was "alliance drift." As European nations became more powerful economically and independent politically, American and European interests were not always parallel, and U.S. leadership was questioned. Mindful of the Soviet threat, many Europeans harbored doubts about the credibility of American security guarantees because of Moscow's enhanced conventional and nuclear military power. Also, because of U.S. experiences in the Vietnam war, and later in Lebanon, many Europeans grew uneasy about the U.S. government's capacity for good judgment in foreign affairs.[28]

The Middle East and the Persian Gulf were areas where cross-cutting political purposes complicated American defense policy. The United States remained committed to the defense of Israel, which continued to be its most reliable friend in the region and de facto military ally. Problems arose, though, because American interests in protecting Gulf shipping and containing Soviet influence in the region required cooperation from local Arab states that, with the exception of Egypt, remained technically at war with Israel. At war or not, all Arab states felt compelled by internal and regional political pressures to distance themselves from Washington because of its strong ties to Israel. It was partly for this reason that even Arab states friendly to the United States rejected U.S. requests for basing rights that would have facilitated American efforts to protect oil shipments in the Persian Gulf.

Problems were most pronounced when the U.S. Congress considered selling Arab states advanced military technology. Viewing Saudi Arabia as a potential threat to Israel, Congress frequently felt obliged to impose restrictions on these sales that Arab governments found objectionable. AWACS early-warning aircraft in Saudi Arabia, for instance, had to be jointly manned by U.S. and Saudi crews to ensure that the planes' electronic monitoring systems were not used against Israel. Likewise, American F-15 fighters were sold to the Saudis, but absent the external fuel tanks that would have extended their range. Thus, when an Iraqi aircraft attacked the U.S. frigate *Stark* in the Persian Gulf, the Saudi planes, had they been so authorized, could not have pursued the attacker.

On the threshold of the 1990s, then, the context of American defense policy had changed dramatically from that which had prevailed several decades before. As other nations prospered and acquired sophisticated military capabilities, the relative position of the United States in military, economic, and political power declined.[29] American strategic superiority fell by the wayside. Emergent regional powers acquired enough military capability to command greater respect than the United States customarily granted when contemplating the use of military force in the Third World. There were new centers of economic power that prevented the United States from exerting a decisive influence on international trade and finance.[30] And the Western alliance's very success in deterring Soviet expansion in Europe fostered disunity over the nature and urgency of the Soviet threat. Finally, cross-cutting security issues involving threats to Western interests outside of Europe made it difficult to formulate consistent, mutually reinforcing U.S. defense policies that enjoyed allied backing.

THREATS FACING THE UNITED STATES

External threats facing the United States can be categorized as military or economic. The primary military threat in the 1970s and 1980s was still posed by the Soviet Union, whose preferences on how international, economic, and political systems should be ordered, and how they should function, conflicted sharply with American ideas on freedom, prosperity, and morality. By the end of the 1980s, four developments in the Soviet military threat were most pronounced: the growth of Soviet military capabilities, the marked improvement in the quality of Soviet weaponry, Moscow's propensity to project military power beyond its borders, and its increased ability to translate its military capabilities into political power. Although troops were withdrawn from Afghanistan and forces were reduced somewhat in East Europe, in other respects the reforms associated with glasnost and perestroika have yet to impact significantly on these developments.

After the 1962 Cuban missile crisis, in which American threats backed by U.S. strategic superiority and local conventional superiority prevailed, the Soviet Union rapidly expanded its nuclear and conventional military capabilities and vastly improved its ability to project military power to influence regional conflicts and local insurgencies. From 1972 to 1982, while U.S. defense investment fell 20 percent, comparable Soviet investment rose 50 percent. Cumulative Soviet military expenditures from 1976 to 1985 far surpassed those of the United States. In those years the estimated dollar costs of Soviet military programs were one-third larger than U.S. defense outlays.[31] In 1986 the Soviet military effort consumed about 15 to 17 percent of the country's GNP; military research and development, which was 20 percent of total Soviet defense outlays, came to about 3 percent of the Soviet Union's GNP.[32]

These substantial defense investments yielded the Soviet Union a commanding military presence. By the late 1980s the USSR had 1,418 fixed and mobile intercontinental ballistic missile launchers, capable of delivering about 6,500 nuclear warheads against the United States and its allies. It had nearly 1,000 submarine-launched missiles, with a little over 3,000 warheads; 553 launchers for intermediate-range nuclear forces to deliver about 1,400 warheads; 862 bombers; 5,200 tactical aircraft; 211 divisions; an operational antisatellite system; some 9,000 surface-to-air missile launchers; 100 antiballistic missile launchers; 1,049 principal combat vessels; four aircraft carriers; 373 submarines; and 1,756 aircraft dedicated to naval aviation.[33]

Because of its long-standing technological inferiority, the Soviet Union had usually opted for quantity and had made many incremental modifications in its weapons systems instead of striving for state-of-the-art sophistication. But while the United States still maintained impressive leads in electronic sensors, guidance technology, and high-speed computers and associated software, the overall quality of Soviet military technology improved remarkably. Advances in guidance systems made Soviet SS-18 ICBMs theoretically capable of destroying 65 to 80 percent of the U.S. Minuteman ICBMs in a preemptive strike. Moscow meanwhile increased the hardness of its own missile silos and deployed new, less vulnerable, mobile ICBMs. It developed the Blackjack, a sophisticated new strategic bomber. And, although it trailed an impressive American lead, Moscow pursued cruise missile technology in a serious way. The Blackjack, for example, was tested with a new air-launched cruise missile (ALCM). Sea-launched cruise missiles (SLCMs) and ground-launched cruise missiles (GLCMs) were also developed.

With these developments, Western analysts noted "progressive consistency" between Soviet force posture and strategic doctrine. In the Soviet view, the best way to deter war—even nuclear war—was to confront adversaries with enough military capability to fight and win if deterrence failed. But for many years the Soviet Union's lack of nuclear capability left major gaps between what its doctrine demanded and the strategic missions its forces could perform. Western analysts worried in the 1980s that Moscow's notable military achievements had narrowed this gap considerably, to the degree perhaps that the USSR might enjoy "escalation dominance." That is, Soviet leaders, in expectation that they would have superior residual striking power after a preemptive strike, might assess more confidently their ability to make U.S. leaders back down in a crisis.

Soviet conventional military power would have been less provocative had it not grown in tandem with a more activist Soviet foreign policy and bolder attitudes toward using military force far from home.[34] The Brezhnev doctrine offered, in Soviet minds, a theoretical justification for intervention by arms to preserve socialism. This idea initially seemed to apply only to Eastern Europe, but with enhanced power projection capabilities, Moscow employed military intervention to raise new bulwarks against American influence in the Third World. With improved airlift and sealift capabilities, it intervened with Cuba in Angola and Ethiopia, where it established logistics and reconnaissance bases for its forces in the Indian Ocean. It airlifted Cuban troops and rendered direct military assistance in support of South Yemeni radicals, sent thousands of military advisers and advanced antiaircraft missiles to Syria, backed Vietnam's invasion of Cambodia, and began maintaining strike aircraft in Vietnam. It also periodically engaged Pakistani forces on the Afghanistan border, where the United States funneled arms and supplies to the Afghan resistance.

None of this implied that the Soviet Union could project more military power than the United States. The Soviet navy had no aircraft carriers resembling U.S. supercarriers; indeed, it was unclear whether their newest carrier under development in the late 1980s would even approach U.S. *Nimitz*-class carriers in capability and firepower. As one analyst observed, "The power of Soviet military force continued to wane as distances from the USSR increased."[35] Of course, the United States was most disadvantaged militarily near the Soviet border, as in Iran and the Persian Gulf.

Many U.S. clients also suffered from chronic political instability and military insurgencies that called for American military and economic assistance and tested U.S. commitments and political resolve. The Philippines, a key U.S. ally and home of essential U.S. air and naval bases, confronted possibilities of right-wing coups and a troublesome Marxist insurgency, as did El Salvador, which was important because of its proximity to Marxist Nicaragua and the Costa Rican and Honduran democracies. With direct U.S. military assistance, Guatemala also confronted a protracted leftist insurgency.

Central America in these respects posed sharp dilemmas for the United States. Whether insurgencies there were directed by Cuba and the Soviet Union or indigenous uprisings that Moscow and Havana could exploit, it was not in the U.S. interest to have hostile governments in the region that opposed U.S. policies and offered footholds for Cuba and the Soviet Union. Nor was it beneficial for the United States to be identified with anti-Soviet authoritarian regimes whose ruthlessness inspired Marxist and other anti-American movements. That the region was contiguous to U.S. territory made the dilemma worse, since this increased chances that the United States would intervene directly and reinforce anti-American sentiments in the region.

Nicaragua, given its strong ties to Cuba and the Soviet Union, was a special concern. Although Moscow was careful not to provoke the United States by giving the Sandinista government advanced offensive weapons, and at times actually pressed the Sandinistas for political moderation, the prospect of "another Cuba" in Central America generated alarm, as well as controversy over the precise nature of the Nicaraguan threat and what should be done about it. By various controversial means the United States also provided humanitarian and military assistance to the "Contras," the anti-Sandinista insurgents. Since the Contras had little hope of defeating the Nicaraguan army, the overriding question was whether the Sandinista government would topple from internal political and economic weaknesses before the United States applied military force directly.

A relatively new political development, Islamic fundamentalism, posed unorthodox, yet significant, challenges to U.S. interests in Southwest Asia and the Persian Gulf. Ayatollah Khomeini's messianic brand of Shiism sought to eliminate both Western and Russian influence in the Persian Gulf and throughout the Middle East. The United States, in Khomeini's eyes the "Great Satan," bore the brunt of Iran's hostility. While utterly pragmatic at times, as when it secretly dealt with the Reagan adminstration for arms, Iran and its followers in the Muslim world objected essentially to what the United States was, rather than to what the United States did in any specific sense. From their perspective, Western culture—in particular American culture because of its ubiquity—constituted a direct and "aesthetically loathsome" threat to Islam.[36] Khomeini therefore strove to demonstrate that Islam could be purged of American influence.[37]

Considerable American interests hinged on the outcome of the Iran-Iraq war because the balance of power in the region would have shifted dramatically with an Iranian victory. Although that has not happened, growing Sunni fundamentalism, in combination with long-standing Arab resentments over U.S.-Israeli relations, has already made joint military exercises in the region problematic and

U.S. basing rights nearly impossible to attain. NATO also is affected since Turkish domestic politics increasingly are influenced by conservative Muslim religious movements.

The United States also remained vulnerable to disruptions in supplies of oil and minerals. On the other hand, during the mid 1980s the United States was somewhat less vulnerable to disruptions in oil supplies than it had been during the 1970s. The availability of new resources from the North Sea and Mexico, combined with global recession and diminished demand, took oil issues off the front burner. United States dependence on foreign oil nonetheless grew, as the lowest prices in decades made it unprofitable for domestic producers to develop American reserves. At the heart of the matter was the fact that between 52 and 55 percent of the world's proven oil reserves were in the Persian Gulf region—Saudi Arabia alone having 25 percent—where war and unpredictable politics generated potential for disruptions in supply at reasonable prices.[38] Although the United States imported only 2 to 4 percent of its national oil requirements from the Gulf, this was not true of U.S. allies and major trading partners. Western Europe imported 20 percent of its oil from the region, Japan 56 percent, and South Korea 74 percent. There was growing concern, therefore, that the oil vulnerability problem had been treated too lightly, since faster economic recovery would have brought increased demand and a tighter market in which even small shortfalls in supply or threats of shortfalls could have provoked speculation, panic buying, and another "energy crisis." In that event, it would matter little that the United States was far less dependent on oil from the Persian Gulf than Europe and Japan, since instability in the price or supply of Gulf oil would have made all oil more expensive, and the Western and Japanese economies were so interdependent.[39]

Strategic minerals were another vulnerability (see table 1). Four minerals—chromium, cobalt, manganese, and platinum-group metals—were the greatest concern because they had no readily available substitutes, and there were risks of disruptions from civil disturbances, strikes, unfriendly political action,

Table 1. U.S. Dependence Upon Foreign Sources for Critical Raw Materials

Raw Material	1950	1970	1985	2000
Aluminum	64%	85%	96%	98%
Chromium	NA	100	100	100
Copper	31	0	34	56
Iron	8	30	55	67
Lead	39	31	62	67
Manganese	88	95	100	100
Phosphorus	8	0	0	2
Potassium	14	42	47	61
Sulfur	2	0	28	52
Tin	77	NA	100	100
Tungsten	NA	50	87	97
Zinc	38	59	72	84

Source: Lester Brown, *The Global Politics of Resource Scarcity,* Overseas Development Council, Development Paper 17 (April 1974), pp. 20–21.

and regional hostilities involving the countries that supplied them.[40] Because self-sufficiency in strategic minerals would have been too costly, the United States relied on the free market and emergency stockpiles to ensure adequate supply. But it would have taken 100 years at the prevailing spending rates to reach U.S. stockpile goals.[41] Meanwhile, U.S. vulnerabilities increased as domestic sources declined and supply hinged more tightly on politically unstable nations and the Soviet Union.

SELF-PERCEPTION

To understand how American leaders perceive the U.S. role in the international system, it is necessary to sketch briefly that role to date.

For most of its 200 years, the United States tended to play a minor or passive role within the international system, on the assumption that such a course would most effectively promote its national security. During the first 100 years of its existence, the United States tried to remain free of entangling alliances and disengaged from the balance-of-power politics practiced by the major European states.

When the United States did become a major actor in the international system, it always felt the need to do so under the guise of moral self-righteousness. Although in many cases the United States was acting primarily to enhance its economic interests, some form of moral justification was always explicitly or implicitly invoked. Thus, when the United States wrestled

control of Cuba and the Philippines from Spain, it referred to its Christian responsibilities toward the pagans. Similarly, the United States entered World War I to make the world safe for democracy and attempted to free the post–World War I period of secret diplomacy. Finally, during the period between the world wars, when the American people discovered that the so-called merchants of death had profited from the war, the United States again vowed to avoid involvement in the international system to the maximum extent possible. Not even Hitler's blitzkrieg attack on Poland could induce the United States to become active in the world arena. It took the Japanese attack on Pearl Harbor to shake the American populace from its isolationist lethargy.

With one exception, the experience of World War II completely changed the American perception of the appropriate U.S. role in foreign affairs. In the immediate postwar period, the United States saw itself charged with containing monolithic communism whenever and wherever it appeared outside the Soviet orbit. To accomplish this task, the United States was willing to apply its economic, political, military, and paramilitary resources all around the globe. The nation that had remained disengaged from world politics now ringed the communist world with alliances, poured hundreds of billions of dollars into military and economic assistance to noncommunist regimes, intervened covertly in countries from Guatemala to Iran, attempted to influence the outcome of elections in such widely diverse nations as Italy and the Philippines, employed military force without war (for political purposes) on more than 200 occasions, and fought two long, bitterly divisive, and costly wars on the Asian mainland.

The one element that remained constant in U.S. post-World War II defense policy was its strong moral component. The conflict with the Soviet Union and its allies was depicted as a fight against godless atheists in the Kremlin. Military and nonmilitary intervention was justified in terms of defending freedom, championing democracy, and liberating captive peoples.

With their overwhelming economic and military strength and a sense of moral self-right-eousness, the American people and many of their leaders felt that there were no limits to their capacity to influence events around the globe. This "arrogance of power" eventually led "the best and the brightest" into overextending the nation in Vietnam, bringing about a dramatic change in American self-perception.

By the close of the 1960s, the United States realized that there were limits to its power, and consequently to its ability to influence events around the globe. While the United States could certainly provide for its own security needs, it could not single-handedly preserve the freedom and independence of noncommunist governments throughout the world. Nor was such a state of affairs vital to American national security. This new perception was given its clearest expression by President Richard M. Nixon on Guam on 3 November 1969. In what later become known as the Guam or Nixon Doctrine, the Republican president proclaimed that although the United States would honor all the commitments it had made in the quarter of a century since the end of World War II, its allies, outside of Western Europe and Japan, would henceforth bear the primary responsibility for their own security. The United States would provide some assistance to these nations, but in the final analysis, they, not the United States, would determine their own fates.[42]

At about the same time, the United States began to perceive that it was not engaged in a zero-sum struggle with a monolithic communist enemy. As the 1960s drew to a close, it became clear to U.S. policy makers that the split between the Soviet Union and the People's Republic of China (PRC) was real, and that the many other Marxist governments and parties around the world often acted independently of both communist giants. Moreover, the United States shared certain common interests with both the USSR and the PRC and considered nationalism, not ideology, to be the dominant motive in the behavior of those nations.

Accordingly, President Nixon and his national security adviser, Henry Kissinger, began to move the United States in the direction of a limited form of détente with the Soviet Union, recognition of the communist government in Beijing as the legitimate rulers of China, and improving trade and cultural relations with other communist governments. These policies were quite successful. Détente with the Soviet Union led to the SALT I treaty in 1972, the Vladivostok Accords of 1974, the Helsinki Agreement of 1975, and SALT II in 1979. Recognition of the PRC and full diplomatic relations with the Beijing government took effect on 1 January 1979.

Throughout the early part of the 1970s, while the United States was moving away from its role of world policeman, there were many who wished to see it return almost to its pre-World War II isolationist posture or "fortress America" strategy, and to reemphasize the moral component of its national security policy. In 1972 these neoisolationists succeeded in helping Senator George McGovern capture the Democratic presidential nomination. McGovern's campaign theme was "Come Home, America," and to make sure that Americans stayed home, the South Dakota senator proposed a 40 percent reduction in the size of the defense budget, which was already 10 percent below its pre-Vietnam level.[43] Similarly, other neoisolationists in Congress repeatedly attempted to circumscribe the ability of the executive branch to employ military force overseas. The War Powers Act of 1973 limited to sixty days the president's power to use the armed services outside the United States. The legislature also used the power of the purse to prevent the commander in chief from intervening militarily in such areas as Angola and Indochina.

The neoisolationists were defeated in the 1972 presidential campaign. Throughout the 1976 Carter campaign the candidate railed against a foreign policy that was contrary to what he believed were America's long-standing beliefs and principles. As candidate Carter noted on 6 October 1976: "We've lost in our foreign policy the character of the American people."[44] Once in office, he set out to define a new policy with a strong emphasis on human rights.[45]

The 1970s were years in which Americans

sought to rebuild the consensus on the country's proper role in international affairs that the U.S. experience in Vietnam had shattered. Americans were no longer willing to assume the role of world policeman, but neither were they ready to withdraw into isolation. After the Iranian hostage crisis and the Soviet invasion of Afghanistan, President Carter revealed publicly late in his administration that he thought his initial assessment of Soviet intentions had been mistaken. He also proclaimed, in what became known as the Carter Doctrine, that any attempt by an outside power to gain control of the Persian Gulf "would be regarded as an assault on the vital interests of the United States," and that "such an assault would be repelled by any means necessary, including military force." Shortly thereafter, the U.S. Rapid Deployment Force (RDF) was conceived with the explicit purpose of intervening militarily in the Gulf region. Also, after campaigning on a platform of cutting the defense budget and making human rights the foundation of his foreign policy, President Carter pledged to increase defense spending by 3 percent annually in real terms and not to pursue human rights at the expense of relations with U.S. friends and allies.

President Reagan entered office on a groundswell of support for his confrontational tone and his commitment to reassert U.S. leadership in foreign affairs. Popular backing for his defense buildup grew, and there were initial indications that a new "paradigm shift" had reestablished a bipartisan foreign policy consensus.[46] But when the Reagan administration sought to implement its ideas, U.S. foreign and defense policies again became major sources of partisan conflict. As one study suggested, President Reagan may have won the 1980 election "in spite of his foreign policy stance, not because of it."[47]

The Reagan administration received popular backing when U.S. F-14s destroyed two Soviet-made Libyan aircraft in self-defense over the Gulf of Sidra; when U.S. forces, in the largest U.S. military operation since Vietnam, made short, but unexpectedly hard, work of invading the Caribbean island of Grenada; and when U.S. Marines helped to evacuate trapped Palestinian and Syrian fighters from Beirut after an Israeli siege. Nor was there much objection when U.S. aircraft bombed Libya in retaliation for that country's support of terrorism. But there was uneasiness when U.S. military advisers were dispatched to help El Salvador fight communist insurgents; when several hundred Marines deployed as an "interposition force" in the Lebanese civil war were killed by a terrorist's car bomb; when the administration used force to aid the Lebanese government in that country's civil war and lost two A-6 aircraft to Syrian missiles; and when, after the Iraqi attack on the USS *Stark*, it extended U.S. naval protection to Kuwaiti oil tankers transiting the Persian Gulf. In light of these experiences, the American public in the 1980s was more conservative to be sure, but not more interventionist, especially when military intervention promised to be prolonged or indecisive.

President Reagan's election and that of his successor, George Bush, therefore did not recreate consensus on America's role in world affairs. American foreign policy elites fell roughly into three groups: those whose basic concerns were Soviet expansionism and reasserting U.S. military power; those who had a predominantly North-South orientation and stressed problems of global poverty and inequitable distribution of resources; and those who emphasized domestic problems and preferred that the United States avoid involvements in other nations' affairs.[48] This fractured political elite weakened the reserve of domestic political backing for military involvement, encouraged American adversaries to bank on an evaporation of U.S. resolve, and made some U.S. friends and allies apprehensive about the credibility of American commitments.

INTERDEPENDENCIES

As discussed above, the U.S. perception of the appropriate role it ought to play in the international system underwent a complete reversal after World War II. Nowhere was this change more evident than in the American attitude toward alliances. Between the Revolutionary War and World War II, the United

States had heeded almost scrupulously President Washington's advice to remain free of permanent or entangling alliances. It even fought its wars alone. The War of 1812, the Mexican War, and the Spanish-American War were all conducted without the assistance of other nations. The United States even entered World War I and World War II for its own reasons, rather than because of formal alliance commitments. After World War I, the Senate refused to ratify the Treaty of Versailles and thus effectively kept the nation out of the collective security arrangements of the League of Nations.

In the post-1945 period, however, the United States actively sought to become involved throughout the world. Before the war came to a close, it took the initiative in founding the United Nations and was primarily responsible for those provisions in the UN charter that provided for collective security through the use of multinational military force, if necessary. Then, in response to what it perceived as Soviet expansionism, the United States initiated and joined a number of regional alliances.[49] The aim was to "contain" Soviet expansionism. In the Rio Treaty of 1947, the United States joined with twenty Central and South American nations to form a multilateral pact that prohibited intervention by foreign states in Latin American affairs and provided for consultations among the nations with regard to the external threat. While the Rio Pact could be considered a normal outgrowth of the Monroe Doctrine and an expression of traditional U.S. concern about its own hemisphere, the North Atlantic Treaty Organization (NATO) Pact of 1949 marked a sharp change from previous practices. The NATO pact was an open-ended, multilateral, peacetime alliance between the United States, Canada, and Western European nations that committed the United States to consider an attack on any member nation as an attack on itself. In addition, the NATO pact provided for the establishment of a permanent multinational military force and the basing of American forces in and around the European continent. Unlike some of the other post-war alliances, NATO has persisted and now has sixteen member states.

NATO was primarily a response to Soviet actions in Czechoslovakia, Berlin, and Greece. However, the communist takeover of mainland China in 1949, the Sino-Soviet Pact of 1950, and the North Korean attack that same year caused the United States to focus on the communist threat to Asia as well. In 1951 the United States signed bilateral mutual defense treaties with Japan and the Philippines and a trilateral pact with Australia and New Zealand (the ANZUS treaty). In 1953 and 1954 the United States entered into bilateral arrangements with South Korea and the Republic of China (Taiwan), respectively. In 1954 the United States, along with France, Britain, and seven Asian nations, signed the Manila Pact, which created the South East Asia Treaty Organization (SEATO). Although not as demanding as the NATO treaty, this pact pledged the signatories to assist one another when their peace and safety were threatened. In 1959 the United States completed its "ring around the communist world" by concluding bilateral agreements with Iran, Pakistan, and Turkey. In addition, it became a silent partner in the Central Treaty Organization (CENTO), which formally consisted of Iran, Iraq, Turkey, Pakistan, and the United Kingdom.

The alliances that the United States put together so carefully in the 1940s and 1950s eroded throughout the 1960s in both form and substance. The first to show signs of coming apart was SEATO. Although it was not officially disbanded until 1977, SEATO began to disintegrate much sooner. In 1962 Laos was removed from SEATO's area of concern when the country was declared neutral by international agreement. Cambodia dropped out of the alliance in 1964 after breaking diplomatic relations with the United States. Moreover, in 1965, when the United States began to intervene massively in South Vietnam, it did so with no visible support from its SEATO allies. Finally, the other major powers, France and Britain, dropped out of SEATO in 1966 and 1967, respectively, and Pakistan formally withdrew in 1972.

CENTO officially lasted until the overthrow of the Shah of Iran in 1979. However, its fate was sealed in 1967 when Great Britain announced its plan to abandon all interests east of Suez, pulling its security forces from the Persian Gulf in 1971. The bilateral treaty between the United States and Taiwan was officially abrogated by the Carter administration in late 1978, but actually began to unravel when President Nixon visited Beijing in May 1972.

NATO still endures, but it, too, has suffered some severe strains over the past three decades. In 1966 France withdrew militarily because of its concern about U.S. domination of the alliance, particularly U.S. control over the use of nuclear weapons by NATO. A decade later Greece took the same step because of its difficulties with Turkey over Turkish occupation of Cyprus. During the late 1960s many of America's NATO allies became disenchanted when the United States redeployed troops from Europe to the Southeast Asia theater. Alliance members also became concerned when the United States concluded strategic arms agreements with the Soviet Union in 1972, consulting only minimally with its NATO allies, and when the Americans sent military supplies from the NATO stockpile to Israel during the 1973 Middle East War. There was some fear among the NATO allies that agreements with the USSR could undermine American resolve to use U.S. strategic nuclear weapons to defend Europe, while U.S. aid to Israel might have resulted in a cutoff of oil supplies to Western Europe by some Arab states.

As the 1970s came to a close, however, NATO appeared to be experiencing a revitalization. Faced with growing Soviet military strength, the members of the alliance pledged to increase defense spending by 3 percent a year in real terms for the foreseeable future. Moreover, they pledged to move toward greater standardization, interoperability, and cost sharing in their force structure. In addition, the United States, having substantially cut back its military forces in the Pacific after the end of the Vietnam War, once again placed primary regional emphasis both on the allocation of resources within its defense budget and on the development of its force structure for the defense of Europe.

A fundamental problem in the NATO alliance was that political centers in Western Eu-

rope and the United States shifted, Europe's moving to the left and the United States' moving right. The consequences were asymmetrical perceptions of the Soviet threat, accompanied by feelings among many Europeans that American leadership was not necessarily in their best interests. With an eye toward bolstering its export economy and securing raw materials, Western Europe expanded trade and financial dealings with the USSR, despite Moscow's "adventurism" in the Third World. President Reagan, meanwhile, sought to restore American leadership with a more aggressive anti-Soviet tone, which many Europeans found unnecessary and frightening.[50]

The resulting differences of opinion between the United States and its European allies found expression in numerous issues—as when Washington tried unsuccessfully to secure European sanctions against Moscow for its invasion of Afghanistan. With the European shift to the left, there also developed a well-coordinated anti-American movement, especially among younger Europeans who had not experienced the allied unity of World War II or the postwar transatlantic consensus on the Soviet threat.[51] For some in this generation, in view of President Reagan's initial hard-line stance on arms control and his greater willingness to use military force, the United States seemed nearly as aggressive as the USSR. Indeed, as the United States Information Agency reported, a wide margin of Europeans believed that Soviet General Secretary Mikhail Gorbachev had done more for peace than President Reagan.[52]

Also, the Reagan administration received only qualified European support in mustering unified action against Libya in 1986. U.S. F-111s were allowed to strike Libya from bases in Britain, but France and Spain refused the bombers permission to overfly their territory. Feeling vulnerable to terrorism, Italy released a suspected Palestinian terrorist leader after American aircraft forced his Egyptian plane to land at an Italian air base. Many in the United States were also bitter when NATO ministers rejected American requests for more assistance in the Persian Gulf to safeguard oil and counterbalance Soviet military and political influence in the region. By 1987 there was growing concern that resentment toward Europe would grow stronger if the U.S. Navy sustained more casualties in the Gulf escorting oil tankers bound for Europe—especially if the oil in the tankers then fueled European factories that helped put Americans out of jobs.

From Europe's perspective, NATO's exclusive military function was to defend against a Soviet attack; in this respect the alliance was deemed to be an inappropriate forum for addressing "out of area" problems like the Persian Gulf and state-sponsored terrorism. Toward these ends, European members of NATO preferred bilateral, not collective, agreements with the United States that were developed case-by-case according to individualized interests. But from many Americans' viewpoint, Europe's reluctance to offer assistance left as alternatives only U.S. unilateralism and isolationism.

These problems within the NATO alliance were not lost on Moscow, which by various strategems sought to draw Western Europe away from the United States, capitalizing on the region's longing for détente and exploiting its reservations about American leadership. Throughout the 1980s, arms control controversies gave Moscow leverage; although, after occasionally heated debates and persistent European misgivings, alliance unity prevailed. Whether each weathering of these controversies left NATO weaker or stronger was debatable, but certainly the outcomes that were obtained were preferable to the rancor and discord that there might have been. With INF and short-range missiles on the negotiating table, British and French cooperation grew unusually close, and France, in the midst of its own nuclear buildup and determined to exercise more influence over Western arms control positions, played an increasingly active role in NATO decision making, something it had not done since it withdrew from NATO's integrated military command in 1966.[53]

Among many observers in the United States, isolationists in particular, there was also a feeling that Europe was not assuming its fair share of the defense burden. In 1978 NATO ministers agreed to increase annual defense spending on conventional forces by 3 percent after

inflation, but only the United States, Britain, and France ever met this goal; defense spending in Belgium, Denmark, and the Netherlands actually decreased in 1983. A central problem was that most European nations did not believe their economies could sustain higher defense spending in addition to their commitments to social welfare. Declining European exchange rates with respect to the dollar also made American-built weapons more expensive and thus less affordable. Many Europeans, however, simply disagreed that their contribution to the alliance was disproportionately small. American security, they pointed out, depended on European security; Europe imposed a military draft on its young and the United States did not; Europe had three and a half million personnel on active duty and the United States had a little over two million; Europe provided facilities for NATO military bases; and, finally, it was argued, it was cheaper to base U.S. troops in Europe than to remove and maintain them in the United States.[54]

Basing rights, too, were a troublesome issue. Polls showed that most Spaniards did not want American bases on their soil; and the Spanish government demanded a nearly complete U.S. withdrawal from facilities that U.S. officials claimed were necessary to defend southern Europe.[55] The future of U.S. bases in Greece and Turkey was also unsettled, particularly in Greece where it was widely believed that the United States favored Turkey in that country's disputes with Greece over Cyprus and mineral rights in the Aegean Sea.

ANZUS, the U.S. alliance with New Zealand and Australia, was also troubled. Relations between New Zealand and the United States were strained severely when New Zealand banned nuclear arms and nuclear-powered ships from its territory, in effect disallowing many U.S. naval vessels from calling there. As in Europe, this "anti-nuclear allergy" stemmed in part from growing "skepticism about America's foreign policy motives."[56] U.S. officials, angered by New Zealand's policy, responded that the United States no longer felt obliged to come to New Zealand's aid.[57] By the late 1980s, the United States had six, perhaps only five, bona fide alliances remaining:

NATO, the Rio Pact, the doubtful ANZUS Pact, and bilateral agreements with Japan, Korea, and the Philippines.

The arrangements nonetheless signaled which interests the United States considered vital. In themselves, however, they did not restrict or alter the American worldview or strategy. Rather, they were a reflection of them. Just as the "pactomania" of the late 1940s and 1950s was a reflection of a "containment" policy directed toward curbing or "containing" Soviet expansionism, the smaller number of more troubled alliances in the 1980s gave evidence of more limited U.S. security objectives and of the difficulty of maintaining alliance unity after preserving more than forty years of peace with the Soviet Union. Equally significant was the fact that many pressing threats to U.S. interests by this time fell outside existing alliance structures—a further indication of broad changes in the international system that had altered the nature of threats to the United States and the means for addressing them.

National Objectives, National Strategy, and Military Doctrine

The United States has six principal national security objectives: to preserve its independence, free institutions, and territorial integrity; to protect U.S. and allied vital interests abroad; to shape an international order in which U.S. freedoms and institutions can survive and prosper; to promote democratic institutions around the world; to promote growth in the world economy; and to prevent hostile powers from dominating other economic-industrial centers.[58]

These objectives have narrowed substantially in the wake of the post-Vietnam reassessment of America's role in the world. As discussed above, prior to the debacle of Southeast Asia, the primary objective of American national security policy was to contain or prevent the spread of communism in any area of the globe. American policy makers did not make much of a distinction between those areas that were essential and those that were merely desirable; nor did policy makers make much of a

distinction between communist movements controlled by the Soviet Union and those independent of it.

Generally speaking, U.S. leaders perceive three distinct threats to the security and economic well-being of the United States and its allies. The first is the challenge posed by the arms buildup of the Soviet Union and its Warsaw Pact allies. Second are the various forms of instability in the Third World that could be exploited by such outside powers as the Soviet Union. And third are potential disruptions of the global economy that could seriously jeopardize the economic health and well-being of the United States and its allies. The most pressing issue in this third area is energy.[59]

The current objectives of American national security policy are likely to remain essentially the same for the foreseeable future. But the means of achieving those objectives are likely to be subject to continuous debate, and thus are more susceptible to change. Indeed, the whole post-World War II American defense policy debate has been a struggle over how to achieve national security objectives more efficiently.

Battles over differing views of how best to achieve national security objectives were fought in the executive and legislative phases of the annual defense budget process. There was also input from congressional "watchdog" agencies like the General Accounting Office (GAO), Office of Technology Assessment (OTA), Congressional Budget Office (CBO), and Congressional Research Service (CRS). Included, too, were studies from research corporations ("think tanks") specializing in defense matters, and advice from private consultants.

Normally, the Joint Chiefs of Staff (JCS) and the military departments support increased capabilities, while the Office of Management and Budget (OMB) and the Arms Control and Disarmament Agency (ACDA) contend that lesser levels would be quite acceptable. The Office of the Secretary of Defense (OSD) and the Department of State normally take a middle-ground position, with OSD leaning more toward the maximum end of the spectrum and the State Department favoring the minimum pole. Within Congress, the armed services committees normally support the JCS positions, while the appropriations and budget committees favor the middle ground. Minimum deterrence, with the relatively smaller expenditures that such a posture entails, often draws strong support from some members of the foreign relations and international affairs committees.

Outside government, research groups represent nearly every shade of opinion on defense issues, ranging from advocacy of unilateral disarmament on the one hand to nuclear superiority and space-based strategic defenses on the other. Those typically favoring a reduced or more passive defense effort include the Institute for Policy Studies, the Committee for National Security, the Center for Defense Information, the Federation of American Scientists, the American Association for the Advancement of Science, and the Arms Control Association. Those that usually favor increased preparedness or more aggressive approaches include the National Strategy Information Center, the Committee on the Present Danger, the American Security Council, and High Frontier. In between these extremes stand the Brookings Institution and the American Enterprise Institute (AEI). The former usually favors making incremental changes toward a smaller or reoriented force, while the latter generally supports small changes in the opposite direction.

These nongovernmental organizations express their dissent primarily through the publication of periodicals. For example, the Center for Defense Information publishes the monthly *Defense Monitor*; Brookings, a series called *Studies in Defense Policy*; and AEI, the monthly *Foreign Policy and Defense Review*. In addition, most of these groups issue an annual analysis of the current defense budget and often supply expert witnesses for sympathetic congressional committees.

The ideas of these groups often enter directly into the defense debate and occasionally form the basis on which the issues are examined within the Congress. However, their overall impact upon policy is diluted because their positions are often contradictory. For example, a congressman who quotes a Brookings study supporting the elimination of a particular program will likely find a colleague citing an AEI study that draws the opposite conclusion.

In addition to these nongovernmental research groups, others, such as the RAND Corporation, the Institute for Defense Analyses (IDA), and the Hudson Institute, engage in research projects commissioned by various bureaucratic elements within the Defense Department itself.

IDEOLOGY, CULTURE, AND CAPABILITIES

The approach nations take toward the international system is generally a mixture of their ideology, culture, and capabilities. However, for each nation, the relative importance of each of these three factors is markedly different. Ideology and culture have had a relatively large impact in determining the objectives the United States pursues in the international arena.[60]

In the minds of Americans, the United States is more than just the world's first new nation, it is the world's first democracy and the first nation in the history of mankind that has devoted itself to improving the lot of the common man. As such, many Americans consider the country morally superior to other nations. Moreover, in the American view, peace is seen as the natural state of affairs, and wars are caused primarily through the abuse of power. Just as power has to be restricted at home, so it must be restricted in international affairs. Similarly, just as the United States prospered at home through a laissez-faire economic policy, so the international system would flourish through free trade. To put it bluntly, in American ideology, economics is good and politics is bad. Therefore, using power and force within the domestic or international system can be justified only by appealing to some higher moral principle. Thus, the United States claimed that it entered World War I not for the quite legitimate purpose of protecting itself from a European continent dominated by Germany, but because the Germans had engaged in unrestricted and morally reprehensible submarine warfare, and therefore deserved to be punished. Even in the post–World War II period, American support for realpolitik (policy guided by national interest and power considerations) could be gained only by disguising it as idealpolitik (policy guided by moral principle).

Finally, because of the impact of ideology and culture, when the United States finds it necessary to use its military power, it is usually plagued with a sense of guilt. Thus, after every major war, the reasons for the nation's involvement have been reinterpreted. These revisionist histories have certain common themes: the conflicts in which the United States became involved did not, in fact, threaten its security interests; the United States became involved primarily because the politicians saw a threat where none really existed; and this illusion was promoted by propagandists who aroused and manipulated public opinion, by civilian and military bureaucrats concerned with promoting the interests of their own organizations, and by bankers and industrialists who benefited from the struggle.

Americans traditionally attempt to assuage this feeling of guilt in two ways. First, they withdraw from the international system and focus on problems at home. As noted above, this was the theme promoted by Senator George McGovern toward the end of the war in Vietnam. Second, to ensure that the policy makers will not become too involved internationally again, restrictions are placed upon their ability to involve the United States overseas. The Ludlow Amendment after World War I, the Bricker Amendment after Korea, and the Congressional War Powers Act after Vietnam were similar attempts to restrain policy makers from overextension in international politics.

In the post-Vietnam period, ideology and culture remained significant factors in justifying continuing U.S. international involvements. However, this moral justification was put in proper context: the United States no longer pretended that moral principle was the primary driving force behind the country's security policy. Rather, it was recognized that economics and politics required the maintenance of a large military establishment and the occasional use of force. As energy and other forms of economic interdependence grew, the American standard of living was tied more closely than ever to the country's ability to influence developments abroad by power politics.[61] This often demanded that the United States associate with regimes that did not share America's democratic values or its regard for human rights. It also required that Americans be willing to use military force for economic reasons. International politics did not permit the United States the luxury of ideological purity.

The Vietnam War, however, did change the country's perspective on containing communism. Anticommunism once served as a useful justification for full-scale global involvement and the use of military force in such places as Korea, Vietnam, the Dominican Republic, and the Middle East. But in the late 1980s Americans were more discriminating. With the idea of monolithic world communism exposed as a myth, Americans were skeptical of the need to oppose communists actively at every turn. They dreaded another prolonged, indecisive conflict in the Third World and the domestic turmoil and economic hardships that would accompany it. They demanded more thoughtful consideration of whether U.S. vital interests were truly at stake before U.S. forces were engaged.

Nicaragua was a case in point. After Vietnam, many Americans doubted that Nicaragua was a serious enough threat to justify U.S. military involvement. They also questioned whether it was right for the United States to decide what form of government another country should have. Others, who anticipated "falling dominoes" in Central America, feared that U.S. failure to act decisively would lead to more serious threats later at the United States' southern border.

NATIONAL STRATEGY

Although not specifically stated in any one document, the American national strategy has been to employ creative diplomacy to direct the country's national assets toward achieving its national security objectives. United States military capabilities have provided an essential backdrop from which American diplomats have been able to negotiate beneficial international accords from positions of strength. The United States has given hundreds of billions of dollars in economic and military aid and manipulated access to its technology and its markets as tools to influence other states. And when creative diplomacy has failed, or seemed too unpromising, military force has been used.

Within the American political system there was basic agreement on this overall strategy. But the previously mentioned lack of consensus among American political elites on how the United States should conduct its foreign affairs caused significant disagreement over the manner and extent to which diplomatic efforts, economic leverage, and military power should be applied. Some observers favored almost complete reliance on moral suasion and "quiet diplomacy." Others were willing to apply economic sanctions. And those who advocated a more aggressive approach frequently divided on whether force should be applied incrementally or decisively, and on whether force should be used at all if certain restrictive criteria were not met. Secretary of Defense Weinberger, for example, sought to apply six criteria in deciding whether American forces should be used. According to Weinberger, there should be: vital American interests at stake; a clear intention of winning; well-defined political and military interests; a continual willingness to reevaluate and assess the size and composition of the forces necessary to do the job; no other reasonable alternative to force—that is, force should be the last resort; and there should be reasonable assurance that the military will have the support of the American people and Congress.

Some in the Reagan administration, like Secretary of State George Shultz, took exception to these criteria. They considered them overly restrictive and an impediment to negotiating from strength. In 1983, for example, Shultz was more willing to use military force in Lebanon than Weinberger and much of the U.S. military establishment. Many opponents of the use of force believed that American partisanship in Lebanon had outstripped the U.S. military mission there, and that U.S. interests in the country, beyond self-defense, were insuf-

ficiently compelling to warrant more aggressive U.S. action. They also felt that public and congressional support was too weak to sustain such a military effort.

DOMESTIC DETERMINANTS

Over a century ago, the French political philosopher Alexis de Tocqueville observed that the institutions and processes of American democracy make it difficult to achieve excellence in foreign policy. Tocqueville noted that "foreign politics demand scarcely any of those qualities which are peculiar to a democracy; they require, on the contrary, the perfect use of almost all those in which it is deficient." Nonetheless, democracies like the United States can and do successfully pursue policies designed to protect their national security. Such policies and strategies are strongly affected by domestic factors. In the case of the United States, the principal factors are its political system, economic system, geography, public opinion, and national strategy.

The Political System. The primary domestic determinant of U.S. national strategy is the nature of the American political system. Even in the area of national security policy, powers are shared by the executive and legislative branches of the federal government. Through its power of the purse, its confirmation powers, and the prerogatives to declare war and raise an army and navy, Congress can restrict the type of strategy that the president can develop. It can affect policy directly, for example, by prohibiting aid to certain countries such as South Africa, or by banning military operations, as in Central America. In addition, it often has an indirect, but important, impact in that the president and his advisers must take into account the effect that a particular action will have on the Congress and how they will respond to congressional questions about particular situations.

The courts can have an impact on defense policy and national strategy. For example, the Supreme Court refused to allow President Truman to seize the steel mills in Youngstown, Ohio, during the Korean War. During the war in Southeast Asia, the courts heard several challenges from reservists who argued that they had been called up illegally because no national emergency had been declared. And in a case unrelated to foreign policy, the Supreme Court upheld a lower court ruling that Congress could not overturn an executive branch decision by concurrent resolution (one passed by a simple majority, not a two-thirds vote as required to override a presidential veto to pass legislation that has already been vetoed by the president).[62] Legal experts immediately suggested that this ruling weakened the War Powers Act because it cast doubt on Congress' authority to compel the president by concurrent resolution to remove American forces engaged in hostilities outside the United States.[63]

A second characteristic of the political system that has affected national strategy is the fact and timing of elections. Foreign policy decisions, such as when to strive in earnest for arms control and when to arrange a summit conference, are often timed for maximum impact upon upcoming elections. Neither is the deployment of U.S. troops unaffected, as when Republican members of Congress expressed concern to President Reagan that keeping U.S. troops in Lebanon could be a liability in the 1983 elections.

Concerns about challenges in the primary or general elections can have a great impact upon policy makers' decisions on issues such as the size of the defense budget or aid to nations that have large ethnic constituencies in the United States. For example, in 1976 President Ford reduced the defense budget by $7 billion from prior projections in order to keep his election year budget below $400 billion. That same year the "Greek lobby" in Congress prevented the executive from giving military aid to Turkey.[64]

The openness of the American political system is a third factor affecting national strategy. Not even the most serious and delicate national issues can be kept secret. Negotiating positions, force-planning doctrines, and crisis action plans are normally revealed and thus debated openly in the Congress and the media. For example, on 23 July 1971, the *New York Times* carried an article outlining the U.S. negotiating position one day before it was scheduled to be presented to the Soviet Union, and on 3 August 1977, the *Washington Post* sum-

marized the minutes of a National Security Council meeting that concluded that the Carter administration would concede one-third of West Germany to a Soviet invasion rather than seek increased defense spending.[65]

The U.S. system of checks and balances is the final factor in the political system impinging upon strategy. It normally prevents any radical changes in strategy, even if such changes are necessary to meet new or different international requirements. The advantage within the American political system is always with those seeking to preserve the status quo. New policies can be killed by bureaucratic inertia, denied funding within the Congress, amended, filibustered, and even challenged in court.

The Economic System. As discussed above, one of the objectives of American national security policy is to maintain an environment in which U.S. companies have access to overseas markets for trade and investment. This objective arises from two American beliefs: first, that unrestricted free trade will do for the international system what laissez-faire economics did for this nation; and second, that the U.S. standard of living depends upon the ability to secure certain raw materials, invest overseas, and have access to foreign markets.

There is no doubt that the American economic system and its underlying philosophy play a role in determining national strategy. The United States would not stand idly by while a raw material cartel undermined the country's economy. However, it is not true, as some have argued, that the strategic behavior of the United States is primarily determined by the interests of the American economy. In fact, the United States often has acted contrary to its own best economic interests. For example, the United States poured over $200 billion and two million troops into Southeast Asia from 1964 to 1972, but did not intervene in Indonesia during its 1965 revolution, despite the fact that the latter area had many more raw materials than the nations of South Vietnam, Cambodia, and Laos combined. In the Middle East, the United States has consistently supported Israel even though the U.S. and Western economies are dependent on Arab oil and the cooperation of Arab states is needed for the defense of the Persian Gulf. In fact, during the 1973 war between Israel and Egypt, the United States continued to send massive amounts of aid to Israel after the Arab nations had embargoed American oil. For nearly three decades after World War II, the U.S. government severely restricted trade with the Soviet Union, mainland China, and Eastern Europe despite great pressures from the business community that clamored for access to these large markets.

Geography. The United States is essentially an island nation. Over 60 percent of its border is shoreline. Although it has neighbors directly on its northern and southern borders, these nations have never posed a threat to U.S. national security. Moreover, the orientation of America has always been more east-west than north-south. Its potential opponents lie overseas, and the majority of its trade has always been overseas, not overland.

Thus, for the greater part of this century, the United States has regarded a maritime strategy as the best hope of providing for its national defense. For example, during the 1930s, the U.S. Navy was among the three strongest in the world, while the Army ranked seventeenth. The maritime strategy, which owed its intellectual rigor to Alfred Thayer Mahan, dictated that the United States control the seas in order to ensure prosperity in peacetime and victory in war. Controlling the seas required a large navy and suitable overseas bases. This maritime strategy meant that even when it demobilized much of its navy between the Spanish-American War and World War I and between World Wars I and II, the United States still maintained a comparatively large naval force.

Many have argued, quite convincingly, that, in the age of intercontinental ballistic missiles and huge air transports, maritime strategy is no longer important, and that geography should no longer be a determinant of U.S. strategy. Yet such traditions die hard. When confronted with a crisis, U.S. policy makers almost instinctively turn to naval forces. In most cases in which military forces were employed for political purposes in the post-World War II period, naval units were the chosen instrument.[66] Recent U.S. military involvements in Lebanon, Grenada, and the Mediterranean continue to bear this out.

The top priority of the Nixon-Ford administration in the area of conventional forces was to rebuild American naval capability so that the United States could maintain maritime superiority. One of President Ford's last acts in office was to present to the Congress a five-year shipbuilding program that would have built 157 ships at a cost of $50 billion.[67] When President Carter cut this program in half, he was heavily criticized. Moreover, to prevent the building of a $2.5 billion nuclear-powered aircraft carrier in FY 1979, Carter took the unprecedented step of vetoing the entire FY 1979 defense authorization bill. Nevertheless, the Carter administration spent the largest portion of its defense budget on the Navy Department in FY 1980: the navy received $44 billion, while the air force received $39 billion and the army $34 billion.

One of President Reagan's foremost priorities upon entering office was to counter growing Soviet "blue water" and power projection capabilities. His administration also sought to change U.S. naval strategy from one that would protect sea lanes to one that would destroy the Soviet fleet in its home waters. The administration therefore submitted an ambitious shipbuilding program that by 1988 was to produce a 600-ship navy centered around fifteen carrier task groups and four missile-armed battleships. When President Carter left office the navy had 479 ships; by late 1982 under Reagan it had 514.[68] In five years out of the seven-year period 1981–87, for example, the navy enjoyed the largest share of the U.S. defense budget, in FY 1987 receiving almost $105 billion, with deployable ships numbering 567.[69] The exact direction that the Bush administration will take on strategy in a period of constrained resources is as yet unclear.

Public Opinion and National Will. One of the greatest paradoxes of the American political system is the fact that the public is generally uninformed about national security issues, yet public support is necessary to implement national strategy. Moreover, uninformed, mobilized public opinion can influence critical congressional action either against or in support of the president in a crisis.[70]

In January 1979, 77 percent of the American people could not identify the participants in the SALT talks, yet many senators up for reelection in 1980 were concerned that their position on the SALT II treaty might send the wrong message to their constituents.[71]

Generally speaking, public opinion sets limits or boundaries on national strategy. The American public is not particularly concerned over whether the United States pursues a maritime or continental strategy for its conventional forces, or a counterforce or countervalue strategy for its strategic nuclear component. The American people nonetheless set broad limits on how much of their resources ought to go to defense, on how much the United States should allow the military balance to shift in the Soviet Union's favor, and—especially—on sending their young to fight in foreign wars.

On specific issues, such as aid to Israel or Turkey, special or single interest groups can have a great impact on policy. The existence of certain groups within the American public has affected American strategy in areas like the Middle East and eastern Mediterranean. For example, as former President Ford notes in his memoirs: "The Israeli lobby . . . is strong, vital, and healthy."[72]

National will becomes a factor when Americans are asked to make sacrifices of blood and treasure to support specific policies. A change in the national mood in the late 1960s was the dominant factor in forcing the United States to attempt to negotiate its way out of the Vietnam War, end the draft, and cut defense spending.

As the "Vietnam hangover" receded, the willingness of people to sacrifice again for national security increased. By the end of the 1970s, support for defense spending reached an 18-year high, and a majority of Americans stated that they would support military involvement by U.S. troops in Western Europe.[73] In the mid 1980s, however, the outward swing of this pendulum lost momentum. The public's willingness to continue funding the Reagan defense program at the same levels dropped considerably, and calls for a more equitable distri-

bution of responsibilities among Western nations and Japan were increasingly heard. The public was pro-defense but apprehensive that the Reagan administration had no real political strategy to guide U.S. defense policy and that it had thrown money at defense problems without achieving commensurate returns in security.

Other Factors. The United States is a large, technologically advanced, comparatively wealthy, and politically stable nation with a highly educated populace. All of these characteristics have had an impact upon U.S. national strategy. Because of its size and wealth, the United States has had little choice but to help maintain the balance of power. Its advanced technology has enabled it to maintain rough military parity with the Soviet Union even though its force size and weapons inventory are considerably smaller, and even though it devotes a smaller portion of its resources to the task. American political stability has enabled the country to focus on external threats to national security without having to devote significant resources to countering internal threats. Moreover, its great wealth has allowed it to spend vast sums on national security since the end of World War II without seriously neglecting the social needs of its people.

FORCE-EMPLOYMENT DOCTRINE

The force-employment doctrine of the United States is spelled out annually in the report of the secretary of defense to Congress. This document, which is known throughout the government as the posture statement, is presented to Congress in January of each year as a justification for the current Department of Defense (DoD) budget. From time to time throughout the year, the doctrines set forth in the posture statement are expanded upon or clarified by speeches and other public statements of the president and other members of the national security apparatus. Nonetheless, the annual posture statements remain the basic source for U.S. force-employment doctrine.

In theory, national security objectives, policy, force structure, and employment doctrine should be interdependent. The force structure ought to be assigned to support the prescribed policy. On the other hand, the policy is not created in a vacuum. At any given time it is controlled by the forces already in existence or the forces the nation is willing to develop and procure. In practice, the fit among policy, structure, and doctrine is rarely perfect; however, these elements are usually connected, albeit loosely.

In their first months in office, administrations normally develop a statement of national security policy objectives to be used as a basic guide in formulating force posture throughout the duration of the administration. The national security policy objectives and assumptions are set forth in a presidential directive (PD). Within the Defense Department, the objectives and assumption of the PD are operationalized in a comprehensive program document. In the Carter administration this document was called the consolidated guidance (CG). In the Reagan administration it was the defense guidance (DG). This document, which was prepared annually by the assistant secretary of defense for program analysis and evaluation (PA&E), was circulated in draft form throughout the Pentagon in January and February of each year and then presented to the president. Although both PDs and CGs were classified documents, there were usually enough references to them in posture statements and public utterances of administration officials to reveal their contents.

The military forces supported by both the Carter and Reagan defense program budgets were to be configured for both deterrence and war fighting. Indeed, as Secretary Weinberger reported to Congress, there was "little disagreement" between the Reagan administration and its immediate predecessor over policies and strategies.[74] Principal differences did arise, however, from different judgments about how to fund these programs at levels adequate to achieve stated objectives as quickly as possible. As Weinberger also reported, the Defense Department sought to maintain capabilities to perform the following key missions: nuclear deterrence; defense of vital interest in NATO, Northeast Asia, and Southwest Asia; protection of the sea lanes of communications; and

power projection.[75] For both the Carter and Reagan administrations, deterrence of nuclear war was the fundamental objective of U.S. national security policy. This required that the United States have the capability to "persuade potential adversaries that the costs of attacking the United States will exceed any gain they could hope to achieve."[76] Although the Reagan administration labeled this approach to deterrence "flexible response," the strategy was much the same as the Carter administration's "countervailing strategy." Both formally acknowledged the existence of limited nuclear war-fighting options in U.S. strategic planning. This concept was not entirely new. Since the early 1960s the keystone of U.S. strategic nuclear policy had been an assured retaliatory or second-strike capability, the ability to inflict unacceptable damage upon an enemy who might attack the United States first. Although for many years it was presumed that U.S. strategic targeting focused on Soviet urban and industrial centers, strategic nuclear planning and nuclear forces actually had been "keyed to attacking Soviet nuclear forces, possibly preemptively, since the outset of the nuclear era."[77] It was during the Nixon administration, with the Schlesinger Doctrine, that the Defense Department began speaking openly about the need to multiply targeting options, to develop capabilities for controlled or limited nuclear exchanges, and to attack heavily protected Soviet military targets in "counterforce" strikes. From 1960 to 1987 the target list for U.S. nuclear weapons grew from 4,100 to 50,000 targets "as each side expanded its nuclear forces to offset the other side's expansion."[78]

What was new about the countervailing strategy was that it dropped such concepts as balance, sufficiency, or essential equivalence as force-sizing criteria. Previously, the United States configured its strategic forces not only so they could carry out their missions, but also so they would be perceived to be at least equal to those of the country's principal adversary, the Soviet Union. For example, in 1978, Secretary of Defense Brown told Congress that he could not see how we could do otherwise than to insist on and maintain essential equivalence with the Soviet Union in strategic offensive capabilities.[79] By "essential equivalence," he meant the achievement of four general conditions: that the Soviets do not see their strategic nuclear forces as usable instruments for political leverage, diplomatic coercion, or military superiority; that nuclear stability, especially in crisis, is maintained; that any advantages in force characteristics or configuration enjoyed by the Soviets are offset by other U.S. advantages; and that the U.S. force posture is not in fact (and is not perceived to be) inferior to that of the Soviet Union.

Achievement of the countervailing strategy also required the attainment of four general conditions. First, the United States must have forces in sufficient numbers and quality that they can: survive a well-executed surprise attack (first strike); react with the timing needed to assure the necessary deliberation and control; penetrate any enemy defenses; and destroy their designated targets. Second, the United States must have the redundancy and diversity built into its forces to insure against the failure of any one component, to permit the cross-targeting of key enemy facilities, and to complicate the enemy's defenses as well as his attack. Third, American forces must have targeting flexibility. That is, they must be capable of covering, or being withheld from, a substantial list of both hard targets (missile silos, command bunkers, and nuclear weapons storage items) and soft targets (cities and industrial sites). Finally, the United States must also possess a survivable command, control, and communications network; weapons with high accuracy and low yield; and some measure of civil defense evacuation capability.

As were those of previous administrations, the force employment doctrines of the Carter administration for both nuclear and nonnuclear forces were attacked as being both too demanding and not demanding enough. Some critics of the strategic doctrine advocate a "finite" or "minimum" deterrence posture, arguing that deterrence can be achieved through the maintenance of a much smaller force—for example, 100 land-based and 400 sea-based missiles. Those holding this view note that one Poseidon submarine contains enough fire power to destroy the 50 largest cities in the USSR. Proponents of minimum deterrence usually feel that it is sheer folly to talk about conducting limited nuclear wars. In their view, once the nuclear threshold is breached, the dreaded holocaust will occur.[80]

Those who maintained that Carter's doctrine for strategic nuclear forces was not demanding enough argued that superiority, not equivalence, is the only sure way to deter the Soviets or to win a nuclear war with them. Proponents of nuclear superiority are uncomfortable with the current Soviet lead in the number of missiles, and the total throw-weight and destructive power of their forces. They feel that the Russians are likely to try to exploit their advantages diplomatically and militarily. These individuals note that Soviet military writers constantly talk about conducting and winning nuclear wars and that the Soviets have invested substantial resources in civil defense.

When the Reagan administration entered office, its chief complaint with U.S. strategic force employment doctrine was that a significant gap existed between what American forces might be called upon to do in war and what they were actually capable of doing; hence the administration's strategic modernization program. This included development of the MX/Peacekeeper ICBM, the Trident II D-5 SLBM, the B-1B bomber, the Advanced Technology (Stealth) Bomber, and improved survivability of Command, Control, Communications, and Intelligence (C^3I) systems.[81] In another departure, the Reagan Defense Department stressed the importance of considering Soviet perceptions when assessing the credibility of the U.S. deterrent. Because Soviet strategic doctrine called for nuclear war-fighting capability, the Reagan administration reasoned that an optimally credible U.S. deterrent demanded forces that could deny Moscow its objective: if the Soviets thought in nuclear war-fighting terms, then the U.S. had to address the Soviets in those terms.[82] Many critics of this approach took this to mean that nuclear war had been "conventionalized" in the administration's mind, and that the U.S. was drifting toward an acceptance of the idea that a nuclear war could be fought and won.[83] President Reagan maintained, however, that nuclear war should never be fought and could never be won.

Nothing contributed more to this controversy than President Reagan's call in 1983 for a research program to explore the feasibility of space-based and ground-based ballistic missile defenses that, as the President put it, would make nuclear missiles "impotent and obsolete." This initiative amounted to a "radical rejection" of established American nuclear thought, which held that maintaining the prospect of "assured destruction" was the best way to deter nuclear war. Critics of the President's Strategic Defense Initiative (SDI) issued a range of charges, arguing that effective defenses could not be built, and that even if defenses could be built, their vulnerability to Soviet countermeasures would render them ineffective. Analysts then split on the question of whether the complications and uncertainties attendant to the introduction of imperfect defenses would strengthen or weaken deterrence.[84] Some held that complicating strategic planners' calculations with defenses would make planners more doubtful of striking successfully and would thus strengthen deterrence; others speculated that defenses of uncertain capability could just as easily lead to miscalculations and weakened deterrence. And some worried that SDI's tremendous cost—a trillion dollars by some accounts—would deplete funds for other important elements of U.S. force posture.

Broadly speaking, the general purpose, or conventional, forces of the United States are likely to be called upon to handle three types of operations. Their primary mission is to conduct, along with NATO allies, a large-scale, intense, conventional war in Central Europe against a blitzkrieg attack by the Warsaw Pact. Second, U.S. non-nuclear forces must be capable of responding effectively and simultaneously to a minor war or contingency in the Persian Gulf to protect oil fields and shipping in the region. Third, they must also have sufficient capability to intervene successfully in other areas, perhaps in contingencies similar

to those the United States encountered in Grenada, Lebanon, and Vietnam.

The Carter administration's handling of force employment doctrine for conventional forces was criticized largely on two counts. On the one hand, as with its strategic forces, it was charged with not doing enough to maintain the balance in Central Europe. Proponents of this view pointed to the advantages of the Warsaw Pact in tactical nuclear weapons, personnel, tanks, tactical aircraft, and armored vehicles.[85]

On the other hand, the "NATO-first" strategy was criticized for "putting too many eggs into one basket." Proponents of this view argued that since the American people never have been willing to pay in peacetime the full cost of providing the forces necessary to support the nation's military strategy, the United States ought to compensate, as it has in the past, by developing flexible forces—forces capable of being used in more than one place and for many purposes. In their view, the force employment doctrine of the Carter administration would have brought about the worst of all possible worlds. The NATO emphasis was not sufficient to offset the Warsaw Pact buildup, while the lack of flexibility prevented the United States from employing its military forces effectively to achieve its objectives in non-NATO areas like the Arabian (or Persian) Gulf.[86]

For its part, the Reagan administration took issue with what it thought was Carter's "excessive" focus on the NATO front. Reagan's analysts assumed that war with the Soviet Union would spill over quickly into other theaters. They therefore denounced Carter's "one and one-half war" assumption (planning for one major and one lesser war to be fought simultaneously) as inadequate for force planning. On the contrary, Secretary Weinberger held, U.S. forces must meet the demands of a prolonged worldwide war that would entail concurrent reinforcement of Europe and deployments to Southwest Asia and the Pacific, as well as the support of other areas.[87]

Three Reagan concepts of national strategy proved controversial. One, which became known as the Reagan Doctrine, was the idea that the United States should actively support anticommunist insurgencies in attempts to "roll back" communist gains in the Third World. The second concerned proposals to confront Moscow with the risk of an American counteroffensive in the event of conventional war in Europe. Initially referred to as "horizontal escalation," the basic tenets were included in the maritime strategy. It was designed to threaten the Warsaw Pact's flanks and destroy the Soviet Navy at its source: in essence, to threaten assets that are as important to Moscow as the ones Moscow is attacking.[88] Critics called this plan a dangerous extravagance that went beyond mere containment.[89] They argued that it was fraught with unnecessary potential for nuclear escalation and that U.S. forces, even with the administration's military buildup, would still lack the capability to do what would be demanded of them. Thus, although President Reagan entered office criticizing the gap between Carter's doctrine and U.S. force levels, his administration confronted the same charge.[90] The third concept, competitive strategies, attempted to address this by trying to match enduring U.S. strengths against enduring Soviet weaknesses.

The Defense Decision-Making Process

Within the executive branch of the federal government, decisions affecting national security objectives, strategy, policy, and force employment are made in two principal forums: the National Security Council (NSC) system and the defense budget process. The goal is to develop the force structure that supports the policy of a given administration. The best way to accomplish this is to ensure that the military experts make meaningful inputs, but do not dominate the process, so that civilian leaders maintain control. When such a situation prevails, it can be referred to as a civil-military balance.

The National Security Council System. The president's key tasks in managing foreign and defense policies are to "control policy in a large intermeshed bureaucracy filled with enthusiastic, ambitious people who are eager for power;" to "shape purposeful, informed, and coherent policy;" and to "communicate policy for effective implementation."[91] The National Security Council is the body that was created by law in 1947 to accomplish these purposes.

The NSC organization varies from administration to administration, and within administrations over time. The discussion of the NSC under Presidents Reagan and Carter is illustrative and representative of a process whose basic outlines have remained fairly constant. The same is true of the budget process discussed below; details change from administration to administration, but the main lines remain in place. As indicated in figure 2, the Reagan NSC system was divided into four main parts: the council itself and four senior interagency groups (SIGs). These SIGs were chaired, respectively, by the secretaries of state, defense, the director of central intelligence, and the secretary of the treasury. Occasionally, too, ad hoc SIGs were created, and these generally were chaired by the president's assistant for national security affairs. Then there was the NSC staff. And, finally (not shown in figure 2), a number of subordinate interagency groups (IGs) were often created as needed, allowing the NSC staff to deal with specific issues.[92]

President Reagan's use of this structure varied. Initially, he appointed several additional members to the NSC and allowed regular NSC staff members to attend meetings. But as the size of the meetings grew, Reagan resorted to a smaller body, the National Security Planning Group (NSPG), which included only the NSC's statutory members and a few hand-picked participants. Over time, the SIGs and the IGs also fell into disuse. In another important development, the NSC's size expanded to nearly that of Henry Kissinger's under President Nixon, which was the largest NSC on record. In 1985 the Reagan staff numbered more than fifty, almost twice as many as there were at the administration's beginning, this number heavily weighted with military officers.[93] Likewise, the input of Reagan's assistants for national security affairs also varied. Richard Allen, the president's first national security adviser, dealt with the president through the senior White

Figure 2. The Reagan Administration's National Security Council Structure

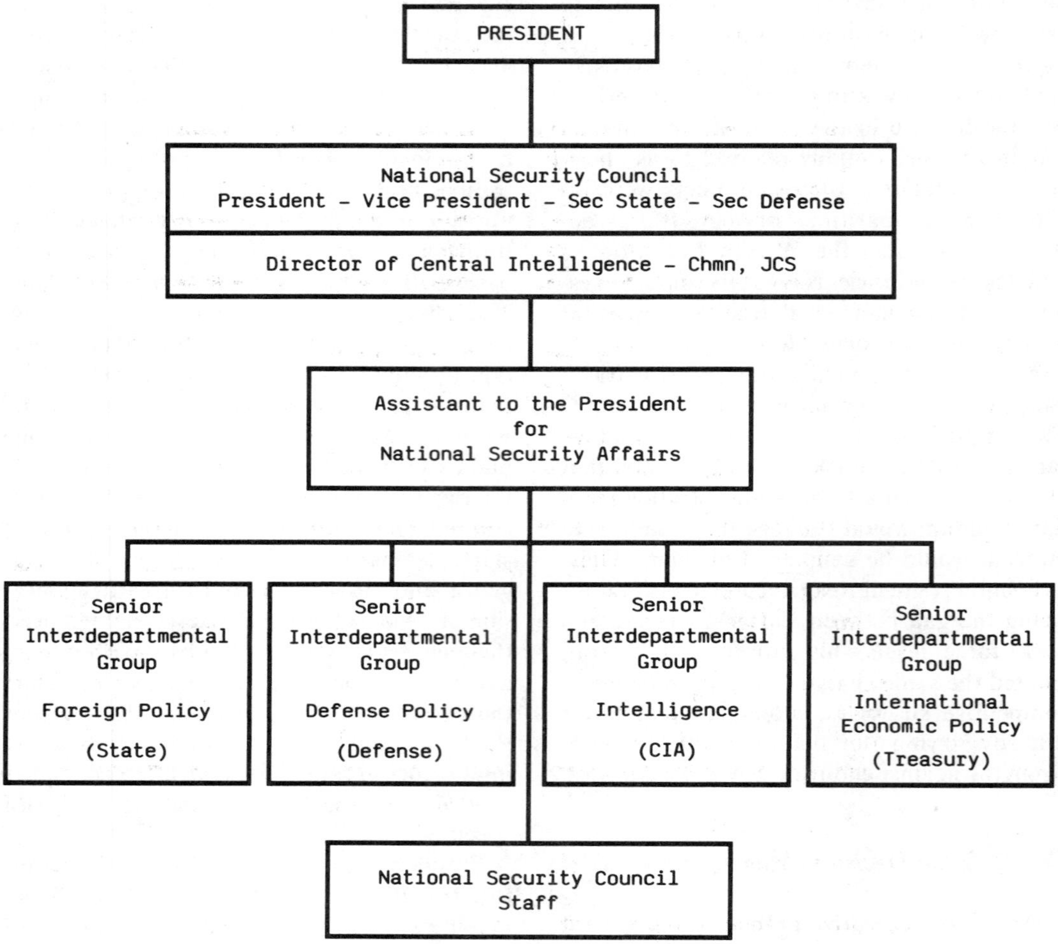

```
                    ┌─────────────────────────────┐
                    │          PRESIDENT          │
                    └─────────────────────────────┘
                                  │
    ┌─────────────────────────────────────────────────────────────┐
    │              National Security Council                        │
    │   President - Vice President - Sec State - Sec Defense        │
    ├─────────────────────────────────────────────────────────────┤
    │       Director of Central Intelligence - Chmn, JCS           │
    └─────────────────────────────────────────────────────────────┘
                                  │
              ┌───────────────────────────────────┐
              │   Assistant to the President       │
              │            for                     │
              │   National Security Affairs        │
              └───────────────────────────────────┘
                                  │
```

Senior Interdepartmental Group Foreign Policy (State)	Senior Interdepartmental Group Defense Policy (Defense)	Senior Interdepartmental Group Intelligence (CIA)	Senior Interdepartmental Group International Economic Policy (Treasury)

```
                    ┌─────────────────────────────┐
                    │   National Security Council  │
                    │            Staff             │
                    └─────────────────────────────┘
```

House staff; but William Clark, a longtime friend and associate of the president, had more direct access, as did Robert McFarlane, Vice Admiral John Poindexter, and Frank Carlucci.[94]

It is fair to say that Reagan's relative lack of interest in foreign affairs and his loose management of the NSC contributed to the "Iran/Contra" affair, in which funds derived from arms shipments to Iran were covertly, and perhaps illegally, funneled by the NSC to Nicaraguan rebels in support of the Reagan Doctrine. Reagan's habit was to delegate considerable authority in the management of foreign affairs; and under this arrangement the NSC drifted into operational roles normally reserved for intelligence agencies.

Issues or problems for NSC consideration can be proposed by a civilian or military member of the national security bureaucracy, with presidential approval sometimes being required before the issue is placed into the NSC process. In the Carter administration, the process began with the promulgation of a presidential review memorandum (PRM), which defined the problem, set a deadline, and assigned it to either the Policy Review Committee (PRC) or the Special Coordination Committee (SCC). In addition, if the issue was assigned to the PRC, the PRM designated the chairman. (As indicated in figure 2, the SCC was always chaired by the assistant to the president for national security affairs, while the chairmanship of the PRC rotated according to the issue area.) Normally, policy issues without short-term deadlines were analyzed by the PRC, while "short-fuse," or crisis, issues and arms control questions were handled by the SCC. In 1977 and 1978 President Carter approved the promulgation of forty-four PRMs, two-thirds of which were handled by the PRC. A list of these presidentially directed studies for 1977–78 is contained in table 2; even though issues change over time, this table is included as an example of the kinds of questions considered by the National Security Council.

The PRM was first analyzed by an interdepartmental or ad hoc group headed by someone at the assistant secretary or deputy secretary level. For example, the interdepartmental group that worked on PRM-10, the comprehensive review of U.S. military force posture, was headed by the deputy assistant secretary of defense for national security affairs, while the ad hoc group working on PRM-2 was headed by David Aaron, the deputy assistant for national security affairs. When the interdepartmental or ad hoc group completed its work, it forwarded its recommendations to the PRC or SCC for review. After holding a formal PRC or SCC meeting on the subject, a committee recommendation was made to the president. On some occasions Carter accepted the recommendations as presented, on others he consulted with individuals on the NSC staff before making a decision, and on still other occasions he convened a meeting of the full NSC.[95] Most of the decisions were made by means of the first two methods. In his first two years in office, the president held only ten meetings of the full NSC. When the president decided on a course of action, a presidential decision (PD) was promulgated. A list of these directives for 1977 is included in table 3 as an example of the kinds of national security decisions made by a president in a given year.

Formally, the NSC system provides for an almost ideal civil-military balance. The chairman of the Joint Chiefs of Staff (JCS) is an adviser to the NSC itself and in the Carter administration participated in all the meetings of the PRC and SCC. In addition, representatives of the JCS and the individual military services had an input into the analyses of the interdepartmental and ad hoc groups. However, the council itself, the PRC, the SCC, the interagency committees, and the interdepartmental groups were all chaired by civilian leaders. None of the groups within the NSC was under the control of a military officer.

Despite the appearance of a civil-military balance within the Carter administration's

Table 2. NSC Studies, 1977–78: A Representative Sample

PRM	Subject	PRM	Subject
1	Panama	26	ABM treaty review
2	SALT	27	Chemical warfare
3	Middle East	28	Human rights
4	South Africa and Rhodesia	29	Review of classification
5	Cyprus/Aegean	30	Terrorism
6	MBFR	31	Export control of U.S. technology
7	International summit	32	Civil defense
8	North/South strategy	33	Science and technology in developing countries
9	Review European issues	34	U.S. policy in North Africa
10	Net assessment force posture	35	International communications policy
11	Intelligence structure/mission	36	Soviet/Cuban presence in Africa
12	Arms transfer policy review	37	Chemical weapons
13	Korea	38	Long-range theater nuclear capabilities and arms control (C)
14	Philippine base negotiations	39	Economic implications of a Middle East peace settlement
15	Nuclear proliferation	40	Military survey teams
16	Nuclear testing	41	Review of U.S. policies toward Mexico
17	U.S. policy: Latin America	42	(Sensitive subject)
18	Law of the sea	43	(Sensitive subject)
19	Micronesian status	44	Export of oil and gas production technology to the USSR
20	Cooperation with France		
21	Horn of Africa		
22	National integrated telecom protection policy		
23	Coherent U.S. space policy		
24	People's Republic of China		
25	Arms control in Indian Ocean		

Table 3. Presidential Directives:
A Representative Sample

PD/NSC	
1	Establishment of presidential review and directive series/NSC
2	The National Security Council system
3	Disposition of national security decision memoranda
4	The law of the sea policy review
5	Southern Africa
6	Cuba (not circulated; limited access)
7	No information available
8	Nuclear nonproliferation
9	Army special operations field office in Berlin
10	Instructions for the tenth session of the Standing Consultative Commission
11	Micronesian status negotiations
12	U.S. policy in Korea
13	Conventional arms transfer policy
14	Disposition of national security action memoranda and national security decision memoranda
15	Chemical warfare
16	Law of the sea
17	Reorganization of the intelligence community
18	PRM-10
19	Intelligence structure and mission
20	SALT
21	Policy toward Eastern Europe
22	ABM treaty review
23	Standing Consultative Commission
24	Telecommunications protection policy
25	Scientific or technological experiments with possible large-scale adverse environmental effects and launch of nuclear system into space

NSC, in reality the impact of military participation was reduced. Indeed, many important issues were handled outside the formal NSC apparatus. Thirty PRMs were issued during Carter's first six months in office, seventeen of these in his first week as president. Subsequently, the president relied less and less on formal mechanisms to reach his national security decisions. The main coordinating mechanism for national security affairs turned out to be a Friday morning breakfast in the cabinet room with the president, Vice President Walter Mondale, Secretary of State Cyrus Vance, Secretary of Defense Harold Brown, and presidential assistants Zbigniew Brzezinski and Hamilton Jordan. No member of the JCS was in attendance. As a result, on some occasions, decisions were made without seeking or permitting JCS input. One such case involved the issue of the length of a comprehensive test ban treaty with the USSR. In mid 1978 the president made a decision to accept a Soviet pro-

posal for a five-year ban, apparently without consulting the chairman of the JCS or any other uniformed military officer.[96] (Eventually, on the advice of then Secretary of Energy James Schlesinger, who also had not been consulted, the president changed his position.)

Another case involved the PRM-12 analysis of arms transfers. In making the decision to reduce the volume of American arms transfers, the president and his advisers were influenced by CIA data that appeared to demonstrate that U.S. arms sales were twice as high as those of the Soviet Union. They did not ask for (nor did they receive) a Defense Intelligence Agency (DIA) study that showed that the two figures were not comparable because the U.S. figures included the cost of advisory and support teams, logistic and infrastructure facilities, support equipment, construction, and spares, while the CIA cost data on Soviet arms transfers included only the cost of the major combat equipment itself.[97]

The Defense Budget Process. Figure 3 outlines the defense budget process as it existed during the Carter administration and, with some exceptions, the Reagan administration. In the Reagan administration, the joint strategic planning document issued by the Joint Chiefs of Staff was sent to the Office of the Secretary of Defense (OSD) and integrated into a draft defense guidance (DG) statement (which replaced Carter's draft consolidated guidance). In January a formal DG (the equivalent of Carter's consolidated guidance) was produced. The DG provided the goals, objectives, and guidelines to the military departments and agencies.[98] Next, the services reviewed the DG and prepared program objective memoranda (POMs), which were forwarded to OSD. The secretary of defense issued program decision memoranda (PDMs) to the military services. These PDMs were based upon inputs from the defense review board or DRB (which assessed the policies and strategies of the DG for feasibility and cost-effectiveness) and from the JCS's joint program assessment memorandum (JPAM). The PDMs gave the military services guidance for the preparation of their individual budgets, which then were sent to OSD and the Office of Management and Budget (OMB) for joint review. Upon that review's completion, OSD made program budget decisions (PBDs) and the defense budget was presented to the president, who submitted it to Congress.

As is indicated in figure 3, the consolidated guidance, which in the Carter administration was drafted in January and approved in April, was an extremely detailed programing document. It covered fifteen specific areas of the defense budget and put down in the minutest detail what the military services were to procure in each of these fifteen areas over the next five fiscal years. In fact, some have argued that the consolidated guidance did not provide an explicit policy or a clear strategic underpinning for its programing guidance other than reference back to PD-18 (see table 3) and other policy guidance. By contrast, the policy and planning and programing documents that replaced the consolidated guidance were much more general in nature, but did not attempt to relate force structure to overall national security and policy.

The JCS and the individual services did have the opportunity to comment on a draft version of the consolidated guidance before it was finalized; however, for two reasons, their impact was negligible. First, since there was no separate policy section in the consolidated guidance, it was difficult to challenge on policy grounds. Second, because of time constraints, it was difficult for the services and the JCS to make more than marginal changes in the consolidated guidance. As in most situations, the initiative and upper hand were with the individual or agency that prepared the document, and, when time constraints were added, there was almost no chance for other groups to have any significant impact.

The professional military input to the defense budget process was also weakened by the elimination of the joint strategic operations plan (JSOP). Written in the absence of concern for fiscal constraints, the JSOP contained detailed threat assessments and outlined the forces that the JCS felt were necessary to deal adequately with various threats. While the JCS objective force was about twice the size that

Figure 3. The Carter DoD Management System

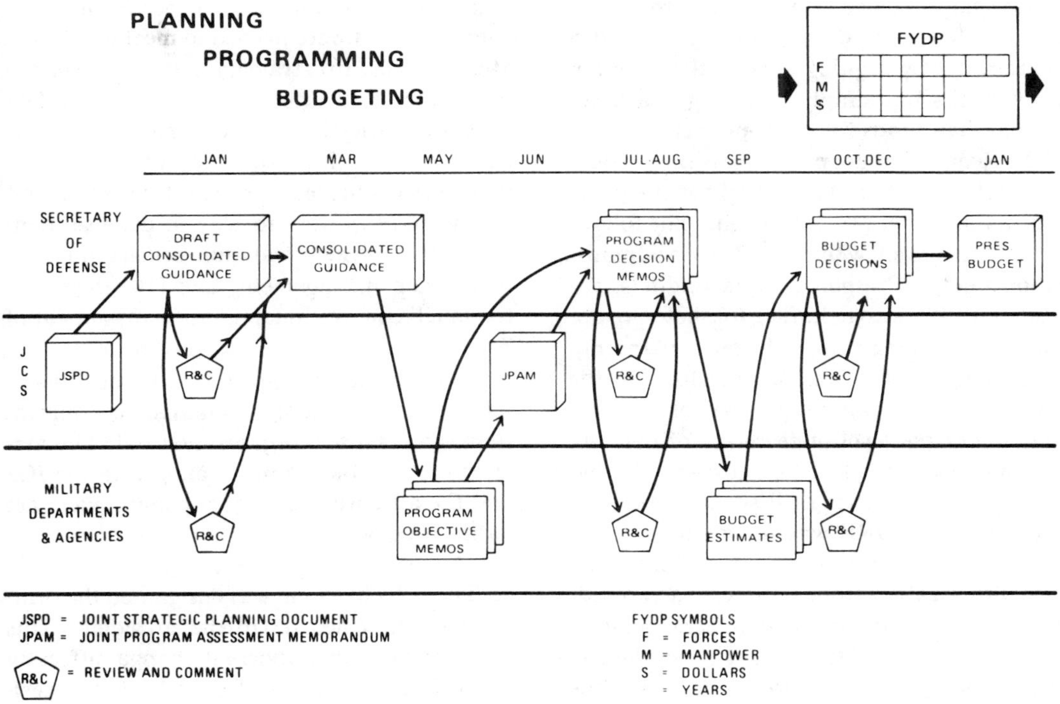

JSPD = JOINT STRATEGIC PLANNING DOCUMENT
JPAM = JOINT PROGRAM ASSESSMENT MEMORANDUM

R&C = REVIEW AND COMMENT

FYDP SYMBOLS
F = FORCES
M = MANPOWER
S = DOLLARS
  = YEARS

could be afforded, it did provide a useful benchmark for the remainder of the process. The Carter administration replaced the JSOP with the joint strategic planning document (JSPD), a short executive summary that described the JCS position on a planning or reduced risk force—that is, a force no more than $10 billion above certain budgetary limits. The difference between the two documents can be illustrated by comparing the JSOP objective force level for navy carriers with the carrier level in the JSPD: the former called for a total of twenty large-deck carriers, while the latter requested only fifteen (the actual level was thirteen).[99]

The chart depicting the budget processes also did not completely take into account the impact of grafting zero-based budgeting (ZBB) onto the planning, programing, and budgeting system (PPBS). While ZBB did not live up to the president's expectations in the Defense Department or other federal agencies, one of the side effects of ZBB in the Pentagon was to diminish further the role of military leaders in the budget process. The ultimate rank ordering, or prioritizing, of defense programs was done not by the services or JCS, but rather at the secretary of defense level. Thus, the secretary of defense could kill a high-priority JCS program not by arguing against the program on its merits but simply by giving it a lower ranking than funds for other projects.[100]

The Reagan budget process was the product of a 1981 evaluation that brought many problems in the Carter process to light. The following changes are a few that the Reagan administration made in response to its findings: the existing PPBS was modified to allow greater emphasis on long-range strategic planning; budgeting authority was decentralized to the services, while stronger management was provided below the level of secretary of defense; new emphasis was placed on cost-savings and efficiencies; the Carter ZBB system was eliminated; and the DRB was restructured to include service secretaries as full members. Also, with authorization from Congress, a two-year budget was instituted. By this arrangement, with one year free of the budget cycle, the Defense Department hoped to devote more time

to broader policy questions and policy management. It was also hoped that the military services would experience greater program stability. Some critics warned, however, that the longer budget cycle would lead to inflexibility in the budget's second year and counterproductive micro-management if OSD officials found time under the new system to formulate more detailed directives.[101]

The most significant organizational changes in the Reagan Defense Department were the result of a three-year study by the presidentially appointed Packard Commission on Defense Management, which reported many serious problems. Briefly, the commission cited the following difficulties: (1) the JCS was dominated by the services, which maintained "an effective veto" over nearly every JCS action; (2) joint military advice took too long to prepare and frequently offered unclear recommendations when issues affected more than one service; (3) there was inadequate quality among personnel assigned to joint duties because the services attached disincentives to such duty; (4) combat commanders had weak authority over their service components and limited influence over personnel and resources; (5) combat commanders lacked authority to specify chains of command that were needed to meet their operational goals; (6) strategic planning took too much time and attention from Defense Department officials; (7) the numerous defense agencies were inadequately supervised; (8) there was confusion over the roles that the service secretaries were to play in defense management; (9) there was unnecessary duplication of top management; and (10) there was too much congressional micro-management of defense matters.

In response to the shortcomings documented by the Packard Commission, Congress passed a defense reorganization bill. The major provisions of this bill dealing with the JCS and the authority of combat commanders are outlined below.

1. The JCS chairman was designated the principal military adviser to the president. This was an extremely important change, affecting the nature and quality of the advice the presi-

dent receives from the military. Under prior law, the *corporate* JCS was designated the principal military adviser. This arrangement, however, often resulted in recommendations to the president that were watered down to facilitate consensus among the Joint Chiefs. The new arrangement provided that the president get military advice principally from one military officer, the JCS chairman; but also that the chairman be required to submit to the president the JCS's dissenting views to ensure that the chief executive is exposed to the full range of advice.

2. The JCS chairman was required to submit fiscally constrained strategic plans to the president. Because under the previous system the JSPD was promulgated without much consideration of constraints on resources, the JCS role in the PPBS was often relegated to a marginal status. By requiring JCS planning to take finite resources into account, the new legislation would compel them to establish priorities, address difficult trade-offs, and produce more realistic planning objectives.

3. The term of office for the JCS chairman was set to end no later than six months after the beginning of a new presidency. Here the idea was that since the JCS chairman was to be the president's principal military adviser, each new president should have the opportunity to choose that adviser early in his first term. To avoid having one officer in the nation's most senior military position for too long, the term of the JCS chairman was limited to six years, or a maximum of eight years with a presidential waiver.

4. The position of JCS vice-chairman was created. This four-star officer would serve as the second-ranking military officer and assume the JCS chairman's responsibilities in the event of the chairman's absence.

5. The president and the secretary of defense were authorized to place the JCS chairman in the chain of command between the secretary of defense and combat commanders. It is important to note, however, that orders issued by the chairman must be initiated and authorized by the secretary of defense; that is to say, the JCS chairman was not authorized to issue commands of his own that were not approved be-forehand by the secretary. This very important measure was included to safeguard the principle of civilian control over the military.

6. The authority of combat commanders was also strengthened and expanded. In essence, combat commanders were given full operational authority over all forces assigned to them. Under prior law, these commanders did not have authority over joint training or over any aspect of support and administration, as these were prerogatives of the individual services. Thus, unified commanders had only very limited authority over commands below them, but in time of conflict they would nonetheless have been responsible for those commands' performance. The change provided here gave unified commanders authority over planning, logistics, training, and support as required for the accomplishment of their missions. It also allowed them to select key subordinate officers, another prerogative formerly enjoyed by the individual military services.

THE CONGRESS

Congress is involved in the defense decision-making process in two principal ways. First, it votes on funds for the defense program. Second, it places some restrictions on how the military power of the United States can be used. It can do this through the appropriations process or through separate substantive legislation.

In the post-Vietnam period, the Congress attempted to play a more active role in the defense decision-making process. During the Nixon-Ford administration, the legislative branch of the federal government tried to apply a brake to the activist national security policies of the administration. The legislators attempted to accomplish this goal by pruning over $50 billion from the defense budget requests of the executive, by restricting the areas of the world to which military force could be applied, and by limiting the time (under the War Powers Act) that the president could employ U.S. military forces overseas.

After President Carter took office, some elements in the legislature tried to prod the executive branch into doing more in the area of national security. Congress used its power of the purse to push the executive into acquiring a nuclear aircraft carrier, the XM-1 main battle tank, and the MX mobile ICBM, while cutting other programs. And, after the Soviet invasion of Afghanistan in 1979, the second strategic arms limitation treaty (SALT II) with Moscow was withdrawn from consideration because of its certain prospect of defeat in the Senate.

The conservative tide that swept the country in the late 1970s generated much support in Congress for the Reagan administration's commitment to rebuild America's defenses. There was some dissatisfaction over how Reagan proposed to allocate funds, along with impatience over his initial reluctance to engage in arms control, and uneasiness over his penchant for using military force; but Reagan's popular appeal made Congress hesitant to challenge him. As his unusually long "honeymoon" with Capitol Hill ended, congressional oversight of defense programs intensified, as did congressional activism against them.

Congressional activism increased noticeably in the latter part of the Reagan presidency. After disclosures of covert U.S. military aid to Nicaraguan rebels, Congress prohibited the use of U.S. funds for the purpose of overthrowing the Nicaraguan government. It prevented grants of anything but "humanitarian" aid to the rebels, later reversed itself, and then, upon learning of possible illegal U.S. assistance, imposed a moratorium on all aid to the rebels until an accounting of the administration's activities could be made. In arms control, Congress cut funds for the U.S. antisatellite (ASAT) program and blocked funds for testing ASATs against objects in space. It also mounted stiff opposition to the administration's reinterpretation of the 1972 antiballistic missile (ABM) treaty. In other areas, congressional opposition caused President Reagan to modify or cancel arms sales to Saudi Arabia; and when U.S. forces were sent to Lebanon, congressional threats to activate the War Powers Act forced the administration into a legislative compromise.

Although it is difficult to measure the exact degree of influence the legislature has on defense policy, it is reasonable to conclude that congressional impact has been spotty, but with occasional significance—as with aid to the Contras, arms sales, and threats of confronta-

tion over the War Powers Act. Congress has been handicapped because direct legislative efforts to influence policy are subject to presidential veto, but also because members are rarely willing to assume the degree of responsibility for policy outcomes that overriding a presidential veto entails. Members fear the political impact of their votes, particularly when there is a possibility that they could be portrayed as "soft on communism" or undermining national security. Moreover, intense lobbying by the president frequently works.[102] Congress, therefore, has been most effective through its power over appropriations, its ability to bargain and compromise with the president, and its ability to establish implicit parameters for acceptable executive action.

BUREAUCRATIC POLITICS

Prior to the pioneering work by Graham Allison and others on the Cuban missile crisis of 1962, decisions affecting national security or defense policy were thought by many to involve very little bureaucratic politics. As Allison himself noted, it is the U.S. public's perception that it is un-American to play bureaucratic politics with national security. Americans need to believe that defense decisions are made by the president unilaterally and rationally.[103]

Since the first publication of Allison's analysis, however, many people have come to view bureaucratic politics as the primary determinant of national security policy outcomes within the American political system. What Allison refers to as the rational and organizational models, and what John Steinbruner calls the cybernetic model, are thought by others to have almost no bearing on the outcome of the policy process.[104]

The truth, as in most cases, lies somewhere between. Bureaucratic politics do affect all decisions, even those involving vital national security interests. However, rational, organizational, and cybernetic factors are also involved. The mix of these factors depends upon such things as the type of decision, the backgrounds and experience of the players, and the extent to which the president takes an active interest in an issue.

For example, political considerations are normally more important in choosing contractors for individual weapons systems than in deciding on force-employment doctrines. Choices made by individuals acting within the policy processes of the executive branch are affected by both domestic and international considerations. Chief among the domestic considerations is the impact of certain key members of Congress. Basic decisions are made and weapons contractors are chosen with an eye to their potential reception on Capitol Hill. In addition, defense decisions are often influenced by their impact upon domestic economic policy. For example, because the defense budget is controllable, it can be used relatively easily to affect such things as the money supply, the size of the deficit, and the rates of employment and inflation. Policy makers thus often vary the amount spent on defense in response to such domestic factors and quite independently of international events.

A second domestic influence upon defense decision makers is the mass communications media. Adverse comments by writers and columnists in such widely read newspapers as the *Washington Post*, *New York Times*, and *Wall Street Journal* influence the decision-making process. In addition, leaks to the media before a final decision is made often have an impact on the final product. It is no accident that the secretary of defense begins each work day with a review of *Current News*, an in-house compilation of news items of interest to the Defense Department.

External influences such as alliances also affect choices made by U.S. policy makers. President Carter's pledge to increase the size of the U.S. defense budget by 3 percent a year in real terms was induced by pressure from NATO allies. Decisions on forward deployments of U.S. forces in Europe and the Pacific and on strategic and intermediate-range nuclear arms control were strongly affected by American membership in NATO, the U.S. defense treaty with Japan, and the de facto U.S. alliance with Israel. Another example of external pressure was Kuwait's request in 1987 for Soviet protection of its ships in the Persian Gulf, used by Kuwait as leverage to secure a greater commitment from Washington.

Disputes among bureaucratic agencies on national security are normally resolved the same way as domestic disputes—that is, through negotiation, bargaining, and compromise among the agencies concerned. Some contentious issues do reach the president for a final decision, but this is the exception rather than the rule. Disputes among the services are normally resolved within the JCS system through compromise. Conflicts among the military and civilian elements of the Defense Department are normally resolved through the intervention of the secretary of defense or his deputy, while disputes among the Defense Department and other agencies are resolved through the NSC system.

Which actors prevail in policy disputes is a result not only of the individual's power base and access to the key decision makers, but also of his or her skill in exploiting these resources and his or her expertise in the area. In the 1950s the views of Secretary of State John Foster Dulles usually prevailed in serious disputes among the agencies. During the Kennedy-Johnson years Secretary of Defense Robert McNamara was the dominant figure. Henry Kissinger, the executive assistant for national security affairs and later the secretary of state, was clearly the key actor in the Nixon-Ford era. Secretary of Defense Harold Brown appears to have been the first among equals in the defense policy processes of the Carter administration.

In the Reagan administration, policy was often the product of disputes between Secretary of State Shultz and Secretary of Defense Weinberger. Shultz initially opposed the less restrictive (or "broad") interpretation of the 1972 ABM treaty, for example, and Weinberger supported it. The president split the difference by deciding with Weinberger, but ruling that Shultz's interpretation would continue to be observed. Shultz lost to Weinberger when President Reagan decided to withdraw from Lebanon, and when the president determined that the United States would no longer observe constraints imposed by the SALT II strategic arms control agreement with the USSR.

Throughout the post–World War II period, the personalities and backgrounds of key decision makers have had a profound impact upon the defense decision-making process. Indeed, as noted above, the personality of the individual, rather than the office per se, has determined the key actors in different administrations.

The president is usually the key actor in the policy process. Even if he himself does not make a decision, he sets the broad guidelines and the tone or atmosphere in which the decisions are made. His presence is felt throughout the process. The impact of the personality and ideological background of the chief executive was vividly demonstrated in the case of President Carter.

With less background and fewer preformed ideas about national security matters than any of his immediate predecessors, Carter nonetheless put his stamp on the policy process and policy outputs. He wanted an "open administration," and, even in the area of national security policy, he attempted to maintain this commitment. Similarly, throughout his administration, Carter held weekly breakfast meetings with his national security advisers and met more frequently with the Joint Chiefs of Staff than any recent president.[105]

Carter took office feeling that he had a moral obligation to keep his campaign promises and to do something about what he perceived to be a dangerous arms race. The impact of these two factors can be seen in the outputs of his defense decision-making process. Early in the administration, as part of an attempt to fulfill campaign promises, the B-1 was cancelled, a Korean troop withdrawal was announced, a slowdown in the rate of growth in defense spending was undertaken, a human rights policy was proclaimed, and an attempt was made to reduce the volume of arms sales to Third World countries. The president's moral imperative to slow the arms race was reflected in his comprehensive proposal to the USSR in March 1977 for a 20 percent cutback in existing levels of strategic offensive weapons and a complete freeze on modernization and testing.[106]

Idiosyncratic factors evidently played a prominent role in President Reagan's policymaking style. The president allowed his secretary of defense to manage the Pentagon with virtually a free reign. Unlike Nixon and Carter, Reagan displayed little interest in policy details

and, with his loose management style, delegated great authority to subordinates, whose infighting often kept policy making at a standstill. Reagan's deep sense of loyalty to his team, moreover, often prevented him from "knocking heads" to get policy moving.

Nonetheless, personality and position, while important, are often constrained by systemic and other realities. The Soviet buildup forced President Carter to back away from his campaign promise to cut $5 to $7 billion from the defense budget, while rapidly rising inflation and large congressional cuts made it difficult for him completely to fulfill his promise to the country's NATO allies to raise defense spending by 3 percent a year in real terms. Likewise, concerns over the budget deficit led Congress to cut back President Reagan's defense effort, leaving many programs underfunded because the administration had expected defense budgets to continue growing.[107]

All presidents must contend with opposition from bureaucratic elements in the government. In part to obtain the support of the Joint Chiefs of Staff for the SALT II agreement, for example, President Carter authorized construction of a multibillion-dollar MX mobile missile system. Another constraint is that in the aftermath of the Vietnam War, it has been difficult for American presidents to consider direct military intervention in the Third World as a viable option. Finally, moral and ethical concerns of certain segments of the American polity limit the president's ability to use covert means to accomplish policy goals, while laws like the War Powers Act make it difficult to use even shows of military force.

Recurring Issues and Defense Policy Outputs

CIVIL-MILITARY RELATIONS

Until World War II, the United States did not have a large standing military force. It maintained a small professional cadre and augmented it during wartime with reservists and conscripts—that is, citizen-soldiers. Since the end of World War II, however, the United States has maintained a large military, first through conscription and now on a volunteer basis.

Not surprisingly, during this same period there has been an intense concern about civil-military relations. This concern has focused not simply on the problem of maintaining effective civilian control, but on the impact of military concerns upon the policy process, for example, the power of the so-called military-industrial complex.

Some analysts, like Samuel Huntington, have argued that the best way to preserve civilian control with a large standing military is through objective means, such as by establishing an autonomous and politically neutral military profession that would be at once self-policing and isolated from society.[108] However, the consensus among Americans is that subjective control is the preferred option—achieving control by civilianizing the military so that it in effect mirrors civilian society. This is accomplished through a rapid turnover in the membership of the armed forces and extensive education programs for careerists, especially those in the officer corps.[109]

The concerns of the American military establishment (except for the National Guard) are primarily external. The professional military compete within the internal decision-making processes to gain personnel and matériel to deal with the external threat. Traditionally, the uniformed military has not reacted favorably to suggestions that it perform even humanitarian domestic roles on a regularized basis because of a fear that performing these functions routinely would degrade combat readiness.

Even in the era of the all-volunteer force, the American military prefers to maintain the citizen-soldier concept and seeks to retain its identity with civilian society. In FY 1981 about 30 percent of the enlisted were minority personnel including roughly 22 percent Black and 4 percent Hispanic. Of the officer force, about 9 percent was Black and 1 percent Hispanic. And, although the percentage of Black officers was still less than the percentage of Blacks in the U.S. population, the percentage of all active-duty officers who were Black more than doubled from 1971 to 1981. Almost 10 percent of the active-duty military force consisted of women, this number remaining proportionately low because women continued to be barred by law from combat assignments.[110]

Noteworthy also is the fact that despite a steady decline in the eligible youth population, the military services in the 1980s consistently met recruiting objectives for the all-volunteer force. The quality of recruits was also higher, an important trend since the growing technological sophistication of American weaponry demands personnel capable of performing more complicated tasks. Of new recruits in FY 1987, 93 percent had earned high school diplomas, compared to 75 percent nationwide and to the 68 percent reported in FY 1980. Likewise, 93 percent also scored average or above on enlistment tests, compared to 65 percent in FY 1980.[111] The American public also held an increasingly positive image of military service and the military in general, another indication that the Vietnam War's traumatizing effects had dissipated somewhat with the passage of time.

WEAPONS ACQUISITION

In FY 1986, U.S. outlays for weapons research, development, testing, and production were a little over $4 billion. And from FY 1981 through FY 1987 these authorizations amounted to over $1 trillion in constant 1987 dollars. From FY 1985 to FY 1987, this included about $7.8 billion for SDI.[112] This represents a significant amount of the nation's resources and will involve a significant commitment of federal expenditures in future years.

Because of the large amount of funds and large number of people involved, there has been great concern over the process by which the DoD buys its weapons. Many people have argued that unnecessary weapons are procured and that poor management practices have driven up costs unnecessarily. Reforms of the process have been suggested by everyone from the General Accounting Office (GAO) to the Harvard Business School.

Policies currently governing the weapons systems acquisition process are contained in directives from OMB and the Department of Defense. OMB establishes the policies to be followed by governmental agencies in management of the acquisition system; analysis of missions; determination of mission needs; setting of program objectives; determination of requirements; planning and budgeting; funding; research; engineering, testing, and development; testing and evaluation; contracting; and production and management control.

OMB specifies that each agency acquiring systems should ensure that the system fulfills mission needs, operates effectively, and otherwise justifies its acquisition; ensure that competition exists between the new system and other similar systems; investigate trade-offs; provide strong checks and balances through testing and evaluation, independent of developers; ensure agency planning built on missions analysis results; develop an acquisition strategy for each program to ensure that competition is encouraged and guidelines are developed for evaluation and acceptance or rejection of proposals; maintain a capability to predict, review, and assess costs for development, testing, and evaluation over the predicted life of the system; and appoint a program manager for each major acquisition program, who is to be given budget guidance and a written charter of his or her authority, responsibility, and accountability.

The key to an effective acquisition process is the agency's ability to determine and develop those needs required to perform its specific tasks based on its mission, reconciled with its overall capabilities, priorities, and resources. To achieve the most effective military posture, each service is required to identify mission area needs and to develop systems to meet those needs at the right time. The essential task is to respond more quickly to threats "while still being assured that the system program doesn't entail unwarranted technological cost, or schedule risks."[113]

The Department of Defense has developed an elaborate process that tries to ensure that it buys only needed weapons at the cheapest possible price. This process has two main steps. The first is to determine whether the mission a new system will perform is needed. In the PPBS, this is accomplished by a justification of major system new starts (JMSNS), which is submitted with a program objective memorandum (POM) in which funds for the budget year are requested. The JMSNS must include the following: an identification of the system's mission and a description of the role the system will play; a description of alternative weapons that will be considered; discussions of the system's technology and affordability; descriptions of its survivability; logistical and manpower requirements; and assessments of whether it can be standardized within other Defense Department components or NATO and of the materials and industrial base it will require.[114]

The second phase involves program reviews by the Defense Systems Acquisition Review Council (DSARC) at four milestones. These milestones are as follows:

Milestone 0—Program need determination.
   a. The JMSNS is submitted by the services.
   b. The secretary of defense states the conditions under which the program may begin, if at all.
Milestone 1—Demonstration and validation.
   a. Concepts, threats, costs, schedules, readiness objectives, and affordability are evaluated.
   b. Authority is given to proceed with a demonstration and validation of preferred system's concepts.

Milestone 2—Approval for full-scale engineering.
   The secretary of defense decides whether to proceed with full-scale development of the system.
Milestone 3—Production and deployment.
   Production decisions are delegated to DoD components if thresholds established at milestone 2 have been met.

Throughout this process, the DSARC normally advises the Defense Acquisitions Executive (DAE) and Procurement Executive (PE), who, in turn, advise the secretary of defense on each milestone decision.[115]

Figure 4 outlines the weapons system acquisition process just described. Obviously this is an idealized version. In reality no program ever flows that smoothly. Requirements often

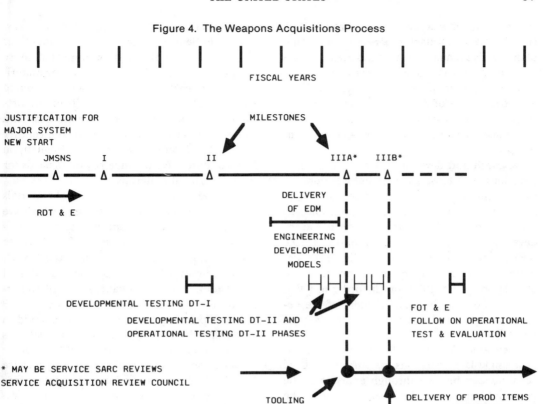

Figure 4. The Weapons Acquisitions Process

change as development continues, and information acquired during one stage of development does (and should) feed back to earlier phases. Specifications change, new components appear, performance does not conform to expectations, retesting is necessary, and other departures from plans are frequent.

An important innovation made at the recommendation of the Packard Commission was the creation in 1986 of an under secretary of defense for acquisition. This reform made one DoD official responsible for ensuring that acquisition processes are efficient and that weapons systems are more uniform throughout the Department of Defense. It also prevented individual services and service secretaries from assuming and executing policy responsibilities for acquisitions without coordination with the rest of the department, as they are wont to do when left to their own devices.[116] Each service therefore now has one senior acquisition execu-

tive who reports directly to the new under secretary, bypassing service secretaries, who no longer have roles in the acquisition process.[117] These reforms were thought necessary partly because of the tremendous cost growth in weapons systems, which by 1981 had reached 14 percent a year. In 1983 and 1984, however, the Reagan administration reduced this to less than 1 percent and in 1985 actually achieved cost reductions of 0.8 percent.[118] In a five-year period the administration also managed to increase competition for new acquisitions by 37 percent.[119]

Except for the need to import strategic materials and a limited number of parts, weapons systems production for DoD is almost exclusively an American enterprise. In FY 1986 there were thirty thousand prime contractors and subcontractors engaged in defense work in the United States.[120] Every state in the Union had some defense-related industry, with the vast majority of weapons systems produced by firms with headquarters or manufacturing plants in five major metropolitan areas: southern California, the San Francisco Bay area, New York, Boston, and Washington, D.C. Moreover, some of America's largest corporations, like Lockheed and General Dynamics, continued to subsist largely on defense contracts.

Research and development of weapons systems for the Defense Department was done almost exclusively within the United States, in both government and private corporations. In FY 1987 planned expenditures on research, development, testing, and evaluation (RDT &E) amounted to 42 percent of the entire defense budget. Total spending for procurement of weapons in FY 1987, on the order of $95.8 billion, came to almost 31 percent of the defense budget, and a little over 2 percent of GNP.[121]

The tremendous impact of the development of a single large weapons system on the U.S. economy can be seen through analyses of the potential benefits to the private sector of the MX mobile missile program proposed in the Carter administration and President Reagan's SDI. If Carter's MX system had been completed as planned, it would have created approximately 130,000 new aerospace and support service jobs nationwide. In California alone the MX would have created 46,000 new jobs and infused $8.5 billion into the state's economy. New York, New Jersey, and Connecticut could have realized up to $1 billion in revenues and 21,000 new jobs. But these figures pale compared to those for SDI, which one observer characterized as the "single largest undertaking ever attempted by mankind."[122] With upper-end costs estimated at $1.5 trillion, SDI will generate a host of skilled and unskilled jobs with prime contractors and small businesses.[123] In 1985, for example, the Department of Defense issued a 28-page list of SDI-related contracts. Total awards among prime contractors were over $1.6 billion. European firms were also awarded some $82 million in 1985 for SDI-related work.

As indicated in figure 5, the United States, unlike the Soviet Union, is highly dependent upon foreign sources to supply the basic raw materials required for defense production. Forty years ago this nation imported more than half of its required supply of four materials; twenty years ago, that number increased to six. By 1985 it depended primarily on imports for about nine of the basic raw materials. And estimates were that by the end of the century the United States would be dependent upon foreign sources for the majority of its needs for thirteen critical materials.

The main U.S. sources of essential materials are Third World countries, some of which are former colonial dependencies that have difficulty running their own industries.[124] Three nations, South Africa, Zaire, and the USSR, account for over half the world's production of chromium, cobalt, manganese, and platinum-group metals, essential to national defense.[125] As Arab petroleum exporters demonstrated in 1973, the withholding of needed materials has the potential for powerful political leverage.

Dependency per se is not necessarily a cause for alarm, however, as long as there is free trade. Concerns arise mainly when high import dependency is linked to only a few suppliers.[126] The United States could lessen its dependence somewhat through such methods as stockpiling, developing synthetics, and substitution of one material or supplier by another; but these measures do not change the essential fact that the United States can be held hostage by some smaller nations. Although the United States has maintained a stockpile of strategic minerals, it would take a hundred years at 1985 spending rates to meet its stockpile goals.[127]

FORCE POSTURE

The military forces of the United States consist of over two million active personnel and over one million ready reservists.[128] They are broken down into three categories: conventional, strategic, and theater nuclear. These forces are stationed on U.S. soil and are also forwardly deployed in many different parts of the globe.

Conventional Forces. Since the end of World War II, and even after the Vietnam War, the United States has stationed large military

Figure 5. Imports of Selected Minerals and Metals (Net Imports as Percentage of 1982 Consumption)

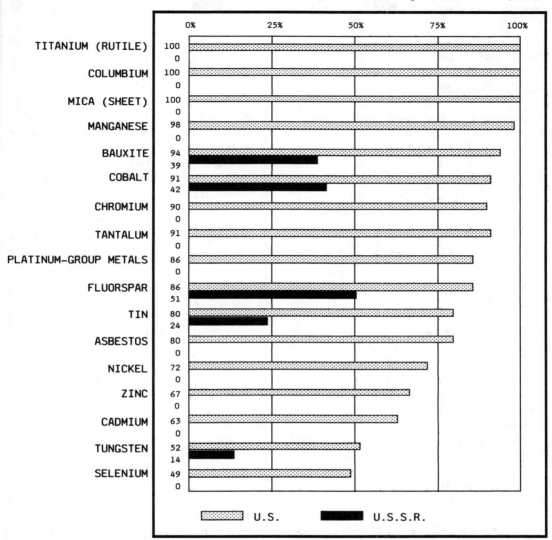

forces abroad, primarily in Europe and the Far East. In FY 1986 the United States maintained approximately 300,000 troops capable of waging full-scale conventional warfare, as well as tactical and theater nuclear war, in Central Europe, mostly in the Federal Republic of Germany. These forces included four army divisions, two armored cavalry regiments, and twenty-eight air force tactical air squadrons.[129]

In the Mediterranean the dominant allied naval force is the U.S. Sixth Fleet, which, like its land and air counterparts, is a force capable of conducting full-scale offensive and defensive operations, including amphibious assaults, on short notice. Throughout the western and northern Mediterranean littoral, the United States maintains approximately 34,000 active-duty military personnel engaged in diverse missions ranging from logistics to intelligence-collecting activities.[130]

The number of U.S. troops stationed in the Far East is not as great, but the geographic area falling under the responsibilities of the commander in chief, Pacific (CINCPAC) amounts to over 50 percent of the earth's surface. In FY 1987 the major units available to the United States in East Asia were two infantry divisions, one Marine amphibious force (MAF), and sixteen tactical fighter squadrons. The primary U.S. Army presence in the region is the Second Infantry Division in South Korea. The withdrawal of this force was announced by the Carter administration in early 1977, but the decision was later reversed, in part because of revised estimates of the size of the opposing North Korean force. Another area of concern is the Philippines, where there is a growing communist insurgency, and where U.S. naval and air facilities are essential to counter the Soviet naval presence in Vietnam.

The U.S. Seventh Fleet rounds out the U.S. force structure in the Western Pacific. Like its counterpart in the Mediterranean, this fleet is a cutting edge of American naval power and is expected to perform the full range of naval operations.

Two other U.S. commands with regional responsibilities, the new Central Command (CENTCOM) and the Southern Command (SOUTHCOM), gained prominence in the 1980s because of growing threats to U.S. interests. CENTCOM, which is responsible for meeting threats in Southwest Asia and the Middle East, was an outgrowth of the Rapid Deployment Force created by President Carter. Among the forces potentially available to CENTCOM were five army divisions, one and one-third Marine amphibious forces, and seven tactical fighter wings.

Because the United States lacks basing rights in the area, few of these forces are physically deployed in the region, although they do engage in periodic exercises with friendly countries there. The navy also maintains three carrier battle groups, one surface action group, and maritime patrol squadrons in the region. Because of threats to shipping and concerns about Kuwait's request for Soviet naval assistance, U.S. naval forces in the area were bolstered and a carrier battle group and a battleship were stationed outside the Straits of Hormuz at the mouth of the Persian Gulf.[131]

SOUTHCOM, the U.S. command for the Western Hemisphere, is responsible for the Ca-

ribbean Sea and waters adjacent to Central and South America. The United States has about 10,000 military personnel in SOUTHCOM, including an army brigade and small air force and naval elements in Panama. There is a naval base at Guantanamo Bay, Cuba, and military advisers are stationed in Honduras, where U.S. forces also hold regular exercises. The steady frequency of these exercises, along with U.S. military assistance to the Honduran government, contributes to a sizable military infrastructure in that country, possibly for future use against Nicaragua.

The majority of U.S. conventional military strength, however, is routinely based in the United States. Of the army's eighteen active divisions, thirteen are based at home, as are two-thirds of the Marine Corps' active divisions.[132] Based at home also are ten Army National Guard divisions and twenty army reserve components; the Marine Corps has one division and one air wing in reserve.[133] The air force has fifteen active fighter/attack wings and approximately twelve reserve wings based in the continental United States.[134] The naval forces of the Atlantic and Pacific comprise approximately 65 percent of the total fleet strength.[135]

Much doubt, however, is expressed about whether the United States has sufficient strategic mobility to transport ground forces based in the United States quickly enough to Western Europe and the Persian Gulf. In FY 1986–87 U.S. airlift capability consisted of about 70 C-5A and 234 C-141 heavy-lift aircraft for intertheater operations, 44 KC-10s for dual airlift and aerial refueling missions, and 217 active C-130 aircraft for intratheater operations.[136] The Pentagon was also installing convertible features on selected wide-bodied civilian aircraft to augment military airlift capabilities.

While optimum speed in reinforcement calls for air transport, it simply is too expensive to airlift heavy forces like mechanized infantry and armored divisions in sufficient numbers to Europe and Southwest Asia.[137] The United States therefore maintains on active status forty-three cargo ships and twenty-four tankers. In preparation for contingencies in the Persian Gulf, the United States also emplaces army and Marine Corps equipment with thirteen maritime prepositioning ships, which are to be kept on station near potential trouble spots.

In view of its security commitments abroad, most analysts agree that the United States lacks adequate mobility, especially considering that U.S. and NATO mobilization might be slow to get started, making the need to transport U.S. forces quickly even greater. Strategic mobility seems even more deficient in view of the high likelihood that crises in Europe and the Persian Gulf would be simultaneous.[138] In that event, CENTCOM's access to strategic lift risks being reduced severely, since European commands, from which CENTCOM would draw its equipment and lift assets, would undoubtedly give highest priority to their own forces.[139] Some analysts, therefore, recommend an across-the-board expansion of U.S. strategic mobility assets, to include airlift, sealift, and prepositioning of equipment.[140] This presents problems, though, because the air force and the navy, which are largely responsible for strategic lift, are interested primarily in acquiring new weapons systems, not the means to transport the Marine Corps and the army.[141] A Command responsible for all forms of special operations was created in 1988 as a result of growing criticism of U.S. military efforts to handle various forms of low-intensity conflict.

Strategic Forces. Since the early 1960s the U.S. strategic offensive capability has been built around three complementary systems for the delivery of nuclear weapons. Referred to collectively as the triad, these systems are land-based ICBMs (intercontinental ballistic missiles), sea-based SLBMs (submarine-launched ballistic missiles), and manned bombers. Missions and targets of all three legs are contained in the single integrated operations plan (SIOP) of the Strategic Air Command (SAC). They are under a single commander in chief, who reports to the secretary of defense through the Joint Chiefs of Staff. In the late 1980s, the ICBM force consisted of 950 Minuteman II and Minuteman IIIs, and fifty MX/Peacekeepers, all based in the continental United States. The fifty MXs are currently based in

fixed silos previously designed for Minutemen. In 1989 the Bush administration announced that in the future the MX would be deployed on railroad cars to enhance their survivability against Soviet attack. At the same time, a decision was made to continue development of a new small ICBM called Midgetman.

The bomber force included about 60 FB-111s, 100 B-1s, and 260 B-52s, deployed for the most part in the continental United States, with one wing based in Guam. About 180 B-52s were armed with nuclear cruise missiles. Meanwhile, research and development has continued on the B-2 "stealth" or deep-penetrating technology bomber.

The navy's fleet ballistic missile submarines, the third leg of the triad, consisted in the late 1980s of thirty-nine ballistic missile Poseidon and Trident submarines carrying a total of 528 Poseidon C-3 and Trident C-4 SLBM launchers. The FY 1987 budget also provided for the procurement of the first twenty-one Trident II D-5 SLBMs, to be "back-fitted" on Trident subs. These missiles were to have both expanded range and sufficient accuracy to be used against hardened targets like Soviet ICBM silos.

Finally, the United States possesses a small strategic defense force. It consists of just 72 active and 198 reserve fighter-interceptor aircraft based in the continental United States, and one deactivated Safeguard ABM missile complex at Grand Forks, North Dakota. The Reagan administration's strategic defense initiative (SDI) would expand strategic defense capabilities significantly.

Theater Nuclear Forces. The United States' stock of tactical, or battlefield, nuclear weapons consists largely of bombs on tactical aircraft and more than 30-year-old 8-inch and more than 20-year-old 155mm nuclear artillery projectiles. These nuclear artillery rounds are being replaced by safer, more reliable versions with greater range. Because of a 1983 NATO decision to improve, but reduce the number of, its tactical nuclear weapons, fewer than 4,600 of these were dedicated to Europe in 1987, with the majority in the hands of U.S. forces and the remainder deployed with NATO allies but subject to American control.[142] Many others were afloat with the navy or deployed in the Pacific, while the remaining weapons were kept in the United States.

As a result of another 1979 NATO decision, the United States began in 1983 to deploy 108 Pershing II ballistic missiles in the Federal Republic of Germany and by the end of the decade 464 Tomahawk GLCMs in Belgium, Italy, the Netherlands, the United Kingdom, and the Federal Republic. These missiles, with their ability to strike military targets in the western USSR, serve essentially two functions. The first is to provide a tangible and reassuring American response to the Soviet Union's deployment of modern Soviet SS-20 intermediate-range missiles targeted on Western Europe. The second and less obvious function is to enhance deterrence of Soviet aggression by convincing Soviet planners that war in Europe is unlikely to remain conventional, and that nuclear exchanges there could spread quickly to Soviet territory.[143] After the American deployment was well underway, however, the two superpowers agreed in 1987 to eliminate all intermediate-range (500–5500 kilometer) missiles in their inventories.

QUALITY OF FORCES

In order for the United States to employ its forces effectively, these forces must possess three characteristics: sufficiency, flexibility, and readiness. At the present time there is some doubt about all three.

Forward-deployed U.S. forces in Central Europe, even augmented by the forces of the NATO allies, are no match for their Warsaw Pact adversaries in a purely conventional (nonnuclear) engagement. To be sufficient to deal with the threat, the United States must be able to reinforce and resupply Europe by air and by sea. In addition, the United States must have sufficient prepositioned materials and war reserves in place on the European continent.

In the mid 1980s, because of budget cuts, the armed services were also confronted with tough choices involving maintenance and support. Between 1980 and 1985 the military budget increased 50 percent above inflation and the Pentagon projected similar growth into the 1990s; but in the mid 1980s funding fell about 26 percent. Rather than addressing

this problem by cutting back on proposed weapons systems, the military opted to postpone planned increases in funding for ammunition, spare parts, base improvements, and personnel.[144] Basically, it treated its planned additional weapons systems, not the vital infrastructure for the weapons it had, as fixed costs. This led to growing concern that military strength would be hollowed out by a lack of funding for support systems essential to readiness and sustainability.

In an ideal world, force posture would be completely responsive to the demands of objectives, strategy, and doctrine. However, in the real world the relationship is more complex and the opposite is often true—that is, the prior existence of a given force posture largely determines doctrine. For example, the bedrock of American strategic doctrine is the triad (three different strategic offensive systems, each of which has unique capabilities that complement the other two, and each of which presents unique problems for any potential attacker). Yet this doctrine was developed after—not before—each of the three legs was built independently, primarily for reasons of organizational enhancement rather than doctrine. Similarly, the doctrine of forward deployment was developed to justify the fact that as a result of the position of U.S. conventional forces at the end of World War II, the Defense Department already had forces permanently deployed outside the United States.

On the other hand, force structure can change to support changes in strategy. For example, the strategy of preparing for a short intensive war on the central front in Europe led to an emphasis on "heavy," or mechanized, divisions in the army and a doubling of the equipment prepositioned in Europe. Likewise, if SDI produces effective ballistic missile defenses, U.S. strategic posture will have changed dramatically as a result of a political decision not to rely on a strictly offensive nuclear strategy, but rather to rely on a mixture of offensive and defensive forces.[145]

ARMS CONTROL

In the post–World War II period, the United States occasionally engaged in negotiations on the control of conventional arms such as the

Mutual Balanced Force Reductions (MBFR) talks in Europe and discussions on the limitation of naval forces in the Indian Ocean. It also sought to limit nuclear testing by way of the Limited Test Ban and Threshold Test Ban Treaties, and tried to control the spread of nuclear weaponry with the Nuclear Non-Proliferation Treaty (NPT). However, its main focus in arms limitation has been in the area of strategic nuclear weapons and, in the 1980s, INF based mainly in Europe.

The United States has concentrated on strategic arms for three reasons. First, these weapons represent the only real threat to the physical security of the United States. Second, given the level of technological advancement in the Soviet Union, there is the expectation that the United States can be matched and offset by the USSR. Thus, the United States could find itself in the position of spending vast sums of money without purchasing any additional security. Third, since the first two factors can also be applied to the Soviet Union, both sides see strategic nuclear weapons as an issue with considerable arms control potential. Therefore, the United States and the Soviet Union concluded three formal strategic arms control agreements: the 1972 Anti-Ballistic Missile Treaty, the 1972 Interim Agreement on Offensive Nuclear Arms, and the 1979 Strategic Arms Limitations Agreement.

Both Democratic and Republican administrations have been committed to maintaining a strategic posture of essential equivalence, or parity, with the USSR. Essential equivalence is defined to be the continuing maintenance of the following conditions: (1) that Soviet strategic nuclear forces do not become usable instruments of political leverage, diplomatic coercion, or military advantage; (2) that nuclear stability, especially in crises, is maintained; (3) that any advantages in force characteristics enjoyed by the USSR are offset by U.S. advantages in other characteristics; and (4) that the U.S. posture is not in fact, and is not seen as, inferior in performance to the nuclear forces of the Soviet Union.[146] In the abstract, this policy has enjoyed nearly unanimous support within the nation as a whole, although some analysts view the prospect of effective ballistic missile defenses as an opportunity for the United States to regain strategic superiority over the Soviet Union.

Although the overall policy of the United States for the past two decades has been to seek strategic arms control agreements with the USSR, there is considerable disagreement within the American political system over the specifics of that policy. At one extreme are those who oppose arms control and who feel that the United States should strive for strategic superiority over the Soviet Union. In their view, the USSR is still bent on world domination and hence will exploit arms control to attain superiority over the United States. At the other extreme are those who feel that national survival depends on arms control and disarmament, and therefore that greater flexibility is needed in negotiating with the USSR. In between these extremes are pragmatists who also promote arms control, but for different reasons: to manage geopolitical competition and achieve stability by managing the arms race and reducing the costs of armaments as much as possible.[147]

No single actor has been able to dominate the arms control policy process. Any treaty must conform to the worldview of the chief executive and simultaneously be acceptable to the Joint Chiefs of Staff, the Arms Control and Disarmament Agency, the State Department, informed public opinion, and the at least sixty-seven senators required to ratify an arms control treaty, each of whom has his or her own perception of the motivations of the Soviet Union and the meaning of essential equivalence.

Strategic arms control between the two superpowers is feasible to the extent that it seems to benefit both sides equally. However, quantitative restrictions are much easier to achieve than qualitative ones, in part because the former are more easily measured and compliance with them is more easily verified. Thus, the two superpowers have agreed relatively easily to halt nuclear testing in the atmosphere, and to limit allowable ABM sites, fixed missile launchers, and ballistic missile submarines. But compliance with qualitative restrictions involving, for example, the ranges, lifting capacities, accuracies, and missions of missiles is more difficult to measure and monitor with high confidence. For example, there is no visual or electronic way to detect with certainty the maximum range of a cruise missile or whether it has a nuclear warhead. SALT II moved into the qualitative area of arms control and thus took twice as long to negotiate as SALT I, even though the basic negotiation principles had been settled beforehand. Moreover, SALT II was subject to a much more rigorous examination by the U.S. Senate. Indeed, the SALT II Treaty signed by President Carter was never ratified. Nevertheless, SALT II did show that U.S.–Soviet agreement on qualitative restrictions is at least possible.

Certain aspects of U.S. strategic force posture no doubt appear threatening to other nations, primarily those that are suspicious of American intentions. Some Soviet strategists suspect that the United States' highly accurate MX, Trident II D-5, and Pershing II missiles; its development of cruise missiles; and its interest in space-based missile defenses indicate an American interest in a preemptive strike, especially since U.S. strategic defenses are expected to perform better against a Soviet missile force that has been "softened up" by a U.S. attack. Similarly, the Soviet Union and its Warsaw Pact allies may have wondered if the forward deployment of large numbers of U.S. land and air forces in Europe and naval forces in the Mediterranean signified some aggressive design on their territories. This no doubt became an even greater concern when the Reagan administration included in its conventional strategy the possibility of a counteroffensive against Eastern Europe. However, some NATO allies, as well as Japan and China, were concerned about the relative decrease in U.S. strategic and conventional capabilities vis-à-vis the Soviet Union. Consequently, they wished to see the United States develop a more formidable posture and increase its forward deployments.[148]

To a certain extent, the force posture currently maintained by the United States is a reaction to the threat perceived from the Soviet force posture. The qualitative improvements in American strategic forces over the past two decades have been primarily a response to the quantitative and qualitative buildup of the strategic nuclear forces of the USSR, while American conventional and theater nuclear forces are sized primarily to deal with a blitzkrieg attack by the Warsaw Pact nations in Central Europe. Indeed, during the post-Vietnam period, the United States drew down its force structure dramatically. Were it not for the rapid Soviet buildup, it is doubtful that a consensus would have emerged in the late 1970s and throughout most of the 1980s on increasing U.S. capabilities.

From the late 1970s through the late 1980s there were a number of important arms control developments. The Soviet invasion of Afghanistan, combined with numerous congressional reservations about SALT II, prevented President Carter from securing congressional approval of that proposed treaty. Both superpowers nonetheless agreed informally to observe SALT II's provisions in the absence of ratification. The Reagan administration, however, after pronouncing the agreement "fundamentally flawed" and charging Moscow with a pattern of noncompliance, finally stopped adhering to the agreement's limitations in 1986. Also, in 1983, when NATO deployed Pershing II missiles and Tomahawk cruise missiles, Soviet negotiators walked out of the INF negotiations and indefinitely postponed strategic arms talks. When negotiations resumed, they were structured in three tiers: one for strategic arms; one for INF; and, for the first time, one for space weapons, because of Moscow's strong objections to SDI. The Reagan administration, however, made SDI the centerpiece of its approach to arms control, calling for jointly managed U.S.–Soviet deployments of strategic defenses combined with deep cuts in offensive strategic arms. President Reagan also sought to interpret the 1972 ABM treaty in a way that would allow tests of defensive technologies in preparation for early deployment of space-based systems. A stalemate thus ensued: Moscow would not consider deep cuts until it could be assured that the United States would adhere to a more restrictive interpretation of the ABM treaty and until agreement could be reached on what manner of tests, if any, a restrictive interpretation would allow. But Washington stood firm in its insistence that SDI not be traded in bargaining for offensive reductions.

After the Reykjavik summit, the greatest potential for progress in arms control was with INF missiles. Moscow surprised NATO by accepting a so-called "Double Zero-Option," which would eliminate nuclear missiles in Europe of *both* long-range INF (capable of hitting targets at 1000 to 5500 kilometers—600 to 3300 miles away) and short-range INF (capable of hitting targets at 500 to 1000 kilometers—300 to 600 miles away) categories. Agreement was finally reached in late 1987 that included an extensive regime of mutual inspections. Even so, this unprecedented opportunity for arms control nonetheless generated concerns among some NATO observers that Europe was sliding toward denuclearization by responding positively to Moscow's initiative; and that, with the Soviet Union's conventional superiority in the theater, denuclearization would put NATO at a distinct military disadvantage.[149]

Given improved U.S.–Soviet relations in the Gorbachev period and the withdrawal of Soviet forces from Afghanistan, the Bush administration has continued the arms control initiatives of the later Reagan years. These efforts have included negotiations on reducing both conventional forces in Europe and strategic arms.

USE OF FORCE

In the post–World War II period, the United States has fought two large and prolonged wars in Asia. From 1950 to 1953, the nation poured a total of over a million people and $50 billion into the fight against the forces of North Korea and the People's Republic of China. (Actual troop strength at any one time peaked at 325,000 in 1953.) In the period from 1964 through 1973, the United States sent a total of over two million citizens and spent some $200 billion in a futile effort to thwart the attempt of the North Vietnamese to expand their control over the rest of Indochina. (Actual troop strength in Vietnam peaked at 579,000 in 1968.)

In addition, since World War II the United States employed its forces over two hundred times in deliberate attempts to influence the behavior of other states without engaging in prolonged contests of violence.[150] These employments ranged from the low-key, but highly publicized, cancellation of a carrier visit to Chile during the Marxist presidency of Salvador Allende to the massive naval blockade of Cuba that brought the United States to the brink of war with the Soviet Union. With the election of Ronald Reagan, the United States employed military force much more conspicuously and more frequently than under Presidents Ford and Carter, although Ford and Carter both had occasion to apply military power in pursuit of U.S. interests. By mid 1987, during President Reagan's incumbency, U.S. military forces were used in the following ways: military advisers were dispatched to El Salvador; navy jets destroyed two Libyan aircraft after being fired upon; an infantry battalion was deployed in the Sinai Peninsula to patrol the buffer zone between Israeli and Egyptian forces; U.S. Marines participated in two multinational peacekeeping efforts in Lebanon, the second of which led to air strikes and naval bombardment against Lebanese factions and Syrian missile sites; combined U.S. air, naval, and ground forces invaded Grenada to deny Cuba another foothold in the Caribbean; U.S. aircraft forced down an Egyptian plane harboring terrorists; air force and navy aircraft bombed Libya; and U.S. naval forces in the Persian Gulf were bolstered in preparation for possible conflict with Iran over rights of free passage. Finally, U.S. counterterrorist units were scrambled repeatedly in response to terrorist incidents abroad.

In fighting its wars in Korea and Vietnam, as well as in using military force as a political instrument, the United States has usually sought limited and rather specific objectives. The primary purpose of sending troops to Korea and Vietnam was to prevent the communist governments in those areas from imposing their will on their southern neighbors by force. Even in the Cuban missile crisis, the United States sought merely to compel the Soviet Union to remove its missiles from Cuba and pledge not to use Cuba as a base for strategic weapons systems.

Similarly, the United States has limited the military means it has used so that they would be commensurate with the objectives sought. In Korea and Vietnam, the United States refrained from using strategic and tactical nuclear weapons, spared the hydroelectric facilities in North Korea and the dams in North Vietnam, and avoided actions that would provoke China and the Soviet Union, even though those countries were actively supplying the forces of North Korea and North Vietnam.

The vast majority of cases in which forces were employed for political purposes involved very limited operations. Often the forces simply provided a presence. Mostly they participated in port visits or exercises. Rarely were armed hostilities used and only extremely rarely did the United States threaten to use or maneuver its nuclear forces, for example, by putting them on a higher alert posture.

In Korea and Vietnam, the level of U.S. involvement was no doubt influenced and limited by the threatened actions of the Chinese and Russians. The United States allowed China to remain a sanctuary in both wars and refused to interdict Soviet supply bases in either Korea or Vietnam because it did not wish to expand the war beyond those areas. Similarly, it was primarily ethical and legal concerns that prevented the United States from destroying such potential targets as dikes and population centers in North Korea and North Vietnam.

In using its forces for political purposes, the United States generally has tried to justify its actions under international law, even if only after the fact or for appearances. Thus, it sought OAS approval for its actions in the 1962 Cuban missile crisis and in the Dominican Republic in 1965. And in Grenada, when it proved difficult to account legally for U.S. intervention, American action was portrayed as a justifiable response to a request for assistance by the Organization for Eastern Caribbean States, whose members felt threatened by Grenada's Marxist, pro-Cuban leanings.

Domestic political pressures and public opinion have had an impact on the use of force

by American political leaders. For example, President Truman's decision to intervene in Korea, as well as those of Presidents Kennedy and Johnson to become involved in Vietnam, were influenced by their fear of the reaction of conservatives in Congress and the public if they failed to take decisive action. Paradoxically, it was the opinion of the public, tired of absorbing high casualties in seemingly futile struggles, that forced Presidents Truman and Johnson to seek a negotiated settlement on terms less than their original objectives may have been in those Asian wars.

Since 1973 the use of American force has been complicated further by the War Powers Act. The act's main purpose was to ensure that the collective judgment of Congress and the president would apply to the introduction of U.S. armed forces into hostilities or situations where hostilities were imminent, and to the continued use of force under such conditions. Every president since its passage has considered the War Powers Act to be an unconstitutional abridgment of his powers as commander in chief, and the act has constrained executive action by confronting presidents with the possibility of an uncooperative Congress at times when national unity was essential. At the same time, although jealous of its prerogatives under the act, Congress has consistently refrained from undercutting the president whenever U.S. forces are engaged. It has either supported executive action outright or sought compromise, as with the 1983 American involvement in Lebanon, when the president and Congress agreed on legislation that allowed U.S. Marines to stay in that country for eighteen months—well over the act's 60-day limit.

One great difficulty, however, is that the War Powers Act has injected into such situations greater uncertainty about U.S. willingness and resolve to use military force. This is especially true in conflicts at the periphery of U.S. interests that have potential for becoming prolonged and costly in American lives, these being circumstances under which the act is most likely to be invoked. Many observers are convinced that this additional uncertainty only benefits America's adversaries, who may be able to plan and adjust their political and military strategies by monitoring publicized legislative-executive debates over the War Powers Act and the American public's reaction to these debates.

Because of its limited duration, the impact of domestic politics and public opinion on the political use of armed force is more difficult to assess. However, there does exist a significant relationship between the popularity of a president and the nation's sense of confidence and the frequency of incidents. Generally speaking, the more popular the president and the higher the people's sense of confidence in him, the greater his flexibility or freedom of choice in responding to threats and, as a result, the more frequent the employment of military force for political purposes.

In Korea and Vietnam, and in the many political uses of U.S. armed forces, the fact that the United States has had a large, technologically advanced military force has made it easier to rely on those forces to achieve policy goals. It is no accident that since the Soviet Union has achieved military parity, the United States has grown increasingly reluctant to employ military force for political purposes.

Conclusion

As the United States moves into the last decade of this century, its national security policy is clearly in a state of flux. Its relative position in the international system and perception of the role it ought to play in that system are changing. Its national security objectives, strategy, force structure, arms control policy, and force-employment doctrine are subjects of intense debate among a somewhat weakened executive, a resurgent Congress, and an informed, but divided, public. The American people, still suffering from the trauma of the Vietnam debacle, are unsure what kind of defense policies they want their leaders to pursue.

The future direction of the defense policies of the United States is difficult to determine with certainty. The only thing that can be said with any degree of assurance is that, whatever they are, these policies will have a profound effect upon the relations among nations. The choices that were open to the United States before 1941 are no longer relevant. Whether it wishes to or not, the United States will remain a major actor in the world arena. But it will need strong and informed leadership to ensure that there is congruence among its perceptions, strategy, policy, force structure, arms control policy, and force-employment doctrine.

Notes

1. Robert Komer, "What Decade of Neglect?" *International Security* 10, no. 2 (Fall 1985): 71.

2. Colin S. Gray and Jeffrey G. Barlow, "Inexcusable Restraint: The Decline of American Military Power in the 1970s," *International Security* 10, no. 2 (Fall 1985): 61.

3. See Lawrence J. Korb and Linda P. Brady, "Rearming America: The Reagan Administration Defense Program," in *Conventional Forces and American Defense Policy*, ed. Stephen E. Miller (Princeton: Princeton University Press, 1986): Gray and Barlow, "Inexcusable Restraint," p. 28.

4. Caspar W. Weinberger, *Annual Report to the Congress, FY 1987*, 5 February 1986, p. 13.

5. William W. Kaufmann, *Defense in the 1980s* (Washington, D.C.: Brookings Institution, 1981), p. 4.

6. Komer, "What Decade of Neglect?" p. 82.

7. U.S. Department of Defense, *Soviet Military Power, 1987* (Washington, D.C.: Government Printing Office, 1987), p. 7; Caspar W. Weinberger, *Annual Report to the Congress, FY 1986*, 4 February 1985, p. 15.

8. Weinberger, *Annual Report, FY 1987*, pp. 60-61.

9. U.S. Congress, House, *Economic Report of the President*, 100th Cong., 1st sess., House Document no. 100-2, transmitted to Congress January 1987, p. 331.

10. Weinberger, *Annual Report, FY 1987*, p. 94.

11. U.S. Congress, Congressional Budget Office, "Defense Spending: What Has Been Accomplished," Staff Working Paper, April 1985, pp. iii-iv.

12. U.S. Department of Defense, *Soviet Military Power, 1987*, p. 33; U.S. Joint Chiefs of Staff, *U.S. Military Posture, FY 1987* (Washington, D.C.: Government Printing Office, 1986), p. 463.

13. Weinberger, *Annual Report, FY 1987*, p. 218.

14. Ibid., p. 228.

15. William M. Arkin and Richard Fieldhouse, *Nuclear Battlefields: Global Links in the Arms Race* (Cambridge, Mass.: Ballinger, 1985) p. 56.

16. Weinberger, *Annual Report, FY 1987*, pp. 60-61.

17. Sam C. Sarkasian and William L. Scully, eds., *U.S. Policy and Low Intensity Conflict* (New Brunswick, N.J.: Transaction Books, 1981), p. 4.

18. Eliot A. Cohen, "Distant Battles: Modern War in the Third World," *International Security* 10, no. 4 (Spring 1986): 160.

19. Harold Brown, *Thinking About National Security* (Boulder, Colo.: Westview Press, 1986), p. 210.

20. U.S. Congress, *Economic Report of the President, 1987*, p. 103.

21. Ibid., pp. 21, 47.

22. Robert Gilpin, *War and Change in World Politics* (Cambridge: Cambridge University Press, 1981), pp. 176–85.

23. *New York Times*, 14 January 1987.

24. U.S. Congress, *Economic Report of the President, 1987*, p. 98.

25. *New York Times*, 3 May 1987.

26. Brown, *Thinking About National Security*, p. 216.

27. *New York Times*, 15 June 1987.

28. Donald M. Snow, *National Security: Enduring Problems of U.S. Defense Policy* (New York: St. Martins Press, 1987), pp. 117–19.

29. Gilpin, *War and Change in International Politics*, p. 243.

30. Ibid., p. 233.

31. U.S. Department of Defense, *Soviet Military Power, 1986* (Washington, D.C.: Government Printing Office, 1986), p. 105.

32. Ibid., p. 106.

33. Ibid., p. 37; U.S. Department of Defense, *Soviet Military Power, 1987*, pp. 8–9, 29, 31.

34. U.S. Department of Defense, *Soviet Military Power, 1987*, p. 125.

35. Edward Luttwak, *The Pentagon and the Art of War* (New York: Simon & Schuster, 1985), pp. 93–129.

36. Daniel Pipes, "Fundamentalist Muslims," *Foreign Affairs* 64, no. 5 (Summer 1986): 945–56.

37. Richard Cottam, "Regional Implications of the Gulf War," *Survival* 28, no. 6 (November-December 1986): 483–94.

38. Thomas L. McNaugher, *Arms and Oil: U.S. Military Strategy and the Persian Gulf* (Washington, D.C.: Brookings Institution, 1985), p. 7; U.S. Congress, House Committee on Armed Services, *Defense Authorization for Appropriations for FY 1987, Hearings*, pt. 2, 99th Cong., 2d sess., p. 615.

39. William W. Hogan, "Import Management of Oil Emergencies," Harvard University, John F. Kennedy School of Government, Energy and Environmental Policy Center, June 1980, cited in McNaugher, *Arms and Oil*, p. 7.

40. U.S. Congress, Senate, Committee on Commerce, Science, and Transportation, *Critical Minerals and Materials, Hearings*, 99th Cong., 1st sess., 2 March 1981, p. 84.

41. U.S. Congress, Office of Technology Assessment, *Strategic Materials: Technology to Reduce U.S. Import Vulnerability* (Washington, D.C.: Office of Technology Assessment, 1985), p. 6.

42. Richard Nixon, *U.S. Foreign Policy for the 1970s*, 18 February 1970, p. 27.

43. *Congressional Record*, 24 January 1977, pp. 1–5.

44. Gerald Ford, *A Time to Heal* (New York: Harper & Row, 1970), p. 421.

45. President Jimmy Carter, "Remarks at a Fundraising Dinner for Abraham Beame," New York, 5 December 1978.

46. William Schneider, "Conservatism, Not Interventionism: Trends in Foreign Policy Opinion, 1974–1982," in *Eagle Defiant: United States Foreign Policy in the 1980s*, eds. Kenneth A. Oye, Robert J. Leiber, and Donald Rothchild (Boston: Little, Brown, 1981), p. 35.

47. Ibid., p. 37.

48. Ole R. Holsti and James N. Rosenau, *American Leadership in World Affairs; Vietnam and the Breakdown of Consensus* (Boston: Allen & Unwin, 1984), pp. 108–39.

49. Robert Osgood, *Alliances and American Foreign Policy* (Baltimore: Johns Hopkins Press, 1968); Congressional Quarterly, *Global Defense: U.S. Military Commitments Abroad* (September 1960).

50. Ellen L. Frost and Angela E. Stent, "NATO's Troubles with East-West Trade," *International Security* 8, no. 1 (Summer 1983): 187–89.

51. Brown, *Thinking About National Security*, p. 91.

52. *New York Times*, 15 June 1987.

53. *New York Times*, 22 March 1987; 12 June 1987.

54. Denis Healy, "A Labour Britain, NATO and the Bomb," *Foreign Affairs* 65, no. 4 (Spring 1987): 729.

55. *New York Times*, 8 February 1987.

56. *New York Times*, 14 June 1987.

57. Ibid.

58. Weinberger, *Annual Report, FY 1987*, p. 28.

59. Anthony Lake, "The International Security Environment" (Paper Presented at Senior Conference 17, West Point, N.Y., 15 June 1979), summarizes these threats quite succinctly.

60. This account is drawn primarily from John Spanier, *American Foreign Policy Since World War II* (New York: Praeger, 1973), pp. 7–21.

61. The first secretary to put the issue squarely before the American people was James Schlesinger, in his *Annual Defense Department Report, FY 1976 and 1977*, 5 February 1975, pp. 1–2 through 1–4.

62. Robert F. Turner, *The War Powers Resolution: Its Implementation in Theory and Practice* (Philadelphia: Foreign Policy Research Institute, 1983), p. 108.

63. Ibid., p. 37.

64. Ford, *A Time to Heal*, pp. 302–4.

65. *New York Times*, 23 July 1971.

66. Barry Blechman and Stephen Kaplan, *Force without War: U.S. Armed Forces as a Political Instrument* (Washington, D.C.: Brookings Institution, 1978), p. 38.

67. Donald Rumsfeld, *Annual Report to Congress, FY 1978*, 17 January 1977, p. 190.

68. Congressional Quarterly, *U.S. Defense Policy* (Washington, D.C.: Congressional Quarterly, 1983), p. 412.

69. Weinberger, *Annual Report, FY 1987*, p. 314.

70. Schneider, "Conservatism, Not Interventionism," p. 61.

71. CBS News/New York Times Poll, 23–26 January 1979.

72. Ford, *A Time to Heal*, p. 247.

73. *Public Opinion*, March/May 1979, p. 26.

74. Weinberger, *Annual Report, FY 1987*, p. 37.

75. Ibid.

76. Ibid., p. 32.

77. Donald Hafner, "Choosing Targets for Nuclear Weapons," *International Security* 11, no. 4 (Spring 1987): 136.

78. Ibid.

79. Harold Brown, *Annual Report to the Congress, FY 1979*, January 1978, p. 56.

80. Daniel Seligman, "Our ICBMs Are in Danger," *Fortune*, 2 July 1979, p. 50.

81. Snow, *National Security*, p. 70.
82. Weinberger, *Annual Report, FY 1987*, p. 38.
83. Robert Jarvis, *The Illogic of American Nuclear Strategy* (Ithaca, N.Y.: Cornell University Press, 1984), pp. 65–66.
84. Charles L. Glaser, "Do We Want the Missile Defense We Can Build?" *International Security* 10, no. 1 (Summer 1985): 25; Robert H. Gromoll, "SDI and the Dynamics of Strategic Uncertainty," *Political Science Quarterly* (Fall, 1987).
85. U.S. Congress, House, Committee on Armed Services, *NATO Standardization Interoperability and Readiness*, 95th Cong., 2d sess., pp. 2–3.
86. Jeffrey Record, *Revising U.S. Military Strategy* (Washington, D.C.: Pergamon, 1984), p. 37.
87. Ibid., p. 42.
88. Weinberger, *Annual Report to the Congress, FY 1983*, pp. 11-16.
89. Barry R. Posen and Stephen Van Evera, "Defense Policy and the Reagan Administration: Departure from Containment," *International Security* 8, no. 1 (Summer 1983): 5.
90. Record, *Revising U.S. Military Strategy*, p. 44.
91. National Security Council Memo.
92. *New York Times, The Tower Commission Report* (New York: Random House, 1987), p. 14.
93. James Bamford, "Carlucci and the NSC," *New York Times Magazine*, 18 January 1987, p. 26; *New York Times*, 4 June 1985.
94. *New York Times, The Tower Commission Report*, p. 14.
95. *Washington Post*, 18 February 1979.
96. *Washington Post*, 22, 26 May 1978.
97. Bridget Gail, "The Fine Old Game of Killing," *Armed Forces Journal*, September 1978; *New York Times*, 7 January 1979.
98. Vincent Puritano, Statement before the Subcommittee on Procurement and Military Nuclear Systems of the House Committee on Armed Services, 11 March 1983, p. 10.
99. Interview with OSD official, 1978.
100. "Memorandum for the Secretary of Defense," 10 December 1977, from R. James Woolsey, Undersecretary of the Navy, *Armed Forces Journal*, September 1978, p. 42.
101. Vincent Puritano, "Streamlining PPBS," *Defense/81*, August 1981, pp. 21-28.
102. Turner, *The War Powers Resolution*, p. 116.
103. Graham Allison, *Essence of Decision* (Boston: Little, Brown, 1971), p. 146.
104. John Steinbruner, *The Cybernetic Theory of Decision* (Princeton: Princeton University Press, 1974).
105. *Washington Post*, 18 February 1979.
106. Herbert Scoville, "A Starting Point for a New SALT Agreement," *Arms Control Today*, April 1977, pp. 4–5.
107. *Philadelphia Inquirer*, 3 June 1987.
108. Samuel P. Huntington, *The Soldier and the State* (Cambridge: Harvard University Press, 1957).
109. Morris Janowitz, *The Professional Soldier* (New York: Free Press, 1960).
110. The data in this section were reported in Weinberger, *Annual Report, FY 1983*, p. 176; and Committee on Appropriations, *Department of Defense Appropriations for Fiscal Year 1987, Hearings*, p. 431.
111. Committee on Appropriations, *Department of*

Defense Appropriations for Fiscal Year 1987, Hearings, p. 431.
112. Executive Office of the President and Office of Management and the Budget, *Budget of the United States Government for Fiscal Year 1988, Supplement* (Washington, D.C.: Government Printing Office, 1987), pp. 5–15; U.S. Congress, Congressional Research Service, Foreign Affairs and National Defense Division (Steven A. Hildreth and Alice C. Maroni, coordinators), "The Strategic Defense Initiative: Program Facts," *Issue Brief*, 20 February 1987.
113. Brown, *Annual Report, FY 1979*, p. 100.
114. This material is outlined in Department of Defense, Directive no. 5000.1, "Major System Acquisitions," 12 March 1986; and Department of Defense, Instruction no. 5000.2, "Major System Acquisition Procedures," 12 March 1986.
115. Department of Defense, Directive no. 5000.1.
116. *Inside the Pentagon*, 17 October 1986.
117. Ibid.
118. William H. Taft IV, "Acquisition Reform and National Security," *Defense Issues* 1, no. 42, 3 July 1986, p. 2.
119. William H. Taft IV, "Defense Management and the Packard Commission Report," *Defense Issues* 1, no. 20, 17 April 1986, p. 2.
120. Weinberger, *Annual Report, FY 1986*, p. 125.
121. Weinberger, *Annual Report, FY 1987*, p. 315; U.S. Congress, *Economic Report of the President, 1987*, p. 244.
122. *New York Times*, 19 November 1985.
123. Ibid.
124. U.S. Congress, Office of Technology Assessment, *Strategic Materials*, p. 83.
125. Ibid., pp. 6, 41.
126. U.S. Congress, Congressional Research Service (Leonard Fishman), "World Mineral Trends and U.S. Supply Problems: Resources for the Future," Research Paper R-20 (Washington, D.C.: Congressional Research Service, 1980), p. 7.
127. Office of Technology Assessment, *Strategic Materials*, p. 6.
128. Weinberger, *Annual Report, FY 1987*, p. 320.
129. Weinberger, *Annual Report, FY 1986*, p. 224.
130. Department of Defense, *Worldwide Manpower Distribution by Geographic Area*, 30 September 1985.
131. Weinberger, *Annual Report, FY 1987*, p. 212.
132. Ibid., pp. 155–56.
133. Weinberger, *Annual Report, FY 1986*, p. 178; and *FY 1983*, p. 38.
134. Ibid.
135. U.S. Joint Chiefs of Staff, *U.S. Military Posture, FY 1988* (Washington, D.C.: Government Printing Office, 1987), p. 14.
136. Weinberger, *Annual Report, FY 1987*, p. 237; Joseph Kruzel, ed., *American Defense Annual, 1986–1987* (Lexington, Mass.: Lexington Books, 1986), p. 132.
137. Weinberger, *Annual Report, FY 1987*, p. 236.
138. McNaugher, *Arms and Oil*, p. 75.
139. Ibid.
140. Ibid., p. 201; Record, *Revising U.S. Military Strategy*, p. 95.
141. Record, *Revising U.S. Military Strategy*, p. 93.
142. *New York Times*, 24 June 1987.

143. Department of Defense, *Soviet Military Power, 1987*, p. 41.

144. *Philadelphia Inquirer*, 3 June 1987.

145. See Jonathan B. Stein, *From H-Bomb to Star Wars: The Politics of Strategic Decision Making* (Lexington, Mass.: Lexington Books, 1984).

146. Brown, *Annual Report, FY 1979*, pp. 5–6.

147. Michael Krepon, *Strategic Stalemate: Nuclear Weapons and Arms Control in American Politics* (New York: St. Martin's Press, 1984), p. 15.

148. *New York Times*, 3 June 1979.

149. *New York Times*, 4, 24 June 1987.

150. The data in this section were drawn from Blechman and Kaplan, *Force Without War*.

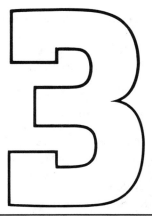

THE SOVIET UNION

Edward L. Warner III

International Environment

As the Soviet Union enters the 1990s, after more than seventy years of communist rule, Mikhail Gorbachev and his colleagues in the Kremlin are bound to view the nation's domestic and international accomplishments with a mixture of pride and very serious concern. During the past half century, their country has weathered the self-inflicted human losses of Stalin's forced collectivization campaign and bloody purges of the 1930s as well as the devastation of World War II. The Soviet Union came back from the very brink of defeat at the hands of Hitler's armies in 1941–42 to become the most powerful nation in Europe and Asia.

The Soviet Communist Party and government have also realized many of the most cherished foreign policy goals of its czarist Russian predecessor. These include: (1) the expansion of the country's frontiers during and immediately after World War II to include the Baltic states, portions of Finland, Poland, Germany, Czechoslovakia, and Romania in the West,

and the southern half of Sakhalin Island and the Kurile Islands in the Far East; (2) the establishment of subservient client regimes throughout most of Eastern Europe in the immediate postwar period; and (3) as the result of sustained efforts since the mid 1950s, greatly increased Russian presence and influence in many other areas, including the Middle East, South and Southeast Asia, and Africa.

The past thirty years have also witnessed a seemingly inexorable expansion of Soviet military power. This buildup has succeeded in establishing the Soviet Union as a coequal with the United States in this critical dimension of power and has helped it promote its foreign policy interests aggressively throughout the world. The Soviets themselves have come to recognize, however, that they may have relied too much on the military dimension of their foreign policy. In the current climate of *glasnost* (translated variously as "public discussion," candor, or openness), Gorbachev and others have repeatedly called for a more balanced foreign policy approach and have

75

called explicitly for restraint in the defense sector.

Yet all is far from well for the Soviet Union regarding both external and internal fortunes. The Kremlin finds itself facing a series of daunting challenges. The last days of enfeebled Leonid Brezhnev and the uncertain interregnums of Yuri Andropov and Konstantin Chernenko in the early 1980s saw a growing accumulation of domestic problems and a perceptible loss of Soviet momentum on the world scene. The Soviet political leadership has come to view these developments with very considerable alarm. Mikhail Gorbachev has succinctly stated these concerns when he has spoken of the grave internal crisis facing the Soviet system and said that nothing less is at stake than whether "the Soviet Union will succeed in entering the twenty-first century in the manner befitting a superpower."[1] Consequently, Gorbachev, having succeeded largely in consolidating his power as the leader of the Soviet Communist Party, is embarked upon a "radical reform program" designed to rejuvenate the lagging economy and demoralized Soviet populace. Under the banner of "new political thinking" he is striving simultaneously to impart new vigor into Soviet relations with allied, uncommitted, and adversary nations.

RELATIVE POWER POSITION

It has become commonplace to attribute the superpower status of the Soviet Union almost exclusively due to its military might. Indisputably, defense efforts enjoy very high priority in the Soviet economy. Moreover, military power has played a critical role in the growth of Soviet influence in the world. Yet Soviet claims to superpower status are not based solely on the country's obvious military prowess.

In aggregate terms the Soviet Union remains one of the world's leading industrial nations. With a gross national product of about two trillion dollars, the USSR ranks third in the world, behind the United States and Japan.[2] It possesses a large, skilled work force and an enormous resource base. The Soviet Union continues to lead the world in several economic categories, including production of iron ore, steel, cement, petroleum, natural gas, lumber, and machinery, and trails only the United States in aluminum production and electric power generation.[3]

Yet the Soviet economy also displays serious weaknesses. Soviet economic achievements are considerably less impressive when computed on a per capita basis. Viewed from this perspective, the Soviet Union, much as czarist Russia did on the eve of the Revolution of 1917,[4] ranks behind not only the United States but also most of the industrial nations of Western Europe and Asia.[5] Moreover, for more than a decade Soviet economic growth has been very sluggish, averaging only some 2 percent per year. This stands in stark contrast to the respectable growth rate of 4–5 percent the Soviet economy enjoyed throughout the 1960s and early 1970s. The USSR has been unable to make the transition from extensive to intensive economic development. Its overcentralized system of planning and management has proven too rigid to manage an increasingly complex economy, to sustain an acceptable rate of economic growth, or to support the timely introduction and absorption of new technologies.

Soviet superpower status also has a substantial political and ideological component. Undoubtedly, the international appeal of the Soviet system has dimmed significantly in recent years as the failure of its economy to adapt to the technological revolution, its ruthless suppression of political dissent, and its manifest difficulties in providing a relatively high standard of living for the increasingly apathetic general populace have become widely known. Nevertheless, the USSR still enjoys substantial influence, particularly in the Third World, as the major influence of the world communist movement and the self-proclaimed champion of the fight against Western imperialism.

THREATS FACING THE SOVIET UNION

The Soviets have a deep-seated and historically well-founded concern about foreign military invasion across their lengthy land frontiers. As Malcolm C. Toon, former U.S. ambassador to the Soviet Union, has noted: "Centuries of invasions from both East and

West have left their mark on the outlook of the Russian people and its rulers."[6]

Soviet concern about foreign invasion is not based simply on bitter Russian historical experience at the hands of such aggressors as the Mongol hordes of Genghis Khan and Napoleon's *Grande Armée*. The regime assiduously keeps alive the memory of several foreign incursions during the Soviet period: the invasion by imperial Germany just weeks after the Bolsheviks seized power in November 1917; the military interventions of Britain, France, the United States, and Japan on behalf of the rival "White" forces who battled the Bolsheviks during the Russian Civil War, 1918–20; border clashes with imperial Japan in 1938 and 1939; and, most significantly, the Nazi invasion and brutal occupation in 1941–44.[7] This "siege mentality"[8] is further intensified by the strong emphasis in Marxist-Leninist ideology on the inevitable hostility of the capitalist powers and repeated warnings about the dangers posed by "capitalist encirclement."

Soviet statements since the end of World War II have left no doubt that the United States has become the USSR's principal adversary. Soviet propaganda has consistently identified the United States as the leading force of "imperialist reaction," dedicated to the defeat of socialism and eagerly poised to attack the Soviet Union at the first opportunity. During the heightened "war scare" of the first years of the Reagan administration, several Soviet leaders and commentators accused the American president of harboring intentions of launching a first strike against the USSR, but Soviet discourse about U.S. intentions moderated substantially in the mid and late 1980s as Soviet-American relations improved.

The only other Western nation that has merited similar Soviet concern has been the Federal Republic of Germany. Periodic Soviet attacks on the "revanchist" goals of the West Germans reflect the deep scars left by two devastating German invasions in this century.

From the mid 1960s until the early 1980s, the USSR often described the People's Republic of China as a significant external threat. In recent years this stance has been softened significantly, but long-term anxieties about the Chinese undoubtedly persist. Soviet concern about China has several roots. These include historical distrust that can be traced back to the Mongol dominance of medieval Russia, racial antipathy, intense rivalry for leadership of the international communist movement, and strongly conflicting foreign policy aspirations, particularly in Asia. This distrust also reflects understandable Soviet anxiety about the long-term threat posed by a mammoth neighbor with whom the USSR shares a 4,500-mile frontier and that has a population of over a billion, a growing nuclear capability, and a suspicious and frequently hostile attitude toward the USSR.

Having noted the Soviet obsession with defense and the threat of foreign invasion, one must not overlook the degree to which the Soviet regime and its czarist predecessors have successfully employed offensive military power to promote their foreign policy interests and forcibly expand their frontiers. Neighboring countries such as Finland, Poland, Bulgaria, and Turkey, to say nothing of the formerly independent Baltic states of Lithuania, Latvia, and Estonia, and more recently, Afghanistan, have periodically been the victims of Russian or Soviet military aggression. The Soviet leaders today almost certainly view the international scene more as an arena of substantial opportunity for the advancement of their interests than as a source of threats to the security of the USSR.

The national security concerns of the leaders in the Kremlin are not limited to external considerations. They also take very seriously the threat of internal political opposition. Their anxieties in this regard include concerns about oppositional political movements and the nationalistic aspirations of several of the minorities within the Soviet multinational state. Soviet spokesmen have traditionally attributed such opposition to the "diversionary activities" of foreign adversaries. Harsh internal security measures to deal with the subversive activities of so-called rotten capitalist elements were especially prominent in the early years of the Bolshevik regime. Fears of "class enemies" were manipulated by Stalin in particular to justify the ruthless suppression of political opposition groups in a series of blood purges in the 1930s.

These fears of subversion and the attendant internal security measures to deal with this threat are still present today, although in much attenuated form compared with the days of Stalin's paranoia and terror. Nevertheless, in the midst of Gorbachev's campaigns for a thoroughgoing *perestroika* (restructuring) of the Soviet political and economic systems and for *glasnost* and *demokratizatsiya* (democratization), the long pent-up nationalist feelings among the minorities in the Caucasus, the Baltic states, and central Asia have burst forth in unprecedented fashion, in some cases with the explicit endorsement of the Party and its senior leaders. The Soviet Communist Party and government, confronting increasingly strident demands for greater political, economic, and cultural autonomy from these groups, are seeking to steer a delicate course that channels their energies into support for the overall reform movement but manages to convince them not to make demands that threaten the directing role of the Communist Party or the political integrity of the USSR.

Despite its determined pursuit of détente with the West in the late 1960s and in the 1970s, the Soviet regime made it absolutely clear that there would be no relaxation of ideological or political controls on the domestic scene. Rather, the Soviet leadership appeared to believe it was precisely in such an atmosphere, with its attendant increased contacts with foreigners and their culture, that the tight social controls were most necessary and thus had to be intensified. In his *perestroika* campaign, Gorbachev has sought through his *glasnost* policy to loosen censorship to a considerable extent as a means to mobilize support for his extensive reform program. The new, more open political and cultural atmosphere under *glasnost* has led to the release of scores of dissidents and has legitimized the public expression of an enormous range of views on virtually any subject. Manuscripts long committed "to the drawer" that could not get past the censor are being published, previously taboo subjects are being debated, and a Soviet brand of investigative journalism has emerged.

SELF-PERCEPTION OF THE SOVIET LEADERSHIP

The Soviet perception of world affairs contains an amalgam of traditional Russian, Marxist-Leninist ideological, and contemporary *realpolitik* elements. Much has been written about the relative weight of the first two factors, especially in relation to Soviet foreign policy. The important thing, however, is to understand that both traditions reinforce Soviet inclinations toward an authoritarian regime at home and expansionism on the world scene.

Both the Russian imperial heritage and the Marxist-Leninist tradition provide support for a highly centralized, authoritarian government and a heavily regulated economy. Both traditions also call for defense of the regime as the most fundamental objective of the state. Both are also marked by strong messianic strains. The Russian tradition included a centuries-old belief that the Russian Empire represented the "third Rome," the successor to Byzantium, with responsibilities to defend and expand the true orthodox Christian faith. Moreover, Russia was viewed as having a special right to exercise hegemony throughout the Slavic areas of southeastern Europe. The imperial tradition was also marked by a paradoxical mix of attitudes to Russia and the West. It combined an almost mystical veneration of things Russian with a nagging sense of inferiority regarding the superior economic and technological achievements of the industrially advanced West.

Up through the late 1970s, Marxist-Leninist ideology provided the USSR, as the leading communist power, with a similar sense of being historically chosen. It also provided an element of long-term optimism by positing that communism will inevitably triumph over capitalism throughout the world. This ideological self-confidence was well captured in Nikita Khrushchev's famous boast that Soviet communism would eventually "bury" the capitalist West. The prolonged stagnation of the Soviet economy since the mid 1970s appears, however, to have eroded significantly Soviet self-confidence about the country's destiny. Soviet leaders and citizens increasingly have become doubtful about the ability of the Soviet communist system to cope with the complex challenges of modernity.

Both the Russian imperialist tradition and Marxism-Leninism have reinforced Soviet tendencies toward an expansionist foreign policy. The czarist pattern of territorial aggrandizement was characterized by the gradual incorporation of contiguous areas along Russia's lengthy European and Asian frontiers through the force of arms. The imperial Russian regimes were not, however, without longer-range ambitions, as evidenced by various diplomatic initiatives and involvement in Western Europe, the Far East, the Middle East, and even Africa.[9] Moreover, it is perfectly reasonable to expect that any twentieth-century Russian government, having industrialized and thus begun to realize the country's immense geopolitical potential,[10] would have broadened its horizons and sought to extend its influence on a global scale.

Some observers nevertheless attribute Soviet expansionist international behavior almost solely to a Marxist-Leninist drive for world domination. This school of thought asserts that the fundamental tenets of Marx and Lenin about the inevitable defeat of capitalism and the global triumph of socialism remain the key to the foreign policy of the Soviet leadership. From this perspective, the leaders of the USSR are viewed as thoroughly committed to a protracted life or death struggle for power and as determined to expand their influence at every possible opportunity.

Regardless of whether one is inclined toward the traditional Russian imperialist or the ideological interpretation of Soviet motivations in the world, there is little doubt that the Soviet leadership today perceives the USSR as a major international actor with a right to be heard, if it chooses, on virtually any issue. Moreover, proud of its status as one of the world's two nuclear superpowers and the recognized leader of the world communist movement, the Soviet leadership is virtually certain to believe that the USSR should continue to play a leading role in world politics throughout the remainder of the twentieth century.

INTERDEPENDENCIES

As befits a superpower, the Soviet Union has an extensive series of treaty commitments. The most prominent of these is the multilateral Treaty of Friendship, Mutual Assistance, and Cooperation signed in Warsaw, Poland, on 14 May 1955. This alliance, commonly known as the Warsaw Pact, commits the Soviet Union and the communist regimes of Poland, Hungary, East Germany, Czechoslovakia, Bulgaria, and Romania to the joint defense of their European territories. Originally conceived as a response to the rearmament of the Federal Republic of Germany and its admission into NATO, over the years this treaty has become a major instrument for the domination of Soviet client states in Eastern Europe.

The common defense commitments of the Warsaw Pact are reinforced by bilateral treaties of friendship and mutual assistance between the Soviet Union and each of the other member states. The USSR has also signed bilateral status-of-forces agreements with East Germany, Poland, Hungary, and Czechoslovakia that provide for the stationing of Soviet troops in these countries. Soviet forces permanently deployed in Eastern Europe include two tank divisions and tactical air formations in the Northern Group of Forces in Poland, five divisions (three motorized rifle and two tank) and a tactical air force in the Central Group of Forces in Czechoslovakia, four divisions (two motorized rifle and two tank) and a tactical air force in Hungary, and nineteen divisions (ten motorized rifle and nine tank) and a tactical air force in the Group of Soviet Forces Germany (GSFG).[11]

There are a number of high-level military and political consultative bodies associated with the Warsaw Pact. All are thoroughly dominated by the Soviet Union. The most important are the Political Consultative Committee (whose membership includes the Communist Party first secretaries, heads of governments, and defense and foreign ministers from each member state) and the Council of Defense Ministers. Both of these bodies convene on average twice a year. The military command structure of the Warsaw Pact is led by the Joint High Command, headquartered in Moscow.

This command is headed by a senior Soviet officer, who serves as commander in chief of the Warsaw Pact. This post is currently occupied by Marshal V. G. Kulikov, who is also a Soviet first deputy minister of defense. The military command also includes a Soviet chief of staff (currently General of the Army A. I. Gribkov), who traditionally serves simultaneously as a deputy chief of the Soviet General Staff. In addition, general officers from each of the member states represent their nations at Warsaw Pact headquarters in Moscow.

The USSR also has close economic ties with the Eastern European communist states, as well as with Cuba and Vietnam, through the Council for Mutual Economic Assistance (CMEA or COMECON). It has sought with only moderate success to use this mechanism to enforce a transnational economic division of labor among CMEA members. Economic relations among these states over the years have been marked by a massive flow of resources from the Soviet Union to its clients through a variety of direct and indirect subsidies. The Soviet "empire," like many other empires before it, is thus being maintained at very considerable expense to the hegemonic power.[12]

The USSR also has bilateral treaties with an array of other states. The oldest is with the Mongolian People's Republic, which has been allied with the Soviet Union since the creation of this vassal state under direct Soviet sponsorship in 1921. Soviet military cooperation with the regime in Ulan Bator is currently governed by a treaty of friendship, cooperation, and mutual aid signed on 16 January 1966, which provides for the permanent stationing of several Soviet divisions in Mongolia.[13] The USSR also has signed other treaties of friendship and cooperation with a number of Third World countries, including Egypt (May 1971), India (August 1971), Iraq (April 1972), Somalia (July 1974), Angola (October 1976), Mozambique (March 1977), Vietnam (November 1978), Ethiopia (November 1978), Afghanistan (December 1978), South Yemen (October 1979), Syria (October 1980), Congo (May 1981), and North Yemen (October 1984). The treaties with Egypt and Somalia are no longer in effect, having been terminated by those countries in

March 1976 and November 1977 respectively after their relations with the Soviet Union had deteriorated severely.

Most of these treaties contain provisions for military cooperation between the parties. All have been accompanied by varying degrees of Soviet military assistance, and, in some cases, the substantial presence of Soviet military personnel. This assistance has become essential to the Marxist-Leninist regimes in Angola, Ethiopia, and Afghanistan, all of which face armed challenges from active liberation movements operating within their borders. These insurgent groups, in turn, are receiving matériel support from the West. The friendship treaty with Afghanistan was invoked by the Soviets in 1979 to justify their invasion that toppled the Amin regime. It was cited as the legal basis to support Soviet occupation of Afghanistan with over 115,000 troops until troop withdrawals began under a UN-sponsored agreement in spring 1988. The prospects for continuation of the friendship treaty with the communist government in Kabul are dubious, given Soviet withdrawal of their forces and a situation in which the survival of the Najibullah regime will be problematical. The twelve treaties of friendship and cooperation remaining in effect, however, provide dramatic evidence of continuing Soviet involvement in Africa, the Middle East, and Asia.

National Objectives, National Strategy, and Military Doctrine

NATIONAL SECURITY OBJECTIVES

The most fundamental security objectives of the Soviet leaders are the defense of the regime and the territorial integrity of the USSR. The bitter experience of the Nazi invasion during World War II and the deep-seated patriotism of the Russian people provide a solid basis for a shared commitment between the Communist Party leadership and the Soviet people regarding the primacy of defense considerations.

The Soviet near-obsession with defense has provided a powerful impetus for the accumulation of military power and for steady expansion of Soviet political and military control beyond the nation's political frontiers. Motivated by what some observers have called a quest for "absolute security," the Soviet government has accorded the highest investment priority to defense for over fifty years. In addition, it has sought to establish and enlarge a territorial buffer, particularly in Europe, between the USSR and its prospective enemies. This drive to erect a *cordon sanitaire* lay behind the establishment of the first Soviet satellite regime in Outer Mongolia in 1921 and the absorption of the Baltic states and eastern portions of Poland, Finland, Czechoslovakia, and Romania in 1939–45. It also lay behind the subsequent westward extension of this buffer zone via the forcible establishment of the "baggage train" communist regimes imposed throughout most of Eastern Europe in the wake of the advance of the Red Army at the end of World War II.

Retention of subservient communist governments throughout Eastern Europe has remained a high-priority Soviet security objective throughout the postwar period. This has been visibly demonstrated in the Soviet Army's brutal suppression of would-be defector regimes in Hungary in 1956 and Czechoslovakia in 1968, and its heavy coercive pressure on a restive Poland in 1980–81, which ultimately precipitated General Jaruzelski's military takeover. The USSR has demonstrated a similar willingness to employ armed force to maintain "friendly" communist regimes in power in neighboring states in Asia, as evidenced by the 1979 invasion of Afghanistan.

This apparent application beyond the previous bounds of Eastern Europe of the so-called Brezhnev Doctrine, which attempts to justify armed Soviet intervention to defend allied "socialist" regimes endangered by "counterrevolution,"[14] initially raised Western concerns that the Soviets might prove willing to expend considerable military effort to preserve other "socialist" Third World governments that have allied themselves directly with the Soviet Union. These Western concerns have been reduced by subsequent failure of the intervention to suppress the Afghan resistance, the ultimate decision to withdraw—leaving their client regime exposed to escalating military pressure, and the public recriminations in

the Soviet media about the decisions to intervene militarily in Afghanistan and earlier in Eastern Europe. In the wake of these events and new Soviet declarations about the rights of Eastern European states to determine their own destinies, Soviet spokesmen have said the Brezhnev Doctrine is "under review."

Soviet national security objectives are not confined to these broadly construed "defensive" concerns. As noted earlier, Russian great power and Marxist-Leninist drives combine to underwrite a strong impulse to expand Soviet influence in areas adjacent to the USSR and throughout the world. Soviet leaders, like their czarist predecessors, have evinced consistent interest in gaining increased influence in Western Europe, the Middle East, and the energy-rich Persian Gulf. Moreover, during the past three decades, Soviet political and military spokesmen have increasingly come to speak about and utilize military power as a primary instrument for the promotion of their state interests.[15] As noted earlier, second thoughts about alleged Soviet overreliance on the military element of their foreign policy have emerged during the Gorbachev period.

The Soviets are intensely concerned about their relative position in the international arena. They regularly assess their overall position in the world in terms of what they call the "correlation of forces" (*sootnosheniye sil*). In Soviet usage, this correlation refers to the overall balance of economic, military, scientific, and sociopolitical capabilities between two competing states or coalitions of states. Soviet analysts frequently calculate the correlation of forces between both themselves and their leading rival, the United States, and between the socialist and capitalist camps.

Soviet commentators have invariably been optimistic in their written characterizations of the long-term trends in the correlation of forces between socialism and capitalism. This optimism reflects the basic tenet of Marxism-Leninism that socialism and communism will inevitably triumph over the capitalist order. From the close of World War II until the early 1980s, the Soviet regime consistently claimed that the correlation of forces was shifting inexorably in favor of the "socialist" states led by the Soviet Union. In recent years, however, these favorable assessments have appeared much less frequently. This is almost certainly due to the fact that the earlier optimistic appraisal has given way to more sober private evaluations of the overall balance during the 1980s. These gloomier judgments likely reflect the combination of a badly lagging Soviet economy, the rise of a more pragmatic and dynamic post-Mao China, a major reassessment of Soviet prospects in the Third World, and the resurgence of a more confident and activist America on the world scene. Soviet leaders are undoubtedly determined to maintain their status as one of the world's two military and political superpowers, but they appear seriously concerned about their long-term ability to do so.

Soviet military experts frequently analyze the narrower military balance, which they describe as the "correlation of military forces and means," between themselves and their prospective enemies.[16] Discussions in this regard range from simple quantitative comparisons of the East-West balance of strategic nuclear or general purpose forces to sophisticated dynamic analyses of relative military capabilities in various scenarios, often using complex mathematical force-effectiveness calculations.[17]

Soviet declarations regarding the state of the military balance and Soviet objectives in the military competition with the West have varied considerably. For several decades, dating as far back as the five-year economic and defense plans of the 1930s, Soviet leaders openly declared their intentions of acquiring military superiority over their prospective enemies. In the late 1950s and early 1960s, Soviet political and military figures often asserted that their military capabilities were in fact superior to those of the West. The most prominent example of such claims was the series of outspoken assertions by Party First Secretary Nikita Khrushchev in the late 1950s that the Soviet Union was superior to the United States in strategic missile strength. These boasts, made against the backdrop of dramatic Soviet "sputnik" satellite launches, helped spur the United States into determined efforts to overcome what was

later revealed to have been an illusory "missile gap."[18] The resultant surge of U.S. strategic missile deployments throughout the 1960s may help explain Soviet avoidance of such bold claims of military advantage since that time.

Over the past decade, Soviet leaders have exhibited increased circumspection in public declarations of their goals in the East-West arms competition. Military figures wrote openly in the 1960s and on into the mid 1970s of the need to attain military-technological superiority over their adversaries.[19] Nevertheless, Soviet claims of the possession of such superiority tapered off significantly in the early 1970s and have virtually disappeared since the latter half of the 1970s. This occurred at the very time when the unrelenting momentum of Soviet arms programs was leading many Western observers to argue that the Soviet Union was, in fact, embarked upon a drive to attain clear-cut military superiority.

Instead, since a pivotal address by Brezhnev at the city of Tula in January 1977, the Soviet declaratory stance has become one of strongly rebutting those Western charges and of asserting that the Soviet Union seeks nothing more than military parity with the West.[20] Gorbachev's "new political thinking" in foreign and defense policy brought a new round of Soviet assertions in the late 1980s that they seek no more than parity in the various military balances with the West. Whatever their public declarations, the combination of military doctrinal incentive, residual siege mentality, and their likely convictions about the political utility of vast military power are such that the Soviet leaders are almost certain to continue to seek to acquire substantial military advantage over their capitalist foes, should that appear attainable.

The Soviet armed forces make important contributions to the fulfillment of the regime's internal objectives as well. The military forces of the Ministry of Defense have infrequently been involved in the maintenance of domestic order. Over the past three decades their activity in this regard has been limited to occasional use in extraordinary circumstances, such as their reported involvement in the forcible suppression of striking workers in Novocherkassk in 1962,[21] in the quelling of rioters protesting food shortages in Rostov in 1963,[22] and in controlling the violence and policing massive nationalist protests in the Armenian and Azerbaijan republics that resulted in the late 1980s from the controversy over the Nagorno-Karabakh region.

The regular troops of the Ministry of Defense may well be called upon more frequently for this type of action in the years ahead, since Gorbachev's policies have raised national expectations that the system will have great difficulty fulfilling. The prime responsibility for maintenance of public order rests with the Ministry of Internal Affairs (MVD) and the Committee of State Security (KGB), both of which have sizable forces organized in regular military formations available for such contingencies. Interestingly, these internal security troops are counted by the Soviets as an element of their armed forces. Nevertheless, the professional military remains a weapon of possible resort if the threat of disorder is particularly acute.

A less dramatic but still significant domestic political role played by the Soviet military establishment occurs in the area of political socialization. Some two million young men are inducted into the Soviet armed forces annually for terms of service of from one and a half to three years.[23] During their stints in the military, these young men are exposed to intensive indoctrination supervised by the political officers of the Main Political Administration, whose organization and activities are discussed below in greater detail. Compulsory attendance at five hours a week of political instruction and mandatory participation in the activities of the Komsomol, or Young Communist League, comprise a determined effort to inculcate desired domestic and foreign policy perspectives. These experiences in the armed forces represent the final phase of a sustained, Party-controlled political indoctrination campaign, begun in nursery and elementary schools, that is designed to meet the regime's long-term objective of developing properly oriented "new Soviet men."

Despite these efforts, senior Soviet commanders and commissars are greatly concerned about the attitudes of Soviet youth. For many years they have complained that as the memory of World War II gradually fades from the collective consciousness, Soviet youth are becoming, in the words of a former deputy chief of the Main Political Administration, Colonel General Dmitrii Volkogonov, "vegetarian pacifists" with little interest in the martial traditions and heroic accomplishments of the Soviet armed forces.[24]

The Soviet armed forces also contribute in various ways to the functioning of the Soviet economy. Soviet troops stationed in agricultural regions of the USSR are regularly called upon to aid in bringing in the harvest. In addition, contingents of the 400,000-strong construction troops, although predominantly involved in the construction of defense-related facilities, have also been employed in building a variety of civilian projects, such as Moscow State University, Sheremetovo Airport, and multistory apartment buildings in Moscow.[25] Both the construction troops and the Ministry of Defense's railroad troops have helped build the Soviet showcase construction project of the late 1970s and 1980s, the new rail line called the Baikal-Amur Mainline (BAM), which runs parallel to the legendary Trans-Siberian Railroad through Siberia and the Far East to the Pacific.

NATIONAL SECURITY STRATEGY

Despite the Soviet penchant for authoritative programmatic statements and the voluminous output of their communities of political commentators and professional military theoreticians, there is no single, publicly available document or group of documents that sets forth Soviet strategy for pursuing national security objectives. It is quite likely that no such document exists even in the inner councils of the Kremlin. Nevertheless, on the basis of the statements of Soviet political and military spokesmen and many defense-related activities of the Soviet government, it is possible to piece together what appear to be the broad guidelines of Soviet national security strategy.

Deterrence, Reasonable Sufficiency, and a Victory-oriented Operational Approach. The central element of the Soviet national security strategy is quite straightforward: the USSR relentlessly improves its large and diverse military forces and then employs these capabilities to protect and advance its interests on the world scene. First and foremost, the Soviet leaders rely upon their massive military power to deter attack on the Soviet Union itself and on its allies and friends. They accomplish this by maintaining a full spectrum of strategic and general purpose forces.

The Soviet leadership assigns the highest priority to the deterrence of nuclear attack. The leaders in the Kremlin clearly recognize the catastrophic damage that would accompany a global nuclear conflict and are determined to avoid the nuclear devastation of the Soviet Union. Over the past three decades, Soviet spokesmen have repeatedly made deterrent threats, directed primarily at the United States and its NATO allies. In recent years, Mikhail Gorbachev and other Soviet spokesmen frequently have asserted that nuclear deterrence is in the long run inherently unstable and dangerous. Thus, they have argued that it should be phased out through a process of nuclear disarmament as soon as circumstances permit. Despite this rhetorical shift, the Soviet approach to deterrence has a decidedly traditional, martial tone. Soviet military and political figures have consistently warned that any state that dares to attack the Soviet Union or its allies will receive a "crushing rebuff" and suffer certain military defeat.

Developments in the 1980s, in particular the "new political thinking" of the Gorbachev period, have brought dramatic changes in Soviet discussions of deterrence. Soviet spokesmen, led by Mr. Gorbachev, claim that their objective in both the strategic nuclear and theater conventional areas is to field forces that are "reasonably sufficient" to provide a reliable defense. With regard to strategic nuclear forces, Soviet civilian and military commentators alike have stated that the reasonable sufficiency—or "sufficiency for defense," as the military prefers to call it—would allow deep cuts in the central strategic arsenals of the superpowers while maintaining rough numerical parity. They have also described reasonable sufficiency in terms of preserving the existing state of strategic stability, or what one Soviet civilian specialist has called the condition of *qualitative parity* between the superpowers.[26] Soviet commentators have defined strategic stability as the prevailing situation, in which both the Soviet Union and the United States have the capability to inflict unacceptable damage in retaliation against the other, even under worst-case circumstances (that is, after the other has launched a surprise, would-be-disarming first strike).[27]

This approach to stability and deterrence represents a direct Soviet appropriation of the *mutual assured destruction* (MAD) concept underlying American deterrence theory during the 1950s and 1960s and long associated with one of its most forceful advocates, former U.S. Secretary of Defense Robert S. McNamara. In fact, Marshal Ogarkov attributed the "unacceptable damage" idea to Mr. McNamara when he first publicly endorsed the concept of a mutual retaliatory stalemate in 1983.

Soviet civilian specialists carrying out strategic nuclear exchange analyses have even adopted the McNamara-Enthoven standard of 400 equivalent megatons (EMT) as the amount of destructive power required in one's surviving retaliatory forces to inflict unacceptable damage on the adversary. According to one recent Soviet article, this damage threshold would involve successful attacks with 400 one-megaton weapons on approximately 200 selected urban centers—attacks that would destroy 25 to 30 percent of the population and up to 70 percent of the industrial capacity of the adversary.[28] Soviet analysts at the Institute for the Study of the United States and Canada (IUSAC) and the Institute of the World Economy and International Relations (IMEMO) reportedly have begun calculating a side's second-strike retaliatory potential in terms of multiples of this 400 EMT value, which they call "McNamaras."[29] A pioneering study produced by a committee of Soviet civilian academics claims that a force of only 400 single-warhead, mobile, land-based ICBMs could inflict a McNamara's worth of retaliatory damage. Consequently, it recommends that this force structure be the long-term objective for both superpowers in the Strategic Arms Reductions Talks (START).[30]

Most Soviet commentators have asserted that a "reasonably sufficient" Soviet strategic force posture would need to be both roughly equal in size to that of the United States and capable of inflicting unacceptable retaliatory damage. Some Soviet civilian analysts have gone beyond this, suggesting that as long as the Soviet Union had a secure second-strike capability that could inflict unacceptable damage, it would not have to be concerned about maintaining approximate numerical parity with the strategic nuclear forces of the United States.[31] This approach is consistent with the ideas set forth in a series of articles by a trio of authors from IUSAC.[32] These authors have suggested that the Soviet Union can adequately provide for its security by undertaking asymmetrical responses to U.S. arms programs that are smaller and less expensive than the initial U.S. force deployments. They argue that U.S. arms initiatives like the massive bomber buildup of the 1950s and the prospective Strategic Defense Initiative (SDI) deployment have been deliberately designed to overstrain severely the Soviet economy as part of a strategy of "economic exhaustion."[33] These authors also argue that the Soviet Union would be well advised seriously to consider making unilateral reductions in its military forces on the path to "sufficient" forces rather than waiting for negotiated reductions. This is, in fact, what Gorbachev proposed in his December 1988 speech to the United Nations.

Unsurprisingly, senior Soviet military figures consistently have rejected the idea that the Soviet Union should settle for numerically inferior strategic forces. Military spokesmen have insisted instead that any reductions in strategic nuclear force levels must be mutual and roughly equal, thus preserving the rough military-strategic parity that currently exists in the U.S.–Soviet strategic balance.[34]

The military are apparently prepared, however, to support policies providing for deep and equitable cuts that preserve both quantitative parity and the existing retaliatory deterrent stalemate. The military leadership appears to have reached this conclusion by the early 1980s, when Marshal Ogarkov repeatedly condemned the continuing buildups of the U.S.

and Soviet strategic arsenals and positively characterized the U.S.–Soviet strategic balance, as noted earlier, as one in which each side had retaliatory forces with the unquestioned ability to survive a first strike and then launch a crushing retaliatory strike to inflict unacceptable damage on the other.[35] Marshal S. F. Akhromeyev appears to have shared his predecessor's views on these matters.[36] In any event, Akhromeyev resigned in December 1988 as chief of the general staff shortly after Gorbachev announced to the U.N. plans for unilateral Soviet reductions in conventional forces.

Despite these dramatic changes in Soviet declaratory policy concerning their objectives with regard to the overall size of strategic nuclear forces, Soviet operational doctrine for the employment of its large and highly capable strategic arsenal almost certainly continues to be directed toward successful war fighting. It commits the Soviet armed forces, should war occur, to carry out a combination of offensive and defensive operations designed to do the best they can to allow the Soviet Union to survive and prevail in any conflict, including global nuclear war. Moreover, Soviet force deployments—from the fielding of large numbers of accurate ICBM weapons, which are increasingly capable of supporting effective "counterforce" strikes against U.S. silo-based ICBMs, to the steady upgrading of their vast array of active and passive defenses, which are designed to limit damage to the Soviet homeland—are consistent with these victory-oriented, war-fighting objectives. These forces would also be employed to carry out extensive strikes against key industrial and political centers throughout an enemy's homeland with the stated objectives of destroying his war effort industries, disrupting his general economic infrastructure, crippling his political-administrative apparatus, and breaking his will to resist.

The Soviets showed little inclination during the 1970s to restrain their strategic programs in the interest of maintaining a stable U.S.–Soviet nuclear deterrent standoff based on mutual societal vulnerability. Although they have been more willing to accept restraints and even substantial reductions in their long-range nuclear strike systems over the past few years (as evidenced in their willingness to accept heavy cuts in their ICBM and SLBM forces in START negotiations), the Soviets continue to maintain large and highly capable attack capabilities adequate to cover U.S. and allied military targets. Nevertheless, Moscow is nowhere near attaining either a position of superiority in the central strategic nuclear balance or a strategic capability that could deny the United States the ability to inflict devastating retaliation against the Soviet homeland, and has little prospect of doing so.

The threat to defeat any aggressor in a general nuclear war remains the cornerstone of Soviet deterrent policy. It is complemented by a clear determination also to acquire the capabilities to fight and win major non-nuclear conflicts in theaters of military operations along the periphery of the Soviet Union. Soviet preparations to fight successfully in such theater conflicts are supported by the combination of a well-developed, combined-arms, force-employment doctrine and a panoply of impressive military capabilities.

Here too, discussions in Moscow since 1987 about "reasonable sufficiency" have broken new ground. Soviet spokesmen have also applied the reasonable sufficiency criterion to theater conventional forces, with particular reference to the NATO–Warsaw Pact balance in Europe. They have muddied these discussions, however, by a simultaneous campaign to characterize their military doctrine and that of their Warsaw Pact allies as "fundamentally defensive."

Initial formulations of reasonable sufficiency in theater warfare simply equated sufficiency with the current Soviet and Warsaw Pact force posture, which they described as adequate "to repulse aggression" and "to ensure reliably the collective defense of the socialist community."[37] Over time, however, the emphasis regarding reasonable sufficiency in the theater has shifted from the present to the future. The Soviets apparently want to reconfigure the military forces of both NATO and the Warsaw Pact so as to preclude a successful surprise attack by either side and ultimately to rule out the mounting of offensive operations alto-

gether. This objective has been described as a cooperative transition to a posture of "nonoffensive" or "defensive" defense—phrases that the Soviets have borrowed from Western European peace and disarmament circles.

Military and civilian spokesmen alike have embraced these utopian objectives, despite the fact that they directly contravene the long-standing offensive tradition in Soviet military-technical doctrine described below. More significantly, the pursuit of these objectives would require the scrapping of the conceptual and organizational innovations introduced over the past decade—innovations designed precisely to support a theater strategic offensive operation fought with conventional weapons in theaters around the USSR.

When pressed for details regarding what a "reasonably sufficient" posture in Central Europe might look like, Soviet civilian analysts readily have admitted that they are in the very earliest stages of exploring this concept. The Soviet civilians who advocate the concept of reasonable sufficiency are seeking to develop a stability concept that can be applied to conventional force balances in ways similar to the "unacceptable damage" threshold that they are using to define strategic stability in the U.S.–Soviet nuclear balance.

In parallel with their discussions of reasonable sufficiency the Soviets have embarked upon a concerted effort to convince the world of the fundamentally "defensive" character of both Soviet and Warsaw Pact military doctrine. Following a meeting of the Warsaw Pact's Political Consultative Committee in Berlin in May 1987, Pact leaders declared that "the military doctrine of the Warsaw Pact member states is strictly a defensive one."[38] Moreover, according to Marshal S. F. Akhromeyev, former chief of the general staff, and Colonel General M. A. Gareyev, his deputy responsible for military doctrine, both the Pact's military-technical doctrine and the structure of Soviet forces, including their doctrinal manuals and training, had already begun to reflect a defensive orientation.[39] The Soviets insist that their military doctrine is now uniquely directed toward the prevention, rather than the conduct, of war.[40]

While the Soviet military leaders praise the "new defensive doctrine," they have also registered a significant reservation. Several senior Soviet military commanders have pointed out that the defensive orientation of Soviet and Pact doctrine does not rule out counter-offensive operations against an aggressor. Thus, Army General A. I. Gribkov, the chief of staff of Warsaw Pact joint forces, said in September 1987:

In the event of an attack, the armed forces of the Warsaw Pact countries will operate with exceptional resolve. While repulsing aggression, they will also conduct counter-offensive operations.[41]

Army General D. T. Yazov echoed this sentiment in October 1987, noting that:

It is impossible to rout an aggressor with defense alone.... After an attack has been repelled, the troops and naval forces must be able to conduct a *decisive offensive* [emphasis in original]. The switch to an offensive will be in the form of a counter-offensive.[42]

This critical caveat that offensive operations are fully consistent with a defensive doctrine allows the Soviet military to develop offensive concepts and capabilities despite their alleged devotion to a "particularly defensive" doctrine.

Senior Soviet commanders have also engaged in a pointed public dialogue with civilian analysts (and possibly a more discreet debate with top political leaders) regarding how the Soviet Union should reduce and restructure its theater forces to meet the "sufficiency objective." Specifically, senior military spokesmen have vehemently rejected the suggestion of civilian experts that the Soviet Union consider substantially cutting its overall troop strength unilaterally, as Nikita Khrushchev had done in the late 1950s, rather than waiting to negotiate mutual force reductions with the West.[43]

In December 1987, Marshal Akhromeyev rejected this approach in general terms,[44] apparently resigning over it a year later. Army General I. Tretyak, commander of the air defense forces, also directly challenged the validity of the civilians' prime example of a unilateral force reduction that allegedly benefited Soviet security. He described Khrushchev's troop reduction in the late 1950s as a "sorry experience . . . [and] a rash step [that] dealt a colossal blow to our defense capacity," and urged that "any changes in our army should be considered a thousand times over before they are decided upon."[45]

Throughout its history, the Soviet Union has confronted a serious "two-front" security challenge due to the presence of hostile, militarily significant adversaries on their extended European and Far Eastern borders. Consequently, Soviet leaders have long adhered to a "two-war" policy in the sense that they have sought to maintain sufficient forces in both theaters with the capability, at a minimum, to defend these areas independently. In the 1980s, they have added extensive preparations for war in a third theater, Southwest Asia, that is, down through Iran to the Persian Gulf.

This "multi-contingency approach," in the language of American defense policy planning, has been increasingly evident since the severe deterioration of Sino-Soviet relations in the early 1960s. Between the mid 1960s and the mid 1970s, Soviet forces facing China in the Far East and Central Asia more than tripled in strength. Soviet forces have expanded modestly since that time and have been steadily modernized despite gradual improvement of Sino-Soviet relations in the 1980s.[46] Many of these forces also threaten U.S. forces in the Far East, as well as Japan and other Asian nations.

This build up has been accomplished at the same time that Soviet forces stationed in Eastern Europe and the western portions of the Soviet Union have also been significantly expanded and upgraded. Preparations for a possible campaign from the Transcaucasus and Central Asia into Iran since the fall of the Shah in 1979 have included the establishment of a new peacetime high command for the Southern Theater of Military Operations (TVD) in 1984, but not a significant expansion of the forces opposite that theater other than the some 110,000 troops who were involved in the unsuccessful attempt to defeat the mujaheddin in Afghanistan.

During the 1970s, the Soviets dramatically improved their ability to project forces by air and sea far beyond the traditional reach of the Red Army in areas adjacent to Soviet territory. In this same period, Soviet military writers have increasingly touted the role of the Soviet armed forces in advancing Soviet foreign policy interests throughout the world. During the 1980s, the growth of these force-projection capabilities has slowed and the military advocacy of such operations has waned. Nevertheless, the cumulative growth in these capabilities and a continuing military interest in the study of "local wars" suggest that a new, lesser contingency objective in Soviet national security strategy has emerged. The main potential for the employment of Soviet military forces in the Third World appears to be focused on the Middle East, with the further possibility of the longer-range projection of Soviet military power into Africa or Southeast Asia as well.

Arms Control. Soviet national security strategy is not confined to the accumulation of military power to support its deterrence and theater warfare objectives. It also includes the utilization of arms control negotiations and military assistance programs of various types to support the achievement of Soviet foreign policy goals.

The Soviets have participated in virtually all of the important international arms control negotiations since the close of World War II. A major objective of this participation has been Soviet determination to gain widespread recognition as one of the world's two leading powers. The USSR has also used these negotiations to seek to sow discord among the Western nations and to support its general claims to peace-loving intent on the international scene.

The Soviet leaders' search for what they call "military détente," which has meant the pursuit of arms control agreements with the West, has been a central element in their broader policy of promoting political accommodations and cooperation with the West. This policy, and the more general political détente approach of which it is an important part, served in the 1970s, and may serve again, as a means of gaining access to Western technology and capital. Soviet arms control efforts have also been designed to foster mutual East-West commitments to avoid nuclear conflict. Despite the clearly stated war-winning objectives of their operational doctrine, Soviet military and political leaders have repeatedly acknowledged the

catastrophic consequences of general nuclear war and are certain to support its avoidance. Talks on limiting and reducing nuclear forces and on creating crisis management tools such as the improved "hot line" between Moscow and Washington are designed to assist in avoiding a nuclear war and to provide some basis for controlling such a war should it occur. The Soviet leaders also seek to use arms control negotiations and agreements to constrain the most threatening military activities of their adversaries while maintaining maximum flexibility for themselves. Arms control efforts in pursuit of these objectives, which are described in greater detail near the end of this chapter, are likely to remain a fundamental element of Soviet national security strategy.

Military Aid to Third World. For nearly seventy years, the USSR has employed military assistance programs to aid factions struggling to gain power and to support friendly regimes in power against internal opposition or international foes. Although there have been setbacks, these programs have frequently proven useful as a means of gaining political influence in the recipient nation and, in many cases, of maneuvering the recipient into a position of dependence on the Soviet Union for economic aid or for maintenance and logistical support of the military equipment provided.

Since the mid 1950s, the Soviets have had considerable experience in this area. Major infusions of military assistance have by no means guaranteed success for the Soviet Union in its dealings with Third World countries. Despite expensive Soviet military aid programs over several years, the USSR suffered major setbacks in its dealings with Indonesia in the mid 1960s, Egypt in the early 1970s, and Somalia in the late 1970s. Nevertheless, the Soviet leaders clearly intend to continue to use this instrument to defend beleaguered Marxist-Leninist oriented client states, to strengthen their ties to Moscow, and to seek to move other countries into the Soviet sphere of influence.

Soviet military assistance programs complement the USSR's growing capacity for long-range power-projection. Arms aid has frequently facilitated Soviet acquisition of basing, staging, and transit rights that are critical to operations in distant areas. Military assistance efforts often result in the establishment of substantial stockpiles of modern Soviet weapons in distant areas such as Libya that could possibly be utilized in short order by Soviet surrogates, such as the Cubans or East Germans, or directly by Soviet military personnel. As noted above, Soviet determination to help defend client states against liberation movements, many of which are assisted by the United States under the "Reagan Doctrine," has generated a strengthening of these Soviet military assistance efforts.[47]

Soviet intentions and actions in these areas have become much less clear under Gorbachev. Heavily engaged in a massive effort not only to restructure radically the stagnant Soviet economy, but also the Soviet political and social system, Mr. Gorbachev appears determined to have the Soviet Union play a more selective and less costly role in the Third World. Consequently, Moscow has focused on improving relations with the larger, more developed regional powers in the Third World such as India, Mexico, Brazil, and Argentina, while clearly seeking to avoid taking on expensive new commitments to underwrite "revolutionary socialist" governments.

Following successful multilateral diplomacy to help facilitate their own withdrawal from Afghanistan, the Soviets have become actively engaged in other multilateral efforts to settle regional conflicts in Cambodia and southern Africa where prominent Soviet clients, the communist governments of Vietnam and Angola, are deeply involved. At the same time, the Soviets continue to provide large amounts of economic and military assistance to these and other "socialist" clients. All in all, regional and internal tensions appear inevitable in the Third World in the years ahead, and Soviet arms diplomacy in the form of the sale of military equipment and the provision of military advisers will remain a significant element of Moscow's foreign and defense policy in these areas.

Domestic Determinants. Soviet national security strategy is the product of many diverse influences. These include not only the aspirations and concerns derived from imperial Russian and Soviet historical experience and from Marxist-Leninist ideology, discussed above, but also the geographical character of the USSR and various aspects of the Soviet political and economic systems.

Character of the Political System. Defense matters are clearly one of the highest priority policy issues within the Soviet system. As such, they are carefully overseen by the top Soviet leadership. Consequently, all key defense decisions are apparently made (or at least reviewed) by the Party Politburo, which sits atop the combined Communist Party and Soviet government hierarchies. The priority of defense matters is also evident in the fact that each time a single dominant Soviet political leader has emerged, he has personally taken charge of defense matters. Stalin, Khrushchev, and Brezhnev all chose to confirm their personal responsibility for defense by assuming the post of supreme commander in chief of the Soviet armed forces.[48] Yuri Andropov and Konstantin Chernenko likely did so as well, and Gorbachev almost certainly occupies this vital post, although there has been no public confirmation of this.

This centralization of authority at the top in defense matters has several important consequences. First, it means that there are no significant checks built into the system once a decision is taken in the Politburo. Second, given the lengthy tenure of the senior Soviet political leaders (Stalin dominated the Soviet political scene from the mid 1920s until 1953, Khrushchev from 1957 to 1964, and Brezhnev from 1964 until 1983), this centralization has provided a pronounced element of continuity in Soviet military policy. Third, the reverse side of this highly personalized pattern is that when a period of leadership transition occurs, it clearly carries with it considerable potential for significant change in defense policy. Consequently, during the struggles for power, which are likely to occur due to the absence of a regularized procedure for leadership succession, the main contenders are virtually certain to be particularly attentive to defense issues.

Conflict over defense matters was evident in the struggle between Khrushchev and Malenkov during the post-Stalin succession in

1953–54, and it appears to have surfaced briefly in 1965 following Khrushchev's political demise.[49] It almost certainly played a major role in the sacking of Marshal N. V. Ogarkov, who lost his post as chief of the General Staff in September 1984 during Chernenko's brief reign as Party leader. Fully aware of this, the constituencies with substantial stakes in defense matters, the professional military and their allies in the defense production ministries, are certain to defend and promote their interests especially actively during such succession periods.

The closed nature of Soviet political processes is another aspect of the Soviet political system that influences both the formulation of Soviet defense policy and our understanding of it in the West. Soviet policy making in all areas, and especially in national security matters, is conducted in considerable secrecy. U.S. suspicions about the strict compartmentalization of defense-related information in the Soviet system were dramatically confirmed in an often-recounted incident that occurred during the early phases of the Strategic Arms Limitation Talks. At that time, the leading Soviet military representative, then Colonel General N. V. Ogarkov, a deputy chief of the General Staff (he later became a marshal of the Soviet Union and commander in chief of the western theater of military operations), asked the U.S. negotiators not to discuss the details of Soviet strategic weapons deployments with Soviet civilian representatives, who, he said, were not knowledgeable about such information.[50] This denial of information to those outside the professional military establishment and a small circle of senior Soviet leaders appeared to persist until at least the mid 1980s.

Under Gorbachev, as discussed in greater detail below, there appears to be an incipient pluralization of the defense policy-making process. This development may be accompanied by somewhat wider access to critical defense-related data for civilian specialists in the Ministry of Foreign Affairs, the Central Committee apparatus, and the institutes of the Academy of Sciences. Their public complaints about access to relevant information, however, suggest that substantial restrictions on such data remain.[51] There is no doubt, however, that a new generation of civilian academics has acquired increased expertise on defense matters through their analyses of security and arms control issues over the past decade.

The consequences of this rather closed policy-making pattern and compartmentalization of defense information are twofold. First, in such an environment, those with access to the controlled information, in this case for the most part officers of the Ministry of Defense, are in an excellent position to wield greater influence in the formulation and implementation of defense policy. The near monopoly of relevant information and expertise in the past was a crucial factor that strengthens the hand of the armed forces on the Soviet political scene. Erosion of this privileged position inevitably dilutes this advantage. Secondly, Soviet secrecy in these matters effectively limits the data available to foreign observers about defense policy making. It compels Western analysts to rely upon a variety of partial sources, including memoir accounts, observable activities such as major weapons deployments, and Kremlinological analyses of defense-related Soviet official publications, to piece together plausible explanations of Soviet defense policy.

The Defense Burden. The Soviet defense effort has long been the primary beneficiary of the Soviet command economy. The extent of this priority has been such that some have been prompted to argue that the accumulation of military power has been the primary social product of the Soviet economic system, while the production of other goods and services is nothing more than necessary social overhead.[52] Although this may be somewhat overstated, there is no doubt that military weaponry has consistently been accorded the highest priority in a host of inputs that are in scarce supply, including direct budgetary support, the infusion of the highest quality equipment, such as advanced computers and machine tools, and the recruitment of talented scientific and technical personnel.

Throughout the Soviet period, the economy has been largely autarkic. Consequently, questions of access to imports or markets for exports have little influence on Soviet foreign or defense policy. In recent years, however, serious difficulties in the functioning of the Soviet economy have surfaced that have altered this situation. These problems include a marked reduction in the rate of economic growth, the prospect of a near-term decline in oil production, continuing poor performance in agriculture (always the economy's weakest area), a sharp decline in investment and labor force growth, widespread corruption, consistently poor worker productivity, and an inability to foster rapid innovation in the USSR's relatively backward technological base.[53]

Many of these problems have been evident for several years. They were almost certainly major factors behind the decision of Leonid Brezhnev and his successors to pursue a "policy of selective economic interdependence" as a key element of Soviet détente with the West since the 1970s.[54] While by no means abandoning their pronounced tendency toward economic self-reliance, the USSR has significantly expanded its involvement in the world economy over the past fifteen years. However, substantial imports of technology, joint ventures in the expansion of motor transport, and major grain imports have failed to reverse the adverse trends in the performance of the Soviet economy. Thus, it appears that Mr. Gorbachev and his supporters have come to the conclusion that the Soviet Union must radically restructure not only its entire economy, but also the political system and the very consciousness of the Soviet people if it is to build a modern economy in the post-industrial era.

These economic difficulties have had a significant impact on Soviet defense policy. Declining overall growth rates in the mid 1970s prompted the leadership to cut back on the rate of growth of defense expenditures as well. In the late 1970s and early 1980s, the Soviet leaders chose to cut back on the growth of capital investment for economic growth and on defense spending while maintaining increasing rates of investment in agriculture and consumer-related industries. Soviet defense spending increased at a rate of 4–5 percent per annum in the first eleven years under Brezhnev (1965–75), but slipped back to roughly 2 percent a year from 1976 to 1985, with the invest-

ment devoted to the procurement of new weapons showing no growth at all over the same period. The rate of growth in the defense budget has remained in the 2–3 percent range.[55]

This reduced rate of growth in defense spending, which continued in the face of dramatic increases in the U.S. defense budget after 1979, prompted increasingly strident demands by senior Soviet military figures, led by Marshal N. V. Ogarkov, then chief of the General Staff. Clearly disturbed by the expanded U.S. defense program and the more assertive Reagan foreign policy, Ogarkov and others spoke often of the growing danger of war and the resultant need for increased Soviet defense efforts.

Perhaps as a result of these outspoken criticisms, the Soviet military has been subjected by the civilian leadership to a number of direct rebukes and symbolic "slights." The most striking of these was, of course, the abrupt removal from office of Marshal S. L. Sokolov, the Minister of Defense, and Marshal of Aviation A. I. Koldunov, Deputy Minister of Defense and commander in chief of the Air Defense Forces, along with several other high ranking air defense personnel in May 1987. These events were precipitated by the much publicized landing on Red Square by Matthias Rust, a young West German aviator, who without Soviet authorization piloted a small sports plane all the way in from Helsinki, Finland. The Rust incident was followed by harsh public criticism of the Soviet military, including unprecedented charges of incompetence and "toadyism" by Politburo member Boris Yeltsin, then First Secretary of the Moscow Communist Party organization. The military continued to be the object of unprecedented public criticism concerning corruption, inefficiency, its failures in discipline, and the harsh hazing of conscripts.

Other less direct but nevertheless significant indications of Party displeasure have included the failure to make either Marshal S. L. Sokolov, the Minister of Defense from December 1984 until May 1987, or his successor, General D. T. Yazov, a full member of the Politburo as their two predecessors had been. (During this same time period, V. M. Chebrikov, the chief of the KGB, historically the institutional rival of the Ministry of Defense, has been accorded full member status.) In addition, there was the conspicuous absence of senior military figures atop the Lenin mausoleum during Chernenko's funeral in February 1985. Moreover, as mentioned earlier, in September 1984 the outspoken Marshal Ogarkov was suddenly relieved of his post as chief of the General Staff, almost certainly a result of his insistent statements regarding the growing American military threat and the need for increased Soviet defense exertions. This move was accompanied by informal explanations from various Soviet sources that Orgarkov's removal had been necessary due to his "un-Partylike" behavior.[56]

Pressures to contain or even reduce defense spending may well have grown as Gorbachev's *perestroika* campaign has failed to produce positive results. Statements of senior military figures have spoken of "doing more with less" and have placed an emphasis on quality rather than quantity in future Soviet defense preparations.[57]

These pressures to ease the Soviet defense burden and the resulting tensions between the senior Soviet political and military leadership will most certainly persist and even intensify over the next several years. This will occur because Gorbachev and company appear determined to devote increased resources to the machine-building and metal-working industries and other selected sectors in an effort to rejuvenate the Soviet economy, while also maintaining high investments in the agricultural, energy, and the light industrial, consumer sectors. Nevertheless, one must keep firmly in mind that although the annual rate of increase in Soviet defense spending over the past ten years has been only half that of the previous decade, defense expenditures have, in fact, increased. Moreover, they have done so from a very large base. They were and have remained some 14–17 percent of a large and slowly expanding gross national product. And even the most determined attention to overall economic expansion in the years ahead is unlikely to produce a substantial reduction in the absolute size of the annual Soviet defense budget.

Geography. The Soviet Union occupies a central geographic position, straddling the continents of Europe and Asia. Spanning approximately 170 degrees of longitude, the USSR directly borders twelve other states and looks out across enclosed seas at an additional seven. Soviet interests and concerns thus range from Norway and Finland in the northwest, through the client states of Eastern Europe, to Turkey, Iran, and Afghanistan in the Near East, Pakistan and India in South Asia, and China, North Korea, and Japan in the Far East. The majority of these frontiers are marked by no significant geographical barriers, thus contributing to the historical perceptions and reality of Russian vulnerability to overland invasion. From this critical "heartland" location, the leaders in the Kremlin, like their czarist predecessors, confront a multitude of challenges and opportunities.

The Soviet Union is richly endowed with natural resources. Its deposits of precious metals, petroleum, natural gas, coal, iron, and several other minerals are among the largest in the world. However, many of these deposits are located in relatively inaccessible regions of Siberia, thus significantly complicating successful exploitation. Another important geographic characteristic is the northerly latitude of the Soviet Union. Most of the country lies above 40° north latitude. Consequently, the amount of arable land available for sustained cultivation is quite small for a country of such vast size, and it has, since the communist takeover, consistently proven inadequate to meet the needs of the nation's people, now numbering more than 270 million.

Public Opinion. The authoritarian character of the Soviet political system is such that until recent years public opinion played no direct role in the shaping of the nation's foreign or domestic policies. The burgeoning of public discussion that has been turned loose by Gorbachev's *glasnost* policy and the emergence of new opportunities for potentially meaningful political participation in the *soviets* (councils) at many levels appears to be changing this dramatically. The state and Party have sought to elicit public support for their reforms by encouraging letters to the media, television "talk" shows, and other means of directly expressing criticism of the past and present and hopefully offering constructive suggestions on how to achieve a better future. The result has been a flood of criticism, including complaints about the military intervention in Afghanistan ("our Vietnam") and the deployment of SS-20 missiles that stimulated the Western offsetting deployments of the Pershing II missile and the ground-launched cruise missiles. Nevertheless, direct public influence on most defense matters is not yet evident. The most prominent exception to this pattern has been the strong pressure to eradicate the cruel hazing inflicted on new conscripts, which has been fueled by several media exposés regarding these brutal practices.

Nationality Issues. Like the czars before them, the Soviet leaders face a significant "nationalities problem." The USSR is a multinational state composed of over 130 national groups. This polyglot population can usefully be divided into two major ethnic groupings: the European nationalities, including the Great Russians, Ukrainians, Byelorussians, Moldavians, Latvians, Lithuanians, and Estonians; and the non-Europeans, such as the Uzbeks, Tatars, Kazakhs, Azerbaijanis, Turkmen, Kirghiz, Tadzhiks, Armenians, and Georgians.

The multinational character of the Soviet state is reflected in the federal structure of the Union of Soviet Socialist Republics, with its fifteen union-republics organized along national lines and a host of smaller, nationality-based "autonomous republics" and "autonomous regions." Yet despite the lip service paid to the rights and traditions of the constituent nationalities, the Soviet leadership long demanded full subordination of these groups to the will of the Communist Party center in Moscow. This Party core has been and remains thoroughly dominated by the Great Russians, with substantial assistance from the other Slavs, notably the Ukrainians and Byelorussians.

Nevertheless, national identities have persisted and during the Gorbachev period have become an increasingly explosive issue. Communal violence has flared up in the Trans-

caucasus where Armenians and Azerbaijanis are locked in an intense and prolonged struggle over the disputed Nagorno-Karabakh region. As noted earlier, a lengthy series of mass demonstrations, strikes, and sporadic outbreaks of violence have forced the imposition of martial law on several occasions. There has also been an unprecedented upsurge of national assertiveness in the Baltic states where officially sanctioned "popular fronts" have demanded greatly increased political and economic autonomy. The Communist Party and Soviet government are clearly being tested severely by these threats to public order and possibly to the very integrity of the Soviet system.

The Soviet nationalities issue presents another, very different challenge to Soviet defense policy due to the pronounced disparities in the population growth rates of the European and non-European groups. The non-European nationalities of Central Asia have produced far higher birthrates over the past few decades, and this disparity is virtually certain to continue. This trend is bound to have significant impact on Soviet economic choices in the years ahead. It has already raised what one author calls the specter of the demographic "yellowing" of the Soviet population as the Asiatic peoples become a larger share of the populace. Moreover, the leaders in Moscow must either succeed in encouraging a migration of the more numerous Asiatics into the labor-short manufacturing centers of the Urals and European Russia or take the necessary steps to expand greatly the industrial facilities of Central Asia.[58]

The increased numbers of Asians in the annual cohorts inducted into the Soviet armed forces has its own direct impact on military matters. Relations between the majority Slavs and the Asiatic and Transcaucasian minorities in particular have long been marked by considerable hostility and not infrequent physical violence. These relationships are likely to be even more hostile as a result of the growing national tensions in the society as a whole. The Soviet military is keenly aware of this problem and has publicly discussed measures to ameliorate these tensions.[59] The growing number of non-Slavic recruits will also likely necessitate major adjustments in assignment policies within the armed forces. Up to this time, Central Asians and other minorities, whose mastery of the Russian language is often very rudimentary, have generally been excluded from most prestigious military career fields, such as service in the Strategic Rocket Forces, the Air Forces, and other crack maneuver units of the Ground Forces. Instead, they commonly make up the majority of the pick-and-shovel soldiers of the Construction Troops. The dramatic increases in the non-Slavic share of the annual conscript cohorts will compel major adjustments in this pattern.

FORCE EMPLOYMENT DOCTRINE

Over the years, the USSR has developed a distinctive style of warfare that reflects a variety of influences. These include imperial Russian military tradition (transmitted to the Red Army by a sizable core of former czarist officers, who were particularly active in the development of Soviet military science in the 1920s and 1930s), geographic factors, the numbers and types of weapons made available by the high-priority defense sector of the Soviet economy, and a unique Soviet approach to theater war that emerged from the "military scientific specialists" working in the General Staff and the prestigious senior military academies in Moscow beginning in the early 1930s.[60]

Soviet leaders devote extraordinary effort to the study of how wars should be prepared for and fought. Much of this work is done by specially trained military officers, holding advanced degrees in military science or Marxist philosophy, in the staffs and academies of the Ministry of Defense. Yet Soviet military writings repeatedly emphasize that it is not the military but the leadership of the Communist Party and Soviet state that ultimately "elaborates and defines" the unified series of views called "military doctrine,"[61] said to set forth Soviet war aims, the probable methods of waging war, the tasks to be performed by the armed forces, and the measures required for the all-round social, economic, and military-technical preparation of the country as a whole for war.[62] Under the influence of Gorbachev's "new political thinking," the Soviets have

made much of the fact that their military doctrine is now oriented, first and foremost, toward the prevention of war rather than toward fighting one.

In the Soviet view, military doctrine has both a sociopolitical and a military-technical dimension. The sociopolitical side is concerned with the probable causes, broad political-economic character, and consequences of war. Officers specially trained in Marxist-Leninist philosophy, who are often affiliated with the Main Political Administration and its Lenin Military Political Academy, are frequent writers on these matters. Soviet civilian commentators also appear to have some license to articulate views on these questions, albeit in the context of the general line approved by the Party leadership.

The military-technical aspect of Soviet military doctrine refers to the study of operational matters. This appears to fall strictly within the purview of the Ministry of Defense. The growth of interest and expertise among Soviet civilian specialists in arms control and defense, noted earlier, raises the possibility that others are beginning to have influence on these operational matters. While they are fully prepared to accord the Party leadership the right to make the final decisions on the nation's military doctrine, the professional soldiers clearly believe that this doctrine should be firmly based upon their expert views on operational matters. This sentiment is vividly captured in the judgment that "military doctrine becomes more scientifically sound, and therefore, more vital, the greater its reliance on the objective evaluations and conclusions of military science."[63]

The USSR has developed a complex taxonomy of military science, the components of which include a general theory of military science, military art, military history, military pedagogy, military administration, military geography, military economics, and military-technical sciences.[64] Groups of uniformed specialists actively research and write in all of these areas. Their work is presented in a host of journals and books that steadily pour out of Voenizdat, the Ministry of Defense's publishing house, and in classified publications such as the General Staff's limited circulation monthly, *Voyennaia mysl'* (*Military Thought*).

Among these disciplines, Soviet work on military art, with its three subcategories (strategy, operational art, and tactics), has the most significant impact on the day-to-day business of the Ministry of Defense. The elaboration of Soviet military strategy, which investigates the preparation for and waging of large scale theater campaigns and war as a whole, is largely done in the General Staff's Military Science Administration and Voroshilov Academy. Its guiding tenets are reflected not only in the operational plans developed by the General Staff's Main Operations Directorate, but also in adjustments in the organizational structure of the armed forces, in peacetime training and exercises, and in the logistics planning that the General Staff oversees.

Operational art, which the Soviets define as that portion of military art concerned with the preparation and conduct of operations at the front and army levels, is developed by both the General Staff and the individual services. The General Staff's Military Science Administration and Voroshilov Academy address this level when it involves coordinated multiservice, combined-arms operations. The operations departments of the services' main staffs and their specialized higher academies work out planning, operational control, and logistics support with regard to their unique spheres of action.

Thus, commanders, staff officers, and academic researchers in the Air Forces are involved, for example, in continuous study of the conduct of independent theater air operations, which combine fighter, fighter-bomber, and bomber elements, to conduct massive conventional or nuclear strikes on key targets in the enemy's rear. Similarly, staff officers and military theorists in the Navy are likely to be continuously refining concepts for mounting operations against U.S. carrier task forces and strategic submarines, while the ground forces seek to affect the manner in which they can introduce follow-on maneuver units to exploit anticipated breakthroughs in the enemy's forward defenses.

Finally, the subcategory of tactics, which deals with the preparation and conduct of operations at the divisional level and below, also has both a combined-arms and an individual service dimension. Work on the former is done in the Voroshilov Academy and probably the Frunze Military Academy as well, while the latter is clearly the business of each of the services and their constituent branches.

Over the years, the Soviet military has worked hard to apply the latest scientific techniques to military problems. Military philosophers and military scientists have been true to the scientific aspirations of their Marxist-Leninist ideology, and have diligently sought to discover Marxist-Leninist laws of war.[65] On a more practical level, the military has developed analytical modeling techniques, designed, for example, to assist in calculating the correlation of military forces to illuminate cost and effectiveness trade-offs in weapons acquisition, to investigate and improve military command and control, to develop optimum tactics for various engagements, and to establish "norms" for optimum rates of advance, firepower support requirements, and general logistics support.

Work on the application of scientific techniques to military problems is apparently conducted in the research bodies attached to the major military academies, the service staffs, and the General Staff.[66] These efforts have produced an enormous body of specialized, highly technical literature, which has not yet been well mined by Western students of Soviet military affairs.[67] Those Soviet analytical efforts that are viewed as particularly useful are likely to find their way to the operating forces in the form of new norms for staffs and commanders to employ in planning and conducting combat operations; computational devices, including computers with programs to solve equations rapidly, facilitating performance of key command or staff functions; and new tactics for accomplishing a given mission.[68]

There is little doubt that military doctrine and its cornerstone, military art, largely shape Soviet military policy. They establish the broad direction of that policy and identify specific operational capabilities to which the Soviet political and military leaders aspire. As such, military doctrine: (1) provides the context in which the General Staff oversees adjustments in military organization, the drafting of war plans and mobilization plans, and the training of troops; and (2) establishes the requirements for the development and procurement of new weapons.

The contemporary Soviet approach to theater war and, to a considerable extent, intercontinental conflict, as well as being embodied in its military-technical doctrine, clearly reflects key elements that were already evident in the Soviet doctrine of massed armored warfare, called the theory of operations in-depth, developed some fifty years ago.[69] These guiding principles include commitments to seize the initiative at the outset of hostilities; to conduct bold offensive operations with massed, armor-heavy forces, including specialized mobile formations for the rapid exploitation of initial battlefield successes; and to operate at high tempo in order to annihilate the enemy's military forces completely. In recent years, the Soviets have devoted greater attention to defensive operations in theater warfare. These continue to be viewed, however, as a temporary form of activity the Pact is forced to employ under unfavorable circumstances, while gathering strength to gain the initiative and mount a decisive counter-offensive. Soviet doctrine calls for all possible offensive and defensive efforts to limit the damage that the Soviet Union itself would suffer in a war. Soviet military theory categorically rejects the dominance of a single weapon or branch of service in the conduct of these operations. It calls instead for the reinforcing efforts of all ground, sea, and air forces to achieve victory via the so-called combined-arms concept.[70]

Contemporary Soviet military writings deal with various facets of complex scenarios for large-scale theater conflicts fought with conventional weapons and for general nuclear war. With regard to a global nuclear war, this literature describes several aspects of the life-or-death clash between the opposing socialist and capitalist systems, including: (1) major theater land and air battles; (2) war at sea; (3) both regional and intercontinental missile and bomber exchanges; and (4) extensive efforts to defend the Soviet homeland. While a compre-

hensive review of these variegated operations is beyond the scope of this study, some of the highlights of the distinctive Soviet force employment doctrine are given below.

Theater War. The Soviets prepare for war fought with both nuclear and conventional weapons in the various theaters of military operations (TVDs) around the Soviet Union. Their scenario for global nuclear war, which was first set forth in the late 1950s and early 1960s, includes major campaigns fought with nuclear weapons in adjacent theaters located in Europe and Asia. These theater campaigns may precede or may be launched simultaneously with the commencement of massed intercontinental nuclear strikes against the main imperialist enemy, the United States. This nuclear campaign in the theater may be fought with nuclear weapons from the very onset of hostilities or it may arise from the escalation of a war begun solely with conventional weapons. In either case Soviet doctrine calls for the employment of several massed strikes throughout the depth of the theater against a combination of military, economic, and political targets.[71] These strikes are to be followed up by combined-arms, air-land offensives along several main axes of attack designed to complete rapidly the defeat of the enemy's military forces, and to occupy his territory.

Beginning in the mid 1960s, but with growing emphasis since the late 1970s, the Soviets have added preparations for conducting what Marshal Ogarkov has called "a strategic operation within a theater of military operations conducted solely with conventional weapons."[72] This would involve the conduct of large-scale, ground-air offensive operations against NATO and, possibly, the People's Republic of China, using only conventional weapons, over a period of many days or even weeks. This war would be fought under the constant threat of nuclear escalation. The USSR says it is prepared to initiate extensive nuclear operations at any time during the conduct of such a conventional war. Consequently, the Soviet military would maintain a high state of nuclear readiness to ensure that it could preempt any enemy attempt to initiate the large-scale use of nuclear weapons. Should such an escalation occur, the nuclear theater offensive would be carried out in the manner described above.

In a large-scale theater war fought without recourse to nuclear weapons, the Soviets foresee a complex scenario. Standard Soviet training depictions of war in central Europe, for example, open with a large-scale NATO invasion that forces the Pact on the defensive in its own territory. Recent Soviet military writings indicate that these defensive operations should be marked by "dynamism and activity." They should feature rapid, bold maneuver, effective use of obstacles and fortifications, and flexible counterattacks by specially configured tank and motorized rifle formations.[73]

The Pact eventually contains and then repels the NATO invader in these scenarios by means of a vigorous counter-offensive. The Soviet concept for offensive operations calls for the massing of their armor-heavy forces along selected main axes of attack in order to carry out a series of simultaneous breakthroughs of the enemy's defenses. These breakthroughs are to be exploited immediately by the continuous introduction of additional echelons that are to advance rapidly into the enemy's rear area. The follow-on forces will be led by specially configured "operational maneuver groups." These division- or corps-sized formations are called upon to break away from the bulk of the second echelon units to pave the way for their advances. The majority of second-echelon formations, in turn, would seek to encircle and destroy the enemy's main formations, occupying enemy territory in a matter of days.[74]

These high-speed advances are to be assisted by the conduct of special "assault landings" in the enemy's rear. A variety of forces, including airborne units, recently created air assault brigades, special forces (*spetsnaz*), and naval infantry formations will move over and around the front lines via transport aircraft, helicopters, and amphibious craft in order to land and seize key facilities and terrain. These attacks are designed to disrupt the enemy's defense efforts severely and to facilitate the advance of second echelon exploitation forces coming over land from the front.[75]

This land offensive fought with conventional weapons is to be supported by an extensive "air operation," integrating attacks by over a thousand fighter-interceptors, fighter-bombers, and medium bomber units; assault landings by the forces noted above; and possibly strikes by conventionally-armed tactical ballistic missiles. These elements will be combined in a series of massed raids conducted over several days in an effort to destroy enemy forces, especially nuclear delivery systems and aircraft, throughout the theater in order to reduce the enemy's nuclear strike potential and gain air superiority in the theater.[76]

In a nuclear conflict, the attacks of these forces would be supplemented by massed strikes of nuclear-armed, operational, tactical missiles and fighter bombers based in the theater as well as longer-range, regional, strategic nuclear missile and bomber forces based in the USSR. These strikes would cover enemy targets located near the battlefield and throughout the enemy's deep rear area.

War at Sea. Primary emphasis in Soviet naval operations will be devoted to efforts to destroy enemy naval combatants, in particular aircraft carriers and ballistic missile submarines capable of striking Soviet forward-deployed forces or targets in the USSR. These efforts will involve coordinated attacks by cruise-missile-equipped surface ships, submarines, and land-based bombers using either conventional or nuclear arms.

Over the past decade the USSR has also developed a concept calling for the employment of combined antisubmarine warfare (ASW) assets—attack submarines, surface ships, and ASW aircraft—in a "bastion defense" or "strategic support mission" to help protect Soviet strategic ballistic missile submarines at sea. These combined ASW operations are designed to protect Soviet SSBNs deployed in the "closed" Barents and Norwegian seas off the northwest coast of the USSR and the Sea of Okhotsk in the Far East from U.S. attack submarines.[77]

The forces of the Soviet navy are also expected to conduct amphibious operations, as noted above, using naval infantry and ground force units in support of land offensives and independently to seize key islands such as Iceland. They must be prepared as well to execute coastal defense operations to deny the enemy the ability to mount successful amphibious assaults on the Soviet Union.

Soviet naval air and submarine forces are tasked as well to interdict enemy sea lines of communication, in particular maritime resupply and reinforcement from the United States to Western Europe, although this appears to be a secondary mission.

Throughout a theater conventional conflict, Soviet submarines carrying sea-launched ballistic and cruise missiles would remain prepared for mounting attacks against key targets in nearby theaters or against critical targets in North America. Those systems committed to cover targets in nearby theaters will be prepared to execute their attacks while the intercontinetal strike forces remain on hold.

Intercontinental Nuclear Warfare. In addressing preparations for a possible strategic nuclear exchange, Soviet doctrine includes a strong predisposition to launch a preemptive strike against U.S. strategic forces if U.S. preparations to commence nuclear operations can be reliably detected.[78] If preemption is not achieved, the Soviet leaders are apparently prepared to employ a "launch on tactical warning" or "launch under attack" tactic, or, failing that, simply to retaliate after absorbing the initial U.S. strike.[79] The USSR could, of course, also initiate a nuclear war with a surprise, would-be-disarming first strike. Although, for obvious reasons, Soviet public statements do not acknowledge such a possibility, their military writings consistently emphasize the value of achieving surprise at the beginning of a war, and their force-modeling literature has explored scenarios beginning with a massive first strike carried out by either of the two superpowers.

Regardless of the manner in which Soviet nuclear operations might begin, Soviet intercontinental and submarine-launched ballistic missiles (ICBMs and SLBMs) and strategic bombers would be employed to strike simultaneously at a wide range of "counterforce" and "countervalue" targets. These targets include U.S. strategic forces (ICBM silos, SSBNs in port, and bomber bases), key military command and control facilities, major groupings of general-purpose forces at garrisons, airfields, and naval bases, and a variety of economic and political objectives, including electrical power systems, stocks of strategic raw materials, and large industrial and transport centers.[80] Although devastating strikes against these targets are considered essential in the "initial period" of a general nuclear war, "final victory" is said to be achievable only with the combined efforts of all arms and services, including major offensives in adjacent theaters and the war at sea.

Soviet doctrinal writings display little interest in the possibility of imposing finely tuned limitations on nuclear warfare for symbolic or bargaining purposes at either the central strategic or theater levels. At the same time, however, this literature does indicate full awareness of possible limitations in terms of targets struck and the numbers and yields of nuclear weapons employed. There is also a potential willingness to consider avoiding nuclear weapons use in secondary theaters, to spare cities located in theaters adjacent to the USSR the Soviet leaders anticipate they will capture, and mutually to avoid strikes on the homelands of the superpowers.[81] This latter possibility of treating the United States and the USSR as sanctuaries during a nuclear war fought in Europe was suggested by Brezhnev to Henry Kissinger during the high-level negotiations in 1972.[82] In recent years, Soviet civilian academics have recognized explicitly the value of both sides mutually avoiding attacks on one another's national command authority as a means to provide a basis for escalation control and war termination.[83]

Moreover, the Soviet military has long favored planning to allow a careful, militarily efficient application of nuclear weapons designed to achieve the desired objectives with the fewest possible weapons and to minimize the disruption of military advances in adjacent theaters that would inevitably accompany substantial nuclear weapons use. Nevertheless, the USSR has publicly rejected U.S. concepts of highly limited nuclear warfare as artificial "rules of the game" and instead continues to embrace the concept of large-scale nuclear strikes that would likely involve, at a minimum, hundreds of nuclear weapons, which are to be employed for maximum military and political effectiveness. Despite this consistent doctrinal antipathy toward small-scale nuclear weapons use, growing Soviet capabilities could, nevertheless, support a wide spectrum of controlled nuclear operations, which the Soviet leadership could choose to employ in a crisis.[84]

The Soviets also assign very high priority to defense of the homeland in order to minimize the destructive effects of enemy attack, to maintain political control by the Communist Party, to reconstitute critical military forces, and to facilitate economic recuperation. Consequently, the Soviets intend to conduct active antiaircraft, antimissile, and antisatellite and other space operations in combination with extensive civil defense measures to reduce the damage inflicted on the USSR by enemy forces that survive Soviet counterforce attacks.

Soviet doctrinal writings are ambiguous as to the likely duration of a general nuclear war. On the one hand, they often speak of the massed nuclear exchanges during the "initial period," which may last a few hours or a few days, as being potentially decisive in determining the final outcome of such a war. On the other hand, they often point out that a global nuclear war might be "protracted" and write of conducting operations over several weeks, or even months, and shifting the economy to a wartime footing for purposes of sustained wartime production and recuperation.

The Defense Decision-Making Process

THE ORGANIZATIONAL SETTING

As described earlier, political power in the Soviet Union is concentrated in the hands of the few who control the Soviet Communist Party. The small group that determines the nation's destiny from atop the twin organizational networks of the Communist Party and the Soviet government clearly exercises control over national security policy as one of its highest priority activities.

In analyzing defense policy making and implementation in the USSR, it is useful to think

in terms of the "decisional trajectory" model developed by David Finley and Jan Triska, two students of Soviet foreign policy.[85] This approach analyzes policy making as a sequence of events beginning with problem identification, then proceeding to information collection and interpretation, the development and analysis of alternative courses of action, decision making (i.e., selection of a course of action), policy elaboration, and, finally, policy implementation. The trajectory aspect of the metaphor is used to indicate that during the course of this sequence, these stages generally take place at successively higher levels of authority on the path upward toward decision and then drop down once again to lower levels during the process of policy elaboration and implementation. When combined with examination of the roles, resources, and tactics of the various organizations and individuals involved, the decisional trajectory model can help us understand the dynamics of Soviet defense policy.

The constellation of organizations in which Soviet defense policy is made includes specialized defense-related oganizations and generalist bodies whose involvement in national security issues constitutes only part of their overall activities. Some of these organs are active across the full range of national security matters, while the involvement of others is limited to a single defense issue area, such as weapons acquisition. The various organizations within the vast Party and government bureaucracies that are engaged in defense policy development, decision making, and execution often serve as arenas for political competition among key individuals and groups interested in shaping Soviet defense policy.

The Politburo. On the Party side, the bodies of note are the topmost elements of the Party bureaucracy, including the Politburo, the Secretariat, and certain departments of the Party apparatus that are formally attached to the Central Committee. The most important of these is the Politburo. This small body, whose exact size varies slightly over time, currently consists of twelve full voting members and nonvoting "candidate" members. It is a generalist organization that exercises ultimate decisional authority on all issues of consequence in the

Soviet Union. It can be presumed to have the prerogative of formally approving all key defense decisions. This places the Politburo at the apogee of the decisional trajectory for such diverse defense matters as the formulation of military strategy, the development and acquisition of weaponry, and, of course, the threat of the actual employment of Soviet military power.

The Defense Council. Although it has ultimate decisional authority, the full Politburo is almost certainly unable to maintain close supervision of defense matters on a regular basis. The highest body with this responsibility is the Defense Council (*Soviet Oborony*). This organization, whose members officially are appointed by the Presidium of the Supreme Soviet under Article 121 of the 1977 Soviet Constitution, appears to function as a defense subcommittee for the Politburo.

The Defense Council is the latest in a long line of high-level councils, or "soviets," with combined civilian and military membership that have supervised Soviet defense matters. Soviet publications have never disclosed its membership beyond announcing that the CPSU's general secretary, first Brezhnev, then Andropov, Chernenko, and now Gorbachev, is its chairman. Gorbachev is very likely joined by other key Politburo figures occupying the most senior Party-state positions: the second-ranking secretary of the Central Committee (if such a position continues to exist); the chairmen of the Presidiums of the Council of Ministers and the Supreme Soviet; those with special responsibility for defense matters, including the minister of defense and the Central Committee secretary supervising defense production; and the head of the KGB and the minister of foreign affairs. Among Politburo members known to have served on the Defense Council in the late 1980s, in addition to Gorbachev, are Ye. K. Ligachev (second-ranking secretary of the Central Committee), N. I. Ryzhkov (chairman of the Presidium of the Council of Ministers), A. A. Gromyko (Chairman of the Presidium of the Supreme Soviet), Army General D. T. Yazov (Minister of Defense), L. N. Zaikov (Central Committee Sec-

retary for Defense Industries), and possibly E. A. Shevardnadze (Foreign Minister) and V. M. Chebrikov (head of the KGB).

Staff support for the Defense Council is apparently given by the General Staff,[86] providing the basis for the regular participation in Defense Council meetings of the chief of the General Staff, who probably has acted as the council's executive secretary. Whatever its permanent membership, other senior Party, government, and military figures almost certainly are invited to attend the deliberations of the Defense Council when issues within their special competence are under consideration.

There is no information available on the activities of the Defense Council. However, memoir accounts of the activities of its predecessors, known variously as the Council of Workers' and Peasants' Defense, the Council of Labor and Defense, and the Supreme Military Council, indicate that it probably serves as the forum in which such matters as significant weapons development and procurement programs, defense budgets, and major force deployments are discussed. These deliberations, carefully orchestrated in accordance with the consensus-oriented style that has apparently marked its proceedings since the Brezhnev period, are likely to culminate in preliminary decisions that are, in turn, considered and almost certainly approved by the full Politburo. During wartime, the Defense Council would very likely provide the nucleus for the formation of a new State Defense Committee, similar to the body of that name created during World War II and which would oversee the overall Soviet war effort.

The Supreme High Command. During World War II the Soviet Union created a General Headquarters, the *stavka* of the Supreme High Command (*verkhovnoe glavnokomandovanie*—VGK), which provided highly centralized strategic leadership for the planning and execution of military operations. Directly subordinate to the small State Defense Committee headed by Stalin, the Stavka VGK included the supreme commander in chief (Stalin), the deputy supreme commander in chief (Marshal Zhukov), and 7–10 other senior military leaders. Various representatives of the *stavka* including Marshals Zhukov, Vasilevskiy, Voronov, Novikov, and others were periodically sent into the field to coordinate personally multifront operations. Critical staff support for the VGK was provided primarily by its "working organ," the General Staff, and by other elements of the Defense Commissariat.[87]

WARTIME AND PEACETIME OPERATION

Most of these organs have been identified by Soviet writers as wartime bodies, and many are reported to have been abolished at the end of the war.[88] There are indications, however, that various elements of the VGK may have been resurrected over the past decade.[89]

The Defense Council could readily serve as a modern-day version of the State Defense Committee. As noted earlier, Brezhnev was publicly identified as the supreme commander in chief of the Soviet armed forces, and Gorbachev almost certainly currently occupies that post. Gorbachev, General D. T. Yazov (the Minister of Defense), Marshal Akhromeyev (Chief of the General Staff until his resignation in December 1988), and possibly Ligachev (second-ranking Central Committee secretary prior to the major Politburo shake-up in September 1988), along with selected members of the Collegium of the Ministry of Defense, discussed below, could readily be called upon to function as the *stavka*, VGK. The General Staff, with its several key staff elements and communications capabilities, appears well prepared to resume its vital planning and execution roles.

Finally, repeated recent Soviet statements regarding theaters of military operations (TVDs) and key personnel shifts indicate that "high commands" (*glavnokomandovaniya*) have already been established in several regional theaters of operations along the periphery of the Soviet Union.[90] In wartime these high commands would operate as intermediate command entities between the Moscow-based VGK and various "fronts" (army groups) in the field.[91] All in all, the USSR appears to be operating today with a peacetime command structure that could rapidly and quite easily be put on a wartime footing (see figs. 1 and 2).

Ministry of Defense. While the Politburo and Defense Council play critical roles in all major defense decisions, they are not involved in the critical day-to-day tasks of gathering and interpreting information, developing and analyzing defense policy alternatives, and implementing the courses of action selected by the senior Party leadership. These activities are largely the responsibility of the various components of the Ministry of Defense and, to a lesser degree, the scientific research institutes and industrial ministries engaged in the design and production of armaments, and a few other specialized Party and government organizations.

The Ministry of Defense has by far the largest role in policy formulation and execution in virtually all aspects of Soviet defense activity. The most important elements in the ministry are its collegium, the General Staff, the five "services" of the armed forces—the Strategic Rocket Forces, Air Defense Forces, Navy, Ground Forces, and Air Forces—and a series of central directorates, including Rear Services, Civil Defense, Armaments, Construction and Billeting, Main Inspectorate, and Cadres (personnel).

The key ministry is run by the Minister of Defense, Army General D. T. Yazov, who is assisted by three first deputy ministers and eleven deputy ministers. The former group has consisted of Marshal Akhromeyev, Chief of the General Staff until December 1988; Marshal V. G. Kulikov, Commander in Chief of the Warsaw Pact; and Army General P. G. Lushev, who apparently has supervised day-to-day administration of the ministry. The latter group includes all the service commanders in chief and the heads of the important central directorates.

The Collegium of the Ministry of Defense. Army General Yazov, his collection of deputies, and the chief of the main political administration (MPA) make up the collegium of the Ministry of Defense (see fig. 3). This collective organ is the most senior of an extensive network of military councils found throughout

Figure 1. Soviet Peacetime Defense Organization

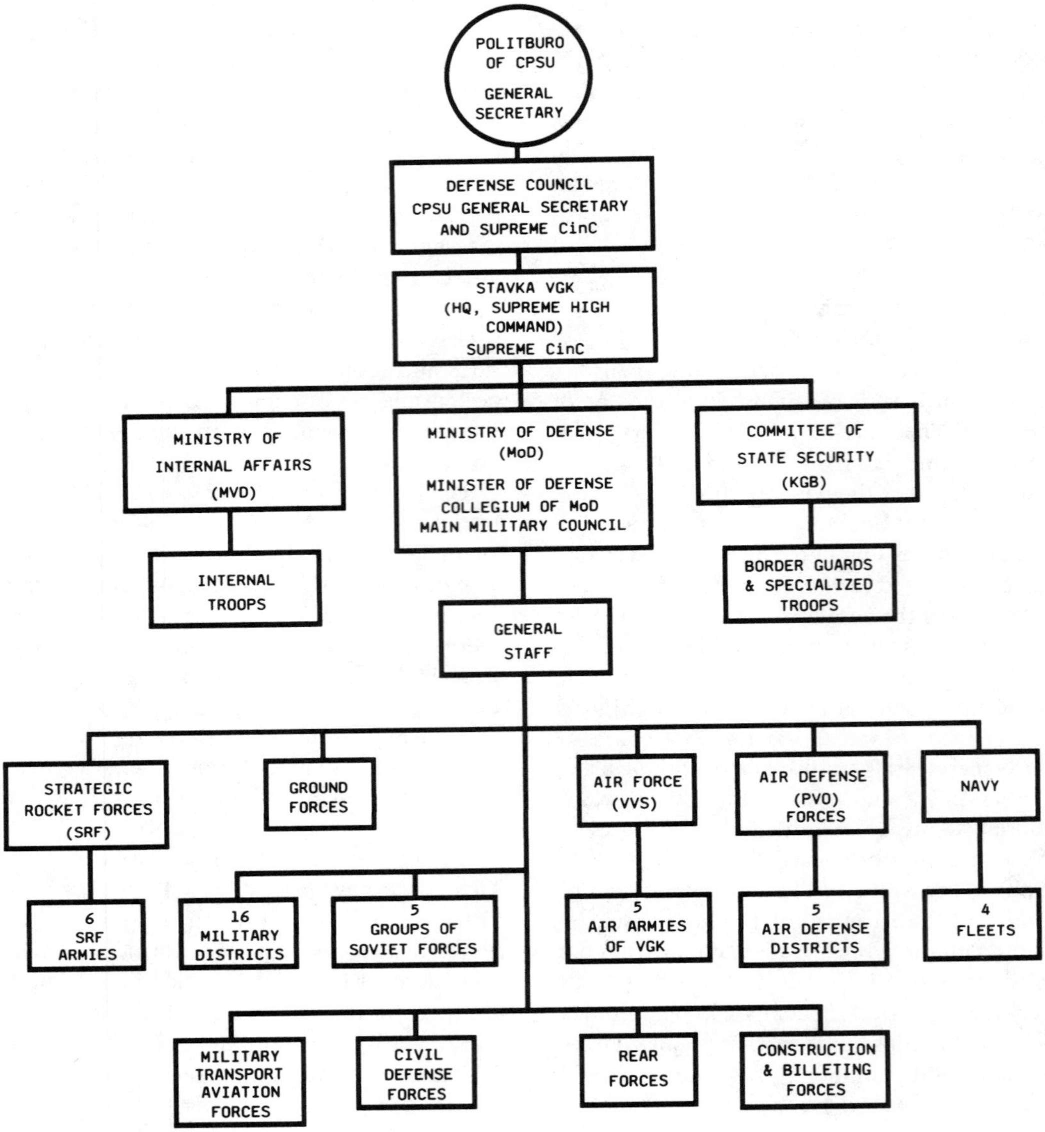

```
                          ┌──────────────┐
                          │  POLITBURO   │
                          │   OF CPSU    │
                          │              │
                          │   GENERAL    │
                          │  SECRETARY   │
                          └──────────────┘
                          ┌──────────────────┐
                          │  DEFENSE COUNCIL  │
                          │ CPSU GENERAL SECRETARY │
                          │  AND SUPREME CinC │
                          └──────────────────┘
                          ┌──────────────────┐
                          │    STAVKA VGK     │
                          │ (HQ, SUPREME HIGH │
                          │     COMMAND)      │
                          │   SUPREME CinC    │
                          └──────────────────┘
```

MINISTRY OF INTERNAL AFFAIRS (MVD)	MINISTRY OF DEFENSE (MoD) — MINISTER OF DEFENSE — COLLEGIUM OF MoD — MAIN MILITARY COUNCIL	COMMITTEE OF STATE SECURITY (KGB)
INTERNAL TROOPS	GENERAL STAFF	BORDER GUARDS & SPECIALIZED TROOPS

STRATEGIC ROCKET FORCES (SRF)	GROUND FORCES		AIR FORCE (VVS)	AIR DEFENSE (PVO) FORCES	NAVY
6 SRF ARMIES	16 MILITARY DISTRICTS	5 GROUPS OF SOVIET FORCES	5 AIR ARMIES OF VGK	5 AIR DEFENSE DISTRICTS	4 FLEETS

MILITARY TRANSPORT AVIATION FORCES	CIVIL DEFENSE FORCES	REAR FORCES	CONSTRUCTION & BILLETING FORCES

the services and the major regional commands—the military and air defense districts, groups of forces, and fleets discussed below. This high-level advisory body apparently serves as a forum for the discussion of key policy issues.

The current minister of defense, General of the Army D. T. Yazov, born in 1923, is a career officer who has served in the Soviet Army since the opening months of World War II. General Yazov was a relatively unknown but steadily rising senior commander until 1987 when he was brought from the Far East to Moscow to become the Deputy Minister of Defense for Cadres. Four months later, General Yazov suddenly vaulted over several other seemingly more qualified candidates to replace Marshal Sokolov as minister of defense in the wake of the highly embarrassing unauthorized flight to Moscow by the young West German Matthias

Figure 2. Soviet Wartime Defense Organization

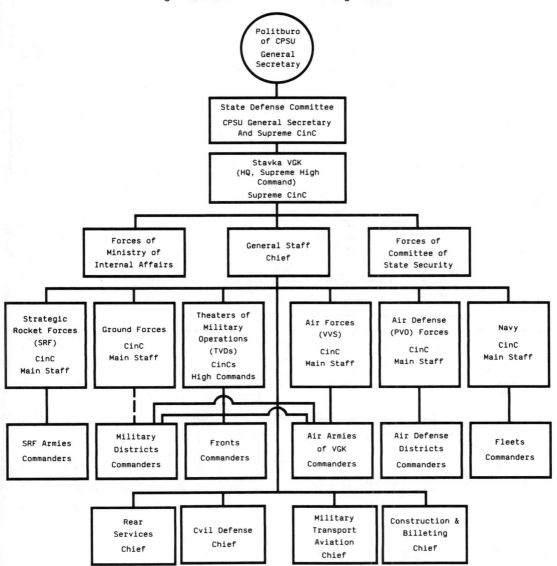

Rust in his small private plane. Yazov's surprise selection for this important post by Gorbachev, as discussed below, suggests that he was viewed as a man who would loyally carry out Gorbachev's *perestroika* campaign to root out corruption and increase efficiency and discipline within the Soviet armed forces. Previous patterns suggest that General Yazov is likely to remain a defense minister for the next several years.

Among the first deputy ministers, Marshal V. G. Kulikov, born in 1921 and now the commander in chief of the Warsaw Pact, is the most senior. He rose to the critical role of chief of the General Staff in 1971 at the relatively young age of 50. He was moved laterally and a little bit downward in January 1977 when he assumed his current position after being replaced by Marshal Ogarkov as chief of the General Staff. During the past twelve years

Figure 3. Collegium of the Ministry of Defense of the USSR, 1988

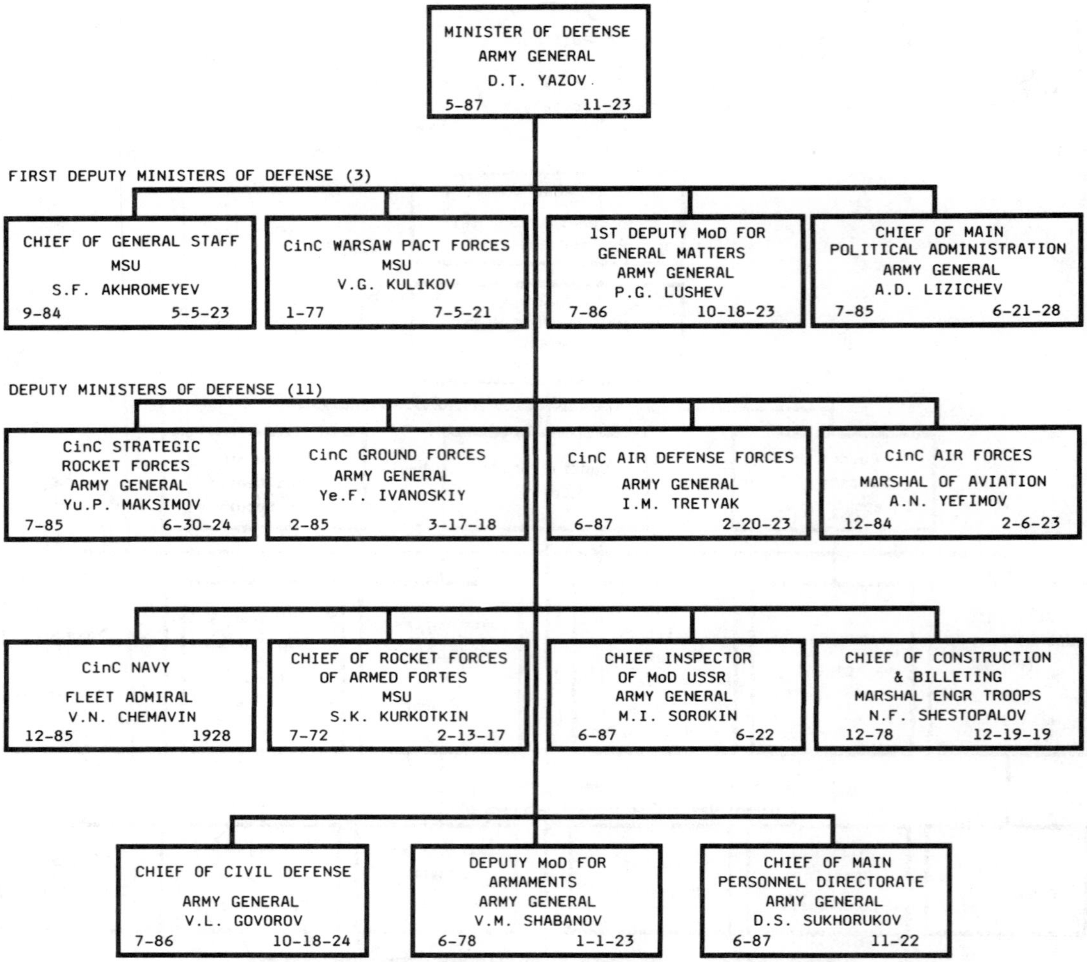

```
                        ┌────────────────────────┐
                        │   MINISTER OF DEFENSE    │
                        │     ARMY GENERAL         │
                        │      D.T. YAZOV          │
                        │  5-87          11-23     │
                        └────────────────────────┘
```

FIRST DEPUTY MINISTERS OF DEFENSE (3)

| CHIEF OF GENERAL STAFF MSU S.F. AKHROMEYEV 9-84   5-5-23 | CinC WARSAW PACT FORCES MSU V.G. KULIKOV 1-77   7-5-21 | 1ST DEPUTY MoD FOR GENERAL MATTERS ARMY GENERAL P.G. LUSHEV 7-86   10-18-23 | CHIEF OF MAIN POLITICAL ADMINISTRATION ARMY GENERAL A.D. LIZICHEV 7-85   6-21-28 |

DEPUTY MINISTERS OF DEFENSE (11)

| CinC STRATEGIC ROCKET FORCES ARMY GENERAL Yu.P. MAKSIMOV 7-85   6-30-24 | CinC GROUND FORCES ARMY GENERAL Ye.F. IVANOSKIY 2-85   3-17-18 | CinC AIR DEFENSE FORCES ARMY GENERAL I.M. TRETYAK 6-87   2-20-23 | CinC AIR FORCES MARSHAL OF AVIATION A.N. YEFIMOV 12-84   2-6-23 |

| CinC NAVY FLEET ADMIRAL V.N. CHEMAVIN 12-85   1928 | CHIEF OF ROCKET FORCES OF ARMED FORTES MSU S.K. KURKOTKIN 7-72   2-13-17 | CHIEF INSPECTOR OF MoD USSR ARMY GENERAL M.I. SOROKIN 6-87   6-22 | CHIEF OF CONSTRUCTION & BILLETING MARSHAL ENGR TROOPS N.F. SHESTOPALOV 12-78   12-19-19 |

| CHIEF OF CIVIL DEFENSE ARMY GENERAL V.L. GOVOROV 7-86   10-18-24 | DEPUTY MoD FOR ARMAMENTS ARMY GENERAL V.M. SHABANOV 6-78   1-1-23 | CHIEF OF MAIN PERSONNEL DIRECTORATE ARMY GENERAL D.S. SUKHORUKOV 6-87   11-22 |

Note: Date of incumbent's appointment to post appears in lower left corner of box and his birth date in lower right corner.

Marshal Kulikov, who is reported to be an aggressive, tough, and somewhat crude leader, has been passed over three times when new ministers of defense were selected, thus suggesting continuing doubts at the highest political levels regarding his suitability for this most important post.

Marshal S. F. Akhromeyev, born in 1923, has been the Chief of the General Staff since the removal of his apparent patron, Marshal Ogarkov, in September 1984. Prior to his December 1988 resignation in the aftermath of Gorbachev's announcement in a United Nations speech of major troop cuts, Marshal

Akhromeyev (whose work had been in the senior staff officer career track rather than as a troop commander) had become an increasingly visible figure on a variety of doctrinal and arms control issues, writing several major articles and making very important substantive contributions in high-level negotiations. In the latter post, he played a leading role in the superpower summits at Reykjavik and Washington and during the closing stages in 1986 of the Stockholm talks on confidence and security building measures in Europe. Marshal Akhromeyev appears to have taken the lead in these doctrinal and foreign policy matters, while

General Yazov has borne the responsibility for the campaign to improve overall performance within the armed forces.

General of the Army P. G. Lushev, the First Deputy Minister of Defense for General Matters, also born in 1923, rose rapidly when he moved in the summer of 1985 from the post of commander of the Moscow Military District to become commander in chief of the Group of Soviet Forces in Germany and then moved again in July 1986 to assume his current responsibilities. In late 1986 and early 1987 he stood in for the ailing Marshal Sokolov, then the minister of defense, leading many to believe he was the leading candidate to succeed Sokolov. This, of course, did not occur when Sokolov was forced into retirement after the Rust affair, but General Lushev remains a powerful and vigorous figure nevertheless.

Another important figure in the senior leadership cadre of the Ministry of Defense is General of the Army A. D. Lizichev, born in 1928, who heads the main political administration of the Soviet Army and Navy. Although General Lizichev is neither a first deputy nor a deputy minister of defense, he is accorded the fifth-ranking protocol position within the ministry, standing behind the first deputies and in front of the deputy ministers of defense. This reflects the importance accorded the MPA, whose political officers, serving throughout the armed forces, are the descendants of the Bolshevik political commissars that were introduced immediately after the revolution. The MPA has operated since 1925 in the unique position of having "the rights of the department of the Central Committee." It is responsible, as discussed in greater detail below, for the political indoctrination of the Soviet officer corps and enlisted personnel.

The General Staff. As the central directing organ of the Soviet armed forces, the General Staff is unquestionably the most important single element in the Soviet military establishment. Its role is well described in the title of a lengthy study by one of its important founding figures, Marshal Boris Shaposhnikov, who called the General Staff "the brain of the army."[92]

Through its many components, including the Main Operations, Main Intelligence, Main Organization and Mobilization, Main Foreign Military Assistance, and Military Science Directorates, the Soviet General Staff plays the dominant role in such diverse undertakings as the formulation of doctrinal concepts, the refinement of Soviet military organization, and the development of mobilization and military contingency plans, as well as the peacetime training and the wartime operational direction of the armed forces.

The General Staff is manned by both a cadre of career staff officers, many of whom spend decades in its directorates, and some of the most promising command figures drawn from all of the services, who usually attend the prestigious Voroshilov Academy in Moscow prior to their posting to the General Staff. During World War II, representatives of the General Staff were sent out to monitor the activities of the staffs of the fronts and armies in the field.[93] It is quite possible that the General Staff continues to reinforce its control today by placing its representatives on the staffs of the high commands of forces, the military districts, the groups of forces in Eastern Europe, and the main staffs of the five services during peacetime.

Directorates of the Ministry of Defense. We do not know a great deal about the role played by the various specialized directorates within the Ministry of Defense such as those for Construction and Billeting, Armaments, Rear Services, Civil Defense, Cadres (Personnel), etc., several of which are headed by deputy ministers of defense.

Each of these directorates is responsible for a particular defense function. The Armaments Directorate, headed by Army General V. M. Shabonov, for example, plays an important role in the management of weapons research, development, and production, while the Civil Defense Directorate, led by General of the Army V. L. Govorov, directs the extensive national civil defense program. Soviet civil defense efforts involve not only a substantial cadre of regular troops assigned to civil defense duties, but also a vast regional network that combines the efforts of local Party and government organizations, economic enterprises, and educational institutions. We also know little about the relationships these bodies have with the General Staff, Minister of Defense Yazov, or First Deputy Minister of Defense Lushev, who is thought to be in charge of day-to-day operations in the ministry as a whole.

The Services and Field Commands. The five services are responsible for the peacetime training and equipping of their various elements. Their activities are overseen by the service commanders in chief (CinCs), who are deputy ministers of defense. These prestigious figures are assisted by military councils, whose members include their several deputy commanders, chiefs of staff, and deputies for political affairs, as well as the main staffs of the services.

The operational responsibilities of the service CinCs and their main staffs in wartime are not clear. The headquarters of the navy, strategic rocket forces, air defense troops, and the air forces apparently exercise operational control over all or portions of their respective forces that have not come under the direction of high commands directing operations in theaters of military operations adjacent to the USSR. The service CinCs would be actively involved in the direction of combat operations as members of the foremost collective military command organ, the *stavka* of the VGK. The service main staffs would likely be involved in directing continuing service training and equipping functions, in providing specialized staff support to the CinCs, and, as an alternative channel of operational command and control, in supplementing the primary command channels run by the General Staff.

In both peace and war, most Soviet forces are deployed and directed by a series of geographically organized field commands. The intercontinental- and regional-range ballistic missiles of the strategic rocket forces, for example, are deployed in several missile armies scattered throughout the USSR. Bombers, longer-range fighter-bombers, and some fighter-interceptor units are assigned to five "shock" air armies of the VGK, four headquartered in the USSR, and the fifth at Legnica in Poland.[94] The surface-to-air missile troops, radar troops, and interceptors of the air defense forces operate in a network of air defense districts throughout the USSR. The tank, motorized rifle, and airborne divisions of the ground forces and their supporting tactical air forces are controlled by the commanders of the sixteen military districts in the Soviet Union (see fig. 4), four groups of Soviet forces in Eastern Europe, and an army in Mongolia.[95]

In the 1980s, the Soviets have apparently begun experimenting with their basic ground force organizational structure and have formed at least two unified or combined-army corps.[96] Some suggest that the Soviets are contemplating a shift to a battalion-brigade-corps structure, along the lines of a recent reorganization of the Hungarian armed forces,[97] as a means to field a "leaner, meaner" force for flexible, rapid-maneuver warfare. For the present, at least, the Ground Forces continue to be structured in the traditional battalion-regiment-division pattern.

In wartime the majority of the divisions from these military districts and groups of forces would operate along fronts moved outward to carry the battle to the enemy in theaters of military operations (TVDs) around the periphery of the USSR. These fronts, consisting of some ten to twenty divisions organized into three to five armies, would, in turn, fall under the control of high commands in the various TVDs. The high commands would carry out operations in accordance with directives from the *stavka* of the VGK in Moscow operating through its working organ, the General Staff.

Four TVD high commands have been organized in peacetime over the past several years. These are the high commands for the western TVD, prepared to conduct war in Central Europe; for the southwestern TVD, encompassing southern Europe from Italy around to Turkey; for the southern TVD, facing Iran, Afghanistan, and South Asia down to the Persian Gulf; and for the far eastern TVD, stretching from Central Asia out to the Far East. These theater high commands apparently develop wartime contingency plans for the employment of ground and air forces drawn from nearby groups of forces and military districts (see fig. 5). Finally, the increas-

Figure 4. Soviet Regional Commands

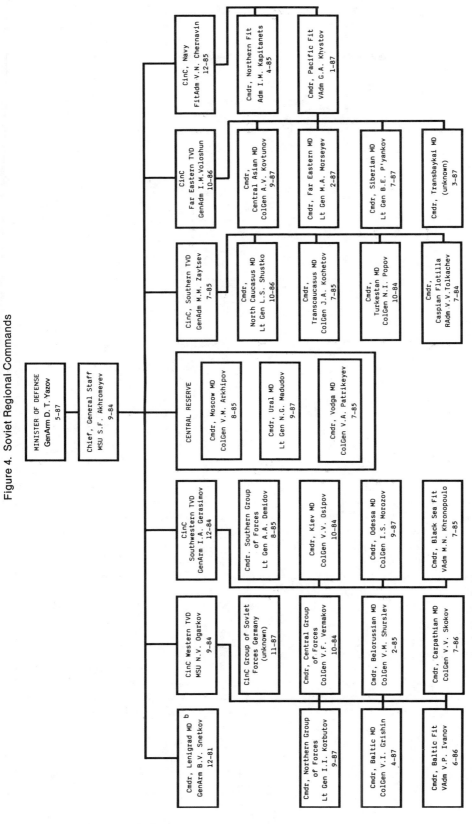

aDate in each box represents first time incumbent was identified in that position.

bIn wartime, the command of the Leningrad MD would likely form the high command of the Northwestern TVD, which does not exist in peacetime, and forces of the Leningrad MD would operate under the Northwestern TVD high command.

107

Figure 5. Soviet Military Districts and Fleets

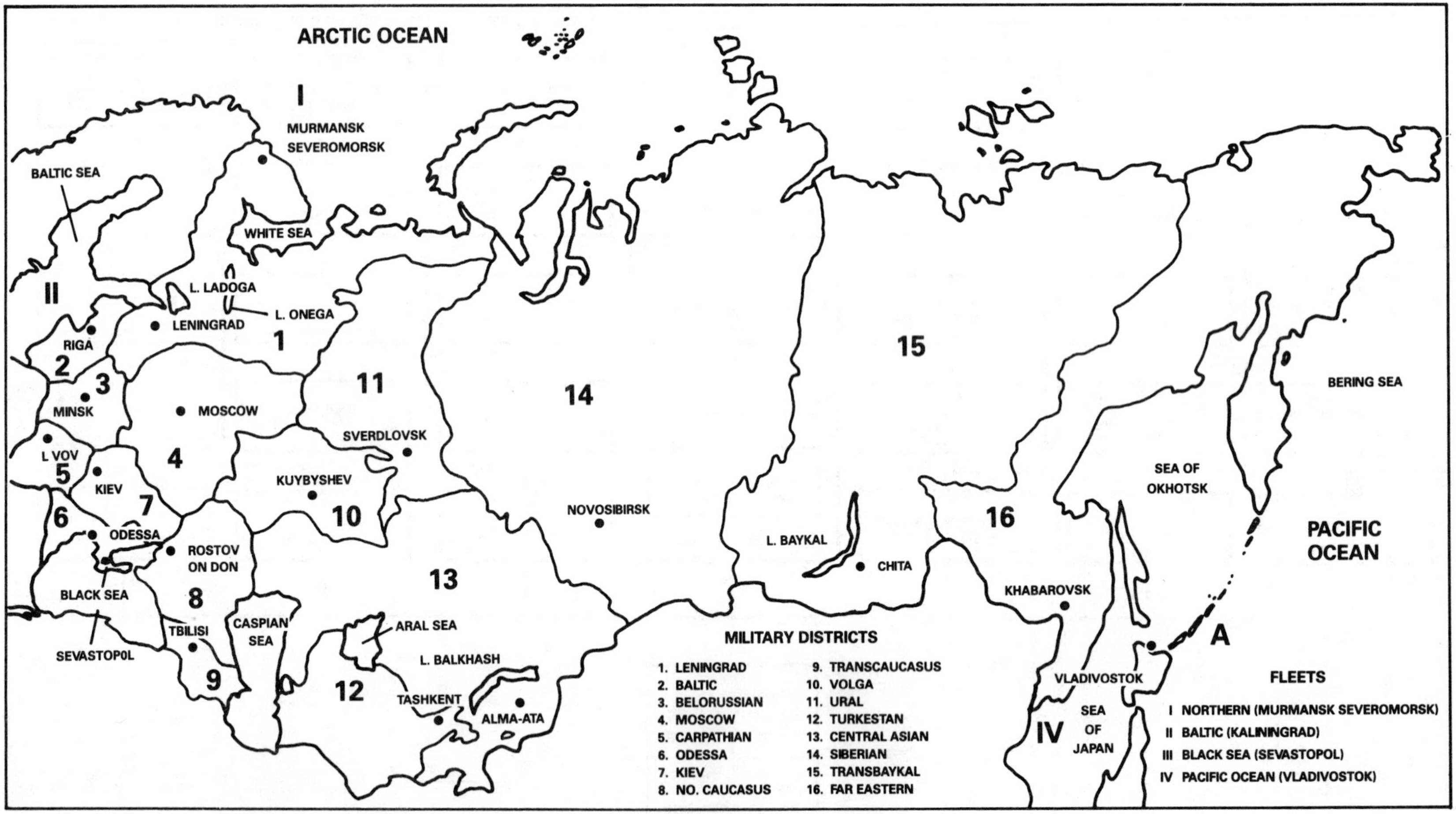

ARCTIC OCEAN

MURMANSK
SEVEROMORSK

WHITE SEA

L. LADOGA
L. ONEGA

LENINGRAD

BALTIC SEA

RIGA

MINSK

L'VOV

KIEV

ODESSA

BLACK SEA

SEVASTOPOL

MOSCOW

ROSTOV
ON DON

TBILISI

CASPIAN
SEA

SVERDLOVSK

KUYBYSHEV

NOVOSIBIRSK

ARAL SEA

L. BALKHASH

TASHKENT

ALMA-ATA

L. BAYKAL

CHITA

KHABAROVSK

VLADIVOSTOK

SEA OF
OKHOTSK

SEA
OF
JAPAN

BERING SEA

PACIFIC
OCEAN

MILITARY DISTRICTS

1. LENINGRAD
2. BALTIC
3. BELORUSSIAN
4. MOSCOW
5. CARPATHAN
6. ODESSA
7. KIEV
8. NO. CAUCASUS
9. TRANSCAUCASUS
10. VOLGA
11. URAL
12. TURKESTAN
13. CENTRAL ASIAN
14. SIBERIAN
15. TRANSBAYKAL
16. FAR EASTERN

FLEETS

I NORTHERN (MURMANSK SEVEROMORSK)
II BALTIC (KALININGRAD)
III BLACK SEA (SEVASTOPOL)
IV PACIFIC OCEAN (VLADIVOSTOK)

Source: Col. William F. Scott, "Soviet Aerospace Forces and Doctrine," *Air Force Magazine,* March 1975, pp. 38–39; compiled by Harriet Fast Scott.

ingly active Soviet Navy is divided into four widely separated fleets, the Northern, Baltic, Black Sea, and Pacific fleets, with headquarters in Severomorsk, Kaliningrad, Sevastopol, and Vladivostok respectively.

OVERVIEW

Within the organizational setting just discussed, the professional military officers of the Ministry of Defense have enormous influence. Although top civilian organizations such as the Politburo and the Defense Council clearly have the right of final decision in all defense matters, the processes of policy formulation, analysis, and implementation in the national security policy area are thoroughly dominated by the Ministry of Defense.

Over the years the military's influence has been reinforced by the fact that the top-level civilian decision makers have had no significant alternative sources of relevant defense information or expertise outside the Ministry of Defense. Consequently, even had the Party leaders been inclined to pursue a defense policy at variance with that recommended by the Soviet military, they would have had considerable difficulty gathering the sensitive information and critical expertise required to develop plausible alternatives. This does not rule out the possibility of dynamic defense policy initiatives sponsored by leading political figures—witness Khrushchev's vigorous attempts to reshape Soviet military policy radically between 1958 and 1964, discussed below. Nevertheless, it underscores the serious obstacles any would-be innovator in this area, acting without the support of the Ministry of Defense, confronted.

This situation has begun to change. Developments in Moscow over the past several years, which are being accelerated by the ongoing debates over reasonable sufficiency and the character of future Soviet defense policy, have begun to challenge this long-standing process. The 1980s have witnessed the emergence of a group of civilian specialists on national security issues with apparently growing ambitions to play a significant role in shaping Soviet military policy. These civilians work largely within the institutes of the Academy of Sciences, in particular its leading foreign affairs institutes in Moscow, the Institute of World Economy and International Relations (IMEMO), and at the Institute for the Study of the United States and Canada (IUSAC). This group includes a number of veteran civilian natural scientists, foreign policy specialists, and a few retired military officers, including Yevgeniy Primakov, Vitaliy Zhurkin, Aleksei Vasil'yev, Roald Sagdeyev, Yevgeniy Velikov, Lieutenant General Mikhail Mil'shteyn, Major General Vadim Makarevsky, and Colonel Lev Semeyko, as well as a rising new civilian generation, including Andrei Kokoshin, Aleksei Arbatov, Andre Kortunov, and Igor Malashenko.

The civilians active in these efforts have acquired their expertise in contemporary defense matters largely through their involvement over the past 10 to 15 years in the study of Western defense policies and of arms control issues. Their work on the latter has increased significantly in recent years as a result of a series of studies produced first under the aegis of the Scientific Research Council on Problems of Peace and Disarmament, established in 1979, and more recently, under the Committee of Soviet Scientists for Peace and Against the Nuclear Threat, formed in May 1983.

Until recently, these civilian specialists concentrated on the analysis of strategic nuclear offensive and defensive forces, an area where useful analysis can be carried out without an extensive background in military affairs. They have, for example, recently produced credible studies on strategic stability between the superpowers under various strategic force reduction configurations and on potential U.S.–Soviet arms interactions should the U.S. deploy a space-based ballistic missile system.[98]

They have turned their attention to the analysis of theater ground force operations as well, an area where the Soviet military has long enjoyed a monopoly of expertise.[99] Owing to the inherent complexities of theater warfare analysis, civilian specialists will have great difficulty producing useful studies of alternative conventional force postures. The Soviet General Staff almost certainly does not look favorably upon receiving analytical "assistance" from a group of civilians on military operational matters, particularly those associated with theater warfare.

One should not, of course, overstate the significance of these developments. The professional military apparently continues to control detailed information on Soviet and foreign military forces and to formulate the military-technical side of Soviet military doctrine. Moreover, the General Staff reportedly provides analytical support to the Defense Council, the subcommittee of the Politburo responsible for defense matters. Nevertheless, Gorbachev is strongly challenging prevailing security concepts and encouraging innovative thinking about these matters. Politburo member Aleksandr Yakovlev and Gorbachev adviser Anatoly Dobrynin have each called publicly for an increased role by civilian international affairs specialists and natural scientists in the analysis of foreign and defense matters and a group of talented and ambitious Soviet civilian academics appears to be stepping forward to accept this challenge.[100]

WEAPONS ACQUISITION

Despite recent changes, the Ministry of Defense continues to dominate the policy preparation and implementation stages in most defense-related matters, although several civilian organizations outside the Ministry of Defense play active roles in these phases of Soviet weapons development and production.[101] The largest organizations in this regard are the various industrial ministries engaged in defense research, development, and production. This group includes nine defense production ministries whose primary products are military equipment and several others that provide important support to the armaments effort.[102] Basic research in defense-related technologies is conducted for the most part within the many institutes of the Academy of Sciences as well as within the research establishments of the Ministry of Defense and the defense production ministries.

The relations between these defense research and production organizations and their steady customer, the Ministry of Defense, usually have been supervised by the Military-Industrial Commission (the "VPK," according to

its Russian acronym) on the government side, and by a secretary specializing in defense production within the central Party apparatus. The occupant of the latter position, possibly still L. N. Zaikov, despite the fact he became the head of the Moscow Party organization in November 1987, has long played, with the help of the Defense Industries Department of the Central Committee, a critical role in personally directing Soviet defense production. Others who have occupied this post include Leonid Brezhnev in the late 1950s, and the long-time "czar" of the Soviet armaments industry, D. F. Ustinov, who held the job from 1965 until 1976 before becoming Minister of Defense.

THE DEFENSE BUDGET PROCESS

Like all of the Soviet system, the Soviet defense establishment operates within the confines of both the recent five-year and annual economic plans for defense. These plans are formulated by the Ministry of Defense and by the key defense production ministries with the assistance of the Military-Industrial Commission, the State Planning Committee (Gosplan), and the Party Secretariat. In the Ministry of Defense, defense budget plans are apparently prepared by the ubiquitous General Staff, which must reconcile the budgetary requests of the services and other elements of the armed forces. Given the generous support that defense spending has generally received since the fall of Khrushchev, this is unlikely to have been a particularly difficult task even in recent years, when the rate of growth in the defense budget has slowed considerably. Just a few years earlier, however, when Khrushchev was determinedly seeking to reduce defense expenditures, this process was almost certainly accompanied by significant interservice conflict in a "scarcity" environment. And should Gorbachev choose to cut back on the growth of defense even more, intensified interservice competition for budgetary support could once again emerge.

After preparation and coordination by the responsible Party and government agencies, the annual and five-year plans must be considered and approved by the Defense Council and ultimately by the Politburo. As noted earlier, for more than twenty years these bodies have consistently been willing to expend steadily increasing amounts on defense. This pattern has persisted despite very substantial Soviet economic difficulties, including a significant decline in the rate of overall economic growth.

In marked contrast to the situation in the Western democracies, there is no meaningful legislative review of the Soviet defense budget or, for that matter, of any other aspect of Soviet political life. Although the bicameral Supreme Soviet is in theory the dominant element in the Soviet parliamentary system, it is convened infrequently and has no impact whatsoever on defense issues. Thus, the shape of the Soviet defense budget is purely the product of politics within the government and Party hierarchies.

The Soviets are amending their constitution to establish a new Congress of People's Deputies, whose 2250 deputies will normally meet only once a year. The Congress will, however, elect a 400-member Supreme Soviet of the USSR from among its members. This body will be in session six to eight months each year. There have been reports that the new Supreme Soviet will establish standing committees to monitor, among other things, Soviet defense and foreign policy. Such legislative oversight was specifically called for by Foreign Minister Shevardnadze in July 1988.[103] This new Supreme Soviet will have the potential for the first time to provide meaningful legislative review of the Soviet defense budget and of many other aspects of the Soviet defense effort. It will remain to be seen if this proves to be the case.

THE IMPACT OF PERSONALITY

Due to the extreme centralization of political power in the Soviet system, a few key individuals have enormous impact on the political process. The personal preferences and idiosyncrasies of these men can be exceptionally important—witness the impacts on Soviet politics of Stalin's suspicious nature, Khrushchev's rambunctious "hare-brained scheming," Brezhnev's conservative, consensus-oriented style, and Gorbachev's dynamic leadership during their respective tenures.

With regard to defense, the styles and per-

spectives of key Soviet leaders have had their effect. Stalin extended his personal domination of Soviet politics into defense matters, where he directly controlled the weapons acquisition process and, during World War II, forcefully supervised Soviet military operations against Nazi Germany and imperial Japan from Moscow. After World War II, he pushed for the acquisition of nuclear weapons and modern delivery systems while insisting on the glorification of his own doctrinal insights gleaned from the war.

Khrushchev's personal preferences and style were similarly important once he had firmly established his political preeminence. His rise to power between 1953 and 1957 was aided critically by his outspoken support of heavy industry and defense spending (in contrast to Malenkov's incipient consumerism) and his personal links with several military commanders with whom he had worked closely while serving as a senior political commissar during World War II. Nevertheless, from the late 1950s until his removal from power in October 1964, Khrushchev engaged in a determined effort to reshape Soviet military strategy and force posture in conformance with his personal views on the dominant role of nuclear-armed missiles, the decreased requirements for large theater ground and air forces, the uselessness of large naval combatants, and, in general, the need to reduce inherently "wasteful and unproductive" defense expenditures.[104] However, due to the determined opposition of the military and like-minded civilian "metal eaters" (as Khrushchev called them), he never achieved his major objectives. Yet the defense policy initiatives that he launched have had a lasting impact on Soviet force posture and military doctrine.

Brezhnev's personal influence on defense policy was less evident. He was obviously proud of his accomplishments as a political commissar during World War II, when he rose to the rank of major general and saw extensive combat along the southern front. During his final years, Brezhnev increasingly sought public recognition for his alleged military prowess by having himself awarded the rank of marshal of the Soviet Union and being publicly identified as the supreme commander in chief of the armed forces and chairman of the Defense Council. Although his "Tula line" declarations heralded a new public emphasis on the non-threatening nature of Soviet military objectives, Brezhnev allowed the military to develop new operational concepts and organizational arrangements for theater warfare without interference and consistently supported an across-the-board expansion of Soviet military power, although this support became less generous in the last few years of his rule.

Mikhail Gorbachev became general secretary with little experience in defense issues. He was too young to have served in World War II and had spent much of his career first as a regional Party leader and then as the Central Committee secretary for agriculture. His exposure to military issues did not begin until he joined the Defense Council after Brezhnev's death in November 1983. Since that time, however, and particularly after becoming the general secretary in February 1985, Gorbachev has undoubtedly been deeply involved in the full range of defense matters. Shifts at the top of the military high command have allowed him to remove several senior military commanders, thus providing him with the opportunity to appoint a new team in the Ministry of Defense.

In the process of his multifaceted *perestroika* ("restructuring") assault on virtually all aspects of the Soviet political and economic system designed to shake the Soviet people out of their sluggish ways, the dynamic Gorbachev has not spared the military. Moreover, Gorbachev, with the assistance of some of his key advisers, became increasingly outspoken in articulating a new approach to Soviet national security policy. Under Mr. Brezhnev, the Ministry of Defense controlled almost exclusively the processes of establishing basic security objectives, assessing external threats, elaborating doctrinal concepts, defining military requirements, developing force programs, and assessing their relative effectiveness. By raising questions about basic national security assumptions and sponsoring a far-reaching debate about crucial aspects of Soviet defense policy under the banners of "new political thinking" and "reasonable sufficiency," as dis-

cussed above—a debate whose participants include for the first time a group of civilian academics as well as the usual military professionals—Mr. Gorbachev is, in Stephen Meyer's phrase, moving to recapture control of the national security agenda.[105]

Gorbachev's new approach includes an ambitious arms control agenda that includes both highly utopian elements and more pragmatic dimensions that eventually could pose a fundamental challenge to the military's long-established views on defense matters. The extraordinary negotiating role played by Marshal S. F. Akhromeyev, then chief of the General Staff, during the Reagan-Gorbachev "presummit" in Reykjavik in October 1986 indicated that, at least with regard to several of the critical issues of deep reductions in nuclear strike systems, Gorbachev appeared to have succeeded in gaining the support of the professional military in this undertaking. The dynamic Gorbachev is likely to be challenged to maintain this support if he pushes the more visionary elements of his arms control agenda, with their implications for very deep reductions and a radical reshaping of Soviet nuclear and conventional forces, while also proceeding with his program for economic revitalization that compels him to continue to limit the growth of, or possibly even cut back, the defense budget.

The marshals have had little choice but to adjust to reduced growth in the defense budget in the late 1970s and 1980s, and, more recently, to the burgeoning discussion of the most fundamental issues of Soviet defense policy. The pressures generated by the fundamental systemic crisis facing the Soviet system and Gorbachev's apparent determination to sponsor significant innovation in Soviet arms control and defense policy are such that the military will be hard pressed to protect its institutional interests and privileges.

Recurring Issues and Defense Policy Outputs

CIVIL-MILITARY RELATIONS

The Soviet military is a significant element not only in the bureaucratic struggles of Soviet politics, but also in the broader aspects of Soviet life. As just discussed, thanks to its near monopoly of relevant information and expertise prior to the Gorbachev period, the military has long wielded substantial influence on the development and implementation of Soviet defense policy. Moreover, in terms of the personnel involved, its far-flung activities, and its vast expenditures, the sheer size of the Soviet defense effort is such that the military establishment has multiple direct and indirect effects beyond the sphere of defense-related activities.

Civilian Control of the Military. Despite the importance of its contribution to the system, the Soviet military has consistently operated under very firm civilian control exerted by the senior Communist Party leadership. This subordinate position has been demonstrated repeatedly. For example, when their performance was deemed unacceptable or possibly politically threatening, civilian leaders have removed the most senior military figures including Marshal Zhukov (1957), Marshal Zakharov (1963), Marshal Ogarkov (1984), Marshal Sokolov (1987), Marshal Tukachevskiy (1937), and several others who were executed in Stalin's deadly purges of the late 1930s.

Most recently, as noted above, the Soviet military has come under substantial public criticism as Gorbachev's generalized *perestroika* assault on Soviet society has gained momentum. This campaign had become increasingly evident in the early months of 1987 and was accelerated significantly following the embarrassing flight of young Mr. Rust and spectacular landing in front of the Kremlin in May of that year. A spate of articles has indicated that the military is in the midst of a process of intensive criticism both from within and without. In the words of one veteran Western observer: "At no other time since the era of Khrushchev a generation earlier, have the political clout, the visibility and the prestige of the armed forces been as low as today."[106]

Led by Army General Yazov, the military leadership began speaking self-critically about the poor state of discipline, training, and combat readiness in the Soviet armed forces. The performance of the officer corps in particular has been strongly condemned by senior military and civilian spokesmen alike. The officers are being called upon to abandon arrogant behavior, "cronyism," and empty "formalistic" approaches to training. They are being exhorted to exhibit instead increased personal responsibility, "exactingness," realistic training, and a genuine concern for the welfare of their men.

The Party leadership, nevertheless, has continued to find it advantageous to encourage the military to play a major role in the indoctrination of Soviet youth prior to their conscription into the armed forces. The Ministry of Defense helps conduct an extensive "military-patriotic education" campaign directed at Soviet young people, the many paramilitary activities of the Volunteer Society for the Support of the Army, Navy, and Air Force (Russian acronym: DOSAAF), and the compulsory civil defense and preinduction training programs conducted within the school system.[107] All of these efforts, although they involve a wide range of Party and government organizations, are directed and actively supported by the Ministry of Defense.

While most of these types of programs have been in existence since the 1920s, their scope was expanded significantly in the late 1960s. At that time, it appears, the Party and the military struck a bargain that brought an expansion of the military-patriotic education effort and the initiation of the compulsory preinduction training programs in exchange for military acquiescence to a one-year reduction in the compulsory service obligation of Soviet conscripts.

These extensive programs, which persist today, reflect the genuine community of interest between the senior Party and military leaderships. Both groups are determined to do all they can to foster intense patriotic commitment to the nation, a proper Marxist-Leninist viewpoint, a sense of discipline, and basic military skills among Soviet youth. Their general desires in this regard are probably intensified by their common perceptions of the need to combat vigorously the unmilitary and apolitical attitudes that have emerged among Soviet urban youth in the past several years.

While the military has considerable impact on the Soviet domestic scene because of the budgetary priority accorded its substantial ar-

mament programs and its broader defense preparedness activities, the military leadership
does not appear to play a direct role in shaping
Soviet domestic policies beyond the defense
sphere. Senior defense figures, including recent Defense Ministers Sokolov and Yazov,
have infrequently commented publicly on nondefense matters. The presence of General
Yazov on the Politburo, albeit as a candidate
member rather than a full member, provides
an opportunity for the minister of defense to be
heard in critical deliberations on the full range
of domestic issues. Nevertheless, there is little
reason to believe that the military plays a leading role in the formulation, analysis, decision,
or implementation of policies with regard to
such matters as economic reform, agricultural
policy, or cultural policy. Its low profile in this
regard reflects a well-established tradition that
allows the Soviet military significant participation and influence in defense matters directly
affecting its corporate interests while discouraging it from involvement in broader issues.

This pattern is reinforced by the fact that
the regime provides significant benefits to the
officer corps in the form of generous pay and
other material benefits, personal security, high
status, and substantial career mobility opportunities, as well as unstinting support of the
nation's defense efforts. One student of Soviet
politics has argued that the military's lack of
involvement in broader societal issues is further reinforced by the fact that, despite its
presence in garrisons, bases, and headquarters
throughout the country, the military is largely a
self-sufficient organization and has only minimal ties with local communities and regional
government and Party organizations.[108]

The military profession has traditionally enjoyed a good reputation in Soviet society. In the
wake of World War II, the standing of the officer corps in the eyes of the general public was
especially high in recognition of its role in repelling the Nazi invaders. By the mid 1960s,
two opinion surveys of Soviet secondary school
students and teachers indicated that the career
of the mililtary officer ranked at approximately the 25 percent level in terms of attractiveness among a wide range of occupations
evaluated.[109] Over the past two decades, the
standing of the Soviet military appears to have
declined somewhat, almost certainly as a result
of the spread of apathy and unmilitary attitudes among a large segment of urbanized Soviet youth. It is precisely this undesirable trend
that has prompted the Soviet military leadership to complain regularly about this development and to devote substantial efforts to try to
propagate a positive view of the role of the
armed forces in the Soviet system.[110]

Main Political Administration. Any review
of Soviet civil-military relations must include a
discussion of the activities of the Main Political
Administration. In the first years of Soviet
rule, the political commissars of the MPA were
assigned two important tasks: monitoring the
political reliability of the officer corps, many of
whom had served in the Russian imperial
army, and indoctrinating both enlisted men
and officers with the proper communist outlook. In the first decade, a third task was
added: the political officers came to share the
responsibilities of the military commanders for
the combat readiness and discipline of their
units.[111]

Over the years, the watchdog function of the
political officers has declined considerably.
This task has largely fallen to the so-called special sections of the KGB, which guard against
espionage and anti-Soviet activity within the
military by means of a network of KGB officers and their informers recruited throughout
the armed forces. Rather than serving as an
alien checking agency within the military, the
political officers of the MPA have become an
integral part of the Soviet military establishment. Political officers today are, in their own
right, career military professionals who have
chosen to pursue the indoctrinational and organizational specialities of the MPA. Their
professional military orientation is reflected in
recruitment patterns. For several decades, the
majority of young political officers has been
drawn from the ranks of junior officers in the
combat services. Since 1971, new political officers have also been supplied each year by the
graduating classes of the MPA's seven higher
military commissioning schools first opened in
1967.

Although the political officers are career

military professionals, they may occasionally find themselves in conflict with line officers. The commanders and their political deputies (*zampolits*) share mutual interests in having units that are well trained, disciplined, and properly politically indoctrinated. Nevertheless, there is bound to be periodic conflict between the commanders and the political officers over a scarce commodity, training time of the personnel that both commanders and *zampolits* seek to utilize.

The political officers must attend to a host of duties: the conduct of political education for all personnel, the maintenance of morale and discipline, individual welfare, the encouragement of technical competence, and the supervision of the operation of the Party and Komsomol organizations found throughout the armed forces. Although many of these activities are likely to be supported by the commanders, the time required may well impinge on the time the commanders would like to devote to improving the military skills and combat readiness of their forces. Friction between commanders and present-day commissars is relatively unimportant, however, and far different from the intense Party-military conflict that has sometimes been depicted in the past.[112]

Military-Political Friendships. Finally, Soviet civil-military relations have often included personal ties between important civilian figures and the senior military leadership. During wartime, in particular, Party politicians often have found themselves in close contact with key military commanders, and political alliances have sometimes emerged. Such was the case with both Stalin and Khrushchev, who developed lasting patronage ties with military officers during the defense of the same city, called first Tsaritsyn, then Stalingrad, during the Civil War and World War II respectively.[113] Over forty years after the end of World War II, these wartime clusterings have lost their significance. One might anticipate a somewhat weaker set of alliance patterns of the same general character to emerge in peacetime between regional Party secretaries and the commanders of the military districts. Regional Party secretaries are, in fact, members of the military

councils of these military districts; yet if Colton is right about the largely autarkic tendencies of the military units, Party-military contacts in the field are not likely to be very substantial.

Personal contacts between senior civilians and key military officers are likely to occur more often and to be more substantive, and thus more important, at the "center" in Moscow. Several memoir accounts testify to the existence of close Party-military working relationships in Moscow, where senior military leaders promote their corporate and individual views on defense matters in routine contacts with key Party and government officials.[114] Western speculation about Marshal Ogarkov's somewhat surprising selection as chief of the General Staff in January 1977 often centered, for example, on rumors of the respect he was reported to have earned from Defense Minister Ustinov in the course of their joint involvement in the Strategic Arms Limitation Talks. Yet a few years later Ogarkov and Ustinov were sharply disagreeing publicly on a host of issues, and eventually Ogarkov was ousted as chief of the General Staff, almost certainly as a precautionary measure to prevent him from succeeding the ailing Ustinov, who died a few months later.

Most recently, Gorbachev's rather surprising choice in May 1987 of Army General Yazov to succeed Marshal Sokolov as Minister of Defense appears to have had an intriguing personal patronage dimension. General Yazov had become the Deputy Minister of Defense for Cadres in early 1987. An article that appeared in *Krasnaya zvezda* on 15 January 1987 revealed that General Yazov, then the commander of the Far East Military District, had spoken bluntly during a large meeting of military officers with the General Secretary (when Gorbachev was visiting the Far East the previous summer) of shortcomings in military discipline within his command. Thus, it appears that General Yazov's initial move to Moscow and subsequent selection to replace Marshal Sokolov is likely to have been the result of his having strongly impressed Gorbachev during this serendipitous meeting that he was the right man to lead a vigorous "restructuring" effort within the Ministry of Defense. It will remain to be seen whether this apparent patronage relationship will tie General Yazov firmly to Mikhail Gorbachev in the years ahead in the face of what will almost certainly be substantial strains over decisions regarding resource allocation, force posture, and arms control policy.

WEAPONS ACQUISITION AND FORCE POSTURE

Over the past six decades, the Soviets have built up a well-entrenched military-industrial complex of organizations engaged in the research, development, and production of armaments. These include research institutes, weapons design bureaus, and production facilities, as well as military, government, and Party bodies that help manage various phases of the weapons acquisition process. Western understanding of the dynamics of Soviet weapons acquisition has increased substantially in recent years.[115] The following observations summarize some of the key aspects of the process.

The dynamics of Soviet weapons acquisition includes a mixture of "demand-pull" and "design-push," developments. In the former case the design and production organs of the defense industrial ministries develop and produce weapons in response to specifications laid down by the armed forces to provide the capabilities needed to meet the operational requirements derived from Soviet military doctrine. There is also clear evidence of "design-push," where armaments are produced as a result of the entrepreneurial initiatives of the major designers, who "sell" their latest weapons ideas to their military customers and key political leaders.

Over the years, the Soviet Union has developed well-established patterns of weapons development. These include widespread use of competitions among two or more design bureaus that extend through the competitive testing of full-scale prototypes; simplicity in the use of austere, uncomplicated, and frequently crudely finished subsystems; and significant conservatism in the development of new weapons, reflected in the high degree of design inheritance from one generation of weapons to another manifested in the frequent use of proven components and incremental changes in design when such changes are made.[116] This general pattern has not, however, kept the Soviets from making significant innovations on a periodic basis as occurred in the 1980s with the development and deployment of the MiG-29 Fulcrum fighter-interceptor and the family of modern air- and sea-launched cruise missiles.

The nine ministries predominantly engaged in weapons production represent the most privileged sector of the Soviet economy. They are supplied with the most advanced equipment, the most talented scientific and technical personnel, priority access to scarce resources, and high status, high pay, and other material benefits for their employees. Many of the key participants in Soviet weapons development and production, including the leading designers, industrial ministers, and Party and government overseers, have spent decades in their senior posts, thus adding the important elements of close personal ties, extensive experience, and continuity to the acquisition process.

There are several links between the design and production facilities of the defense production ministries and their military customers. One of the most important of these is the strict quality control of defense-related products enforced by the military representatives from the weapons directorates of the services who are attached to each major production plant and design bureau.[117]

The systems that emerge from the weapons acquisition process represent a major input into the aggregate of military capabilities fielded by the Soviet Union. The size and quality of this force posture reflect both the predominant design practices that characterize Soviet weapons development and acquisition and the considerable political clout of the Soviet military-industrial complex.

Other factors that influence the character of Soviet force posture include the views of the political and military leadership on the threats and opportunities facing the Soviet Union, their judgments as to the most effective military force deployments to respond to this environment, and the tenets of Soviet military doctrine that help guide the Ministry of Defense, particularly the General Staff, in establishing requirements for both the production and the possible employment of specific military capabilities.

Strategic Nuclear Forces. Since entering the nuclear age in 1949, the Soviet Union has consistently striven to develop and deploy offensive and defensive forces that add nuclear muscle to its military power and could reduce the damage an adversary might inflict in the event of war. In the course of three decades, the USSR has deployed a full spectrum of nuclear weapons with virtually all of its forces, ranging from various tactical weapons deployed by the navy, army, and air force to the multimegaton warheads associated with very large intercontinental ballistic missiles (ICBMs). In the process, two new military services have been created, the National Air Defense Forces (PVO Strany) in 1948 (renamed the Air Defense Forces in the late 1970s) and the Strategic Rocket Forces (SRF) in 1959, whose primary wartime missions would be to defend against bomber and missile attacks and to mount strikes with strategic nuclear missiles.

Soviet strategic offensive nuclear strike capabilities include both regional and intercontinental components. In both cases, these capabilities include a mix of land-based ballistic missiles under the control of the SRF, submarine-borne missiles of the navy, and strategic bombers of the air force's "shock" air armies. The elements of the Soviet strategic triad are not equally balanced in their contributions to Soviet nuclear strike capabilities.

The ICBM component, including third-generation SS-11s and SS-13s, fourth-generation SS-17s, SS-18s, and SS-19s, and fifth-generation SS-25s, provides 60 percent of the Soviet Union's 10,900 intercontinental-range weapons, thus making it the predominant element among the so-called central strategic forces. The submarine-launched ballistic missiles (SLBMs) of the Yankee, Delta, and Typhoon class nuclear-powered submarines armed with the SS-N-6, SS-N-8, SS-N-18, SS-N-20, and SS-N-23 missiles account for some 31 percent of the intercontinental-range warheads, while the air forces' Bear bombers provide the remaining 9 percent of these weapons. The

Badgers, Blinders, and Backfires of the air force and naval aviation account for 71 percent of the regional strategic strike weapons, while the SRF's intermediate-and medium-range ballistic missiles, the older SS-4s and newer, mobile SS-20s (being eliminated under the INF treaty) provide 28 percent, and Golf-class subs carrying the SS-N-5 provide the remaining 1 percent.[118]

Over the years, the USSR has steadily sought to improve both the survivability and the attack effectiveness of its strategic nuclear forces. The quest for survivability has led it to deploy its land-based missiles in successive generations of increasingly harder reinforced-concrete silos, and, in the case of intermediate-range SS-20s and intercontinental SS-25s, in road-mobile configurations. The USSR has also developed the SS-24 ICBM, carrying up to ten MIRVs, which began to be deployed in a rail-mobile configuration beginning in the fall of 1987. It has also deployed SLBMs on increasingly "quiet" submarines that are more difficult to detect acoustically. In the same vein, it has sought to provide a highly survivable command and control apparatus to direct these forces by deploying a host of hardened command bunkers, mobile truckborne, airborne, and trainborne command posts, and highly redundant communications facilities.

The Soviet quest for more effective strategic missile forces has been concentrated on efforts to increase the numbers of warheads carried by missiles and to improve their accuracy. The centerpiece of this effort has been their deployment of increasingly accurate, multiple independently targetable reentry vehicles (MIRVs) on both ICBMs and SLBMs, a process that began in the mid 1970s.

The Soviet MIRV program has been assisted significantly by the development and deployment of large, heavy-payload strategic missiles dating back to the earliest days of Soviet missile development. In the 1950s, the USSR was forced to develop large rocket boosters for its military and space programs in order to compensate for its relative backwardness in both nuclear weapons design and electronics miniaturization. This approach continued in the 1960s with the development of

ICBMs as large as the "heavy" SS-9, which carried either a single large multimegaton warhead or a "triplet" consisting of three reentry vehicles (RVs) dispensed in a cluster pattern without individual independent targeting capability. With the dawn of the Soviet MIRV era in the 1970s, they were able to take advantage of the high-payload capacity, or "throw weight," of their fourth-generation ICBMs, in particular the massive SS-18 and the SS-19, which carry up to ten and six MIRVs respectively.

While the USSR was rapidly expanding its ICBM-borne weapons inventory, it also made major improvements in the accuracy of its missiles. By the late 1970s it had acquired the ability to place at risk a substantial part of hardened U.S. military facilities, the most numerous of which were the fixed silos housing Minuteman ICBMs. Thus, by 1980, the Soviet Union was rapidly achieving one of its highest priority doctrinal objectives, the ability to attack the ICBM component of the U.S. strategic nuclear arsenal effectively.[119]

As it enters the 1990s, the Soviet ICBM force consists of 1,404 missiles: 420 SS-11s, 60 SS-13s, and 126 SS-25s (all carrying single RV equivalents); and 130 SS-17s (four RVs), 308 SS-18s (up to ten RVs), 350 SS-19s (up to six RVs), and 20 SS-24s (ten RVs) within the MIRVed portion of the force.[120] Continuing deployments of the new mobile SS-24 and SS-25 missiles as well as an SS-18 follow-on that may be even more powerful than the current SS-18, will further enhance Soviet ICBM capabilities. The ultimate size of the Soviet ICBM force in the 1990s will depend critically on possible arms control constraints. The new generation mobiles could simply be added to the existing forces or could substitute for current silo-based systems within overall reduced ceilings, should such limits eventually emerge from the Geneva negotiations.

Over the years the Soviet Union has produced several combinations of ballistic missiles and missile-carrying submarines. These include the 350-mile-range SS-N-4 on the diesel-powered Z-V-class submarines and the SS-N-4 and SS-N-5 on the diesel-powered Golf- and

Hotel-classes of subs deployed in the 1950s; numerous Yankee-class nuclear subs (SSBNs) deployed in the late 1960s and early 1970s carrying the 1,750- to 2,000-mile-range SS-N-6; Delta I and Delta II subs with the 4,800-mile-range SS-N-8 added in the mid-to-late 1970s; Delta III SSBNs with the over 5,000-mile-range SS-N-18, which carries three or seven MIRVs, deployed in the late 1970s and early 1980s; and, finally, Delta IV subs with the long-range SS-N-23, carrying four to ten MIRVs, and Typhoon-class SSBNs with the similarly long-range SS-N-20, with six to nine MIRVs, deployed in the mid 1980s.[121]

For a variety of geographical, technological, and logistical reasons, the Soviets have consistently deployed only a small portion of their SSBN force on peacetime patrols at sea where they are capable of launching strikes on short notice against the United States. They maintain an at-sea, day-to-day alert rate of approximately 20 percent of their SSBN force.[122] The Soviet Union apparently continues to count on the occurrence of a period of heightened tensions preceding any major conflict that will allow it to deploy rapidly from their Northern and Pacific Fleet home ports the considerable number of SSBNs in port that are not inoperable due to major refit overhaul. The long range of the SS-N-8, SS-N-19, SS-N-20, and SS-N-23, which allows them to cover targets in the United States from waters near their home ports, gives added credibility to this strategy. However, barring such a force generation during a crisis, the majority of Soviet strategic missile submarines are routinely tied up in port, and thus highly vulnerable.

Once at sea, the vast majority of Soviet strategic missile submarines are reportedly significantly noisier than U.S. SSBNs or attack submarines (SSNs). This makes them vulnerable to possible acoustic detection and attack by U.S. antisubmarine warfare (ASW) systems, an area in which the United States long enjoyed a considerable technological edge. Recognizing this, the USSR has deployed the "bastion" or "enclave" defense approach noted earlier, in which submarines, surface ships, and airborne ASW assets are employed in combination to protect the Delta and Typhoon SSBNs, which can hold U.S. targets at risk from the Barents and Norwegian Seas or the Sea of Okhotsk. Since the early 1980s the Soviets have reportedly deployed some of their SSBNs beneath the polar icecap, where ASW detection and tracking are more difficult, and have developed techniques for launching their SLBMs from this area.

The Soviet long-range strategic submarine force at the beginning of the 1990s consisted of four Typhoon subs, each with twenty SS-N-20s (six or nine MIRVs); three Delta IV subs, each with sixteen SS-N-23s (ten MIRVs); fourteen Delta III subs, each with sixteen SS-N-18s (three or seven MIRVs); four Delta IIs, each with sixteen SS-N-8s (single RV); eighteen Delta Is, each with twelve SS-N-8s; and sixteen Yankees, each carrying sixteen SS-N-6s (single RV).[123] In the years ahead, the number of weapons carried by this element of the Soviet strategic triad will increase substantially with the continuing deployments of MIRVed SS-N-20 and SS-N-23 missiles on Typhoon and Delta IV submarines while Yankee- and earlier Delta-class subs carrying single RV missiles will probably be retired.

The least powerful element of the Soviet long-range strategic arsenal has long been its intercontinental bomber force. Yet with the continuing deployments of modern air-launched cruise missiles (ALCMs) and the likely addition of a new heavy bomber, the Blackjack, this force is in the process of a dramatic expansion. The backbone of the Soviet bomber force remains its Tu-95 Bear, the majority of which were produced in the 1950s. In recent years the USSR has resumed production of the Bear in the form of the "H" model, which carries eight long-range second-generation AS-15 ALCMs with capabilities similar to the U.S. ALCM. Seventy Bear H as well as 95 older Bear A, B, C, and G model bombers carrying two to six gravity bombs or older cruise missiles are still in active service. Eleven prototypes of the new Blackjack bombers have been produced and flight-tested and it appears that substantial numbers of this bomber, which likely will carry modern cruise missiles, short-range attack missiles, or gravity bombs, will have been added to the Soviet central strategic forces by the early 1990s.[124]

The bombers are supported by a modest aerial refueling tanker force of some thirty Bison and twenty Tu-16 Badger converted bombers. These tanker capabilities are being improved significantly with the deployment of the new Midas tanker, an aerial refueling variant of the Il-76 Candid transport aircraft.

The USSR also maintains very sizable regional strategic nuclear forces capable of striking targets in Europe and Asia. Prior to the signing of the 1987 U.S.–Soviet INF treaty, the land-based element consisted primarily of 441 road-mobile SS-20 intermediate-range missiles, each carrying three MIRVs, roughly two-thirds of which were deployed in garrisons in the USSR within range of Western Europe with the remainder covering targets in Asia. In accordance with the treaty, all are to have been dismantled and destroyed by mid 1991. The centerpiece of the bomber component is the Tu-22M Backfire bomber, whose deployment began in the mid 1970s. Some 290 of these bombers are split roughly equally between the air force's "shock" air armies and naval aviation. These newer missile and bomber systems are supplemented by 407 Tu-16 Badger and Tu-22 Blinder bombers in the two regional air armies, and 260 Tu-22 Blinder and Tu-16 Badger bombers in naval aviation. Thirteen older Golf II submarines, each carrying three single RV SS-N-5 missiles, provide a sea-based component for regional nuclear strike operations in Europe and Asia.[125]

Strategic Defense. The USSR has long maintained a large and expensive strategic air and missile defense capability. As the USSR entered the 1990s, the Soviet Air Defense Forces fielded some 9,000 surface-to-air missiles, up to 2,250 fighter-interceptors, and a comprehensive radar early warning and control network. The Air Defense Forces also control the antiballistic missile (ABM) system deployed around Moscow and the co-orbital antisatellite system, which has been operational since the early 1970s at the Tyuratam Space Complex. Since a reorganization in the late 1970s, the Air Defense Forces have also been responsible for training and equipping the mobile surface-to-air missile (SAM) units that provide the ground-based air defense coverage for Soviet ground force units.

Despite enormous exertions to erect a vast antiaircraft defense network, the USSR has only recently begun to erect a defense that would likely be effective against enemy bombers such as the U.S. B-52 penetrating at low levels. At long last, they have begun to correct their chronic low-altitude deficiency through the fielding of: (1) the modern Mainstay airborne warning and control system (AWACS) based on the Il-76 Candid; (2) "lookdown, shoot-down" radar capabilities and improved air-to-air missiles carried on the MiG-31 Foxhound, Su-27 Flanker, and MiG-29 Fulcrum fighters; and (3) new, more effective surface-to-air missiles, the SA-10 and the SA-12A.[126] With the deployment of these systems in substantial numbers, Soviet strategic air defenses will become considerably more effective against aircraft and cruise missiles penetrating at low altitudes. It is not clear, however, that these upgraded air defenses will be highly effective against the U.S. B-1B bomber and air-launched cruise missiles, let alone against the advanced technology ("stealth") bomber or the stealth advanced cruise missiles slated to be added to the U.S. arsenal early in the 1990s.

Soviet ABM and ballistic missile attack warning and tracking capabilities are also being significantly upgraded. These capabilities currently consist of a series of infrared launch detection satellites and eleven older "Hen House" radars located at six sites in the Soviet Union. The latter radars are being supplemented with the construction of a new network of nine large phased array radars (LPARs). When fully operational in the mid 1990s, this network will provide complete 360° coverage around the USSR.[127] One of these, the notorious Krasnoyarsk radar, is located in south central Siberia and oriented northeast, looking across some 4,000 kilometers of Soviet territory. This clearly violates Article VI of the ABM treaty, which stipulates that ballistic missile early warning and tracking radars must be located around the periphery of a superpower's

territory and oriented outward. (The other eight new Soviet LPARs are reportedly sited in conformance with these ABM treaty provisions.) The United States has called this violation to the attention of the Soviet Union, demanding that the Krasnoyarsk radar be dismanted completely. In response, the Soviets announced that work on the radar had been halted in 1987 and offered to convert it into an internationally-manned space tracking facility. On the other hand, they have neither acknowledged that it violates the ABM treaty nor indicated a willingness to dismantle it.

The Soviet Union has a variety of ABM systems under development and actively deployed in the field. The only deployed system is the Galosh complex that has been emplaced around Moscow since the late 1960s. It is currently being improved and expanded from sixty-four to the full one hundred interceptor launchers permitted under the ABM treaty. Two new interceptor missiles, the long-range modified Galosh and high-acceleration Gazelle, both housed in underground launch silos, are being deployed, and a large new phased array "Pill-box" battle-management radar at Pushkino has been added.[128] The Soviets have also developed the ABM-X-3 system, whose original development and testing dates from the early 1970s. Although testing of this system, which includes the Gazelle high-acceleration missile and the transportable "Flat Twin" and "Pawn Shop" radars, reportedly has been halted, it could be deployed to defend a selected region in a matter of several months. On the other hand, emplacement of a series of regional ABM-X-3 radar sites integrated with the existing ballistic missile detection and tracking network would almost certainly take several years. Such a deployment would, of course, represent a violation of the ABM treaty. In light of the obvious Soviet desire so evident in the Geneva negotiations to preserve and even strengthen the ABM treaty, as a means to limit U.S. high technology ballistic missile defense research efforts under the Strategic Defense Initiative, Soviet incentives for "breaking out" from the treaty appear extremely low.

Other strategic defense programs include

antisubmarine warfare efforts and the damage limitation measures associated with the extensive Soviet civil defense program. Soviet acoustic ASW capabilities are, by all reports, grossly inadequate for the task of locating U.S. SSBNs. This shortcoming almost certainly lies behind the decision to reorient the use of these ASW forces to help defend Soviet SSBNs in nearby waters, using the bastion defense concept. Perhaps spurred on by these difficulties, the USSR has investigated a variety of nonacoustic submarine detection means.[129] In the mid 1980s, the Soviets achieved a major advance in the "quieting" of their attack submarines in the new Akula class. Its deployment in substantial numbers in the 1990s will add new uncertainties to the undersea war. Given the magnitude of the U.S. effort in SLBMs and the high priority the Soviet Union assigns to damage limitation, there is little doubt that it will continue to devote substantial efforts to making a breakthrough in strategic antisubmarine warfare.

Soviet civil defense efforts, although supervised by a directorate in the Ministry of Defense, involve the participation of many other organizations, including elements of the Party and government bureaucracies as well as most urban-based economic enterprises and educational institutions. The Soviet Union provides fallout shelters in or near major urban areas for the political and military leadership and a share of the essential work force.[130] Over 1,500 bunkers have reportedly been constructed throughout the USSR to protect more than 175,000 key Party and government personnel.[131] For the protection of the majority of the populace, the Soviet leaders apparently intend to rely upon large-scale dispersal and evacuation, followed by the construction of temporary shelters.

The books and pamphlets published by the full-time Soviet civil defense bureaucracy are generally optimistic about the ability of the Soviet Union to survive and function effectively after a nuclear war. Western analyses are considerably less sanguine in this regard, although it is generally agreed that if circumstances permitted the USSR a week or so to implement the full range of its protective measures, it could appreciably limit fatalities, perhaps to a few tens of millions. These efforts could not, however, prevent the USSR from suffering massive industrial damage.[132]

Theater Forces. The traditional backbone of Russia's military power was its large army, manned by masses of hardy peasants and frequently supported by large concentrations of field artillery. The Soviet Army today continues to reflect its heritage: it is large, its conscript soldiers are tough, and it has impressive firepower, both conventional and nuclear. But it is much more than that, having been fully motorized and equipped with a wide variety of highly effective tanks and armored fighting vehicles, as well as some of the world's most modern tactical missiles, antitank weapons, and mobile air defense missiles and guns. Moreover, it is supported by a large and increasingly capable tactical air arm, whose major elements are fighter-interceptors, fighter-bombers, and armed helicopters. The net result is the world's largest and most powerful standing army, led by a well-trained, dedicated officer corps and prepared to wage armor-heavy, blitzkrieg warfare with considerable air support in various theaters around the Soviet Union.

Plans announced by Gorbachev to be effective early in the 1990s include reduction in the size of the armed forces by some 500,000 troops, withdrawing and disbanding six tank divisions from Eastern Europe. Forces in Soviet Asia and Mongolia would also be reduced "significantly." In terms of military hardware, some 10,000 tanks, 8,500 artillery systems, and 800 combat aircraft would be eliminated.

Prior to any such reductions and as the USSR enters the 1990s, the Soviet ground forces field a total of 214 divisions, of which 52 are tank divisions, 150 motorized rifle divisions, 7 airborne divisions, and 5 unmanned mobilization base divisions. These troops are deployed throughout the sixteen military districts in the USSR, in Eastern Europe, and in Mongolia. Within the Soviet Union, the heaviest concentrations are in the European USSR (the Baltic, Byelorussian, Carpathian, Kiev, Leningrad, Odessa, and Moscow military districts), where 97 divisions are posted, and facing China (the Central Asian, Siberian, Transbaikal, and Far Eastern military districts, plus the army in Mongolia), where there are 56 divisions.[133]

Soviet divisions differ in composition. The largest, best-equipped units are posted with the groups of forces in Eastern Europe. A fully equipped motorized rifle division in Eastern Europe contains approximately 13,000 troops and up to 271 main battle tanks, while a fully equipped tank division is staffed by 11,000 personnel and equipped with up to 328 tanks.[134] Divisions in the USSR are somewhat smaller, with varying numbers of troops and equipment. The seven airborne divisions, all posted within the Soviet Union, are much smaller, numbering approximately 7,000 troops each, equipped with their own specially designed light-armored fighting vehicles and artillery, and supported by military transport aviation (VTA) aircraft.

Not all of the 214 divisions of the Soviet armed forces are fully staffed. There are three degrees of readiness: category 1 divisions are more than 75 percent manned and fully equipped; category 2 divisions are between 50 percent and 75 percent staffed and fully stocked; and category 3 divisions are only 25 percent staffed and, if fully equipped, much of the equipment is obsolete. The category 1 divisions can be brought to full strength in twenty-four hours. The category 2 units can be filled out with mobilized reservists within a few weeks. The category 3 divisions can be brought up to full strength in eight to nine weeks by the mobilization of the extensive reserve system, as was done in the late fall of 1979 to provide the bulk of the troops that invaded Afghanistan.[135]

All of the thirty divisions in Eastern Europe are category 1 and about 20 percent of the divisions in the European USSR are in categories 1 or 2. The vast majority of divisions throughout the remainder of the USSR are apparently in category 3.[136]

In peacetime these divisions, along with their supporting aviation elements, are controlled by the commanders of groups of forces or military districts, who operate under the direction of the General Staff. In time of war, the divisions in all of the groups of forces and most of the military districts would be filled out as necessary with reservists and integrated into fronts composed of four to five combined-arms armies and a tank army—that is, approximately twenty to twenty-five motorized rifle and tank divisions, along with air support elements and a host of combat and support elements—and moved out to conduct offensive operations in adjacent theaters of military operations. The airborne divisions, although an element of the ground forces, appear to fall under the direct control of the minister of defense. In wartime they may be attached to a field command—a front or the high command of a theater of military operations(TVD)—or remain under the direct control of Supreme Headquarters in Moscow.

The level of Soviet investment in defense is amply reflected in the steady improvement in the weapons systems needed to equip this two-million-man army. The latest Soviet main battle tanks (T-64, T-72, and T-80), the BMP fighting vehicle, self-propelled 122-mm and 152-mm howitzers, mobile air defense systems (SA-11, SA-12A, SA-13, SA-14, and SA-16 missile systems and ZSU 23/4 self-propelled antiaircraft gun), and SS-21 and SS-23 tactical missiles are all among the most modern and capable in the world. In addition, the Soviet leaders have taken the prospect of warfare with chemical, biological, and nuclear weapons very seriously, and their forces are extensively trained and equipped to fight in such environments.[137]

In sum, the continuing accumulation of new equipment has significantly increased both the firepower and the mobility of the Soviet combined-arms assault formations to the point where they have a greatly increased capacity to mass the large numbers of armored vehicles and conventional fire support on the main axes of attack needed to meet the armament norms of 3:1 to 5:1 margins of local superiority called for by their conservative military doctrine.[138] Consequently, the USSR is prepared to undertake its multiple breakthrough offensive strategy either relying solely upon conventional firepower or with the support of nuclear weapons.

Soviet tactical aviation is similarly impressive. This force, largely designed to provide support in land battles, is made up of some

4,920 combat aircraft.[139] In recent years, the quality of these aircraft, like that of all the other elements of Soviet military power, has improved dramatically. With the addition in the 1970s and 1980s of third-generation aircraft—the multipurpose MiG-23 Flogger B; the late-model MiG-21 Fishbed J, K, L, and N; the Su-17 Fitter C; the MiG-27 Flogger D; and the Su-24 Fencer—the range and payload capabilities of ground attack aircraft were increased enormously.[140]

The 1980s brought an upgrading of fighter-interceptors to protect ground force formations from enemy air attack with the deployment of "look-down, shoot-down" fighters and the Mainstay airborne warning and control platforms. In addition, beginning in the 1970s, the Soviet Union, clearly emulating U.S. developments of the 1960s, has built up a large force of armed helicopter gunships, including the highly capable Mi-24 Hind A, D, and E, as well as a gunship version of the Mi-8 Hip. These helicopters are equipped for anti-tank and other fire support missions.[141] Moreover, the USSR is on the verge of adding two new attack helicopters, the Mi-28 Havoc and the Hokum, the latter being credited with the capacity to intercept other helicopters.

Soviet fighter, bomber, and helicopter aviation was reorganized in the late 1970s. Today the Soviet Air Forces include the five "shock" air armies of the VGK (the Supreme High Command), the air forces attached to each of the military districts in the USSR and the groups of Soviet forces stationed in Eastern Europe, and military transport aviation. The air forces of the military districts and the groups of Soviet forces include attack helicopters, which are the backbone of a recently resurrected branch of the air force called "Army Aviation." In time of war the vast majority of these armed helicopters, possibly in combination with fixed-wing Su-25 Frogfoot ground attack aircraft, will be directly subordinated to ground force commanders in order to provide close air support to units engaged with enemy forces.

Four of the five air armies of the VGK are positioned to provide support to the high commands of the theaters of military operation in Europe and Asia. The air armies headquartered in Legnica, Poland, and Vinnitsa in the Soviet Ukraine, composed of fighter-bombers, in particular the Su-24 Fencer, fighter-interceptors, and reconnaissance aircraft, are apparently prepared to support campaigns fought with conventional or nuclear weapons in the western and southwestern theaters of operations respectively. The air army headquartered in Smolensk controls the regional strategic Backfire, Blinder, and Badger medium bombers, which can carry out conventional or nuclear strikes throughout the European theater. The fourth theater-oriented air army, headquartered in Irkutsk, controls the full range of fighter-bomber, fighter-interceptor, and reconnaissance aircraft as well as medium bombers. Its units could be employed throughout South Asia and the Far East. The fifth and final air army, headquartered in Moscow, controls the heavy Bear and Bison bombers that are prepared to carry out intercontinental strikes against the United States or to attack major enemy naval formations.[142]

The air forces of the military districts and groups of forces include fighter-bombers, fighter-interceptors, reconnaissance aircraft, transport and attack helicopters, and electronic countermeasures aircraft. The largest of these, the air force attached to the Group of Soviet Forces Germany (GSFG), is reported to have 685 aircraft. The commanders of these air forces serve as deputy air commanders in the military district or group of forces in question.

Many of the aircraft of these air forces, in combination with the fighters, fighter-bombers, and medium bombers of the four regional shock air armies, and possibly conventionally armed tactical ballistic missiles as well, may be employed either in large-scale "air operations" with conventional weapons or in independent efforts to attain air superiority over the main axes of attack or to carry out interdiction attacks against reserve forces, key command posts, and logistics support in the enemy's rear. Close air support for ground forces driving deep behind enemy lines would largely be provided by armed helicopters, and only to a lesser degree by fixed-wing attack aircraft.

Naval Forces. While all of the elements of the Soviet armed forces have steadily increased their capabilities over the past two decades, none has done so more dramatically than the navy. Not only has the navy's nuclear striking power expanded enormously with the deployment of its Yankee-, Delta-, and Typhoon-class nuclear powered strategic missile submarines, but also general naval capabilities have been significantly improved as well. The USSR has attained a genuine blue water capability, based upon a force of 274 modern surface warships of the light frigate class or larger.

These include the first of a new class of large angle-decked Tbilisi-class carriers now undergoing shakedown sea trials, four Kiev-class light aircraft carriers equipped with vertical take-off and landing (VTOL) Yak-36 Forger aircraft; two Moskva-class ASW cruisers; a host of guided missile-equipped Slava-, Kirov-, and Kara-class cruisers; several types of destroyers, including the newer Udaloy and Sovremennyy classes; improved logistics support and amphibious ships, including the Berezina-class fleet oiler and the Ivan Rogov-class amphibious assault transport; and a variety of cruise missile and torpedo-equipped attack submarines, the most impressive of which are the large Oscar-class cruise missile carrier, the high-speed, titanium-hulled Alpha-class attack sub, and the new, very quiet Akula-class SSN.[143] At the same time, land-based Soviet naval aviation has been improved with the addition of the Backfire bomber and the Fencer fighter-bomber.

These new vessels and aircraft have allowed the Soviet Union to increase its visible peacetime presence throughout the world's oceans significantly. More important, they provide the Soviet Navy with greatly enhanced capabilities to fulfill its various wartime missions—mounting nuclear strikes against the United States, neutralizing U.S. carrier task forces, combating American strategic and attack submarines, interdicting the enemy's sea lines of communications, repelling any amphibious assault attempted against the USSR, and conducting amphibious operations along the flanks of its advancing land armies.

Improved naval vessels and aircraft are by no means the full expression of the changing character of the Soviet Navy. Its operational concepts and deployment patterns have also been altered dramatically. These shifts are well captured in the analysis by Michael Mcc-Gwire, a leading Western expert on Soviet naval policy, who describes a steady expansion of the "Soviet maritime defense perimeter" over the past twenty-five years. According to this construct, U.S. carrier and long-range SLBM deployments have compelled the USSR to expand its operations beyond its traditional "inner defense zone." The Soviets have been forced to create an "outer defense zone" that reaches into the North Atlantic, the Mediterranean, the Indian Ocean, and the Western Pacific in order to counter these U.S. strike systems.[144] This process has resulted in a truly ocean-going Soviet naval capability, with obvious potential wartime applications and peacetime uses that have been clearly recognized and increasingly utilized by the Soviet leadership.

FORCE PROJECTION

The USSR has also made significant improvements in its ability to project military power. Its capacity for contiguous force projection—that is, the ability to move military power into areas adjacent to the Soviet Union—is inherent in the extensive theater warfare capabilities discussed earlier. The Soviet moves into Czechoslovakia in 1968 and Afghanistan in 1979, for example, simply involved the application of land and air forces that were trained and equipped to wage theater warfare on the Soviet periphery. Soviet contiguous force projection capabilities have thus grown apace as part and parcel of the steady improvement of theater forces.

The ability to move military forces over long distances well beyond the Soviet frontier is an even more dramatic improvement in Soviet force projection. This has involved the acquisition of new long-range air and sea transport, as well as the development of an embryonic overseas basing infrastructure and the accumulation of greatly increased experience in undertaking such operations. Major developments have been the addition of the An-22 Cock heavy turboprop and Il-76 Candid medium jet transport aircraft in military transport aviation and, on the naval side, the addition of improved transports, including "roll-on, roll-off" ships in the Soviet merchant marine (MORFLOT) and several new vessels that can be used to project power ashore, including the Kiev-class carriers and the Ivan Rogov-class amphibious assault ships.[145] These improved airlift and sealift capabilities are well suited for use by the seven Soviet airborne divisions or by the naval infantry, an 18,000-troop component of the Soviet Navy that is specifically trained and equipped for amphibious assault operations.

Soviet long-distance power projection has been enhanced by the USSR's increased political and military involvement in several Third World countries. These involvements have resulted in significant experience in long-distance movements of troops and equipment, for example, Soviet assistance in air transporting Cuban troops to Angola in 1975–76 and movement of military advisers and equipment by air and sea to such arms assistance clients as Ethiopia, Libya, Vietnam, Iraq, and South Yemen.[146] The latter movements have often been accompanied by the buildup of significant overseas stockpiles of modern Soviet weaponry, which constitute de facto pre-positioned stocks of armaments that might be available to Soviet forces rapidly inserted into these areas in the event of a regional crisis or conflict. More recently, increased Soviet naval operations in the Far East have been accompanied by the expansion and continuous use of Vietnamese port and air facilities at Cam Ranh Bay and Da Nang.[147] This combination of improved long-range transport, increased experience in mounting distant operations, and the development of a support structure of overseas facilities to assist in such activities provides the Kremlin with greatly increased flexibility in the possible use of military power to advance Soviet interests in the Third World, particularly in a symbolic, noncombat manner. Despite these improvements, the Soviet Union

continues to have a very limited capability to project military power into distant areas in the face of armed opposition by a substantial local or rival power.

ARMS CONTROL

The Soviet Union has been a vocal champion of arms control and disarmament for many years. Since the late 1950s, the Soviets have been involved, virtually continuously, in a variety of international arms control negotiations. Within these negotiations and outside them, the Soviets have consistently asserted that they favor dramatic progress toward substantial disarmament.

Mr. Gorbachev has been particularly active on the arms control front, setting forth a continuous stream of proposals, some highly utopian while others have a more pragmatic character. One of the most utopian proposals was Gorbachev's ambitious three-stage plan calling for total global nuclear disarmament by the year 2000 presented in January 1986.[148] Nine months later, in the last hours of the Reykjavik "presummit," Gorbachev took a page from his earlier offer and called for the complete elimination of U.S. and Soviet strategic nuclear arms within a 10-year period.

In 1986 and 1987 Gorbachev was also pressing for less visionary but nevertheless very substantial reductions in nuclear offensive arms. These proposals culminated in the signing of the "double zero," Intermediate-range Nuclear Forces (INF) treaty at the Washington summit in December 1987. This agreement will eliminate all U.S. and Soviet land-based missiles with ranges between 500 and 5500 kilometers by mid 1991. It also provides for unprecedented verification measures, including continuous on-site monitoring of selected missile production facilities and short-notice, on-site challenge inspections.

Mr. Gorbachev's pragmatism has also helped produce substantial U.S.–Soviet agreement on a draft treaty in the Strategic Arms Reductions Talks (START). Due to permissive counting rules for warheads on bombers, the agreed framework for negotiating a 50 percent overall cut (leaving 6000 accountable nuclear warheads) would, in fact, likely reduce the inventories of central strategic weapons—bombers, ICBMs, and SLBMs—held by the superpowers by some 20 percent to 30 percent. In order to conclude such an agreement, the superpowers will almost certainly need to work out satisfactory deals to limit sea-launched cruise missiles and to preserve the ABM Treaty, thus placing some restraints on the testing and deployment of space-based ballistic missile defense systems through the mid 1990s.

By seizing the high ground in proposing major reductions in conventional arms, the Soviets have protected themselves against charges that their press toward the conclusion of agreements significantly reducing nuclear weapons is merely a ploy to make the world "safe" for Soviet conventional superiority. Their moves concerning conventional force reductions have included collective Warsaw Pact proposals first at Budapest in June 1986, then at Berlin in May 1987, and finally in Moscow, New York, and Warsaw in summer 1988. The USSR favors a three-stage process beginning with an agreement to implement asymmetrical reductions in order to eliminate imbalances in selected "offensive" arms, in particular tanks and "strike" aviation, that are deployed in the forces of the member states of NATO and the Warsaw Pact throughout Europe "from the Atlantic to the Urals." Consistent with these objectives is Gorbachev's December 1988 announcement of unilateral, conventional force reductions planned for Europe and Asia by the early 1990s.

The Pact's summer 1988 proposal calls for additional large-scale reductions on both sides and ultimately a fundamental restructuring of the forces of the Warsaw Pact and NATO so that neither side could mount a surprise attack or conduct any large-scale offensive operations. This ambitious proposal is all the more striking because, were it to be implemented, it would mean a complete dismantling of the very conventional blitzkrieg capabilities that the Soviets have worked so long and hard to acquire. It is doubtful that such a possibility can be viewed with much favor by the Soviet military establishment. If faced with the necessity to make substantial ground force reductions, the Soviet military might seek to adapt to this by implementing the "leaner" battalion-brigade-corps structure with which they are currently experimenting, as noted earlier. Proposals for the stage one reductions in selected armaments and their associated manpower are to be discussed in Vienna within the enlarged "Atlantic-to-the-Urals" force reductions negotiations—referred to in NATO as the Conventional Stability Talks—between the seven members of the Warsaw Pact and 16 members of NATO.

The development of arms control policy appears to be an area in Soviet defense policy-making that is open to a wider circle of organizations beyond the familiar lineup of the Ministry of Defense, the defense-industrial organs, and the senior Party leadership. Since contemporary arms control involves extended international negotiations, an important role has been played by the Ministry of Foreign Affairs. In recent years, there has also been a growing involvement of various scientists and scholars connected within the Academy of Sciences, including those discussed earlier who have been active in the discussions of "new political thinking" and "reasonable sufficiency."[149]

Senior representatives from the Foreign Ministry have generally been in charge of Soviet negotiating delegations and, in most cases, have provided the majority of the delegates. This latter pattern was most notably breached in the 1970s during the two lengthy rounds of the Strategic Arms Limitation Talks, SALT I and SALT II, when the military provided two of the six chief Soviet delegates and the defense-industrial sector an additional two.[150] Senior military officers continued to serve as important delegates at the START, INF, and Space/Defense talks in the 1980s. Nevertheless, even in all of these talks, the delegation chief has always been a career diplomat.[151]

A rare example of unusual military prominence in the arms control area occurred at the Reagan-Gorbachev "presummit" at Reykjavik in October 1986 and continued in high-level U.S.–Soviet meetings during 1987 and 1988.

During crucial negotiating sessions between "expert" delegations from both sides, the Soviet team was consistently led by Marshal S. F. Akhromeyev, then chief of the General Staff. His performance has been described by American participants as "tough and decisive," with Akhromeyev apparently being fully in command of the Soviet side in spite of the presence of senior foreign ministry personnel.[152]

Despite the leading role it generally plays in the negotiations process, it is clear that the Ministry of Foreign Affairs is by no means the dominant institution in the formulation of Soviet arms control policy in Moscow. The Foreign Ministry's arms control and disarmament directorate, created in 1986 and headed by veteran negotiator Viktor Karpov, reportedly participates in the development of Soviet bargaining positions in various negotiations. The overall formulation of Soviet arms control objectives and bargaining positions is apparently accomplished in an interagency manner, with key roles played by the Ministry of Defense, in particular, the General Staff, the defense-industrial organs, the Defense Council, and, ultimately, the Politburo.[153]

During the 1970s and 1980s, the major efforts of Soviet arms control policy were focused on the bilateral SALT, START, INF, and Defense/Space negotiations with the United States. The Soviets also played a leading role in the multilateral East-West talks on Mutual and Balanced Force Reductions in Central Europe and on confidence- and security-building measures that were conducted at the Conference on Security and Cooperation in Europe (CSCE) and in the related Stockholm Conference on Disarmament in Europe (CDE).[154]

In all of these negotiations, the Soviets sought to attain both the broad political goals and narrower security-related objectives discussed earlier. With regard to their specific negotiating tactics, despite their repeated calls for agreements based on the "principle of equal security," the Soviets quite unsurprisingly have sought persistently to gain the most advantageous terms possible within the negotiations. They have consistently tried to eliminate or reduce current or projected U.S. attack capabilities that have appeared particularly threatening, such as air-launched, sea-launched, and ground-launched cruise missiles, the MX ICBM, the D-5 SLBM, and the Pershing II INF missiles, while seeking to minimize constraints on their own extensive force modernization efforts. Nevertheless, when confronted by steadfast U.S. resistance to these demands, the Soviets grudgingly have proved willing to agree to compromises that involved reciprocal limits on both sides. Such was the pattern that emerged in the development of the SALT I, SALT II, and INF agreements and that also has been evident in the START negotiations.[155]

THE USE OF FORCE

Since the superpower status of the USSR rests, to a considerable degree, on its massive military power, it is not surprising that the Soviets have frequently used this power to protect and advance their interests on the world scene. As noted earlier, the Soviet leaders, like their czarist predecessors, have employed their armed forces as an effective instrument of foreign policy. They have, for example, used the force of arms to expand the frontiers of the Soviet Union—to absorb the Baltic states and portions of Finland, Poland, Czechoslovakia, Romania, and Japan—and to impose and maintain subservient communist regimes beyond these borders in Mongolia and Eastern Europe. More recently, however, they have failed over a nine-year period to defeat the mujaheddin rebels in Afghanistan, leading to a withdrawal of Soviet forces.

The Soviets have also used their military capabilities in manners other than such straightforward armed intervention. During the Russian Civil War, during the border skirmishes with Japan in the late 1930s,[156] and, of course, following the German invasion in 1941, they were forced to rely upon the Red Army to defend their control of Soviet territory. Moreover, their steadily expanding military capabilities have provided a useful backdrop of Soviet diplomacy and have also been used effectively in the form of peacetime demonstrations, shows of force during crises, and various types of military assistance to woo incumbent governments, to aid insurgent movements fighting to gain power, and to defend Marxist-Leninist regimes already in power against insurgency movements.

The frequency with which the Soviets have employed their military capabilities for foreign policy ends in situations short of armed conflict in much of the post–World War II period was investigated in a study published by the Brookings Institution. This lengthy analysis found that between June 1944 and June 1979, Soviet military units were used as a policy instrument to influence other international actors on 190 occasions. Among these incidents, 158 involved the deliberate manipulation of Soviet forces as a means to coerce other states, while the remaining 32 cases involved cooperative moves in support of other actors.[157]

The various types of Soviet external military involvements are well reflected in their relations with the communist movements in China and Vietnam over the past several decades. In both cases the Soviets provided arms and advisers to these parties when they were struggling to control their nations and again after they had gained power and were at war with major powers—the Chinese with the United States in Korea, 1950–53; the Vietnamese with the United States, 1964–73; and the Vietnamese with the Chinese, 1979. In the Chinese case, Sino-Soviet relations shifted from extensive and close cooperation to bitter conflict, culminating in armed border clashes along the Ussuri River in the spring of 1969. There has been substantial rivalry and tension between the two countries since then, although more recently relations appear to have eased somewhat.[158]

While Soviet military assistance activities have their antecedents in the early years of Bolshevik rule, they have increased dramatically in the past thirty-four years. In the post-Stalin era, the Soviets have come to use arms aid more and more as a means to gain entrée to Third World nations. This development is reflected organizationally in the growth of the Tenth Directorate of the General Staff from an organization established to oversee Soviet defense cooperation with the Eastern European communist allies to a body supervising Soviet military assistance to a host of Asian, African, and Latin American nations.[159]

Soviet military assistance has taken various forms, ranging from small-scale weapons sales to massive arms transfers accompanied by large numbers of Soviet advisory personnel. In some cases, it has led to the direct involvement of Soviet military personnel in regional conflicts, as was the case, for example, with Soviet pilots in China flying with the nationalists against the Japanese in the 1930s and in Egyptian dogfights with the Israelis over the Suez Canal in July 1970.[160]

In the mid 1970s, the Soviets diversified their military assistance repertoire by combining their own efforts with those of their Cuban allies in joint ventures undertaken in Angola and in Ethiopia. In these cases the Soviets apparently provided the arms, air transport, and financial backing to allow large-scale Cuban troop involvements against internal and regional foes—efforts that were vital to the success of their local clients, Neto's MPLA faction in Angola and the Mengistu government in Ethiopia.[161] In Ethiopia, moreover, the successful campaign to drive the Somalis from the Ogaden in 1978 was reportedly planned and directed on the scene by a high-level Soviet military delegation led by the then deputy CinC of the ground forces, General V. I. Petrov.[162]

More recently the Soviets have found themselves providing arms and advisers to help defend embattled Marxist-Leninist regimes threatened by internal armed insurgencies. Cuban mercenaries and Soviet military advisers have reportedly been directly involved in periodic MPLA campaigns in Angola against Jonas Savimbi's UNITA guerrillas, who are backed by the U.S. and South Africa. The Soviets are also providing modern arms to the armed forces of their client states in South Yemen, Ethiopia, Nicaragua, and Vietnam, all of whom face indigenous armed opposition and who are being assisted by the West. (In the Vietnamese case, the armed opposition is found in Cambodia where over 100,000 troops from Vietnam have been seeking to prop up a puppet communist regime since 1978.) More recently, however, Mr. Gorbachev has played

an active role in several major multilateral diplomatic negotiations directed toward resolving
regional conflicts and withdrawing Soviet, Cuban, and Vietnamese forces from the wars in
Afghanistan, Angola, and Cambodia, respectively.

Nevertheless, in an attempt to buttress their
influence in selected regions, the Soviets continue to sell large quantities of sophisticated
weaponry to a few non-Marxist governments
such as India, Syria, and Peru. As discussed
above, Soviet military assistance activities over
the past 20 years have been accompanied by,
and have themselves facilitated, significant improvements in Soviet long-range power projection. The Soviet desire to play an active and often interventionary role in trouble spots in
Africa and Asia has been clearly evident for
many years. Now, however, the Soviet potential
for such involvement has increased substantially. Soviet military and political writings of
the 1970s reflected a growing Soviet interest in
the peacetime political utility of the armed
forces.[163] Thus, in 1974, the minister of defense, Marshal A. A. Grechko, wrote, with
typical hyperbole:

At the present stage, the historical function of the Soviet Armed Forces is not restricted merely to their function in defending our Motherland and other socialist
countries. In its foreign policy activity, the Soviet state
actively and purposefully opposes the export of counterrevolution and the policy of oppression, supports the
national liberation struggle and resolutely resists imperial aggression in whatever distant region of our planet
it may occur.[164]

During this same period the former commander in chief of the Navy, Admiral S. G.
Gorshkov, was particularly outspoken regarding this matter. On numerous occasions,
Gorshkov touted the unique virtues of the
Navy as a means to promote the "state interests" of the Soviet Union on the international
scene. Admiral Gorshkov's claims were not
simply idle boasts. They were accompanied by
the increased manipulation of naval forces in
support of Soviet foreign policy in a wide variety of cases. These included the establishment
of the so-called Guinea Patrol, composed of
two destroyers and an oiler, to support the beleaguered Sekou Toure government in December 1970, the convoy movement of Moroccan

troops to Syria in 1973, and the reactive deployments of Soviet naval task forces to the
Bay of Bengal during the Indo-Pakistani War
in 1971, off Angola in 1973, in the Mediterranean during the Middle East crises in 1967,
1970, and 1973, and in response to the buildup
of U.S. naval forces in the Indian ocean in
1979–80 following the seizure by Iranians of
U.S. embassy personnel in Tehran.[165]

During the 1980s, Soviet military activism in
the Third World tapered off significantly.
While Soviet military sales, particularly to
well-established clients such as India and
Syria, remained very substantial, the military
case for long-range force projection and involvement was infrequently heard during this
period. Mr. Gorbachev's interest in taking on
new commitments has been extremely low.
The Soviets have sought instead to liquidate or
cut back existing commitments in Afghanistan
and elsewhere. Moreover, frequent criticism
has been heard in Moscow about alleged Soviet
overreliance on the military instrument at the
expense of other elements of its foreign policy.
Despite all this, Soviet military sales and assistance as well as other peacetime manipulations
of military power will almost certainly remain
a significant dimension of Soviet foreign policy
in the years ahead.

Conclusion

As the Soviet Union enters the 1990s, it is
one of the world's most militarily powerful nations. For a quarter of a century, its leaders
have been embarked upon a sustained, expensive, across-the-board buildup of Soviet military capabilities, albeit at a somewhat reduced
pace over the past decade. They have derived
considerable benefits from their growing arsenal in terms of increased international prestige
and a repertoire of military activities that has
been used effectively to advance Soviet interests on the international scene. Yet due to its
profound domestic, economic, and political
crises, the overall strength of the Soviet Union
on the international scene is being called increasingly into question. Several Soviet commentators have complained about the Krem-

lin's overreliance on military power in the past and have called for a more balanced foreign policy and reductions in the vast Soviet military machine.

The steady growth in military power noted above does not appear to have importantly strengthened the hand of the military on the Soviet domestic scene. On the contrary, growing criticism is being directed at the military in the context of the massive domestic *perestroika* campaign. The military leadership nevertheless remains an extremely important institutional group with clearly recognized expertise and influence regarding the defense matters for which they are primarily responsible. In combination with their defense-industrial partners, they have ample opportunity to express their own clear preferences regarding Soviet investment priorities.

Yet the final decisions regarding defense matters continue to rest with the senior Party leadership. The sudden removal of Marshal Ogarkov from his post as chief of the General Staff in September 1984 and the sacking of PVO chief, Marshal of Aviation Koldunov, and Defense Minister Marshal Sokolov in June 1987 clearly demonstrate the power of the Party oligarchs when faced with unacceptable military "lobbying" or dramatic and embarrassing failure. Nevertheless, the marshals will undoubtedly continue to seek, defend, and promote their interests, as they define them, albeit in a discreet manner.

In recent years the Soviets have had difficulty in translating their impressive military capabilities into political leverage. While they remain fully capable of using their overwhelming military force, if required, to maintain order in Eastern Europe, Gorbachev and company appear less inclined than their predecessors to do so.

One is less certain about the manner in which the Soviets are likely to use their military power in the future as a means to deal with other neighboring states or in more distant areas. Their intervention in Afghanistan has entailed heavy human and political costs and has by no means assured the survival of a friendly regime in Kabul. A withdrawal of Soviet forces has come after some nine years of

combat with the employment of massive firepower and a variety of tactics. Indeed, there is no indication of increased willingness to resort to the direct use of the armed forces elsewhere beyond their frontiers. Nevertheless, in light of the improvements in Soviet power projection potential discussed above and the virtual certainty that the international political scene will continue to be characterized by a myriad of unstable situations, the potential for the use of military power as a means to protect and advance Soviet interests cannot be ruled out.

Notes

1. Report delivered by M.S. Gorbachev at the Moscow All-Union Scientific and Practical Conference, December 10, 1984, *Pravda*, December 11, 1984.

2. *Handbook of Economic Statistics, 1987* (Washington, D.C.: Central Intelligence Agency, 1987), p. 31.

3. Ibid., pp. 118, 122, 123, 125, 130, 134, 136, 137.

4. This point has been documented in the modernization research of Professor Cyril Black of Princeton University.

5. *Handbook of Economic Statistics*, pp. 31, 32. Today the Soviets and the industrialized nations of the West have been surpassed in GNP per capita by a few of the oil-rich states of the Middle East as well.

6. Statement of Ambassador Malcolm C. Toon, in U.S. Senate, *The SALT II Treaty*, Hearings before the Committee on Foreign Relations, 96th Cong., 1st sess. (Washington, D.C.: Government Printing Office, 1978), part 3, p. 6.

7. The efforts of the Soviet regime to perpetuate popular awareness of the massive suffering of the "Great Fatherland War," as the Soviets call their involvement in World War II, is well captured in the title of Hedrick Smith's chapter on this subject, "Patriotism: World War II Was Only Yesterday," in *The Russians* (New York: Quadrangle, 1976), pp. 303–25.

8. Helmut Sonnenfeldt and William G. Hyland, *Soviet Perspectives on Security*, Adelphi Papers, no. 150 (London: International Institute for Strategic Studies, 1979), p. 9.

9. See Ivo J. Lederer, ed., *Russian Foreign Policy* (New Haven: Yale University Press, 1962).

10. An especially prescient observation about Russia's power potential was made almost 150 years ago by Alexis de Tocqueville, who predicted that Russia and the United States were destined to be the world's dominant powers, with the Russian position resting primarily on its military capabilities.

11. International Institute for Strategic Studies, *The Military Balance, 1987–1988* (London: International Institute for Strategic Studies, 1987), p. 41.

12. Charles Wolf, Jr., et al., *The Costs of the Soviet Empire*, R-3073/1-NA (Santa Monica, Calif.: The RAND Corporation, September 1983); David Albright, "On Eastern Europe: Security Implications for the USSR," *Parameters*, Summer 1984, p. 30.

13. According to the International Institute for Strategic Studies the number of Soviet divisions in Mongolia has varied over the years, moving up from only two divisions in 1974 to a strength of five divisions in 1982 and then back to four divisions in 1987. *The Military Balance, 1985–1986*, p. 29, and *The Military Balance, 1987–1988*, p. 44.

14. The so-called Brezhnev Doctrine justifying Soviet intervention in the "defense" of socialism first appeared in a *Pravda* editorial on 26 September 1968, a month after the Soviet invasion of Czechoslovakia in August 1968. It was repeated by General Secretary Brezhnev at the Polish Party Congress in Warsaw on November 12, 1968.

15. The most outspoken military figure in this regard was the commander in chief of the Navy, Fleet Admiral of the Soviet Union S.G. Gorshkov. From 1965 until his retirement in 1985 he regularly touted the Navy's ability to serve Soviet foreign policy—for example, asserting that "the Navy is, to the greatest degree, capable of operationally supporting the state's interest beyond its borders." See Gorshkov, *Morskaia moshch' gosudarstva* (Sea Power of the State) (Moscow: Voenizdat, 1976), p. v.

16. Ellen Jones, "The Correlation of Forces in Soviet Decision-Making," paper delivered to the 1978 Biennial Conference, Section on Military Studies, International Studies Association, November 1978.

17. For example, Maj Gen I. Anureyev, "Determining the Correlation of Forces in Terms of Nuclear Weapons," *Voennaia mysl'* (Military Thought), no. 6, 1967, pp. 35–45. For a Western commentary on this Soviet approach to the analysis of the strategic nuclear balance, see Stephen M. Meyer and Peter Almquist, *Insights from Mathematical Modelling in Soviet Mission Analysis*, DARPA Report, April 1985.

18. See Arnold L. Horelick and Myron Rush, *Strategic Power and Soviet Foreign Policy* (Chicago: University of Chicago Press, 1966).

19. Cf. Lt. Col. V. M. Bondarenko, "Military Technological Superiority: The Most Important Factor in the Reliable Defense of the Country," *Kommunist Vooruzhennykh Sil* (Communist of the Armed Forces), no. 17, September 1966, pp. 7–14; and *Sovetskaia voennaia entsiklopediia* (Soviet Military Encyclopedia, hereafter cited as *SME*), vol. 2 (Moscow: Voenizdat, 1976), p. 253.

20. At Tula, Brezhnev keynoted a concerted campaign to refute Western assertions that the Soviet Union is seeking military superiority over the United States and its NATO allies and to insist that Soviet military doctrine has a strictly "defensive" orientation. *Pravda*, January 19, 1977. Marshal N. V. Ogarkov, former chief of the General Staff, lent the authority of the professional military to these claims in various public statements and his authoritative article, "Military Strategy," in *SME*, vol. 7. (Moscow: Voenizdat, 1979) p. 563.

21. Timothy Colton, *Commissars, Commanders, and Civilian Authority: The Structure of Soviet Military Politics* (Cambridge, Mass.: Harvard University Press, 1979), p. 251.

22. Harriet Fast Scott and William F. Scott, *The Armed Forces of the USSR* (Boulder, Colo.: Westview Press, 1979), p. 176.

23. For most Soviet draftees, the period of compulsory military service is two years. However, this term is three years for certain naval components, while most deferred students who have received institute or university degrees serve for a year and a half or less. Scott and Scott, *Armed Forces of the USSR*, p. 305.

24. D. A. Volkogonov in *XXVII s'ezd KPSS i zadachi kafedr obshchestvennykh nauk: Materialy Vsesoyuznogo soveshchaniya zaveduyushchikyh kafedrami obshchestvennykh nauk vyschykh uchebnykh zavedeniy* (The 27th CPSU Congress and tasks of the social sciences departments: Materials of an All-Union conference of the leading departments of social sciences in higher educational institutions), *Izdatel'stvo politicheskoy literatury*, Moscow, 1987, p. 129.

25. A. I. Romashko, *Voennye stroiteli na stroikakh Moskvy* (The Military Builders in the Building of Moscow) (Moscow: Voenizdat, 1972).

26. Conversation with A. V. Kortunov, IUSAC, Washington, D.C., January 1988.

27. The growing Soviet literature on strategic stability includes: A. G. Arbatov, A. A. Vasil'yev, and A. A. Kokoshin, "Nuclear Weapons and Strategic Stability," *SShA: Ekonomika, politika, ideologiya* (USA: Economics, Politics, Ideology), no. 9, September 1987, pp. 3–13, and no. 10, October 1987, pp. 17–24; A. Arbatov and A. Savel'yev, "The Control and Communications System as a Factor of Strategic Stability," *MEMO*, no. 12, December 1987, pp. 12–23; A. Kokoshin, "From the Standpoint of New Thinking: Three Major Elements in Stability," *Krasnaya zvezda*, September 16, 1988.

28. A. G. Arbatov, A. A. Vasil'yev, and A. A. Kokoshin, "Nuclear Weapons and Strategic Stability," *SShA: Ekonomika, politika, ideologiya* (USA: Economics, Politics, Ideology), no. 9, 1987, p. 9.

29. Private conversations of the author with A. G. Savel'yev of IMEMO and A. A. Vasil'yev of IUSAC in February and May 1988.

30. R. Sagdeyev, A. Kokoshin et al., *Strategic Stability Under the Conditions of Radical Nuclear Arms Reductions*, Committee of Soviet Scientists for Peace and Against the Nuclear Threat, Moscow, April 1987.

31. I. Malashenko, "Parity Reassessed," *New Times*, no. 47/87, November 1987, pp. 9–10; A. V. Kortunov, conversation with the author, Washington, D.C., January 1988.

32. V. V. Zhurkin, S. A. Karaganov, and A. V. Kortunov, "Reasonable Sufficiency—Or How to Break the Vicious Circle," *New Times*, no. 40/87, 12 October 1987, pp. 13–15; "On Reasonable Sufficiency," *SShA: Ekonomika, politika, ideologiya*, no. 12, December 1987, pp. 11–21; "Concepts of Security—Old and New," *Kommunist*, no. 1, January 1988, pp. 42–50. Zhurkin and Karaganov transferred to the newly formed Institute for the Study of Europe which Zhurkin heads.

33. A. G. Arbatov echoes this concern about an American "competitive strategy" designed to overstress the Soviet economy in "On Parity and Reasonable Sufficiency," *Mezhdunarodnaya zhizn'* (International Life), no. 9, September 1988, pp. 80–92.

34. See Marshal S. L. Sokolov, "In Defense of Peace and the Security of the Motherland," *Pravda*, February 23, 1987; Marshal S. F. Akhromeyev, "The Glory and Pride of the Soviet People," *Sovetskaya Rossiya*, February 21, 1987; Army Gen D. T. Yazov, "The Military

Doctrine of the Warsaw Pact, A Doctrine of the Defense of Peace and Socialism," *Pravda*, July 27, 1987.

35. See Marshal N. V. Ogarkov, *Izvestiya*, September 23, 1983, and "The Defense of Socialism: Experience of History and the Present Day," *Krasnaya zvezda*, May 9, 1984.

36. See Marshal S. F. Akhromeyev, "The Great Victory," *Krasnaya zvezda*, May 9, 1987.

37. Army General D. T. Yazov, *Pravda*, July 27, 1987.

38. On the Military Doctrine of the Warsaw Pact Member States," *Pravda*, May 31, 1987.

39. Marshal S. F. Akhromeyev, "The Doctrine of Preventing War, Defending Peace and Socialism," *Problemy mira i sotsializma* (Problems of Peace and Socialism), no. 12, December 1987, p. 26; Col Gen M. A. Gareyev, "Prevention of War," *Krasnaya zvezda*, June 23, 1987.

40. See, for example, Col Gen M. A. Gareyev, *Sovetskaya voyennaya nauka* (Soviet Military Science), Znaniye, Moscow, November 1987, p. 8; Marshal S. F. Akhromeyev, "Watching over Peace and Security," *Trud*, February 21, 1988; Army Gen P. Lushev, "In Defense of the Achievements of the Revolution," *Mezhdunarodnaya zhizn'* (International Life), no. 8, August 1987, p. 68; "Military Doctrine" and "Military Strategy," in Marshal S. F. Akhromeyev et al., eds., *Voyennyi entsiklopedicheskii slovar'* (Military Encyclopedic Dictionary), Voyenizdat, Moscow, 1986, pp. 240, 714.

41. Interview with Army Gen A. I. Gribkov, "Doctrine of Maintaining Peace," *Krasnaya zvezda*, September 29, 1987.

42. Army Gen D. T. Yazov, *Na strazhe sotsializma i mira* (On Guard Over Socialism and Peace), Voyenizdat, Moscow, 1987, p. 34.

43. Zhurkin, Karaganov, and Kortunov, "Reasonable Sufficiency—Or How to Break the Vicious Circle," *New Times*, no. 40/87, p. 14.

44. Marshal S. F. Akhromeyev, *Problemy mira i sotsializma*, no. 12, December 1987, p. 26.

45. Interview with Gen Ivan Tretyak, "Reliable Defense First and Foremost," *Moscow News*, no. 8, February 21, 1988, p. 12.

46. The defense minister, Army Gen D. T. Yazov, claimed that the Soviets had begun to thin out its forces facing China in January 1968, but Western intelligence sources have failed to confirm that any significant reductions have taken place.

47. Francis Fukuyama, "Gorbachev and the Third World," *Foreign Affairs*, Spring 1986, pp. 715–731.

48. Stalin assumed this position after the German invasion in 1941. Khrushchev apparently did so in the late 1950s or early 1960s as he sought to impose his will on the military regarding doctrinal and budgetary issues. Brezhnev's accession to the post, date unknown, was acknowledged in the course of a routine article in the military press in the fall of 1977.

49. There were signs of disagreement on defense investment priorities within the Brezhnev-led collective leadership that succeeded Krushchev in early 1965. See T. W. Wolfe, *The Soviet Military Scene: Institutional and Defense Policy Considerations*, RM-4913 (Santa Monica, Calif.: The RAND Corporation, 1966), pp. 64–67.

50. John Newhouse, *Cold Dawn: The Story of SALT* (New York: Holt, Rinehart & Winston, 1973), p. 192.

51. See A. Arbatov, "Deep Cuts in Strategic Arms," *MEMO*, no. 4, April 1988, p. 22.

52. This point has been made to the author by William E. Odom and by Robert G. Kaiser in *Russia: The People and the Power* (New York: Pocket Books, 1976), p. 380.

53. Marshall I. Goldman, "Gorbachev and Economic Reform," *Foreign Affairs*, Fall 1985, pp. 56–73; Alice C. Gorlin, "The Soviet Economy," *Current History*, October 1986, pp. 325–328, 343–345; Ed A. Hewitt, "Reform or Rhetoric: Gorbachev and the Soviet Economy," *The Brookings Review*, Fall 1986, pp. 13–20; a special issue on Soviet economic reform in *Soviet Economy*, vol. 3, October-December 1987; and Ed A. Hewitt, *Reforming the Soviet Economy:Equality versus Efficiency* (Washington, D. C.: The Brookings Institution, 1988).

54. John P. Hardt, "Soviet Economic Capabilities and Defense Resources," in *The Soviet Threat: Myths and Realities*, G. Kirk and N. H. Wessell, eds. (New York: Academy of Political Science, 1978), p. 124.

55. Cf. Richard F. Kaufman, "Causes of the Slowdown in Soviet Defense Spending," *Soviet Economy*, Jan-Mar 1985, pp. 9–31; Abraham S. Becker, *Sitting on Bayonets: The Soviet Defense Burden and the Slowdown of Soviet Defense Spending*, RAND/UCLA Center for the Study of Soviet International Behavior, JRS-01, December 1985.

56. See Jeremy Azrael, *The Soviet Civilian Leadership and the High Command*, R-3171-AF (Santa Monica, Calif.: The RAND Corporation, forthcoming), for an excellent review of relations between the senior Party leadership and the Soviet military high command between 1976 and 1986.

57. For Akhromeyev's comments, see Maj I. Sas, "Restructuring Demands Action. Meeting of the USSR Armed Forces General Staff Party Aktiv," *Krasnaya zvezda*, August 13, 1988.

58. Enders Wimbush and Dmitry Ponomareff, *Alternatives for Mobilizing Soviet Central Asian Labor: Outmigration and Regional Development*, R-2476-AF (Santa Monica, Calif.: The RAND Corporation, 1979).

59. Col Yu. Deryugin, interview in *Argumenty i fakty* (Arguments and Facts), no. 35, 1988, p. 16.

60. For an excellent review of these and other factors, see Benjamin S. Lambeth, "The Sources of Soviet Military Doctrine," in *Comparative Defense Policy*, F. B. Horton, A. C. Rogerson, and E. L. Warner III, eds. (Baltimore: Johns Hopkins University Press, 1973), pp. 200–215.

61. Maj Gen S. N. Kozlov, ed., *The Officer's Handbook* (Moscow: Voenizdat, 1971), translated and published under the auspices of the U.S. Air Force, p. 62; "Military Doctrine," *SME*, vol. 3, p. 229.

62. Military Doctrine," *SME*, vol. 3, p. 225; Marshal V. D. Sokolovskiy, ed., *Voennaia strategiia* (Military Strategy), 3d ed., rev. (Moscow: Voenizdat, 1968), p. 38.

63. Kozlov, ed., *The Officer's Handbook*, p. 64.

64. Ibid., pp. 50–61; "Military Science," *SME*, vol. 2, p. 184.

65. See Colonel V. Ye. Savkin, *The Basic Principles of Operational Art and Tactics* (Moscow: Voenizdat, 1972), translated and published under the auspices of the U.S. Air Force.

66. Stephen M. Meyer, "Civilian and Military Influence in Managing the Arms Race in the USSR," in

Robert J. Art et al., eds., *Reorganizing America's Defense* (New York: Pergamon Press, 1985), pp. 44–47. David Holloway, *Technology, Management and the Soviet Military Establishment*, Adelphi Papers, no. 76 (London: International Institute for Strategic Studies, 1971), pp. 6–9. Maj Gen Petro G. Grigorenko reports that he initiated work on cybernetics in the Scientific Research Branch of the Frunze Military Academy in the mid 1950s and created a faculty for military cybernetics in 1959. Petro G. Grigorenko, *Memoirs* (New York: W. W. Norton & Co., 1982), p. 229. For a lengthy description of the extensive military scientific research activities undertaken at the Voroshilov Academy of the General Staff, which are ranked on a par with its teaching activities, see V. G. Kulikov, *Akademiia general'nogo shtaba* (The Academy of the General Staff) (Moscow: Voenizdat, 1976), pp. 178–225.

67. Some good efforts, however, have been made, including Stephen M. Meyer, "Civilian and Military Influence," in Art et al.; Allen S. Rehm, *An Assessment of Military Operations Research in the USSR*, Professional Paper no. 116 (Arlington, Va.: Center for Naval Analyses, September 1963); John Erickson, "Soviet Military Operational Research: Objectives and Methods," *Strategic Review*, vol. V, no. 2, Spring 1977, pp. 63–73; John Hemsley, *Soviet Troop Control* (New York: Brassey's Publishers Ltd., 1982); and Stephen M. Meyer, *Soviet Theater Nuclear Forces*, Parts 1 and 2, Adelphi Papers, nos. 187, 188 (London: International Institute for Strategic Studies, 1983–84).

68. On the use of various norms in Soviet operational planning, see Christopher Donnelly, "The Sustainability of the Soviet Ground Forces," unpublished manuscript, Fall 1987, passim.

69. See Marshal M. V. Zakharov, ed., *Voprosy strategii i operativnogo iskusstva v sovetskikh voennykh trudakh, 1917–1940* (Problems of Strategy and Operational Art in Soviet Military Works, 1917–1940) (Moscow: Voenizdat, 1965), pp. 17–24; John Erickson, *The Soviet High Command: A Military-Political History, 1918–1941* (New York: St. Martin's Press, 1962), pp. 349–354, 404–411; Marshal N. V. Ogarkov, "Deep Operations Battle," in *SME*, vol. 2 (Moscow: Voenizdat, 1976), pp. 574–578.

70. See Col Gen M. A. Gareyev, *M. V. Frunze— voyennyy teoretik* (M.V. Frunze—Military Theoretician) (Moscow: Voenizdat, 1985); Marshal N. V. Ogarkov, "Military Strategy," in *SME*, vol. 7 (Moscow: Voenizdat, 1979), pp. 559–563; Sokolovskiy, ed., *Military Strategy*; and commentaries such as Benjamin S. Lambeth, *How to Think about Soviet Military Doctrine*, P-5939 (Santa Monica, Calif.: The RAND Corporation, 1978).

71. For a superb historical account and analysis of Soviet concepts and capabilities for conducting nuclear war in the critical European theater, see Stephen M. Meyer, *Soviet Theater Nuclear Forces*, Part 1: *Development of Doctrine and Objectives and Soviet Theater Nuclear Forces*, Part 2: *Capabilities and Implications*, Adelphi Papers, nos. 187, 188 (London: International Institute for Strategic Studies, 1983–84).

72. Marshal N. V. Ogarkov, "For Our Soviet Motherland: Guarding Peaceful Labor," *Kommunist*, no. 10, 1981, p. 86.

73. See Lt Gen A. I. Yevseyev, "The Experience of Maneuvering for Concentrating Efforts against Enemy Assault Groupings in the Course of a Front Defensive Operation," *Voyenno-istoricheskii zhurnal* (Military History Journal, hereafter cited as *VIZh*), no. 9, September 1986, pp. 12–23; Maj Gen A. P. Maryshev, "Certain Questions of the Strategic Defensive in the Great Patriotic War," *VIZh*, no. 6, June 1986, pp. 9–16; Col G. Miranovich and Col V. Zhitarenko, "What Makes Defense Strong?" *Krasnaya zvezda*, December 9, 1987.

74. See Phillip A. Peterson and John G. Hines, *The Soviet Conventional Offensive in Europe*, DDB-2622-4-83 (Washington, D.C.: Defense Intelligence Agency, 1983); Christopher N. Donnelly, "The Operational Maneuver Group: A New Challenge to NATO," *International Defense Review*, September 1982, pp. 1177–1186; Major Henry S. Shields, "Why the OMG?" *Military Review*, November 1985, pp. 4–13; John G. Hines and Phillip A. Petersen, "The Warsaw Pact Strategic Offensive: The OMG in Context," *International Defense Review*, pp. 1391–1395; C. J. Dicks, "Soviet Operational Maneuvre Groups: A Closer Look," *International Defense Review*, June 1983, pp. 769–776.

75. See Christopher N. Donnelly, "Operations in the Enemy Rear: Soviet Doctrine and Tactics," *International Defense Review*, January 1980, pp. 35–41; Major Roger E. Bort, "Air Assault Brigades: New Element in the Soviet *Desant* Force Structure," *Military Review*, October 1983, pp. 21–38; David C. Isby, "The Vertical Threat: Air Assault and Airmobile Brigades of the Soviet Army," *Amphibious Warfare Review*, August 1985, pp. 50–54; Mark L. Urban, "The Strategic Role of Soviet Airborne Troops," *Jane's Defence Weekly*, July 14, 1984, pp. 26–28, 30–32; Viktor Suvorov, "Spetsnaz: The Soviet Union's Special Forces," *International Defense Review*, September 1983, pp. 1209–1216.

76. See Phillip A. Petersen and John R. Clark, "Soviet Air and Antiair Operations," *Air University Review*, Mar/Apr 1985, pp. 36–54; Ye. G. Veraka and M. N. Kozhevnikov, "Air Operations," *SME*, vol. 2 (Moscow: Voenizdat, 1976), pp. 281–282; Robert P. Berman, *Soviet Air Power in Transition* (Washington D.C.: Brookings Institution, 1978), pp. 11, 66–73; Chief Marshal of Aviation P. Kutakhov, "The Conduct of Air Operations," *Voenno-istoricheskii zhurnal* (Military History Journal), no. 6, June 1972, pp. 20–28.

77. Michael MccGwire, "Naval Power and Soviet Global Strategy," *International Security*, Spring 1979, pp. 170–173; Robert P. Berman and John C. Baker, *Soviet Strategic Forces: Requirements and Responses* (Washington, D.C.: Brookings Institution, 1982), pp. 62–65.

78. Soviet doctrinal writings spoke openly of such preemption in the 1950s. During the 1960s and 1970s, although they largely avoided explicit references to their intention to strike preemptively, these writings sometimes included highly suggestive euphemisms such as claiming a readiness "to frustrate" or "to nip in the bud" any Western nuclear missile attack. See Edward L. Warner III, *The Military in Contemporary Soviet Politics: An Institutional Analysis* (New York: Praeger Publishers, 1977), p. 151. There have been few Soviet discussions of large-scale nuclear warfare since the late 1970s and thus we have little recent evidence regarding Soviet thoughts on nuclear war initiation.

79. See Marshal N. I. Krylov, "The Nuclear Shield of the Soviet State," *Voennaia mysl'* (Military Thought), no. 11, November 1967, p. 20; Gen S. Ivanov, "Soviet Military Doctrine and Strategy," *Voen-*

naia mysl', no. 5, May 1969, p. 48; Maj Gen N. Vasendin and Col N. Kuznetsov, "Modern Warfare and Surprise Attack," *Voennaia mysl'*, no. 6, June 1968, pp. 46–47.

80. Maj Gen V. Zemskov, "Characteristic Features of Modern Wars and Possible Methods of Conducting Them," *Voennaia mysl'* (Military Thought), no. 7, July 1969, p. 20; Joseph D. Douglas and Amoretta M. Hoeber, *Soviet Strategy for Nuclear War* (Palo Alto: Hoover Institution Press, 1979), pp. 14–33.

81. See Notra Trulock III, "Soviet Perspectives on Limited Nuclear Warfare," in Fred S. Hoffman et al., eds., *Swords and Shields: NATO, the USSR and New Choices for Long Range Offense and Defense* (Lexington, Mass.: Lexington Books, 1987), pp. 53–85.

82. Dr. Kissinger, viewing Brezhnev's proposal as designed to promote the breakup of NATO, did not respond to the Soviet suggestion. Henry A. Kissinger, *Years of Upheaval* (Boston: Little, Brown and Co., 1982), p. 277.

83. Sagdeyev et al., *Strategic Stability Under the Conditions of Radical Nuclear Arms Reductions*, p. 22.

84. For a more complete discussion of Soviet views on limited nuclear war, see Edward L. Warner III, "Soviet Concepts and Capabilities for Limited Nuclear War: What We Know and How We Know It," in Cynthia Roberts et al., eds., *Decoding the Enigma: Methodology for the Study of Soviet Military Policy*, forthcoming.

85. David D. Finley and Jan F. Triska, *Soviet Foreign Policy* (New York: Macmillan Co., 1968) pp. 72–74.

86. There is precedent for such an arrangement, in that Gen Shtemenko writes that while chief of the General Staff in the late 1940s, he was the secretary of the Higher (Supreme) Military Soviet, the precursor of the Defense Council. General of the Army S. M. Shtemenko, *General'nyi shtab v gody voiny* (The General Staff in the War Years), Book 2 (Moscow: Voenizdat, 1973), p. 500. See also John Erickson, "The General Staff: Theory and Practice from the Tsarist to the Soviet Regime," *Soviet Military Digest*, Defence Studies, University of Edinburgh, October 1983, pp. 137–138. Ellen Jones reports that research in Eastern European sources indicates that sections of the general staffs in Czechoslovakia, East Germany, and Hungary act as the secretariats for their respective Supreme Defense Councils, which were established in the 1960s. Conversation with author, October 18, 1983.

87. The best Soviet descriptions of the manner in which Stalin worked with the military in directing the Soviet war effort are found in the memoirs of Marshals Zhukov and Vasilevskiy and General of the Army Shtemenko, all of whom played key roles in the Stavka or the General Staff. See Marshal G. K. Zhukov, *The Memoirs of Marshal Zhukov* (New York: Delacroix Press, 1971), pp. 234–268, 279–289; Marshal A. M. Vasilevskiy, *Delo vsei zhizni* (Cause of a Lifetime) (Moscow: Voenizdat, 1975), pp. 115–602; and General of the Army S. M. Shtemenko, *The General Staff in the War Years*, Books 1 and 2 (Moscow: Voenizdat, 1968 and 1973), passim. An excellent secondary analysis of this process is found in Tommy L. Whitton, "Soviet Strategic Wartime Leadership," conference paper, September 16, 1980.

88. Such was the case for the State Defense Committee and Stavka, abolished on September 4, 1945. Marshal M. V. Zakharov, ed., *50 let vooruzhennykh sil SSSR* (50 Years of the Armed Forces of the USSR) (Moscow: Voenizdat, 1968), p. 477. Stalin, however, appears to have remained supreme commander in chief until his death. Christian Duevel, "Brezhnev Named Supreme Commander-in-Chief of the Soviet Armed Forces," Radio Liberty Research, RL260/77, November 11, 1977, p. 2.

89. For example, Colonel N. P. Skirdo, writing in 1970, stated, "Direct leadership of the Armed Forces *both in peacetime* and in war is exercised by the *Supreme High Command*, the General Staff, and the appropriate military leadership" (emphasis added). Colonel N. P. Skirdo, *The People, the Army, the Commander* (Moscow: Voenizdat, 1970), translated and published under the auspices of the U.S. Air Force, p. 109. Similarly, the discussion of the supreme high command in the *Soviet Military Encyclopedia* notes that this organ can "sometimes exist in peacetime." "Supreme High Command," *SME*, vol 2., p. 113.

90. See Marshal N. V. Ogarkov on TVDs, "For Our Soviet Motherland: Guarding Peaceful Labor," *Kommunist*, no. 10, 1981, p. 86.

91. For the best discussion of the Soviet past and present uses of high commands and theaters of military operations, see Gregory C. Baird, *Soviet Intermediary Strategic C² Entities—The Historical Experience* (McLean, Va.: BDM Corporation, April 30, 1979), Phillip A. Petersen, *The Soviet Conceptual Framework for the Development and Application of Military Power*, Defense Intelligence Report, DDB-2610-36-81 (Washington, D.C.: Defense Intelligence Agency, June 1981), and Edward L. Warner III, Josephine J. Bonan, and Erma F. Packman, *Key Personnel and Organizations of the Soviet Military High Command* (Santa Monica, Calif.: The RAND Corporation, 1987).

92. Shaposhnikov's three-volume classic, *Mozg armii* (The Brain of the Army), published in 1927–1929, is a historical treatise on the role of the Austro-Hungarian General Staff prior to and during World War I, which makes the case for a powerful general staff as a key element of a nation's military power. Earlier, M. V. Frunze, a leading Red Army commander during the Civil War and subsequently the people's commissar of defense, had described the staff of the Workers' and Peasants' Red Army in 1925 as "the brain of the army."

93. These men were members of a Corps of Officers, representatives of the General Staff, a group operating under the control of the Operations Directorate that was in existence only during World War II.

94. *Soviet Military Power, 1986* (Washington, D.C.: U.S. Government Printing Office, 1986), pp. 31, 76; Mark L. Urban, "Major Reorganization of Soviet Air Forces," *International Defense Review*, June 1983, p. 756; *The Military Balance, 1985–1986*, p. 21.

95. The military districts are, in alphabetical order, the Baltic, Byelorussian, Carpathian, Central Asian, Far Eastern, Kiev, Leningrad, Moscow, North Caucasus, Odessa, Siberian, Transbaikal, Transcaucasus, Turkestan, Ural, and Volga. The groups of forces are the Group of Soviet Forces Germany (GSFG) in East Germany, the Northern Group in Poland, the Central Group in Czechoslovakia, and the Southern Group in Hungary.

96. See D. L. Smith and A. L. Meier, "Ogarkov's

Revolution: Soviet Military Doctrine for the 1990s," *International Defense Review*, no. 1, 1987, pp. 870, 872–873, and *Soviet Military Power, 1988*, p. 74.

97. Peter Weiss, "The Hungarian Armed Forces Today," *International Defense Review*, no. 8, 1988, pp. 935–938.

98. See, for example, R. Sagdeyev, A. Kokoshin et al., *Strategic Stability Under the Conditions of Radical Nuclear Arms Reductions*, Committee of Soviet Scientists for Peace and Against the Nuclear Threat, Moscow, April 1987; Ye. Velikov, R. Sagdeyev, and A. Kokoshin, *Weaponry in Space: The Dilemma of Security*, Mir Publishers, Moscow, 1986.

99. See A. Kokoshin and V. Larionov, "The Battle of Kursk from the Standpoint of Defensive Doctrine," *MEMO*, no. 8, 1987, pp. 32–40; A. Kokoshin, "The Development of Military Affairs and the Reduction of the Armed Forces and Conventional Arms," *MEMO*, no. 1, January 1988, pp. 20–32; and A. Kokoshin and V. Larionov, "The Confrontations of Conventional Forces in the Context of Ensuring Strategic Stability," *MEMO*, no. 6, June 1988, pp. 23–31.

100. See A. Yakovlev, "The Achievement of a Qualitatively New Condition of Soviet Society and Social Sciences," *Kommunist*, no. 8, 1987, p. 18; A. Dobrynin, "For a Nuclear-Free World Toward the 21st Century," *Kommunist*, no. 9, 1986, pp. 19, 27–28.

101. For the most comprehensive and insightful account of the Soviet weapons acquisition process, see Arthur J. Alexander, *Decision-Making in Soviet Weapons Procurement*, Adelphi Papers, nos. 147 and 148, International Institute for Strategic Studies, London, 1978/79, and David Holloway, *The Soviet Union and the Arms Race*, Yale University Press, New Haven, 1983, pp. 109–155.

102. The nine defense production ministries and their primary products are: the Ministry of Defense Industry, conventional weapons; the Ministry of Aviation Industry, aircraft and cruise missiles; the Ministry of Shipbuilding Industry, ships and submarines; the Ministry of Electronics Industry, electronic components; the Ministry of Radio Industry, electronic products; the Ministry of Medium Machine Building, nuclear weapons; the Ministry of General Machine Building, ballistic missiles; the Ministry of Machine Building, ammunition; and the Ministry of the Means of Communication, telecommunication equipment.

103. "19th All-Union CPSU Conference: Foreign Policy and Diplomacy," *Pravda*, July 26, 1988.

104. For discussions of Khrushchev's style and beliefs regarding defense issues, see Warner, *The Military in Contemporary Soviet Politics*, pp. 137–146, and Khrushchev's memoirs, *Khrushchev Remembers: The Last Testament* (Boston: Little, Brown, 1974), pp. 18–22, 25–26, 40–42, 46, 50, 540.

105. Stephen M. Meyer, "The Sources and Prospects of Gorbachev's New Political Thinking on Security," *International Security*, Fall 1988, p. 124.

106. Seweryn Bialer, "The Changing Soviet Political System: The Nineteenth Party Conference and After," unpublished paper, September 1988, p. 4.

107. For descriptions of these programs, see Herbert Goldhamer, *The Soviet Soldier: Soviet Military Management at the Troop Level* (New York: Crane & Russak, 1975, pp. 39–88.

108. Colton, *Commissars, Commanders, and Civilian Authority*, pp. 254–255, 284.

109. Ibid., pp. 264, 267.

110. Warner, *The Military in Contemporary Soviet Politics*, pp. 100–102.

111. Colton, *Commissars, Commanders, and Civilian Authority*, pp. 35–44, and E. H. Carr, *Socialism in One Country, 1924–1926*, vol. 2 (Baltimore: Penguin Books, 1970), pp. 432–433.

112. The most prominent advocate of this view has been Roman Kolkowicz, whose most detailed presentation is found in *The Soviet Military and the Communist Party* (Princeton: Princeton University Press, 1967).

113. Stalin's "Tsaritsyn group" included K. E. Voroshilov, S. K. Timoshenko, and S. M. Budenny of the famous First Cavalry Army, all of whom became marshals of the Soviet Union under Stalin's sponsorship. Khrushchev's comrades in arms at Stalingrad included such figures as Marshals V. I. Chuikov, S.S. Biriuzov, and R. Ya. Malinovskiy, all of whom rose to key posts in the Ministry of Defense while Khrushchev dominated Soviet politics in the late 1950s and early 1960s.

114. See *Khrushchev Remembers*; Marshal G. K. Zhukov, *Memoirs of Marshal Zhukov*; Gen S. M. Shtemenko, *The General Staff in the War Years*, Books 1 and 2; and S. Bialer, ed., *Stalin and His Generals: Soviet Military Memoirs of World War II* (New York: Pegasus, 1969).

115. Major works in this regard are Arthur J. Alexander's "Weapons Acquisition in the Soviet Union, United States and France," in *Comparative Defense Policy*, Horton, Rogerson, and Warner, eds., pp. 426–444; and Alexander's *Decision-Making in Soviet Weapons Procurement*; David Holloway, "Technology and Political Decision in Soviet Armaments Policy," *Journal of Peace Research*, no. 4, 1976; John McConnell, "The Soviet Defense Industry as a Pressure Group," in *Soviet Naval Policy*, M. MccGwire, K. Booth, and J. McConnell, eds., (New York: Praeger, 1975), pp. 91–101; and Berman and Baker, *Soviet Strategic Forces*, pp. 74–84.

116. Alexander, "Weapons Acquisition," pp. 430–431; and idem, *Decision-Making in Soviet Weapons Procurement*, pp. 33, 34, 41.

117. Robert Kaiser emphasizes the critical *quality control* function performed by these military representatives in his *Russia*, pp. 378–383.

118. All of these percentages are based on data from the International Institute for Strategic Studies, *The Military Balance, 1987–1988*, pp. 33–34; *Soviet Military Power, 1988*, pp. 15, 45–51; and William Arkin et al., *Nuclear Weapons Databook*, Vol. IV, *Soviet Nuclear Weapons*, forthcoming.

119. The Soviets probably sought to achieve this objective, at least partially, with their third-generation ICBMs by targeting the powerful warheads of the relatively inaccurate SS-9 against the Minuteman launch control centers. The United States countered this possible tactic in the late 1960s by deploying launch control aircraft that can be kept on continuous airborne alert. Berman and Baker, *Soviet Strategic Forces*, p. 53.

120. Arkin et al., *Nuclear Weapons Databook*, Vol. IV.

121. Berman and Baker, *Soviet Strategic Forces*, pp. 93–96, 106–108; *Soviet Military Power, 1988*, pp. 15, 47–49.

122. Stephen M. Meyer, "Soviet Nuclear Operations," in Ashton Carter et al., eds., *Managing Nuclear Operations* (Washington, D.C.: The Brookings Institution, 1987), p. 494.

123. *Soviet Military Power, 1988*, pp. 47–49.

124. Ibid., pp. 50–51; *The Military Balance, 1987–1988*, pp. 34, 207.

125. *The Military Balance, 1987–1988*, pp. 33, 34.

126. *Soviet Military Power, 1988*, pp. 80–82.

127. Ibid., p. 56.

128. Ibid, pp. 55–57.

129. "ASW: Is the US Lead Slipping?" *Armed Forces Journal International*, April 1980, pp. 46–47.

130. *Soviet Military Power, 1988*, pp. 59–61.

131. *Soviet Military Power, 1987*, p. 52.

132. Results of an interagency U.S. government study released by the director of central intelligence in July 1978 and published in *Soviet Civil Defense*, Special Report no. 47 (Washington, D.C.: Department of State, 1978).

133. *The Military Balance, 1978–1988*, pp. 34, 39–45.

134. Ibid., p. 39.

135. Ibid.

136. Ibid.

137. John Erickson, "The Soviet Union's Growing Arsenal of Chemical Warfare," *Strategic Review*, Fall 1979, pp. 63–71.

138. John Erickson, "Doctrine, Technology and Style," in *Soviet Military Power and Performance*, John Erickson and E. J. Feuchtwanger, eds. (London: Macmillan Press, 1979), pp. 20–22; and "Soviet Breakthrough Operations: Resources and Restraints," (London: *Royal United Services Institute Journal*, September 1976), p. 74.

139. *The Military Balance, 1987–1988*, p. 36.

140. Berman, *Soviet Air Power in Transition*, p. 32; William Schneider, Jr., "Trends in Soviet Frontal Aviation," *Air Force Magazine*, March 1979, pp. 76–81.

141. Lynn M. Hansen, "Soviet Combat Helicopter Operations," *International Defense Review*, August 1978, pp. 1242–1246; Christopher N. Donnelly, "The Soviet Helicopter on the Battlefield," *International Defense Review*, May 1984, pp. 559–566.

142. Mark L. Urban, "Major Reorganization of Soviet Air Forces," *International Defense Review*, June 1983, p. 756.

143. *Soviet Military Power, 1988*, p. 85.

144. Michael McGwire, "Soviet Naval Doctrine and Strategy," in *Soviet Military Thinking*, D. Leebaert, ed. (London: Allen & Unwin, 1981).

145. Dennis M. Gormley, "The Direction and Pace of Soviet Force Projection Capabilities," *Survival*, November/December 1982, pp. 266–276; *Soviet Military Power, 1986*, pp. 93–98.

146. David Halevy, "Soviet Airlift in Ethiopia, Aden Reported," *Washington Star*, September 23, 1979, p. 3; Stephen S. Kaplan, "The Historical Record," and Colin Legum, "Angola and the Horn of Africa," in Stephen S. Kaplan, ed., *Diplomacy of Power: Soviet Armed Forces As a Political Instrument* (Washington, D.C.: The Brookings Institution, 1981), pp. 106–107, 195–201, and 570–640.

147. *Soviet Military Power, 1986*, p. 138.

148. Mikhail S. Gorbachev, "Statement by M. S. Gorbachev," *Pravda*, January 16, 1986.

149. The latter group, led originally by the Commission for Scientific Problems of Disarmament and more recently by the Committee Against the Nuclear Threat and for Peace, includes several prominent Soviet scientists, scholars, and members of the academy's social science institutes. Apparently these people are consulted on arms control matters and frequently participate in international conferences such as those sponsored annually by the Pugwash U.S.-USSR Study Group on Arms Control and Disarmament and by several other bilateral and multilateral exchanges with the West. See Warner, *The Military in Contemporary Soviet Politics*, pp. 222-224.

150. The military delegates have included such important military figures as Marshal N. V. Ogarkov and Col Gen N. N. Alekseyev, both of whom were active in SALT I. The defense industry figures included Academician A. N. Shchukin, a leading weapons development scientist, and Petr Pleshakov, then a deputy minister and subsequently the minister of radio industry.

151. The post was held by Deputy Minister of Foreign Affairs V. S. Semyonov from 1969 until 1978 and subsequently by Ambassador V. P. Karpov, who served through the completion of the SALT II negotiations in June 1979, and again in the START and Geneva negotiations throughout the early and mid 1980s.

152. Personal discussions with Ambassador Paul Nitze and Colonel Robert Linhart, who participated in these negotiations in 1986, 1987, and 1988.

153. For discussions of Soviet organizations involved in SALT, see Warner, *The Military in Contemporary Soviet Politics*, pp. 237-244; Raymond L. Garthoff, "SALT and the Soviet Military," *Problems of Communism*, January-February 1975, pp. 21-37; and Thomas W. Wolfe, *The SALT Experience* (Cambridge, Mass.: Ballinger Publishing Co., 1979); Rose E. Gottemoeller, "Decisionmaking for Arms Limitation in the Soviet Union," in Hans G. Brauch and Duncan L. Clarke, eds., *Decisionmaking for Arms Limitation: Assessments and Prospects* (Cambridge, Mass.: Ballinger Publishing Company, 1983), pp. 53-80.

154. Others included negotiations with the United States and the United Kingdom on a comprehensive nuclear test ban, with the United States on an antisatellite warfare regime, limitations on conventional arms transfers, and chemical warfare limits, and participation in the United Nations' continuing Conference on Disarmament in Geneva.

155. For an analysis of the agreed START framework and the remaining unresolved issues in those negotiations, see Edward L. Warner III and David A. Ochmanek, *Next Moves: An Arms Control Agenda for the 1990s* (New York: Council on Foreign Relations, Inc., 1988), pp. 17-65.

156. These were the battles of Lake Khasan in the Far East in 1938 and of Khalgin-gol in Mongolia in 1939, in which the Red Army more than held its own against armed probes by the Japanese Kwantung Army, thus apparently helping convince the Japanese that a full-fledged war with the Soviet Union would not be an inviting prospect. See Erickson, *Soviet High Command*, pp. 494-499, 517-522, 532-537.

157. Kaplan, ed., *Diplomacy of Power*, pp. 27-32. The study represents a follow-on effort to similar Brookings examination of U.S. peacetime uses of force in the post-World War II period. See also Barry M.

Blechman and Stephen S. Kaplan, *Force Without War: U.S. Armed Forces As a Political Instrument*, (Washington, D.C.: The Brookings Institution, 1977).

158. For accounts of the Sino-Soviet and Soviet-Vietnamese military relationships, see Raymond L. Garthoff, ed., *Sino-Soviet Military Relations* (New York: Praeger, 1966); Kaplan, "Historical Record"; William Zimmerman, "The Korean and Vietnam Wars," and Thomas W. Robinson, "The Sino-Soviet Border Conflict," in Kaplan, ed., *Diplomacy of Power*, pp. 67–72, 90–96, 98–105, 107–113, 265–313, 314–356.

159. Oleg Penkovskiy, *The Penkovskiy Papers*, trans. Peter Deriabin (New York: Avon Books, 1966), p. 88; *Directory of USSR Ministry of Defense and Armed Forces Officials* (Washington D.C.: Central Intelligence Agency, 1978), p. 4.

160. Kaplan, "Historical Record," in Kaplan, ed., *Diplomacy of Power*, pp. 170–171; and Ken Booth, *The Military Instrument in Soviet Foreign Policy* (London: Royal United Services Institute, 1973), p. 35.

161. Legum, "Angola and the Horn of Africa," in Kaplan, ed., *Diplomacy of Power*, pp. 570–640.

162. Ibid., pp. 623–626.

163. For a review of these, see William F. Scott and Harriet Fast Scott, *A Review and Assessment of Soviet Policy and Concepts on the Projection of Military Presence and Power* (McLean, Va.: General Research Corporation, 1979).

164. Marshal A. A. Grechko, "The Leading Role of the CPSU in Building the Army of a Developed Socialist Society," *Voprosy istorii KPSS* (Problems of History of the CPSU), May 1974, p. 38.

165. David K. Hall, "Naval Diplomacy in West African Waters," in Kaplan, ed., *Diplomacy of Power*, pp. 519–569; MccGwire, "Naval Power and Soviet Global Strategy," pp. 52–53. For a comprehensive survey of Soviet naval force projection, see James M. McConnell and Bradford N. Dismukes, eds., *Soviet Naval Diplomacy: From the June War to Angola* (New York: Pergamon Press, 1981).

Part Three

EUROPE AND THE NORTH ATLANTIC
The International Environment

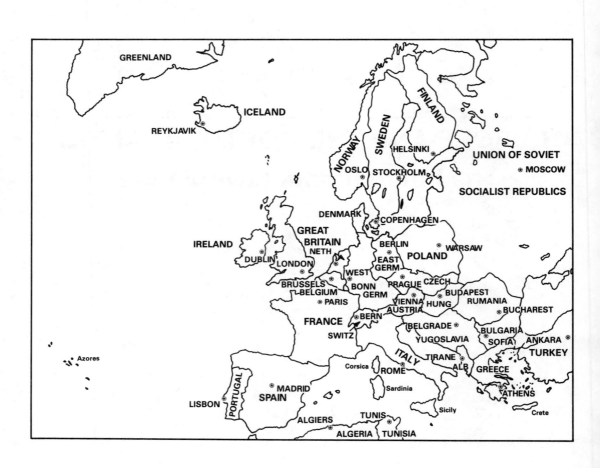

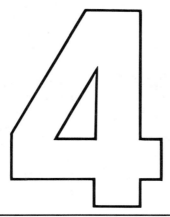

THE FEDERAL REPUBLIC OF GERMANY

Catherine McArdle Kelleher

To omit the Federal Republic of Germany from the list of major military powers in the 1980s and 1990s would be inconceivable. By almost every measure, the Federal Republic ranks as the second power in the Atlantic alliance. Forty-five years after Germany's unconditional surrender in World War II, Bonn compares favorably with London and Paris in the size and capability of its military establishment. The German economic miracle continues, and West Germany has emerged from its state of "political dwarfdom" as a major international actor.

A focus on German defense policy alone, however, suggests as many paradoxes as unquestioned accomplishments in these three decades. All stem from Germany's unique military-political position, which, almost by definition, precludes the formulation of an exclusively German national defense policy.

German strategy and doctrine are founded on the NATO framework; in the words of the 1985 White Paper: "German security policy is a policy of integration in, and commitment to, the Alliance."[1] Although German security rests in the last analysis on the deterrent threat of the American nuclear guarantee, Germany's political rehabilitation was achieved largely through its status as a responsible alliance partner—dependent but equal, reactive to the initiatives of others, yet respected for its sacrifice and responsiveness. This remains true as wider Atlantic interdependence has replaced direct dependence.

Much of this is not surprising, given the circumstances and conditions of German rearmament (table 1). The essential bargain was "no NATO without Germany; no Germany without NATO." Entry into the Western alliance structure—first the proposed integrated European Defense Community, then finally NATO itself—was the essential precondition for restoration of German sovereignty. The German military effort was to be tightly controlled, both to right the military balance vis-à-vis the East and to assure an appropriate military balance in the West. German forces were essential, but only to the maximum levels (500,000) set forth in the separate Western European Union (WEU) treaty.[2] Germany was to

Table 1. Chronology of German Rearmament

Year	Event
1945	Unconditional surrender and demilitarization. Occupation by American, Soviet, British, and French forces.
1948	Breakdown of Four-Power governance. Initial informal discussion on German rearmament.
1949	Federal Republic of Germany established under provisional Basic Law.
1950	First formal discussion of German rearmament within NATO. France proposes European Defense Community (EDC).
1951–1952	EDC negotiations over size, structure, and armament of German forces.
1954	Defeat of EDC. Western European Union (WEU) established as framework for German rearmament within NATO.
1955	Germany enters NATO.
1956	First German forces inducted.
1965	Rearmament completed; twelve divisions assigned to NATO.

be well armed, but was to renounce national production of atomic, biological, and chemical weapons, as well as most major armament classes.

The alliance orientation of German defense policy reflects another central concern: the harmonization and coordination of American and German defense resources.[3] For both states, the involvement of the fourteen other NATO members is essential politically, militarily, and from the perspective of regional balance. But the core of NATO's ability to deter or sustain conflict requires the linking of German and American capabilities. Without this, neither the present form nor the present substance of the alliance could be maintained.

Much of this simply reflects the relative capabilities of these two states.[4] But there are also some basic political axioms at issue. An independent German military capability outside the alliance, or even a significantly lower proportionate German contribution of troops and money, would be unacceptable to most, if not all, of the allies. So, too, would a precipitous decoupling of U.S. forces and any withdrawal of the American political and military guarantee of German security. The only alternative guarantor or protector of the Federal Republic would be a far stronger France or an integrated European defense system, but neither seems presently feasible.[5]

Increasingly, however, there are domestic pressures for a more independent German defense policy, and some international expectations that this may be inevitable. The most obvious are the new challenges raised by the small, strident Green Party. More significant are the interests of some Social Democratic leaders in various alternative defense plans, all non-nuclear and all involving fewer, less well-armed German forces within a looser alliance coalition. More basic still is the increased questioning across the German political spectrum of the necessary congruence of German security interests and those of a global superpower overly tied to the demands of its domestic constituencies—in arms control as in international trade, in the exercise of force as in technology-transfer legislation. It is still uncertain whether these questions will lead to basic policy changes, but such changes cannot be excluded over the next decade. Much, indeed, will depend on the evolution of German-American relations and the rebuilding of Germany's domestic defense consensus in the next several electoral campaigns.

A basic argument of this essay, however, is that there are good reasons why a more independent German defense policy may not emerge. For the present governing elite and most of its conceivable successors, the place of the Federal Republic as NATO's second power ensures most of their foreign policy goals. Political dialogue with the United States is now constant; German access is more automatic than that granted any other ally. Germany's role in NATO is the basis for, and useful operational limit of, U.S. relations with both Eastern and Western Europe. This role provides the best, most credible structure for deterrence and, for most, the only hope of direct conventional defense. And in the short term, it minimizes the political risks to Bonn of achieving continental dominance in conventional forces, still an area of great historical sensitivity.

Finally, it forecloses few options of interest to the Federal Republic in a future as yet unforeseeable. A traditional postwar listing of possible German goals would include reunification, European military integration, nuclear independence, and a return to a looser alliance structure for coalition warfare. More recent versions might also include an improbable extra-European military role (say to ensure oil security) and reduction to a smaller standing military establishment under terms of negotiated arms limitation or stabilization. But whatever the nature of future choices, the Federal Republic's present opportunity for maneuver is substantial. Its centrality in all NATO decisions is assured; costs, programs, and doctrines have long been negotiated, not just imposed. German leadership and initiative are now assumed—as perhaps also is German irritation at failures in the performance of others.

The critical variables, now as throughout Germany's past few decades, seem to be the nature and strength of Germany's American connection and the costs and benefits it imposes. I shall return to this again and again in the following examination of German defense decision making.

International Environment

By most objective measures, the Federal Republic of Germany ranks as a mid-level or second-tier military power in the postwar international system.[6] Like Britain, France, and, in a different way, China, it is a state with major political and military capabilities, a strong regional base, and potential for broader global reach. Germany's non-nuclear status is anomalous—the product of its past, the timing of its rehabilitation (1955), and increasing superpower control over nuclear proliferation. Somewhat discordant, too, is Bonn's constant rhetorical emphasis on the vulnerability of the Federal Republic, its limited room for maneuver, and its exclusively European domain of influence.

Almost from its inception in 1949,[7] the Federal Republic has sought primary identification with the West. The initial relationship showed Chancellor Konrad Adenauer's talent for making a virtue of political necessity. The Federal Republic was, after all, a creature of the Cold War, split among the victors of World War II. The Western powers, and especially the United States, were both occupation

powers and founding fathers. Chancellor Konrad Adenauer understood that in the short run they alone would guarantee German security against internal and external threats and allow German reentry into the postwar international community. Reunification, if it occurred at all, would be a long-term process. It would require a series of dramatic changes not only in the international environment, but also in German political structures and attitudes, which had been bankrupted by Nazism and military defeat.

In the Atlantic framework, the Federal Republic is now the major European partner of the United States. The virtually inextricable involvement of the Federal Republic with the West has proven to be the best means of ensuring and controlling American involvement in German security. This situation has endured since Adenauer's time. For Adenauer's successors, however, the circumstances were hardly propitious (see table 2). On the one hand, there was Gaullist France, formally estranged from NATO's integrated defense and pressing Germany in several respects for a choice between Europe and American alliance. On the other, there was a declining Britain, unwilling to cede the "Anglo-Saxon connection" it had had with the United States throughout the postwar period, and ever chary of German capabilities and intentions.

American expectations of Germany's new role were no less risk laden. In the mid 1960s (and for some still today), the American preference was unquestionably for a junior partner, for a military organization and doctrine "made in America" and an ally willing to accept them. Doctrinal disagreements, such as those over the employment of forces or the control of escalation, were issues for consultation or for education of the Germans, not for joint decision making among equals. Germany was to be America's European debating partner in two respects: first, as a sounding board for American concerns; second, as the medium for indirect continental influence. (The Federal Republic would serve as persuader, example, or threat—primarily in dealings with the French.)

Events and growing interdependence over

Table 2. Principals in West German Defense Policy Making, 1955–Present

Parliament	Coalition Parties	Chancellor	Foreign Minister	Defense Minister
1st (1949–53)	CDU/CSU, FDP, and others	Konrad Adenauer, CDU	Adenauer	
2nd (1953–57)	CDU/CSU, FDP	Adenauer CDU	Adenauer (–1955)	Theodor Blank, CDU (1955–56)
			Heinrich von Brentano, CDU (1955–)	Franz Josef Strauss, CSU (1956–)
3rd (1957–61)	CDU/CSU	Adenauer CDU	von Brentano, CDU	Strauss, CSU
4th (1961–65)	CDU/CSU, FDP	Adenauer, CDU (–1963)	Gerhard Schröder, CDU	Strauss, CSU (–1962)
				Kai-Uwe von Hassel, CDU (1963–)
		Ludwig Erhard, CDU (1963–)		
5th (1965–69)	CDU/CSU, FDP	Erhard, CDU (–1966)	Schröder, CDU (–1966)	von Hassel, CDU (–1966)
	CDU/CSU, SPD (Grand Coalition)	Kurt Georg Kiesinger, CDU (1966–)	Willy Brandt, SPD (1966–)	Schröder, CDU (1966–)
6th (1969–72)	SPD, FDP	Brandt, SPD	Walter Scheel, FDP	Helmut Schmidt, SPD (–1972)
				Georg Leber, SPD (1972–)
7th (1972–76)	SPD, FDP	Brandt, SPD (–1974)	Scheel, FDP (–1974)	Leber, SPD
		Schmidt, SPD (1974–)	Hans-Dietrich Genscher, FDP (1974–)	
8th (1976–80)	SPD, FDP	Schmidt, SPD	Genscher, FDP	Leber, SPD (–1978)
				Hans Apel, SPD (1978–)
9th (1980–83)	SPD, FDP	Schmidt, SPD	Genscher, FDP	Apel, SPD
	CDU/CSU, FDP	Helmut Kohl, CDU (1982–)		Manfred Woerner, CDU (1982–88)
10th (1983–87)	CDU/CSU, FDP	Kohl, CDU	Genscher, FDP	Woerner, CDU
11th (1987–)	CDU/CSU, FDP	Kohl, CDU	Genscher, FDP	Woerner, CDU
				Sholz, CDU

Note: CDU = Christian Democratic Union
CSU = Christian Social Union
FDP = Free Democratic party
SPD = Social Democratic party

the past decades have led to a far more equal and differentiated status. In the Nixon administration some foresaw still greater German sharing of alliance power and responsibility.[8] The Federal Republic would be the explicit synthesizer, coordinator, and, if necessary, "director" of European security efforts and organization. The United States would continue its European deployments, at least for the short run, and remain the alliance leader and general strategic reserve. The Federal Republic would, however, come to have equal decision-making power over issues including nuclear weapons use and arms control negotiations with the Eastern bloc, and would receive fundamental American support for its foreign pol-

icy and economic initiatives. Eventual German possession of nuclear arms and direct military involvement outside NATO would not be precluded, although the United States preferred that such involvement be through the medium of a European force. The final organizational outcome would have to be left to time, and to the progress of German-Franco-British maneuvering. But it might well approach the initial "two pillars" concept put forward by John F. Kennedy or the vision of joint European-American hegemony supported on occasion by the late Bavarian political leader Franz Josef Strauss.[9]

Others under Nixon, and the majority in the Carter administration, favored a more limited division of labor. Within the NATO military framework, Germany was an "almost equal," except, in accordance with Bonn's own preference, in areas involving the direct control of nuclear weapons. Equality, though, involved the assumption of both positive and negative burdens in alliance decision making. Germany had the right to criticize American initiatives, but also the responsibility of proposing alternatives and promoting their approval among Europeans as well as Americans (e.g., on NATO force modernization, reserve readiness, long-range theater nuclear forces, and airborne warning and control systems).

Different expectations about Germany's role have been voiced intermittently by other NATO states. Germany is seen as NATO's most influential European "representative," the source of criticism and correction for a too often preoccupied United States. The specific focus of concerns has varied, largely as a function of European perceptions of either too much American leadership and control in the early 1970s or the diffuse, capricious style of more recent years. A general catalog of recent German criticisms includes: (1) the American obsession with war-fighting requirements rather than the components of the primary deterrence system; Americans who see credible war-fighting capabilities as essential to maintaining deterrence and speak freely of various nuclear and non-nuclear war-fighting options on European soil thus invite the misunderstanding and wrath of Germans and other Europeans, who prefer to emphasize deterrence apart from any war-fighting capabilities per se; (2) recurring American tendencies toward implicit "decoupling" of strategic nuclear forces from the defense of Europe and a limited conception of the "Eurostrategic" balance compared to the European preference for full commitment of U.S. strategic nuclear forces and both nuclear and non-nuclear forces deployed in Europe;[10] and (3) unilateral American actions vis-à-vis the Soviet Union that hinder the pursuit of détente and arms limitations.

Germany is clearly the "once and present king" of Europe, both within the formalities of the European community and outside of it. The German economic miracle in the 1950s (and again in the 1980s) has left Germany in the position of Europe's banker and economic spokesman. Together with France, it has acted to ensure a favorable, but equitable European balance.[11] Germany has also defended broader economic interests and political-economic preferences in a number of diverse arenas outside of Europe, primarily in the transatlantic dialogue with the United States. But there has also been direct economic intervention in Germany's own interests in the turmoil of the Portuguese revolution, the chaos of Chile, the confusion of Turkey and Pakistan, and the continuing Third World debt crisis.

Coexistent with these primary Western allegiances, however, are several special relations with the East. All reflect Germany's unique historical and geopolitical position. All segments of the West German political spectrum support the fullest possible human links to the "other Germany," the German Democratic Republic (GDR or, in German, DDR). Reunification is a major national objective only in the long run; the precedent-breaking treaties of the 1970s formally recognized the existence of "two states in the German nation."[12] The Federal Republic and the DDR remain political and ideological competitors both abroad and at home. Berlin continues to be a symbol painfully open to manipulation, but ties remain: the family relationships revived under the détente of the 1970s, the continuing economic links (however exploitative they appear to other Western states), and unofficial political dialogue. A cautious interweaving of the perceptions of East and West German leaders about the requirements for European security and stability is increasingly evident. Primary alliances and the foundations of national legitimacy lie elsewhere, but the potential for greater intranational identification remains. The determination of both East and West Germany to continue their dialogue despite the deep freeze of Washington-Moscow relations of 1983–85 is proof enough.

Less symbolic, but of perhaps greater short-run significance, are the other German ties to the East. Beginning with Chancellor Willy Brandt's drive for "normalization" in the early 1970s, Germany's *Ostpolitik* has resulted in an increasing German presence in Eastern Europe.[13] In part, it builds on traditional German commercial and economic dominance in the region. It also reflects German support for the "European" policies of Eastern European states, pursued cautiously within the Conference on Security and Cooperation in Europe (CSCE) or the mutual and balanced force reductions (MBFR) framework, and ever mindful of the limits of Soviet toleration. German championing of these causes is relatively low-key, given the political risks and the persistence in some foreign sectors of virulent anti-Germanism.

More troublesome for some in the West has been the evolution of German-Soviet relations. The Adenauer concept was framed in the emphatic anticommunist and anti-Soviet tones characteristic of most Western foreign policies of the mid 1950s. *Ostpolitik* and "normalization" in the late 1960s and early 1970s led to a formal treaty of mutual assurance (1969), myriad new economic and cultural interchanges, including the controversial gas pipeline agreement of the late 1970s, and far more continuous political dialogue.[14] Détente in Europe has been Bonn's primary goal, a process valued both for improving the human landscape in the short term and for the prospect of longer-term European stability.

In the late 1970s there were some in the Christian Democratic Union (CDU) who saw danger in this strengthening of German-Soviet ties. Some cited the precedent of Rapallo, the separate Soviet-German agreement concluded in the 1920s at the expense of the West. Others, most notably U.S. National Security Advisers Henry Kissinger and Zbigniew Brzezinski, proclaimed the danger of Germany being "Finlandized"—creating a less independent Germany subject to Soviet foreign policy preferences. Defenders of German-Soviet ties, particularly those in the Social Democratic Party (SPD) and now the ruling CDU, have stressed the fairly narrow dependencies that have been created on both sides—in long-term loans as in energy supplies, in technology transfers as in the promotion of greater human rights, and in sanctioned emigration of ethnic Germans from the East. They also cite Adenauer's decision in 1955 to open formal relations with the Soviet Union far ahead of any other communist state and in direct contradiction to the German policy at the time of not establishing relations with any state having formal relations with East Germany. His justification was simply that the interests at stake—political, military, and economic—were too important to be ignored or postponed. This argument is seen as even more valid after forty years of military confrontation and arms buildup in central Europe.

The posture of primary identification with the West, but with clear, continuing communication to the East, was at some variance with the broad German consensus through the 1970s on the nature of direct threats to German security. Without question, most Germans saw the direct threat principally to be the Soviet Union and secondarily its Eastern European allies.[15] However, they also viewed a direct Soviet invasion, or even use of direct military pressure, as being a very low probability (see fig. 1). The changing perception of threat among the German population reveals the growing impression that the Soviet Union is not much different than its superpower partner, the United States. To support this view that the USSR does not really pose an imminent threat, some have cited not only the political intractability and resistance in Western Europe to any attempt at Soviet occupation, but also the relative attractiveness to the Soviet Union of the status quo—a Western Europe intact and without the devastation war would entail. Moreover, others doubt Soviet incentives to invade since invasion would forego the easy gains of the détente period in terms of economic support and technological transfers from Western Europe.[16]

Many in West Germany now downplay their status as the European state most exposed and vulnerable to Soviet military and political presence. They stress the slight probability of direct Soviet action, even though should conflict occur, West Germany will inevitably be the battlefield. It is from this perspective that there is now a German debate about whether a capability to counter a Soviet invasion can come only through the involvement of the United States and NATO, or whether there are other

Figure 1. Changing West German Perceptions of the Communist Threat

Question: In your opinion is the communist threat very great, great, not so great, or not to be taken seriously?

Answer	1962	1968	1971	1974	1977	1980	1983	1984
Very Great, or Great	63	48	39	35	41	48	45	47
Not Very Great, Not To Be Taken Seriously	22	29	56	41	40	48	52	53
No Response	5	23	5	24	18	3	3	—

Source: Adapted from EMNID survey, *Meinungsbild in der Bundesrepublik Deutschland zur Sicherheitspolitik* (Opinions in the FRG on Security Policy) [Study Commissioned by the West German Ministry of Defense] (Bonn: Oct. 1984), mimeographed. Taken from Stephen F. Szabo, "The FRG: Public Opinion and Defense" in Catherine M. Kelleher and Gale A. Mattox, eds., *Evolving European Defense Policies* (Lexington, Mass.: Lexington Books, 1987), p. 186.

viable alternatives. In the 1950s and 1960s, when the probability of Soviet action seemed higher, the involvement of the U.S. and NATO was supported by an overwhelming national consensus. The withdrawal of even a small number of U.S. conventional forces occasioned demands for reassurance and remedial action (in 1956, 1962, and throughout the mid 1960s). In the period of "normalization" and increasing strategic parity of the 1970s and 1980s, there was a cooler tone and far less tendency to identify the threat as imminent or exclusively military.[17]

In recent years there has been far more frequent criticism of U.S. force posture and weapons acquisition decisions. Criticism of the Strategic Defense Initiative (SDI), for example, parallels the earlier, negative reaction by many Germans to the deployment of intermediate-range nuclear forces (INF). Far more fundamental, however, are the questions among those on the left in SPD and university and intellectual circles about the continuing negative impacts of U.S. policy choices for German security. German defense policy is said to reflect America's best interests, to be responsive primarily to American calculations

about the necessary role of tactical nuclear weapons, the nature of conventional warfare, and even the need for large standing armies and high military expenditures. From the perspective of Germans on the left of the political spectrum, such dependence on the U.S. contributes to a greater risk of war, to greater chances of confrontation, and even unnecessary provocation of the Soviet Union; such dependence thus undermines "true" German security.

But there is still majority agreement, and governmental insistence, on the inescapable need for an American guarantee of German security in détente and in confrontation, in peacetime and in conflict. As table 3 partially records, the strength of this perception did increase over the low points of the early 1970s, but has declined again in the 1980s.

Soviet attempts to use political means to divide the Federal Republic from its Western allies are seen as a more probable threat. Those on the right (in the CDU and Christian Social Union and in the United States) cite continuing Soviet efforts to use both the carrot and the stick in relations with the Federal Republic. One Soviet tactic is to encourage German op-

Table 3. Confidence in U.S. Commitment to Defend Western Europe

Question 1: "In the event our country's security were threatened by a Soviet attack, how much confidence do you feel we can have in the United States to come to our defense—a great deal, a fair amount, not very much, or none at all?"

	Great Or Fair	Not Much None	DK	Net Confidence
West Germany				
1968	55%	41%	6%	+12
1972	67%	23%	10%	+44
1974	72%	20%	8%	+52
1975	49%	41%	10%	+8
1978	61%	28%	11%	+33
1979	53%	35%	12%	+18
1980	66%	25%	9%	+41
1981	59%	28%	13%	+31

Notes: Wording varies slightly. The 1978 question refers to a "threat to Western Europe's security." The 1975 question refers to "trust" rather than confidence in the United States. The 1974 question refers to a Soviet attack on Western Europe "without involving the United States directly."

"Net confidence" is calculated by subtracting the percentage of "not much/none" confidence from those with "great/fair" confidence.

Question 2: "If our security were threatened by a Soviet attack, how much confidence do you have in the U.S. to do whatever is necessary to defend our country, even if this would risk the destruction of U.S. cities—a great deal, a fair amount, not very much, or none at all?"

	Great Or Fair	Not Much None	DK	Net Confidence
West Germany				
July 1981	48	38	14	+10
Jan 1982	49	39	12	+10
Apr 1982	52	37	11	+15
July 1982	49	39	12	+10
Aug 1983	43	50	7	−7
Nov 1983	41	43	15	−2
July 1984	27	63	10	−36
Dec 1985	40	46	14	−6

Notes: In 1983, the question refers to a direct "attack against the United States itself" rather than to the "destruction of American cities."

Source: Richard C. Eichenberg, *Public Opinion and National Security in Western Europe: Consensus Lost?* (Ithaca: Cornell University Press, 1989): Tables 3.3 and 3.4 (surveys by USIA).

position to important alliance programs, such as debate within alliance countries on the deployment of INF missile systems (1980–83) or the earlier plans to deploy enhanced radiation weapons, or "neutron bombs" (1978–1979).[18] The USSR was more successful in securing German support for completing the gas pipeline, notwithstanding American objections that this would make West Germany dependent on the Eastern bloc for continuing supplies. Simultaneously, Moscow holds out, on the one hand, the prospect of a negotiated "equitable" settlement (e.g., with the agreement in 1987 to eliminate INF missiles from Europe, a proposal to eliminate all short-range nuclear forces as well) or, on the other hand, the threat of a worsening of relations (e.g., a break-off of CSCE contacts or an increase in

the visitor fee for family trips to East Germany).

At least equally unpalatable are Soviet attempts to invoke "the German threat" as a divisive tactic. In the 1950s and 1960s, the rhetorical specter of a revanchist West Germany, inheritor of the Nazi past, provided considerable incentive in Soviet attempts to tighten Soviet–Eastern European relations. *Ostpolitik* efforts of the 1970s, as well as the general improvement of bilateral ties, especially with Poland, have removed most, but not all, of the impact of this Soviet instrument.[19] A nuclear-capable Federal Republic and a competent, ready Bundeswehr as the strongest conventional European force are images that still evoke remembered fear and current suspicion among their European neighbors.

Almost totally unsuccessful now are Soviet efforts to discredit German initiatives in the West. Anti-Germanism remains a potential force among the left in almost all European states, and German economic success is also not the subject of universal admiration, especially among European socialists.[20] Yet the general tightening of Western European political relations and the continuity of Franco-German rapprochement, especially over the past decade, make Soviet claims about a German threat in Europe far less credible to others. Few of the Europeans dependent on German economic leadership are supportive of direct challenges to German preferences, either in NATO or in the European Communities (EC).

From Adenauer onward, German leaders have seen Soviet attempts to weaken the Bonn-Washington link as a major threat. Adenauer repeatedly cited as his nightmare the prospect of a Soviet-American agreement on an acceptable European order, concluded over the head of, and at the expense of, the Federal Republic. Adenauer's fears grew in relation to his declining political power within the CDU and with the advent under Kennedy of a direct superpower-to-superpower approach to the Soviet Union. His demands for reassurance became continuous and his criticism of the new president more strident, language useful to Kennedy's political opponents in the United States. The high point came in the mid 1960s with Lyndon Johnson's insistence on concluding the Nuclear Non-proliferation Treaty (NPT) with the Soviet Union.[21] To Adenauer and Franz Josef Strauss, both then out of power, this was a superpower attempt to impose a "nuclear Versailles," restricting German military options and giving the Soviet Union new rights of control and inspection vis-à-vis the Federal Republic.

In the 1970s, such criticisms became far less frequent and more muted, as Washington pursued a policy of "benign neglect" in European affairs, and Bonn was caught up in its own initiatives toward the East. German tactics were to underscore the primacy of the American connection and to press German demands through every channel, public and private. Successive German governments, moreover,

favored the development of new integrative structures within NATO to deal with thorny questions and provide for "automatic" decision sharing with the United States. The most dramatic new forums, not surprisingly, were suggested in the area of nuclear control in the 1960s—a NATO nuclear force under a NATO commander, a "Western Four" (United States, United Kingdom, France, and the Federal Republic), and the much-discussed Multilateral Nuclear Force (MLF).[22] None ultimately was adopted, although the NATO Nuclear Planning Group (NPG), established in the late 1960s with assured German participation, achieved a considerable measure of success.

The one point of continuing concern was the risk implicit in Soviet-American cooperation in arms limitation—SALT I and especially SALT II. Chancellor Helmut Schmidt, for example, charged that the 1977–78 SALT II discussions were highly questionable.[23] Issues vital to European security were being discussed without real consultation with the European allies or even much consideration of their interests, particularly in the area of theater nuclear systems. The opposite concern—that insufficient progress was being made by the superpowers on important arms control issues—became apparent when the Carter administration failed to secure ratification of the SALT II treaty and subsequently in the early and mid 1980s when negotiated arms settlements received less emphasis.

An increasing number of the German elite have come to question how much more congruent or predictable the German-American connection could become. Most see the core problems to be the U.S. decision-making process (e.g., extensive interagency bargaining and the confused, sometimes unstable, institutional links in the American system) and competing U.S. interests in other areas of the world (e.g., Asia and the Pacific). The trauma the Watergate scandal imposed on American alliance leadership during the Nixon administration, the repeated communications crises of the Carter administration, the frequently surprising statements of the Reagan administration on nuclear war-fighting, and its long attempts to "stonewall" on arms control negotiations all strengthened these arguments. In broad outline, the theme was the same as that pushed by the first postwar leader of the SPD, Kurt Schumacher.[24] Only Germany could define and further German national interests; the solutions could not be wrung from a policy of fixed alliances with West or East, or even, perhaps, from one primarily based on military strength.

There is, however, an elite group, particularly in the left wing of the SPD, that sees independent German-Soviet ties as an equally valuable counter, particularly in combination with continuing *Westpolitik*, or Western-oriented policy. Statements by former Chancellor Willy Brandt and SPD member Egon Bahr, for example, suggest *Ostpolitik* as an antidote to unwelcome superpower agreement or an unwarranted sacrifice of German interests in an international game in which Germany has only veto rights. Whatever the subject—trade, arms control, or a final political settlement of the World War II legacy—attempts to bargain for, but also about, Germany are to be resisted.

A final threat, widely perceived among the German elite, if not by the mass public, is that stemming from the Germans themselves. Critics on the right see the source most simply as a flawed national character. Perhaps the most dramatic expression is found in Adenauer's reaction to the 1954 failure of the European Defense Community, which would have totally submerged German military units in a European whole:

I am 100 percent convinced that the German national army, to which Mendes-France [then French premier] is forcing us, will be a great danger to both Germany and Europe. When I am no longer here, I do not know what will happen to Germany if we have not yet succeeded in creating a United Europe. The French nationalists would rather [have] a Germany with a national army than a united Europe—so long as they can pursue their own policy with the Russians. And the German nationalists think exactly the same way; they are ready to go [i.e., pursue their own independent policy] with the Russians.[25]

On other occasions, Adenauer also cited the fatal German fascination with *Schaukelpolitik*, the playing off of East and West so successfully pursued by Bismarck in the 1870s.

The contemporary critique by the political right focuses in Germany, as elsewhere, on the threat posed by unprecedented economic prosperity and declining popular willingness for civic duty or national service.[26] In simplest terms, West Germans, like all Western peoples, are "too fat to fight." This is asserted whether the targets are unkempt conscripts or unruly students, welfare cheaters or domestic speculators.

The internal threats judged most dangerous by most Germans in the 1970s and at present cluster around the preservation of civic order. The attribution of the particular source of risk is again often dependent on the ideological orientation of the commentator. Those on the right see the danger as the continuing, sometimes violent, demonstrations of students, antinuclear protestors, squatters, environmentalists, the unemployed, and "marginal groups." First and foremost, however, is the threat of terrorism, domestic and international, as epitomized by the activities of the Baader-Meinhof gang and the Red Brigade.

Those on the left are more likely to find the sources of threat in the repressive, constricting nature of the existing German society and state. They point to the widespread popular panic about terrorism and the resulting programs of the 1970s and 1980s to curtail civil liberties in order to capture terrorists or deter terrorist activity. Their arguments focus on the future: at what point will the requirements of internal and external security become so fixed that both individual life and German society in general will be irretrievably transformed?

Both perspectives are articulated most forcefully only at the extremes of the German political spectrum. But both suggest an implicit fear shared by many Germans, all too mindful of the consequences of the chaos of the Weimar period. The threat from outside Germany is at least definable and amenable to partial solution. The threat of an enemy boring from within raises questions and calculations about national identity and national values that few in the German elite are willing to define or able to confront politically.

National Objectives, National Strategy, and Military Doctrine

Given the range of perceived threats, what is the national security strategy of the Federal

Republic? In the short run, it is primarily to seek security against external political threats and military attack through membership in NATO and the closest possible ties to the United States.[27] For this purpose, NATO is only secondarily a 16-member organization. Its essence is the military-political core of the "central front states"—the United States, Britain, Canada, Denmark, the Benelux states (Belgium, the Netherlands, and Luxembourg), and the Federal Republic, plus an informally linked France. This is the basis on which to mount an effective Western deterrence and defense, up to the involvement of strategic nuclear forces.

In the majority German view, the centrality of the United States in this effort stems from a number of sources, most obviously U.S. military and political preeminence. On the other hand, the United States may have lost its strategic advantage or superiority in an age of Soviet-American nuclear parity. U.S. economic dominance has faded even in terms of America's potential for wartime mobilization. The claims of the United States regarding overall technological superiority have also declined because of successive challenges from Western allies and from the Soviet Union. Chancellors and ministers have commented recently on the sorry readiness levels of some American units in Germany and on problems of equipment and morale.[28]

Yet for most of the German elite, the U.S. military capability remains the last and best guarantee of German security. American forces, both conventional and nuclear, offset Soviet military power. The more than two hundred thousand U.S. troops stationed on German soil are living proof of American commitment to the integrity of the Federal Republic; so, too, are the approximately four hundred thousand U.S. American military dependents. Further, the substantial numbers of tactical or "theater" nuclear forces (TNF) in West Germany constitute at least one indicator of American willingness to threaten and, if necessary, to initiate escalation to general nuclear war—a commitment seen as essential to deterrence.[29]

Of significance, too, is the parallel involvement of the other central front states in maintaining a multilateral military presence on German soil (fig. 2). The size and capabilities of the seven national contingents vary considerably; their deployments clearly reflect the early stratification of occupation force assignments. The fifty thousand or so French troops are stationed in Germany under a separate Franco-German agreement concluded in 1966. Together, these national commitments provide, first, an equalizing and legitimizing framework for German national capabilities, and, second, multilateral guarantees for the U.S. security commitment.

The German elite now sees détente policy—efforts to relax tensions and reduce threat levels—as the second major pillar of a national security strategy.[30] Indeed, according to the 1985 White Paper: "The security policy of the Federal government is inseparably linked to serious efforts to achieve détente, arms control and disarmament. This policy renounces coercion, endeavors to prevent military conflict and to settle matters peacefully, and is committed to the promotion of peace."[31] But the clear principle was established in the 1970s by Brandt and Schmidt: defense without simultaneous efforts to reduce the threat, and thus the need for defense, is self-defeating and politically unacceptable.

From this perspective, the long-term answer to German security dilemmas lies in steps to limit the level of military capability on both sides of a divided Europe.[32] Suggestions run the gamut from the full-scale disengagement model first proposed by Germans and others in the 1950s to the more contemporary idea of a series of small cuts or even mutual confidence-building measures (CBM) that will enhance perceptions of stability; such measures include mutual notification between the NATO and Warsaw Pact countries of major exercises and the exchange of observers of such maneuvers. A surprisingly broad popular consensus, too, supports arms limitation. People are often critical of strategic arms control negotiations, but support them nevertheless as an essential process. They welcome the discussion of a wide range of initiatives—the work in the Conference on Security and Cooperation in Europe (CSCE), the UN Special Session on Disarmament (SSOD), and the Conference on Disarmament in Europe (CDE).

Figure 2. Force Deployments on German Territory

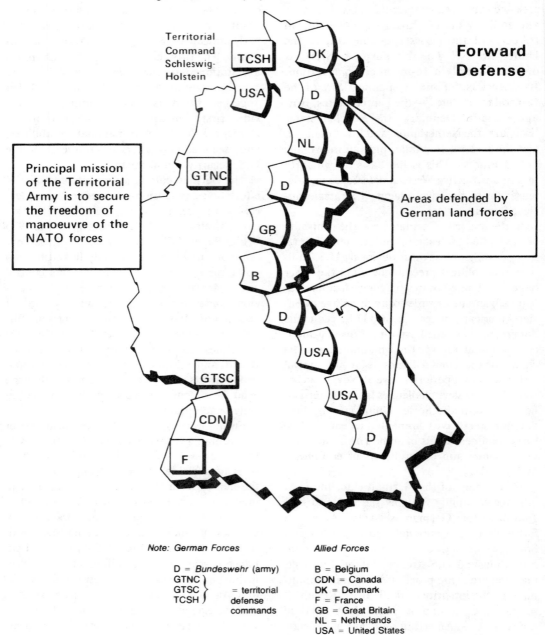

Territorial
Command
Schleswig-
Holstein

**Forward
Defense**

Principal mission
of the Territorial
Army is to secure
the freedom of
manoeuvre of the
NATO forces

Areas defended by
German land forces

Note: German Forces   *Allied Forces*

D = *Bundeswehr* (army)   B = Belgium
GTNC ⎫   CDN = Canada
GTSC ⎬ = territorial   DK = Denmark
TCSH ⎭   defense   F = France
          commands   GB = Great Britain
                                NL = Netherlands
                                USA = United States

In the 1970s this consensus was reflected in a number of official debates and decisions.[33] Popular support for arms control negotiations has been widespread, even when results—as in the talks on Mutual and Balanced Force Reductions in Europe—have been mostly atmospherics, with little tangible progress. Promises of future talks are seen by many on the left and in the center as long-term investments in avoiding misperceptions and increasing European dialogue, if not actually increasing integration between East and West.

Perhaps the most dramatic evidence of this basic argument came in the context of the INF debates of 1979–80.[34] Chancellor Schmidt had initiated the call for new force deployments, citing the gap in the spectrum of deterrence revealed by Soviet deployments of mobile SS-20 intermediate-range missiles. The NATO allies had set up a special High-Level Working Group (HLG) to consider various force options and deployment possibilities. Under direct, continuous pressure from within his own SPD-FDP governing coalition, Schmidt also had to make acceptance contingent on simultaneous efforts to limit these forces. The vehicle was a special group (the Special Consultative Group, or SCG) directed both to consider the arms control impacts of these new weapons and to prepare for negotiating mutual reductions with the Soviet Union. Only in this manner, it was argued both in the Bundestag and outside it, could the West work toward long-term stability in Europe, and avoid setting off yet another upward spiral of the East-West arms race. Success was not assured, but without this effort there would have been no Western INF deployments.

Both strands of the present German national security strategy, however, leave a number of basic questions unanswered. In some measure, this reflects the judgment of German political leadership that a degree of ambiguity is prudent. An equally or even more significant reason is to be found in the unique dilemmas of priorities and modalities imposed by the special position of the Federal Republic. As expressed by several German scholars, the Federal Republic is struggling to create a new type or "model" of security policy, one that acknowledges the demands of both national responsibility and international interdependence.[35]

First, in relation to traditional defense policy, it is clear that reliance on the United States for its primary security has always left the Federal Republic with significant costs and doubts. The most basic of these turns on the level and form of national military forces, depicted in table 4. At one level, these must be sufficient to meet the political conditions of the U.S. guarantee: the demonstration of continu-

Table 4. German Armed Forces, 1986–87

Branch of Service	Troops
Army	
Total strength	485,800
Conscripts	228,850
Organization	
Field Army	340,800
3 corps	
12 divisions	
6 armored	
4 armored infantry	
1 mountain	
1 airborne	
Territorial Army	49,400
Navy	
Total strength	36,300
Conscripts	9,450
Air Force	
Total strength	108,700
Conscripts	38,100
Reserves	
All services	770,000

Source: International Institute for Strategic Studies, *The Military Balance, 1986-1987* (London: IISS, 1986).

ing German (and European) efforts to sacrifice for their own defense. It was under this congressional requirement that U.S. forces were first sent to Europe, and this is the core of the recurring alliance debate about equitable burden sharing.[36] For the first decade of rearmament (1955–65), the Federal Republic was allowed to set the pace and scope of its military development. Thereafter, Washington pressed forcefully for German forces of up to the maximum strength of 500,000 set in the Western European Union Treaty of 1955. At present, the Federal Republic provides over half of NATO's central front land forces, about one-third of the combat aircraft, and almost all of the Baltic naval forces.[37] Moreover, it holds the second largest effective reserve force pool, the second largest force of nuclear-capable launchers and platforms, and the greatest European capacity for rapid defense expansion and general economic mobilization.

There are many within the alliance who would like to see the Germans take on more burdens. Characteristic opposition was sounded by Defense Minister George Leber in a 1975 response to reports of American interest in a 600,000-man Bundeswehr:

There are many arguments against that. It is not as if the Federal Republic of Germany led a charmed life—

not from an economic perspective either—and could afford everything. But more importantly if the Germans were to increase their army while others were to reduce theirs, inner-European problems would arise with certainty, because of the excessive weight that such a German army would then have in a circle of the Western European military powers. And I must preserve Europe from that.[38]

The American definition of sufficiency leaves some of Bonn's basic political worries unanswered. Adenauer's initial fear was that sufficiency would entail a permanent situation in which an oversized German commitment would make Germans the purveyor of cannon fodder for the alliance. Every German soldier might mean less allied effort or more specialization of advanced military functions (e.g., the 1956 plan by the chairman of the U.S. Joint Chiefs of Staff, Admiral Radford, for reduction to small American "atomic units" attached to allied forces).[39] Sufficiency, therefore, has to be interpreted as a commitment to forces of equal armament, organization, and readiness. Moreover, it was American forces that set the standard that all alliance forces should eventually reach. The Federal Republic suffered only one categorical disadvantage (no direct possession of nuclear munitions), but this is true of most other states as well.

German fears about the implications of the sufficiency standard took on a somewhat different character in the 1960s and early 1970s. The most public of them concerned sufficiency as a justification for the withdrawal of American forces and the "Europeanization" of central front defense. Adenauer and his CDU successor, Ludwig Erhard, consistently opposed American reductions of even relatively limited size as a weakening of the basic security guarantee. Efforts to legislate cuts through a series of "Mansfield Amendments" in the U.S. Senate (efforts to reduce U.S. troop strength in Europe by Senator Mike Mansfield, then Majority Leader in the Senate, later U.S. ambassador to Japan) met similar, if less dramatic, resistance. What was in dispute was the prospect of an arbitrary American reduction that would disturb deterrence or undermine public confidence. At the same time, however, the Erhard (CDU) and Kiesinger (CDU-SPD) governments were willing to accept the stripping

of American units of manpower needed to support operations in Vietnam, and in 1973 the Brandt government (SPD) agreed to the re-equipping of Israel from U.S. stocks in Germany. Present German reactions to American force changes are far more restrained, but changes are also less frequent or severe.

Worries continue about another interpretation of sufficiency—that laid down in NATO's doctrine of flexible response. American pressures for a greater conventional buildup began under the Kennedy administration in the wake of the Berlin crisis of 1961–62.[40] The Federal Republic was the ally most responsive to the challenge, and accelerated its buildup by more than 25 percent. It was far less supportive of U.S. demands for greater reserves and for sustainability, and it consistently criticized American scenarios for a conventional war in central Europe of up to ninety days' duration. Along with the other allies, the Federal Republic finally agreed to flexible response as official NATO doctrine, set down in NATO's MC 14/3 of 1967—a NATO Military Committee document outlining the alliance commitment to the doctrines of flexible response and forward defense. But unofficial German policy opinion (as well as many defense leaders) remained critical of lengthy war-fighting scenarios as represented, for example, in the "extended conventional exchange" concept.[41]

The German stance stemmed in part from a more pessimistic assessment of the East-West conventional balance than that current in Washington in the mid 1960s and the 1970s.[42] Unspoken German fears—that the invoking of the American guarantee would come too late, if at all—were fundamental to this. The dread was of a defense first, for example, at the Rhine, leaving a substantial part of Germany to suffer cycles of occupation, then liberation.[43] As a condition of alliance membership, the Federal Republic had insisted from the outset on the absolute principle of forward defense. This meant formal alliance adherence to the defense of German territory as close as possible to the borders of East Germany and Czechoslovakia and as soon as possible after the onset of conflict.

Added insurance came through Bonn's policy, begun in the 1950s, of encouraging settlement and plant location as close to the border as practicable. By 1979 estimates showed that at least 25 percent of the West German population and industrial plant were within 100 kilometers of the demarcation line.[44] Should conflict occur, the military and human costs of these policies would be great, particularly when added to massive westward movements of refugees from East Germany and elsewhere. But in German eyes, this policy in peacetime added another component to deterrence. It was a credible indicator that neither Soviet "salami tactics" (e.g., a "grab" for Hamburg or a limited invasion probe) nor an attempt at a negotiated settlement on the basis of de facto occupation or control (tried by the USSR in the 1950s and early 1960s against several Berlin enclaves) would be left unanswered.

Divergences in German preferences about the timing of nuclear weapons use still remain, but the official debate is largely conducted in vague verbal formulations. American political leaders tend to talk in terms of days—of nuclear weapons use "as late as possible." The German political leadership, now the CDU, suggests that it may instead be a question of hours, the preferred formulation being "as early as necessary." As a concept, flexible response is sufficiently vague—at least in peacetime—to accommodate both points of view.

There is also far more explicit reference to the fear of American "decoupling." Under strategic parity, the argument in Bonn goes, the United States will be far more willing to accept (1) war termination following a nuclear war in Europe that leaves the U.S. homeland unscathed, or (2) a short conventional war in which American forces are attacked but no escalation to nuclear weapons occurs. The German ruling elite rejects both options as contrary to the core bargain of the alliance and ultimately to the long-term security of the United States itself. Any suggestion should be rejected that admits the possibility of (1) a "Euro-strategic" balance separable from the U.S. commitment to European defense, or (2) provision of Soviet and American "sanctuaries" that would leave the superpowers unscathed in the event of European conflict.

The causes for this insistence are to be found in both elite and mass attitudes to defense policy in general. All agree that the principal bulwark of German security is a policy of credible, effective deterrence. At the simplest level, this rests on a fundamental belief akin to that underlying the American "massive retaliation" doctrine of the 1950s. The best deterrent is the specter of total nuclear war resulting almost automatically from the first use of nuclear weapons. Any doctrine that allows the possibility of (1) limited nuclear weapons use (e.g., selected nuclear options in any number), or (2) limiting the effects of nuclear war (i.e., the neutron bomb or any other "clean" nuclear devices) undercuts deterrence. The low risk of Soviet action against Western Europe will remain so only if the Soviet Union is convinced of both the certainty of American involvement and the probability of rapid escalation to a strategic nuclear exchange.

A related attitude cluster concerns the impossibility of an adequate conventional effort by the NATO states. The factors cited parallel those mentioned in connection with nuclear war—the devastation to the German population and property and the dread of additional suffering in an occupation-liberation cycle as efforts are made to roll back gains made by invading forces. Moreover, there would still be the possibility of either side initiating a nuclear war. The more knowledgeable also point to the uncertainty introduced by an autonomous French nuclear force as a contribution to deterrence. (Officially, France's *force de frappe* is to be used as soon as French borders, if not French deployments in Germany, are threatened.)[45] Others, especially on the political left, point simply to the large number of nuclear weapons available for use by American, German, and other allied forces.

The central argument is not new: that the West and Germany itself will not (and perhaps cannot) accept the economic, political, and social burdens required for a conventional mobilization of the needed magnitude. Defense policy analysts point to the experience of the past—the continuing failure to meet any of the conventional improvement goals, let alone the ambitious 96-division level at NATO's outset.[46]

Even in times of direct crisis—Berlin in 1958–59 and 1961–62, Czechoslovakia in 1968—the central front allies have made only marginal increases in force levels or allocation of national resources for defense. The final assertion is always that the Federal Republic cannot mount such an effort alone or bear an even more inequitable burden than at present. German sacrifice would make no essential difference and might risk major economic disadvantage, foreign political charges of revived German militarism, and widespread political disaffection in West Germany.[47]

The less specific public attitudes seem related to the low probability accorded the outbreak of European conflict and to an understanding of national security as having both economic and political requirements. Prevalent images are of the cutbacks higher defense expenditures would impose on domestic prosperity in general and social welfare rights in particular.[48] As in the Weimar period, this would both lessen support for the government and strengthen internal dissidents.

Somewhat paradoxically, there is another German fear of at least equal intensity: that the United States will use nuclear weapons too quickly in Germany's defense.[49] In the 1950s this fear surfaced in the emotional *Ohne mich* (Without me) campaigns against nuclear armament. Mass marches at Easter, a continuing stream of appeals from intellectuals and scientists, and attempts to organize antinuclear plebiscites characterized the rearmament debates.

After a period of relatively limited activity, the antinuclear movement revived in intensity in the 1970s in Germany and throughout Europe.[50] The debate had various sources: (1) an unclassified systematic study by a respected scientist, Carl Frederick von Weizäcker, on the effects of nuclear conflict on the Federal Republic; (2) the strength of antimilitarism among European youth movements; and, finally, (3) the controversy over the neutron bomb (i.e., ERW or enhanced radiation weapons that maximize initial radiation while minimizing blast effects). Their use would be against tanks or troop concentrations. (If used

in populated areas, opponents note, there would be large numbers of human casualties with much less damage to buildings and other structures.) The December 1979 decision to base extended-range Pershing and ground-launched cruise missiles on European soil provided an opportunity for opponents to assert and to win allegiance to an "alternative view." The left wing of the SPD was particularly active, acting in concert with organized groups in the Benelux states, in Scandinavia, and in England. The high point of the movement came in 1981–82; after actual INF deployments began in late 1983, support and organization fell off sharply.

At its serious core, the antinuclear movement raised two damaging questions. The first emphasized the inability of the German government to control the decision to use nuclear weapons, even those stationed on its own soil or earmarked for its own "dual-capable" systems[51] (i.e., weapons systems capable of carrying either nuclear warheads or non-nuclear, conventional munitions). As presently configured, German forces closely resemble those of the United States in terms of equipment with dual-capable weapons across the tactical spectrum. Warhead release will come only in times of NATO-defined crisis, and it will be implemented only after authorization by the president of the United States and by the NATO and national decision makers designated in still-secret NATO guidelines. In short, the United States retains control over nuclear weapons assigned to West German units. What direct influence the Federal Republic will have in an actual conflict is unclear.

A second question is whether, even in peacetime, the Federal Republic will bear the political costs of American decisions to acquire more or new nuclear weapons systems for European deployment. As was forcefully argued in February 1979 by the influential SPD leader Herbert Wehner, the levels of nuclear destructive power already possessed by East and West are awesome.[52] Further Western acquisitions and nuclear modernization programs will perpetuate, if not accelerate, the arms race and result in "defensive" Soviet counteracquisi-

Table 5. FRG Operations and Maintenance Expenditures and Investment Trends, 1970–1984 (Billions of German Marks)

	1983	1984	1970	1971	1972	1973	1974	1975	1976	1977	1978	1979	1980	1981	1982
Total outlays (EP 14)	19.4	21.4	24.3	26.8	29.9	31.2	32.4	33.5	35.4	37.1	39.4	42.6	44.4	46.8	47.8
Operating															
Personnel	9.3	10.5	11.8	13.5	14.0	14.4	15.1	15.8	16.5	17.6	18.7	18.8	19.4	19.8	19.8
O&H	1.9	2.3	2.7	3.0	3.0	3.1	3.1	3.3	3.4	3.5	3.5	3.8	4.2	4.3	4.3
Other[a]	2.9	3.2	3.7	3.7	4.4	4.7	4.9	5.0	5.2	5.5	5.9	6.1	6.4	6.9	7.0
Total	12.8	14.8	16.9	18.5	20.9	21.8	22.4	23.4	24.4	25.5	27.0	28.7	29.5	30.7	31.1
% of Total Budget	66.0	69.1	69.5	69.0	69.9	69.9	69.1	69.7	68.9	68.7	68.5	67.3	66.4	65.6	65.2
Investments															
Procurement	3.9	3.5	4.2	4.8	5.4	5.7	6.4	6.6	7.2	8.0	8.8	10.6	11.1	11.9	12.1
RDT&E	1.1	1.2	1.3	1.4	1.4	1.4	1.6	1.6	1.7	1.8	1.7	1.5	1.7	1.8	1.9
Military construction	3.9	3.5	4.2	4.8	5.4	5.7	6.4	6.6	7.2	8.0	8.8	10.6	11.1	11.9	12.1
Other[b]	1.6	1.9	1.9	2.1	2.2	2.3	1.9	1.9	2.1	1.9	1.8	1.8	2.1	2.3	2.6
Total	6.7	6.6	7.3	8.3	9.0	9.4	9.9	10.2	11.0	11.6	12.3	13.9	14.9	16.1	16.6
% of Total Budget	34.5	30.8	30.0	31.0	30.1	30.1	30.6	30.3	31.1	31.3	31.2	32.7	33.6	34.4	34.8

Source: Joerg F. Baldauf, "Implementing Flexible Response: The U.S., Germany, and NATO's Conventional Forces." Dissertation, Massachusetts Institute of Technology, February 1987.

[a]For example, fuel, food, rental of data transmission lines, etc.   [b]NATO infrastructure, etc., purchase of real estate, vehicles for administrative purposes, etc.

Table 6. The Evolution of FRG Defense Budgets from Fiscal Guidance to Actual Outlays, 1970–1984

	1970	1971	1972	1973	1974	1975	1976	1977	1978	1979	1980	1981	1982	1983	1984
Mid-range financial plan for budget year t-2 (billions) in price levels of budget submission[a]	19.5	20.9	23.3	25.6	27.8	30.5	32.7	33.7	34.4	36.3	38.1	40.0	43.1	46.8	49.5
Government's budget submission to Parliament (billions)	20.4	21.9	24.5	26.6	27.6	29.9	31.4	32.4	34.3	36.1	37.7	41.2	43.8	46.1	48.0
Percentage change from mid-range plan	+4.6	+4.8	+5.2	+3.9	-0.7	-2.0	-4.0	-3.9	-0.3	-0.6	-1.0	+3.0	+1.6	-1.5	-3.0
Budget law (billions)	19.2	21.8	24.5	26.4	28.9	31.0	32.9	32.9	35.0	36.7	38.5	42.1	44.3	46.7	47.8
Percentage change from submission	-5.9	-0.5	0	-0.8	+4.7	+3.5	+1.6	+1.5	+2.0	+1.6	+2.1	+2.1	+1.9	+1.3	-0.4
Actual outlays in year t (billions)	19.4	21.4	24.3	26.8	29.9	31.2	32.4	33.5	35.4	37.1	39.4	42.6	44.4	46.8	—
Percentage change from budget law	+1.0	-1.8	-0.8	+1.5	+1.5	+0.6	+1.4	+1.8	+1.1	+2.7	+2.3	+3.4	+0.2	+0.2	—

Source: Joerg F. Baldauf, "Implementing Flexible Response: The U.S., Germany, and NATO's Conventional Forces." Dissertation, Massachusetts Institute of Technology, February 1987.

[a]Since the mid-range plan of t-2 is calculated at price levels of December of t-3, the figures had to be converted to the same price levels as used in the budget submission (December 31 of t-2). GNP deflators were used for this conversion, as provided by the Budget Division of MOD.
1970–1984 average annual increase/decrease of government's budget submission over mid-range financial plan: −0.4%.
1970–1984 average annual increase/decrease of Parliament's budget over government's budget: 1.0%.
1970–1983 average annual increase/decrease of actual outlays over budget law: 1.2%.

tions. The result will be even greater reliance on nuclear weapons and their almost automatic employment in the event of war.

It is in this context that détente receives the greatest elite support as the best hope for long-term German security. Nuclear arms limitation on a realistic mutual basis is the next step to stabilizing European détente, and therefore is a primary domestic political requirement. However deemed necessary, the acquisition of a new weapons system must be evaluated within this framework. Moreover, there now seems good and sufficient reason to examine the nuclear-based strategy of the alliance and ask "How much is enough?"

Many in the German elite contend that this view of détente and arms limitation is fundamentally different from that pursued by the United States. Their criticism is two-edged. The original Kissinger-Nixon concept of détente in the early 1970s was overly optimistic, with what proved to be a fatal fascination for (1) a series of progressively more comprehensive global arms control regimes, (2) "bargaining chip" deployments, and (3) attempted linkage of political incentives in Europe to constraints on Soviet behavior elsewhere. Equally flawed in the opposite direction were the formulations of the Carter administration, particularly after the Soviet Union's invasion of Afghanistan, and those more intensely pressed by the early Reagan administration. Détente cannot be an arbitrarily defined, stop-and-go process, affected by national threats and punishments and hostage to events that do not critically affect fundamental Western interests. Moreover, the American electorate must be brought to value arms limitation on its own terms, not just as something "given" to the Soviet Union or subject to reconsideration every four years.

Left unanswered, however, are a number of troublesome issues of process and substance. After the prolonged debates of the 1970s and 1980s, there are still widely differing conceptions, even among proponents, about the requirements and priorities of détente. Even SPD circles that now press for the "second wave" of détente seem to have a relatively vague concept of the process to be followed or the concrete goals to be specified. Opposition critiques obviously come from a number of sources. There are those on the German far right who argue that détente is wishful thinking or the start of the "self-Finlandization" process discussed above.[53] Commentators outside Germany trace the roots of détente to the unusual stability and calm in Europe of the 1970s and the USSR's ability to exploit this. They postulate that any dramatic interruption of détente—such as the invasion of Poland or some other Eastern European country—will limit elite attribution of benefits and popular expectation of a continuing process of stability and increasing mutual confidence.

These arguments are often given greater weight in the face of the radical critique of defense efforts launched by the left.[54] Critics stress the nonproductivity of defense investment, the automatic conjunction established between government and defense industries, and the economic exploitation involved in a system of military conscription. True national security, in this view, lies in the satisfaction of individual economic and social rights and the guarantee of a new quality of life. Neither goal can be met by a highly militarized society or a state that is required by its principal ally to sacrifice more and more national resources for Western defense against what is viewed as a slight or nonexistent Soviet threat. In this formulation, it is the United States that thus constitutes a grave threat to German national security and that, by its emphasis on military preparedness and war-fighting capability, may undermine long-term prospects for détente and European stability.

Proponents of détente are somewhat less sure in their formulations of how it is to be maintained or expanded. In strategic arms limitation, however flawed its approach, it is the United States that is the principal Western negotiator with the Soviet Union. Coordination and consultation with the European allies is assumed, but direct involvement in the negotiations is to be avoided. West Germany can warn, stimulate, and maneuver; however, a greater public role than this raises questions of intra-European balance and about Germany's special political and military vulnerabilities.

Moreover, the task of achieving consensus within the NATO alliance on the balance to be struck between defense and détente is clearly formidable. At what point will the efforts toward détente and arms limitation be judged to have adequately served the goals of stability, even if no East-West agreement results? At every stage will not the potential for limitation (real or perceived) appear to domestic publics, if not to political elites, to outweigh the tactical advantages of deployment? Might this not extend to all new weapons systems, even conventional ones, that can be defined as upsetting the existing balance and thus undermining progress toward détente?

One further issue is the past division of labor in NATO, in which Germany and the other European allies have tolerated independent U.S. actions and decisions outside the NATO area so long as these did not directly affect the U.S. guarantee or involve European resources. Increasingly assertive German demands that the United States do nothing to damage European détente result in an expanded agenda for transatlantic bargaining. The potential for continuing domestic German disagreement and Soviet political manipulation appears substantially increased; and the level at which the benefits of détente would be outweighed by the costs to Western political and military capabilities is uncertain, if not indefinable.

At the level of detailed proposals, the question of realistic bargaining strategies becomes even more difficult. The immediate German agenda seems to emphasize three points: (1) the timing and specifics of "central strategic"—ICBMs, submarine-launched ballistic missiles, and long-range bombers or cruise missile carriers—and European-based nuclear arms limitations cannot be left to unilateral American decision; (2) limitations ought to transcend a purely American definition of security requirements by taking European concerns into account (e.g., Germans reject any distinction between strategic and tactical or battlefield nuclear weapons that does not acknowledge linkages among them as part of an overall deterrent); and (3) there must be transatlantic risk sharing in terms both of final limits and negotiating trade-offs. This means, for

example, that European-based nuclear systems, whether American, German, or other, should be considered not as separate capabilities, but rather as parts of "integrated force packages" that would also include some central system elements. How an equitable balance across such aggregates would be calculated is left for future negotiations.

Bonn's assertion of more autonomous policy in these areas has also stimulated major American criticism and questioning. At a superficial level are the mistaken charges of "pacifistic" leanings among Europeans.[55] More serious is the analysis of the inherent contradictions between Bonn's stress on the indivisibility of arms control and the relative divisibility of détente. Often heard, too, is the charge that Germany is more interested in dialogue per se than in results.

This leaves German policy makers with perhaps the most fundamental dilemma of all in balancing defense and détente policies. German anxieties about the American position stem in part from continuing disagreements with the Carter, Reagan and Bush administrations. But they also reflect the increasing German conviction that the United States pursues, and will always pursue, a different set of interests and values. Even with increased coordination, the probabilities of long-term convergence on arms limitations, let alone on steps toward a more stable détente, are at best very low, and will perhaps decline still further in coming years.

Minorities in the Federal Republic argue that the point of divergence is already here, and that the implications for Germany's continued reliance on NATO must be drawn.[56] Most in the German elite at present will admit only to the existence of these dilemmas. Perhaps, as in the past, the passage of time alone will mute the issues and sanction, if not resolve, apparent contradictions.

The Defense Decision-Making Process

Not surprisingly, the German defense decision-making process is finely attuned to American policies and to decisions within the NATO framework.[57] Many of the critical decisions immediately after World War II were made by the Western founding fathers. The Adenauer government could achieve at most only delay or marginal change. The three decades since rearmament have underscored the importance of German-American consultation for agenda setting, bargaining, and even the revocation of previous alliance considerations. In many respects, the German defense decision-making process is as constrained as German defense policy. It is circumscribed by the same lack of a separable national profile; external actors and preferences penetrate German deliberations at every stage. The framework for maneuver and change is fairly narrow. Day-to-day expertise and analytic independence have developed slowly, with considerable encouragement, pressure, and training from the United States. It was not until the early 1970s, for example, that autonomous German defense-planning staffs began to play a major role in the internation studies within NATO (e.g., those set by NATO's Nuclear Planning Group) or to develop national options in the areas of manpower, training development, and equipment management.

External influence over the policy process is made more salient by the often unfocused domestic political debate in these areas that was the norm prior to the political mobilization that surrounded the INF debates of the early 1980s. As in most European states, the level of elite interest in defense issues was often low and quite sporadic. The parliamentary system added three more constraints: strictly organized, infrequent public debates; tight party discipline; and the inherent advantages accruing to proposals initiated by the government. Before the pressures generated by the prospects of INF deployment and the emergence of the Greens, public hearings were almost unknown; cabinet debate was, and still is, confused by the principles of both the "primacy" of the chancellor and ministerial "responsibility" for functional areas. Outside of the sizable civilian and military defense bureaucracy, the form and substance of defense questions were usually of major concern to only a handful, including party defense experts, a few defense

correspondents, and involved defense intellectuals.

It is clear that the INF debates critically changed both the scope of legitimate discussion of defense and the number of groups and institutions who feel that defense is an area of continuing concern. They also led to a significant increase in the amount of information easily and regularly available from nongovernmental sources. What is less clear is whether these changes are permanent and whether new issues will provide a new basis for mobilization. So far, the U.S. Strategic Defense Initiative (SDI) has not proved a sufficient issue to rally opposition; and continuing INF deployments passed almost without comment, the anti-INF movement having been disbanded following the deployment decision in December 1983. Mobilization by groups outside the regular political process remains negligible.

Indeed, as Helga Haftendorn and her colleagues have argued, debates over security policy in the political arena also suffer generally from overbureaucratization and fragmentation (see fig. 3).[58] Both the Foreign Office and the Ministry of Defense (MoD) have major staffs to implement their somewhat overlapping responsibilities. The new organization of the chancellor's office allows for a third major competitor from time to time. Added to the usual problems of coordination engendered by bureaucratic competition and partial information are the difficulties injected by simultaneous negotiations and coordination with external organizations such as NATO staffs and political authorities. A final overlay is frequent communications with various American authorities, military and political leaders actually present in Germany; official representatives in Bonn and at Supreme Headquarters, Allied Powers Europe (SHAPE); and those in Washington. Not only are there frequent official "bilaterals," but also constant informal discussions and information sessions.[59]

The result, too often, is a decision-making system mired in details, overloaded with communications, and relatively unresponsive to immediate political shifts or unfamiliar events. Unlike the United States, Germany has only a few extra-governmental sources of elite exper-

Figure 3. The German Ministry of Defense

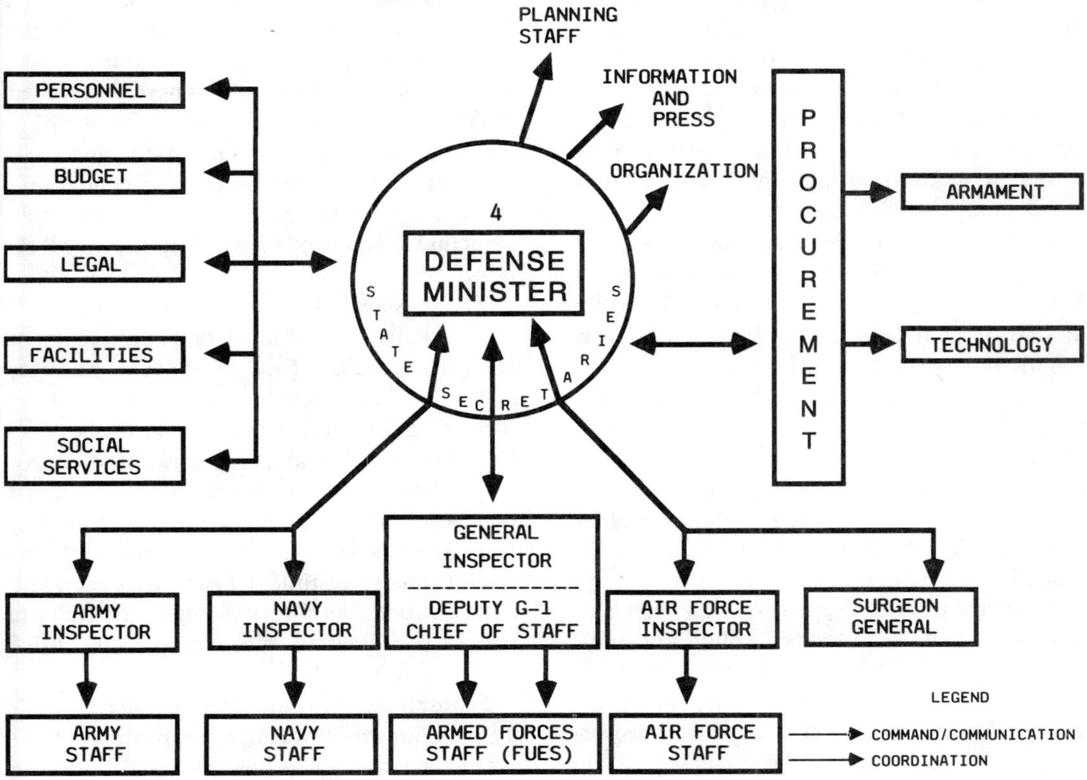

tise that can be mobilized easily or that have credibility or legitimacy. Parliamentary skill is too often limited to a few "assigned" party experts; general expertise is somewhat limited even within the MoD, let alone within the more traditional diplomatic circles in the Foreign Office. There are only a handful of external research institutes concerned with security issues, and even fewer that do not have a systematic progovernment or antigovernment stance. Indeed, until the 1970s, national defense analysis by the media was relatively rare. This has changed since the emergence of the INF issue.

These are criticisms that can be leveled in some measure at the defense decision-making process in most advanced industrialized democracies with the exception of the United States.[60] What is striking about the German case is the contrast between the size and expense of the defense effort and, until recently, the relatively limited scope of public attention

to (and participation in) defense decision making. The lack of a separate national policy is one factor, but it is not the only explanation.

The only circumstances under which the scope of defense decision making expands are those that also make informed, open debate difficult or politically risky. Over the past three decades, this type of debate has generally concerned four different types of issues: (1) nuclear armament and control (1956, 1958, 1962, and 1979–83); (2) maladministered, costly weapons acquisitions (e.g., the F-104 fighter in the 1960s and the "Tornado" multirole combat aircraft in the 1980s); (3) ministerial malfeasance (e.g., Franz Josef Strauss in 1962 and Manfred Wörner in 1983); and (4) "excessive" NATO "requirements" in armament and force structure (e.g., the level of German concurrence with President Carter's target of a 3 percent real increase in defense spending).

More often than not, the cabinet has already

completed preliminary discussion and its first move is to restrict debate. The reaction is an intensified challenge, often spilling over to the extraparliamentary parties or to the public at large. In all but a few cases, the chancellor controls the outcome, but only after private compromise and usually some compensating action in another, perhaps unrelated, sector or issue area. The furor then trails off, to lie relatively dormant until the next spark.

However constricted the present system, it nonetheless represents a considerable evolution from that first established in the early 1950s. In rearmament as in most matters, the personality and preferences of Konrad Adenauer were then critical.[61] In the view of many, the chancellor was "a complete civilian," interested in rearmament only as an instrument to gain Germany's political rehabilitation and integration with the West. Military argument divorced from political calculation was of little importance to him, despite the best efforts of successive defense advisers, civilian and military. What he believed crucial was to retain full control of all German foreign and military affairs in his own hands, and to restrict involvement and information to the smallest possible official circle.

The first steps toward a separate defense policy-making structure were taken by Franz Josef Strauss, defense minister under Adenauer from 1956 to 1962.[62] Ambitious, brash, hard-driving, and well-schooled in defense questions by the U.S. occupation authorities, Strauss soon pulled the Defense Ministry through its initial organizational confusion and contradictions. His aim was always to establish the primacy of the minister—in both external alliance negotiations and domestic discussions. He sought a dominant role in the determination of nuclear doctrine, recruitment practices, and troop levels. His battles with the opposition SPD were legion; he was always good for colorful press copy because of his sweeping pronouncements on all issues of Western defense and civilization.

In the last analysis, however, Strauss remained dependent on Adenauer. He needed the chancellor's support for particular decisions like the acquisition of nuclear-capable weaponry and the extension of Bundeswehr recruitment. Strauss, on the other hand, served as Adenauer's "trial ballooner" or "point man" for public controversy at home and abroad. The outcome was that Strauss never succeeded in developing a ministerial system for planning and analysis or for continuing interagency coordination with the MoD's primary competitor, the Foreign Office, which had, and still has, principal responsibility for "international affairs."

The present system of German defense decision making received much of its impetus from Helmut Schmidt, first as defense minister (1969–74) and then as chancellor.[63] Like Strauss, Schmidt brought to his MoD tasks ambition, considerable expertise, and a proclaimed faith in professionalism. He also faced far fewer battles with critical allies and domestic opponents over basic defense issues. He enjoyed far more latitude to foster discussion and analysis, both within the Ministry of Defense and in coordination with the Foreign Office and other involved agencies.

Schmidt also was accorded greater flexibility in organization within the ministry. For example, he created a new personal planning staff, set up a special "expert" commission on force structure questions for the 1980s, and attracted a number of promising military and civilian staffers to ministry service. These, plus numerous smaller changes, were then consolidated, albeit at a lower level, by Schmidt's successor, George Leber of the SPD.

Schmidt faced some process constraints similar to those Strauss had confronted. The perennial question reemerged of the preeminent authority of the Foreign Office in international affairs not directly concerned with military specifics—such as in positions on arms limitation, NATO policy guidelines, and bilateral relations. Despite successive challenges, Schmidt and his planning staff gained little exclusive control.[64] The minister also found himself in several continuing battles with the top military leadership. In one case, Schmidt was charged with "politicizing" the military, or creating "SPD generals." He, in turn, suggested the need for greater "professional" responsiveness to the policy shifts set down by the new SPD-Free Democrat (FDP) coalition, and for continuing adherence to ministerial discipline regarding public criticism by serving officers.

As chancellor, Schmidt sometimes pursued a similarly activist role in reforming the defense decision-making process. Security policy coordination found new resources in the chancellor's office; the chancellor took a more forceful leadership role in the cabinet, the smaller Federal Security Council (a cabinet committee), and the still smaller meetings of the relevant ministers (usually foreign, defense, and finance). But Schmidt was constrained by both political and operational realities. He had to preserve the careful political balance within his coalition. As foreign minister, the FDP's Hans-Dietrich Genscher took a harder, more pro-American posture, while, at least initially, Defense Minister Hans Apel was the rising star of the SPD and enjoyed considerable support from its more détente-oriented left wing. Moreover, electioneering and times of economic crisis meant that Schmidt's usual role (and that of the cabinet in general) was basically one of approving postures already negotiated by the Foreign Office or the Ministry of Defense.[65]

The role of Manfred Wörner as defense minister in the Kohl government extended many of the best aspects of Schmidt's reforms. The central staff of the minister took greater responsibility in the formulation and negotiation of broad security policy. Wörner's specific background in defense issues, his understanding of emerging problems (improved conventional defense, extended air defense, and anti-tactical ballistic missile, or ATBM, defense) contributed to new international respect and to some national recognition. Yet problems that plagued earlier ministers recurred, such as a major scandal about a serving officer that showed lax internal standards and a failure of ministerial oversight, some costing problems, and the difficulties of achieving organizational coherence.

Wörner's appointment in 1988 to the post of NATO Secretary General (the first German to fill this position) led to his replacement in the defense ministry by Rupert Scholz, a constitu-

tional lawyer who clearly has not shared his predecessor's expertise in security issues. For example, soon after assuming office, he discovered that his order to ban future aerial shows (in the wake of the tragic crash in a 1988 air show at the American air base at Ramstein) was not legally binding since decisions concerning air transportation lanes still fall under the post–World War II Allied arrangements (in this case under American jurisdiction). Scholz was replaced in 1989 by Gerhard Stoltenberg. Indeed, thirty years after rearmament, the position of defense minister in the Federal Republic remains one of the most complex and sensitive in any Western democracy.

The role of the military leadership in the defense decision-making process has not really expanded with the greater legitimacy now accorded the Bundeswehr in general. The organizational structure of the defense ministry is, of course, designed to ensure civilian control and is somewhat parallel to that in the United States. The defense minister has the "power of command" over the armed forces in peacetime.[66] In a "state of defense," this power passes to the chancellor, and operational wartime command passes to the designated NATO commanders. The formal role of the chief of staff of the federal armed forces (Generalinspektur der Bundeswehr) is to serve as "military adviser to the Minister and the Federal Government." Together with service chiefs of staff (army, air force, navy, and health), he acts in the name of the Bundeswehr Defense Council. The respective chiefs function officially both as leaders and as administrative heads of their ministerial divisions.

Informally, the visible participation of the military leadership in decision making was highest in the first decade of rearmament. One clear reason was Adenauer's use of "good generals," especially the honored Hans Speidel and Adolf Heusinger, to gain acceptance of the new Bundeswehr.[67] His targets were both internal and external. Internally, he pursued the support of former military officers and more conservative (or nationalistic) groups. Externally, he looked for support from the victorious allied military, which were respectful of German tradition and experience. Another reason was simply the force of the personalities and personal experiences involved. Those accepting higher command in the fledgling Bundeswehr had been major figures in World War II, and had already emerged from both the postwar de-Nazification process and relegitimization under the Federal Republic. They had little to lose and perhaps much to gain in publicly pointing out mistakes in, say, NATO's nuclear weapons employment doctrines after private persuasion on these issues had failed.[68]

There are still major factions of the German political spectrum, however, that view an active military role as inappropriate, if not dangerous. Moreover, if the Bundeswehr is basically analogous to other state agencies and institutions, it must and will follow their pattern.[69] The result is often as fragmented and bureaucratic an approach to defense decision making as that in the Foreign Office or elsewhere (see fig. 4). The resultant lack of coordination, short-sighted incremental decision making, sensitivity above all to budget constraints, and loyalty to the "usual" and "that invented here"—all are to be expected of, and perhaps preferred by, the civilian leadership within the ministry and the broader political elite.

Particular insights into these process characteristics can be gleaned from even a brief survey of German defense spending patterns (tables 6 and 7). The allocation of resources to

defense and within the defense establishment is unquestionably the most visible phase in the decision-making process and one of the most hotly contested inside and outside the ministry. To be sure, only the indirect traces of major acquisition decisions or doctrinal shifts are discernible. But budgetary analysis does capture the essential trends and allows an estimate of the operating ground rules for decision making.

As analyzed by Richard C. Eichenberg, German postwar defense budgeting exhibits three major process characteristics.[70] The first is the significance of time, in terms of bargaining within the MoD and the relative strength of MoD claims on total governmental resources. In constant dollars, defense spending built to a high in the first decade of rearmament, then underwent a decade of perturbation and returned to its former levels (fig. 5). Despite preferred party images and electoral rhetoric, CDU- and SPD-led coalitions have indulged almost equally in high levels of expenditure. Both appear equally constrained by the rearmament-replacement cycle (as the SPD discovered from 1975 to 1982) and American pressure for greater alliance burden sharing (evident in the Kennedy push of the early 1960s and the Carter initiatives of the late 1970s).

The differences in levels also appear to be a function of the total amount of resources avail-

Figure 4. Institutional Structure for Arms Control and Security Policy Decision Making

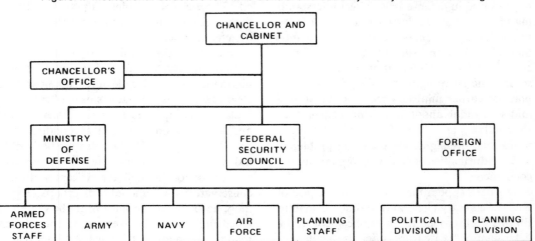

Figure 5. German Defense Spending by Party in Power (Billions of 1970 Deutschmarks)

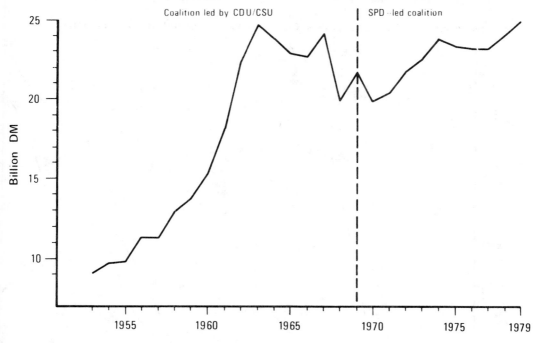

Source: Eichenberg, "Defense-Welfare Tradeoffs in German Budgeting."

Note: Includes defense budget, stationing costs of allied troops, and civil defense outlays, but not federal border guards or Berlin assistance.

able to the central government. Eichenberg found that of all changes in ministerial spending, those in the MoD pattern were most closely correlated with change in overall federal spending. Moreover, the dip in spending in the mid 1960s corresponds closely to that imposed by the "Erhard recession" on all federal expenditures. The budgetary solution imposed spending ceilings and established relatively fixed ratios between the money available to the MoD and other ministries over five-year (and eventually fifteen-year) ministerial planning cycles.

Most critical differences and some contradictions are evident in the shifts between budget categories over time (fig. 6). In the initial rearmament phase, the major share went to procurement, to "equalize" German armaments with the most modern deployed by other allies. As shown in table 7, the total shares claimed by the army and the air force were almost equal, despite very different manpower

levels (350,000 versus 100,000). The battles over budget shares consumed considerable attention in the period 1956 to 1960, when the final terms of buildup were fixed.

Most surprising, perhaps, is the steady upward curve of personnel costs. From 1956 to 1966, this reflects the accretion of military and civilian manpower within the new MoD. Thereafter, it typifies a situation faced by most European states. Soldiers, even conscripts, are now to be paid wages comparable to those of civilian workers, with the same benefits and cost-of-living pay increases. Since the interrelation has been fixed legislatively, these costs have risen as steeply as personnel outlays in other governmental agencies. Moreover, without costly additional perquisites (e.g., officer universities), the Federal Republic would not have been able to overcome severe shortages of junior officers and NCOs. Nevertheless, demographic trends through the end of the century will force hard choices on the Federal govern-

Figure 6. Three Categories of West German Defense Spending (Budget Authority)

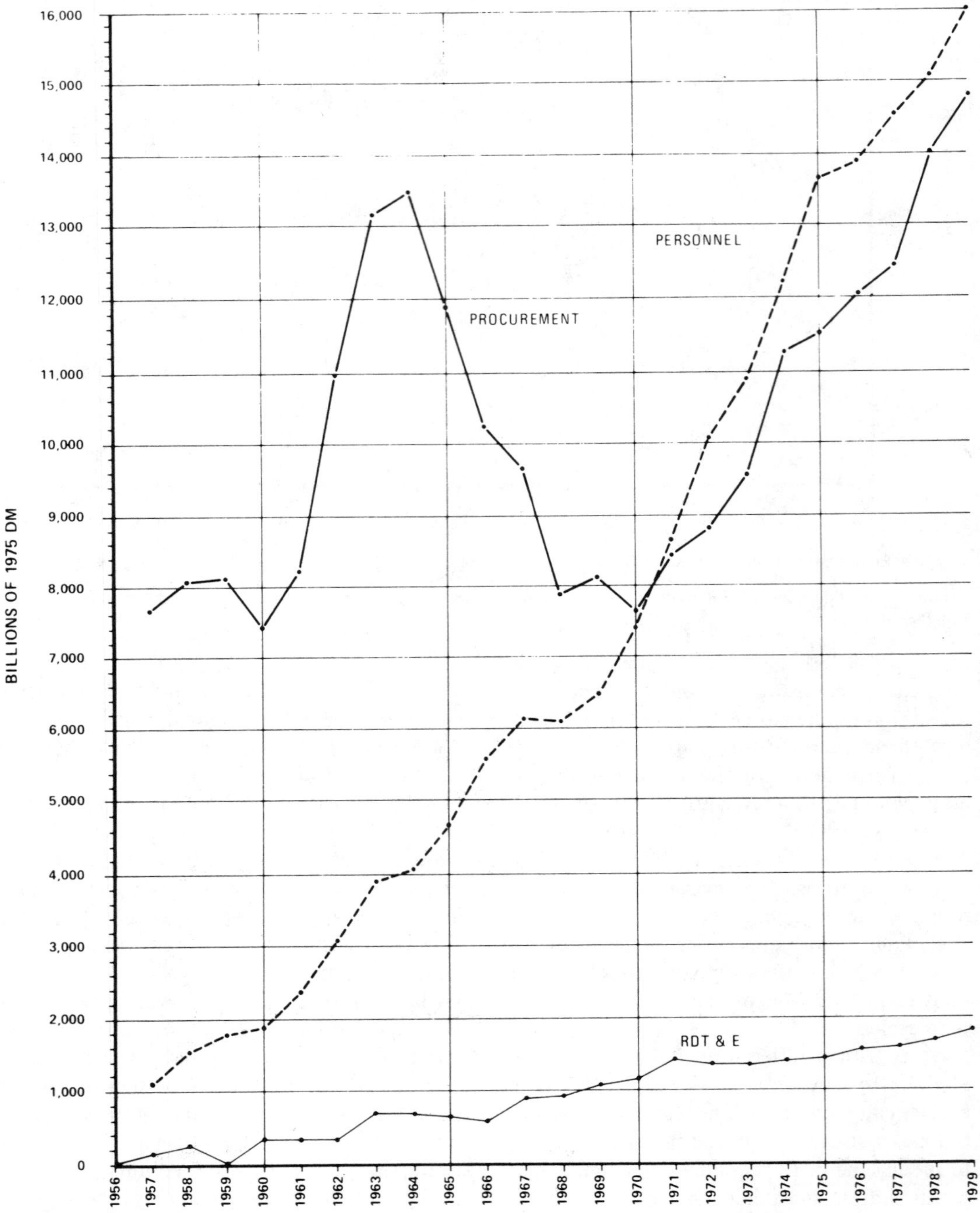

PERSONNEL

PROCUREMENT

RDT & E

BILLIONS OF 1975 DM

16,000
15,000
14,000
13,000
12,000
11,000
10,000
9,000
8,000
7,000
6,000
5,000
4,000
3,000
2,000
1,000
0

1956 1957 1958 1959 1960 1961 1962 1963 1964 1965 1966 1967 1968 1969 1970 1971 1972 1973 1974 1975 1976 1977 1978 1979

Source: Eichenberg, "Defense-Welfare Tradeoffs in German Budgeting."

Table 7. Total Weapons Procurement Costs for the Bundeswehr by Service Category, 1957–69 (Millions of German Marks)

Year	Army	Navy	Air Force	Other	Total
1957/58	1539.8	262.3	553.1	39.9	2395.1
1958/59	601.8	599.8	1097.3	46.2	2345.1
1959/60	1042.3	462.9	702.8	46.0	2254.0
1960a	745.9	386.2	901.6	33.9	2067.6
1961	987.1	464.3	1414.8	73.7	2939.9
1962	1473.7	634.1	2075.5	85.8	4269.1
1963	1559.3	593.4	2630.5	83.6	4866.8
1964	1475.9	885.7	1572.6	78.4	4012.6
1965	1325.1	691.7	1158.5	64.7	3240.0
1966	1271.7	550.1	739.5	122.1	2683.4
1967	1652.1	742.7	1107.5	73.5	3575.8
1968	1177.1	589.0	1236.5	46.7	3049.3
1969b	1477.1	456.7	1575.1	72.9	3581.8
Total	16328.9	7318.9	16765.3	867.4	41280.5

Source: Bundes Presse- und Informationsamt, *Weissbuch 1970: Zur Sicherheit der Bundesrepublik Deutschland und zur lage der Bundeswehr* (Bonn, 1970), pp. 197–98.

aReflects shortened fiscal year (April–December 31).
bEstimated costs.

ment. The necessary outlays for anticipated weapons systems procurement will compete with the increasing costs of personnel-related spending.[71]

This steady increase in manpower costs is made more difficult by a related development: heightened public assertion of a defense-spending ceiling. The trends reflected in public attitudes (see table 8) suggest a general acceptance of whatever the existing defense expenditures are or have recently been. True to its rhetoric, the membership of the CDU/CSU is somewhat more in favor of increased spending, but not by an overwhelming percentage. Incrementalism is clearly the dominant strategy in terms of public acceptance as well as the rules of intraministry harmony.

Recent studies indeed suggest that much of the bargaining about marginal changes takes place within the MoD itself, and often at fairly low levels. The budget total for defense has already been more or less set in the federal five-year planning budget and is strictly monitored by the Ministry of Finance. Unless there are other surprises like the disastrous cost over-runs in the production of the Tornado multirole combat aircraft, it will remain relatively fixed. The amount of interagency bargaining or horse-trading is limited by the lack of a clear executive coordinating body (other

Table 8. Should Defense Spending Be Decreased, Kept the Same, or Increased?

	Decrease	Keep Same	Increase	Don't Know
1967	41	37	8	14
1968	27	35	16	22
1969	31	36	16	17
1971	38	46	12	4
1972	38	38	11	13
1973	35	39	10	17
1974	34	42	9	15
1975	38	42	10	11
1976	27	47	13	13
1977	27	50	12	11
1978	27	58	11	4
1979	27	59	10	3
1980	22	58	17	3
1981	34	52	14	1
1982	34	54	10	1
1983	35	52	12	2
1984	39	50	9	1

Source: Richard C. Eichenberg, *Public Opinion and National Security in Western Europe: Consensus Lost?* (Ithaca: Cornell University Press, 1989): Table 6.1 (surveys by the Federal Ministry of Defense).

than the cabinet, where finance plays a strong role) and a strong tradition of parliamentary oversight. Further, a good portion of social welfare expenditure occurs at the state level where it does not compete directly with federal expenditure for defense. This compartmentalization of expenditure and the principle of ministerial autonomy are, and will almost certainly remain, sacrosanct.

This leaves the leverage in the hands of actors outside the Federal Republic. Whether the forum is bilateral negotiation with the United States about appropriate burden sharing or the annual NATO planning exercise symbolized by national responses to the NATO Defense Planning Questionnaire (DPQ), there are areas for the exercise of constraining influence by foreign military and political actors. NATO "requirements" may be (and often have been) cited when domestic negotiations need additional support or a service finds a major project under unfriendly fire, although the role of the Foreign Office, the Chancellor's Office on occasion, and always the Ministry of Finance must still be reckoned with.

Clearly, however, the German role in allied decision making is far more assertive than in the past. This is partly the result of experience: the Federal Republic has taken a leading role in the Euro-group deliberations on budgetary projections, in the formulation of the NATO Long-Term Defense (Improvement) Program, and in production consortia (as for the Tornado). Moreover, changes in the domestic economy as well as the growth of a domestic defense industry have placed real constraints on German abilities, not to mention willingness, to act as the alliance's foremost supporter of cooperative projects. As the 1980s have shown, a German chancellor can now argue publicly about the fair share borne by specific allies and demand equal consideration for German economic strains.

Recurring Issues and Defense Policy Outputs

What are the specific outputs of defense decision making? How are these different from those produced by processes more distinctly national in character? I will examine, in varying degrees of detail, four critical issue areas: civil-military relations, weapons acquisition, force structure decisions, and perception of the utility of force.

CIVIL-MILITARY RELATIONS

Central to any discussion of German defense policy, present or future, is the evolution of civil-military relations since the first days of rearmament.[72] The reasons are obvious: the legacy of Prussian military tradition, the unique role of the military in the downfall of the Weimar Republic, and the still controversial issue of military responsibility for the crimes of Nazism, within Germany and in external conquest. The defeat of German militarism had been a primary war aim of the West. For the Europeans in particular, the principal issue in rearmament was how to restore the best in the German military experience without also threatening the beginnings of West German democracy or the reestablishment of European order. In the words of Franz Josef Strauss: "The new German army was to be strong enough to threaten the Russians but not the Belgians."[73]

The basic answer was the concept of *Innere Führung* ("inner leadership," i.e., the citizen in uniform) as the core organizing element of the German armed forces. As worked out in the early 1950s principally by Count Wolf von Baudissin, the basic principles explicitly rejected the two most troublesome civil-military models of the past.[74] The first was that of the incipient state-within-the-state, in which the autonomous, aristocratic military establishment set its own standards and loyalties without necessary regard for an overriding political authority or democratic ethic. This was an extreme or romantic interpretation of the "Prussian system," founded on the basis of self-sacrifice, self-imposed duty, loyalty to discipline, and Spartan simplicity. The individual and the institution were to be indistinguishable, with the highest achievement seen as service to the state, but not necessarily the existing government (as in the Weimar period of the 1920s and early 1930s). The second rejected model represented perhaps the opposite of the first model: the politicized, submissive military of the Nazi period. Hitler attempted to break the "Prussian system" by systematically changing the basis of professional authority to one dependent on the Nazi party, and ultimately on loyalty to himself alone. His creation of "people's generals" (such as Rommel), his establishment of the Waffen-SS as a rival organization, his constant probing of military loyalty—all were elements leading to a redefinition of organiza tional competency, discipline, and professional responsibility (a departure from the "only obeying orders" mentality).

As it has evolved over the past twenty-five years, *Innere Führung* has emphasized civilian supremacy in several different respects. As noted above, the authority of the elected political leadership—the minister and the chancellor—is unquestioned, in crisis as in peacetime. More importantly, the soldier is viewed equally as a citizen, with rights and responsibilities to be respected by the military establishment and with a future existence not defined by his present military career. His tasks involve a personal decision regarding the ethics of his profession and his own choices within broad guidelines on behavior vis-à-vis subordinate and superior, ally and adversary. It is a system designed to recognize rights to unionize and to pursue freedom of conscience, to achieve political legitimacy without either unnecessary submission or arrogance.

Not surprisingly, the achievements of the *Innere Führung* program have not always matched these ideals. A major initial difficulty was finding people to implement and administer it. The problem was not inadequate leadership (that had been solved by rigorous screening by politicians and citizens); it was the fact that the majority of lower and middle officer ranks had served during World War II in the German armed forces, the Wehrmacht. Even a decade of civilianization seemingly had not prepared them to make such a radical adjustment or to move from theory to operational practice. Those who supported the program most strongly were, or were perceived to be, outsiders or loners, perhaps even those who had never understood the requirements of military tradition.[75]

A related source of difficulty was the expectations of the West German population as a whole. Again, two rather different conceptions were involved whose requirements were neither congruent nor subject to compromise. The first conception was that of the traditionalists who saw unionization or direct political education, civilian dress, and training for a later second career as alien to the best of German tradition. They found comfort in the adverse reactions of older officers, such as General Al-

bert Schnez, the army inspector from 1969 to 1971, who repeatedly challenged his minister and the SPD-FDP government on these issues.[76]

The second strand was a virulent antimilitary reaction, particularly among the first two postwar generations which found strong echoes in the anti-INF demonstrations. In this perspective, armed forces are largely antithetical to the ideal of a democratic society or a nonmilitaristic Germany. Those attracted to the military profession are viewed as either dupes or antidemocrats, or perhaps people who cannot make it "outside." Conscription is seen as little better than forced labor or exploitation by the state. For those holding these views, the concept of patriotic service had been irretrievably damaged by Nazism.

These views received strong support from external sources during the first decade or so of rearmament that began in the mid-1950s, especially from the Soviet Union and Eastern Europe. All of the emotional baggage of Nazism was attributed by Eastern Bloc propaganda to West, rather than East Germany. The Federal Republic was almost always described as "revanchist," ready to march again. More subtle, but equally painful, were a number of incidents in the West: Eisenhower's refusal to shake General Speidel's hand despite his NATO command, the integrated NATO staff's negative reaction to German uniforms, and the popular demonstrations in France and Holland against "rehabilitated" officers from World War II.

The passage of time has blunted many of these difficulties.[77] The prewar military generation has now largely passed from active duty. Toleration, if not acceptance, is now assured to the Bundeswehr by the vast majority, abroad as at home. Education in *Innere Führung* principles is now a regular and legitimate component of military training at all levels. Moreover, the civil-military problems of other Western military establishments—especially the French and American—have brought new understanding of some of Germany's own past dilemmas.

Still at question, however, is where the limits of individual responsibility truly lie in state service. Over the past two decades, ministerial discipline has been imposed on a number of critical voices within the Bundeswehr by both the left and the right. In each case, the critic proclaimed his right of conscience to bring his case before the public and has cited the parallels in German history.

Even individual interpretations of military tradition have become matters of controversy, most dramatically within the Bundeswehr, but also in the larger political context. As the 1979 White Paper statement of principles shows, the organizational response to the dilemmas reflects more caution and careful balancing than leadership or suasion, moral or political. Paraphrasing from the 1979 White Paper, tradition in the Bundeswehr: (1) cannot be anything except what is justified under the Constitution; (2) must not be allowed to contradict the values and standards of the social system; (3) must be in relation to peace; (4) must not be restricted to the history of the Bundeswehr, given the need to advance values compatible with a liberal, republican, and democratic society; (5) must not be allowed to concentrate solely upon events and figures in military history; (6) must subscribe to understanding among nations and to overcoming chauvinism; (7) must not be allowed to degenerate into traditionalism—an uncritical clinging to the past at the expense of the present and future; (8) is incompatible with the governing image of the enfranchised citizen who engages in private debate and free decision; (9) calls for sympathy from the civilian population, requiring continuous exchange between military members and their fellow civilian citizens; and (10) is also a question of patience with growth of the new democratic tradition taking place over a long period of time.[78]

A cause of even greater uneasiness for some is the questionable congruence of civilianization, especially in the exercise of authority and in dress and personal style, with the requirements of professional efficiency and the hierarchy of command. Here Germany has done at least as well as other allied governments facing the same challenges (Holland, France, and, to a degree, the United States). But there are still major gaps and discrepancies, providing ammunition for attacks from all sides.

These issues may well become more significant as the Bundeswehr confronts the demographic squeeze of the 1990s.[79] Until now, it has conscripted only 80–85 percent of each eligible class, and conscripts in the 1970s constituted only 45 percent (220,000) of total active manpower. Successive legislation has also made it relatively easy to gain a Bundeswehr exemption on grounds of religious or ethical conviction, the numbers of conscientious objectors steadily increasing through the 1980s.

Projections foresee a growing deficit in the 1990s (fig. 7). The immediate impact will be felt in the number of available conscripts, but parallel effects can be expected in the ranks of both the short-term volunteers (two-to-fifteen-year enlistees) and regular forces (officers and senior NCOs). There are a number of remedial actions—plans for a longer conscript term (eighteen months), greater financial and career incentives for volunteers, and a change in the conscript-enlistee ratio. However, some outside the government argue that these alone will not support maintenance of a 495,000-man Bundeswehr. At issue are what type of military organization is deemed necessary by German society, and what sacrifices, if any, must be made to preserve the painfully crafted political character of the present Bundeswehr. At present, it is yet another issue that is foreseeable, but not yet on what the political elite believes to be the unavoidable political agenda. The external alliance issue remains moot especially as long as the United States continues to suffer manpower shortfalls and does not reinstitute the draft. But the question of the political and economic price to be paid for maintaining present force levels is one fraught with internal political risk.

WEAPONS ACQUISITION

The basic outlines of German weapons acquisition have already emerged in the earlier portions of this essay. The Federal Republic began rearmament with virtually no capability for national weapons production.[80] Moreover, under the terms of the Western European Union (WEU) treaty, it was specifically prohibited from the manufacture on German soil of any system judged to have "offensive capabili-

Figure 7. Available versus Required Conscript Manpower

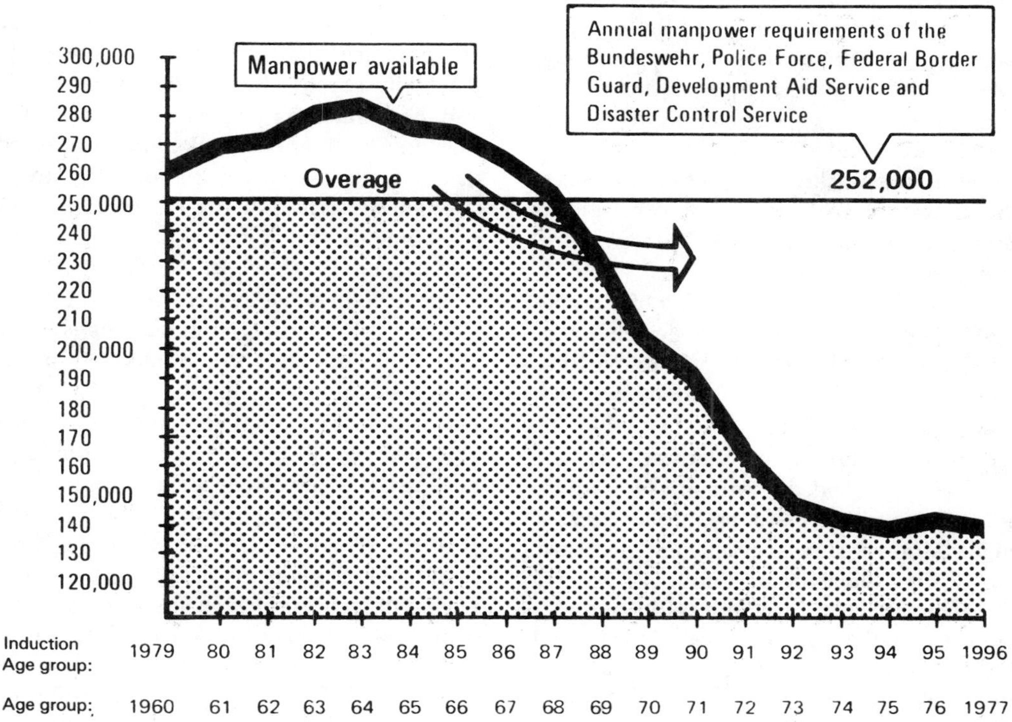

Source: *White Paper*, 1979, p. 226.

ties." The initial equipment for the Bundeswehr came from allied, principally American, stocks already deployed in Europe.

The intervening decades have seen first gradual, then wholesale, lifting of the WEU restriction. Virtually the only one of significance to remain is Adenauer's "voluntary" renunciation of atomic, biological, and chemical weapons on German territory.

This outcome reflects not only Germany's clear alliance status, but also the care and caution Bonn has continually exercised in this sensitive area.[81] The scope of autonomous production in major weapons classes is painstakingly defined; many German weapons emerge from coproduction or licensed production arrangements. Unquestionably, the economies of scale in high technology manufacture are a major reason. But so, too, is Bonn's continuing determination to avoid unnecessary symbols of national independence, and to secure as much military integration as possible. The major na-

tional programs that do exist, such as the Leopard tank, often represent an alternative to desired coproduction as in the failed main battle tank (MBT) program with the United States.

Under these conditions, Bonn's continuing pressures for greater rationalization and standardization of weapons production within NATO have been consistent. Germany is one of the most vocal advocates of the "two-way street" concept of greater transatlantic sharing of contracts and technological development initially supported by the Carter administration but then allowed to fade. German willingness to allow German industries to participate in SDI research is only the latest phase of this pattern. However, the demonstrable successes of German joint efforts have been few, even within the European framework.

As shown in figure 5 above, weapons procurement has proceeded in two cycles. According to the 1979 White Paper, a total of 48 billion DM (about \$20–25 billion) went to weapons purchased from 1970 to 1979, with an additional 13 million DM (more than \$5 million) for research and development.[82] The stated budgetary goal since the latter part of the 1970s has been to insure that at least 30 percent of each budget is devoted to capital expenditure; these include all types of purchases, at home and abroad, as well as construction contracts for military facilities, infrastructure, and housing.

What will be the future direction of German acquisition policy? All available evidence suggests that there will be a more "national" approach, even in the latest co-production effort, the European fighter program in the 1990s. There are suggestions that even these plans will be further stretched out with present equipment being in use for perhaps another decade. Defense Minister Hans Apel suggested as early as 1981 that the Federal Republic, even in more affluent days, probably could not continue major purchases of tanks, aircraft, and ships in the light of inflation and cost overruns.[83] Just as in the recession of the mid 1960s, the solution will be in a less ambitious acquisition schedule and perhaps more reliance on the maintenance and progressive improvement of deployed systems.

There would seem to be little chance of relying on external markets or direct sales. The United States is seen by a number of German analysts to have returned to a policy of "buy American." Most of the European states are under the same pressures as the Federal Republic: high unit costs, a commitment to preserve domestic employment, and an interest in a strong national technological base. The 1976 aircraft "sale of the century," the selling of both the F-16 and the Tornado, has also raised questions about how to manage the next transition to a new generation of weapons in a projected period of constrained economic growth and strong, competing domestic claims.

Foreign military sales are also constrained in a number of ways.[84] The Federal Republic now ranks as the fifth largest arms supplier in the world, but lags by a considerable margin behind the United States, the Soviet Union, France, and Britain. In contrast particularly to the latter two states, its policies have been quite circumspect and mindful of existing regional arms balances in the light of continuing left-wing criticism at home and considerable sensitivity abroad. Moreover, the 1981 public and parliamentary opposition to prospective sales to Saudi Arabia and Chile introduced a new element to sales calculations, the strength of domestic criticism toward the purchasing government. The failure of Schmidt to deliver fully on his promises to the Saudis, despite German oil dependence, is a strong precedent.

The expectation, therefore, must be of an arms policy somewhat more national in orientation, but following familiar lines. The German interest in alliance standardization remains strong, if only because the connections between the persistent alliance mismatches and German national security are relatively clear cut. There are also indirect benefits to be calculated, as in the credit for transfer of obsolete equipment to Greece and Turkey under a complicated NATO burden sharing arrangement. But there will be new economic constraints and a far more cautious German approach to coordination and coproduction.

THE FORCE POSTURE OF THE FEDERAL REPUBLIC

The present force posture of the Federal Republic is remarkably like that negotiated in the first rearmament debate. Personnel levels are perhaps the most stable component: 70 percent for the army (*Heer*), with 50 percent of all conscripts; 22 percent for the air force (*Luftwaffe*), with 30 percent of all conscripts; and 8 percent for the navy (*Marine*), with 20 percent of conscript manpower.[85]

Many of the questions treated in other chapters regarding the fit between doctrine and structure are relatively less important in the German case, given the Federal Republic's pervasive alliance orientation. All of Germany's tactical air capability, for example, is under NATO command (2nd and 4th Allied Tactical Air Forces). All German land forces are major assigned elements under NATO's northern and central commands. At a minimum, this implies a connection with the planning and doctrine of the alliance. In operational terms, it means relatively constant communication and joint exercises with other Western forces deployed on German soil. There are also particularly strong bonds—some fostered, others more informal—between German and American forces.

The amount of perturbation and challenge in force posture policy clearly reflects the size and degree of integration of the three services. The army unquestionably was the hardest hit by the manpower uncertainties of the 1970s and shortfalls in junior officers and NCOs. Its manpower situation then stabilized, and the changes in pay and recruitment practices have garnered higher performance marks from both national and alliance authorities. Nonetheless, it is faced with the huge training and administrative responsibilities associated with inducting approximately 50,000 conscripts every quarter. And planning for the likely shortfalls is an obvious burden, whatever the political rhetoric.

The army's twelve divisions have felt the greatest external pressure for increased efficiency and therefore organizational change. A rough measure of this is the number of major changes in American army divisional organization (three). The Germans have been somewhat more resistant to precipitous shifts, but generally have followed suit eventually. The most recent plan has involved measures (1) to improve combat efficiency, (2) to increase the army's "tooth-to-tail" ratio (i.e., the ratio of combat troops support forces), and (3) to increase the number of trained personnel available for reserve duty and to improve unit training for cadre divisions readily expandable in times of tension.

In many respects, it is the German air force that has been the closest counterpart of an American service. In part, this reflects a planned similarity; much initial pilot training was conducted in the United States in close connection with similar American units. Specific technological requirements beyond those of either army or navy units constitute another parallel element, with a third being constant interaction within the NATO tactical air commands.

The navy has maintained perhaps the most autonomous profile. Its missions are largely confined to Baltic defense and North Sea security, with a small mixed force of naval air support, fast frigates and shallow-draft submarines. Pressures to expand the scope of naval operations continue, both from within Germany and from the navies of its allies. But for the foreseeable future, it will probably continue to operate in the area of "German defense" set down in legislation, with principal attention given to the coastal defense function.

The fourth "regular" service is the health services, organized under its own service *Inspektur*. Its function is "preventive medicine, medical care, and the treatment and evacuation of casualties." It will remain under national command even in wartime and will render support when possible to both civilians and the medical services of the other NATO forces.

The final element within the German defense establishment is the territorial army (TV), organized under the army to provide for home defense under national command in wartime. The TV was a stepchild of the Bundeswehr establishment, understaffed and underequipped. Continuing NATO pressure for greater reserve capabilities has led to new plans for establishing cadre divisions with more modern equipment. Moreover, there will be a strengthened ready reserve force and a more extensive program of reserve duty training. Some twelve home defense brigades will reach close to full strength in a period of heightened warning. All in all, perhaps a million troops can be mobilized in the first two weeks of conflict.

PERCEPTIONS OF THE UTILITY OF FORCE

In discussing German perceptions of the utility of force, an analyst begins with a largely hypothetical framework. No German regular forces have been used in combat since the end of World War II. There have been no instances of direct use of force on the central front; indeed, German forces are deployed at some distance from the East German or Czechoslovak border to prevent accident or incident. By Four Power agreement (the United States, Soviet Union, Britain, and France), they also have been excluded from any functions directly related to the successive Berlin crises. The only use of German force came in the freeing of a captured German plane in Mogadishu, Somalia, and this was undertaken by the special antiterrorist unit of the federal border police, a separate paramilitary organization.[86]

There are few in Germany, or within NATO in general, who are dissatisfied with the stability that restraint on West German use of force implies for the central front. A number of German analysts also note that this posture avoids confrontation between East German and West German troops, obviating attacks on East German forces and cities. Although the separation of the two German states, in many senses, has increased with time, the East German leadership may have similar concerns about the potential for attacks on Germans in the West. But for at least some West German observers, how East German forces would be used is a question that cannot really be answered confidently until conflict occurs.

West Germany has steadfastly refused to allow its troops to become involved outside the European "zone of German defense." Perhaps the most dramatic confrontation came in the mid 1960s, when President Lyndon Johnson pressured Bonn to send at least a token force to Vietnam. Chancellor Erhard responded that this was beyond the spirit of the German Constitution; moreover, it would have constituted an intolerable political and psychological burden for German forces and German society.

In recent years, there have been some renewed calls in the United States for greater German participation in the maintenance of a favorable international order. The security of the Persian Gulf and, thus, of European oil supplies, has been emphasized as an issue of particular significance for Germany. More or less serious schemes have been a German naval presence in the Gulf, direct German support for an alliance rapid-deployment force (RDF), or even the inclusion of some German units in an American-led RDF.

Most German political leaders have rejected all of these suggestions for the same reasons as were given in the mid 1960s. Despite their increasing self-confidence and assertiveness in

NATO affairs, most of the German political elite believe the cost of extra-NATO involvement will still be too high. They have offered a number of alternatives: (1) substantial economic assistance to two Western "anchors" in the region, Turkey and Pakistan; (2) the assumption of "host nation" support duties as well as certain unspecified functions in Europe to allow greater American flexibility; (3) increased diversification of energy imports and utilization, and (4) increased diplomatic links with the Gulf states. The Federal Republic has argued in bilateral and NATO discussions that, taken as a package, these constitute a fair share toward stabilization of the Gulf region and alleviation of energy vulnerability.

For the foreseeable future, German reluctance to expand the scope of its force commitments will almost certainly continue. There are obvious technical and economic constraints; German forces, for example, cannot be projected beyond national borders without relying on other states. The most important limitations will still be political and psychological, in terms of domestic constituencies as well as external allies and adversaries. Even in the case of an energy embargo, the range of nonmilitary instruments available to any future German government would seem considerable.

The pivotal question would seem to be the degree of importance American leadership will attach to direct German participation. Under present conditions, the question has not really been raised. And there is good reason, now as in 1965, to expect German resistance, if not direct opposition to external involvement of its military forces. One solution often discussed is formal expansion of NATO's area of responsibility. But this would be highly questionable, given present alliance politics and West German ambivalence, left and right.

Epilogue

This essay has focused on what seem to be the underlying contradictions of postwar German defense policy. The Federal Republic is the second NATO power in all but direct nuclear capability, yet it has no separable national defense profile. Its forces are among the most numerous and most effective in the West, yet the structure and doctrine of the Bundeswehr reflect alliance compromise and American political necessity more than they do German conceptions and choices. Finally, the Federal Republic is now clearly a power with global impact. But its defense policy remains firmly anchored in the requirements of the central front, and it is likely to remain so.

There is no necessity for speedy resolution of these contradictions. In many respects, they reflect the basic German-American bargains under which rearmament was sanctioned. The present international order is permissive; it is hard even to imagine a systemic challenge that would force greater congruence, much less a radical reorientation, of German national security efforts.

The critical variable would seem to remain the strength and durability of German-American relations. These relations have already withstood a number of major shifts and substantive disputes, including the present levels of domestic questioning on both sides. Yet the basic issues are (1) the convergence of national interests in a preferred European order, and (2) the benefits to both of linking national security resources and defense strategies. The agreements of the past are now challenged on several sides: by the new significance attached to the question of strategic defense by the United States and the primacy that many in the Federal Republic seem to accord to the maintenance of European détente, whatever the longer-term outlook or the global context. These challenges will be all the more intense if present projections of diverging economic policies and financial preferences prove correct.

Much will depend, as it always has, on the perception of long-term mutual benefit in the relationship. There is much to build on in terms of both direct cooperation and in indirect networks of communication. What happens next will be the major issue on Bonn's implicit political agenda—and it may be hoped, on Washington's as well—for the foreseeable future.

Notes

1. Federal Republic of Germany, Federal Minister of Defence, *White Paper, 1985: The Situation and the Development of the Federal Armed Forces* (Bonn: Federal Minister of Defence, 1985), p. 5.

2. This and the later historical discussions are drawn from my book *Germany and the Politics of Nuclear Weapons* (New York: Columbia University Press, 1975).

3. See the essays collected by Wolfram Hanrieder in his *West German Foreign Policy, 1949–1979* (Boulder, Colo.: Westview Press, 1980), especially those by Hillenbrand, Wörner, and myself.

4. By German calculation, for example, in 1985 the total defense expenditures of the NATO states were divided as follows: United States, 71 percent; FRG, 7.5 percent (including Berlin expenditures); France, 6 percent; United Kingdom, 7 percent; Italy, 2.9 percent; Holland, 1.2 percent; Canada, 2 percent; with the remaining 2.4 percent split among the rest. The figures reflect total U.S. spending. See *White Paper, 1985*, pp. 105–06.

5. See the essays by Ann-Marie LeGloannec, John Roper, and Stephen Szabo in Catherine M. Kelleher and Gale A. Mattox, eds., *Evolving European Defense Policies* (Lexington, Mass.: Lexington Books, 1986).

6. Kelleher (*Germany and the Politics of Nuclear Weapons*, Epilogue) suggests one measurement scheme; Bellini and Pattie, a related one.

7. The best treatment in English of the initial period is Robert McGeehan, *The German Rearmament Question: American Diplomacy and European Defense after World War II* (Urbana: University of Illinois Press, 1971).

8. See here the related treatment in my essay, "Germany and NATO: The Enduring Bargain," in *West German Foreign Policy*, ed. Hanrieder, pp. 43–60.

9. See the essays of Kissinger, Uwe Nerlich and Pierre Hassner in *NATO: The Next Thirty Years*, ed. Kenneth Meyers (Boulder, Colo.: Westview Press, 1980).

10. Perhaps the earliest full statement of the "decoupling theme" is Andrew J. Pierre's "Can European Security Be Decoupled from America?" *Foreign Affairs*, July 1973, pp. 761–77.

11. See the essays in *Evolving European Defense Policies*, ed. Kelleher and Mattox.

12. The principal treaty was, of course, the Treaty on the Basis of Relations, or the so-called Basic Treaty between the Federal Republic and the German Democratic Republic, signed in December 1972. The original source of the recognition was Chancellor Willy Brandt in 1969. See Gebhard Schweigler's *National Consciousness in Divided Germany* (Beverly Hills, Calif.: Sage, 1975).

13. *Ostpolitik* is usually defined as FRG relations with the Soviet Union and East European states other than the DDR. The relevant treaties here are: (1) the German-Soviet treaty of August 1970, (2) the German-Polish treaty of December 1970, and (3) the German-Czech treaty of 1973. These together with the Berlin Four Power Agreement of October 1970 and the Basic Treaty of 1972 constitute the legal foundation for

Bonn's "normalization" program. See on this Michael Kreile, "Ostpolitik Reconsidered," in *The Foreign Policy of West Germany: Formation and Contents*, ed. Ekkehart Krippendorff and Volker Rittberger (Beverly Hills, Calif.: Sage, 1980), pp. 123–46.

14. See Kreile, "Ostpolitik Reconsidered," pp. 134–39.

15. Compare contrasting chapters in the official *White Paper, 1985*: "The Foundations of Security," pp. 3–10 and "Developments in World Politics," pp. 11–13 with "The Military Threat Posed by the Warsaw Pact," pp. 41–64.

16. For a contrasting view, see Christian Potyka, "Die vernachlassigte Offentlichkeit", in *Sicherheitspolitik*, ed. Klaus-Dieter Schwarz, 2d ed. (Bad Hunnef-Epel: Osang Verlag, 1976), pp. 365–78.

17. See the *White Paper, 1985*, p. 9, for the formulation of "arms control and disarmament" as being "integral parts of the German security policy for stable peace."

18. See my article on LRTNF, "The Present as Prologue," in *International Security*, Spring 1981; and Alton Frye, "Nuclear Weapons in Europe: No Exit from Ambivalence," *Survival*, May/June 1980, pp. 98–106.

19. See Kreile, "Ostpolitik Reconsidered", pp. 123–46; and Wolf-Dieter Karl, "Entspannungspolitik: Der Weg von der Konfrontation zur Kooperation in den Ost-West Beziehungen," in *Sicherheitspolitik*, ed. Schwarz, pp. 127–50.

20. For a brief synthesis of these arguments, see Frieder Schlupp, "Modell Deutschland and the International Division of Labour: The Federal Republic of Germany in the World Political Economy," in *Foreign Policy of West Germany*, ed. Krippendorff and Rittberger, pp. 33–100.

21. See Kelleher, *Germany and the Politics of Nuclear Weapons*, pp. 296–301.

22. For further details on these various alternatives and the evolution of the German position, see ibid., chapters 7, 9, and 10.

23. See Schmidt's famous Alistair Buchan Memorial Lecture of October 1977, reprinted in *Survival*, January-February 1978, pp. 2–10.

24. For further details, see Lewis Edinger, *Kurt Schumacher: A Study in Personality and Political Behavior* (Stanford: Stanford University Press, 1965).

25. As reported in *Der Spiegel*, 6 October 1954, pp. 5–7.

26. For a more detailed development of this theme, see Catherine M. Kelleher, "Mass Armies in the 1970's: The Debate in Western Europe," *Armed Forces and Society*, Fall 1978, pp. 3–30.

27. For a further development of this theme, see Kelleher in *West German Foreign Policy*, ed. Hanrieder, pp. 43–60.

28. See the comments by then Minister Matthofer and then Chancellor Schmidt reported in press accounts through the spring, summer, and fall of 1980 and translated in the Foreign Broadcast Information Service, *Daily Report: Western Europe*.

29. See *White Paper, 1985*, "The Balance of Forces," pp. 48–61. For a previous, more concise statement of the German interpretation of the role and potential of European-based TNF, see Federal Republic of Germany, Minister of Defence, *White Paper, 1979*

(Bonn: Federal Minister of Defence, 1979), pp. 107–10 and 125–27.

30. See Helga Haftendorn's discussion in her "West Germany and the Management of Security Relations: Security Policy under the Conditions of International Interdependence," in *Foreign Policy of West Germany*, ed. Krippendorff and Rittberger, pp. 7–31.

31. *White Paper, 1985*, p. 134.

32. See "Developments in World Politics," *White Paper, 1985*, pp. 11–13 and "Arms Control and Disarmament," pp. 21–40. Cf. *White Paper, 1979*, pp. 42–43 and 55–84.

33. See the various essays on both processes in the volume edited by Helga Haftendorn, Wolf-Dieter Karl, Joachim Krause, and Lothar Wilker, *Verwaltete Aussenpolitik: Sicherheits-und-entspannungspolitische Entscheidungsprozesse in Bonn* (Cologne: Verlag Wissenschaft Politik, 1978).

34. See Kelleher, "Present as Prologue," for further details.

35. See Krippendorff's introductory essay to *Foreign Policy of West Germany*, pp. 1–5.

36. See McGeehan, *German Rearmament Question*.

37. *White Paper, 1985*, pp. 110–13.

38. As quoted in Walter F. Hahn, *Between Westpolitik and Ostpolitik* (Beverly Hills, Calif.: Sage, 1975), p. 70.

39. Kelleher, *Germany and the Politics of Nuclear Weapons*, pp. 49–56.

40. Ibid., chapter 6.

41. Ibid., chapter 8.

42. See, for example, the discussion of the Soviet threat in the first two white papers under Schroder in 1969 and under Schmidt in 1970.

43. See the further discussion of this throughout Kelleher, *Germany and the Politics of Nuclear Weapons*.

44. For this reason alone, the report of columnists Evans and Novak that in the summer of 1977 the Carter administration was considering defense along the Weser-Lech perimeter occasioned immediate Bonn protests and criticisms.

45. See the essay by Alan Ned Sabrosky in this volume.

46. This was the original goal set at the Lisbon conference of 1952. See McGeehan, *German Rearmament Question*, for further details.

47. See the comment by Defense Minister George Leber quoted above.

48. See below for a report of empirical results on "guns versus butter" achieved by Richard C. Eichenberg in his doctoral dissertation on this topic, "Defense-Welfare Tradeoffs in German Budgeting," submitted to the Department of Political Science, University of Michigan, June 1981.

49. An example of the somewhat inflammatory popular commentary on this issue is a 1981 *Stern* article by Wolf Perdelwitz, "Die versteckte Atommacht," 19 February 1981.

50. See Kelleher, "Present as Prologue."

51. The decision rules are left unpublished, in part for reasons of what the Germans view as "credible deterrence." For discussion of earlier demands for a national veto right, see Kelleher, *Germany and the Politics*

of *Nuclear Weapons*, chapter 8, and my essay on the broader tactical C³I problem in NATO in *Managing Nuclear Operations*, ed. Ashton Carter, John Steinbruner, and Charles Zraket, (Washington: Brookings Institution, 1987), pp. 445–69.

52. The Bundestag debate on these issues took place in March 1979, but Wehner and others had been raising questions in the fall of 1978. On this, see the discussion in *The Modernization of NATO's Long-Range Theater Nuclear Forces*, prepared by the Congressional Research Services for the House Committee on Foreign Affairs (96th Cong., 2d sess.), 31 December 1980.

53. This is not the position of the CDU centrists, as is clear from, for example, the essay by Defense Minister Manfred Wörner in *West German Foreign Policy*, ed. Hanrieder, pp. 37–42. But see the remarks attributed to Richard Allen in the *New York Times*, 29 March 1981.

54. See John Vinocour's report on then Chancellor Schmidt's criticism of these groups, *New York Times*, 5 April 1981.

55. Compare the somewhat different evaluation developed by Martin Muller in *Verwaltete Aussenpolitik*, ed. Haftendorn et al., pp. 167–89.

56. See the convergence between demands of the far left and far right in, say, the *Stern* interview given by the retired Luftwaffe Colonel Alfred Mechtersheimer, "Atomarer Selbstmord und Umwegen," 3 April 1981, pp. 74ff, and the successive platforms of the Green party before it entered the Federal Parliament.

57. This account relies in large measure on the work of Helga Haftendorn in *Foreign Policy of West Germany*, ed. Krippendorff, and with her associates in *Verwaltete Aussenpolitik*, and on my essay on German defense decision making in *Reshaping America's Defenses*, ed. Robert Art, Vince Davis, and Samuel Huntington (New York: Pergammon-Brassey, 1985).

58. *Verwaltete Aussenpolitik*, ed. Haftendorn et al.

59. See Hillenbrand's discussion in "Germany and the United States", in *West German Foreign Policy*, ed. Hanrieder, pp. 73–91.

60. Clearly this is reflected in the various national essays in this volume.

61. On Adenauer's system see Wolfram Hanrieder, *West German Foreign Policy, 1949–1963* (Stanford: Stanford University Press, 1967), and the one volume of Adenauer's own memoirs published in English: *Memoirs* (Chicago: H. Regenery, 1966).

62. Strauss is clearly one of the most colorful and controversial figures in postwar German political life. His works in English include *The Grand Design* (New York: Praeger, 1965).

63. Schmidt has also published two major books on defense policy, both available in English: *Defense or Retaliation* (New York, Praeger, 1962), and *The Balance of Power* (London: Kimber, 1971).

64. Haftendorn, "West Germany and the Management of Security Relations," p. 12.

65. *Verwaltete Aussenpolitik*, ed. Haftendorn et al., p. 13, lists a few interesting exceptions from the early 1970s.

66. *White Paper, 1985*, p. 165.

67. Kelleher, *Germany and the Politics of Nuclear Weapons*, chapters 1 and 2.

68. Ibid., pp. 215–18.

69. See the special collection of essays edited by Ralf Zoll on German civil-military relations published in *Armed Forces and Society* 5 (Summer 1979): 523–686.

70. See Eichenberg, "Defense-Welfare Tradeoffs in German Budgeting."

71. For a discussion of these issues, see Brenton C. Fischmann, *West German Defense Planning for the 1990s: Strategic Consequences for NATO*, CSIS Interim Report (Washington, D.C.: Center for Strategic and International Studies, 1988).

72. The literature on German civil-military relations, prewar and postwar, is substantial. In addition to the sources cited in *Armed Forces and Society* 5 (Summer 1979): 523–686, there are numerous political texts—e.g., from the right, Dieter Portner, *Bundeswehr und Linksextremismus* (Munich: Olzog, 1976), and from the left, *Anti-Wehrkunde: Basistexte zur politischen Bildung*, ed. Ulrich Albrecht, Henning Schierholz and Joseph H. Helmut Thielen (Darmstadt: Luchterhand, 1975).

73. In interview accounts in the 1960s, my sources cited the French as the Europeans to be soothed. Other sources attribute this remark to Adenauer and to Schumacher.

74. See Wolf, Graf von Baudissin, *Soldat fur den Frieden* (Munich: S. Piper, 1969).

75. Compare, on this point, Wilfrid von Bredow, *Die unbewaltigte Bundeswehr* (Frankfurt: Fischer Taschenbuch Verlag, 1973), and Wido Mosen, *Bundeswehr: Elite der Nation?* (Neuwied: Luchterhand, 1970).

76. More recent incidents, reflecting the generational change, have involved "left" critiques of governmental decisions—e.g., the "Bastian" affair of 1979.

77. *White Paper, 1985*, pp. 297–313.

78. *White Paper, 1979*, pp. 197–99. The 1985 White Paper notes, however, that controversies have arisen regarding the Bundeswehr tradition among some parts of the populace. As a result, the 1965 directive, "The Bundeswehr and Tradition," was replaced by "Guidelines for the Understanding and Fostering of Tradition in the Bundeswehr," and a working group was established in 1983 to draft a Joint Service Regulation. See *White Paper, 1985*, pp. 311–12.

79. See the *White Paper, 1979*, p. 226, for data on projected available vs. required manpower figures, and the discussion of the demographic problem and suggested solutions in the *White Paper, 1985*, pp. 284–85 and 396–404.

80. The actual restrictions are contained in the various protocols modifying the "Brussels Treaty," the Western European Union treaty, reprinted in U.S. Senate, Committee on Foreign Relations, *Protocols on the Termination of the Occupation Regime in the Federal Republic of Germany*, 83rd Cong., 2d sess. (1954), executives I and M.

81. See the range of critiques cited in the excellent bibliography attached to *Foreign Policy of West Germany*, ed. Krippendorff and Rittberger.

82. *White Paper, 1979*, p. 275.

83. Quoted in *Frankfurter Allgemeine Zeitung*, 15 March 1981.

84. See U.S., Senate, Committee on Foreign Relations, *Protocols*.

85. *White Paper, 1985*, p. 237.

86. The Frontier Police are a separate "third force" under the control of the Ministry of Interior, although this special antiterrorist unit, GSG9, operated under direction from the chancellor as well.

Other References

Brauch, Hans Gunter. "Arms Control and Disarmament Decisionmaking in the Federal Republic of Germany: Past Experience and Options for Change." In *Decisionmaking for Arms Limitation: Assessment and Prospects*. Edited by Hans Guenter Brauch and Duncan L. Clarke. Cambridge, Mass.: Ballinger, 1983, pp. 131–74.

Haftendorn, Helga. "Der Abrustungsbeauftragte—zur Organisation der Abrustungspolitik in der Bundesrepublik." *Politische Vierteljahresschrift*, vol. 13: 2–38.

———. *Abrustungs-und-Entspannungspolitik zwischen Sicherheitsbefriedigung und Friedenssicherung*. Dusseldorf: Verlagsgruppe Bertelsmann, 1974.

———. "Das aussen-und-sicherheitspolitische Entscheidungssystem der Bundesrepublik Deutschland." *Aus Politik und Zeitgeschichte: Beilage zur Wochenzeitung das Parlament*, No. 43 (1983).

———. *Security and Détente: Conflicting Priorities in German Foreign Policy*. New York: Praeger, 1985.

———. "West Germany and the Management of Security Relations: Security Policy Under the Conditions of International Interdependence." In *The Foreign Policy of West Germany: Formation and Contents*. Edited by Ekkehart Krippendorff and Volker Rittberger. German Political Studies, vol. 4. London and Beverly Hills, Calif.: Sage, 1980, pp. 7–31.

Haftendorn, Helga; Karl, Wolf-Dieter; Krause, Joachim; and Wilker, Lothar. *Verwaltete Aussenpolitik. Sicherheits-und entspannungspolitische Entscheidungsprozesse in Bonn*. Bibliothek Wissenschaft und Politik, vol. 20. Cologne: Berend von Nottbeck, 1979.

Hebel, Stephan. "Eine Denkfabrik fuer Beamte und Parlamentarier." *Frankfurter Rundschau*, 21 April 1986, p. 21.

Hill, Roger. *Political Consultation in NATO*. Canadian Institute of International Affairs Wellesley Papers 6 (1978). Toronto.

Kelleher, Catherine McArdle. "Defense Organization in Germany: A Twice-told Tale." In *Reorganizing America's Defense: Leadership in War and Peace*. Edited by Robert J. Art, Vincent Davis, and Samuel

P. Huntington. McLean, Va.: Pergamon Brassey's International Defense Publishers, 1985.

———. "The Defense Policy of the Federal Republic of Germany." In *The Defense Policies of Nations: A Comparative Study*. Edited by Douglas J. Murray and Paul R. Viotti. Baltimore, Md: Johns Hopkins Univ. Press, 1982.

Krause, Joachim and Wilker, Lothar. "Bureaucracy and Foreign Policy in the Federal Republic of Germany." In *The Foreign Policy of Germany: Formation and Contents*. Edited by Ekkehart Krippendorff and Volker Rittberger. German Political Studies vol. 4. London and Beverly Hills, Calif.: Sage, 1988, pp. 147–70.

Lunn, Simon. "Policy Preparation and Consultation within NATO Decisionmaking for SALT and LRTNF." In *Decisionmaking for Arms Limitation: Assessment and Prospects*. Edited by Hans Gunter Brauch and Duncan Clarke. Cambridge, Mass.: Ballinger, 1983, pp. 259–74.

Mayntz, Renate and Scharpf, Fritz W. *Policy Making in the German Federal Bureaucracy*. Amsterdam and New York: Elsevier, 1975.

Meier, Reihard. "Political Party Foundations in Bonn." *Swiss Review of World Affairs* 31 (Feb. 1982), pp. 25, 27, 29.

NATO Handbook. Brussels: NATO Information Service.

Phillipp, Udo. "Der Verteidigungsausschuss als politisches Instrument." *Wehrtechnik*, No. 4 (1977).

Rittberger, Volker, ed. *Abrustungsplanung in der Bundesrepublik: Aufgaben, Probleme, Perspektiven*. Baden-Baden: Nomos Verlagsgesellschaft, 1979.

———. *Neue Wege der Abrustungsplanung. Organisationsprobleme und Reformoptionen im internationalen Vergleich*. Baden-Baden: Nomos Verlagsgesellschaft, 1981.

Schafer, Friedrich, *Der Bundestag: Eine Darstellung seiner Aufgaben und seiner Abreitsweise*. Oplanden: Westdeutscher Verlag, 1975.

Shearer, Richard E. "Consulting in NATO on Nuclear Policy." *NATO Review*, October 1977.

Sloan, Stanley R. "Arms Control Consultations in NATO," In *Decisionmaking for Arms Limitation: Assessment and Prospects*. Edited by Hans Guenter Brauch and Duncan Clarke. Cambridge, Mass.: Ballinger, 1983, pp. 219–36.

Yost, David S. and Glad, Thomas C. "West German Party Politics and Theater Nuclear Modernization since 1977." *Armed Forces and Society* 8, No. 4 (Summer 1982): 525–60.

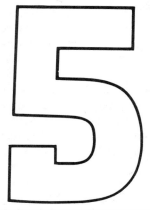

THE GERMAN DEMOCRATIC REPUBLIC

Peter N. Schmitz

World War II left virtually nothing of the German Reich and its diabolic regime that had come very close to dominating the world militarily. The German nation still existed after the war, but its statehood remained a question mark for a considerable time. Many Germans draw this clear distinction between the terms *nation*, or people, and *state*, the legal entity. In particular, West German leaders are prone to refer to East and West Germany as two German states in one German nation. A bone of contention between the United States and the Soviet Union, the two powers that emerged reinforced from the war, Germany's fate became a function of a new East-West confrontation, resulting in the division of Europe and establishment of the respective power spheres of the two superpowers.

Forty-three years after World War II, the Federal Republic of Germany (FRG) ranks as the second power in the Atlantic alliance.[1] And certainly the German Democratic Republic (GDR) has to be considered second in the Warsaw Pact by almost every measure. To include

the GDR in the list of the major military powers of today would, however, be inappropriate. As the smaller in every respect of the two political Germanys, it lacks the economic and demographic base to raise and support a major military force. And yet, the GDR has a unique politico-military position in the Warsaw Pact, which in many respects mirrors the unique position of the FRG in NATO.

The GDR, the former Soviet Zone of Occupation, covers an area a little less than half as big as the FRG. To put it into perspective for the American reader, the Federal Republic is about the size of Wyoming, and the GDR of Virginia. With sixteen million inhabitants, the GDR is far less densely populated than the Federal Republic with its some sixty million citizens. The inner-German border stretches over 1,360 km, from the Baltic Sea at Lübeck to the province of Thuringia, where it meets the Czechoslovak border. The term *inner-German border* is understood as a dividing line *within* the German nation, dividing it into two separate states. Germans use *inner* rather than

Table 1. Comparative Fact Sheet

	GDR	FRG
Geographic area (square miles)	41,000	96,000
Population (millions)	16.7	61.7
GNP ($ billions)	89	679
Defense expenditures ($ billions)	7.6	23.6

inter because the former carries the meaning of *within* Germany whereas the latter implies a line *between* two states, suggesting a more permanent division of the German nation. In the East, the well-known Oder-Neisse Line marks the border with Poland.

The GDR has managed its own economic miracle, albeit within the inevitable constraints of the socialist economic system. Although East Germans continually complain about the shortfalls of the Marxist-type planned supply and production process, they are envied for their standard of living by all their comrades of the socialist "brother countries," including the Russians.

German industriousness has prevailed whether under socialist-totalitarian or republican-democratic conditions. The economic miracles of the two Germanys were created out of the rubble of the war. Certainly the GDR has become an economic power with increasing weight vis-à-vis the Soviet Union and considerable influence in the Eastern bloc economic organization, the Council for Mutual Economic Assistance (CMEA or COMECON).[2] Since the late 1960s the GDR has been the ranking trading partner for the USSR. Economic cooperation with the Soviet Union has played a major role in their bilateral relations. The GDR's optical, electronics, machinery, and chemical industries are supremely efficient. Like the FRG, the GDR has emerged from a status of political dwarfdom, if not pariah existence, to that of an internationally acknowledged actor. But the GDR is certainly not a major actor in the world as a whole, due to its rather limited room for maneuvering, which is closely controlled by Moscow. In military capacity the GDR has risen from a low standard with ill-equipped, poorly trained, and unreliable paramilitary organizations to a level where, according to most observers, its 174,000-man army of first-rate units is second only to the Soviet Red Army in terms of high-quality weaponry and combat potential. It may be true that in the 1950s the officers and men of the East German armed forces thought themselves lucky if their socialist comrades in the other Warsaw Pact armies returned their salutes (as was also the experience of West German officers and men in the early years after their integration with NATO staffs). Today the East German armed forces stand high "in the service of proletarian internationalism," having helped the GDR to advance to second power in the Warsaw Pact.

In contemporary reflections by historians and political analysts, particularly those in West Germany, it is asked time and again whether cementing the division of Germany by integrating the two parts into the two opposing military alliances of NATO and the Warsaw Pact was inevitable. Explanations attempting to blame the swift identification with the West of West Germany and its rearmament as the major inhibitions to achieving unification with East Germany in the early 1950s will remain sheer speculation. Only Soviet leaders at the time could tell about their intentions concerning postwar Germany. Yet certainly those leaders' perceptions of Germany's strategic position in the expanding East-West power struggle did not differ much, if at all, from the Western war allies' perceptions. A rearmed Germany with her 1937 borders was (and is) certainly as inconceivable to Poles and Czechoslovaks as to the Danes and Dutch, to the Russians as well as to the French, British, and Americans, even if that Germany were to pledge its neutrality. Historical memories may be short-lived, but Germany's existence from 1871 to 1945 as one unified state at the core of Europe threatened its immediate and even distant neighbors, if not the whole world, once too often.

The Russians, having paid by far the heaviest toll to German expansionism, were much better prepared than their Western wartime allies to swallow their share of the spoils of victory. Controversy and bickering in the Roosevelt administration about Germany's postwar fate made it difficult for the mightiest of the "Big Three" to take the lead in the many wartime discussions and conferences devoted to planning the allied occupation of Germany. Great Britain's Winston Churchill probably had the clearest and most reasonable image of what should be undertaken not just with the shattered Germany but also with war-splintered Europe as a whole. But he must have had a hard time identifying and reacting to what was the leading opinion at any given time in Washington, the more so because the ailing U.S. president appeared to waver among the many advisors seeking to influence him.[3]

Roosevelt did not share either Churchill's anxious concern about the order of postwar Europe or his suspicions of Stalin's intentions. Roosevelt and his administration failed to recognize the basic divergences within the wartime coalition. American policy was geared toward cooperation with the Russians, even though it clearly saw Stalin's drive for hegemony and social and political transformation in Europe. The United States showed, most observers agree, considerable naïveté in dealing with the Soviet Union.[4]

The USSR acted quite differently. Since 1942 the three allies had had plans for a division of Germany to ensure a lasting peace in Europe. In wartime conferences, Stalin time and again had called for decisions regarding postwar Germany. For differing reasons the Western Powers were, however, cautious and slow in deciding that issue. Stalin, by contrast, had formulated his aims step by step along with each success on the battlefield. He entered the last rounds of the war and the immediate postwar phase with a clear overall concept. Anticipating a bipolar power constellation, this concept was dictated as much by Soviet security concerns as by power politics, and it was inevitably interwoven with ideological strings. "This war is unlike those in the past; whoever occupies a territory will force his own social system upon it. Everyone will introduce his own system as far as his army advances," Stalin told a Yugoslav delegation in April 1945.[5] Accordingly, after the Red Army had marched into Poland (July 1944), Romania (August 1944), and Hungary (September 1944), Stalin implemented a policy of Sovietization and suppression. The other states of the newly acquired Russian buffer in Europe had to fall in line too, from Finland to Albania.

In Germany, the fighting had not even stopped when on 30 April 1945, a group of ten German communists arrived in the East via a Soviet military plane at Frankfurt an der Oder. The head of the delegation was Walter Ulbricht, who began immediately to introduce the communist and Soviet system in that part of Germany conceded to Stalin as the Soviet Occupation Zone.[6] In the shadow of the bayonets of the Soviet occupation armies and under Soviet military rule, the installation of a communist regime in the Soviet Zone of occupied Germany went on steadily. When we regard the origins of the GDR's security policy, we have to bear in mind that an important part in the scheme of a communist takeover of state power is to establish internal security as soon as possible. The evolving communist power apparatus has to be guarded and secured against the so-called counterrevolutionary enemy. Security policy in communist terms means foremost the safeguarding of the Party and its *nomenklatura*, the ruling elite. It is not surprising, then, that as early as 1945 the Soviet Military Administration permitted the arming of the Volkspolizei "People's Police," soon numbering some 45,000 men in its occupation zone, while in the occupation zones of the Western powers the efforts of the victors to disarm "their" Germans did not spare even hunting equipment and antique weapons.

The denazification commissions in the Western zones suspected almost every German, and Nazi Party members in particular, regardless of their positions in the organizations of the Third Reich, to be guilty until they could prove otherwise. The Russians also purged political and administrative institutions at all levels of "Nazis," and substituted communists, or at least cooperating "comrades." Soon afterward, however, they became rather lenient about further denazification. They had been careful not to accuse and condemn the whole German people for Nazi crimes. And once power was with the communists, they could reach out to the population to win support for the radical changes in political, social, and economic conditions intended by the USSR and the Ulbricht group. A minimum level of tolerance and cooperation by the population was necessary. Ulbricht knew that German communist power could not be supported forever by Soviet bayonets. Both the Soviet Union and the German communist leaders wanted to develop a stable and viable system in East Germany. From the Soviet perspective, "their" part of Germany had to play a prominent, if not the most important, role among the "sovietized" Eastern European countries in the Soviet postwar security system.

Both Germanys are creatures of East-West antagonism. Both are very susceptible to any change in superpower relations, and the relative degree of their sovereignty or independence in policy making is sensitive to highs and lows in the East-West climate. Complex as German-German relations have become since the start of West German *Ostpolitik* (the policy of détente and improved and expanded relations with Eastern European countries) in the 1970s, its intermeshing of political, economic, and social strings offers the USSR, in particular, a host of opportunities to pull them roughly or gently, to play the détente tune, or to coerce East German *Abgrenzung* (demarcation) from the Federal Republic. Both Germanys are too small to balance the scales in East-West relations, yet their geopolitical (and more so geostrategic) positions in their respective coalition systems are too important to allow them to retreat from center stage.

The East German leaders have always known only too well that the GDR would never be allowed a maverick role within the Warsaw Pact like Romania, and that they never would get the chance to try to defuse an internal crisis on their own, as the Polish leaders have. Moscow cannot genuinely loosen its hold over the GDR without facing the loss of its influence in all of Eastern Europe. As one observer put it: "The Soviets are so intent on maintaining their position in East Germany that the greatest risk of Soviet attack on Western Europe today is from a panicked Soviet response to rebellion in East Germany."[7] Rebellion in the GDR appears to be unlikely, however, as there is no serious reason for Soviet panic about it. There was no Western intent to interfere in Soviet suppression of unrest in Eastern Europe in the 1950s and 1960s, when there was Western military superiority. Why should the USSR now fear Western intervention in similar cases when it can easily fend off any military pressures?

Also, the East Germans have learned their lessons. Any attempt at fighting the system or challenging Soviet predominance has resulted in forcible suppression, less freedom, and less economic well-being. Again mirror-imaging the Federal Republic's situation, experience suggests that the more reliable the GDR presents itself as being to the USSR and its Eastern European socialist brother countries, the more little freedoms it can gain in playing on its special and profitable relations with the FRG. Just as the Federal Republic does not want to create any doubt about its staunch role in the Western alliance, so it is with the GDR in the East if it is to remain active in *Ostpolitik* and *Deutschlandpolitik* ("Germany policy," or German-German relations).

East German leaders face a multiple dilemma. The mutually exclusive aims in West German policies under continuing East-West antagonism, strong adherence to its "camp" and reunification in freedom, are not the themes of East German policies. Like all the communist governments forced upon Eastern European countries by the Soviet Union, the ruling Party functionaries in the GDR are only too aware of their dependence on Soviet policies. Although the theory of communism was originally developed by Germans (Marx and Engels), the real German communists of today, leaving aside the opportunists, have always realized their absolute outsider and lasting minority position in German society, even after decades of efforts to educate the GDR's population in socialism.[8] Despite the Berlin Wall and the cruel fortification of the border, East Germans have never stopped "voting with their feet"—a continuing exodus of Germans from the GDR—confronting the regime time and again with painful and embarrassing incidents. The prison fence around the GDR may attract too much of the world's attention. Yet the fortification inward of the "state border" with the Federal Republic remains necessary in the eyes of the GDR's rulers to ensure the survival of the "first socialist state of the German nation,"[9] illustrating at the same time, however, its immediate fragility.

After more than a quarter century since the Berlin Wall was erected, despite the favorable development of German-German relations during the 1970s and 1980s, the GDR still justifies the Wall as the "anti-fascist bulwark that has made peace in Europe more secure." A journal published by the ruling Sozialistische Einheitspartei Deutschlands (SED) recently even celebrated the erection of the Wall as "luck for the peoples of Europe and of the world" because in the SED's view the Wall had resulted in a more realistic policy of the West, thus opening the way in the 1970s for the Quadripartite Berlin Agreement, the Basic Treaty between Bonn and East Berlin, and the Helsinki Final Act. Erich Honecker, later Ulbricht's successor to ultimate power in the GDR, directed the erection of the Berlin Wall in August 1961. On the occasion of the twentieth anniversary of the Wall, he justified it as having prevented a military attack on the GDR by the West.[10] The GDR leadership apparently still sees no other choice than to maintain its prison image at the expense of the GDR's international reputation.

International Environment

The GDR was constituted in 1949, the same year as the Federal Republic of Germany. In 1954 the office of Soviet High Commissioner in the Soviet Occupation Zone disappeared and the Soviet Union declared the GDR a sovereign state. By the treaty of 20 September 1955 the GDR became free to determine issues of domestic and foreign policy, including relations with the FRG. The parties to the treaty also solemnly confirmed that the relations between them were based on full equality, mutual respect of sovereignty, and noninterference in internal affairs.[11] On the other hand, the Brezhnev Doctrine, proclaimed by Leonid Brezhnev as justification for Soviet intervention in Czechoslovakia in 1968, asserts a Soviet right—even "duty"—to intervene in "defense" of socialism in Marxist-Leninist states in jeopardy. Beyond the obvious political limitations imposed on the sovereignty of all Eastern European countries by the Brezhnev Doctrine, the GDR's right of self-determination in state affairs remains subject to the provision of the June 1945 Four Powers Agreement at Potsdam among the victorious World War II allies—the United States, the Soviet Union, Great Britain, and France. Provisions of the Potsdam Agreement remain legally in force until a peace treaty with Germany, in the boundaries of 1937, is finally negotiated. The USSR has been careful to retain the maximum of those provisions vis-à-vis the GDR, since that ensures its continuing right to interfere in the internal and external affairs of the GDR. The Soviet declaration of March 1954 therefore included the provision that the USSR would retain functions in the GDR related to the guarantee of security under the Four Powers Agreement at Potsdam. The "Treaty of Sovereignty" between the Soviet Union and the GDR of September 1955 made no explicit reference to the question of security, but reiterated the Soviet reservation regarding rights the USSR retains in the GDR. The 1964 Treaty of Friendship and Mutual Assistance between the two countries also contained an article referring to Soviet rights based on the Potsdam Agreement.

Nine days after the Federal Republic signed the North Atlantic Treaty on 5 May 1955, eight Eastern bloc countries, including the GDR, signed a treaty in Warsaw founding the Eastern bloc's own military alliance. The creation of the Warsaw Pact was portrayed by its signatories as essentially a response to the Federal Republic's membership in NATO, an idea socialist propaganda "sold" rather successfully to the world. But there may have been other reasons for concluding the Warsaw Pact. The Soviet Union certainly had in mind that this treaty would be a means of improving military cooperation and defense posture in its sphere of influence. A multilateral organization under firm Soviet control would enlarge Soviet influence beyond existing bilateral agreements with the Soviet satellite states. The Warsaw Pact also enabled the Soviet Union to improve coordination of the foreign policies of the pact countries. The treaty obliges signatories to consult on all important international issues that touch upon their common interests, "guided by the interest of furthering world peace and security."[12]

For the GDR leadership, one more restriction on their already very limited political flexibility made little difference. Yet membership in the Eastern alliance opened the way for recognition of the GDR's sovereignty by the other socialist countries, and, even more, gave legitimacy to establishing the GDR's own army. The Soviet Union may not have been too enthusiastic about paving the way for rearmament of a satellite whose unrest only two years previously had required Soviet tanks to maintain the socialist regime. But the USSR may have been in urgent need of a new military treaty in Eastern Europe.[13] On 15 May 1955, only one day after conclusion of the Warsaw treaty, the allied treaty with Austria was signed, which would have eliminated the legal basis for stationing Soviet forces in Hungary and Romania under the peace treaties signed with those countries in 1947. Under these treaties the Soviet Union maintained the right to retain such forces on the territory of both states as were necessary to ensure communications with the Soviet army in the Soviet occupation zone of Austria. This clause became obsolete with the conclusion of the Austrian State Treaty, since allied forces were obliged to leave Austria within ninety days of its ratification. It was not in the Soviet

Union's interest to lose its military footholds on its Balkan flank, and the Warsaw Pact accordingly created a new legal basis for the stationing of Soviet troops in Hungary and Romania. A year later the Hungarians might have had a chance to win their freedom in the 1956 uprising had there not been "friendly" Soviet troops in Budapest.

Throughout its development, the GDR has felt threatened or beleaguered in at least three different ways. First, in the early 1950s the Ulbricht regime was threatened by its own instability. It lacked any public support and was hardly able to provide the population with the bare minimum of day-to-day living essentials. Ulbricht's Soviet guarantors saw nothing wrong in looting a state they were allegedly helping to its feet. It needed the uprising of 17 June 1953 to convince the Russians of the dangers of continuing to insist on "reparations." In the early 1950s Ulbricht also had reason for concern about his and his state's future when his political godfather, Stalin, appeared to toy with the GDR—using it as a pawn in an elaborate game—in an apparent effort to prevent a West German alliance with the Western powers. Nevertheless, Ulbricht remained true to Stalin and his successors, more dedicated than any other Party leader behind the Iron Curtain. In the late 1950s and in the 1960s Ulbricht became a respected ally of Khrushchev and Brezhnev, supporting efforts to contain those symptoms of deviation and disobedience that surfaced in Yugoslavia, Albania, Poland, Hungary, Romania, and Czechoslovakia.

Second, each sign of unrest in the socialist camp has threatened the GDR regime because of its potentially destabilizing effects. Shifts within the Eastern bloc have been magnified seismically in their impact on the GDR. Honecker reacted to the events in Poland in the late 1970s and early 1980s just as his predecessor Ulbricht would have done. The prospect that Polish unrest would shake the foundations of the SED and the state apparatus was highly worrisome for Honecker, making him and GDR officialdom the harshest critics of the Polish workers' Solidarity organization. One commentator noted: "As was true during and after the Prague Spring of 1968, East Germany

Table 2. Chronology of East German Armament

1945	Arming of the People's Police (Volkspolizei) approved by the Soviet Military Administration (SMAD).
1946	The Volkspolizei numbers 45,000 men; another 3,000 German Frontier Police (Deutsche Grenzpolizei) deployed in garrison.
1948	SMAD orders the creation of military cadres later named the Garrisoned People's Police (Kasernierte Volkspolizei).
1949	Creation of the German Democratic Republic.
1950	The Kasernierte Volkspolizei numbers 70,000, the Grenzpolizei 18,000, the Transport Police 11,500, and a guard corps under the Ministry of State Security 5,000 men. In addition, there are some 80,000 nonmilitary police.
1955	Warsaw Pact signed.
1956	Official creation of the National People's Army (Nationale Volksarmee, or NVA) and of the Ministry for National Defense.
1961	Building of the Berlin Wall.
1962	Conscription introduced.

rode out the shock waves of threatened change in the socialist bloc more through a policy of Soviet-inspired orthodoxy than through the promise of flexibility and accommodation."[14] Alfred Grosser speculates that Ulbricht's strong opinion may have played a role in 1968 when the Soviet leaders decided upon military intervention in Czechoslovakia despite the hesitant attitudes of the other Warsaw Pact members.[15]

East German participation in the invasion was, however, largely symbolic and may have served domestic purposes more than solving the actual problem in Prague. Final proof of utmost loyalty on part of the GDR may have been needed to convince the USSR of the advantage of having a fully combat-ready and operationally deployable East German army at its disposal. Soviet restrictions on the establishment of East German forces, although formally decreed in 1956, had been in effect far longer, not least because of the shock to the USSR of the 1953 uprising. Another signal went to the GDR's own population. The 1968 events clearly demonstrated what would happen in the event of any analogous "East German Spring."

In the perception of the GDR's leaders, their beleagueredness also stems from a third source—the harsh and unfriendly international environment, the threat from the West, and West German "imperialist machinations" in particular. Just as the GDR is the "westward outpost of the socialist camp in defending the achievements of socialism," so the Federal Republic is the "spearhead of capitalist imperialism" in SED propaganda. The GDR is the "bastion of peace . . . in the struggle against West German imperialism and militarism, and its aggression policy."[16] Was it not the Federal Republic that rather successfully imposed diplomatic isolation on the GDR? West Germany's "Hallstein Doctrine" of the 1950s and 1960s threatened as sanctions the breaking of West German diplomatic and economic ties against any country recognizing East Germany. East Germany won diplomatic recognition only when normal relations with Western countries were established as a result of détente between the superpowers and the Federal

Republic's own *Ostpolitik* of the early 1970s. Even today the GDR has an open list of demands with respect to its claim to full sovereignty and identity. In particular, it asks that the Federal Republic finally recognize a separate GDR citizenship and agree to the exchange of ambassadors (instead of the present permanent representatives in Bonn and East Berlin). Both demands are unpalatable to the Federal Republic, however, since their acceptance would mean conceding that the GDR is politically as much a foreign country as any other. This would clearly contradict the Basic Law of the Federal Republic of 23 May 1949, which does not differentiate between West and East Germans, but asserts the will of the German people as a whole to preserve its national and state unity. Hence the West German difficulties in dealing permanently with a second state in what is seen as one German nation.

THE THIRD WORLD

The Third World has been an area of special interest in the GDR's foreign policy since the early 1960s. "It was in the Third World that East Germany sought to breach the diplomatic isolation imposed by the West German Hallstein Doctrine."[17] The efforts of the GDR to expand its diplomatic recognition concentrated on nonaligned Third World countries and international organizations, while the Federal Republic tried energetically to prevent such recognition. Over the years the establishment of trade missions in a few countries was all the GDR had achieved. The Hallstein Doctrine and the threat of Western economic sanctions were in effect until the late 1960s, when the Federal Republic's new *Ostpolitik* was adopted. With the GDR's accession to the United Nations in 1973, its basic difficulties in obtaining international recognition were largely overcome.

The ideological concept of socialist internationalism also obliged the GDR to do its best to export socialism into areas where decolonization appeared to have left power vacuums and a loss of political, cultural, and economic direction or orientation. Joining efforts with other Eastern European states and the Soviet Union, the GDR concentrated first on educational and cultural support in the developing countries. "Friendship Brigades" of teachers and skilled workers have taught basic mechanical and engineering skills in a fashion similar to Western development aid providers. What has been different, however, are the accompanying ideological education efforts in socialism, the preaching of anti-imperialistic solidarity to the recipients of socialist development aid, and continuous attempts to align those states with the socialist camp and against the West. More significant in the GDR's Third World policy, however, is its provision of military aid to African and Asian countries. That the GDR was also involved in rendering support to "national liberation movements and progressive forces" became apparent soon after the expulsion of Soviet military advisers from Egypt in 1972. In 1971 the SED Central Committee instructed Defense Minister Heinz Hoffmann "to take steps to raise military relations with Third World countries to the same level as economic, scientific-technical and cultural relations, which are already intensively cultivated."[18] According to various Western sources, by early 1977 not less than twenty-two African and Middle Eastern states had received military aid from the GDR, either in the form of arms, or of arms and training. Most were countries where for whatever reason the USSR could not get directly involved. While the international military activities of the GDR first concentrated on sub-Saharan Africa, today the estimated deployment list of some 2,300 East German military advisers includes North Africa and the Middle East as well.

In the author's view, there is insufficient evidence of a GDR military presence in Asia or Central America at present, but there certainly have been contacts in the past with Vietnam, North Korea, Laos, India, and Peru. The GDR is reluctant to acknowledge officially military activities outside the Eastern bloc. When asked in 1981 by a foreign journalist whether any East German troops were stationed outside East Germany, Honecker replied that he knew of none, except, perhaps, troops engaged temporarily in maneuvers.[19] Some Western sources suspect, however, that the GDR supplies far more military aid to the

Table 3. GDR Military Presence Abroad

Algeria	250
Angola	500
Ethiopia	550
Guinea	125
Iraq	160
Libya	400
Mozambique	100
South Yemen	75
Syria	210

Third World than any other Warsaw Pact country apart from the Soviet Union.[20]

THE SOVIET "ALLY"

The division of Germany is at the heart of the East-West divide in Europe, and both German states are in the front line. Just as it is doubtful whether the Western alliance would survive the withdrawal of the Federal Republic, it may be even more doubtful whether Soviet control of Eastern Europe could be maintained without the GDR as its bulwark. It is remarkable that of all the more developed Warsaw Pact states, the GDR is the one that has existed the longest without serious domestic trouble. Even the 1953 demonstrations were a small-scale affair compared to the events in Hungary in 1956, in Czechoslovakia in 1968, and in Poland in the 1980s. In light of these experiences, however, the Soviet Union cannot exclude the possibility that one day there may be trouble once again in the GDR.

So far, the GDR has proven to be a very loyal Soviet ally. It has been more successful than any other Eastern European member of the Warsaw Pact in maintaining its internal stability. Erich Honecker, chairman of the SED, appears to be a well-established leader of the party and state, with respected authority not only within his own Party apparatus, but also among Party leaders in the other Eastern European countries. In his long career he has successfully managed the two most important and closely interwoven policy fields for the GDR: relations with the Kremlin and the German-German connection. Continuity and calculability vis-à-vis Moscow seem to guide Honecker's policy. Continuity may almost be inevitable for a man of his experience and competence after being in office since 1971. Calculability, in the eyes of his Russian supervisors, is certainly vital in his position at a time when he is using some of the flexibility or greater freedom of action offered by a prolonged transition period in the Kremlin leadership. Surely a signal went to the Soviet leadership when Honecker appointed Colonel General Heinz Kessler to follow Hoffmann as defense minister when the latter died in late 1985. Having been the deputy defense minister and head of the main political administration since 1978, Kessler is a purely political general. His tenure in the highest military position in the GDR emphasizes political control of the East German armed forces and is thus reassuring to Moscow.

Honecker's careful maneuvering found approval with both the Soviet leadership and the Federal Republic even at critical times for the GDR's relations with the two states—the transition period in the Kremlin after Brezhnev's death, the transition from thirteen years of social-liberal to conservative rule in the Federal Republic, and the prelude and aftermath of the Soviet walkout in 1983 from the Geneva negotiations on intermediate-range nuclear forces (INF) and subsequent chill in the climate of East-West relations.

This is not the place to analyze and argue about the motivations that may have guided Soviet policy toward the GDR since the INF deployments in NATO began in late 1983. It was not the arrival of the first cruise missiles at Greenham Common in Britain, but rather the vote of the Federal Republic's Bundestag in favor of deployment and the subsequent arrival of the first Pershing II missiles on West German territory that led to the Soviet walkout in Geneva. An unprecedented Soviet propaganda campaign aimed at European, and specifically West German, public opinion, together with political pressure, had not succeeded in preventing the start of the INF deployments in Western Europe. Yet amazingly, and against the expectations of many political commentators, the USSR did not try seriously to use the GDR and German-German relations as leverage against the Federal Republic. It has been rather tempting at times for both the Soviet Union and the GDR to use inner-German relations for political influence on the Federal Re-

public. Because of West Germany's strong interest in maintaining relations with the GDR out of humanitarian concern for GDR citizens, even little issues may take on a political character. At the same time, there are a host of bilateral understandings and agreements that have been, and could again be, exploited by the GDR in attempts to exert influence on West German decisionmaking. The GDR has not made concessions in German-German relations for humanitarian reasons alone. It has also been lured by the prospect of the cash flow it receives in West German currency from such concessions.

In his intriguing analysis of the handling of the INF issue by the Soviet Union and the two Germanys, the British diplomat Roland Smith concludes that "the pressure on the Federal Republic from the Soviet Union contrasted strikingly with the behavior of the GDR. . . . Chairman Honecker did not announce any East German countermeasures against the Federal Republic."[21] Honecker said that "the European system of treaties, including the Basic Treaty on relations between the GDR and the FRG, has sustained serious damage as a result of this decision" of the FRG Bundestag to go ahead with the deployment of new, intermediate range U.S. missiles.[22] Smith views this statement as different from the Soviet line and points to some surprising East German actions in the immediate aftermath of the Geneva walkout, which obviously matched Honecker's words. There appeared to be an East German attitude quite different from the Soviet policy line in the sphere of international (rather than specifically intra-German) relations too: "The GDR made very clear her lack of enthusiasm for the stationing of additional Soviet missiles in East Germany as part of the Soviet response to Pershing deployment" (i.e., the forward deployment of shorter-range "Scaleboard" missiles on GDR territory). Joined to a considerable extent by Hungary, as well as Romania, the GDR seemed to follow a cautious, but distinct, line "aimed at trying to preserve as much as possible of the fabric of East-West relations."[23] Reinforcing this impression was a speech delivered in October 1986 by the SED's chief ideologist, Kurt Hager, which was subsequently printed in the Party organ *Neues Deutschland*, the GDR's version of *Pravda*, where its appearance effectively identified the speech as having met with Party approval. Hager said that in light of the extensive worldwide armaments buildup, the policy of securing peace would rank by all standards above the historic class struggle between capitalism and socialism. According to Hager, the GDR subscribed to a "policy of active dialogue" with the aim being a "worldwide coalition of rationalism, realism, and of good will. The recognition of the legitimate security interests of the respective sides requires an international policy based upon rationalism and responsibility, arrangement and restraint."[24] Remarkable as well is Hager's statement that in war no side would be able to secure victory because of the large stockpile of nuclear weapons and the perfection of conventional arms. This insight has apparently not yet reached Moscow, however, or at least not dawned upon those responsible for the formulation of Soviet military doctrine.

The rather unexpected relative freedom of action in the GDR's recent policy line may have been due to divided counsels in the Soviet leadership stemming from the series of deaths and consequent changes in party chairmen since Brezhnev. Under Gorbachev in particular, the Soviet Union has realized the fragility of its Eastern European empire and the eventual price it might have to pay to maintain rigid control in the post-Brezhnev era. Whether the USSR is following a more sophisticated policy of Warsaw Pact "unity in differentiation"[25] remains to be seen. Signs of liberalization in Eastern Europe are as yet sparse. Gorbachev may, however, feel more obliged than his predecessors to allow his satellite states some degree of autonomy. Apparently he keeps Western public opinion well in mind, and he may also recognize Soviet inability to prevent the Eastern European countries from having contacts with the West. Honecker's rather forthcoming policy during the critical phase in East-West relations after the Soviet walkout and before the subsequent Soviet return to the Geneva talks also bore dividends in terms of needed low-interest credits from the Federal Republic.[26] As is true with other Eastern Euro-

pean countries, the GDR pays economically for the political orientation imposed on it and has also become more vulnerable to the shocks experienced by the world economy, while remaining less well equipped than the Soviet Union to deal with the consequences of worldwide recession.[27]

ECONOMIC POLICY

In the 1970s the GDR had high debts to the West and large trade deficits with the USSR. The GDR achieved a remarkable turnaround, reducing its indebtedness and making considerable savings of energy and raw materials with very little loss of economic growth. It did this through a combination of organizational changes in industry, binding obligations and financial incentives for plants and *Kombinate* (large combinations of industrial units), and enhanced control mechanisms. The reduction by half of the GDR's hard currency debts in less than five years (to about $5 billion) by the mid 1980s was due to a switch in imports from the West to the East, increasing the trade deficit with the Soviet Union while conserving Western hard currency. Such purchases from the USSR and other socialist countries are made in exchange for crude oil, natural gas, and raw materials vital to industry.

Despite some positive aspects, the economic future of the GDR may be rather uncertain. To expand deliveries to the USSR in fulfillment of its obligations will call for more imports from the West, including expanded reliance on intra-German trade. To earn hard currency from the West to pay for its imports, the GDR relies largely on a narrow range of petroleum products and consumer goods. But oil prices have plunged, and in consumer goods there is increasingly stiff competition from the Far East. As is the case with the other Eastern European countries, much of the economic future of the GDR will depend on what happens in COMECON. Originally conceived as an instrument for both political and economic harmonization and integration, some forty years later COMECON has provided institutional justification for a fundamental shift in trade among member countries and, above all, a tightening of the close links between each individual Eastern

European country and the USSR. This evolution has gone hand in hand with a constant increase in the structural difficulties of the Eastern European economies, so that the most basic question raised today is that of the success of the market-oriented reforms, or mini-reforms, undertaken in these countries, or even the possibility of introducing real reforms in them at all.[28]

It appears in this respect that Gorbachev's Soviet Union is poised to be the pacemaker, an almost revolutionary change in the Soviet attitude toward liberalization of East European economic systems. In the past, the USSR used to have its foot on the brake whenever attempts were made in East Europe at even the slightest liberalization of the rigid structures of the socialist economies. Along with *glasnost* and *perestroika* (openness and greater allowance for some restructuring in Soviet society), Gorbachev's Soviet empire now appears to be the spearhead of reform of state and Party, politics and economics—preaching reform to reluctant non-believers in the central committees of the East European states.

Compounding the GDR's economic problems are high defense expenditures, which consume between 7 and 8 percent of GNP. The GDR has seen the most steady growth in its defense expenditures of all Warsaw Pact countries aside from the USSR. From 1970 to 1984 military costs rose at a steady average annual rate of 1.3 percent, and the GDR still has the fastest growth in military costs. In absolute terms the GDR's defense expenditures are surpassed only by Poland, but the Poles also have higher force levels to maintain.

Another threat to the GDR's economy arises from demographic developments. As in the Federal Republic, the population size has shown a declining trend due to fewer and fewer births. In addition, the population is drained by emigration, although with few exceptions the GDR only allows the elderly to migrate to the West. Indeed, allowing them to depart relieves the GDR from having to pay for their social security. The age structure of the GDR appears at first glance to be favorable economically: almost 65 percent of the population are of working age, 19 percent are children, and only 16 percent are retired. But 53 percent of the GDR's population are women, who already represent 49 percent of the total work force.[29] Because there is no reservoir of additional workers to tap, productivity increases have to be achieved by making better use of all resources, working more effectively, better motivating the work force, and modernizing and automating, or by combining all of these approaches. Motivation of the work force may be improved by allowing more privatization in an otherwise very socialist economy, a route such other communist countries as Hungary and China have embarked on, reportedly with success. The GDR leadership could initiate its own *perestroika*, opting for at least some structural changes. Industrial automation would require a lot of investment capital, however, preferably in Western currencies, an asset the GDR has always been short of. Nevertheless, the GDR is the "Golden West of the East." In terms of productivity per head, the GDR outranks all other Warsaw Pact countries. In 1985 each GDR inhabitant produced the equivalent of $10,440 worth of purchasing power. That amounted to about 25 percent more than in the USSR, with its $7,560 per head, and almost equaled the productivity of the United Kingdom.[30] According to GDR reports, national income has been increasing by more than four percent, meeting economic plan goals.[31]

If he is successful, Gorbachev's revolutionary reform ideas and the proclaimed "new thinking in foreign policy" may spell hitherto unknown degrees of flexibility and latitude for the Eastern European countries in their relations with the West. A sudden dynamism appears to be rocking world communism. Either by coincidence or through the interrelations of events, a new leadership in the Soviet Union has embarked on pragmatic changes and reforms of the society and economy with far-reaching consequences. At the same time tendencies toward political and economic change and cautious liberalization have also become noticeable in Eastern bloc countries like Poland, Hungary, and even in Czechoslovakia. In China, a generation after the end of the radical "cultural revolution" of Mao's Red Guard students, today's students demonstrate for democracy in the streets of Beijing. In Vietnam, a "little Gorbachev" and a group of reformers have replaced the aged triumvirate of the Revolution's "Old Men," and, as in China, the new leadership appears determined to establish better relations with the capitalist world and to restructure its ailing economy.[32]

In the GDR, however, few if any changes have been noticed. Whereas in other Eastern bloc countries communist parties somewhat defensively feel challenged by the sudden changes originating in the Soviet Union, the aging GDR leadership seems to have had little difficulty accommodating to the current winds of political diversification in the socialist quarter. The attempts at modernization and reform in the USSR, as well as in other staunchly socialist societies, have apparently been triggered by economic difficulties. By contrast, the GDR regime has fewer internal pressures for change. Indeed, East Germans may well muzzle their aspirations for political liberalization in return for the relative economic prosperity they enjoy. They are perhaps only too aware of their special position in the Eastern bloc, realizing that the Soviet Union's objective in its policy toward East Germany will not change at all, no matter how conciliatory Gorbachev may appear in dealing with the other satellite states. Careful maintenance of the status quo will be essential to the Kremlin, keeping its most important ally under the closest possible control, and not allowing any potential for destabilization there. What Smith has said of intra-German contacts is certainly applicable to the entire policy spectrum of the GDR: "The Soviet Union is evidently unwilling simply to leave the East German leadership to be the best judges of their own interests."[33]

The USSR may for whatever reason have tolerated Honecker's cautious, but distinct, distancing of the GDR from the Soviet line after the initial INF deployments in the Federal Republic. But Honecker is also clearly aware of his limits. During a friendly meeting with the FRG's Chancellor Helmut Kohl on the eve of Andropov's funeral, for example, Honecker accepted an invitation to visit the Federal Republic, but he subsequently had to bow to So-

viet pressures, postponing his visit until finally, in 1987, he obtained Soviet blessings. German-German relations are still to a great extent hostage to issues and forces beyond the two Germanys and thus far from becoming normalized.

What will happen after Honecker dies or retires? He and most of those in the leading positions in Party and state belong to the revolutionary vanguard that established itself during the foundation years of socialism in East Germany. Even if they were flexible enough to cope with the evolutionary changes in socialism, abroad and at home, their age will require a transition to a younger GDR leadership. Such a change may not necessarily spell the beginning of a "Gorbachev way" for the GDR. Honecker, it seems, has been deftly maneuvering his own men into line to take decisive posts in the Politburo. Thus, he could retire one day from his position as Party leader and perhaps stay on as head of state without losing much of his influence. Honecker's candidate for the top Party post is reportedly the Central Committee's current secretary for military and security policy, Egon Krenz. Interestingly, Honecker held this position for fourteen years before he became the secretary general of the SED.

Whether Honecker and his men or a "little Gorbachev" will be in charge in the GDR, sooner or later East German leaders may face a situation in which Gorbachev's complaint will be theirs too: "Between the people, who want these changes, who dream of these changes, and the leadership, there is an administrative layer, the apparatus of the ministries, the Party apparatus, which does not want alterations, and does not want to be deprived of certain rights connected with privileges."[34] The SED, like all ruling communist parties, will have to prove itself by providing efficient managers to adapt the economy and the Party apparatus to the conditions of the late twentieth and early twenty-first centuries. Even the most monolithic communist state cannot escape the challenges of political diversification, pluralism in socialism, differentiation in societies, and the economic necessity of reforms. Those in power will have to choose whether to try once again to suppress the "people's dream of alterations" in the system of Party and state or to opt for change and reform.

National Objectives, National Strategy, and Military Doctrine

To speak of national objectives and national defense strategy in the case of the GDR may be too narrow an approach. The GDR's Defense Law of 1978 refers basically to Article 51 of the UN Charter, but it closely links national defense with Marxism-Leninism, proletarian internationalism, the defense of socialism within the Warsaw Pact framework and the "Treaties of Friendship, Cooperation and Mutual Assistance" concluded with the USSR and other socialist countries.

Neither the Defense Law nor the Constitution refers to defense as being of the nation or the German people. Nor do they mention inalienable qualities or rights such as freedom or the rule of law. Instead, emphasis is on the defense of "socialist achievements" and of the "socialist state" in a socialist community based upon "the principles of socialist internationalism." Certainly the GDR leadership would run into major ideological problems if it claimed the German people or the German nation and its territory as subjects to be defended; even the Federal Republic has some difficulty explaining to its citizens what national defense means for a divided nation where the two parts oppose each other.

The founding fathers of the Federal Republic placed the highest value on freedom, individual liberty, and the rule of the law. The oath taken by soldiers in the West German Bundeswehr obliges them to defend the right and the freedom of the German people in a divided fatherland. For the GDR leadership, on the other hand, socialism is the embodiment of the utmost possible achievements for its people (and all people), even if forced upon them. Despite the GDR leadership's claims of socialism as a German national virtue, it cannot build a national identity upon it. In contrast to other communist-ruled countries, where the citizens are first Poles or Hungarians and then commu-

nists, doctrine in the GDR ranks socialism first and nationality behind it. In other socialist countries socialism may concern only the form of the state and not national identity, but in the GDR the two problems are linked inseparably because the state justifies its existence only by its socialist nature. In its exposed geopolitical situation, and aware of the fragility of socialism as the only pillar of the state, the GDR leadership sees hardly any other choice than to focus on the GDR's role as a wheel in the system of socialist internationalism that will eventually overcome the bourgeois imperialists and their capitalism and, true to Marx's ideals, national boundaries as well. The preamble of the Defense Law of 13 October 1978 states:

The GDR, in close alliance with the USSR and the other states of the socialist community, as well as in concurrence with all peace-loving forces of the world, pursues the goal of banning war once and forever from the lives of the peoples. . . . Safeguarding peace and the socialist achievements of the people, guaranteeing of the inviolability of state borders, including air space and territorial waters, and maintaining the territorial integrity and sovereignty of the GDR and all states of the socialist community require from the GDR the organization of the state's defense.[35]

But as a purely Soviet product, the East German Army does not formulate its own broad military doctrines.

The linkage of the GDR's defense with that of socialism becomes even more apparent from the GDR's Constitution of 7 October 1974. Significant in this sense are the sentences in Article 7: "In the interest of keeping the peace and safeguarding the socialist state, the army fosters close brotherhood-in-arms with the armies of the Soviet Union and other socialist states," and, "a basic precondition for the strength of the home defense of the GDR is the close brotherhood-in-arms of the army with the armies of the Soviet Union and other socialist states resting on the principles of socialist internationalism."[36] The latter sentence from the Constitution's Article 7 has become part of the Defense Law. The military oath clearly reflects the state's commitment of its military potential to the defense of socialism, and thus to the regime rather than country or people: "I swear: to be always ready, side by side with the Soviet

Army and the armies of our socialist allies, to protect socialism against all enemies and to risk my life for the achievement of victory." Despite all the ringing of peace bells and praises of détente and peaceful coexistence in Eastern bloc propaganda, it has to be borne in mind that all such phrases still reflect the basic premise underlying Marxist-Leninist socialism: the continuing class war with capitalism. The GDR's working class is also not relieved "of the need to respect and fulfill the objective law of providing a military guarantee of revolutionary progress through its own measures and endeavors."[37] The sense of a 1976 statement by Defense Minister Heinz Kessler becomes more obvious in conjunction with an observation in 1975 by the previous defense minister, Heinz Hoffmann:

What is the role . . . of military force in determining the victory or defeat of a revolution in the period of transition from capitalism to socialism? Does such a revolution come about without a shot being fired? Can it achieve bloodless victory? So far, in truth, history has witnessed no case in which a socialist revolution was led to victory without guns speaking their message of power, or at least being aimed and loaded.[38]

Hoffmann stressed the army's role as an instrument of ideology and its importance for the supreme ideological aim of spreading socialism throughout the world: "The duties of socialist armed forces nowadays extend far beyond the frontiers of the individual socialist country. . . . They demand that in case of war we should fight alongside our brothers-in-arms for socialism and communism, risking our own lives for victory."[39] Hence, quite in contrast to the Federal Republic's consistent policy of avoiding military involvement outside NATO, the GDR's leadership sends German soldiers all over the world, offering military aid wherever and whenever it seems warranted by the promise of furthering socialism.

A paradox the GDR must contend with is its difficulty with the idea of a German nation. The GDR's armed forces use the attribute "national" ("National" People's Army or NVA) without ever referring to a specific nation or people. Nor are the defense laws, the soldiers' oath, and military doctrine linked to the German nation or people. But to defend only "in-

ternational socialism" leaves a void that needs to be filled. This can be seen in the GDR's choice of almost the same uniforms and insignia for the NVA as those used by Hitler's Wehrmacht. Uniforms, goose-stepping, martial parades, and a host of medals, awards, and banners link the NVA with the German militarism of the past, a militarism the GDR still claims exists in the Federal Republic and which it allegedly fights relentlessly. Neglecting logic, the GDR denies any connection with German history other than those parts that fit into the Marxist view of events. In Marxist eyes, evil in German history is credited to the West German "capitalists' and militarists' tradition." The GDR sees itself in the tradition of the peasant uprisings of the sixteenth century, of the liberation wars against Napoleon, and in the resistance to Hitler (but only so far as it originated with the political left). The NVA considers itself the heir to the ideas and ideals of Prussian Army reformers and reveres Clausewitz.

In self-portrayal the GDR cherishes its role as the "bastion of peace in the struggle against West German imperialism and militarism."[40] Its forces not only defend socialism's western border in Europe, but also "carry high responsibility vis-à-vis the whole socialist camp," as expressed in the Constitution and the Defense Law. The feeling of being constantly beleaguered, foremost by the "aggression policy and the revanchism originating from the FRG," may well have put the leaders of the GDR on the defensive. The theme of aggression from the Federal Republic is constantly reiterated to maintain that the GDR is "a bulwark of peace insurmountable by imperialism." True to the supranational ideological foundation of its defensive function, the GDR's leaders can only define ideological threats: "Because ignoring of historical facts, a disposition for aggressive adventurism, and great power strife are typical of German imperialism, our Party and State leadership have oriented themselves from the very beginning toward the creation of an effective system of socialist home defense."[41]

The Party leadership wanted armed forces that were both combat-ready and politically reliable. From the time of their origins in the Volkspolizei ("People's" Police), the East German armed forces were thus entrusted only to men who were considered ideologically steadfast. This criterion had absolute priority over military qualifications. Willi Stoph, the first minister of national defense from 1956 to 1960, had been a corporal in the Wehrmacht and became an economic expert in the highest echelons of the SED apparatus before turning his skills to the development of the NVA. Heinz Hoffmann, his successor until 1985, had his only military experience during the Spanish Civil War in 1936, when he commanded a battalion of the International Brigades. Both Stoph and Hoffmann were also members of the Politburo of the Central Committee of the SED and, therefore, shareholders in the ultimate decision-making body of Party and State. Heinz Kessler, defense minister since 1986, is also thoroughly politically oriented and will sooner or later become a Politburo member.

In the first years of the rearmament of East Germany, the Party leadership hardly attempted to "convert" members of the new armed forces to the regime's ideology, let alone the top ranks. Passive acceptance of the communist system among the rank and file appeared to suffice. Passivity and even hostile behavior in Volkspolizei cadres toward the regime during the 1953 uprising (and even more so during the events in Hungary in 1956) quickly convinced the Party leadership of the need to shore up its authority within the armed forces. "The Hungarian uprising sent a shock wave through the East German Party leadership. They realized that if a Budapest-type uprising broke out, much of the East German military might stand on the side of the rebels."[42] Political organs as well as a Party organization were created throughout the armed forces. A political apparatus stretching from the SED Central Committee down to company level was established and a policy of intense politicization was pursued throughout the NVA. As a result of this politicization, "the regular officer could no longer sit back and ignore the political issue; he was now expected to share the blame for shortcomings. Evidence of political reliability became increasingly important for officers seeking promotions, and a part-time ideological course was introduced. The course, mandatory for all officers and NCOs, requires a final examination. The results are entered into an individual's record and are said to play an important role in determining his next assignment."[43] The Party extends its influence to all aspects of command in the NVA. As expressed by Defense Minister Hoffmann in 1977, the Party "helps" to reinforce and encourage individual leadership, to analyze in depth what has been achieved in education and training, to understand and implement troop leadership as socialist leadership of human beings, and to assess attentively the effects of commanders' decisions on the thinking and behavior of the soldiers.[44] The SED's omnipresence in the NVA is also manifested by the high number of party members among officers (99 percent, by far the highest percentage of any Warsaw Pact army).[45]

Today the primary vehicles for forming a positive attitude in the military toward the Party are two closely interlocking components: the main political administration of the NVA and the SED Party organization.[46] The major instrument for Party indoctrination and control is the main political administration in the Defense Ministry, headed by a deputy minister for defense. Within the ministry it has the authority of an SED Central Committee department, and as such is directly responsible to the SED's Central Committee. Charged with direction of all political work within the NVA, it controls the large network of "politorgans" from the Defense Ministry down to the company level, extending both horizontally and vertically throughout the NVA. *Politoffiziere* (political officers), "an offshoot of the tradition of Red Army commissars,"[47] are the chief agents of political work on all levels and serve as deputy commanders of units, schools, and military regions, with staffs consisting of numerous officers with full-time duties in political work.[48]

This elaborate organization contributes substantially to the political reliability of the armed forces and also ensures the primacy of policy vis-à-vis the military, a principle that socialist functionaries hold as high as democratic

politicians. The military leadership serves entirely at the pleasure of the Party. Indeed, it
would contradict the Party's doctrine if the
GDR's military were to strive for a special role
or status, or even form a system within the system. The GDR's Defense Laws of 1961 and
1978 state that the GDR's defense "has its firm
basis in the socialist state and social order, in
its growing political and economic strength,
and in the public's political awareness and
readiness to protect and defend socialist
achievements." The defense system rests, as
Defense Minister Hoffmann put it, "on the political power exercised by the working class under the leadership of its Marxist-Leninist Party
in alliance with the class of collective farmers,
with the intelligentsia, and with other actively
employed citizens."[49] The Federal Republic
follows its military reformers' ideal of "the citizen in uniform." The GDR's goal appears to be
"the worker and peasant in uniform." The approach may be different, but both East and
West German concepts share the aim of ensuring the subordination of the military to civil
control and authority.

In the early 1980s it appeared as if the role of
the military in the GDR were increasing, reflecting developments in the Soviet Union at
that time. Around the Ninth Party Congress in
1981, more military personnel entered the Politburo and Central Committee of the SED; at
least seven generals are now members or candidates, and Congress proceedings have featured
an elaborate military ceremony "symbolizing
growing militarism in East German society," as
one commentator has noted.[50] Introduction of
mandatory two-year paramilitary training in
the ninth and tenth grades of school lends further support to this observation. It is also noteworthy in this context that a considerable
number of NVA generals are found in the state
apparatus. Generals hold positions, *inter alia*,
as deputy ministers for external trade, civil engineering, and traffic. The minister of the Interior and his three deputies are generals, and
three more work in this bureaucracy. The minister of state security is of course a general, and
so are his three deputies. Recent estimates put
the number of the general officers of the NVA
at about 150, a corps that exceeds by far the

requirements of commanding a 175,000-man
army, but may indicate the high number of
plainclothes jobs for generals in the Party and
state.[51] It remains to be seen whether the GDR
will continue the course of apparently increasing militarization of the state. Such militarization has somewhat different implications in the
GDR than it would in the West. Far from
threatening the regime, high ranking military
officers are among the staunchest supporters
of Party rule and, as such, help tighten the
Party's grip on the state and its institutions.

The Defense Decision-Making Process

The NVA has to be seen not as an impartial
instrument of the state for its external defense
but rather as a tool of the SED. Defense Minister Kessler has written that "like the Soviet
Union's Communist Party, so also the Socialist
Unity Party of Germany follows the Leninist
principle that the undivided leadership of the
army by the party of the working class and its
Central Committee is an objective law governing the construction of socialist armed
forces."[52] The GDR's Constitution and the Defense Law contain no reference to the Party,
but it is clear in practice, as Kessler says, that
it is not the state organs provided for by law,
but rather the "leadership of the working class
and its Marxist-Leninist Party," (i.e., the key
institutions and figures of the SED), that make
the decisions in defense policy.

It was noted earlier how narrow the margin
of policical maneuverability is for the leaders
of the GDR. Dependence by the GDR's socialist state structure and its ruling party on big
brother in Moscow has a preponderant influence on all questions regarding defense of the
GDR. Aside from the clearly Soviet-dominated
(e.g., in organization and planning of forces
within the Eastern alliance) decision-making
machinery of the Warsaw Pact, bilateral relations between the USSR and the GDR have
even greater weight as a determinant that limits "national" decision making for defense in
the GDR itself. The huge contingent of Soviet
troops and their privileged status on East German territory constitute a constraint that re-

duces the capacity for maneuver and change in the GDR's defense posture.

Thomas M. Forster has pointed to the crucial difference of the troop stationing agreement between the USSR and the GDR in comparison to those with other Warsaw Pact countries. As noted, in all bilateral understandings with the GDR, the Soviet Union has made maximal use of its rights under the Potsdam Agreement. That mathematically every forty-four square miles of GDR territory is occupied by a Soviet division is certainly sufficient reason for GDR leaders to ensure that they are attuned to Moscow. But the USSR has always preferred to create a legal framework, even after having initially established a Soviet presence by the use of force. Soviet attempts to justify legally the invasion of Afghanistan are the most recent example of this pattern. The 1957 troop stationing treaty with the GDR in fact infringes almost completely on GDR sovereignty with respect to defense decisions. The agreement reflects in even greater detail than other treaties and declarations about the GDR's sovereignty the unilateral Soviet prerogative to interfere in the GDR's affairs. Article 18 of the stationing agreement reads: "In case of any threat to the security of the Soviet troops stationed on GDR territory, the Supreme Command of Soviet Forces in the GDR may take measures to eliminate it in consultation with the GDR government and with due regard to the situation arising and to measures taken by state authorities of the GDR."[53] Forster is certainly right in concluding that this provision entitles the Soviet Union, through the commander in chief of the Group of Soviet Forces in Germany, to declare a state of emergency throughout the GDR whenever it would suit Soviet purposes. There are, of course, other areas, however limited, for the GDR leadership to exercise its own decision-making machinery, even if only to gear the state to the ultimate requirements of defense policy for the communist empire. As in all totalitarian regimes, there is an amazing tendency to create laws and legal titles for an organizational jungle of decision making that would hardly work if the letter of these laws were followed.

As mentioned earlier, the most powerful instrument in a communist system is the politburo of the Party's Central Committee. Its general secretary is the focus of power. In the GDR, Erich Honecker has held this top post in the SED since 1971. Born in 1912, he belongs to the "old guard" that took part in the transformation of East Germany into a communist state. From 1957 until his accession to the top position in the Party he was responsible for military and security policy within the SED leadership. Not suprisingly, his expertise is brought to bear today in two other top organs directly concerned with the GDR's security policy, inasmuch as Honecker is also the chairman of the Council of State and of the National Defense Council.

The Council of State is a "parliamentary" body established by the GDR's Constitution that has authority, particularly in emergencies, to make decisions about the ultimate defense of the country. The National Defense Council is the corresponding government body that will, in practice, function as an emergency government. As chairman of this body, Honecker serves as the commander in chief of the NVA. But in case of crisis or war, this authority would pass to the Soviet commander in chief of the Warsaw Pact's joint forces and, in turn, to the Soviet defense minister and the Soviet Communist Party leadership. The approximately dozen members of the GDR's National Defense Council, who have never been named openly, are appointed by the Council of State. The National Defense Council, which includes mostly those members of the Politburo with competence in national security questions, can, according to the Defense Law, order total or partial mobilization if it deems this "necessary in the interests of national defense because of a situation of jeopardy." The prime minister; the ministers for national defense, interior, and state security; and the Central Committee's secretary for military and security policy, together with top functionaries responsible for the economy, are among those who sit on the National Defense Council. The chief of the main staff of the NVA, who is also one of the seven deputy defense ministers, at the same time serves as the secretary of the National Defense Council. To complete the list of players in the defense decision-making process, there are the Council of Ministers, which is the "parliamentary" cabinet, and the Ministry for National Defense. The heads of these organs, the prime minister and the defense minister, are both members of the Politburo and of the National Defense Council.

Despite the democratic parliamentary pretenses of the Constitution and the Defense Law, it becomes fairly obvious where power in the defense decision-making process really lies. Indeed, clout is in the hands of a few Party functionaries who run the SED Central Committee and its Politburo and who have accumulated posts in the various organizations more or less formally involved in decision-making. They maintain not only the primacy of politics vis-à-vis the military, but also ensure the Party's command and control over the state and its military. They are the key figures who issue the guidelines, instructions, and orders for the planning and organization of the GDR's national defense, and they check and supervise the execution of their decisions. At the same time, of course, the Party leadership understands that it must keep in step with the Kremlin. Ultimately, the important contours of East Berlin's defense policy are drawn in Moscow.

Recurring Issues and Defense Policy Outputs

FORCE POSTURE

In Moscow's view certainly the northern triangle of its domain, shaped by the GDR, Czechoslovakia, and Poland, remains geostrategically the most essential. "The GDR and Czechoslovakia form the westernmost spearhead of Soviet power, and Poland is the country providing access. In the strategic calculus of the Warsaw Pact (i.e., the Soviet Union) the GDR plays a leading role because of these geostrategic conditions."[54] The GDR provides the USSR with a base for defense as well as for offense. It provides the locus for the Group of Soviet Forces in Germany (GSFG), it serves as a logistic base as well as a supplier of arms, and

it is the springboard for political subversion of the Federal Republic of Germany.

In the event of war, the GDR would also serve as springboard for the Soviet tactical air armies in their attempt to breach NATO's air defense belt, and for the Soviet shock armies forcing their attack through the north German Plain, and out of the *Thüringer Balkon* (Thuringian Balcony) around Erfurt toward the Rhine-Main industrial complex around Frankfurt. From the GDR's Baltic coast facing Denmark, Warsaw Pact amphibious forces would simultaneously set out to seize the Baltic approaches and to establish bridgeheads in Schleswig-Holstein. This scenario roughly outlines the most likely initial development of a Warsaw Pact conventional aggression scheme as derived by NATO planners from the deployment of Soviet and Warsaw Pact forces in the Eastern European central front states. The GSFG (see table 4), with its twenty-one divisions and tactical air power of some 1,200 combat aircraft at its disposal, "represents the greatest concentration of power in a small space anywhere."[55]

The Soviet forces in East Germany also represent the largest concentration of Soviet troops outside the USSR. They are stationed in that part of the GDR that represents the frontline deployment center of the joint forces of the Warsaw Pact on land. This fact illustrates the strategic importance that the opposing military alliances of East and West attribute to the GDR. When the GDR signed the Warsaw Treaty on 14 May 1955, there were officially no East German Armed Forces. The People's Police, established in 1948 and subsequently equipped with tanks and artillery, had been

Table 4. The Group of Soviet Forces in Germany (GSFG). Headquarters: Zossen-Wünsdorf

Ground Forces
10 Armored Divisions
9 Mechanized Infantry Divisions
1 Artillery Division
1 Air Assault Brigade
1 SS-12/22 Missile Brigade
2 SCUD Missile Brigades
5 Artillery Brigades
5 Attack Helicopter Regiments

considered part of the *Nationale Bewaffnete Kräfte* (national armed forces) since 1952. In September 1955 the constitution of the GDR was amended to clear the way for the creation of the *Nationale Volksarmee* (National People's Army, or NVA), whose cadres came from the *Kasernierte Volkspolizei* (Garrisoned People's Police, or KVP). By the late 1960s, NATO intelligence considered the NVA as part of the first strategic echelon of the Warsaw Pact forces. The GDR's operational forces had reached a level of efficiency that would permit their immediate involvement and deployment in Soviet-led "front" operations of the Central Group of Troops (CGT) facing NATO's central region between Denmark and the Alps. Yet beyond reaching a certain level of combat efficiency, the NVA had also passed a litmus test of political reliability when it participated in the military intervention in Czechoslovakia in 1968 "to secure the socialist achievements" there.

Today Warsaw Pact planners regard the six divisions of the NVA land forces as a national army group that could either fight on its own or be assigned to higher Soviet formations. In either case, frontline troops would be available to march on the Federal Republic. In his standard work on the East German Army, Forster also includes a contingency for the NVA that seems, however, rather remote: "Should the political situation persuade the Soviet leaders that they could achieve their political ends by limited military action, it is possible that the NVA would be thrown in on its own. But its logistic dependence on the Soviet Army would enable the latter to keep it on a short leash at all times."[56]

The 39,000-man NVA air force is principally involved in air defense tasks, for which it is fully integrated into the Soviet air defense network. Its missile and antiaircraft artillery units, as well as the bulk of its operational aircraft, would be assigned to this mission. To a limited extent, it could give support to offensive operations on land.

The 15,000-man NVA navy cooperates closely with Polish naval forces and the Soviet Baltic Fleet in the peacetime mission of "guarding the Baltic Sea." In wartime, their joint mission would be to secure the coastal flank of the invading communist armies and give them support from the sea, including amphibious operations and logistic support.[57]

As with other Eastern European states, the GDR's military is only indirectly involved in fiscal negotiations over the defense budget. These decisions are generally made in the context of the Soviet-dominated Warsaw Pact structure. In the final analysis, defense expenditures are a topic for discussion between the political leadership of the Soviet Union and that of the GDR. Thus, the primary means of

---

Table 5. Operational Armed Forces of the German Democratic Republic

NVA			
Army			
2 armored divisions			
4 mechanized infantry divisions			
		Total:	120,000
		(conscripts 18 months service:	71,500)
Air Force			
2 air divisions (some 380 combat aircraft)			
		Total:	39,000
		(conscripts 18 months service:	15,000)
Navy			
Some 170 vessels			
		Total:	15,000
		(conscripts 36 months service:	8,000)
Frontier Troops			
		Total:	47,000
		Overall Total:	221,000
Reserves			
Army:	330,000		
Air Force:	30,000		
Navy:	40,000		
Total:	400,000		

influencing the size of the military budget is for NVA commanders to use their contacts with Soviet colleagues, who, in turn, may use the Soviet military's influence in the civil-military decision-making process in the Kremlin to make demands on the GDR's political leadership.[58]

WEAPONS ACQUISITION

The close ties between the military of the GDR and the Soviet Union are also reflected in NVA procurement of weapons and major equipment. Having no significant arms production capability of its own, the GDR equips its forces almost exclusively with Soviet weaponry. The GDR manufactures, as end-products, handguns, and other small-caliber automatic weapons. According to Forster, the GDR also produces components for heavy weapons, as well as light and medium military aircraft and naval vessels including mine-layers, anti-submarine warfare boats, and landing craft.[59] Moreover, the GDR has developed considerable capability in the production of military supplies, non-combat vehicles, and electronic, optical, and communications equipment for its own use and for export to other Warsaw Pact armies.

Forster gives plausible reasons why the GDR, compared to other bloc countries, produces only few armaments: "One is that, even before the war, the area [of the GDR] contained far less heavy industry than Western Germany, and the dismantling of factories and removal of plants to the Soviet Union immediately after the war made domestic armaments production unthinkable in the early period of GDR rearmament."[60] Another reason was that the Potsdam Agreement forbade German rearmament, in East and West. It remains somewhat unclear why, in contrast to the Federal Republic and other bloc countries like Czechoslovakia and Poland, no major arms industry was developed after the GDR began to rearm as part of its responsibility as a member of the Warsaw Pact. Also unclear is whether it was the GDR's own decision not to build up such an industry, or whether this decision was forced upon her by the Soviet Union.

Reliance on Soviet arms supplies by the GDR and other satellite states in effect forces the standardization of major equipment in the Warsaw Pact. The logistical advantages are obvious. Moreover, the advantages of being the sole source for acquisition of major weapons systems in the Warsaw Pact lie with the Soviet Union. She holds a monopoly, solely determining military specifications of equipment, its production rates, delivery schedules, and, of course, the price tags. Western observers are not quite sure whether long delays in the introduction of Soviet-made equipment into East European armies is due to reluctance on the part of the Soviets to trust their most modern arms to their allies, or whether it is due to caution by Warsaw Pact states concerned with meeting the resultant financial burdens of such acquisitions. The fact that occasionally non-member states can acquire the most modern Soviet arms long before Warsaw Pact states themselves suggests that the delays are due more to financial reasons than to Soviet distrust of their allies.[61] Close ties between the military elites of the Soviet Union and the Warsaw Pact countries are a very important influence on military budgets. Still, the argument of distrust cannot be entirely disregarded.

The Warsaw Pact has never adopted a scheme of sharing nuclear operations as has occurred within NATO. NATO's pattern of cooperation between nuclear powers and non-nuclear allies (i.e., the U.S. providing nuclear warheads for allied delivery systems in case of war under an intricate scheme of specific consultations for the eventual deployment of these weapons) has never really been seriously considered in the Warsaw Pact. Soviet nuclear weapons, forward based in the GDR and other Warsaw Pact countries, are intended exclusively for use by Soviet crews, even though other Pact states also have "dual-capable" (both conventional-and nuclear-capable) ballistic missiles and aircraft.

PARAMILITARY FORCES AND CIVIL-MILITARY RELATIONS

The overall 174,000 personnel in the GDR's regular forces are not, however, the total standing combat potential of the GDR. Although claimed to be paramilitary units, the 47,000-

man Frontier Troops must be calculated among the operational forces of the GDR. The Frontier Troops fall under the Ministry of Defense and are organized, trained, and equipped like light motorized infantry units. Their commander is also a deputy defense minister. The tasks of the Frontier Troops exceed by far those of a frontier police in the Western sense, and in the final analysis they clearly have the military function of defending the GDR's western border.[62] The reason why the GDR maintains that the Frontier Troops are separate from the NVA and not part of its regular forces may be seen in the Vienna talks about Mutual and Balanced Force Reductions in Central Europe, which have thus far considered only "regular forces."

The Frontier Troops are massed along the inner-German border, with eighteen regiments in three command sections. One regiment each is deployed at the Polish and Czechoslovak borders. Their task is to man and maintain the inward-pointing fortifications destined to prevent *Republikfluchtige* (fugitives from the republic) from crossing the border to the West. That Frontier Troops are also needed at the borders with "socialist brother states" (Poland and Czechoslovakia) flies in the face of GDR propaganda, which glorifies the border fortifications and the Frontier Troops as the defense of the "Workers' and Peasants' Paradise" against Western "border provocations." The reality is that without the Frontier Troops in the east and south of the GDR, fugitives from that "paradise" might well seek their way to the West via Poland or Czechoslovakia.

The ruthless Frontier Troops, with their orders to prevent border crossings to the West, if necessary by shooting the fugitives, remain the single most disturbing issue in the relations between the two Germanys. Year after year numerous incidents at the inner-German border indicate the unbroken desire of many GDR citizens to leave behind the "socialist achievements" of the GDR even at the risk of their lives, and many have already been killed by the bullets of Frontier Troops. Time and again soldiers of these units try their luck in attempts at escape when they are alone or can avoid surveillance by their comrades. Border patrols

and guard tower crews always come in pairs, one watching the other and with orders to shoot his comrade should he try to escape. Another attempt of the regime to prevent the Frontier Troops from taking advantage of their proximity to the West is to recruit only Party members or conscripts who have earned a voucher from the SED's youth organization, the *Freie Deutsche Jugend* (FDJ). Defense Minister Hoffmann often called the Frontier Troops the "Guard of the National People's Army." If the Warsaw Pact one day marches westward, certainly the Frontier Troops would form two elite divisions at the forefront.

Although a conscript army, the NVA also has a huge potential to augment its strength with reservists. The London-based International Institute for Strategic Studies lists about 400,000 personnel as reserves, 330,000 of them army. Reservists have up to three months' call-up per year to a total of twenty-four months' reserve commitment for officers, and twenty-one months for other ranks. The NVA reserve is grouped into two categories, one for mobilization purposes and the other for rear services.[63]

A look at the structure of military command in the NVA reveals the surprisingly high proportion of senior ranks and officers in particular, which is characteristic of all Warsaw Pact forces.[64] Officers represent about 15 percent of the total strength of the NVA. That percentage exceeds the combined officer and noncommissioned officer strength of the West German Bundeswehr, which has a force nearly three times as large as the NVA (see table 6).

Forster is certainly right in stating that the quality of command and military reliability are enhanced by the number of well-trained commanders.[65] But too many chiefs and too few Indians can also cause problems in terms of military efficiency, even in highly specialized

Table 6. Comparative Rank Ratio

	Bundeswehr	NVA
Officers	26,000 (6%)	26,700 (15%)
NCOs	35,000 (7)	35,200 (20)
Other	430,000 (87)	112,100 (65)
Total	495,000 (100)	174,000 (100)

services like the air force and navy. In Western eyes a "chiefs-to-Indians" ratio of one to two in a conscript army appears rather strange (let alone the cost of such a force), and is probably justified more by the need to ensure political reliability than by military efficiency. Further description in detail of the NVA is unnecessary here; it suffices to say that it constitues the first strategic echelon troops in the Warsaw Pact. The focus here rather is on features of a state that has become more and more militarized thanks to socialist military education and the military considerations that dominate all layers of the GDR's society.

Various paramilitary organizations play a prominent role in that scheme. They include the People's Police alert units and Transport Police, falling under the Ministry of the Interior; the Workers' Militia; and to a limited extent the Society for Sport and Technology (GST). There is also a guard regiment of about 7,000 men under the Ministry for State Security (MSS) tasked with protection of government buildings and personnel. Except for the GST, all paramilitary organizations are equipped with armored personnel carriers, light artillery-like mortars, and antitank and antiaircraft guns (see table 7).[66]

The Workers' Militia may have the potential to grow from 3,000 regulars in peacetime to 500,000 men in wartime. Originally designed as Party troops for a civil war, they have meanwhile increasingly taken on the character of a territorial army, of which about half, 250,000 men, could be called upon at any time.[67] As their full name, "Combat Groups of the Working Class," implies, they correspond to the old Marxist concept of a "working class under arms." They are the "Party's army." Command and control extends from the SED Politburo's National Security Commission and the security department of the Central Committee to the SED regional committees and their district committees. The Party's First Secretaries at district and regional levels are also chairmen of the "operational directorates," to which the commanders and commissioners of all military and police units in the district belong. These First Secretaries are themselves in command of the combat groups.[68] The Ministry of the Interior and its subordinate People's Police authorities have some competence in matters of training, equipment, and deployment. In Forster's judgment, the combat groups, "compared with the militias of other Warsaw Pact states . . . are of considerable military value."[69] Membership in the combat groups is meant for men between twenty-five and sixty. It is supposed to be voluntary, but there are legal and other provisions for maintaining recruitment levels and reminding individuals of their duties.[70]

Civil defense, as "the concern of every citizen," is regarded in the GDR as an inseparable part of national defense. Under the minister of defense, the director of civil defense, an active duty general officer is tasked with organizing "the protection of the public, the economy, vital facilities and cultural values against the effects of both military aggression (especially weapons of mass destruction) and natural catastrophes. Civil Defense also has the duty to prepare and deploy manpower for rescue, salvage, and urgent repair work and to execute measures to help maintain state, economic, and social activities."[71] The GDR Council of Ministers prescribes all basic civil defense measures at the national level. The comprehensive concept of civil defense in the GDR from top to bottom ensures that all ministers, directors of economic bodies, industrial combines, enterprises and institutions, and the chairmen of cooperatives are in charge of civil defense within their respective spheres of responsibility. The chairmen of local councils have responsibility for local civil defense and are entitled to give instructions and coordinate within their territorial domains. Compulsory service can be introduced for civil defense tasks if needed, calling on all men between sixteen and sixty-five, and women up to sixty.[72] Civil defense personnel also fulfill some of the func-

Table 7. East German Paramilitary Formations

1 guard regiment (Ministry for State Security)	7,000
People's Police alert units (Ministry of Interior)	12,000
Workers' Militia	500,000
GST (Society for Sport and Technology)	450,000

tions of territorial defense, supporting Warsaw Pact armed forces by ensuring their operational freedom of movement. Forster mentions that there are civil defense staffs under military command in both urban and rural districts, manned by NVA, People's Police, and Party officials with a strength of about 3,000. Other sources put the number of full-time military members of the civil defense organization at 15,000.[73] The civilian members, two-thirds of them female, have combat suits and are equipped with infantry weapons. Courses in civil defense have to be taken in school in grades nine and ten. As in the Soviet Union, civil defense protection measures are directed primarily at providing shelter for the *nomenklatura*, the Party and government bodies.

The police forces under the Ministry of the Interior are much more militarized than in any Western country. I look here in particular at the People's Police alert units, a force of about 12,000 men. There are also 8,500 Transport Police personnel, who, strangely enough in Western eyes, are armed with machine guns and antitank launchers.[74] All twenty-one People's Police alert units (a unit is about equivalent to battalion strength) are uniformly trained and equipped, and some training is done at NVA schools. In their own view the members of the alert units are "fellow-soldiers in green uniform," whose training is designed to create political and military qualifications for optimum combat readiness. "Service in the alert units is military service."[75] Despite this official self-understanding of the People's Police alert units as a military arm to ensure domestic security as part of the "effective protection of the workers'-and-peasants' state," Forster observes, the government evidently has a poor opinion of the political reliability of its workers. The deployment pattern of the alert units is normally one unit to each of the GDR's regions; but the key industrial regions of Leipzig, Halle, and Magdeburg (with their large worker populations) have two units each, and the Police Presidium in East Berlin has three units. After the experience of the 17 June 1953 uprising the GDR leadership apparently sees the threat of disturbances as coming primarily from these areas.[76]

The paramilitary training organization GST is officially defined as a "socialist mass organization of the GDR, whose whole activity is aimed at developing the competency and defense-readiness of the general public, and particularly the young."[77] The GST has to be considered an integral part of the GDR's national defenses. The GST leadership reports of its task: "By helping to educate defense-conscious socialist patriots and proletarian internationalists, and by popularizing the concept of defense-readiness, defense-efficiency, and defense-potential among the workers and all sections of the public, the GST has turned itself into *the* socialist defense organization of the GDR."[78] The GST is managed by a central board consisting of active or reserve NVA officers, the chairman being a high-ranking general officer. Training and financial planning are in the hands of the Ministry for National Defense. Paramilitary sports like target practice with small firearms, parachuting, and even flying, are pursued by the almost half a million members. The GST not only prepares individuals for mandatory service in the NVA, but also represents a reservoir of volunteers. The four-year course is divided into basic training for all members as well as training for NVA careers; the courses are structured for young people of both sexes betwen fourteen and twenty-five years old. Membership is voluntary, and many of the about 70 percent of active members have joined because of the interesting, cost-free activities offered, which certainly attract young people in particular. On the other hand, the activities of the GST are closely coordinated with the schools, with vocational training organizations, and with the SED youth organization (FDJ) in such a way that membership in the GST and qualifications therein reflect the "normal" educational process prerequisite for social and professional advancement. The GST and working-class combat groups are among the never-ending calls of the totalitarian communist system on individuals of all age groups so that virtually no citizen can avoid the Party's influence and control.

Under the Marxist concept of a "working class under arms" everyone has to be a work-

Figure 1. Command Structure of the National Peoples' Army (NVA)

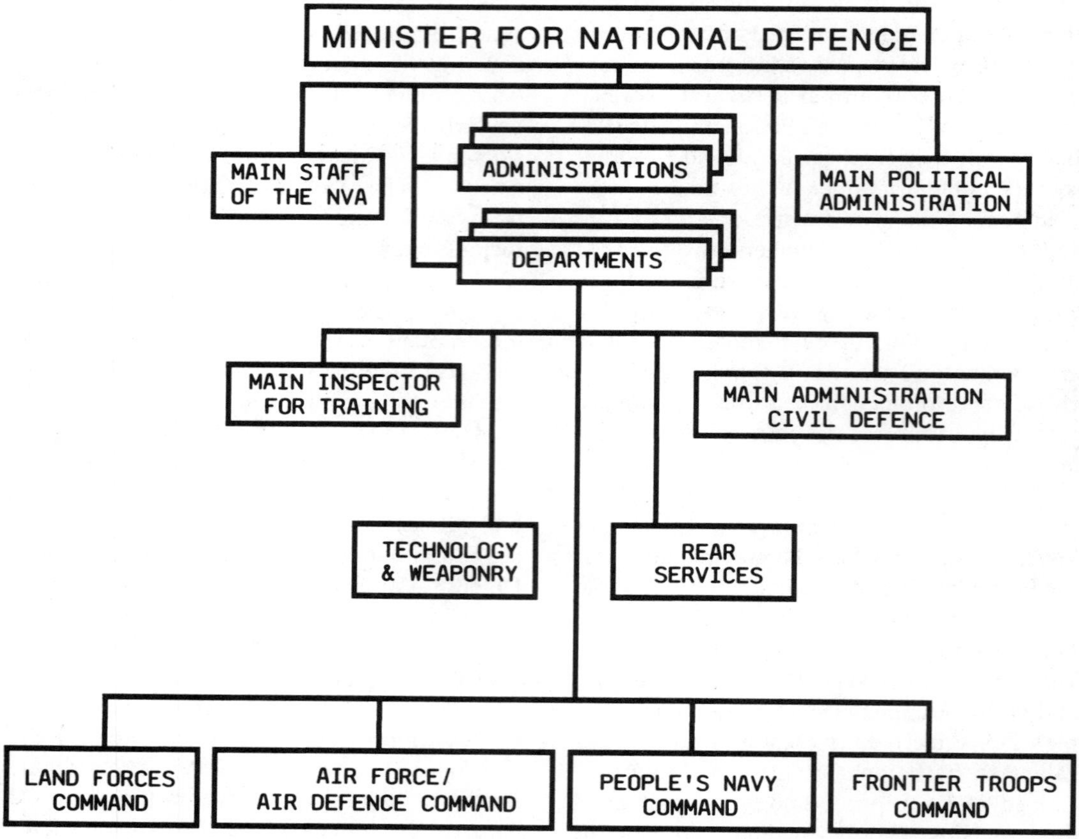

ing-class fighter following the instructions of the Party "to defend the GDR and her socialist achievements at all times, weapon in hand, and to lay down (his) life for her," as the oath of the working-class combat groups claims.[79] In the words of Defense Minister Hoffmann, the system of national defense of the GDR "is a complex of multifarious agencies and institutions, conditioning and complementing one another. They include the NVA as the keystone of national defense, the territorial and civil defense forces, the instruments for the economic underpinning of defense, the social organizations for socialist military education, the command organs and much else."[80]

The alteration of the GDR's constitution in 1955 also laid the foundations for the introduction of conscription, which is only logical for a "working class under arms." But the draft was only established as late as January 1962, about

four months after the erection of the Berlin Wall (when the danger of losing many of the future draftees by escape to the West had been reduced considerably).

Despite intense political indoctrination, particularly of the younger generation, starting almost at kindergarten age, service in the NVA is not an agreeable obligation to most young men in the GDR. Although thoroughly indoctrinated about its debt of honor to serve socialist ideals and defend socialism loyally, the youth of the GDR appear to be less than willing to endure the hardships of military service. Although GDR citizens acquiesce when faced with conscription, they tend to have little motivation or enthusiasm, not unlike most conscripts elsewhere. The trend toward a more independent-thinking youth is also apparent under socialist rule.

A small but growing factor in East German

society, and among the youth in particular, is religion. The Protestant churches are attracting more young people to the Christian message of peace and brotherhood. What may count for the young is that the churches are places where ideas can be exchanged without the strictures of official doctrine. "Swords into Plowshares," a veritable peace and disarmament movement, has emerged. Advocating disarmament not only of the West but also of the East will, however, lead almost inevitably to clashes with the Party. Party doctrine holds that threats to peace emanate exclusively from the West, and that the Warsaw Pact armies exist only to guarantee peace and, if necessary, to fight the "just" war to defend "socialist achievements."[81]

ARMS CONTROL

It may be presumptuous to speak of an arms control policy of the GDR as if the GDR had one in its own right. Probably more appropriate would be the notion that Moscow assigns a certain role in its overall arms control policy to the GDR as well as to the other satellites.

The GDR has played its part, as have the other bloc states, in closest concert with the Soviet Union in the 35-member Conference on Security and Cooperation in Europe (CSCE), follow-on conferences to the CSCE, the Mutual and Balanced Force Reductions (MBFR) talks in Vienna where it has regularly taken its turn as the speaker for the Warsaw Pact countries, the UN Committee on Disarmament (CD) in Geneva, and the Stockholm Conference on Security, Confidence Building Measures and Disarmament in Europe (CDE). The GDR sees its place among the "countries of the socialist community" as pursuing a "consistent policy of peace and disarmament" while "rebuffing imperialist aggression, which meets the interests of all peoples and all of progressive humanity."[82] In the words of former Foreign Minister Fischer: "The socialist states, the Soviet Union above all, strongly favor definite steps to restrain the arms race and promote disarmament."[83]

The commitment to supporting Soviet initiatives on arms control and other issues is underscored by Fischer's comment that "the most important factor of success of our people both on a national scale and in the international sphere is our fraternal alliance with the Soviet Union."[84] More recently the GDR has tried to create the impression that it can take positions in the field of arms control and disarmament on its own initiative. In fact, GDR advocacy of de-nuclearized zones in Europe is really an old idea the Soviets have supported for years. The GDR proposes creation of a de-nuclearized corridor in Central Europe composed essentially of the two German states, and likewise a zone free of chemical weapons on both sides of the inner-German border. Such concepts also find favor within the FRG's Social Democratic Party (SPD). Many observers in the Federal Republic as well as among NATO allies consider this to be an unholy alliance between the major opposition party in the Federal Republic, the SPD, and the GDR's state party, the SED. Although the GDR leadership may have a genuine interest in arms control and disarmament, these concepts bear too much of a Soviet stamp to be taken seriously as independent initiatives of the GDR. As a practical matter, both German states depend heavily on their respective alliances and on the leading powers in each, making it rather difficult for any German state to make independent initiatives in arms control and disarmament. On the other hand, the GDR did not display the usual (and expected) enthusiasm for Soviet weaponry when the USSR responded to American deployment of the Pershing II in the FRG by deploying nuclear missiles of its own in the GDR. Honecker's somewhat reserved attitude toward these deployments on GDR soil differed markedly from expectations, but it would be wrong to infer from this that the GDR could take an independent position in arms control and other security issues. Here again both German states are in a very similar position. Their moves are closely watched, maybe even more closely by their allies than by their opponents.

Notes

1. See Catherine Kelleher's chapter on the Federal Republic of Germany in this volume. The chapters about the two Germanys complement each other in many ways and should be read together.

2. COMECON's members are Bulgaria, Cuba, Czechoslovakia, the GDR, Hungary, Mongolia, Poland, Romania, the USSR, and Vietnam.

3. For readers with a particular interest in the role of the Western powers in forming postwar Germany, Alfred Grosser's *L'Allemagne de notre temps* is recommended. A German translation has been published under the title *Geschichte Deutschlands seit 1945* (Munich: Deutscher Taschenbuch Verlag, 1981). More academic, yet very concise, is the treatment of this subject by Norbert Wiggeshaus, "Von Potsdam zum Pleven-Plan: Deutschland in der internationalen Konfrontation, 1945–1950," in *Anfaenge westdeutscher Sicherheitspolitik, 1945–1956*, ed. Militärgeschichtliches Forschungsamt (Munich and Vienna: Oldenbourg Verlag, 1982).

4. Wiggeshaus, "Von Potsdam zum Pleven Plan," p. 16.

5. Ibid., p. 11, quoted from Milovan Djilas, *Conversations with Stalin*.

6. Grosser, *Geschichte Deutschlands*, pp. 105–6. Also Helmut Baerwald and Rudolf Maerker, *Der SED-Staat* (Cologne: Verlag Wissenschaft and Politik, 1963), p. 1.

7. Jonathan Dean, "How to Lose Germany," *Foreign Policy*, Summer 1984, p. 61.

8. In the Federal Republic, in a "revolutionary situation," with protracted unemployment approaching 10 percent, the communist movement steadily loses supporters, while conglomerations of unrealistic romantics such as the Greens have gained and maintained an influential parliamentary role.

9. Formulation in the GDR's constitution of 1968; the present constitution of 1974 reads differently: "The GDR is a socialist state of workers and peasants."

10. *Süddeutsche Zeitung*, 25 July 1986.

11. Grosser, *Geschichte Deutschlands*, p. 412.

12. Jens Hacker, "Die Vertragsorganisation des Warschauer Paktes und die Rolle der DDR," in *Die NVA der DDR im Rahmen des Warschauer Paktes* (Munich: Bernhard and Graefe, 1980), pp. 10–11.

13. Ibid., p. 11.

14. Arthur M. Hanhardt, "The German Democratic Republic," *Current History*, p. 369.

15. Grosser, *Geschichte Deutschlands*, p. 413.

16. Helmut Bechheim, *NVA der DDR im Ostpaktsystem* (Bonn: Selbstverlag/Dissertation, 1980), p. 128.

17. Hanhardt, "German Democratic Republic," pp. 370–371.

18. Quoted in Thomas M. Forster, *The East German Army* (London: George Allen & Unwin, 1980), p. 99.

19. Hanhardt, "German Democratic Republic," p. 388.

20. Forster, *East German Army*, p. 98.

21. Roland Smith, *Soviet Policy towards West Germany*, Adelphi Papers, no. 203 (London: International Institute for Strategic Studies, 1985), p. 6.

22. Ibid., p. 26.

23. Ibid., p. 28.

24. *Süddeutsche Zeitung*, 7 November 1986.

25. *The Times* (London), 5 July 1986.

26. In 1983 one of the most vociferous critics of East German violations of human rights and of West German concessions to the GDR, Franz-Josef Strauss, prime minister of Bavaria, served as the mediator for securing a one billion DM credit for the GDR. That it was Strauss who channeled this loan gave rise to considerable speculation in the Federal Republic and was the cause of some irritation among the staunchest members of his party.

27. Ferry de Kerkhove, "The Economics of Eastern Europe and Their Foreign Economic Relations Examined at NATO Colloquium," *NATO Review*, June 1986, Brussels, p. 17.

28. Ibid.

29. *Süddeutsche Zeitung*, 28 July 1986.

30. *Süddeutsche Zeitung*, 13–14 December 1986.

31. *Die Welt*, 7 October 1986.

32. *Der Spiegel*, January 1987, p. 91.

33. Smith, *Soviet Policy*, p. 20.

34. *The Independent*, 18 December 1986.

35. Hacker, "Vertragsorganisation des Warschauer Paktes," p. 49. In my interpretation of the original German texts quoted by Hacker I have tried to translate almost literally, at the expense of style. But the formulation of laws hardly follows good diction in any country.

36. Ibid., pp. 48–49.

37. Forster, *East German Army*, p. 29.

38. Ibid.

39. Ibid., p. 30.

40. Heinz Kessler, "Soldaten der Sozialistischen Revolution," *Neues Deutschland*, 1 March 1969.

41. Ibid.

42. Dale R. Herspring, "Civil-Military Relations in Poland and East Germany: The External Factor," *Studies in Comparative Communism* 11, no. 3 (Autumn 1978): 230.

43. Ibid.

44. Forster, *East German Army*, p. 160.

45. Herspring, "Civil-Military Relations," p. 231. Herspring notes that in 1975 Party membership among officers was 90 percent in Bulgaria, 80 percent in Hungary, 65 percent in Poland, 90 percent in Romania, and only 75 percent in the Soviet Union.

46. Ibid., p. 105.

47. Forster, *East German Army*, p. 162.

48. For an exhaustive description of the political organization within the NVA, see ibid., pp. 159–172.

49. Ibid., p. 105.

50. Hanhardt, "German Democratic Republic," p. 124.

51. *Soldat und Technik* (Frankfurt: Umschau Verlag, 1986), pp. 644–45.

52. Forster, *East German Army*, p. 29.

53. Ibid., p. 82.

54. Bechheim, *NVA der DDR*, p. 124.

55. Forster, *East German Army*, p. 82.

56. Ibid., p. 84.

57. Ibid.

58. Herspring, "Civil-Military Relations," p. 233.

59. Forster, op. cit., p. 181.

60. Ibid.

61. For example, the more sophisticated Soviet tactical aircraft have not yet been observed in Warsaw Pact air forces, although in service with the Soviets since the early 1970s. By contrast, the Soviets have already offered India and Syria the late technology type fighter aircraft MiG-29.

62. For a detailed description of the tasks and organization of the Frontier Troops, see Forster, *East German Army*, pp. 122–44.

63. International Institute for Strategic Studies, *The Military Balance, 1985–1986* (London, IISS, 1987), p. 33. See also Forster, *East German Army*, pp. 65–66.

64. Forster, *East German Army*, p. 121.

65. Ibid.

66. IISS, *Military Balance, 1985–1986*, pp. 33–34.

67. Forster, *East German Army*, p. 148.

68. Ibid., p. 150.

69. Ibid.

70. Ibid., p. 152.

71. Defense Law of 13 October 1978, quoted in ibid., p. 146.

72. Ibid., pp. 146–147.

73. Wilfrid Dissmann, "Bewaffnete Organe in der DDR," *Informationen zur Deutschlandpolitik der CSU* 16 (September 80): 3.

74. IISS, *Military Balance, 1985–1986*, p. 33. Forster, however, gives the strength of the People's Police alert units as 18,000. He gives no precise figure for the Transport Police.

75. Forster, *East German Army*, p. 143.

76. Ibid.

77. *Militärlexikon* (East Berlin: *Militärverlag der DDR* 1973), p. 201. Quoted in Forster, *East German Army*, p. 152.

78. Quoted in Forster, *East German Army*, pp. 152–53.

79. Ibid., p. 152.

80. Ibid., p. 141.

81. Hanhardt, "German Democratic Republic," p. 368.

82. Oscar Fischer, "The Foreign Policy of the GDR," *International Affairs*, March 1981, p. 72.

83. Ibid., p. 68.

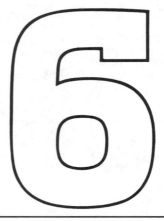

FRANCE

Alan Ned Sabrosky

History is a merciless judge of those who forget the lessons of geopolitical power and entrust their interests exclusively to international goodwill or the skill of their diplomacy.[1] France, for one, does not. As David Yost has noted, "[national] rank and independence have been enduring preoccupations of French statecraft,"[2] and under the Fifth Republic France's "defense policy has been seen [by Paris] as one of, if not *the*, most important instrument to achieve the objectives of French foreign policy."[3] This remains as true under François Mitterrand as it was for his more conservative predecessors.

The central role of military power in world politics, however, has not meant the subordination of broader national interests to the dictates of defense. Military power is properly seen in France as a means to an end, not an end in itself. As a consequence, changes in French ambitions, political priorities, and na-

tional goals have wrought changes in French strategy and have contributed to the subsequent restructuring of the forces required to execute that strategy. Discontinuities, inconsistencies, and ambiguities have certainly not been avoided in their entirety; perfection is at best an elusive ideal in any human endeavor. But there has been in France a remarkably consistent appreciation of the fact that the defense policy of any nation ultimately must be judged in terms of its ability to link military power to political purpose. This means that a country's strategy, doctrine, and force posture must not only be logically consistent with one another in a purely military sense; they must also be directed toward, and consonant with, the attainment of clearly identifiable and operationally defensible goals. The fact that armed forces have both political and military utility, with the former being more important than the latter over time, is apprehended with particular clarity by key French decision makers. What those decision makers have wrought, and why, will be discussed in this chapter.

International Environment

"Any policy," Jean-Pierre Marichy observes, "is conditioned by ideas and ideologies—and no more so than in defense matters."[4] Another French commentator puts it somewhat more metaphysically, asserting that "the defense of a nation is not only the elaboration of a strategy and the acquisition of the means necessary [to execute it], it is also and above all the existence of a 'spirit of defense' that rests on the will to defend essential values."[5] It is all too easy to exaggerate the significance of such intangible considerations, of course. Yet in the case of France at least, it is all too evident that they play a major role in that country's assessment of the international environment and its options therein.

Both French policies and French ambitions have their roots in (a) a complementary set of foreign policy assumptions that define the parameters within which French defense policy is formulated, and (b) France's own historical experience in the post-World War II era. In the former instance, there are actually two separate subsets of foreign policy assumptions of varying significance. First, there are the externally oriented assumptions that bipolarity is inherently unstable, that power is diffusing throughout the world (albeit in a more complicated fashion than was once believed to be the case), and that, as Dominique Moisi says: "Of all the European countries, France is today the only one to insist on the status of a 'mini-superpower' and to conduct itself in that fashion."[6] Second, internally oriented assumptions emphasize the significance of France's *mission civilisatrice* (or, more modestly, its unique role in the world), the overriding importance of preserving national sovereignty even when collaborating with other nations, and the fundamental role of military power—and especially an independent nuclear capability—as the principal guarantor of status and security in the modern world. These assumptions have to-gether produced a near-dogmatic belief in "France's responsibilities as a major power with an independent, lucid and constructive contribution to make . . . in the world community."[7]

Further, France's approach to defense and foreign affairs is strongly influenced by its own recent historical experience with allies and adversaries alike. It also reflects a conscious (and not entirely successful) effort to overcome psychologically the legacy of defeat in the opening days of World War II, as well as of the successive defeats in Indochina and Algeria, reinforced by the debacle at Suez in 1956. From the French perspective, in fact, history has taught the twofold lesson that allies can be as unreliable as adversaries are implacable, and that France must have an independent capability to safeguard its interests and security if it wants to avoid being little more than a pawn on the diplomatic chessboard.[8] Indeed, more than one observer would endorse the view that France combines "an almost pathological compulsion to maintain the ability to act independently" with "unrivalled skills in concluding alliances which left them [the French] relatively free from permanent constraints."[9]

Geopolitical reality, however, has the occasionally distressing quality of requiring a reconsideration (if not a reformation) of even the most closely held and cherished elements of national mythology. Power and preferences must be coordinated well if policy is to be effective and security is to be enhanced. The status of a global middle power (albeit with limitations) that desires to be first among equals (after the two superpowers) defines the limits of France's capabilities and prospects. How those capabilities are put to use and their implications for French defense policy are shaped by the role France has assumed within the Western community and its interpretation of the contemporary international security situation.

Since 1945 three possible roles have been open to France within the Western community, each of which has different implications for French strategy, doctrine, and force posture. First, France can attempt to pursue its cherished independent role in all essential respects in either a global or a European context. Second, it can assume an Atlanticist posture, co-operating with other Western European nations and the United States as part of a general Western security community. Third, it can adopt a European stance, associating itself with one or more Western European nations, without the participation (formal or informal) of the United States.[10]

The clear-cut adoption of any one of these roles would certainly clarify France's defense options. Unfortunately, Paris has found itself unable to make any definitive choices that would provide it with both status and security at an acceptable cost. The notion of Western Europe as a center of power with France at its head is appealing, but France seems unable to find the central organizing principle necessary to make it a reality. The Atlanticist course of action has such a principle, embodied in the North Atlantic Treaty Organization, but U.S. membership ensures France's subordination—de facto if not de jure—in any such arrangement. France's unwillingness to countenance that subordination, coupled with the presumed unreliability of the United States in the aftermath of Dien Bien Phu (1954) and Suez (1956), has resulted in both an aversion to overt dependence on the United States and the adoption of an independent course of action in world politics in general.[11]

The first step in that direction of any significance in foreign and defense policy was taken by General Charles de Gaulle. As president of France, de Gaulle exercised a significant influence on the course of French policy. His so-called grand design of independence, prestige, and continental leadership eventually gained widespread acceptance in France. In many respects, it served to give the French people both a degree of unity and a renewed measure of self-esteem, which had been badly shaken in the preceding years. Nor was his policy without substance. De Gaulle's proposal for a "triumvirate" of the principal Western powers and his later withdrawal from the integrated military structure of NATO, for example, had a common point of departure: the aim of "elevating France to the publicly recognized position of a great world power."[12] When a prominent Gaullist wrote in 1978 that "a great foreign

policy cannot be constructed without the help of a conceptual key that permits one to decipher the nuances and the subtleties of international realities,"[13] he was both defining the purpose of Gaullism and alluding to its success.

What is even more noteworthy is not that a Gaullist foreign and defense policy could have been proposed in the aftermath of successive military defeats and amidst political discontent within France itself; it is that the basic principles of Gaullist foreign and defense policy retain considerable appeal even today, notwithstanding the fact that France has had a socialist president for nearly seven years. Today, as under de Gaulle and his non-Gaullist successors, France essentially asserts its claim to the same degree of diplomatic freedom of maneuver accepted by the United States and the Soviet Union for themselves. The notion that France is both an autonomous power and a military power has been underscored in various forums and reiterated by numerous members of the government, both before and after the 1986 elections produced a conservative majority in the National Assembly and brought Jacques Chirac to the premiership. Further, this worldview did not change after the 1988 elections even though the conservatives lost their majority. A great power, as France defines that term, can only have activist and interventionist foreign and defense policies.[14]

This consistency in French preferences for an independent role rather than a more circumscribed European or Atlanticist one has regrettably not corresponded to reality. By the time Mitterrand assumed office in 1981, the increasing precariousness of "independence" had become all too apparent to some French analysts, one of whom concluded acerbically that "independence no longer exists in a world where interdependence and dependence are the rule."[15] This interpretation becomes even more pointed in the military sphere, where few among even the most ardent advocates of French independence in world politics seriously believe that "France alone" can safeguard itself and its vital interests in all circumstances.

The result of these factors is a French approach to world politics that has grudgingly acknowledged both France's ultimate dependence on the United States for its own security and the importance of cooperating with other Western European countries in order to enhance the security of Europe as a whole. Yet, at the same time, France has clung to an assertive independence whenever actual or perceived threats to French interests or slights to French ambitions have occurred, as evidenced by French hostility to the punitive strikes against Libya in 1986.[16] This French desire to have the game both ways—that is, to act independently when possible and to rely on others when necessary—has continued to promote the "equivocation" noted by David Yost,[17] reflecting an implicit attempt to rationalize an otherwise seemingly inconsistent set of French foreign and defense policies and actions.

Rationalization can go only so far, of course, and a series of developments coming to a head in the early 1980s provided the Mitterrand government with a powerful incentive to reconsider the paths taken by France in the preceding years. In retrospect, it appeared that the decade of the 1970s had been the harbinger of an era of change, presaging the later establishment of new balances of power and new relations of forces.[18] Some constants remained: China continued to grow into the great power it will be in the next century; Japan remained an industrial giant with relatively little political-military influence and less ability to underwrite its own security; Europe was still an economic consortium lacking a unified defense and foreign policy apparatus and dependent upon the United States for its overall protection; and the rest of the world—the presence of certain rambunctious states such as Israel and Iran notwithstanding—was largely handicapped by instability, vulnerability, and economic need.[19]

These relative constants, however, paled in French eyes when contrasted with the changes that were of concern to France. This is because the changes involved the three countries of greatest importance to France—the Soviet Union, the United States, and the Federal Republic of Germany—and in each instance, the direction of the change aroused varying degrees of uneasiness or apprehension within the French government and national security community at large. The changes being initiated in the Soviet Union in the name of *perestroika*, for example, appeared promising, if they succeeded in altering the fundamental character of that state. But the Soviet attempt at reform was dividing the West in the face of a continuing accumulation of Soviet military power and ongoing Soviet initiatives to divide Western Europe from the United States. In the case of the latter country, American policy during the 1980s seemed to be long on rhetoric and short on sophisticated execution, reawakening lingering reservations in France about the constancy of U.S. policy and the robustness of American security guarantees—including at least the possibility of a partial withdrawal of U.S. forces from Europe. Compounding these concerns were perceptions of American tactical clumsiness juxtaposed against improved Soviet tactical skills acquired in Afghanistan.[20]

Of greater significance for France than developments in the superpowers have been actual or feared changes taking place in the Federal Republic of Germany. France's attitude toward West Germany in the post-1945 period reflects a curious admixture of political confidence and military apprehension. Indeed, the unusually close linkage that conventionally exists between France's foreign and defense policies has made the contradiction between them in the matter of Franco-German relations both more astonishing and more detrimental to the formulation and implementation of a realistic French defense policy.[21] France has simultaneously seen the Federal Republic as a "stable security shield for France"[22] and acknowledged only slightly veiled warnings (such as that made by former President Giscard in 1974) about the need to guard against "other [nonnuclear] powers that might threaten French soil."[23]

As the 1980s unfolded, latent fears about a possible resurgence of militarism in Germany (united or not) were replaced by a more immediate and far more serious problem: the specter of German neutralism, prompted by pacifist movements in the Federal Republic and more pragmatic considerations among Germans who favored some form of reunification and were increasingly disinclined to look forward to being the battlefield in some future war on the Continent. There was no sense of immediacy about this problem; even an adroit initiative by General Secretary Gorbachev to exchange some form of German unity for a complete withdrawal of all foreign troops from both Germanies would take years to implement. But France takes a longer view of security affairs than is the case with some Western countries, and the prospect of a "power vacuum" along its eastern border, with American influence in the decline and Soviet influence on the Continent in the ascendancy, hardly constitutes a reassuring augury of the future. Something had to be done.

It is an interesting testimony on French national security policy that something was done. That something definite was contemplated was not immediately obvious to most Western observers, as the initial policy pronouncements of Mitterrand's government reflected an unusual degree of ambiguity due to the coexistence within the Socialist Party's leadership of the Fourth Republic's "Europeanism" and the 5th Republic's "Independent" approach.[24] Yet there is no ambiguity in Mitterrand's belief that socialist France has a mission in the world, coupled with "a clear perception of the dangers presented by a changing world"[25] and the need for new initiatives to come to terms with this state of affairs.

The least controversial of these initiatives has entailed a continuation and an extension of France's participation in various peace-keeping activities abroad. The most obvious of these activities evolved as a function of France's membership in the United Nations, and specifically France's participation in the UN peace-keeping force in Lebanon. A critical element in the French determination to assign contingents to that force was the French belief that "an active peace-keeping role" is important if France is to remain a viable permanent member of the United Nations Security Council.[26] Far more interesting in terms of cooperative French involvement in international security affairs is France's participation in the Multinational Force (MNF) in Beirut (1983–84), re-

gardless of the ill-fated outcome of that venture. Although undertaken outside of the context of both the United Nations and NATO, the presence of French forces alongside of contingents from the United States, Italy, and the United Kingdom reflected both a more flexible attitude on the part of France toward such enterprises, and a return to the sort of great power interventionism characteristic of France's "golden age" as a world power. Qualifying such an assessment, of course, is the obvious fact that France has an historical interest in Lebanon—an interest that manifested itself in France's successful resolve to be the last of the intervening powers in the Multinational Force to withdraw.[27] Last, but certainly not least, was France's decision to take the de facto lead within the Western European Union (WEU) in its "naval peace-keeping mission" in the Persian Gulf in 1987, building on its existing substantial naval presence in the Indian Ocean. Whether the French involvement in this operation would be sustainable in the event significant casualties were incurred remains to be seen.[28]

More far-reaching than a more elaborate role in international peace-keeping activities has been France's growing military involvement with the integrated military structure of NATO. French relations with NATO have been rather complex for more than two decades. In 1966, of course, France announced that it would withdraw the following year from NATO's integrated military organization, but not from the Atlantic Alliance as a whole—a distinction that I suspect would have seemed somewhat forced to NATO's founders. Nevertheless, that decision ostensibly reflected France's agreement with the broad political principles enshrined in NATO, but not with what Paris saw to be the infringement of national sovereignty implicit in the alliance's common defense organization. This intriguing reading of what the very concept of collective defense entails had a less abstract foundation as well—France's general unwillingness to subordinate French policy to that of the United States, which France saw to be dominating the NATO alliance. As Marianna P. Sullivan has observed, "the subordination of French defense policy to that of the United States when the latter's responsibilities expanded globally as those of France contracted was not easily tolerated by a nation that regarded itself historically as a great power."[29] These French concerns proved to be remarkably enduring attributes of France's foreign and defense policy process.[30]

The net effect of these considerations placed France in an ambivalent position with regard to NATO. The French, and especially the Gaullists and their political counterparts, found dependence on U.S. protection to be particularly galling. Yet there remained an equally strong suspicion in most French political circles that "NATO had not outlived its utility."[31] Thus, France abstained from NATO's Defense Planning Committee, the Nuclear Defense Affairs Committee and its Nuclear Planning Group, and the Eurogroup, although French "observers" occasionally appeared. At the same time, however, France collaborated with selected NATO countries (other than the United States) on an ad hoc basis for the development and production of various weapons systems, and became a member of the Independent European Program Group (which included ten members of the Eurogroup) for similar cooperative efforts on a larger scale. France also maintained observer and liaison staffs at NATO headquarters in Brussels and elsewhere, accepted officers from all NATO countries, including the United States, at its Senior Service Colleges, and permitted units of the French armed forces to participate with increasing frequency in maneuvers with military units of other NATO members. Even the French Army's II Corps, which remained outside of the integrated NATO military structure, was "stationed in Germany under a status agreement reached between the French and German governments. Cooperation with NATO forces and commands . . . [had] been agreed between the commanders concerned."[32]

Mitterrand's government soon found it prudent to expand the network of cooperative undertakings between France and the NATO military allies further. To be sure, the essential French precepts of autonomy and independence would not be sacrificed in the name of cooperation. At the outset, French participation in the affairs of the integrated NATO military command "would be restricted to conventional forces" in the event deterrence failed, and would require "French forces . . . [to] remain grouped under national command and in directions or zones covering national territory" if they did become engaged in hostilities in concert with NATO forces.[33] In 1981 Premier Pierre Mauroy reaffirmed that position, as did the minister for external affairs, Claude Cheysson, asserting both France's unwillingness to rejoin NATO's integrated military structure and its essential loyalty to its Atlantic Alliance allies.[34] Cheysson's views seemed particularly promising; as Alex Gliksman concluded: "Cheysson's message is that of pragmatism and continuity: the fulfillment of old commitments and loyalty to the NATO alliance. . . . *With regard to NATO and Europe, Cheysson's position is an advance upon that of Giscard*"[35] [italics added].

Precisely how "advanced" the position of socialist France had become soon became apparent. French participation in NATO planning and exercises grew, usually with an eye to "avoiding most of the more politically visible and more military ones."[36] After 1986 even the more visible military activities became more common.[37] The creation of the Force d'Action Rapide (Rapid Action Force) in 1983 [discussed in detail later in this chapter] was intended in part to give France greater capability to intervene quickly in a European conflict. The redeployment northwards of the headquarters of the III Corps (based in France) from St. Germain to Lille in 1983–84 was widely interpreted to signify a greater French willingness to support NORTHAG (NATO's Northern Army Group) in the event of hostilities. More flexible operational plans reportedly were under consideration by French headquarters to facilitate France's participation alongside its NATO allies. French participation in an integrated airborne early warning network was formalized, and the French Air Force's tactical aviation was for all practical purposes operationally integrated into NATO's 4th ATAF (Alllied Tactical Air Force) if hostilities occurred, at least for the support of French forces. And the removal of the TNW (Tactical Nuclear Weapon) control from the French First Army served to emphasize a reappraisal of the automaticity of the engagement of those systems if war occurred.[38] These and other French actions were seen to be indicative of the reassociation (not reintegration) of France with the members of the integrated military structure of the alliance.

Equally interesting in political terms was the growth of "Europeanist" sentiment during Mitterrand's tenure, paralleling the increase in the "Atlanticist" predisposition signified by France's closer military cooperation with NATO—both of which served to attenuate in fact, if not in name, France's adherence to the "independent" role preferred by de Gaulle and his immediate successors. What constituted a "Europeanist" orientation for France was philosophically different from that of many other countries, given the prevailing French preference for "unilateral action and bilateral agreements . . . [rather than] multilateralism as a way of conducting foreign policy."[39] This qualification notwithstanding, it seems clear that, in Dominique Moisi's words, "France's new orientations vis-à-vis Europe are clearly pro-European";[40] that they may have emerged as a function of necessity rather than of choice makes no practical difference. Mitterrand himself emphasized this new orientation as early as 1983, arguing that it was important for Europeans to "regain confidence in themselves" by moving "toward a system of collective defense."[41] Mitterrand clearly did not intend that system to replace NATO, but there was a potential collateral benefit that did not go unnoticed abroad. As Robert Grant put it: "It is possible that only progress in European defense cooperation can provide the necessary enthusiasm for any French government to overcome the obstacles in the way of continuing to modify gradually the doctrinal principles that still give French defense policy its strongly nationalistic character."[42]

The "Europeanist" sentiment that had emerged (or, to be precise, re-emerged, given the position of the Fourth Republic after 1945) during the years when France had a Socialist Party government waxed after the conservatives regained control of the National Assembly and Jacques Chirac assumed the post of premier following the 1986 legislative election. Chirac himself spoke of the need to create a "European awareness about the demands of their defense," and laid out five basic principles for a "European Defense Charter"—one of which entailed the continued need for a "strategic coupling with the United States."[43] Other, perhaps more predictable, principles included the primacy of nuclear dissuasion in the maintenance of peace in Europe, the global character of the threat confronting the West, the importance of maintaining a defensive capability appropriate to meet that threat, and the utility of "realistic and verifiable [arms control] agreements."[44] Paralleling this conceptual formulation came a series of discussions and evaluations of the prospects for bilateral undertakings—the preferred French style, as noted earlier—with selected European countries, particularly the United Kingdom and the Federal Republic of Germany.[45]

The shift in the French orientation toward the Federal Republic during the 1980s constituted something approaching a "diplomatic revolution" in modern European history. The two countries each had an interest in moving closer to the other in political-military terms, despite the aforementioned French ambivalence about the future of Germany and German interest in some form of reunification, whose realization would inevitably constrain or circumscribe France's ability to realize its own ambitions. There is much truth to the argument that "since the late 1940s, the debate on the appropriate constitution for a Franco-German alliance has been inseparable from the dual aspirations of both France and the Federal Republic to pursue policies of reconciliation, while preserving national claims on independence or reunification."[46] There was also little doubt that the character of relations between France and the Federal Republic of Germany would influence whatever approach France took toward Europe and, to a lesser extent, Germany's attitude toward the United States.[47] Complicating everything was the growing sense in French policy circles that the German people were becoming "fatigued," and thus unreliable in the protracted engagement with the Soviet Union.[48] There were also those who remained unconvinced that close ties to West Germany were wise, as evidenced by Jacques Amalric's declaration that "the Federal Republic is at the same time our ally and our glacis, our friend and a former defeated enemy that must be controlled, in agreement with the USSR if necessary."[49]

These and other reservations were certainly not without some merit, and they were reinforced by somewhat more pragmatic arguments to the effect that any Franco-German military interplay properly ought eventually to include the United Kingdom as an equal participant.[50] But the perceived need to act on improved Franco-German relations "before German neutralism expanded any further"[51] overrode the principal reservations about that enterprise. On 1 March 1986 President François Mitterrand and Chancellor Helmut Kohl reached an accord on a number of security-related matters, including provision for joint maneuvers and training programs and plans for the employment of the French "Rapid Action Force" in Germany if the latter country should be attacked. The accord was seen to represent "France's reconciliation with West Germany and the close political alliance between the two countries, which has become a central feature of both French and West German foreign policy."[52] Three months later the French and West German defense ministers initiated preparations for a meeting later in 1986 to resolve outstanding issues on the coproduction of various weapons systems in conjunction with a programmatic review of existing French armaments policy.[53] And in March 1987 Europe was treated to the intriguing and by no means commonplace sight of France and the Federal Republic making a joint proposal to the Stockholm Conference on European Disarmament.[54]

The culmination of the current round of Franco-German military discussions and undertakings occurred in January 1988, following joint Franco-German maneuvers in September 1987 (Operation "Bold Sparrow," in which approximately 20,000 men and 500 AFVs—armored fighting vehicles—from the French Rapid Action Force functioned as the backup for the German II Corps) and the December 1987 Soviet-American agreement eliminating intermediate-range and short-range missiles in Europe. Key elements of the new understanding between Paris and Bonn included the creation of an integrated Franco-German brigade whose command would rotate between the two countries (the first commander is to be a French general) and the establishment of a Franco-German "Defense and Security Council" at the ministerial level to discuss defense-related issues of concern to the two countries. Anticipating these developments and signaling an end to French ambivalence about Germany (at least for the present), Chirac observed in October 1987 that "France would never consider its neighbors' territory a glacis. . . . The engagement of France would be immediate and without reserve. There cannot be a battle of France and a battle of Germany."[55] For the time being, at least, World War II was finally over for France.

Last, but certainly not least insofar as French concerns with independence and status in the world at large continue to persist, there is France's complex set of relations with various African countries, principally those former colonies that are now part of the French Union. France's relations with NATO and, increasingly, with Europe in general and West Germany in particular, undoubtedly attract more attention outside of France, and are certainly more important in terms of French security. But in the Gaullist lexicon, as well as in that of its non-Gaullist supporters, security and status are inextricably linked, and France's role in Africa is often seen as a more significant bellwether of French status than what France does in Europe.[56]

In Africa, France is what may be termed a postcolonial power that has assumed a neocolonial role, although in a somewhat restrained sense. The French commitment to a number of African countries is based on a complicated blend of historical involvement, contemporary security, and economic interests, as well as the genuine (if self-imposed) French need to act like a truly independent power of consequence in the world. It is quite appropriate to state that "the repertoire of French policies and activities related to Africa is impressive in its variety."[57] Even more impressive than the variety of French actions in Africa is the scope of that involvement. France currently has defense agreements with eight African countries, including Cameroon, the Ivory Coast, the Comores Islands, Djibouti, Gabon, the Central African Republic, Senegal, and Togo. It also has technical military assistance agreements with approximately two dozen countries on the African continent, some 1,300 military advisers in approximately the same number of countries, and stations more than 11,000 men from all services in eight African countries on either a permanent or a rotating basis.[58] Moreover, as the French interventions in Zaire and the Central African Republic demonstrate, France has clearly designated part of its own Rapid Action Force for service in that part of the world should contingencies requiring French involvement occur there.[59] Joint exercises between French forces and those of various African countries are taking place with increasing frequency.

In sum, it is still appropriate to conclude that the French, as Chief of Staff General Guy Mery stated, have "many friends in Africa who trust us and who expect a great deal from us,"[60] and that France fully intends to meet their expectations. As John Chipman once wrote: "Because it is to the mutual benefit of all parties, the Franco-African security system which now exists is likely to remain in place, even if occasionally modified, at least until the end of the century."[61] The fact that France can intervene as it does in Africa and structure the security system there that it has in place, its association with South Africa notwithstanding, is a measure of its success in this regard and a testimony to the adroitness of French diplomacy. These factors help define the parameters within which France's national military objectives, strategy, and doctrine are debated and formulated.

National Objectives, National Strategy, and Military Doctrine

The relations that normally exist among goals, strategy and doctrine are complex and subject to misinterpretation. In the case of France, however, they have been remarkably consistent over time, once one understands the assumptions on which French foreign policy is based and the implications of these assumptions for French defense policy. To a considerable extent, in fact, France's foreign policy has defined the objectives and specified the principles governing the articulation of an appropriate strategy. The latter, in its turn, has dictated both the appropriate means (or force structure) and the preferred employment doctrine for them.[62] The process certainly has not been without some flaws in conceptualization or execution. Yet France has done better than many other countries in this respect, perhaps because, as Edward Kolodziej has suggested, "France's military doctrine went beyond narrow considerations of battlefield use of military force. . . . [It was intended] to strengthen France's internal and external position in competing with other states [and] . . . responded to changes in France's foreign and domestic environment."[63]

In accordance with the assumptions underlying French foreign policy and France's role in world affairs, the French defense establishment has traditionally been tasked with the execution of four general operational missions. These are to (a) secure France at home and French interests abroad, (b) participate in the defense of Europe in the event of another continental war (for example, in case of a Soviet/Warsaw Pact attack) in conjunction with other members of the Atlantic Alliance in accordance with France's own rules of engagement, (c) permit France to act as an independent power outside of Europe as a means of underwriting French prestige, and (d) join in international peace-keeping missions, under the auspices either of the United Nations or of an appropriate regional intergovernmental organization (for example, the Western European Union), or as part of a multinational effort with comparable powers (for example, the Multinational Force in Beruit).[64] The precise priority given to a particular mission at a given point in time was somewhat flexible, of course, as was the selection of the appropriate instrument to carry out that mission, as demonstrated by the evolution of French defense policy under the Fifth Republic.[65] In general, however, these missions reflected the input and interplay of considerations of security and status, of pragmatism and prestige.

FRENCH STRATEGY: A NEVER-ENDING TALE

France's national strategy and military doctrine are both guided by, and modified in accordance with, changes in the priority given to these missions. In the broadest sense, French defense policy as a whole during the Fifth Republic has tended to conform to the general principles laid down by General de Gaulle, occasional deviations therefrom notwithstanding. Those precepts entailed "freedom of decision with respect to the employment of its [France's] forces, cooperation with allies and recourse to nuclear weapons to defend its vital interests."[66] The fact that France's freedom of action was sharply restricted by the realities of France's position in the world, that cooperation with allies occurred erratically because Paris insisted that it take place only on France's own terms, and that recourse to nuclear weapons would mean the certain destruction of France's tangible interests and assets in defense of its intangible pretensions—all have found relatively little support in French strategic circles until recently. Indeed, many Frenchmen believed that it was only by adhering to these precepts that France had been able to achieve (or, perhaps, to retain) a measure of respect in the international community and a degree of influence over what transpired therein.[67]

To say this does not mean that French defense planners, policy makers, and analysts have adhered rigidly to a single strategic doctrine. On the contrary, the French literature on this subject is remarkably open, candid, and sophisticated—more so, in certain respects, than that in some other countries.[68] More to the point, however, is the fact that in the years since de Gaulle first came to power, French national strategy—regardless of its precise formulation—has been linked explicitly to the French armed forces in a more general context. That is, in France, it is correct to say that "tactical nuclear and conventional forces have been developed as adjuncts to the strategic nuclear forces,"[69] and that these [secondary forces] are "closely linked in the *manoeuvre nationale de dissuasion* (national deterrent maneuver) which could bring about the employment of the strategic nuclear forces."[70] And for France, the latter constitute what Charles Hernu, Mitterrand's minister of defense in 1982, called "the final argument."[71]

Even the employment of a "final argument" is necessarily informed by the existence of a proper strategic concept. The first such concept to be put forth was based on the idea of *sanctuarisation totale* (total sanctuary). The initial operationalization of the *sanctuarisation totale* as a basis for French strategic planning saw the appearance of a "fortress France" mentality. That which was seen to be worth preserving was France itself, and secondarily French interests overseas, regardless of the fate that might befall those countries with which France was associated. Thus, only direct threats to the territorial integrity and sovereignty of France would have to be deterred, or fought if deterrence failed. In its initial incarnation, it included the notion of *la défense tous-azimuts* (all-around defense). This was a declaratory policy that denied the existence of any specific threat to France and insisted instead that France must be prepared to ward off an attack from any direction. This fascinating notion rapidly gave way, however, to a more explicit recognition of the threat posed by the Soviet Union, a recognition that crystallized in the aftermath of the Soviet invasion of Czechoslovakia in 1968.[72]

This change in threat perception, on the other hand, did not alter either the priorities assigned to the French armed forces or the basic doctrine for their employment. In both respects, pride of place was given to the Force Nucleaire Strategique (FNS) (strategic nuclear force), first called the *force de frappe* (strike force) and later renamed the *force de dissuasion* to emphasize its deterrent function. Whether it was seen as a "strike force" or a "deterrent force," it was clear that to French planners "strategic nuclear forces constitute[d] the foundation of the French assertion that France's security problems . . . [had] been separated from those of her allies through the creation of a French 'sanctuary'."[73] The primary objective of the FNS was therefore to deter attacks against France itself. If that deterrence failed, the French—in accordance with the accepted precepts of their own somewhat limited version of the doctrine of massive retaliation—would attack the aggressor's population and industrial centers with all of the military resources at their disposal. Second to the FNS were the Forces d'Intervention (intervention forces), renamed the Force de Manoeuvre (field force) in 1964. These included both a five-division regular army, with supporting air and naval general purpose forces, and a light airborne/air transportable force. The former was deployed in France and in the southwestern part of the Federal Republic of Germany, whereas the latter—although largely based in France—was organized for use in Africa and in other parts to be safeguarded. Third and last were the forces of the Défense Opérationnelle du Territoire (DOT), including approximately one hundred regiments of varying strength and reliability, plus supporting units, intended for internal security as well as a source of replacements for the regular forces during wartime.[74]

The origins of this ambitious and explicitly self-centered strategy are as obvious as its flaws. To a considerable extent, the concept of a *sanctuarisation totale*—and especially the extraordinary notion of *la défense tous-azimuts*—reflected de Gaulle's personal irritation with the United States and Great Britain for their refusal to countenance France's proposal for a Western "triumvirate" more than it did a rational appraisal of France's capabilities and options.[75] In a certain sense, de Gaulle essentially decided to take France out of a political-military game in which the other players would

not acknowledge it as an equal whose opinions were worth considering, and defined French strategy accordingly. Militarily, the likelihood that France could be a "sanctuary alone" in the event of an East-West war is actually as improbable an idea as that of "France alone" in a world of competing superpowers—a notion that even the Gaullists dismissed in all but the most limited sense of the term.[76] The fact that a France that truly saw any other power as a potential threat was also a France no other nation could truly trust could have but one meaning. This was that the strategic consequences of the attempt to implement a strategy of *sanctuarisation totale* were a prescription not for independence and security but for isolation and an unprecedented degree of insecurity and vulnerability should war occur—or even threaten—between the opposing superpowers and their allies.[77]

On the other hand, the concepts of *sanctuarisation totale* and *la défense tous-azimuts* (to focus on the more extreme doctrine) did have certain advantages for a power such as France, even if they do not seem to be compelling in an absolute sense. Politically, they did emphasize French independence in a polarized world and a degree of nonalignment in the essentially East-West power game.[78] The fact that neither that independence nor that nonalignment may have been wholly attainable or realistic does not necessarily diminish their symbolic value to Gaullist France. Militarily, it would have been difficult for France to have upgraded all of its armed forces at the same time in the 1960s, especially when one considers the political and economic liabilities of the Algerian war still being borne by France in those years. Thus, given the prevailing French belief that another non-nuclear war on the Continent was extremely unlikely to occur, it made good strategic sense for France to concentrate on an independent nuclear force, with its attendant political appeal to the French people. Finally, the associated doctrine of massive retaliation was certainly not without its adherents in the United States and elsewhere, especially when one is dealing with a relatively limited strategic nuclear capability. This is particularly applicable in the Western European context, where it has been remarked that "the firebreak between TNWs (theater nuclear weapons) and national strategic forces is not so clear-cut as it is for Americans."[79] That is, when it is all too likely that the battlefield will be one's own national territory either at the beginning of a war or shortly thereafter, a European alternative to massive retaliation is much more difficult to formulate persuasively than is the case with the United States.[80]

Nevertheless, the advent of the 1970s saw a number of developments that forced a reconsideration of French strategic thinking.[81] Soviet-American relations seemed to be improving in the early days of détente, and the French generally recognized that a continuation of that process would quickly erode whatever leverage an independent "fortress France" strategy might give Paris in the game of nations. That this détente coincided with a continuing Soviet military buildup in Europe was no less disturbing to French defense planners, who tended as a matter of principle to take a more cautious view of the emerging era of superpower amity than was the case with many Americans. Further, the economic and technological costs of France's independent approach to matters of defense had been high, and—while unlikely to become absolutely prohibitive in the near term—were certain to increase in the future. There was also a growing sense of the limitations associated with an independent nuclear force developed, maintained, and enlarged at the expense of other arms. There is an inevitable complementarity between nuclear and conventional forces going beyond the latter's function as a "tripwire" to bring the nuclear forces into play, as Defense Minister Yvon Bourges later acknowledged. To link the defense of France solely to the strategic nuclear force was unsound in both political and military senses. Even the doctrine of massive retaliation was attacked (albeit indirectly) as a reflection of "a policy of all or nothing" that "in reality . . . would be scarcely credible" in the evolving strategic balance of power.[82]

Having found itself in a dilemma reminiscent of that of the United States in the mid to late 1950s, although for rather different reasons, the France of President Valéry Giscard d'Estaing undertook a comparable redefinition of its defense policy and its military establishment. At the strategic and doctrinal level, two principal changes occurred. First, the idea of France as a *total* sanctuary was replaced (admittedly in a rather tentative and hesitant manner) by the concept of the *sanctuarisation élargie* (enlarged sanctuary, or enlarged security area). This meant that French forces would now be expected to engage an opponent in areas approaching France—the classic *bataille de l'avant* (forward battle)—in place of the earlier "fortress France" notion implicit in the concept of the *sanctuarisation totale*. Second, the nuclear-heavy doctrine of massive retaliation was modified to take into account the deployment of French tactical nuclear weapons. The latter—described by France as "prestrategic nuclear weapons" to emphasize their relation to the FNS (strategic nuclear force) and to distinguish their employment from similar weapons in the NATO arsenal in accordance with the doctrine of flexible response—would be fired in a single salvo against an aggressor approaching France's borders as a "final warning" to halt before the FNS would be engaged. More attention was also given to conventional forces, which were reorganized to facilitate their ability to match different types of threats in different conflict situations in Europe and the Third World.[83]

The political and military implications of Giscard's dual shift in French defense policy were considerable. The strategy of *sanctuarisation élargie*, in the words of one astute observer, meant "no more and no less than closer cooperation with [France's NATO] allies."[84] It certainly implied France's willingness (or acceptance of the unavoidable need) to participate in a NATO battle against the Warsaw Pact, whether or not France was formally a part of that alliance's integrated military organization, even if France itself was not under attack or in imminent danger of being attacked by Warsaw Pact forces. This point was not lost on the Gaullists and their sympathizers, for whom "the new strategic concepts tended to place battlefield confrontation above deterrence and [who] were thought to sacrifice the autonomy of French military policy in the name of European solidarity within the [NATO] alliance."[85]

The impact of this redirection in strategy on the French military establishment was equally profound and was first reflected in the Loi de programmation, 1977–1982. This program outlined four French defense objectives in accordance with the new strategy and doctrine: (a) to maintain France's nuclear capability at the level required for it to remain credible, (b) to provide France with a balanced mix of nuclear and classical (conventional) forces, (c) to increase the level of operations, and (d) to devote more resources to the well-being of those military personnel required for the more extensive strategy to be operationalized.[86]

The new program obviously meant that the strategic nuclear force would not only be retained, but also would be revitalized in keeping with the French notion of dissuasion through nuclear sufficiency.[87] The overseas intervention capability would be retained in fact, if not in name, with its principal components—the Eleventh Parachute and Ninth Marine divisions—keeping their original missions.[88] But the major change required to support the strategy of the *sanctuarisation élargie* was a significant augmentation of the conventional forces assigned to European missions, with the army and navy being the principal beneficiaries. Indeed, two of the principal goals of the new program were to upgrade the entire army to the qualitative level of the intervention forces and to enhance the ability of the navy to do more to protect France's ballistic missile submarine (SNLE) force. It was believed that the resulting defense establishment would give France the more flexible and balanced force structure it would require to function effectively in the evolving international order.[89]

An element of uncertainty with respect to the direction French strategy would take was injected into the equation by the electoral victory of the Socialist Party in the 1981 election, something that was compounded when President Mitterrand included four members of the French Communist Party (PCF) in his first cabinet. That uncertainty turned out to be unwarranted, at least insofar as it reflected concerns about the alignment of France with the West. As the Mitterrand government's defense program took shape, elements of continuity as well as of change appeared. Yet the net effect, ironically enough, was that a government of the left moved closer to the Western security community, whose integrated military structure France had abandoned under de Gaulle, and increased "the probability of French participation in any conflict in Europe" along the lines initiated by Giscard.[90]

The elements of continuity in the Mitterrand approach entailed a reaffirmation of the basic political-military precepts of de Gaulle and his conservative successors. One was the profound belief in the status and autonomy of France as a "special country" with an historical mission in the world. This included a reiteration of France's retention of "the widest possible freedom to determine the level, timing, and character of French external commitments . . . [something that had become] a virtual dogma of French life."[91] A second element of continuity was the certainty that possession of and reputation for the effective use of military power was the principal determinant of influence in global affairs. Shortly after the Socialists came to power, Defense Minister Charles Hernu stated bluntly that "in a dangerous and unpredictable world, having military wherewithal at our disposal is the ultimate insurance, the ultimate rampart of national independence."[92] Third, the Mitterrand government shared its predecessors' ambivalence about France's principal allies within the Atlantic Community—the United States, the United Kingdom, and the Federal Republic of Germany—for a variety of historical and political reasons. It also explicitly rejected Giscard's formulation of the concept of the *sanctuarisation élargie* and its implicit espousal of a form of French "extended deterrence" in Western Europe, asserting "that the FNS cannot be extended to cover France's allies."[93] Finally, France retained its long-standing reservations about the significance of the NATO doctrine of "flexible response," with its potential for making Europe a localized battlefield in any East-West con-

2

19

self would adopt such a doctrine, for the pragmatic reason that the French "tactical nuclear
component is modest in numbers . . . and is
destined to be used in a single blow, after
which, in the absence of peace, [France] would
have to resort to . . . its strategic forces."[94] As
before, while reaffirming the importance of
"the equality of the alliances to which it has repeatedly stated its loyalty," France kept to itself
the sole responsibility to determine when, or
even if, that step would be taken, in accordance with the dictum that "a great country
stands alone when it must make the decisive
choices."[95]

These elements of continuity ensured the existence of a measure of stability at the levels of
policy and (to a lesser extent) strategy in
France's approach to defense-related matters,
some of which quite obviously did not precisely
arouse enthusiasm among the other members
of the Atlantic Alliance. The changes initiated
by Mitterrand involved the establishment of
defense priorities and the adoption of operational and programmatic initiatives commensurate with those priorities.

It was obvious to Paris from the outset that
drastic budget increases were unattainable, for
a variety of political and economic reasons.
Choices would therefore have to be made
among many theoretically desirable programs
if France was to reaffirm its autonomy, maintain a capacity for independent action, and increase its net military power in a fiscally prudent fashion. One could not do everything
simultaneously, and any significant attempt to
modernize the defense establishment in a cost-
effective manner implied giving precedence to
some initiatives, improving the organizational
framework of the military, and accepting some
personnel reductions in some part of the overall force structure.[96]

The priorities set by Mitterrand were to (a)
enhance the credibility of the nuclear forces,
(b) strengthen France's ability to meet its implicit commitments to the Atlantic Alliance
without relinquishing control of its own forces,
and (c) improve the French military's capacity
to conduct out-of-area operations. Precisely
what programs would be initiated were largely

debated in 1981–1982 (with some decisions being made during that time); the key decisions
were set forth in the Loi de programmation,
1984–1988, labeled "The French Five-Year Defense Plan: A Comprehensive Blueprint for a
Modernized Nuclear Deterrent and Increasingly Versatile Conventional Forces."

Unlike some documents issued by some governments, the title of this plan actually captured both the letter and the spirit of what the
architect of socialist France's defense policy intended to do. The principal elements of this
defense plan included (a) a "progressive increase in real defense spending"; (b) "continued emphasis on the nuclear deterrent," including the modernization of all components
of the strategic and tactical nuclear forces; (c)
a "reorganization of conventional forces," to
include increases in mobility and firepower as
well as a reform of the reserve force structure
in the army; (d) "strong overseas power-projection [capability] and prepositioning [of personnel and matériel]," including the establishment of the Force d'Action Rapide, a French
version of the American rapid deployment
force with the capability to act either in Europe
or in the Third World; and (e) a "sustained
R&D [research and development] effort" to
permit France's military to be as technologically competitive as possible.[97] Throughout,
there was a sense of irony, in that "the [1984–
1988] Military Programme Law, the first from
a Socialist government, should so clearly spell
out that the principal threat to France emanates from the Soviet Union."[98] The engagement of France in the event of a NATO-War-
saw Pact war was certainly not a foregone
conclusion. But it was generally understood at
the time that the "formation of [the] Rapid
Action Force and the movement of the III
Corps . . . to Lille in northern France . . . to
block the traditional Belgian-North French
plain invasion route are good indications that
the [French] republic is concerned about Western and not just French security."[99]

Regardless of the relative attention devoted
to French and Western security concerns, one
thread of continuity runs through French strategic and doctrinal thinking since the first
French atomic test in 1960: this is the enduring

importance of nuclear weapons in French defense planning.[100] Indeed, to speak of French defense policy at any point over the past three decades is to speak of the *force de dissuasion*, a situation that shows no sign whatsoever of changing, regardless of actual or declared changes in the French attitude toward other countries or to the prospect of becoming engaged in another European war. This is largely because of the enduring French belief that only nuclear weapons can underwrite French security and ensure that other countries will "give it [France] its rank in the concert of nations."[101] Some, of course, may consider that self-assessment to be overdrawn. But it cannot be denied that France's strategic and pre-strategic (that is, tactical) nuclear capability at least gives it the opportunity (to use David Yost's formulation) of equivocating forcefully.

Exactly how one equivocates, forcefully or otherwise, in a confrontation with other nuclear-armed states is not something well understood in any country, as a perusal of the literature on strategy makes abundantly clear. In the case of France, the operational rationale underlying its strategic nuclear force throughout its existence has been the principle of proportional deterrence.[102] This is in many respects a "poor man's principle" of deterrence, which is commonly associated with the nuclear forces—present or projected—of middle powers. It reflects a belief in the presumed rationality of a potential aggressor, such that the latter would be deterred by the threat of nuclear retaliation inflicting damage certain to exceed whatever gains conquest might produce. There is neither a claim to strategic parity with respect to the probable threat of force nor even an attempt to approach such a capability with respect to the superpowers. There is simply an acceptance of the attainability of a degree of strategic sufficiency that, as Pierre Gallois put it in the specific case of France, entails only "being capable of instilling in a would-be aggressor the fear of reprisal great enough to make the stake represented by France, a relatively modest stake, a prize that cannot be coveted with impunity."[103] The image of a "nuclear scorpion" comes readily to mind.

More important than the theory of deter-

rence on which the French strategic nuclear force is based, however, is the question of its actual employment. That is, when, and under what circumstances, would it be unleashed against the putative aggressor? One such case would obviously be a direct attack against France itself. In this case the French strategic nuclear force would punish the aggressor for its presumptuousness. A more likely contingency would be in the event of an attack (almost certainly from the Warsaw Pact) that subjected France and NATO Europe to a similar threat. Although the French have maintained that the primary function of their strategic nuclear force is to safeguard France, they have also tended to argue that the existence of the French nuclear force also serves the interests of NATO Europe by increasing the risk of escalation that an aggressor would have to consider in addition to the U.S. response.[104] When only France is threatened, Paris would clearly be the sole judge of the need to use its own strategic nuclear forces. Even in the case of a threat to both France and NATO Europe, however, the French strategic nuclear force would be launched when the French leadership believed the attacker had crossed the so-called "critical threshold of aggressiveness." This is the point at which France would believe that it had no other choices left except battlefield defeat or unconditional surrender. Moreover, the French decision would be made independently of the United States and the other allies, *regardless of whether or not NATO itself concurred in the French decision*.[105] France, in short, claims for itself the right to act for other countries that it denies to them with respect to France.

There is admittedly some sound basis for the French position as outlined above. The USSR obviously cannot be certain that France would not act in accordance with its declaratory policy and use its *force de dissuasion* as a *force de frappe* if deterrence failed, even if the United States and the other NATO countries argued for restraint or even surrender. This in itself may add to Soviet uncertainty and thus truly enhance the general deterrent posture of NATO as a whole. The fact that France, unlike the United States and Great Britain, to a certain extent shares the Soviet predisposition to acknowledge both the deterrent and the war-fighting roles of nuclear weapons cannot have escaped the attention of the Soviet leadership or be reassuring to it.[106]

Here, as elsewhere, however, there is an-other side to the coin. It is distinctly possible that Soviet uncertainty with respect to France's probable reaction in time of war may induce Moscow to strike the relatively vulnerable French nuclear forces at the beginning of a general offensive, or even in the midst of a par-ticularly intense crisis in East-West relations. This would have the effect of pulling most, if not all, of France's nuclear "teeth," simultane-ously inflicting substantial losses on France's population and industrial base (depending, of course, on the scope of the Soviet attack), thereby making a mockery of French "inde-pendence" and the *force de dissuasion*. In such an eventuality, the French nuclear force would have been a magnet precipitating an attack that might otherwise not have occurred—the precise opposite of what it was intended to ac-complish. The very credibility of the concept of proportional deterrence, after all, lies (as Graeme Auton once remarked) in "its automa-ticity, that is, its affinity to the American mas-sive retaliation doctrine of the Eisenhower years."[107] Ironically, France appears to have adopted and largely retained a doctrine that—if credible to any potential adversary—would invite murder.

FRENCH STRATEGY RECONSIDERED

These and similar inconsistencies (obvious and otherwise) in French nuclear doctrine gen-erally exceed in importance operational ques-tions such as the prudence of deploying the "Rapid Action Force" into Germany in any event of war, or the sustainability and inter-operability of French forces in concert with those of NATO. They also necessarily invite questions about the validity of the rationale underlying the French fixation on a national nuclear force. And on reflection it appears that Wolf Mendl was correct when he wrote that "one suspects that there is a far more prag-matic basis to French [strategic] policy than its theoreticians would have us believe."[108]

That basis, I am convinced, lies in the dual character of France's strategic nuclear force. As noted previously, every military instrument of national policy has both military and politi-cal functions, and the French strategic nuclear force is no exception.[109] To acknowledge the existence of a political rationale for the *force de dissuasion*, of course, requires one to see even its military rationale in a particular light. It has come to be widely accepted that France's strategic nuclear force actually plays two mili-tary roles. One is to give France the option of *acting* like a power in the world, exerting influ-ence and employing conventional forces in ways and in places that might otherwise not be possible. The second, which usually receives greater attention, is to deter the Soviet Union from attacking or threatening the national ter-ritory and sovereignty of France itself.

There is some objective basis for both of these roles, especially the former, at least if France is dealing with (a) nations that do not possess nuclear weapons of their own, and (b) issues that do not call into play the interests of the superpowers themselves, with their atten-dant strategic nuclear arsenals. Had the French possessed their own atomic weapons in 1954, for example, they would doubtless have used them in a final effort to save their be-sieged garrison at Dien Bien Phu, precisely as they appear to have hoped the United States would do for them in the stillborn "Operation Vulture."[110] It is equally likely that, in 1956, a nuclear-armed France would have resisted out-side pressure from both the Soviet Union and France's then-recalcitrant American "allies" to withdraw from Suez. This resistance could have taken the form of giving Moscow the op-tion of exchanging Russian cities for French ones, and perhaps precipitating a World War III, in defense of Cairo and the Egyptian army—something Russian decision makers would be especially loathe to contemplate. Both of these examples are illustrative of a car-dinal French principle regarding nuclear weapons and foreign policy. This rule is that a state that lacks nuclear weapons can be told to cease and desist if it should act solely in de-fense of its own interests outside of its national territory. A state with its own nuclear arsenal, however, would rarely be asked to do so and cannot be compelled to refrain or to withdraw in most instances at an acceptable cost to the third party. That France may misapprehend the situation does not alter the impact of this point of view on French defense policy in general, and on France's national nuclear force in particular.

Despite the perceived utility of the *force de dissuasion* as a facilitator of French military intervention abroad under certain circumstances, its more important declared military role involves the application of the aforementioned concept of proportional deterrence to France's military relations with the Soviet Union (and, perhaps, with any other country that might someday threaten France proper). Many considerations affect this role's definition and prospects for success. In the final analysis, however, the key issue is whether the French contribution would matter if the Soviet Union decided to throw its military forces against Western Europe—or would even dissuade the USSR from pressing an attack on France.

As is so often the case in military affairs, there is no definitive resolution to this problem. It is difficult even to address this question in terms of different scenarios; as an adviser to former Defense Minister Hernu once remarked: "We French do not tend to reason in terms of scenarios because they do not have much bearing with [*sic*] reality and tend to make one talk in terms of use rather than in terms of deterrence."[111] At a minimum one can acknowledge that France has deployed a strategic and tactical nuclear force whose aggregate capabilities cannot be discounted out of hand, and which is informed by a doctrine whose relative ambiguity may give rise to what has been called a "positive uncertainty factor" that may enhance deterrence by complicating Soviet calculations.[112]

On the other hand, it seems prudent to assume that *any* Soviet decision to invade Western Europe would necessarily have taken account of the possibility that the conflict ultimately could result in a strategic nuclear exchange between the superpowers—the classic "central sanctuary" war. Any Soviet leadership contemplating that step would also have to have concluded that the political-military objectives to be secured, the potential gains to be realized, or the dangers to be averted, were worth both the risk of such an exchange and the losses the USSR would incur if it took place. Otherwise, the Soviet attack would almost certainly not occur as a matter of deliberate policy. It should be readily apparent that a Soviet leadership that would not be deterred by the strategic nuclear capability of the United States is highly unlikely to be deterred by the far less significant damage that might be inflicted by France's handful of manned bombers, IRBMs, and SLBMs, even if they survived to strike a blow. As suggested earlier, the probability that they would *not* survive to do so is extremely high in the context of a general European war.

There is only a marginally better basis for supposing that an independent national nuclear force under French control would be able to accomplish the lesser (in European terms) objective of inducing the USSR to refrain from attacking France itself, regardless of the fate of the remainder of Western Europe. At the most general level, there is much to be said for the argument that "it remains difficult to imagine any circumstances in which it would serve French interests actually to carry out the 'anti-cities' retaliatory threat" if deterrence failed in the first place.[113] More specifically, it would require an extraordinary degree of self-restraint for the French leadership to observe Soviet columns rapidly cutting their way through NATO forces toward French territory and still to withhold their nuclear weapons in the hope that the USSR would not violate France's territorial integrity. It would require even greater self-restraint for the Soviet forces to make such an approach and continue to refrain from striking the French nuclear installations on the assumption that the French would resist the temptation to launch the *force de dissuasion* against Soviet targets. It should be readily apparent that such mutual self-restraint is all too unlikely, given the probable parameters of a European war. Yet even if that mutual self-restraint did occur, the net effect would be to leave France devoid of its former partners, dependent on the USSR in all key respects, and utterly bereft of the status and prestige to which it now clings so adamantly. Surviving as a larger version of Finland can hardly conform to the ideals upon which the Fifth Republic was founded and those it has espoused with such intensity over the years.

These and related questions about the military utility of the *force de dissuasion* suggest that there has been an undue tendency in many discussions to place too much emphasis on its military role. The obvious corollary is that far more attention needs to be given to the political dimension of the *force de dissuasion*, which, I suspect, is a far more useful guide to understanding France's commitment to its less than overwhelming nuclear arsenal.[114]

In the first place, there is the fact that the possession of an independently controlled national nuclear force is widely seen in France (and in many other countries as well) to be synonymous with that country's prestige, status, and autonomy in the world. Unless the French come to believe that such considerations are irrelevant or anachronistic, it is virtually certain that France will retain and continue to modernize the *force de dissuasion* even if no actual or potential military threat to France existed or could be envisioned by the most pessimistic French defense planners. The retention of that independent French nuclear capability would be dictated by France's domestic and international political concerns, the overriding importance of which must not be underestimated.

Second in importance to status in French eyes is the diplomatic leverage seen to be implicit in the very existence of a national nuclear force. It is generally conceded that even de Gaulle recognized that the diplomatic value of a French strategic nuclear force probably exceeded its military utility, and his successors do not seem to have forgotten that lesson.[115] A strong consensus exists in France in support of Pierre Dabezies's contention that France's "nuclear force gives her some freedom of action and . . . ensures that she cannot be ignored."[116] It must be conceded that there is at least some truth to the wry comment of one French writer to the effect that the fact that France is the only European country to have "landbased missiles capable of reaching Soviet territory" has not resulted in France's being "handicapped in her relations with the Soviet Union."[117] In fact, a fair assessment of Soviet-French relations would probably conclude that the opposite situation actually obtained.

The third political aspect of the *force de dissuasion* is related closely to the question of European security and the position that France believes itself to merit within the European community writ large. As noted earlier, developments within and outside of Europe throughout the 1980s have resulted in a more cooperative stance between France and both NATO and the Federal Republic of Germany, among other countries. Looking more to the future, however, being the only European power to possess an independent nuclear force (excluding the extra-continental British force, which is linked to that of the United States) implies that the evolution of any European political union could easily mean that "France would constitute the nucleus of an . . . independent system of common security."[118] That such a development would enhance French status and increase the likelihood that France would dominate such a policy is usually left unspoken, but it is difficult to believe that the French (or anyone else, for that matter) are ignorant of the implications of their own strategy and view of the world on this subject.

CONSTRAINTS ON FRENCH STRATEGIC CHOICE

The influence of perceived threats and preferred roles on French strategic choice is apparent from the preceding discussion. Yet it should be equally apparent that other factors within France itself have also been significant in the past and are likely to have a major impact on the retention or possible redefinition of French strategy and doctrine in the future. Given the general consensus that exists on defense-related matters among the principal French political parties (the Communist Party [PCF] being the obvious exception),[119] four such factors merit our attention. They are: (a) France's geographical position, (b) the state of the French economic and technological base, (c) French public opinion, and (d) the political stability of France as a nation.

The most obvious constraint on French ambitions and strategies is that which is not readily amenable to change, whatever the preferences of some in the French policy community might be. This is the geographical location of France. In general, as Pierre Gallois has remarked, "France has [a] specific role to play [in the nuclear age] which is defined by her continental position and the limited resources at her disposal to defend the security of that position."[120] As with the real estate market, location can be the most important potential consideration in strategic choice. In this instance, France's continental position places demands on French defense planners aggravated by that country's relative vulnerabilities, but moderated by the existence of the Federal Republic of Germany (and NATO forces stationed on German territory) as a buffer—in fact, if not as a canon of French policy—between France and the most likely source of a military threat to France. Granted, the respite (in both spatial and temporal terms) such a buffer zone offers France is much more limited today than would have been the case even when France was still a member of NATO's integrated military structure. But the fact that *some* respite is possible allows French planners to formulate a strategy, articulate a doctrine, and prioritize their forces in a way that simply would not be possible if France were located in the same geostrategic situation as, for example, the Federal Republic of Germany.

In today's security environment, of course, both possession of and direct access to key strategic raw materials are of at least as much importance as a nation's geographical position, and probably more so. The fact that France lacks sufficient quantities of at least one key strategic resource—oil—and has no direct contiguous access to other sources of oil is a critical shortcoming, alleviated to a certain degree by France's domestic nuclear energy program and the development of the North Sea oil fields. Nonetheless, this particular deficiency means that France is a continental power that must act as both a "continental" and a "maritime" power (as both terms are generally understood in strategic circles today) to secure both its position and its resources.

The former dictates some general war capacity for deterrence and, if deterrence fails, for defense. The latter necessitates the possession of substantial power-projection capabilities to give France the potential to undertake offensive operations overseas—independent of foreign assistance—with reasonable prospects of success. These are difficult for a middle power such as France to achieve simultaneously.

This consideration is underscored by France's economic and technological situation. The French economy is by no means insubstantial, nor is its economic system notably inefficient; even the so-called economic giant of Europe, West Germany, has had its lackluster times. Good economic news in 1986–87, most notably a decrease in oil prices and a decline in the value of the U.S. dollar, partially alleviated French budgetary concerns and permitted a real increase of 4.8 percent in the defense budget the following year.[121] Such good years, however, are by no means commonplace in the French experience. Complicating conditions further for French defense planners is the fact that both weapons systems and skilled personnel are becoming more expensive to obtain, while France's efforts to maintain the broad-based military establishment required by its self-defined interests and objectives and the strategy it has chosen strain the limited financial resources available to the French government to the utmost.[122] This is particularly apparent with respect to the extremely expensive research and development programs required if France wishes to continue to try to be as competitive as possible in weapons system development and deployment. Limited assistance may be obtained from other countries, and cooperative ventures with other nations can alleviate difficulties to a certain degree.[123] Yet a reoccurrence of earlier recessions could force French defense planners to make some very difficult choices between what they would *prefer* to have in consonance with France's ambitions, and what they *can* have in the harsh light of economic and budgetary realities.[124]

Much the same state of affairs exists in the field of technology. French technology is by no means antiquated, although in some respects (for example, nuclear weapons technology)

France continues to lag behind the superpowers. Yet France's defense industry has made an international name for itself in other areas, employing over 400,000 people either directly or indirectly in the "big three" industrial sectors: aerospace, electronics, and the Délégation générale pour l'Armement (DGA), which produces the lion's share of the equipment used by the French army and navy. France is the only Western European country to field a competitive air superiority aircraft, its Exocet missile acquired a well-deserved reputation in the 1982 Anglo-Argentinian South Atlantic War, and the unfolding French space and satellite program is particularly ambitious.[125] Yet despite these achievements—and it would be most unwise to underestimate them or the technological and industrial base that has produced them—there persists the far more demanding problem of overcoming other existing technological shortcomings and forestalling the still-impending technological gap of considerable dimensions relative to the most advanced industrial states. That this *is* a problem that must weigh heavily on French planners is due in no small measure to the goals that France has set for itself in the world. There is an enduring verity in the conclusion reached by one French strategist to the effect that France has the financial and technological capacity for both nuclear deterrence and internal security (within the limitations outlined above) but lacks a similar capacity to conduct independent conventional operations anywhere for a sustained period of time without at least some external assistance.[126] The fact that France's self-proclaimed independence both requires it to have the capacity it lacks and contributes to the existence of that inadequacy is illustrative of the dilemma that has confronted the French defense community throughout the 1980s. It remains to be seen if France's more cooperative attitude toward West Germany and NATO as a whole is able to resolve this dilemma without compromising France's long-standing preoccupation with autonomy.

To a certain extent, that dilemma is moderated somewhat by the existence in France of what Alan Gliksman has termed that "broad-based consensus on defense policy and its requirements"[127] that cuts across most party and class lines, particularly with respect to the maintenance of an independent national nuclear force. Yet the existence of a general consensus does not mean that changes have not taken place in the French public's view of the world over time. For example, as table 1 indicates, the principal threat perceived as confronting France in recent years has been terrorism—increasing from 61 percent in 1984 to 79 percent in 1986. Concurrently, however, concern about what might be called "attacks by special weapons" (chemical and biological; nuclear)—never very great—declined somewhat, while apprehension about what the French term "economic aggression" fell off precipitously from 51 percent to 19 percent and fear of a conventional attack dropped from 22 percent to a mere 6 percent. The world may still be a dangerous place in French eyes, but the source of the danger appears to lie elsewhere than in the ambitions of militarily threatening states.

One reason for this particular rank-ordering of French threat-perceptions can be discerned in the changes that have occurred in the identification of the four principal national threats to world peace, as depicted in figure 1. In 1970 allegedly "threatening nations" included a rather diverse set of countries, with the United States outranking the Soviet Union by a hefty margin. The latter rank-ordering had significantly changed by 1983; and by 1986 the three highest-ranking threats—Iran, Libya, and Syria—all had particularly close ties to various terrorist groups, with the Soviet Union not far behind. Paralleling the shift in perceived threats and threateners, and reflecting upon

Table 1. Principal Perceived Threats to France

Source of Threat	1984	1986
Terrorism	61%	79%
Chemical or biological attack	30	22
Nuclear attack	27	19
Economic aggression (e.g., boycotts)	51	19
Conventional attack, followed by occupation	22	6

Source: Jean-Paul Le Bourg, "Opinion et Défense en 1986," *Armées d'Aujourd'hui,* 117 (February 1987): 15.

Note: Multiple responses were permitted; columns do not sum to 100%.

Figure 1. Nations Perceived as Threatening World Peace

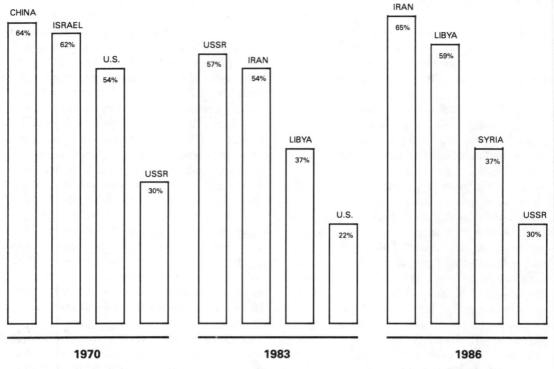

Source: Jean-Paul Le Bourg, "Opinion et Défense en 1986," *Armées d'Aujourd'hui*, 117 (February 1987): 15.

Note: Multiple responses were permitted; totals do not sum to 100%.

the departure of the United States from the "first four threateners," have been the changes taking place in French preferences for alternative security roles, as shown in table 2. The decline in those with "no opinion" from 1979 to 1986 is suggestive of choices being made during a decade of change—although a period of change that did not appreciably alter two posi-

Table 2. Public Support for Alternative Security Roles for France

Security Alternatives	1979	1986
Western alliance	47%	61%
(Europe only)	(28)	(23)
(Europe and the United States)	(19)	(38)
Alliance with the U.S.S.R.	2	3
Independence/neutrality	30	27
No opinion	21	9

Sources: Jerome Jaffre, "France Looks to Europe," *Public Opinion* (March–May 1979), p. 17; Jean-Paul Le Bourg, "Opinion et Défense en 1986," *Armées d'Aujourd'hui*, 117 (February 1987): 18.

tions: disinclination to ally with the Soviet Union, and support for a strictly independent role. What is intriguing is the fact that support for closer ties to the Western Alliance rose to a commanding 61 percent—but it did so *not* in its "Europe only" variant, in which France might hope to play a dominant role, but in conjunction with the United States as well, in an association France cannot hope to lead. This shift in attitude toward the United States may well be the most interesting development during Mitterrand's tenure. Indeed, even when those polled were forced to choose only between the two superpowers, as presented in table 3, the French choice of the United States is clear—and a complete reversal of the position in 1959. These and similar shifts in public opinion are certainly not cast in stone, but they do both parallel and reflect shifts in policy stances that have occurred in the 1980s—and

Table 3. Support for Rapprochement

Rapprochement with	1959	1985
United States	16%	62%
Soviet Union	59	4
Neither/no opinion	25	34

Source: *Wilson Center Security Digest,* March 1986, p. 2.

they may well portend additional shifts in the years to come.

What was once described as the current (and apparently enduring) predisposition of the French to "remain jealous of their national autonomy"[128] has clearly been moderated to a certain degree by a greater inclination to associate with the United States and (in a different context) the Federal Republic of Germany. What has not altered over the past decade—indeed, has become even stronger than before—is the impressive reservoir of popular support for the French national strategic force. This support, it is worth noting, had not always been present. During the 1960s, in fact, there was much public opposition to the *force de dissuasion*. By the early 1970s, however, public opinion shifted sharply in favor of the *force de dissuasion*, to the point where today support for it constitutes one of the "stable poles" in French views on defense-related issues.[129] When Mitterrand assumed office, approximately 63 percent of the French electorate considered the *force de dissuasion* to be an essential element of the French defense effort—a three-to-one majority of those expressing an opinion. By 1986 supporters of the *force de dissuasion* had increased to 69 percent of the electorate, representing nearly a *four*-to-one majority on that position. Somewhat complicating the ostensible linkage between policy and public opinion, however, is the fact that the *force de dissuasion* is notably ineffective against the principal perceived threat to France noted in table 1—terrorism—and that the public's propensity to see the *force de dissuasion* used is much less striking than support for its existence. Some 59 percent would threaten to use nuclear weapons if—and *only* if—France itself were attacked with nuclear weapons. But only 13 percent believed that France should use its own nuclear weapons in

the case of aggression against France whether or not the attacker employed nuclear weapons—which is what French strategy says France should be prepared to do—and only 11 percent would threaten the use of the *force de dissuasion* in the event of an invasion of West Germany, something rather different than might be expected from the recent evolution of Franco-German relations.[130] Clearly, some inconsistencies need to be sorted out between French policy, French strategy, and French public opinion.

As in most political democracies, public opinion in France can be said to set "general constraints"[131] on the formulation and implementation of its defense policy. As in the early years of the *force de dissuasion*, however, when the French government proceeded with the deployment of its nuclear force in the face of considerable public opposition, those constraints are not necessarily binding. But in general, French policy—and the views of the principal political parties on matters of defense—tends to accord with the predispositions of the majority of the electorate. This may well account for both the continuity in French defense (and foreign) policy throughout the tenure of the Fifth Republic, and the decline of the single "outlier" in this respect: the French Communist Party. Interestingly enough, not even communist voters seem openly enthusiastic about a military alliance with the Soviet Union (or even some form of rapprochement with that country), as evidenced by the insignificant percentage of the overall electorate depicted in tables 2 and 3 in support of those positions. But the Communist Party's independent stance[132] has not sufficed to bring it to power, or even to keep it in place as part of a governing coalition of the left.

Finally, it is readily apparent that political stability and societal cohesion are essential for the effective formulation and implementation of any defense policy by any country. Yet it is precisely those conditions whose existence constitutes an enduring concern in the case of France, even if it is a concern rarely translated into political reality. More than in many other Western countries, class and party divisions in France are particularly strong, even when there exists a strong overall policy consensus (for example, on the importance of the *force de dissuasion*). What tends to create disorder are differences over which party should guide France—that is, who should rule. This is owing in no small measure to fairly specific differences in the party's domestic agendas. Even when a single party dominates, consensus is absent; within the Socialist Party on matters of defense and foreign policy, for instance, factions exist supporting stances ranging from an "ultra-Gaullist" emphasis on "independence, neutralism, and nuclear defense" to a "pacifist" preference for disarmament and the abolition of all military blocs.[133] The conservative victory in the National Assembly in 1986 that elevated Jacques Chirac to the post of premier created potential for a divided government unprecedented in the history of the Fifth Republic, producing a form of what the French called "cohabitation" that at least ameliorated differences in defense matters. The elections of 1988 will doubtless provide some answer to the question of "who should rule," as well as some indication of the degree to which French political will to act in accordance with France's ambitions is translated into votes at election time. Yet there remains an abiding suspicion outside of France that there was an underlying element of truth to the suggestion that the events of 1968 dramatized "the vulnerability of France's political system to disorder."[134] This may continue to be indicative of potential long-term political fragility, superficially belied by France's relative power and political assertiveness.

THE FUTURE OF FRENCH STRATEGY: THE NEED FOR CHOICE

The last-mentioned reservation notwithstanding, continuity rather than change continues to be likely with respect to France's doctrine and strategy, at least as declared. That is, France's leadership will continue reasserting France's independence in the world, the importance of its national nuclear force as a guarantee of that independence as well as of French sovereignty, and France's ability to act as a power of consequence in the world, *even if reality requires France to move closer to the*

United States, West Germany, and NATO itself. As Yost has suggested, under Mitterrand, "Gaullist policies that pretend fully to assure France's security are nonetheless still pursued. . . . Official responses . . . proposals (e.g., flexible response, civil defense) suggest that proportional deterrence will persist with little change."[135]

Both this continuity and the anticipation of the need for some hard choices, on the other hand, became evident in the Loi de programmation d'équipement militaire, 1987–1991— the first to be prepared under the Mitterrand-Chirac government of "cohabitation." All of the basic tenets of the Fifth Republic are present, including espousal of "the willingness of France to remain independent . . . [and to maintain] the rank of a great power," the capacity to counter "threats to the Central European theater," and "the maintenance of the French presence in the world," modified only by the need to oppose terrorism—France's greatest perceived threat.[136] Despite its apparent reiteration of precedent, however, this particular *loi de programmation*—which passed the National Assembly by a vote of 536 to 35 (a mandate by anyone's standards!)—gives obvious precedence to nuclear systems (for example, the M5 missile, the Hades replacement for the older Pluton TNW, and the nuclear-capable Mirage 2000 series) within a defense budget predicated on 11 percent real growth in 1987 and 6 percent real growth per annum in following years.[137] Conventional forces would not be utterly neglected, to be sure, but a distinct change from the attempt of the Mitterrand regime to create and to maintain a more balanced force can be discerned.

Even with this shift in emphasis, an ever-latent dilemma has edged closer to the surface. Threat-perception and ambition have impelled the French government toward expansion of its defense establishment and continued modernization of all elements of that establishment. Economics and demographics, on the other hand, argue for retrenchment and a compromise of that ambition in the interests of geostrategic pragmatism. It is all too likely that the continuous real increases in defense spending needed to modernize France's forces adequately because of the actual or impending obsolescence of so many systems will exceed France's capacity to provide those increases. So much is needed—a new SLBM to reduce the vulnerability of the SSBN force; replacements for systems ranging from aircraft carriers and both SSBNs and SSNs; main battle tanks and attack helicopters—that prudent analysts may well wonder if the effort that will surely be made will suffice to provide everything actually needed.

Indications are that reach will exceed grasp in this instance, and that the choices that France will have to make in terms of the type of defense establishment it maintains and equips will properly have to be informed by choices made on a number of political and strategic issues. Several such decision points can be readily identified. Prominent among them are the view of autonomy versus cooperation with other countries in matters of defense; doctrine for the nuclear forces; the attitude to the definition of a strategic "sanctuary" to be protected at all costs, including the use of the *force de dissuasion*; the feasibility and desirability of maintaining a truly balanced force; the proper area of employment of the Rapid Action Force; and—of greatest long-term importance—whether West Germany is, in its essence, an ally, an enemy, or a liability. All of these are significant, although how France assesses Germany will have a disproportionate influence on what France can do or be, at least in Europe.

Traces of choices having been made on certain of these issues are already becoming visible, as evidenced by some of the decisions France has made as noted earlier in this chapter. One is that the retention of an effective *force de dissuasion* remains of critical importance; all nuclear systems will be upgraded, even at the expense of conventional forces other than the Rapid Action Force. The concept of an "extended sanctuary" beyond the borders of France in Europe is becoming a reality in fact if not in name, reinforced by withdrawal of control of TNWs from the French First Army to emphasize more centralized control over those weapons. West Germany has come to be seen as an ally of sorts, if only to

preclude the possibility of its becoming a liability that might deteriorate at a later point into an enemy. And France will accept some form of circumscribed autonomy in Europe, while retaining an activist and independent stance in the Third World, as evidenced by French naval activities in the 1987–88 Persian Gulf crisis. How far these evolve under the 1988–92 *loi de programmation* and its successors in the aftermath of the 1988 elections in France remains to be seen.

The Defense Decision-Making Process

In general terms the French defense policy process encompasses three principal stages: (a) *planification* (the determination of what is desirable for an adequate long-term defense, given the government's identification of ambitions, interests, and objectives); (b) programmation (the identification of what is possible in the middle term, usually formulated in terms of five years); and (c) budget (the specification of what can be done in the short term, usually a single year).[138] When appropriate, a procedure termed the "Rationalization of Budgetary Choice" (RCB) is used to "clarify . . . essential options" by identifying and prioritizing alternatives for inclusion in a five-year plan and subsequent allocation to particular annual budgets.[139] The underlying assumption is that the requirements defined in each stage of the process will shape the next stage, thus ensuring not only continuity of planning but also a high degree of congruence among strategy, force posture, and available defense-related resources utilized as effectively as possible.

Reality, of course, rarely coincides perfectly with design. In the case of France, however, the degree of fit is remarkably close. For a variety of historical, constitutional, institutional and personality-dependent reasons, the defense decision-making process in the French Fifth Republic clearly approximates the classical "rational actor model" to a greater extent than is the case with any other Western country of consequence.[140] The actual policy output can be somewhat uneven,[141] to be sure. Yet there remains little doubt that the defense decision-making process in contemporary France is characterized by much the same "high degree of coherence and consistency"—to say nothing of relative success—that is commonly attributed to France's performance in foreign affairs in general,[142] changes in France's domestic and international security environments notwithstanding.

The French defense policy process has been aptly described as an admixture of "parliamentary impotence and executive dominance," at least in theory.[143] Conceptually, there is no question about the extent to which effective power in this process resides in the executive branch, and specifically with the president of the republic. In most instances, the president is constitutionally and practically the one who has "supreme responsibility" in defense matters, is "the lone judge on the eventual use of nuclear weapons," and "personally exercises the power of decision and control on the use of the armed forces in the event of war."[144] Until the 1985 elections and the ensuing period of governmental "cohabitation," it was also clear that the National Assembly, unlike the Congress in the United States, lacked the ability to pose any serious threat to the paramount position of the president and his staff in the defense policy process. The situation obviously became far more complicated after 1986, moderated only by the general consensus on the broad precepts of defense and foreign policy that did exist between the supporters of President Mitterrand and Premier Chirac. Nonetheless, as a general principle, it is quite correct to acknowledge that "defense is considered a 'reserved domain' of the French president,"[145] regardless of the party in power. Thus, "independence under the watchful guardianship of the president of the republic is repeatedly proclaimed . . . and a Mitterrand as much as a de Gaulle defends foreign and defense policy as a reserved presidential sector."[146] This relatively "limited" role of French parliamentarians in these spheres is reinforced by the fact that oversight "hearings and fact finding missions . . . are not a normal part of the French parliamentary system."[147] Nor does public opinion conventionally influence policy decisions greatly. As Pierre Lellouche has indicated: "When defense is debated in France (as was the case . . . with the adoption of the 1984–1988 Military Program Law), this is done in an atmosphere of near-total [public] indifference, as long as the sacrosanct national deterrent force is preserved and modernized."[148]

Two developments have reaffirmed the essential reality of presidential dominance of the defense policy process by enhancing the overall position of the executive branch therein. One is the codification of that process into the three-stage sequence of *planification-programmation-budget* noted earlier. The other is the flexibility built into the various planning documents themselves, particularly the Loi de programation, 1984–1988 and its successor, the Loi de programme d'équipement militaire, 1987–1991—a change in nomenclature that significantly reduced the proportion of actual defense expenditures included in the five-year planning document for which the government could be held somewhat accountable. The concentration of power in the presidency, however, does not imply that it has become easier for outsiders to understand, if only because of differences in their political cultures. On the contrary, the complexity of the defense policy process within the executive branch itself is considerable, due in no small measure to the durability of a defense policy process in France that "has much more in common with the centralized, secretive, executive-dominated British system . . . than with the pluralistic [American system]."[149]

Yet if the formulation of French defense policy is centralized at the highest level, its execution is not. At the most general level, it is accurate to say that the prime minister is only "an agent of the President" on these matters, and that the defense and foreign ministers have only a "restricted freedom of action" in the implementation of presidential decisions.[150] When the prime minister is from a different party than the president, of course, as occurred after the 1986 elections, the situation becomes more fluid. Administratively, however, responsibility for the actual implementation of defense policy decisions devolves on (a) the General Secretariat of National Defense, and (b) the Ministry of National Defense.[151] A functional portrayal of the central administration of French defense policy appears in figure 2; the defense organization itself is in the Gendarmerie (a paramilitary national police force) and Military Justice, and the offices of the inspector general of each of the individual services and the Gendarmerie, all of whom report directly to the minister of national defense independently of their respective chiefs of staff. Supplementing these activities, a new Scientific Defense Council was established in 1986

to advise the minister of national defense, the secretary of state for defense, and the deputy-general for armaments—the functional equivalent of the Defense Science Board in the United States.[152]

Each of these organizations or agencies has its own particular function. Those in the first set are principally concerned with the administration of the armed forces, whereas those in the second set deal with the operation of the military. Of the former, the Ministerial Delega-

Figure 2. Central Administration of Defense

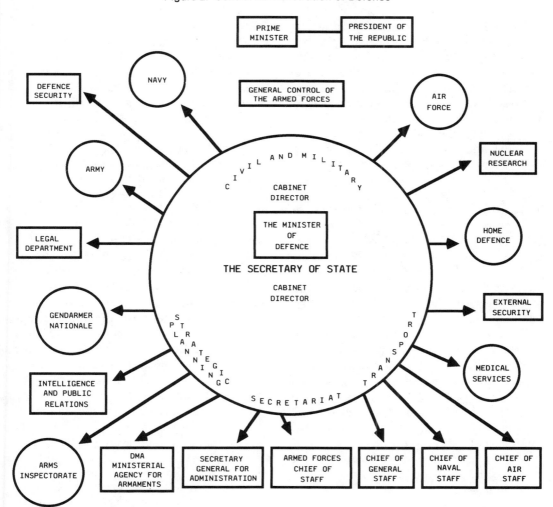

Source: Jean-Pierre Marichy, "The Central Organization of Defense in France," in Martin Edmonds, ed., *Central Organizations of Defense* (Boulder, Colo.: Westview Press, 1985), p. 55.

tion for Armaments (DMA) has the most influence. It has what are called state missions and also industrial missions. The state missions include the types of weapons system planning, procurement, and research and development (R & D) functions one would normally associate with a governmental agency of this variety. The DMA is supported in the execution of these missions by a number of technical/operational divisions and administrative boards. The industrial missions, on the other hand, are a singularly French phenomenon that requires the DMA to function as part of the general armaments industry—a military-industrial complex in fact as well as in name.[153] Indeed, cooperation and coordination between the public and private sectors of defense-related industries—sectors whose spheres of influence overlap to a considerable degree in practice—are both extensive and cordial. This has reduced both administrative workloads and the incidence of industrial noncompliance with policy requirements and procurement obligations. Both the character and the implications of this special relationship have been well summarized by Arthur J. Alexander, who observes that dealings "between the French government and [defense] industry are on an intimate basis, with a great deal of administrative discretion practiced by executive agencies. . . . [A] sense of partnership pervades the relationship . . . [that] reduces the need for official regulation and surveillance."[154] This sense of partnership has facilitated the evolving privatization of French defense industrial activities in recent years.

Primary responsibility for the operation of the armed forces falls under the purview of the chiefs of staff.[155] There are four chiefs of staff, three of whom head their individual services (army, navy, air force) and are generally responsible for their material and operational readiness. In addition, there is also an armed forces chief of staff, whose general responsibility to the minister of national defense for the overall readiness of the French armed forces makes him *primus inter pares* on the Committee of the Chiefs of Staff in peacetime. In wartime, he becomes chief of the chiefs of staff, with the three service chiefs available as his

deputies for specific operations. All of the service chiefs, however, enjoy the right of direct access to the minister of national defense on matters related to the normal operation of their respective services. Regular meetings of the Committee of Chiefs of Staff (usually on a monthly basis), with the minister of national defense presiding, deal with matters affecting the defense establishment as a whole. Finally, a Supreme Council composed of senior general officers deals with service-specific matters.

Despite the normal coherence and general efficiency of the French defense policy-making process, there are a number of constraints that inhibit its functioning, partially compromise the quality and quantity of its output and, in the words of one scholar, "constitute virtually permanent [and potentially detrimental] aspects of the defense policy process in France."[156] First, the anomalous position of France within the Atlantic Alliance has necessarily reduced France's access to American financial and technical assistance, and thus to much of the most advanced U.S. defense technology, although France's participation in the Independent European Program Group, bilateral undertakings with other European members of NATO, and the activities of the U.S. private sector have been mitigating factors. At least in the technical aspect of defense, however, the commitment to "France alone" has entailed more burdens for French planners than would have been the case if France had wholeheartedly adopted either an Atlanticist or a European role. It remains to be seen whether, to what extent, and how quickly this state of affairs may be altered as a function of France's closer association with West Germany and its more positive attitude toward reassociating itself with NATO (but *not* rejoining it), including the United States.

Second, the actual administration of French defense policy is less efficient in some respects than its architects would wish it to be, or outsiders might expect of it. Part of the problem lies in the existence of various intra-organizational conflicts of interest within the ministry of national defense itself. These include differences in the managerial emphases of the armed services; intraservice rivalries that tend

Figure 3. French Defense Organization

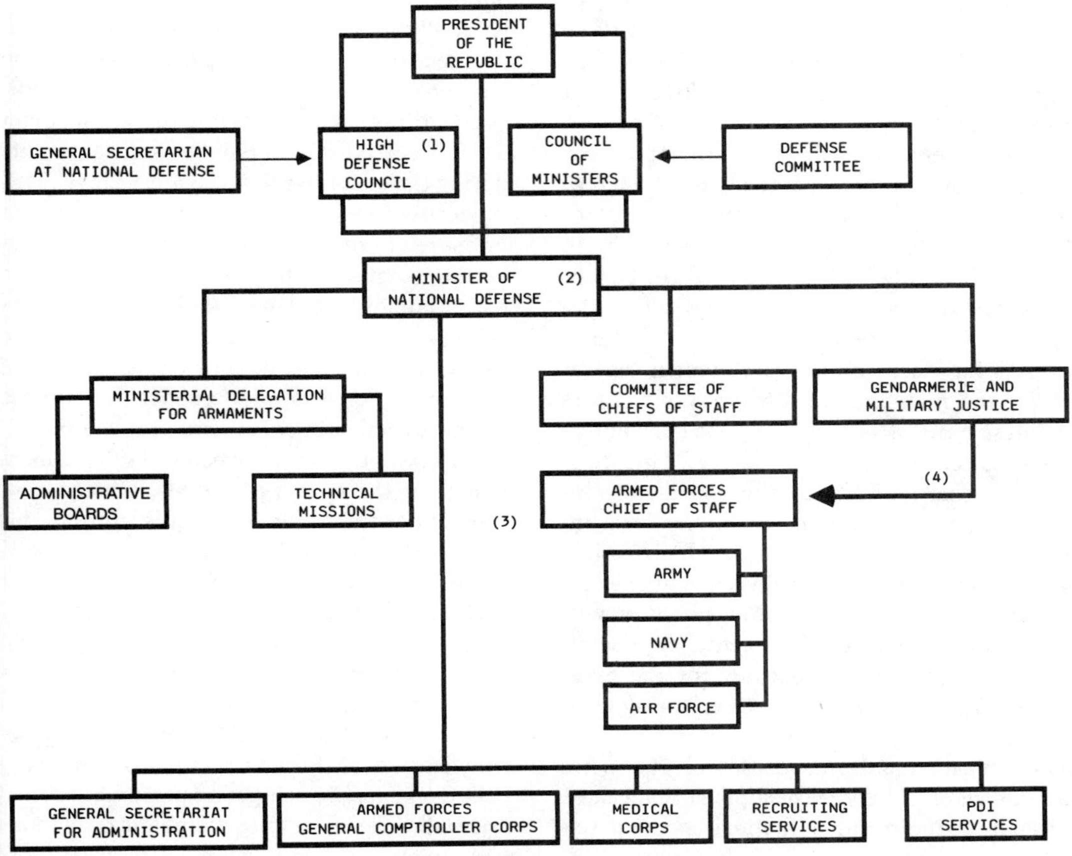

LEGEND:

OPERATIONAL / ADMINISTRATIVE
ADVISORY / STAFF SUPPORT
RIGHT OF ACCESS
WARTIME RELATIONSHIP

NOTES:

(1) CONSISTS OF PRIME MINISTER, MINISTER OF NATIONAL DEFENSE, MINISTER OF FOREIGN AFFAIRS, MINISTER OF THE INTERIOR, MINISTER OF FINANCE, AND THE SECRETARY GENERAL FOR NATIONAL DEFENSE.

(2) SERVES ON HIGH DEFENSE COUNCIL, COUNCIL OF MINISTERS; DIRECTLY RESPONSIVE TO PRESIDENT AND RESPONSIBLE FOR DEFENSE ESTABLISHMENT

(3) EACH MEMBER OF THE COMMITTEE OF CHIEFS OF STAFF HAS INDEPENDENT ACCESS TO THE MINISTER OF NATIONAL DEFENSE

(4) GENDARMEIRE PART OF ARMED FORCES DURING WARTIME

Source: Ministry of National Defense, *White Paper on National Defense*, chaps. 1–2.

to pit the army against both the air force and the navy; and interservice rivalries that are especially pronounced in the army.[157] There is also the more fundamental administrative problem posed at all levels by the ubiquitous French civil service. The civil service in France is, in a certain sense, closer to the British than it is to the U.S. model, being not only powerful but also well trained and professional—something the American civil service would do well to attempt to emulate. Yet while such a bureaucratic apparatus promotes administrative continuity and facilitates the implementation of policies and programs it endorses, it may also—like all bureaucracies—delay or kill initiatives that it opposes.[158] Inflexibility at any of the three stages in the *planification-program-mation-budget* sequence, as well as in the actual implementation of them, necessarily flaws the process as an integrated whole. The French bureaucracy is in a position to do just that, if it so chooses.

Third, there is the question of finance—that is, of resources that can actually be devoted to national defense in both a relative and an absolute sense. Manpower costs are increasing in France as in other Western countries. Higher manpower-related costs mean either higher defense budgets in an absolute sense or reduced outlays for research and development, operations, and maintenance (the areas of France's greatest need) if outlays are kept constant or increase to an inadequate degree. This difficulty is compounded by the continually increasing cost of operations, including those under way in the Persian Gulf, which—when added to manpower-related costs—further reduces the funds available for procurement. This problem is particularly acute for general-purpose forces, and especially for the manpower-intensive army, given the enduring precedence assigned to the retention and modernization of the nuclear forces. It also has an impact on the degree of support that can be given by the government to research and development in the public sector, one-third of whose funds are devoted to defense-related research projects.[159] As figure 4 shows, real increases in defense outlays from 1981 to 1987 hardly suffice to avoid some hard choices. Indeed, the real increase in 1987 barely managed to offset the *decline* in real defense outlays that occurred from 1982 to 1986. Compromises obviously have to be made somewhere if France is to have what it considers to be an adequate defense at a politically acceptable and budgetarily feasible cost.

Somewhat balancing these pressures for compromise are certain assets, intangible and tangible alike, on which those charged with the planning and implementation of France's defense policy can draw. The French preoccupation with autonomy in world politics, albeit somewhat circumscribed by the aforementioned adjustments under way in French policy, still gives France's decision makers considerable resilience in the face of external opposition or criticism. Indeed, such criticism is usually counterproductive, at least from the perspective of foreign governments, as the United States learned once again when it criticized France for its refusal to allow American aircraft based in Great Britain overflight rights during their punitive strike against Libya. This is because foreign criticism tends to produce a measure of popularly supported official recalcitrance that virtually guarantees that France will adamantly pursue whatever policy provoked opposition, simply to demonstrate France's status as a power of consequence in the world. Nor is domestic opposition outside of the normal political process of much significance (except, perhaps, when it results in mass risings in the streets of Paris!). On the contrary, a perusal of the French literature in this field suggests that French defense officials, uniformed and civilian alike, present their cases and dismiss their critics with a degree of aplomb rarely encountered in the United States and some other Western countries. Tangible assets include a reasonably robust economy relative to many other countries; the sophistication of French technology in many areas; a generally competent and stable industrial labor force, despite the political divisions and union activism that reflect France's class and party structure; and a relatively young, well educated and technically competent population, particularly when contrasted to countries such as West Germany and Great Britain.

The extent to which various French governments have had to make compromises, these assets notwithstanding, can be discerned in the various program laws passed over the past decade. For example, the Loi de programmation, 1977–1982 was intended to implement a long-term decision (*planification*) to move to a strategy based on the concept of the *sanctuarisation élargie* (enlarged sanctuary), a doctrine approximating some form of flexible response, and a greater degree of emphasis on reorganized and upgraded general purpose forces. Yet bureaucratic and budgetary forces combined to make the future more like the past than might have been anticipated by someone contemplating the potential budgetary implica-

Figure 4. Evolution of the Defense Budget (Constant Francs: 1981 = 100)

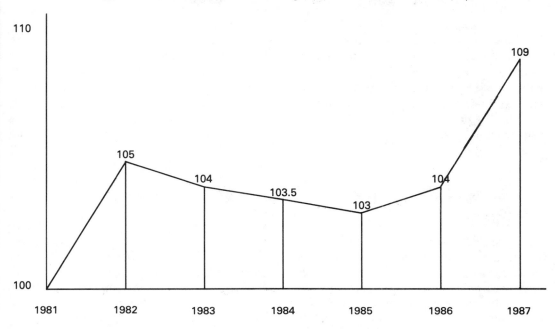

Source: "Les Grandes Données du Budget 1987," *Armées d'Aujourd'hui*, 117 (February 1987): 28.

tion of the *sanctuarisation élargie* and "flexible response" for French defense policy.[160] Mitterrand's own Loi de programmation, 1984–1988 had the objective of reaffirming French autonomy, enhancing France's aggregate power, and modernizing the French defense establishment while realizing some budgetary savings. The priorities contained therein were to enhance the credibility of the nuclear forces, strengthen France's capability to meet its implicit commitments to the Atlantic Alliance without rejoining the alliance's integrated military structure, and improve the capacity for out-of-area operations. Improvements were realized in some respects, such as organization and deployment, and some major procurement decisions were made (for example, to develop the SX mobile land-based missile and to harden existing IRBM [intermediate-range ballistic missile] silos). But the decline in real defense budgets noted in figure 4 required a reduction in personnel strength (especially in the army) that raised questions about the readiness of the remaining forces. More to the point, the first program law put into effect by the government

of "cohabitation" between Mitterrand and Chirac suggested that here, too, France's reach had exceeded its grasp. The new Loi de programme d'équipement militaire, 1987–1991 was put into effect even though its predecessor still had two years left to run. Many of the earlier decisions were continued, but it was clear that increased emphasis would be given to all types of nuclear forces. Other procurement decisions were delayed or deferred.[161]

On balance, it seems certain that French ambitions will continue to guide French defense planning and have a major influence on those decisions affecting the structure, composition, armament, and deployment of the French armed forces. The process itself is virtually certain to remain centralized, and power will continue to be concentrated in the office of the presidency, although internal compromises may well be necessitated at a procedural level by domestic political developments. It is also all too likely that the outcome of that process will continue to be uneven, just as "the history of military program-laws under the Fifth Republic is one of great accomplishments—but also of delays, cutbacks, and outright cancellations in equipment programs."[162] The clash of overcommitment at the level of *planification* with rigorous planning at the level of *budget* has not altered appreciably in recent years and is unlikely to change greatly in the future. This is the almost inevitable consequence of a defense policy dictated more by French pretensions than by French capabilities. It represents a challenge of considerable significance for the French government.

Recurring Issues and Defense Policy Outputs

Despite France's difficulties, the outcome of this complex interaction of role selection, threat perception, strategic choice, and defense decision-making process is a relatively large and remarkably sophisticated military establishment that is active in a surprisingly diverse set of issues and areas in the world. Five specific resultants of this interplay will be examined here: France's (a) current state of civil-military relations, (b) force posture, (c) weapons acquisition system and arms trade, (d) arms control and disarmament policy, and (e) use of force abroad.

CIVIL-MILITARY RELATIONS

The multifaceted role of the armed forces in the French defense decision-making process is suggestive of the complex place held by the military in French society as a whole. For a variety of historical and cultural reasons, the French military (and particularly the army) is seen by different groups as embodying both the spirit of the nation and a potential threat to the constitutional order of the Fifth Republic. Historically, the armed forces have been the guardians and the instruments of French grandeur, and an integral part of society. This is reflected today in the broad-based support for the *force de dissuasion* and the espousal of the primacy of military power in world politics. But at other times in France's past the armed forces have been used by various governments or the so-called ruling classes to suppress the "common people" at home and to oppress in-

digenous colonial peoples abroad. The notion that the military, or at least the professional officer corps, is at heart the repository of reactionary political forces represents this perspective. The activities of the "Secret Army Organization" (OAS) and the abortive coup d'etat during the Algerian crisis provide reasonably recent reminders of this particular concern.

The affirmative view of the armed forces is, not surprisingly, most popular with present and former members of the officer corps, as well as with the aristocracy and bourgeoisie. It finds the greatest degree of political support in the right-of-center political parties. Conversely, the more critical view of the French military is particularly common among enlisted men, the working classes, and the intelligentsia. Not surprisingly, the communists and (to a lesser extent) the socialists tend to adhere to this position, although many of them serve in all ranks—enlisted and commissioned alike—of the armed forces. But class and party lines are not clear discriminators in this regard, and both perspectives exist—indeed, sometimes coexist—at all levels of French society.

It is the ambiguous character of civil-military relations in France that, more than any other single factor, dictates the model of military service in the Fifth Republic. That model is neither one of selective service (as practiced in many countries in Western Europe and elsewhere) nor of an exclusively all-volunteer or professional force (what the French call the *armée de metier*). It is instead a form of "national service" or "national conscription" that was adopted in 1959 and today provides approximately one-half of the personnel in the regular armed forces.[163] In this system "a draftee serves for one year. He then goes into the active reserve for four years and spends the next thirteen in the general reserve."[164] And while it is true that there "is relatively little conscientious objection"[165] to a form of national service with approximately three-quarters of those who are eligible to be drafted each year supporting such service, this support for national services in its current form is by no means constant, as the trends in figure 5 illus-

Figure 5. Support in France for National Service

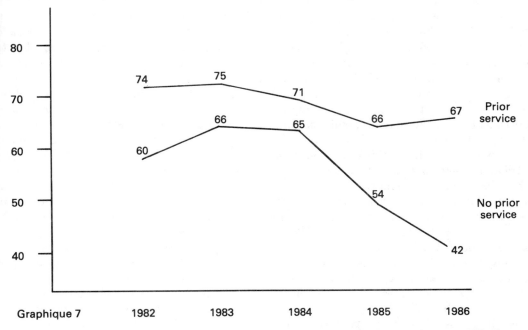

Graphique 7

Source: Jean-Paul Le Bourg, "Opinion et Défense en 1986," *Armées d'Aujourd'hui*, 117 (February 1987): 18.

trate. The decline in support among those who have yet to enter the national service system has occurred as the imminence of direct military threats to France has receded. This trend may turn out to be especially troublesome for French defense planners over the long term. Approximately 29 percent of those polled in France in 1986 also believed that one year of national service was too long a time to spend in uniform.[166] Although by no means a majority, this is indicative of the appearance throughout Europe of growing public pressure to reduce both the human and the financial costs of a military service whose utility is increasingly coming to be questioned.

Despite these reservations, the existing system of national service—which is seen as a means of resolving the conflicting perspectives on the position of the military in French society—was adopted and persists for three basic reasons. First, budgetary considerations make national conscription popular with any French government. Short-term conscripts cost less, in terms of pay and benefits, than either long or short-term volunteers in an advanced industrial society. Second, the career military remain favorably predisposed to this form of military service. This is partly because national conscription allows the armed forces to avoid manpower shortfalls or manpower-driven force reductions by the simple expedient of calling up the annual cohort of French youth. But they are also supportive of this system because the career military see service in the armed forces as a means of forging a sense of national identity and allegiance to France among the conscripts, many of whom come from what the professional military would consider to be "politically suspect origins." And, finally, national conscription is endorsed by the left for the opposite reason to the career military. That is, the left sees national conscription as a leavening influence on the military establishment that helps alleviate fears of an all-volunteer force that might eventually become an instrument for supression of the left.[167]

The existence of such a broad base of support for the concept of national service does

not, however, mean that it has escaped criticism from France's political parties, as reflected in the polls mentioned above. On the
contrary, the fact that such a high proportion
of the French armed forces is composed of conscripts serving a single year on active duty has
engendered criticism from both political
wings. The left essentially lobbies for a reduction in the length of mandated service, an improvement in pay and working conditions, and
the right of military personnel (or at least the
conscripts) to unionize and engage in collective
bargaining with military "management."[168]
For its part, the right (along with many professional soldiers) tends to believe that a single
year of service is simply too short in an era of
increasingly sophisticated military technology.
There is also some concern about the potential
unreliability (in both political and military
senses) of the conscripts, especially in the event
of civil strife in France or an intervention in
some part of the Third World. Compounding
this concern is the fact that conscripts—by
law—cannot be deployed overseas without the
prior approval of the National Assembly unless
they volunteer for such service. To hedge
against that possible unreliability and to have a
viable instrument for power projection abroad,
while retaining the national conscription
model of military service for its acknowledged
advantages, the French government maintains
some forty-four regiments (each equivalent in
strength to a U.S. battalion) for overseas service. Some of these regiments are composed
entirely of volunteers; others are not. These
units are concentrated in the French Foreign
Legion (all of whose personnel are volunteers)
and Rapid Action Force, in which "[all] of the
officers and men are either long-service professionals or recruits who have signed waivers allowing the government to send them overseas
without parliamentary approval."[169] These formations, plus some overseas garrisons, are the
French government's implicit "ace in the hole"
for dealing with militarily demanding and politically sensitive situations at home or abroad.
There has also been a continuation of earlier
efforts to make the armed forces in general
and the army in particular more popular with
the public by having them engage in a wide

range of what would be called "civic action
programs" in the United States, especially in
areas outside major urban centers. Doing so, it
is apparently reasoned, may help soldiers and
civilians alike to think better of one another, to
their mutual benefit as well as to the benefit of
France itself.

These countervailing tendencies are likely to
persist as long as the system of national conscription remains in effect, regardless of which
party rules or shares power in Paris. Nor is
there any indication that this model of military
service will be replaced in the foreseeable future. Calls to significantly reduce the term of
national service, or to emulate the American
and British models by adopting an all-volunteer force, are equally likely to persist and to be
largely unsuccessful. The political barriers to
significant changes are simply too great to permit the French government to replace the system of national conscription, regardless of its
inefficient and uneconomical use of personnel.
The flaws in national conscription are simply
not considered to be sufficiently great, insofar
as French opinion is concerned, to overcome
the liabilities associated with the alternatives to
the manpower equivalent of the *force de dissuasion* in the French military mythology.

FORCE POSTURE

A perennial question when appraising the
defense policy of any nation, as Paul Viotti
once pointed out, "is whether doctrine guides
the evolution of force posture or . . . the converse is true."[170] In the case of France, as suggested earlier, doctrine tends to be the "driver,"
notwithstanding periodic changes in priorities
or occasional programmatic modifications.
The sequential linking of doctrinal change to
alternations in force posture does not always
operate well, of course. But to a remarkable
extent, especially for a Western country,
"France's doctrine [has] responded to changes
in France's domestic and foreign environment
[and has shaped the French armed forces ac-
cordingly]."[171] I have already discussed how
changes in France's foreign and domestic environments have altered French strategy and
doctrine. The question to be addressed here is
the cumulative effect of those changes on

France's military force posture today, and what they portend for the future.

To address this question, I shall examine five principal aspects of France's force posture. They are: (a) aggregate trend data on defense efforts, including the projected impact of the Loi de programme d'équipement militaire,1987–1991; (b) the nuclear forces, strategic and tactical alike; (c) the general forces, with specific reference to the reorganization and redeployment of the army, and the creation of the Force d'Action Rapide (FAR), France's version of the American rapid deployment force; (d) the reserve and paramilitary forces; and (e) the future direction of trends bearing directly on French force posture.

In the first place the aggregate trend data on French defense efforts presented in table 4 depict the same pattern that appeared in the 1970s, persisting throughout the 1980s. This is a substantial allocation of human, financial, and material resources in an absolute sense, and less of a relative effort than might be anticipated if one took France's proclaimed ambitions and objectives at face value. This remains particularly apparent when one compares French defense efforts with those of its closest and less overtly ambitious neighbors: Great Britain (the only other nuclear-armed Western European country) and the Federal Republic of Germany. On the other hand, it is clear that France's considerable outlays for defense have given that country one of the largest and most sophisticated military establishments in the world, with a reasonably well balanced mix of forces unmatched in overall nominal capability except by the two superpowers.[172] Coupled with France's national service system, the result is a French defense establishment of nearly 547,000 active duty personnel, of whom approximately 45 percent are one-year conscripts. The increasing trend toward a more professional force that has occurred while retaining the national service system is reflected in the decline in the proportion of the total force composed of conscripts from the 1979 high of 54%.[173]

Nevertheless, these efforts, while sufficiently impressive in an absolute sense, simply do not seem commensurate with what would be required to lend substance to France's claim to be the leading power in Western Europe, capable of acting independently in world politics and professing to stand immediately behind the superpowers in the eyes of the world. Table 4 clearly shows the price France has paid in terms of its defense effort under Mitterrand, modified by increased efforts during the 1986–87 government of "cohabitation" between Mitterrand and Chirac. Relative to the FRG and Great Britain, moreover, France's efforts are somewhat less impressive, except in terms of the size of its active-duty armed forces. French defense outlays in current dollars have tended to be slightly less than those of Britain.[174] One would have expected a country with France's global designs to do rather more for its own defense than is actually the case. Certainly, a defense effort more appropriate for that design— that is, one considerably greater than that made by either Great Britain or West Germany—would have produced a military establishment whose size and capabilities would be more in keeping with France's declared role, strategy, and doctrine.

French decision makers are hardly unaware of the need to rectify some of the most glaring inconsistencies between proclaimed ends and available means. Mitterrand has attempted— not entirely successfully—to maintain the strategic nuclear force while upgrading the overall military establishment. The recent Loi de programme d'équipement militaire, 1987–1991, and particularly the 1987 defense budget, in

Table 4. Trends in French Defense Efforts

Category	1981	1984	1986	1987a
Military personnelb	504.6	464.3	557.5	546.9
Defense outlaysc	23,867	20,212	24,230	29,260
Per capita outlaysd	444	370	435	N/A
Outlays as percentage of GDP	4.2	4.1	3.5	N/A

Source: International Institute for Strategic Studies, *The Military Balance, 1987–1988* (London: IISS, 1987), pp. 60, 212.

a1987 estimated only.
bIn thousands; regular/active-duty personnel only.
cEstimates based on current exchange rates in U.S. $ million.
dIn current dollars, without controlling for inflation.

many ways represent a reaffirmation of classical Gaullist views on the primacy of the *force de dissuasion*, strategic and "pre-strategic" (that is, tactical) alike, as the sole guarantee of France's "survival and . . . independence."[175] It is worth emphasizing that the size and utility of the *force de dissuasion* are "not determined in relation to the force level of potential adversaries."[176] Instead, it is presumed to have both intrinsic and extrinsic value to France by virtue of its very existence.

That existence, it should be noted, is more than nominal. Occasional disparaging remarks (largely from outside France) to the contrary notwithstanding, the *force de dissuasion* has at its disposal a strategic triad of nuclear-powered ballistic missile submarines (SSBNs), land-based intermediate-range ballistic missiles, and manned bombers, complemented by an increasingly wide and sophisticated mix of tactical nuclear weapons. The result is a force with an exceptional degree of diversity and operational flexibility, manned by some 27,500 personnel from all branches of the armed forces, including the Gendarmerie.[177] All of these forces are being modernized as part of the Loi de programme d'équipement militaire, 1987–1991.

The first leg of France's strategic triad to become operational was the manned bomber force, now considered its most vulnerable component. It now consists of twenty-two Mirage IV-A strike aircraft configured to carry a single sixty-kiloton AN-22 gravity bomb apiece, plus fifteen Mirage IV-P's carrying a single ASMP 100–150 kiloton air-to-surface missile with a maximum range of 300 kilometers. Three more Mirage IV-A's are being converted to carry the ASMP, with six additional Mirage IV-A's in reserve as reconnaissance aircraft. Support is provided by eleven KC-135F tankers for in-flight refueling, as well as four Transall C-160 Astarte airborne command and communications aircraft. The decision to proceed with the development and deployment of the ASMP air-to-surface missile represented a belief that it was strategically and budgetarily necessary to extend the useful operational life of the manned bomber part of the triad.

The second part of the strategic triad consists of the land-based intermediate-range ballistic (IRBM) force based in silos on the Plateau d'Albion in southern France. This force, organized under the aegis of the First Strategic Missile Group, has at its disposal eighteen IRBMs in individual silos; initial plans to deploy nine additional IRBMs were never realized. Early in the 1980s, the older SSBS S-2 missiles (capable of delivering a single 150-kiloton warhead a distance of approximately 1,800 miles) were removed, and the silos were retrofitted with the new SSBS S-3D/TN-61 missiles, each of which carries a single 1-megaton thermonuclear warhead for an estimated range of 2,200 miles. It is intended to harden the IRBM silos as part of the Loi de programme d'équipement militaire, 1987–1991, now in force.

Pride of place within the French strategic nuclear force, however, belongs to the ballistic missile submarine force. There are two principal reasons for making the submarine "the principal element in French deterrent strategy."[178] One is the relatively greater potential survivability of the SSBN force if deterrence should fail. The other is its significantly greater contribution to France's aggregate strategic striking power. The SSBN force currently consists of six nuclear-powered ballistic missile submarines. One SSBN is equipped with the new MSBS M-4/TN-70 missile, capable of delivering six MIRVed 150-kiloton warheads to a range in excess of 2,800 miles. The five remaining SSBNs have the older MSBS M-20/TN-60 missile, carrying a single 1-megaton warhead for some 1,900 miles. It is intended to retrofit these submarines during their refits with either the MSBS M-1/TN-70 missile or an improved version (the MSBS M-4/TN-71) with a range of approximately 4,000 miles. It has been decided to proceed with a "new generation" submarine, intended to be France's seventh operational SSBN. This vessel is projected to be of some 13,000 tons displacement, to carry a new MSBS M-5 missile with as many as twelve MIRVed warheads and more range than the MSBSM-4/TN-71 missile, and to be in service by 1994. The intent is to be able to have three submarines "on patrol at any one time."[179]

Although less ambitious than the design of the strategic nuclear force, there also exists what might best be called a "second level" of the *force de dissuasion*. This is a diverse and growing array of nuclear weapons systems at the disposal of all three French services that other countries would call "tactical" but that France (as noted earlier) terms "pre-strategic" nuclear weapons because of their place in French doctrine. Whatever the ambiguity in their nomenclature, however, there can be no ambivalence about either the objective capabilities of these weapons systems or the French determination to modernize them. The fact is that the 1987 defense budget increased outlays by more than 40 percent over the previous year's level for these systems. The current "dean" of the French "pre-strategic" force is the Pluton, a relatively short-range (about seventy-five miles) missile carrying a single 15 to 25 kiloton warhead. The Pluton first became operational in 1974; at present, thirty Pluton launchers in five regiments are operational. A replacement for the Pluton, called the Hades (the names may be suggestive in these instances!), is scheduled to become operational in the 1990s. The Hades will carry a single warhead of from 20 to 60 kilotons, have a range of approximately 220 miles, and is likely to be deployed in considerably larger numbers—perhaps as many as one hundred launchers, suggesting a growing French interest in these systems.

Complementing these French army systems are the assets of the navy and the air force. The former has some thirty-eight Super Etendard carrier-based aircraft, each of which is configured to carry one (and perhaps two) AN-52 15-kiloton weapons. The air force has forty-five Jaguar and thirty Mirage IIIE land-based attack aircraft, with differing operational ranges but the same payload as the Super Etendard. The navy plans to equip its aircraft with ASMP air-to-surface missiles as soon as possible, while the air force intends to deploy at least eighty-five Mirage 2000-N aircraft—also configured to carry a single ASMP apiece—in place of its existing assets by the 1990s. France also has the declared capability to "produce neutron bombs in several

months"[180] following a decision to do so, but has apparently declined to exercise that option for the present.

The combination of strategic and "pre-strategic" nuclear weapons systems described above certainly gives France an impressive nuclear array at its disposal. In-place force modernization programs can only enhance that capability in the future. Indeed, it has been suggested that "by [the] mid-1990s French nuclear forces, strategic and tactical, will be able to cover 956 targets [simultaneously]—more than enough to make the republic's nuclear forces credible."[181] There is also a clear determination to continue considering a variety of damage-inflicting and damage-limiting options to ensure (insofar as that can ever be done in a nuclear conflict environment) that sufficient nuclear forces would survive an opponent's first strike to make that course of action unappealing to any potential aggressor. It is worth noting that these programs and plans do not intend to supplant any existing force types, but rather to improve or to complement them. For example, an assessment of the IRBM force concluded that even a proposed SX mobile land-based missile would not totally replace the fixed IRBMs at the Plateau d'Albion.[182]

Yet there are problems as well. Three of the six SSBNs now operational will reach the end of their effective sea-going lives in the 1990s; the remaining three will do likewise in the first decade of the next century. Replacing six SSBNs (or even some of them) with state-of-the-art boats will be an extremely costly exercise. The increasing range of the "pre-strategic" systems—especially the aviation assets equipped with the ASMP air-to-surface missile—is on the verge of blurring somewhat the distinction made in French doctrine between those systems and the more strictly defined strategic systems. The diversity of French "pre-strategic" systems also raises doubts about the relevance of French employment doctrine for them. It is difficult to see how one could coordinate the declared "single salvo" or "final shot across the bow" of army-controlled surface-to-surface missiles and both land-based and carrier-based aviation, with either gravity bombs or stand-off air-to-surface missiles, and have any hope of accomplishing what French doctrine says those forces should do. Foreign programs such as the U.S. strategic defense initiative (SDI) also cause French planners concerns. If SDI induces the USSR to develop its own strategic defenses, the long-term consequences may be counterproductive for France.[183] Clearly, the future holds many uncertainties for the architects of the *force de dissuasion* and the theology of autonomy it has been intended to underwrite.

The not unexpected reaffirmation of support for the *force de dissuasion* has not meant a decline in support for conventional forces, all of which receive real budget increases in the Loi de programme d'équipement militaire, 1987–1991 and the 1987 defense budget. When presenting the 1987 defense budget to the National Assembly, Defense Minister Giraud made a point of asserting that "France should equally have at its disposal the conventional means to discourage any hostile action for which a nuclear riposte would not be considered justifiable."[184] In practical terms, beyond adjustments in declared policy and doctrine, this has entailed a reorganization of the army—the third such action within a decade—a redeployment of some major French army headquarters and formations, and some major procurement decisions to modernize all of the services. The dual objectives of these measures were to increase France's capability to act "effectively in support of her Atlantic Alliance commitments" and to provide a credible rapid deployment force for service in either Europe or the Third World.[185]

Not surprisingly, given its size and status within the French defense establishment as a whole, the army has continued to be the principal beneficiary of ongoing force modernization efforts in the conventional sphere. The initial reorganization began in 1976–77; it was intended to create a ground force structure that would have a larger number of smaller maneuver formations than had existed previously, with an enhanced capability to conduct mechanized operations. A sequel, which was essentially completed in 1982, continued that process, increasing the number of armored and infantry divisions (which, in the French army,

have the strength of a reinforced American brigade). The most recent reorganization eliminated the 4th and 6th armored divisions from the force structure; created two "new" divisions, the 4th airmobile and the 6th light armored; and converted the 12th and 14th infantry divisions into light armored divisions.[186] The army's force structure in 1978 and in 1987 is presented in table 5. The deployment of the principal headquarters appears in figure 6. Major garrisons are located in Germany (including the Berlin garrison): 53,000 personnel; the overseas dependencies: 22,000 personnel; and contingents in Africa and the Middle East in support of various treaty and international commitments: 11,000 personnel. Personnel for these garrisons are, of course, drawn from all services, including the Gendarmerie, although the army invariably supplies the largest component.[187]

One sign of an increased French willingness to meet its Atlantic Alliance commitments was the deployment northwards of the headquarters of the III Corps from St. Germain to Lille, along the Belgian border. Far more significant, however, was the creation in 1983 of France's rapid deployment force—the Force d'Action Rapide (FAR). France has traditionally designated certain units for an intervention role abroad, of course, above and beyond the all-volunteer French Foreign Legion. But the FAR has a broader mandate. As John Chipman relates: "The establishment of this new intervention structure was an attempt to reconcile France's African (and Middle East) military vocation with the need to be able to come to the aid of France's allies in Europe."[188] The result was a force of five divisions dedicated to the FAR mission (a rather different situation than that of the U.S. Central Command), totaling 47,000 personnel and a diversity of capabilities. The order of battle of the FAR, including its principal matériel inventories, is depicted in figure 7.[189]

This is clearly an ambitious undertaking. It remains to be seen how effective the FAR will be, or the extent to which it can be equipped adequately without unduly penalizing the remainder of the army. Certainly, programs such as the new main battle tank will compete with

Table 5. Divisional Force Structure

Unit Type	1978	1987
Field army headquarters	First Army	First Army
Corps headquarters	I Corps	I Corps
	II Corps	II Corps
		III Corps
Armored divisions	1st, 3rd, 4th, 5th, 6th, 7th, 10th	1st, 2nd, 3rd, 5th, 7th, 10th
Mechanized divisions	8th	—
Light armored divisions	—	6th, 12th, 14th
Airmobile divisions	—	4th
Marine divisions	9th	9th
Infantry divisions	14th, 15th	8th, 15th
Alpine divisions	27th	27th
Parachute divisions	11th	11th

Sources: Francis Carjean, "Armée de terre," Défense Nationale, February 1979, pp. 146–49; D. C. Isby and C. Kamps, Jr., Armies of NATO's Central Front (London: Jane's Publishing, 1985), p. 127.

the FAR's requirement for expanded airlift and sealift. All will compete with the need for enhanced sustainability and more extensive training of all personnel. As with the *force de dissuasion*, questions persist about the degree of linkage between design and execution over the long term.

Like that of the army, the navy's position in the defense establishment continues to be augmented, reinforced by the visibility of French naval forces in the Persian Gulf crisis. For many years, however, the principal purpose of the French fleet was to deploy and to protect the SSBNs of the *force de dissuasion*. All of that began changing in the late 1970s. The French navy retains its original mission and gives precedence to it. But it has also accepted a wider range of tasks normally associated with the sea control and power-projection missions of a major naval power. Specifically, the French navy is charged with (a) participating in the *force de dissuasion*; (b) securing the maritime approaches to France and its overseas territories; (c) securing France's access to resources and its essential lines of communication; (d) conducting operations in support of French interests, especially along the Mediterranean littoral; and (e) carrying out what former Minister of National Defense Yvon Bourges once described as "the essential mission of giving, by its presence in the world, an impression of France's status."[190]

The naval forces available to France are both impressive in an absolute sense and reasonably compatible with at least some of the missions they are expected to be able to exe- cute—at least in concert with other states. Independently, however, one has a lingering sense that the French Navy is obliged to apply the naval assets of a middle power to the commitments expected of the truly global power France once was, and would like to be in fact as well as in claim. In the late 1980s, nonetheless, the French navy had some 69,000 personnel assigned to five principal naval commands. In addition to the aforementioned SSBN force, it had seventeen operational attack submarines, three of them of the nuclear-powered Rubis class. It also operated forty-five principal surface combatants, including two conventionally powered (and aging) attack carriers, one helicopter carrier, one cruiser, sixteen destroyers and twenty-five frigates. Rounding out the navy are thirty-five minor surface combatants, fifty-two amphibious craft, and sixty-three auxiliaries. The fleet air arm has at its disposal 122 combat aircraft (including the nuclear-capable Super Etendard strike aircraft) and twenty-four armed helicopters, plus auxiliary aircraft. There are also smaller contingents of French marine commandos and naval base defense personnel. Planned acquisitions are extensive, and include at least four additional SSBNs, twelve frigates, and two nuclear attack carriers. France's first nuclear-powered attack carrier is intended to displace approximately 35,000 tons and carry 35–40 aircraft. It was laid down in 1986, and should enter service in the mid 1990s. French naval planning for the future is clearly proceeding apace.[191]

Finally, the French air force now has some 96,000 personnel, organized into Air Defense,

Figure 6. Major Unit Headquarters

4th Armoured Division (Nancy)
6th Armoured Division (Strasbourg)

Artillery: 9 RAMa (F3) (Trier)
Engineers: 13 RG (Trier)
Support: 1 RCS (Trier)

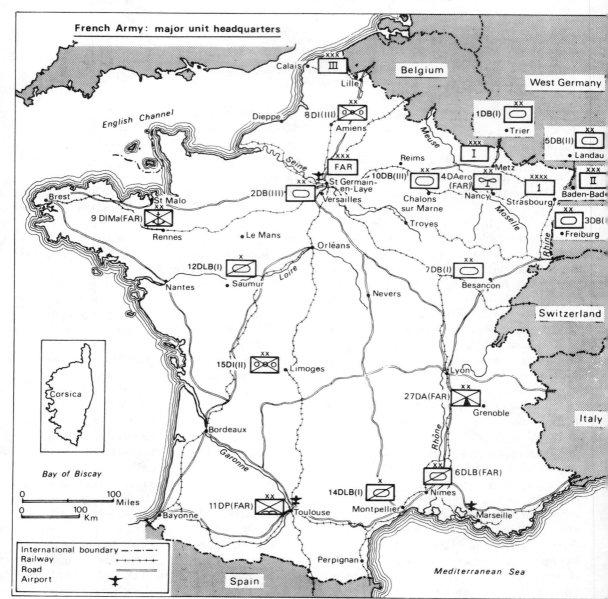

Source: D. C. Isby and C. Kamps, Jr., *Armies of NATO's Central Front* (London: Jane's Publishing, 1985), p. 127.

Figure 7. Order of Battle of the Force d'Action Rapide (FAR)

```
┌──────────────────────────────────────┐   ┌─────────────┐   ┌──────────────────────┐
│         GENEREAL STAFF               │   │     FAR     │   │  LOGISTIC BRIGADE    │
│      AND COMMAND POSTS               │   └─────────────┘   │     6,500 MEN        │
│        COMMUNICATIONS                │                     │   2,000 VEHICLES     │
│  RITA SYSTEM AND SYRACUSE STATIONS   │                     │    (in wartime)      │
└──────────────────────────────────────┘                     └──────────────────────┘
```

4th AIRMOBILE DIVISION

1 command and maneuver
helicopter regiment
1 airmobile support regiment
3 combat helicopter regiments
1 airmobile combat regiment
with:
6,400 men
1,500 vehicles
240 helicopters comprising
    (80 Puma transports, 90 Gazelle
    anti-tank helicopters
    with HOT missiles, 30 Gazelles
    with 20mm cannons
    and 40 observation helicopters
48 Milan launchers
30 Mistrar launchers
12 120mm mortars

6th LIGHT ARMOURED DIVISION

1 command and support regiment
2 armoured regiments
2 infantry regiments with VAB APCs
1 artillery regiment
1 engineer regiment
with:
7,500 men
1,750 vehicles
72 AMX 10RC
340 APCs
24 VAB HOT*
48 Milan launchers
36 Mistrar launchers
24 towed 155mm howitzers
12 120mm mortars

11th PARACHUTE DIVISION

2 command and support regiments
1 light armoured cavalry regiment
6 infantry regiments
1 artillery regiment
1 engineer regiment
with:
13,000 men
2,800 vehicles
36 ERC 90 Sagaie
168 Milan launchers
Mistral launchers
36 120mm mortars

9th MARINE INFANTRY DIVISION

1 command and support regiment
2 armoured regiments
2 infantry regiments with VAB APCs (+ one
motorized infantry regiment in peacetime)
1 artillery regiment
2 engineer companies (one regiment in wartime)
with (in peacetime):
8,000men
1,700 vehicles
72 ERC 90 Sagaie
340 VAB*
120 Milan launchers
Mistral launchers
24 towed 155mm howitzers*
24 120mm mortars

27th MOUNTAIN DIVISION

1 command and support regiment
1 light armoured regiment
6 infantry regiments or battalions
1 artillery regiment
1 engineer battalion
with:
9,000 men
1,550 vehicles
36 ERC 90 Sagaie*
108 Milan launchers
Mistrar launchers
24 towed 155mm howitzers*
36 120mm mortars

**Force
d'Action
Rapide
(FAR)-
organization
and
equipment**

*Equipment scheduled
for delivery

Source: International Defense Review, August 1987, p. 1024.

Tactical Air, Air Transport, and Training Commands, equipped with approximately 520 combat aircraft in addition to training and transport aircraft and helicopters. Air defense assets include twelve fighter squadrons, twelve SAM squadrons equipped with Crotale missile-firing and radar batteries, and some 300 batteries of 20mm antiaircraft artillery. The air defense system has been fully automated, but it remains true that "France is particularly vulnerable to low-altitude air attack, owing to a lack of effective detection means."[192] Tactical air assets comprise ten fighter/ground attack and three reconnaissance squadrons, plus six squadrons operationally subordinate to the Transport Command. Air transport assets additionally encompass twenty-one fixed wing and five helicopter transport squadrons. Finally, the Training Command disposes of more than 430 aircraft, some of which are obsolescent combat aircraft that could be pressed into active service in a secondary role if necessary. Projected acquisition programs for these operational commands include the Mirage-2000 series fighter and strike aircraft, F-1CR fighters, training and transport helicopters, light transport aircraft, and improved airborne detection and air-defense assets.[193]

Like most countries, France includes both paramilitary forces and reserves within its defense establishment. The principal paramilitary force is the Gendarmerie Nationale. In peacetime this force of some 90,000 personnel reports to the Ministry of the Interior. In wartime the Gendarmerie reports to the armed forces chief of staff and functions for all practical purposes as part of the French army. Upon mobilization the Gendarmerie approximately doubles in strength in order to execute its primary missions of maintaining order within France and of defending French territory against hostile incursions.[194]

The impact of reserve mobilization on the deployable strength of the Gendarmerie is suggestive of the role of reserves in the French armed forces as a whole. As is the case with other advanced industrial societies, France maintains an extensive organized reserve system. It makes use of a substantial number of trained reserves to bring its regular armed forces to full strength in wartime. At present, upon mobilization, reserves would provide 52 percent (305,000 personnel) of the army, 28 percent (28,000) of the navy, and 37 percent (58,000 personnel) of the air force.[195] France also employs a second tier of reserves for home defense. The old French reserve system, called the Défense Opérationelle du Territoire (DOT), was once composed largely of fourteen reserve divisions with regular cadres assigned to them in peacetime to facilitate operations. That system was abandoned in the mid 1980s. In its place France has created seven combined-arms defense zone brigades and twenty-three combined-arms territorial regiments with greater mobility and a more realistic use of available resources.[196]

It should be readily apparent from the preceding discussion that French defense policy is in the midst of a number of interesting initiatives, some of which it can control and some of which are hostage to external events. All, however, will bear on the type of force posture France attempts to maintain in being. A critical area is the impact of the internal requirement to replace a major part of the SSBN force in the next decade, and the external challenges posed by the emergence of strategic defense systems in the 1990s and beyond on the *force de dissuasion*.[197] There is no doubt that France will devote whatever resources are necessary to maintain what the French consider to be a credible strategic (and pre-strategic) nuclear capability. A nation that sees status and security to be so inextricably linked, both to one another and to the *force de dissuasion*, is highly likely to forswear the preeminent guarantor of those objectives. Less certain is France's ability over the long term to devote the resources required for it to develop the conventional force structure capable of fulfilling other missions as well. Emerging technologies, as other countries have found, may help in some ways, but they can also be a double-edged sword.[198] Budget constraints are formidable, and one has the impression that all of the compromises and readjustments of program design and execution have not yet been made.

WEAPONS ACQUISITION AND THE ARMS TRADE

For a military establishment to be truly capable of fulfilling its country's expectations, it is obviously necessary for its doctrine and force posture to be congruent with one another. But it is also necessary for it to be sufficiently well armed and equipped to be able to carry out its assigned missions. This requires a country either to produce or to have ready access to whatever military matériel its defense establishment needs.

In the case of France, the combined dictates of political autonomy and military necessity made it essential for the country to become largely self-sufficient in terms of weapons system research, development, and production. Independent powers, by France's definition, simply cannot afford to be dependent on others for the means of their own security. This is because such dependence implies a potential political vulnerability to the supplier that France considers to be unacceptable. American opposition to the French desire for a national nuclear force, in particular, compelled France to develop the full panoply of weapons systems technology essentially on its own, with all of the financial and operational costs associated with that effort. Finally, the French decision to withdraw from NATO in 1967, and France's unwillingness to participate in the Eurogroup collaborative weapons research and development consortium when it was first formed because of its ties to the United States, reinforced these tendencies toward self-sufficiency in the production of defense matériel—tendencies that ongoing policy reassessments in France have yet to alter appreciably.[199]

The net effect of these factors has been the development in France of a defense industry unmatched in effectiveness and productivity in Europe. France not only produces some of the most advanced weapons systems and associated technology in the world, but it is also the only Western European country to have an independently developed and comprehensive nuclear weapons research and development program capable of producing a wide range of warheads, delivery vehicles, guidance systems, and propulsion systems for both strategic and tactical purposes. France also independently produces the entire range of conventional weapons and other matériel needed by its armed forces.[200]

The fact that the French defense industry has developed that independent production capability does not mean that France abjures cooperative armaments research, development, and productive efforts with other countries, at least as long as the United States is not directly involved in the enterprise—an attitude that is so deep-seated in France that much will be needed for it to be moderated. With that exception, however, French participation in collaborative efforts on either a bilateral or a multilateral basis has been extensive and continues to grow, if not always without discord. French membership in the so-called Group of Six for defense industrial cooperation and in the aforementioned Independent European Program Group are the most noteworthy examples. Less extensive cooperative ventures in which France has participated, however, have already registered considerable achievements. Among the most wide-ranging arrangements to date are those with Great Britain. These have resulted in the development and production of the Jaguar fighter-bomber, the Martel AS-37 and AJ-168 air-to-surface missiles, and the Puma and Gazelle tactical assault and armed liaison/transport helicopters, among others. France has also engaged in cooperative efforts with other Western European countries. Prominent among them are ventures with the Federal Republic of Germany for the production of the HOT and Milan antitank and the Roland surface-to-air missiles, and the Alpha Jet training and light attack aircraft; the development of a new minesweeper of L'Eridan class with the Netherlands; the Otomat naval surface-to-surface missile and the ATR twin turboprop transport in development with Italy; and the NH-90 surface attack and tactical transport helicopter being developed in concert with Italy, West Germany, and the Netherlands—established partners in bilateral efforts. Not all such enterprises have gone well, to be sure. The attempt to develop a main battle tank in tandem with West Germany collapsed in 1982, and France withdrew in 1985 from a five-nation attempt to develop the Eurofighter. And at least one of the limits of France's defense industry was acknowledged to have been reached when France agreed to purchase three Boeing E-3A AWACS aircraft in 1987, with delivery to occur by 1991.[201]

From the French perspective, France's increasing level of participation in the cooperative development of weapons systems does not invalidate its fundamental belief in the importance of an antonomous defense capability in all respects. Most of the major and secondary weapons systems employed by the French armed forces are of French origin and manufacture, and impressive advances in space technologies are also being registered. This situation is unlikely to change in the future, if France has anything to say about it. But it is also recognized in France that international cooperation in the development and production of sophisticated weapons systems is essential in an increasingly complex and interdependent world, even for a country such as France, if only for increased economies of scale. Necessity, it seems, can be an ever more demanding taskmaster, notwithstanding the domestic constraints on France's willingness to cooperate with other countries. Indeed, recent decisions to proceed with the privatization of many of the largest French defense contractors (thereby facilitating joint development efforts with private concerns in other countries), to increase coproduction activities, and to consider both the possibility of technological exchanges (for example, German tanks for French helicopters) and selective foreign arms purchases[202] simply reflect a growing awareness of the implications of that necessity.

Less openly discussed in many circles than French cooperation in the design and production of armaments in Western Europe is the growing importance of arms sales abroad to the well-being of the French defense industry. By the mid 1980s, France had become the third largest arms exporter in the world, with over 80 percent of its exports going to Third World countries.[203] French arms sales in Africa in particular are often seen as a relatively low-profile form of intervention that provides

France with both a presence and a degree of leverage that it might otherwise not posssess. They also provide a basis for more direct French intervention in support of a good customer/client, especially in the former French colonies. Examples of French arms sales agreements with selected foreign countries (either completed or contracted) include the export of (a) Agosta-class diesel electric attack submarines to Spain; (b) helicopters of various classes to Spain, the Congo, Gabon, Nigeria, India, and Japan; (c) Mirage 2000 interceptors to India; and (d) landing craft to Senegal.[204] Earlier contractual arrangements involved an even greater diversity of weapons systems.[205]

There remain a number of actual or potential disadvantages to such extensive arms sales, however useful they may be to the health of the French arms industry. The most obvious liability is that French arms sales in the Third World, and particularly in Africa and the Middle East, mean that those countries in which France might have the greatest occasion to intervene will be better able to defend themselves against France and to resist French influence than might otherwise have been possible. Occasional French arguments to the effect that knowing the characteristics of one's own weapons helps French forces to defend themselves better seem something less than compelling. The fact that such arms sales continue to reflect short-term domestic and balance-of-trade concerns rather than long-term security interests, and may therefore be strategically counterproductive, has not gone unnoticed in French circles.[206] But it is equally clear that an avenue of escape from that dilemma (which, it should be noted, exists for more than one other Western country) is not readily apparent.

ARMS CONTROL AND DISARMAMENT POLICY

The conflict between economic interests and security concerns inherent in France's arms sales throughout the Third World has its parallel in France's approach to the problem of arms control. That approach is shaped by five factors widely considered to be relevant in France, albeit different parties occasionally ascribe different degrees of importance to one or more of them. These factors are: (a) the belief that

France's own forces, nuclear and conventional alike, threaten no one; (b) the certainty that actual or potential threats to French security and French interests do or may exist, within Europe or outside of it; (c) the conviction that arms control may be a means to enhanced security for France, but that it is not an end in itself whose attainment has any particular intrinsic value; (d) the view that arms control, in the sense of arms reductions, must be undertaken first by the superpowers, particularly when it pertains to nuclear weapons; and (e) the distinction that is made between vertical proliferation (the acquisition of additional weapons systems of a certain category by states that already possess systems of a similar class) and horizontal proliferation (the acquisition of weapons systems previously absent from a country's arsenal), especially with regard to nuclear weapons.[207]

The political-military implications of these considerations are all too apparent in France's approach to problems of arms control and disarmament in an increasingly more heavily armed world. Instead of making the usual distinctions between nuclear and non-nuclear systems, France has traditionally adhered to a geographical distinction between "existing nuclear zones, that is to say those already covered by the nuclear deterrent, and those that are not."[208] In the case of nuclear-free zones, which largely encompass the Third World (excluding the Middle East and South Asia, because of the Israeli and Indian nuclear capabilities presumed widely to exist), France's official policy is to refrain from introducing nuclear weapons technology (or technology with potential applicability to nuclear weapons) where such technology does not already exist. France also purports to encourage countries that do not now possess nuclear weapons to refrain from acquiring them elsewhere or developing them indigenously. In exchange for that self-restraint, France reaffirms its "guarantees" that it (a) "will not use nuclear weapons against them or on their territory [against a third party]," and (b) "will give them access to the peaceful uses of atomic power"—that is, to what has been called civilian nuclear technology.[209]

There are a number of rather obvious prob-lems with this approach to the issue of nuclear non-proliferation. One is that no nation truly believes that another will exercise unilateral self-restraint when its own interests—especially its actual or perceived vital interests—appear to be threatened. Certainly, few automatically assume that France would acquiesce in defeat rather than escalate, as the United States acquiesced in the Vietnam War, if it had the option of escalation at its disposal. France's willingness to request the use of atomic weapons by the United States in 1954 in an effort to "save" its beleaguered garrison at Dien Bien Phu,[210] coupled with the fact that the French decision to acquire nuclear weapons in the first place reflected in part a reaction to France's forced withdrawal from Suez in 1956, cannot be entirely reassuring to some countries in some parts of the world.

Second, even if France did not intend to use its own nuclear weapons against or on the territory of a non-nuclear Third World country, French restraint does not automatically imply security for the latter. Such forbearance on the part of France, after all, is no guarantee against coercion by another nuclear-armed state, or even by a more powerful conventionally armed country. Pakistan learned in 1971, for example, that the political encouragement and military self-restraint of the United States were inadequate assistance during its war with India. Any non-nuclear country in the Middle East engaged in a conflict with Israel must also be mindful of the fact that victory could be both transitory and more costly than defeat if the Israelis resorted to nuclear weapons to stave off conventional disaster regardless of calls for restraint the superpowers might make. There is no reason for other Third World countries to assume that a militarily weaker country such as France would demonstrate greater fidelity, or that either diplomatic support or conventional military assistance from France would suffice in such a situation. Thus, like France itself in the late 1950s and afterwards, a legitimate concern for security—with or without a corresponding interest in status—independent of what other countries might promise or provide could lead many nations in the Third World to want to emulate

France's own example and develop a national nuclear force, even if of modest proportions.

Third, and perhaps most important, is the fact that French policy toward the export of civilian nuclear technology may well facilitate, if not encourage, the realization by Third World countries of such ambitions. There is a very real potential contradiction between the declared French opposition to the introduction of nuclear weapons into non-nuclear zones and France's equally clear willingness to provide countries within such zones with nuclear technology for ostensibly peaceful purposes. India's detonation of its own "peaceful" nuclear device made it all too apparent that it is extremely difficult for a donor country adequately to police the way in which a recipient nation makes use of such technology without violating the latter's sovereignty to what most countries (and especially France itself, if it were the object of such attention) would consider to be an unacceptable degree. The provision of civilian nuclear technology may even precipitate an attack by a regional adversary of the recipient nation, as demonstrated by the Israeli attack against the French-supplied Iraqi nuclear reactor.[211] Both suggest that a somewhat different approach by France to the problem of nuclear proliferation and the transfer of nuclear technology may be warranted.

With respect to the existing nuclear zones in general, and to Europe in particular, French decision-makers have as a matter of principal tended to declare that two conditions need to be met before effective arms control can become a reality: (a) that the superpowers should take the lead in reducing their own strategic arsenals and (b) that the disparity in conventional forces favoring the Soviet Union and the other Warsaw Pact countries needs to be eliminated. Only when these preconditions have been met will it be possible to proceed seriously with more general and comprehensive arms control and disarmament programs involving other concerned countries, such as France itself. Adherence to, or at least advocacy of, these principles led France to approve the SALT process in general (if not the specific terms negotiated); to reject the MBFR (Mutual and Balanced Force Reductions) talks in

Vienna as counterproductive, on the grounds that almost any MBFR agreement that might be reached in that forum could only worsen the existing imbalance of forces in Europe; and to support reductions in theater nuclear forces, so long as those belonging to France (and to Great Britain as well, for consistency's sake) are neither explicitly nor implicitly part of any accord reached. The French, in short, have encouraged others to negotiate, while France itself abstains.[212]

As with most things, French practice has not conformed precisely to French assumptions and preconditions. Any undertakings that might affect adversely the theater military balance in general and the position of the French nuclear *force de dissuasion* in particular, have been opposed adamantly. Indeed, French participation in any program or negotiations to control nuclear weapons in Europe has continually been asserted to depend on the prior reduction of both international tension and conventional force levels in Europe. Achieving these objectives, in fact, underlay French support for the Helsinki Treaty of 1975 and France's proposal for the "Conference on Disarmament in Europe" (CDE), proposed by France to "increase confidence-building measures" and "improve the balance of military potential" in Europe "from the Atlantic to the Urals" (ATTU)—a proposal and a term that have come into their own.[213] A less obvious, but nonetheless significant, consideration in the French position is an appreciation of the fact that any East-West arms control undertaking of which France is not a part is something of a double-edged sword, especially if it involves bilateral understandings between the two superpowers. That is, any reduction in superpower strategic or theater nuclear arsenals necessarily enhances the marginal utility of the *force de dissuasion*. But if the effect of an accord that produces such a reduction in Soviet and American nuclear arsenals also brings the two superpowers closer to one another in diplomatic terms, that increase in amity between Moscow and Washington might well reduce France's own diplomatic maneuverability and diplomatic freedom of action in the world. As in the heyday of détente in the early 1970s,

France prefers relations between the Soviet Union and the United States to be peaceful, but not too close.

This ambivalence came home to roost with a vengeance in the aftermath of Mikhail Gorbachev's so-called "peace offensive" in 1986, and particularly following the signing of the Soviet-American accord on Intermediate-range Nuclear Forces (INF) in 1987.[214] The "peace offensive" itself was viewed with some reservations, incorporating as it did in the French view a potential "double [political and strategic] snare" that might divide the West without reducing the fundamental basis of East-West tensions.[215] Even before the fact, the possibility of a bilateral Soviet-American INF treaty was described rather pejoratively as "a new Munich," portending "a fatal decoupling between America and Europe."[216] Somewhat later, Mitterrand and Chirac, as well as their defense and foreign ministers, concurred in general (albeit with some minor differences) on the implications of a "zero option" Soviet-American INF treaty. The concept was found largely acceptable, although it was noted that it would be necessary to pay very close attention to the implications of the accord for the theater conventional balance. For its part, France will not be a party to any negotiations affecting its own strategic nuclear forces (which essentially have theater-specific capabilities or orientations in any case), but it does favor the "denuclearization" of the Continent, except for the nuclear forces of Great Britain and France—and, of course, those based on the national territory of the Soviet Union proper.[217] Thus, France will continue to enhance its own nuclear force. The fact is that France's seeming indifference to what it refuses to consider a legitimate problem may be counterproductive in the long run. On the other hand, this concern does not appear to be widely felt in France.

USE OF FORCE

The French preoccupation with the military trappings of status and France's ambivalent attitude toward arms control are reflected to a certain extent in the use of the French armed forces for political purposes. France's foreign commitments exceed those of any other country except the superpowers, as does its employment of its armed forces in various capacities in support of those commitments.[218] France has tended to assign considerable importance to having a reputation for the effective employment of its non-nuclear forces abroad in selected situations, a perspective that found partial expression in the creation of the Force d'Action Rapide. Consciously or not, this concern reflects a certain logic on France's part. France's interpretation of its own status in world politics necessitates having both the capability and the willingness to employ force when challenged, especially when that challenge is directed at one of the far-flung commitments that France as a power of consequence in the world must have. The only way in which such willingness actually can be demonstrated is to use that force occasionally. In fact, the primacy assigned to the *force de dissuasion* has made the occasional employment of conventional forces outside of metropolitan France all the more significant, if only as a symbol of France's determination to fight when challenged—a determination that might well extend to the *force de dissuasion* itself.

Under the governments of the Fifth Republic, France has used its armed forces overseas in four separate capacities, excluding more limited counterterrorist or hostage rescue operations.[219] First, France has used its navy to provide an active military presence or show of force in certain parts of the world. The naval squadron deployed to North Africa early in 1980 was widely seen as indicative of a demonstration of support for French interests there. The maintenance of major naval forces in the Indian Ocean and the deployment of naval assets into the Persian Gulf when events associated with the Iran-Iraq war began to affect shipping in those waters further exemplify this role. Second, French forces (particularly from the army) perform relatively passive functions in countries with which France has military assistance agreements. In this capacity they serve as advisers, instructors, technical specialists, and coordinators for a wide range of civic action programs from road building and related engineering tasks to public health and medical assistance. Third, France uses its military in support of international (that is, United Nations) or multilateral peace-keeping operations. Fourth and finally, France employs its armed forces abroad unilaterally in explicit support of French interests, especially in Africa, supporting friendly governments or intervening to create a favorable political situation.[220]

The third and fourth categories are perhaps of the greatest interest in the present context, simply because they provide the greatest test of the reliability and the efficiency of French forces under the most adverse conditions they are likely to encounter short of a battle in defense of France itself. As indicated earlier, France maintains that participating in international and multilateral peace-keeping operations is both the obligation and the mark of a great power. The U.S. appeal for contingents to police the cease-fire being negotiated in Lebanon in 1978, for example, provided the basis for France to deploy a composite light infantry battalion to southern Lebanon on rotating four-month tours of duty. French participation in the Multinational Force (MNF) in Beirut from 1982 to 1984 likewise signified France's willingness to engage in selected peacekeeping operations outside of the auspices of the United Nations. Despite incurring substantial losses in a single incident in 1983, French involvement in Beirut outlasted that of the United States, Italy, and Great Britain.[221] The fact that both of these endeavors occurred in a country in which France has maintained a considerable interest over the years, may, of course, underscore the selectivity of France's participation in such ventures more than anything else.

It is in Africa, however, that the French use of force for political ends has been most notable in a variety of ways. Indeed, French intervention in Africa has been sufficiently visible that some have described France as a neocolonial power or de facto Western gendarme in that region. The most enduring French intervention has been in Chad, beginning in 1968 in support of the local government, followed by subsequent interventions in 1978 and 1980 against a combination of domestic unrest and

unfriendly Libyan activity along the northern border of Chad—an involvement that has continued through 1987.[222] Supportive actions of a less time-consuming nature occurred in the Red Sea (1983–84), Tunisia (1980), Mauritania (1977–80), Zaire (1977, 1978), Djibouti (1974–77), and Gabon (1964), among other places.[223] A somewhat different basis for French military intervention occurred in the case of the overthrow of the self-proclaimed Central African emperor Bokassa I (1978), which reliable sources report "was arranged and orchestrated by France and carried out in the presence of French troops."[224] In this instance, it seems, French interests were seen to be better served by overthrowing a government rather than maintaining the status quo, as France has usually been inclined to do.

In each case French interventions appear to have been characterized by a judicious linking of military means to political ends. Neither domestic opposition nor foreign displeasure seems to have had a discernible effect on French actions. Perhaps the only exceptions to this general rule have been former President Giscard's abortive suggestion concerning a unilateral French intervention into Lebanon in advance of the UN force, and the militarily insignificant, albeit politically misbegotten, sinking of the Greenpeace ship *Rainbow Warrior* in the South Pacific with its attendant political costs to France—and particularly to certain French officials. French forces also tended to acquit themselves very well in these interventions, perhaps because Paris deployed elite units into especially demanding situations. Whether standard conscript forces would do as well in similar situations, or even in a battle for France itself, cannot, however, be inferred from these events.

Further, French interventions seem to have been motivated by a combination of three factors, whose relative importance certainly varied in specific cases. One factor is a clear and consistent desire to secure France's traditional interests in the Third World, and specifically in Africa. The second factor is to allow France to demonstrate an ability to exercise influence independently of the superpowers, especially in areas where it would be politically extremely difficult for other Western powers (and particularly the United States) to act. The third factor is the least tangible but in many respects the most important. This is that French interventions provide an opportunity to enhance the grandeur of France.[225] The general acclaim France received following its rescue operation in Zaire, for example, was itself the best reward France could have been given for its efforts, and the hope of receiving it may well have contributed to the French decision to act in the first place. Certainly, it was in keeping with past manifestations of French ambitions and interests. The situation attending the French involvement in Beirut was more ambiguous, to be sure, with a grudging pride at having outlasted the United States mingling with a sensitivity to French casualties—a foretaste, perhaps, of limits on public tolerance for the use of French forces abroad emerging more sharply at some point in the future.

There is every indication, however, that France intends to retain its traditional reliance on the selective use of force abroad as an instrument of policy, and to continue to enhance its capability to conduct such interventions when dictated by the appropriate combination of circumstances. It is readily apparent that France's interventions have been politically impressive. It is equally apparent that they have highlighted continuing operational shortcomings, particularly with respect to airlift and logistical support.[226] Steps are being taken or planned to rectify many of these shortcomings, of course, but here again resource constraints may impede the realization of well-crafted designs. In many respects, despite manifest improvements in the 1980s, France's commitments and interventions continue to underscore what has been called "the basic traditional dilemma of France's defense policy—high objectives and limited means."[227]

The Defense Policy of France in Retrospect

It is difficult not to be impressed with the breadth of French strategic thinking, as well as by the extent to which French strategy has shaped that country's force structure and employment doctrine. It is also difficult not to be aware of the extent to which strategy, force structure, and employment doctrine alike are at the service of a policy whose interests and objectives continue to mirror a political ideal whose attainment may well exceed French capabilities, its adjustments of recent years notwithstanding. France remains an "overachiever" in the community of nations, with a remarkably sophisticated strategic culture, an ingrained capacity to be disputatious in international affairs, and a demonstrated ability to link power to purpose more consistently and more effectively than any other Western power of consequence in the post-1945 era. Given what France has accomplished with its relatively limited resources under four very different presidents of the Fifth Republic, one might easily wish that U.S. defense policy had been directed and managed as well. Although "Gaullism," as practiced in varying ways by all of the presidents of the Fifth Republic, is at best a mixed blessing for the Gaullist state itself, there remains much truth to the argument that "France possesses a flexibility of military options unmatched by any other Western nation. . . . Only a very bold or exceedingly stupid aggressor would challenge the French military by attempting to invade French soil."[228] Few other nations can have that said of them.

The decade of the 1980s, on the other hand, has seen an attenuation—but not an outright rejection—of France's deeply held preference for a truly independent role in all aspects of world politics, or at the least one that permits it to lead Western Europe as a genuine center of global power. As observed earlier in this chapter, circumstances required that adjustments be made. These adjustments did not entail precisely a shift in policy orientation from independence to interdependence, as the title of one recent work suggests.[229] It was rather the acceptance of a qualified independence that is a temptation to interdependence. Even that modified interpretation of France's adaptation to the changing world of the 1980s would find something less than wholehearted acceptance in France, particularly from conservatives. To those for whom "France alone" was dogma rather than doctrine, the net effect of Mitterrand's security policy is clear: "France . . . [was] reduced to play[ing] a simple role of an extra in East-West relations."[230] French socialists, not surprisingly, do not share that view.

Regardless of the point of view one takes on what France has become, the 1986–88 period of Mitterrand-Chirac government of "cohabitation" has been an odd period. Whether it has been an interregnum, an interlude, or a stage in the progressive reorientation of France's role in the world remains to be seen. France may remain "the last of the truly 'global' European powers,"[231] or decline to join the ranks of the "merely" European middle powers, for whom even the pretension to a form of global reach (at least in political-military terms) is a thing of the past. In the short term, the government may reaffirm the basic decisions made and priorities in defense set during 1986–87, codified in the Loi de programme d'équipement militaire, 1987–1991, or it may produce yet another change of direction or emphasis to be laid out in a new five-year program.[232]

The perennial question remains whether any middle power can truly be said to have an independent ability to safeguard its own vital interests, much less the coherent defense policy such a capability would imply. At the very least, the impending obsolescence of critical elements of French nuclear and conventional forces alike (due to age and technological change) will require an extensive force-modernization program merely to avoid a relative decline in France's disposable power. It is all too true that a failure to modernize "will negatively affect French prestige and political standing,"[233] yet the resources required for that comprehensive program of force modernization simply may not be there. For France, however, being a power of consequence in the world has never been solely, or even principally, a matter of tangible assets possessed or resources allocated to defense; the intangibles have always mattered more. Early in Mitterrand's tenure, it was suggested that "to conduct its foreign policy, France has chosen to utilize the only assets which a medium-sized power can possess: consistency of policies,

firmness of principle and respect for international law. . . . The big question is how far one can go in making accommodations with pragmatism without betraying fundamental commitments."[234] The same can be said of the defense policy of France. In both areas, the answer remains elusive.

Notes

1. Alan Ned Sabrosky, "America's Choices in the Emerging World Order," *International Security Review*, Fall 1979 p. 247.

2. David S. Yost, *France's Deterrent Posture and Security in Europe, Part I: Capabilities and Doctrine*, Adelphi Papers, no. 194 (London: IISS, Adelphi Paper 194, 1984/85), p. 1.

3. Ibid.; see also John Baylis, "French Defense Policy," in *Contemporary Stategy: Theories and Policies*, ed. John Baylis et al. (New York: Holmes & Meier, 1975), p. 287, and James Bellini, *French Defense Policy* (London: Royal United Services Institute, 1974).

4. Jean-Pierre Marichy, "The Central Organization of Defense in France," in *Central Organization of Defense*, ed. Martin Edmonds (Boulder, Colo: Westview Press, 1985), p. 44.

5. Nicolas Vannier, "Défense: Les Propositions de l'opposition," *Solidarité Atlantique*, January 1986, p. 3.

6. Dominique Moisi, "L'Épreuvé de la realité," *Politique Etrangère* (1986), p. 317. See also Wolf Mendl, *Deterrence and Persuasion: French Nuclear Armament in the Context of National Policy, 1945–1969* (London: Faber & Faber, 1970), pp. 15–16; Yves Laulan, "Une Defense asservie," *Contrepoint*, no. 27 (1978), p. 44; and Valéry Giscard d'Estaing, "La Défense de la France," *Défense Nationale*, July 1976, pp. 8–9.

7. David S. Yost, *France's Deterrent Posture and Security in Europe, Part II: Strategic and Arms Control Implications*, Adelphi Papers, no. 195 (London: IISS, 1984/85), p. 61. See also Michael David, "Réflexion sur la notion d'indépendence nationale," *Armées d'Aujourd'hui*, no. 117 (February 1987); Robert S. Wood and Steven T. Ross, "France: Eurocentrism and Independence," in *Evolving European Defense Policies*, eds. C. M. Kelleher and G. A. Mattox (Lexington, Mass.: Lexington Books, 1987), p. 245; Otto Pick, "Themes and Variations: The Foreign Policy of France," *The World Today*, October 1980, p. 404; and Alan Ned Sabrosky, "French Foreign Policy Alternatives," *Orbis* (Winter 1976), pp. 1432–1435.

8. This is examined in Roger Morgan, "The Foreign Policies of Great Britain, France, and West Germany," in *World Politics: An Introduction*, ed. James N. Rosenau, Kenneth W. Thompson, and Gavin Boyd (New York: Free Press, 1976), p. 164.

9. Pick, "Themes and Variations," p. 398.

10. Sabrosky, "French Foreign Policy Alternatives," and Guy Doly, "Sécurité de la France et Union européenne," *Politique Etrangere* (March 1978), pp. 279–80.

11. For discussions of the issues and problems involved in a European security association independent of the United States, see David Watt, "The European Initiative," *Foreign Affairs* (March 1979), p. 577; Jean Klein, "France, NATO, and European Security," *International Security* (Winter 1977), esp. p. 42; Jeane-Louis Burban, "Le Parlement européen et les problèmes de défense," *Défense Nationale* (February 1978); Wynfred Joshua and Walter F. Hahn, *Nuclear Politics: America, France, and Britain*, Washington Papers, vol. 1, no. 9 (Beverly Hills, Calif.: Sage, 1973); and Marianna P. Sullivan, *France's Vietnam Policy: A Study in French-American Relations* (Westport, Conn.: Greenwood Press, 1978), p. 7.

12. Elliott R. Goodman, "De Gaulle's NATO Policy in Perspective," *Orbis* (Fall 1976); Sabrosky, "French Foreign Policy Alternatives," pp. 1430–32; Sullivan, *France's Vietnam Policy*, chap. 1; and Charles Micaud, "Gaullism after De Gaulle," *Orbis* (Fall 1970), p. 657.

13. Jacques Chirac, "France: Illusions, Temptations, Ambitions," *Foreign Affairs* (April 1978), p. 499.

14. Steven T. Ross, "French Defense Policy," *Naval War College Review* (May–June 1983), p. 29; Giscard d'Estaing, "La Défense de la France," pp. 7–8; Louis de Guiringaud, "Trois Aspects de la politique étrangère de la France: Défense, détente, désarmament," *Défense Nationale* (March 1978), pp. 11, 22; Dominique Moisi, "Mitterrand's Foreign Policy: The Limits of Continuity," *Foreign Affairs* (Winter 1981–82); Robert Grant, "French Defense Policy and European Security," *Political Science Quarterly* (Fall 1985), esp. pp. 412–15; J. Marcus and B. George, "The Ambiguous Consensus: French Defence Policy under Mitterrand," *The World Today* (October 1983), p. 372; D. Bruce Marshall, "Mitterrand's Defense Policies: The Early Sequels," *Strategic Review* (Fall 1981); Lord St Brides, "Foreign Policy of Socialist France," *Orbis* (Spring 1982); and Peter J. Berger, "The Course of French Defense Policy," *Parameters* (September 1982), pp. 22–26.

15. Doly, "Sécurité de la France," p. 265.

16. See, for example, Michael Dobbs, "U.S. Failure to Consult Said to Influence France," *Washington Post*, 24 April 1986; and Arnaud de Borchgrave, "The Candid Jacques Chirac Ignites Controversy in Europe," *Insight*, 24 November 1986.

17. David S. Yost, "French Defense Budgeting: Persistent Constraints and Future Prospects" paper presented at the Biennial Meeting of the Section on Military Studies of the International Studies Association, Kiawah Island, S.C., 8–10 November 1978, p. 35.

18. Doly, "Sécurité de la France," p. 265.

19. Jean François-Poncet, "Speech of May 3, 1979, to the National Assembly on Foreign Policy," *Journal Officiel*, 4 May 1979, p. 2; Marcel Merle, "Le Systeme mondial: Realite et crise," *Politique Etrangere*, (May 1978), pp. 499–500; François de Rose, "The Future of Salt and Western Security in Europe," *Foreign Affairs* (Summer 1979), p. 1067; Pierre M. Gallois, "French Defense Planning: The Future in the Past," *International Security* (Fall 1976), p. 22; and John Cairns, "France, Europe, and the Design of the World," *International Journal* (Spring 1977).

20. Grant, "French Defense Policy," pp. 415–17; Robert S. Rudney, "Mitterrand's Defense Concepts: Some Unsocialist Earmarks," *Strategic Review* (Spring 1983); and François Heisbourg, "Europe-Etats Unis: Le Couplage strategique menace," *Politique Etrangere* (January 1987).

21. Marc Ullman, "Security Aspects in French Foreign Policy," *Survival* (November–December 1973), esp. p. 267; Baylis, "French Defense Policy," pp. 289–90; and Mendl, *Deterrence and Persuasion*, p. 33.

22. Grant, "French Defense Policy," p. 416.

23. *Le Monde*, 26 October 1974; and Raymond Barre, "Discours prononce au Camp de Mailly le 18 juin 1977," *Défense Nationale* (August–September 1977), p. 9.

24. Wood and Ross, "France," p. 245; and Marcus and George, "Ambiguous Consensus," p. 372.

25. Marcus and George, "Ambiguous Consensus," p. 372.

26. International Institute for Strategic Studies, *Strategic Survey, 1978* (London: IISS, 1978), pp. 22–23.

27. The participants in the multinational force (MNF) in Beirut may have been well-intentioned, but the execution of their mission was deficient in both political guidance and military authority.

28. All countries represented in the naval force in the Persian Gulf are democracies, and as such are extremely sensitive to military as well as to civilian casualties, although not to the same degree. France, for example, may have somewhat more resilience and staying power in this respect than, for example, the United States.

29. Sullivan, *France's Vietnam Policy*, p. 7.

30. Walter Schutze, "Défense de l'Europe ou défense européene: Les Institutions," *Politique Etrangère* (June 1978), pp. 662–224; Denise Artaud, "De Wilson a Carter: Mythes et réalités de la politique américaine en Europe," *Défense Nationale* (January 1979), p. 60; and Yves Laulan, "Europe: L'Appel aux armes," *Contrepoint*, no. 29 (1979), p. 29.

31. Sue Ellen M. Charlton, "European Unity and the Politics of the French Left," *Orbis* (Winter 1976), p. 1462.

32. International Institute for Strategic Studies, *The Military Balance, 1978–1979* (London: IISS, 1978), pp. 16, 17; and Frederic M. Anderson, "Weapons Procurement Collaboration: A New Era for NATO?" *Orbis* (Winter 1977), pp. 973–77.

33. Berger, "Course of French Defense Policy," p. 24; Yost, *Capabilities and Doctrine*, p. 9.

34. Ross, "French Defense Policy," p. 29; Grant, "French Defense Policy," p. 411; Alex Gliksman, "Socialist France and Defense," *National Defense* (September 1981); and Emanuel de Margarie, "France," *Washington Post*, 24 April 1986.

35. Gliksman, "Socialist France," pp. 21–22.

36. Yost, *Capabilities and Doctrine*, pp. 9–10; and Ross, "French Defense Policy," pp. 35–36.

37. *Wilson Center Security Digest*, March 1986, p. 1.

38. David C. Isby and Charles Kamps, Jr., *Armies of NATO's Central Front* (London: Jane's Publishing, 1985), pp. 106–7.

39. Pick, "Themes and Variations," p. 402.

40. Moisi, "Mitterrand's Foreign Policy," p. 356.

41. Michael Dobbs, "French Leaders Revive Vision of European Security System," *Washington Post*, 27 December 1983.

42. Grant, "French Defense Policy," p. 426.

43. Chirac, "Cinquantenaire de l'IHEDN: Vers un espirit de défense européen?" *Armees d'Aujourd'hui*, no. 116 (December 1986–January 1987): 7.

44. Ibid.

45. Jerome Paolini, "Politique spatiale militaire français et cóoperation européene," *Politique Etrangère* (February 1987), pp. 435–49; and "Entente Militaire," *Economist*, 14 March 1987, p. 48.

46. Jonathan Story, "The Franco-German Alliance within the Community," *The World Today* (May 1980), p. 209.

47. Marcus and George, "Ambiguous Consensus," p. 375.

48. See A. Frisch, "Vues réalistes sur l'Allemagne," *Défense Nationale* (April 1984); and Jacques Vernant, "Qui a peur des mauvais Allemands?" *Défense Nationale* (March 1983).

49. Jacques Amalric, "Un Pavé dans l'Elbe," *Le Monde*, 22 May 1985.

50. *Wilson Center Security Digest*, p. 1.

51. Ibid.

52. Paul Lewis, "Paris-Bonn Military Accord Is Reached," *New York Times*, 2 March 1986.

53. David Marsh, "Paris, Bonn Plan Crucial Arms Talks," *Financial Times*, 18 June 1986.

54. "France-RFA: Démarche Commune," *Armées d'Aujourd'hui*, no. 118 (March 1987): 7.

55. Howard Cody, "Paris, Bonn Broaden Military Cooperation," *Washington Post*, 13 January 1988.

56. See John Chipman, *French Military Policy and African Security*, Adelphi Papers, no. 201 (London: IISS, 1985), p. 1.

57. Alexander Rondos, "A Widening Role," *Africa Report* (September–October 1979), p. 4.

58. Chipman, *French Military Policy*, pp. 20–26; International Institute for Strategic Studies, *The Military Balance, 1987–1988* (London: IISS, 1987), p. 64.

59. Chipman, *French Military Policy*, pp. 15–24; Pierre Lellouche and Dominique Moisi, "French Policy in Africa: A Lonely Battle against Destabilization," *International Security* (Spring 1979), pp. 109, 111–15.

60. Gen. Guy Mery, "Address to the Institute for Advanced Studies in National Defense, April 3, 1978, on 'France's Defense Policy' " (French Embassy Report 78/68, Washington D.C., 1978), p. 4.

61. Chipman, *French Military Policy*, p. 43.

62. P. Lacoste, "Problemes contemporains de politique et de strategie navale," *Défense Nationale* (October 1978), p. 48.

63. Edward Kolodziej, "French Military Doctrine," in *Comparative Defense Policy*, ed. Frank B. Horton et al. (Baltimore: Johns Hopkins University Press, 1974), p. 257.

64. Yvon Bourges, speech of 15 June 1978, quoted in Gerard Vaillant, "Defense en France," *Défense Nationale* (August–September 1978), p. 165.

65. Peter J. Berger, "The Nuances of French Defense Policy," *Parameters* (September 1981); Ross, "French Defense Policy."

66. Wood and Ross, "France," p. 255n; Jean Klein, "La Gauche français et les problèmes de défense," *Politique Etrangère* (May 1978), pp. 7–11.

67. Isby and Kamps, *Armies of NATO's Central Front*, p. 115.

68. See, for example, Pierre Gallois, *The Balance of Terror: Strategies for a Nuclear Age* (Boston: Houghton

Mifflin, 1961); Raymond Aron, "La Force de Dissuasion et l'Alliance Atlantique," *Défense Nationale* (January 1977), pp. 37–38; and Kolodziej, "French Military Doctrine."

69. Yost, *Capabilities and Doctrine*, p. 48.

70. Ibid., p. 3.

71. Quoted in *Le Figaro*, 30–31 January 1982.

72. Sullivan, *France's Vietnam Policy*, pp. 14–15; Baylis, "French Defense Policy," p. 301.

73. Yost, *Capabilities and Doctrine*, p. 4.

74. Lellouche and Moisi, "French Policy in Africa," pp. 116–17.

75. Bellini, *French Defense Policy*, p. 49.

76. The classic statement of this position remains that of Michel Debre, "La France et sa défense," *Revue de Défense Nationale* (January 1972), p. 7.

77. Edward Combaux, "French Military Policy and European Federalism," *Orbis* (Spring 1969), pp. 147ff. presents the essential arguments.

78. Sullivan, *France's Vietnam Policy*, pp. 14–15; Baylis, "French Defense Policy," pp. 301ff.

79. Graeme P. Auton, "Nuclear Deterrence and the Medium Power: A Proposal for Doctrinal Change in the British and French Cases," *Orbis* (Summer 1976), p. 372.

80. It is sometimes forgotten in the United States, but not in Europe, that a collateral benefit of flexible response is that it allows the United States some additional time to terminate the war short of a Soviet-American nuclear exchange, while Europe is the battlefield upon which that time is being bought.

81. Flora Lewis, "Paris Military Parade Reflects New Strategy," *New York Times*, 15 July 1977.

82. Yvon Bourges, as quoted in *Défense Nationale* (January 1979), p. 182.

83. Berger, "Course of French Defense Policy," p. 24; Robert Ropelewski, "French Emphasizing Nuclear Weapons," *Aviation Week*, 2 August 1976; International Institute for Strategic Studies, *Strategic Survey, 1976* (London: IISS, 1976), pp. 67–69.

84. Richard Woyke, "The Process of Change in French Defense Policy," *Aussenpolitik* (January 1977), p. 10.

85. Gallois, "French Defense Planning," pp. 27–31; Klein, "La Gauche Francais," p. 23.

86. For a discussion of this plan, see Jacques Tine, "France's Military Effort in the Lead-up to the Eighties," *NATO Review* (June 1979), esp. p. 11; and *Défense Nationale* (February 1979), p. 146.

87. Yvon Bourges, as quoted in *Le Monde*, 10 November 1977.

88. The 9th "Marine" Division is an army formation, continuing the heritage of the old colonial troops, with only a limited amphibious capability.

89. Gen. Guy Mery, "Une Armée pour quoi faire et comment?" *Défense Nationale* (June 1976), p. 16; Lellouche and Moisi, "French Policy in Africa," p. 128n; and Mery, "France's Defense Policy," pp. 15–20.

90. Michael C. Dunn, "Mitterrand's France Shapes a Nuclear Defense," *Defense and Foreign Affairs* (July 1983), esp. pp. 13, 32; and Yost, *Capabilities and Doctrine*, p. 12.

91. Wood and Ross, "France," p. 245; and Pierre Lellouche, "France and the Euromissiles: The Limits of Immunity," *Foreign Affairs* (Winter 1983–84), esp. pp. 323–24.

92. Quoted in *Le Figaro*, 30–31 January 1982.

93. Grant, "French Defense Policy," p. 422; Marcus and George, "Ambiguous Consensus," p. 376.

94. Charles Hernu, quoted in *Le Figaro*, 30–31 January 1988; Berger, "The Course of French Defense Policy," p. 24; and private correspondence with French government officials in 1982–83.

95. *Le Figaro*, 30–31 January 1988.

96. Joel Stratte-McClure, "Stagnant French Defense Budget Adds New Impetus to Export Sales and International Cooperation," *Armed Forces Journal International* (June 1983); and Wood and Ross, "France," pp. 248–51.

97. François Heisbourg, "Défense et Sécurité Extérieure: Le Changement dans la continuité," *Politique Etrangère* (1986), esp. pp. 384–85; Dunn, "Mitterrand's France"; and Stratte-McClure, "Stagnant French Defense Budget."

98. Marcus and George, "Ambiguous Consensus," pp. 374–75.

99. Ibid.

100. See W. L. Kohl, *French Nuclear Diplomacy* (Princeton: Princeton University Press, 1971).

101. Mery, "Une Armée pour quoi faire et comment," pp. 13–14.

102. For discussion of this concept, see Mendl, *Deterrence and Persuasion*, pp. 15–16; Gallois, "French Defense Planning," p. 25; and Auton, "Nuclear Deterrence and the Medium Power," pp. 373–76.

103. Pierre Gallois, "The Future of France's *Force de Dissuasion*," *Strategic Review* (Summer 1979), p. 37.

104. Pierre Hassner, "A NATO Dissuasion Strategy: A French View" in *NATO and Dissuasion*, ed. Morton A. Kaplan (Chicago: University of Chicago Press, 1974), p. 97.

105. Roy C. Macridis, "French Foreign Policy" in *Foreign Policy in World Politics*, ed. Roy C. Macridis, 5th ed. (Englewood Cliffs, N.J.: Prentice Hall, 1976), p. 109.

106. Walter F. Hahn and Wynfred Joshua, "The Impact of SALT on British and French Nuclear Forces," in *Contrasting Approaches to Strategic Arms Control*, ed. Robert L. Pfaltzgraff, Jr. (Lexington, Mass.: D. C. Heath/Lexington Books, 1974), p. 154.

107. Auton, "Nuclear Deterrence and the Medium Power," p. 374.

108. Mendl, *Deterrence and Persuasion*, p. 16.

109. For summaries of these functions, see Hahn and Joshua, "Impact of SALT on British and French Nuclear Forces," pp. 155–56.

110. For a summary of "Operation Vulture," see Bernard B. Fall, *Hell in a Very Small Place* (Philadelphia: J. B. Lippincott, 1966), pp. 293–314.

111. Private interview, Washington D.C., 17 March 1983.

112. Ibid.

113. Yost, *Strategic and Arms Control Implications*, p. 21.

114. For an enduring discussion of the French understanding of the political utility of military power, especially with respect to the *force de dissuasion*, see Baylis, "French Defense Policy," pp. 287–91.

115. *Politique Etrangère* (February 1987), p. 473; Heisbourg, "Défense et Sécurité Extérieure;" Yost, *Capabilities and Doctrine*, part 1.

116. Pierre Dabezies, "The Defense of France and the Defense of Europe," *Defence Yearbook, 1974* (London: R.U.S.I./Brassey's, 1974), p. 116.

117. De Rose, "Future of SALT," p. 1066.

118. Gallois, "French Defense Planning," p. 31.

119. Pierre Dabezies, "French Political Parties and Defense Policy: Divergences and Consensus," *Armed Forces and Society* (Winter 1982); Wood and Ross, "France," p. 246; and Heisbourg, "Défense et Sécurité Extérieure."

120. Quoted in D. Bruce Marshall, "Recent Developments in French Strategic Doctrine," paper presented at the Biennial Meeting of the Section on Military Studies of the International Studies Association, Kiawah Island, S.C., 8–10 November 1978, p. 9.

121. Kenneth R. Timmerman, "France: More Money, but Hard Choices in Defense," *Journal of Defense and Diplomacy* (February 1987).

122. Isby and Kamps, *Armies of NATO's Central Front*, p. 107; Alan Gliksman, "Mitterrand: Directions for the French Military," *National Defense* (January 1982), p. 26. Marcus and George, "Ambiguous Consensus," p. 377.

123. See, for example, "Saudi Arabia Says It Funded French Missile Program," *Wall Street Journal*, 27 January 1984.

124. Grant, "French Defense Policy," p. 420.

125. "Technology the French Way," *Economist*, 17 November 1984; "French Plan for Joint Satellite Operations," *Jane's Defence Weekly*, 18 October 1986; Judith Miller, "Mitterrand Urges Plans for Space," *New York Times*, 4 July 1986; and Amy Bodnar, "France Orbits Commercial 'Spy' Satellite," *Armed Forces Journal International* (April 1986), p. 34.

126. Doly, "Sécurité de la France," p. 279.

127. Gliksman, "Mitterrand," p. 27.

128. Jerome Jaffre, "France Looks to Europe," *Public Opinion* (March–May 1979), p. 17.

129. Jean-Paul Le Bourg, "Opinion et Défense en 1986," *Armées d'Aujourd'hui*, no. 117 (February 1987): p. 18; Institut Français de l'Opinion Publique, "Opinion de Défense" (8 September 1981); Jean-Marc Lech, "L'Evolution de l'opinion des français à travers les sondages de 1972 à 1976," *Défense Nationale* (August–September 1977), pp. 51, 54, 56.

130. Le Bourg, "Opinion et défense," p. 16.

131. Morgan, "Foreign Policies of Great Britain, France, and West Germany," p. 167.

132. Michael M. Harrison, "A Socialist Foreign Policy for France?" *Orbis* (Winter 1976), esp. pp. 1489, 1495.

133. David S. Yost, "The French Defense Debate," *Survival* (January/February 1981), p. 22.

134. Combaux, "French Military Policy," p. 145.

135. Yost, *Capabilities and Doctrine*, pp. 2, 40.

136. Minister of National Defense Andre Giraud, "Consensus sur la loi de Programmation," *Armées d'Aujourd'hui*, no. 119 (April 1987): 5.

137. Ibid.

138. Marichy, "Central Organization of Defense in France," and Henri Beauvais, "Planification et programmation dans les armées," *Défense Nationale* (May 1978), esp. pp. 53–54.

139. Marichy, "Central Organization of Defense in France," pp. 39–40.

140. For a classic discussion of this model and its

implications for the decision-making process, see Graham Allison, *Essence of Decision* (Boston: Little, Brown, 1971), chap. 1.

141. Yost, "French Defense Budgeting," pp. 13–16.

142. Morgan, "Foreign Policies of Great Britain, France, and West Germany," pp. 168–69.

143. Yost, "French Defense Budgeting," pp. 17–22.

144. France, *White Paper on National Defense* (1973), vol. 2, chap. 1, pp. 7–8.

145. Berger, "Course of French Defense Policy," p. 22.

146. Wood and Ross, "France," p. 245.

147. Mirichy, "Central Organization of Defense in France," p. 61; Edward Kolodziej, "Measuring French Arms Transfers: A Problem of Sources and Some Sources of Problems with ACDA Data," *Journal of Conflict Resolution* (June 1979), p. 197.

148. Lellouche, "France and the Euromissiles."

149. Yost, "French Defense Budgeting," pp. 22, 34–35.

150. Morgan, "Foreign Policies of Great Britain, France, and West Germany," p. 165.

151. France, *White Paper on National Defense*, pp. 8–9.

152. "Un Conseil Scientifique de la Défense," *Armées d'Aujourd'hui*, no. 116 (December 1986–January 1987): 7.

153. Bellini, *French Defense Policy*, ch. 4.

154. Arthur J. Alexander, "Weapons Acquisition in the Soviet Union, the United States, and France," in *Comparative Defense Policy*, ed. Frank B. Horton et al. (Baltimore: Johns Hopkins University Press, 1974), esp. pp. 438–42.

155. Marichy, "Central Organization of Defense in France."

156. Yost, "French Defense Budgeting," pp. 1, 23–34.

157. Marichy, "Central Organization of Defense in France," p. 39.

158. Jacques Isnard, "Rethinking French Defense," *Manchester Guardian*, 24 August 1974; Stanley Hoffman, "Toward a Common European Foreign Policy?" in *The United States and Western Europe*, ed. Wolfram Hanrieder (Cambridge, Mass.: Winthrop, 1974), p. 83.

159. Stratte-McClure, "Stagnant French Defense Budget."

160. Yost, "French Defense Budgeting," pp. 6–13.

161. See the discussion of the Loi de programme d'équipement militaire 1987–1991 in *Armées d'Aujourd'hui*, no. 116 (December 1986–January 1987).

162. Yost, "French Defense Budgeting," pp. 6–13.

163. Jacques Vuillemin, "Le Service national en question: Service gagnat!" *Armées d'Aujourd'hui*, no. 119 (April 1987).

164. Ross, "French Defense Policy," p. 31.

165. Ibid.

166. Le Bourg, "Opinion et Défense," p. 18.

167. Michel L. Martin, "Conscription and the Decline of the Mass Army in France, 1960–1975," *Armed Forces and Society* (May 1977), pp. 392–93.

168. This is a common phenomenon in advanced industrial societies. See, for example, the discussion in Anthony S. Bennell, "The Effectiveness of Supplementary Military Forces," in *Supplementary Military Forces: Reserves, Militia, Auxiliaries*, ed. Louis A. Zurcher and Gwyn Harries-Jenkins (Beverly Hills, Calif.: Sage, 1978), esp. pp. 64–65.

169. Isby and Kamps, *Armies of NATO's Central Front*, p. 134; Wood and Ross, "France," p. 252; Lellouche and Moisi, "French Policy in Africa," p. 128n.

170. Paul R. Viotti, "Introduction to Military Doctrine," in *Comparative Defense Policy*, ed. Frank B. Horton et al. (Baltimore: Johns Hopkins University Press, 1974), p. 190.

171. Kolodziej, "French Military Doctrine," p. 257.

172. A review of the evolution of the strategic forces of the principal countries in various editions of *The Military Balance* is especially instructive in this regard.

173. International Institute for Strategic Studies, *The Military Balance, 1987–1988* (London: IISS, 1987), p. 60.

174. Ibid., pp. 60, 64, 212.

175. "Priorité aux forces nucléaires," *Armées d'Aujourd'hui*, no. 117 (February 1987): 30. See also Yost, *Capabilities and Doctrine*, pp. 18–28.

176. Mery, "France's Defense Policy," p. 13.

177. IISS, *Military Balance, 1987–1988*, pp. 60–61; "Priorité aux forces nucléaires," pp. 30–32.

178. Marcus and George, "Ambiguous Consensus," p. 372.

179. Gliksman, "Mitterrand."

180. Grant, "French Defense Policy," p. 423.

181. Wood and Ross, "France," p. 250.

182. Jean-Louis d'André, "Le plateau d'Albion: Pilier de la dissuasion," *Armées d'Aujourd'hui*, no. 116 (December 1986–January 1987): 87.

183. Michael Dobbs, "French Defense Minister Steps Up Attack on SDI after U.S. Visit," *Washington Post*, 18 December 1985; Jerome Dumoulin and Dinah Louda, "Why France Can't Decide about Star Wars," *Washington Post*, 20 February 1986.

184. Quoted in "Le Reenforcement nécessaire des forces conventionnelles," *Armées d'Aujourd'hui*, no. 117 (February 1987): 33.

185. M. Darfen, "Le Point sur la réorganisation de l'Armée de terre," *Défense Nationale* (April 1984); Yost, *Strategic and Arms Control Implications*, p. 1.

186. IISS, *Military Balance, 1987–1988*, p. 61; Isby and Kamps, *Armies of NATO's Central Front*, esp pp. 122ff.; Darfen, "Le Point sur la réorganisation de l'Armée de terre."

187. The exceptions are the naval commands in the Indian and Pacific Oceans.

188. Chipman, *French Military Policy and African Security*, p. 15. See also Marcus and George, "Ambiguous Consensus," p. 374.

189. Recall that French marines in the classical sense of the term are in the navy and not in the 9th Marine Division of the army.

190. *Défense Nationale* (August–September 1978), p. 169; Stephan S. Roberts, "French Naval Policy outside of Europe," paper presented at the Bicennial Meeting of the Section on Military Studies of the International Studies Association, Kiawah Island, S.C., 8–10 November 1978.

191. R. J. L. Dicker, "French Navy Programs Present and Future," *International Defense Review* (October 1982); *Armées d'Aujourd'hui*, no. 117 (Feb-

ruary 1987); *International Defense Review* (June 1987); IISS, *Military Balance, 1987–1988*, pp. 61–62.

192. Yost, *Capabilities and Doctrine*, p. 58; Robert Salvy, "The Air Defense of France: Plugging the Low-level Gaps," *International Defense Review* (May 1983).

193. Isby and Kamps, *Armies of NATO's Central Front*, pp. 167–70; *Armées d'Aujourd'hui*, no. 117 (February 1987): 40–41; IISS, *Military Balance, 1987–1988*, pp. 62–63.

194. Isby and Kamps, *Armies of NATO's Central Front*, p. 164; *Armées d'Aujourd'hui*, no. 117 (February 1987): 42; IISS, *Military Balance, 1987–1988*, p. 64.

195. Bennell, "Supplementary Military Forces," pp. 50–54; Gérard Vaillant, "Vers une adaptation de notre système des réserves?" *Défense Nationale* (March 1979); IISS, *Military Balance 1987–1988*, p. 60.

196. Yost, *Capabilities and Doctrine*, p. 61; Isby and Kamps, *Armies of NATO's Central Front*, p. 162; Pierre Michel, "La Nouvelle Orientation de la défense opérationnelle du territoire," *Défense Nationale* (January 1978).

197. Jean de Gelard, "New Approach for French Nuclear Force," *Jane's Defence Weekly*, 14 December 1985.

198. Marc Giacomini, "Missions et capacités futures de l'armée de terre," *Armées d'Aujourd'hui*, no. 118 (March 1987).

199. The decision to withdraw, of course, was made by De Gaulle in 1966.

200. For detailed descriptions of the technical characteristics of various French weapons systems, consult the various publications on these topics in the *Jane's* series.

201. *International Defense Review* (April 1987).

202. Timmerman, "France," p. 61.

203. Frank Barnaby, "France Arms the Third World," *World Press Review* (August 1982), p. 53; David B. Ottaway, "Angry Arabs Diversify Sources of Supply," *Washington Post*, 14 May 1984; International Institute for Strategic Studies, *The Military Balance, 1986–1987* (London: IISS, 1986), pp. 209–11; J. Arben, "The French Socialists Confronted with the Problem of Arms Exports," *Defense Analysis, 1986*, esp. p. 310.

204. IISS, *Military Balance, 1986–1987*, pp. 209–211.

205. International Institute for Strategic Studies, *Military Balance, 1979–1980*, (London: IISS, 1979), pp. 103–07.

206. Jacqueline Grapin, "Des armements pour quoi faire?" *Défense Nationale* (January 1978).

207. "Commentaire," *Politique Etrangère* (February 1987), pp. 461–73; Yost, *Strategic and Arms Control Implications*, pp. 35–61; Wood and Ross, "France," p. 250; and Mery, "France's Defense Policy," pp. 9–15.

208. Mery, "France's Defense Policy," p. 11.

209. Ibid.

210. Fall, *Hell in a Very Small Place*, pp. 293–314.

211. The Israeli attack on the Iraqi reactor has been described incorrectly as "preemptive." It was not; that term applies only to an action attempted to forestall a certain attack whose military execution has already commenced. That was not the case in this instance.

212. "Commentaire," *Politique Etrangère* (February 1987), pp. 461ff.; Pierre Lellouche, "SALT and European Security: The French Dilemma," *Survival* (January–February 1980); Wood and Ross, "France," p. 250; *Le Monde*, 13 June 1986, p. 1.

213. *Le Monde*, 13 June 1986; Mery, "France's Defense Policy," p. 14.

214. Charles François, "L'Equilibre nucléaire en Europe," *Armées d'Aujourd'hui*, no. 119 (April 1987): 13.

215. Pierre Lellouche, "La France et l'option zero: Réflexions sur la position français," *Politique Etrangère* (January 1987), pp. 161–166.

216. Leo Hamon and Jacques Kosciusko-Mouzet, "Reflexions sur la politique étrangère de la France," *Politique Etrangère* (January 1987), pp. 181–82.

217. *Politique Etrangère* (February 1987), pp. 461–73.

218. Renaud Dubow, "La Présence des forces armées outre-mer," *Armées d'Aujourd'hui*, no. 116 (December 1986–January 1987); Chipman, *French Military Policy and African Security*, p. 20.

219. *Défense Nationale* (February 1978), pp. 146–47, 158.

220. See Chipman, *French Military Policy and African Security*, for the French experience in Africa in particular.

221. Isby and Kamps, *Armies of NATO's Central Front*, p. 166.

222. Ibid.; Marcus and George, "Ambiguous Consensus," p. 376; E. J. Dione, Jr., "France's Soldiers Ordered to Widen Control in Chad," *New York Times*, 28 January 1984; Howard Cody, "France Sends More Troops to Aid Chad," *Washington Post*, 10 February 1987.

223. Michel L. Castellon, "Low-Intensity Conflict in the 1980s: The French Experience," *Military Review* (March 1985), esp. p. 69; and Isby and Kamps, *Armies of NATO's Central Front*, p. 166.

224. Ronald Koven, "French Troops, Negotiations Pushed Bokassa off Throne," *Washington Post*, 22 September 1979; and IISS, *Strategic Survey, 1978*, p. 15.

225. Dennis Chaplin, "France: Military Involvement in Africa," *Military Review* (January 1979), esp. p. 45; and Lellouche and Moisi, "French Policy in Africa," p. 33.

226. *Politique Etrangère* (May 1978), p. 619; and IISS, *Strategic Survey, 1978*, p. 16.

227. Lellouche and Moisi, "French Policy in Africa," p. 128.

228. Wilfred L. Ebel, "The French Republic," *Military Review* (August 1979), p. 50.

229. Robin F. Laird, ed., *French Security Policy: From Independence to Interdependence* (Boulder, Colo.: Westview Press, 1986).

230. Jean François-Poncet, "Quatre ans de politique étrangère socialiste: Le Mirage évanoui," *Politique Etrangère* (1986), p. 446.

231. *Journal of Defense and Diplomacy* (November 86), p. 62.

232. Timmerman, "France," p. 61.

233. Ibid., p. 62.

234. Marie-Claude Smouts, "The External Policy of François Mitterrand," *International Affairs* (Spring 1983), p. 167.

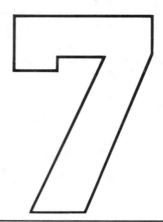

THE UNITED KINGDOM

David Greenwood

The United Kingdom is a great power in reduced circumstances. This has been its position for at least a generation. But like the heads of the country's aristocratic households, with whom fate has dealt similarly, British governments have displayed a remarkable talent for keeping up appearances. So much is apparent from scrutiny of the nation's peacetime order of battle. Not that it is all just for show, as Argentina's General Galtieri learned to his cost in the Falklands conflict in 1982.

On any realistic assessment the country is a middle-rank European power, standing below both the Federal Republic of Germany and France according to many indices of military capacity. Yet the British voice is heard on global security issues even where the influence the United Kingdom can exercise is negligible. The national self-perception is emphatically not that of a "mere" regional actor. Britain's defense effort is concentrated on the North Atlantic and Western Europe, with posture and provision settled more or less exclusively within the Atlantic Alliance framework. Policymakers look beyond these horizons, however, at least when voicing aspirations in declaratory pronouncements.

The British defense organization, too, is on the grand scale, despite the fact that the nation cuts a less formidable military figure than hitherto. Until very recently three service bureaucracies, each imbued with its own traditions and attentive to its own priorities, competed for resources under central supervision, but not effective central authority. It is only the insistent pressure of financial and manpower constraints, necessitating tighter management, that has brought about change of late. Nevertheless, "balance" is the main characteristic of the present-day service structure. A small strategic nuclear force is complemented by comprehensive conventional capabilities in all three branches of the armed forces, which continue to receive near-equal shares of annual appropriations. The Royal Navy no longer has attack carriers or a fully fledged amphibious warfare capability, but in all other respects the United Kingdom retains a balanced fleet.

Over the years the British Army has undergone much restructuring, but it remains a true all-arms force. Short of combat planes and fast jet pilots though it may be, the Royal Air Force has (and plans to have) the wherewithal to perform the full spectrum of tactical air missions.

Whether British governments will for much longer be able, or wish, to maintain across-the-board competence, together with an armaments base that permits self-reliance, though not self-sufficiency, is an open question. Much depends on the performance of the economy and the exact makeup of successive administrations. The former will affect the scale of provision, the latter its pattern. Among Conservatives there is resistance to speculation about, and no disposition to effect, radical change in that pattern. The Labour, Liberal Democrat, and Social Democratic parties are, however, each committed to some reshaping of the defense effort, especially with respect to nuclear capabilities.

International Environment

That the United Kingdom nowadays rates as a medium power in an essentially regional setting is generally acknowledged, albeit reluctantly and not unreservedly. The reluctance is understandable in the light of history, as is the fact that it is tinged with regret. After all, prior to and during World War II the British claim to great power status was incontestable. Moreover, it seemed for a time in the later 1940s that, while clearly unable to aspire to superpower stature, the nation might establish for itself a special position no more than one level below the United States and the Soviet Union in a national global pecking order. Indeed, the international community actually accorded such recognition when the United Kingdom became one of the permanent members of the UN Security Council. British policy makers were certainly not in doubt at this time about where they wished the country to stand. Decolonization proceeded, but it was accompanied by assumption of an active post-Imperial global role. A leading part was taken in fashioning postwar European security arrange-

ments. And wartime atomic weapons development was continued. All these testify to a distinctive self-image.

There was, however, little hope that the United Kingdom could carve out a permanent special niche. The decisive acts of postwar diplomacy were the construction of a European alliance with demanding mutual obligations, expressed in the Brussels Treaty of 1948, and the achievement of an American commitment to Western Europe's defense with the signing of the North Atlantic Treaty and the establishment of NATO, initiatives in which the imperatives of interdependence prevailed over the impulse to independence. To be sure, tension between the demands of these European and Atlantic affiliations and those of worldwide obligations dominated British policy making through the 1950s and into the late 1960s. Vestiges of it are still discernible. Yet there was never much doubt how the tension would be resolved. Western European and North Atlantic concerns assumed greater significance as wider global aspirations steadily receded.

Because of changes in strategic circumstances and the United Kingdom's relative economic position, the nation not only has relinquished its great power standing for "club membership" in NATO (and, since 1972, in the European Communities), but it also cannot properly count itself more than an "ordinary member" of these fraternities. This is evident from the summary statistics in table 1, which show selected indicators of the British defense effort in relation to those of Britain's allies and partners. On one measure—defense spending as a percentage of gross domestic product (GDP)—the United Kingdom ranks above all other Western European countries except Greece. But more than anything else this reflects the expense of all-volunteer forces and a large equipment budget in an economy with an indifferent growth record. On the other measure—actual defense outlays and defense expenditure per head—the British figures are on a par with those of France and West Germany (and, of course, far below those of the United States).[1]

Two related questions invite consideration. First, how does Britain perceive the threats

Table 1. Selected Defense Expenditure Statistics, 1985

	Total U.S. $ (billions)	Per Capita U.S. $	Percentage of GDP
Greece	2.4	237	7.1
United Kingdom	22.6	401	5.2
Turkey	2.3	47	4.4
France	20.1	365	4.0
Belgium	2.6	259	3.3
Federal Republic of Germany	19.8	324	3.3
Portugal	0.6	63	3.2
Netherlands	3.8	261	3.1
Norway	1.7	410	3.1
Italy	9.3	162	2.7
Denmark	1.2	239	2.3
Spain	3.6	97	2.1
Canada	7.4	290	2.2
United States	266.6	1,115	6.9

Source: Statement on the Defence Estimates, 1986 Cmnd 9763 (London: HMSO, 1986: Fig. 8, p. 41).

and challenges to its security (and values) in the Atlantic Alliance setting? Second, in what ways are decisions about posture and provision still affected by "rank consciousness" or reluctance to settle for "ordinary membership" in NATO?

THREAT PERCEPTIONS IN THE ALLIANCE SETTING

Of these questions, the first is the easier to answer, at least in principle. As a member of NATO, the United Kingdom subscribes to the general alliance assessment of "the threat." What is that assessment? What is the contemporary Western view of the aims and assets of the Soviet Union that forms the essential frame of reference for British policy choices?

No truly authoritative analysis exists, strange though that may seem. The final communiques of NATO's regular ministerial meetings are couched in stereotyped language that is singularly uninstructive. The frequent pronouncements of the supreme commanders have to be recognised for what they are: the evaluations of senior officers whose dual obligation is to keep the potential adversary's capabilities under review and to keep politicians, parliaments, and public opinion in NATO states aware of the need to match those capabilities. As for the international staffs in Brus-

sels, "hawks" and "doves" contend there, as they do in national capitals.

Some view of "the threat" clearly does animate Atlantic Alliance members. Otherwise they would dismantle the organization. Yet it evidently is not a hard-line perception of a permanent antagonist, unambiguously hostile, with alarmingly superior forces. It is, rather, a more complex appreciation, encompassing numerous judgments about aspirations, intentions, and capabilities. Impressionistic evidence suggests that if there *were* an "agreed assessment," it would run along the following lines.

Quite what the Soviet Union's basic *aspirations* are is hard to discern. In the content and language of Moscow's rhetoric, however, ideological currents run strongly. Since long-run policy goals derive from these fundamental impulses, the presumption must be that they remain at odds with Western liberal democratic values.

Under the heading of *intentions* (meaning short- or medium-term policy objectives) a distinction has to be made between political conduct and possible military activity. On the political plane, much Soviet behavior, under Gorbachev as under his predecessors, suggests that East-West détente is an instrument of diplomacy, to be wielded as opportunity offers in the promotion of state interests. At the same time the Soviet Union clearly acknowledges shared interests with the United States and its allies, not least in avoiding nuclear war and regulating nuclear arms competition, while the West has sought to allay Soviet fears arising from perceptions of insecurity and to establish such structures of cooperation as exist, for example, in economic relations. The ambiguity or ambivalence here is problematical. But one thing is obvious: as yet the basis for presuming generally beneficent intent is fragile. Thus, NATO countries wisely combine flexibility in the exploration of arms control opportunities and the development of commercial ties with firmness of commitment to the maintenance of countervailing military power. In the military sphere itself, since a more or less stable equilibrium exists at present, there is no solid foundation for suggestions that "the Russians are coming" on NATO's central front (or else-where). But the absence of a direct, immediate threat of aggression does not justify complacency. There is a sense in which the Russians as the preponderant military power in Europe have already arrived. Furthermore, it is evident from recent events outside Europe that, should the commitment of Western powers ever appear to be in doubt, the Soviet Union would probably extract strategic benefit from military advantage.

Much hinges, therefore, on assessment of the balance of military *capabilities*: at the intercontinental level; at the continental strategic level (which is where Soviet intermediate- and medium-range ballistic missiles enter the reckoning); and at the European theater level (where shorter-range nuclear systems and conventional forces are relevant). Is the "Soviet threat" in these areas thought to be increasing, diminishing, or staying more or less the same?

Rigorous measurement is impossible. There are structural asymmetries at each level, not to mention qualitative differences. It is practicable, however, to gauge the direction of change by rough-and-ready calculation. On this the consensus is that Soviet and Warsaw Pact capabilities have been steadily improving relative to those of the Western powers. At the intercontinental strategic level, there is "essential equivalence" and, by a judicious blend of doctrinal refinement, force modernization, and arms control negotiation, the superpowers will, one must hope, keep it that way. At the continental strategic level, it is the view of the United Kingdom and other European members of NATO that the Soviet Union enjoys an advantage: there is particular concern about the threat posed by, and the inadequacy of the West's defenses against, tactical ballistic missiles. In general, the balance of European theater forces is thought to have swung in the Warsaw Pact's favor. That is why NATO launched a conventional defense improvement program in 1985.

On the basis of this sort of analysis, right-wing politicians in Britain (and elsewhere) argue that NATO's force levels are barely adequate, and that the alliance may be courting disaster. In fact a much more decisive superiority would probably be necessary before even a reckless Soviet leadership would contemplate use of arms to upset the European status quo. It should be added, though, that the perception of a shifting balance itself confers benefits on the Soviet Union, both in Europe and (perhaps more significantly) elsewhere.[2]

What the assessment does support is the notion that existing dispositions for deterrence and defense need to be kept in good repair. NATO must also exercise due vigilance against the possibility of the Soviet Union acquiring options that would disturb strategic stability. Efforts to buttress the "partnership" elements in interbloc relations and to develop confidence-building measures in Europe are worth making, but only against the background of continuing and prudent military provision.

It is in such terms that decision makers in the United Kingdom construe the external threats to national security. It is a nicely judged evaluation, and one that accounts for both the care British governments have taken to sustain Britain's contribution to NATO during successive reviews of the defense program and the cautious British approach to various East-West negotiations.

What of internal threats? Have defense policy makers and planners in the United Kingdom had to pay attention of late to domestic challenges to the nation's sense of security (and cherished values) in addition to those posed by the political and military power of the Soviet Union and Warsaw Pact?

In two quite different ways, they have. In the first place, as in many other Western European countries, there has been concern about the problems that Martin Hillenbrand recognized when arguing that "the health of the Western Alliance can be no better than the economic and resulting social and political strength of its various component countries."[3] Accordingly, politicians have approached the allocation of resources to defense with a clear understanding that committing funds to military purposes beyond economic capacity, or to the detriment of key social programs, could be as damaging as inadequate provision. In other words, they have recognized that how judiciously the budgetary balance is struck between defense and other things may be as important to security (broadly defined) as the actual sums allotted. The United Kingdom has not, however, been beset by economic distress and political turbulence on a scale sufficient to cause serious anxiety about the state's social stability.

The nation's only internal security problem is the situation in Northern Ireland. This has had (and continues to have) a direct and significant impact on defense decision making. Yet it is really a law-and-order problem writ large, and the armed forces are engaged in a policing task under the rubric of military aid to the civil power. Even though the present "troubles" began back in the 1960s, the situation is designated "the Northern Ireland emergency"; and the idea that troops might have to assume permanent responsibility for domestic peacekeeping is anathema to the authorities, as it is in public opinion.

Has the United Kingdom genuinely come to terms with the fact that it now ranks as a medium power in a regional setting? Are British policy makers content, not only to accept the kind of threat assessment that has been outlined, but also to make an "ordinary member's" contribution to NATO? Or is the nation's "distinctive self-image" still influential in program decisions, and, if so, why and how? Brief remarks on these matters are now in order.

SELF-IMAGE AND STATURE

As has been suggested already, over the past thirty years or so British governments and the British people have become reconciled to the United Kingdom's inability to maintain the status of a major world power. At the same time the imprint of what Kenneth Waltz has called "hard residuums of national habits and deep-set attitudes towards international affairs" remains discernible in the approach to defense choices.[4] The station in international political life for which British decision makers regard the country as suited, and which they hope it can occupy, is that of a leading regional power. Evidence of the influence of this "rank consciousness" is apparent in the structure and deployment of the armed forces and in the substance and tenor of debate about options for the future.

Looking back over the British defense experience since 1945, the adjustment in the national self-perception can be seen to have taken place in five phases: (1) In the immediate aftermath of World War II, it appeared that a special position one rung below the superpowers might fall naturally to a state armed with nuclear weapons that was determined to play a leading role within NATO and to discharge several post-Imperial global responsibilities. (2) In the first half of the 1950s, although it was apparent that there would be difficulty in sustaining this stance, it was in fact formalized: in 1954–55 the United Kingdom joined the South East Asia Treaty Organization (SEATO) and signed the Baghdad Pact, leading to the formation of the Central Treaty Organization (CENTO); an unprecedented commitment was made to the peacetime stationing of forces in Europe, under the aegis of the Western Europe Union (WEU); and the government embarked on development and production of thermonuclear weapons and a ballistic missile delivery system. (3) There followed a decade, 1955–64, in which policy makers lacked a firm sense of direction, prompting Dean Acheson's celebrated comment that Britain had "lost an Empire but not yet found a role."[5] (4) Not until a fourth phase, covering 1965–74, was a decisive reshaping of the defense effort and reordering of priorities effected through a succession of defense reviews in which all but the last traces of worldwide involvement were progressively eliminated, permitting consolidation of Britain's commitment to the defense of Western Europe.[6] (5) In 1974–75 and again in 1981 there were further extensive and thorough reviews of the defense program and budget, involving further contraction of the military effort (including some diminution of the quantity and dilution of the quality of forces contributed to NATO).[7]

In the first half of the 1980s, thanks to an alliance-wide interest in contingencies outside the NATO area and a burst of national self-satisfaction with the way the services had done their stuff in the Falklands War, there was a brief interval during which some asked whether concentration on Western Europe and the North Atlantic might not have gone too far. But the phase passed.

Having said all that, in present provision and plans for the future, the influence of a distinctive national self-image is still apparent. Retention of influence and prestige within NATO is seen to depend on possession of a particular kind of military establishment and on payment of a "club subscription" that, in its comprehensiveness, if not its scale, stands higher than that of any other European member of the alliance. Thus the United Kingdom makes (and, at the time of writing, plans to continue to make) significant and high-quality contributions to NATO's order of battle at sea, on land, and in the air; in all three elements of the NATO triad (conventional forces, theater nuclear weapons, and strategic nuclear capabilities); and to the ready forces in each of the alliance's major command areas (Atlantic, Channel, and Europe).

Moreover, there are *some* traces of Britain's former position as a state with substantial worldwide interests—for example, occasional naval deployments to the Pacific and Indian Oceans and the presence of ground and air force contingents in Belize, Cyprus, the Falklands, Gibraltar, and Hong Kong. More important, perhaps, discussion about future program possibilities is characterized by continuing emphasis on retention of the distinctive elements in the British defense effort: some strategic nuclear capability (to which only the Labour Party is seriously opposed), comprehensive and balanced conventional forces (with ships of high quality and the most advanced land and air systems), and the "spread" of the investment in Europe and the North Atlantic. In the 1990s, as hitherto, the part the United Kingdom will seek to play in international security affairs is that of a "major power of the second order."[8]

There could, though, be further redefinition of the appropriate role for Britain. Because of financial and manpower constraints, it is becoming increasingly difficult year by year to sustain all-round competence and commitment in a credible way, i.e., with units up to strength and equipment up to date. If budgetary stringency continues, "keeping up appearances" may become impracticable. This is not the place for detailed consideration of what changes might be wrought if further defense

reviews are necessary. Suffice it to say that prevailing notions of what is an acceptable scale of provision could be set aside and the pattern of provision might undergo modification, for example, through reassessment of the priority accorded to the ground and air forces' contribution to NATO's central front vis-à-vis the national investment in maritime forces.[9]

Limited adjustment to present plans would not, of course, transform national perceptions (or aspirations) concerning Britain's role and stature. But even modest change might mean abandoning any pretense to a leading position among the European members of the alliance. Substantial diminution in the defense effort, or radical reshaping, would make it legitimate to ask whether the United Kingdom's standing had not become that of a "major power of the third order," ranking alongside Italy rather than France and West Germany.

What seems most likely is that there will be further marginal changes in the scale of British defense dispositions, with limited structural modifications. Planners may have to wrestle with the choice between preserving a distinctive across-the-board contribution to NATO or defining a feasible specialized contribution. They may have to ask what the United Kingdom's role in NATO should be, much as their predecessors had to ask questions about Britain's role in the world.

The foregoing discussion provides a foundation for more specific analysis. Attention must now be directed to the determinants of policy, posture, and provision; to procedural matters; and to some of the principal features of the current and planned future defense effort and issues arising in debate about it. The obvious point of departure is elucidation of the United Kingdom's security objectives, of the defense strategy derived therefrom, and of the main parameters of military doctrine for the implementation of that strategy.

National Objectives, National Strategy, and Military Doctrine

There is an appealing logic and clarity about the idea that states decide on their aims, devise an approach to the attainment of desired ends, and develop appropriate concepts of operations for their armed forces in a systematic progression. It would certainly seem the rational way to do things. But reality is not like that. Objectives may not be clearly delineated and of those that are, some do not find expression in firm goals but remain as loosely defined aspirations. In making policy proper ("a flow of purposive action over a period of time" in John Garnett's formulation), nations have difficulty in achieving complete consistency.[10] Choice of a becoming security posture is a troublesome business too, given the pressures that impinge on decision making about force structures, levels, equipment, and deployment. Even if a country is successful in investing its defense arrangements with a certain coherence, there may be problems over provision of the resources of manpower, matériel, industrial capacity, technical ingenuity, and organizing ability necessary to sustain them.

On this reasoning, understanding of the basic determinants of the United Kingdom's defence program and budget, which is another way of defining the subject matter of this section, is unlikely to be advanced by speculation about some imaginary "rational deductive" construct that links objectives, strategy and doctrine in British official thinking. For in practice there is probably no such thing. It is more instructive to identify the judgments and assumptions underlying the current national defense effort as they relate to aspirations, policy, posture and provision.[11]

ASPIRATIONS

Much of what can be said about fundamental aspirations has been anticipated in earlier remarks. British defense decision making is rooted in concern with security and status. Security connotes freedom to order the nation's affairs according to its own interests and values, implying freedom from fear of invasion, intimidation, or coercion. The only military challenges that appear seriously to threaten Britain are those posed by the Soviet Union. The values that infuse the Soviet system, and which Moscow is committed to propagate, are regarded as antithetical to those of Western democracies. More immediately, the Soviet Union and its allies present a potential military

threat to Western Europe. The only practicable response to these challenges is countervailing power, expressed in political cohesion and matching military might, provided within the framework of the Atlantic Alliance (and, in certain respects, the European Communities). Considerations of stature, or prestige, enter the reckoning because the United Kingdom aspires to cut a certain kind of figure in international affairs: that of a leading regional power with a global vision.

POLICY

The central objective of policy is to help deter aggression against either the United Kingdom itself or its European allies. National and regional security are regarded as inseparable. At the same time it is recognized that credible deterrence is dependent upon continuing association with the United States, given the link this implies to American strategic power. However, total reliance on the United States entails certain risks. Successive governments have therefore judged it prudent to maintain a semi-independent strategic retaliatory force. It is acknowledged, nevertheless, that dissuasion by the threat of punitive retaliation lacks credibility for many (if not most) contingencies. To deter attack by conventional forces, NATO needs the capacity to mount a robust defense at least sufficient to deny Warsaw Pact forces a quick and easy victory. Indeed, a conventional warfighting strategy is considered essential to the maintenance of deterrence, not to mention its desirability should deterrence fail. Hence the substantial British contribution to the alliance's conventional strength.

Retention of extraregional influence is desired too, despite the fact that the United Kingdom's imperial disengagement is all but complete. To some extent this stems from a desire to be more than an "ordinary" European power. To some extent it is a simple consequence of past involvements, disengagement having left a legacy of minor responsibilities that policy makers feel cannot, or should not, be wholly set aside.

Recurring tension between the competing pulls of independence and interdependence is discernible in these judgments and assumptions. There is also a separate tension field in the policy arena, generated by the imperative of preserving security through maintenance of adequate forces and the incentive to do what can be done to enhance security through arms control.

Under the latter heading, the United Kingdom participates in several disarmament forums under UN auspices and has been responsible for important initiatives in some of them. The national commitment "to pursue negotiations in good faith on effective measures relating to cessation of the nuclear arms race" and to actual nuclear disarmament is, however, a nominal one for all practical purposes. Nor does the United Kingdom pay more than lip service to the desirability of general and complete disarmament.[12]

On the other hand, there is a genuine interest in progress toward regional arms control agreements, because it would serve British interests to moderate the intensity of the military confrontation in Europe and establish a military balance there at a lower level of forces, always provided this can be done on the basis of "undiminished security." What has been achieved in the Conference on Disarmament in Europe (CDE) and in the discussions on Mutual and Balanced Force Reductions (MBFR) is, however, strictly limited. The emphasis in British (and NATO) policy is therefore firmly on the side of maintaining the allied apparatus for deterrence and defense. Accordingly, it is pertinent to ask how NATO views the task of countering the perceived political and military threat from the Soviet Union and Warsaw Pact countries. To what concepts of operations and to what strategic and tactical doctrines do member nations subscribe? What sort of stance has been taken in Europe and the North Atlantic? And what, therefore, are the foundations of the defense posture assumed by the United Kingdom as a member of the alliance?

POSTURE

Deterrence and defense rest on the ability to counter any form of aggression in an appropriate and credible manner. The wherewithal must exist to meet a conventional attack with a conventional riposte, at least in the first instance (and preferably for as long as possible). At the same time NATO's strategy of flexible response embodies the notion of graduated escalation. If the ability to sustain a conventional defense were in question, governments would threaten the use of theater nuclear weapons. Such a crossing of the nuclear threshold would pose the risk of escalation to the use of strategic weapons. The concept of the NATO triad is thus central to the alliance posture.

On the weight to be assigned to the different elements in the triad, the formal NATO position is that substantial conventional capabilities are the sine qua non of flexible response. The United Kingdom accepts this view. Clearly, the effectiveness of an initial conventional defense is crucially dependent on warning. Alliance doctrine supposes that any aggression in Western Europe or the North Atlantic would be preceded by "political warning time" during which redeployment and reinforcement of frontline forces could be undertaken. Put another way, it is thought unlikely that any Warsaw Pact attack would be sudden or that it would take NATO by surprise. This, too, accords with British thinking.

Though committed to the idea of graduated escalation, neither the United Kingdom nor any other NATO country discounts the possibility that the protagonists in a European conflict might not resort to nuclear weapons. This produces a double burden. In the first place, there is a requirement for conventional forces in being and forces in place adequate to withstand the shock of a Warsaw Pact attack—that is to prosecute a "short war" of great intensity. If the period of conventional warfare should be protracted, however, there is the need to provide for the "long war": to think about sustenance, including the movement of men and matériel from the United States, and hence about reserves and forces to protect air and sea lines of communications (SLOCs) both within the theater and between Europe and North America.

How does the United Kingdom's contribution to NATO's order of battle fit into this postural framework? The roles of maritime forces are related to safeguarding "forward areas at sea" and protecting the SLOCs. Ground and air forces—principally 1 (British) Corps and Royal Air Force, Germany—are earmarked for assignment to the Supreme Allied Commander, Europe (SACEUR), to implement, alongside allies, operations for "forward defense" in northwestern Europe. Assigned missions for maritime forces are, principally, surveillance and presence in peacetime, antisubmarine warfare and mine countermeasures in the event of hostilities. The allotted task of 1 (British) Corps is to defend its slice of NATO forces' "layer-cake" dispositions by fighting a succession of tactical blocking engagements and conducting whatever combination of counterpenetration, counterattack, and counterstroke maneuvers might be necessary to halt and repel the invader. The priority missions for the United Kingdom's tactical air power, in addition to air defense, are medium- and long-range attack on targets such as Warsaw Pact airfields and supply lines, with some aircraft tasked for closer support and others withheld to provide a capability for nuclear strikes.

Year-by-year decision making on defense is greatly facilitated by the existence of the frame of reference provided by the alliance's posture and doctrine. At the same time, it is no secret that there are differences of view among the NATO nations about (1) how the flexible response strategy should be implemented, (2) whether the linkages between the different elements in the triad are sound, (3) how the balance between "short war" and "long war" capabilities should be struck, and (4) whether there *is* a danger of sudden or surprise attack, assumptions about warning time notwithstanding. Where the United Kingdom stands on some of these issues can be considered in due course. For the moment other matters take precedence. Why the United Kingdom provides what it does to the NATO order of battle is implicit in the foregoing discussion of the alliance's force posture. To illuminate the rationale of what is provided, and how much, an examination of decision makers' judgments and assumptions about what constitutes appropriate provision is in order.

PROVISION

Whereas fundamental aspirations and decisions about policy and posture are framed in the light of the international environment and a nation's sense of its place in it (with special

reference to perceived threats), ideas about "appropriate" provision for security tend to reflect what sort of defense effort the state's domestic resources and competences permit it to mount. Put another way, it is in settling military provision that governments' choices are most affected by internal influences. D. Hazel and P. Williams have suggested that in the United Kingdom three kinds of judgment are influential in this context: (1) those that determine the political choice about the scale on which resources should be committed to security purposes as opposed to other claims on the national budget; (2) those that impinge on the allocation of resources within the defense establishment, i.e., among the services; and (3) those made within the individual services about (for example) what warships are most suitable for what missions, how field-force formations should be structured and equipped, and the performance characteristics required of combat aircraft.[13]

On the allocation of resources to defense, a key guideline reflected in the current and planned future program is that the share of GDP so allotted should not be significantly greater than that assigned by Britain's European allies. Whether approximate parity in defense/GDP proportions is a rational criterion for deciding the size of the defense effort is debatable. The fact is that nominal equality of sacrifice with other European states is as much, if not more, than politicians are prepared to ask of the electorate. (Provision on this scale is, of course, broadly acceptable to the allies.)[14]

Regarding the division of funds among the services, it has already been stated that importance is attached to the maintenance of balanced forces with a more or less full range of capabilities. Possession of all-round military competence is, among other things, one of the main bases of Britain's claim to a special status among the European members of the Atlantic Alliance. Thus, over the years little or no consideration has been given to the idea of collectively balanced forces that was propounded when NATO was first established (requiring and permitting imbalances at the national level). Having said that, of late there has been a notable revival of interest in the idea of a division of labor among the allies—with states specializing in different roles and missions for the benefit of the alliance as a whole—and British policy makers have cautiously welcomed this development.

Several specific judgments and assumptions about individual service force levels, structures, equipment, and deployment underlie the current program and budget. It is appropriate to spell them out in some detail, so far as the three principal elements in the national order of battle are concerned.

The first is that the United Kingdom should continue to provide substantial ground forces for the European theater. The British Army of the Rhine (BAOR) has rarely mustered its nominal strength of 55,000 men and is costly in foreign exchange. But no major reduction has been seriously contemplated. Political and military judgments combine to make the force level virtually sacrosanct. A crucial consideration is the commitment under the Paris Agreements of 1954. This is not just a matter of adherence to a formal treaty. The rationale of the original undertaking remains valid. The British army presence in Germany helps reassure those who would be apprehensive if the West German armed forces were the only substantial European contingents on the central front. A large contribution also entitles the United Kingdom to a prominent voice in alliance counsels and confers a claim to leading command positions. (In addition, since 1968 it has been assumed that to reduce the Rhine army's strength would be ill-advised while negotiations on mutual force reductions are under way, as they still are.) As for the force structure, planning for the 1990s presumes that armament norms, existing ratios of armored units to mechanized infantry and the like require little change. In choices about equipment, although the current program embodies provision for more light antitank weapons and antitank missiles, armor retains its prominent place in the divisional structure, both to match Warsaw Pact tank capabilities and to provide the means for counterattack and, if appropriate, bold counterstrokes.[15]

The key judgment underlying current and planned naval provision is that it is essential to have a balanced fleet, including some ships of high quality, many less capable general purpose surface units, and a variety of smaller vessels. The operational justification for such a force structure lies in the flexibility it affords, making it feasible to cope with whatever Soviet challenges may be presented in the eastern Atlantic. This is true whether one considers wartime missions (acquiring sufficient "sea control" to safeguard transatlantic SLOCs) or the provision of peacetime presence (to forestall any Soviet efforts at intimidation). Also, a balanced fleet is one thing other European members of NATO lack; it therefore differentiates the United Kingdom from its European partners (and, incidentally, validates retention of residual global aspirations).

The critical assumptions underlying the configuration of the Royal Air Force are similarly rooted in regard for flexibility and versatility, against the background of the inexorably rising cost of advanced systems. The presumption is that only sophisticated aircraft are capable of operating in modern air warfare. Given budgetary constraints, however, only relatively few of the requisite quality can be acquired. Therefore, the argument runs, it is necessary to procure versatile, multirole aircraft. Yet these, by their very nature, are the most expensive. This is a vicious circle, from which there is no obvious escape when mission priorities necessitate emphasis on the most demanding tasks and hence the most complex (and costly) systems. It is this position in which the United Kingdom finds itself, however. Current tactical air doctrine ascribes prime importance to (1) the offensive counterair mission (attacks on enemy air bases undertaken to suppress the threat to NATO's own air capabilities and ground formations) and (2) interdiction (attacks on the adversary's "follow-on forces" and supply lines).

In each of the services' major mission programs, existing assumptions about structure are regarded as virtually immutable. Procurement of new equipment is thus based primarily on a "replacement" philosophy. The predisposition is to replace existing weapons with superior—but essentially similar—systems, like succeeding like. This is one of the most significant assumptions made about provision. Among other things, it means that new technologies tend to be evaluated, and therefore adopted, only to the extent that they are compatible with the existing structure and organization of the armed forces. Opportunities to carry out some missions differently, to dispense with others, and generally to alter mission priorities may be overlooked as a result of the inclination so fostered to focus more or less exclusively on improvements at the margin.

This is not the place to pursue the implications of the "replacement" philosophy, or indeed of other determinants of the size and shape of the defense effort. The United Kingdom's security objectives, strategy, and doctrine have been illuminated, albeit from an oblique perspective; and that is as far as the exposition here needs to go. There are certain glosses to be added, however, principally to facilitate comparison with other countries' arrangements.

OTHER OBSERVATIONS

An obvious first question is: what part, if any, do ideology and culture play in the determination of objectives (or the means chosen to pursue them)? Decision makers in the United Kingdom would resist any assertion that they play a significant role, arguing that over the years British defense and overseas policy has been animated by practical concern for "the national interest" rather than enthusiasm for propagation of a particular set of values. In one respect they would be right. Pragmatism earned Britain the tag "perfidious Albion," and more than one statesman has acknowledged an inclination to fashion policy according to whatever suits the nation's purpose for the time being. In two respects, though, they would be wrong. Underlying policy, there is a definite commitment to certain ideas or values—such as the virtues of democracy on the Western model, respect for individual freedoms and "the open society"—that the nation seeks not only to protect, but also to promote and extend. In addition, the United Kingdom's participation in disarmament and arms control negotiations, and the general tenor of

debate about chemical, biological, and nuclear weapons, testify to some respect for humane, Christian values.

Various questions concerning the extent of consensus and controversy on security matters also suggest themselves. Does one find broad agreement on policy goals? Are there major disputes about force posture? Is the scale or pattern of provision for defense an issue in party politics? Public opinion has been directly influential on very few defense policy choices in recent years. Apathy has something to do with this. More important is the fact that defense and overseas policy is an area in which the government of the day carries authority and exercises leadership. This is not to say that popular attitudes have had *no* influence on planning. For example, defense has been subject to the (indirect) effect of insistent pressure for less public spending and for allocation of larger shares of expenditure to health, education, welfare, and other social security programs. Nor does acknowledgement of governments' authority in international political affairs mean that they have absolute freedom of maneuver. Quite the contrary: they must act within limits set by their sense of what the public will stand.

Looking at electoral politics, until the early 1980s defense was rarely a salient issue. No formal accord existed among the principal parties. But the importance of NATO and the need to pay an appropriate "club subscription" were common ground. There was agreement, too, on most force-postural questions. Although some debate took place within the political community, topics like the role of nuclear weapons in alliance doctrine, or "short war" versus "long war" theses, or force-structure priorities received only cursory or intermittent attention. Consensus began to break down, however, during the period leading up to the general election of 1983. It was shattered during the campaign itself, and there has been no sign of reconstruction since. The main political parties now hold significantly different positions on several central issues, notably nuclear matters (and related arms control questions) and alliance doctrine (ideas of "defensive deterrence" having found favor with the Labour, Liberal Democrat, and Social Democratic parties).[16] [Similarly, ideas such as "nonprovocative defense" and non-nuclear "defensive defense" have found favor in the Social Democratic Party in West Germany and other left-of-center parties in northern Europe—Eds.]

In the defense establishment, of course, there has always been argument about strategy and doctrine. Behind the facade of consensus that political convenience and constitutional propriety require, there is constant controversy on matters of policy, force posture, and provision. No substantial studies have been written exposing the bureaucratic politics of British defense comparable with the work of P. Hammond, W. Schilling, and G. Snyder on overall program issues or that of Ingemar Dorfer on particular procurement decisions.[17] But there is indirect, fragmentary evidence to confirm that major choices do generate disagreements (sometimes profound ones) and that there are strong constituencies for certain courses. Furthermore, each service bureaucracy is naturally inclined to "fight its own corner" as and when necessary. None of this, though, amounts to more than the legitimate contention of opposing viewpoints and priorities. If the air force, backed by the aerospace industry lobby, presses the case for greater emphasis on maritime patrol aircraft rather than surface ships or submarines for antisubmarine warfare tasks, this is likely to ensure full exposure of the merits of the alternatives rather than degenerate into a bout of "no-holds-barred" institutional infighting among the services.[18]

DOMESTIC DETERMINANTS

There is one serious disadvantage to the analytical approach to elucidation of national objectives, strategy, and doctrine that has been adopted here. No easy differentiation is possible between (a) external influences on policy like the state's place in the international environment and its relations with adversaries and allies and (b) internal influences, such as military, economic, technological, or psychosocial capacities. From one standpoint, of course, this shortcoming can be counted a merit. In practice, external and internal inputs to the decision-making process are inextricably interwoven: differentiation for expository convenience can be misleading. On the other hand, to facilitate comparison of the British situation with that in other countries, there is value in a brief examination from this perspective of the essential domestic determinants of policy, force posture, and provision.[19]

Economic factors have to be given pride of place (if that is what it is) in such a scrutiny. For the United Kingdom they have been influential in at least four different senses (and still are). First and most fundamentally, in some degree a nation's economic philosophy determines who its friends are. In this sense, the United Kingdom's Atlantic and European affiliations are the natural ones for a state that favors a "mixed economy." Second, when developing these connections in the late 1940s, British statesmen were (among other things) ensuring reasonable provision for security, despite relative economic weakness. The acknowledgement of interdependence originated in a practical recognition of the country's inability to sustain a fully independent role in world affairs, and the wisdom of this assessment has been borne out by events. It is in the actual evolution of the defense effort since 1945 that the impact of economics in a third sense is evident: general and specific resource constraints have been directly instrumental in prompting the significant transformation that has taken place.[20]

Despite the diminution in the scale of the British defense effort (according to the familiar indicators of military stature) and the contraction in its geographical scope, the nation retains more or less balanced forces whose equipment is kept reasonably up-to-date; and a high proportion of the armed forces' systems and matériel continue to be procured from domestic industry. This last characteristic is the clue to the fourth sense in which economic factors enter the United Kingdom's defense calculations. Having a comprehensive armaments base (for which there is support from economic, social, and technological policy interests) has been, and seems likely to continue to be, influential so far as the pattern of the defense effort is concerned. The point here goes beyond registering the familiar fact that from time to time procurement choices are determined by employment considerations or a desire to preserve a stake in some area of high defense technology. The contention is that having all-round research, development, and production competence means the existence of a structure of interests and incentives for the maintenance of all-round military capabilities.[21]

The technological theme in this argument is worth an additional gloss. It is arguable that the case for the adoption of concepts of operations in which greater emphasis might be placed on simpler, more rugged warships or combat aircraft gets less than a fair hearing in the United Kingdom because the country is wedded to high-technology solutions to defense equipment problems for reasons that have little to do with military effectiveness. The point cannot be pursued here. But the idea that nations "live up" to their technological competence may be worth some attention from students of comparative defense policy.

Of the other domestic determinants of security arrangements that invite mention with facilitation of comparative studies in mind, geography deserves a brief word. Although not highlighted thus far, it would be wrong to overlook how the United Kingdom's dispositions and priorities reflect the strategic location of the British Isles. The nation stands at the western end of NATO's northern flank and forms the southern part of the Greenland-Iceland-Faeroes-Scotland gap, which is the key "choke point" on the Soviet Northern Fleet's access route to the North Atlantic and to NATO's potentially critical sea lines of communication. The European end of that (and the interface with the intratheater sea lines) is the United Kingdom itself, which is therefore the key "rear area" for Allied Command Europe. Nor does it fulfill this role only with respect to reinforcement and resupply. It is from the comparative safety of bases in England that much of NATO's tactical air power might be expected to operate in the event of actual hostilities on the European continent.

Drawing the relevant "strategic maps"—either in this fashion or literally—can enhance understanding of any state's defense policy. It is not too far-fetched to say that the United Kingdom's present-day objectives, strategy, and doctrine could be inferred directly from reflection on (a) the familiar cartographer's representation, showing the British Isles as continental Europe's offshore islands; and (b) the sort of view of the country's geostrategic setting that Geoffrey Kemp produced more than a decade ago.[22] What is equally true is that until the later 1940s, it was only necessary to examine a political map of the world—showing the Dominions, colonies, and other dependencies of the British Empire and Commonwealth, depicted, usually, in an arresting shade of red—to acquire a sound overall appreciation of why the United Kingdom defined its security priorities on a global scale, and made its naval and military dispositions accordingly.

Aspirations, policy judgments, and assumptions about what constitute a becoming force posture and "appropriate" provision—all framed by the state's perception of its place in the international environment and the threats it faces—are the essential inputs to the United Kingdom's defense decision making. In a simple world it might be permissible to proceed from this point to consideration of outputs, to what British governments do and plan to do in defense given these circumstances. Yet no student of national security affairs would make the mistake of supposing that the institutions, personalities, and procedures of the planning, programing, and budgeting apparatus can be regarded as "black boxes" or mere ciphers or formalized routines. Quite the contrary: in the United Kingdom, as elsewhere, some insight into how decisions are taken is a prerequisite for full understanding of the decisions themselves.

The Defense Decision-Making Process

British institutional arrangements for defense policy making and planning are best illuminated, in the first instance, by examination of the organizational structure and bureaucratic procedures. To complement an account along these lines this section also includes a review of constraints that have impinged on decision makers recently and those likely to operate in the future.

STRUCTURE

Enumeration of *all* the institutions and agencies that could be said to be engaged in the defense decision-making process is out of the question. It is necessary to simplify matters, for manageability's sake. This is most conveniently done by consideration of (1) the central organization of the Ministry of Defence itself, which must obviously be the focus of attention; and (2) some of the main "other participants," ranging from the body to which the secretary of state for defense is formally accountable (Parliament, especially the House of Commons) to those that simply seek to influence program and budget choices (e.g., interest groups).[23]

Florence Nightingale wrote of the nineteenth-century War Office that it was "a very slow office, an enormously expensive office, a not very efficient office and one in which the minister's intentions can be entirely negatived by all his sub-departments and those of each of the sub-departments by every other."[24]

No doubt it would be possible to find some people with experience of the present-day Ministry of Defence prepared to voice similar sentiments. However, most would probably acknowledge that, since the introduction of a "new model" organization in 1985, central direction has been greatly strengthened.

An earlier structural reform had sought to achieve this, but with only limited success. In 1964 that exercise brought together a small coordinating Defence Ministry and three virtually autonomous service departments (Admiralty, War Office, Air Ministry) to form the consolidated Ministry of Defence, with a nominally strong central staff element and three nominally subordinate single-service organizations (the Navy Department, the Army Department, the Air Force Department). To these there was added, later, a separate apparatus—the Procurement Executive—to deal with all equipment acquisition. Redrafting of the organization charts did not, however, immediately transform decision making; nor did

it produce substantial manpower savings. Moreover, the service departments retained considerable de facto autonomy and—in the defense reviews of 1964–68 and 1974–75, for example—senior officers and officials frequently behaved as though animated more by a determination to protect their own projects and priorities than by a commitment to fashion the "right" program. The minister's intentions were not "entirely negatived"; but they were occasionally frustrated.

Hence the reexamination of the structure that took place in the early 1980s and yielded the "new model" organization established in January 1985. Under these arrangements, depicted in figure 1, the individual service departments were stripped of their separate policy and planning staffs and a new unified defense staff was formed, under the day-to-day direction of the four-star vice chief of the defence staff. Along with the three single-service chiefs, now left with only executive staffs, this officer reports to the chief of the defence staff, the government's principal military adviser.

On the civil side, all officials concerned with long-term financial planning, resource allocation, and the scrutiny and control of expenditure were brought together in an integrated Office of Management and Budget (OMB), under the second permanent under secretary of state. Together with the chief scientific adviser and the chief of defence procurement, this official reports to the permanent under secretary of state, the top civil appointment in the hierarchy.[25]

Even under this setup, though, the single-service chiefs and their departments are not completely dominated by the central bureaucracy. After all, these organizations remain important sources of technical expertise in their respective domains, and the locus of responsibility for day-to-day administration and accounting; and it is to the service rather than to the ministry that the personnel of the armed forces regard themselves as owing allegiance.

Regular consultation with other government departments is, obviously, a key feature of decision making in defense: thus the first category of "other participants" in the process to be considered must be the cabinet colleagues

Figure 1. The Higher Organization of the Ministry of Defense

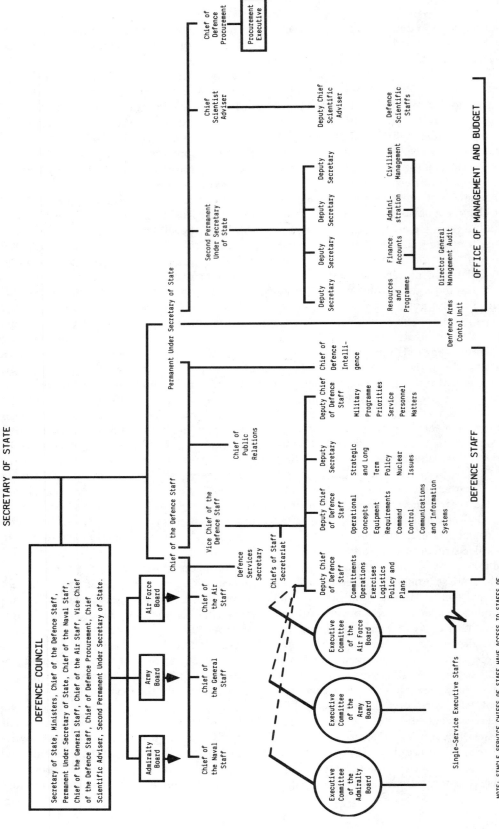

SECRETARY OF STATE

DEFENCE COUNCIL

Secretary of State, Ministers, Chief of the Defence Staff,
Permanent Under Secretary of State, Chief of the Naval Staff,
Chief of the General Staff, Chief of the Air Staff, Vice Chief
of the Defence Staff, Chief of Defence Procurement, Chief
Scientific Adviser, Second Permanent Under Secretary of State.

Admiralty Board

Army Board

Air Force Board

Chief of the Naval Staff

Chief of the General Staff

Chief of the Air Staff

Chief of the Defence Staff

Permanent Under Secretary of State

Vice Chief of the Defence Staff

Chief of Public Relations

Chief of Defence Intelligence

Defence Services Secretary

Chiefs of Staff Secretariat

Deputy Chief of Defence Staff

Commitments Operations
Exercises Logistics
Policy and Plans

Deputy Chief of Defence Staff

Operational Concepts
Equipment Requirements
Command Control
Communications and Information Systems

Deputy Secretary

Strategic and Long Term
Policy
Nuclear Issues

Deputy Chief of Defence Staff

Military Programme Priorities
Service Personnel Matters

Second Permanent Under Secretary of State

Deputy Secretary

Deputy Secretary

Deputy Secretary

Deputy Secretary

Resources and Programmes

Finance Accounts

Admini- stration

Civilian Management

Director General Management Audit

Chief Scientist Adviser

Deputy Chief Scientific Adviser

Defence Scientific Staffs

Chief of Defence Procurement

Procurement Executive

Denfence Arms Control Unit

DEFENCE STAFF

OFFICE OF MANAGEMENT AND BUDGET

Executive Committee of the Admiralty Board

Executive Committee of the Army Board

Executive Committee of the Air Force Board

Single-Service Executive Staffs

NOTE: SINGLE SERVICE CHIEFS OF STAFF HAVE ACCESS TO STAFFS OF
VICE CHIEF OF DEFENCE STAFF, CHIEF OF DEFENCE INTELLIGENCE
AND CHIEF OF PUBLIC RELATIONS

Note: Single-service chiefs of staff have access to staffs of Vice Chief of Defense staff, Chief of Defense Intelligence, and Chief of Public Relations.

of the secretary of state for defence. External defence being an aspect of foreign policy, the defence minister clearly works particularly closely with the foreign secretary. Because of his concern with the well-being of the nation's armaments manufacturers, necessitating an interest in domestic industrial policy, he must (or should) also have good lines of communication with the Department of Trade and Industry. (Conversely industrial capacity, employment and regional policy considerations regularly cut across security policy preoccupations). In the internal security field, links with the Home Office are obviously important, not least where questions of military aid to the civil power are involved. Finally, all of the secretary of state for defence's responsibilities are discharged, as one experienced official has put it, "to the accompaniment of a running dialogue with the Chancellor of the Exchequer about the cost of the defence budget and the ability of the economy to sustain it."[26]

Of the institutions outside government with power or influence vis-à-vis the defense program and budget, a clear distinction should be drawn between those with formal power and those that do no more than exercise influence (or try to do so). The elected chamber of Parliament, the House of Commons, is of paramount importance under the first heading. In the United Kingdom the executive governs subject to its ability to command a majority in the House of Commons. In this sense, all its decisions require parliamentary consent. But there is a particular discipline associated with the Commons' control of the purse. And so far as defense is concerned, there is a need to carry the House of Commons in the vote not only on each year's budget (the defense estimates) but also on annual legislation regarding each service. Yet these are formal powers, for to reject outright what the administration proposes is to take an extreme course in British politics, possibly precipitating a general election. In practice, therefore, the House of Commons can, in normal circumstances, only "influence the Government . . . by the strength of the argument which it brings to bear . . . in debate and otherwise."[27] A corollary is that special significance attaches to the role of certain parliamentary committees. Two are particularly noteworthy: the Defence Committee, which acts as interlocutor with government on defense program and budget issues (and whose periodic reports are, incidentally, an invaluable source of information and analysis); and the Public Accounts Committee, which acts as Parliament's watchdog on the actual use of resources (and has also produced many illuminating reports over the years).[28]

In relation to these core components of the "structure" (the Defence Ministry, other government departments, and Parliament), which are the key positions, how far can the idiosyncrasies of a particular occupant affect the decision-making process?

First and foremost it is obvious that the top political appointment, that of defence secretary, is a crucial one and that a strong-minded and strong-willed holder of the post can make his mark on the defense program and on defense management. The Conservative Duncan Sandys certainly did that in the late 1950s. Following his *Outline of Future Policy*, planning took off in several new directions, driven by little more than the minister's conviction that these were the right directions (although, in retrospect, they appear to have been totally the wrong ones). Sheer force of personality seems to be the only explanation for the episode, the minister taking free rein to indulge his penchant for asking fundamental questions and answering them himself, in defiance of professional advice.[29] In the second half of the 1960s Labour's Denis Healey managed a no less decisive reshaping of the defense effort, establishing the main contours of policy for the next decade and more. However, his was an entirely different method of working. The Healey style involved extensive consultation, but of an informal nature, and with the emphasis on ad hoc groups, personal communication, and private advice rather than regular meetings of formal committees.[30] At the same time, the minister's personal imprint is discernible in all that was done during his tenure of office, and in the way in which things were explained in the Defence White Papers of the period. In fact, at this time, "there is no point in seeking a focus of policy decision-making anywhere in the

Ministry . . . outside the office of the Secretary of State."[31] In the 1980s two Conservative ministers "made their mark." The first was John Nott (1981–82), who conducted the 1981 defense review in the teeth of some skepticism, if not outright opposition, from the chiefs of staff, but delivered (in his policy statement *The Way Forward*) a blueprint for the nation's defenses that remains broadly valid.[32] The second was Nott's successor, Michael Heseltine (1983–85), who antagonized many at the ministry with his no-nonsense managerial style, but must be given credit for putting the bureaucratic house in order, for instituting a broad range of measures aimed at getting better value for money in defense, and for taking his responsibilities with regard to defense industrial policy sufficiently seriously to make them a matter over which he would resign his office.[33]

On the military side, the office of the chief of the defence staff can count for as much or as little as the incumbent wishes. In the mid 1960s, Lord Mountbatten used his immense personal prestige to considerable effect in minimizing interservice squabbling during the childhood and adolescence of the newly consolidated ministry. In the mid 1970s, Field Marshal (now Lord) Carver played an important part in preventing the 1974 Defence Review from degenerating into either indiscriminate application of the law of equal misery among the three services or uncritical slaughtering of the least sacred cows in the equipment program. In the later 1970s, Marshal of the Royal Air Force Sir Neil Cameron fluttered the dovecotes of the ministry by insistence on a more imaginative assessment of new technological opportunities, and more systematic appraisal of medium- and longer-term program possibilities generally, than the machinery then in being was accustomed to making. But these are the only recent holders of the highest uniformed appointment in the United Kingdom to have projected any kind of image other than that of unobtrusive military counselor. Nor has any individual service chief emerged from the shadows into the popular, or the political, limelight in recent years. The last to do so was Admiral Sir David Luce, who resigned from the post of chief of the naval staff in 1966 in protest against cancellation of the first of a new class of attack carriers.[34]

Under no circumstances would the top civil servants of the Ministry of Defence enter the limelight. Be that as it may, the permanent under secretary occupies a powerful position and may, indeed, have the decisive voice on many issues, especially if the minister is unassertive and the chief of the defense staff self-effacing. Likewise on weapons acquisition decisions, short-term political and military appointees may be reluctant to fly in the face of the advice of the chief of defence procurement and the chief scientific advisor. Yet perhaps no single mandarin within the ministry is as influential year in and year out as the Treasury bureaucrat who writes the script for the "running dialogue" the secretary of state for defence holds with the chancellor of the exchequer, namely the official charged with oversight of public expenditure (including the defense budget). This is because, anticipating a thesis to be elaborated later, expenditure *is* policy; in reality, the budgeting process is the central mode of defense decision making.[35]

Lying outside "official circles" are those "other participants" in defense decision making who are able to exercise limited influence on selected issues. The most important are interest groups, whose activities may include (1) direct consultation with the authorities on certain matters, (2) the lobbying of Parliament, and (3) efforts to shape public attitudes. The number of such groups involved in defense affairs in the United Kingdom is fairly small, and most that show a direct concern play generally supportive roles. This is not to say that they wield no influence. Those representing economic interests (certain manufacturers' associations and organized labor in defense-related industry and defense-dependent localities, for instance) clearly do bring effective pressure to bear from time to time, while the veterans organizations invariably get a hearing on welfare questions like pensions.

Protest movements seeking to effect substantive change in security policies have had mixed fortunes. The best known, the Campaign for Nuclear Disarmament (CND), enjoyed considerable visibility in the 1950s and 1960s and was instrumental in the 1960 Labour Party Conference's rejection of an official policy statement and adoption of a unilateralist resolution. But that 1960 conference decision was reversed a year later, and throughout the 1960s and most of the 1970s, the CND languished. It returned to prominence in the later 1970s and 1980s, however, as the leading organization of a self-styled "peace movement" dedicated to the cause of nuclear disarmament and urging on British politicians the renunciation of such weapons. The campaigners were especially active in the early 1980s, using techniques of intellectual persuasion and active protest, the latter directed principally against (a) the emplacement in Britain of American cruise missiles (at Greenham Common and, later, Molesworth) and (b) the decision to acquire Trident submarine-launched ballistic missiles for the United Kingdom's own strategic nuclear force. The dissent played a part in persuading the Labour Party finally to espouse unilateral nuclear disarmament.[36]

Exerting a more significant, if less spectacular, influence on defense decision making in the United Kingdom are the attentive publics in specialist research institutes and some academic centers who make it their business to analyze policy options. These can generate solid and articulate support for, or opposition to, the Defence Ministry's policies and practices. However, with the exception of one or two organizations allied to the peace movement, they do not as a general rule initiate debate on radical departures in policy, although occasionally an analyst's thesis, dismissed as misguided or impractical at first appearance, turns up in official pronouncements at some later stage.

PROCEDURES

Organization charts show how things would work if it were not for the personalities involved. This is only one of their shortcomings, however. Knowledge of the formal institutional structure involved in an activity like defense policy making and management may be necessary, but it is not sufficient for understanding of the decision-making process. It must be matched by an appreciation of the bureaucracy's procedures, particularly planning, programing, and budgeting. This is certainly true in the United Kingdom, where, for all practical purposes, settling the program and budget is the central defense decision-making process.

Reflection on the nature of budgeting confirms that, in fact, this is generally and necessarily the case. For budgeting is not bookkeeping. It is the act of "systematically relating the expenditure of funds to the accomplishment of planned objectives"[37] or "the translation of financial resources into human purposes."[38] Government budgeting is the setting of national priorities. It involves the balancing of claims on resources for security goals against those for personal consumption, industrial investment, social infrastructure, and social services. Defense budgeting entails the refinement and elaboration of security priorities, i.e., deciding what is to be done and what resources are to be allotted to what military purposes over time. That this must be the heart of the business is self-evident, for every policy choice has expenditure implications and every budgetary allocation registers some decision about policy, force posture, or provision. In a phrase: expenditure *is* policy.[39]

How, then, are resources allocated to defense and within defense in the United Kingdom? Essentially there are four stages: (1) Assessment of the resources likely to be available for all purposes, public and private, military and civil; (2) Decisions regarding the proportion of available resources over which government should take command, by taxation or borrowing, to finance all collective provision; (3) Decisions about the allocation of those resources among competing claimants, viz., the defense effort and civil expenditure programs; and (4) Decisions on the content of the defense program, viz., the size and shape, equipment and deployment of the armed forces, both frontline and support elements.

For present purposes the main emphasis can be given to the third and fourth stages, particularly the fourth. But it is important to be aware of the context in which defense decision making takes place. It is also important to recognize that resource allocation procedures in practice are concerned with on-going programs and, therefore, with whether more or less should be assigned to public rather than private ends (stage 2); with whether the balance among public sector outlays should be altered (stage 3); and with whether this or that element in the national order of battle should be strengthened or run down, this or that weapon system developed and produced (stage 4). In short, most decisions are made in incremental or marginal terms. Only exceptionally is an entire line of expenditure open to outright severance or massive extension.

A further and equally important point is that, in the United Kingdom as elsewhere, examining or imagining new possibilities, making plans, monitoring progress on present policies, and mulling over past experiences are activities that go on continuously and simultaneously. Formal resource allocation, geared to the annual budget cycle, does not require the compression of choices into one cosmic operation. Rather, the yearly routine constitutes a bringing together, for overall appreciation and adjustment (if necessary), of numerous decentralized choices and decisions. In the United Kingdom the focus of this routine is the annual Public Expenditure Survey, a government-wide exercise that encompasses the first three of the four stages of budgeting, and hence the allocation of resources to defense.

Each year the Treasury orchestrates a complex operation in which, first, a medium-term assessment of economic prospects is made. To adopt a well-worn metaphor, this is to establish how large the national cake is expected to be and leads naturally to consideration of how it should be sliced. The second stage is concerned, to continue the metaphor, with where the initial cut of the knife should be made, determining how much the state gets and how much private citizens or private enterprise keep to use as they will. Settled at this juncture are the burden of taxation and the extent of borrowing (or redemption of debt) on the one hand, and the overall public expenditure total on the other. The size of the latter figure emerges after discussion of (a) general economic factors plus the government's overall political and social strategy and (b) the amount needed to accommodate at least the minimal

bids of spending departments. These deliberations take place under the auspices of a Public Expenditure Survey Committee (PESC). Hence, the shorthand term for the process: the PESC procedure. They merge imperceptibly into exchanges concerned with the third stage: apportionment of the total public expenditure figure among competing claimants, including the decision on how much should be allotted to defense as opposed to other things. This is the core of the public expenditure review exercise. It yields a set of projections for all government spending, analyzed according to programs (reflecting functions or objectives) and stretching to a three-year distant planning horizon, which is published in a Public Expenditure White Paper. The figure for aggregate (intended) defense spending in this document becomes the point of reference for all subsequent defense decision making. The defense program is a rolling program; each annual review cycle is based on the inherited program.[40]

The crucial question can now be addressed: how is resource allocation within defense conducted? How are defense priorities set? How is the breakdown of the program total decided upon? More specifically, how are decisions made about endorsement or amendment of the program-in-being, as a matter of routine or in special circumstances (and including the incorporation of weapons research, development, and production choices)?

Obviously, in an organization as large as the Defence Ministry, there are several loci of decision making. There has to be suboptimization, or a factoring out of the problems that arise in settling the precise composition of the defense effort. Simplifying brutally, the broad pattern of priorities is sketched by the central policy staffs in the light of the nation's security objectives and the part military power can play in pursuing them, thus defining the desired defense effort. These ideas lie behind any special studies that may be conducted, and equipment proposals are evaluated against this background. Outside the domain of special studies and major equipment proposals, the service departments enjoy substantial autonomy. Provided their decisions are consistent with the policy blueprint, they enjoy freedom of maneuver in making numerous decentralized choices. Equipment acquisition is formally centralized, under the aegis of the Procurement Executive, but there is some de facto delegation. Good accounts of procurement procedures exist elsewhere. For present purposes, it is sufficient to note that their main characteristic is a sequence of phases and thresholds (from concept formulation to the introduction of a system into service) providing ample opportunity for both analysis and adversary politics. The procedures go as far as institutional arrangements can to ensure that only equipment that is both necessary and cost-effective attracts funding.[41]

Resource allocation within defense is, however, about more than just how much more or less should be allocated for purposes that are exclusively the concern of a single service, or whether to include a new weapons system in a given program. Indeed, priority setting involves questions of deployment and force structures, and it is occasionally necessary to ask whether it is worth maintaining some capability at all. Because issues like these arise regularly, and require careful investigation when they do, special studies must be considered part of the regular machinery of decision making. But it is in special circumstances that such exercises come into their own (e.g., whenever the entire defense program comes under scrutiny, as it does when a change of government takes place or when a government in office is impelled to respond to change in economic or strategic conditions). Major defense reviews of this sort are the occasion for fundamental reconsideration of defense's place in national priorities and for associated reconsideration of security priorities.

Examples of such set-piece reviews are the exercises conducted by the Labour government in the mid 1960s, first in 1964–66, when the party entered office "after 13 years of Tory misrule" (as they put it), and again in 1967–68, a review foreshadowing concentration of the defense effort on Europe and the North Atlantic; the "extensive and thorough" review of 1974–75, also conducted by an incoming Labour administration, which led to reduction of the British contribution to the protection of NATO's flanks (especially the southern); and the Conservatives' midterm review of 1981, a courageous attempt to bring commitments into line with resources, which is remembered for the decision to run down the surface fleet.[42]

CONSTRAINTS

What now of the principal constraints policy makers and planners have confronted in the past and may be expected to face in the future? Most students of the United Kingdom's security affairs would nominate budgetary limitations as the most persistent and pervasive influence. Following the sequence of analysis just used in discussing resource allocation, the argument runs as follows: (1) Because of the British economy's poor growth record (and uncertain growth prospects) the resources available for all purposes have not been sufficient of late (and do not seem likely to be sufficient in the 1990s) to allow the nation to enjoy high consumption, undertake substantial industrial investment, maintain a welfare state able to satisfy even basic social security expectations, *and* sustain the kind of defense effort that yields not only a reasonable sense of security within the international system, but also the status to which this erstwhile great power aspires. (2) Their predecessors having countenanced a steady increase in the share of GDP absorbed by the state for collective provision, all governments taking office since the early 1970s have sought to contain the growth of public expenditure as a whole. (3) Against that background and faced with rising entitlements under various social security schemes and diverse pressures on other civil programs, successive administrations, even Mrs. Thatcher's Conservative governments, have regarded the defense effort as an area for economies.

The experience of the first and second Thatcher governments, formed in 1979 and 1983 respectively, is instructive. Honoring a domestic pledge to restore defense to its proper place in national priorities and an alliance pledge to increase spending by around 3 percent each year (after inflation), they planned on rising budgets, but had to conduct one full-scale defense review (in 1981), abandon the 3 percent commitment (in 1985), and project falling real outlays for the later 1980s.

If growth prospects improve and civil public spending programs continue to be squeezed, budgetary constraints may, of course, become less pressing. That there will inevitably be less money for defense in the 1990s is not, therefore, a completely foregone conclusion. But there is another side to the economic facts of defense. In the foreseeable future, as in the past, it does seem inevitable that, because of rising costs, the British will get less defense for their money (as will most other countries). On the manpower side, an improvement in pay relative to civilian alternatives could be required to preserve manning levels in the all-volunteer forces. In addition, more money may be needed for expenditures to mitigate the effects of "turbulence" on service families. On the equipment side, as noted earlier, a set of interlocking vicious circles operates. Technological innovation is sought so that existing missions can continue to be performed effectively in the face of the protagonist's new challenges. Thus, each generation of weapons systems must be more complex than the last. As a result, both initial acquisition and overall lifetime costs go higher. To accommodate higher unit costs, quantities are reduced. This limits the scope for learning and scale economies (i.e., the decreases in the cost of individual units that come when large numbers are produced), adding a further twist to costs. And the prospect of fewer units serves as an inducement to make each one do more—that is, to require multirole or general purpose capabilities, which entails building systems of even greater complexity and expense. Budgets are, therefore, increasingly taken up with fewer and fewer costly but complicated items.[43]

Nor is it wholly a matter of costs. Keeping both regular and reserve formations up to strength could become more problematic for the United Kingdom as time goes by. Although demographic trends are not as unfavorable as in the Federal Republic of Germany, there could well be difficulties with recruitment and retention in the 1990s. In striving to keep the forces' equipment up to date, account has to be taken of the erosion of the United Kingdom's, and Western Europe's, technical competence and competitiveness in certain areas.

Inability to contemplate development of some of the most advanced systems already acts as a constraint on program choices.

Economic constraints on decision making may be the most evident and tangible, but they are not the only ones. In practice, each of the judgments and assumptions about policy, force posture, and provision reviewed in the previous section is a constraint on year-to-year programing and budgeting. Options for neutralism on the Swedish model, or a quasi-independent stance under the North Atlantic Treaty such as France has adopted, simply do not enter the policy reckoning. Neither unilateral efforts at doctrinal innovation nor radical force-postural alternatives are seriously contemplated. Nor do British decision makers spend time speculating about reintroducing conscription or about following the Canadian experiment in service integration, while concern for the defense industrial base sets some limit to the enthusiasm with which collaborative procurement opportunities are pursued. In sum, although policy makers and planners are most conscious of how budgetary stringency constrains choice, in fact they operate within a much more complex framework of explicit and implicit limitations on their freedom of action.

Recurring Issues and Defense Policy Outputs

The outcome of the defense decision-making process is the current program and budget. In the financial year 1986–87, for example, the United Kingdom planned to devote some £18.5 billion (about $27 billion) to military purposes, fractionally more than had been spent, in cash terms, in the previous year. Projections for public expenditure as a whole incorporated provision for additional cash in succeeding years. Making allowance for inflation, however, the appropriation for 1986–87 represented reduced funding, a trend to continue throughout the rest of the decade.

What exactly was this money to be spent on? How have the British resolved, at least for the time being, the complex choices involved in settling the size, shape, equipment and deployment of their armed forces? Answering these questions will elucidate the United Kingdom's security priorities as expressed in the allocation of resources to functions. It makes sense, then, to consider any changes already incorporated or implicit in the program or likely to occur because current intentions are the subject of controversy. It is instructive also to note certain institutional features of the planned defense effort: specifically, how decision makers envisage acquiring the arms and mustering the armed forces for it. Expectations about the outcome of arms control negotiations invite attention too. Nor would an essay of this sort be complete without some remarks on the circumstances in which, rather than contemplating force reductions, the United Kingdom might feel impelled to augment its defense effort either to bolster deterrence in Europe or with actual operations in mind. In short, there is a crowded agenda for this final section.

THE CURRENT PROGRAM AND BUDGET

The defense program is most usefully illuminated by examination of the functional analysis of defense expenditure and personnel. Each year, data on the outlays and manpower associated with particular defense purposes are set out in the United Kingdom's *Statement on the Defence Estimates* (the annual Defence White Paper). Detailed figures are revealed only for the immediately forthcoming year, but fragments of evidence and informed inference allow observations to be made reaching further ahead. The functional divisions used in the *Statement of Defence Estimates, 1986* and the main values for what was then the first year slice of the program (1986–87) are shown in table 2. The following paragraphs consist of summary comment on each of the individual programs.

The *strategic nuclear force* is the least manpower-intensive and the least expensive of the major mission programs. But it represents the most potent single element in the national order of battle: four nuclear-powered ballistic missile submarines (SSBNs), each armed with sixteen Polaris missiles, which from the mid 1990s will be succeeded by four new, British-built boats carrying sixteen American Trident

D5 ballistic missiles apiece. This independent capacity for nuclear retaliation has a dual rationale. It is a contribution to the overall deterrence posture of the Atlantic Alliance, which, because it is a European force, is thought to count for more than its present or planned future destructive power might suggest (though that is not negligible). It is also a national deterrent of last resort. Moreover, symbolizing as it does the United Kingdom's status as a nuclear power, the presumption has been that it yields political as well as military utility, conferring prestige and some influence.[44]

Navy general purpose combat forces account for about 26 percent of expenditure directly attributable to mission programs (and about 14 percent of the total defense budget). The fleet consists of around 150 warships, providing the means to conduct a varied range of operations at or from the sea. Although lacking attack carriers (and before long, perhaps, amphibious warfare ships too), it is in all other respects a balanced fleet; and the intention is that it should remain so. Put another way, with the single exception of power-projection missions, the Royal Navy has and will retain *some* competence in all aspects of naval warfare. Its roles and missions derive from NATO's maritime strategy, while the flexibility that a balanced fleet confers is regarded as a worthwhile asset in its own right, not least as insurance against the unforeseen.

According to table 2, *European theater ground forces* accounted for 28 percent of the total bill for 1986–87 frontline, and for over 45 percent of uniformed, manpower. In fact 100,000 of the 300,000 members of the British armed forces serve with the program's three main components: the Berlin garrison is 3,000 strong; the British Army of the Rhine and Home Forces muster 55,000 and 42,000 respectively. (In addition these formations employ some 28,000 civilians in the United Kingdom and Germany.)

The troops stationed in *Berlin* consist of infantry and some support units. As part of the symbolic Western presence in the precarious enclave, they play a political role compared with which their military mission is relatively unimportant. Although not without political

Table 2. Functional Analysis of British Defense Expenditure and Manpower, 1986–87

Program	Expenditure[a] m	Percentage of Total	Manpower Service	000s Civilian
Nuclear strategic force	658	3.6	2.0	4.0
Navy GP combat forces	2,625	14.2	42.4	12.8
European theater ground forces	2,814	15.2	100.2	24.3
Other army combat forces	204	1.1	15.0	6.9
Air force GP forces	3,687	19.9	60.2	8.9
Mission programs total	9,988	54.0	219.8	56.9
Reserves and auxiliary formations	358	1.9	2.9	2.9
Research and development	2,327	12.6	1.0	24.0
Training	1,257	6.8	63.2	15.6
Equipment support and related facilities (U.K.)	983	5.3	8.0	56.6
Other support functions	3,184	17.2	35.8	45.0
War stocks and miscellaneous expenditures	382	46.0	—	—
Support programs total	8,491	46.0	110.9	144.1
Grand total	18,479	100.0	330.8	201.0

Source: Statement on the Defence Estimates, 1986, Cmnd. 9763-II (London: HMSO, 1986): tables 4.3A and 4.3B, pp. 24 and 25.
[a]Defense estimates (case allocated).

significance, the business of the principal British ground forces on the European mainland— the *British Army of the Rhine*, comprising one corps (the combat element) and support units—is to carry conviction in performing assigned military missions. The key fighting formations are three armoured divisions, with places in the "layer-cake" dispositions to which NATO's troops would deploy in the event of actual or threatened hostilities. Once brought up to full strength by reinforcements and reserves, they would be responsible for mounting there a conventional "forward defense" in the first instance, calling on theater nuclear weapons if the process of controlled escalation that is the essence of the alliance's flexible response strategy were to be implemented. The combat elements of *Home Forces* consist of both regular troops and Territorial Army (TA) units, some for reinforcing the British Army of the Rhine, some for special reinforcement tasks (especially on NATO's northern flank), and some for defending the United Kingdom itself.

No major changes are envisaged in either the essential force structure or the force levels of this key component of the national defense effort. However, minor "adjustments" could be made, particularly in the "special reinforcement tasks" assigned to the United Kingdom Mobile Force (UKMF).

In striking contrast to earlier times, *other army combat forces* (i.e., those stationed out-side Europe) account for less than 10 percent of the army's strength in the current program (and about 1 percent of the total defense budget). These forces now consist of the Hong Kong garrison (mainly Gurkha troops); the Cyprus garrison plus contingents serving with and supporting the UN Forces in Cyprus; a battalion in Gibraltar; a battalion group in Belize; and another battalion group with support units constituting the Falklands garrison. Their budgetary burden is trifling compared with their political and strategic value.

There is nothing trifling, however, about the cost of the *air force general purpose combat forces* program—the fifth, last, and most expensive of the budget's major mission categories—which encompasses all the Royal Air Force's frontline squadrons and immediate support. That is because the United Kingdom maintains, and is modernizing, a tactical air arm with all-round competence. Its roles, derived from NATO's concepts of operations for defense of the North Atlantic and Western Europe, include maritime and overland strike (i.e., the delivery of nuclear munitions) and attack (non-nuclear) weapons; offensive support of ground forces, including intimate close support and shallow (or battlefield) interdiction; air defense of the United Kingdom and surrounding sea areas, and of assets and forces in Germany (or elsewhere); maritime patrol, surveillance in peacetime, antisubmarine operations in war; and reconnaissance, complementary to the strike/attack, offensive support, and maritime roles. In addition to over thirty squadrons of combat planes for these tasks, the RAF's fixed-wing inventory includes numerous transport and training aircraft. There are also rotary-wing squadrons for supporting ground troops, for search and rescue, and for communications duties. In fact, the United Kingdom has the means to cover the full spectrum of tactical air missions, including deep interdiction and long-range offensive counterair operations.

All the funds budgeted for defense *could* be apportioned among the five mission programs, because the whole of defense expenditure is ultimately directed to provision of frontline capabilities. But this does not happen in fact. To be serviceable for force planning purposes, a functional analysis of expenditure should attribute to a particular purpose those costs (and only those costs) that are "assuredly and inescapably bound up with having that function . . . in the overall programme and budget" or, putting it another way, "the sums which one could certainly expect to save if the function . . . were dropped from the programme."[45] This rules out exhaustive attribution. Consequently, in British budgetary practice the costs assigned to mission programs include only those inextricably associated with, indeed inseparable from, the performance of operational tasks (i.e., those that are an integral part of having the capability "on the books"). Other support activities are costed independently in six further programs (see table 2). Brief remarks on each are in order.

Volunteer reserves and auxiliary formations represent a modest claim on the budget, and in the late 1980s fewer than three thousand service personnel were ascribed to this program. This number is misleading, however, for it refers only to those engaged full-time in running the formations in question, which themselves muster some two hundred thousand in the regular reserves and around seventy thousand in the Territorial Army. This manpower is an important component of the British defense effort, since the army in particular depends upon the incorporation of individual reservists and volunteer units to achieve its wartime strength. This program could, therefore, be regarded as provision for part of the "teeth" of that effort rather than the "tail."

Each of the remaining line items in table 2 is, however, much more clearly "support": two of them are concerned with personnel-related functions, the other three with procurement-related activities. Under the former heading the 1986–87 defense estimates record funding of £1.25 billion (about $1.9 billion) for training and more than £3 billion (about $4.5 billion) for other support functions, which include not only the higher direction of defense and the armed forces, but also service pensions. Training in the United Kingdom is predominantly organized along single-service lines, a pattern which there is no strong impulse to change, although some "rationalization" has taken place in recent years. Rationalization by integration of service efforts has been tried with some of the other support functions, but such subprograms as "local administration, communications, etc." and "family and personnel services" remain largely single-service responsibilities.

Under the procurement-related support heading falls, first, outgoings for research and development—that is, fundamental research and systems development work, conducted partly in industry, partly in the government's own establishments. A continuing high and broadly based commitment to research and development will remain a feature of British defense provisions for as far ahead as one can see. Since 1984 there has been a renewed interest in cooperative technology projects and collaborative acquisition arrangements, especially with other Europeans under the aegis of the Independent European Programme Group (IEPG). However, participation in such ventures presupposes sound national competence in most, though not all, areas of military technology. A second program embraces the overheads of equipment support and associated facilities in the United Kingdom. In 1986–87 these comprised (1) Her Majesty's dockyards and other establishments of the Royal Navy's support organization, (2) the counterpart British Army setup, and (3) the Royal Air Force's maintenance units, depots, and other facilities. Having undergone considerable reshaping in the 1970s, including a general paring-down in post-1974 Defence Review exercises aimed at "trimming the tail without blunting the teeth" of the armed forces, these organizations were slimmed further in the 1980s under "privatisation" and "contractorisation" programs. Finally, the presence in the functional analysis of the item "War and Contingency Stocks" serves as a reminder that armed forces are powerless without ammunition and other consumables (on which, incidentally, the United Kingdom spent heavily in the mid 1980s, partly to restore stock levels depleted in the Falklands War, partly by way of response to the NATO drive to improve the sustainability of allied forces).

CHANGE AND CONTROVERSY

Planning in defense means looking to a ten-year distant horizon and beyond. Accordingly, within the current program certain changes are already foreshadowed, while for the later years neither the scale nor the pattern of provision is finally settled (because critical choices have yet to be made and are indeed the subject of controversy).

The short-term prospect is a period of contraction in the British defense effort. As noted, allowing for inflation the 18.5 billion pound appropriation for 1986–87 represented reduced funding compared with the previous year; and further diminution was envisaged for 1987–88 and 1988–89—to be precise, a 6 percent decline in the defense budget's value in real terms.[46] No doubt officials have made the prudent assumption that stringency may continue into the 1990s.

Around the turn of the decade, therefore, the cash allotted to the Ministry of Defence may amount to £20 billion ($30 billion) or thereabouts. However, to finance the forward program fully—to pay for everything the ministry would like to do and has plans to do—it has been estimated that some £25 billion ($38 billion) might be required. In other words there is a funding gap that will somehow have to be bridged.[47]

Where might the burden of adjustment fall? Of what was going to be done, what is it that will not be done? It may not be necessary to axe programs to the full extent of the financial shortfall. The Ministry of Defence believes that it can partially bridge the gap through a drive to get better value for the taxpayer's money: by reorganizing itself, by introducing greater competition in the supply of goods and services, and by "contracting out" certain support services to the private sector. But it does not believe that difficult decisions can thereby be avoided altogether.[48]

With a Conservative administration calling the shots at least until 1991/92, the burden of adjustment will likely fall exclusively on the United Kingdom's contributions to NATO's conventional (non-nuclear) forces. That is because the Conservatives are totally committed to the Trident acquisition, a procurement that will impose heavy demands on the budget, thereby crowding out provision for other purposes. If succeeded by a Labour government, the Trident project—and other nuclear capabilities too—might be abandoned. Whether the whole of the resultant "savings" would then be applied to buttressing the country's non-nuclear forces, however, is an open question. Some Labour spokespersons say that they would; others argue that, under Mrs. Thatcher, civil programs have been starved of resources to such an extent that it is these that must have first claim on funds released by Trident's cancellation. What happens if the divided Center parties attain office—or hold the balance of power in a "hung" Parliament in the mid 1990s—is yet harder to fathom. Trident might be scrapped; but here, in the middle of the British political spectrum, there are wide differences of opinion about the nuclear elements in the national order of battle.[49]

The politics of Trident are the key to the economics of defense in the 1990s. But even if the Polaris successor system is abandoned, the Ministry of Defence could still find itself in a squeeze between the upper millstone of tightly drawn cash limits and the nether millstone of rising real costs in defense. Certainly it is difficult to see how the United Kingdom can make a major contribution to enhancement of the West's non-nuclear forces in the years ahead, notwithstanding the nominal support that has been given to NATO's conventional defense improvement initiative. More likely, and well nigh certain if Conservative governments rule throughout, is the prospect of a progressive dilution of the quality—and, maybe, a diminution of the quantity—of the country's current contributions to the alliance.

MANPOWER AND WEAPONS ACQUISITION

The outputs of the defense decision-making process in the United Kingdom have been considered in terms of roles and functions because that is what illuminates security policy priorities most sharply. Resources are allotted to defense not simply to raise armed forces and purchase arms but to fulfill strategic purposes. At the same time it *is* sailors and ships, gunners and guns, airmen and aircraft that the money is actually used to buy. It is appropriate, therefore, to look briefly at arrangements and prospects for obtaining the manpower and acquiring the equipment for the British defense effort, whatever its prospective size and shape.

Present plans envisage that the strength of the United Kingdom's armed forces will remain at around 320,000 overall (Navy: 67,500; Army: 160,000; Air Force: 92,500). All will be voluntarily recruited; and even if the services are beset by manning problems, there is no likelihood of a return to conscription. Whether intake and retention targets will in fact be met is uncertain. Of the factors to which recruitment is sensitive, some should be generally favorable (from the services' standpoint). The labor market outlook for the United Kingdom in the medium term is one of continuing high unemployment, and forces' pay will not be allowed to get out of line with remuneration in comparable civilian occupations. On the other hand, a service career is not what it used to be. Contraction in the geographical scope of the defense effort means that the opportunity for travel to exotic places is no longer an inducement. Nor is the opportunity to learn a trade the attraction that it once was, because of developments in civil industrial training. Furthermore, it appears that nowadays fewer people are willing to accept the kind of regulation of social and recreational activities that is, and will remain, a feature of service life.

It is sometimes suggested, however, that the factors most influential with potential recruits (and those contemplating reengagement after initial enlistment) are the esteem in which the armed forces are held in society at large and the congeniality of the working and domestic environment. On this argument the United Kingdom ought to have fewer manpower problems. The military profession necessarily stands apart from the rest of society because units may be physically isolated and because distinctiveness is important for *esprit de corps*. But there is no great sense of alienation among the armed forces, nor are they themselves regarded as a separate "state within the state." Management styles in the services have become less rigid and hierarchical, the blurring of old "officers and men" distinctions being particularly noticeable in functions with a high technological content. On the domestic side, considerable attention has always been paid to personal welfare matters in the British armed forces (helped by the individual's association with ship, regiment, or squadron wherever possible); and the general standard of housing and other facilities that service personnel enjoy compares favorably with that in other European armed forces.

The acquisition of arms for the services is undertaken, as has been noted, by the Ministry of Defence's Procurement Executive. The procedures involved are complex, but coherent, as has been explained.[50] In 1986–87 over £6.5 billion (about $9.8 billion) was budgeted for production of new equipment and spares, and over £2 billion ($3 billion) for research and development. In both areas the United Kingdom is highly self-reliant, but not wholly self-sufficient. In fact over the past few years there has been some erosion of the domestic armaments base. The effect has been to make the United Kingdom anxious to arrest the process, hence the greater disposition to participate in cooperative ventures that permit preservation of the nation's stake in (or access to) relevant technologies at acceptable cost. But there has also been a contradictory impulse: to cling to what is left, and therefore to remain prepared to contemplate independent national development and production if the "right" collaborative opportunity does not present itself. It is impossible to predict in which future procurement choices the one or the other influence will prevail. Suffice it to say that a momentum for more cooperative solutions is building up, partly in response to general pressures for the more effective use of resources, partly because of particular pressures on the eastern side of the Atlantic for "rationalization" of the European armaments base. At the same time neither general economic conditions in the United Kingdom nor employment prospects in some of the regions and localities where defense-related industries are sited will make it easy for governments to participate in collaborative projects where the British share of the work is quite modest. Having said that, faced with the stark choice between, on the one hand, giving lower priority to preservation of jobs and competence and, on the other, standing aside completely from major cooperative ventures, the United Kingdom would probably opt for the former.[51]

ARMS CONTROL OR ARMED CONFLICT?

Few commentators would dispute this essay's emphasis on the British defense effort as a contribution of capabilities to NATO—an alliance whose reason for being is to deter aggression. To say that, however, is to prompt two final questions. Does the preoccupation with armed forces and armaments mean that no hope is entertained of security through arms control? Does the commitment to deterrence mean that no British decision maker envisages employment of the country's forces in armed conflict (other than in the defense of Europe should deterrence fail)?

At the level of aspirations—and declaratory policy—the United Kingdom has high hopes, if not great expectations, of arms control. Mrs. Thatcher's governments have consistently registered support for the American stance in U.S.-Soviet negotiations on nuclear and space weapons (albeit subject to reservations on some matters); for efforts to conclude a Comprehensive Test Ban (CTB); for the search for agreement in the long-running talks on Mutual and Balanced Force Reductions (MBFR); and for the attempts being made in the Conference on

Disarmament in Europe (CDE) to define confidence- amd security-building measures.[52] At the same time there is anxiety that a U.S.-Soviet deal might explicitly or implicitly constrain the United Kingdom's freedom of maneuver with respect to its own strategic nuclear force, and great caution has been shown in the MBFR talks and the CDE.

Thus, the short answer to the first question posed is that, at the practical policy level, some hopes *are* entertained. But the British approach to arms control is tempered by realism. That, it can be argued, is no more than prudence requires. A more cynical judgment would be that what really animates the United Kingdom in arms control endeavors is, not so much a desire for enhanced security through acceptance of mutual restraints, but rather the opportunity to set some bounds to the growth of Soviet military power without loss of freedom of action for itself and its allies.

Answering the second question is more problematic. Formally, the only circumstances in which the active use of substantial military force would be contemplated by the United Kingdom are in the event of a failure of deterrence in the NATO area. Virtually all elements in the national force structure have assigned roles and missions derived from the alliance's strategy, and they are equipped and deployed accordingly. To be sure, when great attention was being paid to possible contingencies outside the NATO area in the early 1980s, some measures were set in hand "to improve the capability of the Services to operate world-wide"; but even then, as now, only limited thought was given to the possibility of their employment in intervention actions and the like.[53]

Reflection on recent history counsels caution, however, when it comes to the obvious inference that active employment of forces is unlikely, if not inconceivable, in the foreseeable future. In the first place, when explicit reliance on deterrence for all contingencies was espoused by British planners in the early 1950s, it coincided with a period of intense activity for general purpose forces in fulfillment of extra-European commitments, prompting Richard Rosecrance's remark that the British "had a marvellous doctrine for other people but they applied it to themselves."[54] Global obligations loom less large now, of course. But the use of forces outside the NATO area—if not under alliance auspices, at least in concert with allies—is still required from time to time (for example, in the Gulf in the later 1980s). In the second place it is noteworthy that, even since the concentration of the defense effort on Europe and the North Atlantic, there have been occasional instances of the active use of force for strictly limited national ends. Warships mounted the Beira patrol as part of sanctions enforcement against Rhodesia and were in action during the fisheries disputes with Iceland in the mid 1970s. Ground and air forces have operated (and still do) in Belize. In 1982 considerable resources of all three services were mustered to oust the Argentinian invader from the 7,000-mile-distant Falkland Islands.[55] Lastly, the Northern Ireland "emergency" *is* an internal security operation, even though it is conducted under the rubric of military aid to the civil power.

However, enumerating these instances tends to reaffirm the original assertion rather than contradict it. With the single exception of the Falklands operation, all are comparatively minor policing tasks (in relation to the scale of the national defense effort as a whole). Nor does one really expect the British armed forces to be called upon to fire shots in anger during the next decade other than in contexts such as these (with the possible exception of peace-keeping operations under United Nations auspices).

Summary and Conclusion

It has been shown that the United Kingdom inhabits an international environment in which there are challenges to its security and within which the nation is conscious of its status. The perceived threats to security are almost exclusively those posed by the Soviet Union and its Warsaw Pact allies; and the response to them has been framed within an Atlantic Alliance setting, for the defense of the realm is judged to be inseparable from that of the NATO area as a whole and possible only by

acknowledging interdependence. At the same time there is a residual independent streak in the British psyche of which one manifestation is the diverse form of the country's contributions to the alliance.

Against this background, national objectives, national strategy, and military doctrine have been appraised. The basic judgments and assumptions that lie behind the state's aspirations, actual policy, the force posture it has chosen to assume, and its provision for defense quite clearly derive from NATO's goals, strategy, and concepts of operations. However, the United Kingdom would like to cut a certain figure in alliance, and particularly European, circles; and this is evident in the commitment of forces to each of the three components of the NATO triad (strategic nuclear, theater nuclear, and conventional arms), in all three elements (sea, land, and air) and within each of the three alliance command areas (Atlantic, Channel, and Europe).

National aims and assumptions are inputs to the defense decision-making process. In the United Kingdom this involves an institutional structure whose core is the newly centralized apparatus of the Ministry of Defence and a set of bureaucratic procedures for management of the "rolling" defense program and budget.

The obvious frame of reference for consideration of defense policy outputs is the ministry's current program and budget, whose content, and possible changes, have been discussed. As it happens, analysis along these lines brings the argument full circle. The composition of the present and planned defense effort displays the emphasis on NATO, and the desire to make a distinctive contribution to the alliance is also manifest. So, too, is the fact that, as time goes by, the country will find it harder and harder to make ends meet.

In short, defense dispositions are now made, and will continue to be made, in accordance with the United Kingdom's prevailing self-image, that of a great power in reduced circumstances. Not that "keeping up appearances" is likely to be a feasible policy, beyond the short run. In the not-too-distant future, the United Kingdom will almost certainly have to abandon the pretense of all-round competence.

That will amount to a final, some would say overdue, acknowledgement that things are no longer what they used to be.

Notes

1. International comparison of defense efforts is, of course, a hazardous undertaking. For a discussion of some of the problems, see *The Meaning and Measurement of Military Expenditure*, SIPRI Research Report no. 10, (Stockholm: Stockholm International Peace Research Institute, 1973 (SIPRI)). For data permitting broader comparisons than those in table 1, see the International Institute for Strategic Studies' annual compilation, *The Military Balance*.

2. For an "official" assessment of the East-West military balance, see *NATO and the Warsaw Pact: Force Comparisons* (Brussels: NATO Information Service, 1984).

3. M. J. Hillenbrand, "NATO and Western Security in an Era of Transition" *International Security* 2, no. 2 (Fall 1977): 21–22.

4. K. N. Waltz, *Foreign Policy and Democratic Politics* (Boston: Little, Brown, 1967), pp. 7, 161–62.

5. On the foregoing, see D. Greenwood, "Defence and National Priorities since 1945," in *British Defence Policy in a Changing World*, ed. J. Baylis (London: Croom Helm, 1977).

6. For a detailed analysis of the British defense experience in the third and fourth phases, see D. Greenwood and D. Hazel, *The Evolution of Britain's Defence Priorities, 1957–76*, Aberdeen Studies in Defence Economics (ASIDES), no. 9 (Aberdeen: Centre for Defence Studies, 1977–78).

7. On the 1974–75 exercise, see ibid, and the references in note 42 below. On the 1981 review, see D. Greenwood, *Reshaping Britain's Defences*, ASIDES no. 19 (Aberdeen: Centre for Defence Studies, 1981).

8. The phrase occurs, significantly, in the *Report of the Review Committee on Overseas Representation*, Cmnd. 4107 (London: HMSO, 1969), p. 22. (I am indebted to my colleague Jim Wyllie for this reference.)

9. There is further discussion on such points later in this essay.

10. J. C. Garnett "Some Constraints on Defence Policy-Makers," in *The Management of Defence*, ed. L. W. Martin (London: Macmillan, 1970) p. 30.

11. See D. Hazel and P. Williams, *The British Defence Effort: Foundations and Alternatives*, ASIDES no. 11 (Aberdeen: Centre for Defence Studies, 1977–78), whose analytical framework this is.

12. The quoted phrase is from Article VI of the Non-Proliferation Treaty (NPT), which came into force in 1970.

13. Hazel and Williams *British Defence Efforts*, pp. 13 and 14.

14. For data and interesting argument on the burden-sharing issue generally, see G. Kennedy, *Burden-Sharing in NATO* (London: Duckworth, 1979), and P. Foot, *Problems of Equity in Alliance Arrangements* ASIDES no. 23 (Aberdeen: Centre for Defence Studies, 1982).

15. See the brief remarks on "NORTHAG's New Concept," in *Statement on the Defence Estimates, 1986*, Cmnd. 9763-I (London: HMSO, 1986), p. 33.

16. See D. Greenwood, "Economic Constraints and Political Preferences," in *Alternative Approaches to British Defence Policy*, ed. J. Baylis (London: Macmillan, 1983), and C. Coker, "Naked Emperors: The British Labour Party and Defence," *Strategic Review*, Fall 1984, pp. 39–50.

17. W. Schilling, P. Hammond, and G. Snyder, *Strategy, Politics and Defence Budgets* (New York: Columbia University Press, 1962); I. Dorfer, *System 37 Viggen* (Oslo: Universitatsforlaget, 1973), and id., *Arms Deal: The Selling of the F16* (New York: Praeger, 1983).

18. But see C. Mayhew, *Britain's Role Tomorrow* (London: Hutchinson, 1967), and B. Reed and G. Williams, *Denis Healey and the Policies of Power* (London: Sidgwick & Jackson, 1971), for suggestions of infighting in the 1960s.

19. For an essay specifically directed to "determinants," see J. Baylis, "Defence Decision-Making in Britain and the Determinants of Defence Policy," *Journal of the Royal United Services Institute for Defence Studies* 120, no. 1 (March 1975): 42–48.

20. See D. Greenwood, "Constraints and Choices in the Transformation of Britain's Defence Effort since 1945," *British Journal of International Studies* 2, no. 1 (April 1976): 5–26, for details on this point.

21. For a useful survey of the defense industrial base, see the second part of R. Angus, *The Organisation of Procurement and Production in the United Kingdom*, ASIDES no. 13 (Aberdeen: Centre for Defence Studies, 1979).

22. G. Kemp, "The New Strategic Map," *Survival* (March-April 1977), map 6.

23. For fuller accounts of the present central organization, see *The Central Organisation of Defence*, Cmnd. 9315 (London: HMSO, 1984). On the earlier setup, see R. M. Hastie-Smith "The Tin Wedding: A Study of the Evolution of the Ministry of Defence, 1964–74," *Seaford House Papers* (London: Royal College of Defence Studies, 1974). On "other participants," see Baylis, "Defence Decision-making."

24. Letter to Sidney Herbert, 1859, cited in Hastie-Smith, "The Tin Wedding," p. 27.

25. Details from Cmnd. 9315 (cited note 23 above).

26. Hastie-Smith, "Tin Wedding," p. 38.

27. First Report from the Select Committee on Procedure, Session 1968–69, *Scrutiny of Public Expenditure and Administration*, House of Commons Paper 410 (1968–69), Evidence, appendix 1, para. 3, p. 237.

28. For students of British defense policy, the Defence Committee's reports and accompanying minutes of evidence are invaluable. An outstanding example is its Third Report of Session 1984-85, *Defence Commitments and Resources and the Defence Estimates, 1985–86*, House of Commons Paper 37 (1984-85) (in three volumes).

29. Baylis, "Defence Decision-making," pp. 42–43.

30. Ibid.

31. M. Howard, *The Central Organisation of Defence* (London: Royal United Services Institute, 1970), p. 39.

32. *The United Kingdom Defence Programme: The Way Forward*, Cmnd. 8288 (London: HMSO, 1981).

33. Heseltine resigned from the cabinet in January 1986 because of differences with colleagues over the relative merits of a European or an American "rescue" of the ailing Westland helicopter company.

34. There is an account of the episode in Mayhew, *Britain's Role Tomorrow*.

35. See H. Heclo and A. Wildavsky, *The Private Government of Public Money* (London: Macmillan, 1974), for a superb analysis of the Treasury's role in managing public expenditure (and hence public policy making).

36. See P. Foot, *The Protesters*, CENTREPIECE 4 (Aberdeen: Centre for Defence Studies, 1983).

37. A. Schick, "The Road to PPB," *Public Administration Review* 26, no. 4 (December 1966): 27.

38. A. Wildavsky, *The Politics of the Budgetary Process* (Boston: Little, Brown, 1964), p. 1.

39. This argument is set out more fully in D. Greenwood, *Budgeting for Defence* (London: Royal United Services Institute, 1972), which also contains a fuller exposition of the procedures described in the next few paragraphs of this section.

40. For an official description of the PESC procedure, see *Public Expenditure White Papers: Handbook on Methodology* (London: HMSO, 1972). But cf. Heclo and Wildavsky, *Private Government*.

41. For details and discussion see the second report from the Defence Committee, 1981–82, *Ministry of Defence Organisation and Procurement*, House of Commons Paper 22 (1981–82) (in two volumes).

42. On the 1964–66 and 1967–68 exercises, see Greenwood, *Budgeting for Defence*. For a full exposition of the 1974–75 review, see the second report from the Expenditure Committee, 1974–75, *The Defence Review Proposals*, House of Commons Paper 259 (1974–75) and "Setting British Defence Priorities," two articles in *Survival* 17, no. 5 (September-October 1975), the first by the minister who conducted the exercise, the second by the present writer. For evaluation of the 1981 undertaking, see Greenwood, *Reshaping Britain's Defenses*.

43. L. Freedman, *Arms Production in the United Kingdom: Problems and Prospects* (London: Royal Institute of International Affairs, 1978), p. 13.

44. There is an extensive literature on all aspects of Britain's strategic nuclear deterrent. See, for example,

L. Freedman, *Britain and Nuclear Weapons* (London: Macmillan, 1980); J. McMahan *British Nuclear Weapons: For and Against* (London: Junction Books, 1981); D. Greenwood, *The Trident Programme*, ASIDES no. 22 (Aberdeen: Centre for Defence Studies, 1982); and M. Chalmers *Trident: Britain's Independent Arms Race* (London: CND Publications, 1984).

45. Greenwood, *Budgeting for Defence*, p. 50.

46. *Statement on the Defence Estimates, 1986*, Cmnd. 9763-I, (London: HMSO, 1986), para. 503, p. 40.

47. On the "funding gap" thesis, see the present writer's chapter in *Public Expenditure Policy 1985–86*, ed. P. Cockle (London: Macmillan, 1985), pp. 101–20, and his evidence to the House of Commons' Defence Committee in the material cited at note 28 above.

48. *Statement on the Defence Estimates, 1986*, Cmnd. 9763-I.

49. See Greenwood, "Economic Constraints," and D. Hobbs, *Alternatives to Trident*, ASIDES no. 25 (Aberdeen: Centre for Defence Studies, 1983). Some of the Labour Party's ideas appear to be derived from *Defence without the Bomb*, Report of the Alternative Defence Commission (London: Taylor & Francis, 1983).

50. See above and the work cited at note 41.

51. On NATO-wide and intra-European arms collaboration, see K. Hartley, *NATO Arms Co-operation* (London: Allen & Unwin, 1983), and T. Taylor, *Defence, Technology, and International Integration* (London: Frances Pinter, 1982).

52. See chapter 2 in the *Statement on the Defence Estimates, 1986*, on Arms Control.

53. *The Way Forward* (cited note 32 above), P. Foot *Improving Capabilities for Extra-European Contingencies: The British Contribution*, ASIDES no. 18 (Aberdeen: Centre for Defence Studies, 1981), and id., *Beyond the North Atlantic: The European Contribution*, ASIDES no. 21 (Aberdeen: Centre for Defence Studies, 1982).

54. R. Rosecrance, *Defence of the Realm* (New York: Columbia University Press, 1968) pp. 178–80.

55. On the Falklands operation, see L. Freedman, "The War of the Falklands, 1982," *Foreign Affairs* 61, no. 1 (Fall 1982): 196–210, and the official *The Falklands Campaign: The Lessons*, Cmnd. 8758 (London: HMSO, 1982).

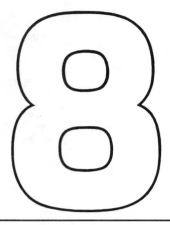

ITALY

Joseph C. Rallo

International Environment

The postwar defense posture of Italy was clearly conditioned by foreign policy cues provided by the United States. Domestic political chaos, erratic economic performance, and the absence of any Euro-centered defense alternative ensured that Italy's attention would be directed inward along avenues delineated by its American protectors. National defense objectives replicated this reality and gradually assumed an unquestioning coincidence with NATO-defined goals. Until the early 1970s the United States and NATO formed the twin pillars of Italian foreign and defense policy.

Italy is currently engaged in a reappraisal of what previously had been accepted as the external underpinning of its foreign and defense policy. Although diminution of American global leadership precipitated this review, Italy's dogged pursuit of international stature results from more diverse sources. Key among these is the geopolitical potential for Italian leadership in the Mediterranean region. The

longevity of the various Craxi coalition governments lent coherence and a sense of permanence to this foreign policy thrust, which also garners support from a public increasingly satisfied in an economic sense and desirous of securing an optimistic future through political stability.

This emerging Italian reorientation, though, does maintain one constant thread from its postwar stance, which is essentially the acknowledged inability to pursue foreign and defense objectives unilaterally. Quite simply, some form of partnership is essential to Italy, with the certainty previously achieved by reliance on America now slowly being replaced by a similar commitment to the inchoate concept of European unity. Indeed, much of the opaqueness over the direction, strength, and shape of Italian defense policy results from the uncertainties associated with this substitution process.

Notwithstanding this uncertainty, the Italian perception of the threat to be offset through a reinvigorated and nationally driven defense policy continues to be denominated in East-West terms. The need to address this threat, not only through continued adherence to NATO, but also by strong support for increasingly coordinated European security efforts is clearly articulated in Italy's 1985 *Libro bianco della difensa*.[1] The gradually converging security views of the major Italian political parties have tempered the postwar dilemma of how to accommodate a multiparty system with a strong Communist Party to a security posture grounded securely on adherence to the Western alliance. Indeed, that convergence has also allowed the government greater latitude to deal with a multiplicity of policy options that a few years ago would have been outside the realm of possibility. A multiplicity of actors was also a response to the fascist era with its structured, personal, and extremely secretive leadership style. This maturation in the Italian sense of problem-solving efficacy has been manifested in Italy's newfound resolve to assert itself more widely within the Mediterranean area. Italian guarantees of Maltese neutrality and peacekeeping efforts in Lebanon join with Italy's call for a regional naval force posture integrating French, Spanish, and Italian units to offset present and anticipated Soviet augmentations in that littoral region. When coupled with the imminent development of an Italian rapid deployment force to deal with Mediterranean-based contingencies, Italy's determination to assume a leading role in the region becomes clear. The coincidence of this policy thrust with the reduction of American naval assets in the basin has ensured that the Italian reorientation will be favorably received in the United States.

National Objectives, National Strategy, and Military Doctrine

Postwar Italian foreign and defense policy has passed through three clear stages. In each of these the Italian inability to attain the stature of the other major European members of NATO has generally been attributed to difficulty in managing competing internal processes. In turn, this has resulted in a passive, dependent outlook requiring external partners around which to structure initiatives. This traditional assessment fails though to acknowledge the success that Italy has enjoyed over the past forty years in attaining economic and defense goals, apparently without the commensurate need for sacrifice inferred by internal shortcomings. As Robert Isaak has noted: "Italians consciously perceive their weakness as a source of strength when it comes to bargaining for what they want."[2] In a very subtle fashion, then, the need for partnership becomes a source of leverage as Italians convince others of the need to sustain objectives that could not be attained in the absence of such assistance. Both Joseph La Palombara and Luigi Barzini would recognize this adaptation of internal bargaining mechanisms to external affairs.[3] This Italian bargaining style subtly changes the issue of dependence from a relationship to be avoided to one that must be cultivated in order to conserve and strengthen scarce domestic assets useful in later negotiations. To pursue this assessment one must approach the Italian desire for postwar partnership as a search, not merely for a protector, but rather for a sympathetic champion to protect and pursue what Italy views as its optimal national policy path. That pursuit of rational foreign policy independence was paralleled by the path of military doctrine, where a static and defensive posture was gradually transformed into an instrument capable of assuming the tasks required of an emerging regional power.

One may term the first period of Italy's postwar policy as one of rebuilding in the aftermath of World War II's societal disruptions. The distance and insularity of Italy from the Soviet Union and Central Europe ensured that any perceived threat radiating from East-West relations would remain indirect in nature. This is not to suggest though that the threat was chimerical. Indeed, much of the immediate history of postwar Italy revolved around the potential challenge to stability suggested by a popular Communist Party whose control over labor unions was a promising vehicle for political dominance. The Italian search for internal stability thus gravitated naturally toward the institutional regime being initiated by the

United States to restructure global affairs after the termination of the war. Italian membership in NATO (1949) and the Common Market (1958) is indicative of this first-stage concern with the immediate need to stabilize the fabric of society prior to attempting more radical programs. In aligning itself with external economic, military, and institutional partners, Italy began to utilize the leverage essential to the success of its longer-term objectives. Italian inputs into these organizations consisted of presence rather than of substance, since in neither economic nor military terms was Italy's short-term potential of much significance. Yet while Italy was a net recipient of aid from NATO and the EEC, even at this early date, both organizations recognized the need to enfold Italy securely into the Western alliance. Its strategic location as the anchor of the southern European democracies and the specter of domestic instability combined to ensure that Italy assumed an importance to both organizations far in excess of its direct contributory potential.

The second stage may be characterized as transitional, building on the advances of the first period and permitting policy options consistent with, rather than dependent on, the strategies of other major Western actors. The sympathetic foreign policy stances of NATO and the EEC during the 1950s and 1960s supported Italy by enabling its European posture to be viewed in Washington as pro-alliance and therefore pro-American. The undisputed global military, political, and economic dominance of the United States was sustained through American control over diverse international organizations newly tasked with the pursuit of global order. The IMF, GATT, OECD, and NATO buttressed a global structure that, while supportive of American goals, also enabled Europe to pursue its essential task of rebuilding. Any potential challenge to long-term American hegemony was amply compensated by the short-term stability engendered through this ordering process. Italian progress during this second period was essentially due to the structure and opportunity afforded by this global patchwork of institutions, which enabled Italy to offset the fragility of an internal

system where governments changed approximately every eight months.

The Italy that emerged from this second period was far different in tenor and outlook from its postwar predecessor.[4] Economic decisions taken in the 1950s to move the Italian infrastructure toward export-oriented manufacturing, consistent with limited natural resources and favorable geographic position, bore fruit in the 1960s.[5] Throughout that decade, a favorable balance of payments became the norm. By 1971 agricultural employment had dropped from 42.2 percent to 17.2 percent, while employment in industry rose from 32.1 percent to 44.4 percent.[6] Yet this modernization in the means and manner of production created turmoil in a society still uncertain as to its role in the transition process. Together this industrial reorganization and those societal disruptions were further buffeted by the 1973–74 oil crisis, which also endangered traditional party-labor relations. Especially troubled was the Christian Democratic (DC) Party, whose southern political base continued to remain isolated from these development plans. Emigration of youth from the south to the industrial north continued to denude the DC both of electoral support and of its traditional base for recruiting party workers and candidates.

The final period may be termed one of reorientation as stability engendered by earlier programs now allowed the Italian government greater leeway in choosing partners and policies for the future. The ability of government to cope with internal changes in this third period was affected by turmoil in the international environment, now tenuously grounded on American global preeminence. American withdrawal from even a partial gold standard in 1970 was merely a precursor to a spate of events that signaled a more equitable, albeit less certain, distribution of power and responsibility in Western economic and defense sectors. Europeans began to question the now dated bargain of accepting secondary status to the United States in return for some measure of stability, and found it wanting. Clearly, the decreasing primacy of the United States required compensating adjustments, especially for Italy, which had assumed American leadership to be long-term, if not permanent, in nature. Perhaps West Germany and France might contemplate unilateral action as a response to these realignments, but Italy was certainly not in a similar position.

As European and American defense and economic objectives began to diverge, the institutions established to fulfill those goals began to drift apart, not only in their objectives, but also in the questions being asked. The NATO "two-way street" (the notion that the United States not only be a seller of arms, but also a buyer of European-manufactured military hardware) was asymmetric—so favorable to the United States that some referred to it as close to being a "one-way street." Although this asymmetry might begin to be redressed through an increase in conventional spending, was the underlying defense posture engendered by that spending consistent with the goals envisaged by Europe? For Italy, this process of questioning occurred when its postwar rebuilding was completed, when political and economic stability were assured and when the need to rely so completely on the United States was no longer clear. Thus, the reorientation within Western Europe toward defense and the economy allowed the Italians the opportunity and the luxury of being able to take part in a venture that clearly mirrored their own domestically generated plans.

The election of President Ronald Reagan may have signaled for some a need for Europe finally to make a choice. Economic and defense tensions between the United States and Europe had progressed to the point where they could no longer be characterized as resulting from the process of "cooperative competition," or dismissed as merely a normal and recurrent by-product of alliance interactions. SDI, technology transfers, and trade embargoes were but the surface manifestations of the increasing dichotomy between European and American policy outlooks. For Italy, the resurgence of Europe provides the partner that is essential to its own plans. Overcoming the uncertainty of this new orientation is the vision of an Italy once again dominant in the Mediterranean region. Lest one assume that this suggests a reversal of the Italian bargaining method that has been so successful since World War II, keep in mind that Italy could still play the dominant Mediterranean role, if need be, under continued American auspices, regardless of how its relations with the rest of Europe evolve. This three-decade transformation in Italian political and military outlooks, then, grants substance to the possibility of a nationally derived security policy complementing the benefits derived from pursuit of a rather unique bargaining style.

Italian doctrine on the use of force continues to be defined in terms of the threat emanating from Warsaw Pact forces to the north. Yet while the five defense tasks assigned to the military have remained constant over the past thirty years, several changes have occurred both as to the priority of respective missions and to the doctrine required for their successful implementation. Clearly it has been the Soviet buildup of forces and capabilities in the Mediterranean that has refocused NATO and Italian attention away from the central front and toward the less secure and more volatile southern region. Alliance support for an Italian counter to this force buildup suggests the inability of either Greece or Turkey to undertake that task. Such NATO support has enabled the buildup to be perceived as alliance-mandated, while simultaneously seen by Italians as supportive of national goals that might have been impossible in the absence of that nexus. The need to increase mission capability was a major motive behind the three 1975 supplementary budgets (discussed below), allowing each of the services to identify and procure systems consistent with its long-term defense goals. Italy's perennial and passive NATO role was being transformed in a fashion designed to be consistent with, and supportive of, national defense objectives. Yet since this new emphasis appears to favor the navy over the army, internal power realignments will ultimately determine its final shape and success.

The emerging Italian sense of increased competency in defense matters is reflected in changes in Italy's operational doctrine since

1951. The original "600 series" identified doctrine for the 1950s as a static posture based on selected fortified army positions designed to blunt an attack from the north. Subsequent reports, culminating in the "900 series" for the 1980s, have transformed Italian operational doctrine into an all-service mission based on mobile, specialized forces. The forces are designed to contain an attack, thus allowing a subsequent counterattack to regain and perhaps expand on any lost territory.[7] Although the "600" through "900" series statements still identify the northeast frontier as the focal defense point, that emphasis is substantially eroded by the more formal description of specific missions assigned to each of the services. Yet the role of northeast defense retains its visibility since it continues as the primary mission of the army, by far the largest single component of the armed forces.

Five defense missions are to be fulfilled by Italian forces, with each encapsulating certain logistic and operational peculiarities. The distance and insulation of parts of the Italian mainland would hamper any external reinforcements, thus requiring that these missions, although linked to NATO plans, also be capable of being effected solely by Italian forces. A brief discussion of each area is instructive to illuminate Italian thought on force employment, structure, and doctrine.

NORTHEASTERN DEFENSE

The Gorizia and Monfalcone corridors have traditionally been viewed as the preferred invasion routes for continentally based forces. The complexity and insularity of that territory require that sufficient forces be permanently based in the region with the capability of performing diverse and often very specialized tasks. To accomplish these requirements the Italian military has stationed twenty brigades in forward defense positions within the 4th and 5th army corps, with the 3rd corps a reserve headquartered in Milan.

Consistent with the operational doctrine enumerated in the "900 series," these forces are highly mobile and equipped with M47 and M60 tanks. Specialized demolition tasks in support of these mobile units are to be performed by an alpine brigade specifically trained to make use of the hilly terrain to create obstacles to any forward enemy advance. Extensive use of TOW and Milan missiles, helicopters, and other air assets is also contemplated. Notwithstanding these plans, severe shortcomings limit the ability of Italian forces to carry out these missions. Principal among these is the obsolescence of the M47 and M60 tanks, whose replacement is not expected until the 1990s. The government's own estimate is that fully 50 percent of current units are no longer field capable. This has led to its conclusion that "forces in place can only guarantee northeast defense for a limited period of time."[8]

SOUTHERN DEFENSE OF THE SEA LINES OF COMMUNICATION (SLOCs)

Italy continues to be extremely dependent on imports and receives nearly all essential goods and materials through its numerous Mediterranean ports. Stretching nearly 3,700 km (2,200 miles), the Mediterranean is accessible only through three routes—the Straits of Gibraltar, the Suez Canal, and the Dardanelles. NATO control of these points by land- and sea-based air power is relatively assured against surface threats. Rather, it is the threat of submarines, protected from detection by the noisy subsurface conditions of the Mediterranean, that poses the major threat to the SLOCs. Soviet submarines regularly stop at Tartus, Syria, and it is possible that attack submarines also accompany Soviet surface units on their increasingly frequent port calls to Tripoli, Libya.[9]

Italian doctrine for Mediterranean and SLOC defense is tightly wedded to NATO forces and infrastructures. In a NATO-derived scenario, Italian air and maritime forces would

Table 1. Italian Active Duty Personnel

	Army	Navy	Air Force	Grand Total
Officers	20,415	5,075	7,490	
NCO's	29,500	8,364	31,360	
Enlisted	221,390	29,768	26,259	
Total	271,305	43,207	65,109	379,621

be placed under command of the relevant alliance commander. In case of a purely Italian matter, involving, for example, guarantees in support of Maltese neutrality, each service would operate individually under overall direction of the defense secretary general (SMD). The core of the Italian Mediterranean fleet, based in Taranto, are the surface units of the 2nd and 4th naval divisions, as well as two submarine groups. They are assisted by Tornados and helicopters based in Bari. Recently Italy's ability to fulfill this maritime mission has been greatly enhanced with the introduction of what is planned as the navy's first in a series of modern aircraft carriers. The *Giuseppe Garibaldi*, which became operational in July 1985, is a 13,600-ton craft capable of carrying six antisubmarine warfare (ASW) helicopters (SH-3D) and six STOVL (short takeoff and vertical landing) aircraft (AV-6 Sea Harriers) for air defense.[10] While incapable of replacing U.S. Mediterranean-based carriers, the introduction of the *Garibaldi* presents a real, albeit limited, power-projection potential for Italy throughout the entire southern littoral region. The introduction of the Sea Harrier into the maritime inventory would also alter navy-air force relations, since only the latter is allowed by law to operate fixed-wing aircraft. Offsets to induce air force agreement to navy plans might include assignment of air force personnel to operate carrier-based planes or air force oversight of all training essential to pilot preparation. Parliamentary attempts have been made to solve these interservice rivalries and finalize trade-offs. For example, in 1989 Parliament authorized the navy to fly fixed-wing aircraft (most likely a Harrier "jump jet" variant) from its carriers. The navy must be careful in pursuing these aims, since any enhancement of the forces assigned to it or of the primacy it wants placed on the southern mission would probably come at the expense of the northeast defense zone and the army.

AIR DEFENSE

Unlike the clear conflict between the army and navy over which defense mission (northeast or Mediterranean) should be given primacy, there is no similar problem for the air force. Its mission is defined as air defense and air interdiction in support of both NATO and national ground and air assets. Clearly the air force position requires forces to support elements for both the northeast and Mediterranean missions, thus ensuring that resolution of the priority contest between the other two services will redound to its benefit.

Yet recent evolutions in air force doctrine suggest that its preference might be to side with the navy in the interservice debate. Current reliance on the F-104 for the air intercept role is expected to be phased out by the 1990s, when its replacement, the European Fighter Aircraft (EFA), becomes available. The recent introduction of the Tornado in a dual-purpose bomber/fighter role has permitted the air force to extend its zone of southern operations deep into the Mediterranean. Clearly the Tornados complement any interdiction role envisaged for the navy's new carrier and also for the developing Italian rapid deployment force. There is no comparable combat mission for the air force in connection with the army's mandate in the northeast.

Of greater importance for the air force are the defense implications of its two multinational cooperative ventures in the aerospace field. The Tornado and the EFA are, or will be, produced by a consortium desirous of reducing reliance on American products as well as increasing the visibility of Europe's growing and lucrative arms production capability. Both political and military offsets are contained in the agreements to build and buy such jointly produced aircraft. Although Spain is involved in both ventures, Italy is the primary partner whose defense interests and mission utilization of these craft are southern in focus. It appears probable, then, that in any future division of defense labor, whether NATO- or Europe-derived, Italy will be given greater responsibility for the Mediterranean region. Capability must follow doctrine if this defense mandate is to have meaning. In this fashion the air force and navy outlooks complement political decisions on Italian armaments cooperation with other European members of NATO and blur the army's traditional leading role in defense matters.

TERRITORIAL AND CIVIL DEFENSE

Although these final two tasks are primarily oriented toward domestic contingencies, they do anticipate events whose resolution would entail use of military force. Territorial defense is described as dual in nature: to protect the state's integrity, with the exception of the northeast defense sector, and, in case of attack, to augment all defense sectors and protect interior lines of communication. It is this latter task that has assumed primary importance and is the training mission stressed for the reserve units that would implement it.

While several distinct types of units are assigned to territorial defense, it is the role of the carabinieri that is of central importance. Acknowledged as an elite paramilitary police force, its role in case of attack on Italian soil is to reinforce the 4th and 5th army corps in the northeast with two carabinieri battalions, the 7th and 13th.[11] These forces constitute a quick-response, mobile force particularly suited for use against parachute, guerrilla, or limited naval infantry landings. In containing such units, the carabinieri would essentially be protecting the lines of communication essential to the army's ability to fulfill its northeast defense function. This use of elite, quick-response forces is being taken one step further with the development of a rapid deployment force.[12] Originally designed for military operations and disaster relief, current plans envisage two separate and specially trained units for each role. The military *Forza di Intervento Rapido* (FoIR) is designed as a mobile force that may be inserted and indefinitely sustained in support of Italian foreign policy objectives. The Italian military role in the 1983 multinational peacekeeping force in Beirut, Lebanon, would now be viewed as a mission to be undertaken by the FoIR. The civilian counterpart to the FoIR is the *Forza di Pronto Intervento* (FoPI), designed as a quick-response force to assist in natural disasters such as the volcanic eruptions in Sicily in 1985. Drawn from all the services, these units are ready to move in sixteen hours and are expected to be on the accident site within twenty-four hours. The future viability of the FoIR and the FoPI is contingent on three factors: whether a permanent, unified all-service command structure can be established; whether the services view their participation as role-enhancing or as another drain on already limited budgets; and the relevance of the FoIR in supporting an increased Italian role in the Mediterranean, including the need to protect the SLOCs in case of interruption of Middle East oil shipments.

It is necessary here to inject a short note with respect to Italy's position on the development and use of nuclear, biological, and chemical weapons (NBC). Italy is generally acknowledged as having little or no interest in independently acquiring intermediate or strategic systems. Financial, operational, and intraparty ideological grounds may all be cited in support of that assessment. The 1985 *Libro bianco* clearly states that Italian policy on NBC issues is consistent with NATO doctrine, and therefore purely defensive and deterrent in nature.[13]

This is not to dismiss the interest of certain Italians in attaining a limited nuclear capability to bolster the more general desire to be accorded co-equal status with other major European states. The clearest indicator of this desire was in the aftermath of India's 1974 detonation of a "peaceful" nuclear device and prior to Italy's ratification of the 1968 Non-Proliferation Treaty (NPT). The Italian ambassador to the International Atomic Energy Agency, Achille Albonetti, strongly criticized the NPT in an article in *Politica e strategia* and laid out his own estimate of the cost of a nuclear capability for Italy.[14] The outcry engendered by his article, as well as pressure brought to bear on Italy by other European signatories to the NPT, finally resulted in Italian ratification of that document in April 1975. This laid the question of an independent Italian nuclear capability to rest, at least for the time being.

Recently two factors have caused the question of Italian nuclear capability to be raised again. Italian support for basing U.S. intermediate-range nuclear missile forces (INF) at Comiso, Sicily, was not only politically important, but also put forces in place so that the perennial NATO issue of "two-key" control could now be raised in the Italian context. Second have been the various Western European Union assessments that a European strategic capability, perhaps initially based on British and French forces, is integral to the successful emergence of a united Europe.[15] Although too early to discuss realistically, the Italian penchant for partnership might suggest Italy's support, tacit or otherwise, of such a Euro-nuclear policy. But until that option becomes reality, if ever, the Italian position will continue to be a non-nuclear one consistent with its signing of, and continued support for, the NPT.

The Defense Decision-Making Process

After decades of political instability, manifested in nearly fifty postwar governments, there is of late an almost palpable feeling in Italy that enough is enough. Terms such as *polarized pluralism* and *imperfect two-party system* have become shorthand for describing the apparently permanent features of instability in Italy. The October 1985 resignation of the Craxi government over the hijacking of the Italian ship *Achille Lauro* was initially seen as yet more evidence of this. Yet the almost immediate reversal of Craxi's decision and the continuation of his government underscore very real changes, which call for reappraisal of the perceived instability of domestic Italian politics.

The party divisiveness inherent in a fragmented electoral system based on proportional representation, although still present, is no longer as pronounced as it was even a few years ago. The inability of the Communist Party (PCI), the second largest party, to portray itself as a viable alternative to the ruling Christian Democrats (DC) negated the possibility of the PCI playing an opposition or "alternate" role. The demise of the ideological fervor engendered by the student and union movements of preceding decades, as well as public aversion to leftist-associated terrorism, effectively defused any popular movement toward inclusion of Communists in the government. Although the DC continued as the majority party and remained in control even during the era of revolving governments, it was also increasingly associated in the public mind with the chaos that seemed endemic to Italy. The net effect

was a DC apparently unable to cope with the day-to-day problems of governing and a PCI lacking the legitimacy to play a more direct and constructive role in pursuit of stability. Incapacity offset by a lack of capability in the two major parties seemed to signal continued immobilization at governmental levels with a concomitant long-range impact on Italian planning, particularly in defense and foreign policy.

It was at this point that the seemingly innocuous 1983 decision was reached to appoint Bettino Craxi, leader of the minor Socialist Party (PSI), which had won only 11 percent of the vote, as prime minister. This decision was viewed as a "no-lose" situation by the politically embattled DC. If Craxi proved a failure, the DC could disavow him and continue to search for a successful formula after this breathing space. Conversely, as the majority partner in government, any success should redound to its credit and be translatable to the electoral arena at the following election. The Communists were likewise supportive of the Craxi appointment, feeling they could only gain from the political experiment of a center-left government, whose failure might actually trigger the long-awaited opportunity for a PCI-PSI coalition.

The fatal flaws in the reasoning of the two major parties were the assumptions that Craxi would be a compliant partner and that the internal dynamics of the PCI and the DC would support efforts to mold the coalition government toward their own objectives. In reality, neither of these assumptions proved to be correct. Craxi proceeded to solidify control of his party by eliminating potential rivals on either ideological or personal grounds. His ability to project a sense of competence was aided by a rapidly improving economy, in turn increasing Craxi's freedom of maneuver with respect to the major party blocks. Yet, notwithstanding Craxi's very real political and survival talents, it was disarray in both the left and right parties that provided him with the time required to secure an independent stature in the eyes of government leaders and, more important, at the public and international levels.[16]

The June 1985 death of the PCI leader

Enrico Berlinguer ushered in a period of internecine ideological feuding over the proper role of the Communist Party, especially in domestic matters. Alessandro Natta, Berlinguer's successor, gained substantial support for his drive to continue moving the PCI's platform toward the more acceptable social democratic formula found elsewhere in Western Europe. Although strongly supported within the party hierarchy, Natta's proposals were quickly denounced by more ideologically driven members. While recognizing the need for change, this faction was unwilling to pursue the rather benign alternative of social democracy, preferring instead a "third path," as yet undefined, but decidedly more sympathetic to traditional PCI values and objectives.[17]

The disarray in the PCI was matched by similar activity within the still powerful, but faltering, DC. The current DC leadership believes that the only way to resurrect its electoral fortunes is to strengthen central party control by lessening local autonomy. In so doing, their party secretary, Ciriaco De Mita is incurring the wrath of local leaders whose base of support is the ability to trade promises for votes and who feel that these changes are designed only to enhance his own personal power base. Yet his efforts have generated the support of older leaders who recognize the need to reorient the party if it wishes to avoid assuming secondary status behind a PSI-PCI coalition.

The outcome of these intraparty realignments plays a key role in the current reformulation of Italian defense policy. The clear sense in Italy that government alone is responsible for economic policy pushes solutions to the party level where trade-offs result in the perpetuation of inefficiencies and the maintenance of control by traditional groups. The dynamism of Italian defense firms when compared to the rest of the industrial infrastructure has made their role in domestic economic planning scenarios increasingly visible and party control over their future direction extremely attractive.

The central role of the defense industry is but one manifestation of Italy's "hidden economy," where the opportunity for resource distribution serves to redirect public awareness

away from inefficiencies and toward participation in this parallel income source. Traditionally notorious have been the *cassa integrazione*, paying 80 percent of unemployment salaries indefinitely, and the *scala mobile*, which indexes salaries to the current inflation rate. Although pensions remain low, their ease of vesting and outpacing of the inflation rate has also caused them to be a net drain on government resources. The dimensions of this alternative economy are suggested by current estimates that it represents 20 percent of Italian GNP and accounts for 2.5 million full-time and five to six million part-time workers.[18] Many of these individuals are civil servants whose lax work schedules allow them to hold other employment in the afternoons, when their offices operate under severely reduced manning requirements. The existence of these alternative income sources appears to ease the relevance of public opinion polls concluding that "unemployment is the greatest concern" to the individual today.[19] Coincidentally, this preoccupation with economic matters serves to diminish public interest in, and appreciation of, defense matters. One Italian analyst concludes that this low interest level in spite of the availability of information "indicates that people simply don't care very much about these [defense] issues."[20]

Economics, defense, and party politics also interact as a result of one of Italy's perennial problems—the southern, or *Mezzogiorno*, region. In spite of private, national and even regional assistance measures, Italy's south remains economically primitive in comparison to the north and culturally deprived in relation to the rest of the country. Migration of young workers to northern industrial areas has exacerbated this split, as few return home. There are also two other employment outlets of interest to southerners that have immediate defense implications. Public service positions, including prefectures, judgeships, and administratorships, are filled by southerners in numbers far exceeding their percentage of the national population.[21] The second option is military service, where southerners, with their relatively conservative social backgrounds, continue to dominate, especially in elite formations such as the carabinieri.[22] For these two groups, career stability is identified with government service and not with the entrepreneurial spirit more prevalent in the north. As a result, efforts to restructure the south in a more dynamic fashion have met with little success. The 1983 decision to allow the United States to base intermediate range nuclear missile forces at Comiso and the recent agreement to build a bridge from Sicily to the mainland may well be viewed as efforts by the DC to reinvigorate support in its traditional southern stronghold. The transition toward greater Italian defense emphasis on the Mediterranean strongly suggests that change may be forthcoming in spite of local elite desire to maintain the status quo. The implications of the imposition of modernity on a staunchly traditional area with few assets, resources, or attractions remain less clear.[23] The strategic location of the south makes resolution of this issue more than a simple matter of internal concern.

Responsive to American political direction and cues, the Italian defense system shares many similarities with its U.S. counterpart. The Italian president serves both as commander in chief of the armed forces and as chairman of the Supreme Defense Council, ensuring oversight of the military as well as related political-technical defense concerns.[24] Yet the potential for the president to exercise unitary or personal control over the military is severely constrained by traditional and constitutional restrictions ultimately dictating that defense policy will be a collaborative product.[25] In addition to the president, other civilian officials with major defense policy roles include the prime minister, senior cabinet members, and members of Parliament. The factionalism inherent in postwar Italian governments ensures that the individuals in these positions will mirror party positions on defense matters, resulting in a competitive bargaining process on any issue, no matter how slight or insubstantial. The actual defense organization is under the civilian leadership of the minister of defense, who administers two separate, but complementary, branches. The first, charged with military operations, is arrayed under a military defense secretary general (SMD), whose pri-

mary function is to assure coordination and joint action by the three service chiefs. Separate heads of the army, navy, and air force in turn administer forces functionally—operations, national defense, and training/education.[26]

The second branch, also under the SMD, is responsible for the administrative and research aspects of defense policy. Formal coordination between these two branches occurs primarily through the SMD and his coordinating committees for each branch: the Armed Forces Supreme Board and the Chiefs of Staff Committee.[27] The latter committee also serves as the major advisory body for the minister of defense and plays a particularly important role as regards the financial ramifications of proposed military policies. Consistent with the need to meet NATO and national defense requirements within a perennially constrained budget, a decision was reached in July 1984 to create a Defense-Industrial Committee designed to: allow defense participation in commercial "dual use" research and development projects; integrate studies on defense outputs and national economics; and inquire into the relation between exports of goods and the imports of technological processes to the Italian military effort.[28]

NEW ACTORS IN THE DEFENSE CYCLE

Italian deference to NATO policy to establish the rationale for its own national decisions has also served to insulate the actual defense decision-making process from all but a few government officials. Simultaneously, this symbiotic relation between alliance and state processes has ensured a less than coherent defense policy output because of the gap between NATO pronouncements and Italian capabilities. Although changes designed to lessen Italian dependence on NATO cues are contemplated, any fundamental modifications in defense decision making must await identification of the military tasks that Italy is willing to undertake. Consistent with that focus is the concurrent need to match more perfectly the allocation of resources with tasks.

Still, the close identification of national policy with NATO requirements has selectively redounded to Italy's benefit. The circularity of the NATO-member requirements process allows Italian objectives to be characterized as alliance mandates, thus further insulating the defense planning process from public and more than cursory parliamentary scrutiny. In a period of limited funds and tightly circumscribed military ambitions, this insularity has allowed defense planning to maintain some coherence and longevity in spite of the instability and often mercurial nature of successive Italian governments. The ability of recent governments to radiate a sense of purpose and resolve that is no longer chimerical has been translated into a desire to open the defense decision-making process to more actors. The first real opportunity to break into that closed cycle occurred with the 1983 debate and decision on INF deployments in Italy. After consulting traditional national defense bodies, Prime Minister Francesco Cossiga then transferred responsibility for the final decision to parliament. The reasoned, parsimonious discussion in both houses convinced many in and out of government that increasing the number of participants in future defense deliberations need not lead to political acrimony.[29] It also served to stimulate public awareness of security and defense matters, but this newfound interest quickly receded after completion of INF deployments in Comiso, and the previous concern with the more prosaic issues of jobs, wages, and inflation resumed. Still, Parliament's foray into defense stimulated a latent awareness that domestic economic matters and military spending could no longer be treated as discrete issues. In this fashion Parliament has gradually assumed a greater role in the process, requiring, in turn, that defense deliberations and decisions rest on a foundation other than a simple division of the budget spoils by the three services.

Roberto Aliboni and his colleagues have argued that a limited defense budget requires that expenditures be matched against missions in a fashion that allows one to assess whether funds are being expended as efficiently as possible. The inability of the three service branches to work together in support of any spending objective suggests that an agency out-side the defense establishment might best perform the requisite oversight function. Their suggestion that, based on its budgetary review responsibility, the defense and foreign affairs committees of Parliament assume that role responsibility, while innovative, is also quite consistent with the apparent trend to expand the groups involved in the process.[30]

Yet the actual defense budget cycle presents very real obstacles to the implementation of Aliboni's suggestions. The annual preparation for the defense budget cycle clearly underscores the interpenetration of national and NATO objectives. In October the SMD begins to formulate the next fiscal year's defense requirements based on the budget of two years prior. From January to March, the central budget office and the SMD respectively prepare their binding and discretionary requests based on the actual allocations of the previous year. Discretionary requests are then offset by the amount of funds assessed under the NATO 3 percent requirement, as well as by fluctuations in national economic performance as manifested in the previous budget. Binding requests are similarly channeled through appropriate ministerial review before being added to the discretionary figures in March to form the final defense budget for review by the Chiefs of Staff Committee. Until this juncture, monetary requests are based on outlays of previous budget years. At this point, the requests of the various service planning boards for personnel, operations, and research and development are received and allocated funds based on the lire totals previously agreed upon in March. After passing through the central budget office once again, the final budget request is approved by the cabinet and then passed by September to Parliament. The absence of any mechanism like that in the U.S. Congress allowing legislative inputs and review of the proposed budget prior to its formal presentation has resulted in a rather cursory review of the entire proposal rather than intensive inquiry into specific requests and proposals.[31] Several Italian commentators view this formal process as a means of minimizing outside involvement once defense mission elements determine their needs within tacitly understood spending boundaries. They conclude that while NATO and national defense commitments are taken into consideration, the real agenda of the review process is to ensure the "elimination of the worst inefficiencies, [and] the operational survival of forces and income."[32]

The outcome, then, is a budget process that minimizes nonmilitary inputs and ties expenditures to past outlays (augmented by special spending laws that are motivated politically rather than by actual requirements), all within very strict spending parameters. Absent interest or ability on the part of Parliament to increase its oversight role, the insularity of this closed process militates against moving spending limits outside tightly constrained existing limits. An opportunity to realign this balance may be suggested by the increasingly acknowledged interrelation of defense procurement with the ability of the Italian commercial infrastructure to enhance its newly won competitiveness in global markets. To allow Parliament to widen its review function to include defense as well as commercial factors of production is to base its role enhancement on matters within its competence, but also singularly important to the political parties' electoral fortunes. The Committee of Industry for Defense, formed in July 1984, strongly suggests the first tentative efforts to bring new actors, already strongly entrenched in government commercial circles, into the defense procurement process.

THE ECONOMICS OF FORCE RESTRUCTURING:
THREE SPECIAL SPENDING LAWS

Although the defense missions assigned to Italy have remained essentially identical throughout the postwar period, the character of the forces entrusted with implementing those tasks has been radically altered. The need to remold the Italian military to redress glaring shortcomings in combat effectiveness, and also to meet a domestic consensus that mandated strict financial accounting in a policy area whose importance was not manifestly clear to all, was first discussed in 1969.[33] Since 1975 major modifications have been designed to remedy three vital shortcomings, whose effect had been to render the Italian military

wholly inadequate for any role excepting that of civilian defense. In so doing, emerging Italian defense policy has not only become more acceptable domestically, but is also now capable of fulfilling national objectives, thereby permitting foreign policy options demanded by a stabilizing and optimistic governmental structure.

The first shortcoming impeding Italian defense planning was the separation in identity and even the defense objectives of the three military services. Stature, funding, and personnel were dependent on how the national defense mission was framed. The army-navy split over the centrality of the northeastern defense area versus the possibilities of the Mediterranean littoral served as the focal point for this debate. The ambiguity of the air force position was regularly confirmed as it supported the sister service whose position was closest to its own immediate needs. Each service continued to define its force requirements in view of its own mission orientation, minimizing any sense of unified or even coordinated planning. Since the annual defense appropriation essentially replicated that of the previous year, any monetary increases were service specific and based on service recommendations.

A second problem arose from the aforementioned interservice rivalries, but coalesced around the issue of spending. Prior to 1975, budgetary allocations to Italian forces were based on the number of personnel in each of the three services. The incongruity of an Italian military totaling half a million, approximately equal to those of France, Britian, and West Germany, yet with a budget of less than one-half of those states, led to a major reappraisal.[34] An additional factor prompting this reappraisal was the effect of inflation on allocation of available resources. Although the actual defense budget in 1975 was 2,450 billion lire, inflation reduced its real value by more than 10 percent to 2,200 billion lire. If fixed and discretionary expenses for personnel, adminstration, and reserve forces were eliminated, about 10 percent or 260 billion lire, was left for infrastructure and force improvements. Yet even this amount was deceptively high since major efforts were under way to increase the pay and benefits of the average soldier. From 1972 to 1977 these measures increased net expenditure per soldier from 670,000 lire to 1,200,000 lire.[35] The effect of these factors meant that in 1975 the Italian military was overmanned, undertrained, and marginally equipped to perform even the most basic of its NATO or nationally derived tasks.

The final shortcoming of the Italian military in the mid 1970s related directly to the amount of funds earmarked for defense. Italian per capita spending in NATO was lower by a large margin than that of any other members except Luxembourg, Portugal, and Turkey. Defense spending as a percentage of GDP over the 1974–83 period averaged 2.5 percent, once again substantially less than that of all major and even some minor NATO members. Perhaps most dramatically in a decade when Western defense outlays tended to move upward to offset increased personnel costs, the percentage of the Italian budget devoted to defense decreased from 8.07 percent in 1975 to 4.00 percent by 1984.[36]

The combination of these three factors engendered major defense reforms designed to offset the problems created by interservice rivalry, outdated personnel policies, and falling budgets. The thrust of the ten-year plan announced in 1975 was to reduce the quantity of the military in favor of qualitative improvements, including substantial support for upgrading personnel and matériel. Political agreement on the proposals was ensured by casting this reorganization in terms compatible with the ongoing transition of the Italian industrial base to a technological stance consistent with a tertiary economy directed toward civilian commercial as well as defense exports.[37] The qualitative improvements in forces and matériel, enhancing the effectiveness of the Italian military in the eyes of NATO allies, were the inducement that ensured that the service chiefs would agree to the proposals, even at the cost of half their personnel.

Two aspects of this reorganization effort are of central importance. First was the passage of three special laws from 1975 to 1977 designed to provide funds for each service to purchase what its respective 1974 *Libro Bianco* had

deemed essential.[38] Easing parliamentary passage of these rather substantial appropriations, each averaging 1,000 billion lire over ten years, was the explicit agreement that expenditure of these sums would be consistent with the longer-term objective of supporting the domestic ability to provide the technologically advanced products central to a defense reorientation. The navy's agreement to spend only about 40–50 billion lire of its total on foreign products is indicative of this understanding and consistent with the plans of its two sister services.[39]

Second are the very real problems being encountered by the cutbacks and reductions mandated by the 1975 plan. The 1982 decision to extend the time allotted for the reorganization from 1985 to 1991 is indicative of the obstacles that have been encountered.[40] The army in particular has been dramatically affected by proposals that have required the following changes in its previous operating style: (1) elimination of recruit training centers and reassignment of training responsibility to the battalion level; (2) monthly rather than quarterly call-up of conscripts to ease the training burdens imposed on more experienced soldiers; (3) reduction of the field army by one-third now to comprise a force of twenty-four brigades, including one paratroop brigade and five alpine units; and (4) abolition of regiments and their replacement by brigades to assist the transition to operational flexibility.

The ultimate objective of this reorganization effort is to allocate funds more expediently through the increased unification of service elements by redefinition of mission tasks. The proposed interservice rapid deployment force is indicative of this trend and perhaps a precursor of other joint ventures.

DECISION MAKING AND THE DEFENSE
INDUSTRY

Italian firms have become very creative in their pursuit of export-oriented marketing opportunities. Particularly noteworthy is the "club" concept, pioneered by naval firms to diminish competition between Italian companies in pursuit of foreign sales opportunities. The "Trieste Club" joins ten firms in a unit that has primary responsibility for the majority of Italian surface ship contracts. Over the past ten years Italian firms have advanced to the point where they now hold 40–50 percent of the global market in naval system sales for key sectors such as frigates and corvettes.[41] The aerospace sector has taken a different, but also successful, route to profitability through the use of coproduction or licensing agreements, principally with American or other European firms. Italian firms such as Aeritalia specialize in certain production aspects of aerospace systems and then utilize this expertise as an entree to lucrative multinational consortia.

Notwithstanding their successes, Italian defense firms continue to suffer from an inadequacy of research and development funding and, indeed, lack of interest by the military services in providing more capital for this purpose.[42] The government estimates that Italian dependence on foreign processes is about 20 percent of the end value of such products.[43] Although national procurement policies are "Buy Italian" in nature, the limits imposed by the scarcity of research and development funds translate into production specialization and cooperative ventures as keys for defense industries. Dismissing suggestions of intra-alliance division of labor as politically unworkable, Italian firms continue to strive to enhance their consortia roles through an acknowledged expertise in certain stages of production cycles.[44] The impact of limited research and development funds is greatly ameliorated by purchases from the United States, with Italian firms concentrating on their design utilization and translation into products for the Italian sales market.

In July 1984, 1,000 million lire (about $1 million) was appropriated to pursue a seven-year building plan for research and development in cooperation with other states.[45] Among the most important joint ventures in the military field are: (1) The AM-X (about $470 million), a light tactical fighter built in cooperation with Brazil, designed to be capable of replacing the G-91 and F-104G. This new platform is designed to be multimission-capable and sympathetic to the bomber role of the Tornado and the air intercept role of the F-104. (2) The EH-101 (about $300 million), an antisubmarine warfare (ASW) helicopter built by the Italian firm Augusta in conjunction with Britain's Westland, designed to replace the SH-3D presently in service with both countries' forces. The EH-101 is expressly designed to offer a commercial version of the craft, which accounts for the interest and support of the minister of industry in the project. (3) CATRIN (about $226 million), a mobile information transmission system for the army, designed to assist in battle management. Like the EH-101, the CATRIN is dual-purpose capable to ensure its easy adaptation to the commercial market to meet needs in the area of, among others, disaster relief. This is an all-"Italian" project. (4) The European Fighter Aircraft (EFA). In cooperation with France, West Germany, Britain, and Spain, Italy is designing an air interceptor capable of replacing the F-104 in the 1990s. The anticipated initial order for the Italian Air Force is about 165 fighters. The EFA will be ready at a time when the F-16 is to be replaced. If the EFA continues on schedule, it should remain far ahead in anticipated market availability date of its major American competitor, currently named the Advanced Technology Fighter (ATF). (5) The Linea Carri. The short-term use of this new tank is to substitute for the M-47 currently used in eight of the thirty Italian armored battalions. An additional Bren-carrier version is also contemplated to augment the flexibility and mobility of attached infantry units. Also as part of this project is the performance upgrade of the Leopard tank, especially in the areas of firing rate, armor, and ammunition characteristics. Long-term plans anticipate replacement of the M-47 in the remaining twenty-two Italian battalions with a third generation vehicle to be produced in conjunction with NATO/IEPG work on a parallel project. An armored personnel carrier, the Italian made VCC-1, is also being introduced with the express purpose of replacing the aging U.S.-produced M113s.[46] (6) The A-129, a light helicopter to be used for close-in ground support of infantry units. Armament will include missiles and rockets. The A-129 is designed primarily for the army, with the contract already awarded to Augusta. The first successful flight of the A-129 was in September 1983, and it entered active service in 1987. Its initial successful production and multiple uses in a variety of commercial and military modes aroused interest among other countries in its purchase. It is exceedingly likely that the A-129 is being designed with the objective of sharing production responsibilities with other firms or states under the overall guidance of Augusta. (7) The NATO Frigate (NFR). A joint venture among eight NATO members, including France, to design and build a multipurpose frigate was announced in April 1984. Italian approval of project participation was agreed in March 1983, and given the major role of Italy's industries in this shipbuilding sector, its responsibility in the final product should be substantial.

While a current listing of Italian projects is interesting, two particular factors should be noted. First is the express Italian effort to ensure that essentially military projects are dual purpose in nature and thus easily adaptable to the commercial sales market. While increased export revenue is one result, it is the blurring of the traditional Italian distinction between defense and commercial industries that is of longer-term significance. The research and development fund shortage imposed on Italian defense firms by constrained national budgets can be eased by such dual-capacity outlooks. Similarly, the political base of support for military outlays is widened, given the benefits to the national, rather than simply the defense, industrial infrastructure. Second, each of these projects is designed to replace an existing product that has been purchased from the United States. The implications are obvious, but nonetheless interesting. If these projects are completed, then a situation much like that with the Tornado should arise, where a European alternative to an American product, albeit more expensive, commands the ultimate sale. The offset for increased price is the direct infusion of jobs, resources, and expertise into the Italian industrial infrastructure. Conversely, if the projects fail or falter, the Italians are still free to pursue bilateral arrangements with American or European firms to secure their needs. Italy's traditional bargaining strategy, pleading the need for economic assistance to ensure the political stability integral to EEC and NATO futures, should once again stand it in good stead. Yet certain constraints are still evident, given the Italian domestic context that will affect Italy's ability to achieve these proposed objectives.

Recurring Issues and Defense Policy Outputs

CIVIL-MILITARY RELATIONS

The fascist formula that subordinated military instruments to the will and whim of a single civilian leader ensured that Italy would not replicate that experience when formulating its post-war defense structure. But neither could Italy assume the separateness between state and military made possible by the stability inherent in the American system. An Italian compromise has emerged gradually that permits independence of the military from direct civilian control, while ensuring effective oversight because of the competing defense policies of the major party groups. It is from the interplay of the Communist Party (PCI) and the Christian Democrats (DC) that one gains a sense of the current status of civil-military relations in Italy.

Ciro Zoppo suggests that the PCI has played a major role in military reorganization, even though not officially in government, for two reasons.[47] First is the PCI assertion that democratization of the armed forces is essential if Italy wishes to move closer to the objectives articulated in its constitution. This desire does not mean that the PCI is supportive of unionization for the military. Rather, its position is that working conditions, including military punishment, must be consistent with the need for discipline rather than simply for the purpose of maintaining an artificial hierarchy based solely on military traditions.[48] Second has been the intense PCI effort through membership on parliamentary committees to inhibit the use of military units to suppress internal protests against the state. The PCI was particularly incensed by several incidents involving rightist senior military officers in the

1960s and 1970s and sought corrective action through its oversight function on parliamentary committees where membership is based on seat totals, thus ensuring substantial inputs by its members. Key among these efforts was the reorganization of military intelligence to separate personnel and operations involved with externally directed counterespionage from those directed at internal actors and groups. While the former remained within the Defense Department, the latter were placed under the Ministry of the Interior. These efforts were aided by the domestic conditions of unrest and the political experiment of détente, which enabled the PCI to capitalize on public perceptions that it was the party best able to direct these changes. These efforts were simultaneously at the expense of the ruling DC, whose close connections to the military were commonly perceived as creating symbiotic relations that benefited both actors. This closeness was particularly evident in elite formations such as the carabinieri, in which 98 percent of the personnel were career troops rather than conscripts. The dual-purpose role of the carabinieri as a military as well as national police force magnified, often out of reasonable proportion, its use in quelling internal disturbances. The carabinieri's success in stamping out terrorism in the early 1980s and its losses in the perpetual fight against the Mafia have recently been translated into changing public perceptions of the threat it poses to a democratic society, a shift that might, in turn, redound to the benefit of the DC.

DEMOGRAPHICS AND MANPOWER

Over the past ten years, Italy has undergone major shifts in military recruitment, training, and retention patterns. In the early 1980s the decision was reached to continue the existing system based on a comprehensive draft of limited duration, augmented by a cadre of skilled individuals who exchange longer service terms for special training opportunities. This rejection of the American all-volunteer model was on political, rather than military, grounds. Major party groups felt it essential that a primarily national defense force reflect the class and social character of the state as a whole.[49]

At present, conscription accounts for the overwhelming majority of Italian military personnel. At seventeen, men are enrolled on the relevant call-up rosters. They are physically and mentally tested the following year. Those selected may choose a twelve-month obligation in the army or air force or eighteen months in the navy. Parliament is presently discussing a bill that would require a twelve-month service obligation notwithstanding the service chosen. Conscientious objector status and deferment for schooling are possible, but the diminishing national birth rate has recently made it more difficult to qualify for either of these options.[50] Burgeoning university enrollments as a result of the loosening of admissions requirements in the aftermath of the student disturbances of the 1960s have also increased scrutiny of temporary or permanent deferment petitions.

The financial cutbacks in defense spending accomplished in the mid 1970s dramatically affected the process of recruit training and raised questions about the military effectiveness of Italian forces as a whole. Recruit training centers were closed to save money, requiring conscripts to be trained in military skills at the battalion level by soldiers only slightly more experienced than themselves.[51] With minor exceptions, each service currently follows a training pattern based on three consecutive cycles: basic, advanced, and specialization consistent with particular NATO or national defense tasks. The primary exception to this pattern is the air force, whose abundance of sophisticated systems leads it to seek, through competitive testing, volunteers willing to enlist for two to six years in return for advanced training and education, often in a skill area that may later be translated into a lucrative civilian position upon discharge.

This effort to increase longevity (and, inferentially, competence) in the armed forces has been especially apparent in the role and training envisaged for noncommissioned officers (NCOs). Following legislation enacted in 1983, NCO training proceeds in three stages after an initial tour of three and a half years has been completed: (1) one year of training at the appropriate NCO academy in Viterbo (army), Taranto or La Maddalena (navy), or Caserta (air force); (2) a qualifying period of varying length in an area of specialization; and (3) an apprenticeship on the job consistent with the technological requirements of that speciality. At the conclusion of this training cycle, the individual is assigned to the regular service with the rank of sergeant major or its naval equivalent.[52]

In comparison, officer recruitment is exclusively based on successful completion of the program, usually four years in length, offered at one of the service or speciality academies: navy (Livorno), air force (Pozzuoli), or army (Modena and Rome, or Turin for advanced courses). Cross-registration agreements with civilian universities allow course and concentration options not possible within the relatively narrow and technologically oriented service school curriculum. Plans developed in 1984 are presently being implemented to allow pursuit of a *laurea* (Bachelor's degree) in previously neglected fields such as information science, law, economics, and political science. Advanced schooling, generally at the 10–13 year point, is offered within most specialities and is modeled on the American example, which emphasizes global and political matters as one attains higher staff level positions. The culmination of the education cycle is the nine-month course at the Center for Advanced Defense Studies in Rome, which includes formal classes, war gaming and study trips in Italy and abroad for its varied student body, drawn from all three services as well as the carabinieri and diverse national police forces.

Italy's ability to meet its military tasks through a conscript-based system will face severe testing in the very near term. Although reserve officer programs of three to five months duration have been used to provide cadre forces at a fraction of the cost of active duty personnel, minimal entrance requirements and unevenness of training make their combat or even military usefulness questionable. A September 1981 parliamentary proposal to include women in the draft foundered. Indeed, the problems facing the Italian military will only become worse in the next few years. Like West Germany's, the Italian birth rate continues to decline, with shortfalls becoming no-

ticeable into the 1990s. By the turn of the century, manning shortfalls are expected to reach 93,000 out of an annual desired force total of 300,000.[53] Although salary and benefits are much improved as a result of the personnel reductions of the mid 1970s, they still continue to lag far behind even modest targets. As an example, base housing availability for officers and NCOs continues to meet only some 80 percent of demand. Retirement pay, a major longevity inducement for American forces, remains low and is buffeted by Italy's perennially high inflation rate. Reserve pensions and benefits are in even worse straits, minimizing any incentive to augment one's civilian career through limited military duty.

These shortfalls, and perhaps an Italian propensity to democracy, have led to the introduction of a representative system that combines in varying degrees the role of ombudsman and union official. These soldier representatives concern themselves with the working conditions, career options, and morale of all levels of personnel. Popularly, though separately, elected by all ranks, representatives are arrayed in three hierarchical layers, the uppermost of which has direct access to both the chief of the General Staff and Parliament.[54] Biannual voluntary elections, first instituted in 1980, appear popular, with over 93 percent of eligible personnel taking part. It is unclear whether this system is designed to ease the lot of the conscripted soldier or to pave the way toward a volunteer force by enhancing the benefits required to support it.

WEAPONS ACQUISITION

Italian defense production is dependent on the more than two hundred public, mixed ownership, and private firms whose primary contractual obligations are military in nature. These small and medium-sized companies produce the bulk of Italian military needs. In addition, of approximately 52,000 civilian workers, 22,000 are directly involved in engineering tasks for upkeep and repair of military equipment, with about 18,000 distributed throughout Italy to oversee the needs of specific units and commands.[55] Of their forty offices, thirty-one are tasked to meet army needs, nine for the navy, and none for the air force, which is expected to deal directly with civilian firms to meet its requirements.[56] The remaining 30,000 workers are dispersed throughout the various military units to perform logistical and maintenance functions more complex than those possible under field conditions. The tasks entrusted to these civilian defense workers have gradually been limited, because of their higher labor costs, to the point where they now perform only very specialized functions. Consistent with the 1975 reorganization thrust, a new division of labor is slowly emerging, with military personnel focusing on frontline readiness and civilian workers concentrating on longer-term, more sophisticated procedures. It is anticipated that the armed forces will be able to perform 70–80 percent of their own repair and maintenance work in the near future.[57]

The industrial infrastructure backing this direct civilian defense network numbers about 8,000 firms with in excess of one million employees. Of these, 200 public and private firms and 80,000 workers are the primary production actors, accounting for 2 percent of all Italian manufacturing employees and 4 percent of national manufacturing output. Although dedicated to the needs of Italian national defense, these firms, taking a lesson from their successful counterparts in France and Britain, are finding that Third World markets are increasingly important to their ability to maintain a domestic industrial infrastructure for production of military goods. These foreign markets have increased dramatically from the 1970s and today account for upward of 2.5 percent of all Italian exports. Indeed fully 60% of Italian military-industrial output is destined for export, with the remainder meeting strictly national needs.[58]

Central to this discussion is the nature of the dependency created by Italy's role as a transformer of proven Western technology to meet the weapons requirements of Third World purchasers. Unlike Britain and France, which to a great extent have sufficient capacity to generate their own technological and process developments unilaterally (although at extreme cost), Italy acknowledges that it is R and D scarcity that has caused it to procure these processes from foreign suppliers.[59] Indeed, Italy traditionally heads the list of Western states that import weapons and processes, with its leading supplier being the United States.[60] Conversely, Italy's major clients are rather volatile Middle Eastern and African states whose purchases for regional use have been paid for by oil revenues. Thus either end of the production stream presents enormous problems for the status of Italian arms-dependent sectors if disruptions were to occur. Arms for oil has been a consistent contractual relationship for France and has increasingly played a similar role for Italy. Yet the Italian decision not to pursue nuclear energy, unlike the dedicated French effort to become the leading Western state in this regard, underscores the fragility of an Italian infrastructure based on volatile ties, with little if any offset recourse if those ties were to be disrupted. The apparent reluctance of the Italian government to support the United States over its 1986 Libyan raid to retaliate for terrorism is quite understandable in light of its geographic proximity to, and contractual dependency on, Middle Eastern purchasers.

Italy's growing stature in the global arms market, then, stems largely from its ability to obtain foreign technology and processes, tailor them to export markets, and sell the product free of the political entanglements associated with purchase from one of the traditional manufacturing powers. Three distinct steps—acquisition, transformation, and transfer—simultaneously reflect the strengths and pitfalls of Italy's capability in a period when foreign markets, especially in the Middle East, are contracting. Recognizing what will be short-term shifts in market composition, Italy seeks to minimize dependence on external acquisition of technology by increasing indigenous R and D through European-oriented consortia. Enhancement of domestic production opportunities would simultaneously lessen the chance that its suppliers, principally the United States, might restrict sales through extraterritorial application of technology transfer restrictions on national security grounds. Indigenization for Italy does not carry with it any sense of lessened commitment to its NATO re-

Table 2. Italian Trade in Major Conventional Weapons, 1985

Recipient	Quantity	Weapon
Developed World		
Greece	25	A-109 Hirundo Helicopter
	30	G-222 Transport
	20	Model 300C Helicopter
Portugal	12	A-109 Hirundo Helicopter
Spain	24	AB-412 Griffon Helicopter[a]
	200	ASPIDE AMM (air-to-air) SAM (surface-to-air) Missile
Turkey	40	AB-205 Helicopter[a]
	2	G-222 Transport
Third World		
Argentina	15	Palmaria 155mm SPH
Burma	4	SF-260M Trainer
Ethiopia	11	SF-260-TP Trainer
Iraq	2	A-109 Hirundo Helicopter
	5	AB-212 ASW Helicopter[a]
	224	ASPIDE AAM/SAM
	60	Otomat-2 ShShM (ship-to-ship missile)
	4	Lupo Class Frigate
	6	Wadi Class Corvette
Kenya	24	Otomat-2 ShShM
Libya	210	Palmaria 155mm SPH
	4	Wadi Class Corvette
Malaysia	4	Lerici Class Minehunter
Nigeria	12	MB-339A Jet Trainer
	25	Palmaria 155mm SPH
	2	Lerici Class Minehunter
Peru	4	SH-3D SeaKing Helicopter[a]
	96	ASPIDE AAM/SAM
	96	Otomat-2ShShM
Saudi Arabia	1	SH-3D SeaKing Helicopter[a]
	200	VCC-1 Armored Personnel Carrier (APC)
Singapore	30	S-211 Trainer
Somalia	6	S-211 Trainer
	100	M-47 Tank
Sudan	12	AB-212 Helicopter[a]
Syria	18	AB-212 ASW Helicopter[a]
	6	CH-47C Chinook Helicopter[a]
	12	SH-3D SeaKing Helicopter[a]
Thailand	48	ASPIDE AAM/SAM
U.A.E.	30	A-129 Mangusta Helicopter
	4	MB-339A Jet Trainer
	6	SF-260-TP
	21	OF-40 Tank
Venezuela	10	A-109 Helicopter
	8	G-222 Transport
	4	S-61R Helicopter[a]
	5	Type 42M Patrol Craft (PC)
Zimbabwe	10	AB-412 Griffon Helicopter[a]

Source: SIPRI Yearbook, 1986 (Stockholm: Stockholm International Peace Research Institute, 1986), pp. 359–418.

[a]Denotes American product under license to an Italian firm.

sponsibilities, but rather a desire to promote an environment where sales are pursued because of Italian, and not American, foreign policy objectives. Yet a main attraction of Italian products has been their use of proven American technology, albeit in a tailored design. To diminish Italian-American defense relations is to place in jeopardy these underlying and essential commercial ties. Balancing the symbiotic tensions in each of these three pro-

duction steps is therefore central in assessing the potential for greater Italian control over Italy's security. By choice, developments will be channeled within parameters established by arms control talks, which Italy strongly supports. Italy's posture on START, INF, and CSCE, to identify a few, is to hold closely to the positions and objectives articulated by alliance partners. In this fashion Italy's quest for security independence retains its pro-NATO, pro-

American, and pro-European qualities, notwithstanding the increasingly contradictory stances of these Western actors. Whatever the outcome of this interplay, it appears that Italy has fortuitously positioned itself to effect its national goals with a minimum outlay of resources.

Notes

1. *Libro bianco della difensa 1985* (Rome: Ministero della Difensa, 1985), vol. 1, p. 10 (hereafter *Libro bianco*).

2. Robert A. Isaak, *European Politics: Political Economy and Policy Making in Western Democracies* (New York: St. Martin's Press, 1980), p. 131.

3. Joseph La Palombara, "Parental Relationships in Italian Government," in *European Politics*, ed. Mattei Dogan and Richard Rose (New York: Macmillan, 1971), pp. 513–26; Luigi Barzini, *The Italians* (New York: Atheneum, 1964).

4. Gian Enrico Rusconi and Sergio Scamuzzi, "Italy Today: An Eccentric Society," *Current Sociology* 29, no. 1 (Spring 1981) pp. 1–161.

5. David M. Wood, *Power and Policy in Western European Democracies*, 3d ed. (New York: John Wiley & Sons, 1986), pp. 132–38.

6. Rusconi and Scamuzzi, "Italy Today," pp. 14–15.

7. "Everybody's Behaving Out of Character," *The Economist*, 28 September 1985, pp. 48–50.

8. "Strong Man of Europe," *The Economist*, 12 October 1985, p. 16.

9. Alain Dauvergne, "Italy's Secret Strength," *World Press Review* (excerpted from *Le Point-Paris*), May 1983, pp. 30–32.

10. Humphrey Taylor, "Nine Nations Assess Economic and Security Issues," *Public Opinion*, August-September 1983, p. 54.

11. Sergio A. Rossi, "Public Opinion and Atlantic Defense in Italy," in *The Public and Atlantic Defense*, ed. Gregory Flynn and Hans Rattinger (London: Croom Helm, 1985), pp. 175–220, at 192.

12. P. A. Allum, *Italy—Republic Without Government?* (New York: W. W. Norton, 1973), p. 157; Gianfranco Pasquino, "The Italian Army: Some Notes on Recruitment," *Armed Forces and Society* 2, no. 2 (1976), pp. 205–17.

13. Ciro Zoppo, *The Defense and Military Policies of the Italian Communist Party*, P-6012 (Santa Monica, Calif.: *Rand* Corporation, 1977), p. 9.

14. Rusconi and Scamuzzi, "Italy Today," pp. 16–19; 89–106.

15. *Libro bianco*, vol. 1, p. 6.

16. Ibid, p. 44.

17. Thomas H. Etzold, "The Soviet Union in the Mediterranean," *Naval War College Review* 32, no. 4 (July–August 1984), pp. 4–22.

18. "Italian Navy Awaits Parliamentary Approval for Aircraft on Giuseppe Garibaldi," *Jane's Defence Weekly*, 7 September 1985, p. 465; *International Defense Review* 18 (September 1985), p. 1386.

19. *Libro bianco*, vol. 1, p. 54.

20. Ibid., pp. 56–60.

21. Ibid., pp. 55–56.

22. Gian Luca Devoto, "Italy's Armaments Program and Nuclear Proliferation," *Lo spettatore internazionale* 11, No. 4 (October-December 1976), pp. 285–93; Maurizio Cremasco, "A New Model of Defense for Italy," ibid. 17, no. 3 (July-September 1982), pp. 231–43; Steven Baker, *Italy and the Nuclear Option* (California: Arms Control and Foreign Policy Seminar, 1974).

23. "Missile Diplomacy: Europe Prepares," *New York Times*, 2 April 1987, p. 3.

24. Stephen P. Koff, "The Italian Presidency: Constitutional Role and Political Practice," *Presidential Studies Quarterly* 12, no. 3 (Summer 1982), pp. 337–51.

25. Luigi Caligaris, "Italian Defense Policy: Problems and Prospects," *Survival* 25, no. 2 (March 1983), pp. 68–76; Roberto Aliboni, Maurizio Cremasco, Franca Gusmaroli and Stefano Silvestri, "Defense Policy and Defense Expenditure Decision-making," *Lo Spettatore Internazionale* 15, no. 2 (April 1980), pp. 167–79; Cremasco, "New Model of Defense for Italy," pp. 231-243.

26. *Libro bianco*, vol. 1, p. 61, table 7.

27. Ibid., vol. 2, appendix 8.

28. Ibid., vol. 1, pp. 79–80; vol. 2, appendix 14.

29. Caligaris, "Italian Defense Policy," pp. 74–76.

30. Aliboni et al., "Defense Policy and Defense Expenditure Decision-making," pp. 167–79.

31. *Libro bianco*, vol. 2, appendix 13.

32. Aliboni et al., "Defense Policy and Defense Expenditure Decision-making," pp. 167–79.

33. *Libro bianco*, vol. 1, pp. 65–75.

34. "The Revised Italian Defense System and the Re-organization of the Army," *Italy: Documents and Notes* (Rome: Presidency of the Council of Ministers 26, no. 1, 1977), pp. 3–17.

35. Ibid., p. 8.

36. *Libro bianco*, vol. 1, pp. 91–95, tables 8–12.

37. Gianluca Devoto, "Italian Military Policy," *Lo Spettatore Internazionale* 11, no. 4 (October 1976), pp. 317–28.

38. *Libro bianco*, vol. 1, pp. 66–68.

39. Devoto, "Italian Military Policy," pp. 287–88.

40. *Libro bianco*, vol. 1, pp. 37, 66–68.

41. Sergio A. Rossi, "Italy," in *The Structure of the Defense Industry: An International Survey*, ed. Nicole Ball and Milton Leitenberg (New York: St. Martin's Press, 1983), pp. 214–56.

42. *Libro bianco*, vol. 1, pp. 77–80.

43. Rossi, "Italy," p. 230.

44. Ibid., p. 244, table 7.12.

45. Dennis Culkin, "Italy's Growth as a Major Defense Industrial Power," *Defense and Foreign Affairs*, October 1982, pp. 21–24.

46. Ibid., p. 23.

47. *Libro bianco*, vol. 1, p. 79.

48. Ibid., p. 84.

49. Ibid., pp. 87–90.

50. Pasqualino Verdecchia, "Italian Armor, Past, Present and Future," *Armor*, May-June 1983, pp. 34–37.

51. Ciro Zoppo, *Defense and Military Policies of the Italian Communist Party*; id., "The Left and European Security: France, Italy and Spain," *Orbis* 24, no. 2 (Summer 1980) 289–310.

52. Zoppo, *Defense and Military Policies of the Italian Communist Party*, p. 8.

53. See *Libro bianco*, vol. 1, p. 103, table 7, for 1974-83 comparison of conscripts versus volunteers in total active duty force. The issue of an all-volunteer force has again been raised by a socialist ("Mamma's Boys," *The Economist*, 4 October 1986, pp. 47-49).

54. *Libro bianco*, vol. 2, p. 217, for deferment legislation.

55. Ibid., vol. 1, pp. 106-8.

56. Ibid., vol. 1, pp. 109-11 and vol. 2, appendix 18.

57. Ibid., vol. 2, appendix 19, chart on p. 216.

58. Ibid., vol. 1, pp. 116-17 and vol. 2, appendix 21.

59. Edward Kolodziej, "France and the Arms Trade," *International Affairs* 56 (1980), pp. 54-72; Lawrence Freedman, "Britain and the Arms Trade," *International Affairs* 54C1 (July 1978), pp. 77-92.

60. *SIPRI Yearbook, 1981* (Stockholm: Stockholm International Peace Research Institute, 1981), p. 197.

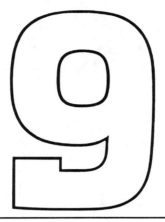

CANADA

Douglas J. Murray

Before examining Canadian defense policy in detail, recognition must be given to what Colin Gray refers to as strategic culture or national style in strategy. Strategic culture means a set of general beliefs, attitudes, and behavioral patterns with regard to nuclear strategy that have a degree of semipermanence, not unlike a nation's culture. The term refers to certain modes of thought and action in regard to the utility of force and is derived from a nation's historical experience, goals, objectives, and self-actualization.[1] Canada possesses a unique strategic culture, composed of the following elements:

First, Canadians can be described as an "unmilitary people" who prefer nonviolent means to military ones to achieve their foreign-policy objectives. C. P. Stacey, a prominent Canadian historian, writes "Canada is an unmilitary community. Warlike her people have been forced to be, military they have never been."[2] Proud of her more than 150 years of military service with no peacetime conscription, Canada has never had a senior military officer later serve as prime minister.[3] The 1987 White Paper on defense summarized this first characteristic: "Canadians tend to approach international relations optimistically, assuming the best of others. Few Canadians feel militarily threatened and most have difficulty imagining anyone as an enemy. While accepting the necessity of a defence effort, we do not expect to have to resort to force of arms to resolve our problems."[4]

But unmilitary does not mean antimilitary or pacifist. Canada supports a strong military but rejects any form of military influence in Canadian society. In many ways, the military operates outside the mainstream of society in Canada. Even though a military career is not necessarily held in high esteem, Canadians respect the man in uniform for what he sacrifices for his nation, and Canadians have sacrificed much. They fought valiantly in two world wars. In World War II, with more than 10 percent of the population in uniform, Canada lost 42,000 soldiers.

Perhaps Canadian history best explains this

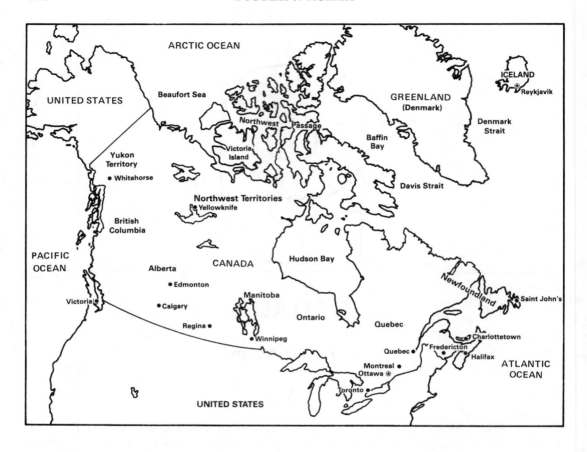

unmilitary society. In Canada, independence came about through an evolutionary, peaceful process rather than a revolutionary, violent one. The keynote was compromise; in the United States, it was confrontation. When Canada made her split from the motherland in 1867, Britain had changed radically from the days of 1776 when the United States revolted. Moreover, Canada, a land of diversity, lives with that diversity and even encourages it. Unlike the United States, Canada never became a melting pot. Today, 40 percent of the nation is English, and 30 percent is French. The remaining 30 percent is composed of twenty-seven European immigrant groups and three different native peoples. Canadians speak two languages and have two cultures and at least four distinct geographical regions.

The impact of this nonmilitary orientation on Canadian defense is significant. "The absence of any deep-rooted military tradition in

this country is probably the single most important factor preventing any collective push for higher spending on national defence," Peter Newman argues.[5] Not only does Canada keep spending down, it does not hesitate to reassess policy and change direction. It puts emphasis now on conventional rather than nuclear deterrence. Since the mid 1960s, Canada has worked to dismantle its nuclear option. Similarly, Canada's nonmilitary orientation finds reflection in a strong position in favor of arms control and in opposition to an antiballistic missile (ABM) system and the military use of space. In the international arena, Canada is content to be the "helper-fixer," the peace-keeper. From the birth of the United Nations and the North Atlantic Treaty Organization (NATO) through the crises in Korea and Suez to the present, Canada has labored hard to curb the great powers by, in the words of two Canadian authors, David B. DeWitt and John

J. Kirton, "consensus, common interests, functional necessity, and international ranking."[6]

The second characteristic of the Canadian strategic culture is that Canada does not have a defense policy in the traditional sense of self-reliance. Canada never has been able to rely solely upon its own resources for its defense. "Canada has always been a country of alliance," J. J. Blais, a former minister of defence, noted in 1983.[7] "There is no external threat which is unique to Canada," declares the 1987 Defence White Paper. "Canada alone cannot assure its own security. As the neighbour of two heavily armed superpowers and as a country that depends on international relationships for its well-being and prosperity, if not for its survival, Canada's security ultimately requires the maintenance of a peaceful international order."[8] Canada has never fought an aggressive war, nor, with the exception of U.S. incursions, one in which its boundaries were directly threatened. Canada has always relied upon alliance for security. It fought wars allied with the British and the Americans. Prior to World War II, Britain was the Canadian protector. Since then, the United States has replaced Britain.

However, Canada has always been able to make a meaningful contribution in its alliances. In the 1950s and 1960s, for example, that contribution was to the North American Air Defense (NORAD) role and in the conventional defense of Europe. In recent years however, the credibility of the Canadian contribution is being questioned because of Canada's reduced NATO commitment in the late 1960s, the size of Canada's defense budget, the shrinking NORAD mission in the 1970s, and reluctance to become involved in missile and space defense systems in the 1980s. Similarly, Canada's unwillingness to field nuclear weapons limits the extent of its contribution to a joint defense effort.

A third factor that has distinguished the Canadian approach to defense is that Canada's armed forces exist primarily to support political and economic policies rather than for military purposes. James Eayrs, a Canadian defense historian, flatly states, "the major

function of the Canadian military establishment has had practically nothing to do with our national security and practically everything to do with supporting and sustaining our national diplomacy. . . . It is exceedingly difficult to choose weapon systems for a military establishment whose function is essentially non-military."[9] Thus, military ties to Europe are attractive only insofar as they secure economic links with the European Economic Community (EEC) or assuage the U.S. desire for greater Canadian involvement in NATO. This factor explains in part why the Canadian Department of External Affairs often dominates policy debate and represented defense issues in the important inner-cabinet committee until the advent of the government of Prime Minister Brian Mulroney. This policy attitude is also reflected in Article 2 of the NATO charter, the so-called Canadian article, which, as drafted by Canada, attempts to mold NATO into something more than a military alliance.

However, the fourth factor, the U.S.–Canadian defense relationship, is without a doubt the most important in understanding the Canadian approach to national security. Canada's geographic position between the two superpowers has simultaneously made it a target in any Soviet attack on the United States and an integral part of any U.S. strategy to defend the continent. The United States penetrates Canadian society at every level. Canadian defense policy and the process that developed it reflect U.S. interests.[10] Efforts since 1945 to reach for multilateral relationships, such as NATO, instead of bilateral ones, such as NORAD, evidence Canada's drive to establish an independent role in defense. The pervasiveness of U.S. influence and the Canadian obsession with eradicating it explain much about Canada's identity crisis and the current thrust of Canada's defense policy.

Finally, the fifth factor, the special nature of Canadian defense policy affects, and is affected by, the structure of the Canadian armed forces. Since 1968, unlike the United States and most Western nations, Canada has had a unified armed force as opposed to separate services. This has a significant impact on the defense decision-making process, as well as a long-lasting impact on the morale and effectiveness of the Canadian military.

International Environment

Canada's position in the international political system is the result of geography, close ties to England and the United States, desire for an independent role on the world stage, and strategic culture. Not a world superpower, Canada is nonetheless more than a minor power. When polled, the foreign policy-making elites of the world ranked Canada with Australia in terms of relative importance and position in the international environment.[11] Canadians would not agree with this perception, however. Particularly since the 1960s, Canada has searched for an independent identity. Canada views itself as a global actor. A series of comprehensive public opinion polls commissioned by the Canadian Department of External Affairs in 1984 and 1985 showed that Canadians believed their government should be an active participant in the world arena. The majority of Canadians polled felt that Canada's influence in world affairs should be focused primarily on finding solutions to the issues of international peace and security and Third World poverty and hunger. They considered the relationship with the United States as the most important, but argued that Canada should be aggressive in developing independent policy positions. Canadians said the relationship with the United States should be "businesslike but neighborly."[12]

In the twentieth century, Canada's position in the international political system has been one of continual transition. A nation that entered the century under the shadow of Great Britain, Canada emerged in 1945 with the potential for a major power status. However, that potential evaporated as Canada decreased its military capability and the European nations recovered from World War II. As Canada stepped onto the world stage after the war, it found itself in the shadow of the world's newest superstar—the United States. In addition, new centers of power, particularly in Asia and Latin America, filled the vacuum created by the war.

Nevertheless, Canada still possesses many elements basic to major power status.[13]

Canada ranks second in size to the Soviet Union, among the world's nations, with an area of 3.8 million square miles. It is among the richest nations in the world, possessing vast amounts of mineral wealth and national resources. It ranks first in the world in mineral exports and third in mineral production, behind the United States and the Soviet Union. It is the largest producer in the world of asbestos, zinc, silver, and nickel and provides the United States with twenty-three of thirty-five materials the U.S. Department of Defense classifies as critical.

Canada is a major producer of hydroelectricity and, unlike most of the Western democracies, is a net exporter of energy. Its gross national product (GNP) is seventh in the world. In total volume of trade, Canada ranks sixth, behind the United States, Japan, the Federal Republic of Germany, France, and the United Kingdom. The value of goods traded between the United States and Canada in 1984 alone was greater than between any two other nations of the world—and remains that way. In fact, the amount of commerce between the United States and Canada is twice that between the United States and Japan and larger than the U.S. trade with the Common Market. Canada is a major food exporter and the second largest wheat producer. In fact, in all but two measures of national power—population and military capability—Canada must be grouped among the major nations of the world.

But with only twenty-five million people, Canada has less than .5 percent of the world's total population and about 10 percent of that of the United States. Significantly, this population is unevenly distributed. One-third of Canada's territory contains less than .3 percent of her population. Nearly 80 percent of all Canadians live within one hundred miles of the U.S. border. In fact, half of Canada's population lives in the southeastern section of the nation near the Great Lakes and the St. Lawrence River. This demographic imbalance governs the direction of Canada's external interests and policy, pointing interests south toward the

United States, and creates a web of economic and social interdependencies between the two nations.

Canada's fiscal year (FY) 1987/1988 defense budget of C$10.3 billion is slightly more than 2 percent of its GNP. The NATO average is nearly 5 percent. In fact, with the possible exception of Luxembourg, no NATO nation spends less of its national wealth on defense than Canada. Its current force of over 86,000 is well trained and professional, but it is also undermanned, often poorly equipped, and considerably overextended. A review conducted by the Canadian government in 1987 concluded

that after decades of neglect, there is a significant "commitment-capability gap." Much of the equipment of the Canadian Forces is already old and ineffective against current threats. Modernization programs have not kept pace with technological change. The navy has too few ships and submarines for Atlantic and Pacific operations and a very limited capability to operate in the Arctic. It could not keep Canadian waterways and harbours clear of mines. The land forces have severe equipment shortages and too few combat-ready soldiers, and the Militia is too small, ill-equipped and insufficiently trained to make up the difference. The air forces suffer from a serious shortage of air transport to move troops and equipment to Europe in times of tension and to sustain them during hostilities. They have too few maritime patrol aircraft. They lack sufficient numbers of modern weapons for the CF-18 aircraft and cannot replace CF-18s lost in peacetime. Nowhere is the gap more evident than in the lack of logistic and medical support for our forces committed to Europe.[14]

The downward trend in Canada's military capability has reversed in recent years, but not to the point where its world position has begun to change. And its perceived military capability has a great impact on Canada's stature in the international environment.

Demography and military power have not helped Canada become a major power, nor has its geography. Canada and the United States not only share a 5,335-mile border, they often share life-styles, ambitions, and outlooks. Many U.S. citizens do not even view Canadians as foreigners, which says something in itself, and Canadians in fact make up the largest foreign population in the United States. At the same time, the United States is the largest foreign investor in Canada. By the beginning of 1982, for example, 80 percent of the total foreign direct investment in Canada came from

the United States, while 15 percent of total foreign direct investment in the United States came from Canada.

The United States and Canada are each other's major trade partners. Some 66 percent of Canada's exports go to the United States and 69 percent of its imports come from the United States. Similarly, 17 percent of all U.S. exports go to Canada, and 18 percent of U.S. imports come from Canada. Each year, nearly thirty-eight million Americans travel north and thirty-four million Canadians go south. A Canadian Parliament study in 1968 documents nearly 6,500 visits back and forth across the border by government officials from the two countries. Nearly two-thirds of Canada's bilateral relations are with the United States.

If Canada were located in South America or Africa, or most any other place, its power position might be enhanced significantly. Perhaps this notion was in the back of U.S. strategist Herman Kahn's mind when he said that Canada was "a regional power without a region."

While the close association with the United States has restricted Canada's power position, it also has in one sense enhanced it, because it has given Canadian decision makers an access to Washington that most other nations do not have, regardless of their power status. This access has enhanced Canada's leverage with other nations; after all, Ottawa seems to have Uncle Sam's ear, particularly on defense issues. The history of Canadian foreign relations reflects an awareness of Canada's special partnership with the United States, as well as an attempt to alter it.

Canada's current orientation toward the international environment, in the words of former prime minister Pierre Trudeau, "is not to imitate great powers by seeking to determine world events, but consists rather in building a just society at home that will serve as an inspiration to others while at the same time permitting Canada to make a distinctive international contribution on the basis of its values."[15] For Canada, that contribution lies primarily in the economic and social spheres. Canadian foreign policy pursues an independent role through developing new markets in the Far East and the Southern Hemisphere, emphasizing U.S.-Canadian dialogue, increasing aid to Third World countries, pushing for arms control at all levels, renewing interest in Latin America and the Caribbean Basin, and strengthening Canadian prestige as a northern or Arctic power.[16]

The election of Brian Mulroney as prime minister in September 1984 did not drastically change these objectives, though the approach is seen to be more cooperative with the United States than in the previous administration. The "third option" of the Trudeau era which called for a more independent role for Canada vis-a-vis the United States, has been set aside. Under the Progressive Conservatives, Canada has gone out of its way to redefine a new relationship with the United States. Even as early as 1982, the U.S. secretary of state began meeting at least four times a year with the Canadian minister of external affairs.

Since Mulroney came to office, these meetings have become institutionalized. Not only have the meetings shown the U.S. and Canadian publics that their leaders care and cooperate, they encourage the two nations' bureaucracies to work together to solve problems. As the Atlantic Council White Paper of 1986 pointed out, "The process has greatly diminished the use of public bullhorn diplomacy, in which some people engaged in the past, and has given quiet diplomacy a chance."[17] In the United States, the office of deputy assistant secretary for Canadian affairs has been reinstituted—Canada is the only nation in the world to be so recognized—and the Bureau of European Affairs has been renamed the Bureau of European and Canadian Affairs. As a result of comparable changes in the Canadian Ministry of External Affairs, cross-border, interagency coordination has improved.

In addition, as pointed out below, meetings of the U.S. president and the Canadian prime minister have become regular events. In short, Canada has made new overtures for cooperation with the United States, and the United States has been doing its homework on Canada in response to them. Underlying and highlighting the current focus of Canadian foreign policy are a Canadian Governmental report on future options; a series of successful summits;

and a reemphasis on Canadian national sovereignty, particularly in the Arctic.

Soon after becoming prime minister, Brian Mulroney directed a comprehensive foreign policy review. This review consisted of a "Green" (or discussion) paper to raise issues and present options, a parliamentary investigation and hearings based on the findings of the Green Paper and public reaction to it, and, based on these findings, a final report titled "Canada's International Relations: Response of the Government of Canada to the Report of the Special Committee of the Senate and the House of Commons" that was published in December 1986.[18] The Green Paper, which appeared in the spring of 1985, received wide circulation.[19] The paper pointed out that in an expanding, highly interdependent world, the international economic environment was changing in ways that put Canadian world competitiveness at risk. The level of debt in the developing world, changing trade and investment patterns, the growth of Soviet military power, and Third World conflicts all challenged Canada's place in the world. If Canada is to be economically secure, it must be internationally competitive.

To enhance Canada's competitive position, the paper maintained, the first priority was to address economic relations, particularly trade relations with the United States. Beyond that, Canada had to work to expand its multilateral economic system and enhance international economic development. While the thrust of the green paper's concern was with international economic issues, national security was not excluded. The paper reemphasized Canada's commitment to collective security and arms control, but raised a series of questions with respect to the direction of Canada's defense policy.

This Green Paper was essentially a draft blueprint of Canada's foreign policy. It set in motion the creation of a special joint committee of the Senate and House of Commons that from June 1985 through June 1986 conducted 61 public hearings across Canada and received briefs from over 500 organizations and more than 600 individuals. Based on this investigation, the special committee issued the report in

June 1986 titled "Independence and Internationalism." It contained 120 recommendations and culminated one of the most extensive analyses of Canadian foreign policy. The blueprint was finalized in the publication of the government's official response in December 1986 that addressed the committee's recommendations. However, even before publication of the 1986 report, Canada undertook efforts to initiate the trade negotiations with the United States that would form the centerpiece of the new foreign policy orientation. In April 1986 the U.S. Congress authorized the United States to enter into these negotiations. In 1988 the agreement on trade was finalized. Indeed, the new free trade agreement represented the broadest trade agreement ever negotiated by the two countries. Covering services as well as goods and investment, it included all major aspects of Canadian–U.S. trade.

No events better dramatize the character of the U.S.–Canadian relationship under the Progressive Conservatives, however, than the series of summit meetings between the two heads of state. The first, held in Quebec City, Quebec, Canada, on 17 March 1985, achieved a number of milestones. Dubbed the Shamrock Summit, since it was between two Irishmen, the meeting resulted in a declaration on trade, the appointment of high-level statesmen to deal with the very contentious issues of acid rain (an agreement on which was signed at the second summit in Washington in March 1986), the reaffirmation of the U.S.–Canadian defense economic relationship, an agreement on a West Coast salmon treaty, and a legal assistance treaty. More important than these specific agreements, however, the Shamrock Summit established a tenor for the future conduct of Canada's foreign policy that would overflow into other areas, particularly defense.

Another major theme of Mulroney's foreign policy, and one that put Canada at loggerheads with the United States, concerned Canadian sovereignty over the Arctic. As the map suggests, Canada is as much a circumpolar nation as a North American one. In fact, 40 percent of Canada's land mass, or 1.5 million square miles, is in the Canadian north. It is no surprise that many Canadians feel that Canada's destiny and the solution to its identity crisis are in the north, politically, socially, and economically. The Mulroney government has taken a number of initiatives toward developing an Arctic foreign policy for Canada.

The concern with the north and sovereignty over it dates from before Mulroney, however. National sovereignty was a major issue for the Trudeau administration. In 1970 Canada passed the Arctic Waters Pollution Prevention Act to exercise functional jurisdiction in the Arctic. The act demanded that nations navigating in these waters recognize Canada's responsibility for the welfare of inhabitants of the area, particularly the Inuit, or Eskimo, and for preservation of the ecological balance. Similar acts were passed in the early 1980s that extended Canada's jurisdiction over the area. At issue with the United States was the Northwest Passage, claimed by the United States as international waters, but claimed by Canada as part of its territory.

In August 1985 the sovereignty question became a public issue when the U.S. Coast Guard, having earlier consulted Ottawa, sailed the icebreaker *Polar Sea* through the Northwest Passage. The ship's passage created considerable furor in Canada. In response, Minister of External Affairs Joe Clark announced in Parliament a number of measures designed to protect and enforce Canada's claim to the north.[20]

The June 1986 Hockin-Simard Report, another name for the special joint committee report discussed above, called for the development of a "coherent Arctic policy." Its nine recommendations on this issue included: development of an Arctic policy; settlement of land claims and development of renewable resources in the north; increased funding for a Canada–USSR exchange program; the development of cooperative arrangements with all northern/Arctic states; special attention to be directed toward relations with Greenland; renewed efforts to get the United States to accept Canada's claim to the Northwest Passage; the submission of the dispute to the International Court of Justice; equipping the Maritime Command with diesel electric submarines; and the demilitarization of the Arctic region.[21]

Nine months later, the Mulroney government response pointed out that the government would accept many of the recommendations, but would modify some, and reject others, particularly the demilitarization of the Arctic. The government further set down a northern foreign policy based on four pillars: enhancement of Canadian Arctic sovereignty; continued modernization of Arctic defenses; further development of the commercial use of the Northwest Passage; and expansion of relations with other polar nations.[22] The issue between the U.S. and Canada over the Northwest Passage was partially resolved in January 1988 when the United States agreed to obtain Canadian consent before using the Arctic waters claimed by Canada; however, the U.S. maintained its position on unimpeded rights to transit.

The Mulroney foreign policy initiatives reflect the new international role and image that Canada would like to project. While this worldview does not reject the goals of the earlier Liberal government, it is one, unlike Trudeau's, that looks more to the north and significantly includes the United States. Both emphases have an impact on the content and structure of Canadian defense policy.

In 1971 a Canadian Defence White Paper described "the only direct external threat to Canada's military security today" as "that of a large-scale nuclear attack on North America."[23] This perception has not changed. The 1987 Defence White Paper repeated the warning: "The principal direct threat to Canada continues to be a nuclear attack on North America by the Soviet Union." This most recent Defence White Paper, the first in sixteen years, expands on the nature of the threat as seen in Canada. It states:

Canadian security policy must respond to an international environment dominated by the rivalry between East and West. These two groups of nations, each led by a superpower, are in conflict—a conflict of ideas and values. . . . It is a fact, not a matter of interpretation, that the West is faced with an ideological, political, and economic adversary whose explicit long-term aim is to mould the world in its own image. . . . This does not mean that war with the Soviet Union is inevitable or that mutually beneficial arrangements should not be pursued. It does mean that unless and until there is concrete progress, the West has no choice but to rely for

its security on the maintenance of a rough balance of forces, backed up by nuclear deterrence.[24]

The greatest divergence between U.S. and Canadian threat perspectives concerns the Third World. While the United States attributes Third World instability to communism and insurgency, Canada attributes it more to poverty and economic underdevelopment.

Until the mid 1950s, geography made Canada nearly immune to invasion. Today, as former prime minister John Diefenbaker put it in a speech to the House of Commons, "Under the irresistible dictates of geography, the defence of North America has become a joint enterprise of both Canada and the United States."[25] Intercontinental nuclear missiles have reduced the two nations to a single target area.

In the Canadian threat calculus, Western Europe has an indispensable role for, as one senior Canadian embassy official in Washington commented, "What would North American defence be if there were no NATO? It would be quite different."[26] Leo Cadieux, former Canadian Minister of Defense, speaking in the House of Commons in December 1968, explained the NATO link this way:

The major threat to the security of Canada and the Canadian people comes from the prospect of an inter-continental nuclear exchange arising out of a conflict of interest or of ideology between the superpowers. The forum where the superpowers' interests most clearly impinge on each other is Europe and hence Europe is the geographic region where Canada's security is most in jeopardy. Thus Canada's security is very closely interlocked with the security of Europe. These are inescapable facts of the world we live in.[27]

On the one hand, Western Europe is the first line of defense for Canada. On the other hand, the ability to defend Canada and the United States enhances the credibility of allied forces to deter attack in Europe. A look at Canada's position on map 2 indicates the importance of geography in defining the threat to Canadian security.

Today, Canadian defense documents describing the strategic environment emphasize an unstable world and continuous erosion of the strategic position and power base of the West. The threat to Canadian security is described in three dimensions: East-West relations; instability in the Third World; and intra-Western and domestic affairs.[28]

The Soviet threat is described in the 1987 White Paper to include not only land-based intercontinental ballistic missiles (ICBMs) but also Soviet bombers carrying air-launched cruise missiles (ALCMs), Soviet submarines penetrating through the Arctic carrying sea-launched cruise missiles (SLCMs), and future space-based threats.

In respect to the second dimension, Canadian strategic thinkers argue that instability in the Third World will become increasingly more important to the national security of the West: "Economic, social, and political frustrations are mounting and, combined with national rivalries, will provide fertile ground for local conflicts detrimental to Western interests."[29]

At the same time, Canadian defense planners warn that economic difficulties within both the Western democracies and the international economic system will tend to exacerbate problems with intra-Western and domestic affairs. These economic difficulties, particularly as they relate to energy, will have an adverse impact on the ability of Canada and other Western nations to defend themselves. Moreover, these Canadian planners point out:

Terrorism has become a worldwide scourge which, although unlikely to threaten the survival of advanced Western democracies, will continue to put at risk both their publics and the exposed vital points of their infrastructures. Terrorism represents a threat also to their ability to maintain law and order without compromising individual freedoms and social well-being.[30]

Canada, in short, does not consider itself immune to the terrorist threat. Joe Clark, Canada's current secretary of state for external affairs, has summarized Canada's world view and place in the international system quite well. He said:

We are respected on the international scene for our faithfulness to moral principles such as the right of peoples to independence and the defence of human rights and of individual and religious freedoms. Our influence is a result of our tolerance, our diversity, and our traditions.

Canada's power stems from its political stability and its economic strength. We have never been an imperial power and we do not seek to impose domination on any part of the world. We are well thought of in the Third World. Our presence in many international organiza-

tions reinforces our ability to influence the course of events.[31]

National Objectives, National Strategy, and Military Doctrine

The history of U.S.–Canadian defense relations in the twentieth century charts a movement from isolationism to interdependence in which both nations abandoned plans to protect only their own borders and adopted realistic attitudes toward collective self-defense. Today, Canadian defense policy is still guided by the commitment to collective self-defense. Brian Mulroney put it best when he wrote: "For Canada, this quest continues to be best pursued through cooperation with our allies. This is a recognition of our common history, our shared interests and our community of values. This unity of purpose is the very foundation of our Alliance, as important to our security as the concrete efforts we undertake to keep the peace."[32]

Though Canada's goal of collective self-defense has remained constant since World War II, two broad periods can be differentiated in the evolution of its defense policy: the era of defense cooperation and convergence of U.S. and Canadian policy (1940–64) and the era of independence and divergence in the two nations' policies (1965–present). However, the election of Mulroney in 1984 and the publication of the Defence White Paper in June 1987 signal a significant variation in the thrust of this second period. While Canadian defense policy has continued to search for an independent role under the Progressive Conservative prime minister, it has also tried increasingly to accommodate U.S. defense policy interests.

CONVERGENCE

The first historical period was marked by the initiation and enhancement of defense cooperation between the two nations. This is the period that Melvin Conant has called the "time of the great compact." It begins with the Ogdensburg and Hyde Park declarations of 1940 and 1941 respectively and includes the establishment of a joint defense plan for North

America during World War II, the creation of NATO, the establishment of the North American Air Defense Command, and the creation and expansion of a defense economic relationship that some have called the North American common defense market.

It had been through the cataclysmic struggle of World War II that Canadians and Americans alike realized that the security of their respective nations and the Western Hemisphere was a mutual problem requiring joint efforts.

That realization gained its first official expression in the Ogdensburg Declaration of 18 August 1940. Originally no more than an unsigned press release on a meeting between Canadian Prime Minister Mackenzie King and President Franklin Roosevelt held at Ogdensburg, New York, the previous day, the declaration has since become "the spirit under which virtually all other security treaties, executive agreements, various understandings, and cooperation relative to or affecting North American security are authorized."[33]

Eight months later, on 21 April 1941, after another meeting, this one at Hyde Park, King and Roosevelt issued a corresponding statement on defense-economic cooperation. The product of these two informal meetings and the accompanying, equally informal, announcements that followed are the foundation for the defense cooperation effort between Canada and the United States that has significantly shaped the nature of Canadian defense policy ever since.

The U.S.–Canadian contributions of 1940–45 were vital for the successful prosecution of the war and laid the foundation for joint defense planning and implementation that continued in the following years. Even more important to establishing a North American defense unit, the war had created within the publics of both the United States and Canada the realization that in matters of defense, the common border joined, rather than separated, their two nations; never again could either nation pursue entirely independent defense policies.

As Soviet political ambitions and the menace arising from them became clearer (highlighted for the Canadian public by the revelation of a Soviet espionage operation in Ottawa), and the realities of a new type of warfare were assimilated (highlighted for the publics of both nations by the Soviet detonation of an atomic device in 1949 and the USSR's development of a sophisticated long-range delivery system a year earlier), the joint defense planning effort shifted to arrangements in the far north. The realization of this new Soviet threat, reinforced by events in Korea in 1950, resulted in the creation of what Samuel Huntington has called a "continental defense system." This system was composed of early warning radar nets—Distant Early Warning Line (DEW), the Mid-Canada Line, and the Pinetree Line—constructed between 1952 and 1958; the North American Air Defense Command (NORAD) established in 1957; the defense production and development sharing agreements (a defense-economic arrangement that evolved between 1958 and 1963); and nearly two hundred other bilateral defense agreements.

In sum, the first twenty-five years of the defense relationship were a remarkably fruitful period. By the beginning of 1964, the U.S.–Canadian defense alliance had grown to a size and complexity unimagined at its inception in 1940. However, this growth would not continue into the latter years of the decade. The concept of a continental defense system would not be challenged, but the orientation would change. This resulted essentially from the fact that the high degree of convergence between the U.S. and Canadian defense policies found during the first period began to break down. Divergence was the result of the evident inability of the Canadian government to accommodate the changes in the North American defense relationship demanded by the new U.S. strategy of flexible response, a strategy designed to meet a new type of Soviet threat.

INDEPENDENCE AND DIVERGENCE

By 1964 the nature of the Soviet strategic threat had changed from bombers to missiles. The Soviet bomber threat projected for the 1950s never materialized, as the Kremlin elected to develop intercontinental missiles as its primary strategic offensive force. In the

1960 U.S. presidential election, in fact, the issue was an alleged missile gap. At the same time the wholesale creation from former European colonies of newly independent nations, to become known collectively as the Third World, set the stage for a type of warfare in which a nuclear arsenal had no rational place. The possibility of guerrilla warfare and of conventional forces fighting limited wars with non-nuclear weaponry began to dominate U.S. defense thinking. The realization that the North American continental defense system developed in the 1950s was irrelevant against the threat of Soviet missiles and equally irrelevant when the values and institutions of the North American continent were to be defended, not in the aerospace over the continent, but in "wars of national liberation" somewhere in the developing world, resulted in the development of a new U.S. defense strategy called flexible response. Although not opposed to the strategy, the Canadians objected to being directed by Washington to change their defense policy to meet that strategy, particularly when such changes resulted in altering Canada's national priorities. Critics argued that Washington, not Ottawa, was making Canadian policy.

The immediate result was the Defence White Paper of 1964, which, surprisingly, proved not to be the statement of an independent defense policy that it reportedly was designed to be. But it did mark the beginning of a period of growing divergence in the history of North American defense. The Canadian search for a defense policy not made in Washington can be divided into three distinct periods, each delineated by a Defence White Paper (1964, 1971 and 1987), under two Liberal administrations—those of Lester Pearson and Pierre Elliott Trudeau—and one Progressive Conservative, Brian Mulroney.

During the first period, a uniquely Canadian defense was sought by emphasizing international interdependence through the performance of peacekeeping missions for the United Nations. It was not very successful.

During the second period, the focus switched to national independence with missions emphasizing Canadian sovereignty. This was more successful and continues today as the

basic rationale for Canada's defense policy. However, the election of Brian Mulroney in 1984 ushered in a third period. The Progressive Conservative prime minister sought to reestablish closer ties with the United States and rebuild the Canadian defense capability, both in support of the national sovereignty role but also in terms of the NORAD and NATO commitments. One of the original results of the Trudeau quest for an independent defense policy was a marked decrease in the military capability of Canadian forces. For example, a significant reduction in manpower was seen, from a peak force in 1963 of 123,000 to 78,000 by 1975. The 1987 Defence White Paper outlined a dramatic effort to reverse this trend.

The 1964 Defence White Paper was strongly influenced by Prime Minister Pearson, who in 1965 also was the architect of the UN peacekeeping force in the Middle East. Pearson asserted that, since the most likely threat to Canadian and North American security would come not from an all-out thermonuclear war in Europe, but from low-level conflict within the developing world, Canada must develop a conventional, mobile, flexible force capable of responding to such conflicts as part of the UN peacekeeping forces. Ironically, however, the 1964 White Paper did not reduce Canada's commitment to NORAD and NATO. It did produce ambivalence. On the one hand, it suggested the need for a new, more independent policy for Canada, directed toward the UN peacekeeping mission, and called for the creation of flexible forces to meet this requirement. However, at the same time, it advocated the maintenance of the existing commitments to both NORAD and NATO, all this at lowered levels of real expenditure.

The ambivalence was short-lived. As early as 1965, the Pearson administration's perceptions of NATO were changing in the light of the French military withdrawal from the organization. Changing also was the attitude toward peacekeeping as a result of the UN Congo operation. The Pearson administration was faced with a dilemma. On the one hand, defense systems acquired at great expense during the period of convergence were becoming obsolete. On the other, the kinds of forces required to fulfill UN requirements set down in the 1964 Defence White Paper were essentially nonexistent.

The dilemma was compounded by a sagging defense budget. During the five years of the Pearson administration, as the result of extensive social programs and inflation, defense appropriations fell from 23.7 to 16.8 percent of the budget and from 4.5 to 2.8 percent of GNP, and the projected savings from the 1968 reorganization of the Canadian forces failed to materialize. The result was a gradual decay in Canada's ability to support its NORAD and NATO missions. In this sense, the Defence White Paper resulted in a defense role for Canada that was neither new nor independent. On the contrary, Canada's role in the defense of North America began to lose credibility if not viability. Pearson's successor would attempt to remedy that by reducing overseas commitments by giving Canadian foreign and defense policies a "Made in Canada" label. These efforts, however, would disrupt the defense consensus between the United States and Canada.

When Pierre Trudeau became prime minister in 1968, few doubted that there would be a significant change in the government's orientation to foreign and defense policies, but no one envisioned the extent of that change. Earlier, drawing a lesson from the expulsion of the UN Emergency Force (UNEF) from Egyptian territory in spring 1967, Trudeau had rejected the thrust of the 1964 White Paper toward peacekeeping and embraced the view that the concern of Canada's defense and foreign policies should be first and foremost Canada and Canadian sovereignty. As a result, the new administration's first act was to order a major review of those policies.

That review, the conclusions of which were reported in the Defence White Paper of 1971, established a new priority for Canada's defense efforts. Peacekeeping was deemphasized, and first priority was again given to the national sovereignty mission. Above all, Trudeau wanted to assure that defense priorities were responsive to Canadian national interests and international developments affecting Canada, not necessarily to the dictates of Washington. The white paper identified four major roles for the Canadian forces: (1) surveillance of Canadian territory and coastlines; (2) defense of North America in cooperation with US forces; (3) fulfillment of agreed-upon NATO commitments; and (4) performance of such international peacekeeping roles as would be found significant. Although Canada thus remained committed to the continuance of the North American defense system and to its modernization, that commitment would not include Canadian involvement in any active missile defense system. The area in which Trudeau's defense policy diverged most from the stated U.S. defense policy of flexible response, however, was NATO.

On 3 April 1969 Trudeau exploded an alliance bombshell by announcing that, although Canada was not withdrawing from the organization and in fact wanted to reaffirm its commitment, it would begin a phased reduction of its NATO forces. Plans were announced for reducing the NATO contingent by 50 percent and identifying a non-nuclear role for the remainder. The defense budget was frozen for three years at C$1.8 billion.

The net result of these reductions was a decrease in the defense capability of Canada—manpower, equipment, money—to support both the NATO and the NORAD missions.

When Brian Mulroney became prime minister of Canada in 1984, one of his top priorities was to address these defense deficiencies. In fact, one of the first actions he took was to send 1,200 troops to Europe to bolster the NATO commitment. However, the initial move to enhance defense had begun before his watch and dates back to a speech in 1975 by James Richardson, then Canadian minister of defense, which indicated that a reevaluation of the defense contribution was under way.[34] The downward trend in defense spending had been reversed with the announcement that major new pieces of equipment would be purchased, including a new fleet of long-range patrol aircraft (LPRA). Defence Minister Richardson observed:

In this fiscal year, 1974–75, the Defence Department will spend approximately $2.5 billion. This is more than $275 million above that appropriated for the previous fiscal year. For next year, 1975–76, the Government will again increase defence appropriations by almost $300 million. This increase in the Defence budget is larger, by itself, than the whole budget of many federal departments. It amounts to about a 12 percent increase and it picks up almost all anticipated inflation. The estimates that we will be submitting to Parliament shortly will indicate a record peacetime defence budget of some $2 billion 800 million.

This substantial increase in the National Defence Budget means that we will be able to maintain the Force at approximately its present strength.

Of particular importance to the achievement of increased military capability, the decision to increase the Defence budget also means that we will be able to proceed with a rational reequipment program.[35]

Three factors in 1975 precipitated the change in defense orientation. The first was considerable criticism of Trudeau's defense policy in the Canadian press and within NATO. The second was a suggestion by U.S. Secretary of Defense James Schlesinger, in a press conference on 16 September 1975, that Canada should assign NATO greater priority than NORAD. Schlesinger stated that he preferred that Canada continue a mix of land and air forces in Europe. The diminished bomber threat meant that the Allies needed tanks to help NATO meet the formidable Warsaw Pact tank threat to West Germany rather than new interceptor aircraft.

The last catalyst for the 1975 change was the Defence Structure Review (DSR) by the Canadian Ministry of Defence, begun in November 1974 in combination with the U.S. Department of Defense's decision, in the same year, to structure its North American air defense force primarily for peacetime surveillance and control, and consequently to reduce the role of manned interceptors and active air defense. These three factors have produced a current Canadian orientation toward defense that suggests agreement with the United States that Canada's contribution to NATO is a vital part of the Western deterrent, that it must be increased, and further, that the time has come to restore to the Canadian armed forces a capability to fight.

When the Progressive Conservative government of Brian Mulroney was elected with an overwhelming majority on 4 September 1984, a new chapter in Canadian defense policy was apparently about to be written. Mulroney and his party had campaigned on a platform that

was highly critical of Pierre Trudeau and the Liberal Party for having let defense "run down." This platform called for both increased spending on defense and a new review of Canada's defense policy. Mulroney promised that, if elected, his government would issue a new White Paper on defense, and he called for a 6 percent a year increase for five years in the defense budget.

In fact, by mid 1985 a confluence of six factors, including the election of Mulroney, had brought Canadian defense policy and the entire defense relationship between the United States and Canada to a crossroads. The five other factors were:

1. The new U.S. emphasis on strategic defense, first reflected in President Reagan's strategic modernization plan, announced in October 1981, and subsequently in the U.S. Air Force's Air Defense Master Plan and the Joint U.S.–Canadian Agreement on Air Defense. In 1984–85, this master plan became the first phase of a new long-range plan for the strategic defense of North America, called Strategic Defense Architecture (SDA) 2000. The first phase addressed shortcomings in the original master plan—specifically, the threat of cruise missiles, particularly sea-launched cruise missiles (SLCMs). Whereas the SDA 2000 Phase One dealt only with air defense, the second phase dealt with air, space, and missile defense and their integration. Associated with this new U.S. emphasis on strategic defense was the activation of the U.S. Unified Space Command on 23 September 1985.

2. The announcement by President Reagan in March 1983 of the U.S. intention to explore new technologies to determine if an effective defense against intercontinental ballistic missiles (ICBMs) was possible. This presidential address created the Strategic Defense Initiative (SDI), also called "Star Wars."

3. A renewed atmosphere of congeniality and mutual respect between the two nations (discussed above), reflected in the annual Shamrock Summits beginning in March 1985 between President Reagan and Prime Minister Mulroney.

4. A significant transformation in the na-

ture of the Soviet threat to North America. Canada's contribution to North American defense had been vital during the 1950s, when the major threat to the continent was from Russian bombers. In the 1960s and 1970s, with the development of ICBMs and SLBMs, the bomber threat receded, and the Canadian contribution to defense became less important, but it now reemerged in the form of the new Soviet Backfire, Blackjack, and Bear H bombers and air- and sea-launched cruise missiles. For the first time in twenty years, North America was seen as vulnerable to an air attack. If it were to respond to that threat, Canada's help would be needed.

5. Shifts in doctrine and demography within NATO. On the one hand, France had begun reducing its land forces. On the other hand, Germany, which has provided over half of NATO's central front land forces—and which has had an active force of 495,000—was finding increasing difficulty manning to that level because of the smaller number of draft-eligible men.[36] In fact, available manpower in West Germany might be cut in half by the end of this century. By 1985 the Bundeswehr had decreased to 478,000.[37] At the same time that a manpower shortfall was seen in Europe because of downward population trends, NATO was calling for an increased emphasis on conventional forces and advocating conventional war-fighting doctrines, like the follow-on forces attack (FOFA). The signing of an arms control agreement in late 1987 to eliminate Intermediate Range Nuclear Forces (INF) in Europe also has had an impact on the NATO allies' conventional commitment. In short, these changes have generated requirements for new air defense systems and overall enhancement of NATO's conventional forces. Canada is expected to contribute its fair share to meeting these requirements.

Singly and jointly, these five factors have created a need for Canada to reemphasize, if not restructure, its defense policy. At present, the ball is clearly in the Canadian court, for these factors create a "window of opportunity" for Canada to increase the level of its defense effort and redefine its defense policy. No guaran-

tee exists that this window will remain open indefinitely. A change in government in either nation could bring to office an administration less disposed to strategic defense or less willing to work with the other government. U.S.–Canadian relations, particularly in the trade area, could cool. Certainly, President Bush's commitment to the level of defense spending, the SDI program, or the defensive strategy that SDI suggests is different from that of his predecessor. The Bush defense budgets are significantly below those of the Reagan presidency. Similarly, the Canadian government's announcement of major reductions in the FY90 defense budget undercuts the major acquisition programs of the 1987 White Paper.

In addition, the nature of the Soviet threat could change again. At present, Canadian participation, if not territory, is required for surveillance, warning, and attack assessment. However, in the future if SDI proves technologically feasible, such tasks could easily, and perhaps more effectively and efficiently, be performed from space-based platforms, negating the need for Canadian territory or participation, especially if Canada continues its current policy of no involvement in missile or space defense.

Reduced need or desire for Canadian participation in North American defense would result, in all probability, in a further reduction in Canadian defense capability and with it in potential economic benefits to Canadian industry derived from new technologies and offsets that would accompany an expanding defense program.

The most significant initiative the Mulroney government has taken to enhance Canada's defense capability was the tabling in Parliament of a new defense White Paper in June 1987. But this broke no new ground in terms of Canada's overall defense policy. It noted:

Since coming to office, the Government has reviewed our defence effort. This review has confirmed that Canadian defence policy, as it has evolved since the Second World War, is essentially sound. That policy will continue to be based on a strategy of collective security within the framework of the North Atlantic Alliance including the continental defence partnership with the United States. Canada will continue to support that strategy through military contributions in North America, in Western Europe, and at sea.[38]

The emphasis on national sovereignty and the search for an independent Canadian role that distinguished the 1971 White Paper were also underlined in the 1987 paper. In the introduction, the prime minister writes:

But just as the Alliance can only prosper through shared effort and a common impulse, so too Canada must look to itself to safeguard its sovereignty and pursue its own interests. Only we as a nation should decide what must be done to protect our shores, our waters and our airspace. This White Paper, therefore, takes as its first priority the protection and furtherance of Canada's sovereignty as a nation.[39]

The minister of defence called the White Paper a "made in Canada defence policy," to be implemented over a 15-year period. In fact, if there is a distinct theme to this paper, it is the idea of a northern foreign policy and the emphasis on the Arctic, and on Canada as a maritime nation requiring a three-ocean navy: "Canadian naval forces must be able to respond to challenges within our own waters, if necessary, denying their use to an enemy. We must also contribute to the collective maritime strength of the Alliance."[40]

The distinctiveness of the 1987 White Paper is in four areas: the delineation of a naval program to give Canada a three-ocean navy capability and the ability to maintain Canadian Arctic sovereignty; the consolidation of the Canadian European commitment and cancellation of the commitment to Norway; the revitalization of the reserves; and, finally, the implementation of an extensive reequipment program to narrow the so-called commitment-capability gap and prevent "rust-out."[41] To achieve these objectives, the White Paper outlines the following tasks:

To Create a Three-Ocean Navy, by: building six new frigates in addition to the six currently under construction and the four destroyers being modernized; acquiring a fleet of 10–12 nuclear-powered submarines to operate in the Atlantic, the Pacific and the Arctic; installing a modern, fixed, under-ice surveillance system in the Arctic; developing new sonar systems and acquiring detection array towing vessels for better underwater surveillance; building minesweepers for the Naval Reserve; and acquiring new shipborne anti-submarine warfare helicopters.

To Reinforce Surveillance, by: purchasing at least six new long-range patrol aircraft; modernizing the existing fleet of medium-range patrol aircraft; maintaining the strength of the CF-18 aircraft and arming them effectively; promoting research, development and deploy-

ment of space surveillance systems; and investigating the installation of synthetic aperture radar in existing aircraft.

To Strengthen Territorial Defence, by: expanding the Canadian Rangers, improving their equipment, training and support; creating new Militia brigades which, together with the Special Service Force and the Canadian Airborne Regiment, will form a new task force; providing new equipment and training for territorial defence; creating within the Militia a military vital point guard to secure key installations across the country; establishing a northern training centre in the High Arctic; and setting up a regional command structure.

To Improve the Credibility of the Canadian Contribution to Alliance Deterrence in Europe, by: cancelling the unsustainable commitment to send a brigade group and two fighter squadrons to northern Norway in order to consolidate commitments on the central front into land and air divisions; prepositioning equipment and supplies for the Canada-based brigade group (5 GBC) which in time of crisis will join the brigade group permanently stationed in southern Germany (4 CMBG); pre-positioning equipment and supplies for the AMF(L) Battalion Group assigned in time of crisis to Northern European Command; re-equipping armoured regiments with new main battle tanks; assuring sustainment of the new army division by 1 Canadian Brigade Group and the new Militia brigades; increasing the personnel strength in Europe to provide land and air Divisional elements and larger logistics and medical support cadres; and providing additional airlift capability.

To Revitalize the Reserves, by: introducing a Total Force Concept, reducing the distinction between the Regular and Reserve forces; assigning the Reserves specific wartime tasks; improving the quality and quantity of training and equipment; increasing the Reserves to 90,000 personnel over time; investigating reactivation of university Reserve officer training programs; and improving Reserve pay and benefits.

To Build a Firmer Foundation for Future Defence, by: providing equitable opportunities in both official languages in the Canadian Forces and the Department of National Defence; expanding the role of women in the Canadian Forces; ensuring that the composition of the Regular and Reserve Forces more adequately reflects the ethnic diversity of Canadian society; strengthening defence industrial preparedness; enhancing the contribution of the Canadian Forces to foreign disaster and humanitarian relief; broadening and extending the Military and Strategic Studies program; replacing the *War Measures Act* with new emergencies legislation; and introducing legislation to establish Emergency Preparedness Canada, the agency responsible for coordinating the civil aspects of Government-wide mobilization planning.[42]

Outside of the usual opposition of the New Democratic Party to Canadian involvement in NATO and NORAD, the White Paper was generally well received. The only really contentious issue was the decision to purchase the nuclear submarines rather than alternative naval enhancements such as additional frigates. For example, a *Toronto Star* editorial called the paper, "a thoughtful but cautious document" and agreed with the decision "to drop Canada's NATO commitment . . . to Norway." Similarly the *Globe* and *Mail* stated, "On the principle, if not necessarily all the details, of Canadian rearmament, the White Paper has scored a solid hit." However, the paper called for the acquisition of cheaper, diesel-powered submarines.[43]

The attitude of the United States, while clearly supportive, has essentially been to wait and see how Canada handles the really critical issue—funding. The estimated 15-year cost of the programs listed above is approximately C$180 billion. To pay this bill, the White Paper calls for an annual increase of 2 percent above inflation beginning with the FY 1987/88 budget baseline or C$10.8 billion. This 2 percent figure, however, (the result of political compromise in the cabinet) is a floor rather than a ceiling, for the amount will provide only annual operating costs and modest capital equipment expenditures. To cover the costs of the really big ticket items, like additional frigates and submarines, which would require a 4 to 5 percent a year increase, the White Paper prescribes a rolling five-year funding plan. Each September the cabinet will conduct an annual review of defense expenditures over the next four years to assess how much the annual budget will need to be increased over and above the 2 percent to pay for particular systems coming due in that time frame. The issue is whether Canada will sustain this level of funding over the entire fifteen years, particularly in light of domestic political pressure to reduce the deficit and curtail inflation. The reelection of Prime Minister Mulroney on 21 November 1988 seemed to insure the same level of defense effort. Publication of the FY90 budget in April 1989, however, revealed significant defense cutbacks to include cancellation of the acquisition of a fleet of nuclear-powered submarines, suggesting that the future of the Mulroney defense enhancements is uncertain. A Conservative Party defeat in the next election could also alter the White Paper plan.

Uncertainty about the success of the acquisi-

tion program detailed in the White Paper should not detract, however, from an impressive list of other defense initiatives undertaken by the Mulroney government prior to the publication of that paper. These included:

1. An increase of 1,200 to reinforce the 4th Canadian Mechanized Brigade (4CMBG) in Germany, which was less than 60 percent manned, well below the 90 percent NATO standard. At the same time, the Canadian Government had agreed to increase the Canadian armed forces to more than 90,000 by the end of the decade. At the end of 1986, Canadian regular forces numbered 86,536.

2. An early effort to eliminate double tasking, whereby the same contingent of Canadian forces tasked to be part of the battalion group for the Allied Command Europe Mobile Force Land was also tasked to be part of the Canadian Air Sea Transportable (CAST) brigade designated for deployment to Norway. In addition, the first major CAST exercise, Brave Lion, with an actual deployment to Norway, was planned and executed in 1986. This exercise demonstrated that Canada could not meet its CAST commitment and led to the recommendation in the White Paper to end it.

3. A commitment to the capital acquisition program begun in 1975 was reflected in the 1985 and 1986 decisions to purchase six new frigates and a low-level air defense system to be deployed with the Canadian forces in Europe. At present, these forces lack any air defense capability, a significant shortcoming among NATO land forces.

4. Expansion of Canada's role as a major center for testing and evaluating weapons systems and training NATO forces. The Mulroney government supported the U.S.–Canadian Test and Evaluation Agreement signed by the Trudeau government in February 1983. Under this agreement, Canada has permitted the United States to test three major weapons systems on or over Canadian territory: the low-altitude navigation and targeting infrared for night (LANTIRN) system (tested in October-December 1983); the U.S. Marine Corps' Harrier aircraft (tested in October 1984); and the

U.S. Air Force's ALCM.[44] The latter test program, which has been particularly controversial in Canada, continues.

The agreement, valid for five years, can be terminated with twelve months' notice by either government; in 1988, it was automatically renewed for another five years. Under the agreement, each year in January, the United States submits an annual forecast of projects that it wishes to conduct in Canada during the following thirty months to Canada for approval. The program has been a major success, enabling the United States to test systems under conditions these systems would face in actual combat operations.

5. Similarly, Canada attempted to persuade NATO to establish an integrated tactical fighter training facility at its World War II-vintage base at Goose Bay, Labrador. In February 1986 Canada signed a multinational Memorandum of Understanding (MOU) governing allied military activity at the base. The purpose of the MOU was to standardize procedures and administration of the various flying operations conducted at the base by West German, British, and U.S. air forces by designating the Canadian Department of National Defence the executive agency for managing all allied training in Canada.

Prior to this MOU, only a series of bilateral agreements were in effect between each of these nations and a variety of Canadian federal agencies. Effective in April 1986, the agreement is for ten years, with the signatories paying all costs associated with their training programs, but sharing costs associated with common services and infrastructure. The Canadian government also made overtures to Spain and Australia to move some of their training operations to Canada.

6. Most significant is Canadian participation in the program to modernize North America's air defenses. A major part of this program is the NWS Agreement designed to upgrade the outdated DEW Line radar sites. The cost of the C$1.5 billion northern warning system will be split, with Canada paying 40 percent and the United States 60 percent. The new system consists of a chain of fifty-two ground radar stations across northern Alaska, the Canadian Arctic, and the Labrador coast. Eleven of the thirteen long-range manned radars will be on Canadian territory, as will thirty-six of the thirty-nine unmanned short-range radars. Canada, which will have complete control over its new radar stations, will be responsible for the overall management and systems integration of the project. Canada also will be responsible for the design, acquisition, and installation of the communications network in Canada, design and construction of all new facilities in Canada, and operation and maintenance of the Canadian sites.

The NWS agreement is part of an overall upgrade program, to include new OTH-B radars along the east and west coasts of the United States and closing down the obsolete Continental Air Defense Integration, North (CADIN)-Pinetree Line in Canada. Overall cost of the modernization effort is C$7 billion, of which Canada will share the cost of shutting down the CADIN-Pinetree site, and the United States will pay 55 percent of the cost of assisting communities affected by the closings.

Under the modernization plan, Canadian crews are expected to man AWACS aircraft and OTH-B sites that cover Canadian territory jointly. In addition, Canada is planning, on a temporary basis, to base CF-18s at forward operating locations (FOLs) in the far north. The plan is to station up to six aircraft at airfields around Whitehorse, Yellowknife, and Frobisher Bay. Support equipment would be brought in for exercises and for deployment in times of increased tensions. The aircraft would not be permanently assigned to these sites, but would be moved there to enhance the air surveillance and defensive role when international conditions dictated. Further, the plan calls for the construction of dispersed operating bases (DOBs) for AWACS aircraft in Canada.

In 1987, the United States and Canada signed six agreements that implemented this air defense modernization plan. These included: 1) an agreement by which the United States will contribute half of the $180 million U.S. required to construct five fighter and three AWACS FOL bases in Canada on which

Canadian firms will do all construction; (2) an agreement to implement the 60/40 percent U.S.-Canada cost-sharing formula on the NWS and to transfer its management to Canada; (3) an agreement whereby Canada will contribute 20 percent of the manpower to the OTH-B radar program and in return receive data on a real-time basis; (4) an agreement to permit two Canadian aircrews to fly on board US AWACS aircraft; (5) an agreement recognizing the 55/45 percent cost sharing formula to pay the $65 million bill to close the seventeen obsolete CADIN-Pinetree radars; and (6) a cost sharing reconcilitation agreement to deal with accounting procedures.

7. Reaffirmation of the U.S.-Canadian Defense Production and Development Sharing Agreements. At the Shamrock Summit of 1985, both nations agreed to strengthen the North American defense-industrial base, reduce trade barriers, improve joint access to information relating to defense procurement, facilitate a freer exchange of technical knowledge, and establish procedures to control the transfer of technology to potential adversaries. The two nations further agreed to periodic progress reports on the status of the agreements and the effort to enhance them.

The first report was completed in September 1985. Among major accomplishments listed, the most important was a MOU that addressed the exchange of technical information to facilitate access for qualified contractors of each country on an equally favorable basis to unclassified data and procedures to safeguard information exchanged. Commitment to the agreements was restated and emphasized in the SCEAND Report on NORAD and by President Reagan and Prime Minister Mulroney at the summit in Washington in March 1986.

New efforts have been made on both sides of the border to increase defense-economic cooperation. Just one example is the creation in November 1985 of the Canadian-U.S. Aerospace Defense Advanced Technology (ADAT) Working Group. The purpose of the ADAT group is to implement the MOU signed at the Shamrock Summit. The group has become an important player in the U.S. Air Defense Initia-

tive (ADI), which includes Canadian participation to develop new air defense technologies, including space systems. One such system is Teal Ruby, a space-based infrared satellite to detect and track bombers. In 1987 alone, the Sharing Agreements' Steering Committee worked on more than eighty projects entailing joint development.

8. Renewal of the NORAD Agreement. The 1986 SCEAND Report on North American defense had recommended the following actions: that the NORAD agreement be renewed for five years; that Canada increase its defense spending from 2.1 percent of GNP to 3.8 percent; that no clause prescribing Canadian non-involvement in an ABM system be included (this clause, which had been inserted in the 1968 renewal, was removed in the 1981 renewal); that Canada and the United States increase their naval cooperation in patrolling the Arctic Ocean; that Canada create a national space agency and undertake a military space program; and that Canada purchase AWACS aircraft and take part in SDA 2000, Phase 2.

On 21 March 1986 the agreement was renewed for five years without the ABM clause. The United States had been opposed to reinserting the ABM clause, arguing that the Ballistic Missile Defense (BMD) clause in the NORAD agreement would be redundant, since the United States was already bound by the ABM treaty. Further, the U.S. government argued that to include the clause would imply a lack of commitment to the ABM treaty. The Canadian concern with the ABM clause was addressed in press statements following the signing of the agreement, in which President Reagan and Prime Minister Mulroney both pointed out that the NORAD agreement was fully consistent with provisions of the ABM treaty.

The above initiatives undertaken by the Canadian government clearly support Mulroney's claim that his administration wants to enhance defense. Added to this list could be the reorganization of the cabinet committee decision-making process that for the first time puts the minister of defence on the all-important Priorities and Planning Committee. Nevertheless, the Canadian government has fallen short in two areas.

First and most important, though promised in the 1987 Defence White Paper, the government has yet to increase defense spending significantly. In fact, in the budget tabled in May 1985, the Progressive Conservatives proposed spending less on defense than their Liberal predecessors had planned to spend. Similarly, in February 1987, the Canadian finance minister cut the defense budget by C$200 million, which, in effect, eliminated the 2 percent increase in 1987. The bottom line, despite the rhetoric, is that defense spending remains at about 2.1 percent of GNP. The problem, of course, is the Canadian economy, particularly the inflation and the unemployment rates.

Second, Mulroney announced in September 1985 that the Canadian government would not favor a government-to-government effort in support of SDI. He did leave the door open for private companies and institutions to participate, however, and supported the concept behind SDI, stating that his government believes that SDI research by the United States is both consistent with the ABM treaty and prudent in light of significant advances in Soviet research and deployment of the world's only existing ballistic missile defense system.[45]

Canada's defense strategy today is the product of the nearly fifty-year history traced above. During the first twenty years, the strategy depended upon a system of collective cooperation, manifested first in NATO and then in NORAD. During the next thirty years, the focus shifted toward a more independent strategy, manifested first in international peacekeeping and then in concern for national sovereignty. Today, each historical role survives and helps define the strategy, force posture, and defense budget of Canada. The Canadian Subcommittee on National Defence of the Standing Senate Committee on Foreign Affairs underlined this point in its May 1983 report. The committee wrote:

In the 1971 White Paper on defence, *Defence in the 70s*, the commitments of the Canadian Armed Forces were listed as the protection of Canadian sovereignty; the defence of North America; contributing to the North Atlantic Treaty Organization; and peacekeeping. In the 12 years since the defence white paper was published, nothing has happened to render any of these general commitments inappropriate. Indeed, nothing indicates that Canada may soon be able to abandon any of them.[46]

MILITARY ROLES

The election in 1984 and reelection in 1988 of the Progressive Conservatives and their 1987 Defence White Paper have not significantly changed this assessment. This section will examine these roles and associated issues and problems faced by the Canadian armed forces in achieving them.

The most basic role of the nation's military—and listed first among priorities for Canada's defense—is the protection of Canada and Canadian national interests. But both at home and abroad, at least until the summer of 1985, this role received little formal attention. Budget and force structure allocations had been inadequate to meet both the NORAD and NATO missions. This was a fundamental issue, for Canada is a nation whose security is built upon a collective defense. As Nicholas Tracy points out, "the essential means to the end of protecting Canada's Arctic jurisdiction is the preservation of a secure alliance of Western Europe and North America."[47] The 1987 Defence White Paper, however, challenged this conclusion.

Emphasis on national sovereignty originally grew from Trudeau's efforts to find a distinctive Canadian defense policy. The assessment was that Canadian forces on and near national territory existed primarily for the protection of Canadian interests, but that these interests were, however, political and economic, rather than strategic or military.

While encompassing such functions as support for civil law enforcement agencies, promoting unity and identity, and emergency relief and search and rescue operations—each of which the Canadian forces fulfill quite well—the focus has been on territorial integrity and jurisdictional authority. The emphasis springs from the fact that Canada is a circumpolar power with jurisdiction over strategically important lines of communication and claims to great mineral and energy wealth. The need to protect this jurisdiction was highlighted for the Canadian public as early as 1969 by the unobstructed passage by the U.S. oil tanker *Manhattan* through the Northwest Passage.

During the 1970s, Canada undertook a number of measures to expand its rights to waters surrounding its land mass. In 1970 Canada extended its definition of its territorial waters from three to twelve miles, which made the Northwest Passage a territorial rather than international waterway. In 1970 Canada passed the Arctic Waters Pollution Prevention Act, which established a 100-mile pollution-control zone in the Arctic. The act affects the continental shelf off Canada and oil and gas exploration and drilling activities. In 1977 the declaration of a 200-mile fisheries zone and a 200-mile exclusive Economic Zone gave Canada rights to manage resources, control pollution, and oversee maritime research.

The difficulty is that none of these claims has been accepted by either the United States or the Soviet Union; and while no major threat of incursions exists at present, the potential for conflict is not insignificant. This fact was demonstrated clearly by the passage of the U.S. Coast Guard icebreaker *Polar Sea* in August 1985. The *Polar Sea* incident set off a wild debate in and out of government and resulted in a so-called "secret plan" for the defense of the north,[48] a series of government actions (outlined above), and the planned construction of the world's most powerful icebreaker.

What the *Polar Sea* passage of 1985 and the *Manhattan* passage of 1969 indicated was that Canadian forces must develop a strategy and capability to supervise and enforce Canada's claims. The problem was that these tasks had not been urgently pursued in the past.

Implementing national sovereignty requires forces that are able to do the following things: sea and air surveillance; challenge or demonstration once a violation is detected; and reinforcement once the challenge has been identified. Today, Canada lacks the sea denial forces to accomplish these tasks.

The various programs outlined in the 1987 White Paper, particularly those to enhance Canadian naval forces, are designed to address this shortfall. Nevertheless, until these programs come on line, Canada's ability to enforce its sovereignty will be limited. However, prior to publication of the White Paper, Canada had already decided to construct six new patrol frigates and upgrade its destroyers. Another bright spot among existing Canadian forces is the new long-range patrol aircraft Aurora, and in response to the *Polar Sea* incident, the Canadian Department of National Defence (DND) increased Arctic flights. Unfortunately, not enough of these highly capable aircraft are available, and they can neither defend themselves nor attack surface targets. Canada currently has only eighteen Auroras to patrol 59,000 miles of coast. If one of these patrol planes is grounded, 25 percent of air antisubmarine resources on the West Coast is lost.[49] The 1987 White Paper addressed this by calling for the acquisition of at least six more LRPAs.

In addition to the air presence, Canada maintains a Northern Headquarters at Yellowknife and Whitehorse. In total, fewer than 1,000 military personnel are spread out in the entire northern area, including those at Alert and DEW radar sites. In addition, another 1,200 cadets and poorly equipped volunteer rangers are available. With this level of capability, not surprisingly, a weather station erected by a Nazi submarine crew in 1943 on the Northern coast of Labrador went undetected for thirty-eight years, and was located only after the DND received an inquiry about its existence.[50] Fortunately, the outlook for the future is good if the various maritime modernization programs are implemented.

Against the Soviet Union, Minister of Defence J. Gilles Lamontagne wrote in 1983, "our basic security has, and will for the foreseeable future, continue to rest on deterrence of nuclear attack provided by the strategic retaliatory forces of the U.S., which, to the extent that they deter an attack on the U.S. itself equally deter one against Canada."[51]

Like that of the United States, Canadian defense strategy today is built around the concept of deterrence—both nuclear and conventional. However, for a nation that does not possess any offensive nuclear weapons and, in fact, has rejected the use of nuclear weapons of all types for itself, Canada must contribute to nuclear deterrence by protecting the nuclear strike capability of the United States. Since 1958 this mission of North American defense has been accomplished through Canada's membership in NORAD, which today has the following three primary missions: air defense; ballistic missile warning and attack characterization; and space surveillance and defense. Of these missions, Canada takes part principally only in the first, air defense.

Since the mid 1960s, Canadian defense policy has eschewed involvement in any form of ABM defense system. In fact, in the past, such nonparticipation was a condition for Canada's continued membership in NORAD. Similarly, Canada has been reluctant to become involved in space defense, originally opposed changing the name of NORAD to North American Aerospace Defense Command in the 1970s, and has been critical of President Reagan's "Star Wars" initiative announced in March 1983. To be sure some Canadians, particularly in the industrial sector, would like to see Canada become more involved in the space mission, in large part because of industrial benefits and technology transfers that would occur.

But the reduction of Canada's participation in space surveillance, by phasing out its Baker-Nunn camera (used to track satellites visually), and creation in the United States on 23 September 1985 of a separate Space Command, whose forces will take over much of the space role from NORAD, greatly limit the potential contributions of Canada in space. Until Canada signs up to the missile and space missions, air defense will be Canada's primary mission in the North American defense role.

Today, although the United States is encouraging Canada to do more, Canada contributes approximately 10 percent of the cost of NORAD (derived from the fact that the Canadian population is approximately one-tenth that of the United States). In 1985, for example, Canada paid C$664 million, while the United States paid C$6,799 million of the NORAD bill.[52] At present, nearly 7,000 Canadian personnel are assigned to NORAD, and a Canadian is always vice commander of

NORAD. In 1986, 46 of the 187 NORAD headquarters uniformed personnel were Canadian. Canada at present contributes the following to the North American defense mission: twenty-one radars of the DEW Line; twenty-four radars of the Pinetree Radar Line; two Regional Operations Control Centers (ROCCs) at North Bay, Ontario, that perform air surveillance, identification, and control of interceptors over Canadian airspace; one squadron of CF-18s; an extensive network of communications facilities; and a Baker-Nunn space surveillance camera at St. Margaret's, New Brunswick.

The Baker-Nunn camera and Pinetree Line are scheduled to be deactivated; the number of CF-18 interceptor squadrons is expected to be increased to three, with two squadrons at Cold Lake, Alberta, and one at Bagotville, Quebec; and the DEW Line will be replaced by the North Warning System (NWS), expected to be fully operational by 1992. The NWS is part of the air defense modernization program, in which Canada is a significant partner.

In light of the renewed Soviet bomber and cruise missile (both air- and sea-launched) threats and the U.S. interest in strategic air defense, Canada's role and commitment to NORAD and North American defense continue to be crucial elements in its defense policy.

Canada's contribution to conventional deterrence lies principally in its commitment to Europe and NATO. Canadian Forces Europe (CFE) consists of 5,400 conventionally armed regulars: 3,200 in the 4CMBG, 1,440 at headquarters, and 760 in the First Canadian Air Group. The Mulroney government has increased the ground forces by 1,200, and the land element is augmented by a brigade group of 2,400 troops stationed in Canada. Significantly, these 2,400 troops must be airlifted to Europe to make the Fourth Mechanized Brigade a self-supporting unit.

In addition, Canada is committed to send a battalion to Europe to support the Allied Command Europe Mobile Land Force, or AMF(L). Stationed at Lahr and Baden-Soellingen, West Germany, the Canadian land forces are committed to the central front, where a Warsaw

Pact offensive is considered most likely. The force serves an important political purpose in demonstrating to the West Germans Canadian resolve to defend Europe. A highly professional force, the CFE participates in the yearly NATO joint exercises and usually does quite well. However, CFE suffers from obsolete equipment and is undermanned. Reinforcements would have to be flown in, but as a recent Canadian Senate Report noted, the Canadian Air Transport Group is facing block obsolescence by 1990.[53]

The First Canadian Air Group, also based at Baden-Soellingen, is composed of three squadrons of CF-18s. Traditionally, these forces have had a conventional air-to-ground role. But the fifty-four new CF-18s equipped with Sparrow and Sidewinder missiles, will be able to take on air-to-air roles as well, provided existing munitions shortfalls are met as promised by the 1987 Defence White Paper. In addition, two CF-18 squadrons stationed in Canada are earmarked for deployment to NATO in time of crisis. In 1988 the Canadian government reactivated the First Canadian Air Division, which includes these five squadrons committed to the central front.

Up until the publication of the 1987 White Paper, the Canadian Air Sea Transportable (CAST) force of nearly 4,000 men was stationed in Canada but ready for European deployment. The CAST was earmarked to reinforce northern Norway, a potentially important contribution in view of the fact that Norway does not permit U.S. forces to be stationed on its soil. However, Canada's inability to meet the CAST commitment, demonstrated in the Brave Lion exercise in fall 1986, led the Canadian government to announce the elimination of the CAST in the 1987 White Paper. Forces committed to Norway are now earmarked for consolidation with the forces already stationed in Central Europe. Canada also provides the Allied Command Atlantic with twelve old destroyers with Sea King helicopters, three obsolete diesel submarines, and two long-range maritime-patrol squadrons (LRPA).

In addition to providing forces, Canada plays a major role in providing training sites and opportunities for its European allies. A very close training association exists not only with the United States but also with West Germany. On any given day, in fact, more German tanks may be in Canada than Canadian tanks. This is a very important contribution to the allied defense effort.

With the exception of the increase of 1,200 ground troops, the size of the Canadian contingent in Europe has remained relatively stable during the past ten years, though Canada has taken major steps toward modernizing the CFE. Modernization measures have included the acquisition of new trucks, armored personnel carriers, Leopard tanks, a new fighter aircraft and, most recently, the decision to acquire 250 new tanks to replace the Leopards.

While a 1982 report by the Canadian Senate Subcommittee on National Defence called for an increase in Canadian troop levels in Europe, initially to 7,800 and ultimately to 10,000 (the number before the 1969 Trudeau reduction), most of the debate within the Canadian national security community centered, not on the size of the Canadian contingent to NATO, but on where it was to be deployed and how it was to be used. The 1987 Defence White Paper has resolved this debate for the time being.

Finally, before closing this discussion of the Canadian NATO commitment, a few words should be said about the political dimension. Canada supports the U.S. strategy of flexible response, though its contributions are directed only toward the third leg of the NATO triad of strategic nuclear, tactical nuclear, and conventional weapons. Canada has supported the effort to achieve a 3 percent increase in defense spending, and in the past has met, or come close to, that goal. She has also supported the Intermediate Nuclear Force (INF) decision of December 1979, as long as the decision to deploy GLCMs and Pershing IIs was linked to an arms control initiative.

Similarly, despite much vocal opposition at home, the Trudeau and Mulroney administrations permitted the testing of cruise missiles over Canadian territory. Where a divergence has arisen between the United States and Canada on NATO policy, the difference in viewpoint has centered on out-of-area issues or on the Third World. In these cases, this difference sometimes results from a Canadian view of a U.S. failure to consult adequately with Canada. For example, Canada opposed U.S. action in Grenada. The fact is that Canada has a somewhat different view of NATO than the United States. Thus, while the United States tries to separate NATO policies from North American defense policies, Canada prefers to treat them as a single entity. In fact, a former Canadian Ambassador to NATO has proposed that NORAD and NATO be combined.[54] NATO for Canada, after all, is the multilateral balance to bilateral military policy dominance by the United States.

Secondly, for Canada, NATO is more than a military alliance. Pursuant to Article 2 of the NATO Charter (the Canadian Article), economic and social interests are also to be pursued by the organization. Canada has not completely discarded this objective. As Joe Clark, Canadian secretary of state for external affairs, stated at the opening of the ministerial meeting of the North Atlantic Council in 1986: "NATO is not only a defensive alliance, of course. It is the primordial instrument of Western political consultation, more so today even than at the time of the Ottawa Declaration that NATO issued 12 years ago."[55]

PEACEKEEPING

While it has the lowest priority, peacekeeping is still an important role for the Canadian armed forces—and a unique part of the nation's security policy. Continued participation by Canada in peacekeeping operations under UN auspices is a manifestation of the Canadian belief that such operations bring stability to the international environment while promoting peace and regional security. In the years since World War II, Canada has engaged in more than two dozen peacekeeping missions, involving nearly 80,000 personnel. Of this number, 78 have died while performing peacekeeping operations.[56]

Today, Canada is involved in seven UN-sponsored peacekeeping activities: the UN Force in Cyprus (UNFICYP), where 515 regular and reserve personnel have joined troops of other nations to keep the peace between Greek and Turkish Cypriots; two separate missions in the Middle East—the UN Truce Supervisory Organization (UNTSO) in which 20 Canadian officers assist in observing and maintaining the 1948 truce between the major belligerents, and the UN Disengagement Observer Force (UNDOF) composed of 220 Canadian communication, logistics, and technical personnel; a Canadian representative to the seven-nation Participating Nations Advisory Group in Korea; and the UN Military Observer Group in India-Pakistan (UNMOGIP), to which Canada provides airlift support twice yearly; the United Nations Good Office Mission in Afghanistan and Pakistan (UNGOMAP) where Canadian forces contributed to monitoring the Soviet withdrawal from Afghanistan; and finally, the UN Military Observer Group to which Canada is providing communications support as well as making up part of the 320-man officer observer corps monitoring the Iran-Iraq ceasefire. In addition, in 1986 Canada committed nearly 150 troops and nine helicopters to the non-UN force responsible for monitoring the Egyptian-Israeli peace agreement in the Sinai Peninsula and has offered its services in Namibia and Central America.

Canada's defense policy today is a response to Canadian perceptions of the international environment. It is manifested in the four commitments discussed above, restated in the 1987 Defence White Paper. In the words of a Senate subcommittee report:

To a large extent, the four commitments can be seen as a continuum. Peacekeeping operations may prevent a situation from growing into a general conflict, which would present a direct threat to Canada. The contribution Canada makes to NATO serves to provide forward defence of its territory, institutions, and way of life, together with guarantees of assistance in the event of a direct threat to this country or continent. Contributing to the defence of North America helps to maintain the deterrent capability of U.S. forces and to extend their defensive umbrella over Canada in a form and a fashion consistent with Canadian sovereignty. As for the protection of Canadian sovereignty, it is simply the basic element of the total defence effort.[57]

The Defense Decision-Making Process

The Canadian defense decision-making process involves an interaction of diverse political and economic actors and interests, taking part in a well-developed, sophisticated, and highly centralized national decision-making structure, which is influenced by a variety of bureaucratic, nongovernmental, and non-Canadian participants.[58] The United States, not surprisingly, has a significant role in this process.

Canada's federal, parliamentary government has created a defense decision-making process characterized by a dominant executive, a constrained legislature, a small number of principal participants centered on the cabinet, and limited input from the media, interest groups, and the general public.

The unified Canadian armed force also results in a highly integrated defense establishment. Unlike the defense organization in Washington, in which a separate civilian staff (the Office of the Secretary of Defense) oversees a number of individual military service staffs, the civilian and military bureaucracy in Ottawa is integrated into a single defense staff. The civilian-military decision line in Washington is hierarchial or vertical; in Ottawa, it is lateral or horizontal.

Finally, transnational and transgovernmental actors introduce into the defense process participants outside the formal governmental decision chain, whose interests may in fact be contrary to those of Ottawa. Significantly, U.S. influence is frequently manifested through these participants.

From a U.S. perspective, the most important consideration for understanding the defense structure of Canada and its impact on Canadian defense policy is a realization that this structure exists within both a parliamentary and a federal form of government. Unlike in the U.S. presidential system, in which power is divided between the executive and legislative branches—the president and the Congress—power in Ottawa is channeled through Parliament to the cabinet and focused on the prime minister. Two decades ago, James Eayrs, Canada's preeminent military historian, wrote:

Politics in Canada have produced governments of extraordinary longevity. They have also produced small and feeble oppositions to the debility of Parliament and the aggrandizement of the Executive. The Cabinet stands supreme and with his Cabinet (his, for he makes

it and may break it) the Prime Minister enjoys a preeminence other parliamentary systems seldom provide.[59]

Today, that statement is even more descriptive. The prime minister and his cabinet are the final arbiters of power in the authoritative allocation of resources in the Canadian political system. Defense policy in Canada is ultimately made in the interaction between the prime minister and his cabinet. In this interaction, the minister of defence and the department he heads do not enjoy the preeminence that their counterparts in Washington have. (The position of the prime minister and cabinet in the overall government structure is depicted in figure 1.)

THE PRIME MINISTER AND STAFF

Canada's prime minister, an elected member of the Parliament, is the leader of the majority party in Parliament's House of Commons. He is directed by the constitutional ruler (the governor general, who represents the queen of England) to form the government. As long as the electorate keeps the prime minister's party in the majority in the Parliament, decisions and policies of the prime minister and his cabinet of about forty ministers cannot be overturned.

A series of reforms introduced by the Trudeau administration enhanced the power of the prime minister and his cabinet. The reforms enlarged the size and decision-making status of the Office of the Prime Minister (PMO) and the cabinet secretariat, or Privy Council Office (PCO), and expanded the cabinet committee system in order to give the cabinet a modicum of independence from the permanent civil service. In general, the PCO deals with policy and administration, while the PMO deals with policy ramifications and political strategy—somewhat analogous to the functions of the U.S. Executive Office of the President and White House Office, respectively.[60]

The secretary of the cabinet advises the prime minister and oversees the operation of the Policy and Expenditure Management System (PEMS). Reforms introduced by the Mulroney administration in the PEMS process have placed increased responsibility on the PCO.

Figure 1. Canada's Overall Government Structure

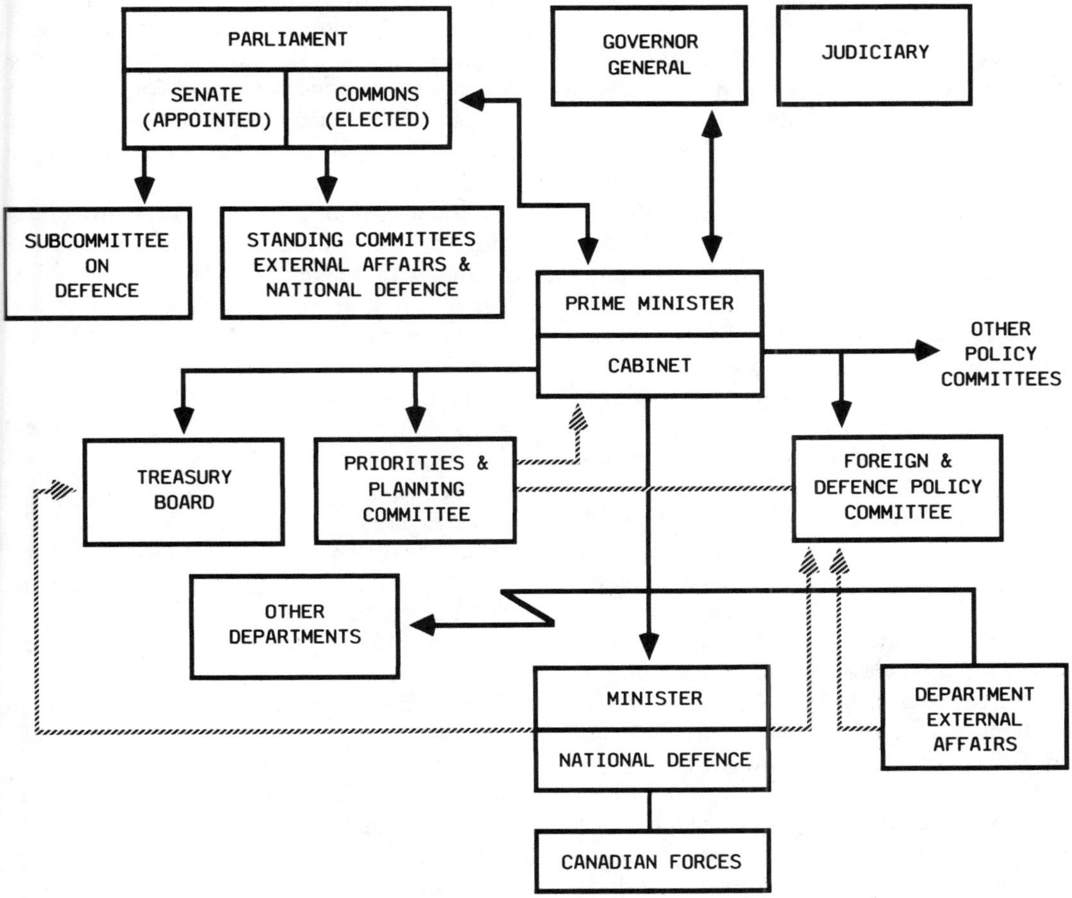

Source: NDHQ

The PMO is concerned primarily with political activities. It provides political advice and strategy on what the government is about and how well it is performing, and advises the prime minister on major policy issues. The PMO is headed by the principal secretary to the prime minister, who, as in the case of other individuals in this office, is a political appointee and not a member of the regular civil service.

CABINET COMMITTEE SYSTEM

The Canadian political system has been described as a government by cabinet committees, in which the central architect is the prime minister. Under Trudeau, the cabinet commit-

tee system was expanded and its influence enhanced.[61]

The system, an extension of the cabinet itself, has evolved over more than forty years in response to the growing complexity of government. It makes possible a decentralized decision-making process that can progressively review and screen issues and prepare them for presentation. In fact, all issues are examined in detail by the cabinet committee before ratification by the full cabinet. The growth of the cabinet committee system has paralleled the growth in power and influence of congressional committees in the United States.

The similarity is not surprising, for their functions are not dissimilar. On the one hand, cabinet committees resemble the White House and Executive Office of the U.S. president in that they give the political executive more control over the bureaucracy and ministers. On the other hand, however, because they perform review and oversight functions, they resemble U.S. congressional committees. In the Canadian decision-making process, if a proposal survives the cabinet committee system, it has a very high probability of becoming law, just as does a bill in the U.S. congressional committee system.

The exact number of committees and their composition have varied by prime minister, as each has structured the system to meet his own needs. Trudeau, for example, set up a total of thirteen cabinet committees. His successor, John Turner, had ten cabinet committees. When Brian Mulroney first became prime minister, he eliminated the Foreign Defense Policy Committee in order to signal a greater role for defense and to bring defense issues directly to the committee he chaired—Priorities and Planning. However, he later recreated the committee because of the cabinet workload.

Membership on these committees is overlapping and consists of cabinet ministers appointed by the prime minister. In addition, under Trudeau each of these formal ministerial committees had an informal mirror committee composed of the deputy ministers of each department. Deputy ministers represent the highest level of the civil service. While the ministerial committee reflects the political dimension, its mirror committee reflected the bureaucratic dimension.

These mirror committees, which were abolished by the Turner government, performed a vital function in the decision-making process by serving as a clearing house for issues and resolving those not requiring referral to the cabinet committees. They were great facilitators, serving as a link between the cabinet committee and individual departments.

Their functions continue through less formal, ad hoc coordinating mechanisms, including the Coordinating Committee of Deputy Ministers, chaired by the secretary to the cabinet, and the deputy ministers' luncheon, which meets monthly to discuss issues and is attended by the deputy ministers and associate ministers of departments.

Before concluding this review of the Canadian cabinet and the cabinet committee system, two points must be noted concerning the minister of defence (MoD). First, his role in the past was greatly circumscribed throughout the process. He was not a member of the most significant committee, Priorities and Planning, or chairman of the cabinet committee dealing with defense. In every case, the MoD was second to the minister of external affairs, reflecting the importance placed on the economic, as opposed to the military, dimensions of foreign policy. This second-class status of the MoD was changed by Mulroney. The MoD now sits on the Priorities and Planning Committee and is vice chairman of the Foreign and Defence Policy Committee. To be sure, the MoD always has the prerogative of circumventing the committee system and taking an issue directly to his colleagues in the cabinet. However, this practice is not common or recommended.

The second point relates to the fact that not only is Canada a parliamentary system like Great Britain, it also is a federal one like the United States. In fact, the Canadian provinces have considerably more power than do the U.S. states. As Thomas Hockin, a political commentator on the Canadian scene, notes:

While in the United States most policy bargains are struck in the congressional committee system, the type of bargaining which is most central to the Canadian federal system takes place between federal and provincial governments.[62]

Federalism not only affects the decision-making process directly but also is a factor in the selection of cabinet members. A prime minister, in selecting his cabinet, must be concerned not only with the qualifications of potential members in their fields, but, more important, with the geographic regions of the nation that they represent. His cabinet has to be balanced in terms of the provinces, regions, and religious, ethnic, and linguistic groups of the country.

As a result, expertise in defense matters is not necessarily a major qualification for selection of the minister of defence. Further, unlike his counterpart in Washington, the Canadian minister of defence is an elected member of the legislature and as such, like a member of the U.S. Congress, must be responsive to his electorate. The U.S. secretary of defence, appointed by the president, has no such constituency. The Canadian minister of defence must, in part, evaluate any proposal in light of the desires of his constituents, who elected him. The cabinet decision-making process is summarized in figure 2.

THE DEPARTMENT OF NATIONAL DEFENCE

Although the Canadian defence establishment is headed by the minister of defence (MoD), the MoD does not become involved in the daily management of the Defense Department. This task is handled by the deputy minister of defence (DMoD) and the chief of the defense staff (CDS). These three individuals—the MoD, the DMoD, and the CDS—form a very close working team that is responsible for overall control and management of Canada's defense forces. While the DMoD is the senior civilian adviser to the minister, the CDS is the senior military adviser. In addition, in August 1985, to further enhance defense, and reduce the workload on the MoD, Mulroney restored a cabinet position that had been vacant since 1967 by appointing an associate minister of defense. While the MoD was to be concerned with policy, the associate MoD would oversee defence construction projects and daily operations.

The relationship between the MoD, associate MoD, and the DMoD is unique and highly personalized. Richard Neustadt uses the term duopoly to define such a system. Describing the relationship in Britian between high-ranking civil servants (the deputy ministers) and elected political officials (the ministers), the minister is concerned with the political sphere beyond the department itself, primarily the cabinet, its various committees, other ministries and agencies of government, and the Parliament. His focus is outward.

The deputy minister, on the other hand, is concerned with the bureaucratic or administrative sphere within the department. His focus is inward, on the center of government. He is the senior civilian adviser to the minister on all departmental affairs of concern or interest to the government and to the central agencies of government. He ensures that all policy direction from the government is reflected in the administration of the department and in military plans and operations.

The chief of the defence staff, a four-star general officer, is the highest-ranking military man in the defense organization. He is responsible for the operational command and control of the Canadian Forces. As the military commander, his role and function is like that of the chairman and each of the respective chiefs of the U.S. Joint Chiefs of Staff. Each commander of Canada's four major commands—Maritime, Mobile, Air, and Communications—as well as Commanders of the Canadian Forces Europe (CFE), the Training System, and the Northern Territory, report to the CDS and, through him, to the DMoD and MoD. The chain of command is direct.

The DMoD and CDS are assisted in the management of the Canadian National Defence Headquarters (NDHQ) by the vice chief of staff and his deputy. The vice chief functions as the chief of staff of the headquarters, while the deputy chief acts as the J-3, or deputy chief for operations. The DMoD and the CDS translate and implement defense decisions coming from the cabinet through the MoD. The two serve as policy advocates up and down the chain of command.

The working relationship that the two maintain with each other, and with the MoD and the rest of the staff, is best described as collegial. They must work closely together. In fact, the acts of Parliament that established these offices give them distinct powers that cannot be shared legally but must be shared informally if the system is to work.

The relationship between the DMoD and the CDS is a manifestation and reflection of the integration of the civilian and military staffs; this integration characterizes and distinguishes the organizational structure of the NDHQ. Along with the unification of the Canadian armed forces, the integrated staff has resulted in a single staff agency responsible for each functional area. Canada's system is unlike

Figure 2. Process of Cabinet Approval

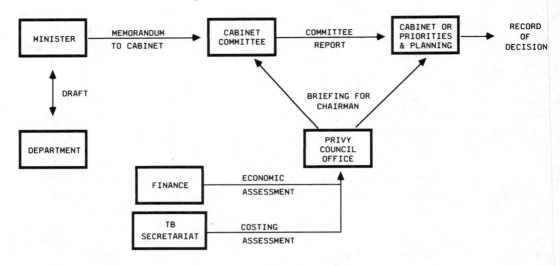

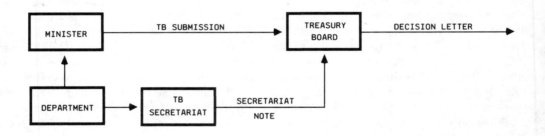

the U.S. system, in which a department for each functional area is repeated for each service and then again at the secretary of defense level.

Development and coordination of policy and programs within Canada's NDHQ occur through a hierarchical committee system that includes the Defence Council, the Defence Management Committee (DMC), the Armed Forces Council, the Program Control Board (PCB), and the Audit and Program Evaluation Committee.[63]

As depicted in figure 3, the organizational structure of the Canadian Department of National Defence (DND) is greatly simplified, compared with the U.S. structure. Under the integrated office of the DMoD and the CDS are four assistant deputy ministers (Policy, Personnel, Matériel, and Finance) and the deputy

chief of staff. All but the assistant deputy minister for personnel are civilians, but each has a three-star military deputy. Similarly, the assistant deputy minister for personnel has a civilian assistant. The assistant deputy minister for policy is the number three civilian in the ministry and is responsible for defense planning and programing functions. Combining the functions of the U.S. under secretary of defense for policy and the assistant secretary of defense for programs and evaluation, his office is responsible for the Defence Program Management System (DPMS), examined below. The primary functions and responsibilities of other deputy ministers are summarized in their titles, as may be seen at figure 3.

The deputy chief of staff is on an equal organizational level with the assistant deputy ministers. He is the focal point through which the

Figure 3. National Defence Headquarters

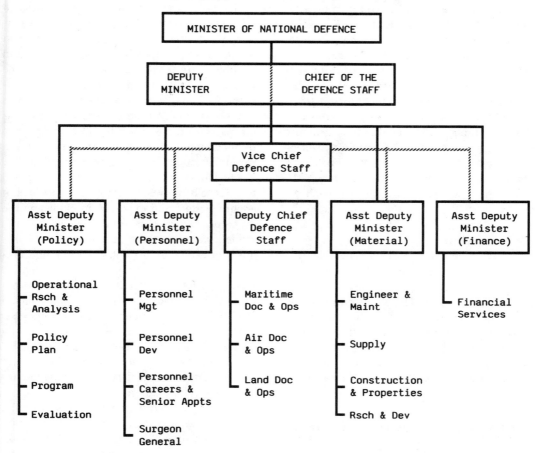

interests, needs, and requirements of each operational command are introduced into the national decision-making process. He reports to the CDS on all operational matters and to the vice chief of defence staff on nonoperational concerns. He guarantees that policy, commitments, and requirements are compatible with operational capabilities and the existing force structure. He oversees planning, programing, and employment of this force structure.

Reporting to the deputy chief of staff are the four branches responsible for doctrine and operations of the major commands and the reserves. These branches are the NDHQ points of contact for each operational command. In this sense, they function like the individual service and department (army, navy, and air force) staffs in the U.S. system.

Thus, for example, if a new requirement is identified in the field, perhaps for a new fighter, patrol boat, or tank, it will be validated at the respective command headquarters (Winnipeg, Manitoba, for Air Command; Halifax, Nova Scotia, for Maritime Command; and St. Hubert, Quebec, for Mobile Command). If the requirement is approved, it will be sent by the command's staff to the appropriate doctrine and operations branch for review and coordination with other branches and possible inclusion in the defense program process. In addition, commanders of the major Canadian commands are members of the Defence Management Council, an NDHQ panel that reviews and approves programs for incorporation into the annual defense program.

In the field, the Canadian armed forces are

organized into functional and regional units. These include the functional commands (Maritime, Air, Mobile, Communications, CFE, and Training) and regions (Atlantic, Eastern, Central, Prairie, Pacific, and Northern). The 1987 Defence White Paper has indicated that in order to "simplify and strengthen Canada's defence structure" a regional command structure will be set up under the commander of Mobile Command. Under this new structure the commander of Mobile Command "will be responsible for assisting civil authorities coordinating militia support, and overseeing the operation of army mobilization in each region."[64]

THE PARLIAMENT

As might be expected in a parliamentary system, the role of the legislative branch in the development of Canadian defense policy is limited. Traditionally, the House of Commons and the Senate (which, like its British counterpart, the House of Lords, is an essentially powerless, unelected body) have had a supporting role in the policy process. As one member of the Conservative Progressive Party in Ottawa points out:

Defence issues are seldom if ever debated in any detail in the House or its Standing Committee on External Affairs and National Defence [SCEAND]. . . . For nearly a 20-year period there has not been a serious debate in Parliament on defence. Certainly there are discussions, but they are short-range, piecemeal, more concerned with particular domestic benefits rather than with long-range, strategic, and overall policy implications for the armed forces and the defence of the nation.[65]

Thus, for example, during the period 1972–80, SCEAND did not conduct a single hearing on defense matters or issue a single report on the subject, aside from addressing the renewal of NORAD. It was content merely to discuss the yearly defense estimates.

Within the House of Commons, defense issues are the purview of SCEAND. Under new rules of Parliament, issued in 1986, SCEAND has been divided into two committees: the Standing Committee on Defence and the Standing Committee on External Affairs and International Trade. The former has seven members.

Essentially, House of Commons involvement in defense matters is one limited to criticism from opposition parties during debates—particularly during the daily question period, in the form of questions to the MoD—and from backbenchers (rank-and-file members of the House of Commons in contrast to frontbenchers, who are government ministers or leaders of the opposition) of the government party during party caucuses. Parliament also serves to publicize issues and sensitize the public to controversial aspects of the defense program.

The House of Commons' inactivity in regard to defense issues results in part from its lack of adequate staff and expertise to challenge the executive and in part from the government's tendency to dismiss the views of parliamentarians. For example, in 1969, the Standing Committee in the House conducted an extensive study and issued a detailed report on the nature of the Canadian military commitment to NATO, but its recommendations were ignored. However, since 1980, a resurgence of activity on defense has been seen in both Houses of Parliament, in part because the government has indicated that it desires a parliamentary input on certain issues.

A renewed interest in defense policy by the Canadian Senate has resulted in the creation for the first time of a special subcommittee on defense. Created in June 1980, this has become one of the most active of the Senate committees and has produced a number of excellent in-depth studies of the Canadian armed forces.

The increased activity by House and Senate committees is healthy, for it enhances public debate on defense. Furthermore, Prime Minister Mulroney has encouraged members of parliamentary committees to become more involved in analyzing government policies and requesting briefings from the government. However, this movement toward greater involvement should neither be interpreted as a change in the relative power position of Parliament in matters of defense nor be compared with congressional assertiveness in the defense area in Washington. In the Canadian system, the legislature will always have a secondary role.

OTHER GOVERNMENT DEPARTMENTS

The analysis to this point has centered on key participants in the Canadian political system who are concerned with the defense decision-making process. In addition to these participants, others within and outside the government have a lesser role in the process.

Within the government, particularly in the area of weapons acquisition, participants include the Department of Supply and Services (DSS), the Department of Industry, Science and Technology, the Department of Regional and Industrial Expansion (DRIE), and, within the Department of External Affairs, offices under the minister of trade.

DSS is the procurement agency for the Department of Defence. The Department of Industry is responsible for industrial benefits and for spreading them across the nation. Offices under the minister of trade deal with developing export trade and assisting Canadian manufacturers to this end. The Defence Programs Bureau within the Ministry of External Affairs administers Defence Production and Development Sharing Programs in Canada. The Department of External Affairs, particularly the secretary of state for external affairs, influences the defense process in a number of ways.

DEFENSE INDUSTRY

Canada has a so-called "military industrial complex," whose impact on the decision-making process is affected by a number of factors: (1) the Canadian defense industry is small compared with that of the United States; (2) it competes chiefly for subcontracts; (3) it is primarily export-oriented; (4) Canadian defense contractors are frequently subsidiaries of, or substantially owned by, U. S. companies; and (5) as a result, much lobbying derives not so much from Canadian companies as from U.S. multinational businesses.

Major Canadian industrial interest groups include the Canadian Manufacturers Association, the Air Industries Association of Canada, and the Canadian Shipbuilding and Ship Repairing Association. More than 100 Canadian and foreign companies are in the Air Industries Association alone. One aspect of the lobbying effort of these interest groups is unique.

Unlike the U.S. experience, in which a lobbying effort, if successful, often results in enhanced military capability through acquisition of new systems, in Canada, the result may just be more business for the Canadian firm, with no increase in Canadian military capability. The reason is that the Canadian firm usually is lobbying for a share of a defense contract that may not be for a Canadian system, or, if it is, may have only minimal returns with respect to increasing Canadian military capability. This is another illustration of a point made earlier—that the primary purpose of the Canadian defense effort is as much economic as it is military.

THE PUBLIC ROLE

The nonmilitary orientation of the Canadian people, as well as the nature of the defense decision-making process, have resulted in a very limited role for the public and the media in formulating Canadian defense policy. This does not mean that the public does not support the military. It does imply, however, that, with one exception, the public is not a force that can be mobilized easily to take a position on defense.

The exception involves nuclear weapons, since the media and the public take part actively in the defense debate when nuclear weapons issues are involved. This debate has occurred at least three times, as follows: in the early 1960s, over deploying nuclear-armed BOMARC (Boeing-Michigan Aeronautical Research Center) missiles in Canada, an issue that brought down the Conservative government of John Diefenbaker; in 1983, over the issue of testing U.S. air-launched nuclear cruise missiles (ALCMs) over Canadian soil; and in 1985–87, over the Reagan SDI program. A similar public debate has occurred over the nuclear-powered submarine acquisition, although these boats will not carry nuclear weapons. More often, however, Canadian public concerns are with domestic and economic issues.

Canada's then associate minister of defence, in a speech before the Conference of Defence

Associations in January 1986, identified the following factors to explain the relatively low priority given defense issues by the Canadian public: fading public knowledge of war and its causes; lack of interaction with the armed forces during peacetime; misperception or misunderstanding of the threat; the overshadowing of Canadian defense issues by those of the United States; lack of in-depth analysis of defense issues; failure to communicate to the public on those issues; and the high public profile of disarmament and peace groups.[66]

Recently, interest in defense issues has increased, generated in part by Soviet actions in Afghanistan and Poland, the Falklands War, Lebanon, and Grenada, and in part by the cruise missile and SDI debates and television shows proposing that Canada adopt a policy of neutrality. This increased interest in defense issues probably will not excite Canadian voters, however, to the extent of determining the outcome of political contests. Despite the hype, a Gallup poll in May 1986 showed that 56 percent of Canadians are opposed to Canada's withdrawal from either NATO or NORAD and to adopting a policy of neutrality.[67]

Similarly, the impact on the decision-making process of "think tank" organizations and academic institutions does not compare with that in the United States. Organizations of this type, such as the Canadian Institute for International Affairs and the Canadian Institute for Strategic Studies, do exist; but they function primarily to educate the public on defense and serve as centers for debate or discussion. One organization that has done an extensive amount of in-depth defense analysis that does have an impact is the Operational Research and Analysis Establishment (ORAE), headquartered in Ottawa. But this "RAND type" organization is responsible to and is established under the assistant deputy minister of defence for policy and thus does not provide an outside analytical perspective.

With respect to interest groups, both public and private, Kim Nossal says that more than half a million Canadians belong to some type of organization whose primary or secondary objective is defense related.[68] In the arms control area, there are the Canadian Center for Arms Control and Disarmament and the Canadian Institute for International Peace and Security, the former established by Prime Minister Trudeau.

Other interest groups that are concerned with such issues as the well-being of war veterans, allocation of funds for defense, military compensation, the status of reserves, and equipment acquisition include the Royal Canadian Legion, the Royal Canadian Air Force Association, the Navy League, the Naval Officers' Associations of Canada, and the Conference of Defence Associations, an umbrella organization composed of many defense interest groups. Also active is the Business Council on National Issues, which, for example, published a position paper on defense in September 1984 calling for increased spending and manpower.

These organizations have a considerable membership and are listened to by the MoD, but their influence on defense policy has been minimal. In part, this lack of influence is owing to limited resources, in part to the structure of the defense decision-making process, and in part to the fact that their concerns tend to be nonpolitical and directed toward benefits for active duty and retired service people. Many of these organizations are merely social or service clubs. Nossal has summarized quite well the role of the interest groups in the decision process. He writes:

The inability of military associations to influence the direction of Canada's defence policies in the 1970s prompts a more general observation that these groups, despite their close association with policy-makers, are structurally less capable of bringing political influence to bear at both the bureaucratic and political levels than interest associations in other areas of state policy making. These structural deficiencies occur on three dimensions. First, their defense policy functions are heavily diluted by their commitment to social and community roles, and to their other policy functions. Second, their memberships, drawn from both those in government and outside it, are not homogeneous: members of those groups who serve with the Armed Forces or with NDHQ will have different perspectives— and different policy references—than those members in civilian life for whom military affairs are important, but not personally related to the imperatives of bureaucratic health and personal career patterns. Finally, most of these groups have not created the kind of institutional means to press their interests that are favored by other interest associations. Military interest groups remain firmly tied to the bureaucracy, institutionally and financially. But by eschewing a truly autonomous existence, they remain—paradoxically—too close to the policymakers and too far from the public to be able to translate effectively specific interests in policy outcomes.[69]

TRANSNATIONAL ACTORS

A second characteristic of the Canadian defense decision-making system is its penetration by transnational actors. Transnational actors are characterized by their ability to operate outside the formal governmental or national decision channels in the pursuit of common interests that may or may not correspond to those of the national government. They are contenders for power whose input impacts on policy output. Three categories are involved in the Canadian process: multinational, transgovernmental, and coalitional.

The first of these categories, the multinational, involves the large private business corporations that control multifaceted economic empires in more than a single nation. Because of their size and status, they are able not only to circumvent an individual government's regulatory and taxing power, but also to challenge its policy directly. The Canadian defense decision-making process is influenced by a number of these multinational corporations, particularly in the aerospace, electronics, and other high-tech fields.

Transgovernmental participants are the various bureaus, agencies, or bureaucratic organizations, primarily within the executive branch of a nation's government, that in the process of developing or implementing foreign and defense policies of that nation interact daily with similar organizations in other nations. Out of this interaction develop relations with regular lines of communication cutting across traditional and formal government-to-government linkages. The relationship often takes on an existence of its own, with the result that these participants identify more often with each other and with their common interests than with the governments they serve or represent. When this occurs, they become essentially independent actors within the process, often making policy irrespective of their governments. Such transgovernmental actors play a significant role in the development of Canadian defense policy.

As a result of close relations with U.S. military forces, the Canadian military has become the principal transgovernmental actor. In fact, the Canadian military is often able to make its influence felt in Ottawa through its transgovernmental relations with the U.S. military.

The third category of power contenders in the Canadian defense decision-making process is participants in coalitions. Robert O. Keohane and Joseph S. Nye write:

Contacts between governmental bureaucracies charged with similar tasks may not only alter their perspective but lead to transgovernmental coalitions on particular policy questions. To improve their chances of success, government agencies attempt to bring actors from other governments into their decisionmaking processes as allies. Agencies of powerful states, such as the United States, have used such coalitions to penetrate weaker governments . . . [and] they have also been used to help agencies of other governments penetrate the United States bureaucracy.[70]

These coalitions, like the governmental and transgovernmental participants who compose them, take on their own identity, becoming influential actors in the defense decision-making process. In some cases they are institutionalized and become permanent bodies. For this reason, they can be called coalition participants.

Two principal coalitional actors who influence the Canadian defense decision-making process are the Permanent Joint Board on Defence (PJBD) and the Defence Production and Development Sharing Agreement (DPDSA) Steering Committee.

Recurring Issues and Defense Policy Outputs

In the final analysis, the business of defense deals with men, money, and machines—and the strategy or doctrine concerned with their employment and deployment. This concluding section will look at the output of the policy process and the recurring issues this output entails.

THE ISSUE OF UNIFICATION

Perhaps the most distinguishing characteristic of the Canadian defense establishment is that, of all the NATO nations, only Canada has a unified armed force. This uniquely Canadian phenomenon is still a fundamental issue in Canadian defense policy.

Unification must be considered an on-going process, rather than as the single legislative act that created a unified armed force on 1 February 1968. In fact, efforts at amalgamation of the Canadian military occurred after World Wars I and II, but not until the issue of the Glassco Report in 1962 were formal legal steps taken toward unification. The Glassco Commission, established to review the Canadian defense organization, had recommended the integration of the three armed forces to address what it identified as three major shortcomings in Canada's defense policy: too much spending in defense administration and too little spending on military hardware; bureaucratic inefficiencies in the decision-making process; and questions of the degree of civilian control over the military. In 1963 the newly elected administration of Prime Minister Lester Pearson and his minister of defence, Paul Hellyer, set in motion the process that would carry out the Glassco Commission recommendations.[71]

The process of integration can be divided into at least five phases:

Phase One. On 1 August 1964 the positions of chairman of the chiefs of staff and army, navy, and air force service chiefs were abolished and replaced with a single chief of the defence staff (CDS), who was charged with control and administration of Canada's armed forces. This action created a single military chain of command that reported to the minister of defence. It also made the chief of the defence staff the principal and senior military adviser to the minister of defence, responsible for the effective conduct of military operations and the readiness of Canada's forces.

Phase Two. In June 1965, the operations, logistics, personnel, and administrative branches of the three services were integrated under the single executive authority of the chief of the Canadian defence staff. The previous eleven separate commands were reduced to six, most of which combined the missions of two or more services. The autonomy of the three services was maintained, but they would now function as part of one or more of the six integrated commands. These commands include: Maritime, Mobile, Air Defence, Air Transport, Training, and Materiel. Thus, for example, the Maritime Command combined the antisubmarine function and operations of the navy and air force, while the Mobile Command would combine the land responsibilities of the army and the air force.

The first two phases of the unification process are referred to as integration.

Phase Three. On 1 February 1968, complete unification occurred when the three armed services were unified into a single force, identified by a single name (the Canadian Armed Forces), and given a common green uniform. This third phase has been the most controversial over the years, because it eliminated individual service identity.

Phase Four. In 1972 the new National Defence Headquarters created by the reorganization initiatives of the 1960s was restructured by combining the previously separate civilian and military staffs into a single cohesive staff responsible to the minister and deputy minister of defence and the CDS. This reorganization eliminated the parallel and duplicate civilian and military bureaucracies.

Phase Five. This phase began in 1975 and continues today. It is characterized by evaluation, assessment, and a movement, albeit slow, away from complete unification. The first step in this direction was the creation of the Air Command in 1975. Combined under a single command were the former Air Transport and Air Defence Commands and tactical air units deployed in Europe and attached to the Maritime and Mobile Commands. Once again, three separate environments could be identified—air, land, and sea. The most recent step was the decision by the Mulroney government in 1985 to permit distinctive uniforms once again for each of these three environments.

The Pearson administration set in motion the unification process for economic, operational, political, and professional reasons. Economically, unification was the Canadian formula for obtaining "more bang for the buck": by reducing support forces, such as logistics, recruiting, and pay, and creating a variety of economies of scale, it provided a means of reducing defense expenditures while meeting military requirements and increasing the capital equipment budget. Operationally, unification increased effectiveness by ending competition among the individual services thus enhancing their ability to conduct increasingly interdependent operations involving sea, land, and air forces. On the political level, there were at least six chains of command reporting to the defence minister, whereas other departments had a single pyramid structure. Minister of Defence Hellyer wanted to eliminate this decentralization by creating a single group of experts under him. Unification would also highlight to the rest of the world a Canadian identity distinct from the United States and other NATO nations. The process would be one more way for the new administration to signal its efforts to develop an independent defense policy, while at the same time improving the policy process and the minister's control of it. Finally, unification was intended to create better and more equitable employment prospects for military personnel by standardizing career planning. Unification would create a broader base from which to identify and assign the best qualified individuals. Assignments would be determined on individual ability and not be constrained by individual service interests or personnel policies.

Today, more than twenty years since the unification process began, debate continues over its merits. In 1979, to fulfill a campaign pledge, the Conservative government of Prime Minister Clark established a task force to review the process. When the Liberals returned in 1980, they initiated a review of the task force's assessment. The conclusions of both

studies were mixed. On the one hand, a number of economies of scale were attained and a single process for equipment acquisition evolved. For example, the armed forces were able to reduce the number of supply depots and training centers, to implement a single, data-automated pay system and a computerized personnel management system, and to create single intelligence, communications, logistic, and recruiting systems. Headquarters was streamlined, eliminating the many tri-service committees and the resulting intense interservice competition for limited resources at senior levels. In short, unification resulted in a more flexible and streamlined organization, with a marked reduction in parochialism.

On the other hand, demonstrating that the cost savings programed as a result of unification actually occurred is difficult. Furthermore, some observers have argued that operational effectiveness has been affected, particularly in the logistic and support areas. For example, the creation of a common support force has resulted in a reduction in environmental experience and expertise among logistic and combat support forces. Requiring a technician to serve one tour working on army equipment, another on aircraft, and a third on ships not only increases training requirements, it can also impact on the competence and expertise of that technician. This negative impact does not occur, however, among operational forces who remain in one environment (land, air, or sea) for most of their careers. Thus, the brigade commander is not required to command a wing or captain a ship.

Perhaps the biggest drawback to unification, and one widely criticized, concerns the individual service identity crisis. Again, this drawback is particularly felt with support forces, who not only cannot identify with a single service but also, unlike the operations people, cannot even identify with a particular command or unit. The lack of service identity, highlighted by the common green uniform, created morale problems. For this reason, a relaxation exists in wearing of distinctive service emblems and badges and in the use of the terms army, air force, and navy. Further, in

1985 the decision was made to return to separate uniforms. Both Conservatives and Liberals have made recommendations to give each service more individual identity.

The difficulty with an accurate assessment of whether unification has achieved its four stated objectives is that since unification a number of other events have occurred that have affected the status of the Canadian forces. For example, the overall reduction in the effectiveness of the Canadian armed forces in the late sixties and seventies was more the result of drastic cuts in defense spending without a commensurate decrease in missions, and of equipment obsolescence, than of unification. An internal assessment in the DND in 1979 summarized this point quite well:

It is almost impossible to assess, let alone to quantify, the results of unification because the Canadian Forces are now quite different both qualitatively and quantitatively from those that existed in the early 1960s. . . . Indeed, it is rather like asking what one has gained from 10 years of marriage. There is no basis for comparison—life has changed.[72]

This author feels that while the debate on merits of unification will continue and further assessments will be made, the process of unification is today a reality in the Canadian defense establishment that will continue irrespective of the administration in office. To be sure, there will be modifications, particularly in the area of service identity, but the overall integrated structure will remain.

BUDGET

If the Canadian military is to modernize its existing force structure and realize the programs identified above, substantial funds will be required. In fact, limited defense funding is one of the major obstacles to Canada's assuming a greater role in both NORAD and NATO.

The Canadian military suffers from a strategy-force mismatch or commitment-capability imbalance. The Canadian armed forces have more missions than the men, money, and equipment required to support them. The Canadian Business Council on National Issues addressed this mismatch in its 1984 report on defense, concluding:

In order to meet our commitments in a fully effective manner, the Government of Canada, beginning in 1985–86, should strive to increase the defence budget by six percent in real terms per annum for a period of at least 10 years, with a view to maintaining the budget thereafter at that level with appropriate adjustments for inflation.[73]

The reality is that over this time frame, notwithstanding the 1987 Defence White Paper, the Canadian defense budget is projected to grow by only 2 percent a year, or one-third of what is required. Until more significant growth occurs, the status of the Canadian forces is not likely to change much; likewise, new policy initiatives will be similarly budget constrained.

In a number of ways, the Canadian defense budget is unique in comparison with that of the United States and with those of other Canadian government departments.

First, the Canadian defense budget can be described as a formula budget. Rather than basing the expenditure level on what is needed to meet a defined threat, the defense budget is determined through the use of a political formula established by the Canadian cabinet. Many critics of the level of Canadian defense expenditures argue that this formula is based on the cabinet's assessment of what level of funding is needed to meet the allies' demands—neither more nor less.

To be sure, the formula has changed. In the mid 1960s it was based on a 2 percent increase per year for five years. In the 1970s the formula called for a 7 percent increase for five years. Since 1979 the NATO goal of 3 percent after inflation has been the basis for the formula; and in 1985 the Canadian minister of defense announced that the formula would be a 2 percent increase after inflation through the end of the decade. This 2 percent increase was not met in 1987–88, but to carry out the 1987 White Paper proposals a 2 percent formula was reaffirmed in 1987, but set aside in 1989 as part of a significant reduction in government spending. Concomitantly, a yearly review was decreed to determine supplemental amounts to cover new acquisition programs undertaken in the coming years. The U.S. defense budget also has a politically targeted real percentage growth figure that the U.S. Congress can adjust, but that figure is used by the U.S. Department of Defense as a guide for, or a limit to, funding levels that are initially based on service needs and threat assessments. Such is not the case in Canada.

Second, the Canadian defense budget process is considerably more autonomous than those of other departments and even the U.S. defense budget. The defense budget is a multiyear fiscal plan, with Parliament authorizing annual funding. However, because of the nature of the cabinet system of government, in which allocation decisions are made and essentially ratified within the executive branch of government, and because the Treasury Board, Canada's equivalent of the OMB, will generally defer to DND as long as the budget amount does not exceed the formula, DND has more flexibility and autonomy in shaping its budget.

Further, as one official in the Treasury Board secretariat commented, "DND is more trusted and while it must obtain Treasury Board approval to move money from one account to another, this approval is pro forma and usually never denied."[74] This fact is reflected in the small number of people outside DND, estimated by some to be less than a dozen, who become involved in the defense budget process. Within the Treasury Board secretariat, the staff that analyzes the defense budget is among the smallest.

To say that the Canadian DND has more autonomy or flexibility is not to say, however, that it can effect significant changes within the budget from year to year. First, the cabinet formula must be met. Second, as is the case with the budgets of other nations, many of the components are relatively fixed or locked in. The capital account, for example, has been the one since 1975 that has reflected the most change. The reason is that in the early 1970s, it was the component that was most depleted, taking 100 percent of the budget cuts in the Trudeau years. Thus, in readdressing the level of defense expenditures in 1975, the first account to receive attention was the capital account—the one that determines the equipment that the armed forces will have. Initially, the formula

prescribed that the capital account would grow by 12 percent a year until it reached 20 percent of the budget. But when the 3 percent NATO budget was adopted, use of the formula meant that the only part of the budget that was growing significantly was the capital account. Yet flexibility within this account is limited because unless a significant increase is shown in overall funding, most of it is locked in to existing equipment acquisitions such as the CF-18s and patrol frigates, which together equal half the account.

ARMS CONTROL

If collective security is one pillar on which Canadian defense policy rests, arms control is the other. Arms control is an integral part of the Canadian strategic culture. Canada currently sits at every multilateral disarmament forum. The Assistant Deputy Minister for Political and International Security Affairs capsulized this point in testimony before the Canadian Parliament in October 1985:

> The constance of Canadian security policy since World War II has been Canada's reliance on alliance and on defence cooperation with the United States and western Europe as the basis for securing Canada from threats of political coercion or military attack. Defence and deterrence, however, have been complemented by Canada's active support for arms control and disarmament efforts which contribute to strategic stability at the lowest possible level of armament and forces.[75]

Being neither a nuclear power nor a major military power, Canada's contribution to arms control has been to encourage compliance among the nuclear powers, generate new arms control initiatives for creating an arms control regime, and enhance verification methods and technology. For example, before leaving office in 1983, former Prime Minister Trudeau undertook a pilgrimage to the capitals of the major powers to encourage the creation of a common approach between the East and West.[76] Today, Canada is involved in a variety of verification programs, including a seismic monitoring program at Yellowknife.

Canadian initiatives in the arms control arena date back to the 1940s, if not earlier. A participant with the United Kingdom in assisting U.S. efforts to develop the atomic bomb during World War II, Canada was among the first nations after the war to reject nuclear weapons development and encourage the peaceful use of nuclear energy. As the world's largest supplier of uranium and bulk radioisotopes for agricultural, medical, and scientific uses, and the fifth largest manufacturer of nuclear power reactors, such as the CANDU (Canadian Deuterium Uranium) nuclear reactor, Canada has achieved a prominent place and reputation in nuclear technology. Canadians believe this place and reputation give them a special responsibility and opportunity to limit the proliferation of nuclear weapons by controlling the export of nuclear materials and technology for peaceful uses. Thus, for example, Canada only sells nuclear materials, equipment, and technology to nations that comply with International Atomic Energy Agency safeguards.

Canada has been a member of every negotiating disarmament body that the United Nations has sponsored. In 1975 Canadian and Swedish diplomats were instrumental in getting a consensus report at the First Review Conference of the Nuclear Nonproliferation Treaty. In 1978 Canada proposed an end to producing fissionable material for nuclear weapons as part of a fourfold strategy to stop the arms race. Since 1973 Canada has been an active participant in the Mutual and Balanced Force Reduction (MBFR) negotiations to reduce conventional forces in Europe, and a stalwart in reaching agreement on measures contained in the Final Act (an arms control forum dealing with conventional arms limitations in Europe) of the Conference on Security and Cooperation in Europe. Canada has also been a strong supporter of the 1979 NATO dual-track decision (a 1979 NATO decision to link the deployment of INF forces and arms control) on theater nuclear forces in Europe and of the 1987 INF Treaty.

The Mulroney government has continued to emphasize arms control as one of the linchpins of its foreign and defense policies. Canadian Ambassador for Disarmament Douglas Roche outlines the Canadian government's "Programme of Action" that set the following objectives:

negotiated radical reductions in nuclear forces and the enhancement of strategic stability; maintenance and strengthening of the non-proliferation regime; support for a comprehensive test ban treaty; negotiation of a global chemical weapons ban; prevention of an arms race in outer space; and the building of confidence sufficient to facilitate the reduction of military forces in Europe and elsewhere.[77]

To achieve these objectives, the Canadian government has focused its efforts in the following three areas: encouraging compliance with existing arms control treaties; building confidence between East and West; and developing verification mechanisms.[78] The first two of these efforts are pursued through bilateral and multilateral consultations, and meetings.

Canada's role in developing verification mechanisms is notable. Operating with an annual budget of C$1 million, the Department of External Affairs Verification Research Division develops systems to verify a comprehensive test ban, a global chemical convention, and prevention of an arms race in space. In addition to a C$3.2 million upgrading of the seismic facility at Yellowknife to enhance research into monitoring a comprehensive test ban, if negotiated, Canada is developing a variety of verification programs, such as the Paxsat projects designed to assess the feasibility of space-to-space and space-to-earth sensing to verify a treaty prohibiting weapons in space if negotiated.

Canada's influence on the course of arms control and disarmament is not as great as it once was, and some would argue that its ability to persuade the superpowers is considerably overrated. Nevertheless, Canada's efforts in multinational and binational forums to highlight the importance of arms control are not insignificant, and its expertise and knowledge in the verification arena are important.

OTHER RECURRING ISSUES

The fundamental recurring defense issues for Canada are the nature and extent of its defense commitment to North American security and specific priorities required to meet that commitment. Canada has three options with respect to defense.

The first is the neutrality option—to reduce Canada's defense force to a very small territorial force, to pull out of NATO and NORAD, and rely on the U.S. deterrent and strategic forces for national security. This "free rider" option has been advocated by members of the New Democratic Party, but it is unlikely to be exercised, however. The reasons are: military (who would enforce Canadian sovereignty?), political (leverage in Washington and NATO capitals would be lost), and economic (defense-economic ties with Europe would be lost by withdrawal from NATO and the United States might abrogate the defense production and development sharing agreements).

The inescapable fact is that Canadian claims in the Arctic, highlighted by the passage of the U.S. Coast Guard icebreaker *Polar Sea* in 1985, will need to be enforced one way or the other, necessitating a significant financial commitment. At present, Canadian involvement in NORAD helps meet some of these requirements. Withdrawal from NORAD would mean that Canada would have to go it alone. Harriet Critchley wrote in her brief to the SCEAND committee investigating the NORAD renewal issue: "Our participation in NORAD contributes significantly to Canada's defence in terms of a scale of surveillance and air defence capabilities which we do not possess ourselves—nor, I would argue, could we provide for ourselves."[79]

The dependence of Canada on NORAD assets to establish sovereignty is highlighted by ramifications of closing the CADIN-Pinetree radar sites in mid Canada, which will essentially eliminate the ability to detect and identify noncompliant aircraft throughout southern Canada. This also would have been the case in the northern United States if the United States had not earlier developed a shared military-civilian system called the Joint Surveillance System (JSS).

Canada has no such system at present. The Department of Transport is building civilian radars, but because of limited funding, these do not meet military requirements: they can only track compliant aircraft.[80] As the sovereignty question indicates, if Canada were to exercise this first option, it would essentially be abrogating its ability to defend itself and its nationhood. L. D. Clarke, chairman and chief executive officer of SPAR Aerospace Limited, summed it up well in his SCEAND testimony when he said:

> Canada is a great country—worth defending. It shares the continent with a world power—which means it could abdicate its defence responsibilities with a certain degree of impunity. To do so would greatly diminish its greatness—there is no recorded case in history of a great nation remaining so once it becomes a vassal—no matter how benign the vassalage.[81]

The second option open to Canada is to *continue the existing level of effort*. While not favored by any of Canada's NATO allies, this option is clearly the easiest choice, for it is the status quo. The problem with this approach, however, is that it has resulted in a Canadian military that is underfunded, underequipped, and undermanned. Furthermore, it propagates a strategy/force mismatch that undercuts the capability of the Canadian forces to do any one job well. As the former chief of the Canadian Defence staff, General Theriaut, points out: "As I contemplate the overall situation which faces us: the size of our country, the expanse of the surrounding seas, our varied commitments in Canada and overseas, I cannot help but feel that we are spread awfully thin."[82]

The third option is to either increase the level of defense spending to match the mission requirements and the strategy as specified in the 1971 and 1987 White Papers, or reduce these requirements. If the former path is taken, Canada would, at a minimum, have to double its current defense budget. As Canadian defense analysts Joseph T. Jockel and Joel J. Sokolsky pointed out in 1986, Canada would have to acquire at least twelve patrol frigates, more Auroras, more submarines, more CF-18s, and extended radar coverage of the southern Canadian area to fill the hole left by shutting down the CADIN-Pinetree radar line. In addition, manpower would have to be increased to meet central front requirements in Europe.

This third option is the one outlined in the 1987 Defence White Paper. The mission requirements have remained and the decision is to increase the defense budget. However, as indicated above, the issue now is whether the cabinet will approve expenditures over the next fifteen years to sustain this option. So far it has not done so.

Issues that relate to both Canada and the United States are more difficult to address or resolve than the issues discussed so far, not only because they involve both nations but because of their complexity. The first of these issues, around which many of the others cluster, is the question of space. Most specifically, the issue is the U.S. Strategic Defense Initiative. SDI, it must be remembered, is primarily a research endeavor, one that even the U.S. government is not certain will become a reality. The promise of SDI is that it will be a catalyst in creating a new strategy other than mutual assured destruction (MAD). If a new strategy evolves and an ABM system is developed, all aspects of strategic defense become critical, and with them, Canada's role in North American defense.

Even if Canada were not to take part in SDI, if an ABM defense system works, it will demand defense in space and in the atmosphere, the latter being very difficult without Canadian support. The one and only connection between SDI and the North Warning System, often lost in the SDI rhetoric, is that a defense against ICBMs is irrational if we cannot also defend against bombers and cruise missiles.

From the Canadian perspective, there are two issues related to space. First, does Canada wish to become involved in the research, development, and implementation of space-based systems? And second, what level of resources does it wish to commit to this effort? The technological and economic benefits that would follow from becoming involved in SDI are significant. As L. D. Clarke writes:

The emergence of a Canadian defence interest in space coincides with an increasing awareness of the important advantages that accrue to industry from participation in the design and development of advanced communications, surveillance, and computer applications. Not only do defence programs provide challenging tasks for many of our brightest and best engineers, but also the advances in technology derived from this work subsequently can enhance Canadian industry's ability to serve both domestic and export requirements for commercial applications. Thus, in addition to the direct economic benefits to our high technology industries, there are extensive indirect benefits.[83]

The fear in Canada is that failure to become involved in SDI research will result in exclusion of Canada from other areas of space research, areas vital not only to the Canadian economy but to Canadian sovereignty as well. For example, Canada is participating in Teal Ruby, a 1.4 ton infrared satellite designed to detect enemy bombers through the heat emissions of their engines. While not now part of SDI, or even of the SDI organization, it could potentially be included under the SDI umbrella, particularly for budgetary reasons. Canada must become involved in space, as the SCEAND reports points out, but how to do it without becoming involved in SDI?

The second question deals with the extent to which Canada wants to be involved in the actual operations and C^3 (Command control and communication) connected with space-based systems. At present, Canada is involved primarily only in the air defense mission of NORAD. A commitment to become involved in space operations would entail involvement in other missions as well, such as missile defense (ABM and SDI) and space defense (antisatellite or ASAT). In this case, Canada might become an integral player in the Unified Space Command as well.

This raises a second cross-border issue—the organization of the new Space Command and its relation to NORAD. The issue is complex and multifaceted, entailing both intraservice and interservice bureaucracies and rivalries. On the one hand, the issue involves debate within the U.S. Air Force on how and where space fits into the air force mission, and the proper level of funding for space programs. On the other hand, an intraservice discussion has arisen over who controls certain defense, air, and space assets.

At the time of this writing, many of these issues have been resolved on the U.S. side. In October 1986 the U.S. Joint Chiefs of Staff reaffirmed that the commander of the Unified Space Command, composed of the air force, army, and navy, would also be commander of NORAD, thus ensuring that NORAD and the

Unified Space Command will be under a single four-star general officer. While this decision had been made a year earlier, the Joint Chiefs decided to look at the issue again in 1986. Discussions had taken place on separating Space Command from NORAD—the air defense mission from that of missile and space defense.

Such a separation could have diminished Canada's role in North American defense, particularly if it elected not to take part in missile and space defense. While at present Canada's position within the NORAD structure will not change—a Canadian serves as NORAD's deputy commander and Canadian personnel are integrated throughout the organization—Canada's place within the Unified Space Command will depend on its decision to become involved in space and missile defense.

A third issue involves the future direction of the defense development and defense production sharing agreements (DD/DSPA), the importance of which was affirmed at Quebec in March 1985. However, serious obstacles still need to be addressed, among them the defense trade imbalance in favor of the United States; Canadian demands for large offsets (a recent U.S. report indicates that Canada is the world's leading recipient of industrial offset benefits); and the existence of various economic obstacles to trade, such as small business set asides, buy U.S. and buy Canadian provisions, potential restrictions on Canadian firms preventing them from installing or servicing Canadian equipment sold to the United States, and an unwillingness to transfer technology.

The decision by the Mulroney government on SDI, while permitting Canadian industrial involvement, will threaten that involvement if some of the issues noted above are not resolved. For one thing, U.S. firms might not be willing to subcontract an SDI project to Canada because of Mulroney's position on SDI. Similarly, Canadian firms could find themselves at a competitive disadvantage, in light of three recent Memorandums of Understanding between the United States and West Germany, the United Kingdom, and Israel on SDI.

In conclusion the issues delineated here are not all those on the Canadian defense agenda.

They are, however, those upon which the future direction of Canadian defense policy will depend, as well as the course of U.S.–Canadian defense relations. For this reason, policy makers in the United States must understand the defense policy of Canada.

Notes

1. Colin S. Gray, "National Styles in Strategy: The American Example," *International Security* 6, no. 2 (Fall 1961): 21–47.

2. C. P. Stacey, *The Official History of the Canadian Army in the Second World War*, vol. 6 (Ottawa: Queen's Printer, 1955).

3. Peter C. Newman, *True North Not Strong and Free: Defending the Kingdom in the Nuclear Age* (Toronto: McClelland and Stewart, 1983), chap. 1.

4. Canadian Department of National Defence, *Challenge and Commitment: A Defence Policy for Canada* (Ottawa: Minister of Supply and Services, 1987), p. 89. Hereafter referred to as Defence White Paper 1987.

5. Newman, *True North*, p. 25.

6. David B. DeWitt and John J. Kirton, *Canada as a Principal Power* (New York: John Wiley and Sons, 1983), p. 57.

7. Extracted from notes for an address by the minister of national defense, J.J. Blais, to the Americas Society Conference, 17 November 1983, pp. 11–12.

8. Defence White Paper 1987, p. 3.

9. James Eayrs, "Military Policy of Middle Powers: The Canadian Experiences" in *Canada's Role as a Middle Power*, ed. J. King Gordon (Toronto: Canadian Institute of International Affairs, 1966), pp. 69, 84.

10. An example of the influence was cited by J.J. Blais, then minister of defence, in November 1983 in a speech to the Americas Society. He said: "[An element] which continues to play a part in the development of Canadian policy is the tendency for American Political debate and sometimes electoral rhetoric to spill over the border into Canada. Where in the nineteenth century, this once tended to marvelously concentrate our defence debate, today it makes the problem of resolving or even focusing upon Canadian defence issues much more difficult and complex. On the one hand, the American debate tends to swamp the Canadian leaving the average Canadian more familiar at times with the vices and virtues of the MX missiles or the deployment of troops to Central America than with the rebuilding of the Canadian Navy or the commitment of troops to Norway in the event of war" [p. 9].

11. When asked in 1975 to name "another country with roughly the same power and influence as Canada," well over half of a group of seventy-one foreign experts replied "Australia" (30 percent), "Sweden" (16 percent), or another comparable power (13 percent). A third of the respondents cited nations traditionally ranked as great powers—"France" (10 percent), "United Kingdom" (7 percent), or "Japan" (4 percent). Lyon and Tomlin, 1979, p. 57.

12. P. H. Chapin, "The Canadian Public and For-

eign Policy," *International Perspectives: The Canada Journal on World Affairs*, January/February 1986.

13. Statistical information presented in this section is drawn from the following sources: U.S. Department of State, Bureau of Public Affairs, *Background Notes on Canada*, March 1983; *World Almanac and Book of Facts* (New York: Newspaper Enterprise Association, 1986); International Institute of Strategic Studies, *The Military Balance, 1985-1986 and 1986-1987* (London: IISS, 1985, 1986); and interviews.

14. Canadian Department of National Defence, *A Synopsis of the Defence White Paper* (Ottawa: Minister of Supply and Services, 1987), pp. 8-9.

15. Bruce Thordarson, *Trudeau and Foreign Policy: A Study in Decision Making* (Toronto: Oxford University Press, 1973), p. 97.

16. For a closer examination of these foreign policy initiatives, see Franklyn Griffiths, *A Northern Foreign Policy*; Dewitt and Kirton, *Canada as a Principal Power*; Stephen Banker, "The Changing OAS"; and John D. Harbon "Canada and Brazil: Comparing Two Hemispheric Grants," *International Perspectives: The Canada Journal on World Affairs*, May-June 1982, pp. 20-16; and D. R. Murray, "The Bilateral Road: Canada and Latin America in the 1980's," *International Journal* 37, no. 1 (Winter 1981-82): 108-31.

17. Willis Armstrong and Louise Armstrong, *U.S. Policy toward Canada: Guidelines for the Next Decade*, Policy Project of the Atlantic Council of the United States, 1986, pp. 4-5.

18. A similar process was to occur in the area of defense.

19. *Competitiveness and Security: Directions for Canada's International Relations* (Ottawa: Minister of Supply and Services, May 1985).

20. Among the measures announced were: immediate adoption of an Order in Council establishing straight baselines around the Arctic archipelago effective 1 January 1986; immediate adoption of a Canadian Laws Offshore Application Act; initiation of talks with the United States on Canadian claims in the Arctic on the basis of full respect for Canadian sovereignty; an immediate increase of surveillance overflights by Aurora long-range patrol aircraft; immediate planning for Canadian naval activity in the eastern Arctic in 1986; immediate withdrawal of the 1970 reservation to Canada's acceptance of the compulsory jurisdiction of the International Court of Justice; and the construction of a Class 8 icebreaker (*House of Commons Debates*, 10 September 1985, pp. 6462-67).

21. See Gerold Graham, "An Arctic Foreign Policy for Canada," *International Pespectives* March-April 1987, p. 12.

22. Ibid. p. 11.

23. Canadian Department of National Defence, *Defence in the 70s: White Paper on Defence* (Ottawa: Information Canada, 1971), p. 25.

24. Defence White Paper 1987, pp. 10-11.

25. Department of External Affairs, Ottawa, *Canadian Weekly Bulletin*, 4 March 1959, p. 1. The same point was made in the Defence White Paper, 1987, which stated: "Because of our geographic position, Soviet strategic planners must regard Canada and the United States as a single set of military targets no matter what political posture we might assume. Even in the unlikely event that the United States alone were at-tacked, geographic proximity and common interests would ensure that the effect on Canada would be devastating" (p. 10).

26. Interviews.

27. Melvin A. Conant, *The Long Polar Watch: Canada and the Defense of North America* (New York: Harper & Brothers, 1962), p. 432. Similarly the Defence White Paper 1987 states, "Canada's security in the broader sense is inseparable from that of Europe. There is nothing new in this reality. The presence of Canadian armed forces in Western Europe contributes directly to the defence of Canada, and, what is more ensures that we will have a say in how key security issues are decided."

28. Canadian Department of National Defence, *Defence 1981, Defence 1982*, (Ottawa: 1982 & 1983).

29. *Defence 1981*, p. 6.

30. Ibid., p. 8.

31. Joe Clark, *Power and Influence: The Making of an Active Foreign Policy* (Printed copy of speech given in Montreal, Quebec, 12 February 1986), p. 2.

32. Defence White Paper 1987, p. II.

33. Stanley W. Dzuiban, *Military Relations between the United States and Canada, 1939-1945* (Washington D.C.: U.S. Government Printing office, 1958), p. 3.

34. James Richardson, address given in Ottawa on 17 January 1975 (mimeographed), p. 15. In many ways the themes of this speech and the points outlined would be repeated in the Defence White Paper 1987. Thus the reemphasis on defense that the Conservatives heralded in their 1984 election campaign and manifested in the 1987 White Paper actually had its roots in 1975 in this speech by Richardson.

35. Ibid., pp. 3-4.

36. International Institute for Strategic Studies, *The Military Balance 1983-1984* (London: IISS, 1983), p. 145.

37. International Institute for Strategic Studies, *The Military Balance, 1985-1986*.

38. Defence White Paper 1987, p. 89. The two papers are essentially alike in the definition of the threat, the commitment to strategic and conventional deterrence, the perception of the critical importance of the European or NATO link, the rejection of any form of neutral option, and the statement of the four fundamental roles and the importance of arms control.

39. Defence White Paper 1987, p. ii.

40. Ibid., p. 49.

41. "Commitment-capability gap" refers to the fact that Canada does not have the capability to meet all of its worldwide commitments. "Rust Out" refers to the "unplanned and pervasive deterioration in the military capabilities of the Canadian Forces." See Defence White Paper 1987, chap. 6.

42. Quoted from a synopsis and summary of the Defence White Paper 1987.

43. These newspaper quotes are from an extensive analysis done by Canada Defence Information Service and contained in a special issue of *Press Roundup* 16/87 done on the Defence White Paper 1987. See this publication for a complete analysis of the media response.

44. For more information on this agreement, see Canada, Standing Committee on External Affairs and National Defence, *House of Commons Debates*, 3 October 1985.

45. From a mimeographed transcript of remarks by Prime Minister Brian Mulroney on 7 September 1985 in Ottawa.

46. Canada, Subcommittee on National Defence of the Standing Senate Committee on Foreign Affairs, *Canada's Maritime Defence* (Ottawa: Minister of Supply and Services, 1983), p. 27.

47. Nicholas Tracy, *Canada's Foreign Policy Objectives and Canadian Security Arrangements in the North*, ORAE Extra-Mural Paper No. 8 (Ottawa: Department of National Defence, 1980), p. 16.

48. For an interesting discussion of the sovereignty issue, see the following: Kevin McHugh, *The U.S.-Canadian Strategic Relationship: Canada's Commitment to Joint Defense*, ACSC Report #86–1680, 1986; Franklyn Griffiths, "Arctic Authority at Stake," *Toronto Globe and Mail*, 13 June 1985, p. 7; Armstrong, 1986; Mary Janigen, "A Secret Plan for Free Trade and Sovereignty," *Maclean's*, 11 November 1985, pp. 14–19; and Russ Laver, "A Secret Plan for Defending the North," *Maclean's*, 11 November 1985, pp. 20–21.

49. Senate Committee *Report on Maritime Defence*, pp. 34–35.

50. Newman, *True North*, p. 152.

51. J. Gilles Lamontagne, *Statement on Defence Policy*, March 1983.

52. See the SCEAND Report on the Report of the Standing Committee on External Affairs and National Defence, *NORAD 1986*, Minutes of Proceeding and Evidence of the Standing Committee First Session Thirty-Third Parliament 4th Report, chap. 2, for these and other figures. For example, eight-two Canadian officers are assigned to other NORAD facilities in the United States, and sixty-two Americans are assigned to NORAD installations in Canada. Data for the analysis that follows is drawn from the SCEAND Report, the Canadian Senate Report on *Canada's Territorial Air Defence*, January 1985, and interviews.

53. Canada, Senate, Special Committee of the Senate on National Defence, *Report on Military Air Transport* (Ottawa: Senate of Canada, 1986). In the foreword to the report, Senator Paul Lafond, committee chairman, writes, "Air Transport Group's fleet lacks numbers, is over-utilized, and suffers from increasing obsolescence." This is the fourth Senate report on the status of Canadian defense. The costs of implementing its recommendations are estimated by Senator Lafond to be C$3.8 billion, of which $1 billion would come from the DND budget. An increase in defense spending of 1 percent GNP (from 2.06 to 3.0) would be needed to fund the recommendations of all four reports.

54. John G. Halstead, "A Canadian View of NATO", at Johns Hopkins University, Washington D.C., 14 September 1983 presentation. Also see id., "Canada's Security in the 1980's: Options and Pitfalls," *Behind the Headlines* 41, no. 1 (1983).

55. Joe Clark, speech at the opening of the ministerial meeting of the North Atlantic Council, Halifax, 29 May 1986 (mimeographed), p. 1.

56. See Rod Byers, *Parliament and Defence Policy, Preparedness or Procrastination*, ed. Brian MacDonald (Canadian Institute of Strategic Studies, 1983), p. 70 and Paul Korning, "Role of Peacekeepers Now Proudest Tradition of Canadian Military," *The Globe and Mail*, September 30, 1988, p. A3.

57. Senate Subcommittee Report, 1983, p. 27.

58. For a more detailed explanation of transnational actors, see Robert Keohane and Joseph Nye, *Power and Interdependence: World Politics in Transition* (Boston: Little Brown, 1977).

59. James Eayrs, *Northern Approaches* (Toronto: Macmillan,1961), p. 3.

60. For a detailed discussion of these two offices, see *Apex of Power: The Prime Minister and Political Leadership in Canada*, ed. Thomas A. Hockin, 2d ed. (Toronto: Prentice Hall, 1977).

61. Both Trudeau and Mulroney wanted to increase the effectiveness and power of the cabinet system. If Trudeau did this by expanding the system, Mulroney has attempted to do it by streamlining the system. Mulroney realigned responsibilities, reduced the number of cabinet committees, consolidated several spending envelopes, and reduced and simplified the cabinet papers system. In addition, the ministries of state that had been created by Trudeau and abolished by Turner, his successor, were not reinstated. The latter were executive-type agencies to the cabinet and were under a minister of state who chaired one of the policy committees and was responsible for that policy envelope. Under Mulroney the functions of the ministries of state are now performed by the three traditional central agencies, which together are responsible for providing ministries and cabinet committees with required analytical and secretarial support. These central agencies are the following: the Treasury Board secretariat, which as the "chief accountant" monitors the status of the financial envelopes and the efficiency and management of existing programs and new proposals; the Privy Council Office, which emphasizes process facilitation and policy advice; and the Department of Finance, which is responsible for monitoring and assessing the impact of proposals on the overall economy. For a discussion of these Mulroney changes, see Ian Clark, *Recent Changes in the Cabinet System Decision-Making System*, Internal Publication of the Government of Canada, 3 December 1984.

62. Hockin, *Apex of power*, P. 203.

63. The Defence Council is the senior advisory body to the minister of national defence (MoD). Chaired by the MoD, its members include the deputy minister (DM), chief of defence staff (CDS), vice chief of defence staff (VCDS), the commanders of MARCOM, MOBCOM and AIRCOM, the assistant deputy minister of policy (ADM(POL)), and the deputy chief, defence staff (DCDS). Weekly meetings include intelligence and operations briefings, review of cabinet meetings and actions, briefings on current developments, and open discussions of current issues. In addition to Defence Council meetings, the DM or CDS periodically present special briefings to the minister, which normally are attended only by those involved in the issue under discussion. Furthermore, the DM and the CDS meet frequently in private sessions with the minister lasting a few minutes to a few hours. The Defence Management Committee (DMC) is co-chaired by the DM and the CDS. Its membership include the VCDS, the three environmental commanders, the DCDS, and each of the assistant deputy ministers. Meeting biweekly, the DMC reviews a wide variety of matters affecting the armed forces and matters requiring the minister's approval, such as new programs. The Armed Forces Council is chaired by the CDS; members include

the three commanders, the VCDS, the DCDS, and the ADM for personnel. Using an informal approach, and meeting at the call of the chairman or when the three functional commanders are in Ottawa, its agenda focuses on military matters affecting the armed forces primarily. It is the forum in which the commanders and senior staff officers provide policy advice to the CDS. Defence Minister Beatty has strengthened its role. See Lt. Col. D. L. Bland, "The Armed Forces Council and the Defence Policy Process," *Canadian Defence Quarterly* (Winter 1986–87): 26ff. A "Daily Executive Meeting" convenes at 0830 each day and is composed of the senior staff. Called the DEM, or daily prayers, it includes daily operations and intelligence briefings and discussions on issues for the day. Functional commanders are expected to attend if in Ottawa. The DEM is quite significant, for it reviews and sets the day-to-day agenda at the highest level in the Department of National Defence. The Program Control Board (PCB) is chaired by the VCDS; membership includes the ADMs for policy, personnel, matériel, and finance, the DCDS, and others in the acquisitions process. The PCB is responsible for allocation of resources and is as-,sisted by a series of subcommittees. Its recommendations go to the DMC and then to the Defence Council. The Audit and Program Evaluation Committee is the newest committee. Chaired by the VCDS, it is responsible for overseeing internal audits and program evaluations. It also reviews commanders' monthly operational readiness reports and the performance measurement system. It recommends follow-up action. For one of the most comprehensive analyses of the Canadian defense organization see Douglas Bland, *The Administration of Defence Policy in Canada 1947 to 1985* (Kingston, Ontario: Ronald and Frye Company, 1987).

64. See Defence White Paper 1987, p. 70, for more details.

65. Interviews.

66. Harvie Andres, speech to the Conference of Defence Associations, Ottawa, 10 January 1986 (mimeographed) p. 27.

67. *Ottawa Citizen*, 26 May 1986, p. A3.

68. Kim Richard Nossal, "On the Periphery: Interest Groups and Canadian Defence Policy in the 1970s," paper presented to Conference on Domestic Groups and Foreign Policy, Ottawa, 10–11 June 1982.

69. Ibid., p. 27.

70. Keohane and Nye, *Power and Intedependence*, p. 34.

71. For a detailed analysis of the unification process and the politics associated with it, see David P. Burke, "The Unification of the Armed Forces" *Revue Internationale d'Histoire Militaire*, no. 51, (1982); Vernon T. Kronenberg, *All Together Now: The Organization of*

the Department of National Defence In Canada, 1964–1972 (Toronto, 1973); DND, *Task Force on Review of Unification of the Canadian Armed Forces: Final Report* (Ottawa: Queen's Printer, 1980); and David P. Burke, "Canada Armed Forces Unification Revisited", paper presented at the International Studies Association Convention, Anaheim, Calif., 29 March 1986.

72. Canada, Department of National Defence, "Integration/Unification: A 1979 Perspective," paper prepared for the minister of defence, 1979, p. 15.

73. Business Council on National Issues, *Canada's Defence Policy: Capabilities versus Commitments*, September 1984, p. 54.

74. Interviews.

75. Allan Sullivan, ADM for Political and International Security Affairs, Department of External Affairs, testimony before House Standing Committee on External Affairs and National Defence, Minutes/Proceedings Thirty-third Parliament, 1984–85, 1st sess., issue no. 30, 1 October 1985, p. 30:10.

76. The ten principles that Trudeau hoped both East and West would accept included the following: agreement that a nuclear war cannot be won; agreement that a nuclear war must never be fought; desire to be free of the risk of accidental war or of surprise attack; recognition of the dangers inherent in destabilizing weapons; acceptance of the need for improved techniques of crisis management; awareness of consequences of being the first to use force; interest in increasing security while reducing cost; commitment to nuclear nonproliferation; recognition of each other's legitimate security interests; and realization that security strategies cannot be founded on the political or economic collapse of the other side. This "third track" approach of the prime minister made little impact and was seen by some as harming NATO solidarity. Within a few months of this peace initiative, Trudeau was out of office.

77. Douglas Roche, *Signals of Hope: Canada and the International Year of Peace*, address at conference, "Canada, the World, and the Future," University of Alberta, Edmonton, 10 March 1986, reproduced copy of speech, p. 6.

78. Ibid., p. 7.

79. Canada, Standing Committee on External Affairs and National Defence, Brief #26, p. 4.

80. Canada, Senate, Special Committee on National Defence, *Canada's Territorial Air Defence* (1985), p. 33.

81. Canada, Standing Committee on External Affairs and National Defence, Brief #63, p. 1.

82. Address by the Canadian CDS, General G.C.E. Theriault, to the CDA, 10 January 1986.

83. Canada, Standing Committee on External Affairs and National Defence, Brief #63, p. 5.

Part Four

EAST ASIA AND THE PACIFIC

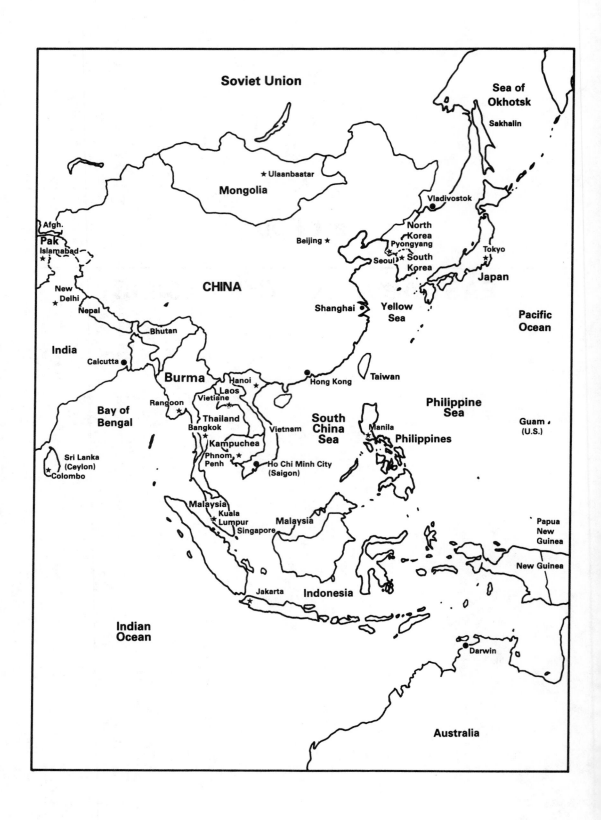

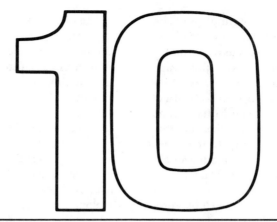

THE PEOPLE'S REPUBLIC OF CHINA

William R. Heaton, Jr.

Over the past decade there have been dramatic shifts in China's perceptions of the international environment and modernization requirements; government policies are increasingly reflecting these shifts. The architect of many of these changes, Deng Xiaoping, has characterized them as a "second revolution," which "is an unprecedented thing in China's history of thousands of years."[1] Military modernization may not have the same priority as other areas. Nevertheless, the Chinese consistently assert that achieving military modernization is very important, and they plan to devote considerable resources to it.

China's "second revolution" has significant implications for defense policy. While many of Deng's desired reforms have yet to be implemented fully, there have been fundamental changes in strategic thinking and organization. In other words, the politics of defense policy is now part of the "revolution." Among the key changes that will be considered in this chapter are: (1) China's shift from a policy of implicit strategic alignment with the United States and the West in the late 1970s and early 1980s to one of greater independence—though not actual equidistance—from the two superpowers; (2) China's new emphasis on modernization, which has led to the reform and revitalization of China's political institutions and corresponding reform of the economy which, in turn, has led to more rapid economic growth, greater emphasis on the development of science and technology, greater interaction with the West, and potentially increasing power and influence in East Asia; and (3) China's major restructuring of its armed forces with emphasis on creating a leaner and more professional military establishment.

International Environment

Chinese perceptions of the international environment are affected by historical experience, Marxist-Leninist ideology, and calculations of the balance of power. Each of these contributes to a composite view that is reflected in Chinese nationalism and in China's posture and behavior in the international community.

China's historical experience imparts the image of threat both from neighbors and distant powers. Traditional China was the "middle kingdom," surrounded by less sophisticated and usually less powerful civilizations. While there was much interaction with foreign cultures, the Chinese never seem to have developed a concept of equality with other races and civilizations. But neither did the Chinese seem to feel a particular need to reach out and civilize their neighbors. The Great Wall was built in an attempt to keep the barbarians out. The principal defense objective of the Chinese was to prevent invasion by the northern barbarians, a policy that might work for one or two centuries at a time but would ultimately fail, as the establishment of the non-Chinese dynasties attests. Beginning with the era of Western expansionism in the sixteenth century, but particularly in the nineteenth, China's perceptions of threat expanded to include Europe, America, and Japan.

The growth of modern Chinese nationalism was directly influenced by the West. Chinese leaders speak of a "century of humiliation" beginning with China's defeat by Britain in the Opium War in 1842 and an ensuing prolonged period of occupation, "unequal treaties," and foreign oppression. Westerners also brought industry and ideas, which, together with the bitterness, sowed the seeds of nationalism and revolution. The movements of Sun Yat-sen and the Kuomintang (Guomindang—the Chinese Nationalist Party) and even the Chinese communist movement had their origins in the onslaught of the West. Perhaps the success of the Chinese Communists over other political movements in China stems from their greater ability to harness this strong anti-foreign nationalism.

The desire to be secure against threat, domination, and humiliation by foreign countries, while true for all countries, is especially salient in China's case. China blames its own perceived economic and technological backwardness on foreign aggression. As former Party General Secretary Hu Yaobang told the British

Royal Institute of International Affairs in London in June 1986: "Having suffered untold hardships under foreign aggression and the scourge of repeated wars for more than a century, China has not yet completely lifted itself from poverty and backwardness."[2]

Given China's historical experience, it is not surprising that China's present leaders place a great deal of emphasis on independence and security. Hu, in a typical statement, told his London audience that "past experience tells us that if China attaches itself to or enters into alliance with a certain big power, it will not only be subjected to the control of others, unable to hold its own destiny, but also jeopardize its own development to the detriment of world peace and stability. Therefore, we are determined to remain independent in our foreign relations."[3]

China's historical legacy has contributed to the strong desire among China's leaders to secure territorial integrity, to modernize and strengthen the economic and social system, and to build national power. Chinese leaders have disagreed and even waged struggle over how these goals should be achieved, but the goals themselves remain paramount.

The historical legacy also represents a profound paradox for Chinese perceptions. While China has feared, resented, and even hated the West (and Japan), China has also admired and learned from the West. In many respects, modern Chinese history may be conceived as the struggle by China to cope with the West. From the time of the self-strengthening movement of the late Qing dynasty to the contemporary reforms of the Chinese Communists, Chinese leaders have been trying to find ways to adopt Western technology and methods without accepting Western values. It has not been an easy path. With respect to the modernization of defense, for example, many of the same issues that faced Chinese reformers in the 1860s also confront Chinese reformers today.[4]

In addition to historical images that color Chinese perceptions, the role of Marxist-Leninist-Maoist ideology should not be underestimated. Chinese communist theoreticians assert that Mao's contribution was to "integrate the universal principles of Marxism-Leninism with the concrete practice of the Chinese revolution."[5] Maoist ideology—like any other extensive body of official dogma—is reinterpreted by the leadership in accordance with existing policy. During Mao's lifetime, he and his supporters emphasized rapid social change of the variety epitomized by the Cultural Revolution. Mao's successors now discredit the Cultural Revolution, but cite Maoist principles to explain their own approach, which includes capitalist-style economic incentives that Mao would likely have abhorred.

Chinese leaders argue that they will continue to adhere to socialism whatever the course of political and economic reform. Their ideological worldview has resulted in a strong rejection of what they term Western-style democracy. An authoritative "Commentator" article in the Party theoretical journal *Hongqi* (Red Flag) put it this way:

> Socialist democracy is not capitalist democracy nor individualistic democracy but a democracy for the majority of people. It can be separated neither from dictatorship over our enemies nor from centralism based on democracy. . . . We should not . . . pursue capitalist liberalization. Pursuing capitalist liberalization in our country is equal to following the capitalist road, which will inevitably do great damage to the political situation of stability and unity and the four modernizations program.[6]

The idea that "only socialism can save China" underwrites an essentially authoritarian (some would argue, totalitarian) political system. Chinese perceptions of the international system reflect their own system of government. The desire to build ties with communist and socialist parties in other countries, and even a continuing desire to maintain "moral and spiritual ties" with illegal communist insurgencies in southeast Asia are only one manifestation of this system. With respect to defense policy, the adherence to Maoist dicta on "people's war" in developing strategy is another manifestation of the powerful influence of ideological precepts.

Chinese perceptions are further influenced by calculations of the balance of power. China perceives itself to be a very large, but economically weak, Third World developing country, geopolitically located to be both a continental and sea power. It is a tribute to China's ability to manipulate the symbols and psychology of

power that when both the Soviet Union and the United States were trying to draw China into their respective systems of security relations, China, "through careful consideration, drawing lessons, and summing up experience," decided to "adhere to its basic principles of independence, safeguarding peace, nonalignment, seeking no hegemony, and opposing both big and small hegemonism."[7]

Chinese calculations of the balance of power, as expressed in official statements, have undergone noticeable shifts over the past few years. During the Cultural Revolution China's posture toward both superpowers was one of strong hostility; China also strongly endorsed revolutionary struggle in developing countries. In the 1970s China shifted to a position of alignment, though not alliance, with the West, calling for a "united front" against Soviet hegemonism, a policy that reached its high point in the late 1970s and early 1980s. Since the early 1980s, Chinese statements have shifted once again. China's present orientation was well expressed by former Premier Zhao Ziyang's report on government work at the fourth session of the Sixth National People's Congress in March 1986, which stated that China's ten basic principles of foreign policy include the provision that "China will never attach itself to any superpower, or enter into alliance or strategic relations with either of them. China continues to seek the steady development of Sino–U.S. relations on the basis of strict adherence to the principles established in the joint communiques between China and the United States, and a true improvement in Sino-Soviet relations through the removal of . . . obstacles by concrete actions."[8]

In summary, Chinese perceptions of the international environment are a composite of unique historical, ideological, and statecraft factors, which may be stated fundamentally as follows: (1) China has an historical mandate to reclaim its pride and honor in the international community after a long period of humiliation. Modernization is a prerequisite to gaining the power necessary to fulfill this mandate. China prefers to avoid war, and believes a period of peace and stability is necessary if it is to accomplish modernization. (2) In the Chinese view, the world is evolving from a bipolar to a multipolar system. This gives China greater opportunities and flexibility in achieving modernization. (3) China's modernization requires extensive ties with the West, particularly in economic, scientific, and technological areas, but China feels more akin to Third World developing countries with socialist orientations than with modernized capitalist systems. (4) While an underlying sentiment that peace and stability require socialism will remain at the core of Beijing's worldview, China will shift and adjust its policies according to its perceived interests, with the primary goal being independence from outside powers and freedom from entangling alliances or other entangling relations.

National Objectives, National Strategy, and Military Doctrine

China shares with other nations the fundamental objectives of securing its borders from attack, establishing domestic order, and securing a better life for its citizens. It shares with other communist systems the objective of maintaining the rule of the Communist Party. But China is perhaps unique in that in one decade many of its fundamental policies for achieving these objectives have been dramatically reversed.

Officially, Chinese objectives are expressed in their formulation of "four modernizations"—agriculture, industry, science and technology, and national defense. But the most important "modernization" is that of the political system. Since the third plenum of the eleventh Central Committee in December 1978, the event the Chinese Communists hail as the beginning of their "second revolution," there has been a significant overhaul of the leadership. The Chinese are rapidly moving away from the charismatic style of Mao's rule toward a much more institutionalized and bureaucratic system. People recruited for political office are judged on the basis of expertise, particularly in science and technology, rather than on more abstract ideological constructs. Older

leaders are gradually being retired and new leadership promoted.

In the economy, Maoist strictures about the elimination of inequality and the promotion of "self-reliance" have given way to capitalist-style market incentives that allow some to get rich. The introduction of "responsibility systems" in rural areas has resulted in an economic boom that has fueled a much more rapid growth of the economy. There has also been some easing of restrictions on cultural expression. While many of these policies have proven controversial among the leadership, there can be no question but that they have substantially affected China's growth and prosperity.

Thus, China is hopeful that it can continue to maintain conditions that will allow it to continue to modernize. According to official pronouncements, the greatest danger to China's progress, and to the world in general, stems from the confrontation and rivalry of the United States and the Soviet Union.[9] Arguing that China requires a long period of peace in order to achieve modernization, Chinese leaders assert that it is, therefore, necessary to reject the manipulation of the superpowers. Chinese leaders point to their own diplomatic achievements over the past several years as examples of how national objectives can be achieved through peaceful means.

For example, Chinese leaders claim that the successful negotiations with Britain for the return of Hong Kong to Chinese control in 1997 were a major achievement in the goal of national reunification. Negotiations with Portugal over Macao yielded similar results. They argue that this approach should also be useful in achieving reunification with Taiwan, but they have not renounced the use of force in the Taiwan case.[10]

Chinese formal pronouncements assign hegemonism of either superpower equally odious status, but Chinese behavior, in fact, indicates greatest concern with the Soviet threat. Nevertheless, there have been significant changes in the Chinese approach to this threat. In the late 1970s and early 1980s China actively called for a "united front against hegemonism," which essentially called for joining with the West against the Soviet Union. The Soviet invasion of Afghanistan and support for the Vietnamese invasion of Cambodia were deemed direct threats to Chinese regional interests. Additionally, the rapid growth of Soviet military power in East Asia and the Pacific increased the threat to China's security.

But in the early 1980s this "united front" approach began to be modified according to China's more independent stance. Changes in China's approach may be attributed to several factors. Chinese public commentary suggested that Soviet internal problems lessened the threat to China. Among these were the failing Soviet economy and a changing Soviet leadership. Additionally, the Soviet Union was overextended with problems in Poland and Afghanistan and would not threaten China. Another reason may have been a Chinese perception that the military buildup of the Reagan administration in the Pacific, independent of Chinese overtures for a united front, would act as a check on overt Soviet aggression. Moreover, problems over Taiwan and other issues with the United States caused some internal dissention among Chinese leaders and seemed to preclude close, cooperative security relations with the United States.

The new Chinese approach has been to offer an improvement in economic and cultural relations with the USSR, and to reduce greatly the level of hostile rhetoric, but without abandoning its three conditions for a restoration of normal relations. China insisted that the Soviets agree to withdraw forces from Afghanistan and cease support of the Vietnamese occupation of Cambodia. Under Gorbachev, the Soviet Union has continued to improve the tone of its relations with China, and trade and cultural exchanges have been expanded. In a significant speech in Vladivostok in August 1986, the Soviet general secretary offered to withdraw some Soviet forces from Mongolia as a means of improving ties with China. Deng responded that a more serious issue for the Chinese was the Cambodia problem and demanded greater Soviet concessions on this issue. The Soviet decision to withdraw some

troops from Mongolia and all troops from Afghanistan, along with the Vietnamese announcement of withdrawal from Cambodia, paved the way for a Sino-Soviet summit in 1989. Nevertheless, in coming years, the two sides will continue to differ on some issues.

There is likely to be no return to the kind of cooperative ties between China and the USSR that existed in the early 1950s. Chinese leaders have expressly disavowed this possibility. Constant reminders of who constitutes the most serious threat to China's security are improvements in Soviet military capabilities, including expansion of the Pacific Fleet, upgrading Soviet capabilities and facilities at Cam Ranh Bay in Vietnam, and (prior to U.S.–Soviet agreement in 1987 for the removal of all INF missiles on a global basis) the stationing of SS-20s east of the Urals.

In spite of improving ties, the Soviet political challenge to China is substantial. Besides forging an alliance with Vietnam and supporting Vietnam's invasion of Cambodia, the USSR has developed good relations with Chinese adversaries such as India. More recently, the Soviet Union has decided to export more modern weapons to North Korea and has with some success begun to woo Pyongyang from Beijing's orbit. While the Chinese express confidence that they can withstand these various kinds of pressures from the USSR, there will be lingering suspicion and hostility toward Moscow's perceived attempts to limit China's influence and prestige.[11]

As has been repeatedly stated by Chinese leaders, they not only hope to avoid war in order to devote more resources to modernization, but also to base the modernization of national defense on improvements in the other three of the "four modernizations." The People's Liberation Army (PLA), for example, is expected to make a substantial contribution to modernization in other areas. According to Monte Bullard and Edward O'Dowd: "The PLA's economic role now provides very concrete support to the modernization of the Chinese economy."[12]

Since the mid 1980s, national strategy and military doctrine have received increased public attention in China. For example, in July 1986 Chinese media reported that a "Seminar on National Defense Strategy for the Year 2000 and Systems Engineering" had been convened in Beijing, with over one hundred experts from the military services and civilian community participating. This type of gathering is apparently unprecedented. Reports from the conference indicated that participants debated the nature of the international system (bipolar or multipolar), the relevance of Western strategic concepts for China, the influence of economics, and other relevant subjects. One journal suggested that such conferences "may become a new form of providing consultative services to the leadership for policy making."[13]

Officially, Chinese military doctrine is termed "people's war." Its precepts were developed in the 1930s and broadened through experience gained in fighting the Japanese and in the Chinese civil war. In the mid 1960s, Lin Biao argued that the "people's war" idea was relevant to all Third World countries struggling for liberation. Depending on one's point of view, the popular image created by the Maoist legacy was either one of small handfuls of guerrillas struggling for victory against a vastly superior foe or one of hordes of foot soldiers sweeping down to overwhelm a technologically superior smaller force. In fact, the reality of "people's war" was considerably more complex. The basic problem Mao faced was how to defeat an enemy objectively stronger than China, a problem still relevant to Chinese strategy and doctrine today.

According to one view, "people's war" is a "broad outlook rather than a particular plan," which is not limited war but a total mobilization approach. Central to the concept is its resort to mobilization, protraction, and its defensive flavor.[14] In 1978 then Chinese Defense Minister Xu Xiangqian observed that in any likely future conflict China would confront an enemy possessing superior military technology and better arms. China would wage a war of attrition, and "everyone will be a soldier, every village a fortress and every place a battlefield." Chinese forces would defend key points, would prevent enemy forces from moving into Chinese territory unchecked, and would systemat-

ically lead them to battlefields of Chinese choice to wipe them out piecemeal. Such a protracted conflict would gradually change the balance of forces between China and its enemies.[15]

In fact, one of the striking features of contemporary Chinese defense policy is that, in spite of major revisions of Chinese perceptions of the international system and in China's methods for achieving its strategy of modernization, basic Chinese strategy and doctrine concerning the total nature of warfare have changed very little. Most observers agree that this central feature of "people's war" has remained fairly consistent. The addition of "under modern conditions" has to do primarily with how and where battles will be fought and the quality of the forces by which the war will be conducted. According to one group of Chinese academics studying strategy, "the successful historical experience of using 'millet plus rifles to defeat the enemy's aircraft and artillery' is no longer an eternal truth under all circumstances."[16]

Paul Godwin observes that the strategic revisions that have occurred in the past few years are designed to disrupt and defeat a Soviet invasion of China before it can achieve deep penetration. The Chinese have decided to defend their cities rather than surrender them to invading forces in order to maintain freedom of maneuver. This fundamental revision of traditional Maoist strategy requires that Chinese planners now give greater attention to military operations that will be successful in the early stages of a war. Chinese exercises over the past few years indicate a commitment to a more forward defense of China, especially in the industrial areas of the northeast.[17]

The addition of the principle of "under modern conditions" has also had the effect of increasing the role of military professionals in the formulation of strategy; this is probably why there is now increasing emphasis on "active defense" (rather than letting in invaders so as to "swallow them in a people's war") and a greater emphasis on combined arms. Ellis Joffe and Gerald Segal argue that those doctrinal modifications have already begun to produce results that would greatly raise the costs to any potential attacker.[18] Harlan Jenks, in a review of the relations between Chinese doctrine and the actual threat, observes that there are strong implications for weapons systems modernization. Specifically, China must develop improved air and air defense systems; reliable, survivable nuclear second strike capabilities; forces capable of conducting forward defense of land and sea frontiers; and Command and Control Communications and Intelligence (C³I) systems.[19] Paul Godwin agrees that a modernization of military technology is necessary in the "people's war under modern conditions" context, but also points out that severe limitations and constraints in resources will be an impediment to weapons modernization, and that, therefore, traditional doctrines are likely to have considerable staying power.[20] It is also significant to note that since the founding of the People's Republic of China, weapons modernization has always had a high priority, no matter what the composition of the leadership or particular ideological campaign at any given time. The high priority given to national defense industries and nuclear weapons, not to mention the development of aircraft, tanks, and a full range of other weapons, bears ample testimony to the Chinese commitment to weapons modernization. China may lag behind the West and the Soviet Union in technological applications, but there can be no question about the tremendous resources expended to maintain and improve military capabilities.

Further evidence of this modernization is China's gradual development of a "blue water" naval capability. The PLA navy has begun conducting port calls with neighboring countries in an effort to "show the flag" and has conducted passing exercises with the U.S. Navy. Chinese naval vessels were also involved in the ICBM tests in the Pacific in 1980. Additionally, China is expanding its SSBN capability.

The impact of modernization of strategy is also reflected in various Chinese commentaries on strategy. In February 1986, for example, Li Desheng, former commander of the Shenyang Military Region and now political commissar of China's new National Defense University, spoke on the need to change Chinese strategy

in accordance with the evolution of the world situation. Li stated that China must switch from a strategy of "fighting an early, major, and nuclear war" to a strategy of "building a regularized and modernized revolutionary army during a period of peace." Li characterized this shift as "fundamental."[21]

Also relevant to national strategy and military doctrine is the Chinese calculus of deterrence. Allen Whiting's study of the Chinese use of force summarizes the Chinese approach thus:

1. The worse our [Chinese] domestic situation, the more likely our external situation will worsen.
   a. A superior power in proximity will seek to take advantage of our domestic vulnerability.
   b. Two or more powers will combine against us if they can temporarily overcome their own conflict of interest.
   c. We must prepare for the worst and try for the best.
2. The best deterrence is belligerence.
   a. To be credible, move military force; words do not suffice.
   b. To be diplomatic, leave the enemy "face" and a way out.
   c. To be prudent, leave yourself an "option."
   d. If at first you don't succeed, try again, but more so.
3. Correct timing is essential.
   a. Warning must be given early when a threat is perceived but not yet imminent.
   b. The rhythm of signals must permit the enemy to respond and us to confirm the situation.
   c. We must control our moves and not respond according to the enemy's choice.[22]

Steve Chan, applying the concept of "coercive diplomacy" developed by Alexander George, has examined the use of military force by China. Five distinct phases of Chinese action were found: (1) probing, (2) warning, (3) demonstration, (4) attack, and (5) détente. Chan also found that the Chinese emphasize centralization of the decision-making process, so that local commanders are prohibited from carrying out actions without central approval.[23] A study by Edward Ross of China's "defensive counterattack" against Vietnam in 1979 indicates that China followed similar patterns there.[24] China's armed forces continue to put pressure on the Vietnamese border and also challenge the Vietnamese navy over islands in the South China Sea. In the spring of 1987 China warned India that building tensions could produce an armed clash, though both sides seemed to want to avoid such a clash. Consequently, whether or not China's "calculus of deterrence" will be modified remains to be seen.

An important component of China's strategy and doctrine has to do with nuclear weapons. During the Maoist period Chinese propaganda disparaged the applicability of nuclear weapons, calling the "atom bomb of Mao's thought" more powerful than the nuclear weapons of the reactionaries and the revisionists. Some Chinese leaders also claimed that China would be much more able to survive a nuclear attack than other countries. Nevertheless, as Jonathan Pollack has pointed out: "No Chinese military program was accorded a higher priority during the 1960s than the acquisition of an independent nuclear deterrent."[25]

The Chinese continue to place a high premium on the development of nuclear weapons. According to the International Institute of Strategic Studies in London, China has deployed six ICBMs, sixty IRBMs, and fifty MRBMs. It is also testing and will soon deploy two Xia-class SSBNs, each of which may have sixteen launch tubes.[26] William Tow, citing various Western analysts, states that by the end of the century the Chinese could have about 150 strategic nuclear delivery vehicles with multiple, independently targeted warheads.[27] The Chinese have also conducted maneuvers involving the simulated use of tactical nuclear weapons.[28]

The importance China attaches to its nuclear deterrent is reflected in its leaders' denunciations of the U.S. Strategic Defense Initiative (SDI). Chinese statements condemn SDI on the basis that it will provoke a new arms race between the superpowers. Privately, however, Chinese strategists express their real concern that SDI would potentially undermine China's own nuclear deterrent. Though China would like to benefit from technological spinoffs from SDI research, it is likely that it will continue to oppose any move toward deployment of SDI.

Concerning national objectives, strategy, and doctrine, we may conclude that: (1) China will likely continue to strive to build its power and prestige, particularly in the region. China

will view the Soviet Union as its primary adversary. (2) Chinese strategy accepts that major war is unlikely and that China has time to devote resources to the economic foundation upon which military power is predicted. China will modernize both its nuclear and conventional forces as resources permit. (3) China's doctrine of "people's war under modern conditions" will be maintained; gradual defense modernization will not cause this concept to be abandoned, but it will be flexibly interpreted as incremental improvements in force posture occur.

The Defense Decision-Making Process

In recent years, considerable light has been shed on how decisions are made in China. The substantial reform and reorganization of the Party and government bureaucracies have permitted more insights into what goes on, though in many areas we still have little information.

Unlike in most Western countries, where there has been a sharp separation of civil and military authority, the distinction in China is blurred. The development of Chinese communism was inexorably linked with its military power. The communist leaders fuse civil and military roles. Consequently, defense decision making in China must be broadly construed.

Defense decisions are ultimately Party decisions. From the 1930s, when Mao stated that "political power grows out of the barrel of a gun" and that "the Party must always control the gun; the gun must never be allowed to control the Party," Chinese leaders have remained acutely aware of the relations between political power and military force. Like Mao, Deng Xiaoping has written extensively on the role of the military; while Deng has retired from other formal positions in China, he retains the chairmanship of the Party Central Committee Military Commission (CMC), suggesting the importance of this role.

The political reforms initiated by Deng and carried out since 1978 seek to replace the charismatic style of Mao with a more institutionalized and legal style. The position of Party chairman was abolished in 1983 and the office of general secretary established. Other reforms such as the creation of an Advisory Council, the reorganization of the Central Committee, the restructuring of the State Council, and a host of other changes have been implemented. In an effort to reform defense decision making, Deng pushed for the establishment of a State Military Commission that would take over some of the responsibilities of the CMC, though the membership of the new State Military Commission was identical. Thus far, the new commission does not appear to have assumed its intended role, though eventually it could become influential.

Not only are these institutions undergoing reform, but the leadership is also changing. Deng is trying to push Party elders into retirement and establish mechanisms for orderly succession. He has been successful in getting many older leaders to retire, and several younger people are being groomed for future leadership. As part of the reform several Politburo members whose primary careers have been military have been retired. This raises the potential that the military will have less voice in future policy decisions.

While the Politburo retains ultimate decision authority, Deng himself has the final word on issues of his choosing. He chairs both the party and state military commissions. In an effort undertaken in the fall of 1987 to strengthen the PLA command and control authority and to prepare for the eventual succession to Deng, the 13th Party Congress named Party General Secretary Zhao Ziyang the "First Vice Chairman" of the Party Military Commission. Since that time, Zhao has become more involved in military matters.

The government organs most directly relevant to defense policy making are the Ministry of Defense (MND) and the Commission on Science, Technology, and Industry for National Defense (NDSTIC). Little is known about the MND, though its former head, Zhang Aiping, was widely known as a strong proponent of defense modernization. Qin Jiwei, former commander of the Beijing Military Region, replaced Zhang in 1988. Under Qin, an expansion was expected beyond the MND's traditional role of budgeting, training, and in-

dustrial coordination and planning.[29] One section, the Foreign Affairs Bureau, usually has served as point of contact between the PLA and foreign military representatives. According to some accounts, however, it often acts more as a barrier than as a conduit. The NDSTIC has the unenviable task of overseeing the defense research and development effort as well as presiding over the often cumbersome and unwieldy overlapping bureaucracies that deal with defense.[30]

Apart from the formal structures by which decisions are made and implemented, however, there are informal processes. There is a tendency in the Western media to lump Chinese leaders into two groups, conservatives and moderates. These categorizations are inherited from earlier analysis. During the Cultural Revolution, the Chinese categorized leaders into two types: revolutionaries and counterrevolutionaries. Some Western observers, apparently influenced by the Chinese categories, decided that the revolutionaries were radicals and the counterrevolutionaries were moderates. With the victory of Deng and his supporters at the third plenum in 1978 the new dichotomy that emerged was between the reformers, or moderates, and the conservatives.

According to this analysis, the reformers want more rapid change while the conservatives are not anxious to move rapidly, fearing that Party authority will be undercut. When applied to defense decision making, this analysis suggests that the reformers want rapid modernization, professionalization among the armed forces, a more rigid bifurcation between civil and military institutions, a repudiation of Maoist ideological principles dealing with the armed forces, and other key changes. The conservatives believe that Mao's teaching on maintaining strong links between the army and the masses is vital and that overly rapid professionalization poses some risks to maintaining these links. They also believe that the armed forces should retain a prominent voice in cultural expression, a view generally rejected by the reformers. Moreover, conservatives are afraid morale in the military will be undermined if reforms such as retiring senior officers and eliminating their privileges are adopted.[31]

The conservative-reformer dichotomy is somewhat useful in understanding divisions among the leadership on some issues, but it is not the whole story. The essence of Chinese policy making is *guanxi*, the network of personal loyalties and ties that pervades decision-making structures. People are promoted into leadership roles not because of their consensus on policy questions, but because of their personal ties. For example, there is strong evidence that Hu Yaobang took exception to some of Deng Xiaoping's policies, yet as Deng's protégé, he was promoted to high level positions. One of the charges made against Hu that contributed to his removal was that he was overly zealous in promoting his protégés to higher level positions. Other senior leaders have their own *guanxi* networks in the Party. Thus, the making of defense policy reflects both personal loyalty networks and diverging views.[32]

A review of strategy and policy decisions over the years suggests that informal coalitions develop and change as leaders change. As was noted previously, much of the debate since the founding of the PRC has been over how to deal with the superpowers, and this debate has been associated with the formation of groups.[33] Since the third plenum of the eleventh Central Committee in 1978, Deng Xiaoping and his reform coalition have largely held the upper hand, though there have been compromises and shifts. Between 1978 and 1982, Deng concentrated on removing from power those leaders, including Party Chairman Hua Guofeng, who were most closely associated with Mao's approach. During that period, policy shifted from close cooperation with the United States on security issues to greater divergence, probably because of differences with the United States on Taiwan. In the view of some, Deng was willing to discard his previous flexibility on Taiwan and take a firmer line toward the United States because he needed greater support for his domestic policies.[34]

Since 1982 Deng and his supporters have continued to press for reform, but have been opposed on occasion by some other senior Party leaders, and have continued to make compromises. Concerning defense policy issues, this has resulted in some apparent incongruities. For example, while China and the United States were in the process of working out some military technological transfers and sales to China, the Chinese blocked a port call by U.S. naval vessels in 1985 because of the U.S. policy of neither confirming nor denying the presence of nuclear weapons on the vessels. The decision to obstruct the visit reflected internal debate over defense relations with the United States. The difficulty Deng has had in arranging for his succession as chairman of the Military Commission is another example of internal division.

The central point to be made here is that security policy decisions are influenced by the forces at work in the broader political spectrum. Over the past decade the principal trend in China has been a move by Deng and his reformist supporters to overhaul the entire system. This has resulted in struggles for power and influence and consequent turns and twists in Chinese policy, but with the main trend being gradual success by the reformers. With this perspective in mind, it is now useful to consider what some of the key decisions have been.

REFORM AND MODERNIZATION

Besides the broad strategic issues discussed above, the principal focus of defense decision making has been the modernization of the People's Liberation Army. The principal goals of the reformers have been: (1) making the armed forces a more effective fighting force by enhancing professionalism; (2) reducing the size of and consolidating the armed forces so as to make them leaner and less costly; (3) improving technological capabilities so as to upgrade weaponry and improve combat capabilities; and (4) enhancing ideological and political training in the armed forces so as to insure adherence to Party leadership by the troops.

With respect to professionalization, decisions made by the reformers are beginning to have a profound effect. In the years since 1982, a series of steps have been taken to reduce the political role of the armed forces. At the Party Congress of Delegates in 1985, for example, seven senior members of the Politburo who were career military officers resigned. At the

13th Chinese Communist Party (CCP) Congress in the fall of 1987 only two career officers remained on the Politburo, Vice-Chairman of the Central Military Commission Yang Shangkun (who was elected President of the PRC in April 1988), and Qin Jiwei, former commander of the Beijing Military Region who became defense minister in April 1988. Even more military leaders resigned from the Central Committee, reducing military representation on that body to a new low of around 16 percent; this compares with a high point of slightly over 50 percent in 1969 and 22 percent in 1982. These actions underscored the reformers' intentions of making it clear that the military would be subordinate to the political leadership. Undoubtedly, many key military leaders supported the decision to reduce the PLA's role, favoring increased military professionalism over the heavy involvement in politics now seen as a burdening legacy of the Cultural Revolution.

The system of military education, devastated during the Cultural Revolution, is also being rehabilitated. Beginning with the newly created National Defense University at the top, down to basic level training for soldiers, new emphasis is being placed on military training and education.[35] Educational requirements are being implemented for officers, and a separate noncommissioned officer corps is being established. Much more emphasis is being placed on technological and managerial skills, and promotions are being made contingent on their mastery by military personnel. The question of restoring military ranks, which were abolished in 1965, was strongly debated and was repeatedly postponed, possibly because deciding who should get what rank was overly controversial. Rank and insignia were finally restored in 1988. Additionally, the noncommissioned officer (NCO) corps, abolished in 1964, was restored in 1986, and a number of the military academies began training NCOs. As part of the move for professionalization, new research institutes are being developed to study strategy, technology, research and development, and other features of modern defense.[36]

There have been fundamental changes in the size and organization of the armed forces.

Beginning in the early 1980s a series of reforms were begun to reduce the size of the armed forces. In 1982 the Railway Engineer Corps and the Capital Construction Corps were transferred from the PLA to local administration, reducing PLA size by 500,000. Subsequently, various local forces and troops garrisoning the frontiers or under different garrison commands previously considered to be part of the PLA were transferred to local administrations, local frontier guards, garrison divisions, and the People's Armed Police. In 1985 it was announced that the PLA would reduce its size by one million personnel, or about 25 percent of its overall strength, over a two-year period. A year later several articles said that the troop cuts were proceeding ahead of schedule. A report in January 1986, for example, said that 800,000 troops had been demobilized, and also indicated that half of the one million troops being demobilized were officers.[37]

The cuts in size corresponded with a major reorganization. All service arms with the exception of the strategic missile forces (formerly the 2nd Artillery), were incorporated into the General Staff Department, thus reducing the command organs of the different service arms. The number of military regions was reduced from a total of eleven to seven to streamline organization and make more weapons available in each area. The right to command service arms was transferred from the center to military regions. For example, tank units under the Armored Force Command were placed under the military regional commands while the Armored Force Command was converted to a department under the General Staff Department.[38] Additionally, the field army system has been abolished, and the PLA's main force units have been converted to group armies consisting of the various arms of service.[39] According to various accounts, this will enable PLA commanders to conduct combined arms operations more effectively. Moreover, the reductions have actually resulted in better-armed troops in sensitive areas such as along the Sino-Soviet border.

Chinese sources claim that manpower reductions and reorganization have enabled cuts in the defense budget to be made. China's official news agency said the defense budget had been cut from 22.7 billion yuan (about U.S. $7 billion) in 1979 to 19.1 billion (around U.S. $6 billion) in the mid 1980s. In 1985, for example, defense expenditure amounted to 10.5 percent of the budget, whereas in 1979 it had amounted to 17.5 percent.[40]

In spite of budget cuts, a continuing effort is being made to improve the PLA's technological base and to acquire more modern weapons. As noted above, considerable resources have been devoted to continuing modernization of the strategic nuclear forces.[41] Additionally, China is gradually improving its conventional weapons, with particular emphasis on antitank defense and air defense.[42] A communist newspaper in Hong Kong reported in 1986 that China had begun to employ a new automatic 5.56-mm rifle similar to the M-16, new grenade launchers, several new armored personnel carriers, new tanks, missiles, and aircraft. It also said China was developing new naval vessels, including a small "aircraft carrier."[43] Some of the technology is being acquired from abroad. For example, the United States has announced a program to provide avionics for China's F-8 aircraft and has conducted negotiations with the Chinese on other systems. European countries have also agreed to provide weapons and technology for China. The problems of technology transfer are complex, however. Chinese leaders have repeatedly stated that they do not have the inclination or resources to spend huge sums on foreign weapons. China has attempted to "reverse engineer" some systems with mixed success. ("Reverse engineering" amounts to acquiring a technical system and then trying to reproduce it domestically by breaking it into its components. It is a form of technology transfer, although not usually intended by the provider of the technical system.) Also, some technology transfers—such as those entailed in improving the F-7 aircraft (similar to the MiG-21), and the T-59 tank—are designed primarily to improve the prospect of selling them to other countries.

The acquisition of foreign technology, together with organizational reform throughout China's bureaucracy, has contributed to a reorganization of the weapons acquisition process.

A large and cumbersome weapons bureaucracy has been somewhat reduced, with six ministries of machine building now responsible for most military construction. These ministries are organized vertically, much as in the Soviet system, and answer to the State Council, the Ministry of Defense, and the Commission for Defense Science, Technology, and Industry.

China has entered the international arms market in a major way and earns substantial foreign exchange from weapons sales. As China improves education and training and creates better conditions for the military's ability to absorb technology, technological enhancement of weaponry will continue.[44]

A significant policy decision also has been to divert defense industry production to the consumer sector. In 1978 Deng Xiaoping ordered that defense industries "switch to the production of civilian products without affecting the army." By the late 1980s as much as 50 percent of the value of production by these industries was in civilian goods. Premier Zhao Ziyang argued that since the defense industry had received the state's best scientific and technical resources, it should make a greater contribution to the nation by producing civilian products.[45] An article in *Beijing Review* noted that several defense industries were making major contributions to the economy. The Ministry of Ordnance Industry, responsible for guns, cannons, and munitions, was producing over seven hundred products, including bicycles, cameras, refrigerators, washing machines, and sewing machines. It produced half of the country's motorcycles.[46] At the same time it exported goods worth U.S. $100 million between 1980 and 1985 and planned to increase this to $400 million over the remainder of the decade.[47]

Though technically part of education and training, the improvement of political and ideological indoctrination in the PLA deserves special treatment. It is the nature of communist systems that political reliability in the armed forces assumes a special significance, and in the PLA, political reliability has been a fundamental issue. The PLA General Political Department, responsible for the political commissar system throughout the PLA, has shown signs of obstructionism vis-à-vis some of Deng's reform efforts in the past. The director of the General Political Department (GPD), Wei Guoching, was replaced by Yu Qiuli shortly after the Twelfth Party Congress in September 1982, and various publications produced by the GPD, including the *Liberation Army Daily* (Jiefangjun Bao), were reorganized.[48] Yu has devoted particular attention to seeing to it that political indoctrination in the PLA supports modernization goals. At one forum, for example, he stated that raising the political consciousness of PLA officers would enable them to master advanced science and technology while fostering "a sense of national pride and self-confidence in the future of our country and the cause of communism."[49] In early 1987 the PLA was praised for not succumbing to "bourgeois liberalism," but the *Liberation Army Daily* stressed the need for the army's constant vigilance against such tendencies. Yu was replaced as head of the GPD by Yang Baibing, brother of PRC President Yang Shangkun, just after the 13th CCP Congress in the fall of 1987.

There are, of course, many other areas of defense decision making that could be explored. But the modernization question has become the essence of the process of allocating scarce resources. It is likely, moreover, that allocation of scarce resources will continue to complicate the process of defense modernization well into the 1990s. Decisions over professionalism, reorganization, improved weapons, and ideological indoctrination will be both necessary and difficult and will essentially determine China's capabilities for the remainder of this century.

Recurring Issues and Defense Policy Outputs

The previous discussion of modernization suggests that China's military posture and capabilities are in a state of flux. With this in mind, we can consider some present features of the organization of the armed forces and force posture.

The People's Liberation Army includes ground, air, and naval forces. Its size is being reduced to about 3 to 3.5 million; it is one of the world's largest military forces, yet quite small in relation to China's approximately 1.1 billion people. A revised military service law enacted by the National People's Congress in the mid 1980s established universal obligation for service, but only a small percentage of China's youth actually serve. A decade ago, service in the PLA was highly esteemed and sought after: military service offered prospects for social mobility. This is no longer true. Because of low pay, morale problems, and greater civilian opportunities, most young people would prefer to avoid military service.

Command and control authority over the PLA originates in the Central Military Commission (CMC) chaired by Deng Xiaoping. Immediately under the CMC are the three PLA departments: the General Staff Department, headed by Chief of Staff Chi Haotian; the General Political Department, headed by Yang Baibing; and the General Logistics Department, headed by Zhao Nanqui. Under the General Staff Department come the three service arms: the air force, the navy, and the strategic missile forces. Also under the General Staff Department come the group armies stationed in the military regions, though military region commanders may be gaining greater authority over these forces.[50] As was noted previously, local forces are also being reorganized.

The exact status of the militia is uncertain. Prior to the death of Mao, the militia was deemed a fundamental component of the people's war concept. The training and equipping of the militia was not given much emphasis; however, it did play an important political role.[51] In mid 1986 the official Chinese news agency said that the primary militia had been reduced by 80 percent and the number of militia trainees by 88 percent. The report observed that emphasis on militia work had "shifted" from organizing military training to building material and spiritual civilization. Millions of militia members were said to be joining— "helping the poor groups" and "serving the people groups" while others were working on public projects such as fighting earthquakes and forest fires.[52] With the establishment of a new military service law, China also announced the implementation of a reserve system. The relation between the reserves and the militia is uncertain. In December 1985, for example, Deputy Chief of Staff He Qizong stressed the importance of the reserves in mobilization, but made no mention of the militia.[53]

In past years there has been some thought that the organization of China's armed forces could lead to regionalism and powerful warlords in the event of a collapse of central authority. The current reorganizations would appear to make such a situation highly unlikely. Military regional commanders have been rotated or replaced on several occasions in recent years. Additionally, the restructuring of the command and control system would seem to assure that the central authorities now have even greater control than previously, except in specific instances such as the People's Armed Forces (reserves), which have been specifically placed under local control.[54]

Most of China's forces are ground forces. The navy has about 350,000 personnel; the air force, 450,000. Both services require longer enlistments than the ground forces owing to the greater technical skills required. Both the navy and air force are seeking technology transfers from the United States and other Western countries to enhance modernization. Compared with Soviet forces, China's naval and air capabilities are severely limited, and they will likely remain technologically inferior for the foreseeable future; but with technological enhancements, China could make some progress in improving its capabilities vis-à-vis the Soviet Union and other potential adversaries.[55]

POTENTIAL SIDE EFFECTS OF MODERNIZATION

As was noted earlier, one of the principal reforms of the armed forces concerns political indoctrination. This has become a highly controversial issue, since some Chinese leaders have expressed concern that the reforms are contributing to corruption in the military, a problem that in China, as in other communist systems, is to be resolved through political indoctrination. Moreover, the PLA, which during the Cultural Revolution was deemed a model for emulation, has frequently been criti-

cized in the post-Cultural Revolution period for arrogating both property and power to itself. The result of this criticism has been lowered prestige and morale. On top of this, recruitment has been made more difficult because young men and women have better prospects for financial success by staying out of the PLA and making money through private entrepreneurship in village responsibility systems or by working in a service or industry.

Several measures have been adopted to try to cope with these problems. In 1984 and 1985 the PLA conducted a program to negate the influence of Lin Biao and the "Gang of Four" by repudiating their slogan of "giving prominence to politics." (Representative to some extent of the old order under Mao, the "gang of four" was a group that included Mao's wife. Purging the "gang of four" became symbolic for the new regime under Deng of clearing the way for reforms.) The purpose of this effort was to restore revolutionary spirit, but without neglecting material benefit in the PLA.[56] The PLA General Political Department also continued to conduct a campaign to "respect the government, cherish the people, and serve the people wholeheartedly." Efforts to intensify self-criticism campaigns in the PLA were also stepped up.[57]

Since 1985 there has been continued concern about some PLA activities. Yang Shangkun, permanent vice chairman of the Military Commission (and now PRC president), has decried the problems of pornography, corruption, and other unhealthy trends and said that they were having an adverse effect on discipline.[58] Another report decried "sectarianism" in the officer corps.[59] In January 1986 the Fifth All-Army games were suspended since some units had fraudulently recruited athletes.[60] The PLA newspaper reported cases of bribery with money, cigarettes, and wine.[61] An air force rectification campaign revealed problems of watching pornographic videotapes, gambling, graft, embezzlement, and illegal use of Party funds. The report stated:

Certain Party members lacked self-sacrificial spirit and paid no attention to communist ideals. In their eyes, ideals were void, and money was practical. They were willing to sacrifice petty interests, but only for a short time, rather than sacrifice major interests in the long term. Certain company level cadres [officers] did not keep their minds on their work in the grass-roots units. They always dreamed of a transfer to leading organs. Some others attempted to leave the army and work in local units.[62]

This report also decried the tendencies among the lower levels toward favoritism in promotion, transfers, recruitment for Party membership, educational opportunities, and home leave. In late July 1986, the CMC directed that the PLA stop engaging in business activities since about 80 percent of serious investigations and cases concerned the army's involvement in economic activity.[63]

To combat these "unhealthy tendencies," the CMC's Discipline and Inspection Committee directed that a major rectification be conducted within the PLA. This corresponded with a nationwide campaign to purify the Party of graft and corruption. The rectification was first conducted at the higher levels of Party organization within the PLA, and then a second stage was launched at lower levels. Various reports claimed that major successes were being achieved. One report claimed that the "spirit and political consciousness" of Party members was being raised, that party organization and unity within the military was being strengthened, and fraudulent practices were being corrected.[64] Another report stated that fundamental changes within the PLA were being accomplished. Most discipline cases had been investigated and resolved, and many officers had canceled plans to purchase cars, had returned surplus property and gifts, and had strictly abided by rules and regulations.[65]

In July 1986 Yu Qiuli proposed that "Eight No's" be added to the PLA's traditional Three Main Rules of Discipline and Eight Points for Attention. The "Eight No's," designed primarily for officers, include: no beating, scolding, or corporal punishment of troops; no acceptance of gifts from soldiers; no infringement of soldiers' interests; no fines; no alcoholism; no gambling; no reading of pornography; and no cheating. These new rules were seen as necessary to correct past abuses and improve ties between officers and men.[66]

Clearly, the long-term results of this rectification effort and other programs to weed out "unhealthy tendencies" in the PLA remain to be seen. There will also continue to be debate over whether these tendencies result from the PLA's past legacy or whether they should be blamed on the effects of the reforms. Should the problem of corruption grow, Chinese leaders fear that it will undermine other modernization efforts. Consequently, the role of political indoctrination will continue to be extremely important and will be an ongoing issue.

ARMS SALES

Ten years ago, China was an exporter only of small arms to revolutionary movements. Today, arms exports to a wide variety of foreign countries have become one of China's greatest sources of foreign exchange; the PRC now ranks as the world's fifth largest seller of arms. Some estimates indicate that China has earned several billion dollars through sales of weapons to countries such as Iran and Iraq.[67] No longer limited to small arms, Chinese exports include aircraft, tanks, artillery, other heavy weapons, and even "silkworm" missiles to Iran and other Middle East countries and CSS2 IRBMs to Saudi Arabia. Chinese arms export companies hold exhibitions to promote sales. Undoubtedly, China hopes that technological imports from the West will enable it to improve weaponry that can then be sold on the international market.

But the drive to export weapons has resulted in some organizational and bureaucratic problems. Individual ministries have formed corporations to market Chinese weapons. Sometimes they compete with each other, causing confusion and acrimony. For example, the North China Industries Corporation (Norinco), a government authorized point of contact for foreign military sales operated by the Ordance Ministry, competes with other firms set up by other ministries. According to Hong Kong newspapers, personnel in some of these firms include relatives of high-ranking party leaders, who are then able to exploit their connections to undercut Norinco and make tidy profits. The PLA itself established a company, *Baoli*, to sell surplus equipment at a profit. There have been allegations that Baoli has used its advantages to acquire equipment and then sell it abroad at prices below those offered by Norinco. The degree of autonomy to be permitted these various enterprises is a matter still under consideration—and probably some heated debate—in Beijing. In any case, it is highly likely that China will continue its successful and profitable forays into the international arms market.[68]

ARMS CONTROL

Over the past decade China has also come to express more interest in arms control. In part, this reflects China's desire to become much more engaged in various international activities, thereby boosting its status and prestige. But this interest also probably was stimulated by the initial Soviet deployment of SS-20 missiles east of the Ural mountains, and by the U.S. decision to press forward with the Strategic Defense Initiative. In China's view, both pose a threat to China's defense capabilities. Chinese delegations have made it clear that while China would like to take advantage of technological advances made via SDI research, China is opposed to any deployments that could undermine its own deterrent. China also opposed any arms agreement among Western powers that might have allowed the Soviet Union to continue to deploy SS-20 intermediate-range nuclear missiles in Asia. Beyond these specific issues, the Chinese are likely to participate more extensively in the international arms control dialogue in order to seek limits on the superpowers and to enhance China's prestige.

In 1986, then Premier Zhao Ziyang made a speech to commemorate the UN "International Year of Peace" in which he outlined China's approach to disarmament. Zhao, in a first for any Chinese leader, stated that China would not conduct atmospheric nuclear tests. Beyond that, he reiterated a nine-point plan that pledged no first use of nuclear weapons, called on the two superpowers to take the lead in disarming, and called for the complete prohibition and thorough destruction of nuclear and chemical weapons. He also called for a ban on space weapons. Zhao claimed that China was continuing to take measures to reduce its military forces and cut its defense ex-

penditures. He further pledged that China would "support all proposals truly conducive to disarmament."[69] Following the U.S.–Soviet INF missile accord in 1987, China called on the superpowers to make even further reductions.

China's heightened interest in arms control has resulted in several detailed discussions with U.S. arms control officials since 1984. According to former U.S. Arms Control and Disarmament Agency Director Kenneth Adelman, China agreed with the United States 70 percent of the time on arms control resolutions in the UN First Committee. Adelman also indicated that the Chinese were showing much more interest in becoming involved in arms control dialogue with the superpowers.[70] China is not a signatory to the Non-Proliferation Treaty, but, as part of the process of securing a nuclear accord with the United States, Chinese leaders personally pledged that China would not export nuclear weapons or technology. Chinese leaders, including both General Secretary Zhao Ziyang and Premier Li Peng, have expressed support for the U.S.–Soviet INF agreement.

CIVIL-MILITARY RELATIONS

The legacy of China's communist revolution is heavily flavored with the vision of an army closely connected with the people. Mao's writings on protracted war emphasize that the army should never become divorced from the masses. Throughout the period of communist rule, there have been campaigns to "love the army and cherish the people" or otherwise to promote unity. During the Cultural Revolution the army was set up as an institution to be emulated by the people; in some respects, professionalism was seen as making the army separate and aloof. In the post-Cultural Revolution period, the PLA is no longer a favored and respected institution, and the problem of civil-military relations has become more complex.

The leadership now evidently hopes that increased professionalism will enhance the PLA's status. If the military can give a good accounting of itself, then its public image may be improved. Meanwhile, the propaganda apparatus continues to call attention to the ongoing conflict with Vietnam in an effort to point out the sacrifices being made by the army for the benefit of the nation. Additionally, PLA achievements in efforts such as fighting floods and droughts, assisting in various kinds of civilian production projects, and other types of public service are given wide publicity.[71] Also, individual meritorious PLA soldiers are often held up for emulation, both by their fellow soldiers and, on occasion, by the public at large.

Undoubtedly, civil-military relations will be greatly affected by the effort to weed out corruption discussed above. Though the military is probably perceived to be no more inherently corrupt than the Party or other Chinese organizations, because it is more in the public view and has greater mobility and access to vehicles and other resources, the public may be more aware of transgressions by military members than by other government officials. Additionally, because of what is now described as the deplorable role played by the PLA in the Cultural Revolution, it bears a special public image burden. As the PLA returns buildings, facilities, and other property it occupied during the Cultural Revolution, its image is likely to be enhanced. However, continuing reports of corruption within the armed forces will work against PLA respectability.

Related to the problem of image is the problem of recruitment. Because of the implementation of the "responsibility systems" that allow for a kind of market economy in many rural areas, many young people are now able to earn more by staying and working on a local farm or in a local factory than by joining the army. Youths in urban areas are even more likely than their rural counterparts to try to avoid military service, since they prefer better-paying jobs and more prestigious occupational status. The large pool of manpower the PLA has to draft from partially offsets this problem. Without care, however, the army could become the repository of less-qualified youths and even ne'er-do-wells. Partly for this reason, the PLA has implemented a special draft for specialty occupations such as doctors and engineers. Also, it is now requiring that officers have college degrees.

A major issue in civil-military relations is the question of how to absorb demobilized PLA veterans, particularly since half of the million demobilized are officers. The State Council and CMC have been working to resolve this problem through a variety of techniques. The PLA has launched a special drive to give training to PLA veterans that will enable them to find jobs when they are demobilized. The government has adopted the principle that any demobilized veterans will be returned to the local areas where they entered duty, unless they are requested by another area. Most of the burden of finding jobs for these veterans has been placed on provincial and local governments.[72]

Under the PLA reorganization program, about six or seven hundred thousand soldiers will be released from service each year. About 80 percent of these come from rural areas and will return there. If the PLA's training program works, they will be able to contribute new skills and "become a vital new force in the nation's rural construction."[73] However, some of the resettlements have been difficult. Some officers feel threatened because of the loss of special privileges or perks. Some soldiers do not want to return to the rural areas from whence they came and want to find jobs in the cities. There have been reports of special protests and demonstrations by demobilized veterans who complain that they are not able to get jobs and earn a living after leaving the PLA. Also, some areas, which already have unemployment problems, are not anxious to have veterans return, particularly since some veterans—those who have received decorations for meritorious service—are to be given preference in jobs. Consequently, the highest levels of government have held conferences and other meetings to try to persuade both the veterans and local leaders to accept demobilization policies. According to various press accounts, the program is moving along well. Nevertheless, we should expect that demobilizations will provoke some further tensions in civil-military relations.

The Future of Chinese Defense Policy

A review of Chinese defense policy during the communist period suggests several general conclusions. First, Chinese defense policy basically has worked. China has not been invaded, even though it has been almost surrounded by different hostile countries. China has effectively employed the psychological advantage of size and location to be considered a key player in East Asia, even though its objective military capabilities relative to the superpowers have declined. Though there have been ups and downs in the past, China's present emphasis on modernization and stability seems to be working well.

But on specific issues, the picture is more mixed. Beijing's employment of the PLA has been within a pattern of coercive diplomacy—as an instrument to support various foreign policy objectives, such as involvement in Korea in the early 1950s, India in the early 1960s, the USSR in 1969, and Vietnam today. Besides the small, but hot, conflict with Vietnam, conflicts with adjacent states over territorial and, perhaps, other disputes are possible. And China has not ruled out the use of force against Taiwan.

In this context, Chinese strategists are not only reconsidering the role of the use of force, but are also giving greater attention to the relations between the military instrument and other instruments of statecraft. For example, the Chinese decision to stage a naval "show the flag" cruise to Pakistan, Sri Lanka, and Bangladesh in late 1985 suggests that gradual development of a blue water navy is designed not only to enhance military capabilities, but also to increase China's diplomatic leverage. Additionally, the use of military exchanges, weapons sales, training, and other elements of military capability will increasingly be utilized in conjunction with economic and other instruments.

As modernization proceeds in both military and nonmilitary sectors, it is likely to have a substantial impact on thinking about defense policy. Over the next few years, we are likely to see new ideas about how China should achieve its security objectives. Potential new approaches could have an important effect on how China deals with its neighbors, with the superpowers, and with the international community.

The key word in this chapter is modernization. The Chinese Communists have always placed a high degree of emphasis on improving

weaponry; this emphasis will continue. But there are now significant changes in military strategy, doctrine, organization, education and training, and other areas as well. As observed in the preceding pages, there are many difficult challenges raised by the effort to change and improve various aspects of defense policy, including the armed forces themselves. There will unquestionably be some setbacks in China's modernization effort; however, the outlook is for a China that is economically stronger, more confident, and probably more assertive in the international community.

In the 1982 edition of *The Defense Policies of Nations* this chapter placed considerable emphasis on evolving security relations between China and the United States. It warned that misunderstandings based on incorrect perceptions could damage these relations. Fortunately, in the view of this author, perceptions on both sides have achieved a greater degree of realism, and there is no longer the talk of alliances or "card playing" that characterized these relations just a few years ago. (The expression "playing the China card" was used by some in the late 1970s and early 1980s to mean balancing China against the USSR to American advantage in a complex, three-way strategic triangle.) China has embarked on an "independent" course—though one that seeks cooperative relations with the United States and the West—while the United States more accurately comprehends China's regional position. There will be areas of conflict between the two sides, particularly over Taiwan and trade issues, but there will also be broad areas of cooperation. For the United States, China will not again be seen, at least not in the foreseeable future, as a lurking communist dragon menacing and devouring U.S. friends and allies in Asia.[74]

China's test will be in the effectiveness of the reform agenda and whether it can be sustained, especially as new leaders come to the fore. Insofar as China is successful in achieving comprehensive modernization, its interests will also grow and change. Chinese leaders are not likely to forget that a sound comprehensive defense policy is vital, not only to the defense of China against potential aggressors, but also to the exercise of China's regional, and increasingly global, power.

Notes

1. As quoted by Zheng Xinli, "The Second Revolution and Theoretical Development," *Jingji Ribao*, 2 November 1985 (Foreign Broadcast Information Service, *Daily Report* (China), 19 November 1985, p. k9; hereafter FBIS translations are abbreviated as DR/C). This chapter has benefited enormously from the research of scholars and practitioners such as Monte Bullard, June Dreyer, Carl Ford, Paul Godwin, Harlan Jencks, Richard Latham, Jonathan Pollack, Harvey Nelsen, William Tow, and many others. Their contributions are detailed in the bibliographic essay by Richard Latham elsewhere in this volume. For an overview of some current literature, I highly recommend Harlan Jencks, "Watching China's Military: A Personal View," *Problems of Communism* (May–June 1986), pp. 71–78.
2. "Key to Understanding China" (excerpts of a speech by General Secretary Hu Yaobang at the British Royal Institute of International Affairs, 11 June 1986), *Beijing Review*, no. 25, 23 June 1986, pp. 14–16.
3. Ibid., p. 15.
4. For an excellent insight on this question see, John Frankenstein, "Back to the Future: A Historical Perspective on Chinese Military Modernization" (unpublished paper presented to the meeting of the International Studies Association, Anaheim, Calif., March 1986).
5. "On Questions of Party History" ("Resolution on Certain Questions in the History of Our Party since the Founding of the People's Republic of China," adopted by the Sixth Plenary Session of the 11th Central Committee of the Communist Party of China on June 27, 1981), *Beijing Review*, no. 27, 6 July 1981, pp. 10–39; quote is on p. 29.
6. Commentator, "The Four Basic Principles are the Basis of All Policies," *Hongqi* (Red Flag), no. 22. 16 November 1985 (Joint Publictions Research Service (JPRS) CRF-85-027, 31 December 1985, p. 14).
7. Peng Di, "Are There Changes in China's Foreign Relations?" *Liaowang* (overseas ed.), no. 11, 17 March 1986, pp. 3–4 (DR/C, 25 March 1986, pp. a1–4).
8. "Report by Zhao Ziyang, Premier of the State Council, on the Seventh 5-Year Plan for National Economic and Social Development at the opening to the Fourth Session of the Sixth National People's Congress in Beijing," Beijing Television, 25 March 1986 (DR/C, 28 March 1986, p. k24). The obstacles Zhao is referring to are: (1) the stationing of Soviet troops along the Sino-Soviet border and in Mongolia, (2) the Soviet invasion of Afghanistan, and (3) Soviet support for the Vietnamese invasion of Cambodia.
9. For example, see Chen Qiman, "Tentative Discusson on Postwar Changes in International Relations and the Possibility of Winning Lasting World Peace," *Hongqi*, no. 13, 1 July 1986, pp. 20–26 (DR/C, 28 July 1986, pp. a5–14).
10. Zhao's report, DR/C, p. k27.
11. For some analysis of Sino-Soviet relations, see Guo-cang Huan, *Sino-Soviet Relations to the Year 2000*, Atlantic Council Occasional Papers (Washington, D.C., 1976). Also see Gerald Segal, "Sino-Soviet Relations after Mao," Adelphi Papers, no. 202 (London: International Institute for Strategic Studies, 1985); for a comprehensive treatment of Soviet policy in Asia, see *Soviet Policy in East Asia*, ed. Donald S. Zagoria (New Haven: Yale University Press, 1982). Also see Jonathan D. Pollack, "China's Changing Perceptions of East Asian Security and Development," *Orbis* (Winter 1986): 771–94.
12. Monte R. Bullard and Edward C. O'Dowd, "Defining the Role of the PLA in the Post-Mao Era," *Asian Survey*, no. 6 (June 1986): 706–20. The "four modernizations" include agriculture, industry, science and technology, and national defense.
13. Xinhua (Official New China News Agency), 20 July 1986 (DR/C, 22 July 86, pp. k1–3). Zhu Songchun, "Chinese Scholars Discuss Strategy for the Development of National Defense in Year 2000," Liaowang (overseas ed.), 21 July 1986; pp. 6–8 (DR/C, 25 July 1986, pp. k3–8).
14. Harlan W. Jencks, "Chinese Defense Strategy and PLA Modernization" (paper submitted to the SRI International Project on PLA Modernization, 30 August 1984), pp. 7–17; also see Jack H. Harris, "Politics of National Security in China," *Problems of Communism* (March–April 1979): 64–66.
15. Xu Xiangqian, "Heighten Our Vigilance and Get Prepared to Fight a War," *Beijing Review*, 11 August 1978, pp. 5–9.
16. "Reforms Have Brought Five Major Changes to China's Armed Forces," Zhongguo Xinwen She (China News Agency), 27 July 1986 (DR/C, 29 July 1986, pp. k2–4; quote is on p. k3).
17. Paul H. B. Godwin, "People's War Revised: Military Doctrine, Strategy, and Operations," in *China's Military Reforms: International and Domestic Implications*, ed. Charles D. Lovejoy, Jr., and Bruce W. Watson (Boulder, Colo.: Westview Press, 1986), pp. 1–13. See especially pp. 4–8. Also see Godwin's "Changing Concepts of Doctrine, Strategy and Operations in the Chinese People's Liberation Army," *China Quarterly* (December 1987), pp. 572–90.
18. Ellis Joffe and Gerald Segal, "The PLA under Modern Conditions," *Survival* (July–August 1985): 148–49.
19. Jencks, "Chinese Defense Strategy," p. 16.
20. Paul Godwin, "People's War Revised: Military Capabilities, Strategy and Operations" (unpublished paper, Center for Aerospace Doctrine, Research and Education, Maxwell AFB Alabama, July 1984), pp. 6–8. For a somewhat differing view on people's war, see Robert S. Wang, "China's Evolving Strategic Doctrine," *Asian Survey* (October 1984): 1040–55. According to Wang: "China has in fact been modernizing its armed forces along the lines of a strategic doctrine that departs significantly from Mao's people's war approach. This new doctrine emphasizes the importance and interdependence of conventional, tactical nuclear, and strategic nuclear forces in defending China against a potential Soviet attack."
21. *Ta Kung Pao*, 16 February 1986, p. 1 (DR/C, 18 February 1986, pp. w11–12). Also see *Wen Wei Po*, 3 March 1986, p. 2 (DR/C, 6 March 1986, pp. w3–4). For a Chinese analysis of foreign operational strategy see *Liaowang*, 2 June 1986, pp. 46–47 (DR/C, 17 June 1986, pp. k7–11).
22. Allen S. Whiting, *The Chinese Calculus of De-*

terrence (Ann Arbor: University of Michigan Press, 1975), pp. 202–3.

23. Steve Chan, "Chinese Conflict Calculus and Behavior: Assessment from a Perspective of Conflict Management," World Politics, no. 30 (April 1978), pp. 391–410.

24. Edward Ross, "China Punishes Vietnam: Chinese Conflict Management in Perspective" (unpublished paper, Department of National Security Affairs, Naval Postgraduate School, March 1979).

25. Jonathan D. Pollack, "The Logic of Chinese Military Strategy," Bulletin of the Atomic Scientists, no. 34 (January 1979), p. 26. For an interesting Chinese account of the development of their nuclear weapons, see Gu Mainan, "Deng Jiaxian, a Man of Great Merit in Developing the 'Two Bombs,'" Liaowang no. 25, 23 June 1986, pp. 4–8 (DR/C, 14 July 1986, pp. k13–20).

26. International Institute for Strategic Studies, The Military Balance, 1985–1986 (London: IISS, 1985), p. 113.

27. William T. Tow, "Science and Technology in China's Defense," Problems of Communism, (July–August 1985): 26. Also see Tow's "The Interplay of Science and Technology in Chinese Military Modernization," in China's Military Reforms, ed. Lovejoy and Watson, pp. 15–34.

28. Godwin, "People's War Revised," p. 12; Jencks, "Chinese Defense Strategy," pp. 38–9.

29. Cheng Hsiang, "China's Post-Reform National Defense Strength," Wen Wei Po, 17 October 1985, p. 2 (DR/C, 17 October 1985, pp. w1–2).

30. Tow, "Science and Technology in China's Defense," p. 18. Also John Frankenstein, "Chinese Weapons Development: Process, Progress, Program?" in China's Military Reforms, ed. Lovejoy and Watson, pp. 69–90.

31. For some views on the conservative-moderate split, see Joffe and Segal, "PLA under Modern Conditions," p. 154. Also see June T. Dreyer, "China's Military Modernization," Orbis (Winter 1984): 1011–26.

32. An excellent background discussion is Harvey W. Nelsen, "Internal Management in the Armed Forces: Confucian Anachronism or Model for the 1980s?" in The Chinese Defense Establishment, ed Paul H. B. Godwin (Boulder, Colo.: Westview Press, 1983), pp. 139–54.

33. On the history of this debate, see Gregory J. Terry, "The 'Debate' on Military Affairs in China, 1957–59," Asian Survey (August 1976), pp. 788–813; Harry Harding and Melvin Gurtov, The Purge of Lo Jui-ch'ing: The Politics of Chinese Strategic Planning, R-548-PR (Santa Monica, Calif.: RAND Corporation, 1971; Thomas M. Gottlieb, Chinese Foreign Policy Factionalism and the Origins of the Strategic Triangle, R-1902-NA (Santa Monica, Calif.: RAND Corporation, 1977); Michael Pillsbury, SALT on the Dragon: Chinese Views of the Soviet-American Strategic Balance, P-5457, (Santa Monica, Calif.: RAND Corporation, 1976); Kenneth Lieberthal, Sino Soviet Conflict in the 1970s: Its Evolution and Implications for the Strategic Triangle, R-2342-NA (Santa Monica, Calif.: RAND Corporation, 1978).

34. On the development of the Taiwan arms sales issue that led to the 17 August 1982, U.S.-China Joint Communique, see John W. Garver, "Arms Sales, the Taiwan Question, and Sino-U.S. Relations," Orbis (Winter 1983), pp. 999–1035.

35. William Heaton, "New Trends in China's Professional Military Education and Training" (paper presented to the annual meeting of the International Studies Association, Anaheim, California, 25 March 1986). Also see William Heaton, "Professional Military Education in the People's Republic of China," in Chinese Defense Establishment, ed. Godwin, pp. 121–38. For examples of education and training, see the following reports: "Reforms Have Brought Five Major Changes to China's Armed Forces," Zhongguo Xinwe She, 27 July 1986 (DR/C, 29 July 1986, pp. d2–3); Xinhua, 27 July 1986 (DR/C, 29 July 1986, pp. k4–5). More than 1,200 soldiers received master's degrees in military academies between 1978 and 1986, and the number of Ph.D candidates had increased eleven times since 1981, according to Xinhua, 25 August 1986 (DR/C, 26 August 1986, pp. k3–4). On China's National Defense University, see Kai Wang-min and Tai Hsing-min, "A Visit to China's Highest Military Academy," Ta Kung Pao, 2 September 1986, p. 3 (DR/C, 3 September 1986, pp. k1–2).

36. See the remarks made by Yang Dezhi as cited by Ming Pao, 1 April 1985, p. 6 (DR/C, 3 April 1985, pp. w3–4). Also see Zhang Chunting and Zhang Qinsheng, "Beijing's 'Military Salon," Liaowang (overseas ed.), 25 November 1985, p. 11 (DR/C, 5 December 1985, pp. k10–12).

37. There are numerous sources on the Chinese decision to cut troop strength by one million. See, for example the following: Cheng Hsiang, "China's Post-Reform National Defense Strength," pp. w1–2; Xinhua, 30 July 1986 (DR/C, 1 August 1986, pp. k29–30); China Daily, 25 January 1986, p. 1 (DR/C, 27 January 1986, pp. k3–4); Lu Yun, "One Million Soldiers to Modernize," Beijing Review, (28 April 1986), pp. 15–17 and related article, id., pp. 17–19. An interesting interpretation of how PLA manning levels were determined was excerpted from the PRC journal Shehui Kexue (Social sciences) by Inside China Mainland (December 1985), pp. 7–8. The article estimated that China spent $2,000 per serviceman, compared with $126,000 for the United Kingdom, $65,000 in the United States, $41,800 in France, $38,170 in West Germany, and $47,700 in the Soviet Union. By reducing troop strength by one million, the article surmised, China could double its per capita expenditure.

38. Cheng Hsiang, "China's Post-Reform National Defense Strength," pp. w1–2.

39. Xinhua, 31 December 1985 (DR/C, 31 December 1985, pp. k10–11); Also see Tai Ming Cheung, "Ready for Modern War," Far Eastern Economic Review, (7 August 1986), pp. 22–23.

40. Xinhua, 30 July 1986 (DR/C, 1 August 1986, pp. k29–30).

41. "China's Strategic Missile Units Already Have Considerable Strike Capability," Zhongguo Xinwen She, 21 December 1985 (DR/C, 27 December 1985, p. k2).

42. For a discussion of specific weapons systems, see Jencks, "Defense Strategy," pp. 32–5. For an overall picture, see IISS, Military Balance, 1985–1986, pp. 111–15.

43. Mu Chi, "New State of Weaponry in China's Three Armed Services," Ta Kung Pao, 15 February 1986, p. 3 (DR/C, 20 February 1986, pp. w3–4). Also see Yi Jianru and Chen Xiangan, "The PLA Engineering Corps is on the Move," Liaowang, 28 July 1986, pp.

20–21 (DR/C, 15 August 1986, pp. k13–16). Also see Sun Zhenhuan, "Developing the National Economy and Strengthening National Defense Construction," *Zhongguo Jingji Tizhi Zaige* (23 March 1988), pp. 44–45; DR/C, 14 April 1988, pp. 40–42.

44. On technological acquisitions from the West, see Wendy Frieman, "Foreign Technology and Chinese Modernization," in *China's Military Reforms*, ed. Lovejoy and Watson, pp. 51–68. For discussion of technology and modernization in the PLA Navy, see "The Navy Grasps Military Scientific Research, Modern Weapons," *Ming Pao*, 15 January 1986, p. 5 (DR/C, 17 January 1986, p. w6). For the air force, see Cai Shanwu, "China's Air Force Today," *Liaowang* (overseas ed.), 24 February 1986, pp. 19–20 (DR/C, 4 March 1986, pp. k12–14).

45. Chen Siyi and Gu Mainan, "China's National Defense Industry Faces a Historic Turning Point—Sidelights on Zhao Ziyang's Meeting with National Defense Industry Specialists," *Liaowang* (overseas ed.), 10 February 1986, pp. 4–6 (DR/C, 5 March 1986, pp. k13–18). For an extensive discussion of the defense industries, see Richard Latham, "Implications of the Post-Mao Reforms on the Chinese Defense Industries" in *China's Military Reforms*, ed. Lovejoy and Watson, pp. 35–50. In 1986 the PLA Xinxing Corporation hosted a commodities export fair for four hundred army-owned factories with more than 5,000 products on display (China Daily, 14 August 1986, p. 2).

46. An Zhiguo, "Army Aids," p. 4.

47. Xinhua, 28 June 1986 (DR/C, 1 July 1986, p. k29). Also see Xinhua, 7 August 1986 (DR/C, 8 August 1986, pp. k1–2). Xinhua, 14 August 1986 (DR/C, 18 August 1986, p. k3).

48. See Shi Ping, "The New Trends in the Chinese Army," *Kuang Chiao Ching*, 16 March 1985, pp. 8–9 (DR/C, 22 March 1985, pp. w1–2). Xinhua, 26 February 1986 (DR/C, 27 February 1986, pp. k17–18). Also see Zhang Qinsheng and Zhang Chunting, "Reforms and Opening Up Have Brought Profound Changes to China's Armed Forces," *Liaowang* (overseas ed.), 21 April 1986, p. 19 (DR/C, 28 April 1986, pp. k21–24).

49. Xinhua, 26 February 1986 (DR/C, 27 February 1986, p. k17). For background on the General Political Department, see Monte R. Bullard, *China's Political-Military Evolution: The Party and the Military in the PRC, 1960–1984* (Boulder, Colo.: Westview Press, 1985). Also see Richard Nethercut, "Party-Military Relations in China" (paper, Groton, Mass., August 1984).

50. For additional details please refer to the section on China in IISS *Military Balance 1985–1986*, pp. 111–15.

51. For background on the militia, see June Dreyer, "The Chinese People's Militia: Transformation and Strategic Role," in *Chinese Defense Establishment*, ed. Godwin, pp. 155–86. Also see Tom Roberts, *The Chinese People's Militia: Doctrine of People's War*, NDU Monograph 83–4 (Washington, D.C.: National Defense University, 1983).

52. Xinhua, 7 August 1986 (DR/C, 8 August 1986, p. k3).

53. "Central Military Commission Instructs PLA to Build Reserve Units to Boost National Defense," *Ming Pao*, 1 December 1985, p. 5 (DR/C, 3 December 1985, pp. w6–7). Some information on militia reorganization was carried by Xinhua, 13 August 1986 (DR/C, 18 August 1986, pp. k1–2).

54. Xiong Zhengyan, "The People's Army is Undergoing a Strategic Change," *Ban Yue Tan*, 25 July 1986, pp. 14–16 (DR/C, 14 August 1986, pp. k14–16).

55. See, for example, Thomas W. Robinson, "Chinese Military Modernization in the 1980s," *China Quarterly*, no. 90 (June 1982): 231–252, on the "requirements approach" to Chinese military modernization. Also see Douglas T. Stuart and William T. Tow, "Chinese Military Modernization: The Western Arms Connection," *China Quarterly*, no. 90 (June 1982): 253–70.

56. Jiang Siyi, "Thoroughly Negate 'Giving Prominence to Politics:' Do a Good Job of Reforming Political Work," *Hongqi*, no. 14, 16 July 1984, pp. 23–6 (DR/C, 17 August 1984, pp. k4–9).

57. Xinhua, 1 August 1985 (DR/C, 2 August 1985, pp. k1–2). Also see *Renmin Ribao*, 27 October 1985, p. 1 (DR/C, 28 October 1985, pp. k5–7).

58. Xinhua, 28 August 1985 (DR/C, 3 August 1985, pp. k2–3).

59. "Sectarianism in PLA Hampering Officer Readjustments," *Ming Pao*, 12 November 1985, p. 6 (DR/C, 14 November 1985, pp. w1–2).

60. Xinhua, 31 January 1986 (DR/C, 3 February 1986, pp. k14–5).

61. "Military Officers Make Things Easy for Those Who Give Them Money: It Is a Common Practice for Soldiers to Give Gifts," *Ming Pao*, 25 February 1986, p. 6 (DR/C, 26 February 1986, p. w6–7).

62. "PLA Air Force Removes Obstacles to Party Rectification in Grass-Roots Units," *Ming Pao*, 17 March 1986, p. 6 (DR/C, 19 March 1986, pp. w1–2).

63. Shanghai Radio, 29 July 1986 (DR/C, 31 July 1986, p. k37). For an example of PLA business activity, see *China Daily*, 14 August 1986, p. 2 (DR/C, 15 August 1986, pp. k16–17).

64. Xinhua, 6 July 1980 (DR/C, 10 July 1986, pp. k25–26).

65. Xinhua, 4 July 1986 (DR/C, 17 July 1986, pp. k22–24).

66. Beijing Radio, 8 August 1966 (DR/C, 11 August 1986, pp. k1–2); Xinhua, 27 September 1986 (DR/C 29 September 1986, pp. k17–19). The Three Main Rules of Discipline are: (1) Obey orders in all your actions; (2) Don't take a single needle or piece of thread from the masses; and (3) Turn in everything captured. The Eight Points of Attention are: (1) Speak politely; (2) Pay fairly for what you buy; (3) Return everything you borrow; (4) Pay for anything you damage; (5) Don't hit or swear at people; (6) Don't damage crops; (7) Don't take liberties with women; (8) Don't ill-treat captives.

67. Richard Harwood and Don Oberdorfer, "China Now Largest Supplier of Arms to Iran, U.S. Says," *Washington Post*, 26 August 1986, pp. a1, 14.

68. Joffe and Segal, "PLA under Modern Conditions," p. 149. For a general overview, see Anne Filks and Gerald Segal, *China and the Arms Trade* (London: Croom Helm, 1985). In November 1986 the Xinshidai Corporation hosted an international defense technology exhibition in Beijing that featured various Chinese missiles, aircraft, and other heavy equipment. Xinhua, 24 September 1986 (DR/C, 25 September 1986, pp. k16–17).

69. Speech by Premier Zhao Ziyang in Beijing, 21 March 1986. Full translation is available in *Beijing Review*, no. 12, March 1986, pp. 14–16. On the PRC's approach to disarmament, see David I. Salem, "The

PRC, Disarmament and Legal Development: The Link to Modernization" (paper, 1984). Also see Robert G. Sutter, "Developments in China's Nuclear Weapons and Attitudes toward Arms Control," in *China's Military Reforms*, ed. Lovejoy and Watson, pp. 101–10.

70. Transcription of press conference by ACDA Director Kenneth Adelman in Beijing, 31 July 1986.

71. For example, see Qiu Jianhong, "China's Army Takes an Active Part in Economic Construction," Zhongguo Xinwen She, 31 July 1985 (DR/C, 6 August 1985, pp. k1–2).

72. Gai Yumin and Yang Minqing, "Do Placement Work Well to Support the Army's Reform and Reorganization—Answers to *Liaowang* Reporters' Questions by the Responsible Person of the State Council Group for Assignment of Army Cadres Transferred to Civilian Work," *Liaowang*, 23 September 1985, pp. 15–16 (DR/C, 17 October 1985, pp. k18–21). Xinhua, 13 June 1986 (DR/C, 16 June 1986, pp. k11–12).

73. Chen Deyi and Zhou Dinghua, "Former Soldiers Active in Rural Areas," *Beijing Review*, (28 April 1986), pp. 17–19. On the effects of demobilization, see June Dreyer, "The PLA: Demobilization and Its Effects," *Issues and Studies* (February 1988), pp. 86–106.

74. For further reading on this subject, highly recommended is Jonathan Pollack, *The Lessons of Coalition Politics: Sino-American Security Relations*, R-3133-AF (Santa Monica, Calif.: RAND Corporation, 1984).

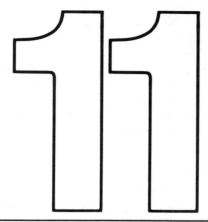

JAPAN

John E. Endicott

In World War II Japan experienced a defeat as traumatic as any experienced by any nation on earth. After rapid, dramatic victories early in the war, the invincible war machine of the empire soon came to a halt, tottered, and collapsed in ruin, accompanied by abject national poverty, near famine, and psychological shock. In rapid succession, Japan was told by U.S. occupation authorities that it would be stripped of its war-making potential and that elements of its militant past would be eradicated. Purges, land and Zaibatsu reform, general programs to democratize the state, and a constitution that renounced war as an instrument of national policy became part of this total postwar experience.

After remarkable progress was made along all these fronts to create an Asian version of Switzerland, it became all too apparent to American officials that more than a weak Japan was needed in long-term competition with Soviet power. This fact became abundantly clear when war on the Korean Peninsula broke out in June 1950, requiring the redeployment of American troops and the creation of a Japanese defense capability to replace U.S. occupation forces.

Two years later, Japan regained its independence; the occupation ended, and on the same day that the peace treaty was signed, a U.S.-Japanese Mutual Security Treaty was initiated that tied Japan's defense—and future—to the West. This security arrangement and the establishment of the Self-Defense Forces became focal points of leftist opposition. Also, soon after independence, in delayed reaction to the events of Hiroshima and Nagasaki and as a demonstration of regained sovereignty, an anti-nuclear aspect was added to the defense picture. Gradually, numerous ideas and concepts were created that surrounded the defense issue in Japan as restraints. Elements such as the three non-nuclear principles (no production, possession, or importation of nuclear weapons), no dispatch of Japanese forces overseas, no "offensive" weapons, and no export of weapons or the equipment necessary for their manufacture became part of Japanese defense

policy. In addition to these policies being debated in the Diet, there was public opposition—even antipathy—to the Self-Defense
Forces. This attitude was at a personal level
and became so keen that defense personnel often commuted to work in civilian clothes to
avoid public contempt. The defense environment of Japan that existed until the late 1960s,
in essence, was not positive. The government,
and especially the Defense Agency, measured
all advances in defense capabilities first in political terms; overall military considerations
were denigrated.

Gradually, changes in how Japan and the
Japanese treat the defense issue are occurring;
a new defense environment is coming into being. Largely due to events since 1969, the Japanese have become more tolerant of the Self-Defense Forces and the Mutual Security Treaty
with the United States. In the international
arena, the spectacle of socialist state fighting
socialist state has destroyed the myth of socialist benevolence, and with it much of the theoretical base for leftist alternative defense policies, such as unarmed neutrality, that were
once considered viable policy alternatives. The
relative decline of U.S. military power in comparison to that of the Soviet Union has also introduced an updated sense of realism, and the
rapprochement between China and the United
States has removed a previously negative aspect of the Japanese defense pact with America. Domestically, over thirty years of "good
work" (disaster relief, civil assistance, etc.) by
the Self-Defense Forces have also paid dividends. Attitudes have changed and are changing. In 1985 as much as 86 percent of the general public supported the existence of the
Self-Defense Forces. While such figures are a
far cry from the militant opposition of earlier
days, a deep-set antimilitary bias still exists
among the Japanese public when it comes to
considering use of the military for national policy objectives. "Peace diplomacy" is still preferred as the method of obtaining national objectives, and only 15 to 20 percent of the
population supports expanding the current
limited size of the Self-Defense Forces.[1]

These are some of the factors that have generally constrained the military in Japan and

have led to the long-term, disproportionate influence of the United States in Japanese
defense policy. The U.S. influence still exists,
and may explain why considerations of
Japan's strategy since World War II often begin
with a statement of the viability of the U.S. defense establishment rather than a review
of Japanese perspectives.[2] Relations between
the United States and Japan in the defense
field are changing at this very moment; an era
of partnership among equals is being approached. The decade of the 1990s will reveal
its degree of realization.

International Environment

Japan is a respected member of the world
economic system, with a GNP, depending on
the source, as large or larger than that of the
USSR.[3] In the economic sense, by almost any
standard, Japan is a superpower: its products,
people, and performance have earned it the
reputation of a heavyweight.

But Japan is not a military superpower.
While possessing considerable actual defensive
power, it has chosen to pursue policies that
strictly limit the use of military force as an instrument of national policy.[4] In fact, although
the Japanese defense budget is the eighth largest in the free world, and Japan possesses considerable military power in relative terms, it
has chosen to concentrate on defensive missions in and about its four Home Islands.[5] In
fact, the term "defensive defense" has become
inseparable from the overall concept of the use
of Japanese military power.

WHAT THREATS EXIST?

Potential threats to Japan are multifaceted.
The Japanese belief in the nonutilitarian nature of military power derives largely from the
complex network of interdependencies between Japan and many nations (see table 1).
Japan's interests are so wide and its dependencies so deep that it is faced with the dilemma
that use of military power in one region might
well create an unacceptable reaction in another. In the main, Japan views its interests as
best served by an international stability that

Table 1. Japanese Dependence on Imports (Raw Materials Imported as a Percentage of Total Individual Imports Plus Domestic Production)

Crude oil	99.8%	Natural rubber	100.0	Cotton	100.0
Coal	73.3	Iron ore	99.5	Soybeans	95.8
Copper	97.5	Pulp	85.5	Wheat	93.8
Bauxite	100.0	Wool	100.0		

Source: Japan, Ministry of Finance.

cannot be created by the use of force. Japan, in essence, is dependent on various states, but chiefly the United States, to maintain an international milieu that supports its continuing efforts for economic development.

An awareness of the security implications of Japan's economic dependence is shared by the Japanese at large and is underscored by polling data in which nonmilitary threats to Japan were seen as most likely "in the next several years."[6] Economic threats, primarily dependence on imported oil, are perceived as the most likely externally produced danger to Japan's stability. This perception is so keenly felt that even after the general negative reaction to the Chernobyl incident, the Advisory Committee for Energy of the Ministry of International Trade and Industry proposed increasing the nuclear energy program from 26 percent of the current energy base to almost 60 percent by the year 2030.[7] Likewise, growing recognition of a military threat does exist. In a September 1981 poll, 69 percent of respondents who felt a threat indicated that the Soviet Union was the source. Other countries that followed were the United States, 6.2 percent, North Korea with 3 percent, China with 2 percent, and South Korea with 1.4 percent.[8] In a 1984 poll, with dissimilar techniques, however, the greatest number, or 43 percent of respondents, indicated that their principal concern when allowed multiple choices, was Soviet deployment of troops in the Northern territories.[9] In a December 1985 poll where respondents were asked to list three nations they dislike, 53.7 percent indicated the Soviet Union, 32.5 percent North Korea, and 18.3 percent South Korea.[10] Japanese who live in Hokkaido, however, demonstrated particular sensitivity to the Soviet threat. In fact, some 80.2 percent in a 1985 survey replied that they felt militarily threatened as compared to 55 percent who felt that

way in 1981.[11] To explain some aspects of these responses, a quick examination of the internal and external threats is necessary.

INTERNAL ASPECTS OF MILITARY THREATS

Since the end of World War II, U.S. occupation, and the creation of the U.S.-Japan Mutual Security Treaty, there has been a degree of mistrust between the political left and political right in Japan—a mistrust that goes far back, it might be added. For years the right has feared a leftist-inspired revolt that could call in help from Japan's socialist neighbors; the left, on the other hand, has feared U.S. unilateral intervention in Japanese internal affairs (a kind of reimposed occupation), as well as a coordinated rightist-sponsored coup that would feature joint military action by the Japanese Self-Defense Forces, U.S. forces in Japan, and selected Korean units from South Korea.[12]

These various threats of intervention were largely the fears or fantasies of the extremist fringes on the Japanese political scene, and an understanding of their mistrust of each other over the past three to four decades does much to explain the responses.

To a much more worrisome degree, however, is the ever present, but limited, threat of urban terrorists belonging to the Sekigun Ha, or Red Army Faction. These extremists—few in number, but resolute and determined—have successfully disrupted commuter traffic when attacking vulnerable communication linkages and gained worldwide attention in firing homemade "bottle" rockets during the Tokyo Summit of 1986. They are significant only to the degree they tie down resources and threaten public figures.

EXTERNAL THREATS

The uniformly high perception of a Soviet threat among the Japanese comes from historic animosity that has existed between the two Northeast Asian powers since the czar and Bakufu clashed over Hokkaido in the mid nineteenth century. More recent events between the two countries have emphasized the irredentist claims of Japan to four islands (Etorofu, Kunashiri, Shikotan, and the Habomais) taken from Japan by the USSR in the closing days of World War II. Continued deployments of combat forces to these islands and a general enhancement of air, sea, and ground capabilities in the Far East to include SS-20 intermediate range missiles, Mig-31 and Mig-23 aircraft, and enhanced naval force projection capability have contributed to a perception of a Soviet military threat at popular and governmental levels.[13] The Soviet invasion of Afghanistan in 1979, the arrest of a former Japanese Ground Self-Defense Force major general on charges of spying for the USSR, and the brutal downing of the Korean Airlines Flight 007 helped to focus the traditional anti-Soviet attitudes of the Japanese public.[14] Even the "peace diplomacy" of the Soviet president has not been able to alter substantially this historic Japanese perception.

The notion of a Soviet "threat" as critically defined by the government of Japan stresses potential rather than actual threat. Clearly, increased Soviet activity throughout East Asia is noted by Japanese decision makers, but the likelihood of actual military attack upon Japan is held to be minimal. The primary threat to national security is still seen in terms of resource availability, especially oil.[15]

While resources remain an area of intense Japanese concern, a survey that focused on issues of political-military concern to the Japanese recorded the greatest concern as "the deployment of Soviet troops on Japan's Northern Territories." Some 42.6 percent of respondents indicated that they had paid some attention to this issue.[16]

In this kind of threat environment, military forces are considered as contributing only partially to the national security needs of Japan. However, the impact of former Prime Minister Nakasone's positive reinforcement of the Self-Defense Forces has been such that public acceptance of the SDF has continued at a high level of over 80 percent of respondents[17] and public discussion of defense issues has reached a new and generally positive mark. Since the threat to security from internal sources is minimal and can be easily dealt with by the current defense establishment (including police), and since the threat from external sources is viewed as less than imminent, the national security needs of Japan are increasingly identified by elements of the government and the defense community as resulting from two factors. First is the changing international situation in and about Japan, especially the Soviet buildup in the Northern Territories. Second is the overall need of the United States to have a defense partner that more equitably shares in the burdens of defense. These national security needs would include technological development, resource availability, assistance to Third World states, and, finally, a military capability to provide a minimum level of deterrence to external attack. Only by achieving progress in all these areas, it is argued, can Japan be secure and compete adequately in the world of the 1990s. Inattention to any one item could expose Japan to a threat possibly as serious as military attack, but this is not considered likely unless regional conditions deteriorate at an unexpected rate.[18]

WORLD VIEW

The interpretation of Japanese national security interests along the lines described above reveals the ascendancy of a particular worldview in the Japan of the late 1970s. This worldview is one that can be called internationalist. It has been in control of the main thrust of Japanese foreign and defense policy since the end of World War II and may remain predominant for some time to come. Its basic objective, as one of the historic worldviews in Japan, is to ensure Japan's development and well-being through interdependency with the outside world, particularly the English-speaking world.[19]

Prime Minister Nakasone's personal commitment to this concept of Japan's interdependency with the rest of the Western world had been made manifest frequently during his tenure since 1982, but especially so by his unqualified support for the controversial Maekawa Report, or "Report of the Advisory Group on Economic Structural Adjustment for International Harmony," of 7 April 1986. Basically, the report calls for necessary economic and social changes to "transform the Japanese economic structure into one oriented toward international cooperation."[20] This report recommends a frontal attack on such areas as housing, agriculture, market access, and industrial structure, placing the prime minister and government, once again, in a leadership role as significant as in any other major period of change in Japan's historic development.

Ever since the restoration of imperial power in the 1860s, this worldview has competed with one that, in contrast, can be called self-reliant. The self-reliant view holds that the key to Japan's success is in introspective and autonomous development. Thus, from this perspective, an independence born of the absence of (or, at least, a minimum number of) dependencies can be created that will produce a Japan able to capitalize on its unique characteristics among states.

Control of foreign policy has alternated over wide periods of time between advocates of these two perceptions. As one might expect, the 1930s and the World War II period witnessed the ascendancy of the self-reliant worldview. Since World War II, the internationalist view, with close ties with the United States and the West, has been dominant.

While the above views did contend with one another prior to World War II, they were primarily held by those with conservative political orientations. After World War II, a third view—that of the political left—rose to considerable power and served as a definite constraint on policy advocated by the two conservative worldviews. This leftist worldview held that since all socialist states were by definition benevolent toward other socialist states, no military power was needed in a Northeast Asia controlled by leftist or socialist states. Calling for unarmed neutrality as the defense policy for Japan, the Japan Socialist party, in particular, led forces that acted as effective restraints on any moves to change the nature of Japan's military forces.

Developments between the socialist states in Asia since the 1960s, and especially during the late 1970s, have completely destroyed the myth of socialist benevolence. In addition to actual hostilies between socialist states, China (PRC) and Japan normalized relations. Chinese leaders chided Japanese socialists for their naïveté in defense policy and endorsed the U.S.–Japan Mutual Security Treaty. Fear among Japanese of being drawn into a war with the PRC because of U.S. "adventurism" evaporated, and with it the effectiveness of the leftist worldview.

The decade between 1976 and 1986 was witness to a dramatic transformation of the defense debate in Japan. The power, even willingness, of the left to control and dampen this debate waned, and the debate over the basic defense orientation of Japan achieved new levels of sophistication. It is, in fact, this lack of traditional leftist restraint (that had existed since World War II) that has led to defense issues being discussed more frankly and realistically by various Japanese without fear of censure or public condemnation. It has led some observers, especially in the Soviet Union, to believe that Japan is about to rearm on a major scale. What is happening in Japan is that the defense issue is returning to the public arena—a healthy and nonprovocative state of affairs in a democratic society.

As a result of the 6 July 1986 election, the opposition parties, but especially the leading Japan Socialist Party (JSP), suffered a major setback at the polls. The Liberal Democratic Party (LDP) gained 300 of the 512 seats on its own; 4 independents joined later, and the New Liberal Club (a 1976 spin-off of the LDP) decided to once again cast its lot with the LDP; thus, another 7 seats were added. As 1986 concluded, 311 of the 512 seats in the Lower House were held by the ruling Liberal Democratic Party. While the outcome cannot be assessed entirely, if at all, in national security terms, the magnitude of the victory will have a further muting effect on the opposition parties and will ensure a greater, more robust, public debate of the defense issues.

The vitality of the internationalist worldview among Japan's elite still seems unquestioned, although it is being put to the test by some U.S. trade policies such as "Super 301." The degree of Japan's interdependence with the world system is not likely to change appreciably over the next decade. Certainly the internationalist view that has directed Japanese policy since World War II is dependent on the continued involvement of the United States in its worldwide defense obligations in the face of a continued Soviet arms buildup. This renewed U.S. commitment and the clear interdependency commitments made by Japan since the war may act to prevent the concept of self-reliance from becoming predominant again in Japan unless a cataclysmic change in the basic stability of the international system occurs. Changes, either economic or political, that threaten Japan's livelihood could force an appeal to other solutions. One such option would inevitably be the self-reliant one. However, even this worldview would need to reflect the dependencies of modern Japan.

BASIC LINKAGES WITH THE INTERNATIONAL SYSTEM

Besides dependencies on resource suppliers, Japan bases its foreign and defense policies on a long-term military reliance on the United States and a general commitment to the United Nations system. Indeed, the U.S.-Japan Mutual Security Treaty is the key to understanding current Japanese defense policy. In a treaty first executed in 1952 and revised in 1960, the United States agreed to assist Japan (after required constitutional procedures) in the defense of Japanese territory. Japan was not required, as in the case of NATO members, to assist the United States if America was placed under attack and Japan was not physically involved. While this is legalistically the case, an implied obligatory relationship has evolved over time. This can be seen in the case of the sanctions questions involving Iran and the Soviet Union, where a high degree of political reciprocity was expected by the United States.[21] What might seem to be a lack of reciprocity in terms of treaty obligation has not, in fact, been upsetting to American officials. In return for the commitment to defend Japan, the United States retains a military presence in

Japan—an invaluable logistics base in the event of involvement in the Korean Peninsula or other Asian areas.

More specifically, Japan depends on the United States for deterrence of nuclear threats or blackmail and actual use of nuclear weapons against Japan. In return, the United States has constantly encouraged the Japanese to develop and maintain a sound conventional capability that would deter insurgency and small- or medium-sized attacks from external sources. Such a capability would make it possible for Japan to defend itself, allowing more time for the United States to react and possibly even to deter aggressive action completely.[22]

As the 1980s end, support for the U.S.-Japan Mutual Security Treaty (MST) continues largely because of Soviet belligerence, the buildup of Soviet forces in Asia, and the collapse of the leftist defense policy alternatives mentioned above. Acceptance of the Mutual Security Treaty reached 71.4 percent of respondents in nationwide polls in 1984,[23] and support for a national orientation toward the West soared to 57.3 percent from 28 percent in 1974.[24] Japan is firmly linked to the United States through its defense relations, not to mention common economic and political objectives. For their part, U.S. officials maintain that Japan—not China—is the principal pillar on which U.S.-Asian policy will be based for the indefinite future.[25]

All, of course, is not in complete accord between the United States and Japan, and some Japanese observers have become increasingly vocal in criticism of various economic and military pressures being applied by Americans to Japan. Pressures on the Japanese to increase their defense effort, to increase purchases of U.S. military hardware, and to develop common sanction policies toward Iran and Afghanistan have worked in some quarters to weaken the confidence that is placed in the U.S.-Japanese relationship. A perceived lack of U.S. resolve during the late 1970s led to increased concern about U.S. credibility. Accordingly, specific doubts as to the commitment of the United States to defend Japan increased somewhat.[26] However, the impact of a stable and special relationship between the two nations' leaders (the "Ron-Yasu" relationship) has benefited an already improving situation.

National Objectives, National Strategy, and Military Doctrine

A consensus on Japan's national security objectives seems to be emerging from the Japanese policy process. In actuality, this new consensus will not differ as much in its substance from the past as in its breadth of support. What is happening is the development of a widened political support base for U.S.–Japan security relations and for the existence of the Self-Defense Forces. Practically all political parties except the Japanese Communist Party (JCP) now support to some degree the fundamental security characteristics advocated by the Liberal Democratic Party since its creation in 1955.[27] While the broadening of the defense consensus is occurring, the articulation of a framework that will perhaps better define the security objectives of Japan is also under way. This framework has often been referred to in the Japanese media as overall, or comprehensive, security. While the exact nature has still to emerge from the consensus-building process, which is slow and demanding, part of the concept can be seen in what the Ministry of International Trade and Industry (MITI) published as a "think piece" in the summer of 1979.[28]

In this preliminary paper by a MITI study commission, a ten-year projection was drafted that outlined the objectives of Japan's broad national security policy. Security policy in itself was seen not only as encompassing military forces in being and deterring aggression by an enemy, but also as including efforts to increase Japan's technological base, assure adequate resources, and realize diplomatic influence. Basic national objectives remained focused on ensuring the economic well-being of the nation within the context of the U.S.–Japan Mutual Security Treaty, but the study did posit defense expenses in the late 1980s and 1990s as roughly 1.5 percent of the GNP.[29]

To give institutional body to the comprehensive security concept, the government created the Council of Ministers Concerned with Comprehensive Security in December 1980.[30] This group meets to discuss items requiring coordination across the government on issues dealing with overall national security.

The pursuit of the concept of comprehensive security, with emphasis on economic well-being, has been dictated by external considerations as much as internal ones, and the genesis of such an economic focus can be seen in the traumatic defeat of Japan in World War II and the humiliation, despair, and abject national poverty brought about because of policies pursued in the 1930s and 1940s by the military elite of that period. As a result of the defeat and the experience of the U.S. occupation, the utilitarian value of military forces per se is still viewed as extremely low; however, Japan is not, after its history of militarism, given over to the pursuit of "pacifistic purity." A pragmatic society has seen that a very efficient military machine, unless supported by a technological and natural resource base of unquestioned excellence, cannot seek security solely by resort to the military instrument. This has not quite become the dogma of the land, but, by 1984, 44 percent of the Japanese thought that the future primary role of the Japanese Self-Defense Forces would be related to the forces' national security mission.[31] Items such as disaster relief, public welfare, and internal security were viewed collectively as important tasks for the military to pursue, but the closest second to national security was disaster relief at 32 percent. The Japanese generally continue to view their national security objectives as economic in nature—objectives that will contribute to the public well-being.

To place such emphasis on economic considerations, however, is not to say that Japan does not have certain key objectives that could be considered secondary goals—goals that would, it is hoped, be achieved through an active diplomacy, not through the commitment of military forces. Such goals in the security field would possibly encompass maintenance of the status quo or political stability on the Korean Peninsula; continuation of the Sino-Soviet competition in Northeast Asia; development of the PRC into a modern state as a foil to Soviet power; a return to normalcy in the Indochina area; maintenance of secure sea lines of communication throughout the world, but especially from the Persian Gulf; extension of profitable economic relations with Taiwan; and return of the four islands held by the Soviet Union.

Most of these desiderata, while generally supportive of the status quo and international stability (except for the irredentist Northern Territories issue), have significant economic bonuses, and to most of these objectives Japan brings economic skill and determination. It may be possible, after a period, to advance a package of economic incentives (development of Siberian resources) that could even cause the USSR to reconsider its intransigence regarding the Northern Territories. Currently, Japan's leverage in connection with most of these objectives is weak. Attempts to use aid as an inducement to the Vietnamese government to alter its policy vis-à-vis Cambodia have proved frustrating.

Unilateral Japanese strategies to further the realization of these policies could incorporate developmental aid in the case of developing states on the Indian Ocean littoral, especially Association of Southeast Asian Nations (ASEAN) states; transfer of advanced technology in the case of the PRC; and the proffering of necessary capital in the case of the USSR.

In none of the above objectives does the military, as presently formulated, play any but the most minor of roles; however, while on a visit to the United States in January 1983, Nakasone, building on the defense policy of former Prime Minister Suzuki Zenko, spoke candidly and forcefully on Japan's defense objectives:

The whole Japanese archipelago or the Japanese islands should be like an unsinkable aircraft carrier putting up a tremendous bulwark of defense against the infiltration of the Backfire bomber. To prevent Backfires from penetrating through this wall should be our first goal.

The second target objective should be to have complete and full control of the straits that go through the Japanese islands so that there should be no passage of Soviet submarines and other naval activities.

The third objective is to secure and maintain the ocean lines of communication. For the ocean, our defense should extend several hundred miles, and if we are to establish sea-lanes then our desire would be to defend the sea-lanes between Guam and Tokyo and between the Strait of Taiwan and Osaka.[32]

THE POLITICAL SYSTEM

Japan's parliamentary system of government has been dominated since 1955 by the Liberal Democratic Party (LDP). For many years this conservative party has captured two-thirds of the seats in the Diet. In July 1986 uncertainties over the implications of a strengthened yen and the international economy combined with popular respect for Prime Minister Nakasone's personal leadership style to produce the largest LDP victory in its history in terms of the number of elected candidates. It did not hurt that secretary general of the LDP, Kanemaru Shin, was an adroit election manager either. He saw to it that the age-old LDP practice of backing too many candidates did not occur, and of the 322 candidates nominated and endorsed by the LDP, 300 were elected.

This overwhelming LDP victory has thus provided us with a Japanese Diet that will lead Japan into the 1990s. In fact, as the Lower House has a four-year term, the majority now possessed by the LDP will remain almost 100 at least until mid 1990. Only through unbridled factional discord within the party, leading to a fundamental split in the LDP—something always possible, but not likely—could the opposition parties hope to challenge current LDP dominance. The repercussions of the 1989 Recruit-Cosmos scandal could bring the LDP as close to notions of coalition government as anything.

However, this is evidence that a significant change has occurred over the past decade in Japan. Even if the LDP were to split and a new array of political parties emerge, the foreign policy-security policy outcome would be acceptable to the United States in almost all cases except, of course, for a communist victory. This latter option is not a serious eventuality.

Gradually, most of the opposition parties (with the JCP the only exception) have come to accept the existence of the SDF and the Mutual Security Treaty with the United States. Even the Japanese Socialist Party, once the most dogmatic of all political parties in Japan, issued a statement from its convention in February 1984 that "The SDF, which is unconstitutional, exists according to laws."[33] The other parties, the Democratic Socialist Party and the

Komeito (Clean Government Party), have adopted foreign and defense policies compatible enough with those of the LDP to allow them to seek coalition with the LDP. In fact, even in the JSP some mention of a coalition with "responsible" conservative forces (meant to imply a splinter group leaving the LDP) had been heard prior to the 1986 election.

In essence, the policy once advocated by the "progressive" (leftist) parties—renunciation of the Mutual Security Treaty, abolition of the Self-Defense Forces, and adoption of the concept of unarmed neutrality—is all but dead.

During the early periods of the Japanese defense debate, the LDP's majority permitted it to press forward with its foreign and defense policies in spite of vociferous attacks from the leftist opposition. Repeatedly the Self-Defense Forces were termed by the political left as illegal and a contravention of Japan's antiwar constitution, especially article 9. Over the years, however, as a result of the repudiation of the concept of socialist benevolence, these parties—the Democratic Socialist Party (DSP), Komeito, the Socialist Democratic Federation, and even the once doctrinaire Japanese Socialist Party—have adopted a new pragmatism that brings them closer to the policy advocated by the LDP. In essence, a consensus that involves all parties of the right, center, and left-of-center—omitting only the Communists—and that supports the security treaty and the Self-Defense Forces, has emerged.[34]

While the political parties evince a new receptivity to the existence of the Mutual Security Treaty and the Self-Defense Forces, the underlying national will or inclination of the Japanese people remains basically against any policy that would result in a greater role for the military (as can be regularly demonstrated by polls taken by the government of Japan and other institutions).[35] Asked if the U.S.–Japan Security Treaty should be abolished and replaced by a strengthened SDF, only 5 percent said yes; 69 percent wanted relations maintained as they currently are; 7 percent held to the old unarmed neutrality concept; and 18 percent had no ideas.[36]

This point is substantiated again in questions related to defense expenditures. Only 14 percent agreed with the idea of a reinforced

SDF, 54 percent wanted the present scale, 18 percent wished to see a reduction, and 14 percent could not make up their minds.[37] Lessons learned by one Japanese generation are perhaps even more emphatically held than those held by the American generation that determined never again to lose a peace or to allow incipient aggression to go unpunished. Indeed, the Japanese public resists any move to use military force in other than defense of the islands (in fact, in a "defensive" defense mode) and any efforts that might weaken civilian control over the military. This is basic and is unlikely to change rapidly.

JAPAN'S NATIONAL STRATEGY

Deterrence of attack through the U.S. security commitment is fundamental to Japanese strategy. If deterrence fails, conflict could take on several forms. If the evolving struggle comes from within Japan and is characterized as indirect, fifth column, or small-scale direct, Japan will attempt to counter it through its own defense resources. If the attack is of major conventional proportions or involves nuclear threats or nuclear weapons use, the United States would be expected to provide the necessary assistance.

Deterrence of a conventional attack through enemy knowledge of probable losses that would be suffered in such an effort will function during the 1980s and 1990s as a most effective part of Japanese strategy. The Japanese have stressed the Self-Defense Forces' capacity to destroy or badly degrade the ability of an enemy to project forces to the Home Islands. Emphasis, in fact, has been placed on efforts to secure lines of communication and "strengthen air-defense capabilities." But in the event of a successful invasion, the Ground Self-Defense Forces (GSDF) have been engaged in modernization programs to "improve mobility and firepower, with special emphasis on upgrading the northern deterrent."[38]

While not officially admitting that the Soviet Union is the primary potential enemy, it was reported that the GSDF regarded the Soviet Union "as the main enemy."[39] Strongly indicative of national concern are the locations of key defensive units in Hokkaido, the creation of a new mechanized division with firepower strong enough to engage a Soviet main battle force successfully, and the general GSDF reorganization to place the bulk of its major hitting power on Hokkaido.[40]

GENERAL ELEMENTS OF JAPAN'S DEFENSE POLICY

In addition to political and overall strategic considerations, there exists another body of extremely important features that control or establish the framework for consideration of defense issues in Japan. Within this general grouping is a subgrouping of elements that either became government policy or were reaffirmed as government policy in 1976 during the tenure of Prime Minister Miki Takeo and his defense adviser, Sakata Michita, director general of the Defense Agency.

NATIONAL DEFENSE OUTLINE (TAIKO)

At the core of Japan's current defense policy is the National Defense Outline, or *Taiko* (see table 2). Subject to considerable pressure from the opposition parties, but aiming to provide the necessary force levels for deterrence or defeat of possible small-to-medium-scale attacks, the government of Japan, after four successive buildup plans (see table 3), chose in 1976 to indicate clearly the size of the Self-Defense Forces. The size and general composition as projected by the *Taiko* would remain fixed as long as the following assumptions about the state of the world remained valid:

1. The United States and the Soviet Union continue to avoid nuclear war as well as conventional war of total involvement.
2. The Soviet Union continues to be occupied with European problems such as NATO confrontation and control of Eastern Europe.
3. There is little possibility of Sino-Soviet confrontation being resolved, although relations may be partially improved.
4. The United States and China continue mutual negotiations to adjust their relations.
5. The situation on the Korean Peninsula generally remains as it is, with no major armed conflict.[41]

The original 1976 White Paper comments:

"Given no major change in the above preconditions, there is little possibility of major armed aggression against Japan; however, the possibility of limited aggression, or of neighboring conflicts spreading to this nation, cannot be denied."[42] It has been over ten years since the *Taiko* was endorsed by the National Defense Council.

Improvements in the nature of the Self-Defense Forces under the above assumptions concentrated on qualitative upgrading of weapons systems, logistical infrastructure, and command and control systems. As of early 1987, the effort to revise these assumptions had only just begun; the Kosaka Commission, an ad hoc advisory commission established by Prime Minister Nakasone, recommended in December 1984 that, in light of the changed international environment, the *Taiko* be reexamined. This was agreed to by the prime minister, and the LDP began to study the matter. Work to revise the "attached tables," which actually indicated the "ideal" force structure needed by the Self-Defense Forces, began in 1986 with an effort to create an "effective defense posture" in the Defense Reform Committee, a special body of the Japan Defense Agency.[43]

THE 1 PERCENT BARRIER

Several other elements of Japan's continuing defense policy were established in 1976 that are perhaps more familiar to Western readers than the *Taiko*. Incorporated into cabinet-level decisions during the tenure of Prime Minister Miki Takeo was the keying of defense expenditures to a fixed percentage point of the gross national product. While it may appear "unstrategic" to fix expenditure levels without reference to a threat by setting the defense level at a ceiling of 1 percent of GNP, given the political environment of Japan, the measure was acceptable to all sides. For those who desired more money for defense, an expanding economy or GNP promised increasing real sums for defense. In bureaucratic terms, the amount, although fixed, was a guarantee that the Japan Defense Agency could at least have a planning figure that would approximate its actual annual budget. For those opposed to large increases in defense spending, the 1 percent fig-

Table 2. The Taiko—National Defense Program Outline Targets

Item	National Defense Program Outline (Standard Defense Force)	Defense Force Strength Attained at the End of FY 1979
GSDF		
Self-defense official quota	180,000 troops	180,000 troops
Basic units		
Units deployed regionally in peacetime	12 divisions	12 divisions
	2 composite brigades	1 composite brigade
Mobile operation units	1 armored division	1 mechanized division
		1 tank brigade
	1 artillery brigade	1 artillery brigade
	1 airborne brigade	1 airborne brigade
	1 training brigade	1 training brigade
	1 helicopter brigade	1 helicopter brigade
Low-altitude ground-to-air missile units	8 antiaircraft artillery groups	8 antiaircraft artillery groups
MSDF		
Basic units		
antisubmarine surface ship units (for mobile operations)	4 escort flotillas	4 escort flotillas
antisubmarine surface ship units (regional district units)	10 divisions	9 divisions
Submarine units	6 divisions	5 divisions
Minesweeping units	2 flotillas	2 flotillas
Land-based antisubmarine aircraft units	16 squadrons	16 squadrons
Major equipment		
Antisubmarine surface ships	approx. 60 ships	59 ships
Submarines	16 submarines	14 submarines
Operational aircraft	approx. 220 aircraft	approx. 190 aircraft
ASDF		
Basic units		
Aircraft control and warning units	28 groups	28 groups
Interceptor units	10 squadrons	10 squadrons
Support fighter units	3 squadrons	3 squadrons
Air reconnaissance units	1 squadron	1 squadron
Air transport units	3 squadrons	3 squadrons
Early warning units	1 squadron	
High-altitude ground-to-air missile units	6 groups	6 groups
Major equipment		
Operational aircraft	approx. 430 aircraft	approx. 400 aircraft

Source: Japan Defense Agency, *Defense of Japan* (1979), p. 86.

ure was a ceiling that promised an end to concern over possible massive and rapid rearmament. The existence of a definite level also assured critics that they would be able to keep tight control over the specific contents of any defense agency budget. No fixed time span was considered for the 1 percent limit; it was to remain in effect "for the interim."[44]

Some critics of the Japanese defense effort contend that this method of determining defense expenditures errs in not considering the threat. As such, they maintain, Japanese programs tend to concentrate on frontline, high-cost equipment with very little logistical backup. This indeed seems to be the case, but it has been the natural consequence of several other policies also pursued by the government: failure to identify a specific threat because of a diplomatic policy that is omnidirectional; a be-

lief by certain segments of the government that no imminent threat exists and that, short of such a threat, efforts should be focused on development of the nation's industrial base; a general reluctance on the part of the public to support any increase in the size of the Self-Defense Forces; and LDP concern with depoliticizing the defense issue.

During negotiations over the fiscal year 1986 budget, Prime Minister Nakasone committed himself to discarding the 1 percent barrier as an unrealistic budget compromise unrelated to strategic concerns. In so doing, he seemed to get out in front of his own party perhaps a bit too much. Some of the "Old Guard" (Miki, Fukuda, and Suzuki) opposed any move to discard it, saying that it had become the popularly accepted principle in Japanese defense policy. Forced into a corner, Nakasone aban-

Table 3. Development of Defense Capability

Item	1st Build-up Plan (1958–60)	2nd Build-up Plan (1962–66)	3rd Build-up Plan (1967–71)	4th Build-up Plan (1972–76)
GSDF				
Self-defense official quota	170,000 troops	171,500 troops	179,000 troops	180,000 troops
Basic units				
Units deployed regionally in peacetime	3 divisions	12 divisions	12 divisions	12 divisions
Mobile operations units	3 composite brigades 1 mechanized combined brigade	1 mechanized division	1 mechanized division	1 composite brigade 1 mechanized division
	1 tank regiment	1 tank regiment	1 tank regiment	1 tank brigade
	1 artillery brigade	1 artillery brigade	1 artillery brigade	1 artillery brigade
	1 airborne brigade	1 airborne brigade	1 airborne brigade	1 airborne brigade
	1 training brigade	1 training brigade	1 training brigade	1 training brigade
			1 helicopter brigade	1 helicopter brigade
Low-altitude ground-to-air missile units		2 antiaircraft artillery battalions	4 antiaircraft artillery groups (another group being prepared)	8 antiaircraft artillery groups
MSDF				
Basic units				
Antisubmarine surface ship units (for mobile operations)	3 escort flotillas	3 escort flotillas	4 escort flotillas	4 escort flotillas
Antisubmarine surface ship units (regional district units)	5 divisions	5 divisions	10 divisions	10 divisions
Submarine units		2 divisions	4 divisions	6 divisions
Minesweeping units	1 flotilla	2 flotillas	2 flotillas	2 flotillas
Land-based antisubmarine aircraft units	9 squadrons	15 squadrons	14 squadrons	16 squadrons
Major equipment				
Antisubmarine surface ships	57 ships	59 ships	59 ships	61 ships
Submarines	2 submarines	7 submarines	12 submarines	14 submarines
Operational aircraft	(approx. 220 aircraft)	(approx. 230 aircraft)	(approx. 240 aircraft)	(approx. 210 aircraft) (approx. 300 aircraft)
ASDF				
Basic units				
Aircraft control and warning units	24 groups	24 groups	24 groups	28 groups
Interceptor units	12 squadrons	15 squadrons	10 squadrons	10 squadrons
Support fighter units		4 squadrons	4 squadrons	3 squadrons
Air reconnaissance units		1 squadron	1 squadron	1 squadron
Air transport units	2 squadrons	3 squadrons	3 squadrons	3 squadrons
Early warning units				
High-altitude ground-to-air missile units		2 groups	4 groups	5 groups (another group being prepared)
Major equipment Operational aircraft	(approx. 1,130 aircraft)	approx. 1,100 aircraft)	approx. 940 aircraft)	approx. 510 aircraft) (approx. 930 aircraft)

Source: Japan Defense Agency, *Defense of Japan* (1979), p. 70.

Note: Numbers of operational aircraft in parentheses denote total number of aircraft including trainers. The number of units is as of the end of each plan period.

doned the drive to exceed the 1 percent barrier in exchange for elevation of the midterm planning estimate (see below) from a Defense Agency internal document to the status of a government sponsored plan. This, in essence, returned the government of Japan to the era of the five-year plans. However, arguments over meeting the pledged rate of defense buildup for the fiscal year 1988 budget have required the government finally to alter the 1 percent guide to read "about" 1 percent and adopt a procedure that places overall defense budget limitations in five-year increments. Any one year can exceed 1 percent, but not the total approved in the five-year plan. In planning the fiscal year 1988 budget, it became clear that expenditures at a 1.004 rate of GNP would be necessary to meet the goals of the five-year plan. With an impressive LDP majority in the Diet, this one percent barrier effectively was broken.[45]

1976 WEAPONS EXPORT POLICY AND NPT RATIFICATION

Two other elements of Japan's current defense policy that were given official sanction in 1976 were the policies toward weapons export and nuclear weapons. The 1976 articulation of policy toward weapons exports came after defense contractors brought significant pressure on the Ministry of International Trade and Industry to review the existing restrictive no-export policy which had been a feature of Japanese policy since 1967. In the wake of a business slump because of the worldwide oil crisis, some business spokesmen advocated a liberalization of export policy to help the economy. Rather than finding a panacea for under-utilized production capability, the defense interest groups found that their efforts had backfired. Indeed, in 1976 the ministry issued updated guidance that not only banned the export of weapons, but also disallowed the export of facilities with which to manufacture weapons. The only exception granted to this ban has been a 1983 decision to respond favorably to U.S. requests to share defense technology when so requested. The other significant policy guideline to be realized in 1976 concerned nuclear weapons and was accomplished by ratification of the Nuclear Non-proliferation Treaty (NPT).

OTHER ELEMENTS OF JAPANESE POLICY

The principles of civilian control, the all-volunteer nature of the Self-Defense Forces, the "no offensive forces" limitation, and the very nature of the rules of engagement should a crisis occur are found in the Constitution of Japan and the basic laws establishing the Japan Defense Agency and the Self-Defense Forces. So restrictive are some of these regulations that General Kurisu Hiroomi, the chairman of the Joint Staff Council in 1978, publicly criticized existing procedures to deal with a surprise attack on Japan, saying that it might be necessary for the Self-Defense Forces to take extra-legal measures to defend themselves if brought under attack.[46]

This critique of emergency procedures cost Kurisu his job, but it did start a general review of existing legislation for possible corrective action. This was published in reports to the Diet in April 1981 and October 1984.[47] Efforts to create a unified command post were redoubled, and basic means of ensuring effective combined operations were completed in the early 1980s. A document on *Guidelines for Japan–U.S. Defense Cooperation* provides for enhanced cooperation in operations, intelligence, and logistics between the Self-Defense Forces and U.S. forces in Japan. Greater capacity for coordinated operations is seen as a result of these guidelines facilitating military-to-military contacts. The joint posture for deterring aggression, responding to any armed attack on Japan, and enhancing Japan–U.S. cooperation in situations concerning the Far East (outside of Japan) are addressed in the guidelines and made somewhat more precise. While only a beginning, these guidelines serve as a basis for achieving significant levels of U.S.–Japanese interoperability.[48]

Japan's grand military strategy, in summary, can be seen as dependence on the U.S.–Japanese Security Treaty and maintenance of a standing defense force that will provide the nucleus around which a larger force can be created if necessary. Accomplishment of this strategy is constrained by the following limitations: no nuclear weapons, no "offensive" weapons, no export of weapons, approximately one percent of the GNP for defense expenditures, strict civilian control, and no Japanese Self-Defense Forces in combat overseas.

There are many who insist that the mere existence of the Self-Defense Forces is a contravention of Article 9 of the Constitution. It is clear that the Japanese government has taken the view that the Self-Defense Forces do not challenge the Constitution but exist because of the basic right of all nations to self-defense, a right reaffirmed by the UN charter. To date, court tests of these views have sustained the government's position, and as the capabilities of neighboring countries' forces improve, the nature of the Japanese defense will of necessity change. Within this context, even defensive nuclear weapons can be defined by the government as constitutionally allowable; however, the nuclear option has been foresworn by adherence to the NPT and numerous affirmations of the three non-nuclear principles.

OTHER DOMESTIC DETERMINANTS

The level of economic and technological development of Japan is, of course, not a factor that limits its defense potential. Japan manufactures, or has the capability to manufacture, most of its defense needs. As has been pointed out in several works, these needs could even include nuclear weapons and appropriate delivery vehicles. In the case of Japan it is, as always, the political factor that has the greatest impact on defense policy. While Japan could produce practically all the weapons needed, this is frequently not done because of questions of economy of scale, technology transfer, or simple political realism. This issue will be treated at greater length later in the chapter.

POPULATION AND EDUCATION

Japan is experiencing a population inversion much like that of the United States. The proportion of the population fifty-five years of age and over will have increased from 16 percent of the labor force in 1975 to 23 percent by the year 2000.[49] As the population ages, the percentage of young people available for military service will decrease. Japan's particular situation, like that of the United States, is complicated by the "all volunteer" nature of service and the generally good state of the economy, which provides ample job opportunities in the private sector. The program of maintaining sufficient manpower is already becoming a problem in the recruitment of second class male personnel. The number needed is significant; the eligible population (18–25) is declining, and short-term service is not attractive.[50] Of course, given

changes now being made in retirement age, there may also be some increase in the average age of personnel in the Self-Defense Forces. Current Ground Self-Defense Forces manning is at 86.7 percent of authorized levels, while the two other services stand at 97 percent for the Maritime Self-Defense Forces and 94 percent for the Air Self-Defense Forces.[51] No attempt is being made to attain full strength at this time.

Despite being less than fully manned, applications for various positions in the military run well above minimum requirements and as long as the service maintains its current profile, manpower will not be a debilitating problem. Rates of competition for available openings at the National Defense Academy run 15:1 for science and engineering and 34:1 for social sciences and humanities. Applications for noncommissioned officer candidate positions for the ground forces have a 14:1 ratio, for the maritime forces, 9:1, and for the air force, 10:1.[52] Such levels of interest from high school graduates are impressive indeed. Since Japan boasts the highest literacy rate in the world and possesses an excellent educational system, there is no constraint on the military from this quarter. Only when military members attempt to attend Tokyo University for postgraduate degrees do problems arise, but the environment there is improving somewhat.

FORCE EMPLOYMENT

Controversy over emphasis on readiness of cadre forces has been a traditional element of the defense debate in Japan. While not exactly a debate on force employment per se, a steady stream of literature over the years has been available from two principal schools of thought that seem to have emerged concerning what Japan's posture should be on a day-by-day basis. The first stresses that Japan needs to stop buying high technology, expensive aircraft, naval vessels, and tanks if the missiles, ammunition, and basic logistical support infrastructure do not exist. One of the most outspoken proponents of this school is Kaihara Osamu. Kaihara frequently makes comparisons between Japan's Imperial Army and current forces. According to Kaihara, the rates of fire even for battles in the late 1930s consumed ammunition at rates unsupportable by the Self-Defense Forces as currently configured.[53] He insists that "the present Self-Defense Force is nothing more than a high-class flying club."[54]

The other school concentrates on creating capabilities for the Self-Defense Forces to perform a wide range of missions. Stressing development of experience with high-quality systems that can be provided with logistical back-up when a "real" threat emerges, this school places emphasis on training a cadre. While proponents of this school advocate the acquisition of ships, planes, and tanks that will match any in the world, they also emphasize the expandable nature of the Self-Defense Forces. In an emergency they can be increased, while at the same time, the industrial base can focus on necessary munitions to fill in the gaps in logistical support. From available data, and the fact that the Standard Defense Force concept was established during Sakata Michita's tenure as director general of the Defense Agency, it would appear that current policy places primary emphasis on the cadre concept rather than on readiness. Until a major threat develops, the Self-Defense Forces will continue to be employed primarily to combat the all too numerous national disasters that plague Japan—earthquakes, tidal waves, typhoons, and fires.

In recent years, the Defense Agency has focused on the problem of inadequate logistic support in response to criticism by domestic and U.S. observers. Fiscal year 1985 expenditure for ammunition procurement was 17 percent more than in fiscal year 1984, for a total of 103 billion yen.[55]

A debate reportedly conducted inside the Self-Defense Forces concerning force employment and the critical tactical question of where to defend Japan was in full swing in late 1980. In a debate reminiscent of the *san sen ron* ("three-line debate") of World War II, the three services contend with each other regarding the role of interdiction and island defense. Where is it best to stop an attacking force—at sea or in the air as it approaches, on the beaches, or through defense in depth? Solutions offered tend to stress the capability inher-

ent in a particular armed service. The Air Self-Defense Force and the Maritime Self-Defense Force favored attacking forces as they approached Japan. The Ground Self-Defense Force stressed mechanized forces that could be brought to bear only after an enemy had landed.

In February 1985 Nakasone made a critical decision to settle this internal debate. The enemy would be met at sea and destroyed. Air and naval interdiction capabilities would be enhanced, and as the GSDF would receive the SSM-1 ground-to-ground missile with a 150-kilometer range, all services would have a role in defeating an enemy at sea. Not all were pleased by this decision. General Nakamura Morio, while chief of staff of the GSDF, attacked the decision saying:

It is naive to think that the enemy can be destroyed on the high seas if sea and air defenses are strengthened. This thinking can be traced to Hayaski Shihei's "coastal defense" strategy advocated in the Edo Period [1603–1867]. In this modern age, the enemy will not attack from the sea only, their attack will be three-dimensional and multilateral. The Sea of Japan is no longer a rampart for Japan. It will be the GSDF that will stop the enemy from landing on Japan. It will be the GSDF that will serve as the core deterrent power.[56]

The Defense Decision-Making Process

Decision-making authority within the Japanese government bureaucracy is so diffuse that it is recognized as a weakness of the Japanese political system. Until 1 July 1986 the system provided for the National Defense Council (NDC) as a special clearing house for defense issues. Under article 62 of the Defense Agency Law, the NDC had to approve long-range planning before the initiation of a plan, budgets, major equipment commitments, and so on.[57] When the Japan Defense Agency presented its budget or major new weapons procurement programs, it did so in the NDC, where the prime minister, deputy prime minister, Ministry of Finance, Ministry of Foreign Affairs, Economic Planning Agency director general, and JDA director had membership. Others were invited as appropriate. These ministries and agencies that composed the National Defense Council, not in any way subordinate to the Japan Defense Agency, considered the request. The power to deny Defense Agency requests represented by membership of the Ministries of Finance and Foreign Affairs on the NDC was considerable. The Japan Defense Agency, a junior, appeared as a suppliant before the council in presenting its major programs. The NDC forum did not have the power of the U.S. National Security Council (NSC). It had only a small professional staff of bureaucratic personnel who concentrated on defense-related studies, and it was not a location of substantive debate for the creation of policy alternatives. In essence, the NDC was not a primary actor but more of a facilitator for interministerial consideration of defense policy that was formulated elsewhere, generally in the LDP, the Ministry of Foreign Affairs, and the Japan Defense Agency. Attempts to make it more like the U.S. NSC had failed, primarily because of political and bureaucratic opposition to such a move.

On 1 July 1986, however, in what was called a "sweeping reform," the Japanese government acted to enhance its capacity to coordinate overall national security policy. To accomplish this new coordinative power—which for Japan is almost revolutionary—the cabinet secretariat and the National Defense Council were reorganized.

In the case of the cabinet secretariat, two offices were created: the External Affairs Office (EAO) and the Internal Affairs Office (IAO). The EAO is charged with coordination of intergovernment positions on externally driven "critical issues,"[58] such as problems arising from trade friction.[59] The National Defense Council was disestablished and a National Security Council was created in its stead. Responsible for the areas once covered by the NDC it is also involved in crisis management for military, economic, and social emergencies. Response to natural disasters and major terrorist threats are also coordinated by the new NSC.

This fundamental reform of the Japanese decision-making process—turning it on end, so to speak—responds to the consistent failure of the traditional Japanese bottom-up, or *renqi*, decision-making process in a modern information-oriented society. It may also reflect the leadership of Prime Minister Nakasone, who was dedicated to administrative reform during his entire term of office, and who sees a need for top-down guidance to establish a new model for Japanese diplomatic initiatives.[60]

While the reform is heralded as facilitating intragovernmental coordination, EAO is not charged with either policy formulation or implementation. One official has noted that EAO deals exclusively with issues such as implementation of the Maekawa Commission Report. Since that report calls for the restructuring of the entire Japanese economy, it would appear that EAO and IAO will be at the very center of things. Whether or not these reforms can succeed will, in large measure, depend on consistent follow-through by top leadership. In essence, the prime minister has just reordered the bureaucratic system to provide the kind of support necessary to move from a weak prime minister system—so characteristic of past Japanese leaders—to a strong system somewhat approaching the U.S. presidential model.[61]

While the decision-making process in the government centers on the NSC for formal presentation of defense budgets, the Japan Defense Agency must work out its draft budgets and major programs in close contact with the Ministry of Finance, the Ministry of International Trade and Industry, and their representatives seconded to the Defense Agency. This, in essence, gives the major ministries a multifold opportunity to influence Defense Agency programs.

Within the Japan Defense Agency itself, decision making is largely handled by what is called the Naikyoku, or Internal Bureaus (see fig. 1). Five bureaus—Defense, Personnel and Education, Health and Medical, Finance, and Equipment—function as the heart of decision making for overall defense policy. Staffed by civilian professionals, these bureaus make all important decisions for approval by the director general or his administrative deputy.

The lack of military officer participation in the Naikyoku has been a long-term source of contention between the military and civilian members of the Japan Defense Agency. While some efforts have been made to introduce mili-

Figure 1. Defense Structure

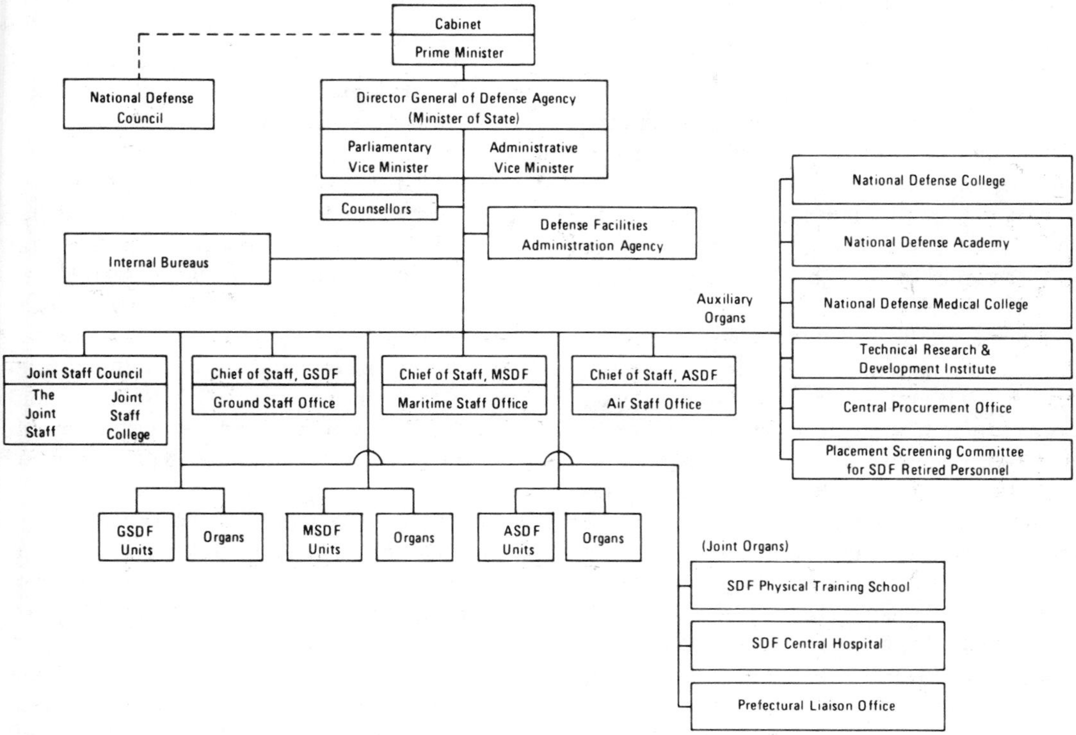

Source: Japan Defense Agency, *Defense of Japan,* 1979

tary officers into the Naikyoku, they have not resulted in changing existing authority patterns. Since some see this issue as a key to the concept of civilian control of the military, it might be a long time before a senior-ranking military officer finds himself assigned to a position of authority in the Naikyoku. This is particularly true since the increased assertiveness of several Japanese generals (especially General Kurisu Hiroomi) has rekindled concern over the adequacy of civilian controls of the military. As graduates of the Defense Academy reach general rank, there is growing concern that competent civilian control will fade. This is brought about by what observers see as a decline in the quality of civilian bureaucrats in the Defense Agency at the same time as the military will be promoting the cream of the Defense Academy system to general. In the near future, it is noted, "the quality of the controllers may be dangerously surpassed by that of the controlled."[62] Attributed, among others, to the former director general of the Defense Agency, Kato Koichi, this concern for civilian control can be seen in the strict management of command authority that rests with the prime minister and runs down through the director general of the Japan Defense Agency to the military commander involved.

The Japanese system, as has been pointed out elsewhere, is undergoing structural reform at the top in the national security arena. This reform will, however, in no way reduce the effectiveness of civilian control of the military.

Recurring Issues and Defense Policy Outputs

CIVIL-MILITARY RELATIONS

The Japan Self-Defense Forces must be given full marks for their efforts to improve relations with the civilian population. Polls reveal that most respondents feel positively about the assistance provided by the military during and after natural disasters. In addition to disaster relief, the services also engage in civil action projects and programs to reduce or moderate the impact of military bases on neighboring communities. Such items as noise abatement and TV-interference compensation to affected housholds are indicative of a defense establishment with a high degree of concern for the civilian sector.

Recent public attitudes demonstrate that the alienation of the military from the rest of the society is ending. Personnel recruiting can be conducted, even in Okinawa, one of the most sensitive environments in all Japan, and for the first time in years, young *Jieitai* personnel have been invited to the coming-of-age ceremony (seijinshiki) in Naha.

As yet, officers of the Self-Defense Forces cannot attend the prestigious Tokyo University (Tohdai) for postgraduate work, but a few Tokyo University graduates are entering the military to become officers. These items are indicative of a general and growing acceptance of the Self-Defense Forces by the Japanese. The military is gaining a place in society—not militarism.[63]

WEAPONS ACQUISITION

The actors of the Japanese weapons procurement systems can be seen as falling into primary, secondary, and tertiary levels of involvement.[64] Primary actors who play an active role from beginning to end include the three services; the Research and Development Division, Equipment Bureau, and Development Division of the Japan Defense Agency; the Technical Research and Development Institute; and, of course, military industrial contractors such as Mitsubishi Heavy Industries and Nippon Denki.

The secondary actors are the Defense and Finance Bureaus of the Japan Defense Agency, as well as politicians who represent certain policy or constituent interests. These secondary actors often resolve conflicts among primary actors and can have a very important role.

The tertiary actors consist of the cabinet and the National Security Council. While these two bodies may not be actively involved during most of the process, they have crucial roles to play if they choose to intervene. (The Lockheed case demonstrated that involvement and direction from above can happen in the Japanese system.)[65]

The first stage in weapons acquisition takes place primarily between the service that has recognized an operational deficiency or requirement and the Technical Research and Development Institute (TRDI). A three-star general is assigned to the TRDI from each service. When the operational requirement is developed, the Defense Agency's Research and Development Division and the TRDI consult to determine if the research will be accomplished domestically or not. At times, decisions to do research in Japan are made just to keep abreast of the latest developments in a particular field. This first decision is subject, of course, to some lobbying from domestic industrial representatives.

If a decision is made to do the research domestically, a research priority is established for the project. This is done by the Finance Bureau of the Japan Defense Agency, with considerable input from the Equipment Bureau. Various industrial candidates are considered for the job on the basis of past performance and need. The word that a contractor is being sought is passed to potential contractors, and a source is selected to do the research. Some political input probably exists at this point if the project is significant in budget terms. If the matter is a routine research decision, however, politicians probably do not get involved.

Once the decision is made to do research, the matter is controlled by the TRDI. As a prototype is created, the TRDI follows the progress and approaches the next decision.

Development Decision. As a prototype comes down the line, the question of its development potential is addressed. Up to this point, the issue has been primarily research oriented, and policy levels of the Japan Defense Agency have largely remained outside the effort. However, the question of development is very much a policy question and receives input from the agency's defense bureau charged with policy determination, the Ministry of International Trade and Industry (MITI), politicians, and business. Also involved are study teams from the individual service concerned, as well as the Defense Agency's Equipment Bureau, which often is closely tied to MITI's wishes. If the equipment concerned is a major item, the influence of MITI is particularly critical.

Basically, what is decided at this point is whether to buy the equipment in question, license-produce it, or produce it domestically, drawing on research already completed in the preceding phase. As can be imagined, contractor pressure for domestic production is usually heavy. Decision criteria usually include such technical questions as the benefit to Japanese industry if a technology transfer is involved and the quality of foreign equipment versus domestic alternatives. Another policy consideration is the question of impact on the U.S.-Japan alliance. The questions of interoperability and standardization of American and Japanese weapons systems have to be addressed and can sometimes weigh quite heavily in the final decision. Besides technical and other defense policy considerations, a final decision includes, as in the United States, the impact of political influence. MITI, various members of the Diet, and leaders in the government can make final recommendations that can have a disproportionate impact on the decision to buy or produce.

If a decision is made to produce the item domestically, agreement as to who will produce which components and accomplish the final assembly is reached between business and the Japan Defense Agency. In most cases the industrial firms handling military orders have already agreed on the division of the contract. However, whether or not such a division takes place is dependent on government concurrence, not just acquiescence. In the event that a decision is made to license-produce, a letter of offer is issued to the foreign producer (probably to the U.S. government) and a reaction is awaited. Production involving Japanese firms is often accomplished with on-site representation of the Japan Defense Agency, thus assuring quality control and facilitating production.

While the capability of the Japanese industrial base to produce a wide range of military hardware is unquestioned, it suffers from a problem of under-utilization.[66] This forces management to seek ways to diversify sufficiently into nonmilitary applications to permit maintenance of a skilled cadre. A former head of the Japanese Defense Committee of the Keidanren captured the frustrations of some producers when he stated that the Self-Defense Forces would change into "bamboo-spear units" unless capital expenditures were increased.[67] Keidanren reported the fiscal year 1983 percentage of defense production of various industries to be: aircraft manufacturing, 77.1 percent; shipbuilding, 4.4 percent; electric communications apparatus production, .92 percent; and vehicle production, .1 percent. Total defense production was only .50 percent of industrial production.[68] With the decision to co-develop and co-produce the FSX support fighter with the United States, a new page in arms technology transfer may be turned. However, the acrimony surrounding this decision—on both sides of the Pacific—will focus all eyes on the future course of such collaboration.

For the time being, the limited nature of the domestic market for military hardware will keep Japanese-produced equipment comparatively high-priced. The quality will remain competitive, but the size of production runs dictates what amounts to continued subsidy through high costs paid by the government.

FORCE POSTURE

The force posture and deployment of the Japan Self-Defense Forces reflect their several roles. The most modern and well-manned ground units are stationed in the Northern Army opposite one of the possible Soviet invasion routes (see fig. 2). And as previously mentioned, this modernization will increase for the GSDF as preparation for the next midterm plan continues. Other forces are assigned throughout the main islands as garrison forces and reflect another role, that of preservation of peace and security in Japan itself. Levels of equipment held by the Self-Defense Forces are reflected in table 4.

Figure 2. Force Posture: Deployment

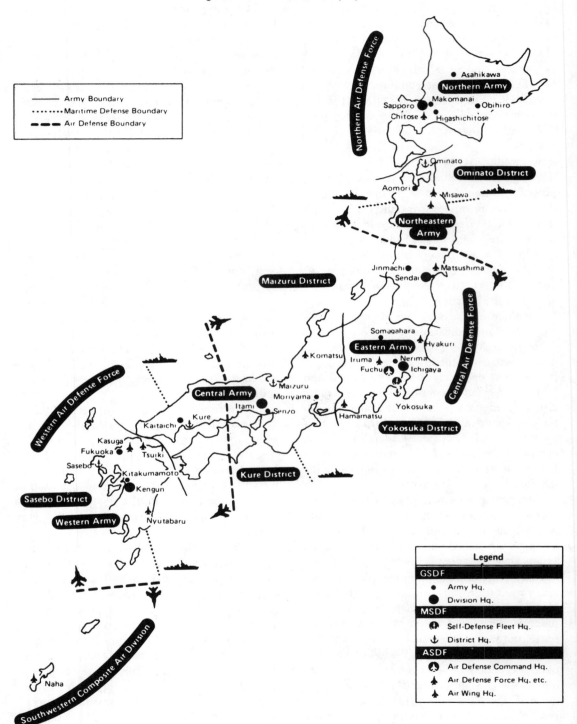

Source: Japan Defense Agency, *Defense of Japan,* 1979, p. 12

Table 4. Self-Defense Forces Equipment

Force	Equipment	Number
GSDF	Recoilless rifles	2,990
	Mortars	1,890
	Field artillery pieces	1,130
	Rocket guns	120
	Antiaircraft guns	140
	Tanks	1,180
	Armored personnel carriers	610
	Hawks	8 groups
MSDF	Destroyer escorts	53 (140,000 tons)
	Submarines	14 (29,000 tons)
	Minelayers	39 (17,000 tons)
	Patrol ships	14 (1,000 tons)
	Transports	9 (12,000 tons)
	Special service ships	31 (68,000 tons)
ASDF	Fighters	250
	Reconnaissance planes	10
	Airborne early warning	10
	Trainers	190
	Transport planes	50
	Reserve planes	31
	Nikes/Patriots	6 groups

Sources: Japan Defense Agency and International Institute for Strategic Studies.

The positioning of forces on separate islands is necessary in Japan because of the dictates of geography and good military tactics, but this does create mobility problems. As to the ability of Japanese forces to defeat an invasion, even Japanese observers cannot agree. It is likely, however, that the forces, as postured in the 1980s, can accomplish the goal set out by Director General Nakasone in 1970: to create a force that can resist small-scale aggression successfully, but one that must ultimately depend on the United States to repel any large-scale and determined invasion.

MILITARY DOCTRINE AND FORCE POSTURE

Military doctrine, as previously pointed out, does not control force posture as such in Japan. Force posture has been largely a political creation and happens to be what can be supported with approximately 1 percent of the GNP. The coming decade will see a growing capability on the part of the Japanese to act as a cohesive force in resisting aggression, but for the near term, focus will remain on equipment and building up a cadre force as determined in the 1976 *Taiko.* The doctrine, as such, should be related to the characteristics of the Standard Defense Force as defined in the 1976 White Paper:

Japan's defense forces are peacetime in nature. On the whole, they should be well balanced and flawless, rather than capable of handling a specific, imminent threat of invasion. The necessary characteristics of such defense strength are listed below.

First, all defense functions must be arranged with no flaws so that minimum action can be taken against any conceivable type of aggression with conventional weapons. If any functional defect existed, counteraction in that particular field of operations would be impossible, leaving an aggressor a free hand.

Our defense capability therefore requires all functions and data necessary for air, sea, and land defense, including command and communications and the various auxiliary functions that supplement them, with no defects.

Second, these functions must be organized and systematized in accordance with Japan's topography, so that immediate defensive action can be taken systematically against any invasion of our land, air, or sea space. Proper balance and effective combination of combat units and logistics support are necessary for an integrated defense capability against aggression.

Third, during peacetime, high-quality volunteers must be enlisted and thoroughly trained to maintain personnel capacity. Emphasis must be placed on the SDF's positive cooperation in public welfare, taking prompt relief and rescue action in case of natural calamity or major disaster. This also requires an even geographic distribution of units, and necessary equipment and facilities must be kept in good condition.

Standard Defense Forces as such must include the following capabilities:

First, data-gathering in nearby air space and straits must be maintained at higher levels than in other fields.

Since Japanese military power is limited to self-defense and is based on a peacetime conception of the general international situation, it is extremely important to have efficient detection of military activity around Japan and to be able to deal flexibly with any changes.

Second, the defense forces must be capable of responding quickly and effectively to indirect aggression (large-scale internal disturbances or uprisings caused by agitation or intervention of one or more foreign powers), invasion of air space, or other unlawful military activity against Japan.

Third, the defense forces must be prepared to counter any potential small-scale attack that would be likely to come by surprise. Therefore, logistics support such as personnel, equipment and ammunition supply and other functions must be ensured on an emergency-response level.

Fourth, the development of operational functions and equipment must be effectively compatible with the Japan–U.S. security arrangement for smooth cooperation with forces.

Fifth, the defense forces must be capable of smooth expansion and strengthening should the government find this necessary due to changes in the international situation.

Should the international environment undergo some

drastic change, this concept of defense would, of course, require reexamination.[69]

ARMS CONTROL

Japan is committed to all aspects of arms control, both conventional and nuclear. In the conventional area, this commitment is clearly demonstrated by Japan's example of unilateral control. As pointed out previously, the government of Japan follows a program that prohibits the export of weapons as well as the facilities with which weapons are produced.

The three principles of no-weapons export that constitute government policy were reiterated in 1976. This policy strictly delimits the export of weapons and is overseen by the Ministry of International Trade and Industry. Under this policy, exports are prohibited to communist states (weapons and equipment on the Japan, U.S., and NATO Coordinating Committee (COCOM) List), to states subject to UN sanctions, and to any state involved or about to be involved in conflict.[70] The government of Japan has, in essence, decided not to export anything that can be defined as an instrument of death. It is one of the most effective arms control measures in the international community.

NUCLEAR ARMS CONTROL

Japan ratified the NPT in 1976 and disavows any intent to produce nuclear weapons. Additionally, since the government of Prime Minister Sato, it has followed an explicit policy of not permitting the introduction of nuclear weapons, not manufacturing them, and not possessing them.

The antinuclear feeling of the Japanese people was first actively revealed in the early 1950s when the fishing vessel *Fukuryu Maru* was unlucky enough to receive fallout from US nuclear tests at Bikini Atoll.[71] This event acted as a catalyst to create an outpouring of antinuclear feeling, which has moderated somewhat over the years, but not much.

In addition to the NPT and the three nonnuclear principles, the antinuclear weapons bias of the Japanese people has been reflected by government actions with regard to SALT and talks for general disarmament. The government of Japan has endorsed the SALT process between the two nuclear superpowers but has been on the fringes of the negotiations. Prior to the U.S. determination to halt consideration of the ratification of SALT II as a result of Soviet involvement in Afghanistan, the Japanese government was concerned that in SALT III greater emphasis be placed on the question of regional nuclear balances.

In the meetings of the Committee on Disarmament (CD) in Geneva, under the auspices of the United Nations, Japan has consistently advocated general and complete disarmament and has made several proposals along this line regarding nuclear disarmament.[72]

USE OF FORCE

Japan has not employed its defense forces in actual hostilities since their creation as a National Police Reserve. The government of Japan has even resisted efforts to involve the military in operations on behalf of the United Nations, taking the position that Japanese armed forces cannot be used overseas except for the defense of Japan. National opinion is still probably far from permitting such a use of the Self-Defense Forces.

The 1980s started on a very uncertain note. The erosion of respect for the norms of international diplomatic behavior, continued adventurism of nonstate and some state actors, and the spectacle of Soviet forces being employed outside the traditional areas of Soviet military presence collectively set a disturbing tenor for the decade. Prime Minister Ohira was so shocked over the use of Soviet forces in Afghanistan that he termed the Soviet pressure in the northern islands of Japan "a potential threat."[73] This was followed by a statement by General Takeda, chairman of the Joint Staff Council, that called for a fundamental reassessment of the midterm operations estimate for planning.[74] Implicit in his statement was an increased emphasis on readiness, as well as a possible telescoping of the equipment objectives reflected in the midterm planning estimate, which listed objectives to 1984. By February 1980 the reaction to Soviet moves in

Afghanistan had resulted in the two important LDP defense policy formulation committees, headed by Sakata Michita and Genda Minoru, endorsing a goal for Japanese fiscal year 1981 of .92 percent of the GNP for defense. They also went on record as supporting an annual increase of .2 percent until the 1 percent figure was reached.[75]

The efforts set the tone for the decade, leading to the realization in September 1985 of the first formal Midterm Defense Program in thirteen years[76] and, in December 1986, of a budget decision by the government that would raise the defense spending level by 11 percent to 1.004 percent of GNP. This, of course, technically broke the 1 percent barrier for the first time since the cap was implemented in 1976.[77]

To base an evaluation of future Japanese defense policy on single-point analysis would fail to recognize the complex multidimensional nature of defense policy in Japan. While spokesmen for the Defense Agency often tend to capture the ear of eager U.S. reporters, they speak for an agency with only a moderate amount of domestic bureaucratic power. It does not compare with the power of countervailing bureaucracies in the Japanese system, such as the Ministries of Finance, International Trade and Industry, and Foreign Affairs. Moreover the patronage enjoyed by the Defense Agency from Prime Minister Nakasone ended in 1987. In an era of limited economic growth, the demands of other sectors of the Japanese government will have to be balanced with those of the Defense Agency. Alternative energy development, development of sophisticated technology for Japan's industrial base, and assistance to selected states of the Third World may take precedence, in certain instances, over increased emphasis on the military element of national security.

Summary

Japan's military might is disproportionate to its economic power. This has given rise to the criticism from elements in the United States that Japan does not pull its weight in defense matters. Such may be the case, but one must also ask what the United States has received in return from its relations with Japan. It has received a forward base from which it may be possible to operate in the event of renewed hostilities in Korea, an advanced logistical and industrial system that may be called upon in times of emergency, and a base for stability in Northeast Asia (stability that has been enhanced over the past three decades by the absence of a well-armed and highly feared Japanese military). While some portions of Japan's former colonial empire may not mind a militarily strong Japan, there are others, especially Korea, that do not forget the suffering of the colonial era.

Now that the seeds of democracy and civilian control of the military have had an opportunity to develop and take root, an increased military posture for Japan may not have the same immediate connotations as in years gone by. Regardless of this, it will be many years and will require a fundamental realignment of the basic assumptions of the Japanese polity before the military is once again given a substantial role in the determination and the attainment of Japanese policy. When that time does come, professional military officers in Japan will look more like their colleagues in the United States than their Japanese predecessors. It may be possible to forecast a significant Japanese naval presence in the North Pacific as the century nears its conclusion, but to imagine large military forces with missions on the Asian continent seems unjustified.

In any event, Japanese defense policy will continue to evolve as a product of a complex and multifaceted system of pressures—political, economic, and social, external and internal. External pressures will be accommodated in the context of a cooperative policy with Japan's principal ally, the United States. Internal pressures will continue to reflect the fundamental changes that have occurred in Japan's political system since World War II. The creation and maturation of new political constituencies ensure that whatever Japan's response, it will be within the framework of a stable and democratic society.

Notes

1. See especially U.S. International Communication Agency (USICA), "Japanese Public Opinion Relevant to US–Japanese Security Relations," *USICA Research Memorandum*, 13 June 1979. Also, an *Asahi Shimbun* poll released 25 March 1980 revealed a figure of 25 percent willing to support a strengthened Self-Defense Force.

2. For example, p. 1 of *Summary of the Defense of Japan*, by the Japan Defense Agency and released by the Foreign Press Center, Tokyo, Japan, begins with a review of the U.S. factor.

3. *Japan Times*, 19 December 1979.

4. "In conformity with the spirit of Japan's Constitution, Japan's defense power is limited to purely exclusively defensive purposes," Japan Defense Agency, *Defense of Japan* (1979). Also see "Basic Policy for National Defense," as provided by cabinet action of 1957, Japan Defense Agency, *Defense of Japan* (1979), p. 64.

5. On the 1982 defense budget, see Japan Defense Agency, *Defense of Japan*, 1985 (Tokyo: JDA, 1985), p. 153. See, too, *Business Japan*, July 1979, p. 57. According to the *Nihon Keizai*, 29 August 1979, the Japan fiscal year budget request was 2,295.9 billion yen. Also see *Nihon no Boei* (1979), p. A-23, for a comparison of worldwide defense spending.

6. USICA, "US–Japanese Security Relations," p. 5.

7. *Nihon Keizai*, 19 July 1986, p. 5.

8. Hasegawa Tsuyoshi, "Japanese Perceptions of the Soviet Union: 1960–1985," (National Council for Soviet and East European Research, Washington D.C., 1986), p. 56.

9. *Boei Antena*, August 1985, p. 31.

10. *Jiji Press*, 14 December 1985.

11. Hasegawa, p. 59.

12. Interview with Nathaniel B. Thayer, Johns Hopkins School of Advanced International Studies.

13. Japan Defense Agency, *Defense of Japan* (1979), p. 2.

14. *Asahi Shimbun*, 19 January 1980.

15. See especially Kubo Takuya on the Soviet threat, in *Asahi Shimbun*, 15 October 1979 (evening). He makes a distinction between "potential threat" and "manifest threat."

16. Japan Defense Agency, *Defense of Japan* (1985), p. 313.

17. Ibid., p. 181.

18. On comprehensive security, see *Tokyo Shimbun*, 21 March 1979; *Nihon Keizai*, 8 August 1970; and *Nikkeiren Times* 26 July 1979.

19. For another interpretation of Japan's self-image, see Herbert Passin's "Socio-Cultural Factors in the Japanese Perception of International Order," in Japan Institute of International Affairs, *Annual Review*, especially pp. 69–71.

20. *Maekawa Report*, Provisional Translation in *The Brookings Institution, JCIE Tokyo Seminar*, 1–6 June 1986, Supplementary Reading.

21. *Japan Times*, 19 December 1979.

22. USICA, "Japanese Public Opinion: The Self-Defense Forces and Security Links with the U.S.," *USICA Research Memorandum*, 7 April 1979, p. 3.

23. *Boei Antena*, August 1985, p. 2–36.

24. *Jiji Press*, December 1985.

25. See the 6 March 1980 interview with Assistant Secretary of State Richard Holbroke in *Yomiuri*.

26. USICA, "Credibility of the U.S.," *USICA Research Memorandum*, 27 August 1979, p. 7.

27. Even the Japanese Socialist Party, in the face of intense leftist opposition, is slowly moving away from its traditional revisionist policy. Moves to minimize policy differences with the Komeito to enable joint campaigning in the forthcoming Upper House elections (June 1980) have been striking. See *Asahi Shimbun*, 17 October 1979; and *Yomiuri*, 24 October 1979.

28. *Nihon Keizai*, 25 July 1979.

29. This represents an extrapolated figure derived from the 1990 7 percent of GNP rate for national security, which would include defense, economic cooperation, and development of technology (Nihon Keizai, 25 July 1979).

30. Japan Defense Agency, *Defense of Japan* (1985), p. 58.

31. Ibid., p. 182. The rates show 13 percent for domestic security, 32 percent for disaster relief, and 4 percent for community programs.

32. *Washington Post*, 19 January 1983, and Tokinoya Atsushi, *The Japan–U.S. Alliance: A Japanese Perspective*, Adelphi Papers (London: Institute for Strategic Studies, 1986), p. 5. These comments relating to the "unsinkable aircraft carrier" were mistranslated (the actual phrase should have been "big carrier"), and a political reaction resulted in Japan.

33. *Kupdo*, 28 Fesbruary 1984.

34. *Asahi Shimbun*, 1 March 1980, and *Mainichi*, 3 March 1980.

35. USICA, "U.S.–Japanese Security Relations," p. 5.

36. Japan Defense Agency, *Defense of Japan* (1985), p. 183.

37. Ibid., p. 185.

38. Ibid., p. (1976), p. 79.

39. *Asahi Shimbun*, 9 July 1986.

40. *Gunji Kenkyu*, June 1986, pp. 42–49.

41. Japan Defense Agency, *Defense of Japan*, (1979), p. 70.

42. *White Paper*, 1976, pp. 38–39.

43. *Nihon Keizai Shimbun*, 28 October 1986, p. 2.

44. Japan Defense Agency, *Defense of Japan* (1976), p. 79.

45. *Wall Street Journal*, 30 January 1986, p. 3.

46. Research Institute for Peace and Security, *Asian Security* (Tokyo: Research Institute for Peace and Security, 1979), p. 172.

47. Ibid., p. 165.

48. Japan Ministry of Foreign Affairs, *Guidelines for Japan–U.S. Defense Cooperation*, 28 November 1978; and Research Institute for Peace and Security, *Asian Security*, 1979, p. 173.

49. Nakagawa Yatsuhiro, "Japan's Defense" (Manuscript, spring 1980), p. 5.

50. Japan Defense Agency, *Defense of Japan*, (1985), p. 138.

51. Ibid., p. 278.

52. Ibid., (1986), p. 279.

53. See especially Kaihara Osamu, "Japan's Military Capabilities, Realities and Limitations," *Pacific Community*, pp. 129–42.

54. Ibid., p. 139.

55. Japan Defense Agency, *Defense of Japan* (1985), p. 293.

56. *The Japan Times*, 30 January 1986, p. 3.

57. John Endicott, *Japan's Nuclear Option* (New York: Praeger, 1972), p. 65.

58. *The Japan Times*, 29 June 1986, pp. 1-2.

59. *Sankei Shimbun*, 17, 18, 19, 22, 25 September 1986, an informative series on the External Affairs Office.

60. Ibid., 22 September 1986, p. 4.

61. *The Japan Times*, 29 June 1986, pp. 1-2.

62. *Japan Economic Journal*, 21 May 1986, p. 7.

63. USICA, "Self-Defense Forces and Security Links with the U.S.," p. 3.

64. This short summary of the weapons acquisition process represents a synthesis of material found in Sungjoo Han's excellent account, "Japan's PXL Decision: The Politics of Weapon's Procurement," *Asian Survey*, August 1978, pp. 769-84, and in the work by Kaihara Osamu, *Nihon Boei Taisei no Uchimaku* (Tokyo: Jiji Press, 1977). Conversations with members of the Naikyuko and long time observers of the Japanese scene are also reflected. See especially Reinhard Drifte's *Arms Production in Japan* for an excellent analysis of the industry itself (Boulder, Colo.: Westview Press, 1986).

65. See especially Kaihara's *Nihon Boei Taisei no Uchimaku*.

66. *Nihon Keizai*, 1 April 1980.

67. *Mainichi*, 25 May 1976.

68. Defense production data are from Drifte, *Arms Production in Japan*, p. 24.

69. Japan Defense Agency, *Defense of Japan* (1976), pp. 39-40.

70. John Endicott and William Heaton, *Politics of East Asia* (Boulder, Colo.: Westview Press, 1978), p. 226.

71. Jijimondai Kenkyujo, *Gensuikyo* (Tokyo: Jijimondai Kenkyujo, 1961), pp. 1-2.

72. Endicott, *Japan's Nuclear Option*, pp. 51-52.

73. *Asahi Shimbun*, 5 February 1980.

74. *Yomiuri Shimbun*, 31 January 1980.

75. *Nihon Keizai*, 31 December 1986, p. 4.

76. Japan Defense Agency, *Defense of Japan*, (1986). p. v.

77. *Nihon Keizai*, 31 December 1986, morning ed., p. 4.

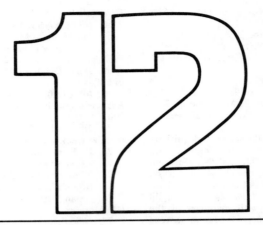

REPUBLIC OF KOREA

William E. Berry, Jr.

In almost all analyses of potential global "hot spots," the Korean peninsula ranks very high. The reasons for this ranking are fairly obvious. Both the North Korean Democratic People's Republic of Korea (DPRK) and the South Korean Republic of Korea (ROK) are heavily armed, and the hostility between the two is extremely real, as evidenced by the Korean War of 1950–53. In addition, four great powers have interests on this peninsula that sometimes conflict. The purpose of this chapter is to determine how both international and domestic factors influence the formulation of ROK defense policy.

International Environment

There are few countries where geographical factors are considered more important to the formulation of national defense policy than is the case with the Republic of Korea. Seoul, the unquestioned political, economic, and cultural center of the country, is less than thirty miles south of the 38th parallel dividing South Korea from North Korea, making it impossible to trade space for time if the North should launch another attack like that of June 1950 initiating the Korean War.[1] This sense of geographic vulnerability has been and remains a major factor in the shaping of South Korean security relations with the United States as well as the ROK and U.S. military strategies and force deployments.

In addition to these geographical considerations, great power involvement in Northeast Asia also influences South Korean defense policy. The United States, the Soviet Union, Japan, and the People's Republic of China (PRC) all have political, military, and economic interests on the Korean peninsula. Because of this involvement, many Koreans are concerned that regardless of the efforts made to provide for national defense, South Korea could well find itself a pawn in great power machinations on or near the Korean peninsula.[2] These concerns have increased in the past ten years because of the military buildup in North Korea and the enlarged Soviet military presence in Northeast Asia.[3]

From the South Korean point of view, the major military threat, without question, emanates from North Korea. This is not to suggest there is no concern with the Soviet buildup, because there is. But the military might of the North, the palpable hostility between the two Koreas, treaty relations between North Korea and its two major allies (the USSR and the PRC), and the fact that a peace treaty between the belligerents at the end of the Korean War has never been signed exacerbate the fears of South Korean political leaders and public, focusing their attention on the peninsula.

There are strong arguments to support the South Korean–U.S. contention that North Korea is one of the most militarized countries in existence.[4] The North, with a population of approximately twenty million, maintains an active military force estimated at 838,000, including 750,000 in the army, 35,000 in the navy, and 53,000 in the air force. In addition, North Korea has a regular army reserve of over 500,000 veterans who receive over 500 hours of training on an annual basis. Perhaps even more ominous than these troop figures are the twenty-two brigades of commandos, estimated at approximately 100,000 men, whose primary function would be to infiltrate the South to attack population centers and both supply and command and control lines in the rear areas.[5]

According to the International Institute for Strategic Studies, North Korea spent over $4 billion on defense in 1984.[6] Because economic figures are difficult to obtain for North Korea, various experts estimate that the North spends between 10 and 20 percent of its GNP on defense.[7] The Korean People's Army comprises the bulk of military manpower and the largest percentage of the defense budget. The army's emphasis is on armored forces and firepower, and both the quantitative and qualitative improvements made in the past few years are impressive. There are over 3,000 tanks in the inventory with the bulk of them being T-54s, T-55s, and T-62s. To transport its troops, North Korea has obtained over 1,100 armored personnel carriers, including the BTR-50 and BTR-152, which have the capacity to carry ap-

proximately twenty soldiers each. Artillery pieces number more than 4,600 guns, ranging from towed guns and howitzers to self-propelled weapons having a range of 15–17 miles. The army maintains more than 11,000 mortars including the 82mm, 120mm, 160mm, and 240mm varieties. It also employs the Soviet surface-to-surface missiles known as the FROG 5 and 7, which have sufficient range to reach Seoul when fired from North Korean territory.[8] This is not in any way an all-inclusive list of North Korean firepower and equipment, but is representative enough of its substantial capabilities to make clear the South Korean concern, particularly since many of these forces and weapons systems are forward-deployed near the 38th parallel.

The North Korean Navy includes 20 vintage submarines that have both torpedo and mine laying capabilities. In addition, there are about 350 fast attack and coastal defense craft in the inventory and 90 amphibious landing craft, each capable of carrying ninety personnel. The North Korean Air Force has over 800 combat aircraft, although many of these are of the MiG 15, 17, and 19 variety, which are getting quite old. There are also 160 MiG 21s, the main Soviet fighter aircraft in the 1960s. Many of these more modern aircraft are stationed within five minutes flying time of Seoul. The air force also maintains over 250 An-2 transport aircraft, which could be used to transport troops, including the commandos, into the South.[9]

Within the past couple of years, North Korea has been able to obtain 87 Hughes helicopters on the international market despite U.S. efforts to prevent this. These helicopters are very similar to those in the South Korean fleet, and are a source of concern to the South because they could be camouflaged so that they appear to belong to the South Korean Air Force.[10] In 1985 the Soviet Union agreed to sell the North approximately 40 MiG 23 aircraft, which represented a major change in Soviet policy as well as a qualitative improvement for the North Korean Air Force. The USSR was apparently reacting to the U.S. agreement to provide the F-16 to the South.[11]

This brief description of North Korean military forces in being, defense expenditures, and weapons systems available is impressive from a military perspective. It becomes even more ominous for South Korea when considered in conjunction with perceived North Korean force deployments and strategy and North Korea's relations with the Soviet Union and, to a lesser extent, the People's Republic of China. The conventional wisdom in both South Korea and the United States is that if the North Koreans launch another attack on the South, they would use the two major invasion routes taken in 1950. Approximately 50 percent of North Korean forces are within a few miles of the demilitarized zone (DMZ) at the 38th parallel. Being so deployed, they likely would be able to launch a sizable invasion without the mobilization that would warn the South of an impending attack. Such an attack also would be facilitated by the North Korean decision in 1985 to move armored units much closer to the DMZ from their previous billets more than 100 miles further north and to build underground storage shelters within approximately 15 miles of the DMZ, which contain an estimated 65 percent of North Korea's combat supplies. Recent U.S. military analyses have predicted that if the DPRK decides to attack, the ROK and U.S. forces would have no more than twelve hours notice, and perhaps not that long.[12]

In this scenario, North Korean military units would try to open gaps in the South Korean–U.S. ranks by concentrating artillery fire on selected parts of the line so that armored forces and infantry could break through. If successful in this effort, the North Koreans could make a drive on Seoul before the United States had the opportunity to send reinforcements. This strategy is sometimes referred to as the "three-day war strategy," since, if carried out according to plan, Seoul would fall within the first three days of the war, leading to the likely collapse of the South.[13] In addition to capturing Seoul, the North Koreans would try to envelop the South's army and destroy as much of it as possible.[14] Achieving this result would compel the United States to face the reality of having once again to engage a major military force in a land war in Asia.

Since July 1961 North Korea has had bilat-

eral Treaties of Friendship, Cooperation, and Mutual Assistance with both the Soviet Union and China.[15] Both of these treaties have provisions committing the contracting parties "immediately [to] render military and other assistance by all means at its disposal to the other party subjected to armed attack." As the Sino-Soviet split became more pronounced, North Korean leader Kim Il-Sung became very adept at playing the two sides off against each other to the advantage of his country. However, by the middle of the 1970s, the Soviet Union had become concerned over Kim's unpredictable behavior and reduced to a trickle the military assistance provided. Apparently, the USSR also feared that weapons or technology given to the North Koreans might find their way into Chinese hands.[16]

Nevertheless, by the 1980s there has been another shift in trilateral relations, with Kim attempting to move closer to the USSR. Most likely, a major reason for this North Korean policy shift is the desire to acquire more modern military equipment from the Soviet Union, which is in a better position to provide such equipment than are the Chinese. Whatever the reasons, there have been some recent high-level visits between Moscow and Pyongyang, and the USSR has agreed to sell MiG 23s to Kim and to discuss the possibility of advanced tank and helicopter sales as well.

It is not possible to predict with any degree of certainty what future relations will be between North Korea and its two major allies. From the South Korean perspective, however, the important factors are that North Korea has built up its own military capabilities, has a military strategy that threatens the very survival of the South, and has improved its military relations with the Soviet Union as the latter is becoming a more dominant military power in Northeast Asia. South Korea has attempted to meet this threat by maintaining its security ties with the United States, increasing its own military strength, and improving its relations with other countries in Asia.

SOUTH KOREAN–U.S. SECURITY RELATIONS

In October 1953 representatives of the United States and South Korea signed a Mutual Defense Treaty that went into effect in November 1953.[17] Article III stipulates that each country accepts that an external attack in the Pacific on either of their territories under their respective administrative control "would be dangerous to its own peace and safety and declares that it would act to meet the common danger in accordance with its constitutional processes." Article IV provides for American land, air, and naval forces to be stationed in South Korea. When this treaty was ratified by the U.S. Senate, an "understanding" was included stating that the treaty was only applicable if an external armed attack were directed against the South.[18] Presumably, the Senate intended to ensure by this understanding that the treaty would not be applicable if South Korea launched an attack against North Korea.

South Korean political leaders have remained apprehensive about the American commitment to come to their assistance ever since the treaty went into effect. The Senate reservation expressed in the referenced "understanding" partly explains this concern, but more important is the clause in Article III that each country would act "in accordance with its constitutional processes." The Koreans wanted the United States to commit to an automatic response in case of attack, but such a commitment has never been made in the South Korean case. Therefore, the presence of American ground forces deployed along the likely invasion routes provides the next best guarantee that the United States will respond immediately to an attack south across the 38th parallel.[19] The "trip-wire" nature of these American soldiers' presence is so important because the ROK views this presence as a major deterrent against another North Korean invasion. In this particular case, it is the psychological element of deterrence that is deemed important, both to reassure the South and deter the North.[20]

Korean anxieties about the American commitment increased substantially during the Nixon administration. President Nixon was influenced by both domestic and international pressures as far as his views on American troops in Korea were concerned. Domestically, public opinion and the mood of the Congress opposed continuation of the U.S. role as "policeman of the world," a role the United States had assumed in the period leading to the involvement in the Vietnam war. Congress demanded that military budgets be decreased and American forces abroad be reduced. Internationally, Nixon was influenced by his own desires to improve relations with China. A reduction in the American military presence in Asia was perceived as a means to this end.

During a trip to Asia in July 1969, the president indicated on several occasions that American allies must assume more of the responsibility for achieving peace within the region. The United States could play a role in this endeavor, but the individual countries would have to do more.[21] At the conclusion of this trip, Nixon released a statement on Guam that has come to be known as the Nixon Doctrine.[22] Briefly, this doctrine contained three main principles. First, the United States would keep its treaty commitments. Second, the nuclear umbrella would continue to be extended to those countries deemed vital to American security interests. Third, and most important as far as the troop issue is concerned, the United States would furnish economic and military assistance, but the country directly involved would be responsible for providing the actual manpower for defense. What this meant essentially was that the United States would consider providing air and naval support to an ally, but the ground forces would have to come from the country itself.

In August 1969 President Park Chung Hee and President Nixon met in San Francisco. The joint communique issued at the conclusion of this meeting was significantly different from that issued after Park's meeting with Lyndon Johnson in 1968.[23] Rather than the pledge to offer "prompt and effective assistance to repel armed attacks" that his predecessor had made, Nixon agreed only "to meet armed attack against the Republic of Korea in accordance with the Mutual Defense Treaty between the Republic of Korea and the United States."

In 1971 Nixon began to reduce the ground presence in Korea by withdrawing the 7th Infantry Division. After this withdrawal, only the 2nd Infantry Division remained. The U.S. military presence had been reduced from approximately 60,000 troops to 40,000 by this action.[24] Because of the deterrent value attributed to the American presence, the Korean government was profoundly disturbed by the Nixon decision. As a result, President Park launched a major effort in the early 1970s to increase the industrial capabilities of his country so that South Korea would become as self-sufficient as possible in the production of military hardware. Quite obviously, Korean confidence in American reliability was shaken by the Nixon troop withdrawal decision. The latent fears always just below the surface in bilateral relations were exacerbated by this action.

When Gerald Ford succeeded to the presidency in 1974, he attempted to reassure American allies in Asia that the United States intended to remain a regional power. On his return from the Vladivostok meeting with Leonid Brezhnev, Ford stopped in Seoul to consult with Park. The joint communique they issued is instructive in that Ford stated that the United States would remain an Asian power, but more specifically because of the wording he used in reference to the U.S. ground forces in South Korea.[25] Ford reverted to the language used by Johnson in 1968, pledging "prompt and effective assistance to repel armed attack against the Republic of Korea." He went on to state directly that "the United States had no plan to reduce the present level of United States forces in Korea."

At the conclusion of a subsequent 1975 Asian trip, Ford attempted to clarify his Asian policy further. In a speech delivered in Hawaii, he outlined his "Pacific Doctrine" and made specific reference to South Korea. The fifth tenet of this doctrine stated that peace in Asia would be difficult to achieve as long as existing tensions remained high on the Korean peninsula. To reduce these tensions, the United States intended to maintain close ties with South Korea, to include the retention of American military forces there.[26]

Secretary of State Henry Kissinger attempted in a 1976 speech to develop more specifically what the Ford administration's Asian policy was. Kissinger warned against unilateral troop withdrawals from the region as threatening the security of allies and reducing

American influence. Concerning Korea, he stated that the United States "will not undermine stability and hopes for negotiation by withdrawing forces unilaterally."[27]

Ford and Kissinger were attempting to reassure American friends and allies in Asia that the United States intended to remain an Asian power even though this country had not been able to prevent the communist victories in Indochina. It is clear that Ford and Kissinger believed that the retention of combat ground forces in South Korea was a signal of American intent to remain an Asian power. While these reassurances were welcome in Seoul, doubts still remained because of previous policy shifts from one administration to another. In other words, Korean political leaders were not certain what the long-term U.S. policy on the troop question would be, and their anxiety level increased as it became clear who the Democratic nominee for president in 1976 was.

As early as 1975, candidate Jimmy Carter indicated he would withdraw American ground forces from Korea if he became president.[28] The Korean reaction was more muted than might have been expected because in 1975 it did not appear Carter would win the Democratic nomination, let alone the presidency, and because campaign rhetoric is not always translated into policy. Carter proved the Koreans wrong on both counts. After becoming president, he directly addressed the troop issue. The president believed that the approximately 32,000 U.S. ground troops in Korea could be removed over a four-to-five-year period, allowing South Korea time to prepare its own forces. Carter did anticipate, however, that American air and naval support would remain in Korea for a long time.[29]

During the spring of 1977, the administration prepared Policy Review Memorandum 13. This document contained the various arguments being considered at that time on the troop withdrawal plan. Although granting that the strategic balance had shifted in favor of North Korea since 1970, it concluded that after a five-year period of withdrawing American ground forces, South Korea could defend itself adequately if U.S. air, air defense, naval, and logistic support continued.[30] In May 1977 Presidential Decision 12 was sent to the Departments of State and Defense ordering them to implement Carter's planned withdrawal.[31]

There were several reasons for the Carter decision. First, he did believe that because of quantitative and qualitative improvements in South Korean forces and equipment, U.S. ground forces were no longer necessary to maintain stability. Second, what he described as "strategic considerations" had changed from the late 1940s and early 1950s in relations between the United States and the Soviet Union and between the United States and China.[32] Although he did not say so, presumably the president was referring to the improvement in U.S. relations with both China and the Soviet Union and deteriorating relations between the two communist giants. In this view, these changing "strategic considerations" had reduced the possibility of a repetition of the North Korean invasion in June 1950. This kind of thinking was exactly what the South Koreans feared: events outside the country, and over which they had little control, directly affecting the defense of the South. Third, South Korea had developed a strong economy and was approaching the time when it could provide for its own defense.[33]

There were other reasons for Carter's decision. The new president desired additional flexibility in how or if the United States would respond to an attack against South Korea. If American forces remained deployed along the major invasion routes, his choices were limited. Also, Carter had campaigned to cut the defense budget; reducing the forces overseas was a means to accomplish this pledge. Finally, the president stressed human rights during the campaign and in his first months in office. He found many of the practices of the Park regime offensive, and he wanted to distance himself and the country from Park.[34]

The Korean response to the withdrawal plan was predictable. Even opposition political leaders supported the retention of the U.S. forces. Park indicated strongly that the United States would have to make major contributions to the South Korean force improvement program so that his forces could provide for the

national defense. In 1977 it was estimated that Korean industry was actually supplying 50 percent of the equipment used by the South's military. In negotiations during the summer of 1977, the United States agreed to contribute approximately $1.5 billion during the course of the five-year force-improvement program, primarily through Foreign Military Sales (FMS) credits.[35] This assistance would be valuable in South Korea's effort to expand its own defense industries. Nevertheless, Korean skepticism about the validity of the U.S. commitment reached one of its highest points since the end of the Korean War during the first years of the Carter administration.

In actuality, less than one combat battalion was removed from Korea. The withdrawal plan was never popular with many in the U.S. Congress and military, and when an intelligence reassessment was conducted in 1978, the remaining support largely disappeared. Prior to this reassessment, the balance of forces between South Korea and North Korea was estimated as indicated in table 1.[36] While the North had some definite advantages in this comparison, such as more combat aircraft and superior naval forces, the disparity was not perceived in the Carter administration to be so great that Kim Il-Sung could be confident of victory if he launched an attack. Geographical features favored the South as far as defensive positions were concerned, and the South Korean Air Force had more modern aircraft. Also, the Korean military experience in the Vietnam War had provided recent battlefield training that the North Koreans did not have.[37]

An intelligence reassessment began in the summer of 1978 involving the Defense Intelligence Agency, the Central Intelligence Agency, and the assistant chief of staff for intelligence, U.S. Army. This reassessment focused on the military capabilities of North Korea, and the results were announced in June 1979 by Congressman Les Aspin, a member of the House Select Committee on Intelligence.[38] After reviewing the new intelligence data, Aspin and others reached the following conclusions: the North had achieved a numerical superiority on the ground to accompany its numerical advan-

Table 1. Korean Military Force Comparison

	1970		1977	
	ROK	DPRK	ROK	DPRK
Personnel				
Active forces	634,000	400,000	600,000	520,000
Reserve forces	1,000,000	1,200,000	2,800,000	1,800,000
Maneuver divisions	19	20	19	25
Ground balance				
Tanks	900	600	1,100[a]	1,950
APC	300	120	400[a]	750[a]
Assault guns	0	300	0	105[a]
Anti tank	(deleted)	(deleted)	(deleted)	24,000
Shelling capability				
Artillery/multiple rocket launchers	1,750	3,300	2,000[a]	4,335[a]
Surface-to-surface missiles (battalions)	(deleted)	(deleted)	1	2–3
Mortars	(deleted)	(deleted)	(deleted)	9,000
Air balance				
Jet combat aircraft	230	555	320[a]	655[a]
Other military aircraft	35[a]	130	200	320
AAA guns	850	2,000	1,000[a]	5,500[a]
SAMs (battalions/sites)	(deleted)	(deleted)	2	38–40[a]
Navy combat vessels	60	190	80–90[a]	425–50[a]

Source: U.S. Congress, Senate Committee on Foreign Relations, *U.S. Troop Withdrawal from the Republic of Korea,* a report by Senators Hubert H. Humphrey and John Glenn, 95th Congress, 2nd Sess., 9 January 1978, p. 27.

[a]Approximations. Actual figures may be greater.

tages in the air; the number of North Korean divisions had increased from a projected twenty-nine in 1977 to thirty-seven in 1979; and the number of its tanks and armored personnel carriers had grown by 35 percent and 20 percent respectively.

As a result, the gross ratio of South and North Korean forces had changed significantly between 1977 and 1979, as table 2 indicates. While these figures were disconcerting to Aspin, he found additional cause for concern in how these forces were deployed. Previously, military analyses believed the North was dedicated to a forward defense concept in which forces would be deployed along the 38th parallel and then reinforced if necessary from rear areas. Such reinforcement requires time and could be detected by various surveillance means. However, the new intelligence data indicated that rather than a forward defense deployment, the North more than likely had assumed a defense-in-depth posture. This new posture could allow North Korea to launch an attack without the reinforcements required under forward defense. This capability would permit the North to attack without the time delay required for reinforcements and the con-

Table 2. Ratio of Forces: North Korea and South Korea

	DPRK:ROK Ratio	
	1977 Estimate	1979 Estimate
Ground forces manpower	0.9:1	1.1–1.2:1
Tanks	1.5:1	2.1:1
Artillery	1.9:1	2.3:1
Armored personnel carriers	1.9:1	2.3:1

Source: U.S. Congress, House Committee on Armed Forces *The Impact of Intelligence Reassessment on Withdrawal of U.S. Troops from Korea: Hearings Before the Investigations Subcommittee,* 96th Cong., 1st Sess., 21 June and 17 July 1979, p. 3.

comitant warning period for the South. Because of the importance of geographical factors so critical to South Korean defense, such a capability could well be devastating.[39]

Confronted with opposition from the Congress, his own military, and the Park government, plus the new intelligence data, President Carter reevaluated his troop withdrawal plan. To assist in this effort, he included Korea on his itinerary for an Asian trip scheduled for the summer of 1979. In an exchange of toasts with President Park, Carter emphasized the importance of U.S.–South Korean relations and stressed that the American military commitment to Korea's security was "strong, unshakable, and enduring."[40] In the joint communique, the American president was more specific about this commitment. He promised "prompt and effective assistance to repel armed attack" against the South and assured President Park that "the United States nuclear umbrella provided additional security for the area." Specifically relating to the withdrawal plan, Carter pledged that "the United States will continue to maintain an American military presence in the Republic of Korea to ensure peace and stability."[41] Although this statement was somewhat nebulous, the implication was that the ground forces would not be removed. Richard Holbrooke, Assistant Secretary of State for East Asia and Pacific Affairs, made this point more explicitly in his testimony before the House Investigations Subcommittee after the president returned from Korea.[42]

Finally, on 20 July 1979 President Carter announced that the withdrawal plan was being held in abeyance.[43] Although Carter did not completely abandon his plan, he postponed further consideration of withdrawal until well after the 1980 presidential election. More important, he attached a condition to any subsequent consideration of this issue: some sign that North Korea was willing to help reduce tensions between the Koreas. Any future withdrawal decision would not be a unilateral action on the part of the United States.

The Carter policies on the troop issue and also on human rights violations in Korea had reduced bilateral relations to one of their lowest levels. When Ronald Reagan succeeded to the presidency, he made it clear that he opposed any U.S. troop withdrawal because he believed a withdrawal would work against American political and security interests. Chun Doo Hwan, who became president in 1980 after the assassination of Park in October 1979, was one of the first foreign leaders to visit the new U.S. president in February 1981. The timing of this visit was no accident. President Reagan was attempting to send a clear signal to Chun that the United States was a reliable ally and could be depended upon. Specifically in reference to the American ground forces, President Reagan stated in the joint communique that the United States "had no plans to withdraw U.S. ground combat forces from the Korean peninsula."[44] This pledge was reiterated on Reagan's visit to Korea in 1983 and Chun's second trip to the United States in 1985.

Although there is no question that U.S.-South Korean relations have improved during the Reagan years, there still remain some irritants involving security issues. Trade and other economic problems are beyond the scope of this chapter and will not be discussed at any length. As noted previously, however, South Korea began to build up its heavy industrial capabilities in the 1970s during the Park administration. Part of the reasoning behind this decision was the concern over the viability of the U.S. commitment after the enunciation of the Nixon Doctrine and the withdrawal of the 7th Infantry Division.

To accomplish this industrial development, the Korean government began efforts to redirect investment into capital- and technology-intensive industries. Between 1974 and 1979, almost 75 percent of investment was allocated to heavy machinery, electronics, shipbuilding, and steel production.[45] Unfortunately for South Korea, the international recession of the late 1970s and early 1980s reduced the foreign demand for many of these products. This reduction in demand occurred at the same time that Korea gained the capability to meet almost 100 percent of its conventional weapons demand.[46] As a result, by the mid 1980s the utilization of the defense industrial plant had declined to approximately 50 percent of capacity. South Korean sources estimated that the South needed to export a minimum of $500 million worth of military hardware per year to maintain sufficient production capacity.[47]

The U.S. Arms Export Control Act and the International Traffic in Arms Regulations limit the third country sales of defense items produced outside the United States with U.S. assistance, technical data, manufacturing license, or coproduction agreements. In order to protect U.S. defense industries, safeguard defense technologies, and limit weapons proliferation, the United States has been reluctant to grant Korean requests to export weapons produced in Korea with some form of U.S. assistance. Statistics have tended to support the South Korean argument that the United States severely limited the third-country sales Korea is permitted to make. In 1981–82, for example, South Korea requested American approval for $55.4 million in sales, of which $1.7 million was granted. In 1983 the figures were $49 million requested with $4 million approved; for 1984, $31 million requested but only $870,000 approved.[48]

Actually, these statistics are somewhat misleading. If one examines the actual number of requests rather than the value of the weapons, the U.S. approval rate is much higher. The conclusion to be drawn is that lower-value weapons and equipment are approved for sale much more frequently than the high-value items. Third-country sales are not a major problem affecting bilateral relations, but Korean officials almost always make this topic an agenda item for the annual Security Consultations Meeting.

Another defense issue involves the different perceptions of the threat that sometimes exist between Washington and Seoul. For the U.S. military forces stationed in Korea, this difference does not pertain. Their training, strategy, and deployments are designed to deter a North Korean attack and defeat it if it occurs. However, many U.S. policy makers far removed from the peninsula view the primary threat differently than the South Koreans on some occasions. From a superpower perspective, particularly during the Reagan administration, the most serious threat in Northeast Asia is the increased Soviet military presence in the region; for South Korea, it remains the threat from North Korea.

In the future, as Korean economic and military capabilities increase, it is possible that the United States will request that South Korea accept additional military missions to meet the Soviet threat. One such mission might involve air defense, particularly against Soviet Backfire bombers flying over the Sea of Japan. Korean aircraft could scramble against these flights and thereby reduce the potential danger to merchant shipping in the area and U.S. ba-

ses in the Philippines. Another possible mission would be for South Korea to lay mines in the Korean Strait (Tsushima Strait) and thereby restrict the movement of Soviet surface ships and submarines.[49] From the Korean perspective, neither of these potential missions would be acceptable if they resulted in the reduction of the South Korean and American capability to deter North Korea. Again, this is not a major problem between the two allies now, but bears watching in the years ahead.

Another potential irritant involves command relations in Korea. In 1978 the command structure was reorganized with the creation of the Combined Forces Command (CFC), a combined U.S.–South Korean military command. As has been true since the end of the Korean War, an American army general exercises operational control over U.S. forces and almost all Korean combat units. The long-term viability of this command relationship has been questioned by scholars from both countries. Gregory Henderson argues that having an American general command Korean forces reinforces the impression that the United States dictates Korean policy, which in turn lends additional credence to radical Korean students such as those who led anti-American demonstrations attacking President Chun and his American connection.[50] On the Korean side, Ahn Byung-Joon believes that South Korean military forces must be commanded by a Korean if these forces are to remain a viable deterrent in the years ahead.[51]

In sum, Korean-American relations have evolved into one of the most stable bilateral alliances the United States has. There is no question that the vast majority of Koreans value the importance of both the Mutual Defense Treaty and the continuing U.S. military presence. For example, in late 1983, a Korean Gallup nationwide poll of 1,500 individuals revealed that 88.1 percent of those interviewed believed that the withdrawal of U.S. ground forces would invite an attack by North Korea.[52]

Despite the fact that anti-American sentiments have been more widely expressed by radical students, it is clear that security relations remain extremely important as a foundation block for Korean defense policy.[53] During the 1986 Asian Games in Seoul, the U.S. Seventh Fleet deployed thirteen warships in and around the Korean peninsula to indicate American support and to serve as a warning to North Korea not to interfere with the games.[54] The Korean people appreciate such gestures and assistance.

SOUTH KOREAN RELATIONS WITH OTHER REGIONAL POWERS

South Korea and Japan established normal diplomatic relations in 1965, but these relations have remained strained during most of the intervening years.[55] The brutal Japanese colonial occupation of Korea from 1910 to 1945 is primarily responsible for the ill feelings many Koreans still have for the Japanese. Although the Japanese prime minister and South Korean president have exchanged official visits in an effort to improve relations, difficult issues remain. Included among these issues are trade problems, differences over Japanese economic assistance programs to South Korea, the manner in which Japanese textbooks refer to the Japanese occupation of Korea, and the treatment of approximately 750,000 ethnic Koreans living in Japan. In addition to these issues, there is widespread resistance to Japanese cultural influences, and many Koreans believe that to be "truly Korean" requires a rather substantial expression of anti-Japanese sentiment.[56] While relations are improving, there are still many problems to be resolved that will take time.

In military relations with Japan, South Korea faces a dilemma. On the one hand, many Korean political and military leaders believe that Japan should spend more of its resources on defense to improve its capabilities. On the other hand, there is concern with what Japan might do with these increased capabilities. In this instance, the historical legacy of Korean-Japanese relations is an important factor. More important, however, is the Korean concern that if Japan became a more powerful military actor in the region, the United States might see this development as an opportunity to reduce its own military presence in Northeast Asia.[57] The possible implications for U.S. forces stationed in the South are not something

the Koreans want to encourage. In sum, the possibility for increased Japanese-Korean security cooperation in the near future seems to be minimal at this time.

The Asian Games in Seoul provide a good example of the state of Korean-Japanese relations. Most South Koreans had expected the Asian Games and Olympics to provide the same economic and political benefits that the 1964 Olympics in Tokyo provided to Japan; there is respect in Korea for Japanese accomplishments, particularly Japan's economic growth and development. However, the greatest sense of accomplishment for many Koreans in the Asian Games was that South Korea finished well ahead of the Japanese team and second only to the Chinese.[58] This sense of satisfaction at beating the Japanese was certainly one of the major highlights of a very successful hosting of the games for Korea, but also serves as a good example of the somewhat tenuous relations between the two Asian neighbors.

South Korea has no diplomatic relations with the People's Republic of China, primarily because of the political and security ties China has established over the years with North Korea. Yet, there is no question that the Chinese strategy of "walking on two legs" (i.e., a more flexible, less one-sided policy) has provided opportunities for expanded economic and political contacts between South Korea and China.[59]

Economically, the indirect trade between the two countries increased to approximately $800 million by the mid 1980s, with most of this trade passing through Hong Kong. The estimated trade level for 1985 ranged from $800 million to $1 billion. By comparison, Chinese-North Korean trade totaled about $530 million.[60] In many ways, the economies of South Korea and China are complementary in that Korean technology and its economic model for development are important for the Chinese as they attempt to modernize their country. By the same token, access to the China market is very important to the Koreans, particularly for the heavy industries that have been functioning below capacity in recent years.

Political contacts have primarily involved negotiations for the return of Chinese aircraft and ships flown or sailed to the ROK by Chinese defectors and the exchange of athletic teams and other representatives. In the past six years, there have been five defections, the most significant of which was the May 1983 hijacking of a Civil Aviation Administration of China (CAAC) passenger plane. What made this incident so significant was that the Chinese requested direct negotiations with official representatives of the South Korean government, and this request was addressed to "the Republic of Korea," the first time that China had referred to the South by its official name. When the representatives did meet, it was the first official contact between the two governments, and the issue was resolved to the satisfaction of both.[61]

Since 1984 athletic exchanges have become routine, and as indicated previously, China participated in the 1986 Asian Games in Seoul and in the 1988 Olympics. South Korean representatives also have attended conferences held in Beijing such as the 1983 training course sponsored by the United Nations Development Program and the Food and Agricultural Organization.[62]

Political and security relations with North Korea restrict how far China can go in its contacts with South Korea, as does the Sino-Soviet competition for influence with Kim Il-Sung. For the South, a favorable outcome is to have China exercise a moderating influence on North Korean policy decisions. There is some evidence to suggest that China has tried to exercise such influence on the issue of U.S. forces in South Korea. As will be discussed later in this chapter, North Korea has made the removal of the American military presence a precondition for substantive talks on reunification of the peninsula. In late 1983, Party Chairman Hu Yaobang visited Pyongyang and allegedly advised Kim that rather than making the troop withdrawal a precondition for negotiations, it might be a wise policy to call for the beginning of a withdrawal while the talks progressed.[63] This is not to suggest that this proposal would be acceptable to the South, but only that it is the type of influence South Korea would like China to use.

There is little likelihood of improved South

Korean relations with the Soviet Union, particularly in the next few years. The Soviet shooting down in 1983 of a Korean Airlines jetliner with the loss of all the passengers and crew exacerbated the hostile attitudes toward the Soviet Union already evident within the society. The closer military relations between the USSR and its North Korean allies, including the decision to make available MiG 23s, provides additional support to the argument that there will not be much improvement in South Korean relations with the USSR in the foreseeable future.

One issue that has offered a litmus test of sorts to these relations is the Soviet Union's participation in the Seoul Olympics. There had been a few athletic exchanges between the two in recent years, and obviously South Korea wanted the Soviets to participate. The Soviets would have found it difficult not to send a team because of its boycott of the 1984 Olympics in Los Angeles. To boycott successive Olympics would have been devastating to the Soviet sports program and would have made the selection of a Soviet site for future games highly unlikely. Therefore, even though North Korea adamantly opposed Soviet participation, the Soviet Union ultimately saw no attractive choice but to take part, regardless of the effects on its North Korean ally.

This chapter has focused thus far upon the international environment, particularly South Korea's security ties with the United States and its relations with Japan, China, and the Soviet Union. The following section will examine what South Korea has attempted to accomplish domestically as far as defense capabilities, strategies, and force deployments are concerned and outline the defense decision-making process at work within the Korean government.

National Objectives, National Strategy, and Military Doctrine

According to some of the most recent statistics available on the South and North Korean gross national products and defense spending, the South's economy is approximately 4.5

times larger than that of the North. South Korea's GNP in the mid 1980s was slightly more than $80 billion while that of the North was estimated to be $16–$20 billion.[64] Because of this tremendous disparity in economic performances, South Korean expenditures for defense in the range of 6–7 percent of GNP, which have been the norm in the 1980s, would require North Korea to allocate between 27 and 31 percent of its GNP for defense just to stay even in real terms.

If the present trends in economic growth continue until the mid 1990s, the South will have an economy six times larger than the North. Therefore, continued defense spending of 6–7 percent in Seoul would require expenditures between 36–42 percent of GNP in Pyongyang.[65] A major conclusion to be drawn from these statistics is that as time goes by, South Korea will continue to be in a more advantageous position than North Korea regarding defense spending because of the comparative strengths of the two economies. Even though the North devotes more of its economy to defense than just about any other country, its political leaders will be hard pressed to compete with the South in the years to come.

Since 1976, South Korea has been spending more in real terms on defense than has North Korea, and the gap continues to widen.[66] An important question is whether or not there is sufficient support in the South to continue funding defense at these levels (6–7 percent of GNP). The answer appears to be that the government will be able to continue such expenditures primarily because the threat from North Korea is perceived to be very real by a large majority of the South Korean people. Numerous infiltration efforts and incidents such as the 1983 Rangoon bombing in which several South Korean cabinet officers and presidential advisers were killed in the Burmese capital by North Korean commandos reinforce this support. This level of defense spending has not adversely affected the economy by significantly reducing the consumer goods available or by reducing investments to the extent that the defense budget would be challenged seriously. Further, South Korea is increasingly able to produce more of its own military equipment, including high-technology items such as the F-5 fighter and a medium-range tank.[67] This type of production increases the ability of the South to be as independent as possible, which is popular with the people.

Whether the current and projected defense-spending ratios are stabilizing or destabilizing from the South Korean perspective is an interesting question. On the one hand, it can be argued that as the South becomes stronger militarily, there will be an increased reluctance in the North to initiate an attack. On the other hand, North Korean leaders may believe that to wait before attempting to reunite the peninsula under their control would be unwise because the correlation of forces is moving against them, and they must act soon or not at all.

The predominant ROK national security objective has been and remains to deter an attack by the DPRK. The comparative economic advantages just outlined enable the ROK political leaders to expend increasing amounts of scarce resources to help achieve this objective. U.S.–ROK security relations are at the very heart of South Korean deterrent efforts, and these relations appear to be on sound footing for the present and foreseeable future. South

Table 3. Comparison of North and South Korea Military Expenditure (Millions of 1979 Dollars)

Year	North Korea	South Korea	Ratio South/North
1968	1,398	1,195	0.85
1969	1,366	1,289	0.94
1970	1,655	1,368	0.82
1971	1,952	1,499	0.77
1972	2,266	1,537	0.68
1973	1,980	1,596	0.81
1974	2,341	1,827	0.78
1975	2,079	1,978	0.95
1976	2,236	2,409	1.08
1977	2,489	2,727	1.10
1978	2,521	3,184	1.26
1979	2,405	3,154	1.31
1980	2,665	3,431	1.25
1981	2,676	3,276	1.22
1982	2,523	3,399	1.35
1983	2,598	3,612	1.39
Cumulative			
1968–83	35,150	37,381	1.06
1976–83	20,113	25,102	1.25

Source: Charles Wolf, Jr., et al., *The Changing Balance: South and North Korean Capabilities for Long-Term Military Competition,* p. 43.

Korea also has attempted to improve its relations with the PRC in the hopes that the Chinese will exercise a moderating influence on their North Korean allies. As will be discussed subsequently, the two Koreas from time to time have attempted to establish a series of formal contacts between themselves, albeit many of these efforts have been more for propaganda purposes than actual efforts to reduce tensions on the peninsula. As long as the mutual suspicion, hostility, and enmity between the ROK and DPRK remain at current levels, deterrence will continue as the overwhelming ROK national security objective. In order to meet this threat, the ROK and U.S. have designed a military strategy they hope will be successful.

SOUTH KOREAN–U.S. MILITARY STRATEGY

The best guess of the likely North Korean offensive strategy was outlined earlier in this chapter. Suffice it to say here that South Korea and the United States must be prepared to defend against the "three-day war strategy" designed to overrun Seoul and defeat the South Korean military in that short period of time. On the other hand, a major problem could well develop for North Korea if its military forces were unable to achieve a quick victory. One American expert on North Korean capabilities estimates that with resources and manpower currently available, the North could sustain offensive operations for approximately ninety days. Beyond those ninety days, North Korea would need resupply from its major allies.[68] A further complicating factor for the North is that the longer the war lasts, the more time the United States, and perhaps other countries still under the United Nations Command, have to reinforce their military units on the peninsula.

Because of the geographical factors and North Korean deployments, the South Korean–U.S. defense strategy is based on the forward-defense concept that has been in effect at least since 1973. What this means essentially is that Korean and American ground forces would engage invading units as close to the DMZ as possible and then rely upon massive firepower to drive them back. Components of this massive firepower would be fighter and fighter-bomber aircraft based in Korea as well as units from Japan, the Philippines, and from the Seventh Fleet. Artillery and anti-armor weapons assigned to South Korean and U.S. ground units would be employed, and sustained bombing attacks using B-52 aircraft from Guam would be devastating against massed North Korean invading forces.[69] In this regard, geographical features work to the advantage of the South because the natural invasion corridors are relatively narrow and can be defended well. This circumstance would create bottlenecks, making the invaders more susceptible to bombing attacks. This concentration of strong points along a line two to five miles south of the DMZ is designed to stop a North Korean attack on the ground while South Korean and U.S. air forces gain control of the air.

During 1984 President Chun stated that South Korea had adopted a new strategy quite similar to the follow-on-forces-attack (FOFA) concept developed in NATO, whereby South Korean forces would strike deep into North Korea to disrupt supply lines and communications as well as reinforcements moving south.[70] Another important factor in the defense of South Korea concerns the possibility that the United States has placed nuclear weapons in the South. The U.S. neither confirms nor denies such a presence, although the American columnist Jack Anderson, writing in 1983 and allegedly quoting official sources, reported that there were 133 nuclear bombs, 94 nuclear artillery shells, and 21 nuclear demolition mines deployed in South Korea.[71] Whether or not this report is accurate, the fact remains that North Korean leaders include this possibility in their calculus of whether or not to attack.

"Team Spirit" is an annual joint military exercise designed to address logistical problems and to increase the deterrent value of U.S.–South Korean security ties. In 1984, for example, 147,300 Koreans representing all services participated in this exercise as did 60,050 U.S. troops, many of whom were transported to South Korea from the United States along with their equipment.[72] This exercise, which generally lasts from the beginning of February to the end of March, provides the opportunity for extensive training under battlefield conditions and improves the logistic support the United States is committed to supply in case of a contingency. The two allies also have announced plans to increase war reserve stockpiles stored in the South, particularly ammunition and petroleum supplies. These plans will increase South Korean capabilities to fight without immediate resupply from outside sources.[73]

In sum, South Korea, along with its American ally, has allocated resources, deployed forces, and implemented strategies that should cause any rational leadership in North Korea to think very seriously before initiating another attack on the South. If deterrence fails, South Korea and the United States would inflict extreme punishment on the attacking North Korean forces and more than likely prevent them from achieving anything that could be construed as a political or military victory.

The Defense Decision-Making Process

Since the formation of South Korea in 1948, its government has been characterized, with only brief exceptions, by strong executive leadership, with the president frequently being a military man who seized political power. Chun Doo Hwan certainly fit this description in that he seized power through a military coup in August 1980 not long after the assassination of Park Chung Hee in late 1979. Contributing to this executive dominance in South Korea is the traditional Korean proclivity to expect the population to give practically unopposed support to the strong leader.[74] Recognizing that military men (who are used to giving orders and having them obeyed) serve as president in a country with a political culture that stresses the need for public obedience is very important to an understanding of how the defense decision-making process works in South Korea.

The 1980 Constitution, which Chun had written to usher in the Fifth Republic, provides numerous examples of the broader constitutional powers a South Korean president exercises in comparison with his American counterpart.[75] Article 48 allows the president to

conclude and ratify treaties and to declare war. He may issue presidential decrees deemed necessary to enforce the law and, according to articles 50 and 51, may suspend the rights and freedoms of the people and take "special measures" with respect to the legislative and judicial branches of government. He may declare martial law under Article 52, although he must lift it if a majority of the National Assembly so dictates. Article 57 provides that the president has the authority to dissolve the National Assembly if there is sufficient "cause to believe such a dissolution is necessary for the security of the state and the interests of all the people." Finally, Article 62 stipulates that the president will appoint the prime minister with the consent of the National Assembly.

This review of executive powers is instructive in understanding how powerful the South Korean presidency can be and how effectively the president and his closest advisors can dominate the foreign policy process, particularly defense policy formulation. President Chun and his advisors, almost all of whom are graduates of the Korean Military Academy and current or former high-ranking military officers, were without question the major actors in making defense policy with other agencies within the executive branch (such as the Ministry of Foreign Affairs) playing largely a supporting role.[76] President Roh Tae Woo, also a former general as well as close advisor to Chun, has continued this executive dominance in defense policy-making. This is not to suggest that there are no differences of opinion or challenges to executive authority, because there are, as will be evident in a later section of this chapter. What this review does suggest is that there is a high degree of consensus among the South Korean people concerning the threat that permits a strong president a relatively free hand in defense policy making.

The executive branch also dominates the legislature to the extent that one Korean expert has referred to the National Assembly as little more than a "debating society."[77] This domination derives not only from the constitutional powers listed above, but also because of the electoral system by which representatives to the National Assembly are selected. The members are elected through a combination of direct vote by their constituents and a proportional representation system that clearly favors the dominant political party.

The February 1985 election to the National Assembly provides a good example of how this system works. In that election, the Democratic Justice Party (DJP), Chun and Roh's party, received 35.2 percent of the popular vote, which translated into 87 Assembly seats in the 276-member legislature. The major opposition party, the New Korea Democratic Party (NKDP), formed only three weeks before the election around the leadership of Kim Dae Jung and Kim Young Sam (the most influential of the anti-Chun forces), won 29.4 percent of the popular vote and 68 seats.[78]

Korean electoral law stipulates, however, that the political party that wins the largest percentage of the popular vote is awarded 61 additional seats. As a result, the Democratic Justice Party (DJP) enjoyed a comfortable 148-seat working majority that allowed President Chun to dominate the National Assembly, thanks in part to tight party discipline within the DJP. The NKDP has been able to increase its number of legislative seats through coalition building to approximately 100, but still is limited in its legislative role.[79] In short, the strength of the president and his political party has diminished the National Assembly's ability to act as a check on presidential dominance of the defense decision-making process and actually has contributed to it by acting as a rubber stamp for executive initiatives.[80] While Roh has proposed to redraft the National Assembly electoral law, many of the new president's democratic reforms remain to be implemented.

A major political issue in South Korea, instructive due to the manner by which it was resolved, involved how the current president was elected. This issue has important implications for future national defense policies. Article 39 of the Constitution provides that the president shall be elected indirectly through an electoral college, and Article 45 limits the president to a seven-year term of office, with the incumbent prevented from seeking reelection. Beginning early in 1986, the New Korea Democratic Party, the Democratic Justice Party's strongest rival, organized a petition drive among the population demanding changes in the electoral system, specifically that the people elect the president directly.[81] The government has opposed this petition effort, and violence has occurred as a result, with a most serious incident happening at Inchon in May 1986.[82] Roh's success as a presidential candidate in persuading Chun to revise the national Constitution and hold direct elections cleared the way for relatively peaceful elections on December 16th. Student rioting in the summer of 1987 probably pressured Chun finally to abandon the electoral college system, but for Chun's Democratic Justice Party, the election was a success. For the first time in South Korean history, a democratic transfer of power had taken place. Chun had become the first ROK leader to transfer power peacefully. Roh emerged as a clear victor, garnering over 36 percent of the popular vote, compared to 27 and 26 percent respectively for the next two contenders.

In review, the defense decision-making process in South Korea is dominated by a relatively small group of men in the executive branch, the majority of whom have come from a military background. The National Assembly has not performed an oversight function of any significance because of constitutional provisions that establish a strong presidency and election laws that have worked to the advantage of the dominant political party, the Democratic Justice Party. Although the New Korea Democratic Party was successful in effecting a change in the electoral system that allows the direct election of the president, Chun still handpicked his successor and may even continue to play a powerful role behind the scenes. If this scenario of executive dominance pertains, then it is probable that South Korean defense policies, strategies, and force deployments will remain constant in the foreseeable future, but the possibility of serious political turmoil clearly could disrupt this assessment.

Recurring Issues and Defense Policy Outputs

REUNIFICATION EFFORTS

Beginning in the early 1970s and continuing until the present, there have been efforts initiated by both North and South Korea to hold talks on reunification, although frequently these initiatives have been more for propaganda purposes than as serious offers to reunite the peninsula. In 1971 the North and South Korean Red Cross organizations proposed talks to discuss the problem of divided families. These talks, beginning in September 1971, were the first official contact between the two Koreas since the division of the country in 1945.[83]

In July 1972 officials from both Koreas met, and at the conclusion of a series of meetings, they announced agreement on a number of points that became known as the "historic communique." This document contained three general principles. First, unification should be an internal Korean matter settled without external intervention or interference. Second, unification was to be achieved through peaceful means rather than force. Third, unification was to be pursued regardless of differences over ideologies, political systems, or other factors. To facilitate increased contacts, each side agreed not to slander the other or to undertake armed provocations. They pledged to establish a "hot line" between Seoul and Pyongyang and agreed to assemble a South-North Coordinating Committee for further discussions.[84]

Kim Il-Sung proposed in March 1973 that South Korea and North Korea join together to form the Democratic Confederal Republic of Koryo to accomplish reunification. Included in this proposal, however, was the provision that all foreign military forces were to be removed from both countries, which obviously was directed specifically at U.S. military forces in South Korea. This proposal was unacceptable to the South, as were several others, and the talks broke off by the end of 1973.[85]

The Sixth Congress of the Korean Workers' Party, the North Korean communist party, officially adopted the concept of the Democratic Confederal Republic of Koryo in late 1980, a plan almost identical to Kim's 1973 initiative, which also called for the immediate withdrawal of the U.S. forces. At least in part to counter this effort, Chun Doo Hwan formally proposed to the South Korean National Assembly in January 1982 that it write a "constitution for a unified Korea" to be submitted to the North as the basis for negotiations.[86] Because of mutual distrust, neither of these efforts really furthered the cause of reunification.

A major reason for these failures is the different reunification goals and processes on the part of South Korea and North Korea. South Korea has adopted a more incremental approach, calling for the gradual integration of the two countries, with cultural and economic contacts occurring first and actual political negotiations later. North Korea has favored more dramatic steps, with the goal of near-term reunification being foremost. The South has emphasized security and stability as preconditions, while the North's major precondition has been the removal of U.S. forces. In simple terms, South Korea has stressed "peace first, unification later" while North Korea has emphasized "unification first, peace later."[87] The North's position on the removal of U.S. forces as a precondition has made any agreement very difficult.

In addition to these bilateral efforts, there were also other proposals in the early 1980s addressing reunification. In late 1983 Prime Minister Zhao Ziyang of China suggested to the United States, at the initiative of North Korea, that three-way talks be held involving the United States, South Korea, and North Korea. During his visit to Seoul in 1979, President Carter had made a similar recommendation, but it was unacceptable to the North at that time. By 1983, North Korea had changed its position, at least in part because of the bad publicity it received as a result of the Rangoon bombing incident, but the United States and South Korea refused.

Instead, the Reagan administration suggested four-party talks that would add China to the discussions, and South Korea demanded that North Korea apologize for the Rangoon incident before any discussions could be held.[88] Although these talks did not come to fruition, the North's proposal was significant for two reasons. First, it included South Korea as a potential negotiator for the first time; second, North Korean leaders no longer listed U.S. troop withdrawal as a precondition for the negotiations. As suggested earlier, this change on the troop issue may represent an example of China exercising a moderating influence on North Korea, but it is impossible to be sure of this.

Just when both bilateral and multilateral negotiations seemed at a dead end, an act of nature intervened. In September 1984 torrential rains inundated Seoul, causing major flooding in some areas. North Korea offered relief assistance, and to the surprise of many, probably including Kim Il-Sung, South Korea accepted.[89] The delivery of relief supplies and the slight improvement in bilateral relations provided the impetus for discussions on several levels, including the resumption of the Red Cross talks that had been suspended in 1973, economic talks, discussions between legislators from both countries, and interactions among representatives of the respective Olympic committees.

The Red Cross discussions resumed in May 1985 after a 12-year hiatus and focused primarily on efforts to reunite some of the many families separated during the Korean War. These efforts culminated in September 1985 when a hundred members of separated families from both North and South Korea traveled to the respective capitals, where families were reunited in sixty-five of the one hundred cases. Relatives of the remaining thirty-five could not be found.[90] In addition, dance troupes from both countries and representatives of the press participated, so that there was wide coverage of these events. There is no question that family reunions, mail exchanges, and other forms of personal contact would help to alleviate some of the tremendous suffering caused by family dislocations. Progress toward these goals remains slow, primarily because of political factors on both sides, but there is the possibility that Red Cross efforts can provide confidence-building measures that may lead to improvements in other direct contacts too.

Both sides worked together to establish an economic cooperation committee in November 1984 to address economic relations. In many ways, the economies of North and South Korea are complementary, as evidenced by the North's natural resources, which are needed in the South, and South Korean technology needed in the North. Despite this complemen-

tary nature, progress has been slow. The South has proposed that trade ties between the two countries be encouraged as the first stage, whereas North Korea has emphasized joint exploration for additional raw materials in the North.[91] North Korea interrupted these talks early in 1985 when the "Team Spirit" exercise was announced, but they were resumed in June 1985.[92] They were stopped again as a protest against Team Spirit in 1986 and have not made significant progress in achieving increased economic cooperation.

The South Korean National Assembly proposed in June 1985 that legislators from the two countries meet together to write a new constitution that would provide the framework for reunification efforts.[93] This meeting occurred the following month, the first time legislators had met with each other since the division of Korea. Once again, however, an impasse occurred when South Korea continued with its insistence that a constitution be written first, while North Korea demanded that the first step be a nonaggression pact.[94] The troop issue is very much involved with this difference in priority. From the North Korean perspective, if a primary goal is to remove U.S. forces from South Korea, a nonaggression pact, followed by a possible peace treaty, makes sense because such an arrangement would remove the major South Korean justification for the retention of these forces. On the other hand, South Korea does not want to agree to anything that jeopardizes this retention. No further progress has been made in resolving this fundamental difference.

An effort was made in 1983 and 1984 to form one national team to participate in the Los Angeles Olympics, but the Soviet boycott of those games and the North Korean decision to follow suit ended this attempt. Subsequently, North Korea demanded that the 1988 games be co-hosted, with half of the events in Pyongyang and the other half in Seoul. This proposal was not only unacceptable to South Korea, but also to the International Olympic Committee (IOC).[95] IOC President Juan Antonio Samaranch interceded in the effort to resolve this dispute, and the two Korean Olympic Committees met on occasion at the IOC headquarters. In June 1986 Samaranch suggested that a possible compromise would be what he called "a distribution of the games," whereby North Korea might host a few events and share a couple of others such as the road cycling race, which could begin in Pyongyang and end in Seoul.[96] In any event, North Korea found itself embarrassingly isolated on this issue; its two primary allies, China and the Soviet Union, chose not to boycott the Olympics hosted by South Korea.

There have also been reports of meetings between high-ranking officials from both countries for the purpose of arranging a summit between the South Korean president and Kim Il-Sung. Chang Se Dong, the director of the National Security Planning Agency, formerly the Korean CIA, and Ho Dam, a member of the Korean Workers' Party Secretariat, allegedly met twice in September 1985.[97] These meetings have been denied by both sides, but speculation continues that they did occur. There would be political risks involved for both the South Korean president and Kim if a summit were held, but there also would be political benefits. For Kim, a meeting with Roh and improved relations with South Korea could be important in legitimizing the succession of his son, Kim Jong-Il, to the supreme leadership position in North Korea. (The succession issue will be discussed in the next section of this chapter.) For Roh, a meeting with Kim might allow him to mute some of the domestic critics who call for an accord of some sort with the North. Suffice it to say at this point that these high level discussions, if in fact they occur and lead to a summit, would surpass the other negotiations that have been outlined.

Since the division of the Korean peninsula, there have never been so many official contacts between the two governments as there have been in the past few years. Whether these talks will pave the way for eventual reunification remains to be seen. Both sides are trying to use the negotiations to further their national interests and achieve their own goals, goals that frequently are in conflict with each other, as evidenced by the different positions on the nonaggression pact. South Korea is not going to agree to something that threatens its security, particularly anything that would jeopardize retention of U.S. forces on its soil. Similarly, the North has resisted participation in quadripartite talks, because if China negotiates with South Korea, this contact would amount to tacit recognition of the South, legitimizing the division of the peninsula and impeding reunification efforts. Based on these observations, there is little likelihood that the current negotiations will lead to an early solution of the Korean problem. Nonetheless, there is more movement at present than has been true before, which is encouraging.

NORTH KOREAN SUCCESSION

Political succession in South Korea already has been addressed from the perspective of why this event is important for present and future security considerations. The succession issue in North Korea is perhaps even more important and merits analysis. During the Sixth Congress of the Korean Workers' Party in 1980, Kim Il-Sung, the dominant political leader since the country was formed, announced that his son, Kim Jong-Il, would be his successor. Thus, the first hereditary succession in a communist system appeared imminent.

The Congress did not officially endorse this succession plan, but it did elect Jong-Il to three powerful positions that provide him with the power base so critical if he is to be successful. These positions are: the second-ranking Korean Workers' Party secretary (outranked only by his father); the fourth-ranking member of the Politburo and its presidium (outranked only by his father and two veteran revolutionaries too old to be a challenge); and the third-ranking member of the Military Commission (outranked only by his father and O Jin U, the North Korean defense minister). The two Kims are the only individuals to hold all three of these powerful positions.[98]

It is important to consider why the elder Kim selected his son as his successor. A variety of reasons have been suggested by experts on North Korean politics. First, Kim does not want what happened to Stalin, Mao, and other communist leaders after they died to happen to him. By choosing his son, he can perpetuate the political system he developed and ensure that his legacy remains venerated by his people. Second, there just weren't that many other eligible contenders, primarily because Kim had eliminated many of them through purges over the years. Plus, Kim had a son he could turn to, whereas Stalin and Mao did not.[99] Third, Kim Jong-Il has proven himself to be capable of governing the country, at least in his father's eyes. He took the lead during the 1970s in developing the Three Revolution Team movement that is designed to "revolutionize" the use of technology, culture, and ideology within the society. He also has played a leading role in institutionalizing the Chuch'e principle of national self-reliance his father initiated many years ago.[100]

Regardless of the steps that both father and son have taken to enhance the legitimacy of the succession, there is no guarantee that it will be smooth. Unquestionably, Kim Jong-Il will operate from a very strong position both within the party and the military because of the actions taken by the Korean Workers' Party in 1980. However, North Korea is approaching a very difficult period, particularly with its economic development. Major decisions will have to be made that will not be popular with all segments of the population. Kim Il-Sung has been successful in controlling dissent by various means, but it remains to be seen how much success his son will have in similar efforts.[101]

How long Kim Il-Sung lives during the succession process is also important. If he lives for a few more years, and if he chooses to transfer all power to his son during the time he has left, then the chances of a peaceful transition are improved. If he dies suddenly before the transition is completed, then there may be more problems. Reports in 1986 of Kim Il-Sung's death and the resulting confusion until the reports were proven incorrect support this argument.[102]

Another interesting issue to raise is how the Soviet Union and China will react to the new North Korean leader. Clearly, both of them object to the hereditary succession for ideological reasons, but more importantly because the current Soviet and Chinese leaderships have attempted to downplay personality cults. It also will be interesting to learn how Jong-Il will attempt to structure North Korea's relations with its two major allies. His father has been quite successful in playing one off against the other while trying to maintain North Korean flexibility. This has not been an easy task and certainly will not be for his son either.

Finally, what are the possible implications of the succession process for the security of South Korea? There are many variables involved that make speculation risky, but at least two scenarios are worthy of mention. Kim Jong-Il may attempt to reach some sort of rapprochement with the South that would lead to improved bilateral relations and possibly peaceful reunification in the future. This was the rationale given for the reported high-level discussions between leaders of the two countries in 1985. Another possible scenario is that Jong-Il may attempt to offset domestic opposition to his rule by initiating a military adventure against South Korea. Based on worst-case planning, the South must continue its high state of readiness for fear the second contingency occurs. Determining how the succession in the North will develop will remain difficult, but the security implications for the South are taken very seriously by its political leaders and people.

CIVIL-MILITARY RELATIONS

At the conclusion of the Korean War in 1953, the United States devoted much of its effort in the South to building up the South Korean military forces so that the North Koreans would not attempt to unify the peninsula by force again. The United States was very successful in this effort, and the Korean military became a dominant factor in the Korean political process.[103] Whereas the boundaries between civilian and military duties and responsibilities are clearly distinguishable in the United States, they became blurred in South Korea and the military became a much more dominant factor than was the case in earlier periods of Korean history.[104]

As long as the threat from North Korea remains widely accepted and credible, the majority of the South Korean people have been willing to accommodate the preferential treatment accorded to the military, even though this violates the very strong Confucian cultural traditions in the country that place the military at a much lower level in the societal hierarchy. Conscription remains generally acceptable because of the threat and the need to maintain a large standing army. However, there have been some indications that other forms of military training are coming under attack, primarily by the more radical students. South Korean college students are required to participate in one week of military training during their second year. In April 1986, for example, two students set themselves on fire to protest this training, which they and their supporters termed "a mercenary education for U.S. imperialists."[105] Incidents of this kind are not common, but they are symptomatic of the inherent tension that exists for many people in the South between Confucian tradition on the one hand and the practical reality of the dominant military role in the country on the other.

This tension manifests itself in two other major issues that had confronted the Chun regime. The first of these involves the popular perception among Koreans that former President Chun did not have political legitimacy because he seized power in August 1980 through a military coup and then manipulated the election in February 1981 to extend his rule. Some opponents condemned Chun, holding him responsible for the bloody suppression of the 1980 Kwangju riots. Critics maintained that he came to power through the use of force and had employed both covert and overt coercion to ensure his position. Further, they criticized him and his family for enriching themselves through illegal activities in the intervening years.[106] Roh's credibility, while bolstered by his victory in the December 1987 presidential election, is considered by some to be damaged by the role he played as commander of the military police during the 1980 Kwangju riots. Among those who share these sentiments, the Reagan administration is faulted for the close support it provided to Chun. These criticisms are a major cause of the anti-American demonstrations that have become more frequent in South Korea during the past two years.[107]

The second source of tension involving the current regime derives from the slow pace of political liberalization. There is no question that the South Korean economy has grown and developed dramatically during the 1970s and on into the current decade. But government critics point out that concomitant political growth and development have not occurred. Chun, like most of his predecessors, argued that the North Korean threat mandates that South Korea cannot tolerate a political system based entirely on Western democratic principles, because such a system would appear weak to the North and could precipitate an attack. Roh, given his close connections to Chun and military background, may have similar sentiments, although he has promised to "demilitarize" the government. Kim Dae Jung, Kim Young Sam, and other opposition leaders have countered by pointing out that Israel and the Federal Republic of Germany are confronted with similar external threats, but still have democratic government systems.[108] The political reality is that as the economy has expanded, a large middle class has developed, which is now putting more and more pressure on the government to liberalize the political system.

It is important to keep anti-government and anti-American demonstrations in proper perspective. Those who are demonstrating represent only a very small percentage of the population and are mostly students. The United States and the U.S. military forces in the country are looked upon respectively by most as a good ally and an important deterrent to North Korean aggression.

ARMS CONTROL

As far as conventional weapons are concerned, there is little prospect that significant progress will be made between the DPRK and the ROK as long as political relations remain so hostile. Both countries desire to acquire or produce the most modern weaponry possible. The Soviet agreement to provide MiG 23s to the DPRK and the U.S. decision to sell F-16s to the ROK are recent examples of weapons system escalation. The fact is that the Korean peninsula is one of the most heavily armed areas in the world and will most likely continue to be so on into the future.

There has been some progress on reducing the possibility that the peninsula will become the scene of a nuclear confrontation. In December 1985 the DPRK became a signatory to the Nuclear Non-Proliferation Treaty (NPT), which provides that those countries not possessing nuclear weapons will neither produce these weapons nor accept them from another country.[109] Signatory countries are subject to inspections by the International Atomic Energy Agency. The ROK became a signatory in 1975, at least in part because of pressure from the United States. Since both Koreas have nuclear energy programs, signature of the NPT is important as a restraint on either side choosing the nuclear weapons option.

Conclusion

The Republic of Korea faces a basic dilemma in present and future security considerations. It has been extremely successful in developing its own economy and increasingly is able to supply the sophisticated military equipment so essential to the defense of the country. South Korean military forces are highly trained and skilled soldiers who will give a good account of themselves in any contingency. In this regard, time is definitely on the South's side. The North Koreans will have an increasingly difficult task matching South Korean military growth and development. Serious questions also pertain to the effect the succession issue will have on political stability in North Korea. The South Korean–U.S. alliance is better established at the present than it has been at any time since the Mutual Defense Treaty went into effect in 1954. The U.S. rapprochement with China is another factor in South Korea's favor, because the North Koreans cannot now be as certain of Chinese support that was so critical during the Korean War.

What, then, is the basis of South Korea's dilemma? In bilateral relations, South Korean political leaders and the population in general can never be absolutely certain that U.S. policy will not change from one administration to the next, on the troop issue in particular. The Carter decision has not been forgotten. In addition, there is a further complicating factor to the continuation of the American military presence. It is true that the vast majority of South Koreans want these forces to remain into the foreseeable future because of their deterrent value. There also is a rather widespread sentiment, however, that it was the superpowers who were responsible for the division of the country in 1945, and that as long as the USSR and the United States are so deeply involved on either side of the 38th parallel, the possibilities for peaceful reunification are reduced.

On the domestic political front, the Chun government had not been able to establish its legitimacy among the people. Support from the Reagan administration had been very important to President Chun, but this support also contributed to increased anti-American sentiment among some South Koreans. President Roh faces the same dilemma. There are those who continue to be concerned that if the United States does not continue its involvement and exert whatever moderating influence it can, President Roh may also become repressive and justify this repression, as Chun did, in terms of the increased security threat. What this suggests is that the most substantial challenge to South Korean security may no longer come just from the North, although this is a real threat that cannot be ignored. The more serious threat may well be the lack of political growth and development in South Korea, which could lead to widespread political instability in the years ahead and provide the North with an opportunity that would not normally be there. It is in the best interests of the Republic of Korea to ensure that this does not happen.

Notes

1. Taek-Hyung Rhee, *U.S.–ROK Combined Operations*, p. 15.

2. Jong-Chun Baek, "Problem for an Alternative Strategy of Conflict Resolution in the Korean Peninsula," *Asian Perspective* 8, no. 1, (Spring–Summer 1984): 120–21. This feeling of lack of control was also expressed to the author on numerous occasions during his assignment in the ROK between 1984 and 1986.

3. Sang-Seek Park, "Korea in the World: Major

Sources of Threat in Northeast Asia from a Korean Perspective," *Korea and World Affairs* 8, no. 4, (Winter 1984): 777–80.

4. See paragraph 3 of the annual Security Consultative Meeting held in Washington, D.C., on 7–8 May 1985.

5. International Institute for Strategic Studies, *The Military Balance, 1985–1986* (London: IISS, 1985), pp. 126–27, and Larry A. Niksch, "The Military Balance on the Korean Peninsula," *Korea and World Affairs* 10, no. 2, (Summer 1986): 257–58.

6. IISS, *Military Balance, 1985–1986*, p. 126.

7. For the lower figure, see ibid., p. 126. For the higher figure, see Niksch, "Military Balance on the Korean Peninsula," p. 255. For an intermediate estimate of 14.6 percent, see *Asian Security, 1985*, (Japanese Research Institute for Peace and Security), p. 105.

8. IISS, *Military Balance, 1985–1986*, p. 127, and Niksch, "Military Balance on the Korean Peninsula," pp. 255–56.

9. IISS, *Military Balance, 1985–1986*, p. 127, and Niksch, "Military Balance on the Korean Peninsula," p. 257. See also *Far Eastern Economic Review* (hereafter *FEER*), 5–11 March 1982, pp. 26–34.

10. For some background on the Hughes helicopter diversion, see *International Herald Tribune* (hereafter *IHT*), 16 July 1985, p. 1.

11. *IHT*, 15 August 1985, p. 4, and *FEER*, 20 June 1985, pp. 32–34.

12. Niksch, "Military Balance on the Korean Peninsula," p. 261, and *FEER*, 1 December 1986, pp. 29–31.

13. Young Choi, "The Korean Military Strategy in the 1980s," *Asian Survey* 25, no. 3 (March 1985): 346.

14. Niksch, "Military Balance on the Korean Peninsula," p. 264.

15. Copies of these two treaties are available in *Korea and World Affairs* 10, no. 2 (Summer 1986): 425–29.

16. *FEER*, 20 June 1985, pp. 32–34.

17. Treaties and Other International Agreements Series (hereafter TIAS), 3097, vol. 5, part 3, 1954, pp. 2368–76.

18. Ibid., p. 2375.

19. Claude A. Buss, *The United States and the Republic of Korea: Background for Policy*, p. 139.

20. For a good discussion of the psychological aspect of deterrence, see John F. Reichart and Steven R. Sturm, *American Defense Policy*, p. 150.

21. *Department of State Bulletin* 61, no. 1574 (25 August 1969): 143.

22. For a copy of the Nixon Doctrine, see "U.S. Foreign Policy for the 1970s: A New Strategy of Peace," A Report to the Congress by Richard Nixon, 18 February 1970.

23. The joint communique, dated 22 August 1969, is found in U.S. Congress, Senate Committee On Foreign Relations, *United States Security Agreements and Commitments Abroad: Republic of Korea, Hearings before the Subcommittee on United States Security Agreements and Commitments Abroad* (hereafter Symington Hearings), 91st Cong., 2d sess., part 6, 24–26 February 1970, p. 1725.

24. Buss, *United States and the Republic of Korea*, pp. 143–44.

25. The joint communique, dated 22 November 1974, is found in *Department of State Bulletin* 81, no. 1852 (23 December 1974): 877–78.

26. Ford's Pacific Doctrine can be found in the *Department of State Bulletin* 72, no. 1905 (29 December 1975): 913–16. The specific reference to Korea is on p. 915.

27. Kissinger's speech, delivered in Seattle on 22 July 1976, is found in *Department of State Bulletin* 75, no. 1938: 217–26. Specific references to Korea are found on pp. 221 and 223.

28. U.S. Congress, Senate Committee on Foreign Relations, *U.S. Troop Withdrawal from the Republic of Korea*, a report by Senators Hubert H. Humphrey and John Glenn (hereafter the Humphrey and Glenn Report), 95th Cong., 2d sess., 9 January 1978, p. 1.

29. *Public Papers of the Presidents: Jimmy Carter, 1977*, book 1, p. 343.

30. Humphrey and Glenn Report, p. 20.

31. Ibid., p. 20.

32. *Public Papers of the Presidents, Jimmy Carter, 1977*, book 1, p. 1018.

33. Ibid., pp. 1018–19.

34. For a good discussion, see Franklin B. Weinstein and Fuji Kamiya, eds., *The Security of Korea*, pp. 81–84. See also Frank Gibney, "The Ripple Effect in Korea," *Foreign Affairs* 56, no. 1 (October 1977): 167–68.

35. *FEER*, 10 June 1977, p. 10.

36. Humphrey and Glenn Report, p. 27.

37. Ibid., p. 28.

38. U.S. Congress, House Committee on Armed Forces, *The Impact of Intelligence Reassessment on Withdrawal of U.S. Troops from Korea: Hearings before the Investigations Subcommittee* (hereafter Intelligence Reassessment Hearing), 96th Cong., 1st sess., 21 June and 17 July 1979, p. 3.

39. Ibid., p. 6.

40. *Department of State Bulletin* 79, no. 2029 (August 1979): 15.

41. All of these quotes are from Ibid., p. 16.

42. Holbrooke's testimony is found in Intelligence Reassessment Hearing, p. 77.

43. *Department of State Bulletin* 79, no. 2030 (September 1979): 37.

44. Joint communique dated 2 February 1981, *Department of State Bulletin* 81, no. 2048 (March 1981): 14. For additional coverage of the Chun visit and the implications, see *FEER*, 6–12 February 1981, p. 18.

45. Chung-In Moon and Kwang-Il Baek, "Loyalty, Voice, or Exit? The U.S. Third-Country Arms Sales Regulations and R.O.K. Counterwaiting Strategies," *Journal of Northeast Asian Studies* 4, no. 1 (Spring 1985): 23.

46. *New York Times*, 1 April 1982, p. 6.

47. Moon and Baek, "Loyalty, Voice, or Exit?" p. 25.

48. *New York Times*, 1 April 1982, pp. 6, 32–33.

49. Larry A. Niksch, "South Korea in Broader Pacific Defense," *Journal of Northeast Asian Studies* 11, no. 1 (March 1983): 94–97.

50. Gregory Henderson, "Why Our Good South Korean Friends Turn Against Us," *Fayetteville Observer-Times*, 6 July 1986, p. F3.

51. Byung-Joon Ahn, "The Republic Of Korea and the U.S.," *Korea and World Affairs* 9, no. 1 (Spring 1985): 8.

52. *Korea Herald*, 4 July 1984, p. 1.

53. On recent violent, anti-American student demonstrations, see *New York Times*, 31 October 1986, p. 20.

54. *FEER*, 2 October 1986, pp. 42–44.

55. The Treaty on Basic Relations between the Republic of Korea and Japan, dated 22 June 1965, is available in *Korea and World Affairs* 10, no. 2 (Summer 1986): 429–31. Article III states that the ROK government is "the only lawful Government in Korea."

56. For a good article on Japanese-Korean relations, see *FEER*, 29 November 1984, pp. 51–54.

57. For two Korean expressions of this concern, see Sung-Joo Han, "South Korea's Policy towards the United States," *Journal of Northeast Asian Studies* 2, no. 3 (September 1983): 27, and Soong-Hoom Kil, "South Korean Policy toward Japan," ibid., p. 43.

58. For a good article on the sense of nationalism evident at the Asian Games, see *FEER*, 30 October 1986, pp. 40–41.

59. On "walking on two legs," see Jonathan D. Pollack, "U.S.-Korean Relations: The China Factor," *Journal of Northeast Asian Studies* 4, no. 3 (Fall 1983): 23. What this term means is that the PRC indicates there is no change in policy on the official level and that it only deals with the DPRK, while in reality the PRC tacitly recognizes that the ROK is becoming a more influential player in Northeast Asia.

60. For the 1984 PRC-ROK trade statistics, see *International Herald Tribune*, 4–5 May 1985, p. 8. For 1985, see *FEER*, 6 November 1986, p. 49. The Chinese–North Korea statistics for 1984 are included in Pollack, "U.S.-Korean Relations," p. 28, no. 25.

61. Byung-Chul Koh, "China and the Korean Peninsula," *Korea and World Affairs* 9, no. 2 (Summer 1985): 275.

62. Ibid., p. 276.

63. *FEER*, 17 January 1985, p. 27.

64. Charles Wolf, Jr., Donald P. Henry, K. C. Yeh, James H. Hayes, John Schank, and Richard Sneider, *The Changing Balance: South and North Korean Capabilities for Long-Term Military Competition*, p. 56.

65. Ibid., pp. 56–57.

66. Ibid., p. 43.

67. Ibid., p. 4, Research Institute for Peace and Security, *Asian Security 1984*, Tokyo, pp. 122–23.

68. Niksch, "Military Balance on the Korean Peninsula," p. 266.

69. Ibid., pp. 270–71.

70. Research Institute for Peace and Security, *Asian Security 1985*, Tokyo, p. 103.

71. *Asian Security 1984*, p. 126.

72. Ibid., p. 104.

73. Niksch, "Military Balance on the Korean Peninsula," p. 276,

74. Whan Young Kihl, *Politics and Policies in Divided Korea: Regimes in Contest*, pp. 119–20.

75. For a copy of the 1980 Constitution, see Harold C. Hinton, *Korea under New Leadership: The Fifth Republic*, pp. 176, 203.

76. Chul Koh Byung, *The Foreign Policy Systems of North and South Korea*, pp. 114–15.

77. Ibid., p. 115.

78. *FEER*, 28 February 1985, pp. 43–44, and *IHT*, 19 February 1985, p. 1.

79. For a good article on the composition of the DJP, see *FEER*, 13 March 1986, p. 25. For the NKDP coalition-building efforts, see *FEER*, 18 April 1985, p. 46.

80. Young O. Yoon, "Policymaking Activities of the South Korean National Assembly," *Journal of Northeast Asian Studies* 5, no. 1 (Spring 1986): p. 33.

81. *IHT*, 25 February 1986, p. 5.

82. *IHT*, 16 May 1986, p. 5.

83. Chin-Wee Chung, "South-North Korean Relations," *Korea and World Affairs* 6, no. 1 (Spring 1982): p. 118.

84. Ibid., p. 118.

85. Ibid., p. 119.

86. Pyong-Choon Hahm, "Korea's Unification Policy and Its Implementation," *Korea and World Affairs* 6, no. 1 (Spring 1982): pp. 20–21.

87. Whan-Kihl Young, "Evolving Inter-Korean Relations," *Korea and World Affairs* 9, no. 3 (Fall 1985): pp. 460–61.

88. *Asian Security, 1985*, p. 107, and *New York Times*, 12 January 1984, p. 3.

89. Ibid., pp. 108–9, and *IHT*, 1 October 1984, p. 1.

90. *FEER*, 10 October 1985, p. 22, and *IHT*, 23 September 1985, p. 1.

91. *FEER*, 29 November 1984, pp. 17–18, and *Asian Security, 1985*, pp. 109–10.

92. On the influence of Team Spirit exercises on the various negotiations, see *IHT*, 10 January 1985, p. 4, and *FEER*, 24 January 1985, pp. 13–14.

93. *IHT*, 3 June 1985, p. 4.

94. *IHT*, 24 July 1985, p. 5.

95. *FEER*, 5 September 1985, pp. 15–16.

96. *FEER*, 9 October 1986, pp. 42–43.

97. *FEER*, 5 December 1985, pp. 46–47, and *IHT*, 17 December 1985, p. 5.

98. Byung-Chul Koh, "Political Succession in North Korea," *Korea and World Affairs* 8, no. 3 (Fall 1984): p. 566.

99. Ibid., pp. 569–70.

100. Yung-Hwan Jo, "Succession Politics in North Korea," *Asian Survey* 26, no. 10 (October 1986): 1095–96 and 572.

101. For a good article on potential differences within the DPRK political leadership, see Aidan Foster-Carter, "Reading the Entails of the Pyongyang Goat," *FEER*, 29 August 1985, pp. 28–30.

102. *Washington Post*, 17 November 1986, p. 1. The identity of those responsible for these rumors and the possible reasons for their actions remain unclear as of this writing.

103. Edward A. Olsen, "The Societal Role of the ROK Armed Forces," in *The Armed Forces in Contemporary Asian Societies*, ed. Edward A. Olsen and Stephen Jurika, Jr., pp. 88–89.

104. C. I. Eugene Kim, "Civil-Military Relations in the Two Koreas," *Armed Forces and Society* 2, no. 1 (Fall 1984): 20–21.

105. *IHT*, 29 April 1986, p. 1.

106. *Washington Post*, 17 August 1986, p. 1.

107. For an example of criticisms of the "Chun-Reagan Dictatorship," see *IHT*, 7 April 1986, p. 1.

108. For the reference to Israel, see the *FEER*, 10 April 1986, p. 21. For the Federal Republic of Germany, see *Washington Post*, 17 August 1986, p. 28.

109. *IHT*, 28–29 December 1985, p. 2.

Part Five

OTHER REGIONS

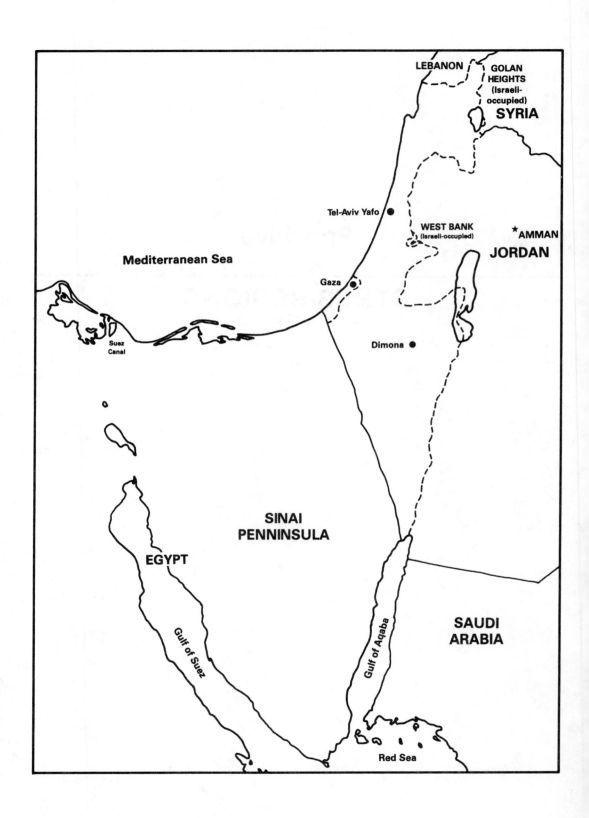

LEBANON

GOLAN
HEIGHTS
(Israeli-
occupied)

SYRIA

Mediterranean Sea

Tel-Aviv Yafo ●

WEST BANK
(Israeli-occupied)

★ AMMAN

JORDAN

Gaza ●

Dimona ●

Suez
Canal

SINAI
PENNINSULA

EGYPT

SAUDI
ARABIA

Gulf of Suez

Gulf of Aqaba

Red Sea

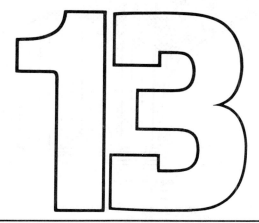

ISRAEL

Bard E. O'Neill

"Small nations do not have foreign policies; they only have defense policies."—Moshe Dayan

"I can, perhaps, define national security as serving and ensuring the basic values of the people of Israel in the State of Israel. At the top of the list of priorities of these basic national values, I would put life itself. . . ."—Avihu Ben Nun, Chief of Planning, Israel Defense Forces

International Environment

Despite its small size, Israel's formidable military capabilities qualify it as a mid-level power in the global context and the preeminent power in the Middle Eastern region. During its thirty-eight years as a state, Israel's defense policy has been determined primarily by threats emanating from its international environment. The self-perceived role of Israel is to be a state wherein all Jews will be welcome and secure. Ironically, the fulfillment of that role in

Palestine has continuously generated violent opposition from many quarters in the Arab world (for reasons that will become clear as we proceed), a reality that has created an acute and pervasive sense of insecurity. The threat perceptions that account for this insecurity are, in turn, the product of a crucial interplay of historic, geographic, and demographic factors.

THE CREATION OF A JEWISH STATE

The declaration of Israel's statehood in May 1948 was the culmination of a long, arduous, and frequently violent struggle on the part of Jews to create an independent state in the area of their ancient biblical kingdoms, consisting of the territory that now makes up Israel, the West Bank, the Gaza Strip, and parts of western Jordan (see figure 1). The main impetus behind this enterprise came not from the small Jewish community that had resided there since the time of the Roman conquest in 63 B.C., but rather from European Jews who were part of the Diaspora (i.e., the Jews who had dispersed

Figure 1. The Evolution of the State of Israel

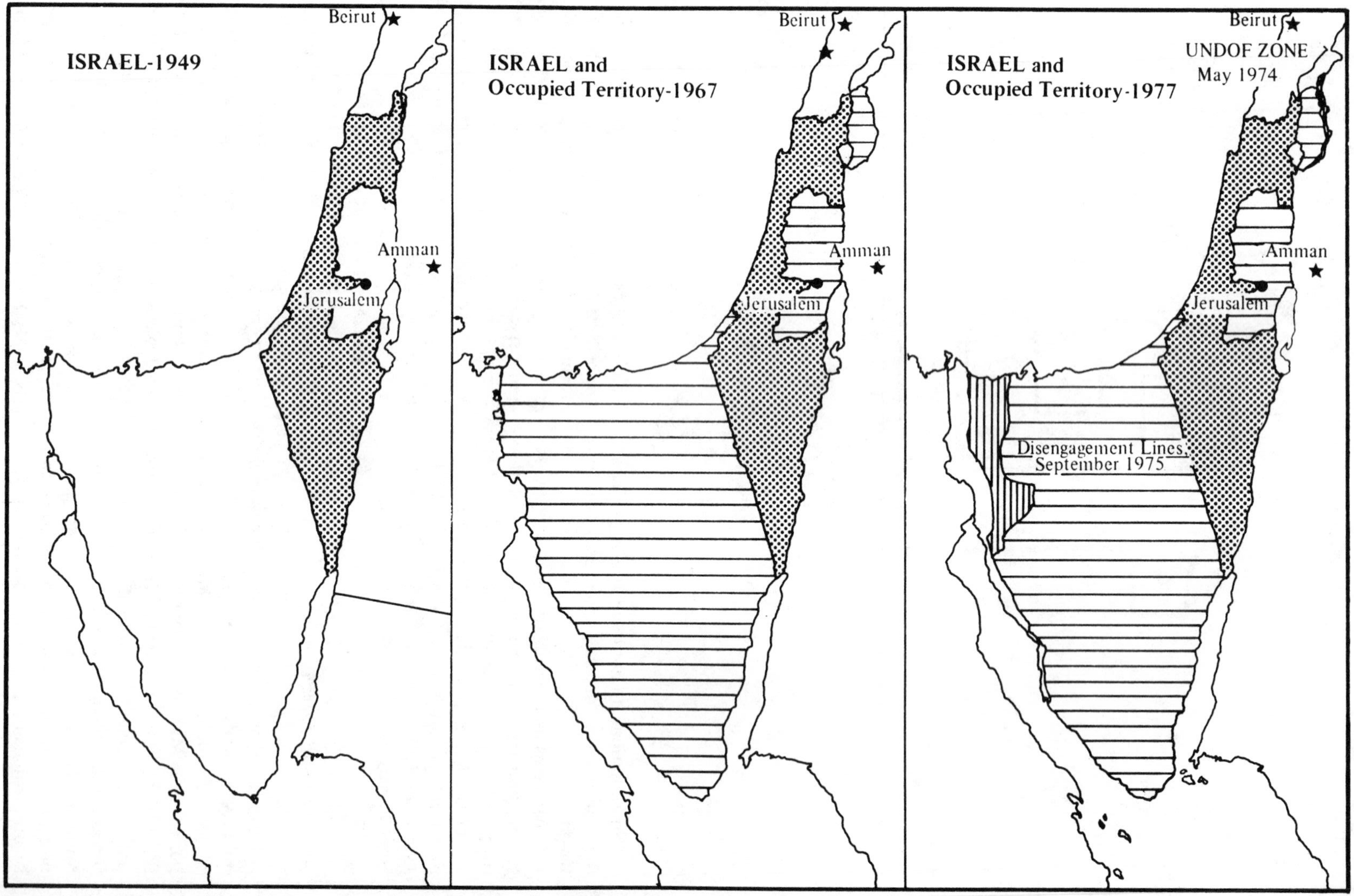

ISRAEL-1949

Beirut

Amman

Jerusalem

**ISRAEL and
Occupied Territory-1967**

Beirut

Amman

Jerusalem

**ISRAEL and
Occupied Territory-1977**

Beirut

UNDOF ZONE
May 1974

Amman

Jerusalem

Disengagement Lines,
September 1975

throughout the world commencing with the Babylonian exile and subsequently under the Roman Empire and thereafter). Although the Jews had never abandoned hope of one day returning, their interest in Palestine remained largely religious until the emergence of a nationalist movement among Eastern European Jews in the latter half of the nineteenth century. A conjunction of two political trends accounted for the new political activism of the Jews: the rise of nationalism in Europe and increased discrimination and violence against them in eastern Europe, particularly Russia.

Both nationalism and anti-Semitism led a number of Jews to conclude that the security of the Jewish people could never be assured unless they attained a national home. The most prominent proponent of such thinking, an Austrian by the name of Theodor Herzl, wrote a major pamphlet entitled *Der Judenstaat* (The Jewish state), in which he made the case for a Jewish national state. Inspired by Herzl, Jewish nationalists met in Basel, Switzerland, in August 1897 and endorsed the aim of creating a Jewish home. Whereas Herzl had not indicated the location of such a home, the Basel conferees proposed that it should be in Palestine. Moreover, they established the World Zionist Organization (WZO) as the major instrument for its actualization. In the years between the Basel conference and World War I, the Zionists expanded their organization internationally, encouraged settlements in Palestine, set up a national fund to buy land, and made intensive, albeit unsuccessful, efforts to persuade the major powers, especially Turkey, which controlled Palestine, to adopt policies favorable to the achievement of their ultimate aim.

When the British consolidated power in the area during the war, they too were subjected to Zionist pressure. Motivated by a desire to secure Jewish support for the war, the British government engaged in talks with two important British Zionists, Dr. Chaim Weizmann and Lord Lionel Walter Rothschild. Although the British had previously agreed to an Arab demand for postwar independence in the Arabian peninsula (except Aden) and the area of

Palestine, Lebanon, Syria, and Iraq, their support was subject to reservations and exclusions of territory because of concern for French interests. Shortly thereafter the British added to the confusion generated by their imprecise pledges to the Arabs by dispatching a letter to Lord Rothschild on 2 November 1917 (known since then as the Balfour Declaration) in which they indicated that Britain viewed with favor the establishment of a national home for the Jews in Palestine as long as it did not prejudice the civil and religious rights of the non-Jewish communities located therein. Pursuant to its objective of creating a Jewish state, the World Zionist Organization stepped up its support for immigration to Palestine, thereby incurring resistance from the Arabs, who feared losing their lands. This led to intermittent violence between the Jews and both the British and local Arabs, whose own sense of nationalism was stirring.

The accomplishments of the Zionists during this period were limited not just by Arab and British opposition, but also by a failure to gain the support of a large segment of European Jewry, which rejected Zionism on various religious, ideological, and practical grounds. Most of this Jewish opposition to Zionism was soon shattered by Adolf Hitler's ascent to power in Germany and his adoption of virulent and violent anti-Semitic policies. The monumental act of genocide known as the Holocaust obliged many previous skeptics in the Jewish community to conclude that the campaign for an independent Jewish state deserved active and immediate support. As a consequence, political and material backing from international Jewry rose substantially.[1]

As Jews continued to arrive in Palestine, Arab resentment increased. Although several commissions of inquiry reviewed the problem, a viable solution remained elusive. When World War II began, the British government quickly found itself preoccupied with survival and therefore postponed any major decision. In the aftermath of the war, a weakened Britain, beset with severe economic difficulties, decided to transfer to the United Nations what seemed to be an unsolvable problem. After several months of intensive and skillful lobbying by the Zionists, the U.N. approved a partition plan on November 29, 1947, that made provision for both Jewish and Arab states.

When both the Palestinians and other Arabs rejected this decision, fighting ensued between the two sides. Anticipating continued violence in the absence of a UN plan to implement the partition, the Zionists seized the initiative by acquiring weapons and training the forces necessary to defend their community and to sustain the state that would be established when the British withdrew in May 1948. As things turned out, the Palestinian Arabs proved unable to mobilize and organize the capability necessary to negate the partition plan. When a poorly coordinated (but nonetheless threatening) intervention of regular Arab military forces failed, the Jews took control of the Negev Desert in the south and the western Galilee sector of the north, thus making the state far more defensible than had been the case under the partition plan.

THE LEGACY OF THE HOLOCAUST

Two aspects of the Holocaust left a lasting impression on those who would be charged with the responsibility for formulating national security policy for Israel in the years ahead. First, the Holocaust focused attention on the basic question of physical survival. Unlike their counterparts in other states, Israeli leaders believed that it was inadequate to define security as the safeguarding of political values and structures and a way of life; for them, security had come to mean the very existence of a people.[2] Second, the experience of the Holocaust led to the further conclusion that physical security was too important to be left to others, since, even in moments of extreme peril, sympathetic friends might be indecisive. From the Jewish point of view, this was a painful and costly lesson that had been learned from the unwillingness of the Allies in World War II to undertake any serious measures for relief and rescue at the height of the Holocaust, even when such measures would not have conflicted with their military objectives or required the use of military power.[3]

DEMOGRAPHIC AND GEOGRAPHIC VULNERABILITY

Although the Arabs were greatly demoralized by the outcome of the 1948 war, they pledged themselves to the eventual eradication of the Jewish state. Inasmuch as the Arabs enjoyed a fifty to one manpower advantage (32.3 million to 650,000), such hostility was of no small concern to Israel. The fears that it engendered were further magnified by the geographic facts of life. In the words of one scholar: "Israel's geo-strategic position until June 1967 was a strategist's nightmare."[4] Surrounded by four belligerent Arab states and vulnerable to a blockade from the sea, it was "a state under siege."[5] The total area of Israel was close to 8,000 square miles, and the length of its borders was 615 miles on land and 159 miles by the sea. There were no natural obstacles along the land borders.

In the south, Israel is contiguous to Egypt's Sinai peninsula, a barren and sparsely populated region (see figure 2). Because of its large size and terrain, and Egyptian control of the few obstacles that could impede an invading force, the Sinai was conducive to the massing and movement (in the northern and central sectors) of large forces not far from Israeli population centers. Although the mountainous southern part of the peninsula was not suitable for the movement of modern military forces, it was still important, since the location of Sharm el-Sheikh near the Strait of Tiran allowed it to control shipping in the Gulf of Eilat.

Another area adjacent to Israel is the Gaza Strip, located in the northernmost part of the Sinai and running some twenty-six miles along the Mediterranean coast. Originally intended as part of the Palestinian Arab state, it was occupied by Egypt in 1948 and placed under a military government. Its pre-1948 population of 70,000 swelled to 261,000 as the result of an influx of refugees from the fighting. In 1948 it served as the main base of the invading Arab armies and for attacks on the western Negev. By 1952, it had become a staging area for unorganized guerrilla attacks on Israeli settlements. Three years later, these attacks were

Figure 2. The Egyptian Border: Sinai and Gaza

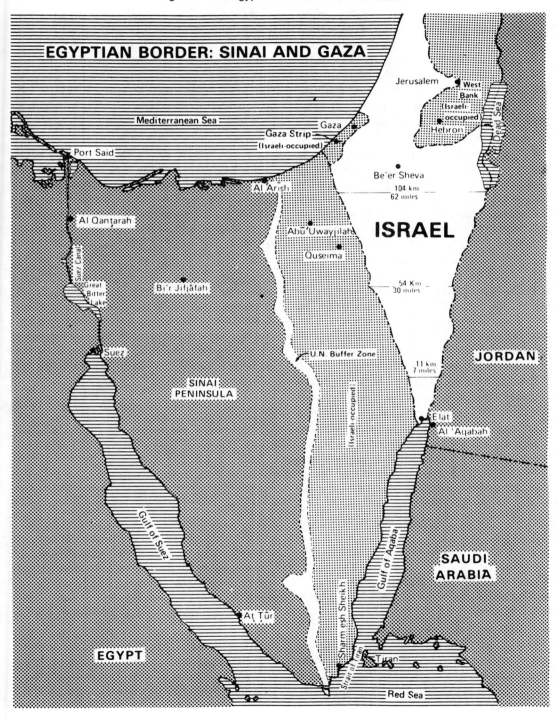

placed under the control of Egyptian military intelligence and increased considerably.

From a security point of view, the border with the West Bank poses the most serious problem. Like the Gaza Strip, the West Bank was to have been part of the Palestinian Arab state, but during the fighting in 1948, it fell under the control of Jordan. Formally annexed to Jordan in 1950 despite objections from the Arab League, it was seized by Israel in 1967. Since the West Bank is next to the narrow waist of Israel, which at one point is only nine miles wide from the Mediterranean coast to the border, it was possible that a surprise attack by Jordanian armored forces might cut the country in two, thereby severing vital north-south lines of communications. Aside from that, almost all of the heavily populated and industrialized central section of Israel was within Jordanian artillery range. Furthermore, the West Bank could be (and eventually was) a base for periodic guerrilla attacks against Israel, occasionally supported by the Jordanian army. The city of Jerusalem, meanwhile, was surrounded on three sides by Arab forces and thus was vulnerable to being quickly isolated from the rest of Israel (see figure 3).

Finally, in the north Israel is bordered by the Golan Heights, which overlook the Hula Valley and northern Galilee (see figure 4). After 1948 the Syrians heavily fortified the area and from time to time shelled Israeli settlements below. Regardless of who was to blame for such incidents, Syrian military activity reminded the Israelis that both Israel's citizens and vital water resources in the north were vulnerable to a potential Syrian military attack from the heights.[6]

National Objectives, National Strategy, and Military Doctrine

NATIONAL SECURITY OBJECTIVES

While there is no precise, overall codification of national strategy, much less a detailed longer-term plan for the orchestrated use of resources to attain political aims, several interrelated elements have been discernible since the leaders of the new state moved to grapple with a host of formidable problems, including the consolidation of political control, economic development, social integration of immigrants from diverse backgrounds, and the provision of national security.[7] The most salient of these elements is the overriding emphasis placed on security and its corollary objectives, namely, the pursuit of peaceful acceptance of Israel by its Arab neighbors, the commitment to become as self-reliant as possible in defense, and the maintenance of a strong military establishment.

In establishing priorities, Israel's first prime minister, David Ben-Gurion, saw "no alternative for Israel but to grant a central status to considerations of national security."[8] The centrality of security, as Dan Horowitz has pointed out, is an outgrowth of an essentially pessimistic view of various ideological and political persuasions. Such pessimism is rooted in the belief that survival involves not just the safeguarding of the state but, more important, the physical existence of all Jews in Israel as well. This conception, which derives from the painful historical experiences of the Jews described in the previous section, is reinforced by the "strategic data" of the Arab-Israeli conflict. In Horowitz's words:

> As a result of these data Israeli security conceptions have emphasized Israel's narrow security margin, resulting from a quantitative inferiority in population and resources and a lack of strategic depth. It is against this background that we must see the Israeli tendency to worst-case analysis as a guiding line in the formulation of foreign policy, which in these circumstances tends to be subordinated to the needs of security policy.[9]

THE ULTIMATE GOAL

The primacy accorded to security policy can be seen in all aspects of national strategy, beginning with its long-term goal of achieving peace with the Arab states. By peace, Israel does not have in mind agreements to avoid the use of force; instead, peace is conceived to be the full normalization of relations (i.e., diplomatic representation and international links in the areas of communications, trade, culture, travel, and so forth) with its neighbors. Only the actualization of peace along these lines, Israelis believe, can yield meaningful security. However, since Arab bellicosity has relegated

Figure 3. The Jordanian Border

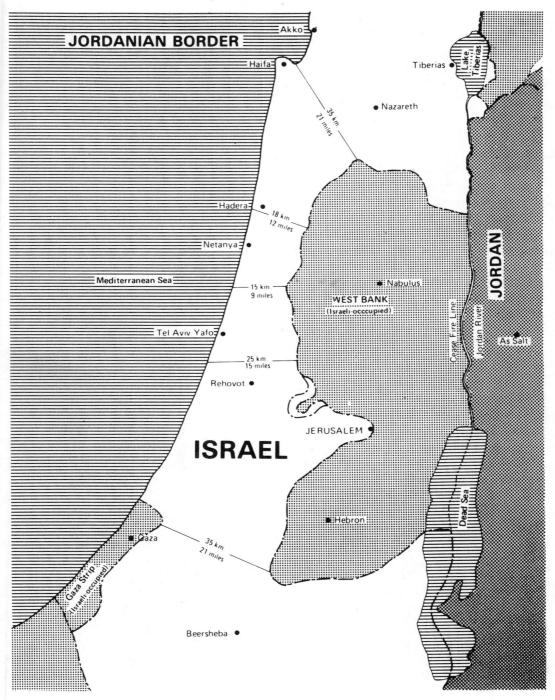

Figure 4. The Syrian Border

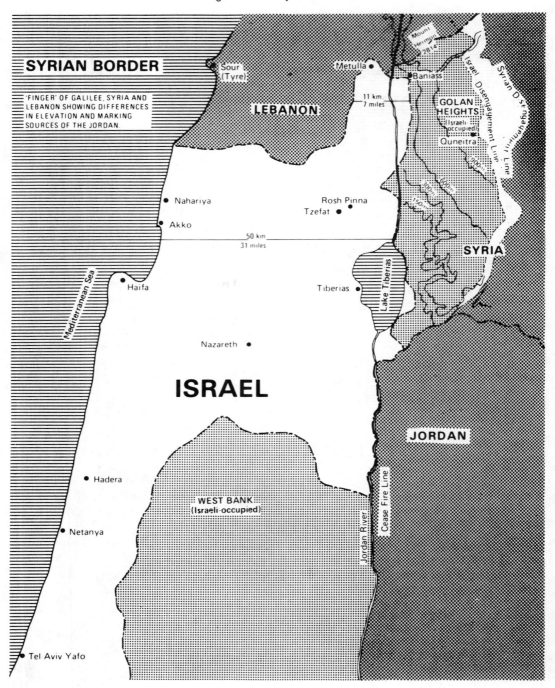

SYRIAN BORDER

'FINGER' OF GALILEE, SYRIA AND
LEBANON SHOWING DIFFERENCES
IN ELEVATION AND MARKING
SOURCES OF THE JORDAN.

Sour
(Tyre)

Metulla

Mount
Hermon
2814'

Baniass

11 km.
7 miles

GOLAN
HEIGHTS
(Israeli
occupied)

Israeli Disengagement Line

Syrian Disengagement Line

LEBANON

Quneitra

Nahariya

Rosh Pinna
Tzefat

Akko

50 km
31 miles

SYRIA

Mediterranean Sea

Haifa

Tiberias

Lake Tiberias

Nazareth

ISRAEL

JORDAN

Hadera

WEST BANK
(Israeli-occupied)

Netanya

Jordan River

Cease Fire Line

Tel Aviv Yafo

the goal of peace to a long-term pursuit, Israel has been compelled to concentrate its efforts on the more proximate objective of ensuring the physical security of Israel's land and people. Israeli leaders understand that military victory alone cannot bring peace, but they have calculated that eventually the Arabs will become convinced that Israeli military strength makes the destruction of Israel improbable, and thus will come to terms.[10] As of 1987, only one Arab state, Egypt, had fulfilled this expectation. Accordingly, Israel has continued to focus its assets on the overriding aim of guaranteeing survival of the state. In pursuit of this aim, both a pragmatic foreign policy and military strength are emphasized.[11] As far as military strength is concerned, Israel stresses a capability that either will deter Arab attacks by posing potentially high costs and the prospect of few gains in the event of war or that will enable it to defeat enemy forces if deterrence fails.

SELF-RELIANCE

An intermediate strategic objective, greatly influenced by the Holocaust, the 1948 war, and a number of events thereafter, is to be as self-reliant as possible where security is concerned. This commitment notwithstanding, the realities of international politics and Israel's own limitations necessitate a considerable degree of flexibility. Although originally preferring a policy of nonalignment vis-à-vis the great powers, Israel found that Soviet policies, such as growing support for the Arabs and restrictions on the emigration of Jews, were inimical to its interests. Consequently, by the early 1950s, Israel had, in effect, aligned with the West. The shift toward the West marked a return to the policy of seeking the support of one great power that had been pursued in relation to Great Britain during the mandate but that had been dropped in the period following independence. By reverting to a policy of obtaining the support of one Great Power, Israel stood to benefit in three ways: first, the legitimacy of Zionism would be increased; second, the military and economic sectors could acquire badly needed material assistance; and third, the Arabs might come to realize that violent opposition to Israel was no longer a sensible policy.[12]

As things turned out, the concrete payoffs of aligning with the West were slow in coming. Therefore, the assurance of physical survival continued to rest on armed strength and self-reliance and the associated need to enhance the country's economic and military capabilities. In the economic sphere, this meant that educational, technical, and human resources had to be marshaled for development. As the years went by, the impressive achievements of the Israeli economy became a mainstay in the drive for self-reliance, albeit at substantial cost to a civilian sector that was simultaneously called upon to pay the costs of absorbing new immigrants.

The economic efforts directed toward self-reliance worked out reasonably well until the Soviet decision to provide Egypt with arms in 1955 stimulated an already fledgling arms race. From that point onward, Israel's dearth of national resources and heavy industry compelled it to look abroad for sophisticated (and expensive) equipment, first to France and then, after the 1967 war, to the United States. Over the years, Israel's dependence on, and linkages to, the United States steadily grew, to the point where in the mid 1980s it was receiving $3 billion a year, nearly half of which was military aid. That periodic political disagreements between the two countries had no appreciable effect on this trend was evident in the signing of a November 1981 memorandum of understanding providing for joint naval and air exercises, and cooperation in military research and development, as well as American use of Israeli medical facilities and the establishment two years later of a joint political military group (JPMG) for consultations about common threats posed by the Soviet Union and its clients. The JPMG and its subcommittees institutionalized relations between mid-level defense officials on both sides, thus helping to raise American-Israeli cooperation to its apogee.[13]

Although welcoming the obvious advantages of the closer American connection, some members of the defense establishment have warned

that Israel might be drawn into East-West conflicts that were not in its interests. Even more
importantly, they have asked whether self-reliance might be undercut if Washington's increased leverage eventually reduced Israel's
decision-making flexibility during crises. Although Israeli leaders are aware that absolute
self-reliance is unattainable, they have sought
to minimize foreign dependence as much as
possible through a combination of foreign and
domestic policies. Externally, the Israelis have
been able to alleviate their heavy international
debt to some extent through German reparations and private contributions from international Jewry. Internally, they have accepted a
steep level of taxation, the allocation of a high
percentage of the GNP for defense purposes,
and the disruptive effects of an extensive military reserve system. In addition, to reduce
costs and to further self-reliance, Israel has established a sophisticated defense industry that
produces, modifies, and maintains military
hardware.[14]

MILITARY POWER AND SECURITY

Maintaining a strong military capability as
the centerpiece of national strategy has required not only money and weapons, but
organizational acumen as well. In fact, in its
formative years, organizational considerations
were accorded a very high priority. On 31 May
1948 a government order was issued establishing the *Zvah Haganah Le Israel* (Zahal), or, as
it is known in English, the Israeli Defense
Forces (IDF).[15] The largest of several Jewish
underground military organizations, the Haganah, became its foundation.

The overriding organizational task during
the incipient years of the IDF was to transform
the segmented units of the 1948 war into a cohesive and modern military force capable of
engaging regular armies equipped with aircraft, armor, and artillery. Accordingly, the existing situation, wherein brigades tended to operate in regions from which their troops were
recruited, was rejected. Despite opposition
from left- and right-wing parties seeking to
maintain their own armies, Prime Minister
Ben-Gurion prevailed in a determined effort to
create a single military force. Structurally, the

leadership opted for a unified command in
which there would be one general headquarters and a chief of staff commanding all the
military branches. New units were no longer
recruited on a local basis or confined to single
areas of operations; and the country was divided into three major areas of command—the
north, central, and south. At that point, also,
a tradition of appointing young chiefs of staff
was established (the first two were in their early
thirties).

To cope with the demographic disparity vis-
à-vis the Arabs, Israeli strategy stressed continued immigration. Cognizant that success in
this endeavor would still leave Zahal far short
of the number of recruits required for a large
standing army, Yigal Yadin, the first chief of
staff, devised a universal reserve system in
which every citizen was transferred to a reserve
unit after completion of his mandatory tour of
regular duty. Upon entering the reserves, individuals were to continue training, sometimes
up to forty-five days a year, and to advance in
rank until age fifty-five. Large military exercises were held to test the reserve system. In
light of its small regular army and sizable reserve components, Zahal became a veritable
citizens' army.[16] Because of the time required
to mobilize and deploy the reserves, a premium
was placed on advance warning from a high-
quality intelligence apparatus. Furthermore,
management of such a complex system required the IDF to devote considerable effort to
the education and training of a new generation
of officers.

Although military capability was upgraded
by organizational and educational policies,
there was trouble when it came to weapons acquisition. The Western powers were reluctant
to provide arms (the United States, in fact,
refused to supply arms). Hence, the Foreign
Ministry—then in charge of foreign weapons
procurement—scrambled to obtain whatever
arms it could, rather than wait until preferred
weapons might become available. This had
three notable effects: first of all, it led Israel to
hoard and accumulate arms; second, it stimulated greater efforts to acquire equipment
abroad; and third, it reaffirmed the wisdom of
having a domestic arms industry.[17]

The effort to obtain advanced weapons abroad finally paid dividends in the mid 1950s. After strenuous efforts by the defense ministry and the IDF, close ties were established with France. As a consequence, the IDF was able to acquire up-to-date weapons for the first time, weapons that shortly thereafter were employed against Egypt in what was to be the first of several postindependence wars that left their mark on national strategic thinking.

THE 1956 WAR

Trouble with Egypt was precipitated by incidents along the Gaza Strip border. In response to alleged Egyptian aggressive activities, Israel carried out large-scale reprisal attacks. One of these, which took place in February 1955, was a reaction to decisions by Egypt's President Gamal Abdel Nasser to seek advanced weapons and to sanction attacks inside Israel by Egyptian-trained guerrillas.

By the summer of 1956, the interjection of major power interests made a bad situation worse. Disconcerted by Egypt's purchase of Soviet arms via Czechoslovakia and its recognition of communist China, the United States withdrew an offer to help finance Cairo's main development project, the Aswan Dam. In reaction, Nasser nationalized the Suez Canal, a move that resulted in British and French collaboration with Israel. As fall approached, Israel became increasingly concerned about guerrilla raids and the arms being shipped to Egypt. When Egypt moved to form an alliance with Jordan and Syria, there was trepidation that, in time, the balance of power in the area might shift in favor of the Arabs. To preclude any serious threat to Zahal's ability to defend the state, Israeli leaders decided to act before Egypt consolidated its military strength and the new alliance.

After coordinating with Britain and France, Israeli forces invaded the Sinai in late October. Besides the objectives of eliminating guerrilla bases and decimating Egyptian military power, Israel hoped to compel Egypt to conclude a peace settlement on Israeli terms and to acquire strategically important territory. By early November, an Israeli military victory was all but confirmed by the withdrawal of Egyptian forces westward over the canal; however, in the course of the next few months, American pressure, Soviet threats, and the possibility of sanctions by the United Nations forced Israel to relinquish its gains and France and Britain to accept Egypt's nationalization of the Suez Canal. Though obviously unhappy with this turn of events, Israel nonetheless had achieved some of its other aims. Large amounts of Egyptian military hardware were destroyed, and the Strait of Tiran was opened to Israeli shipping. In addition, the United States declared, inter alia, that it was prepared to exercise the right of freedom of navigation through the Strait of Tiran and to join with other nations to secure this right.[18]

The relative ease with which Zahal moved across the Sinai in the 1956 war testified to the improving military capability of Israel. Although the war gave Israel over ten years of peace, it did little to alter basic national strategy, especially the elements of self-reliance and commitment to a powerful IDF.

As noted above, despite Egypt's defeat in the field, international pressure forced Israel, Britain, and France to yield their territorial gains and accept Nasser's nationalization of the Suez Canal; and Nasser's successful defiance of "imperialism" made him a hero in the minds of Arabs throughout the Middle East. Motivated by (and taking advantage of) his new stature, the Egyptian leader sought to assert his leadership in the Arab world through diplomacy, propaganda, subversion, and, in the case of Yemen, military force. This preoccupation with Pan-Arab matters did not allow Israel to rest easily, however. Since aspirations for Pan-Arab leadership were hardly compatible with accommodating the perceived common enemy of the Arabs, namely Israel, there was no modification of the professed long-term Arab aim of destroying the Jewish state. In spite of Nasser's orientation toward Arab affairs, Israel could never be sure that Egypt and its allies would not one day turn their attention to the "Zionist problem." And, because the Egyptians and the Syrians were being equipped, trained, and advised by the Russians, the longer-term possibility of a military move could not be ruled out. In short, the Sinai war did not eliminate Israeli fears about the future, particularly since geostrategic vulnerabilities along the borders had not been rectified.

In view of this situation, Israel devoted considerable time, effort, and resources to analyzing and adjusting military doctrine and modernizing Zahal. Since the defense establishment was unable to acquire all the weapons it desired, the IDF depended increasingly on improvisation and its own technical knowhow. In addition to enhancing its conventional capability, Israel also channeled resources into nuclear research and development.

THE 1967 WAR

In the spring of 1967, Israel's military capability was again tested when Nasser arbitrarily closed the Strait of Tiran, requested UN peacekeeping units to leave the Sinai, and augmented his military forces there. While Israel mobilized its reserves and the daily costs of this undertaking mounted, the Western powers procrastinated over whether or not to send ships to open the strait. Frustrated by the inaction of the West, concerned about the Arab military threat, and enticed by another opportunity to redress the unfavorable geostrategic situation that had existed for nineteen years, Israeli generals argued for a swift preemptive attack. Once approval was given by Prime Minister Levi Eshkol, a dawn air attack all but eliminated the Egyptian air force. Following this decisive blow, the IDF moved with alacrity to seize the Sinai and the Gaza Strip from Egypt, the West Bank from Jordan, and the Golan Heights from Syria, thereby dramatically changing Israel's geostrategic environment.

The seizure and occupation of the three Arab territories posed a dilemma for Israeli strategists. On the one hand, the indefinite retention of the areas brought over one million Arabs under Israeli control. Aside from the potential problems of ruling an antipathetic population, Israel had to contemplate the long-term effect on its democratic political ethos that indefinite rule without equal rights might have. On the other hand, an expeditious re-

turn of the territories to Arab control would mean going back to the disadvantageous geographic circumstances that prevailed before the war, something that security planners were loath to do, particularly after the Arab leaders met at a summit in Khartoum during August 1967 and resolved that there would be no recognition of, or settlement and negotiations with, Israel. The policies adopted by the Israeli government were consistent with existing national strategy. The magnitude of the Israeli victory in 1967 left few doubts about the military superiority of the IDF. Yet the Arabs did not seek the peace that Israeli leaders had long hoped they would. Instead, the major Arab states demanded the return of all occupied areas and a restoration of Palestinian rights. While confining their main efforts to the diplomatic arena, the Arab states began the slow process of refurbishing their armed forces.

It did not take long for Israel to realize that the war had increased, rather than mitigated, Arab hostility. Nowhere was this more evident than in Arab support for commando and terrorist attacks against Israelis by the Palestinian guerrilla organizations that had proliferated after the war. Although many of these groups were controlled by Arab states, others, such as Al Fatah, were independent. The stated purpose of the Palestinian groups, many of which coordinated their activity through an umbrella organization called the Palestine Liberation Organization (PLO), was to expunge Zionism. From the Israeli point of view, the support of the guerrillas (known collectively as the *fedayeen*—"men of sacrifice") by the Arab states appeared to be yet another indicator of their determination to annihilate the Jewish state. This, in turn, had the effect of reconfirming major elements of national strategy.

As in the past, security remained the most important consideration. Unlike in the past, the conditions for providing security, particularly the geographic ones, were vastly improved. Aside from removing various threats that could have been posed by nearby Arab forces, the occupation gave the Israelis defense in depth for the first time and provided natural defensive barriers (e.g., the Jordan River and the Suez Canal). Moreover, it enabled the IDF to build dispersed new bases and facilities. The dispersal of air bases was especially important given their vulnerable prewar concentration in a few areas due to Israel's small size. Retention of the Sinai allowed Israel to construct four new air bases and a number of smaller airfields.

The security value of the territories to Israel increased as a result of fedayeen attacks along the borders, particularly the border with Jordan. Through the establishment of fortified settlements and military outposts, Israel was able to engage Palestinian guerrilla units (though not urban terrorists) in relatively open terrain a good distance from Israel's heartland.

There was no gainsaying that retention of the territories strengthened Israel's military capability and thereby enhanced overall national security. Thus, while Israel indicated a willingness to return large portions of the territory and population, it insisted on controlling other areas for security reasons.[19] The degree of Zahal's military superiority that resulted from this new situation accentuated the importance of deterrence in Israeli strategic thinking. Although still committed to a strong war-fighting capability, the security establishment came to believe that the Arabs would be deterred from starting a major war because they would suffer unacceptable costs while having little chance of achieving their aim of destroying Israel. What Israel did not count on was the Arab states conducting a major war for limited aims.

THE 1973 WAR

Israel's refusal to return to the 1967 borders eventually led Nasser's successor, Anwar al-Sadat, to begin preparations for war. Although Nasser's initial attempts to dislodge the Israelis from the territories had been primarily diplomatic, by 1968 his despair with the continued impasse led him to approve of intermittent hostilities against IDF units along the canal. As Israeli casualties from artillery and commando raids began to rise in 1969, the cabinet approved air strikes deep inside Egypt. Unable to contain the Israeli Air Force, Nasser finally agreed to a cease-fire in the summer of 1970. In September the Egyptian president died of a heart attack.

Shortly after assuming power, Sadat was confronted with an internal threat from the left. In the spring of 1971, he eliminated this opposition and then turned his attention to the dispute with Israel, promising to wage a "battle of destiny." Much to his displeasure, he found that the Egyptian military was in no condition to engage Zahal. Consequently, he appointed a new defense minister, who was charged with preparing the armed forces for a war with Israel. Meanwhile, Sadat relied on diplomatic efforts to bring pressure to bear on Israel, albeit with little effect. By the spring of 1973, Sadat became convinced that a limited war was the only way to create a new diplomatic situation that would eventually lead to a return of the occupied territories. Hence, he moved to obtain Syrian agreement to join the conflict. While the plans and preparations for war were being finalized over the summer, Egyptian diplomats went about lining up Arab and Third World support.

On 6 October 1973, the Arab armies attacked the IDF on both the southern and northern fronts, inflicting heavy casualties and achieving limited, but politically significant, territorial gains.[20] Despite some very tense moments early in the conflict, especially in the north, where Syrian forces drove to the doorstep of northern Israel, the IDF eventually routed the Syrians and threatened to do likewise to the Egyptians.

In spite of their eventual military success, the Israelis were shocked by the war, particularly by the Arab ability to gain strategic surprise and to achieve initial military objectives. In retrospect, the close call in the Golan Heights was of special concern.

The October War had the effect of underscoring once more the basic elements of national strategy. The improved military capability of the Arabs, coupled with their continued disinclination to recognize Israel, accented the stress on national security. In fact, Israel became preoccupied with security matters as it sought to ascertain why things had gone so badly at the beginning of the conflict. One outcome of the postwar assessment was a decision to upgrade military strength substantially through doctrinal changes, reorganization, improved training and maintenance, greater discipline, and a massive arms acquisitions program. A factor that played a key role in the renewed attention to arms acquisition was the belief that the dramatic rise in postwar oil revenues would enable the Arabs to rebuild their forces with huge quantities of costly, sophisticated equipment. Another factor was the realization that the West's dependence on oil made it more responsive to the Arabs. During the conflict, the Europeans refused to sanction the transit of supplies to Israel for fear of provoking the Arabs, and immediately after the war, both the Europeans and the Japanese endorsed the Arab demand that the occupied territories be returned.

The shift by Europe and Japan provided further impetus for an already greater emphasis on self-reliance that derived from perceived American hesitation in resupplying Israel. Whatever the truth in the debate over whether or not the United States deliberately held up supplies, Israel experienced some anxious moments when the first few days of fighting reduced its inventories. In light of this, Zahal committed itself to acquiring enough arms to wage a prolonged war without depending on any outside source.

From the Israeli standpoint, the war also reinforced the strategic importance of the territories. Although the Arabs argued that the war proved that territory could not provide security in an era of missiles and long-range artillery, Israeli generals drew the opposite conclusion when they asked themselves what would have happened without the defense in depth provided by the Golan Heights and the Sinai.

THE SADAT INITIATIVE

As time went by, the Israeli assumption that the Arabs would accept Israel only when they could not defeat it was partially vindicated. The reason for this was, of course, Sadat's gradual move toward an accommodation with Israel. Following acknowledgement that Israel's destruction was not a realistic aim because of American security pledges, Sadat astonished the world with a trip to Jerusalem in December 1977. Two years later a treaty was signed between Israel and Egypt, but only after very difficult negotiations. Although Israel finally achieved a degree of long-sought-after acceptance and legitimacy, the Arab states (except the Sudan and Oman) and the PLO bitterly castigated Sadat, with some calling him a traitor. As a result of this continued hostility, the essential ingredients of national strategy were not questioned. Moreover, when the Likud Party came to power in Israel in 1977, a new dimension was added to national strategy, which in time would prove to be a major reason for the decision to go to war in Lebanon in 1982. This new dimension was the Likud's expressed goal of retaining the West Bank and Gaza Strip because they were considered part of Eretz Israel (the land of Israel from biblical times). How this goal affected Lebanon is discussed below.

OPERATION PEACE FOR GALILEE

Israel's most recent war with the Arabs started with air attacks on Beirut on 4 and 5 June 1982.[21] These were followed with a major invasion on 6 June involving all branches of the IDF. Although dubbed "Operation Peace for Galilee," it soon became apparent that the political goals of the war transcended the aim of securing the citizens of northern Israel from possible attack by the PLO, which had been building up its stocks of conventional armaments (e.g., mortars, artillery, tanks, etc.) in southern Lebanon. The concern over bombardments of northern towns and settlements had resulted in intermittent air and commando raids against PLO facilities since 1968, as well as periodic search-and-destroy missions by regular forces, the largest of which was Operation Litani in 1978.

While such military activity reduced the PLO threat, it never eliminated it, largely because many PLO fighters exfiltrated northward during combat and reinfiltrated southward after the fighting, events during and after Operation Litani being a case in point. Although the frontier had been quiet for almost a year due to a cease-fire arranged through American diplomatic efforts in 1981, Israeli preparations to cross the border were evident to many observers (including this writer) who visited the northern areas. Hence, when the June 1982 assassination attempt against Israel's ambassador in London by the anti-Arafat Abu Nidal group triggered Israeli air attacks and the invasion, it came as no surprise to those who had been monitoring events.

While Israel's move against the PLO in southern Lebanon could be explained by its traditional preoccupation with physical security, its rapid drive north and its siege of Beirut suggested that factors other than security had entered into strategic calculations. Foremost was the Likud government's ideological goal of retaining the West Bank. The principal architect of the invasion, Defense Minister Ariel Sharon, believed that the destruction of the PLO's military and political infrastructure would eviscerate its influence in the West Bank and thereby facilitate Israel's plans to spread settlements and consolidate control there. Sharon and his supporters further believed that the turbulent situation in Lebanon could be stabilized by reducing, if not eliminating, Syrian influence and by backing the emergence of a strong Maronite Christian president, Bashir Gemayel.

When the fog of war finally cleared, Israel found itself in an unenviable position. Although the IDF had moved to the outskirts of Beirut in a matter of days, it had engaged in some costly battles with Syrian ground forces, which many analysts felt could have been avoided if the initial aim of securing southern Lebanon to a point forty kilometers north had been adhered to. Moreover, as the rapid movement of Israeli forces gave way to a prolonged siege of Beirut, the IDF opted for heavy artillery and air bombardments of PLO areas of the city in order to avoid the casualties that would be entailed by house-to-house combat in an urban labyrinth, a decision that, not surprisingly, galvanized both international and domestic criticism. To make matters worse, following an evacuation of PLO fighters from Beirut, Israel's Maronite allies entered the Palestinian refugee camps of Sabra and Shatila in mid September and proceeded to slaughter civilians there. The IDF was blamed because it

had allowed the Maronites access to the area and, in February 1983, a commission of inquiry recommended the dismissal of several officers, as well as the defense minister.

For over two years after these events, the IDF remained bogged down in southern Lebanon and managed to alienate most sectors of the Lebanese population. As casualties increased from guerrilla and terrorist attacks carried out by various Lebanese groups, especially the Shiites, public and military morale in Israel eroded noticeably. Dispirited by the experience in Lebanon and the loss of his wife, Prime Minister Menachem Begin resigned in the fall of 1983. But, it was not until new elections were held and a coalition government led by the Labor Party's Shimon Peres was formed a year later that Israel withdrew its forces to a narrow security strip along the border.

In retrospect, the political tally sheet of the 1982 war was hardly impressive. Although the PLO's military and political apparatus in the south was destroyed and the organization was engulfed in both internecine and inter-Arab conflicts, Arafat continued as a political force in the area and the PLO's influence in the West Bank was not expunged. Furthermore, the alliance with the Maronites backfired, as Bashir Gemayal was assassinated and succeeded by his brother, Amin, who not only distanced himself from Israel, but also proved incapable of keeping order among the Maronites, to say nothing of Lebanon as a whole. Finally, Syria gradually reestablished its presence and influence in Lebanon. Perhaps the most poignant summary of the war came from two of Israel's most respected military commentators, Ze'ev Schiff and Ehud Ya'ari, who wrote:

It was a war for whose meager gains Israel had paid an enormous price that has yet to be altogether reckoned; a war whose defensive rationale belied far-reaching political aims and an unconscionably myopic policy. It drew Israel into a wasteful adventure that drained much of its inner strength, and cost the IDF the lives of over 500 of its finest men in a vain effort to fulfill a role it was never meant to play. There is no consolation for this costly, senseless war. The best one can do now is to learn its lessons well.[22]

One outcome of the process of studying the war's lessons was a return to the narrower and more familiar conceptualization of national security that, as we have seen, centers around the existence of the Jewish people and state rather than political expansion.

MILITARY DOCTRINE AND FORCE STRUCTURE

In view of the high priority all Israeli governments have accorded to security and military strength, the nexus between national strategy on the one hand and military doctrine (i.e., the guiding principles for the application of military force) and force structure on the other has been inherently close and self-evident over the years. In part, this is due to the fact that the same historic, geographic, demographic, and economic factors that have played such an important part in determining national strategy have also influenced military doctrine and force structure. Since the events on the battlefields during Israel's wars have been equally important with respect to the evolution of doctrine, the military aspects of those wars require more direct attention at this point.

The Formative Years: 1948–1955. According to Maj. Gen. Israel Tal, in the early 1950s two basic assumptions guided Israeli strategists who consolidated doctrine and planned for future hostilities: one was that the destruction of enemy forces bestowed only a temporary advantage on the IDF in view of Arab material and human resources; the other was that captured territory would be difficult to hold because of international opposition. Thus, conquered territory was viewed as conferring a strategic advantage and a bargaining chip for peace negotiations.[23] The recognition of the enemy's capability to rebuild following a defeat, the advantages the Arabs had by virtue of their numbers and resources, and the importance of territory led Israeli strategists to fashion a doctrine and force structure that would fully exploit the advantages of the Jewish community, notable for its high motivation, organizational abilities, and education. The effects of these attributes were felt as early as the War of Independence.

To offset the Arab advantages during the War of Independence, Israeli military leaders found it necessary to mobilize the entire war potential of the Jewish community. In the absence of strategic depth, border settlements came to play an important role, namely, containing enemy advances until regular units could be transferred to their areas. To assure quick movement and concentration of power, a unified command structure was adopted. Once forces were concentrated against the Arabs, the problem of how to cope with the enemy's greater firepower had to be solved. The Israeli answer was to maximize surprise by following the strategy of the indirect approach: that is, doing the unexpected in space, time, and direction. Because of the success in this undertaking, both the indirect approach and flexibility in planning and operations became essential ingredients in IDF military doctrine.[24] On the tactical level, this meant placing a high premium on competent middle- and lower-echelon commanders who were willing and able to adjust to changes on the battlefield (as opposed to adhering slavishly to textbook plans and standard operating procedures).

During the early years of statehood, the principle of transferring the war to the enemy's territory as quickly as possible through highly mobile, deep-penetration operations also became part of military doctrine. To do otherwise and engage the enemy inside Israel was considered too costly in view of the state's small size and concentrated population and economic assets.

The force structure that emerged from the War of Independence was primarily infantry-oriented; air and naval components were small. Between 1949 and 1953, it underwent a number of organizational changes, the most important of which was the previously discussed institution of the reserve system. Border settlements retained their role as a first line of defense until the reserve could be mobilized.

The main instrument of attack remained the infantry. It was to receive fire support from tanks that functioned as mobile artillery. Accordingly, the pace of advance was necessarily dependent on the speed of infantry movements; little thought was given to the use of armor as a spearhead.

When Moshe Dayan became chief of staff in 1953, he did not alter the infantry's central role. Nevertheless, he did place great emphasis on the further development of an offensive spirit. Although he subscribed to the indirect approach, Dayan recognized that it could not be used in all cases. Thus, he saw to it that the IDF was trained for direct assaults on fortified positions. Whether following the direct or indirect approach, Dayan believed in attacking forcefully and aggressively, even if it resulted in somewhat higher casualties.[25]

The emphasis on offensive spirit could be seen in the policy that the IDF adopted to deal with guerrilla attacks. Instead of responding with similar types of actions, as had been done from time to time, the IDF carried out reprisals against military targets. The purpose was to deter future attacks by increasing the costs to the Arab states and demonstrating to the Arab governments that their armies could not prevent retaliatory measures.

Whether dealing with guerrillas or planning for the possibility of conventional warfare, the IDF continued to accord primacy to the infantry despite entreaties from commanders of the armored corps, who wished to operate in large concentrations rather than as small ad hoc groups supporting the infantry. It was only in the last few days prior to the 1956 war that Dayan suddenly reversed course and approved the use of tanks in large formations, a change of thinking that proved more successful than had been anticipated.[26]

During Dayan's tenure, the air force was treated much the same way as the armored corps, in that its principal mission was to protect and support the infantry. Given the importance of the reserve components in the IDF, the air force was to ensure that mobilization met little interference and that aid was given to contain enemy advances until mobilization was completed.[27] From the air force point of view, the successful accomplishment of such objectives was contingent on the ability to perform two important missions: the achievement of air superiority (by striking enemy air units on the ground if possible) and the interception of enemy aircraft threatening Israel. To fulfill these missions at a reasonable cost, the air force opted for compact fighter-bombers in lieu of more expensive and less flexible bombers.[28]

In addition to the missions noted above, the air force also acquired primary responsibility for the defense of Israel's coastline. While the navy provided support in this undertaking, major importance was not assigned to its activity. In fact, the primary strategic maritime objective, maintaining Israel's lines of communication with the outside world, was given to the merchant marine.[29] The role of the navy continued to be circumscribed after the Sinai war.

Mobility, Firepower, and Quick Victory: 1956–66. The Sinai war influenced military doctrine and force structure in a number of ways. The swift Israeli drive across the Sinai indicated that rapid military victory was attainable (Dayan believed that such a victory was imperative in order to avoid external political or military interference). The strategy of the indirect approach, deception, and surprise once again emerged as key elements of success. Although the advantages of preemptive attack also became apparent, it was not until the postwar Arab military buildup that "it became a principle to deliver the first blow whenever a threatening situation developed as a result of the concentration of regular Arab forces in the proximity of [the] borders."[30]

The roles of the various components of the IDF were affected significantly by the war. In view of the new stress on combining mobility and firepower, the armored corps replaced the infantry as the principal instrument for decisive action; consequently, it was enlarged, personnel of higher quality were recruited, and extraordinary gunnery standards were established (and achieved).[31] Since the other land forces were tasked with supporting the armored corps, they were mechanized.

Like armor, the air force's star rose as a result of the Sinai campaign. Because of the key part that allied air superiority played in the Israeli victory, Israel augmented its aircraft inventory through the acquisition of French Mystères and Mirages and devised new programs to enhance the quality of its pilots. Successful efforts were also made to modify aircraft to suit local conditions and to shorten their turnaround time by improving maintenance procedures.[32] Within the air force, meanwhile, there was an increasing belief that the force should be committed first and foremost to the offensive. As the air force commander, Ezer Weizman, continually importuned: "Israel's best defense is in the skies of Cairo." Such thinking led to detailed planning of operations to catch the Arab air forces on the ground before takeoff.[33]

Unlike the armored and air force components of the IDF, the importance of the navy was not significantly upgraded. Yet, even though there were few improvements in the navy force structure, it was called upon to support the doctrinal principle of quickly transferring the battle to the adversary's territory by blockading enemy ports in time of war.

The Vindication of Doctrine and Force Structure: 1967. As the fateful spring of 1967 approached, the IDF's doctrine and force structure were oriented toward swift, intensive operations inside enemy territory, led by armored and air force units. Though constantly alert to the opportunity for conducting indirect attacks, the IDF was prepared for direct assaults on the Soviet-inspired deep linear defense posture of Egyptian forces in the Sinai. Where it was impossible to outflank the enemy, Israeli doctrine called for heavy armored attacks along a narrow front near the center of the adversary's defense system. The air force was to attack antitank defenses, provide close support, and disrupt the enemy's rear areas. Heliborne operations would also be used for the last-named purpose. Should armored units arrive earlier than the mechanized forces, they would be encouraged to attack immediately in order to prevent the opposition from reorganizing.[34]

Israeli military doctrine was implemented in 1967. In the midst of mounting tensions that had their origins in border hostilities during the fall of 1966, the Soviets misled Nasser with exaggerated reports about an Israeli buildup against Syria. This brought a series of Egyptian moves described earlier (closing the Strait of Tiran, requesting evacuation of UN forces, and increasing forces in the Sinai). After some hesitation following the mobilization of their forces, Israeli leaders finally initiated hostilities. Consistent with the strategy of the indirect approach and the principles of attacking first and transferring the war to enemy territory, the

IDF began operations with massive, devastating, and simultaneous predawn attacks against Egyptian airfields by aircraft sweeping in from several directions. Taken by surprise, the Egyptian air force was obliterated. As the air attacks were taking place, Israeli armored units launched a general offensive against Egyptian land forces. Shortly thereafter, Jordanian artillery opened up against Jerusalem, and ground units seized part of the city. The Israelis responded with a counterattack that hurled the Jordanians back and engaged them at several points along the front. Although the Syrians entered the war with air and artillery attacks, the Israelis adhered to the principle of dealing with the strongest opponent first by adopting a defensive posture against the Syrians until offensive operations were completed on the Egyptian and Jordanian fronts.

Within four days, a combination of direct and indirect attacks in the Sinai had routed Egyptian forces and enabled the IDF to achieve all of its objectives. Though the air force received much of the credit for the success of the Sinai battles, the speed and thoroughness of victory was also due to other factors, including the quality and leadership of Israeli commanders, swift maneuvers in the field, excellent intelligence, good communications, and impressive logistics support. By contrast, the Egyptian forces fared poorly in all these areas, thus undercutting otherwise courageous efforts in a number of specific situations.

Though the sea battles were of secondary importance, it should be noted that the outnumbered Israeli Navy took to the offensive early in the war; as a result of these naval operations, Egyptian missile boats and submarines were prevented from inflicting any appreciable damage.

Though intense, the battle for the West Bank and Jerusalem was over within fifty hours. Once again, the expeditious accomplishment of military objectives was due largely to the air-armor tandem.[35] Much the same was true on the Golan Heights, where the Israeli commander, Gen. David Elazar, relying on the strategy of the indirect approach, mobility, and envelopment, put Syrian forces to flight within two days.[36] The magnitude of the Israeli military victory was aptly summarized in *Paris Match*, 24 June 1967, by Gen. Andre Beaufre, one of France's leading strategic thinkers:

In these three campaigns the Israeli armed forces demonstrated their high quality from the uppermost to the most modest levels. Such a series of successes rules out the idea of an accidental stroke of good luck.

Sinai three days, Jordan two days, Syria two days—this decidedly is systematic lightning war.

The recipes used are all well known: Surprise, resolve and speed, air superiority, a large degree of decentralization of command, ardent troops unencumbered by the complex of rigid and inhibited actions that still prevail all too often in the European, and even the American armies, a simplified logistics system. The utmost of maneuver is thus made possible. . . .

All this was known. But perhaps never before has an execution been seen that was so close to perfection; nor has a victory that was more rapid and more complete.[37]

The Interplay of Offense and Defense: 1968–72. It is somewhat ironic that the same war that vindicated major elements of military doctrine also had the longer-term effect of undermining some of them. Although the offensive orientation that stressed speed, mobility, and the like proved its worth, the strategic depth provided by the newly occupied territories engendered some important defensive warfare inclinations. Nowhere was this more true than in the Sinai, where Israel established a quasi-static defense line along the Suez Canal (the Bar Lev Line), manned by small numbers of troops who were charged with holding the line during a conflict while the rest of the IDF gathered forces for a counterattack.[38] With the passage of time, the newly acquired defensive depth raised questions about the need for the kind of preemptive attack that was decisive in June 1967. As things turned out, Israeli military commanders remained committed to the notion of striking first, but found their arguments overruled by political leaders in the hours just before the 1973 war. Though international political considerations (i.e., fear of negative U.S. reaction) were cited as the overriding reason for not attacking first, it must be recognized that there was no anxiety that Israel faced an immediate nearby threat, as in 1967. The difference, of course, was the existence of the Sinai buffer zone.

The vulnerability of the Bar Lev Line had become apparent one year after the 1967 war, when Egypt began the so-called war of attrition, a combination of artillery attacks and commando raids along the canal designed to inflict substantial casualties on Israeli forces. The IDF's first reaction was to relieve pressure along the canal by carrying out deep commando raids against lightly defended targets inside Egypt. The military purpose of this offensive riposte was to demonstrate that Israel could dictate its own terms of fighting and compel Egypt to withdraw forces to the rear. When this brought a lull to the fighting, the IDF undertook a crash program to shore up the canal fortifications.

In June 1969 Nasser recommenced the war of attrition. Since intensified commando attacks failed to bring an end to the fighting, the Israelis resorted to air attacks, first along the canal and then deep inside Egypt. At this point, the Soviet Union came to Egypt's assistance by building a formidable air defense system in the areas of important targets and cities, and, in some cases, directing defensive operations and flying missions. As the Egyptian air defense network gradually moved toward the canal, the Israeli Air Force began heavy round-the-clock bombing of air defense installations. After gaining the upper hand, Israel reluctantly yielded to American pressure for a cease-fire in the summer of 1970.

Both the 1967 war and the war of attrition left their marks on military doctrine and force structure.[39] The air force emerged from the June conflict as the most important part of the IDF, a development that was underscored by its performance in the war of attrition. As a result, the air force inventory was improved both quantitatively and qualitatively through the acquisition of American aircraft (most notably F-4 Phantoms that had greater range, payloads, and versatility). Moreover, the air force devoted more attention to electronics and counterelectronic warfare following its confrontation with the air defense system installed by the Russians during the war of attrition. Efforts were also made to improve radar control systems through computerization and to upgrade reconnaissance capability. In addition, the fighting gave a major boost to domestic production. The Israeli aircraft industry produced several aircraft of its own, developed its own electronic equipment, and acquired the ability to repair and service all planes in the air force arsenal.[40]

While the 1967 war reinforced the centrality of the armored corps within the land forces, there was more (but insufficient, as it turned out) attention paid to integrating armor with mechanized infantry and artillery. Furthermore, the armored forces had to adjust to the new geostrategic situation by adopting a defensive posture along the Suez Canal. This did not mean that offensive operations were neglected. Indeed, considerable efforts were devoted to planning and training for armored operations across waterways.

As part of its preparation for the future, the armored corps was doubled in size. New tanks were acquired from abroad, and both old tanks and captured Russian tanks were converted and improved by adding new guns, engines, and range finders. All the guns and most of the ammunition were produced in Israel.

As far as the infantry was concerned, the 1967 war convinced the IDF of the need for a unified training system that would mitigate the distinction between elite and regular units. Accordingly, all combat personnel were trained for airborne, mechanized, and counterguerrilla operations.[41]

Although the June war did not alter the lower priority accorded to the navy, the naval force structure underwent a fundamental transformation. The post-June war sinking of the destroyer *Eilat* by Egyptian sea-to-sea missiles and the disappearance of a submarine en route to Israel intensified existing doubts about the utility of large warships in the region, while underscoring the wisdom of a previous decision to produce missile boats. As those boats became operational, they were fitted with Gabriel sea-to-sea missiles produced by the Israeli aircraft industry. Though small submarines were also given attention, the missile boat eventually became the backbone of the navy.[42]

One of the more notable developments after the 1967 war was the substantially greater part the domestic arms industry came to play in improving air, land, and sea forces. Despite the national strategic objective of self-reliance noted previously, Israel had made only modest progress prior to the war. Although Israel still continued to recognize the impossibility of producing all of its weapons and equipment, it nonetheless concluded that greater sacrifices could and should be made in order to decrease its dependence on outsiders, especially during emergencies, the major precipitant being the decision of its main supplier, France, to embargo Israel during and after the war. The outcome was an Israeli commitment to produce as many weapons as feasible, given cost calculations, and, with respect to essential weapons, to proceed even if the price were high. To offset the increased expenditures involved, sales to other countries were emphasized.[43]

The newly flourishing domestic arms industry, together with the qualitative and quantitative improvement of the force structure, the new geostrategic situation, and morale, leadership, and training problems in the Arab armies gave the IDF a clear margin of military superiority through the early 1970s. In fact, Israel's confidence that its military superiority would deter the Arabs from starting a major war was so high that intelligence indicators of impending hostilities in early October 1973 were dismissed. The prevailing assumption was that the Arabs would not go to war because they had no hope of winning. Since the Israelis further assumed that winning to the Arabs would mean the destruction of Israel, little or no attention was paid to the possibility that their adversaries might initiate major hostilities in order to achieve limited objectives.

The October 1973 War: Reappraisal and Rebuilding. It was evident that the Israelis had seriously miscalculated Arab intentions when the Egyptians and Syrians attacked on 6 October 1973. Though this is not the place for a detailed account of the October War, a summary of events is important because of the far-reaching effects the conflict had on Zahal.

Since the Egyptians and Syrians came to realize in their initial planning for the war that destruction of the IDF was impossible, they set tough, but limited, objectives for themselves. The preeminent political goal was to generate a new diplomatic process that would eventually lead to a return of the occupied territories. In order to bring the desired results, the Arabs believed that the passivity of the superpowers would have to be transformed into active pressure against Israel. In Sadat's view, the United States was the key because of the leverage it derived from Israeli dependence on American economic and military assistance.[44] If the United States were to use this leverage on behalf of the Arabs, its interests in the area had to be threatened. In more specific terms, the Arabs hoped to take advantage of both the increasing Western need for petroleum and fears of a superpower confrontation that could result from a gradual escalation of hostilities. Besides creating international pressure on Israel, the Arabs also intended to add internal pressures by inflicting heavy losses on the IDF.

Success on the battlefield was critical for the achievement of these political aims. It was also necessary for creating a psychological climate conducive to negotiations involving Israel. Before the war, such negotiations were inconceivable to the Arabs because of the belief that they would be tantamount to supplication. The only way Arab leaders thought this state of mind could be changed was to redeem their honor and dignity (a very important consideration in Arab culture) through a military success that would leave them in a position of perceived strength.[45] If everything went as planned, there would be another important benefit, namely, an enhancement of the legitimacy of the governments in Cairo and Damascus.

Thanks to an elaborate and brilliant deception plan, as well as a monumental Israeli intelligence failure, the Arabs achieved strategic surprise. During the early fighting, the Arabs were able to inflict costly defeats on the IDF and to achieve significant territorial gains. In the south, the Egyptians crossed the canal, destroyed the Bar Lev Line, and consolidated control of a narrow beachhead running the length of the canal, while in the north the Syrians drove through the Golan Heights. The reluctance of the Egyptians to send their forces beyond their air defense umbrella and into the

Sinai allowed Israel time to mobilize its reserves and concentrate on the perilous situation in the Golan, where the Syrian offensive had advanced within a few miles of northern Israel.[46] The Egyptian minister of defense rationalized his conservative approach with this explanation:

> In order to advance we had to wait for armor to enter the field, then for the mobile anti-aircraft missiles to enter the field, regardless of opportunities that others saw or I saw.
> If I had thrown in my forces after the [opportunities] experts are talking about without adequate defense against the enemy's air superiority, I would have been putting the whole burden on the air force, which would have exceeded its capacity.[47]

Following heavy fighting in the Golan Heights, Zahal went on the offensive and drove halfway to Damascus, a turn of events that brought frantic Syrian appeals to Egypt to relieve pressure by moving forces forward in the Sinai. By the time Egypt responded, Israel had already begun to redeploy units to the Sinai; shortly thereafter, both sides engaged in a massive armored confrontation. When this confrontation checked the Egyptians, the high command in Cairo decided to move additional forces across the canal, thus setting the stage for Israel's use of the strategy of the indirect approach.

Implementing a plan that had been conceived and tested in maneuvers after the 1967 war, the Israelis sent armored columns across the canal. Although the success of this bold stroke was very much in doubt during the early hours, because of stiff Egyptian resistance, the IDF finally secured the crossing point, moved forces across the canal, surrounded the rear of the Egyptian Third Army in the south, and posed a similar threat to the Second Army in the north. At this point, heavy pressure from the superpowers brought an end to the fighting, thus sparing the Egyptians a potentially disastrous defeat.

Despite the favorable military outcome, there was little rejoicing in Israel. The anxious moments and heavy casualties that the IDF experienced early in the war led to a wide-ranging reassessment of military matters that included a critical look at doctrine and force structure.

One of the first elements of doctrine scrutinized after the war was the principle of delivering the first blow. Though eminently successful in 1967, a first strike was eschewed in 1973 because of the aforementioned concerns about the American reaction and the defense in depth provided by the occupied territories. As one of Israel's leading generals put it:

After the Six-Day War, our defense concept changed. Thanks to the strategic depth we no longer clung to the principle of the "first blow," and we also believed that we had reached safe harbors and could allow ourselves to conduct a defensive war. All this was correct insofar as the question of our national existence was at stake, but it was wrong with regard to the possibility of Arab success in gaining limited military objectives. We certainly did not intend to allow the Egyptians and Syrians to conquer the Suez Canal or the Golan Heights from us by force of arms.[48]

Such views notwithstanding, there were reasons to doubt whether a preemptive attack would have been as decisive in 1973 as it was in 1967. To begin with, the Arabs had not only developed and implemented aircraft revetment and dispersal plans, but they had also constructed a massive air defense system against both high- and low-altitude attacks.[49] Furthermore, they were psychologically prepared for a possible Israeli air assault.

As things turned out, Israeli leaders were not convinced that war was imminent until early on the morning of 6 October. Although a decisive preemptive attack was questionable for the military reasons just noted, there was still the possibility of a damage-limiting or spoiling blow.[50] Because Prime Minister Golda Meir took the United States at its word that it would be hard pressed to support Israel if the IDF struck first, she turned aside a first-strike proposal by the chief of staff.[51] Since, in retrospect, many Israeli leaders concluded that not striking first had been a mistake, the principle of preemptive action was once more underscored, despite concerns about possible American opposition and the better preparedness of the Arab states.[52]

The doctrinal emphasis on offensive operations, transferring the battle to enemy territory as soon as possible, dealing with the most threatening enemy first, and following the indirect approach was reinforced by the 1973 war. Early reverses during the hostilities were attributed by many to the defense posture along the canal that enabled the Egyptians to dictate the terms of battle and seize the initiative. The fact that armored forces were dealt major setbacks when they moved against the Egyptians shortly after the fall of the Bar Lev Line did not diminish the preference for offensive operations; indeed, postwar analyses concluded that the failures were due to inadequate preparation, faulty coordination, and poor control and leadership by the southern command. After the containing of enemy advances in the Golan Heights and the Sinai, it was offensives—first into Syria (the most threatening front) and then across the canal into Egypt—that ultimately proved decisive, in that they transferred the initiative to the IDF and allowed it to dictate the terms of battle. As a consequence, the Israeli defense establishment renewed its commitment to offensive warfare. Illustrative of this situation was the serious consideration devoted to a range of offensive options for a future conflict that included the possibility of outflanking Syrian forces by means of invasion through either Jordan or Lebanon, even if these states were avoiding involvement. Other options raised by the IDF were air strikes against the supporting Arab states and amphibious operations against Egypt's long coastline.[53]

The reaffirmation of offensive warfare was also designed to support another element of strategic doctrine that deserves brief mention here—the stress on quick victory. As suggested above, the Israelis were denied a complete military victory on the Suez front because of Soviet and American political intervention (the very sort of thing Dayan had warned against when he was chief of staff). The length of the conflict had given both superpowers enough time to contemplate their responses and enabled them to avoid (though narrowly) a rapid Israeli *fait accompli*. Besides failing to attain a total victory over the Arab armies, the IDF also incurred heavier losses because of the prolonged fighting, a point that brings us to an evaluation of the effects of the war on the tactical aspects of Israeli military doctrine.

On the tactical level, Israeli military doctrine stressed a number of themes prior to the war: initiative and flexibility by local commanders (as long as they achieved assigned objectives), high-quality middle- and lower-echelon commanders, highly motivated personnel trained to use modern equipment, good maintenance, and minimization of casualties.[54] The war had important effects on all of these.

The Agranat Commission, a blue ribbon panel established to analyze all aspects of the war, concluded after an exhaustive inquiry that initiative and improvisation had played a key role in extricating Zahal from a very difficult situation.[55] Yet, at the same time, it reaffirmed the fact that commanders exhibiting flexibility and initiative cannot afford to do so at the expense of the objectives assigned to them, by pointedly noting that a major reason for failure in the Sinai early in the war had been an "erosive deviation" from the objectives the chief of staff had set.[56] On the Golan Heights, by contrast, the adroitness and flexibility of Israeli commanders during both the defensive and offensive phases of the fighting were key factors in battlefield success.[57]

The Golan fighting also demonstrated the importance of middle- and lower-echelon officers of high quality. As the Agranat Commission pointed out, the initiative and resourcefulness of junior and field-grade commanders, who were forced by circumstances into independent and isolated actions, influenced the outcome of the entire campaign.[58] For example, despite being outnumbered twelve to one, the armored corps achieved an impressive twelve-to-one kill ratio.[59] Active frontline leadership was not without costs, however, since 24 percent of those killed in action were officers, a 4 percent rise above 1967.[60]

While the performance of lower-ranking officers was no doubt reassuring to the IDF, the same could not be said of all the major commanders. One of the most significant opinions of the Agranat Commission was that the southern front commander, Maj. Gen. Shmuel Gonen, did not possess the qualities necessary for moving, deploying, reinforcing, and supporting forces in accordance with the strategic aims of a major command. Specifically, Gonen was charged with not preparing thoroughly for the early containment battle (there was no detailed operational plan); failing to ascertain whether his forces had arrived in full and were properly deployed; overlooking the need to review and approve the plans of his commanders; conducting the battle without effective command of his forces, with the consequence that he was not properly informed of developments; hastily moving forces without due regard for whether the objectives of higher command levels were achieved; changing the objectives of his Ugdot ("battle groups") without giving them information about Egyptian and Israeli forces; causing a general erosion of both the objectives and method imposed by the chief of staff; and being impatient to cross the canal before the essential conditions for such a move had been created.[61]

In explaining why it believed Gonen had failed, the commission argued that although he possessed courage and comprehensive professional knowledge and expertise in operations used by Zahal, Gonen was lacking the "special administrative command expertise and know-how . . . required to coordinate the forces of a regional and theater command at the right time and place."[62] What all this suggested, of course, was that the skill and achievements of forces on the tactical level could be undercut by poor leadership at the high command level. While the IDF has always been aware of this, the Agranat critique had the effect of increasing sensitivity to the need for assuring quality and proper preparation for high echelon command as well as for middle and lower levels. To assure that the process for appointing top commanders was as thorough as possible, a permanent committee of commanders was tasked with reviewing the credentials of candidates and advising the chief of staff.

The importance of well-trained and motivated personnel in relation to modern weapons systems and high standards of equipment maintenance was borne out in the October War. For example, the high operational readiness rate (over 90 percent) and the impressive turnaround time for aircraft, which were made possible by both superb maintenance and the renowned skills of the pilots, enabled the Israeli Air Force to average 2,000 sorties per day and to achieve an air-to-air kill ratio of sixty to one.[63] That the armored corps experienced similar success was no doubt due to a demanding training program.[64]

Despite the success of its training programs, the IDF could not rest on its laurels. The Agranat Commission expressed apprehension about a perceived diminution in regimen and discipline, which it felt had created some "grave difficulties."[65] To arrest this adverse trend, greater emphasis was placed on expanding and strengthening training programs.[66]

The final tactical principle of doctrine, the minimization of casualties, was the subject of national attention after the war. According to Trevor Dupuy, the Israelis lost an estimated 2,838 killed, 8,800 wounded and 508 missing in action during the fighting.[67] As bad as these figures appeared, they could have been worse were it not for several decisions made during the conflict. The objective of sparing lives, for instance, was one of the reasons for the adoption of a cautious campaign on the Golan Heights that was marked by the use of close air support and heavy artillery barrages before infantry and armored formations carefully moved through Syrian lines; it was also said to have been one of the factors dissuading the IDF from moving on to Damascus.[68]

The human cost in 1973, together with an estimate that another three-week war involving the use of improved technology might result in a staggering 8,000 casualties, heightened the IDF's concerns about battlefield losses. For the most part, resolution of this problem was viewed as a function of strategic doctrine and force structure. With regard to the former, the emphasis on swift, offensive warfare by concentrated and integrated forces was considered the best way to minimize loses; with respect to the latter, primary reliance on air and armor, supported by mobile artillery and infantry, as well as by the use of advanced weapons (especially precision-guided munitions), was believed conducive to fewer casualties. As one observer put it: "The obsession of Israel's military leaders since 1973, therefore, has been to restore the ability of their aircraft and tanks to operate freely on the battlefield, where those reservist infantry men must venture onto it, to give them the maximum possible chance to survive. More than before, this has meant a concentration on new kinds of weapons."[69]

The implementation of the recommendations of postwar analyses reconfirmed the salient features of military doctrine. Both short-term and, especially, long-term war plans reemphasized familiar principles of strategic doctrine (offensive orientation, surprise, striking first, fighting in enemy territory, quick victory, the indirect approach, and so forth) in addition to the tactical elements discussed above. At the same time, however, it is important to note that, as in 1973, IDF plans and deployment patterns did not rule out defensive operations, at least for a time. On the West Bank, for example, some of the settlements established since 1967 became part of a defensive network designed to impede an enemy thrust until the IDF was mobilized and moved into positions where it could conduct offensive operations if deemed necessary.[70] In the final analysis, the major changes that occurred after 1973 were in the area of force structure rather than doctrine. A major effort was undertaken to improve all facets of the IDF: support functions (intelligence, logistics, and maintenance), combat arms (both regular and reserve components), and weaponry.

The initial scheme for strengthening the IDF was set forth in a 1974 plan called Matmon B, which defined military requirements in such a way that Israel would have the capacity to conduct a rapid, intensive offensive against its neighbors before external powers could intervene.[71] It involved substantially higher manpower levels and "an enormous increase in weapons inventories, accompanied by qualitative improvements of a similar magnitude."[72] To accomplish its aims, the IDF not only stepped up the acquisition of sophisticated hardware abroad, but also encouraged domestic arms producers to expand and increase their output.[73]

In the land forces, the number of tanks rose by one thousand, mobile artillery pieces by several hundred, and armored personnel carriers by several thousand. In addition, antitank weapons were purchased in large quantities from the United States.[74]

The air force capability was also upgraded considerably by adding over two hundred combat aircraft, including American F-4Es, A-4Ns, F-15s, and F-16s. The F-15 was particularly noteworthy in that it generally was considered to be the best fighter aircraft in the world. To cope with the surface-to-air missiles that had caused serious problems in the war, a large number of precision-guided munitions, air-to-surface missiles, and electronic countermeasures were introduced. To extend the combat range of fighter-bombers, old Boeing KC-97 tankers were retired in favor of jet tankers modified from Boeing 707s by the Israeli aircraft industry.[75] Air defense was also improved considerably through the acquisition of improved Hawk surface-to-air missiles, Chaparral antiaircraft missiles, and antiaircraft guns on the E-2C airborne early warning aircraft.[76] Finally, as the well-publicized 1976 raid at Entebbe in Uganda showed, the air force had also developed the ability to control, move, and supply forces from Israel.

Although most of the effort to strengthen the IDF structure focused on the land and air forces, the navy was not neglected. For example, the number of missile boats was increased, Harpoon antiship missiles were ordered from the United States, and Israeli-built reconnaissance aircraft entered service.[77]

Force structure improvements were not limited to the addition of greater and more sophisticated equipment to the arsenals of the land, air, and sea components, since postwar assessments had identified several related issues that needed serious attention. These included requirements for sound intelligence, greater coordination of the combat arms, more efficient mobilization procedures, better maintenance, and improved discipline. After careful analysis, a series of corrective steps was taken with respect to each.

The intelligence issue was considered most critical because of breakdowns at the national and field levels. How an intelligence apparatus renowned for its dexterity could have blun-

dered so badly was a question addressed by the Agranat Commission. Not surprisingly, the answer was that interpretation, not collection, was to blame. Both structural and psychological shortcomings accounted for this.[78]

Intelligence had been structured in such a way that only one agency, Military Intelligence, with a staff that ironically was described as "refreshingly small" just prior to the war, was responsible for interpretation and analysis.[79] Within a unitary structure such as this, the estimates of the Military Intelligence Branch were dominant. As things turned out, the absence of contending views was nearly fatal. The Military Intelligence Branch misinterpreted various Arab moves in the days preceding the outbreak of hostilities. The prewar view of the head of the Military Intelligence Branch, Maj. Gen. Eliahu Zeira, was that a conventional attack was improbable because the Arabs had little chance of victory. As pointed out earlier, the problem with this was that victory had been defined as a successful invasion of Israel rather than just limited gains along the border.[80] Similar opinions were also expressed by other military leaders, such as the 1967 hero Maj. Gen. Ariel Sharon.[81] Judgments like these led both military and academic analysts to dismiss Arab warnings as nothing more than a penchant for rhetorical flourishes that masked a lack of capability.[82]

In light of the consequences and recommendations of the Agranat Commission, Israeli leaders were aware of the need to make improvements in the intelligence apparatus. In an effort to ensure that contending interpretations might be voiced, the capabilities of Mossad, the major external intelligence agency, and the Foreign Ministry were improved. Yet, while both reportedly had channels to the political echelon, the Military Intelligence Branch remained the agency responsible for providing a warning of war.[83] Public commentaries in Israel and periodic discussions with various Israeli military and civilian officials over the past several years have made it clear to this writer that significant doubts persist about whether the problem has been successfully addressed.[84] As far as field-level intelligence is concerned, numerous improvements were made in response to deficiencies identified by both the Agranat Commission and independent observers.

A second major problem, coordination of the combat arms, was manifest early in the war, when Egyptian infantry using antitank rockets played a major role in several Israeli defeats. In retrospect, the Israelis traced their difficulties to a failure to integrate infantry, armor, artillery, and air elements sufficiently on the battlefield. As a consequence, the IDF paid much greater attention than before to preparing its components for combined operations in a future war.[85]

During the war, the IDF also experienced difficulties in three related areas: mobilization, which Chaim Herzog characterized as "hastily improvised"; maintenance of equipment, which reservists complained was often shoddy; and lax discipline, which the Agranat Commission believed was partially responsible for equipment readiness problems, as well as other shortcomings.[86] In response to the first two criticisms, the IDF instituted a number of reforms (e.g., dry storage and better protected and decentralized vehicle and equipment depots located closer to the anticipated battle fronts) and carried out exercises that putatively enabled it consistently to achieve full mobilization in thirty-six hours. While improvements in the area of discipline were more problematic in view of the informality and egalitarian values of Israeli society, there was a discernible tightening up, particularly under Rafael Eitan, who became chief of staff in 1978. Nevertheless, doubts that the IDF had resolved all its difficulties were raised by a 1979 comptroller's report that identified continued deficiencies in the areas of maintenance, safety, discipline, and field intelligence.[87]

As the new decade of the 1980s began, there was a general consensus among analysts that force structure improvements and reforms had left the IDF stronger than ever. Though budgeting constraints stemming from national economic problems and the costs of redeploying from the Sinai to the Negev (as required by the Egyptian Treaty) were forcing cutbacks in a number of areas, there was confidence that the

IDF was able and ready to conduct operations in accordance with existing military doctrine.[88] That doctrine, fashioned in four wars, provided the IDF with what it considered to be a series of consistent and reliable guidelines for the conduct of large-scale warfare on the conventional level. How it was affected by the unusual circumstances of the 1982 war in Lebanon is the subject to which we now turn.

A "Unique" War: Lebanon, 1982. With their three-pronged attack in Lebanon on 6 June 1982, Israeli forces began a contentious war, the impact of which was felt more in the realms of national strategy and political decisionmaking than in doctrine and force structure. The major reason for this was the General Staff's conclusion that the war was *sui generis* because of its unique topographical and sociopolitical contexts. Of all the areas immediately adjacent to Israel, the area of southern Lebanon and northward toward Beirut was least conducive to the quick movement and maneuvering of armored and mechanized land forces because of its mountainous terrain and narrow, twisting roads. Moreover, it rendered such forces vulnerable to commando attacks and ambushes, especially by Syrian units using antitank weapons. While this situation caused many problems and resulted in more casualties than perhaps necessary, the overall military campaign was successful. By 11 June the Israeli Air Force had defeated the Syrian Air Force and the ground forces were consolidating positions south and west of Beirut and astride the Beirut-Damascus highway. Because of these achievements, few questions were raised with respect to doctrine and force structure. Instead, soul-searching was directed to larger questions: i.e., whether the political aims of the war were achievable through the use of military force; whether those aims were honestly articulated at the onset; and whether the moral, political, and human costs incurred during the siege of Beirut and the occupation of southern Lebanon were justified.

The acrimonious debate over national strategy and objectives in the war was not replicated when it came to doctrinal principles. Although Israel's preemptive move did not achieve strategic surprise, it did enable the IDF to transfer the battle immediately to enemy territory and to gain and retain the initiative. While it was obvious that the generally poor leadership and mediocre equipment of the Palestinians and Syria's reluctance to become involved in the fighting also played a key role in Israel's success, they did not detract from the value ascribed to preemption by the General Staff. Likewise, the larger doctrinal emphasis on offensive warfare and rapid victory was reinforced, not only by the predictable American diplomatic intervention, but also by the quagmire the IDF found itself in after reaching Beirut. In getting bogged down and entangled in the Lebanese hornet's nest of bitterly conflicting political and religious groups and by positioning troops in southern Lebanon, the IDF suffered significant casualties, added to the economic costs of the war, strained relations with American military forces that were on a peace-keeping mission, and eventually was forced to withdraw—all within a context marked by national divisiveness and serious morale problems in the ranks. Since the relatively static and defensive nature of the military occupation provided an unwelcome and costly contrast to the positive outcome of the decisive, quick offensive operations that marked the first week of the war, it could not but strengthen the commitment to the latter.

Two other principles of strategic doctrine came into play. The first, attacking the most threatening enemy initially, in this case the PLO forces in southern Lebanon, was successful and received support from the vast majority of Israelis. The second, adhering to an indirect approach where feasible, could also be seen, albeit not as dramatically as in previous wars. While the ground forces advancing northward generally followed a direct course, amphibious operations by the navy were carried out to the rear of PLO units that cut them off from their Beirut command centers, prevented reinforcement, and blocked their withdrawal. In the final analysis, then, the essential elements of strategic military doctrine remained intact. While much the same could be said of tactical doctrine, there was concern in some quarters about the execution of doctrine in the war.

Although definitive analyses resolving different points of view about the IDF's performance in the war have yet to appear, it was clear that emphasis was again placed on initiative, flexibility, and leadership by local commanders, with small-unit officers and noncommissioned officers representing over 60 percent of those killed in action. This notwithstanding, some analysts believed there had been leadership deficiencies at the command level and some erosion at the company and battalion levels. One source of the difficulties was said to be the frequent moving of forces from one command to another and commanders in and out of positions of command. Since these developments contradicted the normal Israeli commitment to unit and leadership integrity throughout a battle, they were criticized by IDF soldiers and officers alike.[89]

The situation regarding the motivation of the soldiers was even less clear in the Lebanon war. Although it was impressive during early battles, motivation began to wane after the first week of the war. At first, the deterioration was generally confined to the officer ranks, with some commanders questioning the political aims of the war. The well-publicized resignation of one of the IDF's best field commanders, Col. Eli Geva, was a case in point. Far more significant was the growing desire to avoid being stationed in Lebanon and the sometimes unprofessional performance in battles during the 1983–84 occupation phase. Once again, however, this situation was attributed to the unusual circumstances of the conflict, especially the lack of public consensus that inevitably infected the IDF, rather than to a diminished commitment to defend Israel against the armies of hostile neighbors. The lesson drawn from all of this was that a prolonged involvement in a hostile environment where the terrain favors the enemy and where Israeli objectives are unclear and controversial will have a negative impact on motivation.

There is no reason to believe that motivational problems adversely affected the technical skills of the IDF. The air force, in particular, was most impressive, as the execution of a sophisticated battle plan involving electronic warfare skills, precision-guided munitions, remotely piloted reconnaissance vehicles, and modern attack aircraft crippled the Syrian air force without the loss of any manned Israeli aircraft. Maintenance of equipment, and particularly logistics support, also received generally high marks.

As in all Israeli wars, the tactical principle of minimizing casualties was very much in evidence, as was clear from decisions to rely on air and artillery bombardments, particularly when advancing on the eastern axis, and the reluctance to deploy ground forces inside heavily populated areas of Beirut. The relatively high casualties that were nonetheless suffered were a product of strategic policy decisions to engage the Syrians, who caused close to 70 percent of the casualties, and to the occupation of southern Lebanon until 1985.[90]

The war in Lebanon did not have a major impact on the IDF's force structure. The major problem was the absence of sufficient leg infantry to secure and facilitate the movement of armored and mechanized units in the difficult terrain of southern Lebanon and the Bekaa valley. Recognition of this problem by the IDF did not alter force-structure thinking in any basic way because of its belief that the important battlefields of any future conflict are likely to be along Israel's other borders, where the terrain is conducive to the use of airpower, armored forces, mechanized infantry, and mobile artillery.

COUNTERINSURGENCY

From its very beginning, Israel has had to cope with terrorist and guerrilla attacks from adjacent Arab states. Since the fedayeen organizations were controlled and supported by the Arab governments, the Israelis established a policy of holding the Arab governments responsible and carried out small-scale reprisals against targets in the Arab states. By the mid 1950s the reprisal actions had taken the form of large-scale operations against military objectives. The purpose was to demonstrate the weakness of the Arab armies and to increase the costs of supporting the insurgents to the point where the Arab regimes would discontinue their support.[91] Although this policy did bring periodic lulls, it did not end fedayeen

raids. The longest period of calm came after the 1956 war. Raids began again in 1966 and played a role in triggering the series of events that culminated in the 1967 war.

After the Arab defeat in 1967, the insurgent threat took on a new, more serious, dimension. Although still receiving assistance from various Arab states, several Palestinian organizations acquired an independent political status. Consequently, the Palestinian resistance became an amalgam of groups under the umbrella of the Palestine Liberation Organization. Some were autonomous (e.g., Al-Fatah, the Popular Front for the Liberation of Palestine, and the Democratic Popular Front for the Liberation of Palestine) and others were controlled by Arab governments (e.g., Sa'iqa by Syria and the Arab Liberation Front by Iraq). Although these organizations differed in terms of ideology, strategy, and tactics and were constantly engaged in internecine power struggles, they shared the common goal of destroying the Israeli state. They also agreed that the only way this aim could be accomplished was by means of a protracted people's war that stressed familiar insurgent techniques (i.e., political organization, terrorism, and guerrilla warfare). Thus, between 1967 and 1970 Israel was faced with guerrilla raids from across the border (especially Jordan), and terrorism and political organization efforts inside the occupied areas (and sometimes within Israel itself). From 1971 until the late summer of 1973, the guerrilla threat receded, but internal terrorism continued. Moreover, a new dimension, terrorist attacks outside the Middle East (transnational terrorism), was added. With a few exceptions, the period after the 1973 war through 1986 was largely one of internal terrorism conducted by groups either inside the occupied territories or infiltrating from Lebanon.

The Israeli policy for coping with this expanded insurgency in the late 1960s and early 1970s was a multifaceted one that went beyond reliance on Zahal. To preclude the insurgents from establishing a wide base of popular support among the Arabs, a series of political and economic steps were taken to restore and improve normal life patterns. The administrative policy of the military government stressed non-interference, a minimal Israeli presence, and freedom of movement in the occupied areas. Economic policy, meanwhile, was designed to improve the standard of living in the occupied areas in order to give the inhabitants a stake in stability.

To deal with guerrilla raids and terrorism, several coercive measures were adopted. The guerrilla threat was handled mainly by the IDF. Besides retaliatory attacks inside Arab states that harbored guerrillas, IDF counter-guerrilla actions included the building of security barriers along the borders, sabotage of economic targets (e.g., the east Ghor Canal in Jordan), interception of seaborne insurgents by the Israeli Navy, and, most important, extensive patrolling by small units along the borders.

The internal terrorist threat was reduced significantly by a skillful blend of carrot-and-stick techniques. Active popular support for the fedayeen was largely neutralized by the aforementioned administrative and economic policies, while terrorists were apprehended by the police and the intelligence apparatus. To put teeth in the antiterrorist program, a number of sanctions were used: curfews, cordon and search operations, detention without trial, deportation, and the destruction of the homes of terrorists and suspected supporters. The military courts imposed long prison sentences on those found guilty of terrorist acts, membership in illegal organizations, possessing unauthorized weapons, and the like.

The response to the problem of transnational terrorism involved both the IDF and intelligence agencies. Since terrorist attacks abroad were frequently planned in Lebanon, the IDF conducted various kinds of punitive attacks against Lebanon, and in 1976 it demonstrated a willingness to respond outside the Middle East with the surprise rescue operation inside Uganda. By and large, however, operations against the terrorists outside the region were carried out by Mossad. Such operations included assassination of Palestinian terrorists and the mailing of letter bombs.

By the mid 1970s, the main elements in Is-raeli counterinsurgency doctrine had become clear. It combined political, economic, and military measures, and different threats were handled with different responses by appropriate arms of the government. In many cases, the actions of Zahal were in line with the offensive orientation that marked its conventional warfare doctrine and operations. The IDF consistently, though not always successfully, sought to deliver hard blows to the fedayeen with search-and-destroy operations and air attacks and to achieve surprise with unanticipated raids (e.g., a heliborne attack against the Beirut airport in 1968 and the 1976 Entebbe operation). The proclivity for the offensive was exemplified by a 1979–80 campaign of continuous air, ground, and naval attacks against Palestinian bases in Lebanon, the previously discussed Operation Peace for Galilee in 1982, and the raid against PLO facilities in Tunisia in October 1984. Although not devoid of problems stemming from occasionally counterproductive policies, such as air and artillery attacks that killed and wounded innocent civilians in refugee camps in Lebanon, the Israeli counterinsurgency campaign was, on balance, successful in reducing violence to manageable levels in the occupied territories and along the borders. Such success was, of course, facilitated by the disunity and organizational ineptitude of the Palestinians and a physical environment that was unfavorable for protracted guerrilla warfare—i.e., a small, open area with a good road and communications systems. With its "armed struggle" contained, pragmatic elements of the PLO redefined their aim in 1974 as a small Palestinian state made up of the West Bank and the Gaza Strip. This move away from the goal of a "secular, democratic" state (i.e., an Arab state) in all of Palestine gave rise to both political and violent strife within the PLO.[92] Its accomplishments notwithstanding, the counterinsurgency campaign could not resolve the problem once and for all, since that required political decisions at the highest level to cope somehow with the intensification of Palestinian nationalism and the increased identification with the PLO that had become apparent in the West Bank and

Gaza Strip by 1979 and continued through the 1980s despite PLO Chairman Yasir Arafat's military defeats, political vacillation, and serious disagreements with Arab governments and rivals in the resistance.

Israel's success in counterinsurgency against the PLO was not matched during the IDF's 1983–84 occupation of Lebanon for several reasons. First of all, the Shiite population, which initially welcomed the Israeli invasion because it drove the PLO out of the south, turned actively against the IDF; second, the IDF's military operations, especially bombardments that killed civilians, intensified the hostility of the Shiites; third, the insurgents received ample moral, political, and material support from Syria and Iran; fourth, of all the areas surrounding Israel, only southern Lebanon provided the kind of terrain favorable to guerrilla warfare; and, fifth the IDF's morale gradually degenerated due to sharp discord at home, increasing recognition that withdrawal was inevitable, and the continued casualties inflicted by guerrillas, some of whom were willing to sacrifice their lives out of religious convictions (others, as it turned out, were coerced by Shiite extremists to go on suicide missions). When all was said and done, the fundamental reason why the Israelis were unable to deal with the insurrection in south Lebanon in the same way they were able to cope with the PLO was that most Israelis believed the Palestinians posed a mortal threat to Israel's existence whereas the Shiites did not. Hence, the public willingness to accept whatever costs were necessary in the PLO case was absent in the Lebanese situation.[93]

NUCLEAR POLICY

While the understanding of Israel's military doctrine and force structure on the conventional and insurgent levels of conflict is enhanced by substantial data and public commentaries by present and former leaders of the security establishment, the general public knows relatively little about nuclear weapons. Even less is known about nuclear war-fighting doctrines, plans, and concepts, given the dearth of verified empirical evidence on the subject. Beyond Israel's stated policy that it

will not be the first party to introduce nuclear weapons into the Middle East, a veil of secrecy and sensitivity has descended. As a result, analyses of the Israeli nuclear weapons questions have been highly conjectural and sometimes contradictory. Disagreement obtains on whether Israel has, or is close to achieving, a nuclear capability, as well as on the political, psychological, and military aims that nuclear weapons might feasibly serve. Although one expert, Alan Dowty, has cast doubts on the existence of nuclear weapons in Israel by pointing out that officially there are no indications that Israel has acquired the ability to separate plutonium from other by-products necessary for the manufacture of nuclear weapons, others (reportedly including the CIA) estimate that the IDF could assemble and deliver between ten and twenty bombs.[94] The seriousness of this possibility has engendered considerable debate and discussion of the possible objectives that such a capability might achieve. In general, the most prevalent thinking is that if Israel does possess nuclear bombs, they are probably weapons of last resort that would be employed to prevent the destruction of Israel if that seemed imminent.[95]

Initially, Israel might state publicly that it has, and is prepared to use, nuclear weapons to defend itself, the aim being to deter an invasion by Arab states by threatening them with devastating losses. Such a pronouncement could also be used to exert pressure on friendly states, such as the United States, to assist Israel without delay, lest the nuclear genie be let out of the bottle. If such moves aimed at deterring a perceived genocidal invasion failed, nuclear weapons might be used to inflict massive losses on any aggressor poised to overrun Israel, a possibility that has been linked to the commitment never again to permit the killing of innocent Jews such as occurred in the Holocaust.[96]

Israelis are well aware that, given the small size of the area, the use of nuclear weapons against invading forces could mean significant collateral damage for Israel. Moreover, if the Arab states acquired a nuclear capability, Israel could quite literally be destroyed. As both a former defense minister and chief of plans of the IDF told this writer, the enemy would only need four or five bombs. It is this ominous reality that may explain Israel's secrecy about nuclear weapons at present, for to acknowledge it possesses them might add new pressures on Arab governments somehow to acquire them. It most surely explains the kind of preemptive attack that the Israeli Air Force made against the Iraqi nuclear reactor at Osiraq on 7 June 1981.

The assumptions that Israel has nuclear weapons and that they are to be used only in response to the most extreme peril leads to the conclusion that the political and military utility of nuclear weapons is severely restricted.[97] The possibility of employing such weapons in a tactical, limited manner on the battlefield (similar to NATO's plans) seems to be negligible in view of the problem of collateral damage in such a small area and persistent efforts to strengthen conventional forces. Yet, how long this situation will continue is a matter for speculation, especially since no less a personage than Dayan questioned whether Israel could continue over the longer term to match an Arab military buildup fueled by petrodollars. If it could not, Dayan suggested that an open reliance on nuclear deterrence might be necessary.[98] Needless to say, should this ever occur, Israel's military doctrine and force structure could be profoundly affected.

The Defense Decision-Making Process

Up to this point, the discussion of Israeli defense policy has focused on the substantive dimensions of defense policy, i.e., national strategy, military doctrine, and force structure. How major decisions have been made with respect to these is a question of institutional setting and process.

THE MAIN ACTORS

The locus of defense decision-making power in Israel has always been the prime minister and cabinet. Within the cabinet, the Ministries of Foreign Affairs and Defense traditionally have exercised the greatest influence; of the two, the Ministry of Defense clearly has been the most important. In fact, for eighteen of Israel's first twenty years, the prime minister served as his own defense minister. Although lacking a legal basis for the making of security policy, Ben-Gurion established a tradition that the minister of defense would deal with grand strategy and security, while the IDF would concentrate on operational matters and execute policy. However, the lines between the two were never clearly delineated, a point criticized by the Agranat Commission in 1975.[99]

In an effort to resolve this problem, a basic law was passed in 1976 that formally vested command in the government and made the minister of defense the highest authority over the IDF and its link to the cabinet. The chief of staff was made responsible to the minister of defense for all Zahal matters. Although in general the defense ministry was to be in charge of technical and administrative matters (military research and development, production or procurement of matériel, and financial planning and budgeting) and the IDF General Staff was to retain responsibility for organization, training, and the planning and execution of military operations, the minister of defense could intervene in all IDF matters by virtue of his role as supreme commander of the IDF.[100] As things turned out, however, the basic law did not eliminate all of the ambiguity related to the powers of the minister of defense.

As far as the main features of the organizational structure of Zahal are concerned, it is composed of a General Staff whose permanent members are the heads of five branches (operations, manpower, quartermaster, planning, and intelligence); the commanders of the ground forces, navy, and air force; and the three area commanders of the ground forces (i.e., north, south, and central commands). The General Staff has control over all IDF branches. Although not separate services, the navy and the air force enjoy a fair degree of autonomy. The General Staff also exercises authority over more than twenty functional commands such as artillery, armor, and training.

The three ground force area commanders have been assisted by a deputy and staff officers for supply, training, manpower, and operations. Area commanders have responsibility for area defense and all ground force installations and combat units in their sectors.[101]

While the prime minister, cabinet, ministry of defense, and IDF have been the most important institutions in the defense decision-making process, other actors have exercised intermittent influence from time to time. Among these have been the Knesset committee on foreign affairs and security, party leadership echelons, and the media.

INSTITUTIONAL INTERPLAY

Major defense policy decisions in Israel are the result of a complex interaction of the actors noted in the preceding section, and the influence of particular institutions in the process has varied over the years. Although precise calculations of relative power and influence are elusive, because of the intermeshing of actors (e.g., party leaders, cabinet officials, and prime minister) and the secrecy that has surrounded defense policy making, several scholars have provided valuable insights and propositions about the decision-making process.

Aaron Klieman, for instance, points out that Israeli policy has been made in a setting where interpersonal relations at the highest level have been more important than bureaucratic considerations.[102] Although the prime minister has always been the pivotal figure in important defense decisions, in view of the authority vested in the office, some prime ministers have been particularly dominant. The most striking example, of course, was the charismatic Ben-Gurion, whose constant preoccupation with security matters motivated him to act as his own minister of defense. While his forceful personality has frequently been cited as the principal factor in his accomplishments, especially the difficult task of unifying the various Jewish military forces after the War of Independence, Ben-Gurion's control of the Ministry of Defense put powerful institutional resources at his disposal, not the least of which were the ministry's wide-ranging contacts with all the key elements of the government bureaucracy.[103] Although the Foreign Ministry's impact on foreign policy issues vacillated over the

years, in the specific area of defense policy it had minimal influence, since Ben-Gurion viewed it primarily as an implementing agency. Moreover, Ben-Gurion sought little advice.[104] In cases where he did, it usually was provided by a small inner circle referred to as a "kitchen cabinet," a few senior officials from the Ministry of Defense, the chief of staff, the director of the Military Intelligence Branch, a few other officers, and the head of the Security Service.[105]

When Ben-Gurion first retired and Moshe Sharett became prime minister in 1954, the cabinet emerged as a key decision-making organ in defense matters. Even though Ben-Gurion returned as prime minister a year later, it was not until Sharett departed the government in 1956 that Ben-Gurion's influence and modus operandi again became dominant. In 1959 Ben-Gurion's reassertion of power in the security sphere was increasingly criticized as "authoritarianism." On 31 January 1961 Ben-Gurion resigned, precipitating a cabinet crisis that lasted several months.[106]

During the crisis, the smaller parties that the Labor Party needed to form a coalition government pressed hard for institutional controls over security policy and for Labor's relinquishment of its monopoly over the major finance, foreign affairs, and defense portfolios. In November 1961, this crisis was resolved through the creation of a ministerial committee on defense; however, since Ben-Gurion resisted interference in the security area, the new committee had little real impact.[107]

The succession of Ben-Gurion by Eshkol in 1963 eventually changed this situation. Membership in the ministerial committee on defense was increased, and the committee became a powerful organ in defense decision making (Eshkol viewed it as being similar to a "war cabinet"). It retained this status until the early spring of 1967, when the entire cabinet again became the main decision-making forum. While other institutions such as the Knesset committee on foreign affairs and security and Zahal exerted pressures on the top leadership through 1967, the cabinet was, in Michael Brecher's words, "the ultimate arena for strategic-level decision-making in policy issues involving party, personal, and institutional conflicts."[108]

Despite the lack of a systematic treatment of defense decision making in Israel in recent years similar in scope to Brecher's impressive work on the earlier period, press reports and academic commentaries on the subject suggest that the dominant role of the prime minister and cabinet has diminished little, even though the 1973 war and the resignation of Golda Meir's government had the effect of subjecting defense policy and the IDF to more public scrutiny and criticism.[109]

The advent of a right-wing government in 1977 did nothing to offset this trend. In fact, its success in negotiating the peace with Egypt seemed to strengthen the hand of the prime minister and cabinet to the point where they continued to implement controversial settlement policies on the West Bank, frequently citing security imperatives, and to set in motion plans for attacking the PLO in Lebanon. The purposefulness, confidence, and capability of the government were especially noteworthy because of the sharp and reasonably extensive criticism emanating from the media and intellectual circles, which centrist and leftist opponents tended to dominate.

The decision making surrounding the war in Lebanon left no doubt about the locus of power. Accounts of critics and supporters alike make it clear that the cabinet, and most especially the defense minister, played a key role. What they disagree on is whether the defense minister misled the cabinet.[110] Despite the acrimonious controversy and political turbulence following the war (i.e., the prime minister's resignation, new elections, and the creation of a national unity coalition), there is no evidence, as of this writing, that the cabinet has yielded control over defense decision making.

Increased outside pressures notwithstanding, it is safe to say that the prime minister, as in the past, remains the final arbiter on major defense policy matters. As far as the interest groups that have influenced security policy deliberations and outcomes are concerned, available studies suggest that the Defense Ministry and the IDF have been the most important over the years. However, the reader should be cautioned that the paucity of detailed data on interest articulation by the IDF has made propositions regarding the relative influence of the Defense Ministry and the IDF necessarily tentative. Furthermore, much of the evidence that does exist must be gleaned from studies of other facets of defense policy, especially those dealing with civil-military relations.

In general, most writers contend that the IDF has wielded considerable influence owing to the high priority attributed to defense matters and the access to the political leadership enjoyed by the chiefs of staff.[111] During the Ben-Gurion years, the IDF seemed to have had more prestige and influence than the civilian component of the Defense Ministry, largely because the prime minister forged a special and close relationship with the chief of staff and the high command.[112] Although Ben-Gurion did not rely on the chief of staff for his principal military advice and the chiefs of staff rarely participated in cabinet meetings, the high command did influence strategy from 1948 to 1955. Such influence no doubt stemmed from the fact that the prime minister selected chiefs of staff who shared his basic views, including the belief that the Arabs were intent on encircling and destroying Israel. Ben-Gurion's confidence in the IDF permitted him to avoid involvement in day-to-day operational matters, a situation that had very important consequences for strategy. As Amos Perlmutter has noted: "Zahal was assigned operational responsibility for many crucial defense policies and, therefore, in its successful pursuit of these operational goals, Zahal's strategy could determine to a large extent the course of Israel's foreign relations. Zahal became identified with national security; and national security became identified with Arab encirclement."[113]

Not all IDF and Ministry of Defense perceptions and policies went unchallenged, however. Between 1953 and 1955, the IDF's hard line toward the Arabs was opposed by Prime Minister Sharett and part of the cabinet. Coincidental with this discord over basic policy orientations there was a struggle between the defense minister, Pinhas Lavon, and the IDF, caused by Lavon's attempt to assert control over operational matters. In the end, Lavon's efforts to reform IDF-Defense Ministry relations came to nothing, in part because he managed to alienate not only the foreign policy moderates but his erstwhile IDF allies as well. In fact, Lavon's IDF opponents went so far as to present false testimony against him before an ad hoc committee investigating a series of espionage failures that had led to the demise of a major Israeli spy ring in Egypt.[114] It is interesting to note that one of the reasons for the IDF's opposition to civilian involvement in operational matters was said to have been its fear that such intrusion would have undercut the doctrinal emphasis on quick and decisive offensive operations.[115]

The return of Ben-Gurion to power in 1955 strengthened the hand of the hard-liners, who immediately began preparations to deal with what was perceived to be an increasing threat from Soviet-armed Egyptian military forces. The prestige of Zahal and Ben-Gurion's allies was enhanced even further by the military success of the Sinai campaign. Parenthetically, it should be noted that one important trend during this time was a tremendous growth in the Defense Ministry's power, due to its deep involvement in the country's scientific, technological, and industrial affairs.

In 1960–61 the politics of defense in Israel were subjected to heavy criticism when Lavon attempted to exonerate himself of any wrongdoing during his previous tenure as defense minister. Although Ben-Gurion weathered a rather heavy political storm, the so-called Lavon affair nonetheless set in motion a public examination of the centralizing tendency evident in the political and economic systems of Israel. This examination continued into the Eshkol administration.

The Eshkol years were marked by acrimonious relations between the prime minister on the one hand and Ben-Gurion and his allies on the other (even though Ben-Gurion had nominated Eshkol as his successor). While the politicians were immersed in various disputes, the IDF's power and influence gradually increased. Efforts by the deputy defense minis-

ter, Zevi Dienstein, to transfer several tasks (e.g., armaments, recruitment, and supply) to the IDF were successfully obstructed by the high command, which feared that accepting responsibility for support functions would adversely affect operational capabilities. More importantly, according to Perlmutter, the chief of staff, Yitzhak Rabin, emerged as the de facto minister of defense. Since Eshkol, who held the defense portfolio, had little experience in military matters, he deferred to Rabin in the formulation of military strategy and, unlike his predecessors, acceded to IDF requests for larger military budgets.

The influence of the IDF during the Eshkol years was obvious during the 1967 crisis. Once Nasser announced the closure of the Strait of Tiran and increased his forces in the Sinai, the IDF moved ahead with military planning, mobilized reserve components, and argued for a preemptive war against Egypt. Following Eshkol's unsuccessful two-week pursuit of a diplomatic solution, heavy public pressure led him, however reluctantly, to appoint Dayan as minister of defense. Since Dayan's views coincided with those of Zahal, the pressure on Eshkol mounted, and he finally reached a decision to go to war. While the principle of civilian supremacy had been upheld, there was no denying that IDF actions and advice had played an influential part in the decision-making process.[116]

Not surprisingly, the overwhelming victory of 1967 added once more to the prestige and influence of the defense establishment, especially the IDF. Yet, while experts agreed that Zahal wielded significant influence, they offered contradictory explanations for such influence. Perlmutter argued that Dayan's continuation as defense minister after the war ushered in a period of notably close relations between the civilians in the ministry and the IDF, mainly because Dayan was an assertive administrator, an acknowledged expert in military affairs, and an inspirational leader. The input of chiefs of staff Bar Lev and David Elazar (1971–74) and other high-ranking officers, many of whom were former colleagues or disciples of Dayan's, was said to have been considerable. In contrast to Perlmutter, Jon Kimche contends that the IDF's influence was due to Dayan's exclusion from matters relating to both national (grand) and military strategy.[117] Yet, although they disagree on the matter of the defense minister's actual influence, both Perlmutter and Kimche conclude that the General Staff became the focal point for military advice to the political leadership following the 1967 war.[118] This state of affairs and its policy consequences were a major theme in a careful examination by Avi Shlaim and Raymond Tanter of the defense policy arena during the 1969–70 war of attrition.

After noting that the balance between civilian politicians and the General Staff shifted noticeably toward the latter following the 1967 war, Shlaim and Tanter investigated the decision to bomb Egypt (in reaction to Nasser's war of attrition in 1969) with respect to the participants in the process and the objectives they wished to achieve. One of the conclusions reached by the authors was that the military had preponderant influence in the making of policy. The General Staff acted as the cabinet's principal source of information and advice and, according to Shlaim and Tanter, this predisposed the cabinet to agree to the military's proposal—the only option presented, as it turned out—to carry out deep-penetration bombing of Egypt as a means of ending Egyptian violence. Although the military aspects of the bombing option had been carefully analyzed by the IDF, such was not the case with regard to the political ramifications. The political and psychological aims were never articulated in an exact manner and did not command a consensus. Likewise, the reactions of the Egyptians and, especially, the Russians were badly miscalculated.[119] Since the Foreign Ministry was almost completely excluded from the decision-making process, both orderly and careful staff work on the costs, risks, and benefits of various options, as well as a regular flow of verified information, were denied the cabinet. Under such conditions, cabinet members putatively relied on their general knowledge, informal conversations, and data gleaned from newspapers in forming their opinions. This led to a situation where short-term military realities shaped Israeli responses, with little or no

attention paid to long-term implications. As Shlaim and Tanter put it: "There was a tendency to act on a day-to-day basis, guided solely by the dictates of military requirements."[120] That the IDF had exercised dominant influence was beyond doubt. That such dominant influence was conducive to formulating security policies that effectively integrated political and military considerations was not.

Although the extent to which these conditions continued after the war of attrition is difficult to determine, the preeminent role of Military Intelligence in the days prior to the October War would seem to suggest that little change had occurred. At the same time, however, Prime Minister Golda Meir's refusal to accede to the chief of staff's preemptive strike option on the eve of the war demonstrated that IDF influence was not always translated into policy.

While it might have been expected that the problems experienced by the IDF in 1973 would have diminished its influence, such was not the case. Indeed, the demise of Dayan and the weaknesses of, and rivalries among, the new leaders—Prime Minister Rabin, Defense Minister Shimon Peres, and Foreign Minister Yigal Allon—enabled the new chief of staff, Mordechai Gur, to exercise greater influence. Indicative of this was his inclusion in the government's delegation for negotiations with the Arabs. In fact, Gur's assumption of political responsibilities and contribution to national security policies rivaled that of Dayan between 1954 and 1957. Moreover, in his role as military advisor, Gur apparently enjoyed a status similar to, if not greater than, that of Rabin under the Eshkol government.[121]

Gur's successor as chief of staff, Rafael Eitan, perpetuated the IDF's strong influence. Widely respected as a combat soldier, Eitan's generally hard line views about the Arabs and support for retention of the West Bank were compatible with those of Prime Minister Begin. Although such views were sometimes at odds with the perspectives of the defense minister, Ezer Weizman, Eitan's leadership qualities and accomplishments as a combat commander had led Weizman to propose him as chief of staff. Although Eitan tended to focus on operational matters until Weizman resigned in May 1980, his fervent support of expanded settlements in the West Bank and his willingness to justify them on security grounds made the IDF a visible participant on the political level.

While Eitan's role was supportive of policy already determined by the prime minister, it entangled the IDF in legal proceedings and made it an object of criticism in national debates. Weizman, in the meantime, played an active role in talks with Egypt, owing to his strong personal rapport with Sadat. Within the military establishment, he was attentive to general strategic issues, managerial concerns and, especially, the future of the Israeli Air Force. The limitations of his influence, nonetheless, were clear. His inability to persuade the prime minister to adopt more flexible policies vis-a-vis the Arabs and to prevent budget cuts in the IDF reinforced Begin's image as a strong-willed leader who acted decisively on high-level security issues.

The eventual appointment of Ariel Sharon as defense minister dramatically increased the influence of the ministry because his views on relations with the Arabs and the disposition of the occupied territories coincided with Begin's, and he pursued their implementation vigorously. Moreover, Begin's respect for Sharon's military expertise made him less inclined to question Sharon's judgments, particularly in the crucial cabinet meetings preceding and during the war in Lebanon. Whereas various assessments of these deliberations may disagree over the intentions, veracity, and honesty of Sharon, they do not dispute the decisive influence he exerted.

With the replacement of Sharon by Moshe Arens, a civilian politician and technocrat, and of Eitan by the more low-keyed Moshe Levy, the influence of the defense ministry and relations between the ministry and the IDF seemed to revert to previous patterns. There was little apparent change during the first two years of the national unity coalition (1984–86). Although former Chief of Staff and Prime Minister Rabin held the defense portfolio and proved to be an active spokesman on defense

issues, he acted within the Labor Party consensus and the coalition agreement. Morever, even if he had wished to pursue an independent agenda (and there is no evidence he did), he would no doubt have been checkmated by his old rival, Prime Minister Peres.

Several general conclusions emerge from this brief overview of the formulation of national security and defense policy in Israel over the years. First, although many actors have played roles from time to time, the prime minister, cabinet, ministry of defense, and IDF have been the most important. Second, while the IDF has concentrated on operational matters, several chiefs of staff have made strong inputs on the national strategic level. Third, the relative impact of defense ministers and chiefs of staff has been determined largely by interpersonal relations at the highest levels. Fourth, the IDF's important role in the policy process is rooted in the centrality of security in the context of national strategy, the continuous hostility of many Arab states, the constant emphasis on military strength, and the omnipresent fear that a major miscalculation could lead to another catastrophe for the Jewish people.

Recurring Issues and Defense Policy Outputs

THE USE OF FORCE

In the years following Israel's fortieth anniversary, there is no reason to believe that security considerations will be any less important than in the past. Although the normalization of relations with Egypt has raised hopes that the Arab-Israeli dispute will be resolved one day, such an accomplishment is a long way off, inasmuch as many Arabs have yet to reconcile themselves to the notion of a Jewish state in the region. Libya and Iraq still call for the displacement of the so-called "Zionist regime," as does the Iranian government under the ayatollahs. While other Middle Eastern states such as Syria, Lebanon, Jordan, and Saudi Arabia may be inclined to accept Israel at some time in the future, such acceptance is contingent minimally on a satisfactory resolution of the Palestinian, Jerusalem, and Golan Heights problems. Unfortunately, only an inveterate optimist could envisage a speedy and comprehensive resolution of these matters, in view of the profoundly divergent positions of the Arabs and Israelis with respect to each.

Leaving ideological commitments to the concept of Eretz Israel aside, security considerations strongly militate against major concessions by Israeli leaders, especially on the West Bank and Golan Heights questions. (Again, the term *Eretz Israel* refers to the idea of a "greater Israel" that would include such territories as Judea and Samaria on the West Bank as well as other areas that were part of biblical Israel.) From the perspective of Israel's defense establishment, a comprehensive withdrawal in the context of belligerent relations with many of its neighbors would be highly imprudent. This creates a dilemma, for as long as the IDF remains in the occupied territories, those Arab governments that seem disposed to reach an accommodation with Israel are unlikely to undertake dramatic diplomatic initiatives involving major concessions. A major reason for this reluctance is, and no doubt will continue to be, the domestic uncertainty that prevails in the Arab world. The combination of socioeconomic underdevelopment, corruption, inefficient administration, and psychocultural disruption that has marked the modernization process in the Middle East has either undermined or threatens to undermine the legitimacy of most Arab governments. The resurgence of Islam in the late 1970s and in the 1980s has been the most notable symptom of this state of affairs. Faced with a recrudescence of Moslem fundamentalism, plus anti-Westernism, sporadic political violence, and endemic domestic divisiveness, there is a high probability that most Arab leaders will continue to perceive substantive concessions to Israel as an invitation to even more internal and external turbulence, which may well lead to their own demise.

The implication of this predicament for the Israeli leadership is painfully obvious. Simply stated, as long as the hostile impasse with the Arabs remains, there can be no diminution of the priority ascribed to security and, as long as violence and bellicosity continue, military force will remain an instrument of statecraft that is used variously to deter, punish, and, if need be, debilitate adversaries whose military strength poses a threat to Israeli military superiority. With respect to the last point, it is important to note that Israel's military superiority notwithstanding, significant interstate hostilities may well be initiated far short of the point where Israel's existence is jeopardized. As in 1973, one or more of Israel's neighbors might opt for a war with the limited aims of regaining territory and inflicting substantial human and material losses on Israel.

From the IDF's point of view, the principal threat is Syria, which has continuously been building its forces pursuant to its publicly stated aim of achieving military parity with Israel. An obvious scenario is an attack in the Golan Heights with the aim of recapturing some territory, possibly Ramat Magshimim and nearby settlements or Mount Hermon and Druze villages in its vicinity. In order to hold recaptured areas, Syria would probably encourage international involvement in the hope of bringing the fighting to an early end. While a limited war such as this could occur at any time, the most dangerous situation would seem to be one in which there is a breakthrough in the peace process that does not involve Syria and that Syria is unable to undermine. Should Jordan emerge as the major interlocutor with Israel, another scenario is possible: namely, an attack on Jordan rather than in the Golan Heights. This, in turn, would raise the possibility of Israeli military support for the Hashemite kingdom of Jordan (similar to that contemplated in September 1970). Less ominous than the use of force in the two scenarios just depicted would be Syrian troop movements in the Golan Heights designed to heighten tensions and compel the IDF to mobilize. The peril here, of course, would be the possibility of escalation to actual fighting, given expected pressure in Israel to preempt.[122]

Aside from the more specific threats posed by Syria, there is concern that a victory in the Iran-Iraq war by either side could pose serious dangers for Israel. An Iraqi success could mean future deployments of battle-tested troops against Israel whereas an outcome favorable to Iran could result in threats to the regimes of moderate Arab states by newly inspired Islamic fundamentalists, an increase in Iranian-backed terrorism directed at Israel, or, in the longer term, to the deployment of Iranian forces against Israel. The concerns about Iran, Iraq, and Syria underscore the point that the IDF's anticipation of the need to use force has not changed.

FORCE POSTURE, WEAPONS ACQUISITION, AND ARMS CONTROL

To cope with potential military threats emanating from what Israelis see as a hostile environment at a time when the IDF is experiencing manpower reductions and budget cuts, Israel will continue to rely (perhaps more than ever) on military forces designed to operate in accordance with the doctrinal emphasis on the offensive—i.e., surprise, speed, transferring the battle to enemy territory, the indirect approach, and so forth. This means that the latest state-of-the-art aircraft and tanks, supported by mechanized infantry and mobile artillery, will remain the centerpieces of the Israeli force structure. To assure adequate quantities of weapons possessing the qualities deemed necessary by the IDF, Israeli production has been (and will no doubt continue to be) stressed, a striking example being the resources committed to building the modern Lavi fighter plane. It remains to be seen how feasible such undertakings are, however, in light of severe economic problems, budget cutbacks, high costs, and American reluctance or inability to provide further subsidies. Especially in view of the cancellation of the Lavi project, Israel's desire to acquire highly sophisticated American equipment is undiminished. To what extent the United States is able to meet Israel's requests is also an issue, given its own budgetary problems.[123]

Further complicating Israel's problems are questions about the personnel who will operate and maintain the weapons systems in the years ahead. Until now, the men and women of the IDF have demonstrated enviable technical skills and proficiency. Whether this can continue at the same high levels will be determined, in no small measure, by how the IDF responds to a series of emerging challenges, including, inter alia, the decline in technologically prepared recruits entering the ranks; the decreasing attractiveness of the military as a profession because of lower pay and fewer opportunities than in the civilian sector; disappointing immigration trends; emigration to the United States; what many perceive to be morale problems associated with the 1973 and 1982 wars and the continued occupation of the West Bank and Gaza Strip; and, most important, budgetary cutbacks. While none of these may be crucial when taken alone, there is some concern that together they could lead to an erosion of quality at a time when that very attribute is being reemphasized as the answer to the military buildup in the Arab world and the challenges of the increasingly complex technological battlefields of the future. The greatest apprehension of Israeli military leaders is not the closure of the quality gap, but the point at which it narrows and combines with the quantitative advantages enjoyed by their adversaries to produce a serious threat to Israel.[124]

Compared to many of the other countries covered in this volume, arms control is not as important in Israeli defense policy calculations. Essentially, this is because of the willingness of the Soviet Union and western powers to sell arms to the Arabs. Moreover, the lack of mutual recognition and the climate of hostility and profound distrust that mark Israel's relations with many Arab states render direct agreements improbable, if not unrealistic. The best Israel can do is exert pressure on western suppliers to refuse Arab requests for military hardware in whole or in part. Although this has met with some success in the case of the United States, as restrictions on sales to Jordan and Saudi Arabia demonstrate, the Europeans are generally unresponsive. This situation, coupled with Soviet arms sales, which Israel is unable to affect, has led some to argue that it might be better if the United States were the major supplier of military equipment to the Arabs because Israel is in a position to influence the particulars of transactions and the U.S. would have continuing leverage over the use of such equipment by the Arabs by virtue of the latter's dependency on the United States for logistics and training.[125] As of this writing, the tendency of the Israeli defense establishment is to reject this idea. Whether this will continue to be so is uncertain.

With meaningful arms control out of the picture for the foreseeable future, Israel's commitment to a favorable military balance will continue to place a great burden on the budget. Whether a troubled economy can manage this problem while simultaneously responding to demands from deprived social groups is an open question. If it cannot and budgetary restraints adversely affect force structure and weapons acquisition, the issue of open nuclear deterrence may surface in spite of Israel's profound reluctance. Should that transpire, an already troubled and volatile Middle East may well enter its most perilous period to date.

CIVIL-MILITARY RELATIONS

In view of Israel's preoccupation with security, its need to maintain strong military forces, the active participation of most of the citizenry in the military and its continuous warfare with the Arabs, the IDF, as noted earlier, has exercised consistent influence in defense policy making and, at times, in other political spheres as well. Since the exercise of that influence has undergone change and since it has been cloaked in secrecy, owing to security considerations and the IDF's reluctance to provide information, civil-military relations is a complicated subject that does not always lend itself to facile portrayals. Accordingly, scholarly writings have had an evolutionary character, with early works, like those of S. E. Finer and Amos Perlmutter, stressing the professionalism of the military and its loyal subordination to civilian authority, and later works, notably those of Dan Horowitz and Yoram Peri, emphasizing the IDF's involvement in politics.

During Israel's formative years, Prime Minister Ben-Gurion laid the foundation for civilian supremacy by disbanding the armed militias that had been associated with various political parties during the pre-independence period. Ben-Gurion believed the military should be a unified, apolitical institution serving the elected government and that it should

be shielded from the political and ideological conflicts of party politics. Despite Ben-Gurion's successful imposition of civilian supremacy and the public's support thereof, the IDF's actual involvement in the political process diverged from his ideal, largely because of its links to the ruling Labor Party. To augment further the civilian control over the IDF and its subordination to the elected national leadership, key military positions were filled with party loyalists; the military was proselytized through a party servicemen's department (which eventually was disbanded because of public opposition) indoctrination with respect to government policies (that were identical to party policies) was carried out by the chief education officer of the IDF; and settlement movements connected to Labor and other left-wing institutions (i.e., the *kibbutzim* and *moshavim*) became a key source of recruits for elite units and command positions. Concurrently, however, there was a conscious effort to preclude other parties from influencing the military by supporting professional autonomy in operational matters and allowing the chiefs of staff to participate in the formulation of strategic policies. The net result, according to Peri, was diffuse support for the political leadership by the military elite and a high level of coordination and understanding between the two.[126]

As the publication of biographies and diaries of the political and military elite revealed new details about the political behavior of the IDF leadership, scholars sought to explain why Israel had avoided becoming a praetorian state and had retained its pluralistic democracy. Dan Horowitz suggested that a schizophrenic society had developed, composed of military and civilian spheres, each with different rules. While Israelis accepted the intrusion of military influence in the security sphere, the military agreed to avoid upsetting the civil rules of the game in domestic politics.[127] In general, this arrangement worked reasonably well until the spring of 1967.

Political deliberations in the tense weeks prior to the June war were marked by a more assertive IDF role that went beyond its normal inputs to the political echelon and intermittent linkages to the Labor Party. Although the generals never challenged the right of the civilian leadership to make the decision to go to war, they aggressively and sometimes acrimoniously exerted pressure on the prime minister and cabinet to approve the initiation of hostilities. In the course of events, military leaders became involved in party issues, as politicians sought them out for information and they, in turn, sought to influence the cabinet. Politicians, meanwhile, engaged in detailed discussions of operational planning. Particularly noteworthy was the IDF's attempt to increase support for its views through proposals that the cabinet be expanded to include other parties and that Dayan be appointed minister of defense. Although IDF leaders had been consulted in the past on the appointment of defense ministers, their involvement in 1967 was more extensive and crucial. This extension of influence beyond policy making and into deliberations on the composition of the government led Peri to conclude that the IDF has interfered with the rules of the game in the political sphere.[128]

The successful outcome of the 1967 war, most notably the retention of the occupied territories, sowed the seeds of another major conflict in 1973 and created a situation that eventually led to a major political intrusion of the IDF into political affairs in the late 1970s. While the grave events of 1973 did not alter civil-military relations in any fundamental way, they did reveal a significant problem regarding the role of the defense minister. Essentially what happened was that during the fighting the generals often disregarded orders given by Minister of Defense Dayan, and some, including the chief of staff, even questioned his authority to interfere in operational matters.

Efforts by Dayan to restore his authority after the cease-fire on the Egyptian front failed to resolve matters in his favor. Dayan, along with the chief of staff and Maj. Gen. Sharon, supported a policy of active and severe retaliation for cease-fire violations, hoping that this would lead to the destruction of Egypt's encircled Third Army and unconditional surrender by Cairo. The newly appointed commander of the southern Command, Maj. Gen. Israel Tal, stoutly resisted efforts to implement the retaliatory measures because he believed they would violate the government's support for the cease-fire agreement. Although Tal was eventually reassigned, Dayan's plan had been thwarted.[129]

More important than the crisis surrounding the defense minister's authority was the adverse impact the war had on the Labor Party. Unable to address social and economic problems and immobilized by a sharp internal rivalry between Prime Minister Rabin and Defense Minister Peres, the Labor Party was also held accountable for the early setbacks in the war. As the Rabin-Peres rivalry intensified, Peres forged strong ties with Chief of Staff Gur, who had longer-term political ambitions. In return for his support for Peres, Gur was able to play a major role in determining the defense budget, received support for his recommendations on promotions, was active in diplomatic aspects of negotiations with Egypt, and at times was openly critical of government political and economic policies.[130]

The next chief of staff's involvement in politics was even more extensive and controversial. Eitan upbraided the civilians for their poor handling of the economy, publicly identified with the Likud's policies in the West Bank on both military and ideological grounds, and went so far as to back the settlement policies of the radical Gush Emunim group.[131] In a celebrated case that came before Israel's Supreme Court in 1979, Eitan's justification of a settlement on security grounds was rejected. In so doing, the court agreed with the testimony of Defense Minister Weizman, who argued that political considerations were the primary motive. The acting president of the court characterized the disagreement between the chief of staff and defense minister as "unprecedented" and questioned whether the chief of staff would implement an order from the defense minister that differed from an order received from the government. An obvious conclusion drawn from this was that the Basic Law of 1975 had not solved the recurring problem of the authority relationship between the chief of staff and defense minister, a point noted earlier.[132]

Available information on Eitan's successor, Moshe Levy, suggests that the chief of staff's political involvement has subsided. Whether this trend will continue and whether the IDF leadership will avoid a major intrusion into the political process in the future have become increasingly important questions in the minds of a number of informed Israelis. While they all agree that, on balance, the IDF has remained a loyal servant of the elected government, despite the constant external threat, the fact remains that precedents have been set for the military's involvement in politics. The probability that this could eventually result in a major intrusion and even a takeover by the military is low because of the strong societal aversion to such a development and because the IDF's reserve system and the early retirement of senior officers militates against the development of a corporate sense that would make the military a sharply distinct subsystem. The possibility of a major intrusion, nevertheless, cannot be dismissed altogether, given the combination of external, social, economic, and domestic problems that Israel will face for the remainder of the decade. Various scenarios depicting the divisiveness, immobility, loss of confidence, and the acute sense of insecurity rooted in a failure to resolve such problems, which, in turn, raises the specter of a national emergency leading to military intervention are, as Peri has shown, not hard to conjure up.[133]

Notes

1. At least some knowledge of the Holocaust is indispensable for understanding the conceptions underlying Israeli national strategy and defense policy. Those interested in the Holocaust will find a sizable corpus of literature. One especially useful account is Nora Levin, *The Holocaust* (New York: Shocken Books, 1973).

2. A former speechwriter for President Jimmy Carter captured the essence of this when he wrote: "For some the word 'security' may be an intellectual construct. For the Jew, security means life. For 2000 years, Jews qua Jews have been the objects of calculated attempts at annihilation. And for 30 years the tiny nation of Israel, populated by the survivors of Hitler's unfulfilled Final Solution, has lived in constant danger of extermination, fighting four major wars, surrounded by 22 hostile Arab countries intent on the goal of a truly final destruction. Only an Israeli Jew can fully understand the psychic scars and strengths that are consequences of this unrelenting pressure; only Israeli parents can know a literal fear for the lives of their children; only a kibbutznik can appreciate the necessity of the 24-hour watch. The state of Israel and, in a broader sense, the Jewish people, have not only walked through the valley of the shadow of death, they have lived in that valley of death." (Mark Siegel, "Security Means Life," *New York Times*, 26 March 1978.)

3. *The Holocaust* (Yad Vashem, Jerusalem: Martyrs and Heroes Remembrance Authority, 1975), pp. 64–65.

4. Michael Brecher, *The Foreign Policy System of Israel* (New Haven: Yale University Press, 1972), p. 65.

5. Michael I. Handel, *Israel's Political-Military Doctrine*, Occasional Papers in International Affairs, no. 30 (Cambridge: Harvard University Press, 1973), p. 1.

6. The geographical vulnerabilities of Israel between 1948 and 1967 are well known to analysts of the Arab-Israeli conflict, and they receive ample attention in the large body of literature on the conflict. Those interested in a succinct accounting of Israeli perceptions of the geostrategic situation may consult the following background papers published by Carta, Jerusalem, in 1974: *Golan Heights; The Gaza Strip; Judea and Samaria;* and *Secure and Recognized Boundaries*. For a more detailed and analytical assessment of this issue, see Saul Cohen, *Israel's Defensible Borders: A Geopolitical Map*, paper no. 20 (Tel Aviv: Jaffee Center for Strategic Studies, Tel Aviv University, July 1983).

7. National strategy is considered here to be the systematic and orchestrated use of economic, military, diplomatic, and psychological capabilities to accomplish major goals and objectives articulated by leadership elites.

8. Dan Horowitz, "Is Israel a Garrison State?" *Jerusalem Quarterly* (Summer 1977): 69.

9. Ibid., p. 68.

10. The recognition that military victory could not by itself resolve the dispute with the Arabs is noted by Maj. Gen. Israel Tal, "Israel's Defense Doctrine: Background and Dynamics," *Military Review* (March 1978): 23.

11. For a discussion of the pragmatic nature of Israeli foreign policy, see Aaron S. Klieman, "Zionist Diplomacy and Israeli Foreign Policy," *Jerusalem Quarterly* (Spring 1979): 99–109.

12. Ibid., pp. 100–103.

13. On the memorandum of understanding and the JPMG, see James A. Phillips, "America's Security Stake in Israel," *Backgrounder* (Washington, D.C.), 7 July 1986, pp. 2–12; Charles R. Babcock, "U.S.-Israeli Ties Stronger Than Ever," *Washington Post*, 6 August 1986.

14. Handel, *Israel's Political-Military Doctrine*, p. 8; Horowitz, "Is Israel a Garrison State?" pp. 71–72. Those interested in the economic costs of Israel's defense effort should consult the following analyses: Fred M. Gottheil, "An Economic Assessment of the Military Burden in the Middle East," *Journal of Conflict Resolution* (September 1974), pp. 502–13; Paul Rivlin, "The Burden of Israel's Defense," *Survival* (July–August 1978), pp. 146–54; Ibrahi, M. Oweiss, "The Israel Economy and Its Military Liability," *L'Egypte Contemporaine*, July 1984, pp. 5–21.

15. Zahal and IDF are used interchangeably in this chapter.

16. For a good summary of the main features of the Israeli reserve system, see Irving Heymont, *Analysis of the Army Reserve System of Israel, Canada, United Kingdom, Federal Republic of Germany*, report pre-

pared for Office of the Director for Planning and Evaluation, Department of Defense (McLean, Va.: General Research Corporation, 1977), pp. 6–15.

17. Handel, *Israel's Political-Military Doctrine*, p. 19.

18. For a succinct account of these developments, see Fred J. Khouri, *The Arab-Israeli Dilemma*, 3rd ed. (Syracuse, N.Y.: Syracuse University Press, 1985), chap. 7.

19. The debate over the disposition of the territories produced a variety of proposals both outside and inside the government. By 1969 a scheme devised by Yigal Allon, known as the Allon Plan, became the unofficial basis of policy. The plan called for a security belt 10–15 miles wide along the sparsely populated edge of the Jordan River, which would be considered Israel's new security frontier. Guarded by a string of paramilitary settlements, the strip would contain fewer than 20,000 Arabs. New towns were to be constructed to overlook the Arab population centers of Jericho and Hebron, and a corridor 4.3 miles wide linking Jordan with the West Bank was to be created. With the exception of Jerusalem and areas near Latrun and Hebron, the area outside the paramilitary strip, which contained most of the Arab population, would either be permanently demilitarized and given an autonomous status or be linked to Jordan, depending on negotiations with the Jordanians. Moreover, Hussein's government would be asked to accept 200,000 refugees from Gaza. Besides providing for defense against conventional attacks—the Jordan River as a natural tank ditch—the Allon Plan, with its paramilitary settlements, was also directed at the problem of guerrilla infiltration. The training of the settlers would enable them to carry out patrolling and other tasks associated with territorial defense. Finally, to the south, Allon's scheme called for a demilitarized Sinai and a new Israeli town near Sharm el-Sheikh, to protect a north-south line to El-Arish, which represented the Israeli withdrawal area. For information on the plan, see Abraham S. Becker, *Israel and the Occupied Palestinian Territories: Military-Political Issues in the Debate* (Santa Monica, Calif.: RAND Corporation, 1971), pp. 27–32; *Le Monde* (Paris), 11 June 1978; and *New York Times*, 18 and 24 June 1969.

20. Not surprisingly, the October 1973 War spawned a vast outpouring of literature. Those who wish to examine it in more detail should find the following useful: D. K. Palit, *Return to Sinai* (London: Compton Russell, 1974); Chaim Herzog, *The War of Atonement* (Boston: Little, Brown, 1975); Edgar O'Ballance, *No Victor, No Vanquished* (San Rafael, Calif.: Presidio Press, 1978); Trevor N. Dupuy, *Elusive Victory* (New York: Harper & Row, 1978), pp. 387–605; Nadav Safran, *Israel, the Embattled Ally* (Cambridge: Harvard University Press, 1978), pp. 476–534; and Mohammed Heikal, *The Road to Ramadan* (New York: Quadrangle, 1975).

21. For overall assessments of the war in Lebanon, see Trevor N. Dupuy and Paul Martell, *Flawed Victory* (Fairfax, Va.: Hero Books, 1986); Ze'ev Schiff and Ehud Ya'ari, *Israel's Lebanon War* (New York: Simon & Schuster, 1984).

22. Shiff and Ya'ari, *Israel's Lebanon War*, p. 301.

23. Tal, "Israel's Defense Doctrine," p. 23.

24. The profound influence of the strategy of the in-

direct approach on Israeli military leaders before, during, and after 1948 is attributed to the eminent British analyst Sir Basil Liddell Hart. On this point, see Brian Bond, "Liddell Hart's Influence on Israeli Military Theory and Practice," *Journal of the Royal United Services Institute* (June 1974): 83–89, and Jac Weller, "Sir Basil Liddell Hart's Disciples in Israel," *Military Review* (January 1974): 13–23.

25. Handel, *Israel's Political-Military Doctrine*, p. 25.

26. Ibid., p. 23. Bond, "Liddell Hart's Influence," p. 25, contends that despite Dayan's reversal, tanks were to be used only in a support role. As things turned out, Israeli armored commanders flouted the high command's orders and achieved major victories.

27. Zeev Schiff, "The Israeli Air Force," *Air Force Magazine*, August 1978, pp. 33–34.

28. Two additional considerations were believed important in the decision not to acquire bombers: one was the relatively short ranges within the potential target area; the other was the burden on Israel's scarce human resources that the larger air and ground crews required by bombers would have created. See Handel, *Israel's Political-Military Doctrine*, pp. 27–28, and Schiff, "Israel's Air Force," p. 34.

29. For a brief summary of the IDFN's evolution, see Lt. Comdr. Ruben Porath, "The Israeli Navy," *U.S. Naval Institute Proceedings*, September 1971, pp. 33–39.

30. Tal, "Israel's Defense Doctrine," p. 27.

31. Yigal Allon, *The Making of Israel's Army* (New York: Universe Books, 1970), p. 65.

32. Handel, *Israel's Policy-Military Doctrine*, pp. 43–45.

33. Schiff, "Israel's Air Force," p. 34.

34. Handel, *Israel's Political-Military Doctrine*, p. 41.

35. Nadav Safran, *From War to War* (New York: Pegasus, 1969), chap. 7.

36. On the successful use of the strategy of the indirect approach in 1967, see Bond, "Liddell Hart's Influence," pp. 86–88; and Weller, "Sir Basil Liddell Hart's Disciples," pp. 19–23.

37. Quoted in Safran, *From War to War*, p. 382.

38. The Bar Lev Line consisted of a series of fortified bunkers connected by a patrol road. It was to receive immediate support from air and artillery and tanks positions a short distance to the rear.

39. On the war of attrition, see Lawrence L. Whetten, *The Canal War* (Cambridge: MIT Press, 1974).

40. Schiff, "Israeli Air Force," pp. 35–36.

41. Handel, *Israel's Political-Military Doctrine*, p. 62.

42. Porath, "Israeli Navy," pp. 36–38.

43. Handel, *Israel's Political-Military Doctrine*, pp. 62–63; Aaron S. Klieman, *Israel's Global Reach* (Washington D.C.: Pergamon-Brassey's, 1985), pp. 21–22. The economic reasons for Israeli arms sales are surmised by Klieman, pp. 56–66.

44. Before and after the war, Sadat repeatedly made this point publicly and in private meetings (several of which this author attended) by saying that the United States held 99 percent of the cards in the bargaining process.

45. The need to redeem honor and dignity was a constant theme before, during, and after the war. For a good illustration, see "Speech of President Hafez al-As-

sad over Damascus Radio and Television," Damascus Domestic Service, 6 October 1973, in *Foreign Broadcast Information Service, Daily Report, Middle East and North Africa*, 9 October 1973, pp. F2–4. Hereafter references will be to *FBIS/MENA* or *FBIS/MEA* (North Africa became Africa when FBIS coverage of all of Africa was added to the Middle East daily report).

46. See *Aviation Week and Space Technology*, 7 December 1974, p. 17. Some critics and observers have faulted this strategy as being overly cautious. Edgar O'Ballance, for instance, is of the opinion that Egyptian forces could probably have seized the Sinai passes by 7 October. See Edgar O'Ballance, "The Fifth Arab-Israeli War, October 1973," *Army Quarterly and Defense Journal* (U.K.) (April 1974): 317; and Robert R. Rodwell, "The Mideast War: A Damned Close-Run Thing," *Air Force Magazine* (February 1974): 40. Other analysts, by contrast, have pointed out that armor and mechanized losses were heavy when Arab forces ventured beyond their air defense cover. See Lawrence Whetten and Michael Johnson, "Military Lessons of the Yom Kippur War," *World Today* (March 1974): 104, and J. I. Koek, "The Middle East Conflict, October 1973," *Army Journal* (Australia) (December 1974): 5.

47. Cited in *Aviation Week and Space Technology*, 7 December 1973, p. 7.

48. Tal, "Israel's Defense Doctrine," pp. 30–31; also see Samuel W. Sax and Avigdor Levy, "Arab-Israeli Conflict Four: A Preliminary Assessment," *Naval War College Review* (January–February 1974), p. 8.

49. Whetten and Johnson, "Military Lessons," pp. 103, 105.

50. For a contrary analysis that argues that a preemptive attack would probably have produced an overwhelming victory similar to 1967, see Kenneth S. Brower, "The Yom Kippur War," *Military Review* (March 1974), p. 33.

51. O'Ballance, "Fifth Arab-Israeli War," p. 320.

52. Bonner Day, "New Role for Israeli Air Force," *Air Force Magazine* (August 1978), p. 38. For a cogent discussion of the military advantages of preemption in a future war, see Steven J. Rosen and Martin Indyk, "The Temptation to Pre-Empt in a Fifth Arab-Israeli War," *Orbis* (Summer 1976): 276–82. In discussions that I had with civilian and military planners in Israel, it became apparent that preemption was viewed as a dubious option in the face of incremental deployment changes by Arab forces surrounding Israel. Although the cumulative effect by such changes might constitute a serious threat, each change by itself might not be sufficient to justify a preemptive attack and the associated risk of adverse international, and particularly American, reaction. Accordingly, preemption would appear to be a viable option only when Arab redeployment had reached a point where the threat to the IDF was obvious.

53. Herbert J. Coleman, "Israel's Shift Toward Long-Range Fleet," *Aviation Week and Space Technology*, 10 March 1975, pp. 15–18.

54. This convenient summary is borrowed from Handel, *Israel's Political-Military Doctrine*, pp. 67–68.

55. *Press Release Issued by the Commission of Inquiry, Yom Kippur War, upon Submission of Its Third and Final Report to the Government and the Defense and Foreign Affairs Committee of the Knesset* (Jerusa-

lem: Ministry of Information, 30 January 1975), pp. 14, 33. Hereafter referred to as *Agranat Press Release*.

56. Ibid., p. 15.

57. See Herzog, *War of Atonement*, pp. 98–105.

58. *Agranat Press Release*, pp. 17–18.

59. Brower, "Yom Kippur War," p. 26.

60. *Armed Forces Journal International* (March 1974), p. 18.

61. *Agranat Press Release*, pp. 22–23.

62. Ibid., p. 22.

63. Brower, "Yom Kippur War," p. 26; Holtz, "Israeli Air Force," p. 16.

64. *Armed Forces Journal International* (October 1973), p. 68.

65. *Agranat Press Release*, pp. 28–30, 33.

66. Gen. Herzl Shafir, head of the General Staff branch, described the training programs in 1974 as "unprecedented in scope." He asserted that the IDF had succeeded in filling all the gaps left by the October war and in preparing all new conscripts. See *Jerusalem Post* (in English), 13 April 1975; in *FBIS/MENA*, 17 April 1975, p. N6.

67. Dupuy, *Elusive Victory*, p. 609.

68. Brower, "Yom Kippur War," p. 27; Sax and Levy, "Arab-Israeli Conflict Four," p. 13.

69. Charles Holley, "IDF Strategy in 1977: Quick, Offensive Fighting," *Middle East* (September 1977): 29. As Holley notes, a primary reliance on the infantry would undoubtedly result in higher losses. See also "Chief of Staff Gur Discusses IDF Plans," Jerusalem Domestic Service (in Hebrew), 24 December 1974; in *FBIS/MENA*, 24 September 1974, p. N5.

70. Former Chief of Staff Mordecai Gur put it this way during an interview in October 1974: "The distances between us and the important centers of the hostile countries are not great. Their armies are concentrated to a major and decisive extent along the borders. This means that if you succeed in finding the right political, strategic and tactical path, you can definitely expect to terminate an engagement by what we term a blitzkreig. There is no reason to assume that a future war must be a long one. I certainly do not accept this." See Gide'on Levari, "Interview of the Month," Jerusalem Domestic Service (in Hebrew), 26 October 1974; in *FBIS/MENA*, 30 October 1974, p. N7. Three years later, Jac Weller, "Armor and Infantry in Israel," *Military Review* (April 1977): 7, observed that "in Israel today, everything is offense oriented." A somewhat contrary view may be found in Charles Wakebridge, "Israel's Changing Military Posture," *Military Review* (June 1976): 6–7. Wakebridge argues that although offensive doctrine may remain and be taught to Zahal, in practice many troops are in a static defensive disposition. That at least some Israelis see defensive actions as a distinct possibility was evident in discussions I had with one top civilian planner, who ruminated about the option of conducting a "surprise defense" in the West Bank. What he had in mind was reliance on the defensive network involving the settlements and an emphasis on creating unforeseen obstacles for an attacking force. Not surprisingly, a ranking military officer evinced some discomfort with this notion when it was broached with him during a later interview. At the same time, however, he conceded that cutbacks in defense spending and draft requirements had increased the importance of territorial defense.

71. Anthony H. Cordesman, "How Much Is Too Much?" *Armed Forces Journal International*, (October 1977), p. 6.

72. W. Seth Carus, "The Military Balance of Power in the Middle East," *Current History* (January 1978), p. 29.

73. Israel's multifaceted and highly sophisticated defense industries turn out a wide variety of products and play a major role in the economy. Those interested in this subject will find the following very useful: *The Israeli Economist* (Jerusalem), February 1986 in Joint Publications Research Service, *Near East/South Asia Report* (hereafter *JPRS/NESA*), no. 86036, 28 March 1986, pp. 46–54 (the variation *JPRS/NEA* also appears because older reports covered Africa rather than South Asia); Edward Duyker, "The Evolution of Israel's Defense Industries," *Defense Journal International*, January–February 1983; and, particularly, Alex Mintz, "Military-Industrial Linkages in Israel," *Armed Forces and Society*, Fall 1985, pp. 3–24.

74. Carus, "Military Balance of Power," p. 30.

75. Holtz, "Israeli Air Force," pp. 15–18. The Israelis lost 37 percent of their fighter and attack aircraft in 1973.

76. In the last half of 1978, a doctrinal debate was reportedly taking place between air force leaders, who continued to stress the traditional missions and leading offensive role of the Israeli Air Force, and ground commanders, who wished to see the air force concentrate on ground support operations. See Day, "New Role for Israeli Air Force," p. 38.

77. Carus, "Military Balance of Power," p. 30; Norman Friedman, "Protecting the Coast Required Revamping Israel's Navy," *Military Electronics/Countermeasures*, February 1983, pp. 89–92.

78. The analysis of the intelligence failure became a fertile topic for social scientists. The following are among the more insightful treatments: Michael Brecher and Mordechai Raz, "Images and Behavior: Israel's Yom Kippur War and the Inevitability of Surprise," *International Studies Quarterly* (September 1977), pp. 461–502; and Avi Shlaim, "Failures in National Intelligence Estimates: The Case of the Yom Kippur War," *World Politics* (April 1976), pp. 348–80. These authors and others address the psychological (e.g., images, attitudes, values, and beliefs of the decision makers) and structural dimensions.

79. *Armed Forces Journal International* (October 1973), p. 47.

80. Arab success was believed to be dependent on Egypt's ability to stage deep air strikes inside Israel. Since this was considered to be beyond Egyptian capability, war was thought to be unlikely. See Shlaim, "Failures in National Intelligence Estimates," pp. 352–53.

81. Sharon provided an insight into Israeli thinking prior to the war when he argued that the IDF presence along the canal left the Egyptians with no line of defense between Cairo and the canal, and that Sadat would not attack because he would not want to fight near Cairo. In more specific terms, Sharon called attention to two factors that he believed would dissuade Egypt from attacking. In his words: "Operations that are the result of a simple drill, they do very well. But where you have to improvise, react to a changing situation, where the commander has to be forward, the kind of fluid situation a river crossing is—that is not one of their strong points. Thus, the Canal becomes a real obstacle for the Arabs. The second reason is the desert. [Sharon crossed the Sinai twice, in 1956 as commander of the paratroopers and in 1967 as the head of an armored division.] A desert crossing is hard. It takes will power. You must conduct a mobile operation, take risks, make fast decisions, use initiative, do things even if contrary to what you were told before. That's not the strong point of the Arab. And you have to be good at close combat fighting, hand-to-hand, night combat. This is one of our strongest points. The Arab soldier doesn't have the psychological structure." (Quoted in *Armed Forces Journal International*, October 1973, p. 70).

82. Ibid., p. 47.

83. See *Agranat Press Release*, pp. 18–19; Sax and Levy, "Arab-Israeli Conflict Four," p. 11; O'Ballance, "Fifth Arab-Israeli War," p. 314; Koek, "Middle East Conflict," p. 13; Cordesman, "How Much Is Too Much?" p. 35; and Schiff, "Israeli Air Force," p. 38. Several officials with whom I discussed this matter have pointed out that Israel's limited resources made it very difficult to have three strong intelligence structures. They made the point that factors other than a major reorganization (i.e., access, coordination, and interpersonal relations) were the key considerations in fostering pluralism. Interviews with Brig. Gen. Yoel Ben-Porat, 10 September 1979; Abraham Lif (Ministry of Defense), 22 October 1979, and Maj. Gen. Manachem Meron, 23 October 1979.

84. Reuven Pedahtzur, "Those Responsible for the National Intelligence Decision" and "Possibility of Improvement," *Ha'aretz* (Tel Aviv), 17, 18 April 1985, in *JPRS/NEA*, no. 85084, 25 June 1985, pp. 68–72.

85. One reason for lack of coordination in 1973 may well have been the encouragement given to each arm to develop its own "philosophy of battle" and the concomitant belief that it could win a war without the help of other arms. See *Armed Forces Journal International*, (October 1973), p. 64. On the efforts to improve coordination, see Weller, "Armor and Infantry," pp. 5–11; and Schiff, "Israeli Air Force," p. 38.

86. "The Middle East War 1973," lecture by Gen. Chaim Herzog, *Royal United Services Institute* (March 1975), p. 5; and *Agranat Press Release*, pp. 11, 19, 28.

87. Hirsh Goodman, "Tank in a Bag," *Jerusalem Post*, 23 March 1979; "Agranat Report: Highlights," *Middle East* (September 1977), pp. 26–27. Goodman describes "dry storage" as follows: "By this method, which is now in extensive use in the IDF, a tank is oiled, greased, fueled up, loaded with ammunition, packed with the crew's equipment and food, dusted off and placed in a gigantic zipper bag. It is then plugged into an air conditioning unit, which keeps the tank and its contents at a constant temperature and as fresh as a daisy for months on end without any running down of batteries, evaporation of fuel or deterioration of ammunition. In times of emergency, all a crew had to do is unzip the bag and drive off to battle." On the comptroller's report, see *Jerusalem Post*, 10 May 1979.

88. *Jerusalem Post*, 9 July 1979. The consistency in Israeli military doctrine is noted by Tal, "Israel's Defense Doctrine," p. 22, where he argues that all military thinking since the 1950s amounted to little more than a series of footnotes to the ideas that crystallized then.

89. Richard A. Gabriel, "Lessons of the War: The IDF in Lebanon," *Military Review*, August 1984, p. 49. A particularly critical assessment of the performance of

commanders in the 1982 war was produced by Col. (Reserve) Dr. Imanuel Wald. Its main points may be found in *Hadashot* (Tel Aviv), 19 May 1986; in *FBIS/MEA*, 22 May 1986, p. 14.

90. For accounts of the military aspects of the 1982 war, see Depuy and Martell, *Flawed Victory*, pp. 98–160; Schiff and Ya'ari, *Israel's Lebanon War*, pp. 109–229; Abraham Zohar, "The Israeli Navy in the 1982 War in Lebanon," *Marine-Rundschau* (Koblenz), March-April 1985, *JPRS/NEA*, no. 85105, 14 August 1985, pp. 64–72. For a cogent assessment of the causes and effects of dissent in the war in Lebanon, see Shai Feldman and Heda Rechniz-Kijner, *Deception, Consensus and War: Israel in Lebanon*, paper no. 27 (Tel Aviv: Jaffee Center for Strategic Studies, Tel Aviv University, October 1984), especially pp. 66–76.

91. Moshe Dayan, *Diary of the Sinai Campaign* (New York: Harper & Row, 1965), pp. 8–9.

92. For an expanded analysis of the Israeli counterinsurgency effort, see Bard E. O'Neill, *Armed Struggle in Palestine* (Boulder, Colo.: Westview Press, 1978), chap. 4.

93. *Washington Post*, 20 and 21 April 1985, 7 June 1985, 31 March 1986; *Christian Science Monitor*, 4 and 6 June 1985.

94. Alan Dowty, "Nuclear Proliferation: The Israeli Case," *International Studies Quarterly* (March 1978), pp. 82–83. In contrast to Dowty, another observer states flatly that a separation plan was completed in 1969. See Special Correspondent, "Israel's Nuclear Weapons: Are They in Safe Hands?" *Middle East* (June 1976), p. 27. The CIA estimate was reported by *Washington Post*, 15 March 1976. Those who are interested in pursuing the matter of nuclear weapons in Israel may wish to compare the following to Dowty's article: Yair Evron, "Israel and the Atom: The Uses and Misuses of Ambiguity, 1957–1967," *Orbis* (Winter 1974), pp. 1326–43; Fuad Jabber, "Israel's Nuclear Options," *Journal of Palestine Studies* 1, no. 1 (n.d.): 21–38; S. Jaishankar, "Israeli Nuclear Option," *India Quarterly* (January-March 1978): 39–53; Robert J. Pranger and Dale R. Tahtinen, *Nuclear Threat in the Middle East* (Washington, D.C.: American Enterprise Institute, 1975); and Steven J. Rosen, "A Stable System of Mutual Nuclear Deterrence in the Arab-Israeli Conflict," *American Political Science Review* (December 1977): 1367–83.

95. The late Moshe Dayan reportedly indicated that a nuclear option should be used only if the country's existence were in danger. See Avraham Schweitzer, "The Importance of the Nuclear Option," *Ha'aretz* (Tel Aviv), 15 March 1976; in *FBIS/MENA*, 16 March 1976, p. N3.

96. Many observers attribute this to the so-called Massada complex, by which they mean a determination to go down fighting rather than submit to destruction. However, since this refers to an act of mass suicide on the part of Jewish defenders about to be overtaken by Romans at Massada in 73 A.D., the analogy is not compelling. This is because the nuclear policy of Israel putatively is designed to destroy the enemy if the state is being overrun. A better analogy might be Samson's act of bringing the temple down on his enemies as he was about to be killed. Hence, it may be more appropriate to refer to a Samson complex rather than a Massada complex.

97. Shai Feldman sets forth the argument for Israel developing an overt nuclear deterrence posture in *Is-raeli Nuclear Deteterrence* (New York: Columbia University Press, 1982). For critiques of Feldman's proposal, see Peter Pry, *Israel's Nuclear Arsenal* (Boulder, Colo.: Westview Press, 1984), especially pp. 109–16, and Alan Dowty, "Going Public with the Bomb," *Society*, January-February 1986, pp. 52–58.

98. As Dayan put it: "We have come to a highly critical point in regard to exploiting manpower. The Arabs have inexhaustible conventional power. In facing the facts we cannot escape emphasizing a specific consolidation of our strength. Not another 1,000 tanks or 200 aircraft; we must confront growing Arab power with deterrent atomic weapons. The Arabs want to destroy us and what will cool their verve is the news that they can expect total destruction. We must bear in mind that we are a state with a population of 3 million. If we keep up the tempo of armament aimed at a conventional balance of power, we shall ultimately find every one of us busy tightening tank treads and maintaining aircraft" (Yediot Aharonot, Tel Aviv, 14 March 1976; cited in *FBIS/MENA* 18 March 1976, p. N7).

99. Amos Perlmutter, *Politics and the Military in Israel, 1967–1977* (London: Frank Cass, 1978), p. 63; *Agranat Press Release*, pp. 25–27; Horowitz, "Is Israel a Garrison State?" p. 70.

100. Richard F. Nyrop, *Israel: A Country Study* (Washington, D.C.: Government Printing Office, 1979), p. 255. Not all experts agree that the Basic Law provided sufficient clarity on the relations among the political leaders, the minister of defense, and the IDF. See, for instance, Peter Elman, "Basic Law: The Army, 1976," *Israel Law Review* (April 1977), pp. 232–42.

101. On the basic organization of the IDF, see Nyrop, *Israel: A Country Study*, pp. 255–57; Edward Luttwak and Dan Horowitz, *The Israeli Army* (New York: Harper & Row, 1975), pp. 94–98. During the 1980s, a new ground forces command (GFC) was established, despite resistance from the area commanders. By April 1984 the first stage of the establishment was completed with the transfer of all aspects of training of the ground forces from the General Staff Military Training Department to the GFC. See Weller, "Armor and Infantry," p. 5, and Jerusalem Domestic Service (in Hebrew), 1 April 1984, in *FBIS/MEA*, 3 April 1984, pp. 16–17. For an appreciation of the policies, interpersonal relations and functioning of the General Staff, see *Ma'ariv* (Tel Aviv), weekend magazine, 20 September 1985, in *JPRS/NESA*, no. 86008, 24 January 1986, pp. 46–53.

102. Klieman, "Zionist Diplomacy," p. 94.

103. Brecher, *Foreign Policy System*, p. 178. Jon Kimche, "Politics and the Israel Defense Forces," *Midstream* (June–July 1974), pp. 31–33.

104. Klieman suggests that the political stock of the Ministry of Foreign Affairs did not improve. After noting its "permanent downgrading," he goes on to describe it as an auxiliary agency with "little voice and even less influence in the actual formulation of policy" (Klieman, "Zionist Diplomacy," p. 96). See also Horowitz, "Is Israel a Garrison State?" p. 70.

105. Brecher, *Foreign Policy System*, p. 175.

106. Ibid., p. 182.

107. Ibid., pp. 182–83.

108. Ibid., p. 185, and Kimche, "Politics and the Israel Defense Forces," p. 34.

109. Between 1967 and 1973, defense policies were conceived and designed by Prime Minister Meir's

"kitchen cabinet" according to Perlmutter, *Politics and the Military*, pp. 63ff.

110. Depuy and Martell, *Flawed Victory*, pp. 151–54 and Schiff and Ya'ari, *Israel's Lebanon War*, pp. 190ff, especially pp. 109–15, 181–94 and 301–8, make the case that Sharon misled the cabinet. For contrary views, see Sharon's rebuttals in *Yedi'ot Aharonot* (Tel Aviv), weekend supplement, 7 June 1985, in *JPRS/NEA*, no. 85124, 25 September 1985, pp. 76–81 and Eitan's comments in *Ma'ariv* (Tel Aviv), 7 June 1985, in *JPRS/NEA*, no. 85112, 4 September 1985, pp. 16–21.

111. See, for example, Perlmutter, *Politics and the Military*, pp. 1–2 and 197–208, and Yoram Peri, *Between Ballots and Battles* (New York: Cambridge University Press, 1983), pp. 271–78.

112. Perlmutter, *Politics and the Military*, pp. 197–98; Kimche, "Politics and the Israel Defense Forces," pp. 33–34.

113. Amos Perlmutter, *Military and Politics in Israel: Nation-Building and Role Expansion* (London: Frank Cass, 1969), pp. 123–245.

114. Perlmutter, *Military and Politics*, pp. 87–89.

115. The specific issue involved was a Lavon proposal that a national security authority be established to oversee the Ministry of Defense (ibid., p. 91).

116. Ibid., pp. 105–8, 113–14; Perlmutter, *Politics and the Military*, pp. 29, 40–42; and Horowitz, "Is Israel a Garrison State?" pp. 69–70.

117. Perlmutter, *Politics and the Military*, pp. 62–63; Kimche, "Politics and the Israel Defense Forces," pp. 34–35. One high-level officer with whom I talked was of the opinion that Dayan's exclusion was the result of his preoccupation with relations with the Arabs in the occupied territories rather than the actions of others.

118. Perlmutter, *Politics and the Military*, p. 66, indicates that the high command became the exclusive source of advice to the political leaders; Kimche, "Politics and the Israel Defense Forces," p. 35, states that matters concerning military strategy "become the preserve of the High Command."

119. Anticipated reactions in Egypt included demoralization of the Egyptian people and the downfall of Nasser. As for the Soviet Union, there was little thought given to the possibility that Moscow might take command of, and massively rebuild, Egyptian air defenses.

120. Avi Shlaim and Raymond Tanter, "Decision Process, Choice, and Consequences: Israel's Deep-Penetration Bombing in Egypt, 1979," *World Politics* (July 1978): 516.

121. Perlmutter, *Politics and the Military*, pp. 195–98; Peri, *Between Ballots and Battles*, pp. 168–72.

122. On the Syrian scenarios, see interview of the head of the IDF Intelligence Corps, Maj. Gen. Ehud Baraq, by Nisim Mish'al, Eytan Haber, and Moshe Shlonsky, Jerusalem Television Service (in Hebrew), 19 October 1985; in *FBIS/MEA*, 17 October 1985, p. 14; *New York Times*, 29 July 1986; Ze'ev Schiff, "Do Syrians Want War?" *Ha'aretz* (Tel Aviv), 14, 17, 18, 19 March 1986; in *JPRS/NEA*, no. 86048, 16 April 1986, pp. 36–44.

123. For background on the Lavi project and American support, see Duncan L. Clarke and Alan S. Cohen, "The United States, Israel and the Lavi Fighter," *Middle East Journal* (Winter 1986): 16–32; Charles R. Babcock, "How U.S. Came to Underwrite Israel's Lavi

Fighter Project," *Washington Post*, 6 August 1986. Clarke and Cohen question whether U.S. support is in the interests of either country. In the summer of 1986 a Pentagon study group noted that costs of the Lavi were understated and argued that it would be more cost-effective for Israel to drop the Lavi and instead acquire modified F-16s or F-20s from the United States. See C. Robert Zelnick, "The Lavi Aircraft Milestone—Flying High," *Christian Science Monitor*, 19 June 1986. Israel Aircraft Industries argues, by contrast, that the cost of the Lavi is cheaper than acquiring F-16s. See Jerusalem Domestic Service, 27 March 1986, in *FBIS/MEA* 1 April 1986, pp. 16–17. On the linkage of doctrine with budgetry and manpower cuts, see the comments of Maj. Gen. Yosef Peled, who was in charge of training and doctrine, in *Jerusalem Post*, 20 September 1985.

124. The issue of the future capability of the IDF, both quantitatively and qualitatively, has been a major continuing concern that encompasses a broad range of sub-issues. Without question, the most significant problem has been the effects of the 1985–86 budgetary cutbacks stemming from the general economic crisis. Some members of the General Staff have acknowledged the negative impact on the forces under their command. For example, Maj. Gen. Amir Drori, commander of the ground forces, has referred to a long-term process of decline in the army, especially the reserve components, which he attributes to general budget cutbacks and disproportionate allocations to the air force (Drori is one of the opponents of the Lavi project in the IDF). The negative effects of budgetary cutbacks have been felt in other IDF branches as well, according to Defense Minister Rabin. Chief of Staff Moshe Levy's main concern in 1985 was that the principal impact of budget cuts would be felt in the future unless the IDF overcame the tendency to postpone investments in long-term projects because of short term needs. See interview of Maj. Gen. Amir Drori by Ze'ev Schiff in *Ha'aretz*, supplement (Tel Aviv), 16 May 1986 in *FBIS/MEA*, 22 May 1986, pp. 14–15; interview with Defense Minister Rabin, *Bita'On Heyl Ha'avir* (Tel Aviv), in *JPRS/NEA*, no. 86011, 29 January 1986, p. 13; interview with Chief of Staff Lt. Gen. Moshe Levy by Yosi Uzrad and Gay Zohar, Tel Aviv IDF Radio, 16 September 1985, in *FBIS/MEA*, 18 September 1985, pp. 19–110. For more specific information on the budget cuts see Ze'ev Schiff, "The Cuts Were Not Carried Out," *Ha'aretz* (Tel Aviv), 2 and 3 May 1985 in *JPRS/NEA*, no. 85092, 19 July 1985, pp. 4–8; *Jerusalem Post*, 10 July 1985 and 6 January 1986; and interview with Brig. Gen. Nehemya Dagan, IDF education commander, by Yisra'el Zamir, *Al-Hamishmar* (Tel Aviv), 10 January 1986, in *JPRS/NEA*, no. 86020, 18 February 1986, pp. 68–69. The problems associated with the recruitment of personnel with technical skills is discussed by Roman Priester, "The IDF Wants You," *Ha'aretz* (Tel Aviv), 8 June 1984, in *JPRS/NEA*, no. 84118, 1 August 1984, pp. 29–31. The level of Jewish immigration in 1985 was described as "disastrous" by the Absorption Minister and the head of the Jewish Agency Aliya Department, according to the *Jerusalem Post*, 16 May 1986.

Needless to state, American assistance will be crucial in light of Israel's difficulties. To what extent the United States can meet Israel's needs may be influenced, more than ever, by pressures in Washington to reduce its own deficits and budget and by its own military requirements, which are considerable.

125. Ze'ev Schiff, *Israel's Eroding Edge in the Middle East Military Balance*, policy paper no. 2 (Washington, D.C.: Washington Institute for Near East Policy, 1985), pp. 20–23.

126. Yoram Peri, "Party-Military Relations in a Pluralist System, *Journal of Strategic Studies*, September 1983, pp. 51–60.

127. Horowitz, "Is Israel a Garrison State?" pp.

458–65, and id., "Civil-Military Relations in Israel," as cited in Peri, *Between Battles and Ballots*, p. 8.

128. Ibid., pp. 244–51.

129. Ibid.,pp. 251–59.

130. Ibid., pp. 168–72; Perlmutter, *Politics and the Military*, pp. 198–200.

131. Peri, *Between Battles and Ballots*, pp. 266–71.

132. Ibid., pp. 269–70.

133. Ibid., pp. 283–86.

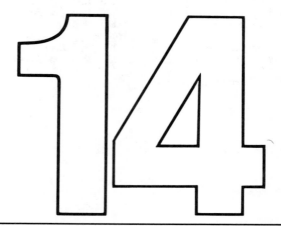

THE REPUBLIC OF SOUTH AFRICA

Mark Veblen Kauppi

The Republic of South Africa (RSA) is the final bastion of white minority rule in sub-Saharan Africa. The ultimate goal of maintaining the political dominance of five million whites over twenty-five million blacks, Asians, and persons of mixed race has created particular threats to national security that go beyond those faced by all states in an anarchic international system that lacks a central authority. The pursuit of racially based political domination and attempts to end it have decisively shaped the objectives, strategy, and development of South African defense policy. Government protestations notwithstanding, this defense policy is basically designed to secure the power and privileges of the white minority. This is the essential starting point for understanding South African national security issues—they must be viewed in a broader political, social, and economic context.

To consolidate white domination, the Afrikaner-based National Party began in 1948 to create systematically an imposing apartheid edifice. Apartheid—the doctrine and policy of racial group separation—was seen as one strategy to maintain white power and Afrikaner national identity. This edifice, confidently expected to have been institutionalized by the 1980s, instead came under severe attack, resulting in a crisis of confidence within the Afrikaner community. While this attack stems from a variety of national, regional, and international sources, the common thread has been opposition to the white racial oligarchy. With the advent of a perceived "total onslaught" against South Africa in the mid 1970s, a multi-dimensional response by the state was deemed imperative. The result was the development of a "total national strategy" that attempted to consolidate and integrate South Africa's domestic, foreign, and defense policies. It is necessary, therefore, to cast our discussion of South African defense policy in the larger context of an increasingly important national security management system. As will be seen, a critical component of this system is the South African Defence Force (SADF), whose enhanced status is both a cause and a conse-

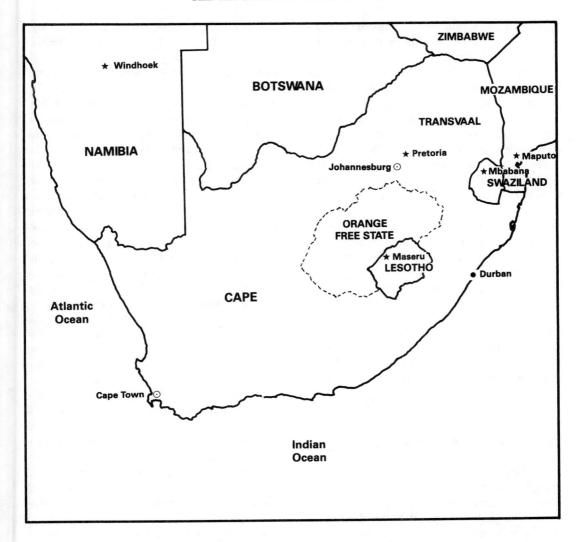

quence of the growing militarization of the South African polity and society.

To students of international relations, South Africa is a fascinating case study, albeit one filled with potential landmines. First, the country dramatically illustrates the internationalization of a state's domestic problems and conflicts. Similarly, South Africa represents a classic example of the domestic sources of a state's foreign and defense policies. Hence, the societal level of analysis is of crucial importance.[1]

Second, observers differ as to how to categorize South Africa. Is it, for example, a restricted democracy or an "unlegitimated police state"?[2] Is it essentially of the First World or of the Third World? On the one hand, South Africa seems to reflect certain characteristics of the Western world. It has a high gross national product (GNP), an impressive standard of living for the majority of whites, functioning public services, opposition parties, and an efficient military establishment. On the other hand, South Africa seems to exhibit certain affinities to many Third World states. As is often the case in less developed countries (LDC), the major threat to national security is internal, not external; defense involves the security forces and police as well as an influential military; and the most serious threats are directed against an ethnic minority that monopolizes all significant political power, in this case the "white tribe of Africa."[3]

Third, information on South African defense policy, particularly the policy-making process, is difficult to come by. The government and military are tight-lipped when it comes to security issues, generally viewing foreign academics and journalists with suspicion.

Finally, with perhaps the exception of the Soviet Union and Israel, few other countries elicit such visceral reactions, if not morbid fascination, from outside observers. Almost every topic is loaded with emotion, colored with moral and ethical overtones, and influenced by value judgments. Defense policy is certainly no exception, given its preeminent role in protecting the existing political order from the violent unrest of the mid 1980s that so riveted the world's attention. Remaining a detached observer, therefore, is not always an easy task. Indeed, much of what is written reflects either thinly disguised admiration for South Africa's military prowess or, conversely, disdain and outrage.[4]

International Environment

The Republic of South Africa can be characterized as a medium-sized world economic power, a regional military-economic Leviathan, and an international political outcast. With a gross national product of around $70 billion, it ranks about twenty-fifth out of 171 nations and is the only country in sub-Saharan Africa that the World Bank classifies as "upper middle-income." While the gross domestic product (GDP) of sub-Saharan Africa as a whole has fallen every year since 1980 and per capita income is 4 percent below the 1970 level, South Africa experienced an average annual GDP growth rate of 3.6 percent between 1970–1982 and 1.8 percent between 1984–1987. South Africa also accounts for approximately two-thirds of the GNP of southern Africa (south of Zaire and Tanzania), and 90 percent of the energy consumption. It has developed a military and security establishment second to none in the region.[5]

South Africa's relative importance, position, and reputation in the eyes of the world community, however, more precisely stem from two sets of factors. First are matters relating to the historical development of South Africa. Ineluctably, race is the recurrent theme. The ethnic makeup of the society is a legacy of Western European exploration and immigration, the importation or immigration of Asians, and the interaction of these groups with indigenous African cultures. The unfolding of this drama, particularly the black-white dimension, has historically been of varying degrees of interest to the outside world. Since World War II, however, the progressive institutionalization of apartheid has created a series of moral dilemmas for Western governments. This is particularly true of Great Britain, given its role as the former colonial power, and the United States, which tends to view South Africa through the prism of its own history of race relations. Among black Africans, South Africa is important inasmuch as it is perceived as representing the final act of the colonial drama.

The second set of factors that accounts for international interest in South Africa is geostrategic in nature: South Africa's mineral treasure chest; its location at the southern tip of the African continent and control of important sea lanes; and Soviet support of national liberation movements and self-professed Marxist-Leninist regimes in Angola and Mozambique.

Taken together, these racial and geostrategic considerations go a long way toward explaining what can only be described as an international fixation on South Africa, a country that otherwise does not play a particularly important international role. The question of how Western powers should balance these concerns has not been easy to answer and is the source of acrimonious debate. Economic and strategic priorities are understandably on the minds of Western policy makers and academic grand strategists. A failure to address the issue of apartheid, however, could threaten these priorities should a black leadership eventually come to power with the perception that the West had given de facto support to the apartheid regime. However a state may happen to weigh the relative importance of each of these considerations will directly influence the country's policies toward South Africa. This in turn will influence South Africa's relations with the outside world. This section briefly examines each of these sets of factors determining South Africa's international status, if not notoriety, beginning with a discussion of racial issues in the context of the historical development of white domination. This brief overview is crucial in setting the stage for subsequent discussion of threats to South African national security and defense strategies devised to deal with these threats.

HISTORICAL DEVELOPMENT OF WHITE DOMINATION

European settlement in what now constitutes present-day South Africa dates from 1652 and the arrival of a small band of intrepid adventurers employed by the Dutch East India Company.[6] In order to provision the company's ships in transit between Europe and the Far East, a resupply station was established at Table Bay at the Cape of Good Hope. Although the Cape settlement was not originally intended to be a colony, a labor shortage led to the importation of slaves from Angola, East Africa, and the Dutch East Indies. Beginning in 1679 German and Dutch settlers lured by the promise of free farmland began to arrive, and new settlements were formed. The number of Europeans increased after 1688, when Huguenots who had fled persecution in France accepted a Dutch invitation to emigrate to the Cape Colony. As settlers moved inland, an all-too-familiar African scene unfolded. Trekboers, or wandering farmers, clashed with native Africans for control of fertile farm and grazing land. As confrontations in the hinterland increased throughout the eighteenth century, so did the fiercely independent Boers' resentment of the efforts of the Cape administrators to control them.

After 143 years of Dutch rule, Great Britain took command of the Cape Colony in 1806 as a consequence of the Napoleonic wars. Relations between the British and Boers were predictably strained, and they quickly deteriorated even further. In 1807 a ban on the importation of slaves to the British Empire was announced,

and in 1828 a law was passed allowing the Coloured population, working virtually as forced labor, to own its own land and move freely within the colony without passes. In response to such actions and other perceived grievances, the Great Trek began in 1836. Six thousand Boers left the Cape Colony and crossed the Orange River to escape British rule. Some settled in the Natal region, where in 1838 nearly seven hundred men, women, and children were killed in battles with Zulu tribesmen. Seeking revenge, a Boer army under Andries Pretorius routed the Zulus at the Battle of Blood River. In 1847 Natal became a British colony with limited self-government. A similar pattern was repeated to the northwest with the creation of the Orange Free State in 1854 and the South African [Transvaal] Republic in 1855. With the discovery of gold in the Transvaal in 1872 and the growing economic instability of the Boer republic, Britain moved to assert full control in 1877. In 1880–81, the Boers rose in revolt and managed to regain self-government. Intrigues against the Boer republics (often encouraged by British mineowners) worsened relations with London. In 1899 the Transvaal and Orange Free State declared war against Britain. Initial Boer victories turned to defeat by reinforced British troops. To combat guerrilla tactics, the British destroyed Boer farms and herded families into what was at the time an innovation—concentration camps. Some 26,000 women and children died from assorted diseases and malnutrition.

The bloody and vicious war lasted until the Boers surrendered in 1902. In return for local self-government, financial aid, and the continued exclusion of blacks from the electoral process, the colonies agreed to acknowledge the sovereignty of the British king. The passage of the South Africa Act in 1909 by the British Parliament led to the creation of the Union of South Africa the following year. A British governor-general would continue to be appointed by the king, and foreign and defense matters lay in the hands of the British. This situation remained basically intact until 1934, when sovereignty was formally transferred from Westminster to Cape Town.

The South Africa Act also created a political

system legitimating the virtual monopolization of political power by whites. Aside from the Cape, where weak protection was provided for the franchise of the black and Coloured population, non-whites were excluded from the electoral rolls throughout the country. In the 1930s the Cape blacks lost their restricted franchise except for the right to elect three white members to Parliament. Land acts resulted in limiting black ownership to approximately 13 percent of the country's area, and legislation further restricted blacks from entering urban areas by granting local authorities the power to refuse work permits and to implement the forcible return of the unemployed to the reserve lands. These actions, however, did not generate any particular international hue and cry.[7] South Africa's association with Great Britain helped to deflect foreign criticism, as the country was viewed in terms of its incorporation into the British imperial system. Despite the resistance of some Afrikaners, South African military forces participated in both world wars; South African delegates attended the Versailles peace conference; and the country joined the League of Nations. Furthermore, other Western powers were understandably reluctant to raise the issue of the appropriateness of white minority rule, given their own colonial empires. The immediate post–World War II era, however, witnessed a dramatic reversal of South Africa's fortunes in terms of its international standing. The Western world had to come to terms with the demand for the universalization of human rights and national self-determination. Colonialism and white domination were condemned by Asians and Africans utilizing the West's own political vocabulary. After having just fought a world war to defeat a regime trumpeting its racial superiority, the West's close association with South Africa proved something of an embarrassment. This international morality was reflected in the charter of the United Nations. The initial reference to human rights is found in the preamble and was, ironically, drafted by South Africa's prime minister, J. C. Smuts. At the very first session of the UN General Assembly, the issues of South West Africa and the treatment of South Africa's Indian population were discussed. This was an indication of what South Africa could come to expect from such an international forum.

As international opinion moved one way, South Africa's domestic policies moved in the opposite direction. With the coming to power of the National Party in 1948, apartheid emerged as a national ideology and political program of the Afrikaner community.[8] The party addressed the problems of how to suppress potential black challenges, assure a white monopoly of organized political power, and maintain Afrikaner identity. In order to secure the legislative foundation for these goals, gaps in the apartheid structure were filled. With little resistance from the white population as a whole, the Afrikaners drafted legislation to organize relations among the races and construct a bureaucratic apparatus designed to oversee the implementation of the new laws. Important measures prohibited mixed marriages and miscegenation, officially categorized each South African by race, set aside residential areas for each racial group, and in 1952 consolidated and expanded the pass laws that resticted access to white areas.[9]

In 1959, at a time when much of Africa stood on the threshold of independence from its colonial masters, Prime Minister H. F. Verwoerd unveiled a sweeping partition plan that was euphemistically termed "separate development." It was hoped that this policy would not only reinforce white political control, but actually increase South Africa's legitimacy in the eyes of the Western world. The cornerstone was the Bantu Self-Government Act. Cloaked in the guise of supporting black nationalism and political rights, this measure called for the creation of eight (later ten) black homelands that would slowly move toward self-government. Each black person was to be legally assigned to a particular homeland even if he or she had never set foot in these tribal preserves. As each homeland became "self-governing," the residents would no longer be citizens of South Africa but rather citizens of the Transkei, Ciskei, and other newly created "countries."[10] In other words, blacks would no longer be disenfranchised but would rather exercise their political voting rights in the newly created homelands. By this strategy, South Africa hoped to mute international criticism of the disenfranchisement of the black majority. It was to be carried out and justified in the name of equality and self-determination, core values of postwar liberalism.[11]

This massive attempt at social engineering required vigorous implementation of influx controls to the cities, bizarre geographic gerrymandering, attempts to encourage tribal identities by resurrecting historical symbols, forced removal of so-called "black spots" located near white areas, economic subsidization of desolate and unproductive homelands, and the creation of transportation networks designed to allow businesses to tap the underemployed black labor market. By classifying workers as "temporary sojourners," blacks were to be kept out of white living areas.[12] Action was also undertaken to deal with the urban concentration of Coloureds and Asians. Application of the Group Areas Act (1950) led to the destruction of long-established Coloured neighborhoods in Cape Town and displacement of the Asian community in Durban. Justification for such policies was not on the basis of something so crude as white racial superiority. Rather, the government claimed that separate development ensured the cultural integrity of the different races. To avoid a white/non-white definition of the situation, the Afrikaner leadership and associated academics argued that a multiplicity of nations existed within the black population. Hence, there was supposedly not a white minority and black majority, but rather a country consisting solely of minorities. Despite the financial cost to the state and the human cost to non-whites forced to be part of the Afrikaner dream, the development and elaboration of the apartheid system continued into the 1970s.[13]

GEOSTRATEGIC FACTORS AND PERCEIVED THREATS

While South Africa's apartheid system has been the object of virtually universal condemnation, Western countries have felt compelled to weigh the moral repugnance of apartheid against South Africa's economic and strategic importance because of an abundance of key minerals and its geographic location. Soviet inroads in southern Africa in the 1970s heightened these concerns. An important aspect of South Africa's foreign policy has been an attempt to convince the West that geostrategic considerations should outweigh any moral qualms concerning apartheid.[14]

South Africa is the world's fourth largest producer of nonfuel minerals. It controls reserves of eleven of twenty-seven critical minerals and, along with the Soviet Union, is the major producer of gold, diamonds, and four minerals with industrial and military application: chrome, manganese, vanadium, and platinum.[15] (See table 1.)

What gives Western strategic planners nightmares is a scenario in which a hostile black government eventually comes to power and cuts off minerals to the West, perhaps aided and abetted by the Soviet Union. A less threatening, but nevertheless disturbing, scenario would be a situation in which a future South African government joins with the USSR to form a cartel and drive up prices to the point where the economic stability and vitality of the West are threatened. There are at least three reasons, however, why such scenarios are unlikely or, with appropriate action, could be avoided.

First, various mineral statistics are generally estimates of presently known reserves that are mined economically; they do not include undiscovered reserves, which undoubtedly exist, or possible functional substitutes. Furthermore, planning and foresight could considerably reduce the West's vulnerability to a mineral embargo and hence reduce the possibility of it ever occurring in the first place. Despite Western handwringing over events in southern Africa, the Reagan administration in 1985 actually suggested selling off part of the strategic stockpile to reduce the budget deficit. Whether this reflected optimism concerning the future of South Africa or a dismissal of the mineral cut-off scenario is not clear.[16]

Second, a cut-off by a black radical government would be doubtful, as any new regime would surely need the income generated from mining operations. In 1982, for example, the South African mining industry accounted for

Table 1. Western Dependency on South Africa and the U.S.S.R. for Selected Nonfuel Minerals

Mineral	S. African 1984 Production (% of world)	S. African 1984 Reserves (% of world)	Soviet 1984 Production (% of world)	Soviet 1984 Reserves (% of world)	Overall Percentage Dependency on S. Africa		
					U.S. (1982–84)	EEC (1983)	Japan (1983)
Platinum	41.1	79	52.5	19	91	100	95
Chromite	31.6	78.4	31.5	12.2	82	92	99
Manganese	14.6	40.7	36.2	36.5	99	99	95
Vanadium	35.3	19.8	29.6	60.4	41	100	70

Source: U.S. Congress, Subcommittee on Transportation, Aviation and Materials, *The National Critical Materials Act 1984* (Washington, D.C.: U.S. Government Printing Office, 1986), pp. 100, 131, 133.

two-thirds of the country's export earnings.[17] Such income would be particularly imperative if the transition to post-apartheid South Africa were violent and the economic infrastructure were severely damaged by war, if there were a flight of domestic capital, and if foreign investment were withdrawn. The rebuilding of the economy and the elevation of the standard of living for blacks would require enormous expenditure of capital. The case of Angola is instructive in this regard: there a Marxist government has continued highly profitable relations with Western oil companies, whose installations have been protected by Cuban troops.

Finally, it is questionable whether Moscow would even suggest that a radical South African government cut off strategic minerals to the West. Owing to the Soviet Union's own domestic economic difficulties, it has been unwilling to bankroll Third World client states, with the exception of Cuba and Vietnam. Soviet advice to "states of socialist orientation" has been to maintain economic relations with the West, not to sever them. Similarly, the Soviet Union itself must operate within the world capitalist system, and hence international economic stability and a West willing to provide high technology also work to Moscow's advantage. Blackmailing advanced capitalist states would undoubtedly lead to a severe and unwanted backlash. Furthermore, despite the hostility between South Africa and the Soviet Union and the South African portrayal of Moscow as the supreme threat, the Anglo-American Corporation and De Beers of South Africa have enjoyed a highly profitable, though unpublicized, arrangement with the

USSR dating back to the late 1950s. In order to dominate the world market, De Beers purchases Soviet diamonds to the tune of $600–$700 million annually. Although the USSR could destroy the South African-controlled diamond market and damage the South African economy, De Beers officials doubt it would wish to end such a profitable relationship.[18]

If one wishes to engage in apocalyptic speculation, a more likely scenario, albeit lacking Soviet machinations, would involve South Africa slowly descending into civil war. As political and economic chaos spread, the flow of raw materials could be interrupted either by work stoppages in the mines or sabotage of the railways linking the mineral deposits in the interior to the shipping ports on the coast. Alternatively, severe international sanctions might lead to an embargo of raw material exports on the part of the South African government as it defiantly prepares for a modern-day version of the Battle of Blood River.

As for the Cape route, its importance is due to the number of ships, volume of goods, and types of commodities that transit through the sea lanes. In 1983, for example, 3,257 ships used the Cape route, including oil tankers too large for the Suez Canal. These tankers carry 60 percent of Western Europe's and 20 percent of U.S. oil requirements.[19] Furthermore, approximately 70 percent of NATO's strategic raw materials travel around the Cape.[20]

The importance of the Cape route is acknowledged by all. What is subject to debate are Soviet intentions. Let us reexamine the scenario in which a pro-Soviet regime comes to power in South Africa and grants Moscow naval installations. Is it realistic to expect that the

USSR would interdict oil tanker traffic? Most analysts agree this is highly improbable if for no other reason than such an action could conceivably precipitate World War III. Let us assume, however, that the USSR is dedicated to preventing oil from reaching the West. The question then becomes, is mounting a naval blockade from South African ports the most efficient means? Hardly. A better policy would be to bomb, sabotage, or occupy the oil fields in the Persian Gulf or interdict the tankers at the Strait of Hormuz. Furthermore, it is unlikely the Soviet Union in the first place would maintain a large naval contingent in the southern African region when the Soviet navy's primary function is defense of the homeland and counteracting the threat posed by U.S. carrier task forces and submarines. Finally, if war did break out, Soviet vessels and facilities would naturally be targets for NATO forces. Not only would African states undoubtedly wish to avoid the extension of a NATO/Warsaw Pact conflict to their homelands, there is also the likelihood that Western forces would sweep the Soviet Navy from the seas in short order.[21] Nevertheless, Western strategic planners are compelled to consider worst case analyses when dealing with mineral and Cape route questions, particularly since the collapse of Portuguese rule and the establishment of Marxist-Leninist regimes in Angola and Mozambique.

Since the rise to power of the National Party, white South Africa[22] has been concerned with four perceived threats—potential or actual—to its national security: internal disturbances, a direct conventional attack from hostile neighbors, guerrilla warfare, and international sanctions. Over the years, the perception of which threat or combination of threats is most dangerous has varied depending upon changing domestic and international circumstances. Three time periods can be discerned.

1948–1960. Internal security was the primary concern during the postwar period as the National Party moved to expand apartheid. Due to black unrest, three successive governments emphasized that the Defence Force's primary responsibility was to help maintain internal security in conjunction with the police.[23] With an increase in black protest throughout the 1950s, stronger security laws were passed. Externally, there was no immediate security fear. But with the rising tide of black African nationalism, the government engaged in preventive diplomacy by attempting to lure Western powers into a formal defense pact with South Africa. In 1951, for example, South Africa suggested the creation of an African Defence Organization as an extension of NATO. The suggestion was not pursued by NATO members. The best Pretoria could do was the Simonstown Agreement with Great Britain in 1955. Although South Africa assumed official control of the British naval base, Britain was to be granted access to it in the event of war. The agreement, terminated in 1975, also resulted in joint South African-British naval exercises and British arms sales.[24]

1960–1974. In the township of Sharpeville on 21 March 1960, police fired on a crowd of blacks protesting the pass laws, killing 69 and wounding 180. From that day forward internal security became an even higher priority for the Afrikaner government. Two organizations deemed a threat to national security were subsequently banned—the African National Congress (ANC), and the Pan Africanist Congress (PAC). A state of emergency was declared, 11,000 persons detained, and harsher security laws passed. Defense expenditure rose from 1 percent of GNP in 1960 to 2.4 percent of GNP by the end of the decade.[25]

Founded in 1912, the African National Congress developed into a mass organization by the 1940s. The ANC originally preached nonviolence and attempted to work within the system. As individuals such as Nelson Mandela and Oliver Tambo rose to prominence, they urged a more militant approach involving civil disobedience while still favoring nonviolent, nonrevolutionary change. With its banning in 1960, the ANC went underground and came to accept the necessity of using violence to achieve the end of white minority rule. Even so, its violence has basically been directed against property, occasionally against the police and military, and rarely against civilians. Its military wing, Umkonto we Sizwe, was founded in 1961. Some of its more spectacular actions included the bombing of Sasol, South Africa's

oil-from-coal refinery, in June 1980, the bombing of the Koeberg nuclear power station in
December 1982, and a car bomb explosion
outside air force headquarters in Pretoria in
May 1983. This latter action killed seventeen
and injured more than two hundred persons.
In the summer of 1986, however, the ANC announced it could no longer guarantee the
safety of "soft targets" and warned it would
"bring the battle to the white areas." ANC political headquarters are located in Zambia,
with other representatives elsewhere in southern Africa, in Europe, and in North America.
Training camps are located in Angola and Tanzania; refugee camps in Botswana and Tanzania. Estimates of the ANC's strength vary,
ranging from 2,000 to 10,000, but such numbers do not capture the breadth of support and
sympathy for the ANC within South Africa.[26]

It is subject to dispute as to how much influence the South African Communist Party
(SACP) has in the ANC. Founded in 1921,
banned in 1950, and reformed in 1953, the
SACP is pro-Soviet and it is estimated that ten
of its members sit on the ANC's thirty-member
national executive committee.[27] The ANC dis-
misses the South African charge that the ANC
is equivalent to the SACP, that the ANC is a
front organization of the SACP, or is even dominated by the SACP. The ANC leadership emphasizes the common opposition of the two
groups to apartheid and repression. Nevertheless, over the years the role of the SACP has
caused some discontent within the ANC not to
mention Western governments. Analysts generally agree that black nationalists—not communists—dominate the organization. The Soviet connection to the ANC is basically one of
convenience. It is estimated that Moscow provides 90 percent of the ANC's weaponry and
channels approximately $80 million a year to
the ANC.[28] ANC officials argue that they will
accept aid from any country willing to provide
it and that the organization's reliance on Moscow is a function of Western countries being
less than forthcoming in the provision of aid.

The Pan Africanist Congress was formed in
1959 by blacks who disapproved of the multiracial approach to political power as pursued
by the ANC and other organizations. Its mili-

tary wing Poqo (Xhosa for "alone" or "pure")
occasionally attacks installations, and it was a
PAC campaign against the pass laws that led to
the events in Sharpeville.[29]

During this time period domestic concerns
were matched by consternation over a number
of regional and international events: further
decolonization of the continent, South Africa's
exiting the British Commonwealth in 1961, a
U. N. resolution calling for the breaking of
diplomatic ties with Pretoria, and growing
Western criticism of apartheid. The policy response was a rapid buildup of the South African Defense Force (SADF) in anticipation of
future challenges. The goal was less to deter a
conventional military threat (a remote possibility) than to handle anticipated guerrilla operations. The Permanent Force expanded from
9,000 to 15,000 between 1960 and 1964, and
the number of individuals undergoing military
training in 1964 was ten times the number in
1960. Military equipment was modernized and
arms expenditures dramatically increased,
and a program to achieve virtual self-sufficiency in weapons was instituted.[30]

By the late 1960s South Africa felt confident
it would be able to handle all perceived internal and external military threats. In order to
reduce further the possibility of guerrilla raids
being staged from regional bases, the "outward policy" of Prime Minister B. J. Vorster
emphasized increased aid and trade with
southern African states, enticing them while
holding the military option in reserve. It was
also hoped that such a policy would improve
South Africa's image in the eyes of the West.
The more benign dimension of the outward
policy, however, was counterbalanced by selective political-military intervention in Lesotho
and military assistance to Rhodesia and the colonial regimes in Angola and Mozambique.[31]

1974–Present. A military coup in Lisbon in
April 1974 was a watershed event, as it led to
the collapse of the Portuguese empire and set
in motion a train of events that brought to
power hostile governments in Angola and Mozambique, opened the door to an expansion of
Soviet and Cuban influence in the region, and
provided havens for the ANC and the Southwest African People's Organization (SWAPO),

Table 2. South African Defense Vote: The Decade of the 1960s

Financial Year	Defense Vote (millions of rand)	As Percentage of Budget	As Percentage of GNP	Percentage Increase over Previous Year
1960/61	44	6.6	0.9	
1961/62	61	10.0	—	38
1962/63	120	—	—	96
1963/64	120	—	—	0
1964/65	230	21.0	—	92
1965/66	219	—	—	—
1966/67	248	19.0	—	13
1967/68	256	—	—	3
1968/69	252	16.1	2.5	—
1969/70	272	16.8	2.4	8

Source: Robert S. Jaster, *South Africa's Narrowing Security Options*, Adelphi Papers, no. 159 (London: International Institute for Strategic Studies, 1980), p. 16.

which for years has sought the independence of South African–controlled Namibia. Following the Portuguese coup, three rival Angolan factions agreed in January 1975 to the formation of an interim government, with a formal transfer of authority in November. The agreement soon collapsed and fighting broke out. In March the Soviet Union stepped up its aid to the Marxist MPLA, and two months later Cuban advisers arrived. In August there was a limited South African incursion into southern Angola, followed by a major SADF operation beginning in October. Lacking Western support and meeting stiff Cuban and MPLA resistance, South Africa eventually withdrew the last of its forces in March of the following year. By that time the MPLA had consolidated control with the help of 12,000 Cuban troops.[32]

Closer to home, South African support for Rhodesia failed to prevent the collapse of white minority rule in 1979. Throughout the 1960s ZANU and ZAPU, two guerrilla organizations, grew in strength. A Rhodesian plan to create a moderate, yet unrepresentative, black government was rejected by the national liberation movements as well as Western governments. As a result of the Lancaster House agreement of November 1980, power was officially handed over to the black nationalist leadership. Robert Mugabe, a long-time opponent of white minority rule, was elected president.[33]

During this same time period the all-important domestic security situation began to unravel. Some of the most serious disturbances

occurred in Johannesburg's black satellite city, Soweto, in 1976. What began as a student protest against inferior black schooling exploded into ten months of violence. Soweto has since become, like Sharpeville, an important symbol of black resistance. While whites were not overly disturbed by Sharpeville, Soweto caused more than a little unease. It also led to the imposition of a mandatory UN arms embargo in 1977.

The 1970s also witnessed the emergence of the Black Consciousness Movement. Its charismatic leader, Steve Biko, argued that before organizational and strategic issues were to be addressed, blacks must free themselves from inferiority complexes stemming from years of oppression and paternalism. Biko died in police custody in 1977, and the movement was banned the same year. The Azanian People's Organization (AZAPO) and the Pan Africanist Congress (PAC) are representative of the black nationalist perspective. Founded in 1978, AZAPO has encouraged political involvement on the part of the black working class, while the PAC favors armed stuggle.[34]

One of the most important developments in recent years has been the establishment of independent black trade unions in 1977. Initially nonpolitical, cautious, and primarily concerned with wage and working conditions, the unions became increasingly politically assertive. In November 1984 a two-day general strike was called in support of township grievances. It was the largest political strike by blacks in South African history. In December of the following year, the newly formed Congress of South African Trade Unions, (COSATU), 500,000 strong, pledged to use its strike power to end the pass laws and emergency rule. Over a million and a half blacks staged a one-day strike in May 1986. The mere existence of so many groups, movements, and organizations illustrates the breadth of opposition to white minority rule. The wide variety, however, also reflects divisions among the opposition, and the government has worked assiduously to encourage these fissures as part of its divide-and-rule strategy.[35]

Not all internal threats to security, however, can be reduced by simply jailing leaders of the black community, banning organizations, and crushing demonstrations. Of particular concern to the authorities has been the rise of seemingly spontaneous violence in townships and homelands that cannot be traced to subversive organizations or outside agitators. Beginning in the summer of 1984, widespread violence in the townships, sparked by school boycotts and rent hikes, led to a strong government response. Over the next two years, at least 1,600 persons died as a result of civil strife. In June 1986 a state of emergency was declared in anticipation of the tenth anniversary of the Soweto uprising. In December the emergency decree was tightened to outlaw virtually all forms of political expression. The number of individuals arrested over the previous six months totaled 22,000. That same year a number of Western countries moved to implement limited sanctions and companies began to pull out of South Africa.

As noted, the genesis of such threats can, ironically, be directly traced to Afrikaner policies designed to maintain white minority rule. The South African government's perception of the source of these threats is quite different, however, and has been consistently detailed in official speeches and government publications. The first line of the 1984 *White Paper on Defence and Armaments Supply* succinctly states the basic proposition: "The major threat to world peace remains the USSR's pursuit of world domination." Through a variety of means the USSR is attempting to undermine South Africa in order eventually to control the

country's natural resources. Moscow is therefore engaged in the purposeful pursuit of "the consolidation of its influence in certain states in Southern Africa" and utilizes Third World countries and national liberation movements for its own purposes.[36] The threat is not seen in terms of direct military confrontations involving major pitched battles. It is more indirect and sinister and involves a "total onslaught" consisting of a variety of techniques utilized by the state's enemies to erode South Africa's security through a persistent war of attrition:

Indirect action in the form of a revolutionary onslaught serves to establish Soviet influence in Southern Africa. The South African Communist Party (SACP) and the African National Congress (ANC), which, for all practical purposes, has been integrated with the SACP and acts as its military wing, are the major elements of the Soviet plan to obtain control of the RSA. SWAPO plays a similar role in Southwest Africa (SWA) in the achievement of Soviet objectives in that region. Several worldwide and regional organizations, of which the United Nations (UN) and the Organization for African Unity (OAU) are the most important, also lend themselves to furthering USSR objectives in Southern Africa by joining the propaganda onslaught against the RSA.[37]

Many outside observers tend to ridicule this analysis, characterizing it as simplistic, distorted, and self-serving. The official government view resurrects the idea of a monolithic communist movement controlled by Moscow whose master plan is carried out by an assorted array of allies, dupes, and subversive forces. South Africa, of course, is hardly the first country to adopt such a perspective. While one may question the validity of such an analysis and even find South African officials who find it overstated, what is important is the fact that such a perception exists in the minds of a significant segment of Afrikaner officialdom. And it is the perception of reality rather than reality itself upon which action is based. Furthermore, there is a tactical utility in laying South Africa's internal and regional security problems at Moscow's doorstep. First, it allows the National Party to pose as the guarantor of white survival, fending off a communist-directed black onslaught. Second, if Western powers accept the logic of the Soviet-directed "total onslaught," Pretoria hopes the West will be less critical of South Africa's domestic and regional policies. To date the West has generally rejected this linkage, voicing concern over Soviet activity in the region but arguing that it is the lack of domestic political reform and Pretoria's military actions against its neighbors that have improved Moscow's standing in southern Africa.[38]

National Objectives, National Strategy, and Military Doctrine

THE TOTAL NATIONAL STRATEGY

Long-term defense, foreign, and domestic objectives correspond to the perceived threats outlined in the previous section: gain Western acceptance of, or at least acquiescence toward, South Africa's domestic policies; create a band of compliant neighboring states in southern Africa; and maintain control over the evolution of South Africa's domestic order.[39]

With the rise of a perceived "total onslaught" in the mid 1970s, the government responded with a call for a "Total National Strategy" (TNS) designed to defend fortress South Africa. The fullest expression of this strategy is to be found in the 1977 *White Paper on Defence.* TNS is described, rather tortuously, as "the comprehensive plan to utilize all the means available to a state according to an integrated pattern in order to achieve the national aims within the framework of the specific policies. A total national strategy is, therefore, not confined to a particular sphere, but is applicable at all levels and to all functions of the state structure."[40] Basic components are political, economic, psychological, technological, and military; all call for coordinated governmental and nongovernmental action in defense of South Africa's national security. As stated in the White Paper, "The defence of the RSA is not solely the responsibility of the Department of Defence. On the contrary, the maintenance of the sovereignty of the RSA is the combined responsibility of all governmental departments . . . and the responsibility of the entire population."[41] TNS identifies the threats to national security, purports to explain their genesis and interdependent nature, and, most important, provides guidance as to the most appropriate response. Impressive as this might sound, in

reality the policy is not quite as integrated as the government claims. Nevertheless, TNS serves as an effective metaphor and is designed to mobilize public support for government programs.[42]

The Total National Strategy, according to Philip Frankel, is a "formulation blending peculiarly South African conceptions of the social and political world with a variety drawn from imported foreign sources."[43] Key among the latter are works analyzing the counterrevolutionary experiences of the United States in Vietnam, the British in Malaya, and the French in Algeria and Indochina. South African strategists have also extensively analyzed the eight-year-long Rhodesian war and are particularly impressed with how Israel has dealt with the Palestine Liberation Organization (PLO). The writings that have had the single biggest impact on the thinking of South Africa's national security establishment are those by two Frenchmen, Roger Trinquier (especially his analysis of the Algerian War) and General André Beaufre. Beaufre's works are standard material assigned at the Joint Defence College attended by South Africa's military elite and hence are deserving of some comment.[44]

Beaufre's strategic view is based on four underlying assumptions. First, following Clausewitz, strategy is "the art of applying force so that it makes the most effective contribution towards achieving the ends set by political policy."[45] Second, strategy, warfare, and social conflict should be viewed in the context of a fundamental clash of wills. Priority should be placed upon the psychological defeat of the enemy as a precondition to material defeat. Third, war in the contemporary age is all-encompassing in nature. In an increasingly interdependent world, political, military, economic, and ideological warfare requires an appropriately integrated strategic response. Military strategy and tactics must be effectively wedded to nonmilitary components of what Beaufre terms a "total strategy."[46] Fourth, the distinction between war and peace has become blurred. Direct confrontation of military forces is only one type of warfare. The world is increasingly witnessing indirect warfare, as exemplified by insurgencies, guerrilla campaigns, and wars of national liberation. It becomes difficult to distinguish internal threats from external threats. Indirect warfare requires an indirect strategy in response. This means that the actual surrender of the enemy due to military defeat is not necessarily the goal. Rather, military actions should be designed to suggest to the enemy that "he should consider as a possible compromise a solution which accords with our political objectives."[47] In the final analysis, according to Beaufre, it is the "moral disintegration of the enemy" that "causes him to accept the conditions it is desired to impose upon him."[48] Similarly, the public must understand the multidimensional nature of threats to national security and be psychologically prepared for the encounter with the enemy. This requires the development of a coherent and well-reasoned ideology attuned to the emotions of the public at large. In dealing with the enemy as well as one's own people, therefore, correct political and psychological analyses are integral parts of the total strategy.

Beaufre's analysis struck a responsive chord in South Africa, particularly his emphasis on insurgent challenges to state authority and the necessity of an integrated response. The driving forces behind the articulation, formulation, and implementation of South Africa's Total National Strategy were Pieter W. Botha and Gen. Magnus Malan, respectively minister of defense and chief of the SADF at the time the 1977 White Paper was written. The following year Botha became prime minister and Malan was named minister of defense.

The most immediate reflection of the TNS was to be found in defense policy and military doctrine. Policies were designed to: improve self-sufficiency in the production of arms; prepare for effective counter-insurgency warfare; enhance conventional capability and increase manpower; support the South African police in the maintenance of internal order; maintain and further develop an efficient intelligence network; and improve operational capability not only within South Africa but also in neighboring states.[49]

To accomplish these goals, a five-year expansion of the Defence Force was approved in

1974. Defense expenditures rose from $933 million in 1974–75 to $2.9 billion in 1979–80. Compulsory military service was extended from twelve to twenty-four months, the total size of all components of the SADF almost doubled from 270,000 to 500,000 between 1974–80, and in 1980 a decision was made to create a South West Africa Territory Force (SWATF). Border security was improved by providing financial incentives to white farmers to move into vulnerable areas and tie them into the Military Area Network (MARNET) to reduce SADF reaction time to cross-border incursions. Spurred on by a 1977 mandatory UN arms embargo, Armscor, the state-run arms agency, dramatically expanded. By the end of the 1970s, Armscor had a budget of over $1 billion, employed 19,000 persons, and utilized 800 contractors.[50]

What has been the public reaction to governmental statements on the Total Onslaught and the Total National Strategy? Does white South Africa believe the government has overstated the extent of the threat and what is required to deal with it? Apparently not. In 1982 a public opinion poll of white South Africans indicated that 80 percent disagreed with the statement that "the Communist threat against the country is exaggerated by the government." Within the Afrikaner community, almost 87 percent disagreed. This same survey also found widespread support for South Africa's policy of regional destabilization: 81 percent agreed that "South Africa should militarily attack terrorists based in neighbouring states," including 86 percent of the members of the Afrikaner-based National Party.[51] The government had obviously made a convincing case in the minds of most white South Africans.

NUCLEAR WEAPONS

Conspicuously absent from official government publications is any discussion of South Africa's nuclear potential. There is a general consensus that South Africa has the capability to design, produce, and deliver a nuclear device. Rich in uranium, South Africa was encouraged by the United States and Great Britain in the postwar period to develop uranium-processing facilities. The United

States in particular allowed access to nuclear technology that aided in the construction of a research reactor. By the mid 1970s, South Africa accounted for almost 14 percent of the uranium output of noncommunist countries.[52] U.S. suspension in 1977 of an agreement to provide low-enriched uranium for two reactors under construction near Cape Town has delayed South Africa's development of a major enrichment facility, which would be necessary to produce weapons-grade fuel. What had caught the attention of foreign governments in 1977 was the discovery by Soviet and U.S. satellites of what appeared to be preparations for a nuclear test in the Kalahari desert. Then in September 1979 a U.S. satellite detected a double flash of light in the South Atlantic, generally indicative of an atmospheric nuclear test. Suspicion has been further increased inasmuch as South Africa has not allowed international inspections of the Valindaba and Pelindaba facilities nor has Pretoria seriously considered signing the Treaty on the Non-Proliferation of Nuclear Weapons. While South African political leaders have been coy on the subject of whether or not they have developed a nuclear capability, military leaders have stated the country is prepared to manufacture nuclear arms if necessary.[53]

Assuming a tactical weapon exists, potential nuclear force employment doctrine is subject to speculation. Nuclear threats and blackmail are unlikely to deter insurgents and it is hard to imagine weapons being used to control domestic disturbances in townships. If, however, the South African leadership is convinced of the possibility of a future conventional onslaught supported and armed by the Soviet Union, a nuclear weapon may perform deterrent and defense functions. It has been suggested that if the survival of white South Africa is threatened, the government might explode a weapon in a remote location as a warning device or even to destroy targets in neighboring states to force the halt of a conventional attack.[54] Within South Africa, a tactical weapon could possibly be used against a concentration of conventional forces threatening major cities.[55] Aside from the possible military utility, one should not underestimate what the possession

of such weapons would mean to the morale, confidence, and resolve of the white South African public.[56] Finally, by keeping the world guessing as to the current status of South Africa's nuclear weapon program, the government may hope to increase its diplomatic leverage with the West, which may be afraid to push the Afrikaners into a corner.

CONVENTIONAL CAPABILITY

According to the 1957 Defence Act, the South African Defence Force is to defend against (1) foreign attack and (2) domestic unrest; (3) preserve life and property; and (4) assist the police in maintaining internal order. Toward these ends, the SADF is composed of a Permanent Force, National Service component, Citizen Force, and Commandos. The Permanent Force consists of the army, air force, navy, medical services, and support institutions. In the late 1980s, the Permanent Force and conscripts totalled 97,000 members.[57] One way to look at the SADF in terms of type of service and available manpower is by distinguishing between the full-time and part-time components: the full-time component (31.9 percent) is comprised of Permanent Force, 9.1 percent (careerists); National Servicemen, 15.6 percent (conscripts); Service Volunteers, 1 percent (white females volunteering one year's continuous service and Coloured and Indian males who voluntarily render continuous service); Auxiliary Service, 1.1 percent (noncombatant males of all population groups); and Civilians, 5.1 percent. The part-time component (68.1 percent) is comprised of a Citizen Force, 47.2 percent, and a Commando Force, 20.9 percent.[58] Even these figures are slightly misleading in that if one compares the number of days per year actually served, the full-time component accounts for 87 percent of service actually rendered and the part-time component only 13 percent after adjusting for deferments and financial constraints.

After fulfilling the national service obligation, an individual becomes a member of the Citizen Force for twelve years (720 days in uniform), the Active Citizen Force Reserve for five years, and then the Commando Force and Citizen Reserves until age sixty-five (the latter three reserve elements are called up only in the event of emergencies). The Citizen Force is well-equipped and highly trained. Its primary roles are: (1) employment in counter-insurgency operations, traditionally in Namibia, or when the full-time force requires assistance and (2) employment during conventional and semiconventional conflicts. As the calling up of Citizen Force units is disruptive of economic productivity, the actual number of days served in recent years has not reached the statutory limit.[59]

After completion of the two-year obligation, one may go directly into the Commandos. This is particularly encouraged if one lives in outlying rural areas, as Commando units play home defense, anti-insurgency, and anti-infiltration roles in remote and border areas. They have become increasingly important as South Africa experiences continual urbanization and the abandonment of white farms along certain stretches of the border. Commandos are also assigned to protect "key national points" such as power plants and command centers.[60]

The overall structure, ethos, and military doctrine of the SADF is a result of commando, citizen army, and British military traditions and the nature of the threats facing South Africa. In the past ten years military doctrine has been adjusted to take into account the changing security situation within South Africa and the region.

The South African Army, little more than a home militia in 1960, is assigned three basic tasks: (1) conventional operations involving use of ground units supported by paratroops and air cover; (2) counterinsurgency operations involving cross-border attacks into "Frontline states" against SWAPO and ANC bases, supply depots, and logistic routes; (black African states in the "front line" against South Africa include Angola, Botswana, Mozambique, Tanzania, Zimbabwe, and Zambia); (3) border area protection involving regular army units and Commando forces designed to curtail infiltration. In the 1986 *White Paper*, the role of the army in quelling township disturbances was prominently featured and justified in a somewhat defensive tone. Army commanders were reportedly less than enthusiastic about utilizing their troops in such a manner, particularly in conjuction with the often undisciplined and brutal South African Police (SAP).[61]

The Army is organized into ten regional territorial commands plus Walvis Bay in Namibia. Its structure and force deployment reflects the internal and cross-border counterinsurgency roles and the need to be prepared for possible conventional confrontations. Due to extended borders and a long coastline, army doctrine stresses area defense as opposed to operating along a front, mobility necessitated by territorial expanse, and the need for fast, hard-hitting, preemptive operations. Two divisions, consisting of armored and semimechanized brigades, are backed by a parachute brigade. The latter is an elite force used in quick strikes against targets in Frontline states and also in counterinsurgency operations. In September 1984 the SADF held its largest military exercise since World War II, Operation Thunder Chariot, which involved 11,000 troops and simulated the repulsion of a conventional attack originating from Namibia.

In 1972 the Reconnaissance Commandos (Recce) organization was established. It has been variously compared to the U.S. Green Berets, British Special Air Service, and the Rhodesian Selous Scouts. The Commandos are tasked with destroying strategic targets such as weapons stores and communications facilities, and creating chaos behind enemy lines. It has been reported that a number of foreigners have been recruited for the Commandos. After the victory of the Patriotic Front in the 1980 Zimbabwean elections, South Africa began to recruit Rhodesian forces. Almost the entire Rhodesian Light Infantry supposedly joined, as did officers from the Selous Scouts. In the November 1981 mercenary attack on the Seychelles, South African military men and mercenaries from Britain, the United States, and other countries were utilized. These foreigners either were (or had been) in the Commandos or regular SADF units.[62]

The South African Air Force (SAAF) is the most effective in Africa despite aging aircraft resulting from the international arms embargo. It seeks to maintain air superiority and plays a critical role in providing close air support for army operations. Army mobility is enhanced by the utilization of air force helicopter squadrons which, despite a shortage, have been important to the success of cross-border operations in southern Angola. Deep interdiction of enemy ground forces is a low priority in low-intensity warfare. Even in the case of Angola, the SAAF has been reluctant to test Soviet-built and supplied surface-to-air missiles (SAMs) and MiG-23s. Indeed, the buildup of sophisticated air defense systems and combat aircraft in neighboring states has been a primary SADF concern for more than a decade.[63] While coastal reconnaissance remains a prime air force function, protection of sea lanes is no longer an objective given the growing obsolescence of long-range Shackleton reconnaissance aircraft and South African reaction to increased Western hostility.[64] SAAF pilots are quite skilled given the fact that they must be extremely careful in training exercises because of the difficulty in replacing aircraft. To increase performance, current jet inventories are basically retooled and modernized.

The South African Navy is essentially designed to protect the 1,500 mile coastline. An earlier blue water capability has all but disappeared. Although lacking maritime air support, it is still the regional power. Patrol craft, armed with Israeli-designed missiles, are important to coastal defense.[65] In 1979 a marine brigade was established primarily for harbor and base protection, reflecting growing concern over insurgency and sabotage.[66] Nine protection unit headquarters have been established, each provided with marine combat units, harbor patrol boats, diving teams, and ordnance disposal teams. As in the case of the army, marine units have been deployed in support of the South African Police in the Western Cape to quell disturbances in recent years.[67]

Simonstown, originally a major British Royal Navy base, has been enlarged and modernized since the mid 1970s. It has been described by P. W. Botha as "the most modern and best equipped naval harbor in the sea area bounded by South Africa, Australia, and the Mediterranean."[68] The harbor can now service all types of ships except the largest U.S. carriers, and overhauls can be undertaken of all submarines and ships up to the destroyer class. A second dockyard now exists owing to expansion work at Salisbury Island in Durban harbor. Given the modest needs of the South African Navy, the expansions were principally undertaken to encourage Western powers to reconsider South Africa's military and strategic significance during a time when the Soviet Union was gradually creating a permanent naval presence in the South Atlantic. Furthermore, following the passage of the 1963 United Nations Security Council arms embargo resolution, South Africa once again lobbied NATO for the creation of a South Atlantic Treaty Organization (SATO), emphasizing the necessity of protecting the sea lanes. While this suggestion was rejected, informal links reportedly exist between NATO and South Africa. A military surveillance center designed to monitor ship and aircraft traffic was built at Silvermine (near Cape Town) and opened in 1973.

With the closing of the Suez canal in 1967, monitoring the increased Soviet ship activity around the Cape became a priority. The radar, computer, and communications equipment was provided by West German, British, Ameri-

---

Table 3. The South African Defense Force

Total Armed Forces
   Regular: 97,000 (67,900 conscripts)
   Term of service: 24 months

Reserves: 325,000
   Army: 146,000, Navy: 2,000; Air Force: 27,000

Army: 75,000; Regulars: 19,900 (12,000 white, 54,000 black and Coloured, 2,500 women)
   National Service: 55,000
   11 territorial commands
   1 corps headquarters, 1 armored division hq, 1 infantry division hq

Navy: 9,000, including 900 marines, 4,500 conscripts
   Commands: Cape Town and Durban
   Bases: Simonstown and Durban

Air Force: 13,000 (2,400 conscripts)
   3 territorial commands
   Training, tactical support, and logistic commands

Medical Corps: 8,000

South West Africa Territorial Force (SWATF): 22,000
   Conscription: 24 months (all races), selective, with Citizen Force (reserve) commitment

Source: International Institute for Strategic Studies, *The Military Balance, 1987–1988* (London: IISS, 1987).

can, French, and Danish companies. Silvermine is reportedly linked to the U.S. naval base in San Juan, Puerto Rico, the Royal Navy in Britain, and also Argentina, Australia, and New Zealand. Its monitoring capabilities supposedly extend north to the Tropic of Cancer and as far as Bangladesh, the Antarctic, and South America.[69]

SWATF. In 1980 South Africa announced the creation of the South West Africa Territory Force (SWATF). Officially, SWATF is meant to be the basis of Namibia's own defense force following independence. It also, however, reduces manpower commitments on the part of the SADF and serves to bolster South African-backed political parties. SWATF is basically a land force designed, according to the Ministry of Defence, "to discourage or repulse semiconventional or insurgency attacks."[70] In 1981, because of manpower shortages, it became mandatory for all Namibian population groups, black and white, to register for military service. By 1985, 51 percent of all soldiers deployed in operational areas (basically in the north) were members of SWATF.

A South West Africa Military School offers leadership courses, but armor, artillery, and parachute training is provided by the SADF. Financial constraints have hampered expansion of SWATF and the building of facilities. Furthermore, as 40 percent of white high school graduates leave Namibia, there are problems in finding qualified leadership material, and hence the SADF traditionally has taken the lead in cross-border and counterinsurgency operations. The SADF also has been engaged in a Civic Action program in which teachers and agricultural experts have been sent to Namibia. The program hopes to win the hearts and minds of locals, but it also has been a way to introduce military forces into various areas and collect intelligence. Following the December 1988 agreement among South Africa, Cuba, and Angola on Namibia's UN-supervised transition to independence, SWATF's future is uncertain.[71]

Police. As the threats to South African national security are as much domestic as international, the South African Police (SAP) is an important component of the defense establishment. The SAP is a semimilitary organization with three branches: uniform, detective, and security. Like the gendarmes in France, it is a national force and distinct from the municipal police. As opposed to the SADF, the SAP has always relied heavily on non-white recruitment to fill the lower ranks. In 1986 the police numbered approximately 45,000, of which about half were non-white. The government's goal for the 1990s is to increase the size of the national police force to 87,000. In 1987 the police budget was increased by fifty percent. Six thousand blacks belong to township police forces, and there are also two reserve forces.[72] The Police Reserve consists of over 15,000 former SAP members who are called up in emergencies. The Reserve Police is a voluntary citizen force made up of people with prior police or military experience. Numbering over 21,000, they assist the SAP by doing routine work and allowing the full-time force to engage in more important activities. In all, the SAP can mobilize over 80,000 persons in the regular and reserve forces during emergencies. In 1986 the government ordered the recruitment of new black police auxiliaries to help control the townships. Aside from aiding regular security forces, the auxiliaries have contributed to conflict between blacks of opposing allegiances.[73]

Prior to the mid 1970s, the SAP played a key counterinsurgency role, being involved in operations not only within South Africa but also in Namibia against SWAPO and in Rhodesia against ZAPU, ZANU, and the ANC. Although the SAP is still active along South Africa's borders, the SADF now handles the major counterinsurgency operations. The Police Amendment Act of 1979 created a border zone of one to ten miles within which the police may conduct warrantless searches of people and property. The SAP was active in suppressing the 1976–77 Soweto uprisings. It was also highly visible during the nationwide disturbances that began in 1984, earning a reputation for brutality and lack of discipline in the townships.[74] The Security Police is also subject to much criticism for allegedly practicing torture and violating human rights. South Africa's myriad of security laws gives the organization broad powers in terms of investigation and interrogation. Between 1963 and 1982, forty-five persons died in the custody of the Security Police, the best known being Steve Biko (head of the Black Consciousness movement) in 1977.[75]

Intelligence Services. Aside from the Security Police, there are two other important organizations engaged in intelligence work: the National Intelligence Service (NIS) and the Department of Military Intelligence (DMI). The evolution of the NIS has been particularly stormy. Its genesis can be traced back to a clandestine organization known as Republican Intelligence formed in the early 1960s. Designed to counter internal resistance movements and help relieve the intelligence burden on the police, it was publicly reconstructed as the infamous Bureau of State Security (BOSS) in 1969 and given the responsibility of supervising military intelligence and internal security operations. The Security Police and DMI were fiercely hostile toward BOSS, both fearing it would further encroach on their respective territories. This is exactly what BOSS attempted to do, given its mandate to investigate "all matters affecting state security."[76] When the Head of BOSS, Hendrik van den Bergh, was appointed security adviser to his old friend Prime Minister Vorster, P. W. Botha, minister of defence at the time, worked to protect DMI's status and mission. Over the years BOSS engaged in all sorts of dirty tricks and high-handedness, including spying on and harassing anti-apartheid groups in London.[77] Van den Bergh was eventually brought down in 1978, in part due to the "Information Scandal."[78] As Botha increased his own power (he became prime minister in 1978), DMI's fortunes rose at the expense of BOSS. That same year BOSS was reorganized and renamed the Department of National Security (DONS), another unfortunate acronym ("opdons" in Afrikaans means "beat up"). Botha assumed the portfolio for intelligence, named a young political science professor the head of DONS, and integrated SADF intelligence experts into DONS operations. All these actions undercut the old guard and, as a result, NIS (the latest designation dates from 1980) no longer enjoys the sort of power it displayed in earlier years.

The intelligence community, however, is still marked by turf battles.[79]

TNS in Action. Space precludes a thorough discussion of the total national strategy. The critical components have, however, involved neutralization of the so-called Frontline states and reform of the apartheid system. The two are inextricably linked: neutralization of South Africa's neighbors reduces the conventional guerrilla (ANC and SWAPO) threat and buys time for restructuring South Africa's domestic order. It also sends a message to domestic and foreign audiences that South Africa can act with tough-minded resolve irrespective of international opinion. The neutralization strategy combines the use of military force with the coercive potential stemming from the economic reliance of southern Africa on South Africa. It is the military destabilization policy that has drawn the most international attention. The two countries that have borne the brunt of the policy are Angola and Mozambique, which hence are worthy of some comment.

Neutralization. Pretoria's actions against Angola stem from concern over the civil war. In August 1975 a small SADF force entered southern Angola to protect workers at a joint Portuguese-South African hydroelectric project and to safeguard two refugee camps. That October a squadron of armored cars moved north to support a UNITA-FNLA attack on Cuban-MPLA forces. There is disagreement as to how many South African troops were involved, figures ranging from 300 to 1500. On 11 November, the official Angolan independence day, some 2000 SADF troops were engaged in fighting. The U.S. Congress, however, banned further aid to anti-MPLA forces on 19 December. This led to a major political and military reassessment on the part of South Africa and a decision was made not to launch an all-out attack on MPLA-Cuban forces. By January the FNLA was all but destroyed, and UNITA retreated to the bush. Two months later SADF forces crossed back into Namibia. Pretoria continued the struggle by aiding hardpressed UNITA forces with supplies and logistics support.[80]

Military incursions into southern Angola became frequent beginning in 1977. The official reason was a forward defense against SWAPO insurgents as required by the total national strategy, but South Africa was quite willing to mete out punishment to Angolan forces whenever the opportunity presented itself. In August 1981 the SADF launched a full-scale invasion of Angola. Clashes with Cuban troops were reported. Official statements to the contrary, the Cuban troop presence actually has been of some benefit to Pretoria, serving as a pretext for footdragging on the implementation of UN Security Council Resolution 435 concerning independence for Namibia. Trumpeting "the Cuban-Soviet-SWAPO threat" and engaging in cross-border operations allowed South Africa time to decide what it wanted to do with Namibia as well as time to structure the internal situation so that any political outcome would be, at a minimum, tolerable to Pretoria.[81]

South Africa's goals and strategy in Mozambique somewhat paralleled those in Angola. The major goal was to deny the ANC military bases and to force Frelimo to drop all but moral support of the ANC. This involved direct military attacks on ANC offices, economic sabotage, and the provision of sanctuary, arms, and logistic support to the Mozambican National Resistance (MNR, or Renamo). Renamo can be traced back to individuals recruited by the Portuguese to fight Frelimo. Renamo was initially aided by the Rhodesian intelligence service and then sponsored by South Africa since 1980. Estimates of its membership range from 5,000 to 10,000. It has no particular ideology or compelling vision of what Mozambique's future should be, but excels in sabotage and destruction.[82]

South Africa also applied pressure on tiny Lesotho by attacking an ANC office in 1982 and threatening to squeeze the economy. Pretoria disapproved of the 1983 decision by Prime Minister Leabua Jonathan to allow North Korea, China, and the Soviet Union to establish embassies and the provision of sanctuary to political refugees fleeing South Africa. In January 1986 an economic blockade of this landlocked country contributed directly to the overthrow of Jonathan by the Lesothian military.[83] Economic destabilization was carried out in 1982 against Zimbabwe, and Swaziland was coerced into signing a secret nonaggression pact with Pretoria in February 1982 in which the Swazis pledged to control or expel ANC members. Botswana claimed in 1984 that it was under similar pressure, and once again South Africa's tools were economic threats and a military strike (in June 1985).[84]

Despite recent economic difficulties, the South African economy is the engine that drives the region. This gives Pretoria a considerable amount of potential leverage. Black states are caught up in a complex web of trade, transport, communication, and labor dependencies: 25 percent of Zimbabwe's trade, for example, is with South Africa, as is 37 percent of Mozambique's.[85]

Owing to the earlier construction of railways from South African ports to the interior, nearly all the trade of Lesotho, Swaziland, and Botswana passes through South Africa. In part because of rebel activity in Angola and Mozambique that has closed down rail lines, approximately 50 percent of Zaire's exports and imports, 55 percent of Zambia's and Malawi's, and 65 percent of Zimbabwe's move through South Africa. Similarly, the electricity distribution system is organized in such a way that South Africa supplies 60 percent of Mozambique's power, 79 percent of Swaziland's, half of Botswana's, and all of Lesotho's. Finally, more than one million foreign blacks work in South Africa, and their remittances home are important sources of foreign exchange for Lesotho and Mozambique.[86]

Given this economic dependence on South Africa, the Botha government in 1979 proposed a voluntary association or "constellation of states" in southern Africa. This economic carrot, however, was rejected by the Frontline states. The destabilization policy was therefore stepped up in 1979 and came to fruition in 1984. In a meeting in Lusaka, Zambia, in February 1984, Angola and South Africa agreed to a cease-fire and the formation of a joint commission (a) to monitor the disengagement of South African troops from southern Angola and (b) to prevent SWAPO incursions into northern Namibia. Pretoria had a number of

Table 4. Southern African Military Balance

Country	Total Armed Forces	Combat Aircraft	Naval Combatants	Tanks	Defense Budget[e] and Year
South Africa	97,000 (325,000 reserves)	366	16 (39)[c]	250	3.29 bn. (87/88)[d]
Angola	53,000[a]	148	11 (12)	540	1.09 bn. (86)
Botswana	3,250	5	0	0	27.29 m (87/88)
Mozambique	31,700	60[b]	0 (25)	250	146.53 m (87)
Tanzania	40,050	29	6 (10)	60	223.42 m (85/86 est)
Zambia	16,200	43	0	60	—
Zimbabwe	47,000	43	0	43	389.62 m (86/87)
Frontline States Total	191,200	328	17 (47)	953	N/A

Source: International Institute for Strategic Studies, *The Military Balance, 1987–1988* (London: IISS, 1987).

[a]Does not include an estimated 28,000 Cuban troops plus 8,000 Cuban civilian instructors/advisers, 500 East German intelligence and security advisers, 950 Soviet advisers and technicians, and an estimated 5,000 North Koreans.
[b]Perhaps only 50–60 percent operational.
[c]Numbers in parentheses refer to patrol craft.
[d]Excludes South African intelligence and internal security budgets.
[e]Billions of dollars for South African and Angola, millions of dollars for all others.

incentives at least temporarily to wind down the war and reduce its extensive commitments to Namibia. Approximately 40,000 troops were stationed in Namibia at the time, $1.5 billion a year was being spent on fighting SWAPO, and $3.5 billion a year was allocated for the entire Namibian strategy. This was at a time when South Africa was experiencing 11 percent inflation, a 20 percent prime interest rate, a weak currency, falling gold prices, and its worst recession in the postwar world. As Prime Minister P. W. Botha stated in Parliament at the end of January 1984, "If there is to be a choice between the interests of South Africa and the interests of South West Africa [Namibia] I will give priority to the interests of South Africa."[87] Furthermore, while there was no question South Africa was willing to bear the military cost of its Namibia operation if deemed necessary to national security, there was some concern over the results of Operation Askari in southern Angola in December 1983. Attempting to preempt a SWAPO offensive, the SADF ran into unusually strong resistance. The tide fluctuated. Twenty-one South African soldiers were killed, the highest total for any military operation since 1976. This was partially due to increased arms to the Angolans from the Soviet Union. Shipments included helicopters, tanks, and antiaircraft missiles. This undoubtedly contributed to a questioning

Table 5. Gross Domestic Product Comparison

Country	Year	Gross Domestic Product (millions of dollars)
South Africa	1986	62,480.0
Botswana	1986	944.0
Angola	1985	4,040.0
Lesotho	1983	388.8
Mozambique	1985	2,550.0
Swaziland	1986	478.0
Zambia	1985	2,330.0
Zambabwe	1986	5,600.0

Source: International Institute for Strategic Studies, *The Military Balance, 1987–88* (London: IISS, 1987); Figure for Swaziland from Central Intelligence Agency, *The World Factbook, 1988* (Washington, D.C.: 1988).

in some government circles of South Africa's open-ended military commitment.[88]

As for Angola, the country is plagued by a number of severe problems caused by drought, civil war, and near economic disaster. By the time the MPLA seized control in 1975, some 350,000 Portuguese had left the country, leaving an unskilled native population. Continuous warfare against UNITA has been a tremendous drain on the economy. Cuban troops, a military necessity, have been an economic albatross, as they have been paid for with hard currency earned from oil operations. By signing the agreement, the MPLA hoped to gain a respite from direct South African military pressure. This in turn would allow the government to concentrate on UNITA, which had been making military gains.

Western hopes that the Lusaka Accord would break the logjam involving independence for Namibia and the removal of Cuban troops were not fulfilled. Suspicion on both sides was deeply entrenched, and the fighting continued. In July 1988, however, Angola, South Africa, and Cuba announced they had ratified an agreement on principles for a disengagement of forces. With the United States continuing to act as mediator, talks began on a timetable for the withdrawal of Cuban troops and the eventual independence of Namibia.[89]

South African pressure in Mozambique yielded results in March 1984 with the signing of the Nkomati Accord. Essentially a nonaggression pact, the accord committed South Africa to end its military support for Renamo; in turn, Mozambique would expel ANC guerrilla forces. Mozambique's official explanation for signing the Nkomati Accord was that South Africa, failing to overthrow Frelimo, was forced to come to the bargaining table. No one seriously accepted this view. The truth is that Mozambique was faced with a cruel combination of war, starvation, and natural disasters. Approximately 100,000 people had died due to a three-year drought, and another four million were threatened with starvation. Guerrillas from Renamo were operating in nine of ten provinces, killing, looting, burning villages and crops, blowing up rail lines, and mining roads. In January 1984 a cyclone destroyed agricultural projects and bridges and flooded entire villages. In certain areas of the country peasants were reduced to bartering. All of these disasters occurred within the context of failed socialist economic policies and a colonial legacy that at independence in 1974 left 93 percent of the population above the age of seven illiterate and unprepared to run the country. At the time of the accord, Mozambique's external debt stood at $1.4 billion. Frelimo estimated that South Africa's undeclared war cost Mozambique about $3.8 billion.[90]

Two years later, however, the agreement was all but dead. Renamo, aided by Portuguese businessmen and elements of the SADF, continued its destructive war against Frelimo. In May 1986 South African helicopter-borne commandos attacked ANC offices and camps in the capitals of Botswana, Zambia, and Zimbabwe. While the attacks were perhaps designed to reassure the white population, they also effectively wrecked the mediation effort of the Commonwealth's Eminent Persons Group.[91]

DOMESTIC REFORM

As noted, a major purpose of the regional neutralization strategy was to buy time for the restructuring of the domestic political and social order. Simultaneously with the deterioration of regional security in the mid 1970s, it became apparent to the white leadership that separate development was failing to work out as planned. International acceptance of the black homelands was not forthcoming, strikes by black workers in Natal erupted in 1973, and the explosion of violence in Soweto in June 1976 had a ripple effect throughout the country. Influx controls failed to stem the tide of people moving into urban shanty towns in search of work, the black elite of the despotically ruled homelands were viewed as collaborators, and South Africa's increasingly sophisticated urban economy was faced with severe problems due to the limited skills and training of the "temporary sojourners."

A restructuring of apartheid to enhance the long-term security of white South Africa hence began. The goals were to secure at least the tacit support of better-off blacks, Asians, and Coloureds, cultivate an image of reform abroad, and redress the growing problem of a lack of skilled workers for the economy. At the same time, however, the ruling National Party had to protect its flanks and maintain the loyalty of the Afrikaner community by cracking down on dissent.[92]

Toward these ends, 1979 marked the beginning of changes in government policy in a number of areas: the ending of the job reservation system for whites, the recognition of certain black and nonracial unions, modifications in the ability of some skilled and economically useful blacks to live and work in white areas, ninety-nine-year leases on township land, and repeal of the Mixed Marriages and Immorality Acts. A government referendum among whites in November 1983 passed by a two-to-one majority and resulted in the creation of separate parliamentary chambers for Asians and Coloureds the following year. Each chamber is ostensibly responsible for affairs within its own community. The 73 percent black majority was excluded. In September 1985 President P. W. Botha hinted at the possibility of restoring citizenship to blacks who were stripped of it by the creation of the homelands. The following month at a National Party congress, Botha announced "I finally confirm that my party and I are committed to the principle of a united South Africa, one citizenship and a universal franchise."[93] Some form of federation or confederation, it was suggested, could be established based on geography and race, and blacks might be admitted to the advisory President's Council. The speech was, however, hedged with qualifications, and critics charged that Botha's proposals were designed to create the illusion of black political participation while maintaining the reality of white domination. The government, however, was still against dismantling the tribal homelands, the granting of political rights to blacks, the abolishing of influx controls, and residential segregation. Further pronouncements were soon forthcoming.

In a January 1986 speech to parliament, Botha stated: "We have outgrown the outdated colonial system of paternalism as well as the outdated concept of apartheid."[94] He announced plans to abolish the most hateful symbol of apartheid, the pass laws, which restrict where blacks can live, work, and travel, substituting national identity papers for all South Africans. An interracial "national statutory council" would be formed to advise the government on new legislation. Influx controls would hence officially end, although under the concept of "orderly urbanization" only those blacks with homes and jobs would be allowed to live in urban areas. In June 1986 the South African Parliament approved a reform package that abolished the pass laws, restored citizenship to 20 percent of the nine million homeland blacks, and gave urban blacks a limited increase in township self-government. Unaffected, however, were laws governing the segregation of schools, hospitals, and residential

areas. Urban anti-squatter laws were actually strengthened.[95] Furthermore, it is important to keep in mind that the dismantling of apartheid does not mean the surrender of white political power. That is the one—and most important—concession the government refuses to make. Even so, extremist whites believed the National Party had already gone too far in its reforms while at the same time the policy changes did little to dampen protest and violence in the townships. As a result the Botha government found itself caught between black unrest and a right-wing white backlash.

The Defense Decision-Making Process

As noted at the outset, the study of South African defense policy must be examined in the broader context of an increasingly important national security establishment designed to cope with the multiplicity of threats stemming from a perceived "total onslaught." The security establishment is composed of six basic elements.[96] First, there are the SADF and the Ministry of Defence. The president is the commander in chief and officially controls the military through the defense minister. The chief of the SADF has traditionally been an army general who works directly with the chiefs of the various branches. He is also chairman of the Defence Command Council, the highest command body. There are three other support groups. The Defence Staff Council is charged with internal management and policy coordination. The Defence Planning Council oversees the defense budget and procurement plans. The Defence Advisory Council serves as a contact point between the military and civilian sectors and includes important industrialists and financiers.[97] Associated with the SADF are service academies, advanced training institutions, and strategic planning groups. Second, there is the intelligence community. The three critical institutions, as already noted, are the Department of Military Intelligence (DMI), the National Intelligence Service (NIS), and the police Security Branch. Third, academics and think tanks occasionally work for the government on an ad hoc basis. Exam-

Figure 1. The South African Defense Force

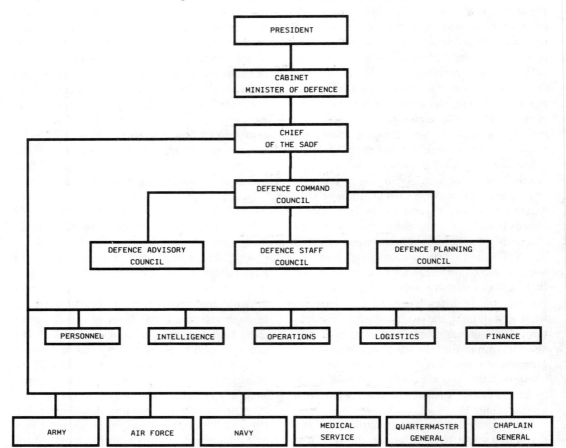

ples would include the Institute for Strategic Studies at the University of Pretoria and the Terrorism Research Centre in Cape Town. Professors at times become actively involved in governmental commissions, engage in contract work, and address government training courses dealing with national security issues. Fourth, the Armaments Corporation of South Africa (Armscor) and its related industries produce weapons and are under the authority of the Ministry of Defence. Fifth, the South African Police (SAP) plays an important role in internal security. Sixth, and finally, there is the State Security Council (SSC) which is generally viewed as the most important institution in South Africa today.

THE STATE SECURITY COUNCIL

Although officially charged with an advisory role to the cabinet, the SSC is perhaps the primary organization in formulating security policy. The following is based on what little information has been made public. Government officials are understandably reluctant to discuss the actual inner workings of the SSC in any detail.

The State Security Council was created by law in 1972 and is formally charged with advising the government on the formulation and implementation "of national policy and strategy in relation to the security of the Republic."[98] Government officials compare it to the National Security Council in the United States.

Since the collapse of South Africa's regional cordon sanitaire in the mid 1970s, however, the SSC has taken on a much larger role than that of merely advising the cabinet. The SSC is the heart of the national security management system (NSMS) and the key institution behind the formulation and elaboration of the Total National Strategy. As a result, it has a sweeping mandate to marshal the resources of South Africa. Defense, foreign, and internal security policies are all discussed within the SSC, and occasionally issues involving the economy, justice, and even critical constitutional matters are also addressed.

The State Security Council is one of four cabinet-level committees. The permanent members are the president as chairman, the defence, foreign affairs, justice, and law and order (police) ministers, and the most senior cabinet member if not holding one of the above portfolios. Also included are the senior civil servants of the Departments of the President, Foreign Affairs, and Justice, as as well as the Chief of the SADF, the commissioner of police, and the head of the National Intelligence Service. It has been reported that the ministers in charge of the three other cabinet committees (economic, social, and constitutional affairs) also attend. As of 1982 observer status was given to the deputy minister of foreign affairs and the SADF's director of military intelligence.[99] The SSC usually meets every two weeks prior to cabinet sessions.

The SSC initially played a desultory role in the national security realm. In September 1975, however, a commission issued a report on what the state needed to do to combat threats to national security. The major recommendation called for the establishment of an integrated national security management system. Events in Angola lent urgency to this recommendation. It was decided that the SSC should take the lead, and an interdepartmental committee suggested that a number of new structures be created to aid the SSC in its expanded responsibilities as the center of the state security system.[100] In 1978 the cabinet agreed to the implementation of the proposals. Aside from the SSC, key supportive institu-

tions of the national security management system are as follows.

The Work Committee provides support by formulating the SSC's agenda, developing position papers and policy alternatives, and making recommendations. It is chaired by the head of the SSC Secretariat and is composed of the heads of most of the departments represented on the SSC, the chairmen of the working groups of the other three cabinet committees, and other departmental heads depending on the issue. The membership usually numbers about eleven, and the committee meets every two weeks prior to the next SSC meeting.

The Secretariat provides the staff support to the Work Committee and SSC, coordinates departmental inputs to the SSC decision-making process, conveys final cabinet decisions to departments, and monitors the implementation of the decisions. It is estimated to have forty-five members drawn from various departments. The Secretariat consists of four branches. The National Intelligence Interpretation Branch provides timely intelligence to decision makers that is received from various organizations such as the police, SADF, NIS, the Department of Foreign Affairs, and lower levels of the national security management system. It also interprets this information and provides finished intelligence reports, which are utilized in the formulation of particular strategies. The Strategy Branch participates in this latter function and also monitors the implementation of policies. The Strategic Communication Branch advises and coordinates government engagement in the "war of words," and the Administration Section handles day-to-day bureaucratic routines. The head of the Secretariat is an army general and it has been suggested that the SADF dominates the staff positions.[101]

Interdepartmental committees coordinate policy planning, implementation, and, according to one author, are generally the source of almost all policy recommendations. They are subordinate to the Secretariat and deal with such topics as manpower, transportation, telecommunications, and the economy. The chairman of a committee is usually a department

Figure 2. The National Security Management System

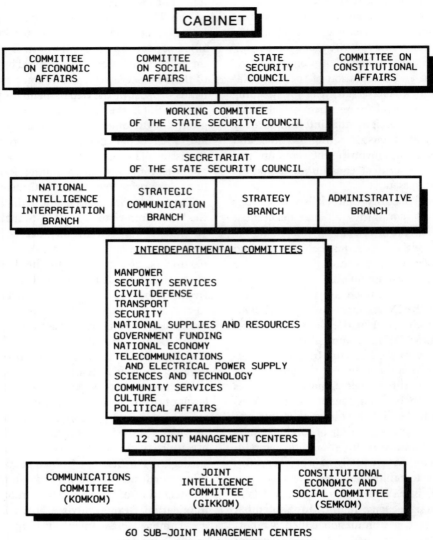

CABINET

| COMMITTEE ON ECONOMIC AFFAIRS | COMMITTEE ON SOCIAL AFFAIRS | STATE SECURITY COUNCIL | COMMITTEE ON CONSTITUTIONAL AFFAIRS |

WORKING COMMITTEE
OF THE STATE SECURITY COUNCIL

SECRETARIAT
OF THE STATE SECURITY COUNCIL

| NATIONAL INTELLIGENCE INTERPRETATION BRANCH | STRATEGIC COMMUNICATION BRANCH | STRATEGY BRANCH | ADMINISTRATIVE BRANCH |

INTERDEPARTMENTAL COMMITTEES

MANPOWER
SECURITY SERVICES
CIVIL DEFENSE
TRANSPORT
SECURITY
NATIONAL SUPPLIES AND RESOURCES
GOVERNMENT FUNDING
NATIONAL ECONOMY
TELECOMMUNICATIONS
  AND ELECTRICAL POWER SUPPLY
SCIENCES AND TECHNOLOGY
COMMUNITY SERVICES
CULTURE
POLITICAL AFFAIRS

12 JOINT MANAGEMENT CENTERS

| COMMUNICATIONS COMMITTEE (KOMKOM) | JOINT INTELLIGENCE COMMITTEE (GIKKOM) | CONSTITUTIONAL ECONOMIC AND SOCIAL COMMITTEE (SEMKOM) |

60 SUB-JOINT MANAGEMENT CENTERS
324 MINI-JOINT MANAGEMENT CENTERS
LOCAL MANAGEMENT CENTERS

Source: Washington Post, 25 December 1986, p. A33.

head assisted by his top aides. Each committee usually includes a representative of the Ministry of Defence.[102]

Joint Management Centers (JMC) operate at the regional level and are tasked with coordinating the implementation and monitoring of national security policies in their areas. Actual implementation is left to local governmental departments. Eleven centers cover the RSA, and there is a twelfth for Walvis Bay. Each center is staffed by approximately sixty officials, with an army or police brigadier as chairman.

Each Joint Management Center has three specialized committees that deal with communications, intelligence, and constitutional, economic, and social matters. Under the JMCs are 60 subcenters that basically coincide with metropolitan regions. The subcenters consist of local military and police commanders and city officials. There are also 324 minicenters corresponding to municipal councils that include civil defense officers, fire chiefs, postmasters, and municipal officials. Even smaller local management centers are in the planning stage. The JMC network collects information at the grass-roots level, identifying potential problems that could escalate into unrest and violence. The information is passed up the line to Byron Place in Pretoria, headquarters of the security management network, where it is collated and interpreted by the committees. Summaries and recommendations are placed before the State Security Council.[103]

The SSC is officially subordinate to the cabinet. As the SSC is the only cabinet committee chaired by the president, however, it can be assumed that the cabinet will agree with SSC recommendations. This leads to the important question of whether the SSC, due to its key role in the national security process, has become the single most important institution in the land, overshadowing the white South African public, Parliament, and cabinet. Based on the available (albeit limited) evidence, the tentative answer appears to be yes. As one scholar concludes, "the SSC has become the court of virtually final resort for a broad range of national issues."[104] It has been suggested, for example, that the SSC has devised the Namibian strategy, authorized military operations in Angola, decided on the provision of military aid to UNITA and Renamo, and approved attacks on ANC offices in Mozambique.

While the SSC may now be the single most influential institution in the South African political system, a number of qualifications and observations are in order. First, given the real and perceived threats faced by South Africa since the mid 1970s, it should not be surprising that the SSC has increased in importance. The enhancement of the SSC's power reflects a pragmatic response to a hostile security situation and meets with the general approval of the Afrikaner political establishment.

Second, it could actually be argued that the SSC represents a broadening, not a restriction, of the number of individuals who participate in national security decision making. Under Botha's predecessor, B. J. Vorster, foreign and defense policies were decided by a handful of cronies. The formulation of the Total National Strategy, however, requires contributions and cooperation from a wide variety of actors and institutions. Under Botha's leadership, expert officials representing a diverse range of civil and military institutions were tapped for key roles, reflecting Botha's preference for a technocratic style of government.

Finally, how closely the actual functioning of the SSC matches the formal description is an open question. Government officials leave one with the impression that decision making is a streamlined, regularized process involving clearly defined roles, responsibilities, and a dedication to teamwork. It is inevitable, however, that such universal factors as personality conflicts, bureaucratic competition, friendships, and a whole host of administrative problems work to undermine the technocratic and streamlined image of the SSC apparatus. Ad hoc decisions involving only a few individuals and informal alliances cutting across bureaucratic boundaries have undoubtedly been made. Furthermore, the SSC is reliant upon a number of departments for the implementation of policy decisions, departments that may have lost some of their authority because of the expansion and enhanced power of the SSC and hence are resentful.

Be that as it may, what a number of South Africans find disturbing is the fact the SSC is part of what appears (particularly since the June 1986 declaration of a state of emergency) to be an increasingly powerful national security management system. The NSMS has been likened to a shadow state administration existing alongside the regular civilian government bureaucracies from the local to the national levels. Various elements of the system are only answerable to similar security bodies higher in the hierarchy, bodies dominated by the military, police, and other unelected individuals. Officials claim that the system only deals with security-related matters and "things that if they are not handled properly, can be a cause of crisis."[105] In contemporary South Africa, however, virtually everything involves security. Hence, JMCs are concerned with water supplies, housing, electricity, the condition of roads, and rent, consumer, and school boycotts. If local officials are not cooperative or slow in the implementation of JMC suggestions, the JMCs can go around the normal political and departmental chain of command by appealing to higher levels of the security system. With a decline in township violence, 1987 witnessed an expansion of the government's "hearts and minds" strategy, which involved extensive use of JMCs.

It has also been alleged that the communication committees of the JMCs do more than simply disseminate information about the work of the JMCs and their subunits, and that they also engage in propaganda and disinformation. In October 1986 it was claimed that officials in the Department of Foreign Affairs and Information (DFAI) and in numerous JMCs had been collecting information designed to discredit individuals and groups opposed to government policy as well as using disinformation to spread disunity among legal black political organizations.[106] The government denied this charge, insisting the security system as a whole is nonpolitical. Critics, however, are worried that the system has in fact encouraged the abandonment of the democratic ideal of a politically neutral military and police force, increased the trend toward governmental secrecy, and contributed to the erosion of constitutional rights in response to a domestic "total onslaught."

BUREAUCRATIC POLITICS

Bureaucratic infighting is endemic both within and among organizations. Disputes and disagreements may be a function of personalities, different organizational missions, a desire to aggrandize power, and disagreement over strategy and tactics. Bureaucratic disputes may, of course, actually be healthy if they contribute to an airing of alternative perspectives and recommendations. While it may be rational, however, from the point of view of an individual bureaucracy to push policy recommendations that enhance the organization's own political power, the pursuit of such narrow

interests could conceivably result in collective disaster for the country as a whole. In the case of South Africa, the likelihood of divisive and counterproductive bureaucratic infighting has been reduced in recent years by several factors. First, there is general agreement amongst Afrikaner officialdom as to the seriousness of foreign and domestic threats to security. Similarly, the general strategy enunciated to deal with these threats—TNS—also has broad elite support.

Second, the enhanced power of the State Security Council and its interagency composition has possibly tended to mute bureaucratic rivalry. Given the lack of information on the SSC, this statement should be treated as a hypothesis rather than as a fact. It is currently impossible to tell whether the SSC has developed a corporate identity that binds together the members into a cohesive group and overshadows their loyalty to the institutions they represent.

Third, in part due to the deterioration of the regional security situation and the resultant high priority placed on the use of force, the SADF has played an increasingly important role and has come to overshadow or dominate other institutions. Indeed, the notions of "total onslaught" and "Total National Strategy" have either been devised or elaborated upon by the military.

Finally, the SADF's relative standing has been further enhanced by the fact that P. W. Botha was a former defense minister and relied heavily on such individuals as General Magnus Malan for advice and counsel. Several observations are required on P. W. Botha's role in affecting the dynamics and structure of South African government. No other individual has had such an impact on the organization of the political and administrative system. The Vorster government has been characterized as slack and inefficient, with decisions made on an ad hoc basis by Vorster and several intimates, but Botha is viewed as the quintessential organization man, enamored of rationalizing the decision-making process and improving its efficiency, performance, and effectiveness.[107] As defense minister, Botha became acquainted and impressed with the management system of the SADF. Compared to the rest of the government and civil service, the military as an institution was viewed as a paragon of professionalism. Upon ascending to the position of prime minister in 1978, Botha began to plan and then implement policies designed to enhance governmental performance. His policies included the reorganization of the cabinet, creation of interdepartmental cabinet committees to devise policy, and establishment of a council charged with advising the government on constitutional and racial matters. Last but not least, this rationalization process worked to enhance the power of the prime minister (and then president), Botha. As Kenneth Grundy summarizes events:

Decisionmaking at the top has been tightened and centralized. P. W. Botha is indispensable to the process. The security establishment exercises an enlarged role, and decisions arrived at are more likely to be enforced and implemented than in the past with interdepartmental coordination the norm rather than the exception. The managerial revolution has arrived in Pretoria, and the vanguard of the revolution has been P. W. Botha and the SADF.[108]

Nevertheless, bureaucratic competition in the past has sometime been fierce and could escalate under Botha's successor. Such competition has particularly been the case, as noted earlier, within the intelligence community.

A certain amount of institutional rivalry also exists between the Department of Foreign Affairs and Information (DFAI) and the SADF/ Department of Defence. It is not simply a matter of the former favoring diplomacy and the latter military force as an instrument of policy. Indeed, the military has been a strong proponent of a "hearts and minds" and "civic action" stategy in Namibia dating back to 1974.[109] Nevertheless, it is to be expected that the military would be more willing to engage in the exercise of force than the foreign ministry simply given its mission. This is best illustrated in terms of regional destabilization. The military believes that weak, and even unstable neighbors are the best guarantee of South Africa's security, and hence punitive cross-border military operations and an "eye for an eye" philosophy are in order. In part, this attitude is a result of the failure of regional diplomatic initiatives such as the "outward policy" of the

1960s and the initially conciliatory approach to the Rhodesian issue in 1974–75. Compared to the DFAI, the SADF is not overly concerned with world opinion and condemnations. While the DFAI may accept the destabilization policy, it is with the understanding that it is designed to pave the way for diplomatic solutions.[110]

Given the veil of secrecy, there is little concrete evidence on particular disputes between the military and the diplomats. It has been reported, however, that the SADF succeeded in persuading the State Security Council to agree to a raid into Angola in 1983 at a time when the DFAI was engaged in negotiations with the Angolan government. Conversely, it had been suggested that Foreign Minister Pik Botha and his colleagues managed to muster enough support to get the government to push for the Lusaka and Nkomati accords in 1984, despite the misgivings of some senior military officials. The South African Police apparently sided with the DFAI on the Nkomati issue. The hope was that the accord would weaken the ANC, whose actions are an internal security threat and hence of primary concern to the SAP. In August 1985, however, Mozambican soldiers overran a Renamo base and captured diaries of the rebel leader, Alfonso Dlakama. The diaries showed SADF generals were still willing to provide military support. South African diplomats attempted to shore up the Nkomati accord, and just before Mozambican President Samora Machel's death in a plane crash in October 1986, they offered to act as brokers between Frelimo and Renamo. SADF officials were not enthused at this prospect. The Department of Military Intelligence, in particular, apparently preferred to topple Frelimo and strike a deal with Renamo.[111]

If strong international sanctions are eventually invoked and the domestic and regional security situations begin to unravel, bureaucratic infighting could increase. While it has become a veritible cliche that external threats increase group unity and coherence, the opposite is also possible, as evidenced by the rise in recent years of right-wing extremist groups in South Africa and the defection of a number of moderates from the National Party. A similar splintering process is also possible within the bureaucratic realm as different policies are recommended to cope with a deteriorating security environment.

Recurring Issues and Defense Policy Outputs

CIVIL-MILITARY RELATIONS

The discussion of bureaucratic politics and the State Security Council touched on the important matter of civil-military relations. As we have seen, since the mid 1970s the SADF has assumed a high profile as a result of its staffing key governmental positions and its conducting military operations against insurgents and Frontline states. Has the rise of the military resulted in a concomitant diminution of civilian power? Are senior SADF officials skeptical of, if not hostile toward, South Africa's domestic reforms? If South Africa's domestic and regional security situations begin to deteriorate, what is the possibility of a coup d'état?

The argument to be made here is that the military does not in fact run South Africa, if "running South Africa" means military control over the decision-making process and the exclusion of civilians. Civilian politicians are still in control, and the president has the major voice in determining policy. Nor is he simply being manipulated by the SADF. Civilian and military officials are not engaged in a bitter power struggle. This is not necessary, as one aspect of the "militarization" of South Africa is the fact that senior civilian officials sympathetic to the National Party already agree with the military on such essentials as the nature of the threats to white South Africa and how to deal with them. P. W. Botha, for example, has always been one of the most enthusiastic supporters of the regional destabilization policy. Furthermore, some of the most hardline right-wing views are to be found within the civil service. In other words, a military mind-set pervades the senior levels of South African officialdom. Pretoria's generals are hence unlikely to seize power, as they currently wield substantial political influence.

This influence is evident not only in government circles, but is also pervasive throughout the society and reflects the growing strength of the military. Several examples make the point.[112] First, military cadet programs are run by the SADF in all government secondary schools and serve as an agent of military socialization. Compulsory training is required for all white males. Some school detachments are affiliated with Permanent Force and Citizen Force regiments and attendance at two-week camps during school vacations is encouraged.

Second, state-owned radio and television networks assiduously work to promote a positive image of the SADF. In 1977 the SADF established its own full-time public relations office, and favorable publicity is also enhanced by censorship laws such as the Defence Act, which prohibits statements that are "calculated to prejudice or embarrass the government or to alarm or depress members of the public." Such acts encourage self-censorship on the part of journalists. In terms of media manipulation, the most notorious example was revealed by the *Johannesburg Sunday Times* in 1980. The SADF had produced a document on how the media could be utilized to undercut parliamentary opposition and criticism of P. W. Botha and the National Party's legislative program. As a result of this disclosure, Botha appointed a SADF board of inquiry, which, not surprisingly, exonerated the SADF. A more direct approach to controlling the media resulted from restrictions placed upon journalists under the June 1986 state of emergency and the strengthening of the decree in December of that year.

Third, Civic Action programs run by the SADF were designed to win the hearts and minds not only of Namibians but also of blacks within South Africa. National servicemen serve as teachers, agricultural experts, medical doctors, and engineers. Programs in townships have not been particularly successful, especially when heavy-handed attempts at political proselytizing were made to portray individuals such as Nelson Mandela, imprisoned leader of the African National Congress, as mere "convicts."

Finally, the military has established intimate

ties with civilian-run industries and companies as a result of the international arms embargo. The most obvious connection is through the state-run Armscor and its affiliated defense industries. But other private firms deal with the military by aiding in stockpiling and strategic reserve programs, as well as cooperating by maintaining secrecy on trade figures, production levels, and sources of supply. In sum, the military's presence and influence is pervasive throughout the country, lending credence to the observation that South Africa is becoming increasingly militarized.

Aside from the fact that the SADF already exerts substantial influence in governmental and societal realms, there are other factors contributing to the military's disinclination to disregard the principle of civilian supremacy. First, the SADF is essentially a civilian force. The career officers and enlisted men of the Permanent Force constitute less than 10 percent of total mobilizable manpower. The military is heavily dependent upon reserves and conscripts called up for their two-year terms of National Service. While it could be argued that the military experience socializes recruits into adopting the national security perspective held by senior members of the Permanent Force (TNS, total onslaught, etc.), the opposite argument can also be made: the large number of conscripts and the civilian bases of the reserves work to undercut the development of a military mentality at odds with the rest of society. Furthermore, the Afrikaner community has traditionally been suspicious of a professional military and tends to feel more comfortable with a *volksleer*, or people's army.

Does this mean a coup will not happen? Of course not. Speculation on possible scenarios for South Africa is a popular pastime, and circumstances can be foreseen that would lead to military intervention. For example, a government might come to power supported by moderates in the National Party and a large segment of the English-speaking population. If it announced it was committed to sharing political power with blacks, the military might conceivably intervene with the blessing of right-wing whites. It is just as plausible, however, that the SADF might back the government

against the right wing. Both scenarios, however, assume the SADF is a monolithic entity and would not be divided on the issue of military intervention. Alternatively, if the country were on the brink of civil war and threatened by foreign military action, the SADF might be given complete control to combat a truly total onslaught. This, however, would hardly constitute a military coup. Informed South Africans are themselves unsure as to the plausibility of such scenarios. While critical of outsiders, who they feel overstate the degree of military influence, they also raise the specter of military intervention as a warning to foreigners not to push too hard for substantive political concessions.

MANPOWER

Since the 1970s, a major concern of the South African government has been to assure that there is adequate manpower to combat foreign and domestic threats. With whites comprising only 16 percent of the population, the basic problem is simply not enough white males. While the influx of white Rhodesians temporarily alleviated the problem, current population projections show the demographic nightmare will only get worse. With increased threats to white rule in recent years, it was inevitable that discussion and debate would intensify over the issue of the utilization of non-white manpower.

The selective employment of blacks in the white man's army is not new, although such actions are taken with doubt, reluctance, and some trepidation. Prior to the twentieth century Afrikaners manipulated divisions among the indigenous population to their advantage and played one tribe off against the other, enlisting blacks to serve temporarily in white-led commando units. As far back as 1795, "Hottentots" and Coloureds were levied for service. Despite white suspicion, non-whites and their various organizational permutations served with distinction over the years. In the Boer War (1899–1902) both the Afrikaners and British coerced or hired non-whites to work as laborers and support personnel. In World War I a volunteer Coloured corps served with the British in East Africa and the Middle East, and blacks enlisted as noncombatant laborers to aid British forces in Europe. They served a similar role in World War II after the usual intense debate within the white South African community. When the National Party came to power in 1948 with its apartheid vision, the non-white units were disbanded as part of the Afrikaner policy of "not arming the natives." In 1963, however, the South African Cape Coloured Corps was reestablished, and it commenced combat training in 1978. That same year it began to be utilized in Namibia. It is estimated that there are over 4,000 Coloureds serving in the army.[113]

By the 1970s it was generally accepted by all but the most right-wing politicians that blacks would have to be utilized in the SADF, albeit principally in noncombatant roles, in order to ameliorate manpower shortages. The result was the establishment of the South African Army Bantu Training Center in 1974. The Center's professed initial ambition was no more than to train blacks for armed guard duty because gun-toting, full-fledged black soldiers made too many whites nervous. In 1975 blacks were for the first time permitted to join the Permanent Force and were given the designation 21 Battalion. The SADF reassured the Afrikaner community that the battalion was officially charged with merely training blacks for noncombatant services. In 1978, however, a company began to train for operational duty, and it has since served in Namibia. Morale is reportedly quite good, and desertion is not a problem. Although the SADF does not provide figures, estimates of the number of black PF members trained for combat range from 1,000 to 1,700, seemingly a relatively insignificant number. In 1978 it was also decided to establish small regional black units based on different ethnic groups and attach them to SADF commands. These units will supposedly form the basis of homeland armies once these "countries" achieve "independence."[114]

According to the 1986 White Paper, the racial composition of the full-time force is as follows: Whites, 76 percent; blacks, 12 percent; Coloureds, 11 percent; Asians, 1 percent. Blacks are generally members of the army,

and, as noted, most serve in noncombatant roles. Those that are armed are confined to the infantry. Armored and artillery units, as well as the air force, are all-white, sophisticated weapons not being trusted to other ethnic groups. Indians who join the SADF are principally found in the navy. Three hundred men annually enter for a service period lasting two years. Along with Coloured volunteers, they comprise 20 percent of the navy's Permanent Force. Coloureds also serve in the Citizen and Commando Forces, comprising 7 percent of the latter.[115]

Why do blacks in particular serve in the white man's army? The basic reason is economic. The unemployment and poverty experienced by young blacks make military service a tempting option, albeit one that leads to social ostracism from their own community. Economic factors also help to explain why approximately half of the South African police force is black.

To meet manpower requirements, the government has admitted that the SADF must in the "future increasingly utilize the various population groups."[116] The unstated fear, however, is that in training and arming non-whites to defend the system, the SADF might actually be helping eventually to undermine it. As army recruiters would hardly be welcome in black townships, initial recruiting efforts might be directed toward the Indian and Coloured communities. It should be recalled that the 1983 constitutional changes were also aimed at enlisting Coloured and Indian support. The response was less than enthusiastic, and it is similarly unlikely that these communities would support militarily a system that has denied them basic rights.[117]

In the 1970s there was some hope expressed that an integrated military would be a model for future racial relations. Indeed, military journals such as *Paratus* make a point of highlighting non-white contributions to national defense. It is continually claimed that non-white recruits are treated the same as their white enlisted counterparts, and that all work toward the achievement of common goals. In the 1980s, however, optimism concerning the

SADF as a social experiment faded in the face of the black unrest that erupted during the decade.[118]

WEAPONS ACQUISITION, PRODUCTION, AND ARMS CONTROL

The South African government does not see arms control agreements as being in its interest and has not expressed any desire to participate in arms control and disarmament negotiations. On the contrary, to counteract threats to South African national security, a major concern has been the establishment and expansion of a domestic arms industry. The impetus for such actions has been UN Security Council resolutions in 1963 and 1977 calling for an international arms embargo. While South Africa has assiduously worked since the mid 1960s to improve arms self-sufficiency in a number of areas, it has also been aided by countries that are willing to violate the spirit and specific prohibitions of the UN resolutions.

The 1963 Security Council Resolution 181 officially called on "all states to cease forthwith the sales and shipment of arms, ammunition of all types and military vehicles to South Africa." Resolution 182, passed in December of that year, extended the embargo to include "equipment and materials for the manufacture or maintenance of arms and ammunition in South Africa." In June 1964 a third resolution reaffirmed the call for an international arms embargo. France, however, abstained on the first and third resolutions. Great Britain abstained on the first and supported the second and third. The United States voted for all three resolutions after having announced its own embargo immediately prior to the first Security Council vote.[119]

What weakened the embargo, however, was the fact that a number of Western countries stated that existing contracts for arms, parts, and maintenance would be honored. Britain pledged adherence to the 1955 Simonstown Agreement (terminated in 1975), which led to the provision of Buccaneer fighter-bomber aircraft, helicopters, and maintenance and parts for Shackleton patrol planes and Canberra bombers. South Africa later managed to pur-chase British Centurion tanks via India and Spain and Tigercat antiaircraft missile systems via Jordan. Dual-use equipment such as the Marconi radar system, trucks, Landrover vehicles, and ICL computers were also supplied to the South African military and police.

France did not adhere to the calls for a total embargo, and replaced Britain and the United States as South Africa's principal arms supplier over the following ten years. Not only did French companies provide weapons, but they also signed licensing agreements allowing for weapons assembly and production in South Africa. Weapons agreements included the Mirage III and F-1 fighter-bomber aircraft, armored cars, helicopters, transport planes, antitank rockets, and three Daphne-class submarines.

Protestations to the contrary, Italy has also been a source of arms. Italian firms have provided jet trainers with British engines (Impala I), strike aircraft (Impala II), light transports, and American-designed light planes and helicopters. West German companies have reportedly provided heavy transport vehicles used by the SADF, engines for missile boats, and have helped to construct factories producing armored vehicles. Furthermore, West German firms were involved in providing technology and specialized equipment to South Africa's pilot uranium enrichment program.

Dual-use items from the United States have also turned up in South Africa. These include Cessna light planes, Swearingen Merlin light transport planes, and IBM computers. Repeated charges have been made that U.S. weapons shipped to third countries have ended up in South Africa. For example, in 1979 it was reported that eleven Bell helicopters built in Italy under American license were exported to Israel, sold to a U.S. company in Singapore, and then sent to South Africa and Rhodesia.[120]

Western countries were reluctant to strengthen the 1963 arms embargo. Following the Soweto riots of 1976 and the death of Steve Biko, however, a second UN Security Council resolution was passed in December 1977 at a time when U.S. and British administrations were pressuring South Africa into a Namibian settlement and domestic reform. As with the 1963 action, there were loopholes. The resolution, for example, called on all states "to review all existing contractual arrangements with, and licenses granted to, South Africa relating to the manufacture and maintenance of arms, ammunition of all types and military equipment and vehicles, with a view of terminating them." Termination of such agreements was, therefore, desirable but not mandatory. A committee established by the Security Council to oversee the embargo has the power only to collect information, not to enforce the resolution.[121]

In conjunction with efforts to circumvent the arms embargo, South Africa has developed its own domestic arms industry. In 1964 the Munitions Production Office was reconstituted as the Armaments Board. In 1968 the parastatal Armaments Development and Production Corporation of South Africa (Armscor) was created. Armscor initially took over state-owned arms factories run by the Armaments Board. It was also tasked with building new factories to produce weapons subject to the arms embargo. In 1976 it merged with the Armaments Board to form the Armaments Corporation of South Africa, the Armscor acronym being retained. Aside from overseeing state-owned companies, Armscor also utilizes private companies as contractors and subcontractors in the production of weapons and component parts. Armscor's subsidiaries produce a wide variety of products.

A board of directors appointed by South Africa's president oversees operations. The chief of the SADF determines requirements and holds Armscor responsible for the fulfillment of its assigned tasks.[122] Armscor initially employed 2,200 workers. By 1980 the number had climbed to 29,000, plus 90,000 in the private sector. Although recent figures are not available, in 1978 the government reported that of Armscor's 19,000 workers, 42 percent were non-white.[123] Expenditures on arms procurement have also risen dramatically over the years from 32 million rands in 1968 and 979 million in 1978 to over 1.5 billion in the late 1980s.[124]

The end result, according to the South African government, is that the country is 95 percent self-sufficient owing to a combination of local design, foreign-licensed production, and embargo violations. Armscor, its subsidiaries, and its network of 1,000 private firms produce approximately 8,000 defense items.[125] In recent years South Africa has actually entered the international arms market. It has displayed its wares in overseas exhibitions in 1982, 1984, and 1986. At the 1986 exhibition in Chile, Armscor unveiled a new attack helicopter (Alpha-XH1), cluster bomb, 20mm cannon, and an aircraft machine gun system. Armscor advertises its products in military magazines, touting some products as "battle tested" and "backed by individualized instruction." Presumably this means SADF personnel will occasionally accompany an arms shipment and provide training.

Armscor does not reveal which countries purchase its arms, but experts claim its clients range from Africa and the Middle East to South America and Southeast Asia. It has been reported that Morocco has purchased the Ratel armored vehicle for use in the Western Sahara, Iraq and Iran have both bought howitzers, Chile has acquired Kukri V3 missiles, ammunition has supposedly been provided to Zaire, and Thailand has expressed interest in long-range howitzers. South Africa now offers for sale about 170 types of ammunition, troop carriers, armored vehicles, ambulances, different types of missiles, mortars, long-range artillery, radio equipment, mobile operating theaters, field kitchens, naval assault craft, advanced combat rifles, parachutes, and uniforms.[126]

Although South Africa claims virtual self-sufficiency in arms production, this is not to suggest that it has produced virtually all of its weapons from scratch. In fact, some Western analysts believe only two indigenous weapon systems have actually been produced: the Ratel armored personnel carrier and the Valkiri 127mm rocket. The latter was designed to counter the 122mm "Stalin Organ" supplied by the Soviet Union to Angola.[127] The vast majority of South Africa's arsenal, therefore, consists of excellent copies and adaptations of existing weapons: the Israeli Galil rifle has

Table 6. Armscor Subsidiaries

Name	Location	Production	Comment
Atlas Aircraft Corp.	Kempton Park Waterkloof Ysterplaat	Aircraft, aircraft engines	Founded in 1964; taken over by Armscor in 1968
Eloptro	Kempton Park	Electro-optical equipment	Since 1978 part of Kentron
Infoplan	Pretoria	Computer service	Founded in early 1980s
Kentron	Pretoria Kempton Park St. Lucia	Missiles, rockets	Founded in 1978 to unite rocket and missile research with related areas
Lyttleton Engineering	Verwoerdburg	Small arms, ammunition	In existence since early 1950s; part of Armscor since 1964
Musgrave	Bloemfontein	Small arms	Manufacture & marketing for civilian market
Naschem	Braamfontein Potchefstroom Lenz	Large-caliber ammunition, bombs	
Pretoria Metal Pressings	Pretoria West Elandsfontein	Small-caliber ammunition	
Somchem	Somerset West Krantzkop	Explosives, propellants	In 1962 constructed as a factory of African Explosive & Chemical Industry (subisidiary of ICI, U.K. & Anglo-American, S.A.); Armscor subsidiary since 1971
Swartklip Products	Cape Flats	Pyrotechnics, grenades	
Telcast	Kempton Park	Castings	Part of Atlas

Source: Michael Brzoska, "South Africa: Evading the Embargo," in *Arms Production in the Third World,* ed. Michael Brzoska and Thomas Ohlson (London and Philadelphia: Taylor and Francis, for Stockholm International Peace Research Institute, 1986), p. 197.

become the R4, the Uzi submachine gun (the Kommando), the Gabriel naval missile (the Scorpion), the French Crotale missile system (the Cactus), the French Magic air-to-air missile (the V3), the Italian Macchi jet (the Impala), the British Centurion tank (the Olifant). Even some of South Africa's proudest achievements look suspiciously like foreign models. The G-5 155mm howitzer was initially acquired from the Israelis, who in turn purchased it from the Space Research Corporation located in the United States. The Alpha helicopter (unveiled in 1986) owes its origins to the French Alouette, and its weapon systems may be copies of those mounted on Soviet Hinds shot down by the SADF and Savimbi's UNITA forces. Even the Cheetah jet aircraft, unveiled with much publicity in July 1986, is an upgraded version of the aging French-built Mirage III. The Cheetah is basically designed to increase the operational life of the Mirage by ten to fifteen years.[128]

Furthermore, South Africa is (covertly or overtly) engaged in arms development with a number of countries, among them Israel, Tai-

wan, South Korea, Chile, and Brazil. The Israeli arms connection has been particularly strong since the 1973 Yom Kippur War. It is surmised that the two countries are also partners in nuclear research, and that Israel helped Pretoria with the alleged September 1979 test blast over the South Atlantic.[129]

What, then, is the bottom line on the question of arms self-sufficiency? Defence Minister Magnus Malan stated in 1985 that South Africa was entirely self-sufficient in terms of weapons conception, design, and development. What was required from the outside world was not military equipment per se, but tools and technical assistance.[130] Analysts tend to find this evaluation overly optimistic. Prior to becoming assistant secretary of state for African affairs in the Reagan administration, Chester Crocker provided an analysis of the issue of arms self sufficiency. He found that import dependency remains particularly strong in the case of fighter and fighter-bomber aircraft. South Africa is also dependent on outsiders for heavy modern tanks, advanced avionic and electronic countermeasures, ships

Table 7. Production of Small Arms and Other Military Equipment in South Africa

Item	Comment
Small arms	
9-mm Mamba pistol	Producer: Viper Manufacturing; small number only
R1 7.72-mm rifle	Version of FN FAL (Belgium; licensed production at Lyttleton since 1961; more than 300,000 produced
R4 5.56-mm rifle	Version of Galil (Israel), which itself is developed from AK-47 (USSR)
Uzi submachine gun (SMB)	Israeli design; produced under Belgian license; license revoked 1962, but production may have continued
MPS 9-mm SMG	Developed in early 1970s
BXP 9-mm SMG	Developed in early 1980s, production not vertified
R5 5.56 carbine	Shortened R4
MG4	Version of U.S. designed Browning M-191-A4
Shotguns	Various types for military purposes
Larger-caliber weapons	
20-mm AA gun	Not confirmed; possibly copy of French gun
60-mm M1 mortar	Produced under French license at Armscor since early 1960s
60-mm M4 mortar	South African-designed improved M1
81-mm M3 mortar	Adapted Hotchkiss-Brandt (France) design, early 1960s
90-mm gun	Unconfirmed; to arm APCs
105-mm gun	Unconfirmed; for Centurion; update, copy of British ROFL7
155-mm field gun	Unconfirmed, for G-5/G-6; possibly U.S. design
Valkiri	127-mm Multiple rocket launcher
Ammunition	
.303-in, 5.56-mm	For small arms, producer: Pretoria Metal Pressings; new
7.62-mm, 9-mm, 12.7-mm, .38-in	machinery delivered from Manurhin (France) in 1974; in production since early 1960s
20-mm, 30-mm, 35-mm	For AA guns
76/62-mm	For OTO-Melara shipborne guns
75-mm rifle grenade	Producer: Naschem
60-mm mortar ammunition	
60-mm M61 bombs	Copy of Hotchkiss-Brandt (France) designs; producers Swartklip, Naschem since early 1960s
81-mm mortar ammunition	
81-mm M61 bombs	
90-mm	For tanks and APCs; unconfirmed
105-mm	For tanks; unconfirmed
155-mm	For field guns, howitzers
Other explosives	
Antipersonnel mine	Copy of U.S. M-18-A1; Armscor
Antitank mine	Naschem, Swartklip
Hand-grenade	Copy of U.S. M-26; Swartklip

Source: Michael Brzoska, "South Africa: Evading the Embargo," in *Arms Production in the Third World,* ed. Michael Brzoska and Thomas Ohlson (London and Philadelphia: Taylor and Francis, for Stockholm International Peace Research Institute, 1986), p. 204.

larger than patrol boats, and perhaps small submarines.[131] When South Africa's own design and production is combined with locally licensed production and international coproduction agreements, Crocker concluded, South Africa exhibits a moderate, and increasing level of self sufficiency. How one defines "self-sufficiency" is, however, a function of the nature and level of the threat. South Africa is essentially prepared to deal with low-level conflict with African opponents and is not faced with the sort of concentrated threat with which Israel must deal. As Crocker notes, however, should South Africa be faced with a great power (Soviet) combat intervention, "there is

no way for local defense industries to produce latest generation ships and aircraft or advanced electronic defense systems. Pretoria must live with the risk of being technologically overwhelmed, while preparing to make such intervention as costly as possible."[132] In particular, a prolonged war of attrition would be beyond South Africa's defense capabilities.

Progress toward self-reliance has, if anything, increased throughout the 1980s. The domestic turmoil that intensified in 1985 and the imposition of limited economic sanctions by Western powers in 1986 has only reinforced this trend. Furthermore, leaving out of account the impetus of threats to national security, the expansion of the South African arms industry is in part a result of the lucrative export market. Ironically, South Africa's economic difficulties in the mid 1980s increased the market for its weapons because of the fall in the value of the rand.

While Pretoria might occasionally have to pay a substantial price in the international arms bazaar to receive what it desires, it has also been willing to do so. What about a stronger embargo? There have naturally been continuous calls for just such action. Even if the embargo were strengthened, it is apparent

there are enough states willing to cooperate with South Africa to undercut the effectiveness of any further collective action. It can be expected in any case that South Africa will continue to increase its level of arms self-sufficiency.

THE MILITARY BUDGET

A final concern to a number of white South African officials has been the financial cost entailed in supporting the military establishment. The dramatic expansion of the size of the SADF and the growth of the armaments

Table 8. South African Sources of Arms Production Technology

Weapon System	Type of Technology	Origin	Start of Design Work
Aircraft			
Impala 1	license	Italy	1966
Impala 2	add-on engineering	Italy/SA	1974
C-4M Kudu	add-on engineering	Italy/SA	1973
Mirage F-1	assembly/license	France	1971
Mirage F-1C	license	France	1971
Cheetah	add-on engineering	France	?
Armour and Artillery			
AML 60/90	license	France	1962
Eland 60/90	add-on engineering	France/SA	1970
Eland 20	add-on engineering	France/SA	1980
Ratel 20	add-on engineering	Belgium/SA	1975
Ratel 20	add-on engineering	Belgium/SA	1981
Ratel 90	add-on engineering	Belgium/SA	1981
Ratel Log	add-on engineering	Belgium/SA	1982
Safire	indigeneous	SA	not produced
Casspir	add-up engineering	SA/FRG	1975
Hippo	add-up engineering	SA	1976
Buffel	add-up engineering	SA/FRG	1978
Samil-100 APC	add-up engineering	SA/FRG	1982
G-5 155-mm	add-on engineering	Canada/SA	1979
G-6 155-mm	add-on engineering	Canada/SA	1985
Missiles			
Whiplash	foreign experts	SA/FRG	not produced
V-3A	add-on engineering	France/SA	1975
Kukri	add-on engineering	France/SA	1979
Ships			
P-1558 Type	indigeneous	SA	1975
Reshef	license	Israel	1978
Selected ordnance			
R1 rifle	license	Belgium	1961
Uzi SMG	license	Belgium/Israel	1955
MG4	license	USA	1964
60/81-mm mortar	license	France	1963
MPS SMG	indigeneous	SA	not produced
Mamba pistol	indigeneous	SA	1976
R4 rifle	add-on engineering	Israel	1977
R5 carbine	add-on engineering	Israel	1978

Source: Michael Brzoska, "South Africa: Evading the Embargo," in *Arms Production in the Third World,* ed. Michael Brzoska and Thomas Ohlson (London and Philadelphia: Taylor and Francis, for Stockholm International Peace Research Institute, 1986), p. 197.

Note: "Add-on engineering" refers to an adaptation of an existing weapons system by changing components, adding features, or taking them away, and trying to incorporate as many home-built parts as possible. "Add-up" means the basic source of technology is not from one specific system, but rather components available from a number of outside sources are put together into a system not available elsewhere.

industry over the past twenty-five years are perhaps the most obvious examples. The occupation of Namibia has also been a financial drain, what with the construction of some forty military bases, the presence of SADF troops, and the arming of 110,000 whites.

The SADF is very sensitive to criticisms of the size of the military budget, and in recent years defense White Papers have attempted to make the case that South African defense spending is neither out of line with that of other countries nor necessarily harmful to the economy, and that expenditures must be adjusted for inflation. Nevertheless, military expenditures more than doubled in real terms between 1973 and 1977. Even drops in military spending have to be treated with caution. For example, the reduced rate of increase in military expenditure as a percent of GNP in 1978/79 was a function of the arms embargo curtailing foreign arms purchases.

Budget figures are also misleading for what they leave out. For example, in the early 1980s, the original figures agreed upon by Parliament were in fact exceeded. Not included in the budget figures are funds assigned to the Special Defence Account, which is designed to provide financing for weapons not yet available. Amounts drawn were more than one-half the regular military budget. The costs involved in undertaking unforeseen military operations are also covered by this account, and in recent years supplementary defense budgets have been required to cover operations in Namibia and elsewhere. The military budget also does not include such defense-related items as the construction and maintenance of military bases, which are paid for by the Department of Public Works, or housing, paid by the Department of Community Development. Nor does it include the cost of maintaining nonmilitary intelligence services and the South African Police. In sum, the financial cost of defending white South Africa is greater than official government figures would suggest.[133]

Conclusion

Most authors who deal with South Africa feel compelled to conclude their analyses with a bit of informed speculation concerning the future. This author is no different, but comments will be suitably circumspect. Given the internal unrest of recent years, an important question is whether the SADF and related security services would be able to handle even more serious disturbances. The answer is undoubtedly yes. The world has only seen the tip of the iceberg in terms of the amount of military force and firepower the SADF could bring to bear on the black population. Townships, for example, have been situated and constructed in such a way so as to maximize the ease by which they can be brought under submission. Homes and business establishments are carefully laid out to make it easier to control rioters and apprehend suspects, hence avoiding the problems associated with a tangled urban labyrinth such as faced by the French in Algeria. Roads have even purposely been made wide enough so that military and police vehicles can easily maneuver. Firepower would not even necessarily have to be employed, as it would be simple to cut off the few roads leading into the townships and weaken the resistance by starvation. Although ghastly to contemplate, such Draconian measures could conceivably be utilized by a desperate white regime. In terms of regional security, the SADF is still more powerful than any coalition of Frontline states armed by the Soviet Union and its allies. To be significantly threatened, South Africa would have to face a dramatic increase in Cuban troops and the introduction of Soviet combat forces willing to engage the SADF directly. This is an unlikely event.[134]

If in the future, however, the SADF no longer plays the twin roles of protector of exclusive white privilege and the bulwark against black majority rule, it will most likely not be due to a military defeat. Instead this would be the result of an Afrikaner political decision to reach a compromise with the black population and such organizations as the ANC. Even if some sort of political accommodation is reached that is acceptable to all parties, it is unlikely that white South Africans would agree to the complete emasculation of the SADF as it is currently structured. Undoubtedly they would demand white control of the SADF during any extended transition to black majority

Table 9. The South African Defense Vote: The 1970s and 1980s

Financial Year	Defense Vote[a] (Million Rand)	As Percentage of Budget	As Percentage of GNP	Percentage Increase Over Previous Year
1970/71	257	13.0	—	
1971/72	317	12.0	2.6	23
1972/73	335	12.0	2.3	6
1973/74	472	13.7	2.6	41
1974/75	692	16.0	3.2	47
1975/76	948	18.5	3.7	37
1976/77	1400	17.0	4.1	48
1977/78	1526	19.0	5.1	9
1978/79	1682	16.6	4.2	10
1979/80	1857	—	5.0	10
1980/81	1890	—	—	2
1981/82	2459	—	—	30
1982/83	3100	20.0	4.0	—
1983/84	4000[b]	—	—	—
1984/85	4950[c]	15.0	—	21 +

Source: Robert S. Jaster, "South African Defense Strategy and the Growing Influence of the Military," in *Arms and the African,* ed. William H. Foltz and Henry S. Bienen (New Haven: Yale University Press, 1985), p. 127.

[a]From official data. Excludes defense spending by other departments, as well as DoD expenditure of loan account.
[b]Derived figure.
[c]Preliminary total.

Figure 3. Comparative Defense Expenditure as Percentage of State Expenditure

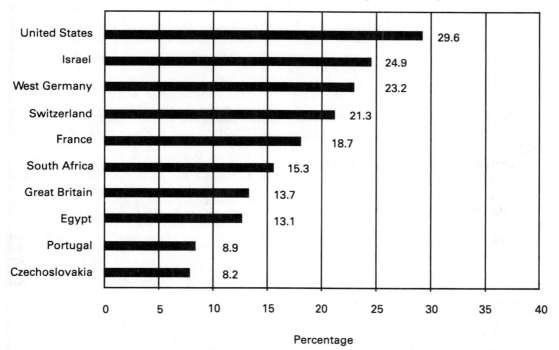

Source: Republic of South Africa, *White Paper on Defence and Armaments Supply, 1986,* p. 25.

rule. Furthermore, if a particular settlement is rejected by various segments of the society (and here one can include more than die-hard Afrikaners), the military would play an important role in maintaining order. If one is optimistic enough to foresee the day in which the SADF becomes a truly multiracial force, it is also possible that the military might come to play a key role as political broker. Politicians of all races may be tempted to enlist the support of the

Figure 4. Comparative Defense Expenditure as Percentage of Gross Domestic Product

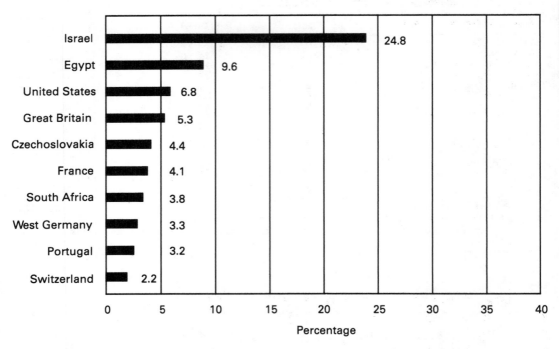

Source: Republic of South Africa, *White Paper on Defence and Armaments Supply, 1986*, p. 26.

SADF for their own partisan purposes. Nor should one assume that such a force and a black South African government would necessarily remain on the best of terms with its neighbors. Unless completely destroyed by a protracted and devastating civil war, South Africa under any government will continue to be a regional power with a great deal of political, economic, and military influence. This will most likely make for a certain degree of regional envy and tension. As events elsewhere since 1945 have shown, apparent ideological compatibility among states does not necessarily make for harmonious relations. The important point, therefore, is not simply that the military is currently a dominant actor. However the future of South Africa unfolds and whichever scenario one wishes to adopt, the SADF will continue to play an absolutely crucial role.

Notes

1. See James N. Rosenau, *Linkage Politics*, (New York: Free Press, 1969); and Peter Gourevitch, "The

Second Image Reversed," *International Organization* 32, 4 (Autumn 1978): 881–911.

2. Leonard Thompson, "What Is To Be Done?" *The New York Review of Books*, October 23, 1986, p. 4; "Third-World Toughs," *The Economist*, 21 June 1986, pp. 15–16.

3. David Harrison, *The White Tribe of Africa* (Berkeley: University of California Press, 1982).

4. Consider, for example, the fierce debate which has raged around the answers to the following questions: Has the presence of foreign companies abiding by the Sullivan principles and the EEC Code of Conduct been a force for black upward economic mobility and encouraged the strengthening of increasingly powerful unions, or have foreign companies created a 70,000 person elite black labor force and undercut black protest by helping to stabilize the economy? Would sanctions and economic disinvestment bring about fundamental political change or simply inflict disproportionately economic hardships on blacks, adversely affect neighboring African countries dependent on the South African economy, and increase South Africa's self-sufficiency? Will further international ostracism contribute to the dismantling of apartheid or reinforce Afrikaner obstinacy and the laager mentality? For recent works on apartheid see Heribert Adam and Kogila Moodley, *South Africa Without Apartheid: Dismantling Racial Domination* (Berkeley: University of California Press, 1986); and Leonard Thompson, *The Political Mythology of Apartheid* (New Haven: Yale University Press, 1985).

5. *World Development Report 1984* (New York, Oxford: Oxford University Press, 1984), p. 221; World

Bank, *Toward Sustained Development in Sub-Saharan Africa* (Washington, D.C.: The World Bank, 1984), p. 1; George T. Kurian, *The New Book of World Rankings* (New York: Facts on File Publishers, 1984), p. 96; *Christian Science Monitor*, 11 May 1988.

6. The following discussion is based on *South Africa: A Country Study* (Washington, D.C.: U.S. Government Printing Office, 1981); and Monica Wilson and Leonard Thompson, *The Oxford History of South Africa*, 2 vols. (New York and Oxford: Oxford University Press, 1969 and 1971).

7. The treatment of the Asian population was raised by India at a series of Imperial conferences following World War I, and the Permanent Mandates Commission of the League of Nations criticized aspects of Cape Town's rule of the former colony of South West Africa which had been placed under South African administration in 1919.

8. Robert M. Price, "Apartheid and White Supremacy: The Meaning of Government-Led Reform in the South African Context," in Robert M. Price and Carl G. Rosberg, eds., *The Apartheid Regime: Political Power and Racial Domination* (Berkeley: Institute of International Studies, 1980), p. 329.

9. Earlier, Section 10 of the Natives (Urban Areas) Consolidation Act of 1945 stipulated that no African was allowed to remain in urban areas for over 72 hours without special permission or a record of long-term residence. In 1956 coloureds were removed from the voting rolls of the Cape.

10. As the Minister of Plural Relations stated in 1978, "If our policy is taken to its logical conclusion as far as black people are concerned there will not be one black man with South African citizenship . . . every black man will eventually be accommodated in some independent new State in this honorable way and there will no longer be a moral obligation on this Parliament to accommodate these people politically." *Rand Daily Mail*, 13 June 1984, p. 10.

11. Price, p. 308.

12. For a graphic description of the life of "temporary sojourners," see Joseph Lelyveld, *Move Your Shadow* (New York: New York Times, 1985), Chapter 5.

13. Implementation of the pass laws and influx controls is estimated to have cost R113 million by the mid-1970s. *South Africa: A Country Study*, p. 108. On the notion of South Africa as a nation of minorities, see the comments of P.W. Botha in *Southern Africa Record*, December 1980, p. 7.

14. For typical arguments, see Foreign Broadcast Information Service (hereafter FBIS), MEA-86-165, 25 August 1986, p. U2.

15. In 1985, South Africa accounted for 55 percent of noncommunist world gold sales, earning South Africa $7 billion. *Christian Science Monitor*, 18 September 1986.

16. T.B. Millar, *South Africa and Regional Security*, Bradlow Series No. 3 (Johannesburg: The South African Institute of International Afairs, 1985), p. 4. See also The Study Commission on U.S. Policy Toward Southern Africa, *South Africa: Time Running Out* (Berkeley and Los Angeles: University of California Press, 1981), Chapter 14; Hanns W. Maull, *Energy, Minerals, and Western Security* (Baltimore: The Johns Hopkins University Press, 1984). On the proposed administration action, opposed by Congress, see "Critics Rap Plan to Sell Off Key Minerals," *The Washington Times*, 7 May 1986, p. 4.

17. Department of Foreign Affairs, *South Africa 1985* (Cape Town: CTP Book Printers, 1985), p. 563.

18. Kurt Campbell, "The Soviet-South African Connection," *Africa Report*, March–April 1986. In December of 1985, a South African cabinet minister went so far as to suggest South Africa and the Soviet Union might form a mineral cartel if the west tightened its economic sanctions, noting "We already work together in the diamond business and we get along very well with the Russians." *Washington Post*, 1 December 1985. In 1981, South Africa produced 9.18 million carats of diamonds, the Soviet Union 8.8 million carats (industrial) and 2.4 million carats (gems). In that same year, South Africa mined 658 tons of gold and the Soviet Union 260 tons. D. Hargreaves and S. Fromson, *World Index of Strategic Minerals* (New York: Facts on File, 1983). On general Soviet views, see also R. Craig Nation, "Soviet Perceptions of South Africa," paper prepared for presentation to the 26th Annual Convention, International Studies Association, 5–9 March 1985, Washington, D.C; and Kurt Campbell, *Soviet Policy Towards South Africa* (New York: St. Martin's, 1986).

19. *South Africa 1985*, p. 317. See also Richard E. Bissell "How Strategic is South Africa?" in Richard E. Bissell and Chester A. Crocker, eds. *South Africa Into the 1980s* (Boulder, CO: Westview Press, 1979), pp. 214–15.

20. John Peel, "The Growing Threat to Freedom and the North Atlantic Alliance," *South Africa International* 9 (October 1978): 79, as cited in Larry Bowman, "The Strategic Importance of South Africa to the United States: An Appraisal and Policy Analysis," *African Affairs* 81 (April 1982): 161. See also Robert M. Price, *Sub-Saharan Africa: National Interest and Global Strategy* (Berkeley: Institute of International Studies, 1978); and L.H. Gann and Peter Duignan, *South Africa: War, Revolution, or Peace?* (Stanford: Hoover Institution Press, 1978), Chapter 2.

21. Richard B. Remnek, "The Significance of Soviet Strategic Interests in Sub-Saharan Africa," in R. Craig Nation and Mark V. Kauppi, eds. *The Soviet Impact in Africa* (Lexington, MA: Lexington Books, 1984), pp. 147–163.

22. In this essay the term "South Africa" is generally used as shorthand for *white* South Africa. In point of fact, persons of all races may see themselves as "South Africans." The usage of the term in this more limited context is not meant as a judgment on the claims and aspirations of blacks, coloureds, and Asians.

23. Robert S. Jaster, *South Africa's Narrowing Security Options*, Adelphi Papers 159 (London: International Institute for Strategic Studies, 1980), p. 5.

24. Ibid., p. 7.

25. Timothy M. Shaw and Lee Dowdy, "South Africa," in Edward A. Kolodziej and Robert E. Harkavy, eds., *Security Policies of Developing Countries* (Lexington, MA: D.C. Heath and Co., 1982), p. 308.

26. Mark A. Uhlig, "Inside the African National Congress," *The New York Times Magazine*, 12 October 1986. Attacks were stepped up in 1981 and numbered less than one hundred a year until 1984. *Washington Post*, 8 July 1986. As the radicalization of black youth in the townships continued, the ANC was forced to adopt a more hardline policy in order to keep pace and maintain its authority.

27. *Christian Science Monitor*, 8 July 1986.

28. Tom Lodge, *Black Politics in South Africa Since 1945* (London and New York: Longman, 1983), pp. 301–04; *CSM*, ibid; Mark Uhlig, "The Coming Struggle for Power," *The New York Review of Books*, 2 February 1984, pp. 27–31; Thomas G. Karis, "Revolution in the Making: Black Politics in South Africa," *Foreign Affairs* 62, 2 (Winter 1983/84): 378–406; Paul Rich, "Insurgency, Terrorism and the Apartheid System in South Africa," *Political Studies* 32 (March 1984): 68–85; Thomas G. Karis, "South African Liberation: The Communist Factor," *Foreign Affairs* 65, 2 (Winter 1986/87): 267–287. On the SACP's military strategy, see Gene Gungushe (Titus), "Our National Democratic Revolution Will Defeat the Enemy," *The African Communist* 94, 3 (1983): 52–69.

29. For a discussion of the PAC, see Lodge, pp. 306–17 and 241–48.

30. Jaster, p. 12.

31. For examples, see Jaster, p. 19.

32. On events in Angola, see John Marcum, *The Angolan Revolution*, 2 vols. (Cambridge, MA: MIT Press, 1969, 1978); Arthur Klinghoffer, *The Angolan War: A Study of Soviet Policy in the Third World* (Boulder, CO: Westview Press, 1980); John Marcum, "Lessons of Angola," *Foreign Affairs* 54, 3 (1975–76): 407–425.

33. On events in Zimbabwe, see Keith Somerville, "The Soviet Union and Zimbabwe," in *Nation and Kauppi*, pp. 195–220.

34. On Black Consciousness and AZAPO, see Lodge, 323–25 and 344–46, and *Weekly Mail* (Johannesburg), 19 September 1986, p. 2. See also Steve Biko, *I Write What I Like* (London: Heinemann, 1979). On Soweto, see Alan Brooks and Jeremy Brickhill, *Whirlwind Before the Storm* (London: International Defence and Aid Fund for Southern Africa, 1980).

35. *Washington Post*, 7 November 1984 and 2 December 1985; *New York Times*, 2 May 1986. Divide and rule includes trying to win over the small black middle class and creating a privileged homeland elite. Mutual hostility exists between Inkatha, a Zulu-based movement headed by Gatsha Buthelezi, and groups sympathetic to the ANC such as the UDF. This is to the satisfaction of the South African government. In May of 1986, Inkatha launched a new labor federation, the United Workers' Union. This action was in part in opposition to the CSATU which would not allow some 200,000 adherents of black consciousness to join. *New York Times*, 1 December 1985 and 2 May 1986. See also "Why Are Activists Murdering Activists?" *Weekly Mail*, 12 December 1986, pp. 10–11; Michael Massing, "The Chief," *The New York Review of Books*, 12 February 1987, pp. 15–22.

36. *White Paper on Defence and Armaments Supply, 1984*. Republic of South Africa: Department of Defence, 1984, p. 1.

37. Ibid. See also Jan A. DuPlessis, "Soviet Blueprint for Southern Africa," *Paratus* 34, 5 (May 1983): 20–21; "Soviet Aggression and Bending of Realities," *Paratus* 37, 1 (January 1986): 30–32, 49. For more balanced views of Soviet activity, see Winrich Kühne, *Die Politik der Sowjetunion in Afrika* (Baden-Baden: Nomos, 1983); Nation and Kauppi, eds., *The Soviet Impact in Africa*; David E. Albright, "The USSR and Sub-Saharan Africa in the 1980s," *The Washington Papers* 101, V. XI, 1983; Michael Clough, editor, *Reas-*

sessing the Soviet Challenge in Africa, Policy Papers in International Affairs No. 25 (Berkeley: Institute of International Studies, 1986).

38. See Flora Lewis, "Pax Afrikaansa," *New York Times*, 25 January 1983.

39. On the notion of creating a "constellation of states," see Robert M. Price, "Pretoria's Southern African Strategy," *African Affairs* 83, 330 (January 1984): 14–17.

40. *White Paper on Defence, 1977*. Republic of South Africa: Department of Defence, 1977. p. 5.

41. Ibid., p. 4. See also two monographs by James M. Roherty, "The International Thrusts of South Africa's Total National Strategy," Center for Naval Warfare Studies, Naval War College, February 1984; and "South Africa's Total National Strategy: The Next Phase," Defense Intelligence Agency, June 30, 1985.

42. Phillip H. Frankel, *Pretoria's Praetorians: Civil-Military Relations in South Africa* (Cambridge: Cambridge University Press, 1984), p. 53.

43. Ibid.

44. Jonathan Kapstein, "Armed Confrontation Builds in South Africa," *Proceedings* 107, 12 (December 1981): 36. According to Frankel, "Total strategy … is essentially Beaufre writ large in the particular context of contemporary South Africa," p. 46. See two works by Beaufre, *An Introduction to Strategy* (London: Faber and Faber, 1963); and *Strategy and Action* (London: Faber and Faber, 1967). A retired South African general believes Frankel overemphasizes the impact of Beaufre on military thinking. "Book Review," *Politikon* 12, 1 (June 1985): 64–68.

45. As cited by Frankel, p. 46.

46. "Action is total and … must prepare … and exploit the results expected from military operations by suitable operations in the psychological, political, economic, and diplomatic fields." *Strategy of Action*, p. 104, as cited by Frankel, p. 48.

47. *Strategy of Action*, p. 115, as cited by Frankel, p. 49. For an interesting series of articles by South Africans on how to deal with modern threats, see Michael Hough, ed., *Revolutionary Warfare and Counter-Insurgency* (Pretoria: Institute for Strategic Studies, University of Pretoria, 1984).

48. *Introduction to Strategy*, p. 24, as cited by Frankel, p. 51.

49. *White Paper, 1977*.

50. Richard Leonard, *South Africa at War: White Power and the Crisis in Southern Africa* (Westport: Lawrence Hill, 1983), p. 18.

51. Deon Geldenhuys, *What Do We Think? A Survey of White Opinion on Foreign Policy Issues* (Braamfontein: South African Institute of International Affairs, November 1982).

52. Robert S. Jaster, "Politics and the Afrikaner Bomb," *Orbis* 27, 4 (Winter 1984): 826–27.

53. Richard K. Betts, "A Diplomatic Bomb for South Africa?" *International Security* 4, 2 (Fall 1979): 97. On the possible shift in Pretoria's stance on the Non-Proliferation Treaty, see *The Christian Science Monitor*, 29 September 1987.

54. Chester A. Crocker, "South Africa's Defense Posture: Coping With Vulnerability," *The Washington Papers* No. 84 (Sage Publications for The Center for Strategic and International Studies, Washington, D.C., 1981); Kenneth Adelman and Albion W. Knight, "Can South Africa Go Nuclear?" *Orbis* 23, 3 (Fall

1979): 642–43; Jack Spence, "South Africa: The Nuclear Option," *African Affairs* 80, 321 (1981): 441–52.

55. Adelman and Knight, p. 643.

56. Betts, p. 107.

57. *The Military Balance, 1987–88* (London: International Institute for Strategic Studies, 1987), p. 137.

58. *White Paper on Defence and Armaments Supply, 1986*. Republic of South Africa, Department of Defence, 1986, p. 4.

59. The average number of camps per member over a three year period was 2.09, the authorized number 3. The average number of days of service over the same period was 87, the authorized number is 120 days over two years. *White Paper, 1986*, p. 5.

60. Ibid., p. 6.

61. Ibid., pp. 14–15. On troops in the townships, see *Washington Post*, 23 October 1985. For an overview of the army, see Norman Dodd, "The South African Army," *The Army Quarterly and Defence Journal* 113, 2 (April 1983): 135–46.

62. Leonard, p. 106.

63. *The Economist*, 30 March 1985, p. 21; *Christian Science Monitor*, 19 August 1986, p. 9. See also the comments by General Constand Viljoen, former chief of the SADF, upon his retirement, in *The Citizen*, 30 August 1985 (JPRS-SSA-85-008, 19 September 1985, p. 127).

64. Helmoed-Römer Heitman, *South African War Machine* (Novato, CA: Presidio Press, 1985), p. 83. It should be noted that this book was released with SADF approval. For another flattering portrait, see Doris Alves, "The South African Air Force in the Early Eighties," *Air University Review* (July/August 1983): 72–79.

65. *Jane's Weapon Systems, 1985–86* (London: Jane's Publishing Co., 1985), p. 80.

66. *South African War Machine*, p. 85.

67. *White Paper, 1984*, p. 9; *White Paper, 1986*, p. 16. See Norman Dodd, "The South African Navy," *Navy International* (January 1980): 38–44.

68. Kapstein, p. 1.

69. Leonard, pp. 134, 153–54. See also *New York Times*, 20 April 1981, p. 12; John Prados, "Sealanes, Western Strategy, and South Africa," in *U.S. Military Involvement in Southern Africa*, eds. Western Massachusetts Association of Concerned African Scholars (Boston, MA: South End Press, 1978), p. 61; Richard E. Bissell, *South Africa and the United States: The Erosion of an Influence Relationship* (New York: Praeger, 1982), p. 57.

70. *White Paper, 1986*, p. 30.

71. Leonard, pp. 104–5; *White Paper, 1986*, pp. 30–32. *Washington Post*, 16 June 1987.

72. *The Washington Times*, 22 September 1986; *Washington Post*, 4 June 1987.

73. Leonard, pp. 118–19; *New York Times*, 11 December 1986; *The Economist*, 29 November 1986, pp. 33–34. In December 1987, 60 black policemen mutinied in Johannesburg and fought a gun battle with riot police, ostensibly due to grievances over working conditions. *Washington Post*, 11 December 1987.

74. Ibid.; *Washington Post*, 23 October 1985.

75. Leonard, p. 121.

76. Leonard, p. 123. See also Gordon Winter, *Inside BOSS: South Africa's Secret Police* (London: Penguin Books, 1981).

77. James Barber, "BOSS in Britain," *African Affairs* 82, 328 (July 1983): 311–328.

78. On the Information Scandal, see Deon Geldenhuys, *The Diplomacy of Isolation: South African Foreign Policy Making* (New York: St. Martin's Press, 1984), pp. 107–20.

79. Kenneth W. Grundy, *The Rise of the South African Security Establishment: An Essay on the Changing Locus of State Power*, Bradlow Series No. 1 (Johannesburg: The South African Institute of International Affairs, August 1983), pp. 12–13.

80. "Minister Discloses Links with UNITA," *Paratus* 36, 10 (October 1985), pp. 22–23.

81. Former National Security Adviser William Clark is said to have offered this linkage in 1981 to the South Africans who saw no reason to disagree. See the testimony of the Assistant Secretary of State at the time, Chester Crocker, in "Namibia and Regional Destabilization in Southern Africa," Hearing before the Subcommittee on Africa of the Committee on Foreign Affairs, House of Representatives, 98th Congress, First Session, 15 February 1983 (U.S. Government Printing Office, 1983).

82. Colin Legum, "The MNR," *CSIS Africa Notes* No. 16, 15 July 1983.

83. *Washington Post*, 21 January 1986.

84. *Los Angeles Times*, 5 April 1984; *Rand Daily Mail*, 14 June 1984. A great deal has been written on the neutralization policy. See Deon Geldenhuys, "The Destabilisation Controversy: An Analysis of a High-Risk Foreign Policy Option," *Politikon* 9, 2 (December 1982): 17–32; Robert S. Jaster, *South Africa and Its Neighbors: The Dynamics of Regional Conflict*, Adelphi Paper 209 (London: International Institute for Strategic Studies, 1986); Simon Jenkins, "Destabilization in Southern Africa," *The Economist*, 16 July 1983, pp. 19–28; T.B. Millar, *South Africa and Regional Security*, Bradlow Series No. 3 (Johannesburg: The South African Institute of International Affairs, 1985); Robert Davies and Dan O'Meara, "Total Strategy in Southern Africa: An Analysis of South African Regional Policy Since 1978," *Journal of Southern African Studies* 11, 2 (April 1985): 183–211; Joseph Hanlon, *Beggar Your Neighbours: Apartheid Power in Southern Africa* (Bloomington: Indiana University Press, 1986).

85. *The Economist*, 16 July 1983, pp. 26–27.

86. *New York Times*, 15 September 1985. In October 1986, South Africa announced that the contracts of Mozambicans working in South African mines would not be renewed. See also Gavin G. Maasdrop, "Squaring Up to Economic Dominance: Regional Patterns," in *South Africa and Its Neighbors: Regional Security and Self-Interest*, Robert I. Rotberg, ed. (Lexington, MA: D.C. Heath and Co., 1985), pp. 91–135; John H. Chettle, "Economic Relations Between South Africa and Black Africa," *SAIS Review* 4, 2 (Summer/Fall 1984): 121–133.

87. *The Sun* (Baltimore), 28 February 1984; "Little Relief in Sight for SA Economy," *Washington Report on Africa* V.II, 4 (December 1, 1983), p. 14; *New York Times*, 5 January 1984; *The Wall Street Journal*, 8 February 1984.

88. Barry Streek, "South Africa's Stakes in the Border War," *Africa Report*, March–April 1984, p. 59. In November 1987, the South African military officially acknowledged that SADF troops fought alongside UNITA forces the previous month, dealing a major defeat to FAPLA (Angolan) forces. *Washington Post*, 12 and 13 November 1987.

89. *Washington Post*, 21 July, and 23 December 1988.

90. "Diplomacy and Destabilization," *Africa*, no. 151 (March 1984): 35; Joanmarie Kalter, "The Economics of Desperation," *Africa Report*, May–June 1984, pp. 19–23.

91. *New York Times*, 20 May 1986.

92. For an earlier example of the Afrikaner ability to adapt to changing circumstances, see Leonard Thompson, *The Political Mythology of Apartheid*, Chapter 6.

93. *New York Times*, 1 October 1985.

94. *Washington Post*, 1 February 1986.

95. *Washington Post*, 24 April 1986.

96. Grundy, pp. 11–17.

97. Frankel, *Pretoria's Praetorians*, p. 4.

98. Geldenhuys, p. 92, citing the law.

99. Grundy, p. 15. Three other de facto members are reportedly from Finance, Constitutional Development, and Planning, Cooperation and Development. Deon Geldenhuys and John Seiler, "South Africa's Evolving State Security System," Paper presented to the Annual Conference of the Section on Military Studies, International Studies Association, U.S. Air Force Academy, Colorado Springs, Colorado, 25–27 October 1984, p. 8.

100. Geldenhuys and Seiler, p. 6. For the most extensive statement by the government on the SSC (and heavily relied upon by academic analysts), see "Press Briefing by the Secretary of State of the State Security Council on 21 September 1983," *Southern Africa Record* 34 (December 1983): 43–50. General van Deventer claimed the SSC has only an "advisory function."

101. Sensitive to such charges, P.W. Botha revealed in September 1983 the supposed departmental composition of the Secretariat: NIS, 56%; SADF, 16%; Foreign Affairs, 11%; Security Police, 11%; Railways Police, 5%; Prison Service, 1%. Geldenhuys and Seiler, p. 11.

102. Robert I. Rotberg, "Decision Making and the Military in South Africa," in Rotberg, ed., *South Africa and Its Neighbors*, pp. 19–20; Geldenhuys and Seiler, p. 12.

103. Allister Sparks, "South Africa's Security Network," *Washington Post*, 26 December 1986, p. 1. As of October 1986, the twelve Joint Management Centers were based in Durban, Kimberley, Pretoria, Port Elizabeth, Bloemfontein, Outdshoorn, Walvis Bay, Johannesburg, Cape Town, Potchefstroom, Pietersburg, Nelspruit. Anton Harber, "The Uniformed Web That Sprawls Across the Country," *Weekly Mail*, 3 October 1986, p. 12; *Christian Science Monitor*, 11 May 1988, p. 1.

104. Rotberg, p. 20.

105. Sparks, *ibid*; and Harber, p. 13. See also the article by Peter Jastrow of the Progressive Federal Party, "The Real Message Is: The Military's Ruling the Country," *Weekly Mail*, 13 November 1986, p. 2. For a rebuttal, see Jannie Geldenhuys, Chief of the SADF, *Weekly Mail*, 14 November 1986, pp. 10–11.

106. See "The Disinformation Scandal," *Weekly Mail*, 31 October 1986, p. 1. Inkatha was also allegedly a target of disinformation. *Weekly Mail*, 7 November 1986, p. 1.

107. See the two articles by Deon Geldenhuys and Hennie Kotze, "Aspects of Political Decision-Making in South Africa," *Politikon* 10, 1 (June 1983): 33–45; and "P.W. Botha as Decision Maker: A Preliminary Study of Personality and Politics," *Politikon* 12, 1 (June 1985): 30–42.

108. Grundy, p. 10.

109. Geldenhuys, *The Diplomacy of Isolation*, p. 143; *White Paper, 1979*; and Jaster, *South Africa and Its Neighbors*, p. 18. It was General P.W. Van der Westhuizen who P.W. Botha sent to Namibia to help reorganize the feuding political parties in the mid-1980s. General Van der Westhuizen, however, also played a more familiar role between 1980–84 when he helped to direct Renamo's activities against Frelimo.

110. Geldenhuys, *The Diplomacy of Isolation*, p. 145.

111. Geldenhuys and Seiler, p. 20; *The Economist*, 25 October 1986, pp. 36–37. The SADF's former chief of intelligence and leading hawk on Mozambique is General P.W. Van der Westhuizen, currently secretary of the powerful State Security Council.

112. The following examples are drawn from Kenneth W. Grundy, *The Militarization of South African Politics* (Bloomington: Indiana University Press, 1986), Chapter 4.

113. Kenneth W. Grundy, *Soldiers Without Politics: Blacks in the South African Armed Forces* (Berkeley: University of California Press, 1983). See also Mathew Midlane, "South Africa," in *World Armies*, ed. by John Keegan (Detroit: Gale Research Co., 1983), p. 530.

114. Grundy, *Soldiers Without Politics*, Chapter 9; Conor Cruise O'Brien, "What Can Become of South Africa?" *The Atlantic Monthly* March 1986, p. 64; Kenneth W. Grundy, "South Africa's Regional Defence Plans," in *South Africa in Southern Africa: The Intensifying Vortex of Violence*, ed. Thomas M. Callaghy (New York: Praeger, 1983), pp. 133–51.

115. *White Paper, 1986*, p. 18; Robert S. Jaster, "South African Defense Strategy and the Growing Influence of the Military," in *Arms and the African: Military Influences on Africa's International Relations*, eds. William J. Foltz and Henry S. Bienen (New Haven: Yale University Press, 1985), p. 141.

116. *White Paper, 1986*, p. 20. Note the use of the term "population groups" as opposed to "citizens"; blacks, coloureds, and Indians are not citizens.

117. A divide-and-maintain-rule policy has also been discussed in terms of the black community. Speculation (if not fantasy) involves possibly enlisting the support of the Zulu-based Inkatha movement that has its differences with the ANC and UDF. What Inkatha thinks of such an idea apparently has not been taken into account. The all-black 121 Battalion based at Mtubatuba (strength of 500–600) apparently launched a drive in 1986 to recruit up to 30 Zulus. *African Defence Journal* 69 (May 1986): 34.

118. Mention should also be made of the End the Conscription Campaign, founded at the end of 1983. The ECC is a broad front of organizations (Black Sash, churches, members of the Progressive Federal Party, the UDF, etc.) united against the use of troops in the townships. Conscription laws as of 1986 allowed for alternative community service only on religious grounds. Objections on moral or ethical grounds are not accepted and can result in a six year prison sentence. See *Cape Times*, 23 September 1985, p. 8; and the comments by a SADF spokesperson in *The Citizen*, 4 September 1985, p. 4, JPRS-SSA-85-008, 19 September 1985, p. 126. In December 1986 the government announced that it was illegal to issue statements that dis-

credited or undermined the system of compulsory military service. *Weekly Mail*, 12 December 1986, p. 3.

119. This and the following discussion is based on Leonard, pp. 132–34, 150–53.

120. Anthony Sampson, "The Long Reach of the Arms Men," *The Observer*, 4 February 1979, as cited in Bissell, *South Africa and the United States*, p. 61.

121. Leonard, pp. 135–36.

122. *White Paper, 1979*, p. 22.

123. Ibid., p. 25.

124. Based on *White Papers* for 1979, 1982, 1984, 1986.

125. *The Washington Times*, 20 March 1986.

126. *The Sunday Star* (Johannesburg), 8 December 1985, p. 4; Johannesburg International Service, 5 September 1985 in JPRS-SSA-85-008- 19 September 1985; *The Washington Times*, 20 March 1986.

127. *The Washington Times*, 20 March 1986.

128. Ibid.; FBIS-MEA-86-136, 16 July 1986, pp. U2-U4; Leonard, pp. 141–42. See also Ian V. Hogg, "Something New from Africa," in *Jane's Military Review*, ed. Ian V. Hogg (London: Jane's Publishing Co., 1983), pp. 128–40. Elsewhere it has been reported the Cheetah is derived from Israel's Kfir fighter. *Washington Post*, 22 February 1987, p. C2.

129. Bissell, *South Africa and the United States*, pp. 18, 36; Aaron S. Klieman, *Israel's Global Reach: Arms Sales as Diplomacy* (McLean, VA: Pergamon-Brassey's International Defense Publishers, 1985); Rita E. Hauser, "Israel, South Africa and the West," *Washington Quarterly* 2 (1979): 75–82. On South African licensed weapon production agreements with France, Israel, and Italy, see SIPRI, *World Armaments and Disarmament, SIPRI Yearbook 1984* (London and Philadelphia: Taylor and Francis, 1984), p. 278. After the Yom Kippur War two dozen black African states cut ties with Israel. In early 1976 defense minister Shimon Peres secretly visited South Africa and later that year Prime Minister Vorster paid an official visit to Israel. A number of commercial and military documents were signed, including one on scientific and technological cooperation that formed the basis for a pooling of information on nuclear research. South Africa also be-

gan to invest in the Israeli arms industry. A lightweight helicopter was produced (the Scorpion), Israeli drones have been used for reconnaissance against guerrillas in the Frontline states, work is reportedly underway in Simonstown on the joint development of a submarine, and small numbers of Israeli advisers have gone to South Africa over the years to advise on guerrilla warfare. Yossi Melman and Dan Raviv, "Has Congress Doomed Israel's Affair With South Africa?" *Washington Post*, 22 February 1986, pp. C1–2. In March 1987, the Israeli government formally admitted to having significant military ties with South Africa. It pledged no new military agreements would be signed, but existing pacts would be honored. Israel was principally concerned over a potential cut-off of U.S. aid. The 1986 *Comprehensive Anti-Apartheid Act* states U.S. aid cannot be given to countries that violate the arms embargo on South Africa. *Washington Post*, 20 March 1987, p. 1; U.S. Department of State, "Report to Congress Pursuant to Section 508 of the Comprehensive Anti-Apartheid Act of 1986: Compliance With the U.N. Arms Embargo" (April 1987). On difficulties in cutting economic links, see *Washington Post*, 20 September 1987.

130. Johannesburg International Service, 5 September 1985, in JPRS-SSA-85-008- 19 September 1985.

131. Crocker, *South Africa's Defense Posture*, pp. 51–52.

132. Ibid., p. 52.

133. SIPRI, *World Armaments and Disarmament, SIPRI Yearbook 1984* (London and Philadelphia: Taylor and Francis, 1984), pp. 109–10. Due to a resurgence in the price of gold in 1987, it was announced that the police budget would be increased by 50 percent and defense spending by one-third. *Washington Post*, 4 June 1987, p. 39.

134. As Defence Minister Magnus Malan stated at the National Party congress in August 1986, "Those who chant loudest in the chorus for sanctions and condemnation should take note—we have not even started to use our muscle and capabilities." *Washington Post*, 23 September 1986.

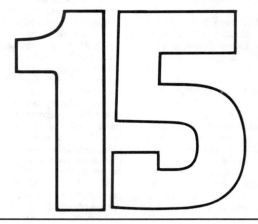

INDIA

Jerrold F. Elkin and Andrew Ritezel

International Environment

Since gaining independence from the United Kingdom in 1947, New Delhi has gained an ascendant power position in the Indian subcontinent, and seeks to attain like status in the Indian Ocean littoral. It presently maintains the world's third largest standing army, fifth largest air force, and eighth largest navy. Defense expenditures for 1987–88 increased to U.S. $9.8 billion, a 23 percent rise over 1986–87 spending levels. Monies allocated to defense constitute nearly 20 percent of total budgetary outlays.[1] Systems acquisition programs focus on weapons of indigenous as well as foreign manufacture. Indeed, India's defense production sector surpasses all other noncommunist Third World states in terms of quantity, value, and equipment diversity.[2]

Acceleration of arms procurement efforts is driven both by instabilities in the South Asian security environment and a desire to achieve recognition as a middle power in the context of global interaction. At the apex of New Delhi's threat hierarchy are two geographically proximate states, Pakistan and China. The increasing effectiveness of Pakistan's armed forces, evidenced by the purchase of U.S. F-16 multirole combat aircraft and possible development of nuclear weapons, raises serious defense issues.[3] Indian disquiet is heightened by the prospect of augmented or closer military linkages between Pakistan and extraregional powers, to include the United States, China, and even the Soviet Union. Pakistan has been the recipient of substantial economic assistance from the Soviet Union, as instanced by Soviet construction of a large steel mill. In the late 1970s, an agreement was reached to expand economic ties. However, Moscow unilaterally terminated this arrangement because of perceived support for Afghan insurgents by Islamabad.

India is concerned that extensive involve-

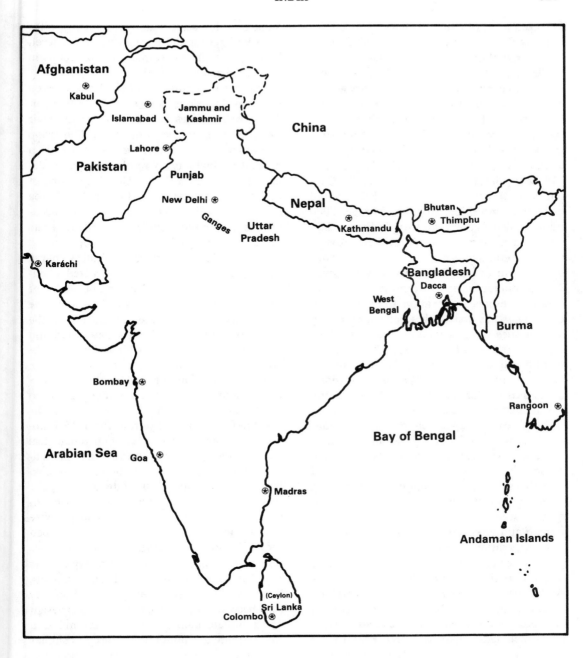

ment in subcontinental affairs by extraregional states could jeopardize its status as the dominant regional power. This, in turn, has led to repeated articulation of the demand that no foreign military bases be established in South Asia. New Delhi also is endeavoring to lessen the disadvantages presented by Islamabad's defense ties with Islamic nations. This undertaking is grounded in the need to prevent third party arms transfers during any future conflict with Pakistan. Policy implementation measures include support for Arab causes in international forums and institution of training programs for West Asian military personnel.

(Assured access to vital primary commodities is an ancillary benefit of Indian endeavors at enhancing relations with Arab states.)

The assimilation of advanced systems into Pakistan's conventional arms inventory greatly complicates Indian contingency planning. Nevertheless, Indian arms acquisition efforts far surpass those of Pakistan, involving such weaponry as Soviet T-72 tanks, BMP infantry combat vehicles, MiG-23/27/Flogger and MiG-29/Fulcrum fighter aircraft, IL-76/Candid heavy transport aircraft, and Mi-25/Hind helicopter gunships; French Mirage 2000 multimission fighters; and Anglo-French Jaguar deep penetration strike aircraft. Absent the unilateral deployment of nuclear weapons by Pakistan (an unlikely circumstance given Indian domestic political imperatives), increasing resource allocation for defense requirements has done little to alter preexisting asymmetries in regional power relations. Thus, a fourth Indo-Pakistani war probably would witness rapid advances by Indian combat units, resulting in the occupation of considerable Pakistani territory before external diplomatic pressure could terminate hostilities.

Such a conflict appeared imminent in January 1987 when India and Pakistan positioned substantial military forces along their common border. The crisis resulted in part from mutual apprehensions (and misjudgments) regarding troop movements during exercises held adjacent to areas of internal unrest *viz.*, India's Punjab and Pakistan's Sind. The Indian exercise, "Operation Brasstacks," was the largest ever conducted by New Delhi, involving nearly one-third of the Indian Army. This, in turn, reflected Chief of the Army Staff General K. Sundarji's desire to enhance combat readiness and interservice coordination (exercise participants included Indian Air Force Western Air Command assets and Indian Navy amphibious units) as well as refine the operational employment of mechanized ground elements. Among the Pakistani responses to "Brasstacks" were the prolongation of its winter exercises followed by the forward deployment of armored and infantry divisions near Indian Punjab. Ultimately, both parties recognized that preexisting policy disputes did not warrant engage-

ment in a full-scale war. Consequently, talks were initiated at the Foreign Secretary level, leading to a phased restationing of troops in peacetime cantonments.[4]

The early months of 1987 also witnessed heightened tensions along the Sino-Indian border as both parties increased materially their force levels near the Himalayas. The troop buildup was occasioned, *inter alia*, by (1) a continuing inability to resolve boundary demarcation issues, (2) New Delhi's granting of full statehood to Arunachal Pradesh, an area claimed by Beijing, and (3) the trading of accusations that Indian and Chinese military units repeatedly executed cross-border operations. This last point is illustrated by India's charge (issued in 1986) that China constructed a helicopter pad in the Sumdorong Chu valley of western Aruchanal Pradesh. It should be noted that platoon-scale skirmishes in the same area during October 1962 escalated into a major conflict in which China's People's Liberation Army rapidly gained the ascendancy.[5]

The humiliation suffered in the 1962 war and Beijing's issuance of an ultimatum (ostensibly dealing with military works on the Sikkim-Tibet frontier) during the 1965 Indo-Pakistani war have had a lasting psychological effect on India's ruling elites. Indian apprehensions respecting Chinese military intentions, including a possible thrust into the Gangetic plain or Indian heartland, contributed to Indian decisions to detonate a nuclear device in 1974, to station mountain divisions trained for high-altitude operations and air force squadrons in border areas, and to expand the regional logistics network. India's satellite launch vehicle development program also may have been actuated in part by a desire to design and fabricate ballistic missiles, serving as a counterpoise to China's ICBM force. A similar motivation (i.e., fear of Chinese military capabilities) may impel the procurement of some conventional weapons systems, such as artillery suitable for mountain operations.

For its part, China has upgraded substantially the logistics infrastructure in Tibet by building roads, an oil pipeline, and a railway. In consequence, Beijing reportedly can support approximately 20 divisions in the border region.[6] Nevertheless, several factors suggest that India readily could withstand a major Chinese attack (although China may prove able to achieve limited military goals, e.g., territorial gains in the Thag La triangle). Thus, the Indian Air Force (IAF) holds sophisticated fighters in its inventory, while China must employ aircraft copied from obsolescent Soviet designs. New Delhi also enjoys a marked technological advantage in armor, anti-tank weapons, and naval systems. In addition, it is likely that operational constraints presented by a Himalayan combat setting would preclude full application of China's numerically superior ground and air resources. Further, Chinese military adventurism (including such indirect action as provision of war matériel to Islamabad during an Indo-Pakistani conflict) well may be inhibited by India's close association with the Soviet Union.

In sum, it appears that India's growing war prosecution capabilities will permit the repulsion of a Chinese offensive in the Himalayas and the rapid defeat of Pakistan. Accordingly, the ongoing procurement of advanced weaponry (including naval, naval aviation, and amphibious warfare systems) demonstrates that India's security concerns are not confined to the subcontinent, but include the Indian Ocean and its periphery. Arms modernization efforts that now make application of military force throughout the region possible may have contributed to the expanded geographic scope of Indian security interests. Indeed, New Delhi's increasing ability to project maritime force at considerable distances from the South Asian mainland likely has revivified earlier aspirations to achieve politico-military paramountcy in the Indian Ocean. This, in turn, would form an underpinning for status elevation demands upon the international community, entailing recognition as a middle power on the order of Great Britain or France.

It should be noted parenthetically that employment of military resources as a status enhancement mechanism is a novel phenomenon for India. In the immediate postindependence period, Indian prestige was grounded in articulated concern with ethical principles of international behavior. New Delhi endeavored to regulate the conduct of other nations, suggesting that its own foreign and defense policies conformed to the highest moral standards. Defeat in the 1962 border war with China led to a rethinking of these policies and a substantial expansion of Indian ground and air forces. Recent years have witnessed a strengthening of naval forces as well, resulting from heightened awareness of threats to India's coasts (with 10 major, 29 intermediate, and 195 minor ports), sea lines of communication, and offshore island possessions and commercial interests. (Among the assets located in India's "exclusive economic zone" are the Bombay High oil field, possessing sufficient petroleum deposits to satisfy nearly two-thirds of domestic requirements; manganese nodules; and traditional fishing grounds.)

Despite its large military arsenal, New Delhi's attempts to gain recognition as the principal Indian Ocean power have been impeded by the presence of American, Soviet, and French naval vessels. Clearly, India can not be characterized as the dominant regional actor if warships from nonlittoral state navies may be positioned in its contiguous waters during crises. In this context, the U.S. aircraft carrier *Enterprise* was deployed to the Bay of Bengal during the 1971 Indo-Pakistani war, an application of armed force intended to restrict the latitude for action by Indian policy makers. Subsequently, Washington has stationed a carrier battle group in the Arabian Sea, upgraded its military installations on the island of Diego Garcia, and organized a Rapid Deployment Force.[7] India is troubled particularly by the prospect of U.S. tactical units being employed against states with which it enjoys significant political or economic ties. Among other efforts to counter U.S. strategic capabilities in the area, the USSR has acquired basing rights in Aden.[8] In consequence, a major power confrontation disrupting India's shipping routes to the Persian Gulf has become an increasingly plausible scenario to Indian policy makers.[9]

New Delhi has launched several diplomatic initiatives to exclude U.S. and Soviet warships from the Indian Ocean. For example, it has supported the institution of an Indian Ocean Zone of Peace; establishment of this legal regime would compel the withdrawal of all extraregional military and naval forces. Further, it has backed the demand submitted by Mauritius for retrocession of the Chagos archipelago, including Diego Garcia.[10] Confirmation of Mauritius' title to Diego Garcia would severely inhibit U.S. operations in these waters. If such undertakings ultimately reach fruition, India well could fill the resulting power vacuum.

Given a history of policy discord, Indo-American adoption of incompatible positions regarding power distribution in the Indian Ocean is far from surprising. However, Indo-Soviet policy disharmony is contrary to expectation, in light of assessments previously advanced by senior U.S. officials that India is little more than a Soviet client state. In fact, disagreements between India and the USSR comprehend several issue areas, including Moscow's occupation of Afghanistan. India's disapprobatory attitude concerning the injection of Soviet troops into South Asia rests on the possible invalidation of its claim to regional politico-military supremacy. Soviet action also induced the United States to conclude a $3.2 billion security and economic assistance agreement with Pakistan. Further, Soviet military pressure increases the likelihood of Pakistan's disintegration, which could (1) compel New Delhi to assume administrative control over a large, hostile Muslim population, and (2) occasion armed confrontation between Indian and Soviet units stationed along a common border. New Delhi's defense requirements are therefore best satisfied by a strong Pakistan (although not one powerful enough to threaten India) serving as a buffer state.

At the same time, however, the Indo-Soviet relationship is marked by considerable mutuality of interest. Moscow views New Delhi both as a counter to China and a useful contributor to efforts at constricting the range of U.S. military activity. In addition, Indian backing of Soviet policy stances (e.g., recognition of the Heng Samrin government in Kampuchea) is most consequential given its leadership role in the Non-Aligned Movement.[11] Conversely, New Delhi views its defense ties with Moscow as a deterrent to third party intervention in future Indo-Pakistani conflicts. Such linkages

also may serve to arrest any Soviet expansionist ambitions in South Asia. The 1971 Treaty of Peace, Friendship, and Cooperation constitutes the juridical foundation of this security relationship. Its terms stipulate that neither state may execute agreements inimical to the other's defense needs and require joint consultation in the event of substantial military threat to either party.

Military sales form a core element of Indo-Soviet interaction, the USSR furnishing some 70 percent of India's arms imports. The signing of purchase agreements has been facilitated by low unit costs, concessionary interest rates, and payment in rupees. (Moscow accepts the rupee as a medium of exchange in all commercial transactions with India. In this way, New Delhi can obtain Soviet crude oil, petroleum products, and other goods without reducing its hard currency reserves. This arrangement in part accounts for Moscow's status as India's second largest trading partner, after the United States.[12]) The attractiveness of Soviet arms packages is further enhanced by Moscow's willingness to (1) permit licensed production of various systems in India and (2) sell increasingly sophisticated weaponry, thereby furnishing a disincentive for arms source diversification. Nevertheless, New Delhi still devotes scarce pecuniary resources to the acquisition of Western combat equipment and looks to the West for the import of advanced technology (nonmilitary as well as military). These states also provide considerable economic aid to India, typically channeled through such multinational bodies as the International Monetary Fund and Asian Development Bank.

Procurement of Soviet and Western weapon systems has greatly improved the combat effectiveness of India's military services. However, the application of such combat assets to external defense missions may be hindered by the intensification of centrifugal sociopolitical forces within India. Thus, the Indian Army has positioned some 200,000 soldiers in the northeastern states (one of the largest troop concentrations in India) to suppress armed insurrection. Robert L. Hardgrave, Jr., observes that "tribal regions of the Northeast remain under a form of quasi-martial law, reflecting both the continuing danger of unrest and the strategically vulnerable nature of the region."[13] The army's counterinsurgency program has two principal components: combat operations (often assisted by the air force) and such developmental welfare activities as expanding transportation and communication infrastructures and providing medical support, including health education as well as diagnostic and curative services. It should be noted that political initiatives by the central government have led to conclusion of accords with militant leaders in Assam and Mizoram. However, the agreement with Assamese student militants appears unstable, as New Delhi may prove unable (or disinclined) to discharge certain of its commitments, e.g., erection of a physical barrier separating Assam and Bangladesh. (Demands for political autonomy, often accompanied by violence, have been advanced in other regions of India as well, to include Punjab and Kashmir. The latter is a likely battleground in future Indo-Pakistani wars, where military success may rest on the active cooperation of the civil population. Most recently, there has been an effort to establish a Gurkha state encompassing the Darjeeling district of West Bengal. The declared objective of the Gurkhaland movement has alternated between secession and statehood within the Indian Union.) In addition to internal security duties, the army has regularly been tasked with riot control. Police and paramilitary units have proven unable to quell growing urban violence, a phenomenon grounded in communal antagonisms and economic inequality.

Aid to civil authority thus constitutes a central army mission element, as evidenced by participation in more than three hundred internal security and violence suppression operations during 1980–83.[14] Concern has been voiced that this mission reorientation could substantially degrade the army's combat readiness. Absent supplemental funding, army resource allocation for domestic task execution implies a concomitant diminution of resources available for external defense measures. Involvement in domestic affairs has impaired the army's organizational integrity as well. For ex-

ample, the 1984 antiterrorist offensive in Punjab generated considerable dissension among the ranks of Sikh military personnel. Approximately two thousand Sikh soldiers were arrested and fifty killed in a series of desertions and mutinies.[15] Further, the ineffectual manner in which state officials responded to terrorism led to the appointment of Lt. Gen. R. S. Dayal (chief of staff, Western Command) as home advisor to the governor of Punjab. Army supervision of the Home Department marked the first time in Indian history that the military had assumed de facto control of a state government. It therefore appears that attention devoted to intrastate conflict not only has affected the army's corporateness and group cohesion, but also may serve to politicize the armed forces.

Additional domestic factors having a detrimental influence on Indian national security include the lack of a high technology base, precluding the indigenous manufacture of advanced military end items; energy resource dependency on foreign states; and insufficient hard currency reserves, limiting the purchase of weaponry from Western sources.

National Objectives, National Strategy, and Military Doctrine

The fundamental security objective held by ruling elites is maintenance of India's territorial integrity, a concern generated by insurgencies in strategically important border regions. This statement is confirmed by examination of issue areas addressed in recent countrywide elections when domestic threats to national unity, rather than external defense, constituted the thematic focus of campaign debate. Nevertheless, the Indian leadership is devoting considerable attention to external security questions. Thus, New Delhi is determined to gain recognition as a dominant regional actor. Goals have been couched in the language of nonalignment. For example, Indian demands that (1) no foreign bases be established in the subcontinent, (2) the Indian Ocean be demilitarized, and (3) South Asian security and political relations emphasize bilateral interaction are clearly intended to limit regional involvement by outside powers. Such arrangements also would preclude formation of military linkages among South Asian states inimical to Indian security interests. Further, New Delhi claims a right to intervene in the internal affairs of neighboring countries if disorder threatens to extend beyond national boundaries (the "Indira Doctrine"). Implementation of this agenda would greatly facilitate creation of a sphere of influence comprising both the subcontinent and the Indian Ocean littoral.[16]

In the future, the geographic scope of Indian defense concerns likely will continue to broaden, encompassing extraregional security matters. Indeed, numerous officials have articulated the view that India will emerge as a global power by the end of the century. In this context, New Delhi's security interests soon may reach to near Earth orbit. India has designed and fabricated satellites and launch vehicles. Policy pronouncements have stressed the peaceful nature of space undertakings. On the other hand, such capabilities could readily be put to military use: reconnaissance satellites; a satellite-enhanced command, control, and communications (C^3) network; and ballistic missiles (assuming an antecedent determination to develop nuclear weaponry, along with improved guidance systems and an ablative heat shield for warhead reentry).

The formulation of defense policy, and consequent distribution of resources among the military services, have not been subjected to meaningful public scrutiny. Parliament customarily endorses Ministry of Defense (MoD) proposals with little dissent or discussion. In consequence, MoD budget debates constitute one of the most poorly attended legislative activities. The tractability of Indian parliamentarians may in part reflect popular apathy (with an attendant absence of pressure on representative institutions) regarding security questions. Such lack of interest well may rest on the failure of the executive to produce a coherent body of statements defining official security doctrine. While commentators frequently call for more thoughtful consideration of military programs by Parliament, it is doubtful that existing deliberative procedures will be modified in the near term.[17]

GOAL ACHIEVEMENT STRATEGIES

Several elements likely enter New Delhi's decision calculus regarding Indian Ocean policy goals. First, India has greatly expanded its arms inventory, focusing on procurement of sophisticated weaponry. This effort is motivated principally by a desire to counter the Sino-Pakistani threat. However, it has also rendered feasible a number of previously unavailable policy choices in the Indian Ocean (based on augmented force projection capabilities). Thus, the Indian Navy's ability to lift battalion-size infantry formations, along with armor and artillery support, may permit execution of violence suppression missions in Sri Lanka. Further, naval units can now successfully conduct antishipping and antisubmarine operations throughout much of the Indian Ocean.

Second, New Delhi has significant commercial interests in the Indian Ocean (e.g., fishing, extractive industries, oceanic trade routes) and enjoys broadened economic relations with Indian Ocean island and littoral states. A novel aspect of India's regional trade relations is the importance assigned to export of weapons and other combat support equipment. Military sales previously were limited to small arms and ammunition; New Delhi presently seeks consumers for light artillery, military vehicles, and electronics systems.[18] Beyond this, India has instituted a modest program of economic and military assistance to regional states. As with arms sales, this undertaking serves to lessen dependence on the Soviet Union and the West, while increasing island and littoral state interaction with New Delhi (a politically acceptable alternative because of India's nonaligned status).[19]

Third, Indian nationals (and persons of Indian descent) residing in neighboring countries have experienced recurrent threats to their lives and property. Difficulties encountered by the Tamil minority in Sri Lanka demonstrate the vulnerability of Indian communities throughout the region. In addition to the ties of citizenship and consanguinity, New Delhi's concern for the welfare of overseas Indian populations rests on commercial opportunities in Indian Ocean states, foreign exchange requirements, and domestic politics. There is no evidence to suggest that New Delhi has influenced second party trade policies by manipulating these communities; nevertheless, they furnish a useful access mechanism for Indian entrepreneurs endeavoring to launch business initiatives. Further, these groups are an important source of foreign exchange, with remittances totaling some $5 billion annually. Finally, the safety of overseas Indians has become a contentious political issue. Thus, Sri Lankan communal violence has precipitated demands by Tamil politicians in southern India that the central government take coercive steps against Colombo.

Fourth, serious defense concerns have been generated by the deployment of extraregional naval forces in the Indian Ocean. Withdrawal of these warships would materially alter the Indian Ocean threat environment, thereby simplifying New Delhi's contingency planning. For example, the Falkland Islands conflict in the south Atlantic has alerted India to the fact that its own offshore island chains may be open to attack. If a littoral state managed to occupy one or more of these possessions, senior Indian Navy officers suggest that support by outside powers would greatly complicate dislodgment operations.[20] Most significantly, removal of American and Soviet naval combatants from the Indian Ocean would allow New Delhi to fill the resulting power vacuum (as the U.S. and USSR filled the void left by Great Britain in the 1960s). This, in turn, would facilitate establishment of sponsor-client security relations with island and littoral states.

Fifth, New Delhi's concentration on Indian Ocean security issues in part arises from the need to limit involvement by West Asian countries (situated on the Indian Ocean periphery) in subcontinental affairs. Islamabad maintains defense ties with a number of Islamic nations. At least one Pakistani infantry division is stationed in Saudi Arabia; servicemen have been seconded to other West Asian military forces as training program instructors.[21] These linkages both increase Pakistani familiarity with advanced weapons systems and enhance prospects for arms transfers during future Indo-Pakistani wars.

Sixth, New Delhi wishes to translate heightened regional influence into acceptance as a major participant in global security and political arrangements. This policy determination is likely driven by prestige and other psychological considerations. India covers a vast land territory and offshore "exclusive economic zone"; possesses substantial natural and human resources; and maintains a large military establishment, as well as a growing industrial base. New Delhi believes it should enjoy a position in the hierarchy of states commensurate with these realities. In this context, various governmental undertakings can be seen as prestige enhancement vehicles. The space program offers a useful case in point. An improved communications capability forms a core objective of space activities. However, nationwide television broadcasting could have commenced in the 1970s (at greatly reduced cost) through off-the-shelf purchase of satellite systems from second parties. It therefore appears that emphasis given to the indigenous manufacture of space hardware is grounded in national pride and strategic concerns, with articulated economic goals as a secondary motivation.

Taken as a whole, this set of factors has impelled New Delhi to seek a dominant power position in the Indian Ocean. Measures adopted to attain regional objectives include: modernization and expansion of naval and naval aviation assets, the coast guard, and air force units performing maritime interdiction roles; Indian Navy visits to foreign ports; provision of defense training and economic and technical assistance to other countries; and other diplomatic initiatives.

The Indian Navy numbers over seventy combatant ships and approximately fifty thousand men. It is the only fleet of an Indian Ocean nation to maintain an aircraft carrier—the INS *Vikrant*, a light carrier of the British Majestic class. The *Vikrant's* naval air force component consists of British Sea Harrier V/STOL fighters and Sea Kings, furnishing a significant antishipping capability. The *Vikrant* is expected to remain in service until 1992; New Delhi has purchased the HMS *Hermes* from Great Britain (to be renamed the INS *Virat*) as a replacement vessel.[22] India is endeavoring to procure such other capital ships as Soviet Kresta-class guided missile cruisers.[23]

Naval air defense resources have been strengthened by the acquisition of Soviet

Kashin-class guided missile destroyers fitted with SA-N-1 surface-to-air and SS-N-2c surface-to-surface missile launchers. The Indian Navy has eight Soviet F-class diesel submarines. These will be supplemented by six Soviet Kilo-class submarines, the first of which was delivered to the navy in 1986.[24] Further, India is acquiring four SSK Type 1500 submarines from West Germany.[25]

Construction of Godavari-class guided missile frigates (an Indian design based on the British Leander-class frigate) forms another element of the navy's modernization program. Modernization efforts also involve procurement of landing craft, supplementing the existing inventory of six Polnocny-class LCTs and four LCUs.[26]

The naval air arm consists of more than thirty-five combat aircraft and twenty helicopters.[27] Airborne maritime reconnaissance operations have been inhibited by the limited number (and subsequent overuse) of IL-38/Mays. The navy therefore may obtain the Soviet TU-142m, a variant of the TU-95/Bear, to meet strategic reconnaissance requirements.[28]

The Indian Navy's ability to discharge regional power projection responsibilities has been enhanced by the establishment of a coast guard. This service has assumed many duties previously assigned to the navy, such as marine search and rescue. Indeed, some Indian journalists now discuss a two-tiered maritime strategy with force projection throughout the Indian Ocean performed by the navy while the coast guard focuses on offshore areas.[29]

The Indian Air Force contributes to power projection efforts as well, with IL-76/Candid transports available for strategic airlift missions. (The IL-76 is a Soviet cargo aircraft, equivalent in payload and performance to the U.S. Air Force's C-141.)[30] Further, Indian Air Force fighter-bombers can be employed in a maritime strike or interdiction role. In this context, a Southern Air Command has been established at Trivandrum, tasked with protecting the southern peninsula and offshore island territories.[31]

Some Southern Air Command assets may be repositioned from the mainland to forward operating locations in the Andaman-Nicobar islands. Such a move, long planned by the air force[32] would (1) substantially increase the ocean area defended by landbased aircraft; (2) make possible attacks against ships transiting the adjacent Strait of Malacca; and (3) permit enemy naval and air forces to be engaged at considerable distances from the subcontinent.

While force projection and defense of sea lines of communication constitute primary navy missions, the navy has been assigned diplomatic tasks as well. Warship visits to foreign countries traditionally have served as influence-building measures, demonstrating the naval power available to national decision makers. New Delhi now utilizes this technique to increase its political influence throughout the region. Thus, the past decade has witnessed naval visits to virtually all Indian Ocean and Persian Gulf states.[33]

The institution of defense training programs also serves to acquaint regional actors with the growing effectiveness of India's armed forces. In addition, foreign student interaction with Indian military instructors (especially in academic or professional military education courses of long duration) could well contribute to a sympathetic view of New Delhi's security policies. The generation of such perceptions would be most consequential, as many foreign trainees have assumed senior positions in their government's military and administrative bureaucracies.[34]

New Delhi has established military training arrangements (although some are no longer active) with extraregional as well as Indian Ocean states. Participating states can be grouped into four categories (with overlapping membership), which suggest ancillary benefits India expects to derive from training efforts. Thus, New Delhi has furnished instruction to servicemen from a substantial number of Commonwealth nations, including Botswana, Ghana, Kenya, Malaysia, Mauritius, Nigeria, Seychelles, Singapore, Sri Lanka, Tanzania, Uganda, and Zambia.[35] India likely hopes that strengthened ties with Commonwealth states may lead to increased support for its policy stances in such organizations as the Non-Aligned Movement and United Nations. Countries with large Indian populations (citizens or persons of Indian ancestry) form a second category of training recipients that includes Burma, Kenya, Malaysia, Mauritius, Oman, Singapore, Sri Lanka, and Tanzania.[36] The conclusion of military training agreements with states in this category has probably been motivated by a desire to ensure the social and economic well-being of these Indian communities. A third category is composed of principal trading partners, such as Iran and Iraq.[37] In this case, New Delhi has likely initiated military training programs both to encourage broadened commercial linkages and to guarantee the availability of critical primary commodities. The final category consists of Persian Gulf states: Iran, Iraq, and Oman.[38] Involvement with states in category four is in part designed to counter Pakistani–West Asian security relations.

Beyond this, New Delhi is contributing significantly to the economic development of several Indian Ocean states. Cooperative efforts focus on reservation of seats for foreign students in medical, engineering, and other technical institutions; in-country provision of technical assistance by Indian experts (e.g., physicians, engineers, accountants, and public administrators); in-country operation of small-scale industrial facilities for training purposes; and execution of economic feasibility studies.[39] Implementation of such measures results from New Delhi's desire to promote its image as a regional patron.

Finally, New Delhi has employed diplomatic initiatives to facilitate achievement of Indian Ocean policy objectives. For example, it has fashioned a consensus among island and littoral states supporting the institution of an Indian Ocean Zone of Peace (IOZP) which would exclude extraregional powers. (It should be noted, however, that IOZP definitions advanced by other Indian Ocean states frequently envision a reduction in the force levels of all navies patrolling these waters, including the Indian Navy. New Delhi does not support such an expansive interpretation of the IOZP concept.) In the early 1970s Sri Lanka was persuaded to introduce this proposal before a conference of the Non-Aligned Movement and the United Nations General Assembly. The IOZP plan was embraced by both organizations.[40] The IOZP has also been endorsed by the USSR. Soviet acceptance could well rest on the assumption that demilitarization of the Indian Ocean remains infeasible, given U.S. hostility toward this arrangement. Additionally, proximity to the region would give Moscow a clear geostrategic advantage if all nonlittoral armed forces were in fact withdrawn.

DOMESTIC DETERMINANTS OF NATIONAL STRATEGY

The Indian public typically manifests disinterest in defense issues. Nevertheless, the exacerbation of ethnic tensions in Sri Lanka has generated significant reaction in southern India, based on emotional association with Tamil separatists. The disinclination of the central government (controlled by northern Indians) to take military action against Colombo has reinforced the perception that political elites remain insensitive to southern sentiments. Such disaffection also demonstrates that segments of Indian society are now directing considerable attention to external security questions. Additionally, calls for a military resolution of Tamil-Sinhalese differences in Sri Lanka suggest that, if necessary, New Delhi could mobilize substantial public support for the expansion of its Indian Ocean combat forces.

It should be noted parenthetically that traditional public disregard of security and foreign policies does not extend to domestic affairs. For example, there has been resistance to imposition of quotas favoring scheduled or lower castes and other disadvantaged minorities. Indeed preferential treatment of specified communal groups has frequently precipitated urban violence, most recently in Gujarat.

The organization of India's economy may also influence its defense posture. India is in transition from a socialist to a mixed economy, emulating Western models. Further, it is seeking increased investment from the United States and EC countries. Greater economic interaction with the West in time could affect a broad spectrum of defense questions, ranging from arms procurement to security alignments.

Defense policy formulation may be affected

by geographical concerns as well. The fact that (1) the subcontinent projects into the Indian Ocean; (2) New Delhi's sea lines of communication pass through these waters; and (3) the Andaman-Nicobar island chain lies adjacent to the Strait of Malacca, a principal oceanic choke point, in part accounts for the establishment of hegemonic regional policy goals.

The subcontinent's varied geophysical features and climate likely constitute another determinant of defense policy. Indian Army personnel must be trained and equipped for operations in mountain, plain, and jungle environments. Indeed, recent exchanges of fire with Pakistani troops have occurred in the Siachen glacier area of Kashmir, at altitudes exceeding 18,000 feet.[41] The Indian Army, a force numbering more than one million men, is thus designed to repel conventional attacks by neighboring states in diverse combat settings.

Finally, demographic factors may impinge upon defense aims. India possesses an impressive human resource base, including one of the largest pools of engineers in the world. Moreover, the increasing proficiency of defense industry workers has allowed India to produce sophisticated weaponry. Nevertheless, there remain profound weaknesses in many industrial sectors, such as electronics. Further, India's huge population suffers from poverty, illiteracy, and disease. Amelioration of these problems ultimately may compel the redistribution of money from defense needs to human services.

MILITARY DOCTRINE

India's security objectives require (1) creation of asymmetrical power relations with South Asian states and (2) a greatly augmented maritime force-projection capability. The first element in this program has been achieved, as New Delhi presently has overwhelming military superiority in the subcontinent. However, if New Delhi hopes to attain Indian Ocean supremacy, additional funds must be devoted to the navy, which now receives only 10 percent of defense outlays. Systems acquisition must focus on advanced, carrier-based strike aircraft; amphibious warfare assets, including large

landing ships and establishment of an independent naval infantry (thereby ending reliance on army personnel with limited training in amphibious operations); and, possibly, a second aircraft carrier to join the *Hermes* (some Indian strategists assert that two such vessels are needed to safeguard the "exclusive economic zone" and monitor local deployments of extraregional navies).

The manner in which New Delhi will employ its combat resources best can be ascertained by examining a given scenario, e.g., a non-nuclear conflict with Pakistan. In the event of an Indo-Pakistani War, the Indian Army's principal goal will be to maximize territorial gains before external pressures terminate hostilities.[42] The army probably will direct the majority of its forces against Pakistani military and urban targets in Punjab. The Indian Army well may execute combined arms operations, supplementing tank formations with mechanized infantry, self-propelled artillery, and assault engineers. If tactics adopted during the 1971 East Pakistan campaign are deemed applicable to the Punjab, the army will attempt to encircle concentrations of Pakistani armor and defensive fortifications.[43] This would isolate elements of the Pakistani Army, disrupting communications and supply links. Destruction of the north-south transportation network in Sind will likely be a secondary army mission; such an undertaking will be facilitated by the ongoing expansion of the logistic infrastructure in neighboring Rajasthan.

In previous Indo-Pakistani conflicts, the civilian population in border regions has supported the Indian Army. Active cooperation no longer may be obtainable in Indian Punjab, as military occupation of this state (resulting from antiterrorist actions in 1984) has alienated important segments of the Sikh community. Indeed, it is possible that such persons would attempt to interrupt the movement of Indian troops and equipment. While instances of sabotage would not preclude the ultimate success of army offensives, they clearly would impede the war effort.

A future war with Pakistan would also witness Indian Air Force raids on command and control centers, Pakistani Air Force main bases, and communication and transportation facilities.[44] The Jaguar, India's principal deep penetration strike aircraft, would perform many of these tasks. Typical Jaguar (and other fighter-bomber) missions reportedly will involve sixteen aircraft, hitting targets in waves of four at 30-second intervals. They may be accompanied by two aircraft equipped for electronic countermeasures, along with four other escorts.[45] The consequent immobilization of Pakistan's armed forces would be followed by strikes against major ground units, likely carried out by Mig-23BNs and Mig-27s (a dedicated ground attack Flogger variant). This attack chronology may be altered by increasingly favorable Indian-Pakistani air force strength ratios which would allow the Indian Air Force to perform close air support and long-range interdiction and counterair responsibilities simultaneoulsy.

The conduct of naval operations in 1971 suggests that the navy will endeavor to blockade Karachi, thereby confining the small Pakistani Navy to this port and preventing the ingress and egress of Pakistani merchantmen.[46] Further, the positioning of Indian Navy vessels in these waters may lessen the prospect of direct or indirect (e.g., the transfer of war goods) intervention by extraregional states.

The development of force-employment doctrine falls within the organizational purview of the individual services. Limited interaction among service headquarters on doctrinal questions evidences a serious problem confronting senior officers, viz., the absence of integrated decision-making structures at upper echelons of the military hierarchy. The civilian leadership is not involved in doctrinal matters; rather, it fashions the broad strategic objectives that determine military planning.

War plans generated by the three services will be modified substantially if Pakistan assembles a nuclear bomb. Several factors indicate that Islamabad is currently endeavoring to fabricate such weaponry. In 1984 a Pakistani businessman confessed in U.S. federal court to the attempted illegal export of high-speed switches used to trigger nuclear explosives.[47] Additionally, China may have provided Pakistan with nuclear arms design information.[48]

Most significantly, Pakistan can now produce weapons grade uranium, employing centrifuge-enrichment technology.[49]

Prime Minister Rajiv Gandhi has declared that Pakistan's apparent willingness to exploit nuclear research for military purposes may compel India to implement like measures.[50] Further, the 1984–1985 Ministry of Defense Annual Report states that Pakistan's pursuit of nuclear capabilities has altered the nature of security threats facing India. Such pronouncements, in concert with (1) detonation of a nuclear device (requiring miniaturization to become a deliverable system) in 1974, (2) refusal to sign the Non-Proliferation Treaty, and (3) possession of unsafeguarded plutonium in considerable amounts, suggest that New Delhi could rapidly deploy nuclear armaments.[51] Indeed, it is doubtful that any Indian government could resist popular pressure for nuclear weapons deployment if Islamabad constructs atomic bombs. Moreover, the Indian military would not accept the neutralization of its conventional superiority over Pakistan with equanimity.

If the subcontinent experiences a nuclear arms race, India (given its greater resource base) probably will surpass Pakistan in warhead production. It would enjoy a marked advantage in delivery vehicles as well. For example, Indian bombers can attack targets throughout Pakistan, while Pakistani aircraft can only reach objectives in northwestern or north central India.

Beyond this, New Delhi readily could translate its civilian space undertakings into an intermediate range ballistic missile program. The addition of nuclear weapons to India's inventory would also yield the following benefits: materially enhanced status in the international community; improved ability to deter low-level threats from extraregional powers; and the prospect of negotiating border questions with China from a position of equality. Furthermore, it likely would not damage Indo-Soviet relations, as New Delhi still forms a useful counter to Beijing.

Increased concern about nuclear conflict in the subcontinent probably has impelled Indian planning staffs to begin formulating a strategy for conducting nuclear war. In this context, the army chief of staff, Gen. Krishnaswamy Sundarji, has declared that military personnel are now being trained and organized to limit physical and psychological damage in the event of a Pakistani nuclear attack.[52] Further, some newly acquired Soviet equipment such as the T-72 tank and BMP Infantry Combat Vehicle may be designed to survive in a nuclear, biological, or chemical (NBC) environment.

The Defense Decision-Making Process

Article 53(2) of the Indian Constitution vests command of the armed forces in the president.[53] However, de facto control rests with the prime minister and cabinet. Such control is strengthened by the absence of a meaningful parliamentary role in the fashioning of national security policy.[54] The views of the prime minister on security questions thus often prove to be decisive.

The cabinet's Political Affairs Committee is the highest policy-making authority on defense matters. The prime minister serves as chairman; other members include the defense minister and the ministers for external affairs, home affairs, and finance. The convention exists that the chiefs of staff should be in attendance when military issues are reviewed, but the service leadership has no established right of access to this body.[55] Further, committee consideration of proposals advanced by military headquarters (usually relating to equipment purchases and conditions of service) is structured in terms of yes/no decisions. The government has failed, however, to establish agencies for independent appraisal of these programs, examining their defense, foreign policy, and economic implications.[56]

The minister of defense is the principal link between the cabinet and service chiefs. As head of the MoD, his responsibilities are manifold and include endorsement, disapproval, or modification of proposals generated by the military; control of public sector industries which manufacture defense items; interministerial coordination; and issuance of public policy statements on national security questions.

Details of finance, administration, and supply are managed by the defense minister's secretariat, led by the defense secretary, a senior civil servant.[57] The execution of ministerial duties is facilitated by two committees: the defense minister's committee, which originates plans and deals with interservice issues; and the defense minister's (production and supply) committee, which oversees defense production efforts. The defense minister, minister of state for defense, deputy defense minister, defense secretary, financial advisor (defense), and service chiefs make up the membership of both committees.[58]

The defense minister's committee at one time constituted the only formal mechanism for incorporating service opinion into the formulation of national security policy. However, since 1974 this body has played a limited role in decision making, being superseded by the "morning meeting" and the committee for defense planning (CDP). The "morning meeting," instituted after the 1962 defeat by China, is held twice each week (or as desired by the defense minister). Participants include the cabinet secretary the ministry of defense secretaries, the science advisor to the defense minister (who superintends a large research and development organization engaged in improving and "indigenizing" military weaponry), and the service chiefs. The "morning meeting" furnishes a vehicle for the exchange of views on defense issues and presentation of collective advice to the defense minister.[59] Nevertheless, substantive decisions cannot be taken at such meetings, given the absence of a fixed agenda or papers circulated for discussion. Further, this arrangement may facilitate treatment of daily events, but clearly is not conducive to long-range planning.[60] The CDP was established in 1978 under the chairmanship of the cabinet secretary and includes the secretary to the prime minister; the secretaries for defense, defense production, finance, and external affairs; the secretary of the Planning Commission; and the three military chiefs. The defense minister does not take part in CDP activities. Evaluation of defense plans drafted by the services is a major committee function.[61]

In addition to the MoD, other ministries

participate in the determination of national security policy. The joint intelligence committee (JIC) serves as a channel of communication between the defense and foreign affairs bureaucracies, and falls within the administrative purview of the cabinet secretariat. This committee had been chaired by an additional secretary in the cabinet secretariat; now two full secretaries head its internal and external wings. The membership includes joint secretaries from the Ministries of Defense, External Affairs, and Home Affairs; the military intelligence chiefs; and representatives of other intelligence agencies.[62] It should be noted parenthetically that the Senior Intelligence Board forms the apex of India's intelligence establishment. The security advisor in the cabinet secretariat presides over this body; members include the chairmen of the internal and external sections of the JIC and the directors of the Intelligence Bureau and the Research and Analysis Wing. Under this arrangement, the services have no intelligence collection responsibilities, but merely process information supplied by civilian agencies.[63]

Activities of the Finance Ministry are also central in defense policy formulation. Budgetary constraints established by this ministry (based on, say, foreign exchange holdings) materially affect the magnitude and direction of defense expenditures. The financial advisor, a representative of the Finance Ministry, works with the MoD on a continuing basis. He enjoys veto authority over weapons purchases, and can so act even after procurement decisions have been reached by the Ministry of Finance and Parliament. Formerly, proposals drafted by senior military officers were referred to the financial advisor and a consensus achieved before submission to the MoD. Such proposals now are referred to the financial advisor through the MoD, which precludes direct interaction between the military and those responsible for allocating funds to national defense.[64]

Service headquarters are affiliated with the Ministry of Defense (manned exclusively by civil servants), but fall outside its organizational structure. Interrelations among the military branches are designed to reinforce civilian political supremacy. Thus, the government has striven to augment the influence of the air force and navy at the expense of the numerically predominant army: each service head is designated a chief of staff (the position of commander in chief of all the services, held by the most senior army officer, was abolished shortly after independence); the chairman of the chiefs of staff committee is the officer with the longest tenure on that body, which often has meant an air force or navy representative.[65]

The chiefs of staff committee decides multiservice issues within its competence and serves as a platform for the joint presentation of advice or problems to the government. Subordinate entities include the joint planning committee, joint administrative planning committee, joint training committee, joint sea-air warfare committee, inter-services equipment policy committee, joint communications electronic committee, joint electronic warfare board, joint signals intelligence board, and the medical services advisory board. Except for the joint training committee and joint signals intelligence and medical services advisory boards, the chairmanship of these bodies is rotational, as is the case with the chiefs of staff committee.[66]

Several Indian military analysts suggest that the failure to incorporate the service headquarters and financial advisor into the Ministry of Defense has had a number of deleterious consequences: lack of an integrated approach to service requirements; isolation of the services from governmental decision loci; triplication of work, whereby the same question is examined independently in a military headquarters, then in the MoD, and yet again in the office of the financial advisor.[67] These analysts also object to the manner in which service recommendations are treated by the MoD and financial advisor. The Defense Ministry often processes service-generated proposals in a dilatory fashion. More significantly, MoD civil servants at all bureaucratic levels typically lack sufficient expertise in military affairs.[68] Nevertheless, such nonprofessionals sit in judgment on service programs, while bearing no executory responsibility.[69]

If a proposal is approved by the MoD, it is

forwarded to the financial advisor. The chief concern of this individual is to effect economy rather than support the legitimacy of service requirements. Further, he can veto a proposal (or approve a truncated version) without being answerable to the defense minister. On the other hand, those excessive budgetary distributions that do occur could be reduced by integrating the financial advisor and MoD, since responsibility for such profligacy would rest solely with the Defense Ministry. Moreover, this arrangement would improve relations between the services and the financial advisor (who still could receive functional guidance from the Ministry of Finance) and help achieve optimal use of available assets.[70]

The efficacy of present national defense committee arrangements also has come into question. While the membership of the defense minister's committee included senior political appointees, the CDP is dominated by civil servants. Therefore, institution of the CDP has served to limit interaction between the military and government leaders. In addition, underrepresentation of military personnel on the CDP weakens the professional underpinning of its determinations. Finally, CDP endorsement of service proposals may be only an antepenultimate step in the decision-making process, since proposals remain subject to time consuming examination in the Ministries of Defense and Finance.[71]

The chiefs of staff committee suffers from structural deficiencies as well. First, this body only has recommendatory, not peremptory, authority and its advice can be disregarded (even in conflict situations) by policy makers. Second, only questions deemed of common concern to all three services are submitted to the committee. If a chief unilaterally determines that his branch should take sole cognizance of a given administrative or operational issue (including force levels and choice of weaponry), then he may place the matter before the Defense Ministry without reference to the chiefs of staff or any other interservice committee.[72]

Critics contend that the higher defense organization has demonstrated an inability to meet wartime requirements. In the 1962 war with China, questions of strategy and tactics were

settled by the prime minister, defense minister, chief of the army staff, and some senior army officers. Multiservice committees, such as the chiefs of staff, joint intelligence, and joint planning committees, proved moribund or ineffective.[73]

The late Air Chief Marshal P. C. Lal asserted that India's higher defense organization made no significant contribution to combat operations against Pakistan in 1965. Gen. J. N. Chaudhuri, army chief and chairman of the chiefs of staff committee, anticipated a Pakistani attack but did not impart this information to the air force or navy. Rather, he considered the impending conflict to be an army affair in which the use of air and naval assets would be incidental.[74] After hostilities began, New Delhi decided to expand the geographical scope of military activity beyond Jammu and Kashmir. The army and air force thereupon drafted separate war plans (without any mutual consultation). According to Lal, air force leaders viewed the fighting in terms of strikes against the Pakistani air force and strategic targets, assigning low priority to close air support for ground forces.[75]

Following the 1965 war, a number of reforms were introduced to facilitate service interaction. For example, air force representation at army commands was strengthened and formed into advance headquarters with control over those units designated to assist land forces. Further, a program of frequent multiservice exercises was initiated.[76] Nevertheless, interservice coordination again was lacking in the 1971 war with Pakistan, especially in the western sector. To illustrate: the naval raid on Karachi harbor and air force strikes against nearby oil installations were conducted as separate operations by individual military branches. The level of cooperation that did obtain was attributable largely to the excellent personal rapport among the then military chiefs.[77] It must be stressed that the services exhibited cooperation (e.g., favorably responding to requests for help), not coordination, during this conflict. These cooperative impulses might have been strained in a war of greater duration than fourteen days. There also was the advantage of a similar absence of coordination among the Pakistani armed forces.[78]

Several suggestions have been advanced for reform of India's higher defense structures, viz., shifting chiefs of staff committee support elements from the cabinet secretariat to the prime minister's office, thereby giving the head of government direct access to professional military opinion; inviting the military chiefs to attend political affairs committee meetings regularly; reorganizing sections within the Ministry of Defense from single service to functional groupings; and authorizing active duty military personnel to fill positions in the MoD bureaucracy.[79]

The structural modification most frequently discussed by commentators, politicians, and both serving and former officers is creation of a chief of defense staff (CDS) post, analogous to that of the chairman of the U.S. Joint Chiefs of Staff. However, there is little likelihood that a CDS will be appointed in the next five to ten years. This assessment in part rests on service opposition, the air force and navy fearing that a succession of army CDS appointees would upset triservice equality and skew resource allocation decisions. Further, MoD civilian bureaucrats perceive the CDS as a status diminution mechanism, based on reduced control over the military. Senior political figures also view the CDS concept with disfavor, concerned that creation of a new center of authority within the military could threaten Indian democracy in exigent circumstances.

The political leadership's hostility toward institution of a CDS forms part of a larger design intended to maintain civilian supremacy over the military, both in terms of symbolism and the actual distribution of power. Thus, for example, the "warrant of precedence" has been adjusted to place ranking generals below cabinet officers. More significantly, the civilian administration traditionally has been reluctant to permit organization of an effective joint staff. The resulting perpetuation of interservice discord necessitates the resolution of contentious security issues at the political level (e.g., removing helicopter assets from air force control, thus permitting the establishment of an army aviation corps).

CONSTRAINTS ON DECISION MAKERS

If New Delhi deems a course of action to be militarily imperative, external pressure likely will not prevent the implementation of requisite measures. For example, the Soviet Union has proven unable to end Indian arms source diversification efforts, despite its status as principal foreign supplier of advanced weaponry. Nevertheless, second party reactions frequently affect Indian policy stances. Thus, New Delhi's reluctance to antagonize Islamic governments well may inhibit its response to provocative measures by Islamabad.

India's uneven industrial capabilities, concentrated in middle technology ranges, form a significant constraint on policy makers. To date, New Delhi has proven incapable of manufacturing sophisticated military equipment, as evidenced by its inability to design and fabricate a supersonic fighter aircraft. Efforts at surmounting technological shortcomings include the incorporation of technology transfer and coproduction provisions in arms procurement agreements. However, licensed production of weapons systems has often increased dependency on foreign suppliers rather than Indian self-reliance. Further, indigenously manufactured weapons typically contain a substantial number of foreign components, for example, the engine, gear box, and communications equipment on the army's "Arjun" main battle tank.[80] Technical problems in arms production are compounded by administrative difficulties. Thus, the air force established a requirement for a multipurpose armed light helicopter in the early 1970s. Design and construction responsibilities were assigned to Hindustan Aeronautics, Ltd. (HAL), a public sector or government firm. However, changes in air force design parameters, inadequacies of HAL's engineering staff, and a dilatory approach to project decision making severely impeded helicopter development. Consequently, New Delhi has been compelled to obtain two squadrons of helicopter gunships from the Soviet Union; reportedly, it seeks to purchase an additional 200 combat helicopters from a Western source (likely the Italian Augusta A-129 or West German MBB Bo-105).[81]

While India possesses a huge population, its

military establishment (an all-volunteer force) has experienced officer recruitment shortfalls in various career fields. For example, the army and air force have failed to attract sufficient numbers of qualified engineers. Thus, in 1982–83, engineering courses at the Indian Military Academy were conducted well below sanctioned strength, fewer than 25 percent of available positions being filled. Among the reasons that have been adduced to explain recruiting difficulties are lack of financial rewards, attractive employment opportunities in business and the civil service, and limited promotion prospects for technical branch officers.[82] In crisis situations, 200,000 army reserve personnel could increase the army's overall manpower levels. However, the nearly 300,000 members of centrally controlled paramilitary organizations (including, inter alia, the border security force, central reserve police, and industrial security police) likely constitute the primary force augmentation base.

Availability of military hardware is another constraining factor, although the Indian military maintains a large and sophisticated arms inventory. The ongoing expansion and modernization of this arsenal have greatly enhanced the effectiveness of combat units. While deficiencies exist in some weapons categories (as instanced by inadequate numbers of heavy machine guns and surface-to-surface missiles furnished to infantry divisions), New Delhi is rapidly rectifying these problems. Thus, artillery regiments presently do not have self-propelled and towed medium artillery pieces comparable to those Pakistan has obtained from the United States. However, India recently concluded a purchase agreement with Bofors, a Swedish munitions firm, for approximately 1,500 FH-77BS 155-mm towed artillery pieces. Contract terms require Bofors to construct one and possibly two manufacturing facilities in India, where this system will be produced under license. Bofors representatives have declared that the value of this contract may exceed $3.5 billion; if so, it would constitute the largest arms order in Indian history.[83] (Consummation of this contractual relationship reportedly was facilitated by the payment of substantial commissions to Indian interme-

diaries and, inferentially, to government officials. Earlier, Defense Minister V.P. Singh was compelled to resign after announcing an investigation into kickbacks associated with the purchase of West German submarines.)

It is unlikely that India's defense industry will meet equipment shortfalls. Domestic industry traditionally devotes inordinate time to the design and production stages of weapon projects. For example, assembly of the air force's new basic trainer, the piston-engined HPT-32, did not commence until nine years after a feasibility study was approved by the MoD.[84] Further, Indian defense plants cannot build systems at the high end of the technology spectrum. Accordingly, some service chiefs have expressed reservations about the government's emphasis on the indigenous manufacture of war goods. Conversely, continued dependence on external sources for advanced weaponry precludes equipment standardization, complicating maintenance and repair. Such dependence also serves to undermine existing self-reliance efforts. Thus, Soviet willingness to construct an infantry combat vehicle manufacturing facility in India effectively terminated India's own development program.[85]

Nevertheless, India's defense industry has enjoyed a number of successes. New Delhi is self-sufficient in light artillery, small arms, ammunition, explosives, and utility vehicles. HAL has produced several variants of the Soviet MiG-21/Fishbed, along with HS-748 transports, and Aerospatiale Alouette III and Lama helicopters. Mazagon Docks, Ltd. (Bombay) has built three Indian-designed Godavari-class frigates, a substantially modified version of British Leander-class vessels.[86]

Fuel reserves may not prove a constraint on wartime operations because of increased domestic oil production (chiefly from offshore drilling sites) and petroleum refining capabilities. Wartime operations may be aided as well by an expanding logistic infrastructure in northern and western India, including pipelines and road and rail networks.

As suggested earlier, another constraint stems from the decision-making process itself. Numerous individuals both within and without the Ministry of Defense can delay consideration of military requests or impede decision implementation. In particular, MoD civilians frequently process service requirements in a dilatory manner, especially those viewed as affecting their bureaucratic interests negatively. Further, the finance minister can change defense priorities by inflexibly adhering to applicable regulations. For example, he can withhold money from a given project because desired allocations exceed a spending category limit, even though overall military outlays remain below prescribed maximum levels.

Mobilization of public opinion to oppose foreign or security policy initiatives is an uncommon circumstance. On the other hand, if the Indian government embraced extremely controversial policies, as in refusing to deploy nuclear weapons should Islamabad produce such explosives or granting concessions to Pakistan and China so that border demarcation questions could be resolved, then considerable public reaction would likely be generated.

Finally, ethical norms are not the constraint they once were, in that Indian defense measures no longer are limited by elevated principles of international morality, although they continue to be justified in these terms. It has been argued, for instance, that New Delhi's apparent disinclination to develop nuclear bombs is grounded in ethical concerns. It seems more likely, however, that this policy determination rests on the perception that Indian security is served better without nuclear weaponry, assuming of course that Pakistani military forces also remain non-nuclear.

Recurring Issues and Defense Policy Outputs

CIVIL-MILITARY RELATIONS

Historically, the Indian military has been apolitical, solely engaged in interest group activity, such as lobbying for increased resource allocations.[87] However, recurrent involvement in internal security and national development tasks has transformed the military into an organization endeavoring to preserve the existing political regime.

The expansion of the military's role in India has not been self-generated; rather, it has resulted from decisions taken by political elites to assign the armed services increased responsibility for internal security. Nevertheless, the military's involvement in suppressing violence—and its consequent concern with secessionism, communalism, and terrorism—may have weakened constraints on the officer corps regarding domestic political undertakings. To illustrate: in 1984 New Delhi charged the army with administering the Punjab state government in order to maintain its control over Sikh extremists. Clearly falling within the ambit of political activity, this mission marked the first time the army has directed the affairs of an Indian state since independence.

The Indian armed forces traditionally have disliked assisting civil authorities in areas other than disaster relief, which, in addition to saving life, constitutes a useful public relations vehicle. In 1972 Lt. Gen. G. G. Bewoor, then general officer commanding in chief, Southern Command, attributed Pakistan's defeat the preceding year to the military's immersion in civil affairs. Bewoor admonished the Indian defense services not to assume such burdens (including civic action and "nation building" tasks) in peacetime, declaring that their *raison d'être* remained protection against external threat.[88]

India's political elites also do not favor extensive interaction between the military and civilians. Thus, the government maintains the cantonment system instituted by the British, endeavoring to insulate the military from civilian influences. Further, New Delhi has organized paramilitary forces (the central reserve police force and the border security force) to limit military involvement in internal pacification duties. The provenance of these policies likely resides in governmental apprehension about politicization of the armed services. Nevertheless, despite an apparent consensus on the inadvisability of using the military in police-type or counterinsurgency operations, such missions in fact have been assigned to the armed forces with increasing frequency. The Indian Army was deployed in support of civil authority on 82 occasions in 1982–83, 96 the next year, and 175 times in 1984–85, most frequently to quell public disturbances.[89]

Various factors account for the acceleration of military participation in civilian affairs. First, centrifugal sociopolitical forces in India have intensified, with a concomitant proliferation of domestic violence. Second, the central government has gained power at the expense of the states. As a result, the central government has had to assume primary responsibility for violence containment. New Delhi maintains two control mechanisms: paramilitary organizations and the armed services. Manifest inadequacies of paramilitary units necessitate greater reliance on the military for restoration of public order.

Continual assistance at the behest of the political leadership, along with a demonstrated ability to execute such missions effectively, may lessen the military's disquiet regarding the propriety of these commitments. Indeed, views articulated by senior officers suggest that aid to civil authority now constitutes an acceptable role for Indian military professionals. In 1983 Gen. K. V. Krishna Rao, then chief of the army staff, observed that the counterinsurgency effort in the northeastern states comprised political and economic as well as military elements. He commended army involvement in regional civic action programs, which included such diverse activities as school and sports grounds construction and distribution of food during drought. He further noted: "These measures have had a great impact and the Army has won the confidence and affection of the people. Taking advantage of the conducive conditions created by the Army, the civil administrations in these states . . . are endeavoring to implement development and social projects."[90]

Operations against separatist elements form one component of a broad spectrum of domestic responsibilities assigned to the military. Principal missions include cantonment administration, disaster relief, maintenance of essential services (e.g., railways and power plants) during labor strikes, counterinsurgency missions in sensitive border areas, and restoration of law and order.

Numerous factors suggest continuation of current domestic activities by the military. To illustrate: riot control missions have proven a useful status enhancement vehicle for the armed forces. The Indian Administrative Service, composed of mid-level and senior government bureaucrats, has long regarded itself as superior to the military. However, increased interaction with the army, based on its expanded role in internal security management, is altering this assessment.[91] Similarly, popular recognition that the military now forms the principal institutional safeguard against social disorder has strengthened its reputation outside government.

The military's political responsibilities have ranged from administering governmental affairs in Punjab to facilitating the dissolution of the Jammu and Kashmir state governments (by providing a threatening presence in the form of a senior officer when state officials were informed of their dismissal).[92] To date, all such measures have been taken at the behest of the authorities in New Delhi. However, an increasing number of military intellectuals and political commentators are disturbed over the prospects of self-initiated action. Lt. Gen. (retired) S. K. Sinha admonishes:

> If the civil administration is reduced to the position of being unable to maintain order on its own, and has constantly to seek Army assistance, the authority of the Government is seriously damaged. Soldiers may start getting the wrong ideas; they may even begin to acquire political ambitions. The frequent use of the Army to quell internal strife carries the germs of politicizing the Army.[93]

Maj. Gen. (retired) S. N. Antia agrees, noting that the military ultimately may perceive itself as the sole vehicle by which India can be governed.[94] Kuldip Nayar, a respected journalist, cautions that "the invisible line between the civil and military set-ups is [being] violated," adding that similar circumstances in other countries have led to military coups.[95]

Despite such concerns, continually increasing military involvement in domestic affairs is by no means certain. Significant constraints on the military's latitude for action in domestic affairs will likely keep such involvement at present levels. Indeed, there are some factors that may well prompt the services themselves to seek assurances from the central authorities that they will not be required to assume further political duties:

1. The magnitude of the external threats facing India (e.g., China and Pakistan) and recognition that expanded internal security responsibilities could degrade combat readiness may discourage military preoccupation with domestic issues.

2. Performance of civil aid functions has had a deleterious impact upon army morale. Soldiers are neither trained nor mentally prepared for police duties; such duties also affect posting and annual leave availability.[96]

3. Mutiny by Sikh personnel has doubtless generated apprehension about the growth of factionalism in the military. Senior officers may therefore be disinclined to accept domestic responsibilities that could exacerbate preexisting ethnic antagonisms among servicemen.

4. The central government is endeavoring to reduce military participation in counterterrorist and counterinsurgency operations. For example, New Delhi has established a new 23,000-man national security guard, specially trained in antiterrorist warfare. However, the ability of the guard to perform tasks more effectively than other paramilitary forces remains uncertain.

5. Usurpation of political authority by the military would require the support both of the Indian Administrative Service, responsible for the orderly functioning of state and district governments, and the Indian Police Service (middle-grade and senior law enforcement officials at the state and district levels). However, it is doubtful that either would countenance a military coup unless the central government clearly proved unable to contain social unrest. Absent such support, the military could not impose its rule without reconstituting administrative structures on a nationwide basis. Similarly, military rule would require the backing of the business community, in which much of India's wealth resides. Business leaders probably would not sanction a seizure of power unless violence and labor unrest disrupted such public sector industries as transportation and energy.

The military has proven to be a vehicle of so-cial integration generating national, secular perspectives in its personnel. The substitution of national attachments for communal (i.e., tribal, ethnic, linguistic, cultural, or religious) identification in part may be an unintended consequence of military service. Common military training, shared hardships, and corporate life in a highly disciplined environment may weaken subgroup loyalties. Further, senior officers have taken active measures to ensure that servicemen view national unity (and, inferentially, military cohesion) as an imperative circumstance. Such measures include trans-community deployment of military personnel, inculcation of national values during recruit training, and the army's establishment of a national integration institute.

Beyond this, the military's participation in civic action programs has strengthened ties between central India and peripheral regions containing significant minority populations. Among the developmental and welfare responsibilities discharged by the military are bridge and road repair, provision of rations and medical support, and reconstruction of housing.

Conversely, army operations have at times alienated minority communities. For example, the 1984 assault on the Golden Temple in Amritsar and subsequent stationing of troops throughout Punjab antagonized many Sikhs. Indeed, the nature and intensity of Sikh reaction to these steps ultimately threatened the army's organizational integrity. As noted earlier, as many as two thousand Sikh soldiers were arrested, and fifty were killed during a series of desertions and mutinies following the Golden Temple attack.

New Delhi periodically has announced plans to alter military recruitment patterns. The overrepresentation of certain segments of society in the armed forces would be eliminated; rather, the number of minority members entering military service would reflect their community's percentage of the national population. Under this arrangement, which has not been implemented to date, Sikh involvement in the military would decrease by 80 percent, from more than 100,000 to 20,000 active duty personnel.

Further, the 1984 Sikh mutiny impelled New

Delhi to accelerate the scheduled deactivation of infantry regiments manned exclusively or substantially by specified communal groups. However, the new chief of the army staff, General Sundarji, has suspended efforts at integrating all army elements. In justifying this step, Sundarji emphasized that only five of the one hundred battalion-size units dominated by Sikhs experienced mutiny or desertion after the Golden Temple attack.[97] Sundarji evidently believes that this approach will restore a sense of trust and confidence to Sikh servicemen, whose loyalty has been subject to intense scrutiny.

WEAPONS ACQUISITION

New Delhi commits approximately one-third of its defense budget to arms procurement.[98] Combat equipment and weaponry are manufactured domestically by nine public sector companies and thirty-six munitions plants. (The involvement of private sector firms in defense undertakings is at present limited to assembly of commercial vehicles and provision of components for state-controlled programs.) Ordnance factory production includes tanks, antitank and antiaircraft guns, rockets, grenades, depth charges, and optical and fire control instruments.[99]

The indigenous fabrication of advanced systems (e.g., the T-72 tank) is typically contingent on conclusion of licensed production agreements with the Soviet Union or Western European states. On the other hand, New Delhi has achieved self-sufficiency in such areas as small arms, mortars, and mines. Continued modernization of the munitions industry forms a central policy objective, as increased self-reliance would lessen (1) vulnerability to political interference, based on threats to suspend or terminate arms deliveries, and (2) spare parts dependence. Self-reliance efforts have met their greatest success in the provision of war goods to the army, which uses a substantial number of low- and mid-technology items. Conversely, air force and navy inventories principally consist of foreign equipment at the high end of the technology spectrum, with some systems coproduced in

India. Consequently, overseas suppliers today receive 40 percent of India's weapon acquisition outlays.

New Delhi is endeavoring to reduce this figure by stipulating technology transfer requirements in purchase contracts. However, its ability to attain mastery of imported technology remains problematic at best. Thus, many systems built under license still employ foreign components, transforming a manufacturing activity into the mere assembly of parts. Indeed, this situation often holds for nominally indigenous equipment. To illustrate: India has made the Shaktiman three-ton truck for twenty-five years, but must obtain its engine block and steering gear from West Germany.[100]

Nevertheless, New Delhi is now attempting to fabricate sophisticated weaponry with only marginal support from second parties. For example, in the 1990s HAL is scheduled to produce a light combat aircraft (LCA) tasked with battlefield air superiority and ground attack missions. Some Indian defense analysts view the LCA effort with skepticism, noting that power plant development and airframe design seemingly have been treated as discreet undertakings by project managers.[101] (HAL adopted a similar approach in developing the HF-24 Marut during the 1960s, largely accounting for this aircraft's poor performance characteristics.)

Such administrative difficulties, along with inadequate engineering and quality assurance resources in the defense industry, have made senior military officers reluctant to accept indigenous weaponry. While these individuals typically favor the purchase of Western equipment, Soviet armaments remain attractive to the civilian leadership, based on lower initial costs, payment in rupees, long-term credits, and guaranteed transfer of technology. In addition, Moscow has demonstrated its reliability as an exporter of military hardware and spares, never threatening to cancel contractual relationships with India because of modified political circumstances. At the same time, New Delhi has obtained several Western European systems in order to (1) avoid dependence on a single arms source and (2) enhance its bargaining leverage with the USSR, forcing the Russians to offer top-of-the-line equipment in military sales packages.

Indian defense production clearly falls short of U.S., Soviet, or Western European standards. In a Third World context, however, Indian capabilities are most impressive. Thus, India coproduces the West German Type 1500 submarine and MiG-27/Flogger, while Pakistan's limited industrial base precludes any licensed manufacture of high performance weaponry. Further, New Delhi now is exporting military goods, especially small arms, to developing nations.

FORCE POSTURE

The Indian Army consists of thirty-one divisions: eighteen infantry, ten mountain, two armored, and one mechanized infantry, along with several independent infantry, mountain, armored, artillery, and parachute brigades. Up to nineteen divisions are probably oriented toward Pakistan (either in a frontline or reserve capacity); the majority of the ten mountain divisions are deployed to counter the Chinese threat, while two or three divisions are tasked with anti-insurgency missions in the northeastern states. In a conflict with Pakistan, as many as five mountain divisions could be transferred to the western sector within one to six weeks.[102]

As noted earlier, the Indian military has experienced difficulties in recruiting sufficient numbers of qualified personnel. Many Indians apparently consider employment in business or civil administration, rather than military service, as a suitable career alternative. Consequently, the army officer establishment has on occasion fallen more than 12 percent below authorized strength levels.[103]

All standard infantry weapons, including light and medium machine guns, antitank guns, antitank rockets, and mortars are manufactured domestically. The infantry's combat effectiveness is being improved through provision of heavy machine guns and night firing equipment. Further, the army is endeavoring to enhance its field communications capability. Mechanized troops are mounted on armored

personnel carriers (APCs), such as the BTR-60 PB and BMP-1 infantry combat vehicles (ICVs). New Delhi's desire to procure advanced APCs and ICVs (an Indo-Soviet purchase agreement for the BMP-2 has reportedly been concluded) suggests that the raising or conversion of additional mechanized infantry units may be contemplated.[104]

The armored corps has more than three thousand main battle tanks, including approximately three hundred Soviet T-72s. The T-72 inventory is expected to double over the next three years; in this context, Moscow has offered to facilitate the in-country production of this weapons system by transferring engine and armor technology, along with the laser range finder fitted on its T-72Ms.[105] The T-72 will serve as an interim main battle tank until an Indian-designed and manufactured vehicle becomes operational, presumably in the early 1990s.

New Delhi's remaining tanks are either obsolete (e.g., the Soviet T-54/55, although it is superior to Pakistan's Type 59 MBT) or obsolescent (the Indian-built Vijayanta). The army has attempted to upgrade the Vijayanta by developing night vision devices and an improved fire-control system. Further, a 130-mm gun has been mounted on the Vijayanta chassis in an attempt to develop a self-propelled medium artillery capability.[106] In addition, the air defense of armored formations is to be strengthened by placing antiaircraft weapons on PT-76 light tanks.

At present, the absence of an adequate self-propelled and towed medium artillery inventory constitutes a principal army weakness. However, this shortcoming in part will be rectified by the impending acquisition of 1,500 Bofors FH-77BS field guns.

The Indian Air Force is the largest air arm in noncommunist Asia, composed of 113,000 personnel and more than seven hundred combat aircraft. Its principal interceptor is the MiG-21/Fishbed. Air defense assets are being supplemented by three advanced aircraft: the Soviet MiG-23 MF/Flogger B air superiority fighter, armed with AA-7/Apex and AA-8/Aphid air-to-air missiles (AAMs); the French

Mirage 2000 multirole fighter, carrying two Matra 550 short-range and two Matra Super 530-D medium-range AAMs; and the Soviet MiG-29/Fulcrum. India's acquisition of MiG-29s marks the first time the Soviet Union has exported frontline fighters to a Third World country before full modernization of its own squadrons and initial deployment to Warsaw Pact forces. (Moscow's willingness to furnish state-of-the-art weaponry is, in part, a reflection of concern regarding New Delhi's arms source diversification effort, as evidenced by the purchase of Anglo-French Jaguars and the Mirage 2000.)

Air force long-range interdiction/counterair missions are assigned principally to Jaguar squadrons. The Jaguar can carry 10,000 pounds of ordnance on underwing and overwing pylons. A number of Jaguars may be equipped with the French Agave radar to enhance maritime interdiction capabilities. The air force also is tasked with providing offensive air support to the army. Consequently, the air force is developing a powerful tactical strike force, consisting of at least three MiG-23 BN/Flogger H and eight MiG-27/Flogger D squadrons, to facilitate rapid advances by ground elements.

The multiplicity and obsolescence of transport aircraft types, along with concomitant difficulties in spare parts acquisition, have degraded operational readiness. The air force is attempting to remedy this situation by updating its airlift resources; it is receiving approximately 100 AN-32/Cline medium transports and a number of IL-76/Candid heavy transports from the Soviet Union.

As with the Indian Army, Indian Air Force deployments evidence a continuing preoccupation with Pakistani military capabilities. For example, most squadrons possessing advanced fighters and fighter-bombers fall under the operational control of the Western and South-Western Air Commands, organizations concerned primarily with the Pakistani threat. Weapons systems held by the Indian Navy already have been discussed in the second part of this chapter. The navy's largest base is in Bombay, with additional major facilities in Vishakapatnam, Cochin, and Goa. It reportedly is also constructing a large (9,000 acre) base at Karwar.

USE OF FORCE

India's traditional security concerns are Pakistan and China. Accordingly, Indian force deployments reflect a perceived need to counterbalance the military power of these states. (Terrain and the potential vulnerability of various military installations and urban areas also affect the disposition of Indian units.) The fundamental decision to position troops opposite enemy force concentrations has in turn governed the formulation of Indian military doctrine. India's armed forces provide a credible deterrent to the Pakistani and Chinese threats. However, the navy remains unable to counter the presence of extraregional naval units in the Indian Ocean fully.

India could rapidly overcome Pakistani opposition in a fourth war unless Islamabad were to enjoy sole possession of nuclear weaponry. A future conflict would probably result in the defeat of Pakistani forces and removal of the military regime in Islamabad (assuming external diplomatic pressures did not compel an early termination of hostilities), resulting in the establishment of a civilian government amenable to Indian wishes. New Delhi might then choose to transmit admonitory messages to Moscow reflecting present concerns about Soviet expansionist ambitions in South Asia. Soviet forces in Afghanistan clearly pose a threat to Pakistan's territorial integrity. Moreover, a materially weakened Pakistan (following military defeat by India, for example) could disintegrate with key western provinces falling under Soviet control or influence.

Enhanced Indian military capabilities serve to discourage any new Chinese attack. A Chinese offensive in the Himalayas could, moreover, require the redeployment of forces oriented toward the Soviet Union, with a concomitant expansion of the logistic infrastructure near the Indian border. Such efforts were not needed to defeat India in 1962. If war with China occurred (a conflict India is unlikely to initiate), New Delhi might seek to acquire such disputed territory in frontier areas as the Aksai Chin.

In the Indian Ocean, the navy and air force probably will not engage in any hostile action against island or littoral states (a policy determination reinforced by the presence of powerful extraregional naval units). Rather, New Delhi will concentrate on alerting regional actors to its growing military prowess in an attempt to foster creation of sponsor-client security ties.

Beyond advocacy of an Indian Ocean Zone of Peace that would control use of the Indian Ocean, particularly naval powers from outside of the region, arms control in the subcontinent is not an issue of high salience. However, some bilateral understandings have been reached, such as an Indo-Pakistani agreement to refrain from attacking each other's nuclear facilities.

Notes

1. "Massive Rise in Indian Budget," *Jane's Defense Weekly*, 30 May 1987, p. 1040.
2. Onkar Marwah, "National Security and Military Policy in India," in *Subcontinent in World Politics*, ed. Ziring, p. 71.
3. The Indian Defense Ministry's annual report for 1984–85 emphasizes Islamabad's "relentless pursuit of nuclear weapons," concluding that "Pakistan has been and remains our principal security concern" (S. Sahay, "A Close Look: Indo-Pakistani Relations," *Statesman* [Calcutta], 9 May 1985, p. 5).
4. Matt Miller, "Tensions Rising Between India, Pakistan," *Wall Street Journal*, 4 March 1987, p. 22; Inderjit Badhwan and Dilip Bobb, "Indo-Pak Border: Game of Brinkmanship," *India Today*, 15 February 1987, pp. 26–32; Dilip Bobb and Inderjit Badhwan, "India-Pakistan Talks: Back From the Edge," *India Today*, 28 February 1987, pp. 40–43.
5. "A Border on the Boil," *Asiaweek*, 10 May 1987, pp. 14–17; "If There is a Military Threat from China, We Are Ready to Face It," *Telegraph* (Calcutta), 22 May 1987, p. 1.
6. V. G. Kulkarni, "Eyeball to Eyeball on the Himalayan Border," *Far Eastern Economic Review*, 9 April 1987, p. 40.
7. G. Jacobs, "South Asian Naval Forces," *Asian Defense Journal*, December 1984, p. 44.
8. Marwah, "National Security," p. 67.
9. Gary L. Sojka, "The Missions of the Indian Navy," *Naval War College Review* 36 (January–February, 1983): 11.
10. G. K. Reddy, "India Wants Islands Free from Big Power Influence," *Hindu* (Madras), 9 February 1982, p. 1.
11. Robert H. Donaldson, "Soviet Security Interests in South Asia," in *Subcontinent in World Politics*, ed. Ziring, p. 184.
12. Salamat Ali, "It's Roubles to Rupees," *Far Eastern Economic Review*, 7 March 1985, pp. 34–35.

13. "The Northeast, the Punjab, and the Regionalization of Indian Politics," *Asian Survey* 23 (November 1983): 1173–74.
14. G. C. Katoch, "Soldiers as Policemen," *Statesman* (Calcutta), 18 January 1985, p. 8.
15. William Claiborne, "Punjab's Sikh Shrine Reopened as Sporadic Violence Continues," *Washington Post*, 26 June 1984, p. A10.
16. Richard Nations, "Pride and Paranoia," *Far Eastern Economic Review*, 16 August 1984, pp. 23–26.
17. See, e.g., Suresh Kalmadi, "Defense Matters Should Be Publicly Debated," *Telegraph* (Calcutta), 15 May 1985, p. 6. The following text section on goal achievement strategies appeared in our "New Delhi's Indian Ocean Policy," *Naval War College Review* 40 (Autumn 1987): 50–63.
18. "India Keen on Arms Exports," *Ceylon Daily News* (Colombo), 8 February 1984, p. 4. India hopes to increase arms exports by means of low unit costs and the absence of political stipulations in sales contracts.
19. R. C. Ummat, "India and the Developing World," *India and Foreign Review* 21 (1 April 1982): 12.
20. K. A. Sidhu, *The Role of the Navy in India's Defense* (New Delhi: Harnam Publications, 1983), p. 115.
21. Shirin Tahir-Kheli, "Defense Planning in Pakistan," in *Defense Planning in Less-Industrialized States*, ed. Stephanie G. Neuman (Lexington, Mass.: D. C. Heath, 1984), p. 216.
22. "Talks for a New Aircraft Carrier," *Statesman* (Calcutta), 14 December 1984, p. 5.
23. Dilip Bobb, "The Message from Moscow," *India Today*, 31 August 1984, p. 51.
24. "India Receives First 'Kilo' Class Submarine," *Jane's Defense Weekly*, 27 September 1986, p. 679.
25. "Military Balance," *Pacific Defense Reporter*, December 1984–January 1985, p. 141; Bobb, "Message from Moscow," p. 51.
26. "Military Balance," p. 141. Navy headquarters is endeavoring to upgrade ASW, electronic warfare, and communications systems as well. Thus, for example, the navy is building a VLF communication facility in southern India, making possible the receipt of messages by submarines at considerable depths ("New Communication System for Navy in '88," *Hindu* [Madras], 19 February 1985, p. 1).
27. "Military Balance," p. 141.
28. "Defense Team Back after Finalizing New Deals with Moscow," *Hindu* (Madras), 2 May 1984, p. 7.
29. See, e.g., Cecil Victor, "Forward Maritime Defense," *Patriot* (New Delhi), 31 May 1985, p. 5. Coast guard assets include ships and fast patrol craft, with Chetak helicopters embarked on offshore patrol vessels; its fixed-wing air component is composed of Dornier 228–100 maritime surveillance aircraft from West Germany (D. Banerjee, "Second Dimension to Coast Guard," *Sainik Samachar*, 29 January 1984, p. 8).
30. A. W. Grazebrook, "Soviet Equipment Lifts India as Military Power," *Pacific Defense Reporter*, April 1985, p. 44.
31. "Modernization a Priority for Indian Defense," *Jane's Defense Weekly*, 18 May 1985, p. 837.
32. See, e.g., Ravi Rikhye, "The Island Scare," *India Today*, 15 May 1982, p. 107.
33. Sojka, "Missions of the Indian Navy," p. 10. Navy overseas port calls are reported in *Sainik Samachar*, a semi-official military publication. See, e.g.,

"Eastern Fleet Ships to Malaysia," 1 July 1984, p. 19; "Goodwill Visit by Naval Ships to Middle East," 27 March 1983, pp. 16–17.

34. For example, a former prime minister of Malaysia served as a cadet at the Indian Military Academy ("Modernized Training at the IMA," *Asian Defense Journal*, February 1983, p. 86).

35. Ibid.; Lt. Col. H. C. Tewari, "India Lends a Helping Hand to Friendly Nations," *Sainik Samachar*, Army Number 1981, pp. 60–61; "Air Force Planning to Train More Pilots," *Patriot* (New Delhi), 20 July 1981, p. 7; "India to Train Seychelles' Army, Navy Cadets," *Sunday Standard* (Bombay), 28 June 1981, p. 5; H. S. Chhabra, "India's Africa Policy," in *Studies in India's Foreign Policy*, ed. Surendra Chopra (Amritsar, 1980), p. 416.

36. "Modernized Training," p. 86; Tewari, "Helping Hand," pp. 60–61; "Air Force Planning," p. 7.

37. Tewari, "Helping Hand," p. 61; "Training at the Torpedo and Anti-Submarine School," *Hindu* (Madras), 9 January 1983, p. 7; H. Kusumakar, "Challenge of Soaring Up in Sky," *Times of India* (Bombay), 18 September 1982, p. 5.

38. Tewari, "Helping Hand," p. 61; "Torpedo and Anti-Submarine School," p. 7.

39. H. S. Chhabra, "India and Africa: Partners in Progress," *New African*, February 1983, p. 55. Recipient states include Bangladesh, Burma, Kenya, Madagascar, Mauritius, Mozambique, Seychelles, and Sri Lanka.

40. Leo Rose, "India and Its Neighbors: Regional Foreign and Security Policies," in *Subcontinent in World Politics*, ed. Ziring, p. 59.

41. Manoj Joshi, "Blood on Throne Room of Gods," *Frontline*, 20 April–3 May 1985, pp. 76–84; "Pak Attack on Siachen Repulsed," *Hindu* (Madras), 12 June 1985, p. 1.

42. A. Balakrishnan Nair, *Facets of Indian Defense* (New Delhi: S. Chand, 1983), p. 37.

43. Ibid., p. 110.

44. Ravi Rikhye, "New Pak Threat to India's Security," *Times of India* (Bombay), 7 January 1982, p. 4.

45. Ravi Rikhye, "The F-16 Again," *Indian Express* (Bombay), 12 January 1983, p. 1.

46. Sojka, "Missions of the Indian Navy," p. 8.

47. Seymour M. Hersh, "A Pakistani Tried to Send Trigger for A-Bomb Home," *New York Times*, 25 February 1985, p. 1.

48. Milton R. Benjamin, "China Aids Pakistan on A-Weapons," *Washington Post*, 28 January 1983, p. 1

49. Suman Dubey, "India, Keeping its Nuclear Options Open, Monitors Weapons Program in Neighboring Pakistan with Concern," *Wall Street Journal*, 26 November 1984, p. 32.

50. "India to Reconsider Nuclear Options," *Business Standard* (Calcutta), 5 May 1985, p. 1.

51. T. V. Paul, "Will India Join the Nuclear Club?" *Asian Defense Journal*, February 1986, pp. 76–78.

52. "N-War Training for Forces," *Asian Defense Journal*, March 1986, p. 130.

53. This section is based on Jerrold F. Elkin and W. Andrew Ritezel, "The Debate on Restructuring India's Higher Defense Organization," *Asian Survey* 24 (October 1984): 1069–85.

54. Indeed, there is no defense committee in the Lok Sabha, the lower house of Parliament. Further, few Lok Sabha members are informed fully on defense issues. This is a truly remarkable circumstance in a country where defense expenditures exceed $7 billion annually. See Chris Smith and Bruce George, "The Defense of India," *Jane's Defense Weekly*, 2 March 1985, p. 366.

55. Air Chief Marshal P. C. Lal, *Some Problems of Defense* (New Delhi: United Service Institution of India, 1977), p. 8; M. L. Thapan, "Higher Defense Control: Fostering a Tri-Service Spirit," *Statesman* (Calcutta), 9 August 1982, p. 4.

56. G. C. Katoch, "Decisions on Defense, I: Civil and Military Bureaucracies," *Statesman* (Calcutta), 28 May 1985, p. 8.

57. Lal, *Some Problems of Defense*, p. 16.

58. P. R. Chari, "The Policy Process," in *Defense Policy Formation*, ed. James M. Roherty, International Relations Series, no. 6 (Durham, N.C.: Carolina Academic Press, 1980), p. 133.

59. Ibid., p. 145.

60. Lt. Gen. S. K. Sinha, "Higher Defense Organization," *Indian Express* (Bombay), 29 February 1984, p. 1; G. Jacobs, "India's Army," *Asian Defense Journal*, September 1985, p. 10.

61. G. C. Katoch, "Integrating Defense, I: A Supreme Commander for Cohesion," *Statesman* (Calcutta), 4 August 1981, p. 5.

62. Chari, "Policy Process," p. 143.

63. G. K. Reddy, "Senior Intelligence Board Being Formed," *Hindu* (Madras), 25 July 1983, p. 1.

64. Lt. Gen. S. K. Sinha, *Of Matters Military* (New Delhi: Vision Books, 1980), pp. 47–48.

65. Stephen P. Cohen, "Civilian Control of the Military in India," in *Civilian Control of the Military*, ed. Claude E. Welch, Jr. (Albany: State University of New York Press, 1976), p. 48.

66. Chari, "Policy Process," p. 145; Sinha, *Of Matters Military*, p. 42.

67. Lt. Col. M. P. Singh, "The Muddled Defense Set-Up Surprisingly Works," *Journal of the United Service Institution of India* 112 (January–March, 1982): 11; G. K. Reddy, "It Is Time to Revamp Defense Command Structure," *Hindu* (Madras), 6 February 1984, p. 1.

68. Despite an inadequate knowledge and experience base, Indian defense secretaries assume duties similar to those of the chairman of the joint chiefs of staff in other countries, e.g., serving as a link between the minister of defense and service chiefs.

69. Sinha, *Of Matters Military*, pp. 33–34.

70. G. C. Katoch, "Military Spending: Need for Integrating Finance," *Statesman* (Calcutta), 22 March 1982, p. 8.

71. Katoch, "Integrating Defense, I," p. 6.

72. Lal, *Some Problems of Defense*, pp. 11–12.

73. P. V. R. Rao, *Defense without Drift* (Bombay: Popular Prakashan, 1970), p. 23.

74. Lal, *Some Problems of Defense*, pp. 34–35.

75. Ibid., pp. 73–74.

76. Ibid., pp. 82–83.

77. G. C. Katoch, "Integrating Defense, II: Unfounded Fears of a Military Coup," *Statesman* (Calcutta), 5 August 1981, p. 1.

78. Sqn. Ldr. N. K. Bhasin, "Need for Closer Tri-Service Integration and Validity of the Integrated The-

ater Concept for the Indian Armed Forces," *Journal of the United Service Institution of India* 109 (April–June, 1979): 141.

79. G. C. Katoch, "Decisions for Defense, II: An Instant Package for Reform," *Statesman* (Calcutta), 29 May 1985, p. 8.

80. G. C. Katoch, "Servitude in Defense: Developing Swadeshi Weapons," *Statesman* (Calcutta), 3 September 1984, p. 8.

81. Shekhar Gupta, "Distress Deals," *India Today*, 15 February 1987, p. 124.

82. Shekhar Gupta, "Asking for More," *India Today*, 31 January 1985, p. 94.

83. "Bofors' Indian Deal Worth Three Times Initial Price," *Jane's Defense Weekly*, 7 June 1986, p. 1023.

84. Smith and George, "Defense of India," p. 370; Somnath Sapru, "Work on Trainer for IAF Begins," *Indian Express* (Bombay), 20 April 1984, p. 8.

85. Dilip Bobb, "Moscow's New Offensive," *India Today*, 31 August 1984, p. 84.

86. "India: Indigenous Programs Flourish amid Defense Modernization," *International Defense Review*, April 1986, p. 435.

87. This section is based on Jerrold F. Elkin and W. Andrew Ritezel, "Military Role Expansion in India," *Armed Forces and Society* 11 (Summer 1985): 489–504.

88. "Pak Army's Civil Role Blamed," *Times of India* (Bombay), 10 September 1972, p. 7.

89. "Misusing the Army," *India Today*, 15 May 1985, p. 7.

90. "Year of Progress," *Sainik Samachar*, 9 January 1983, p. 5.

91. Lt. Gen. S. K. Sinha, "Honor the Soldier," *Statesman* (Calcutta), 25 June 1984, p. 8.

92. Kuldip Nayar, "Why Was the Army Commander Present When Dr. Abdullah Was Sacked?" *Telegraph* (Calcutta), 24 July 1984, p. 1.

93. "Politicizing the Army," *Statesman* (Calcutta), 9 September 1984, p. 5.

94. "Army for Law and Order," *Sunday Statesman* (Calcutta), 29 July 1984, p. 5.

95. Nayar, "Why Was the Army Commander Present?" p. 1.

96. Katoch, "Soldiers as Policemen," p. 8.

97. Brian Cloughley, "Sikh Extremism and the Indian Army," *Jane's Defense Weekly*, 24 May 1986, p. 933.

98. Mohan Ram, "Planes and Boats and Guns-the Bill is Growing," *Far Eastern Economic Review*, 31 May 1984, pp. 26–27.

99. S. P. Baranwal, ed., *Military Year Book, 1984–85* (New Delhi: Guide Publications, 1984), p. 110.

100. Katoch, "Servitude in Defense," p. 8.

101. See, e.g., Kalmadi, "Defense Matters," p. 6. Shortcomings in the LCA development program are further evidenced by India's reported willingness (at least initially) to substitute the General Electric F404 engine for an Indian-designed one.

102. Pushpindar Singh, "India's Defense Perspectives and the Armed Forces," *Asian Defense Journal*, October 1982, p. 14; Giri Deshingkar, "Can Pakistan Take Us On?" *Illustrated Weekly of India*, 5 August 1984, p. 8.

103. Salamat Ali, "In Step with Tradition," *Far Eastern Economic Review*, 31 May 1984, p. 30.

104. Singh, "India's Defense Perspectives," pp. 16–17; "Stronger Defense to Meet Pak Threat," *Hindu* (Madras), 12 October 1984, p. 1.

105. Bobb, "Message from Moscow," p. 51.

106. "An Hour with General Vaidya: The Chief of the Army Staff Speaks on Various Aspects of the Army," *Sainik Samachar*, 8 and 15 January 1984, p. 7.

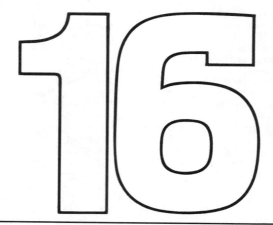

MEXICO

Michael J. Dziedzic

There is particular salience in the study of Mexican defense policy, both from a theoretical perspective and from the pragmatic viewpoint of the policy maker. In the first place, our understanding of comparative defense policy is aided greatly by the study of states that are neither major powers nor members of NATO or the Warsaw Pact. Generalizations derived exclusively from an examination of powerful states may not hold when applied to a Third World country of very modest military means, such as Mexico. Through a consideration of Mexico's policy and process we may come to a broader understanding of the dynamics that govern defense policy. The second justification for addressing this subject is also compelling, especially for policy makers. The security postures of the United States and Mexico are inextricably linked; an insecure Mexico would present enormous challenges for U.S. defense planners. Indeed, Gen. Paul Gorman, former chief of the U.S. Southern Command, has projected that within ten years the president of the United States may focus as much time on affairs in Mexico as on any other security matter.[1]

In spite of the clear policy relevance of this subject, comparatively little has been published about Mexican defense policy, at least until very recently.[2] This dearth of information is attributable to the closed nature of the Mexican armed forces rather than to disinterest on the part of scholars or practitioners.[3] Thus, the purpose of this chapter is twofold. One aim is to assemble available fragments of knowledge on this topic into a theoretical mold suitable for advancement of scholarship on compara-

The author wishes to express particular thanks to Adolfo Aguilar, James Busey, Eugene S. Dziedzic, Robert Stephan, and Paul Viotti for their comments on an earlier version of this chapter. Additionally, the bibliographic essay on the Mexican military written by Howard Colson deserves special recognition. Contained within Colson's comprehensive work are a number of obscure but very useful sources. While the quality of this work has benefited greatly from their suggestions, remaining deficiencies are attributable to no one but myself. Moreover, the views expressed in this chapter are those of the author and are not necessarily representative of any agency of the U.S. government.

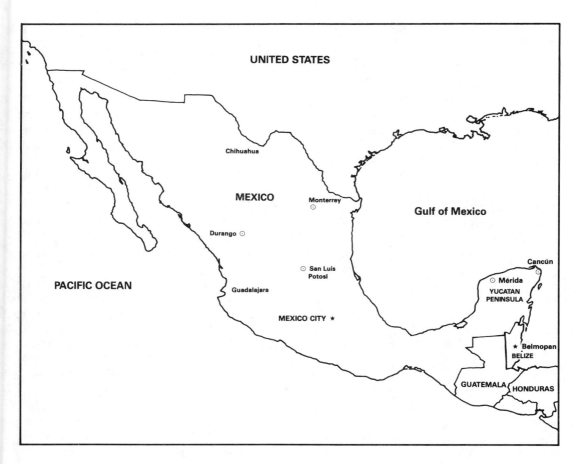

tive defense policy. The second is to deepen our appreciation of defense policy in Mexico itself.

International Environment

Mexico's defense policy has been profoundly influenced by geopolitical circumstances. Former Mexican despot Porfirio Diaz captured the essence of Mexico's situation in his oft-cited lament, "Poor Mexico, so far from God and so close to the United States."[4] Historically, juxtaposition with the United States has been painful and costly for Mexico. As the "Colossus of the North" sought inexorably to fulfill its destiny in westward expansion, Mexico paid dearly. Beginning in 1836 with the secession of the Mexican province of Texas, a chain of events unfolded in which Mexico forfeited *half* its national territory. When the

United States ultimately moved to annex Texas in 1845, conflict with Mexico ensued. In the Treaty of Guadalupe Hidalgo (1848) ending the Mexican-American War, Mexico ceded to the United States all its territory north and west of the Rio Grande River, including the present states of Texas, New Mexico, Arizona, California, Nevada, Utah, and parts of Colorado and Wyoming.

In addition to the humiliation of lost territory, Mexico suffered the ignominy of having its capital city occupied for nearly a year (1847–48). During the defense of the capital, however, the nation was bequeathed a legacy of heroism: the *Niños Héroes* (child heroes), cadets at the military academy in Mexico City who leapt to their death from the parapets of Chapultepec Castle rather than surrender their positions. Their legacy is immortalized in the form of a towering monument adjacent to Cha-

pultepec Castle, just as the bitter loss of territory is kept alive in the breast of every Mexican
school child.[5]

There are Mexican citizens alive today who
can recall U.S. military intervention during
the Mexican Revolution (1910–17). The first
incident in 1914 involved naval bombardment
of the port city of Veracruz in retaliation for the
arrest of several U.S. sailors. The second incursion was precipitated by Pancho Villa's raid
on Columbus, New Mexico. In 1916 Gen. John
"Blackjack" Pershing led a U.S. expeditionary
force in a futile pursuit of Villa across the des-
erts of northern Mexico.[6] Taking these historical experiences into account, it is not surprising to learn that in a nationwide poll taken in
1986 by a leading Mexican newspaper, *Excel-
sior*, 59 percent of respondents viewed the
United States as an "enemy" country, whereas
only 31 percent considered the United States to
be "friendly."[7]

Being situated adjacent to one of the world's
superpowers has also had salutary ramifications. Since an invasion of Mexico would simultaneously threaten the United States, Mexico automatically falls within the security
umbrella of its superpower neighbor. Undoubtedly, an assault on Mexico would be
treated as a precursor to attack on the United
States itself. Consequently, Mexico enjoys the
benefits of a de facto military alliance without
attendant obligations.

While this implicit arrangement is of some
value to Mexican defense planners, it must
also be noted that credible external threats to
Mexican security are lacking. Although the
historical record may give rise to uneasiness toward the United States, the likelihood of hostilities between the two neighbors is extremely
remote. The only scenario that appears to generate any concern within Mexico centers
around a potentially oil-starved United States
seizing control of Mexican oil fields.[8] Even if
such highly extraordinary circumstances were
ever to materialize, it is evident U.S. forces
would be overpowering. Given the obvious futility of confronting the United States, there is
no point in posturing forces for such a highly
unlikely event.

The converse is true of Mexico's neighbor to
the south. To Guatemala, Mexico is the "Colossus of the North." As one well-placed Mexican military officer commented to this researcher in 1982, "Sure they could do some
damage to the oil fields but then we would go
down there and stomp them to death. We are
seventy million and how many are they—a few
million."[9] Given the obvious disparity in power
between the two, there is little point in troubling over a conventional threat from that
flank either. The prospect, however, that Central American insurgency could eventually
constitute a threat to Mexican national security is a somewhat different matter.

The extent to which Mexican officials view
the turmoil in Central America as a serious
threat to themselves is not entirely clear. It is
apparent, though, that they do not share the
apocalyptic vision of certain U.S. policy
makers. Indeed, it is insulting to suggest that a
communist takeover of governments in El Salvador, Honduras, and Guatemala would automatically result in the overthrow of the Mexican regime, like the toppling of so many
dominoes. Since the Mexican "domino" is far
heftier than its Central American counterparts, it is belittling to imply that Mexico is
somehow of their stature. A comment in *The
Economist* reflects this sentiment with characteristic crispness: "Mexico responds to the suggestion with aloofness: only a gringo could confuse the petty dictatorial backwaters of the
Spanish empire with Mexico, whose capital
city alone is more numerous than any one of
them."[10]

The "domino theory" is also flawed from the
Mexican perspective because it implicates the
Soviet Union and Cuba as root causes of Central American unrest. From the Mexican viewpoint, the conflict arises out of indigenous social, economic, and political injustices. Since
Mexico has already experienced its own revolution, there is the view that this will have a pro-
phylactic effect on the spread of insurgency to
Mexican soil. For example, in assessing Mexican policy vis-à-vis the turmoil in Central
America, Jorge G. Castañeda writes, "Mexico
felt it had nothing to fear from left-wing gov-

ernments in the Caribbean Basin. . . . It had learned from the records of Guatemala from 1950 to 1954, Cuba since 1959, and Chile from 1970 to 1973 that left-wing governments would never think of meddling in Mexican politics."[11] Indeed, the revolutionary origins of the present Mexican regime have inclined government officials to be sympathetic toward similar movements in Nicaragua and El Salvador. Caesar Sereseres sums up the Mexican position with the following three premises: "The old order cannot be maintained in Central America; revolutionary change is necessary and inevitable; and it is Mexico's duty to align with the progressive, nationalist forces seeking such change."[12]

It is not revolutionary strife in El Salvador, therefore, that alarms the Mexican policy maker. Rather, it is the prospect that external actors (principally the United States) will broaden the conflict through direct military intervention. Such "internationalization" of the conflict carries with it the prospect of a broader regional conflict that could easily spill over into southern Mexico. Among the adverse consequences could be "increased flows of refugees, a forceful reaction from the Mexican left, or the appearance of helplessness in the face of U.S. 'gunboat diplomacy' close to its southern border."[13] Thus, restraining the United States has become an important objective for Mexico.

Assuming the U.S. response to conditions in Nicaragua and El Salvador is reasonably moderate, Mexican strategists will likely be mollified. Such complacency would be engendered in part by the feeling that Mexico is adequately buffered from such strife by neighboring Guatemala. Unrest in Guatemala itself, however, carries rather ominous implications. It is not merely because the most prolific of Mexico's on-shore and off-shore oil fields are situated in the vicinity of the Guatemalan border. Most troubling is the tendency for Guatemalan insurgency to infect the neighboring state of Chiapas. Proximity is not the only reason for this. Chiapas is one of the poorest states in Mexico, and the inhabitants of that region, mainly Indians, are ethnically of the same stock as the Guatemalans. Indeed, the region historically was included in the Captaincy General of Guatemala and, as Sereseres notes, "To this day Chiapas still seems to have more in common with Guatemala than with the rest of Mexico."[14] Familial and commercial linkages, as a result, are extensive in this region, and the border is especially porous. Thus, unrest originating in Guatemala tends to be contagious.

Chiapas constitutes an especially perplexing security problem because it exposes an inherent contradiction in Mexican policy toward Central America. While Mexican policy makers can perhaps afford to maintain a sanctimonious posture toward social unrest in more distant locales like Nicaragua and El Salvador, such an attitude has worn thin in Chiapas. Grinding poverty, social injustice, and political inefficacy are the norm there as well. It is apparent, therefore, that Mexico is also susceptible to internal unrest; external developments in Guatemala could conceivably sow the seeds of instability in southern Mexico. This is a security concern with which Mexican policy makers have only recently begun to grapple.

The case of Chiapas helps to demonstrate the primacy of internal security matters in Mexican defense policy. While the origins of the problem are partially external to Mexico, the need for a policy response does not arise until the issue becomes a potential threat to internal order. The same is true of Mexican concerns about the "internationalization" of the Central American imbroglio. The fear is that U.S. policy might run amuck in the region and thereby destabilize the constellation of forces inside Mexico itself. Bona fide external threats, however, are lacking.[15] There is little point in preparing for conflicts with either neighbor given the vast disparities in military power, one of which favors Mexico and the other of which does not. Moreover, the circumstances under which a conflict with either the United States or Guatemala could erupt are very difficult to imagine. In the event an outside power should threaten Mexico, there is no doubt the United States would feel compelled to come to its neighbor's defense, for reasons of its own security. Thus, while the U.S.-Mexican relationship has historically been a checkered one, in the contemporary era the U.S. security umbrella has permitted Mexican defense planners to concentrate their energies almost exclusively on internal security matters.

RELATIVE POSITION IN THE INTERNATIONAL SYSTEM

Mexico is a middle-range power capable of exerting moderate influence among states of the Caribbean littoral. Sheer size alone warrants ascribing a degree of clout to Mexico. With seventy-seven million inhabitants (1984), Mexico ranks eleventh in the world.[16] Additionally it is about to capture the distinction of having the world's largest city, with fifteen million people estimated to be living in Mexico City. Its land mass of 760,000 square miles places Mexico fourteenth in the world.[17] These attributes, however, do not translate directly into influence. Hidden within the aggregate figures are certain unenviable statistics. The population growth rate, for example, stands at 2.6 percent (although this is down from a 3.5 percent rate in the 1970s) and arable land accounts for only about 12% of total land mass.[18] Mexico, it is apparent, is a large country, but so are its problems.

A similar pattern persists in the economic realm. The country has the world's fifteenth largest Gross National Product ($173 billion in 1987),[19] but it also has the second largest external debt of any developing country, hovering at around $100 billion. For decades, sustained economic growth in the 6–7 percent range had led observers to speak of the "Mexican miracle." When growth seemed to be faltering in the early 1970s, the discovery of enormous oil fields in southern Mexico and in the Gulf appeared to be the harbinger of even greater prosperity. Beginning in 1974, Mexico became a net exporter of petroleum, and as of 1985 it was the world's fourth largest producer of crude oil.[20] Proven crude oil reserves of 49.3 billion barrels place Mexico fourth globally.[21] Yet, a combination of declining oil prices and economic mismanagement has produced negative growth, triple-digit inflation, and underemployment in the 40 percent range. Approximately a million new workers enter the job market annually, yet job creation has recently averaged less than half that figure. These deficiencies make it difficult for Mexico to translate its economic and industrial strength into tangible influence.

The armed forces of Mexico are small in comparison to the country's size and economic output. Measured in terms of the number of troops per thousand population, Mexico is in 107th place globally (out of 143 nations ranked). If we consider defense spending as a percentage of GNP, Mexico comes in 129th in the world (out of 133 nations ranked).[22] From these figures it is apparent that Mexico does not consider the armed forces to be a vital instrument of foreign policy. To the extent that Mexico has sought to influence events in the region, it has done so primarily through economic and diplomatic means.

NATIONAL ROLE

Traditionally, Mexico has played a distinctly passive role in regional and international affairs. As a state that has suffered deeply from foreign intervention, it has regarded the international environment as an inhospitable place. To insulate itself from further depredations, Mexico has adhered to principles outlined in the Carranza Doctrine (1918) of sovereign equality of states, nonintervention, and peaceful resolution of disputes.[23] This has suited the conservative goals Mexican policy makers have established for themselves. As Ferris explains, "Mexico's foreign policies have largely been formulated to meet domestic political needs and to increase domestic political support for the system. . . ."[24]

Under the influence of Mexico's economic expansion and its subsequent emergence as a major oil power, the country began to adopt a more assertive posture in regional affairs. During President Luís Echeverría's administration (1970–76), Mexico began to chart an independent course that often collided with U.S. interests. Most notable were his support for Marxist Salvador Allende in Chile and his effort to reform the international economic order via a charter on the economic rights and duties of states. These actions were, in part, stimulated by Echeverría's personal desire to place Mexico and himself in a leadership position among Third World states. Additionally, splashy socialist rhetoric in the international realm was a useful palliative against pressure from leftist critics who decried the country's extreme maldistribution of wealth. It was not until the *sexenio* of José López Portillo (1976–82), however, that the country had the accumulated economic clout to give real meaning to its independent foreign policy line.[25]

Mexico was a significant actor in Central American affairs during López Portillo's tenure. The country provided substantial diplomatic and economic support for the Sandinista revolution. This included withdrawing recognition of the Somoza regime in 1978, providing hundreds of technical experts to the new Sandinista government, and supplying Nicaragua's oil needs at concessionary prices.[26] The country also recognized the rebellious forces in El Salvador as legitimate political actors in an August 1981 joint Franco-Mexican declaration. Moreover, Mexico has been one of the driving forces behind the effort to find a negotiated solution to the strife in Central America known as the Contadora Plan. This unusual activism prompted Bruce Bagley to conclude in 1981 that "Mexico has emerged as a major independent actor in hemispheric affairs." He hastened to add, however, that "Mexico's regional power status remains tenuous."[27] With the subsequent collapse of world oil prices, it became apparent how tenuous Mexico's assertive regional role actually was.

Upon taking office in 1982, President Miguel de la Madrid inherited a nearly bankrupt economy as well as a severe legitimacy crisis. The need to pursue painful austerity measures and, simultaneously, an anticorruption campaign left few fiscal resources and little governmental energy to perpetuate the activist foreign policies of preceding administrations. The oil-support arrangement with Nicaragua has been terminated, and no new initiatives have been promulgated. Mexico, however, has continued its support of the Contadora Plan as a means of restraining U.S. policy in the region. The evolution in Mexico's role is captured once again by Bagley, who observed in 1983 that "an economically crippled and militarily weak Mexico appears to have only a limited role to play in the Central American tragedy."[28] The pendulum has swung back, though certainly not completely, toward Mexico's more traditional passive role in regional affairs.

LINKAGES AND INTERDEPENDENCIES

The latitude enjoyed by Mexico in pursuing an independent foreign or defense policy is significantly constrained by its dependence on the United States. While the U.S. has come to rely on Mexico to a greater extent in recent years, relations remain asymmetrical. This is particularly apparent in the economic realm. Although Mexico has become the third largest trading partner of the United States, leverage is clearly weighted in favor of the latter. For Mexico, trade with the United States constitutes 60 percent of its total, while Mexico only acounts for 5.5–6 percent of U.S. trade flows.[29] Between 1982 and 1986, moreover, the enormous burden of servicing the country's $100 billion debt caused Mexico to negotiate three separate bail-out schemes; the quid pro quo has been externally imposed austerity programs.

Relations are not totally one-sided, however. U.S. bankers account for the largest single share of outstanding loans to Mexico. The health of the U.S. banking system, and indeed of global financial markets, depends on Mexico's success at repaying its debt. Until recently, moreover, Mexico had been the largest supplier of U.S. petroleum imports, a position that has both economic and strategic significance for the United States. Thus bilateral economic relations are clearly interdependent. This is especially true for the entire tier of states from Texas to California along the shared border. On balance, however, the relations remain asymmetrical and a significant constraint on Mexico's policy options.

DOMESTIC ENVIRONMENT

Mexico's *economic system* impinges upon its defense policy in a variety of ways. First, owing to a reasonably sophisticated industrial base, including automotive and shipbuilding industries, Mexico possesses the technological resources necessary to sustain a modest arms industry. Second, the country's GNP ranks fifteenth globally. Means are thus theoretically available to sustain a far larger military establishment than currently exists. Historically, however, Mexican defense planners have limited allocations to the defense sector to approximately 0.8 percent of GNP. The reasons for this are political and are explored elsewhere. The point to be made here is that the size of the GNP itself is not a primary constraining factor upon the defense budget.

In another sense, however, resource availability has influenced allocations for defense. A correlation exists between the rapid influx of oil revenues, which took place predominantly during the López Portillo administration (1977–82), and increased spending on defense, especially in the area of weapons modernization. Indeed, Mexico was still a net oil importer during the Luís Echeverría administration (1970–76). At the outset of the López Portillo *sexenio* (1976), oil income totaled a mere $436 million. By the final year of his administration, however, revenues from oil had burgeoned to $16.5 billion.[30] It should be noted in this regard that exploitation of Mexico's oil wealth is the exclusive province of the state-owned oil company, PEMEX. With the decline of oil prices in 1982, and the related economic dislocations that Alden Cunningham has termed the "equivalent of an economic meltdown,"[31] a surplus was no longer available to perpetuate a major modernization effort. Consequently, planned acquisitions of additional Azteca patrol boats, F-5 fighters, and light tanks had to be shelved.

Clearly there is a relation between the status of the economy and military expenditures. Under normal conditions, the armed forces have not commanded a high budgetary priority. In the midst of Mexico's oil bonanza, however, when other constituencies were being handsomely indulged, the armed forces could scarcely have been spurned. Thus the oil windfall made possible a weapons acquisition program not contemplated during normal years. As oil prices declined and the burden of repaying the foreign debt rose, allocations for the armed forces diminished to the point where

major weapons purchases were constrained once again.

Strains caused by continued economic hardships could also profoundly affect defense policy. The current plight of the Mexican economy has raised concerns for the stability of the political order itself. Euphoria generated by discovery of massive oil reserves in the 1970s has been supplanted today by despair over the Sisyphean task of repaying the nation's $100 billion debt. Economic mismanagement and malfeasance by the López Portillo administration were replaced by externally imposed austerity programs during the De la Madrid era. The living conditions of the average Mexican have declined under the combined effects of triple-digit inflation, sluggish or negative growth, aggregate unemployment and underemployment in the 40 percent range, and a plummeting peso. Compounding these grim statistics is the fact that the Mexican government controls 60 percent of the nation's productive capacity. Thus, the government can be held directly accountable for the maldistribution of wealth and economic hardships experienced by the citizenry. It is for these reasons that Cunningham has concluded: "The current financial crisis presents an unprecedented threat to the social and political fabric of Mexico. Support for what has been one of the most stable political systems not only in Latin America but in the entire third world, is in jeopardy."[32]

In spite of the gravity of the economic situation, the capacity of the *political system* to respond and weather the crisis remains considerable. The purpose here is to identify and categorize features of the Mexican political system that have a bearing on the nation's defense policy.

Mexico's political process displays certain trappings of pluralism. Elections are held at regular intervals, presidents transfer power to successors every six years, generals refrain from plotting coups, and journalists ply their trade without obvious government interference. On the basis of these observations, it might seem appropriate to include Mexico among the democratic polities of the world. In categorizing a political system, however, it is necessary to look beyond appearances in an effort to capture the essence of political relationships. After stripping away Mexico's pluralistic veneer, an essentially hegemonic political system comes into view.

To establish the nature of the regime in Mexico, the first step must be to consider the difference between a hegemonic and a pluralistic polity. The presence or absence of elections does not suffice in making such a distinction because electoral processes can be manipulated to deprive the people of a voice. For elections to have meaning, the electorate must be given a choice. For a choice to have meaning, at least two sides must have an opportunity to win political power or to prevail on an issue.

Contestation for office and contestation over policy are irreplaceable features of pluralism. The absence of these features produces a system where power is concentrated at the center. The term "hegemonic" may properly be applied to such a regime.

According to Robert Dahl, hegemonic regimes are characterized by an absence of "permissible opposition, public contestation, or political competition."[33] In such a regime, top executive and legislative positions are monopolized by a narrow governing clique. Elections may be held at regular intervals, but they merely offer the electorate the opportunity to confirm the hegemony of the existing government. Power is not transferred peacefully to factions outside the ruling elite. Nor do those opposed to policy choices of the government possess an effective, constitutional means of registering their concerns.

Since the conclusion of the violent phase of the Revolution and establishment of the *Partido Nacional Revolucionario* in 1929 (the party has been rechristened twice; today it is known as the *Partido Revolucionario Institucional*, or PRI), the official party has never lost a major electoral contest.[34] Indeed, if the official vote tally is to be trusted, the official party candidate has always won the presidency in a landslide. Since the 1934 presidential election, the victorious candidate has garnered between 71.6 percent and 98.7 percent of the vote.[35]

The official party's record in gubernatorial elections is also unblemished; the opposition has yet to occupy the governor's mansion in a single state.[36] The PRI's stranglehold on the national legislature has never been in doubt either, although a minority of the seats are now routinely allocated to opposition parties in the lower house, the Chamber of Deputies. The regime has been so certain of perpetuating its majority in that body that it has allocated 100 of the 400 seats to minority parties in proportion to their share of the national vote.[37] The PRI is not so generous with its opponents in the Senate. Until 1976 no rival party candidate had been seated in that chamber. Even the loss of a single seat in 1976 was not the result of an electoral defeat. Rather, the PRI withdrew its candidate as a result of a political bargain struck with the *Partido Popular Socialista*.[38]

This impressive electoral record demonstrates the futility of opposition to the official party in presidential, gubernatorial, and national legislative races. In the words of former Mexican President Emilio Portes Gil, "No other party will ever win power."[39]

Deference and respect are the watchwords guiding representatives of interest groups in their dealings with government officials. Effective political activists generally seek private consultation with the president or his ministers rather than public confrontation.[40] Especially destructive to one's cause, and potentially to one's person, is direct criticism of the president.[41] Student leaders who violated this norm in 1968, for example, suffered tragic consequences at Tlatelolco (discussed below).[42] In particular, the president seeks to avoid "giving the impression that violent disruption is rewarded."[43] Rather, he wishes to cultivate the notion that all political change originates in the presidency.[44]

The Mexican political context is one in which demands must be channeled through the political center for maximal success.[45] It is, in other words, a corporate system in which functional groups are encouraged to associate themselves either formally or informally with the regime for pursuit of their objectives. Encouragement comes in the form of cooptation and, if that fails, coercion.[46] As described by Judith Hellman, cooptation is "the process by which individuals or groups independent enough to threaten the ongoing domination of a single group or party (in this case, the PRI) are traded small concessions or favors in exchange for moderating their demands and reducing their challenge to the dominant group's control over the system."[47] For intractable elements unwilling to respond to such inducements, the regime's monopoly on the "legitimate" use of force can be employed to remove them from the political scene. It is a venerable tradition, the essence of which is captured in the Mexican phrase *pan o palo* (bread or the stick).

Relations between the state and various interests comprising the Mexican political community are governed by this combination of cooptation and coercion. It is an arrangement that affords the central government a great deal of leverage. The interest group having greatest relevance to defense policy is the military. It is essential, therefore, to consider at some length the place occupied by the armed forces in the political spectrum.

CIVIL-MILITARY RELATIONS

The place of the armed forces in contemporary Mexican politics contrasts dramatically with that of most of their Latin American counterparts. Overt disruption of the political process by the armed forces has been avoided for over five decades, the last serious uprising occurring in 1929.[48] This is especially remarkable in light of Mexico's tempestuous origins. Charles Cumberland, for example, has calculated that "during independent Mexico's first fifty hectic and catastrophic years, over thirty different individuals served as president, heading more than fifty governments."[49] Indeed, conspiracy, rebellion, and coup d'état constitute the leitmotif of the nation's history, reaching a crescendo with the Revolution of 1910–17. The present quiescent nature of civil-military relations stands out not only against the backdrop provided by other nations in the region, but also against Mexico's own historical experience.

The degree of Mexican military involvement in the domestic political process clearly diverges from the Latin American norm, but the nature and extent of this involvement is a subject of some dispute. As Frank Margiotta has noted, two basic schools of thought exist.[50] One asserts that the military in Mexico is apolitical.[51] This position is summarized by Edwin Lieuwen: "By 1958 all the generals of the revolution had either died off or were in retirement, and the post-revolutionary professional officers now in charge of the defense establishment showed no inclination to mingle in politics."[52] The other body of scholarship holds that the military continues to be a central political actor, even though it has abandoned its previous role as the leading agent for governmental change. David Ronfeldt discusses the "residual" political roles of the Mexican military;[53] Margiotta asserts that the military continues to engage in political activity;[54] Needler stresses the political nature of their internal security function, and Williams traces the "resurgence" of the military as a political force since the late 1960s.[55]

In conceptualizing the role of the military it is essential to avoid the false dichotomy that the military is either political if it is running the government or apolitical if it is not. If these were the only two categories available for characterizing civil-military relations, then analysts would agree that the Mexican military today is apolitical. This mode of analysis, however, would conceal more than it reveals. As Needler has noted, "Clearly, the formula that in Mexico the army is non-political constitutes a considerable simplification."[56] The primary reason for this oversimplification is that it is based on a narrow construction of the term *politics*. In this study I take *politics* to mean the authoritative allocation of the scarce values of society.[57] If viewed in this fashion, it is possible to conclude that the Mexican military establishment has a pronounced impact upon politics even though it avoids usurpation of governmental authority.

Virtually all analysts acknowledge that a striking transition has taken place in the political function of the Mexican military since 1917. Ronfeldt states this proposition most persuasively in "The Mexican Army and Political Order Since 1940."[58] In assessing the activities of the military, he concludes that much of its behavior is indeed laden with political content. Among its "residual political roles," Ronfeldt identifies (a) gathering of intelligence, (b) articulation of interests, (c) management of political conflicts, (d) defense of the ruling party during elections, (e) suppression of dissent, and (f) extension of governmental control over isolated regions.[59] Ronfeldt concludes that "the endurance of the established Mexican political system has probably depended significantly—and will continue to depend— upon the army's performance of its residual political roles."[60] Particularly germane to this discussion is evidence that the military routinely involves itself in internal political matters and is not above direct participation in partisan political affairs.

Daily activities of Mexican soldiers range across a broad spectrum, extending from standard training activities to implementation of politically sensitive government programs. One primary function is civic action. In performing this role, the military serves to bring the presence of the central government to remote and isolated corners of the nation. Military involvement in building roads, hospitals, and airports has been well documented elsewhere.[61]

A regional perspective on this role is supplied by the observations of officers who attended the *Escuela Superior de Guerra* (ESG), or Higher War College. As part of this program, officers participate in numerous field trips throughout Mexico. In the Pachuca region, for example, one officer noted that the army distributes water to small villages and communal farms. Elsewhere, in rugged portions of San Luis Potosi, the army disseminates school books to outlying settlements that are otherwise inaccessible.[62] Naval units provide shore patrols and lifeguards for local beaches in the coastal regions of the state of Veracruz.[63] The nature of civic action programs varies according to the needs arising in each state. The overall impact of these activities, in a political sense, is that the military functions as a leading agent through which the government penetrates outlying regions. In this capacity it

serves a political purpose of at least some significance.

The army also constitutes the primary expression of governmental authority in many of these same locations. In Oaxaca, for example: "The 24th Military Zone relies heavily on the employment of *partidas* or small detachments to maintain law and order in isolated areas. Their most common task is to mediate over land disputes that involve small Indian villages. These *partidas* are also called upon to investigate murders and other potentially explosive situations."[64] These examples indicate the military is employed routinely by civilian elites to maintain the authority of the central government whenever local conditions warrant. If the regular government apparatus is unable to cope, the military will be assigned the task of maintaining law and order. Ronfeldt has termed this the "management of political conflicts."[65] Such activity is instrumental to maintaining the capacity of the ruling elite to govern.

In addition to maintaining order and implementing sensitive government programs, the armed forces also enter directly into the electoral process itself. One observer noted how buses were used in 1981 "to transport troops to the towns where PRI candidate Miguel de la Madrid was to visit starting that Friday. . . . The troops were formed up at about 0630 to prepare for the trip. They were in civilian clothes and were to serve as extra guards and crowd fillers. . . . It happens every election year."[66]

Thus, the armed forces appear to take an active role in securing the electoral success of the ruling party's presidential candidate. This is not an entirely new role for Mexican foot soldiers. Betty Kirk cites the support provided by the Mexican Army for official government candidate Avila Camacho on election day, 7 July 1940.[67] That this practice continues today is an indication that the Mexican armed forces are far from being neutral observers of the political scene. This unequivocally removes them from the apolitical category.

An even more stark illustration of military guardianship over the "revolutionary family" took place in the *Plaza de las Tres Culturas*, or

Tlatelolco, in October 1968. The massacre of scores of student demonstrators by army troops is a clear illustration of the military's draconian potential.[68] It is not clear, however, to what extent the Mexican secretary of defense may have been the instigator of this act. The commonly accepted version is that Luís Echeverría, then minister of interior and subsequently president, ordered the army to quell the student unrest. Other evidence exists, however, to suggest that the military may have played a more active, perhaps even dominant, role in resolving this crisis. Needler hints at this in the following passage: "Some observers have even speculated that the strongly repressive line taken by [President Gustavo] Díaz Ordaz toward the student demonstrations of 1968 was in part stimulated by the desire to preempt any military dissatisfaction with a softer attitude."[69] Authors of a study published by the Center for Advanced International Studies at the University of Miami observe, "It appears that the military in Mexico advocated the action against the student" demonstrations.[70] Information collected by this researcher during interviews conducted in 1983 casts even more doubt on the conventional interpretation of this event.

In the words of one American who has been in close contact with members of the Mexican military since the early 1970s: "At the height of the crisis, Díaz Ordaz left town. The Secretary of Defense, General Marcelino Garcia Barragán, consulted with the president's aide concerning how the military should respond to the growing crisis. [Interior Minister] Echeverría was there. He was saying, 'Be kind to the students.'. . . Subsequently, Garcia Barragán had his troops clear the plaza."[71]

A more detailed account was offered by a Mexican military officer who was in a sensitive post at the time. In his words:

The situation was becoming serious, and it was decided that President Díaz Ordaz had to leave town. General Garcia Barragán had arrayed the troops, and he was in the Presidential Palace. Echeverría, who was the interior minister at the time, was down on the street with General Ballesteros. Echeverría began giving orders to move the troops, and General Ballesteros interrupted him saying that General Garcia Barragán was commander of the troops and that these orders would need to be cleared through him. So General Ballesteros

called General Garcia Barragán to explain the situation to him. General Garcia Barragán's response was that Echeverría should keep his hands off Army matters. General Ballesteros then put Echeverría on the phone and that is when Garcia Barragán told Echeverría what he could do. After that the order was given to clear the square. General Garcia Barragán then went to tell Díaz Ordaz that the situation was all clear. Díaz Ordaz was scared because he thought the army was about to tell him they had taken over. When he heard what General Garcia Barragán had to say, he gave him an emotional embrace and told him he was a good soldier.[72]

Although the details vary somewhat, this version portrays Garcia Barragán as the driving force behind the decision to repress student unrest. If true (and further research into this subject would hopefully shed additional light) neither Díaz Ordaz nor Echeverría sought this action. Indeed, the revisionist interpretation indicates Díaz Ordaz was not present when the fateful decision was made. Moreover, Echeverría may have sought to prevent, or at least limit, the use of force against the demonstrators.

Two inferences about the role of the military may be drawn from this event. First, the military would seem to be deadly serious about its role as guarantor of the established order. Though President Díaz Ordaz may have vacillated, the military leadership clearly perceived its mission. The military recognized its duty to maintain the prevailing distribution (i.e., concentration) of power. Rival power contenders who were unwilling to be coopted were dealt with according to the established tradition of *pan o palo*. In this case, the army discharged its responsibilities by smashing a burgeoning student movement.

If the revisionist account is accurate, then the military response to this situation suggests a second lesson about civil-military relations in Mexico. While Garcia Barragán may not have required an order from civilian elites for him to act, neither did he need to be told not to assume the presidency. This would be an indication the military recognizes the outer limits of its role. Once the threat to the established order had been met, the military leadership apparently hastened to reaffirm its fealty to the president. This is an action Mexican military officers cite with pride for they realize that at that crucial moment in 1968 Garcia Barragán was in a pivotal position. That he harbored no intention to depose Díaz Ordaz, and that the military applauded his action, suggests the existence of a boundary the officer corps is loathe to cross.

The preceding analysis has sought to clarify the nature of civil-military relations in Mexico. In large part, the dispute over the political significance of the Mexican military establishment would seem to stem from differing interpretations of the meaning of *politics*. If we take it to mean the authoritative allocation of scarce values, it is clear that the armed forces are indeed highly political. An institution that recurringly involves itself in electoral politics and, when necessary, represses challenges to the established political order can scarcely be considered apolitical.

The political activities described above have one unifying theme: preservation of the existing power structure. Civic action programs extend the reach of the central government into outlying regions. Constabulary duties allow civilian elites to maintain control in trouble spots. Support for the PRI candidate during the presidential campaign clearly is partisan in nature and intended to ensure victory by the dominant political faction over its rivals. The initiative taken by the army at Tlatelolco is undeniable testimony that the military possesses ultimate responsibility for maintaining the political status quo. This set of activities warrants describing the Mexican military as the guarantor of the revolutionary order.

In this role, the armed forces of Mexico do not constitute an independent source of political power. They do not contest the ruling elite for control over the political apparatus. Rather, their function is to ensure that civilian elites comprising the "Revolutionary Family"[73] perpetuate themselves in power. The armed forces, therefore, are an integral and politicized part of the hegemonic regime that is Mexico.

The Defense Decision-Making Process

In Mexico's hegemonic political context, where pressing external security threats are lacking, the decision-making process bears little resemblance to decision making in the United States and other Western democracies.

The conceptual frameworks most commonly employed by scholars and policy makers in their efforts to explain defense decisions have little in common with decision-making processes in Mexico. Typically analysts seek to explain national security decisions either as a product of rational, analytic calculation aimed at maximizing the national interest or as the outcome of political bargaining among contending elites.[74] The first approach, which I shall refer to as the analytic model, places particular emphasis on the *external* constraints that mold security policy.[75] The alternative approach, frequently referred to as the bureaucratic politics model, is especially concerned with *internal* determinants of policy. It accentuates organizational and individual factors that are discounted by the analytic model.[76]

The problem, in sum, is this. In the Mexican context, where the threat to security is predominantly internal to the polity, focus on factors external to the state—as in the analytic model—provides an unsatisfactory basis for explanation. However, in a political system where decision-making power is concentrated at the top rather than being scattered broadly across the political landscape, the bargaining and coalition formation so fundamental to bureaucratic politics may be lacking as well.

In Mexico's hegemonic political system, where internal security concerns predominate, decision making appears to depart substantially from the analytic and bureaucratic political styles. Decision-making processes conform more closely to a pattern of personal interaction known as the patron-client exchange relationship.

THE PATRON-CLIENT MODEL

Patron-client ties constitute a form of exchange relationship that is common in traditional societies.[77] They have also shown a remarkable degree of adaptability elsewhere amidst the processes of modernization, industrialization, and bureaucratization.[78] Any setting, in fact, that is characterized by a persistent, unequal distribution of valued resources and by an absence of dependable legal guarantees for life, wealth, and status will tend to produce patron-client alliances.[79] Under these conditions, relatively powerless clients seek to shield themselves from uncertainties in their environments by affiliating with a patron.

Anthropologists and political scientists have generally identified the presence of patron-client alliances using the following distinguishing characteristics: (1) They are based on an exchange of valued resources where the patron offers security and other benefits to clients in return for loyalty and support for his own objectives; (2) they involve informal understandings rather than legal, binding contracts; (3) they are established between actors of unequal power; (4) they are personal, face-to-face relationships; (5) they are multifunctional, potentially covering any aspect of the lives of the participants; and (6) they persist over time, so long as the two parties have resources of value to offer each other.[80]

Because of the face-to-face nature of these ties, the number of followers that any individual patron can manage is normally fewer than thirty.[81] Once a patron-client cluster exceeds this size, intermediaries or brokers typically arise to extend the scope of the system. Brokers do not have direct control over the resources they dispense; rather, they have access to them by virtue of a personal relationship with a more powerful patron.[82] As the number of brokers proliferates, these patron-client clusters expand into hierarchically arranged pyramids that may eventually permeate society.[83]

The tendency for patron-client relationships to penetrate political and bureaucratic structures is crucial from the perspective of decision-making theory. In the first place, decision makers enmeshed in an informal patron-client network may tend to respond to the expectations inherent in that exchange relationship rather than to the official norms and routines of the bureaucracy to which they formally belong. Additionally, to the extent that a single patron-client network comes to dominate the entire political system, there will be little need for compromise and coalition building during the decision-making process itself. A pervasive patron-client system, once in place, constitutes a built-in "coalition" that the patron simply activates to effect a decision.

Given a hegemonic regime in which interpersonal relations are organized along patron-client lines, the decision-making process may bear little resemblance to the "pulling and hauling" of bureaucratic politics. Authority to set policy would be confided in an individual or a small, closed elite at the top of a pyramidal structure.[84] Legislatures, political parties, the news media, interests groups, and the public at large would have negligible impact on policy formation. Decisions would be made at the top by a handful of participants without regard for the preferences of outside groups. Indeed, only those privy to the inner circles would be aware a decision was imminent.[85]

Centralization of power in a patron-client decision unit contributes to a vertical pattern of interaction. Instead of proceeding sideways in search of supporters, the direction of movement is upward in quest of patronage. Because power is concentrated at the top of the governmental pyramid, efforts to influence policy are made in personal contacts with the president and those high-level bureaucrats who are his confidants.[86]

National security policy making, according to the patron-client model, entails interaction between the head of government and the cabinet minister responsible for the functional area involved (most commonly the defense minister or equivalent). This is in keeping with the dyadic nature of the patron-client relationship. The process itself constitutes an exchange in which the chief executive allocates resources and receives in return the continued loyal support and problem solving activity of the minister involved. After the patron has rendered a decision, his wishes must still be put into action. As with bureaucratic politics, implementation may not always conform to expectations of the decision maker. Once the governmental machinery begins to act, those who are negatively affected become aware that the decision poses a threat to their interests. At this point, they may attempt to mobilize their own sources of patronage to seek an accommodation.[87] This may produce a clash of interests as occurs in the bureaucratic politics process. If this takes place, however, it will be associated with implementation rather than formulation of the decision.

In another crucial dimension, implementation is quite unlike bureaucratic politics. Organizational constraints in the form of standard operating procedures have minimal relevance under the influence of a pervasive patron-client network. The ability of a bureaucrat to carry out tasks is primarily a function of informal exchange relations.[88] As a result, formal operating procedures are not nearly as deterministic as informal bonds of patronage. Ultimately, implementation follows the patron-client network downward through the bureaucracy.

To illustrate Mexico's national security policy-making process, I shall use examples from that country's 1981 decision to purchase a dozen F-5 Tiger II aircraft from the United States. I have examined this decision in considerable detail elsewhere.[89]

STRUCTURE OF THE DECISION-MAKING UNIT

A decision-making unit consists of those individuals who participate in, and have influence over, a decision. Decision units are shaped by the nature of the political context in which they exist. In Mexico, the political system is hegemonic, with power concentrated at the apex of a corporatist governmental structure. The impact of this upon the structure of decision units involved in the F-5 decision was as follows: (1) decision units were small (five or fewer members), and (2) decision units had an *authoritative leader* (an individual who was able to commit the decision unit to action even if every other member had been opposed).

The principal actors involved in the decision to allocate resources for the purpose of upgrading the Mexican Air Force inventory were President José López Portillo and his secretary of defense, Gen. Felix Galvan López. The president played the pivotal role because of his control over military spending. On military procurement matters, the president's authority is absolute. Funds for the purchase of major weapons systems are not contained in the annual military budget. To obtain such funds, the armed forces must petition the president

for an allocation from his fund. Thus, the president was not merely an important player, he was the authoritative leader of this decision unit. No other actor could have allocated these "special funds." Moreover, if the president had decided to deny funding, the secretary of defense would have had no legitimate recourse.

The only other significant player in the decision to allocate resources was the secretary of defense. Galvan began to lobby for a major renovation of the armed forces early in the López Portillo administration, perhaps even before the presidential succession took place. He proselytized the president publicly through the conduct of a joint army and air force maneuver in October 1977. Later, in his Army Day speech of 1979, after the anticipated financing had failed to materialize, Galvan asserted that the military had a right to its share of the national patrimony. While these events may have been orchestrated for public consumption, they nonetheless portray General Galvan as the dominant protagonist in the drive for military modernization.

In sum, the structural features of the decision-making unit that allocated funds for an armed forces modernization program were the following: (1) size: small (including only López Portillo and Galvan López), and (2) distribution of power: authoritative (López Portillo).

As tables 1 and 2 reveal, a remarkably consistent pattern existed throughout all phases of the formulation and implementation of this decision.

One dimension remained consistent throughout: all twelve decision-making units were *small*. While this finding itself is notable, an even closer inspection reveals that in eleven of twelve cases, no more than two significant actors were involved.[90] This pattern is a distinct departure from that which has been

Table 1. Structural Characteristics of
Decision-Making Units during
Decision Formulation

Issue	Size	Distribution of Power
Resource allocation	small	authoritative leader
Aircraft selection (1977)	small	authoritative leader
Aircraft selection (1980)	small	authoritative leader (probably)

Table 2. Structural Characteristics of Decision-Making Units during Decision Implementation

Issue	Size	Distribution of Power
Instructor pilot selection	small	indeterminate
Conversion pilot selection	small	authoritative leader (probably)
Selection of maintenance trainees	small	authoritative leader
Allocation of supplementary pay for trainees	small	authoritative leader
Non-acquisition of munitions	small	authoritative leader
Selection of freight forwarder	small	indeterminate
Sole source procurement decisions	small	authoritative leader (probably)
Construction of a new hangar	small	no authoritative leader
Paint scheme	small	authoritative leader

found to characterize decision-making units in the United States. Glenn Paige, for example, in a study of the U.S. decision to intervene in the Korean conflict, finds that four of six decision-making units had more than ten members, and the smallest unit had five members.[91] It seems reasonable to suggest that decision-making units in Mexico's hegemonic political system are structured differently from those in pluralistic systems.

A clear predominance of *authoritative leadership* was also apparent. Of the ten units for which a determination could be made, six were clearly authoritatively led, and three were probably so structured. Certainly, those units possessing only a single actor were, ipso facto, authoritatively led.

It is worth noting that this authoritative pattern was reproduced throughout various strata within Mexican officialdom. Not only did the president appear as an authoritative decision maker, but the secretary of defense, the MAF's F-5 program manager, and the army comptroller (a lieutenant colonel) also wielded power in this fashion within their own decision-making units. During the implementation of the F-5 decision, for example, General Javier Salinas, the MAF's program manager, had dominion over logistical, technical, and personnel matters, while Lieutenant Colonel Nicolas Bocanegra, the army comptroller, was dominant when it came to finances.

A clear and consistent pattern emerges from this analysis: decision-making units in the case of the F-5 acquisition by Mexico were small and authoritatively led. Paige suggests the significance of this finding for the decision-making process when he claims that "decisions tend to vary with the composition of the decision unit."[92] The composition of units in this case was conducive to a patron-client process.

THE PATRON-CLIENT APPROACH TO DECISION FORMULATION

Ideally, the presence of patron-client interaction would be demonstrated by exposing the exchange that is at the heart of this process. This is normally not possible, however. By its nature the patron-client exchange is informal, unspoken, and implicit. It is understood by the two parties that the patron has bound the client to future, unspecified supportive actions by virtue of his assistance to the client. To fashion indicators for this process, it is necessary to look for phenomena related to the exchange itself. The following set of characteristics should allow observers to examine whether the behavior of decision makers conforms to essential features of the patron-client process: (1) the decision reinforces the bond between patron and client; (2) the decision is a product of private, personal interaction and does not involve public debate aimed at mobilizing supporters outside the patron-client dyad; and (3) the decision-making unit remains small in size, encompassing patron, client, and perhaps a broker. Behavior of Mexican decision makers in the F-5 case was consistent with each of these indicators.

REINFORCEMENT OF THE BOND BETWEEN PATRON AND CLIENT

Every six years, with the inauguration of a new president, the Mexican governmental bureaucracy undergoes wholesale renovation. A legion of new officials is swept into office with the new chief executive. These individuals are personally tied to the president as members of his *equipo*, or team.[93] The military is not exempt from this sexennial process.

The relationship between president and secretary of defense is crucial to the continued dominance of civilian elites over the military establishment. To secure the loyalty of the armed forces, the president must first secure the loyalty of the secretary of defense. This is facilitated through the traditional Mexican presidential practice of appointing a trusted ally to this key post. The secretary of defense, in turn, places loyal subordinates in important command positions. Consequently, the transition to a new president causes a ripple effect within the military as a new team assumes positions of power and influence.

The president's concern for maintaining the support and allegiance of his secretary of defense persists throughout the six years of his administration. It is in this context that the decision to modernize the military can be placed. Viewed as a patron-client exchange, the president's decision to allocate resources for this purpose is explainable as a quid pro quo for securing the fidelity of his senior military commander and thereby the entire military command structure.

Several factors specific to the López Portillo administration reinforce this rather generic assessment. When López Portillo took office, the prospect of enormous revenues from oil sales was palpable, though the actual influx of funds did not begin immediately. As a result, military pleadings for updated hardware would need to be taken more seriously than had been the case during previous administrations. The generals could stoically accept neglect of the military inventory during austere periods; to ignore the armed forces when other sectors were benefiting from governmental largesse, however, would have been to court serious discontent among the military elite.

López Portillo may also have been more favorably disposed toward the military than his predecessor. He may have possessed a different perspective on the utility of its combat capability; certain fragmentary evidence suggests that military backing may have been instrumental in his accession to the presidency.

A variety of published sources recite the uncertainty surrounding the July–December 1976 transition period prior to López Portillo's inauguration.[94] "The question was whether Echeverría would still retain his influence,"

Smith writes, "whether his efforts to perpetuate his power would succeed. He had been scheming, many thought, to impose another *maximato*."[95]

Observations cited elsewhere[96] suggest the armed forces may have played a central role in preventing President Luís Echeverría from installing himself as the "maximum ruler" of Mexico, as Plutarco Calles had done in the 1930s. The period preceding the presidential transition in Mexico, however, is a particularly fertile one for rumormongering. It is, thus, not possible to place great confidence in these reports. If these accounts are eventually shown to have substance, though, the contours of an exchange between military commanders and the president-elect would come readily into focus: the generals prevented Echeverría from retaining power in return for a major modernization program.

These observations are consistent with the notion that decisions to allocate resources to the military in Mexico serve to reinforce linkages between the president and the military hierarchy. Two conditions may account for the enormity of the allocation made by López Portillo: (a) swelling oil revenues made it possible, and (b) Echeverría's putative power grab may have made it necessary. The essential point is that López Portillo, as patron in this decision, was left in a vastly more advantageous position to elicit support for his political goals from the military leadership.

PRIVATE, FACE-TO-FACE DECISION MAKING

One obligatory decision-making rule in a patron-client system is avoidance of public notice. Neither the patron nor the client would benefit from revelation of the intimate details of their relationship. The personal, face-to-face nature of patron-client relationships has been observed so commonly that it constitutes one of the key features by which this exchange relationship is identified.[97] This aspect of patron-client interaction corresponds strongly with the actions of Mexican decision makers in the F-5 case.

Private, face-to-face interaction between López Portillo and Galvan predominated during the resource allocation phase of decision formulation. Funding for the F-5 purchase came from a special presidential fund, the allocation of which was totally at López Portillo's discretion. As noted, Galvan and López Portillo were the only individuals involved. In reaching this decision, the president and secretary of defense generally shunned the spotlight. Certainly their deliberations regarding the allocation of the president's special funds were held behind closed doors.

THE DECISION-MAKING UNIT REMAINS SMALL

The final indicator of the patron-client approach to decision formulation is particularly useful in distinguishing this approach from the bureaucratic politics mode. Since the essence of the patron-client process is an exchange between patron and client, the decision-making unit ought to remain constant in size and small throughout the process. The central dynamic of the bureaucratic politics approach is just the reverse. Decision makers search far and wide for potential allies capable of helping them amass a winning coalition. Nothing of the sort took place during the formulative stage of the F-5 decision.

The three decision-making units involved in formulating this decision never expanded beyond a patron, a client, and (in one instance) a broker. The decision to allocate resources for a modernization program encompassed only López Portillo and his secretary of defense. The selection of the F-5 in 1977 included only Galvan himself as a central figure, although he did secure the president's approval for this decision. The final selection of the F-5 in 1980 included only Galvan and an influential individual who played the role of a broker. None of these decision-making units experienced any expansion during the course of the decision. The remarkable exclusivity of membership in these units constitutes an unambiguous repudiation of the bureaucratic politics approach and a solid endorsement of the patron-client style.

THE PATRON-CLIENT APPROACH TO DECISION IMPLEMENTATION

The pattern of behavior in a patron-client decision-making process ought to be distin-

guishable from other approaches primarily because of the closed, personal nature of this decision-making style. The ramifications of this upon decision implementation are manifold: (1) looking from the top down, effective execution of the decision should be limited only by the extent of the patron's circle of clients, not by bureaucratic procedures; (2) looking from the bottom up, resistance to the decision should begin only after implementation itself has begun, owing to the private nature of decision formulation; and (3) looking at the decision-making unit itself, membership should expand during the implementation phase, to the extent that those seeking to resist the decision have the connections to do so.

IMPLEMENTATION GOVERNED BY PERSONAL RELATIONS

In a patron-client system, implementation is constrained by the limits of the patron's cluster of faithful supporters. If the patron's network of ties is expansive and strategically placed, implementation will be relatively straightforward. If this is not the case, problems will abound. Since the objectives of decision makers were successfully met during execution of the F-5 program, this model predicts we ought to discover intimate, personal interaction sustaining each phase of implementation.

One major task undertaken by the MAF was construction of a hangar, taxiway, and engine test cell for the F-5. In all these matters, General Salinas, the MAF program manager, relied upon a trusted friend and architect. The bonds of friendship between these two individuals were long-standing. General Salinas had known his architect friend when the latter was a young boy. The architect could walk into Salinas' office ahead of a line of generals.[98] The original notion that a new hangar would be needed was born out of a conversation between these two friends, and the execution of that project was entrusted completely to the architect. On friendship alone, the architect began construction of the $4.5 million hangar. If he had insisted on a contract, the project would have been delayed at least four months. Overall, if General Salinas had conformed to U.S. Air Force construction procedures, the hangar would have taken six to ten years to complete, as opposed to the two years it took his architect friend.

INITIATION OF RESISTANCE

To assess whether attempts were made to impede execution of the F-5 decision, it is essential first to consider what objective or outcome was desired by decision makers. Assuming the decision represented a patron-client exchange, the purpose was to cement for the president the loyalty of his secretary of defense. The president exchanged a dozen F-5 fighters (along with a considerable amount of hardware for the army) in return for loyal service from the secretary of defense. This objective could have been undermined if the acquisition had been prevented altogether or if it had been excessively delayed. A high priority was placed on ensuring these aircraft were available to perform in the final Independence Day Parade (16 September 1982) presided over by the López Portillo administration. Any deliberate actions aimed at interfering with the successful performance of the F-5 in the September 1982 air show would have constituted resistance to the decision.

One of the more remarkable aspects of the F-5 decision was the very low incidence of activity that might have distorted the outcome desired by López Portillo and Galvan. This is especially true of the MAF's campaign to ready the aircraft for operations by 16 September 1982. In all phases of execution of the F-5 decision, the behavior of the MAF was compliant with the wishes of decision makers.

A different pattern of activity was exhibited by agencies outside the military hierarchy. The secretary of the treasury reportedly balked at Galvan's attempt to obtain funding for the F-5 acquisition. Additionally, the Interior Ministry would not supply work permits for technical advisers from Northrop and General Electric. This meant these advisers could not officially enter Mexico for the purpose of employment, even though their employer was the government of Mexico. These impediments did not prevent successful execution of the F-5 decision; nevertheless, they are consistent with the expectation that resistance in a patron-client

decision-making process does not begin until the implementation phase itself is under way.

While the behavior of the Treasury and Interior Ministries is consistent with the patron-client model, their actions had little impact on the eventual outcome. When contrasted with the overwhelmingly compliant attitude of the MAF, these attempts at resistance appear insignificant. Conceptually, however, the contrast is very consequential. As maintained above, implementation in a patron-client environment is constrained by the implementor's network of personal supporters. If execution of a decision requires support from agencies beyond the patron's scope of connections, troublesome resistance is virtually assured. The F-5 decision was not seriously afflicted by such impediments for one fundamental reason: it was carried out exclusively within military channels. Moreover, it came to fruition without the awareness or involvement of the public. For decisions not requiring interagency cooperation, absence of resistance is consistent with the patron-client model. It may be that most Mexican national security decisions will fall into this favored category because of the self-sufficiency of the military and the secrecy with which its actions are generally carried out. For all other decisions requiring substantive interaction among discrete patron-client clusters, however, the implementation phase will likely instigate competition and resistance. In the F-5 decision the contrast between the cooperative behavior of the MAF and the obstructionist behavior of the Treasury and Interior Ministry exemplifies this proposition very well.

EXPANSION IN THE SIZE OF THE DECISION-MAKING UNIT

The supposition that unit size will increase during implementation is directly related to the notion that this phase will invoke opposition to the decision. Once political elites become aware that their interests are at risk, they will presumably mobilize resistance to the intended outcome. As noted above, however, implementation of the F-5 decision generated virtually no significant opposition because it was carried out in secret and almost entirely within military channels. There was no need to interact in a significant manner with other patron-client clusters. Expansion in unit size consequently did not take place during the implementation phase of this decision.

The conduct of Mexican officials in formulating and implementing the F-5 decision was consistent with behavior patterns predicted by the patron-client model. The bond between President López Portillo (as patron) and Secretary of Defense Galvan (as client) was solidified by this decision. In return for promising to modernize the armed forces, López Portillo may have received support from the generals for his assumption of power. Mexican policy makers also complied with the decision-making rule that patron-client decisions will be conducted in a private, face-to-face manner. López Portillo and Galvan arrived at decisions to allocate resources and select the F-5 privately and without fanfare. Finally, decision-making units in this case remained small. During the course of this decision, only three individuals played substantive roles: López Portillo (patron), Galvan (client), and a broker. All three aspects of the patron-client approach to decision formulation were fully satisfied.

Mexican officials also conformed to patron-client patterns in the way they implemented the F-5 decision. The first measure of patron-client behavior during implementation entailed use of personal connections to accomplish required tasks. General Salinas exemplified this almost ideally. For construction matters, he turned to a close friend. The second expectation was that resistance would not be manifested until the implementation phase. In those few instances in which Galvan had to step outside his own domain to carry out this decision, he did indeed encounter resistance. This came in the form of Treasury's reluctance to release funds for the purchase and the Foreign Ministry's refusal to grant long term visas for technical advisers to the MAF.

The final indicator of patron-client behavior, expansion of the decision-making unit, was not in evidence. Nevertheless, this finding can be explained within the logic of the patron-client model. Since this decision involved neither interagency cooperation nor public involve-

ment, membership in decision-making units was confined essentially to the MAF and its immediate circle.

These findings strongly support the claim that Mexican decision makers did employ the patron-client approach in making the F-5 decision. This style, moreover, would seem to typify the Mexican policy-making process far more accurately than either the analytic or the bureaucratic political models.

Recurring Issues and Defense Policy Outputs

NATIONAL OBJECTIVES, STRATEGY, AND FORCE EMPLOYMENT DOCTRINE

Mexico has historically avoided developing a formal national security doctrine integrating the role of the military with other elements of national policymaking. This is due primarily to the internal security orientation of the Mexican military and the irregularity with which civilian elites have felt compelled to call upon the armed forces to maintain political equilibrium. Only in recent years has the leadership of the military sensed a need to articulate the contribution it has to make to overall national security. Indeed, no consensus yet exists in Mexico regarding the desirability of adopting an overarching national security doctrine, much less regarding the place of the military within it.[99] Since national security doctrine is presently in its formative stages, only general features have emerged.

The foundation for military doctrine in Mexico is the Constitution of 1917, which stipulates the military is responsible for the internal security and external defense of the country.[100] With regard to its external mission, Mexico has adopted a decidedly defensive posture. As noted earlier, the country has suffered extensively as a result of foreign intervention. In response, policy makers have stressed a moral-legal approach to foreign policy, espousing principles of nonintervention, self-determination, and peaceful resolution of disputes.[101] Accordingly, the military itself has adopted a strictly defensive outlook. This notion is expressed with particular clarity in the following passage cited by Alberto Lozoya, a highly respected Mexican scholar of military affairs:

A nation can employ Armed Forces in two senses: with the aim of aggression or of defense. Mexico has organized its Army along the lines of the second of these aspects, that is to say, in order to guarantee the life of the nation and defend its territorial integrity, sovereignty, and institutions. Our country is not, nor has it ever been, an aggressive nation; on the contrary, it has always sustained the most elevated principles of international rights.[102]

In line with Mexico's defensive philosophy, military strategy has been neither aggressive nor preemptive. Judging from the conduct of Mexican forces during past conflicts, military doctrine would appear to be to limit an aggressor to the periphery of the nation whenever possible and, "wherever he moves inland, oppose his progress and cut his lines with mobile small-unit warfare."[103]

The only major instance in which Mexican troops have been used extraterritorially was during the final stages of World War II in support of allied powers in the Philippines. Mexico's contribution to the allied effort consisted of the deployment of its 201st Fighter Squadron to Pracos Air Force Base in the Philippines in 1945. This contingent, which consisted of 250 volunteers, conducted ground attack operations against Japanese installations in the Philippines and Formosa. Eight Mexican airmen were killed in action.[104]

Nominally, external defense held top priority in the basic textbook used at the military academy until 1952. Up to that time, the primary function was "to guarantee the national territory against all possible aggression," with the secondary task being "to safeguard . . . tranquility and order." Lastly, the military was expected to recognize that "the government has the Armed Forces as its principal means of realizing its duties and making its decisions respected."[105] Lozoya notes a fundamental realignment of these priorities occurring with the revision of this text in 1952. He writes that "the 1952 edition inverts the order of the first and third points. Thus, it mentions in the first place that it is the obligation of the state to attend to the conservation of internal order 'using as support the Armed Forces,' and only in the third place does it say that 'national territory is defended from outside attack by the Army.' "[106] If we take note of the fact that "the state" has been the captive of a ruling elite, or "Revolutionary Family,"[107] since the consolidation of the 1917 Revolution, then this revision would seem to acknowledge the primacy of the military's role as guardian of the ruling elite.

While the emphasis placed on this internal security mission is clear, formal doctrine for its implementation is not. Extrapolating once again from the historical pattern of employment, Mexican presidents have tended to invoke military firepower only after it has become clear that the threat to public order can no longer be contained by police forces.

This reluctance to use military force is apparently motivated by two concerns. First, the soldiery of any nation will normally find it distasteful to perform constabulary functions, particularly if discharging these functions involves firing upon their own populace.[108] Second, Mexican presidents recognize that the army is the one institution potentially capable of usurping power. It is in part for this reason that the budget, manpower, and weaponry of the armed forces have been kept at modest levels. The more that politicians come to rely on the military to maintain themselves in power, the greater must be the allocation of resources to the military sector. This becomes necessary both to purchase the loyalty of the generals and to provide the capacity to address increasing challenges to the regime.[109] A threshold exists beyond which a military establishment can no longer accept the constabulary function, however. If military capabilities and self-confidence have concurrently expanded to the point where it feels itself to be more competent to run the government than the civilian leadership, then a coup becomes likely.[110] Mexican presidents wish to keep the military well below this threshold. While they have been skillful at balancing these trade-offs in the past, the trend in recent years has been in the direction of greater dependency upon the military.

A pattern of escalating reliance upon the armed forces is apparent in the post-World War II era. Military involvement was at its nadir during the administration of Ruíz Cortines (1953–59). José Luís Pineyro observes that during this *sexenio*, "the Army hardly ever left its barracks."[111] The armed forces assumed a more prominent role under López Mateos (1959–64), who was compelled to use force to stifle unrest among various labor unions. Most serious of these was the railway workers' strike, but the military also responded to work stoppages against the Mexican Aviation Company and the telegraph, telephone, and postal service.[112] These incidents were discrete and isolated, however, and did not carry the potential for inflaming other sectors of society or regions of the country.

The student unrest confronted by President Díaz Ordaz (1964–70), in contrast, could have ignited a revolutionary upheaval.[113] Beginning in mid 1968, prior to the Summer Olympics in Mexico City, a series of student demonstrations grew to the point where "as many as 400,000 people" were mobilized and involved in antigovernment activity in the capital city.[114] This situation was especially volatile because student leaders sought to establish linkages with the urban poor and peasant groups; this could have provided a mass following for the movement. There were indications the protests were about to spread to outlying areas, which would likely have overtaxed the responsive capacity of the army. It was at this critical juncture that the army stepped in with overwhelming force to quash the rebellion. Estimates of student fatalities as a result of the "Tlatelolco massacre" vary, but it appears several hundred must have lost their lives.[115]

This tragic event was a watershed in modern Mexican history; apparently Tlatelolco initiated a process of evaluation among military leaders regarding Mexico's national security requirements and the military's role in satisfying them.[116] Tangible evidence that such ferment was taking place is suggested by Secretary of Defense Barragán's comment in his 1970 farewell speech in which he identified the lack of a "war doctrine" as a deficiency in military preparedness.[117] It would be left to his successors, however, to enunciate the rudiments of such a doctrine.

The process of reappraisal continued during the Luís Echeverría administration (1970–76). The primary challenge confronting military

strategists during this *sexenio* was urban terrorism and rural guerrilla activity. The 23 September Communist League conducted a series of kidnappings, assaults, and bank robberies until security forces managed to capture the bulk of its membership in 1974. In the countryside, a 250–500 member guerrilla "army" under the leadership of Lucio Cabañas operated for several years in the impoverished state of Guerrero. The government eventually assigned thousands of troops to the task of eradicating this guerrilla band before Cabañas was tracked down and killed. While national survival was not threatened by this activity, it constituted another challenge to the stability of the regime stemming from troubled domestic conditions.

While José López Portillo was president (1976–82), the armed forces became heavily enmeshed in drug eradication efforts and enforcement of unpopular electoral outcomes (e.g., in Juchitán and Piedras Negras).[118] Moreover, the flood of refugees fleeing the strife in Guatemala began to create security concerns in the state of Chiapas. Clearly, "national security" had come to encompass a broad spectrum of domestic social, economic, and political concerns, as well as regional issues, that could only be addressed effectively through coordinated action of various elements of government. It was perhaps inevitable that Secretary of Defense Galvan López would acknowledge this fact and seek to assert the role of the armed forces in meeting the array of security challenges confronting his country.

In a frequently cited interview published by *Proceso* in 1980, General Galvan expressed the military viewpoint on the meaning of "national security." He asserted, "I understand by national security the maintenance of social, economic, and political equilibrium, guaranteed by the armed forces."[119] This pronouncement by Galvan carries a twofold significance. First, it suggests a certain confidence on his part, for the subject of "national security" had been a heretofore forbidden subject. In the opinion of David Ronfeldt, public discussion of "national security" had been tabu for a variety of reasons: "In their view, national security is a dangerous language nurtured by the great power that has led armed forces elsewhere (notably South America in the 1960s and 1970s) to commit the sins of militarism: exaggerating local threats, criticizing civilian authority, seizing the government, repressing the public, and indulging in arms races."[120] That Galvan would feel secure enough to discuss this issue in public is tacit acknowledgement that the stature of the military has risen over the years. The repeated and growing reliance of a succession of presidents upon the military establishment no doubt had contributed to this development.

Substantively, Galvan's comments have perhaps even greater import. His notion of national security as "the maintenance of social, economic, and political equilibrium" parallels the doctrine of "security and development" emanating from the Brazilian *Escola Superior de Guerra* in the early 1960s. This redefinition of security to encompass the entire range of social, political, and economic developmental issues encouraged the Brazilian military to assume power in 1964.[121] Indeed, another Mexican development paralleling the "Brazilian model" has been establishment of a senior service school for the Mexican Army (the National Defense College) where "high-ranking officers now study national security concepts as an academic subject."[122]

None of this is to suggest that the Mexican military is about to follow its Brazilian counterparts along the perilous path of institutional military rule. The Mexican political system remains far more stable, mechanisms of civilian control over the military are far more firmly entrenched, and Mexican generals have the benefit of hindsight: such attempts in Brazil and Argentina ended with the officer corps thoroughly discredited.

What Galvan's comments do portend, however, is an enlarged military role in dealing with the many critical and enduring issues confronting Mexico. These include the Guatemalan border problem, the drug control challenge, and perhaps future attempts to introduce a measure of pluralism into the body politic. On the basis of a careful review of recent civil-military developments, Williams, for example, concludes, "More military men

are walking the corridors of power in Mexico and their voices have assumed added resonance . . ."[123] The armed forces have become increasingly vital to perpetuation of Mexico's institutionalized revolutionary government. Because of the pivotal military role in maintaining internal security, senior military leaders appear to have assumed a more consequential position in the Mexican political hierarchy.

It is not clear how the President is to accommodate greater military involvement in these issues, especially given the apparent inclination to use the personalistic, patron-client style of decision making. It appears that the gravity and complexity of problems confronting Mexico today may necessitate considerable reshaping of the mechanisms of government. This, fundamentally, is the challenge a national security doctrine must address. *How is the military's role to be harmonized with the contribution of other branches of the Mexican government?* The answer to this question is lacking. Nevertheless, future stability and security for Mexico will be affected in no small measure by the effective blending of the military role into a coherent national security doctrine.

FORCE POSTURE

The size, structure, and distribution of forces in Mexico generally reflect the military's internal security mission. Military manpower authorizations have increased steadily over the years. In 1975, for example, combined strength of all services was 82,000. By 1985 this figure had grown to 129,000. This gradual expansion correlates most closely with population growth in Mexican society and not with either unrest in the region or expansion or contraction in the strength of U.S. or Guatemalan forces. Thus, it is reasonable to conclude that Mexican defense planners have been responsive to internal rather than external trends in establishing the size of their military.

The military command structure is divided between the secretary of national defense, who is in charge of the army and air force, and the secretary of the navy, who oversees naval elements. Although forces under the jurisdiction of the secretary of national defense are by far the more powerful, this bifurcation of command militates against any unified attempt by the armed forces to overthrow civilian authority. Coordination of a military response to external aggression, by contrast, would not be facilitated by this dual command arrangement.

Similarly, the *distribution of forces* is also a function of internal political considerations. The most combat-capable elements of the Army and Air Force are stationed in and around the capital city. Indeed, the presidential guard is uniformly equipped with the most powerful weaponry in the Army inventory. The distribution of remaining forces shows no pattern of concentration toward peripheral or border areas.[124] Rather, ground and air elements not stationed in the Federal District (where a disproportionate number are assigned) are distributed in roughly uniform fashion among thirty-six military zones throughout the nation. These generally coincide with Mexico's states. The exceptions to this are the states of Guerrero, Chiapas, Oaxaca, and Veracruz. All other states have but one military zone. Guerrero, Oaxaca, and Chiapas contain two military zones because they have traditionally been a breeding ground for guerrilla activity. Veracruz receives additional emphasis because of the oil fields located within its boundaries.

The foregoing assessment has provided a broad accounting of force posture in Mexico. Additional data pertaining to the distribution of forces are cited below in individual service breakdowns.

Army. With a strength of 105,000 soldiers, the army accounts for over three-fourths of Mexico's combat forces. These ground elements are organized primarily into three echelons, with brigades being the largest units, battalions and regiments coming next in order of magnitude, and the smallest units consisting of mobile detachments called *partidas*.

As of mid 1980, the Mexican Army consisted of three infantry brigades: the mechanized presidential guard and two infantry brigades. All three are based together in Mexico City. Equipped with World War II–era M-3 light tanks, the presidential guard brigade possesses the heaviest firepower of any unit in the army.

Below the brigade level, there are seventy-five independent infantry battalions and twenty-one cavalry regiments. These units are dispersed among the thirty-six military zones.[125] The zone commander performs a vital role within the Mexican political matrix. Personally designated by the president with the recommendation of the secretary of national defense, these commanders wield considerable clout at the state level. While their chain of command runs to the president through the secretary of national defense, they are expected to work closely with the state governor associated with their zone. As Lozoya describes this role, the zone commander "voices his opinions on the problems of political importance and frequently supports the governor in the application of solutions."[126] If a crisis arises in the state and the president decides to relieve the governor of his position, the zone commander will be ordered to take control until a new governor can be assigned. Thus the zone commander's function is intrinsically political and intimately tied to the internal security mission.

At the lowest echelon of command are the small detachments, or *partidas*. Their purpose is to extend the authority of the government into the countryside, "especially where the Army needs to maintain constant contact with the local populace and improve the security of strategic installations."[127]

During the past decade, the army has begun to modernize its inventory. Particular emphasis has been placed upon mechanizing the infantry and providing cavalry regiments with wheeled vehicles (see weapons acquisitions, below). Heavy firepower is lacking, however. The few light tanks in the army inventory are of World War II vintage. Self-propelled 105mm howitzers are the largest artillery pieces in the order of battle.[128] Recently procured French Panhard armored cars and Swiss Mowag armored personnel carriers have added considerable mobile firepower. Major items in the army order of battle include: forty-five M-3 light tanks (U.S.); forty Panhard ERC-90 armored cars (French); thirty Mowag armored personnel carriers (Swiss); and seventy 75mm and 105mm howitzers.[129] Nevertheless, foot soldiers armed with the newly acquired, indigenously assembled G-3 automatic rifles still account for a considerable proportion of overall firepower.

Navy. While the navy is afforded co-equal status in the military command structure, the 28,000-member service is vastly inferior to the army in terms of manpower and combat potential.[130] This is fitting, given the emphasis placed on maintenance of domestic tranquility by Mexican decision makers. Recent developments, however, have accentuated the need to equip the navy to protect Mexico's offshore interests. Initially, the impetus for expanding naval capability was provided by the declaration of a 200-mile economic zone. This created the need to police fishing fleets operating in the expanded Mexican waters. The second development that stimulated expansion in naval forces was the discovery of vast oil reserves in the Gulf of Mexico.[131] To satisfy these coastal patrol missions, the navy has added dozens of large patrol craft to its inventory since the mid 1970s. The essential character of the Mexican Navy has not been substantially altered, however. It continues to function primarily as a coastal patrol force with only a limited oceangoing capability.

Veracruz, the country's leading port, is the location of Naval Headquarters, the Naval Academy, and other major naval facilities. Remaining naval elements are divided between Mexico's two coasts. Responsibility for protecting the Caribbean coastline is divided among naval units based at Veracruz, Tampico, Chetumal, Cuidad del Carmen, and Yakalpetén. Naval units on the Pacific coast are assigned to bases at Acapulco, Ensenada, La Paz, Puerto Cortés, Guaymas, Manzanillo, Mazatlán, Salina Cruz, Puerto Madero, and Lázaro Cárdenas. Also incorporated within the navy are a 6,500-man marine force and a 500-man air arm.[132] The navy inventory includes: 2 destroyers (Gearing-class) (U.S.); 6 frigates (U.S.); 6 Corvettes (Halcon-class) (Spain); 35 patrol ships (including ex-USN minesweepers); 31 Azteca-class large patrol craft; and 14 river patrol craft.[133] Aircraft in the Naval Air Corps include: three Fokker F-27; one Learjet; eleven Cessna aircraft; eight HU-16 helicopters; five Bell helicopters; and four Alouette helicopters.[134]

Air Force. Organizationally subordinate to the secretary of defense (an army general), the Mexican Air Force is the smallest of the three services, numbering only about 5,500 personnel. Included in the air force is a 2000-man airborne brigade based in Mexico City. The distribution of forces is similar to that of the army. The most combat-capable elements (F-5s and AT-33s) are concentrated in the vicinity of Mexico City, in this case at Santa Lucia Air Base on the outskirts of the capital. Five of the nine air groups in the air force are located at Santa Lucía. In addition to the 7th Air Group containing the MAF's jet fighter aircraft, other elements assigned to the base are the 1st Air Group (light transports and helicopters), the 5th Air Group (light transports and photo reconnaissance aircraft), the 6th Air Group (transports of the C-54/C-118 category), and the 9th Air Group (transports of the C-47 type). Also located in the environs of Mexico City is the 8th Air Group at Benito Juarez International Airport. This unit provides airlift support to the president and other senior officials using primarily Boeing 727 and 737 passenger jets. Remaining operational elements consist essentially of PC-7s assigned to three air groups at six bases throughout the country: The 2nd Air Group dispersed between bases at Puebla and Ciudad Ixtepec, the 3rd Air Group with squadrons at La Paz and Ensenada, and the 4th Air Group split between Cozumel and Mérida. Finally, trainer aircraft are assigned to the Mexican Air Force Academy at Zapopán near Guadalajara. Primary flight training is conducted in the Musketeer Sport III, with the Bonanza F33C used for basic flying training, and the PC-7 used as an advanced trainer.[135]

The Mexican Air Force's frontline fighter is the supersonic F-5, a dozen of which were purchased from the United States in 1981 (one was subsequently lost in an aircraft accident). This aircraft is capable of both air defense and close air support missions, although the lack of an air defense radar system greatly reduces its effectiveness as an interceptor.[136] The Korean War–vintage AT-33s can be armed with rockets or bombs, but their aging condition raises questions about their continued airworthiness. The pending acquisition of 30 additional T-33 aircraft from the US Air Force, along with a sizable package of spare parts, can be expected to rejuvenate this portion of the MAF inventory.[137] The purchase of PC-7 Pilatus Porter aircraft affords the MAF a counterinsurgency capability. The PC-7, although essentially a trainer aircraft, can be outfitted with rockets, machine guns, and two 550 lb bombs.[138]

The air force inventory includes the following aircraft: 11 F-5 (U.S.), 12 AT-33 (U.S.), 55 PC-7 (Switzerland), 9 Boeing 727 (U.S.), 2 Boeing 737 (U.S.), 3 DC-6/7, 2 C-118, 5 C-54, 12 C-47, 8 Arava, 3 Shorts Skyvan, 20 Beech Bonanza F-33C, 34 Musketeer Sport III, and 20 Mudry CAP-10B.[139]

Reserve Forces. Two distinct categories of reserve or paramilitary forces exist in Mexico. One is the Rural Defense Corps, made up of rural landowners, which in the early 1970s numbered some 120,000. The other reserve force consists of "conscripts," youths who upon reaching the age of eighteen are required to undergo drill instruction on weekends for one year. Annually, 250,000 youths complete this obligatory program.[140]

Although the concept of a rural defense force originated with Porfirio Díaz in the 1880s, the present variant is sui generis. Known as *rurales*, Díaz's regional police forces were noted principally for oppressing the peasantry. The contemporary version, in contrast, is essentially a rural self-defense force drawn exclusively from the small landholding class. This force sprang up spontaneously during the immediate postrevolutionary period as a consequence of government-sponsored land reform programs. Peasants who had received parcels of land as a result of the dismemberment of large estates banded together to defend themselves against forcible attempts by former owners to recapture these lands. The federal government helped these peasants de-

fend themselves and was repaid handsomely during the Cristero Rebellion in 1926. Siding with the government against the church and the landed oligarchy, these irregular forces contributed significantly to the defeat of the rebellion. As described by Lozoya: "The help that the social defense groups gave to the Army in this particular campaign was of considerable importance: they served as guides, couriers, and spies; in addition, they formed a guerrilla force with a profound knowledge of the terrain."[141] In 1929 President Portes Gil formalized this relationship through the creation of the Rural Defense Corps under the supervision of the Mexican Army.

The Rural Defense Corps has proven to be a cost-effective means of penetrating and controlling the countryside. In exchange for outmoded carbines and some instruction by regular army members, these unpaid forces have been especially valuable as informants. Lozoya makes this point well, commenting that "the present reason for the existence of these groups is more than anything else political: it provides the government with an extraordinary mechanism of information which results in an immediate knowledge of any subversive activity in any corner of the country."[142] Thus the Rural Defense Corps is clearly an institution whose origins and present raison d'être can be attributed exclusively to a concern for internal political conditions. The system has flourished because of a natural symbiosis between the central government and the landowning peasant. For the peasant, the arrangement is advantageous, because possession of firearms would otherwise be illegal. As a member of the Rural Defense Corps, small landowners acquire the means to defend their property as well as a measure of prestige in the rural community. In exchange, the government elicits the loyal support of an important element in the countryside and a significant hedge against rural insurgency.

"Conscripts," the other component of the reserves, also contribute to the maintenance of internal order, though in a less direct fashion than the Rural Defense Corps. Conscription in Mexico is not a mechanism of manpower accession for the regular army. Rather, it is a form of universal military service for youths not in the armed forces. Upon reaching eighteen years of age, all able-bodied Mexican males are obliged to participate in a one-year program of military instruction. In practice, however, only those from lower-class families are compelled to comply. As noted by Alan Riding, "Few youths from the middle or upper classes ever serve because exemption can be bought for a standard $10 bribe."[143] Steve Wager estimates the number of youths involved to be some 250,000.[144]

Training received by the conscripts, consisting of two hours of drill on Sundays, is of limited military value. These men seldom touch a rifle, and uniforms are never worn.[145] As Lozoya observes, "Needless to say, these men are not truly being prepared to defend the country."[146] The real utility of this program is to provide the government with a means of controlling the populace. Through participation in this universal program, males are registered with the government. Upon completion of the program (or if exempted), each individual is issued a *cartilla* or identification card, which "must be presented when applying for a passport, driver's license, or employment."[147] Summing up the significance of this system for the maintenance of internal order, Lozoya observes: "The military service system in Mexico does fulfill an important political function: it permits the control and classification of the male population. The military service constitutes an effective system of general control over the country."[148]

WEAPONS ACQUISITION AND PRODUCTION

During the late 1970s and early 1980s, roughly coinciding with the latter portion of the Echeverría administration (1970–76) and continuing throughout the López Portillo *sexenio* (1976–82), the Mexican armed forces underwent a substantial modernization program. Prior to that time, much armament was of the same vintage as display pieces commonly found in front of veterans' halls. Indeed, all three services continue to rely on equipment dating from the World War II and Korean War eras (e.g., M-3 tanks, circa 1945; AT-33 aircraft, circa 1950; and Gearing class destroyers,

circa 1945). Nevertheless, all three branches have accomplished a major upgrading of their inventories since the 1970s.

The navy was the first service to benefit from the impetus to modernize. Owing to Mexico's declaration of a 200-mile economic zone in 1972 and subsequent discovery of massive deposits of oil and gas in the Gulf of Mexico, the need to upgrade the navy's coastal patrol capability was apparent early in the 1970s. Acquisitions to satisfy this need have come both from domestic and foreign sources. A shipbuilding program was initiated, with assistance from the United Kingdom, to build Azteca-class (130 tons) and Olmeca-class (40-foot) patrol craft.[149] To date over thirty Azteca patrol boats have been added to the inventory, along with eight Olmeca river patrol craft. Through external sources the Mexican Navy has acquired two U.S.-built Gearing-class destroyers and six Spanish Halcón-class frigates.

The Mexican Army has also felt the impact of modernization. Perhaps the most notable development was mechanization of the cavalry. Horse cavalry regiments completed the transition to wheeled vehicles by the mid 1980s.[150] Mobile firepower was significantly upgraded with the purchase of forty Panhard ERC-90 Lynx armored vehicles from France and the addition of indigenously produced DN III armored personnel carriers.[151] Another major accomplishment for the domestic arms industry was commencement of licensed production of the West German G-3 assault rifle. The semi-automatic G-3, which can fire at the rate of 600 rounds per minute, is to become the standard weapon for the Mexican foot soldier. When full production is achieved, Mexico will be turning out 10,000 of these rifles annually.

Perhaps the most sensational addition during this period was the 1982 acquisition of a dozen supersonic F-5 fighters from the United States. These aircraft, which made their debut in the September 16, 1982 Independence Day parade in Mexico City, are capable of performing both interceptor and close air support roles. Until Mexico develops a network of early warning and ground-controlled intercept radars, however, their air defense capability will be truncated. In addition to F-5s, the Mexican

Air Force added fifty-five Swiss-built PC-7 trainers to its inventory, and has purchased 30 additional T-33 aircraft from the U.S.

Mexico's defense industry has made an appreciable contribution to armed forces modernization. Alisky notes that since 1976 domestic production has grown slightly each year.[152] Production of the DN-III armored personnel carrier at the government-run DINA plant is about a dozen per year. Because of fiscal constraints plans for assembly of M-3A1 armored personnel carriers from imported parts had to be shelved in 1982.[153] The Defense Ministry's Bureau of Military Industry has also experimented with production of rocket launchers since the early 1980s, but development of this weapon has apparently not reached the stage of full-scale production.[154] Mexico's defense industry is capable of limited repair and manufacture of tank parts, but technology for tank production does not exist.[155]

Mexico's naval shipyards are capable of turning out large patrol craft to satisfy a portion of the country's coastal patrol needs. Apparently the bulk of the production is now accomplished in Mexican shipyards, although a few components are still imported.[156]

Mexico's defense manufacturers have contributed the least to modernization of the air force. At present, no military aircraft or major systems are fabricated domestically. Output is limited to certain replacement parts, such as rotor blades for helicopters and electronic equipment (e.g., oscilloscopes).[157]

Mexico's defense planners have followed two guidelines in determining procurement sources for military hardware. The first imperative is to buy Mexican. Within the limits of its technological capacity and economies of scale, Mexico has used itself as a supplier of first resort. To the extent that it must look elsewhere for advanced weaponry, Mexican decision makers have attempted to diversify their sources of supply. At least that has been the outcome of their recent acquisitions. Major weapon systems or arms have been obtained from France, Spain, Switzerland, the United Kingdom, the United States, and West Germany.

This spate of weapons acquisitions coincided with both discovery of vast quantities of oil in southeast Mexico and intensification of civil strife in Central America. Consequently, certain analysts are willing to attribute this extensive modernization effort to external factors. Among these are claims that Central American turmoil may inexorably be heading northward, that Mexican oil fields may be threatened, and that Mexican strategists may wish to add some clout to their diplomacy through acquisition of sophisticated arms. The remark by former Secretary of Defense Felix Galvan López that "the strong are more respected than the weak" is often cited in this regard.[158] Undeniably, these conditions have provided a certain stimulus and a facile rationale for the modernization program. It would be shortsighted, however, to conclude that this defense policy output is explainable exclusively with reference to external considerations.

As noted earlier, revolutionary movements in Nicaragua and El Salvador have elicited more sympathy than fear from civilian elites in Mexico. It should also be recalled that the president is the ultimate decision maker regarding allocations for weapons acquisitions. Historically, the president has been most interested in maintaining the fealty of his senior military commanders. This is particularly true in the face of growing reliance upon the armed forces for maintenance of internal order. A review of the items obtained during this period reveals an emphasis on weaponry useful for internal security as opposed to power projection (a few navy destroyers being a partial exception to this).

To a certain extent, though, this debate may be more a matter of perspective than of substance. From the viewpoint of Mexicanists accustomed to a defense policy driven by internal concerns, the intrusion of external considerations into the policy equation has quite naturally been seen as an extraordinary development. Thus, for those viewing the evolution of Mexican defense policy in isolation, external factors have assumed unusual significance of late. Compared to other countries included in this volume, however, the more remarkable aspect of weapons acquisition in Mexico may be the relatively limited impact that the international context has had on this issue area.

ALLIANCE POSTURE

Mexican defense policy differs markedly from other countries treated in this volume with regard to the propensity, or lack thereof, to enter into alliances. With the exception of the 1947 Rio Pact (formally the Inter-American Treaty of Mutual Assistance), Mexico has avoided entangling itself in military alliances. Even its involvement in the Rio Pact is a vestige of an earlier era and was always more symbolic than real. The Pact itself lacks substance, and Mexico's willingness to participate militarily in any sort of future contingency is doubtful. The country's actual attitude toward collective defense, at least for the purpose of resisting communist advances in the hemisphere, is reflected in its consistent practice of opposing all such American-led efforts (e.g. Dominican Republic, 1965; Grenada, 1985). Thus, Mexican membership in the Rio Pact and another World War II–era carry over, the Joint Mexico–U.S. Defense Commission, is nominal.

It is the avoidance of alliance commitments, therefore, that requires an explanation. Clearly, the absence of a bonafide external threat removes the fundamental impetus for alliance creation. Given the primacy of internal security concerns, however, some might suggest that common cause could be found in some form of anti-subversive partnership with neighboring states. While certain types of collaboration have been possible, such as the purchase of military hardware from the U.S. and participation in associated training programs, it is unlikely these efforts will ever lead to a formal bilateral alliance.

Several powerful constraints impede such an evolution in bilateral relations. One is a divergence in threat perceptions. Mexican civilian elites do not generally subscribe to the view that communist subversion poses a threat to their domestic tranquility. As described earlier, Mexico's revolutionary credentials are counted upon to keep it off the communist hit list. Second, the U.S. constitutes, in the Mexican perspective, a present danger to the nation's economic and cultural independence. By becoming the junior partner in a military alliance with the U.S., Mexico would invite domination in yet another sphere. Third, policy makers in Mexico find foreign policy to be a valuable mechanism for defusing domestic dissent, particularly that emanating from the left. Foreign policy initiatives have served routinely to refurbish the regime's revolutionary image. Inevitably, this translates into an anti-American stance on regional issues and in its voting record in the United Nations. In the Mexican view, a military alliance with the U.S. would certainly undermine the government's revolutionary image.[159] Finally, Mexican strategists may not wish to ally themselves formally with the U.S. out of a fear that this would cause their strategic assets (e.g., oil fields, air fields, the capital city) to be added to Soviet nuclear target lists.[160]

By avoiding encumbering alliances, especially an alliance with the U.S., Mexico has managed to preserve flexibility in its foreign affairs. Indeed, it has carved out for itself a comfortable niche wherein it can even assume a posture of moral superiority for having avoided the taint of involvement in the power politics typically associated with alliances. In reality, of course, the Mexican stance is consistent with classic *Realpolitik*: in the interstices of power, weaker states discover their room for maneuver.

Conclusion

This treatment of Mexican defense policy has set for itself two objectives: one theoretical in nature, the other substantive. With regard to the latter, we have found that Mexican defense policy is driven predominantly by internal rather than external considerations. To understand Mexican defense policy, it is crucial to appreciate the nature of the country's political order and the place of the military within it. Mexico has a hegemonic polity. At the apex of this pyramidal structure stands the president. The central mission of the Mexican armed forces is to preserve this hierarchy. Because the armed forces have faithfully performed this role for many decades, we recognize them as guardians of the existing order and of the elites who manage it. Internal security concerns thus emerge as dominant inputs into the policy equation in Mexico.

The predominance of internal security matters is also the product of an unthreatening external environment. Neither neighbor is a major factor in defense planning because of the enormous disparities of power involved. Mexico is shielded from foreign invasion, moreover, by the geopolitical reality that its superpower neighbor could not tolerate such a challenge to its own security. The Central American conflict does not cause alarm in Mexican policy circles in large part because of the country's own revolutionary mystique.

The litany of domestic security concerns has grown longer and more challenging in recent years. The complexity of these issues demands a coordinated response from political, social, economic, and military sectors. Mexico's embryonic national security doctrine constitutes a step in this direction. The country's future stability will hinge in part upon the degree to which Mexican policy makers are able to harmonize the military contribution to national security with that of other actors.

The principal theoretical dimension of this chapter is related to the features highlighted above. Owing to the minimal nature of the external threat and the centralization of power within the polity, the process by which Mexican defense policy is produced departs categorically from that of other countries treated in this volume. The limited impact of external conditions upon defense policy means that the "analytic" model provides an unsatisfactory basis for explanation. Similarly, any attempt to superimpose the bureaucratic politics model on the Mexican political context would be to put a pluralistic peg into a hegemonic hole. Mexico's defense policy can more adequately be explained as a product of patron-client exchange relationships. Decision units are small and authoritatively led, unlike the unwieldy coalitions that typify bureaucratic politics. The dynamic that governs this process is the exchange of val-

ued resources, as opposed to the quest for a value-maximizing alternative, as is the case with the "analytic" model.

It may be that other countries share with Mexico this combination of a relatively unthreatening international environment and a domestic order that is hegemonic in nature. Under these conditions, the decision-making process ought to bear a resemblance to Mexico's. That is to say, the patron-client "paradigm" may have application beyond the Mexican context, especially, it would seem, in the Third World. Perhaps the theoretical contribution of this chapter can be summarized in the form of a question: "Is Mexico unique, or are the relationships suggested here shared by other countries?" This is a question that can only be answered authoritatively in subsequent comparative studies of the defense policies of nations.

Notes

1. Gen. Paul Gorman, "Defining a Long-Term U.S. Strategy for Central America and the Caribbean" (remarks presented as part of the National Defense University Symposium "Inter-American Security Policy: Political-Economic Dimensions," 13–14 November 1986).

2. The most comprehensive work on the subject of the Mexican military appeared recently. See *The Modern Mexican Military: A Reassessment*, ed. David Ronfeldt (San Diego: University of California at San Diego, 1984).

3. Stephen J. Wager, for example, notes: "There exists no public record of the military's activities, nor are these activities ever debated publicly. Access to military archival records is restricted since most of them remain classified. In addition, current regulations discourage military officers from openly discussing military operations or policies with outsiders." See "Basic Characteristics of the Modern Mexican Military," in *Modern Mexican Military*. Alan Riding provides evidence that the Mexican military is obscure even to civilian authorities. See "Mexican Army amid Rumors, Insists It Steers Clear of Politics," *New York Times*, February 5, 1974, p. 4. A Mexican politician is cited by Riding as proclaiming, "It's impossible for us to know what's going on in the Army."

4. As cited in Hudson Strode, "Alvaro Obregon: The Happy Man with One Arm," in *Revolution in Mexico: Years of Upheaval, 1910–1940*, ed. James W. Wilkie and Albert L. Michaels (New York: Knopf, 1969), p. 128.

5. See, for example, Dennis Volman, "Growing Unease in Relations With U.S.," part 3 of "Mexico: The Ultimate Domino," *Christian Science Monitor*, 31 October 1985.

6. For a succinct account of U.S.–Mexican relations in the mid nineteenth and early twentieth centuries, see Thomas E. Weil et al., *Area Handbook for Mexico* (Washington, D.C.: Government Printing Office, 1975), pp. 66–67, 75–76.

7. "Survey Finds that Most Mexicans Regard U.S. as 'Enemy Country,'" *Philadelphia Inquirer*, 26 August 1986, p. E2.

8. Volman, "Growing Unease."

9. Interview with senior Mexican Air Force officer in Mexico City, July 1983.

10. *The Economist*, 18 April 1981, p. 35.

11. Jorge G. Castañeda, "Don't Corner Mexico!," *Foreign Policy*, No. 60, (Fall 1985), p 78.

12. Caesar Sereseres, in *Modern Mexican Military*, ed. Ronfeldt, p. 201.

13. Ibid., p. 209.

14. Ibid., pp. 202–3.

15. Other analysts who have arrived at the same conclusion regarding the lack of an external threat include Marvin Alisky, "Mexico," in *Arms Production in Developing Countries*, ed. James Everett Katz (Lexington, Mass.: Lexington Books, 1984), p. 248; Wager, "Basic Characteristics of the Modern Mexican Military," in *Modern Mexican Military*, ed. Ronfeldt, p. 100; and Jorge Alberto Lozoya, "The Army Today," *International Journal of Politics* 1 (Summer–Fall 1974): 272.

16. Derived from George T. Kurion, *The New Book of World Rankings* (Facts on File Publications, 1984), and *The Statesman's Year-Book*, John Paxton, ed. 122d ed. (New York: St. Martin's Press, 1986).

17. Ibid.

18. Weil et al., *Area Handbook*.

19. *Mexico Social (1985-86): Indicadores Seleccionados* (Mexico City: AEIO, S.A., 1986).

20. *Basic Petroleum Data Boom: Petroleum Industry Statistics*, vol. 7, no. 1, (Washington D.C.: American Petroleum Institute, 1987), sec. 4, table 2c.

21. Ibid., sec. 2, table 4c.

22. Kurion, *New Book of World Rankings*.

23. Robert E. Scott, "National Development and Mexico's Foreign Policy," *International Journal* 37, no.1 (Winter 1981–82).

24. Elizabeth G. Ferris, "Mexico's Foreign Policies: A Study in Contradictions", in *The Dynamics of Latin American Foreign Policies: Challenges for the 1980s*, ed. Jennie K. Lincoln and Elizabeth G. Ferris (Boulder, Colo.: Westview Press, 1985).

25. Bruce Bagley, "Mexico in the 1980s: A New Regional Power," *Current History* 180, no. 469 (November 1981): 353–94.

26. Ibid.; Bruce M. Bagley, "Mexican Foreign Policy: The Decline of a Regional Power," *Current History* 82 (December 1983).

27. Bagley, "Mexico in the 1980s," p. 394.

28. Bagley, "Mexican Foreign Policy," p. 437.

29. *Comparaciones Internacionales: México en el Mundo* (Mexico City: Instituto Nacional de Estadística, Geografía e Información, 1986), pp 302–3; *1984 International Trade Statistics Yearbook*, Vol. 1, (New York: United Nations, 1986), pp. 835, 1187.

30. Petroleos Mexicanos, *Memoria de Labores*, 1977–82.

31. Alden Cunningham, "Mexico's National Security," *Parameters* 14 (Winter 1984): 56–68.

32. Ibid.

33. Robert A. Dahl, *Polyarchy: Participation and Opposition* (New Haven: Yale University Press, 1971).

34. John Bailey, "What Factors Explain the Decline of the PRI and Will it Continue to Accelerate?" (Issue Paper #9 prepared for the Department of State working group on "Mexico, the Next Five Years," 1985), p. 30; Susan K. Purcell, *The Mexican Profit Sharing Decision: Politics in an Authoritarian Regime* (Berkeley and Los Angeles: University of California Press, 1975), pp. 31–32.

35. Daniel Levy and Gabriel Szekely, *Mexico: Paradoxes of Stability and Change* (Boulder, Colo.: Westview Press, 1983), pp. 68–69.

36. Martin Needler, *Politics and Society in Mexico* (Albuquerque: University of New Mexico Press, 1971), p. 15; W. Tuohy, "Centralism and Political Elite Behavior in Mexico," in *Development Administration in Latin America*, ed. Clarence E. Thurber and Lawrence S. Graham (Durham, N.C.: Duke University Press, 1973), p. 264.

37. Levy and Szekely, *Mexico*, p. 67.

38. Martin Needler, *Mexican Politics: The Containment of Conflict* (New York: Praeger, 1982), p. 87.

39. Ibid., p. 71.

40. Frank Brandenburg, *The Making of Modern Mexico* (Englewood Cliffs, N.J.: Prentice-Hall, 1964), p. 4.

41. Judith A. Hellman, "Social Control in Mexico," *Comparative Politics* 12 (January 1982): 41; Tuohy, "Centralism and Political Elite Behavior," p. 277.

42. Kenneth F. Johnson, *Mexican Democracy: A Critical View* (New York: Praeger, 1978), pp. 4–6.

43. Susan K. Purcell, "The Future of the Mexican System," in *Authoritarianism in Mexico*, ed. José L. Reyna and Richard S. Weinert (Philadelphia: Institute for the Study of Human Issues, 1977), p. 137.

44. Brandenburg, *The Making of Modern Mexico*, p. 5; Roderic A. Camp, *Mexico's Leaders: Their Education and Recruitment* (Tucson: University of Arizona Press, 1980), p. 205; Reyna, 1977, op. cit., p. 162.

45. Judith A. Hellman, *Mexico in Crisis* (New York: Holmes & Meier, 1978), pp. 100–10.

46. B. Anderson and J. D. Cockroft, "Control and Cooptation in Mexican Politics," in *Latin American Radicalism: A Documentary Report of Left and Nationalist Movements*, ed. Irving C. Horowitz, José de Castro, and John Gerassi (New York: Random House, 1969), p. 380; Hellman, *Mexico in crisis*, p. 129; Levy and Szekeley, *Mexico* p. 61.

47. Hellman, *Mexico in Crisis*, p. 100.

48. A. Carillo, "Mexican Political Stability," in *The Caribbean Today*, ed. A. Curtis Wilgus (Gainesville: University Press of Florida, 1964), p. 4; Edwin Lieuwen, *Mexican Militarism: The Political Rise and Fall of the Revolutionary Army, 1910–1940*, (Albuquerque: University of New Mexico Press, 1968), p. 104; Jorge A. Lozoya, *El ejército mexicano, 1911–1965* (Mexico City: El Colegio de Mexico, 1970), p. 48.

49. Charles C. Cumberland, *Mexico: The Struggle for Modernity* (New York: Oxford University Press, 1968), p. 141.

50. Frank D. Margiotta, "Civilian Control of the Military: Patterns in Mexico" (paper presented to the Conference on "Civilian Control of the Military: Myth and Reality in Developing Countries", State University of New York at Buffalo, 18–19 October 1974), p. 2.

51. W. S. Ackroyd, "Professionalization through Military Education: A Case Study of Its Impact on the Political Behavior of the Mexican Army Corps" (paper presented at the 32nd Annual Meeting of the Rocky Mountain Conference on Latin American Studies, Tucson, 23–25 February, 1984); Edwin Lieuwen, *Mexican Militarism*; id., "Depoliticization of the Mexican Revolutionary Army, 1915–1940" (paper presented at the research workshop on "The Role of the Military in Mexican Politics and Society: A Reassessment," Center for U.S.-Mexican Studies, University of California, San Diego, 19–21 March 1984).

52. Lieuwen, 1984, op. cit., pp. 12–13.

53. Ronfeldt, 1976, op. cit.

54. Margiotta, 1975, op. cit., p. 3.

55. Needler, 1971, op. cit., pp. 65–72; Edward J. Williams, "The Mexican Military and Foreign Policy: The Evolution of Influence" (A paper presented to a research workshop on "The Role of the Military in Mexican Politics and Society: A Reassessment" at the Center for U.S.-Mexican Studies, University of California, San Diego, March 1984).

56. Ibid., p. 65.

57. In making this distinction, I am building upon an argument originally advanced by J. H. Garrison, "The Political Dimension of Military Professionalism," in *American Defense Policy*, ed. John Endicott and Roy Stafford, 4th ed. (Baltimore: Johns Hopkins University Press, 1977).

58. Ronfeldt, 1976, op. cit.

59. Ibid., pp. 295–96.

60. Ibid., p. 306.

61. Center for Advanced International Studies, "The Political and Socio-Economic Role of the Military in Latin America" (n.d.), vol. 3, appendix.

62. Trip Report—Tuxpan, Tampico, Ciudad Valles and Pachuca (1981), 22 October 1981.

63. Trip Report—Yucatan Peninsula, Mexico (1981), 8 September 1981.

64. Trip Report—Oaxaca (1981), 23 September 1981.

65. Ronfeldt, 1976, op. cit., pp. 295–96.

66. Trip Report—Escuela Superior de Guerra (1981).

67. Betty Kirk, "Election Day, 1940," in *Revolution in Mexico: Years of Upheaval, 1910–1940*, ed. James W. Wilkie and Albert L. Michaels (New York: Knopf, 1969), p. 266.

68. Ronfeldt, p. 292.

69. Needler, p. 71.

70. Center for Advanced International Studies, "Political and Socio-Economic Role of the Military," vol. 1, p. 41.

71. Interview with American businessman with extensive contacts with the Mexican military, March 1983.

72. Interview with a senior Mexican Air Force official, July 1983.

73. Brandenburg, op. cit., p. 33.

74. See, e.g., Graham T. Allison, *Essence of Decision: Explaining the Cuban Missile Crisis* (Boston: Little, Brown, 1971); Robert Art, "Bureaucratic Politics and American Foreign Policy: A Critique," in *American Defense Policy*, ed. Endicott and Stafford; Robert Art and S. E. Ockenden, "The Domestic Politics of Cruise Missile Development, 1970–1980," in *Cruise Missiles, Technology, Strategy, Politics*, ed. R. R. Betts (Washington, D.C.: Brookings Institution, 1981); Morton H. Halperin, *Bureaucratic Politics and Foreign Policy* (Washington, D.C.: Brookings Institution, 1974); Roger Hilsman, *The Politics of Policy Making in Defense and Foreign Affairs* (New York: Harper & Row, 1971); Samuel P. Huntington, "Strategic Planning and the Political Process," *Foreign Affairs* 38 (1960): 285–99; E. A. Kolodziej and R. E. Harkavy, eds., *Security Policies of Developing Countries* (Lexington, Mass.: D. C. Heath, 1982); Douglas J. Murray and Paul R. Viotti, eds., *The Defense Policies of Nations: A Comparative Study*, 1st ed. (Baltimore: Johns Hopkins University Press, 1982); Richard E. Neustadt, *Presidential Power* (New York: John Wiley & Sons, 1960); John D. Steinbruner, *The Cybernetic Theory of Decision: New Dimensions of Political Analysis* (Princeton: Princeton University Press, 1974); Adam Yarmolinsky, "The Military Establishment (or How Political Problems Become Military Problems)," *Foreign Policy* 1 (Winter 1970–71): 78–79.

75. *Analytic* is used in lieu of the perhaps more common term, *rational*. Following Steinbruner's logic (*Cybernetic Theory of Decisions*, p. 27), this is desirable because of the normative implications inherent in the use of *rational* as a label. Since the purpose here is to describe the process of decision in Mexican security policy, it is useful to avoid terminology that might unintentionally suggest evaluation or criticism.

76. These two models do not exhaust the possibilities that could be suggested. As many as ten different types have been postulated. Cohen and S. A. Harris argue, however, in "Foreign Policy," in *Handbook of Political Science*, ed. Fred Greenstein and Nelson Polsby, vol. 6 (Reading, Mass.: Addison-Wesley, 1975), that basically three "conversion mechanisms" or decision-making models have been propounded: (a) Rationality (or the analytic model), (b) Political bargaining (or the bureaucratic politics model), and (c) Incrementalism/cybernetics. Whatever figure one prefers, the two models considered in this study (i.e., the analytic and bureaucratic politics models) have probably had the greatest impact on the study of foreign and national security policy. Prior to the flowering of the bureaucratic politics approach, for example, Steinbruner (*Cybernetic Theory of Decision*, p. 8) claimed that "the fact is that virtually all analysts use in some way a conception of the decision process derived from the ideal of rational choice." The factor most responsible for loosening the hegemony of the rational or analytic model over the discipline has been the revolution in thinking wrought by the bureaucratic politics school. Contemporary national security analysts, however, often employ a combination of those two models in their conceptual approaches to the subject (see e.g., Kolodziej and Harkavy, eds., *Security Policies of Developing Countries*).

77. The alternative decision making model presented here draws heavily upon Merilee Grindle's work on policy making in Mexico in the area of rural development, *Bureaucrats, Politicians, and Peasants* (Berkeley: University of California Press, 1977). My intention is to extend Grindle's insights into the realm of national security policy. Exchange relations may exist between persons of equal power, wealth, or attainment, or they may occur between individuals of unequal stature. Pa-

tron-client ties belong to the latter category. The bargaining process at the core of the bureaucratic politics model is an example of an exchange between equals.

78. See Arnold Strickon and Sidney M. Greenfield, "The Analysis of Patron-Client Relationships: An Introduction," in *Structure and Process in Latin America: Patronage, Clientage and Power Systems*, ed. A. Strickon and S.M. Greenfield (Albuquerque: University of New Mexico Press, 1972).

79. Grindle, *Bureaucrats, Politicians, and Peasants*; J. C. Scott, "Patron-Client Politics and Political Change in Southeast Asia," *American Political Science Review* 66 (1972): 91–113.

80. S. N. Eisenstadt and L. Roniger, "Patron Client Relations as a Model of Structuring Social Change," *Comparative Studies in Society and History* 22 (1980): 42–77; Grindle, R. R. Kaufman, "The Patron-Client Concept and Macro-Politics: Prospects and Problems," *Comparative Studies in Society and History* (1974); J. C. Scott, "Patron-Client Politics."

81. Scott, pp. 94–5.

82. Grindle; Strickon and Greenfield.

83. Scott, pp. 94–5.

84. Lucian Pye, "The Non-Western Political Process," *Journal of Politics* 20 (1958): 471–72; R. Spaulding, "Welfare Policymaking: Theoretical Implications of a Mexican Case Study," *Comparative Politics* 12 (1980): 422.

85. Grindle, 1977, op. cit.; Purcell, 1975, op. cit.; Susan and J. F. H. Purcell, "State and Society in Mexico: Must a Stable Polity be Institutionalized?" *World Politics* 32 (1980): 194–227; Scott, 1972, op. cit.

86. Grindle, 1977, op. cit., p. 110.

87. Ibid., p. 172; R. Spaulding, "State Power and Its Limits: Corporatism in Mexico," *Comparative Political Studies* 14 (1981): 152.

88. Grindle, 1977, op. cit., p. 58.

89. Michael J. Dziedzic, "The Essence of Decision in a Hegemonic Regime: The Case of Mexico's Acquisition of a Supersonic Fighter" (diss., University of Texas at Austin, 1986).

90. Five decision-making units contained only one major actor: selection of the F-5 in 1977 (Galvan); selection of maintenance trainees (Salinas); resolution of pay problems (Salinas); use of sole source procurement (Salinas); and selection of the paint scheme (Galvan). Six decision-making units contained two major actors: allocation of resources (López Portillo and Galvan); selection of F-5 in 1980 (Galvan and Mr. X—); selection of instructor pilots (Salinas and Lucero); selection of conversion pilots (Salinas and Arcos); non-purchase of munitions (Bocanegra and Salinas); and selection of freight forwarder (Bocanegra and Salinas).

91. Glenn Paige, "The Korea Decision," in *International Politics and Foreign Policy: A Reader in Research and Theory*, ed. James N. Rosenau (New York: Free Press, 1969), p. 467.

92. Ibid., p. 286.

93. Brandenburg, p. 145; Camp, p. 12; Martin H. Greenberg, *Bureaucracy and Development: A Mexican Case Study* (Green Bay, Wis.: D.C. Heath, 1970), p. 2; Grindle, 1977, op. cit., p. 2; Purcell, 1975, op. cit., p. 40; Smith, 1977, op. cit., p. 139; Wesson, 1985, op. cit., pp. 281–82; Edward J. Williams, "The Evolution of the Mexican Military and Its Implications for Civil Military Relations," a chapter in a forthcoming book,

Rod Camp (ed.), p. 1B; title uncertain, to be published by Westview Press.

94. S. Bizzarro, "Mexico's Government in Crisis," *Current History* 72 (March 1977): 102–3; "Mexico's Transition Turns Disorderly," *Business Week*, 6 December 1976, pp. 34; J. N. Goodsell, "Mexico Changes Presidents amid Fiscal, Political Crisis," *Christian Science Monitor*, 29 November 1976, p. 5; Johnson, 1978, op. cit., p. 51; Levy and Szekely, 1983, op. cit., p. 65; S. Loaeza, "La Política de rumor: Mexico, noviembre–diciembre 1976," *Foro Internacional* 17 (no. 4): 557–86; Riding, "Farm Seizure Poses Problems for Mexico," *New York Times* 26 November 1976, p. 10; Smith, 1979, op. cit., pp. 282–98.

95. Smith, 1979, op. cit., p. 297.

96. Dziedzic, 1986, op. cit.

97. Grindle, 1977, op. cit.; Kaufman, 1974, op. cit.; Scott, 1972, op. cit.

98. Interview with Mexican official, August 1983.

99. Ronfeldt, op. cit., p. 34.

100. *Constitución política de los estados unidos mexicanos* (Mexico: Comision Federal Electoral, 1982), p. 93.

101. See, for example, Robert E. Scott, "National Development and Mexico's Foreign Policy," *International Journal* 37, no. 1 (Winter 1981–82): 42–59.

102. Jorge A. Lozoya, "The Army Today," *International Journal of Politics* 1 (Summer–Fall): 284–85.

103. Ronfeldt, 1984, op. cit., p. 33.

104. Weil, et al, op. cit., p. 374–75.

105. Lozoya, op. cit., p. 285.

106. Ibid., p. 285.

107. Brandenburg, op. cit., 33.

108. Ronfeldt, 1984, op. cit., 33.

109. Edward J. Williams, "Mexico's Modern Military: Implications for the Region," *Caribbean Review* 10 (Fall 1981): p. 45; Alan Riding, "Mexican Army, Parading Pride, Raises Concern," *New York Times*, 5 October 1980.

110. Eric A. Nordlinger, *Soldiers in Politics: Military Coups and Governments*, (Englewood Cliffs, N.J.: Prentice-Hall, 1977), pp. 90–93.

111. José Luís Pineyro, "The Mexican Army and the State: Historical and Political Perspective," *Revue Internationale de Sociologie* 14 (April–August 1978): 131.

112. Ibid., p. 132.

113. Ronfeldt, 1984, op. cit., p. 25.

114. Weil, et al, op. cit., p. 348.

115. Riding, 1980, op. cit., reports the figure to be three hundred.

116. Sereseres, op. cit., p. 211.

117. Pineyro, op. cit., pp. 143–44.

118. Williams, undated, op. cit., pp. 10–11.

119. As cited in Ronfeldt, 1984, op. cit., p. 35.

120. Ibid., p. 34.

121. Alfred Stephan, "The New Professionalism of Internal Warfare and Military Role Expansion," in *Armies and Politics in Latin America*, ed. Abraham F. Lowenthal (New York: Holmes & Meier, 1976), pp. 244–60; Williams, undated, op. cit., p. 7.

122. Ronfeldt, 1984, op. cit., p. 39.

123. Williams, forthcoming, op. cit.

124. Weil, et al, op. cit., p. 357, observes that, "The regular disposition of Mexican army and air force units includes no particular concentration along land or sea frontiers."

125. Ronfeldt, 1984, op. cit., pp. 6–7; Sereseres, op. cit., p. 212; Wager, op. cit., p. 91; Lozoya, op. cit., p. 273.

126. Lozoya, Ibid, pp. 274–75.

127. Ronfeldt, op. cit., p. 7.

128. Alisky, "Mexico," in *Arms Production in Developing Countries: An Analysis of Decision Making*, ed. James E. Katz (Lexington, Mass.: Lexington Books, 1984), p. 249.

129. Ibid., p. 248; Wager, op. cit., p. 103; Ronfeldt, 1984, op. cit., p. 8; *Defense and Foreign Affairs Handbook*, (Washington, D.C.: Perth Corp., 1985), p. 431; International Institute for Strategic Studies, *The Military Balance 1986–1987* (London: IISS, 1987), p. 190.

130. Alisky, op. cit., p. 248.

131. Ronfeldt, 1984, op. cit., p. 8.

132. Alisky, op. cit., p. 250; *Army Quarterly and Defense Journal*, op. cit., p. 24; IISS, *Military Balance 1986–1987*, op. cit.

133. Alisky, Ibid., pp. 249–50; *Army Quarterly and Defense Journal*, Ibid., pp. 24–25; IISS, *Military Balance 1986–1987*, op. cit.

134. Alisky, Ibid, p. 250; IISS, *Military Balance 1986–1987*, op. cit.

135. Adrian J. English, *Armed Forces of Latin America: Their Histories, Development, Present Strength, and Military Potential* (London: Jane's Publishing Company, Ltd, 1984); Santiago Flores Ruiz, "Mexico Fashion: An Aerial Poncho," *Air International*, November 1981, pp. 225–50.

136. *Jane's All the World's Aircraft, 1980–81* (London: Jane's Publishing Co.), pp. 397–8; Ronfeldt, 1984, op. cit., p. 9.

137. Alisky, op. cit., p. 255; *Army Quarterly and Defense Journal*, op. cit., p. 24–25; Ronfeldt, 1984, op. cit., p. 9; United States Department of Defense Offer and Acceptance, Case Mx-D-SCA, July 1 1987.

138. *Jane's All the World's Aircraft, 1980–81*, op. cit., Ruiz, op, cit.

139. Alisky, op. cit., p. 250; *Defense and Foreign Affairs Handbook*, op. cit., p. 432; Weil, et al, op. cit., p. 353; *Army Quarterly and Defense Journal*, op. cit., p. 24; IISS, *Military Balance 1986–1987*, op. cit.

140. For an authoritative treatment of the historical evolution and political significance of the Rural Defense Corps, see Alberto Lozoya, op. cit., pp. 278–82.

141. Lozoya, Ibid., pp. 278–79.

142. Ibid., p. 281.

143. Riding, op. cit., p. 4.

144. Wager, op. cit., p. 92.

145. Lozoya, op. cit., p. 277.

146. Ibid.

147. Wager, op. cit., p. 92.

148. Lozoya, op. cit., pp. 277–78.

149. Cunningham, op. cit., p. 62; *Army Quarterly and Defense Journal*, op. cit., p. 25; Ronfeldt, 1984, op. cit., p. 8; Wager, op. cit., p. 103.

150. Wager, op. cit., p. 103; Edward J. Williams, "Mexico's Modern Military: Implications for the Region," *Caribbean Review* 10 (Fall, 1981): 12.

151. Ronfeldt, op. cit., p. 8.

152. Alisky, op. cit., p. 256.

153. Ibid., pp. 252 and 249.

154. Ibid., p. 252.

155. Ibid., p. 248.

156. Ibid., pp. 253 and 259.

157. Ibid., p. 252.

158. Williams, 1981, op. cit., p. 12.

159. For three excellent contemporary discussions of this and other aspects of Mexican foreign policy see M. Delal Baer, "Mexico: Ambivalent Ally," *The Washington Quarterly*, Summer 1987, pp. 103–113; Jorge G. Castañeda, "Don't Corner Mexico," *Foreign Policy* 60, Fall 1985, pp. 75–90; and Elizabeth G. Ferris, "Mexico's Foreign Policies: A Study in Contradictions" in *The Dynamics of Latin American Foreign Policies: Challenges for the 1980s*, ed. Jennie K. Lincoln and Elizabeth G. Ferris (Boulder, Colo.: Westview Press, 1984), pp. 213–227.

160. The notion that strategic considerations might factor into Mexican thinking on such matters was suggested to me by Adolfo Aguilar Zinser.

Part Six

CONCLUDING PERSPECTIVE

DEFENSE POLICY IN COMPARATIVE PERSPECTIVE: A CONCLUSION

Douglas J. Murray and Paul R. Viotti

Within the discipline of political science the comparative study of defense policy is an emerging subfield of study similar in many ways to another subfield, comparative foreign policy.[1] Comparative defense policy cuts across such traditional divisions as international politics and economics, public policy and administration, domestic politics and economics, and comparative political and economic systems. The purpose of this book (as with its first edition) is to contribute to the development of this subfield by constructing a framework within which to study the defense policy of a given state. Accordingly, the core of this work is the collection of individual country-study chapters. In this concluding chapter we combine some of what has been written in this volume with comments made earlier in conferences with our authors. Our aim is merely to illuminate some of the conceptual issues related to the field of comparative defense policy, perhaps creating a better foundation for theory development.

National Objectives, National Strategies, and Military Doctrines

Given an understanding in part 1 of each country study of the international environment within which the state is immersed, one can turn to an examination in part 2 of national objectives, strategies for mobilizing national capabilities for these purposes, and military force-employment doctrines. That strategy and doctrine in fact flow in such a logical pattern from national objectives is an assumption that conforms closely to a rational model of defense decision making. Although such a model is useful for organizing the discussion of strategy and doctrine, "nonrational" factors are treated explicitly in the exposition of decision-making processes that follows in part 3.

A fundamental problem for defense policy makers is formulation of national objectives. At times these may be more implicit than explicit. Even when they are stated explicitly, different objectives may conflict in such a way that pursuit of one may preclude attainment of the others. In other instances there may be considerable uncertainty concerning objectives that should be sought, situations in which competing political factions often conflict. Decision makers would undoubtedly prefer to operate in response to clear-cut sets of objectives, but such simplicity is not typical of the complex world within which defense decision makers usually operate.

As we use the term, *national strategy* refers to the grand strategy of a given state. Successful implementation of national strategy typically calls for some consensus on methodology for the use of economic, diplomatic, military, and other "instruments of policy." A common occurrence in most writing on defense policy is the blending of the meanings of terms such as *strategy* and *doctrine*. Although one can attempt to establish fairly precise analytical distinctions between the two, empirically they are very closely related. Indeed, national strategy and military strategy or doctrine as categories are not mutually exclusive. Nevertheless, we think it useful to treat national strategy and force-employment doctrine as separate categories, even if they do overlap. National strategy is the more inclusive term, incorporating both military and nonmilitary factors; military doctrine, by contrast, is concerned exclusively with the ways and means of employing military forces for either deterrence or war-fighting purposes.

Military strategy or doctrine can be defined as a methodology that describes the environment within which the armed forces must operate and prescribes the methods and circumstances of their employment.[2] The primary function of such doctrine is to maximize the effectiveness of a state's military capabilities in support of national objectives. As such, military doctrine has at least two levels of definition. At the national (or grand strategy) level, military doctrine is concerned with coordinating the separate contributions of the armed services with the diplomatic, economic, and nonmilitary instruments of policy. At a lower level, each armed service also has its own military doctrine governing the employment of the forces under its command.

The traditional focus of military strategy or doctrine was on the use of force in an operational context—maximizing war-fighting capabilites. In the post–World War II era, however, the development of nuclear and other weapons of mass destruction resulted (at least in the West) in a considerable shift in doctrinal emphasis from war fighting to deterrence. (Only recently has there been any evidence of a shift in the opposite direction.) The perceived capability and willingness to use force are crucial to deterrence of war. Paradoxically, however, maintaining a deterrence posture is itself a use of force. Although one may argue that there has been a decline in the operational or active battlefield use of force among the industrial countries, one must also acknowledge the continuing presence of nuclear and nonnuclear arsenals for deterrence purposes as a passive use of force. In short, to the extent that deterrence based on the willingness to use the military instrument has substituted for war fighting, force remains centrally a part of international relations.[3]

A perennial question is whether doctrine guides the evolution of force posture or whether the converse is true. As becomes clear from reading the country studies in this volume, doctrine and force posture are inextricably linked, although one may lag behind the other. Doctrine in the absence of requisite capabilities to implement it can hardly be very useful. On the other hand, acquisition of new military capabilities (as in a technological breakthrough or new access to foreign sources of weapons systems) can inspire new doctrines to govern the use of these new kinds of military forces.

Aside from the rational concern of providing the decision makers of a state with a logical framework or methodology for the acquisition and employment of its armed forces, military strategy or doctrine may also be made to serve several other functions.[4] For example, it may be designed to boost morale in the armed forces, balance domestic political factions, demonstrate adherence by the leadership to the tenets of a particular ideology, develop a popular consensus in support of the state's defense policies, contribute to alliance cohesion, and mislead or threaten adversaries. As a result of these often contending functional objectives, formally stated military strategy or doctrine may not be a true reflection of de facto or informal doctrine operative in a particular state. The analyst must, therefore, delve into the military practices of the country being examined. Indeed, many countries do not even have a formally and publicly articulated military strategy or doctrine, and one must, instead, turn to the body of information on doctrine established in large part by actual practice.

THE SUPERPOWERS

The Soviet Union assigns the highest priority to the deterrence of nuclear war, but has pursued a victory-oriented or war-winning approach to deterrence. With respect to targeting, Soviet declaratory doctrine has assigned highest priority to attacks on the enemy's military forces, but also has emphasized extensive strikes against key industrial and political facilities. In the Gorbachev era, however, there has been a shift in public emphasis to a more "defensive" doctrine with "reasonable sufficiency" as the force posture criterion. Consistent with this thinking, the USSR is planning substantial reductions in general purpose, or conventional, forces to include troops, tanks, aircraft, and artillery.

Soviet defense efforts are focused in two geographical theaters of operation: Europe and the Far East, particularly along the Chinese frontier. Force reductions are planned for both theaters. War-fighting doctrine in these theaters has held that Soviet forces must rely on massed armored warfare, with a commitment to seize the initiative at the outset of hostilities. Victory would be secured through reinforcing efforts of all ground, sea, and air forces—the combined arms concept. Moreover, Soviet forces would be prepared to initiate extensive nuclear operations, including a strong predisposition to preempt any enemy resort to the use of nuclear weapons. According to their long-established force employment doctrine, Soviet strategists would mass their armor-heavy forces along selected main axes of attack and seek to achieve a series of simultaneous breakthroughs of the enemy's defenses.

The United States is also committed to deterring nuclear war, conventional attacks by the Warsaw Pact nations on Western Europe, and smaller contingencies elsewhere, particularly if such conflicts lead to a crisis or conflagration in Western Europe. Certainly the keystone of U.S. strategic nuclear policy has been an assured second-strike capability as being necessary for maintenance of a deterrence posture; however, the United States also has a collateral interest in being able to exercise nonnuclear options or to engage in a controlled or limited nuclear exchange should deterrence fail. Moreover, the Reagan administration placed increased emphasis on strategic defense programs, exploring longer-range alternatives to deterrence based on the threat of assured destruction.

Combining deterrence and war-fighting remains a core concern of American strategy. In terms of "extended deterrence," the United States retains defense commitments in Asia, particularly in South Korea and Japan, but following the end of U.S. involvement in the Vietnam War, emphasis shifted to the European theater, the Middle East, and Central America. Strengthening NATO through both conventional and nuclear force modernization and improving the capacity to deploy U.S. forces to the Middle East have been key American strategic concerns throughout the 1970s and 1980s. Given these world-wide commitments, budgetary concern is expected to continue to be a very important limiting factor on the development of U.S. strategy and forces in the Bush and future American administrations for some years.

OTHER EUROPEAN AND NORTH ATLANTIC COUNTRIES

Although a common focus in security policy studies is on threats and threat perceptions, note should also be taken of the obverse side of the same security coin: perceived opportunities the state may wish to pursue.[5] Indeed, policy makers may see little or nothing in the international environment that would obstruct or otherwise impede the attainment of certain goals. To the contrary, other actors may be supportive of these purposes and be willing to collaborate in a common effort to achieve collective goals.

Decision makers hold certain images of the role their states should play internationally. A substantial change in power position relative to other states inevitably alters these perceptions; however, there is sometimes a considerable lag between changes in the "objective" situation and "subjective" realization (and acceptance) of a new role. Britain is a classic case in point. In the years immediately following World War II, the United Kingdom attempted to retain its global position and even developed its own strategic nuclear force. Britain was finally forced to reduce its overseas commitments, however, withdrawing from east of Suez. No longer a global power, the United Kingdom has retained its close security linkage with the United States, but now has a Eurocentric security focus.

French perceptions of France's international role during and subsequent to the Gaullist period have greatly exceeded what one might have expected from a middle power. France has developed an independent nuclear force, maintained its European-based forces under French national control, and retained the conventional capability for selective intervention in Africa and the Middle East. Thus, France's relative position has been influenced by its self-image, but constrained or moderated by its actual capabilities. In short, as illustrated by the British and French cases, the relative international power position of a given state is a function of both objective and subjective factors.

For its part, the middle-rank position of the Federal Republic of Germany is further limited by the countries that occupied Germany following World War II. Nuclear weapons stationed on West German soil, for example, are under foreign control. Although the FRG contributes substantially to NATO defense in terms of both committed manpower and financial support, the country's offensive capability is severely constrained. Certainly the division of Germany between East and West and the continuing presence of allied troops are continuing reminders that very real external constraints on Germany's military role persist. Nevertheless, the FRG now has the strongest economy in Europe and, for that matter, also maintains the largest European ground force commitment to the NATO alliance. Indeed,

the FRG remains firmly committed to the West for security even as it tries to reduce tensions with the East.

It is interesting to compare the defense policies of East and West Germany. Aside from cultural commonality as two German states in one German nation, both are subject to considerable superpower influence and both are considered to be the leading and most reliable non-superpower members in their respective alliances. At the same time, each not only represents the major threat to the other, but also is viewed with some suspicion by its other allies. In fact, leaving ideological issues aside, one finds a great number of similarities in the defense policies of these two states—the basis for generating a series of hypotheses about the defense policies of divided nations. The chapter on Korea is also suggestive of such hypotheses.

French doctrinal commitment to proportional deterrence (dissuasion) and flexible response would appear to have few escalatory rungs. In the French context proportional deterrence really means minimum or finite deterrence.[6] The earlier French military doctrine of all-horizon defense that was closely tied to a "fortress France" mentality has been modified consistent with French objectives of securing national interests abroad and permitting the country to operate internationally as an independent power. French participation in the defense of Europe is certainly necessary if the country hopes to attain its other objectives. Thus, France has maintained forward deployments of forces in West Germany and has joined in creating a joint French-West German brigade stationed in West Germany. The French have also improved their bilateral military ties with West Germany and other NATO allies, while still remaining outside of the formal, integrated military command structure of the North Atlantic alliance.

Unlike the French, the British are fully integrated with NATO's military command structure, contributing directly to maintenance of the NATO "triad"—central strategic systems, theater nuclear systems, and conventional forces. On the other hand, continuing this commitment at present levels remains a major problem for the British in light of severe resource constraints that preclude major increases in defense spending.

Although British strategic nuclear forces can still be used independently to provide the country with a minimum or finite deterrence against an attacker, they have in fact been closely tied to American nuclear employment plans. Aside from having submarine-launched ballistic missile capabilities, the British navy would also assist other allied navies in a joint attempt to keep the European and Atlantic sea lanes open in the event of war. British deployment of ground and air units in Germany is also a clear demonstration of the country's continuing commitment to NATO's theater nuclear and conventional defense capability. Although British forces have some capability for counterattack, force-employment doctrine puts primary emphasis on "defensive" measures that would blunt any invasion by Warsaw Pact forces. The hope, of course, is that NATO defenses will be strong enough to deter any such attempt. Moreover, the British also have supported various attempts to reduce tensions in Europe by endorsing such confidence-building measures between East and West as mutual notification of military maneuvers and training exercises.

The Germans are painfully aware that in any future European war, Germany would be the primary battlefield. For obvious reasons, then, the country's planners favor a defense posture that would not provoke an attack, but would deter any attempt by adversaries to invade the country. The West Germans have also resisted talk of strategies in which forward-based troops would intially withdraw from the front lines, thus conceding a large proportion of German territory to an advancing enemy. Instead, West German doctrine has maintained a commitment to forward defense that would blunt and, even more important, deter any invasion. Whether allied forces have the capability for a sustained forward defense or whether they would necessarily have to withdraw (in preparation for counterattack or as part of an attrition strategy) remains a subject of considerable controversy. Another matter of concern, of course, is when "tactical" or theater nuclear weapons would be employed. Given that the West Germans maintain the largest ground force contribution to NATO forces in Germany, observers ask whether the allies would necessarily have to escalate to nuclear weapons in the face of the advancing mass of Soviet and other Warsaw Pact forces. In some ways, it is this uncertainty, not only with respect to the threat from the East, but also concerning the nature of the allied response, that explains West German commitment to reduction of tensions through confidence-building measures and arms control on the one hand and the much-heralded Ostpolitik of improved relations with the East on the other.

A country study on East Germany is new with this edition. West Germans frequently refer to there being two German states in one German nation. Be that as it may, presentation of defense policy from both East and West German perspectives contributes significantly to understanding the overall security equation in Central Europe. Just as the FRG is a key member of NATO, so the GDR is a most important part of the Warsaw Pact. Indeed, the context of East German defense decision making is set by the presence of nineteen Soviet divisions and other military forces, which provide the USSR with enormous influence. Moreover, a feeling of being "beleaguered" colors the perceptions of East German leaders.

Also new with this edition are country studies on two other NATO members—Canada and Italy. Large in land area and resources, but small in population and in the size of its economy, Canada presents an interesting example of a country managing its defense relations with an adjacent superpower. Although Canada and the United States are allies in NATO and in North American Air Defense (NORAD), Canada takes a more independent stand on defense matters than one might suppose. To be sure, Canadian perspectives are different. Depending historically upon Britain for their defense, Canada did not develop a strong domestic military tradition, and Canadian officials are prone to avoid the use of force, preferring to look for pacific solutions to international problems. Thus, Canadians have taken pride in their participation in UN peace-keeping activities. At the same time, of course, Canada has also maintained its NATO commitment of ground and air forces deployed in Europe. Indeed, participation in NATO also provides Canada with a multilateral forum for developing its defense policy, allowing somewhat greater flexibility than might be true if Canada's defense relations with the United States were strictly bilateral.

Since the end of World War II, Italy's ties to the United States have been close. Depending on American contributions to their defense and deferring on most security issues to American leadership in NATO, Italian leaders have been less concerned than some of the other allies about charting an independent course on such matters. While Italian military capabilities do not match those of the British, the size of Italy's gross national product now makes it third-ranking in West Europe (behind West Germany and France, but ahead of the United Kingdom). An important country in NATO's southern region, Italy has been strengthening its naval and air forces capable of conducting operations in the Mediterranean. This is in addition to its continuing ground and air force deployments in the north opposite potential Warsaw Pact approaches across neutral Yugoslavia.

THE MIDDLE EAST

Israel is closely tied to the United States for its security. Attempts to reduce this dependence by developing its own defense industries have met with only limited success. Security policy is subject to considerable controversy among Israelis, some favoring greater accommodation with neighboring Arab states and resolution of the Palestinian problem as the best long-term guarantee of security, while others continue to hold to a harder line. Even so, the perception of Israel as surrounded by hostile Arab states is pervasive. In its most extreme form, some have described the Israeli security problem as the "Masada complex" (a reference to the siege mentality exhibited in the first century A.D. when Jewish zealots committed suicide rather than submit to the Romans). With the exception of Egypt, Arab reactions to the legitimacy of Israel as a state have indeed been hostile (or at best skeptical). Without a doubt, this hostility has reinforced Israeli perceptions of insecurity that play such a large part in shaping the country's defense policy. Indeed, Israeli strategy, military doctrine, and force posture have evolved during five wars since 1948. Of all the countries studied in this volume, Israel has the most empirical data available on actual war-fighting capabilities—tests of the viability of doctrine and forces that few other states have faced so frequently.

For their part, Arab leaders resent the great power intervention that resulted in the creation of Israel as a state, particularly since it was imposed on the region with what they regard as insufficient attention to the rights of Palestinian Arabs. Unfortunately, we still have no country-study chapters on the Arab states that we could publish in this volume. Given the extensive treatment that would be required by the common framework we devised, the scholars we contacted argued that the absence of sufficient data precluded such an effort at this time. Although considerable work has been done on civil-military relations and sociological aspects of various Arab military establishments, defense policy per se has not received as much attention. One of our goals for the next edition of this book is to work toward filling this gap in the literature by commissioning at least one Arab country study.

Israel maintains a relatively small regular force, but relies heavily on rapid mobilization of reserves at times of national emergency. Particular emphasis is placed on mobility and, as demonstrated in the June 1967 war, on achieving surprise. Israeli doctrine stresses offensive operations, transferring the battle to enemy territory as soon as possible and dealing with the most threatening enemy first. The country is surrounded by Arab states, but Israel has been able to capitalize on divisions among them. Seizure in 1967 of the West Bank, Golan Heights, and Sinai Desert (including Gaza) provided buffers against Israel's adversaries. Similarly, making a separate peace with Egypt was a clear attempt to neutralize the threat to Israel's western front. Of course, the encirclement of Israel is also offset to some extent by the geomilitary advantage of internal lines of communication that allow for flexibility in the deploying of forces from one front to another and in maintaining logistical support for combat operations on more than one front. Although Israel retains military capabilities in the north, intervention in Lebanon in the early 1980s proved to be costly both militarily and politically.

EAST ASIA

Japan is another middle power subject to constraints on its military capabilities. Like the FRG, Japan has accepted a lesser military posture while embracing a significant economic role. In the Japanese case, defense expenditures have been limited by domestic preference to about 1 percent of the GNP. Reliance upon the American security umbrella has resulted in defense cost savings that have made possible the large-scale aggregate investment of national resources in Japanese industry. It is also true, of course, that the United States benefits from its security relations with Japan. Indeed, apart from American and Japanese contributions to regional stability, the United States also derives considerable leverage from Japanese security dependency upon the United States. This leverage is linked not just to security issues, but also to the entire range of socioeconomic and other nonsecurity issues that constitute the substance of Japanese-American relations.

Japanese security relies on close links with the United States. The Japanese Self-Defense Forces (SDF) are structured to cope with what has been defined as the central problem for Japanese military strategy or doctrine: stopping an invading force. By establishing and maintaining the capability to destroy or badly degrade the ability (of an adversary) to project forces to the Home Islands, the SDF would hope to deter any such attempt. Given this defensive character, Japanese military strategy is further constrained by explicit commitments not to acquire nuclear or other "offensive" weapons and weapons systems, not to sell or otherwise export weapons to other countries, and not to engage in overseas combat operations.

For their part, the Chinese perceive themselves as part of the Third World. Although the military sector is one of the "four modernizations," the other three—agriculture, industry, and science and technology—have even higher priority in Chinese planning. Improvement in China's defense capabilities will undoubtedly occur, but there is little prospect that the country will be anything more than a regional power during the remainder of this century. Even in regional terms, the very real limits to China's capacity for using force were demonstrated in the "punitive" intervention in Vietnam in 1979 and the attempt to influence events in Cambodia in the late 1970s and 1980s. Although China's nuclear weapons and ICBMs pose a continuing threat to other countries (notably the Soviet Union), mere possession of such a capability by no means confers great power or superpower status on China. Even though the country has unquestioned potential, both military and economic, China will likely remain a middle power for the foreseeable future.

Offensively, China does not possess the necessary sea- or airlift capabilities for projection of its forces outside of the region, and the relatively small number of nuclear weapons in China's arsenal and relative inaccuracy of the country's delivery systems severely limit their use in a war-fighting mode. This could change, of course, with improvements in Chinese nuclear weapons systems and increases in numbers deployed, particularly if the United States and the Soviet Union were to adopt an arms control regime that reduced significantly the number of their own strategic nuclear weapons. Nevertheless, given China's relative capabilities and the likelihood that they will not be altered substantially in the near term, the defensive orientation of China's military doctrine will likely remain unchanged.

South Korea is a country with a strong tradition of deference to authority in defense matters. Although the regimes in North and South are markedly different in other respects, decisions on defense matters and other political questions of high salience tend to be highly centralized in both cases. The focus in the Korean country study added to this edition is on the Republic of Korea, but it is also a comparative essay replete with references to similarities and contrasts between North and South Korea. Although its Marxist-Leninist regime places North Korea formally in the "Second World" of communist countries, in fact it shares a level of economic development comparable to many "Third World" countries. By contrast, South Korean economic success has placed it among the "newly industrializing countries," or NICs, a distinction that brings it much closer to "First World" status. Although both countries remain dependent on outside sources of supply for maintaining their military capabilities, the robust economy of the South gives it greater potential for a more self-reliant position.

Coverage of North Korea is an interesting addition to this study for another reason. The succession problem that confronts most Marxist-Leninist states takes a particular turn in North Korea, where transfer of political power (to include control of the military and defense matters) from father to son is a distinct possibility. This contrasts sharply with other Marxist-Leninist states, which deemphasize family connections. As such, North Korea appears to have more in common with more traditional Third World states. Although the position taken by the military on political succession is most important in both North and South Korea, family ties as a determining factor apply only in the North.

THIRD WORLD AND OTHER COUNTRIES

The Mexican case added to this edition stands apart from the others in that the focus of the Mexican military is almost exclusively internal. Although in recent decades the armed forces have avoided any direct intervention in politics that would undermine the ruling political party, the regime rests upon a foundation of active (though usually behind-the-scenes) military support. Indeed, it is the armed forces that provide a guarantee to the status quo. From the Mexican case, then, comes a challenge to the assumption implicit in the framework constructed for all of the country studies in this volume—that the armed forces are created by states primarily to respond to threats coming from the international environment. When such external threats are relatively low, as has been true in the Mexican case, the orientation of the military may be more inward. In fact, the Mexican study suggests that a common purpose of Third World militaries is to assure internal political stability, if not continuity of a particular regime.

Most publications on South Africa have focused either on the country's strategic significance, both in terms of location and mineral wealth, or on the moral repugnance of separation of the races under apartheid. The chapter on South Africa prepared for this volume goes further, shedding new light on the ways and means by which the South African white minority maintains its position of dominance. Like Mexico's armed forces, South Africa's military is preoccupied with domestic concerns, but the offensive character of South Africa's domestic regime of apartheid to neighboring black African states gives rise to external threats. South Africa's armed forces, unlike Mexico's, are thus both outwardly and inwardly oriented. South Africa is also an interesting case because its white minority, which dominates political and economic relations, can be classed as First World, whereas the majority black population has much more in common with the populations of other third world countries—white, black, or otherwise.

The final new addition to this volume is a country study on India. Notwithstanding Gandhian pacifism and moral concern about the use of force (particularly in the early years of national independence from Britain), India has developed a substantial military capability, including the capacity to produce nuclear weapons. A leader in the nonaligned movement since Nehru's days, India wants to be the principal power in South Asia and in the Indian Ocean. It is a unique example of a state that views nonalignment not just as a condition to be maintained, but also as an instrument of policy to be used to attain a regional pattern of dominance. Consistent with this objective, India tries to balance its relations with the superpowers, China, and Pakistan. Although it seems unlikely, achievement of an "Indian Ocean Zone of Peace" free of superpower and other great power presences would, by default, leave India with the dominant naval force in the region.

The Defense Decision-Making Process

LENINIST REGIMES

An understanding of a state's domestic politics is clearly central to the analysis of its defense policy. Indeed, the internal structure of states (including organizational or bureaucratic elements) has a direct impact on the defense decision-making process. Authoritarian regimes, as in the Soviet Union, for example, have made policy centrally, usually without open debate and without much need for compromise to resolve disputes among competing interests outside of government or party. *Glasnost* or "public discussion" in the Gorbachev period has broadened the base for public policy, but decisions continue to be made centrally within the party's politburo. To be sure, there is competition and political compromise within the ruling elite that takes alternative institutional and private views into account, but the domain within which the politics of policy choice takes place has been a relatively narrow one.

Following this "Leninist" model, in China and East Germany, as in the Soviet Union, the highest authority for defense decision making is the politburo. Although there are differences among them owing to cultural and geopolitical factors identified in the separate country studies, similarities make it possible to identify the Leninist model as a separate type. Although the party and its politburo are at the center of defense policy formulation, an array of other institutional actors also make inputs to (and participate in) the defense decision-making process.

The nature of politics within this party and government elite has indeed been the subject of controversy in the West. Indeed, the absence of information about the decision-making process in Marxist-Leninist countries remains a major problem for Western scholars. One "pluralist" view, for example, is that the Soviet military is an interest group that competes for political influence.[7] The Chinese and Soviet country studies in this volume conform fairly closely to this pluralist view. These authors have observed that the "concept of shifting coalitions or informal groups" within the Chinese elite seems "more appropriate" and that Soviet defense policy and, in particular, the Soviet defense budget are "purely the product of bureaucratic politics within the government and party hierarchies." Indeed, as the ruling coalition in the politburo has shifted, Soviet military figures, or the Soviet military establishment as interest group, have not had the degree of influence in the Gorbachev years they enjoyed earlier, particularly in the Brezhnev era.

An alternative interpretation is a more unitary image of military-party relations—that the Soviet decision-making elite is not as factionally divided as the pluralist model would suggest.[8] In this view, party-military relations are not so much an adversary process. Rather, both elements share similar views—a "party-military consensus" on "fundamental issues" and a basic compatibility of "institutional methods."[9] The military is depicted as "an administrative arm of the party, not something separate from and competing with it."[10] Whatever may be the case in the Soviet Union, this characterization of party-military relations certainly is the understanding one gets from reading the East German country study.

Acknowledging that the military is a "political institution," one observer states that

the military's political life is bureaucratic in character, not parliamentarian and not lobbyist. . . .

Personal cliques and coalitions of cliques take shape in bureaucracies, but they differ generically from interest groups. They cannot formalize themselves and thereby institutionalize the pursuit of an interest. In the Soviet bureaucracy, informal cliques and coalitions are established only at great risk; they probably do not extend beyond small face-to-face groups.[11]

Implicit in this critique, of course, is the view that superimposing a Western pluralist model on Soviet (or Chinese and East German) politics is a bias that largely ignores "unique political and cultural contexts"[12] and thus distorts the reality of Soviet defense decision-making processes.

DEMOCRATIC REGIMES

Although there are marked differences among the countries explored in this volume, most of them can be labeled democracies. Political authority and the exercise of power in some are highly centralized, with fewer points of access to those in power, whereas in others, notably the United States, political authority is highly fragmented, with many points of access to those exercising power and making policy choices. In addition to these structural differences, cultural variations are also significant. Thus, decision making in Japan is the often slow-moving politics of consensus building, whereas in Britain open conflict among opposing parties is central to the political process. The impact of culture on political process is striking, particularly when one considers that Japan and Britain have the same formal political structure, a parliamentary regime in a unitary state.

Parliamentary regimes, as in the United Kingdom, West Germany, Italy, Canada, Israel, and Japan, have a fusion of executive and legislative functions such that policy choice is made centrally within the cabinet. (In most parliamentary regimes there is also little, if any, judicial check on the legislature.) There is still considerable debate and compromise both within and outside of the majority party or coalition that controls the government, but most such politics occur within the cabinet or among the members of the governing coalition.

Although the titles vary from country to country, the principal defense decision makers within the cabinet are the prime minister and the ministers of defense, foreign affairs, and finance or treasury. Maintaining a consensus within the majority party is a major task undertaken by these and other cabinet members that typically involves considerable political compromise. The necessity for compromise is underscored, of course, when no single party has a majority of seats in the legislature and the government is composed of a coalition of parties. Although there are exceptions, both the prime minister and the defense minister are usually members of the party in the governing coalition that has the most seats in the legislature.

Although the point has been made that defense policy making in parliamentary regimes takes place primarily within a cabinet composed of ministers from the majority party or from the parties within the governing coalition, note is also taken of the crucial role played by bureaucracies formally subordinated to these government ministers. The career civil service members remain in place even as governments change. More than just a source of stability, these civil servants are repositories of the information upon which the government ministers so heavily depend. Accordingly, as has been widely recognized, bureaucracies play a decisive role in shaping the alternatives among which policy makers are forced to choose. In other instances, of course, career bureaucrats can act as a conservative force by delaying or otherwise obstructing implementation of political decisions they oppose. Appreciation of this bureaucratic role is central to understanding defense policy processes in authoritarian and democratic regimes of all types.

France has a presidential regime with some separation of powers between the legislature and the executive; however, the executive has clearly been the more powerful branch, particularly in relation to defense matters, since the Gaullist Constitution came into effect in 1958. A relatively strong executive, coupled with the fact that the country is a unitary state with ultimate political authority centralized in the national capital, results in a concentration of defense decision making comparable to that in parliamentary regimes. This is reinforced, moreover, by a political culture or tradition of strong bureaucracy centrally directed from Paris.

By contrast, the United States not only has a presidential regime of separation of powers within the central government, but also considerable division of powers between the central government and fifty state and thousands of municipal, county, and other local governments. Although local administrations exist in unitary states, they are usually subordinated to the central government. There is no such subordination in American federalism. Indeed, when the federal dimension is combined with the existence of a strong legislative counterweight to any executive initiatives, the result is a highly fragmented political system, with numerous points of access by interest groups to political authorities operating in a wide variety of places and on various levels. None of this is accidental, of course. Distrust of centralized political power is deeply set in the American political culture, with roots early in the country's history. The rationale for both separating and dividing power—a presidential regime in a federal state—is most clearly expressed in *The Federalist Papers*, especially numbers 10 and 51, written by James Madison.

Although West Germany is also a federal state, with power and authority more dispersed than in other parliamentary regimes, defense decision making is viewed primarily as a national concern and thus is centralized within the cabinet, with inputs received from military elements, a relatively small defense bureaucracy, and opposition parties. A similar assessment is true for Canada, where the New Democratic Party has even called for withdrawal from NATO and NORAD. But in both of these countries, unless associated with weapons acquisition and deployment or nuclear issues, defense is more often than not a non-issue for much of the public. By contrast, in the United States defense procurement and military force deployment are issues that regularly draw the attention and participation of private interests, local officials, state governors, and representatives of both houses of the U.S. Congress. The attempt in the late 1970s and early 1980s by the Defense Department to gain approval for deployment of a new ICBM system (the "MX") in Utah and Nevada is a classic case that clearly illustrates the political milieu within which American defense decision making takes place. Coalitions and countercoalitions of private and governmental actors, federal and state and local officials, and legislative and bureaucratic figures all participated in the process.

Interest-group politics of this sort also exists in the parliamentary regimes already discussed, but usually not to the same degree. Fragmentation of political authority and a political culture that legitimizes the dispersion of power go a long way toward explaining the extreme pluralism of American political processes. Multiple points of access enable interest groups to flourish in a way not possible in democratic regimes with greater concentration of political authority and fewer points of access to those in political power. Interest-group pluralism is by no means unique to American politics, but structural and cultural factors do strengthen the role that interest groups can play. Interest groups are relevant actors in other democratic regimes, but to a somewhat lesser extent.

It can also be argued that the nature of defense policy outputs themselves—decisions and actions—is directly affected by the type of internal political structure and the associated political culture. Thus, in the United States, where political power and authority are highly fragmented, decisions are reached (and almost always implemented) incrementally and as the result of considerable compromise. Although the politics of compromise and incremental choice is also present in parliamentary regimes, as a matter of degree the implementation of decisions and actions taken by these democracies do have a somewhat more comprehensive and coherent character. Certainly this is one inference that can be drawn from the country studies in this volume.

ALTERNATIVE DECISION-MAKING MODELS

In our view more conceptual and empirical work is needed on alternative models and modes of decision making. Although the Leninist model has been addressed, further work needs to be done on other authoritarian styles of decision making, particularly as they are found in Third World settings.

With respect to democracies, some function on the basis of a deep commitment to building consensus, however arduous the task or however long it may take to build the very large majorities deemed necessary. Passing legislation on contentious issues in defense or other issue areas may take many months or even years with considerable compromise along the way, but when these measures finally do come to a vote they are passed by majorities as high as 80 percent or more. By contrast, in other democracies, more prone to conflictual politics, the leading party or governing coalition may push measures through with not many more votes than 50 percent plus one, if that many.

How are these differences to be explained? Is "consensus politics" produced by an underlying political culture prone to compromise and conflict avoidance? By contrast, does the society not only expect conflict and opposing voices to be heard, but consider such discord legitimate—the "stuff" of politics? Apart from political culture, is the "consensus" mode to be found primarily when there is genuine agreement on such major issues as in the relative allocation of national resources between welfare and defense? If there are only marginal differences of opinion in the society and among government leaders on such questions, building consensus by forging compromise on the few points of difference is relatively an easier task than in countries lacking such underlying agreement.

To what extent is a "consensus" or "conflict" mode a reflection respectively of underlying socioeconomic homogeneity or heterogeneity? In other words, is conflict politics more common in societies prone to class conflict because of disparities in the distribution of wealth or opportunity? To what extent do national, ethnic, or racial divisions in a society have any bearing on defense decision making, or are defense issues somehow insulated from the discord produced by these divisions?

Social structure and the value system associated with it can have important influence on defense decision making. In this regard, the Mexico country study addresses the extent to which defense decision making in Mexico conforms to patron-client, vertical patterns of exchange common to many Third World countries. This mode of defense decision making may be more prevalent in the Third World than either the pluralist model of "horizontal" interaction of groups and individuals common to the United States and many other Western

democracies or the Leninist model common to the Soviet Union and other communist countries. Moreover, the patron-client model may have application in some First World countries, such as Japan, that have been able to preserve traditional patterns of social interaction even in a modern industrial setting. Work by Chie Nakane on *Japanese Society*, for example, needs to be extended to see if the same vertical, corporate ties identified in other issue areas also apply to defense decision making.[13]

ORGANIZATION PROCESSES AND BUREAUCRATIC POLITICS

The relevance of organizational processes and bureaucratic politics to understanding how defense policy is actually made has been underscored by the efforts of Graham Allison and others.[14] That defense decisions and actions do not necessarily proceed in a logical sequence from national objectives, strategies designed to coordinate the use of the state's capabilities, and employment doctrines governing the use of force is an argument that flows from their work.

On the other hand, some have cautioned against too heavy a reliance on organizational and bureaucratic variables.[15] To what extent, for example, does focus on organizational and bureaucratic factors obscure the importance of variables external to the decision makers? From this perspective, the specific decisions and actions taken may be shaped by decision makers and organizational perspectives in the "pulling and hauling" and coalition formation of bureaucratic politics, but the general course of policy is more a function of the international environment with which decision makers have to contend. How to account for the effects of individual perceptions in general and for such personalities as a de Gaulle in France, a Gorbachev in the USSR, or a Mao or Deng in China in particular (not to mention other idiosyncratic factors) was a problem that confronted each of our country-study authors. Personalities can and do change, but there often remains a degree of constancy in defense policy that survives alterations in domestic authorities.

Defense Policy and the Level-of-Analysis Problem

If relative constancy in the general course of defense policy is an accurate description applicable to most countries (and not everyone would agree that it is), is this to be explained by the dominance of such external factors as the relative distribution or balance of power within the international system, which usually changes very slowly? Or is relative constancy to be explained by the nature of decision-making processes themselves—that they usually involve incremental or marginal changes from established policy? Is "any policy" really encumbered by all preceding policies, and does it in turn encumber "all succeeding policies?"[16]

In a very real sense, the conceptual issue of how to study defense policy is the relative importance of these different "levels of analysis."[17] More than thirty years ago, the late Fred Sondermann (to whom this book is co-dedicated) grappled with the linkage between foreign policy and international politics.[18] Sondermann noted the importance of the "international system which has profound impact upon the behavior of participants in that system's processes."[19] On the other hand, he also took note of the view that "international politics cannot be understood without a thorough examination of the policies of the states participating in that process" and the "complex web of factors and forces which affect governmental policies."[20]

In other words, how important are distribution of capabilities (or power), degree of interdependence, level of tensions, and other system-level variables as determinants of policy? To rely exclusively on such variables opens one to the criticism of system determinism—that states and other "actors" are mere automatons lacking any capacity for independent action. Ernst Haas describes the problem when he excoriates "determinists" who "see the components (of systems) as relatively unchangeable and arrange them in an eternal preprogrammed dance; the rules of the dance may be unknown to the actors and are specified by the theorist. The recurrent patterns discovered by

him constitute a super-logic which predicts the future state of the system."[21]

On the other hand, instead of focusing on the "system" of states and other actors, some would argue that one will find the dominant variables to be the types of states (or their internal structure, including organizational and bureaucratic factors). Still others would argue that personality and the set of cognitive orientations and perceptions (or operational codes) of individual decision makers are central.[22] To adopt such a position (ignoring external or environmental factors) is, of course, to open oneself to the charge of reductionism. Indeed, as Sondermann observed: "As one progresses down the path toward greater (and narrower) specifity, one does reach points which—however valid and interesting they are in themselves—are rather far removed from the subject of international politics which provided the starting point for one's inquiries."[23]

To say that systemic considerations, the type or structure of states, their associated political cultures, the organizational and bureaucratic dimensions of this internal structure, and psychological variables are all important is not to say very much. Indeed, to say that everything is important begs the more relevant question of the relative importance of the different vari-

Figure 1. The Level of Analysis Problem

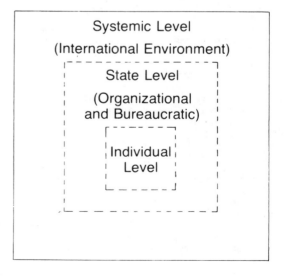

Systemic Level
(International Environment)

State Level
(Organizational and Bureaucratic)

Individual Level

ables in explaining defense decisions and actions. Even more to the point, can we identify the conditions that affect the relative importance of systemic, state, organizational or bureaucratic, and individual-level variables? (See figure 1.)

A theory of comparative defense policy offering explanations and predictions would necessarily be built upon the answers to such questions. Because we do not pretend to have these answers, we do not claim to have provided a theory; our only claim is to have offered a framework for the comparative study of defense policy. We do contend, however, that the variables we have identified will be central to any theory of comparative defense policy, the development of which remains to be accomplished.

Notes

1. Path-breaking efforts in this field were James Rosenau's "Pretheories and Theories of Foreign Policy," in *Approaches to Comparative and International Politics*, ed. R. B. Farrel (Evanston, Ill.: Northwestern University Press, 1966), pp. 27–92; and id., "Comparative Foreign Policy: Fad, Fantasy, or Field?" *International Studies Quarterly* 12 (September 1968): 296–329. Later efforts include Wolfram F. Hanrieder, ed., *Comparative Foreign Policy: Theoretical Essays* (New York: David McKay, 1971); James N. Rosenau, ed., *Comparing Foreign Policies: Theories, Findings, and Methods* (New York: John Wiley & Sons/Sage Publications, 1974); Patrick J. McGowan and Howard B. Shapiro, *The Comparative Study of Foreign Policy: A Survey of Scientific Findings* (Beverly Hills, Calif.: Sage Publications, 1973); and Maurice A. East, Stephen A. Salmore, and Charles F. Hermann, eds., *Why Nations Act: Theoretical Perspectives for Comparative Foreign Studies* (Beverly Hills, Calif.: Sage Publications, 1978).

2. One of us addressed this subject in Frank B. Horton, Anthony C. Rogerson, and Edward L. Warner, eds., *Comparative Defense Policy* (Baltimore: Johns Hopkins University Press, 1974), pp. 190–92.

3. The literature on the use of force and the question of whether it is declining is extensive. A representative sample would include Robert J. Art and Kenneth N. Waltz, eds., *The Use of Force* (Boston: Little, Brown, 1971); Klaus Knorr, "International Coercion: Waning or Rising?" *International Security* (Spring 1977); id., "On the International Uses of Military Forces in the Contemporary World," *Orbis* (Spring 1977); id., "The Limits of Economic and Military Power," *Daedalus* (Fall 1975); Robert Tucker, "Oil: The Issue of American Intervention," *Commentary* (January 1975); id., "Further Reflections in Oil and Force," *Commentary* (March 1975); Stanley Hoffmann, *The Acceptability of Military Force*, Adelphi Papers, no. 102 (London: In-

ternational Institute for Strategic Studies, 1973); Robert Johansen, *Toward a Dependable Peace* (New York: Institute for World Order, 1978); and Barry M. Blechman and Stephen S. Kaplan, "U.S. Military Forces as a Political Instrument since World War II," *Political Science Quarterly* 94, no. 2 (Summer 1979): 193–209.

4. See the discussion in Arnold L. Horelick, "Perspectives on the Study of Comparative Military Doctrine," and Benjamin S. Lambeth, "The Sources of Soviet Military Doctrine," in *Comparative Defense Policy*, ed. Horton, Rogerson, and Warner, pp. 192–216.

5. See, for example, the discussion in Kenneth N. Waltz, *Man, the State and War* (New York: Columbia University Press, 1954, 1959), p. 204.

6. See Graeme P. Auton, "Nuclear Deterrence and the Medium Power," *Orbis* (Summer 1976): 367–99.

7. See Roman Kolkowicz, "Interest Groups in Soviet Politics: The Case of the Military," *Comparative Politics* 2, no. 3 (April 1970): 445–72.

8. See William E. Odom, "The Party Connection," *Problems of Communism* 22, no. 5 (September–October 1973): 12–26.

9. Ibid., esp. pp. 14–17.

10. Ibid., p. 23.

11. Ibid., pp. 24–25.

12. Ibid., p. 23.

13. See Chie Nakane, *Japanese Society* (Berkeley: University of California Press, 1970). For a discussion of patron-client ties, particularly in Third World settings, see James C. Scott, "Corruption, Machine Politics, and Political Change," *American Political Science Review* 63, no. 4 (December 1969): 1142–58.

14. For example, see Allison's "Conceptual Models and the Cuban Missile Crisis," *American Political Science Review* 62 (September 1969): 689–718; and id., *Essence of Decision* (Boston: Little Brown, 1971). Cf. Allison and Morton H. Halperin, "Bureaucratic Politics: A Paradigm and Some Policy Implications," *World Politics* 24, supplement (Spring 1972): 40–79.

15. See Stephen D. Krasner, "Are Bureaucracies Important? (Or Allison Wonderland)," *Foreign Policy*, no. 7 (1972): 159–79; and Robert J. Art, "Bureaucratic Politics and American Foreign Policy: A Critique," *Policy Sciences* 4, no. 4 (1973): 467–90.

16. Fred A. Sondermann, "The Linkage between Foreign Policy and International Politics," in *International Politics and Foreign Policy*, ed. James N. Rosenau (New York: Free Press, 1961), p. 14.

17. An early treatment of the level-of-analysis problem is Waltz, *Man, the State and War*. Cf. Harold Sprout and Margaret Sprout, *Man-Milieu Relationship Hypotheses in the Context of International Politics* (Princeton: Princeton University Center of International Studies, 1956). Another discussion of the problem is J. David Singer, "The Level-of-Analysis Problem in International Relations," in *The International System: Theoretical Essays*, ed. Klaus Knorr and Sidney Verba (Princeton: Princeton University Press, 1961), pp. 77–92. Another treatment is Waltz, "Theory of International Relations," in *Handbook of Political Science*, ed. Fred I. Greenstein and Nelson W. Polsby (Reading, Mass.: Addison-Wesley, 1975), vol. 8, pp. 65–75. Finally, a useful discussion of the issues is Robert Jervis, *Perception and Misperception in International Politics*, esp. chap. 1.

18. Sondermann, "Foreign Policy and International

Politics," pp. 8–17. The article was based on a paper presented to the annual meeting of the American Political Science Association, St. Louis, September 1958.

19. Ibid., p. 13.

20. Ibid.

21. See Ernst B. Haas, "On Systems and International Regimes," *World Politics* 17, no. 2 (January 1975): 151.

22. For one of the best treatments of perceptual factors, see Jervis, *Perception and Misperception in International Politics*. The concept of "operational code" has been developed by Alexander George. See his " 'Operational Code': A Neglected Approach to the Study of Political Leaders and Decisionmaking," *International Studies Quarterly* 13 (1969): 190–222. Cf. Ole Holsti, "The Operational Code Approach to the Study of Political Leaders," *Canadian Journal of Political Science* 3 (1970): 123–57; and id., "The Belief System and National Images," *Journal of Conflict Resolution* 6, no. 3 (1962): 244–52.

23. Sondermann, "Foreign Policy and International Politics," p. 14.

BIBLIOGRAPHIC ESSAYS
GLOSSARY
INDEX

Bibliographic Essays

The United States

Frank L. Rosa

To offer a bibliographic essay on the evolution of U.S. defense policy is, to say the least, a formidable task. This is a result of both the richness and diversity of available sources. The focus of this essay is on the strategic environment that emerged out of World War II and the American response to the perceived threats and dangers. This bibliographic essay is restricted to books, avoiding a comprehensive survey of journal articles, an extensive task in itself. Nevertheless, the books listed in this essay provide a useful starting point, both in comprehending the scope of the policy evolution and in offering source documents for further bibliographic studies.

It is readily apparent in the defense literature that security policy has not developed in an intellectual or political void. The study of American defense policy has been dominated by a debate over the assessment of the international situation. This includes differences over three crucial elements: (1) the nature of the threat, (2) the utility of force in the nuclear age, and (3) the nature of stability in this era. While there are various cross cleavages in this debate, it must be noted that the differences that do exist are substantial. There can be little agreement—or compromise—among those who are committed to their policy positions. They see the world

differently and act in accordance with their world outlook. This is the first concept that students of security studies should grasp.

The Nature of the Threat

A nation's security policy is a reaction to a threat—real or perceived. In American diplomatic history, World War II and the immediate postwar period is a crucial era for understanding the formulation of American defense policy. Certain fundamental assumptions about the world and the appropriate role for the United States were accepted. From this world view emerged a policy of containment toward the Soviet Union, the second dominant power in the postwar period. Containment, as a policy direction, has remained a consistent feature of Soviet-American relations.

An understanding of the policy-making environment, the policy actors, and major policy issues in U.S. diplomacy is relevant to the student of defense policy. An excellent overview is provided by several texts. A standout is *American Foreign Policy: Pattern and Process*, 3d ed., by Charles Kegley, Jr., and Eugene R. Wittkopf (New York: St. Martin's Press, 1987). Kegley and Wittkopf observe a pattern of continuity in American foreign policy behavior. The goals are constant; it is the methods employed to realize them that change.

A pattern of continuity is also observed in *American Foreign Policy: A Search for Security*, 3d ed., by Henry T. Nash (Homewood, Ill.: Dorsey Press, 1985). Especially noteworthy is Nash's discussion of events that shaped the development of American perceptions and, consequently, U.S. policy in the postwar period.

The advent of the nuclear age and the emergence of the United States as the dominant international actor occurred simultaneously. While continuity in American foreign policy has been noted, the evolving nuclear technology has had a major impact on American foreign policy. This thesis is noted in *American Foreign Policy and the Nuclear Dilemma* by Gordon C. Schloming (Englewood Cliffs, N.J.: Prentice-Hall, 1987). Schloming is critical of American policy direction, noting that no administration has achieved a permanent improvement in U.S. relations with the Soviet Union. For this author, the threat of nuclear war is the overriding consideration. Yet, the American policy of containment was conceived as a clear attempt to modify the behavior of the Soviet Union to avoid such an apocalyptic event.

When George F. Kennan developed and advanced the concept of containment in 1946–47, he envisioned the strengths and capabilities of the United States—moral, economic, political, and military—containing the advance of Soviet power. This policy, pursued consistently and coherently, could lead to internal changes within the Soviet Union. This was Kennan's argument; it became the intellectual framework for the Truman administration's response to Soviet actions throughout the world. Rather than it prompting changes in the Soviet system, what emerged was a Cold War between the two dominant powers.

An extensive number of texts have been written on this topic. It must be noted that, on the fortieth anniversary of the "Mr. X" article, the publishers of *Foreign Affairs* issued a retrospective on the containment policy (Foreign Affairs 65, no. 4, Spring 1987). This included Kennan's "The Sources of Soviet Conduct" and excerpts from Walter Lippmann's serial response, "The Cold War." Kennan has also provided an updated assessment, "Containment Then and Now." This retrospective should be the starting point for the serious student of the Cold War. A similar, but expanded, historical review of the period is offered in Terry L. Deibel and John Lewis Gaddis, eds., *Containment: Concept and Policy*, 2 vols. (Washington, D.C.: National Defense University Press, 1986).

The Cold War can be analyzed from two distinct perspectives: an "orthodox" view or a "revisionist" view. Proponents of the "orthodox" theory see the U.S.-USSR Cold War as the inevitable result of the confrontation of two opposed political-economic systems over the power vacuum that emerged in central Europe at the end of World War II. This view of the Cold War is presented in *The United States and the Origins of the Cold War, 1941–1947* by John Lewis Gaddis (New York: Columbia University Press, 1972). This work presents both a descriptive and analytical discussion of this period.

Walter Lafeber offers a detailed examination of this same period in *America, Russia, and the Cold War,* *1945–1984*, 5th ed. (New York: Knopf, 1985), which describes the events of the immediate postwar period and the implications for the last decades of the twentieth century. While accepting the orthodox view of the origins of the Cold War, Lafeber stresses the changes that have taken place in the international environment. These changes—the growth of Soviet power and the increased destructiveness of war—dictate a change in policy to stress diplomacy and negotiation.

The revisionist view of the Cold War, as opposed to the orthodox view, argues that it was the result of either deliberate American policy choices or the inherent structural demands of a capitalist system. The first explanation is advanced by Barton J. Bernstein in *Politics and Policies of the Truman Administration* (Chicago: Quadrangle, 1970) and D. F. Fleming in *The Cold War and Its Origins, 1917–1960*, 2 vols. (Garden City, N.Y.: Doubleday, 1961). The second explanation—structural determinism—is central to Gabriel Kolko's argument in *The Roots of American Foreign Policy* (Boston: Beacon Press, 1969) and to the thesis advanced by William Appleman Williams in *The Tragedy of American Diplomacy*, 2d ed. (New York: Delta, 1972).

The othodox/revisionist debate is based upon different assessments of the motivations behind the policies of the Soviet Union and the United States. A partial explanation for the divergence is found in *Shattered Peace, The Origins of the Cold War and the National Security States* by Daniel Yergin (Boston: Houghton Mifflin, 1979). Yergin presents the concept of the Riga and Yalta axioms—a framework that can be used to view the USSR. The Riga axiom views the Soviet Union as an implacable enemy; the Yalta axiom concedes to the Soviet Union the status of a more traditional great power. With the first, conflict is the norm. The second offers the possibility of accommodation, cooperation, and convergence. This fundamental distinction, often drawn by other authors using different terms, clearly illustrates the impact on policy formulation of perceptions held by decision makers about the intentions and capabilities of the Soviet leadership.

The Commitments

The security policy choices of President Truman in dealing with the crisis situations that developed in Iran, Greece, Turkey, the central European theater, the Korean peninsula, and Indochina set the pattern for American relations with the Soviet Union and America's global role in the postwar era. This pattern and its pursuant commitments were based upon two widely accepted beliefs: first, that the United States must take an active role in international affairs, rejecting any return to the prewar isolationist policy; second, that the greatest danger to world peace and security was communism. The United States, as part of its activist role, must limit the political influence and geographic expansion of the Soviet Union—communism's fountainhead. Clearly, the threat was recognized; the response required of America an expanding peacetime commitment to the security of various regions of the world.

The history of this period is described in Adam Ulam's seminal work, *The Rivals: America and Russia since World War II* (New York: Penguin Books, 1971). Covering the period from 1945 to 1970, Ulam offers a balanced treatment of the foreign policies of the two superpowers for dealing with each other. An updated assessment, dealing with the rise and fall of détente throughout the 1970s and into the first term of the Reagan administration, is provided in *Détente and Confrontation: Soviet-American Relations from Nixon to Reagan* by Raymond L. Garthoff (Washington, D.C.: Brookings Institution, 1985). It is in this period that a serious breakdown occurred in the bipartisan consensus on the goals and means of America's containment policy.

The policy consensus breakdown revolves around the legitimate concern that extensive international security commitments have led to tremendous strains on diminishing American resources with few perceived benefits or improvements in the world situation. In this context, John Lewis Gaddis' *Strategies of Containment: A Critical Appraisal of Postwar American National Security Policy* (New York: Oxford University Press, 1982) is an important contribution to the literature on evolving U.S. national security policy. He offers a basic definition of strategy: "the process by which ends are related to means, intentions to capabilities, objectives to resources." Gaddis highlights the problems of balancing means and ends in the defense strategies selected by the postwar presidents. He analyzes successive U.S. policies through a framework that differentiates between "symmetrical" and "asymmetrical" forms of containment, which he contrasts between a universalistic and particularistic definition of the threat; between a perimeter versus a strongpoint defense; and between a presumption of unlimited and limited resources. The concern over resources and the limits of military power has led to a scaling back of the commitments that the United States has been willing to undertake—especially in the aftermath of the disastrous Vietnam experience.

While President Truman charted the path for America's world role, each subsequent administration contributed something to the further development and expansion of the containment policy. The extensive literature on the problems that faced the United States and the programs advanced to deal with them by postwar presidents provides a ready source of information for the ambitious student of defense policy. Such works offer a more complete picture of the hectic and dynamic nature of the decision-making environment. Additionally, the memoirs, reflections, and political observations of presidents, cabinet officers, and policy advisers are a rich source of material, though some of these works may be self-serving rather than illuminating.

For an understanding of the Truman era, the following works should be noted: Dean Acheson, *Present at the Creation: My Years at the State Department* (New York: Norton, 1969); James F. Burns, *Speaking Frankly* (New York: Harper & Row, 1947); and Harry S. Truman, *Memoirs*, 2 vols. (Garden City, N.Y.: Doubleday, 1955-1956). Assessments of the foreign policy initiatives of President Truman are provided in such works as Timothy Ireland, *Creating the Entangling Alliance: The Origins of the North Atlantic Treaty Organization* (Westport, Conn.: Greenwood Press, 1981); Charles L. Nee, *The Marshall Plan: The Launching of Pax Americana* (New York: Simon & Schuster, 1984); Avi Schlaim, *The United States and the Berlin Blockade, 1948-1949* (Berkeley and Los Angeles: University of California Press, 1983); and William W. Stueck, Jr.,

The Road to Confrontation: American Policy Toward China and Korea, 1947-1950 (Chapel Hill: University of North Carolina Press, 1981).

The Eisenhower era saw a continuation and expansion of the Truman policies. This period is described by the president himself in two works: *Mandate for Change* (Garden City, N.Y.: Doubleday, 1963) and *Waging Peace* (Garden City, N.Y.: Doubleday, 1965). Traditionally, the intellectual driving force of this administration was considered to be Secretary of State John Foster Dulles. The assessment of this particular individual goes the full gambit: John R. Beal, *John Foster Dulles* (New York: Harper & Row, 1956); M. A. Guhin, *John Foster Dulles: A Statesman and His Times* (New York: Columbia University Press, 1972); and Townsend Hoopes, *The Devil and John Foster Dulles* (Boston: Little, Brown, 1973). In a reassessment of the Eisenhower presidency, however, some political analysts today are depicting Eisenhower in a more positive light—recognizing the quiet decisiveness of this president. The following works are representative of this trend: Stephen E. Ambrose, *Eisenhower: The President*, vol. 2 (New York: Simon & Schuster, 1984); Fred I. Greenstein, *The Hidden Hand Presidency: Eisenhower as Leader* (New York: Basic Books, 1982); and W. W. Rostow, *Europe after Stalin: Eisenhower's Three Decisions of March 11, 1953* (Austin: University of Texas Press, 1982).

For further assessments of the international events and crises that occurred in the decade of the 1950s, the following brief sample is offered: Charles C. Alexander, *Holding the Line: The Eisenhower Era, 1952-1961* (Bloomington: Indiana University Press, 1975); Robert A. Divine, *Eisenhower and the Cold War* (New York: Oxford University Press, 1981); and Donald Neff, *Warriors at Suez: Eisenhower Takes America into the Middle East* (New York: Linden Press/Simon & Schuster, 1981).

President Kennedy opened his administration with an inaugural address that pledged "that we shall pay any price, bear any burden, meet any hardship, support any friend, oppose any foe to assure the survival and success of liberty." America's commitment to world security through the containment of communism had reached its zenith. But America was to learn that the cost of such a commitment would be too high—in terms of human costs, expended resources, lost credibility, and the strain on the political and social fabric of the nation. This nation's commitment to the Republic of Vietnam was the catalyst for a reassessment of American foreign and military policy.

The goal of the Kennedy administration was to tailor foreign policy and military capabilities to deal with a broader range of issues and threats. The United States would have the ability to challenge Soviet or Soviet-sponsored aggression in low-intensity conflicts, as well as at the strategic level. Flexible response was the codeword. This was not a new concept. Maxwell Taylor had called for a flexible response strategy in his book, *The Uncertain Trumpet* (New York: Harper, 1960). With Kennedy in office, there was now a presidential willingness to spend more on defense to match the requirements of this new strategy. The strategic policy direction during this period is examined by Laurence Martin in *Strategic Thought in the Nuclear Age* (Baltimore: Johns Hopkins University Press, 1979); and Jerome Kahan in *Security in the Nuclear Age* (Washington, D.C.: Brookings Institution, 1975).

The American strategic buildup caused immediate concern in the Kremlin. Premier Khrushchev responded with a parallel construction program for the long term; the short-term response, however, created the most dangerous superpower confrontation in the nuclear age—the Cuban Missile Crisis. This incident has been analyzed extensively. The preeminent works are Graham Allison's *Essence of Decision: Explaining the Missile Crisis* (Boston: Little, Brown, 1971) and Robert F. Kennedy's *Thirteen Days: A Memoir of the Cuban Missile Crisis* (New York: W. W. Norton, 1968).

On the conventional level, the Kennedy administration increased the number of military advisers to the South Vietnamese government. The pattern of increased involvement leading to the actual American direction of the war effort was set into operation. The American experience in Vietnam has been covered extensively. The notable works are Frances Fitzgerald's *Fire in the Lake: The Vietnamese and Americans in Vietnam* (Boston: Little, Brown, 1972); David Halberstam's *The Best and the Brightest* (New York: Fawcett Crest, 1972); Guenter Lewy's *American in Vietnam* (New York: Oxford University Press, 1978); and Stanley Karnow's *Vietnam History* (New York: Viking Press, 1983).

The argument has been advanced by former advisors within the administration that President Kennedy was planning to withdraw U.S. forces from South Vietnam after election to a second term. Whether this policy reversal was planned or not, an assassin's bullet brutally ended this presidency. The literature on the overall legacy of the Kennedy period is encompassed in several exceptional, though highly partisan, works. These include Roger Hilsman's *To Move a Nation* (Garden City, N.Y.: Doubleday, 1967); Arthur M. Schlesinger, Jr., *A Thousand Days: John F. Kennedy in the White House* (Boston: Houghton Mifflin, 1965); and Theodore C. Sorensen, *Kennedy* (New York: Harper & Row, 1965) and *The Kennedy Legacy* (New York: Mentor, 1969).

The presidency of Lyndon B. Johnson proved to be just as tragic as that of Kennedy; it fell as one of the casualties of the Vietnam War. Johnson entered office with a desire to complete the political and economic programs envisioned in Franklin Roosevelt's New Deal. He sought to create the Great Society as his enduring legacy. His strength was in domestic issues, but it was foreign policy that demanded Johnson's attention. When faced with the real possibility of an imminent South Vietnamese military defeat, he opted to take direct charge of the war effort. It was now America's war.

The Johnson administration sought to put the best possible light on the American efforts in Vietnam. This carefully managed effort was to collapse in the wake of the 1968 Tet offensive. Though a military disaster for the North Vietnamese, it was the United States that lost the most. The administration's credibility was called into question by an increasing number of congressmen, as well as by the American public.

The literature on the Johnson presidency reflects the sadness of the lost dream—of the lost American innocence. This attitude is seen in *The Lost Crusade* by Chester Cooper (New York: Dodd, Mead, 1970); *The Tragedy of Lyndon Johnson* by Eric F. Goldman (New York: Dell, 1968); and *Lyndon Johnson and the American Dream* by Doris Kerns (New York: Signet, 1977). As with other former presidents, Lyndon Johnson gave his view in *The Vantage Point: Perspectives of the Presidency, 1963-1969* (New York: Holt, Rinehart & Winston, 1971).

Subsequent presidents were forced to reassess America's world role. A more forceful Congress and a more wary American public sought limits on U.S. commitments. President Nixon attempted to reduce this nation's commitments without a loss in American power and influence. Containment of the Soviet Union was still accepted; this was to be achieved through diplomatic initiatives rather than force of arms. The Nixon-Kissinger view was that the Soviet leadership could be coopted into the existing international political-economic system. According to Roger P. Labrie in *SALT Handbook* (Washington, D.C.: American Enterprise Institute, 1979), President Nixon's goal was to ensure that by acquiring "a stake in this network of relationships with the West, the Soviet Union may become more conscious of what it would lose by a return to confrontation."

Détente was the new catchword in Soviet-American relations. While moving from one foreign policy success to another—opening relations with the People's Republic of China, the success of arms control negotiations with the USSR, and the finalization of a peace treaty ending the Vietnam War—President Nixon became the victim of a domestic political crisis, Watergate.

The two primary actors in this administration—President Nixon and Secretary of State Henry A. Kissinger—have proved to be prolific authors. The most insightful but cautious works are: Kissinger's *The White House Years* (Boston: Little, Brown, 1979) and *Years of Upheaval* (Boston: Little, Brown, 1982), and Richard Nixon's *RN: The Memoirs of Richard Nixon* (New York: Grosset & Dunlap, 1978). More critical assessments are provided in such diverse works as Seymour M. Hersh's *The Price of Power* (New York: Summit Books, 1983); Roger Morris's *Uncertain Greatness: Henry Kissinger and American Foreign Policy* (New York: Harper & Row, 1977); Tad Szulc's *The Illusion of Peace: Foreign Policy in the Nixon-Kissinger Years* (New York: Viking Press, 1978); and Gary Wills's *Nixon Agonistes* (Boston: Houghton Mifflin, 1970).

It was left to Gerald Ford to explain the necessary, but controversial, decision to pardon President Nixon, and Ford's efforts to continue the policy focus of his predecessor, in *A Time to Heal* (New York: Harper & Row, 1979). President Ford, however, was faced with a more hostile Congress, no longer content to play a secondary role in the formulation of foreign and defense policy.

The election of Jimmy Carter in 1976 set the stage for a return to a more traditional, moralistic policy, consistent with the American character explored by Arthur M. Schlesinger, Jr., in "Foreign Policy and the American Character," *Foreign Affairs* (Fall, 1983), and by George F. Kennan in *American Diplomacy, 1900-1950* (New York: New American Library, 1951).

While continuing to pursue a policy of détente with the Soviet Union, the Carter administration showed a definite North-South orientation. By supporting and advancing the concerns of the Third World, Carter hoped to stabilize this area and increase U.S. influence throughout the developing world. The goals were noble; the actors were sincere; and the policy initiatives were carefully developed. Nevertheless, the Carter presidency seemed unable to wield American power effectively.

There was a crisis of confidence. While President Carter pursued a policy of détente with the Soviet leadership, the Kremlin appeared to be exploiting crisis situations in Africa, the Middle East, and the Far East to advance its own position and undermine that of the United States. The Soviet invasion of Afghanistan proved to be the turning point for relations between the two superpowers. The diplomatic strains were seen as the start of a new Cold War. At this point, the administration acted more decisively, but events in Iran were to prove fatal to the president's reelection plans.

The four years of the Carter presidency are explored in significant works by several of the primary actors in the administration. Zbigniew Brzezinski's *Power and Principle: Memoirs of the National Security Advisor, 1977-1981* (New York: Farrar, Straus & Giroux, 1983) offers an insightful look at some of the significant events, programs, and policies of the Carter years. Brzezinski provides a coherent framework for the analysis of this presidency. In *Hard Choices: Critical Years in America's Foreign Policy* (New York: Simon & Schuster, 1983), Cyrus Vance focuses the reader's attention on the range of tough issues that the Carter administration was forced to tackle. These were the sad consequences of the entire pattern of past American foreign policies. The impact of the Iran hostage crisis on the president is the theme of Hamilton Jordan's *Crisis: The Last Year of the Carter Presidency* (New York: Putnam, 1982). The inner strength of Carter the man is captured in the former president's own book, *Keeping Faith: Memoirs of a President* (New York: Bantam Books, 1982).

It will be left to future political analysts and historians to assess properly President Carter's overall impact on America's status in the world. The electorate in 1980 passed judgment on the policies of the 1970s. Unwilling to accept a reduction in the status or power of the United States, it accepted the Reagan view that more must be done to reexert American influence in the world.

Reagan entered the White House committed to a program of rearming America. The security of the nation called for this. This administration seemed committed to action—even if the United States had to act unilaterally. Some analysts saw the administration overcommitting the United States. This is the view expressed in Kenneth Oye, Robert Lieber, and Donald Rothchild, eds., *Eagle Defiant: United States Foreign Policy in the 1980s* (Boston: Little, Brown, 1983). The assessments of the various articles compiled are often harsh and affected by ideological biases—a problem with many evaluations of an incumbent president's policies. A far better analysis of the events that have occurred during President Reagan's tenure is contained in the annual reports *America and the World*, published by *Foreign Affairs*.

The question being examined once again is the proper extent of the United States' responsibility for the defense of the Western nations and Western world interests. While the United States has sought to maintain free passage in the Persian Gulf, critics have argued that U.S. allies should play a greater role. There are shared interests, but is that proper justification for sharing responsibilities?

The continuing problem is that the interests and world view of the United Sates do not always coincide perfectly with those of the other partners in the Western alliance. The independence of various alliance members is readily apparent. The Siberian natural gas pipeline controversy with Western Europe, the nuclear free zone policy of New Zealand, and the lack of a uniform counterterrorism policy are but a few examples that demonstrate the limits of American power.

Then, is the safest course of action for the United States to act unilaterally to advance its own security interests? In the past, the military and economic weaknesses of the allies led to a greater sense of responsibility and increased commitments by the United States. Each postwar president recognized the security interdependence of the Western alliance. Such a policy approach enhanced the security of all the alliance members. It seems ironic that when a true situation of interdependence among nations more equal in resources and status exists in the West, the security relationship that fostered such an economic and political recovery is called into question.

The Utility of Force in the Nuclear Age

The post–World War II study of American defense policy has been dominated for the most part by the strategic nuclear debate. In this section, I shall limit myself to the subject of nuclear strategy and deterrence theory.

Nuclear weapons opened a new era in the history of man. They confronted humanity with the actual potential for destroying itself. American decision makers and defense policy analysts in the last half of the twentieth century have expressed divergent opinions on the value and projected uses of these "unique" weapons.

Though nuclear power was to usher in a new military age, the traditional factors that influenced the development of military strategy were still relevant. There are three variables through which the evolution of defense policy—both prenuclear and nuclear—can be traced. These are offered by Amos Jordan and William Taylor in *American National Security: Policy and Process* (Baltimore: Johns Hopkins University Press, 1981). They include: (1) international political and military developments, (2) domestic priorities, and (3) technological advances. This provides a convenient framework for assessing the defense decision-making environment.

As Jordan and Taylor have noted in their book, the technological status of a nation can be a prime determinant of the defense strategy that nation can pursue. However, technology is limited by man's ability to adapt and use it to meet his needs. The issue of technology is explored by Paul P. Craig and John A. Jungerman's book, *Nuclear Arms Race: Technology and Society* (New York: McGraw-Hill, 1986).

Immediately after the development of atomic weapons, the accepted military strategy in the United States was to employ the "bomb" as just another weapons system. With emerging awareness of nuclear weapons' potential, the policy of the "use" of nuclear weapons was called into question. Bernard Brodie was one of the first to write of his concerns. Notable among his works are *The Absolute Weapons* (New York: Harcourt, Brace, 1946); *Strategy in the Missile Age* (Princeton: Princeton University Press, 1959); and *Escalation and the Nuclear Option* (Princeton: Princeton University Press, 1966). It was in *The Absolute Weapon* that Brodie first observed that in the nuclear age the primary purpose of the military establishment had changed. Its responsibility was to avert war; "it can have almost no other useful purpose."

In "Atomic Weapons and American Policy," *Foreign Affairs* (July 1953): 525–35, J. Robert Oppenheimer addressed the problems that nuclear weapons created for military and diplomatic strategy. Oppenheimer's approach suggested the possibility that the new technology might have little significance for diplomacy. The destructiveness of these weapons might lead ultimately to their rejection as an instrument of policy. What Oppenheimer saw were the risks inherent in the new technology.

In 1957 Henry A. Kissinger addressed these same concerns in *Nuclear Weapons and Foreign Policy* (New York: Praeger, 1957). His perspective was radically different; he stressed the opportunities of the new technology. While Oppenheimer saw them as purely military weapons, Kissinger saw nuclear weapons possessing three characteristics: (1) military, (2) political, and (3) psychological. They could—and should—play a role in the diplomacy of the United States. In *The Necessity for Choice* (New York: Harper & Brothers, 1960), Kissinger further expanded on the psychological dimension of deterrence. He observed that deterrence required "a combination of power, the will to use it, and the assessment of these by the potential aggressor."

In essence, these two views reflected what could be considered two emerging schools of strategic thought: a "pure" deterrence school that, given the mass destructiveness of nuclear weapons, did not contemplate ever having to fight a war with such weapons, and a deterrence school that advocated development of "war-fighting" capabilities that would both make deterrence more credible and provide options in the event deterrence failed. These two differing views of deterrence were at the heart of the divergent "declaratory" policies of the Truman and Eisenhower administrations. Truman saw nuclear weapons as an instrument of terror and a weapon of last resort. Eisenhower, on the other hand, viewed these weapons as an integral component of America's defense—a weapon of perhaps first resort. The policy issues and debates of this and subsequent periods are covered in the following works: David Alan Rosenberg, "The Origins of Overkill," *International Security* (Spring 1983): 3–71; Fred M. Kaplan, *The Wizards of Armageddon* (New York: Simon & Schuster, 1983); Laurence Freedman, *The Evolution of Nuclear Strategy* (New York: St. Martin's Press, 1983); and Thomas Powers, "Choosing a Strategy for World War III," *Atlantic*, November 1984, pp. 53–64.

Even as early as 1950, there was concern in the American defense community about overdependence on a nuclear arsenal for the defense of the United States. In a formal document, NSC-68, the National Security Council endorsed a massive conventional buildup in April 1950. This policy statement foresaw the need to challenge the Soviet system in ways other than all-out war. Increased conventional capabilities tied to a politically and economically strong Western alliance would offer an additional deterrent to any Soviet aggression. Such a buildup was undertaken in conjunction with the Korean War, but this was a short-lived phenomenon. The Eisenhower administration had opted for a "massive retaliation" doctrine as the most effective—and least costly—defense strategy. Yet the concern with a lack of flexibility in the American strategy was clearly evident.

Flexible response became the declared strategy of the Kennedy and Johnson administrations. The policy direction of this period is examined in the previously cited works by Laurence Martin, *Strategic Thought in the Nuclear Age*, and Jerome Kahan, *Security in the Nuclear Age*. Two strategic approaches were considered at this time—damage limitation and assured destruction. The first sought to achieve a counterforce capability; the second strove for the protection of a retaliatory capability. Ultimately, Secretary of Defense Robert McNamara enunciated an "assured destruction" doctrine. This was seen as a way of achieving stability in strategic relations with the Soviet Union. An explanation of the acceptance of this policy is presented in McNamara's book *The Essence of Security* (New York: Harper & Row, 1968).

Another view of the defense decisions of the McNamara era is offered by Desmond Ball, *Politics and Force Levels: The Strategic Missile Program of the Kennedy Administration* (Berkeley and Los Angeles: University of California Press, 1980). Ball argues that the decisions in the 1961–1962 period resulted more from adversary processes than from rational calculations. He states that the most significant conclusion reached during his research was that force-level decisions were the product of haste and political compromise. The defense doctrine of this era "served as no more than a rationalization for decisions taken on other grounds."

Nevertheless, the defense of the United States was to be ensured by both strategic deterrence and conventional capabilities. Deterrence would be secured by the ability and willingness to launch a catastrophic retaliatory strike against an opponent. Low-threat situations could be handled by conventional forces. Critics of the strategic policy protested the underlying premise of the "assured destruction" concept—the mutual vulnerability of both civilizations. It flew in the face of the primary responsibility of a government to provide for the security of its citizens. This concept sought to stress the element of stability in superpower strategic relations.

Mutually Assured Destruction (MAD)—whether accepted as a doctrine or a condition of the nuclear age—took on a life of its own. It began to drive the military procurement, force structure, and arms control decisions of subsequent administrations. The facade of mutual vulnerability had to be maintained at all costs. It was a visible symbol of strategic stability and the irrationality of nuclear war—at least for the American advocates of a pure deterrence position. This policy appeared to close the door on the "war-fighting" strategies that had been developing simultaneously with the pure deterrence strategies.

The acceptance of MAD restricted U.S. defense options. It limited the prospects for an effective ABM system in the late 1960s and continued to plague the Strategic Defense Initiative of the Reagan administration. Morton Halperin's *Bureaucratic Politics and Foreign Policy* (Washington, D.C.: Brookings Institution, 1974) examines the decisions of the Johnson administration on the development of a limited ABM system. The concern, especially that of McNamara, was centered on the issue of fostering strategic stability with the Soviet Union. Another work, *The Fallacy of Star Wars* (New York: Random House, Vintage Books, 1984), was published in association with the Union of Concerned Scientists. Its concern is what the authors consider to be the destabilization caused by President Reagan's strategic defense concept. What is stressed in these two cases is the attention paid to the maintenance of strategic stability, even at the cost of mutual vulnerability.

The increasing military capability of the Soviet Union throughout the 1960s led to a reassessment of American policy. President Nixon, as he states in his previously mentioned autobiography, accepted the idea of parity with the USSR. He opted for a "realistic" deterrence strategy, which contained four basic pillars. First, assured destruction would have to be maintained—the United States needed a secure retaliatory capability. Second, the president needed flexible nuclear options—a continuation of the Kennedy administration's operational plans. Third, crisis stability needed to be maintained by providing the United States with a variety of ways of countering Soviet activities. This was a continuation of the conventional component of Kennedy's flexible response. Last, it was necessary to maintain perceived equality.

While MAD seemed to preclude the development of formal war-fighting strategies, the matter was far from resolved. Discussions in the strategic field of the 1970s continued to look at the possibility of limited nuclear war options. Secretary of Defense James Schlesinger advocated a more realistic policy based on a greater emphasis on counterforce weapons and targeting. While previous administrations had advocated nuclear options, little had been done to ensure the development of the appropriate war plans or even the necessary weapons systems to implement such a strategy. The intention of this approach was to bolster the deterrence value of strategic forces. This would be achieved by a visible willingness to plan for the use of nuclear weapons.

The real change was to take place in the Carter administration with the acceptance of a "countervailing" strategy. The assessment made by Secretary Harold Brown was that the best chance to deter the USSR would be to initiate a change in U.S. targeting policy. This was publicly announced in Presidential Directive 59 (PD-59). The thrust of this document was to increase the flexibility of targeting policy in order to have the capability to destroy strategic and military targets, leadership and control centers, and industrial and economic recovery targets. These were considered to be the assets most valued by the Soviet leadership. The background events leading up to this policy decision are fully explored in Brown's *Thinking about National Strategy* (Boulder, Colo.: Westview Press, 1983), and Brzezinski's *Power and Principle.*

This countervailing strategy has been continued and expanded by the Reagan administration. Assessments of the defense policies and strategies of this administration are often harsh. This view is reflected in Robert Scheer's *With Enough Shovels: Reagan, Bush and Nu-*

clear War (New York: Random House, Vintage Books, 1983), and Barry R. Posen and Steven W. Van Evera, "Reagan Administration Defense Policy: Departure from Containment," in *Eagle Resurgent: The Reagan Era in American Foreign Policy*, edited by Kenneth Oye, Robert Lieber, and Donald Rothchild (Boston: Little, Brown, 1987). The Posen-Van Evera critique centers on what they consider to be the overcommitment, irrational military construction programs, and the unilateralist tendency of the Reagan administration. A more balanced view is presented in *The Reagan Defense Program: An Interim Assessment* (Wilmington, Del: Scholarly Resources, Inc., 1984), edited by Stephen J. Cimbala.

There is an extensive literature on the evolution of nuclear strategy. The following is a list, by no means complete, of significant works in this area: William Baugh, *The Politics of Nuclear Balance: Ambiguity and Continuity in Strategic Policies* (New York: Longmans, 1984); Lawrence Freedman, *The Evolution of Nuclear Strategy* (New York: St. Martin's Press, 1981); Harvard Nuclear Study Group, *Living with Nuclear Weapons* (Cambridge: Harvard University Press, 1983); Robert Jervis, *The Illogic of American Nuclear Strategy* (Ithaca, N.Y.: Cornell University Press, 1984); Robert J. Pranger and Roger P. Labrie, *Nuclear Strategy and National Security* (Washington, D.C.: American Enterprise Institute, 1977); and Donald M. Snow, *National Security: Enduring Problems of U.S. Defense Policy* (New York: St. Martin's Press, 1987).

In this evolutionary process, the movement toward a war-fighting deterrence strategy and away from acceptance of mutual vulnerability has prompted a caustic debate in the defense community. Colin Gray, "Nuclear Strategy: The Case for a Theory of Victory" (*International Security*, Summer 1979: 54–87), is critical of the MAD position, arguing that "one cannot build a credible deterrent on an incredible action." It is the responsibility of the defense community to design options that a reasonable decision maker would not be self-deterred from ever executing. As a counter, Sir Michael Howard has argued in "Reassurance and Deterrence: Western Defense in the 1980s" (*Foreign Affairs*, Winter 1982/83) that deterrence "can no longer depend on the threat of nuclear war." The stress should be on conventional forces, and in "On Fighting a Nuclear War" (*International Security*, Spring 1981: 3–48), Sir Michael has argued further that victory in a nuclear war is not possible.

The strategic debate has now moved into the conventional force arena. Critics of the current nuclear strategies recognize that threats still exist that require a response or the ability to respond. In "Nuclear Weapons and the Atlantic Alliance" (*Foreign Affairs*, Spring 1982), McGeorge Bundy, George F. Kennan, Robert S. McNamara, and Gerard Smith question the credibility of the nuclear defense of Europe. This strategy, rather than providing security, is putting untold strains on the NATO alliance, and these authors advocate conventional forces capable of defending against a more likely Soviet conventional move against Europe. This argument is developed further in McNamara's "The Military Use of Nuclear Weapons: Perceptions and Misperceptions" (*Foreign Affairs*, Fall 1983).

The response to this argument came from four West Germans—Karl Kaiser, George Leber, Alois Mertes, and Franz-Josef Schulze. In "Nuclear Weapons and the Preservation of Peace: A Response to an American Proposal for Renouncing the First Use of Nuclear Weapons" (*Foreign Affairs*, Summer 1982), the West Germans stress the need for linkage between Europe and the American nuclear arsenal. The acceptance by NATO of the flexible response strategy mandates the nuclear defense of Europe by the United States.

The demands of the strategic environment resulting from reluctance or inability to use nuclear weapons and the public protests that occur when the subject is addressed have prompted a more thorough reassessment of the utility of conventional strategies. Works that deal with this area are: James Fallows, *National Defense* (New York: Random House, 1981); Edward N. Luttwak, *The Pentagon and the Art of War* (New York: Institute for Contemporary Studies/Simon & Schuster, 1984); Jeffrey Record, *Revising the U.S. Military: Tailoring Means to Ends* (Washington, D.C.: Pergamon-Brassey's, 1984); Andrew J. Pierre, ed., *The Conventional Defense of Europe: New Technologies and New Strategies* (New York: Council on Foreign Relations, 1986); and Stan Windass, ed., *Avoiding Nuclear War* (New York: Brassey's Defence Publishers, 1985).

What is evident is that flexible response and the corresponding levels of deterrence—from special forces units to conventional, to theater nuclear, and to strategic nuclear forces—are products of the advancing technology of the twentieth century. Nuclear weapons have given the superpowers the means of deterring an opponent and ensuring the security of the nation. On the other hand, these very weapons have complicated the security environment by opening the real possibility that the ultimate doomsday device has been invented. The utility of nuclear forces, therefore, becomes a real question.

In *The Evolution of Nuclear Strategy*, Lawrence Freedman observed the cyclical nature of debates about strategy. Freedman states that "much of what is offered today as a profound and new insight was said yesterday, and usually in a more concise and literate manner." Indeed, we already have reviewed the debate in the late 1940s and early 1950s over the utility of nuclear weapons and now have come full circle to a debate in the 1980s over essentially the same issue—the utility of nuclear weapons, whether for pure deterrence or for "warfighting": David P. Barash's *The Arms Race and Nuclear War* (Belmont, Calif.: Wadsworth, 1987); Jerome D. Frank, *Sanity and Survival in the Nuclear Age* (New York: Random House, 1982); George F. Kennan, *The Nuclear Delusion: Soviet-American Relations in the Atomic Age* (New York: Pantheon Books, 1983); John B. Harris and Eric Markusen, eds., *Nuclear Weapons and the Threat of Nuclear War* (New York: Harcourt Brace Jovanovich, 1986); Joseph S. Nye, Jr., *Nuclear Ethics* (New York: Free Press, 1986); and James P. Sterba's *The Ethics of War and Nuclear Deterrence* (Belmont, Calif.: Wadsworth, 1985).

Stability in the Nuclear Age

A basic question in the nuclear age is how best to maintain the stability of deterrence relations. There has been an ongoing debate over the stability of deterrence

based on a "mutually assured destruction" doctrine that relies primarily on survivable strategic offensive forces and that provided by a "mutually assured survival" doctrine that calls for heavy reliance on strategic defenses. To provide a credible deterrent force that does not provoke an adversary either into engaging in an arms race or undertaking a preemptive strike is a difficult goal to achieve. The mutual hostility and distrust between the two superpowers complicates this process. Through negotiations, the two sides can hope to establish a dialogue, ascertain intentions, and develop a working relationship.

The desire for stability and dialogue became more important as the Soviet Union began seriously to challenge American nuclear superiority in the mid 1960s. The purpose and goal behind arms control efforts are elaborately described in Coit D. Blacker and Gloria Duffy, eds., *International Arms Control: Issues and Agreements* (Stanford, Calif.: Stanford University Press, 1984); by Richard F. Staar, ed., in *Arms Control: Myth Versus Reality* (Stanford, Calif.: Hoover Institution Press, 1984); by Thomas C. Schelling and Morton H. Halperin in *Strategy and Arms Control* (Washington, D.C.: Pergamon-Brassey's, 1985); and by John H. Barton and Lawrence D. Weiler in *International Arms Control* (Stanford, Calif.: Stanford University Press, 1976).

It is one thing to argue for arms control; it is quite another to achieve an agreement acceptable to both sides. The actual negotiations leading up to an arms control agreement are difficult, tedious, slow, and cautious. Several participants and observers have provided glimpses of this process: John Newhouse, *Cold Dawn: The Story of SALT* (New York: Holt, Rinehart & Winston, 1973); Gerard Smith, *Doubletalk: The Story of SALT I* (New York: Doubleday and Company, 1980); and Strobe Talbott's two volumes—*Endgame: The Inside Story of SALT II* (New York: Harper & Row, 1979) and *Deadly Gambits* (New York: Knopf, 1984). The history and background of the negotiations are found in *Arms Control and Disarmament Agreements: Text and Histories of Negotiations* (Washington, D.C.: U.S. Arms Control and Disarmament Agency, 1980) and subsequent editions.

Conclusions

The superpower goals of total security have been elusive. The very nature of the strategic environment precludes either side from completely solving its security dilemma. The constant fear of the opponent's capabilities and intentions will continue to exist. Deterrence and defense strategies and arms control negotiations by themselves cannot create a climate of mutual understanding. This is the unfortunate consequence of the nuclear age, where an ineffective strategy or a failed policy carries with it such dire consequences. Albert Einstein observed that "the splitting of the atom has changed everything save our mode of thinking and thus we are drifting toward a catastrophe beyond comparison." The problem that continues to face the leadership of the United States and the Soviet Union is how to break out of this situation. This clearly is the dilemma of the nuclear age.

The Union of Soviet Socialist Republics

Kenneth A. Rogers

Why study Soviet defense policy? The answer is obvious. The Soviet Union derives its superpower status primarily from its military capabilities, and it is the military dimension that poses the greatest challenge to Western security. However, understanding Soviet defense policy has not always been an easy task. Churchill once described the Soviet Union as a riddle wrapped in a mystery inside an enigma. While the Soviet Union is somewhat better understood today, obtaining reliable information on Soviet defense policy continues to pose a challenge to the scholar interested in researching this important—and often misunderstood—area of Soviet affairs. This bibliographic essay on Soviet defense policy seeks to provide the foundation for a better understanding of potential sources of information by acquainting the reader with a basic appreciation of the types of primary and secondary sources available to the researcher.

This essay incorporates and expands on the bibliographic essay written by Schuyler Foerster in the preceeding edition of this text. To facilitate gathering information on Soviet defense policy, an appendix listing some of the major libraries, book stores, and addresses of relevant publishers of Soviet defense policy related materials is included. The "Selected Bibliography on the Soviet Military Establishment" by Jerome Martin that follows this bibliographic essay provides the reader with an in-depth listing of available sources on Soviet defense policy.

Understanding Soviet Defense Policy

Over the years, a number of factors have prevented Western scholars from having a firm understanding of Soviet defense policy. One of the primary causes has been a lack of appreciation for such influences on Soviet behavior as history, ideology, domestic affairs, and geostrategic considerations. For example, Russian czarist traditions and events such as the Bolshevik Revolution, Allied intervention during World War I, the Great Patriotic War (World War II), and the development of nuclear weapons, as well as more recent events such as the Cuban missile crisis and Afghanistan, have undoubtedly influenced Soviet military thinking. Some Western scholars state that historical influences have made the Soviets more defensive in nature, while others argue that this has prompted a more aggressive Soviet defense posture.

The exact impact of ideology on Soviet policy has been widely debated. The role of Marxism-Leninism and subsequent modifications by Soviet leaders have undoubtedly influenced Soviet perceptions of the USSR's role in world affairs; which, in turn, has had an impact on defense policy formulation in a number of areas, such as the ability to project power and maintain defense readiness.

Domestic considerations such as leadership personalities, bureaucratic competition, and economic performance have also influenced Soviet defense policy formulation. Individual Soviet leaders can affect Soviet defense policy thinking, as witnessed by the dramatic shifts in Soviet foreign and defense policies associated with Stalin's and Khrushchev's views on nuclear weapons and the role of conventional forces. For example, Stalin did not believe that nuclear weapons dramatically changed the nature of warfare. Hence, he downplayed the role of nuclear weapons, instead preferring to concentrate on conventional forces. In contrast, Khrushchev believed that destructiveness associated with nuclear weapons did dramatically alter the nature of warfare. Hence, he opted for "Peaceful Coexistence" and emphasized the role of nuclear forces over conventional forces in order to reduce the economic burden of defense expenditures on the Soviet economy. Defense policy formulation also can be influenced during periods of leadership succession—as witnessed by the relative stagnation in Soviet policy formulation during the Brezhnev succession. Bureaucratic competition among the various military services, other defense related organizations, as well as competition between the nondefense and defense sectors have occurred, especially during periods of poor economic performance.

Geostrategic considerations such as the stability of Eastern Europe, Sino-Soviet relations, and U.S.–Soviet relations also have had a profound impact on Soviet defense policy. For example, the relative lack of stability in Eastern Europe since World War II undoubtedly has forced the USSR to question the reliability of its Warsaw Pact allies, thus necessitating it to continue to shoulder a large part of Warsaw Pact defense. The Sino-Soviet rift has forced the Soviets to deploy a considerable amount of military resources to the Far East as well as attempt to thwart Chinese influence in the Third World. The state of U.S.–Soviet relations can influence Soviet policy, as witnessed by the massive Soviet military buildup that took place after the Cuban missile crisis, culminating with the USSR reaching parity with the United States during the early 1970s.

Moreover, it is difficult fully to appreciate Soviet defense policy without understanding Western defense policies—especially U.S. policy—since defense policy rarely is formed in a vacuum without regard to outside influences. Hence, an appreciation of others' defense policies will aid the scholar in gaining a more thorough understanding of outside influences that could have an impact on Soviet defense thinking. It is with the realization of the potential impact of these factors that the scholar should proceed in the study of Soviet defense policy.

Ethnocentrism also can cloud our understanding of Soviet defense policy. For example, after World War II many U.S. decision makers believed that the destructiveness of nuclear weapons coupled with increasingly sophisticated technology would prompt Soviet military strategists to adopt defense policies similar to those adopted by the United States. When it was determined that Soviet defense policies did not necessarily conform to what U.S. observers had expected, it was frequently thought that Soviet policy was in its early stages of development and eventually would conform to American expectations. When it became increasingly evident that this divergence in Soviet defense policies from U.S. expectations was not transitory, it was realized slowly that unique Russian and Soviet experiences likely caused Soviet decision makers to perceive events differently. While it is extremely difficult for the Western researcher to view the world from a Soviet perspective, every attempt should be made to suppress ethnocentric biases.

Finally, one of the major problems in understanding Soviet defense policy has been the difficulty of obtaining timely and reliable data from official Soviet sources. While this poses an obstacle to research, it does not prevent the researcher from gaining a basic understanding of Soviet defense policy, since a wide body of primary and secondary sources is available.

Primary Source Materials

One key to researching Soviet defense policy is access to original Soviet source materials. However, many scholars lack adequate knowledge of Russian. In the past, the analysis of primary sources has been the province of a few select scholars who, by virtue of their linguistic ability and experience, were capable of detecting nuances and sharing their insights with other scholars in the field. In more recent years, this problem of access has been lessened somewhat by the substantial amount of translated material available—albeit generally from U.S. government sources. Nevertheless, relying on available translations can pose the risk of missing important material, not gaining a representative sample of Soviet defense thinking, or possibly relying on inaccurately translated material if the translator either makes an error, is imprecise, or incorporates biases. Therefore, whenever possible, cross-checking by re-translating potentially critical passages is recommended.

In addition to language difficulties, other potential problems confront the scholar who is interested in researching original Soviet sources. For example, Soviet sources generally are difficult and arduous to read. The writing style can be ponderous, propagandistic, and excessively ideological. Moreover, because of the secretive nature of Soviet society, sensitive material on Soviet defense policy often has been difficult to obtain, the reliability of the information sometimes has been in doubt, and frequently it has been outdated. Obviously, censorship plays an important role. It restricts not only the availability of information, but also the quality of the published material. Moreover, at times the reliability of some information must be questioned due either to inaccurate data or deliberate efforts at disinformation. Attempts at disinformation are not uncommon, and

the researcher must attempt to cross-check crucial information with as many sources as possible. Another major problem is that by the time defense policy thinking is published in the open Soviet press, it is frequently outdated.

The foregoing discussion is not intended to discourage scholars from researching original Soviet sources. On the contrary, it is intended to outline some of the potential pitfalls so as to enable researchers to make informed choices about available primary source information. Although the reader faces disadvantages in studying the defense policy of a closed society, there is one important point to remember: the Soviet media generally reflect Soviet policy, and a reader can gain insight into Soviet thinking by carefully following responses to specific events. Hence, while censorship can complicate the researcher's task in understanding Soviet defense policy, it does not present an insurmountable obstacle. For example, at times the censor will not delete all sensitive and interesting information. At other times, by understanding the problems associated with pervasive censorship, one can "read between the lines" and sift out valuable information. For example, sometimes Soviet writers—knowing the problems of censorship—will discuss a specific issue historically with the intent of sending a more contemporary message that the author knows would be censored.

RUSSIAN-LANGUAGE MATERIALS

Where should the researcher look for primary source materials on Soviet defense policy? Obviously, there are certain classic Soviet works relevant to the study of defense policy such as V. D. Sokolovskiy's *Voyennaya strategiya* (*Military Strategy*). While these sources provide important information, the researcher must be aware that many of the "classics" are now outdated, and hence less relevant today.

There are numerous Soviet sources that publish materials that at least touch on Soviet defense policy. While it is beyond the scope of this essay to discuss all of these sources, two defense-related publishers merit special mention. One of the most important sources is Voyennoye Izdatel'stvo (Voyenizdat), the Soviet Ministry of Defense publishing house. The researcher can find a variety of books on a wide range of military and defense policy topics in Voyenizdat's output. Two useful sources published by Voyenizdat that are usually readily available are the *Sovetskaya voyennaya entsiklopediya* (*Soviet Military Encyclopedia*), and the *Voyenniy entsiklopedicheskiy slovar'* (*Military Encyclopedic Dictionary*). The former currently consists of eight volumes (a new edition is forthcoming) and provides information on a wide range of Soviet military issues; the latter also is an excellent source, especially for biographical information on Soviet military leaders and definitions of military-related terms. Another Ministry of Defense publishing house, Krasnaya Zvezda, publishes several important defense-related journals that will be highlighted below.

Three of the better-known Soviet military journals are: *Voyenno-istoricheskiy zhurnal* (*Military-Historical Journal*), published monthly by the General Staff of the Ministry of Defense and one of the best Soviet military journals, it provides not only historical examples of Soviet doctrine and tactics, but also insight into more recent policy; *Voyennaya mysl'* (*Military Thought*), a restricted journal published by the Soviet General Staff (a number of the issues from the 1960s and 1970s have been made available by the U.S. government to the public), which highlights the development of Soviet doctrine; and *Kommunist vooruzhennykh sil* (*Communist of the Armed Forces*), published biweekly by the main political directorate, which provides insight into political-military issues.

Four of the five Soviet military services openly publish journals: *Aviatsiya i kosmonavtika* (*Aviation and Cosmonautics*), published monthly by the Soviet Air Force; *Vestnik protivovozdushnoy oborony* (*Herald of Air Defense*), published monthly by the Soviet Air Defense Forces; *Voyennyy vestnik* (*Military Herald*), published monthly by the Soviet Army; and *Morskoy sbornik* (*Naval Collections*), published monthly by the Soviet Navy. Other more specialized military journals include: *Agitator armiy i flota* (*Agitator of the Army and Navy*), *Voyennoye znaniye* (*Military Knowledge*), *Znamenosets* (*Banner Carrier*), *Sovetskiy voin* (*Soviet Soldier*), *Teknika i vooruzheniye* (*Equipment and Armaments*), and *Tyl i snabzheniye sovetskikh voorzhennykh sil* (*Rear and Supply of the Soviet Armed Forces*). In addition, the official Soviet military newspaper, *Krasnaya zvezda* (*Red Star*), is an excellent source for daily information on the Soviet military and can provide useful information on defense-related activities and military personalities. Other Soviet journals and newspapers—while not specifically dedicated to Soviet defense issues—also can prove useful. For example, *Kommunist* (*Communist*), the official journal of the Communist Party of the Soviet Union (translated copies available through the Joint Publications Research Service—JPRS); *Pravda* (*Truth*), the Party newspaper; and *Izvestiya* (*News*), the government newspaper, can provide useful information at times, especially during special military events or military holidays. While the availability of each of the above sources varies, major university libraries and research institutions can usually provide access to many of them.

ENGLISH-LANGUAGE MATERIALS

There is a surprising amount of Soviet material available in English. The Soviet publishing house Progress Publishers produces books on a wide variety of topics, which can be useful for the researcher investigating Soviet defense policy. In addition, there are a number of Soviet journals published in several languages that can provide worthwhile information on defense-related issues: *Soviet Military Review*, published monthly by the Ministry of Defense in Russian, English, Arabic, Dary (or Dari, a language spoken in Afghanistan), French, Portuguese, and Spanish; *International Affairs*, published monthly in Russian, English, and French by the All-Union Znaniye Society; and *New Times*, published weekly in Russian, English, French, German, Spanish, Portuguese, Italian, Polish, and Czech by Trud.

There also is a wealth of translated information available for the researcher interested in primary source materials. One continuing source for major Soviet military writings is the *Soviet Military Thought* series, available from the U.S. Government Printing Office. Translated and published under the auspices of the U.S. Air Force, this series presently consists of twenty-two volumes. In addition, *Soviet Press: Selected Translations*, published bimonthly under the auspices of the Direc-

torate of Soviet Affairs, U.S. Air Force, provides translations of Soviet defense-related articles from a wide variety of Soviet military publications. Another avenue for gaining access to this literature is through publications that routinely screen and translate the Soviet press. Within the U.S. government there are two vehicles for doing this. The most familiar is the Foreign Broadcast Information Service (FBIS) *Daily Report: Soviet Union*, published Monday through Friday, which includes not only translations of the Soviet press, but also Soviet radio and television coverage. The Joint Publications Research Service (JPRS) translates books, articles, and monographs on a variety of subjects. For example, *USSR Report: Military Affairs* provides a readily available source for translations of Soviet military writings. While JPRS reports may not be readily available in some libraries, these reports are accessible through the National Technical Information Service of the Department of Commerce. *The Soviet Review*, published quarterly by M. E. Sharpe, Inc., occasionally provides unabridged translations of Soviet defense-related articles. The *Current Digest of the Soviet Press*, published weekly by the American Association for the Advancement of Slavic Studies, and *Reprints from the Soviet Press*, published biweekly by Compass Publications, Inc., provide a wide variety of translated articles from the Soviet press. In addition, *Pravda* is now available in English and is published daily on a delayed basis by Charles Cox Associated Publishers. Usually, one of these publications is available in major libraries.

To help readers identify relevant Soviet sources on Soviet defense policy, a key research aid to original language sources that is published in English is the four-volume *Bibliographic Indexes of Soviet Military Books* by William F. and Harriet Fast Scott. Over 10,000 Soviet military books and pamphlets have been indexed for the period 1960–84. Volumes for subsequent years are published periodically. They also have published a useful reference source entitled "Soviet Bibliographies and Their Use as Research Aids," which is extremely helpful in identifying Soviet-produced bibliographies, books, and journals. These publications have been published under the auspices of the Defense Nuclear Agency (DNA) and can be obtained as DNA Reports.

Secondary Source Materials

The past few years have witnessed a dramatic expansion in the study of Soviet defense policy in the West, especially since the ambitious Soviet military buildup of the 1960s. This, in turn, has produced a wealth of secondary source material. Researchers must, however, understand some of the potential problems with using secondary sources. For example, Soviet defense policy is rarely viewed by scholars in its totality. More often than not, the literature includes, in recurring publications, articles dealing with more specific aspects of Soviet security affairs. In viewing this literature, the reader must realize that such articles may reflect institutional interests, editorial bias, or policy advocacy on the part of the journal or individual author. The reader can only hope to rectify this inevitable slant in the literature by reading broadly and critically. Although this is true of most policy-related writings, it is especially true of the literature on Soviet defense policy because of the high degree of uncertainty that characterizes our knowledge of the USSR as well as the policy stakes that may exist on any particular issue.

U.S. SOURCES

Within the United States, there is an abundance of material published on Soviet defense issues. Archive materials from a number of sources are available. Moreover, numerous books are published on Soviet military and defense thinking. Among other publishers, Westview Press regularly issues books dealing with Soviet defense policy. The major works will be cited in the selected bibliography on the Soviet military establishment following this essay.

Virtually any Soviet-oriented journal or any journal that deals in any way with international security issues will contain at least an occasional article on Soviet defense policy. Four academic journals do so on a regular basis: *Orbis*, published quarterly by the Foreign Policy Research Institute in association with the Graduate Program in International Relations, University of Pennsylvania; *International Security*, published quarterly by the Center for Science and International Affairs, Harvard University; *Armed Forces and Society*, published quarterly by the Inter-University Seminar on Armed Forces and Society; and *Comparative Strategy*, a journal published quarterly for the Strategic Studies Center, SRI International, by Crane, Russak, & Co. Two additional U.S. journals have consistently opposing perspectives on Soviet defense policy, particularly insofar as these views relate to U.S. defense policy issues: *Strategic Review*, published quarterly by the United States Strategic Institute, and the *Defense Monitor*, published ten times annually by the Center for Defense Information. Both of these organizations conduct research and advocate policy positions in Washington, D.C.; the former tends to adopt a more pessimistic view of Soviet military power as being more threatening, while the latter tends to take a somewhat more optimistic perspective. The "Soviet Aerospace Almanac," published annually in March by the Air Force Association in *Air Force Magazine*, provides a useful research guide to the Soviet armed forces. The "Gallery of Soviet Aerospace Weapons" and articles on Soviet military leadership and organization provide up-to-date information on these important aspects of the Soviet military. In addition, *Aviation Week and Space Technology*, published weekly by McGraw-Hill, frequently provides information on the latest Soviet weapons systems technology.

In addition to journals, there are numerous research institutes and centers that routinely publish articles on Soviet defense policy. For example, the Brookings Institution and the Hoover Institution on War, Revolution and Peace publish occasional monographs that provide analysis of Soviet defense issues. The former tends to take a liberal interpretation of Soviet capabilities and intentions, while the latter takes a more conservative view. The RAND Corporation is an important source for the study of Soviet defense policy. The RAND/UCLA Center for the Study of Soviet International Behavior (CSSIB) periodically publishes monographs on Soviet defense issues through the CSSIB Occasional Paper Series and the recently established CSSIB Joint Reports Series. In addition, the RAND Paper Series publishes occasional monographs on Soviet defense policy

issues. The National Strategy Information Center, Inc., has produced numerous books, agenda papers, and strategy papers on Soviet defense issues. The center presents a wide range of views and provides some good analytical insights into Soviet defense thinking. In addition, the College Station Paper Series published by the Center for Strategic Technology, Texas A&M University, provides excellent analysis on a host of Soviet defense-related issues, such as military strategy and tactics, military personalities, and defense organization. For example, volume 1 of its publication *Organizing for War: The Soviet Military Establishment Viewed Through the Prism of the Military District* is the most up to date and complete work available on the Soviet military districts; and volume 2, *A Directory of Soviet Military District Officials*, provides reliable and timely information on Soviet military personalities.

Other sources address Soviet defense policy more indirectly, dealing with the broader issues of international politics. Yet, they are worth consulting on a regular basis not only because it is difficult to separate defense policy and international issues, but also because Soviet defense policy can often be understood better in this broader context. Articles on Soviet defense issues are occasionally published by a number of journals: *Foreign Affairs*, now published five times a year by the Council on Foreign Relations; *Foreign Policy*, published quarterly by the Carnegie Endowment for International Peace; *International Studies Quarterly*, published quarterly by the International Studies Association; *World Politics*, published quarterly by the Princeton University Press; the *Washington Quarterly*, published quarterly by the MIT Press for the Center for Strategic and International Studies (CSIS) of Georgetown University; *Atlantic Community Quarterly*, published quarterly by the Atlantic Council of the United States and the Helen Dwight Reid Educational Foundation; the *Journal of International Affairs* (originally *Columbia Journal of International Affairs*), published quarterly by the School of International and Public Affairs, Columbia University; *Global Affairs*, published quarterly by the International Security Council; *Arms Control Today*, published ten times a year by the Arms Control Association; and *Proceedings*, published monthly by the U.S. Naval Institute.

A number of U.S. government agencies also publish relevant materials on a recurring basis. The Department of Defense (DoD) periodically publishes unclassified monographs related to Soviet defense policy. For example, *Soviet Military Power*, published annually by DoD, provides a useful and updated look at Soviet military capabilities and latest trends in systems acquisition. The Studies in Communist Affairs Series published under the auspices of the U.S. Air Force can provide in-depth analysis of Soviet defense affairs from a Western perspective. The Defense Intelligence Agency (DIA) and the Central Intelligence Agency (CIA) periodically publish unclassified monographs on Soviet defense issues such as doctrine, strategy, and force development. Congressional hearings and reports can occasionally provide insight into Soviet defense-related issues, especially arms control. The *Department of State Bulletin*, published monthly by the Office of Public Communications in the Bureau of Public Affairs, Department of State, is worth consulting, especially on U.S.–Soviet arms control initiatives. In addition, *Problems of Communism*, published bimonthly by the U.S. Information Agency, and the *Radio Liberty Research Bulletin*, published weekly by Radio Free Europe/Radio Liberty, usually provide insightful analyses and occasionally publish articles on Soviet defense policy related issues. In addition, the DoD and military service schools of the army, navy, and air force publish journals and monographs that occasionally address Soviet defense policy issues: *Air Power Journal* (quarterly), *Military Review* (monthly), *Parameters* (quarterly), *Naval War College Review* (now quarterly), and periodic monographs from the various DoD and military staff and war colleges.

CANADIAN SOURCES

There are a number of Canadian sources that routinely publish analyses of Soviet defense policy. *Soviet Armed Forces Review Annual* (*SAFRA*), published annually by the Russian Micro Project, Dalhousie University, University of Halifax, is a valuable research source for Soviet military affairs. *SAFRA* provides quantitative data on the Soviet military, as well as analysis of events and trends in the Soviet armed forces. SAFRA Papers, occasional papers on Soviet defense related issues, also can provide useful analysis of the Soviet armed forces. *Conflict Quarterly*, published quarterly by the Centre for Conflict Studies, University of New Brunswick, provides occasional Soviet defense-related articles.

EUROPEAN SOURCES

Since each European country has its own litany of publications that pertain to Soviet defense policy, it is beyond the scope of this essay to name them all. Moreover, since the publications outside the United Kingdom are generally published in languages other than English, this essay will focus on British journals. Nevertheless, it is important to remember that other European countries—especially the East European and major West European countries—also publish journals that at least occasionally address Soviet defense and foreign policy issues and are worth consulting if the researcher has the appropriate language capability.

While European publications pertinent to Soviet defense policy undoubtedly suffer from many of the same criticisms that American sources do, there appears to be less of a concern for policy advocacy and hence more of a tendency for objectivity and depth of analysis. Indeed, perhaps the most consistently objective and insightful publications on Soviet defense policy and related international security issues are those published by the International Institute for Strategic Studies (IISS) in London. There are four useful publications from IISS: a bimonthly journal, *Survival*, which includes articles and important primary source documents; occasional Adelphi Papers, a series of monographs on a variety of security issues by single authors; the annual *Strategic Survey*, reviewing the political context and trends for international security of significant events of the previous year; and the annual *Military Balance*, which remains the best unclassified source of national and alliance force postures, including a quantitative assessment of Soviet military strength and defense spending.

There are several additional European journals that merit at least an occasional review: *International Af-*

fairs, published quarterly by Butterworth for the Royal Institute of International Affairs (RUSI), Guildford; the *Journal of Strategic Studies*, published quarterly by Frank Cass & Co., London; *NATO Review*, published bimonthly by the NATO Information Service, Brussels; the *RUSI Journal*, published quarterly by the Royal United Services Institute for Defence Studies, London; *Survey*, published quarterly by Survey Ltd., in association with the Institute for European Defence and Strategic Studies, London; *Soviet Studies*, a quarterly journal on the USSR and Eastern Europe, published by the Longman Group UK, Ltd., for the University of Glasgow, Scotland; and *International Defense Review*, published monthly by Interavia, Geneva. While these journals generally include articles on Soviet military doctrine and organization, *International Defense Review* is primarily devoted to a review of Soviet force-posture and weapons systems issues.

In addition, Defence Studies at the University of Edinburgh, Scotland, publishes periodic analyses of Soviet defense policy.

OTHER SOURCES

There are a number of non-U.S. and non-European sources that can provide useful information on Soviet defense policy related issues. However, frequently they are published in languages other than English. Notable exceptions are journals published in Australia, New Zealand, and South Africa. In addition, some journals in India, Pakistan, and Israel are published in English. Refer to *Ulrich's International Periodicals Directory* (specifically the military section), available in the research section of libraries, for current foreign periodicals that could contain articles related to Soviet defense policy.

CONCLUSIONS

There is a wealth of information available to the scholar interested in researching Soviet defense policy. One problem may be the ability to choose selectively the best source. This essay has attempted to provide the researcher with a better understanding of the potential sources of information that are available, as well as some of the potential pitfalls facing the scholar interested in researching Soviet defense policy.

For the reader just beginning to research Soviet defense policy, it would be beneficial to have a basic understanding of Soviet domestic and foreign policy. There are a number of classic works on the Soviet Union that are worth consulting. These sources are outlined in the selected bibliography on the Soviet military establishment by Jerome Martin that follows this bibliographic essay.

Research Source Guide

This guide to research sources is not intended to be all-encompassing. Rather, it is intended to provide a somewhat geographically distributed listing of some of the available sources for research on Soviet defense policy.

LIBRARIES

There are a number of libraries across the country that can provide useful information on Soviet defense policy. Since it is beyond the scope of this Appendix to list them all, some of the libraries with larger collections of foreign policy and defense-related materials are listed below.

The DoD and military war colleges, command and staff schools, and service academy libraries.

The East: the Ivy League universities, especially Harvard and Columbia; Syracuse University; the Library of Congress (open to the public), and the Pentagon's Army Library (open to U.S. government employees), Washington, D.C.

The Midwest: University of Illinois, University of Indiana, and Ohio State University.

The West: Stanford University to include the Hoover Institution, University of California at Berkeley, University of Southern California, and the University of California at Los Angeles.

BOOKSTORES

There are a number of bookstores that specialize in primary source materials on Soviet defense policy in both Russian and English: Globus Slavic Bookstore, 332 Balboa St., San Francisco, CA 94121; Imported Publications, Inc., 320 West Ohio Street, Chicago, IL 60610; Victor Kamkin, Inc., 12224 Parklawn Drive, Rockville, MD 20852; Victor Kamkin, Inc., 149 Fifth Ave., New York, NY 10010; and Znanie Bookstore, 5237 Geary Blvd., San Francisco, CA 94121.

PUBLICATIONS

Adelphi Papers; The Sales Department, IISS; 23 Tavistock St.; London WC2E 7NQ, UK

Air Force Magazine; Air Force Association; 1501 Lee Hwy.; Arlington, VA 22209-1198

Air University Review (discontinued) and *Air Power Journal*; Air University; Maxwell AFB, AL 36112

Arms Control Today; Arms Control Association; 11 Dupont Circle; Washington, D.C. 20036

Armed Forces and Society; Inter-University Seminar on Armed Forces and Society; Seven Locks Press; P.O. Box 27; Cabin John, MD 20818

Atlantic Community Quarterly; Atlantic Council of the US; 1616 H St., N.W.; Washington D.C. 20006

Aviation Week and Space Technology; McGraw-Hill, Inc.; 1221 Avenue of the Americas; New York, NY 10020

Brookings Institution; Foreign Policies Studies Program; 1775 Massachusetts Ave., N.W.; Washington, D.C. 20036

Central Intelligence Agency (CIA); Unclassified reports available through the National Technical Information Service (see NTIS)

College Station Paper Series; Center for Strategic Technology; Texas A&M University; College Station, TX 77843

Comparative Strategy; Crane, Russak and Co., Inc.; now Taylor and Francis, Inc., 242 Cherry St.; Philadelphia, PA 19106-1906

Conflict Quarterly; Centre for Conflict Studies; University of New Brunswick; Fredericton, New Brunswick E3B 5A3, Canada

Current Digest of the Soviet Press; American Association for the Advancement of Slavic Studies and American Council of Learned Societies; 1480 West Lane Ave.; Columbus, OH 43221-3987

Defense Intelligence Agency (DIA); RTS-2A; Washington, D.C. 20301

Defense Monitor; Center for Defense Information; 1500 Mass. Ave., N.W.; Washington, D.C. 20024

Defense Nuclear Agency (DNA); Washington, D.C. 20305

Department of State Bulletin; Bureau of Public Affairs; Department of State; 2201 C St., N.W.; Washington D.C. 20520

Foreign Affairs; Council on Foreign Relations, Inc.; 58 East 68th St.; New York, NY 10021

Foreign Broadcast Information Service (FBIS); Reports available through the National Technical Information Service (see NTIS)

Foreign Policy; Carnegie Endowment for International Peace; Subscriptions Department; P.O. Box 984; Farmingdale, NY 11737

Global Affairs; International Security Council; 393 Fifth Ave.; New York, NY 10016

Hoover Institution on War, Revolution and Peace; Stanford University; Stanford, CA 94305

International Affairs (Moscow); All-Union Znaniye Society; 14 Gorokhovsky Pereulok; Moscow K-16, USSR

International Affairs; Royal Institute of International Affairs; Butterworth Scientific, Ltd.; Westbury House; Bury St.; P.O. Box 63; Guildford GU2 5BH, UK

International Defense Review; Interavia S.A.; International Center Cointrin, 20; Route de Pre-Bois; P.O. Box 636; 1215 Geneva 15; Switzerland

International Security; Center for Science and International Affairs; The MIT Press Journals; 55 Haywark St.; Cambridge, MA 02142

International Studies Quarterly; International Studies Association; Butterworth Publishers; 80 Montvale Ave.; Stoneham, MA 02180

Joint Publications Information Service; 1000 N. Glebe Rd.; Arlington, VA 22201

Journal of International Affairs; School of International and Public Affairs; International Affairs Bldg.; Columbia University; New York, NY 10027

Journal of Strategic Studies; Frank Cass & Co., Ltd.; Gainsborough House; 11 Gainsborough Rd.; London E11 1RS, UK

Military Balance; The Sales Department, IISS; 23 Tavistock St.; London WC2E 7NQ, UK

Military Review; U.S. Army Command and General Staff College; Fort Leavenworth, KS 66027-6910

National Technical Information Service (NTIS); Department of Commerce; 5285 Port Royal Road; Springfield, VA 22161

NATO Review; NATO Information Service; 1110 Brussels, Belgium. Editions in English can be obtained from: Bureau of Public Affairs (PA/OAP); U.S. Department of State; Room 5815A; Washington, D.C. 20520

Naval War College Review; U.S. Naval War College; Newport, RI 02841-5010

New Times; Pushkin Square; Moscow; GSP 103782, USSR

Orbis; Foreign Policy Research Institute; 3615 Chestnut St.; Philadelphia, PA 19104

Parameters; U.S. Army War College; Carlisle Barracks, PA 17013

Pravda (in English); Associated Publishers, Inc.; 2233 University Ave.; Room 225; St. Paul, MN 55114

Problems of Communism; U.S. Information Agency; 301 4th St., S.W.; Washington, D.C. 20547

Proceedings; U.S. Naval Institute; 2026 Generals Hwy.; Annapolis, MD 21402

Radio Liberty Research Bulletin; RFE/RL; 1775 Broadway; New York, NY 10019

RAND Corporation; 1700 Main St.; P.O. Box 2138; Santa Monica, CA 90406-2138

Reprints from the Soviet Press; Compass Publications, Inc.; 115 E. 87th St.; P.O. Box 12F; New York, NY 10128

RUSI Journal; Royal United Services Institute for Defence Studies; Whitehall, London SW1A 2ET, England

SAFRA; Russian Micro Project; Dalhousie University; University of Halifax; Halifax, N.S. B3H 4H8, Canada

Soviet Military Power; Superintendent of Documents; U.S. Government Printing Office; Washington, D.C. 20402

Soviet Military Review (Moscow); 2 Marshal Biryuzov St.; Moscow 123298, USSR

Soviet Military Thought Series; Superintendent of Documents; U.S. Government Printing Office; Washington, D.C. 20402

Soviet Press: Selected Translations; AFIA/INIP; Bldg. 1304; Stop 18; Bolling AFB; Washington, D.C. 20332

The Soviet Review; M.E. Sharpe, Inc.; 80 Business Park Dr.; Armonk, N.Y. 10504

Soviet Studies; Longman Group UK, Ltd.; Subscriptions (Journals) Department; Fourth Ave.; Harlow, Essex CM19 5AA, UK

Strategic Review; United States Strategic Institute; 265 Winter St.; Waltham, MA 02154

Strategic Survey; The Sales Department, IISS; 23 Tavistock St.; London WC2E 7NQ, England

Studies in Communist Affairs Series; Superintendent of Documents; U.S. Government Printing Office; Washington, D.C. 20402

Survey; Subscriptions Office; 44 Great Windmill St., London W1V 7PA, England

Survival; The Sales Department, IISS; 23 Tavistock St.; London WC2E 7NQ, England

Washington Quarterly; Center for Strategic and International Studies; MIT Press Journals; 55 Hayward St.; Cambridge, MA 02142

World Politics; Center of International Studies; Princeton University; Princeton University Press; 3175 Princeton Pike; Lawrenceville, NJ 08648

USSR: The Soviet Military Establishment

Jerome V. Martin

This selected bibliography is a survey of published works on the military forces of the USSR, with an additional short listing of books on the Soviet Union, the Soviet government, and Soviet foreign policy to provide a background for those readers not familiar with these areas. This bibliography is not all inclusive, but will provide a solid foundation for the study of the Soviet military. The titles below are intended to complement the preceding bibliographic essay by Ken Rogers, which should be consulted for information on primary sources, journals, and materials available from institutes and government agencies.

BACKGROUND ON THE SOVIET UNION

Barghoorn, Frederick C., and Thomas F. Remington. *Politics in the USSR*. Boston: Little, Brown and Company, 1986.

Brzezinski, Zbigniew, and Samuel P. Huntington. *Political Power: USA/USSR*. UK: Penguin Books, 1978.

Dallin, David J. *Soviet Foreign Policy after Stalin*. New York: J. B. Lippincott Co., 1961.

Fainsod, Merle. *How Russia Is Ruled*. Cambridge: Harvard University Press, 1963.

Florinsky, Michael T. *Russia: A History and an Interpretation*. Vols 1 & 2. New York: Macmillan, 1953.

Gregory, Paul R., and Robert Stuart. *Soviet Economic Structure and Performance*. 3rd ed. New York: Harper & Row, 1986.

Hammer, Darrell P. *USSR: The Politics of Oligarchy*. New York: Praeger Publishers, 1974.

Hazard, John N. *The Soviet System of Government*. Chicago: University of Chicago Press, 1964.

Heller, Mikhail, and Aleksandr Nekrich. Trans. Phyllis B. Carlos. *Utopia in Power: The History of the Soviet Union from 1917 to the Present*. New York: Summit Books, 1986.

Hoffmann, Erik P., and Frederic J. Fleron, Jr. *The Conduct of Soviet Foreign Policy*. Chicago: Aldine Publishing Co., 1977.

Hough, Jerry F. *Soviet Leadership in Transition*. Washington, D.C.: The Brookings Institution, 1980.

Howe, G. Melvyn. *The Soviet Union: A Geographical Survey*. Estover, Plymouth, U.K.: MacDonald and Evans, 1983.

LeFeber, Walter. *America, Russia and the Cold War, 1945–1971*. New York: John Wiley and Sons, 1972.

Lydolph, Paul E. *Geography of the USSR: Topical Analysis*. Elkhart Kale, Wis.: Misty Valley Publishing, 1979.

Nove, Alec. *The Soviet Economic System*. 3rd ed. Boston: Allen & Unwin, 1986.

———. *An Economic History of the USSR*, revised ed. Baltimore: Penguin Books, 1969.

Papp, Daniel S. *Soviet Policies toward the Developing World during the 1980s*. Washington D.C.: GPO, 1986.

Pipes, Richard. *Russia under the Old Regime*. New York: Charles Scribner's Sons, 1974.

Reshetar, John S., Jr. *The Soviet Polity*. New York: Harper and Row, 1978.

Riasanovsky, Nicholas V. *A History of Russia*. 4th ed. New York: Oxford University Press, 1984.

Rosser, Richard F. *An Introduction to Soviet Foreign Policy*. Englewood Cliffs, N.J.: Prentice-Hall, 1969.

Rubinstein, Alvin Z., ed. *The Foreign Policy of the Soviet Union*. New York: Random House, 1972.

Shapiro, Leonard. *The Communist Party of the Soviet Union*. New York: Vintage Books, 1978.

———. *The Government and Politics of the Soviet Union*. New York: Vintage Books, 1971.

Skilling, H. Gordon, and Franklyn Griffiths. *Interest Groups in Soviet Politics*. Princeton: Princeton University Press, 1973.

Swartz, Morton. *The Foreign Policy of the USSR: Domestic Factors*. Encino, Calif.: Dickenson Publishing Co., 1975.

Treadgold, Donald W. *Twentieth Century Russia*. 6th ed. Boulder, Colo.: Westview Press, 1987.

Ulam, Adam B. *Expansion and Coexistence*. New York: Praeger Publishers, 1976.

U.S. Congress, Committee on Foreign Affairs. *Soviet Diplomacy and Negotiating Behavior*. Washington D.C.: GPO, 1980.

U.S. Congress, Committee on Foreign Relations. *Perceptions: Relations between the United States and the Soviet Union*. Washington D.C.: GPO, n.d.

Zimmerman, William. *Soviet Perspectives on International Relations, 1956–1967*. Princeton: Princeton University Press, 1969.

GENERAL MILITARY

Alexander, Arthur J. *Decision-Making in Soviet Weapons Procurement*. Adelphi Papers, Nos. 147/8. Winter 1978. London: International Institute for Strategic Studies.

———. *Knowing About Soviet Weapons Acquisition and Strategic Weapons*. RAND Paper P-7247. Santa Monica, Cal: RAND Corporation, 1986.

Baxter, William P. *The Soviet Way of War*. Novato, Cal: Presidio Press, 1986.

Beaumont, Roger. *Maskirovka: Soviet Camouflage, Concealment and Deception*. Stratech Paper Series—SS82-1. College Station, Tex: Center for Strategic Technology, Texas A&M University, 1982.

Becker, Abraham S. *Sitting on Bayonets: The Soviet Defense Burden and the Slowdown of Soviet Defense Spending*. RAND/UCLA/JRS-01. Santa Monica, Cal: RAND Corporation, 1985.

Bonds, Ray. ed. *Soviet War Machine*. New York: Hamlyn Publishing Group, 1977.

Chizum, David G. *Soviet Radioelectronic Combat*. Boulder, Colo: Westview Press, 1985.

Cockburn, Andrew. *The Threat: Inside the Soviet Military Machine*. New York: Random House, 1983.

Collins, John M. *U.S.–Soviet Military Balance: Concepts and Capabilities: 1960–1980*. New York: McGraw-Hill Publishers, 1985.

———. *U.S.–Soviet Military Balance 1980–1985*. New York: Pergamon-Brassey's International Defense Publishers, 1985.

Colton, Timothy J. *Commissars, Commanders, and Civilian Authority: The Structure of Soviet Military Politics*. Cambridge: Harvard University Press, 1979.

Cordier, Sherwood S. *Calculus of Power: The Current Soviet-American Conventional Military Balance in Central Europe*. 3rd ed. Washington, D.C.: University Press of America, 1980.

Cross, Jack L. *Current Soviet Military Commmanders' Articles on Military Affairs, 1964–1979*. College Station, Tex: Center for Strategic Technology, Texas A & M University, 1985.

———. *The Soviet Higher Military Educational System*. College Station Paper No. 4. College Station, Tex: Center for Strategic Technology, Texas A & M University, 1982.

Currie, Kenneth M., and Gregory Varhal, eds. *The Soviet Union: What Lies Ahead?* Studies in Communist Affairs, Vol. 6. Washington: U.S. Government Printing Office, 1984.

Deane, Michael J. *Political Control of the Soviet Armed Forces*. New York: Crane, Russak and Co., 1977.

Erickson, John. *The Russian Imperial/Soviet General Staff*. College Station Paper No. 3. College Station, Tex: Center for Strategic Technology, Texas A & M University, 1981.

———. *The Soviet High Command: A Military-Political History*. New York: St. Martin's Press, 1962 (Reprint by Westview Press, 1984).

———. *Soviet Military Power*. Washington: United States Strategic Institute, 1973.

Erickson, John, et al. *Organizing for War: The Soviet Military Establishment Viewed Through the Prism of the Military District*. College Station Paper No. 2. College Station, Tex: Center for Strategic Technology, Texas A & M University, 1983.

Erickson, John, and E. J. Feuchtwanger. *Soviet Military Power and Performance*. Hamden, Conn: The Shoe String Press, 1979.

Erickson, John, and Lynn Hansen. *Soviet Combined Arms: Past and Present*. College Station Paper No. 1. College Station, Tex: Center for Strategic Technology, Texas A & M University, 1981.

Gabriel, Richard A. *The Antagonists: A Comparative Combat Assessment of the Soviet and American Soldier*. Westport, Conn: Greenwood Press, 1984.

———. *The Mind of the Soviet Fighting-Man*. Westport, Conn: Greenwood Press, 1984.

———. *The New Red Legions*. Westport, Conn: Greenwood Press, 1980.

———. *Soviet Military Psychology: The Theory and Practice of Coping with Battle Stress*. Westport, Conn: Greenwood Press, 1986.

Goldhammer, Herbert. *The Soviet Soldier: Soviet Military Management at the Troop Level*. New York: Crane, Russak & Co., 1975.

Gouré, Leon. *Soviet Civil Defense in the Seventies*. Washington: Center for Advanced International Studies, 1975.

———. *War Survival in Soviet Strategy: USSR Civil Defense*. Washington: Center for Advanced International Studies, 1976.

Green, William C. *Soviet Nuclear Weapons Policy: A Research Guide*. Boulder, Colo: Westview Press, 1986.

Grigorenko, Petro. *Memoirs*. New York: W. W. Norton and Co., 1982.

Hemsley, John. *Soviet Troop Control: The Role of Command Technology in the Soviet Military System*. New York: Brassey's Publishers, 1982.

Jones, David R. *The Military-Naval Encyclopedia of Russia and the Soviet Union*, Vols. 1–50. Gulf Breeze, Fla: Academic International Press; Publication began in 1978 and is ongoing.

———. *Soviet Armed Forces Review Annual*, Vols. 1–9. Gulf Breeze, Fla: Academic International Press, 1977–1986. (Published yearly.)

Jones, Ellen. *Red Army and Society: A Sociology of the Soviet Military*. London: Allen & Unwin, 1986.

Katz, Mark N. *The Third World in Soviet Military Thought*. Baltimore: Johns Hopkins University Press, 1982.

Kaplan, Stephen S. *Diplomacy of Power: Soviet Armed Forces as a Political Instrument*. Washington: The Brookings Institution, 1981.

Kolkowicz, Roman. *Communism, Militarism, Imperialism: Soviet Military Politics After Stalin*. Boulder, Colo: Westview Press, 1987.

———. *The Soviet Military and the Communist Party*. Princeton, NJ: Princeton University Press, 1967.

Kolkowicz, Roman, and Ellen Mickiewicz. *The Soviet Calculus of Nuclear War*. Lexington, Mass: Lexington Books, 1986.

Laird, Robbin F., and Dale R. Herspring. *The Soviet Union and Strategic Arms*. Boulder, Colo: Westview Press, 1984.

Lambeth, Benjamin S. *The Soviet Union and the Strategic Defense Initiative: Preliminary Findings and Impressions*. RAND Note N-2482-AF. Santa Monica, Cal: RAND Corporation, 1986.

Leites, Nathan. *What Soviet Commanders Fear from Their Own Forces*. RAND Paper P-5958. Santa Monica, Cal: RAND Corporation, 1978.

Lewis, William J. *The Warsaw Pact: Arms, Doctrine, Strategy*. New York: McGraw-Hill Publications, 1982.

Meyer, Stephen M. *Soviet Theater Nuclear Forces*. Adelphi Papers, Nos. 187/8, Winter 1983/1984. London: International Institute for Strategic Studies.

Oberg, James E. *Red Star in Orbit*. New York: Random House, 1981.

Penkovskiy, Oleg. *The Penkovskiy Papers*. Garden City, NY: Doubleday, 1965.

Porter, Bruce D. *The USSR in Third World Conflicts: Soviet Arms and Diplomacy in Local Wars, 1945–1980*. New York: Cambridge University Press, 1984.

———. *Prospects of Soviet Power in the 1980's*. Adelphi Papers Nos. 151/2, Summer 1979. London: International Institute for Strategic Studies.

Sallagar, F.M. *An Overview of the Soviet Threat*. RAND Report R-2580-AF. Santa Monica, Cal: RAND Corporation, 1980.

Scherer, John L. *Handbook on Soviet Military Deficiencies*. Minnneapolis, Minn: J. L. Scherer, 1983.

Scott, Harriet Fast, and William F. Scott. *The Armed Forces of the USSR*, 3rd ed. Boulder, Colo: Westview Press, 1984.

———. *The Soviet Control Structure: Capabilities for Wartime Survival*. New York: Crane Russak, 1983.

Schmid, Alex P. *Soviet Military Interventions Since 1945*. New Brunswick, NJ: Transaction Books, 1985.

Shtemenko, S. M. *The Soviet General Staff at War*. Moscow: Progress Publishers, 1970.

Sonnenfeldt, Helmut, and William G. Hyland. *Soviet Perspectives on Security*. Adelphi Papers, No. 150.

Spring 1979. London: International Institute for Strategic Studies.

Soviet Military Power. Washington, D.C.: U.S. Government Printing Office. (Published yearly by the Department of Defense since 1981.)

Valenta, Juri, and William C. Potter, eds. *Soviet Decision Making for National Security*. Boston: Allen & Unwin, 1984.

Warner, Edward L. *The Military in Contemporary Soviet Politics: An Institutional Analysis*. New York: Praeger, 1977.

Weiner, Freidrich. *The Armies of the Warsaw Pact Nations*, 3rd ed. Translated by William J. Lewis. Vienna: Carl Uberreuter Publishers, 1981.

Whetten, Lawrence L., ed. *The Future of Soviet Military Power*. New York: Crane, Russak & Co., 1976.

Wolfe, Thomas W. *Soviet Power and Europe, 1945–1970*. Baltimore: Johns Hopkins University Press, 1970.

Yepishev, A. A. *Some Aspects of Party-Political Work in the Soviet Armed Forces*. Moscow: Progress Publishing, 1975.

Zey-Ferrell et al. *Initiative and Innovation in the Soviet Military*. Occasional Paper No. 6. College Station, Tex: Center for Strategic Technology, Texas A & M University, 1984.

THE *SOVIET MILITARY THOUGHT* SERIES TRANSLATED AND PUBLISHED UNDER THE AUSPICES OF THE U.S. AIR FORCE BY THE U.S. GOVERNMENT PRINTING OFFICE.

1. *The Offensive*
2. *Marxism-Leninism of War and Army*
3. *Scientific-Technical Progress and the Revolution in Military Affairs*
4. *The Basic Principles of Operational Art and Tactics*
5. *The Philosophical Heritage of V. I. Lenin and Problems of Contemporary War*
6. *Concept, Algorithm Decision*
7. *Military Pedagogy*
8. *Military Psychology*
9. *Dictionary of Basic Military Terms*
10. *Civil Defense*
11. *Selected Soviet Military Writings: 1970-1975*
12. *The Armed Forces of the Soviet State*
13. *The Officers Handbook*
14. *The People, The Army, The Commander*
15. *Long-Range Missile-Equipped*
16. *Forecasting in Military Affairs*
17. *The Command and Staff of the Soviet Army*
18. *Fundamentals of Tactical Command and Control*
19. *The Soviet Armed Forces: A History of Their Organizational Development*
20. *The Initial Period of War*
21. *Tactics*

STRATEGY AND DOCTRINE

Berman, Robert P., and John C. Baker. *Soviet Strategic Forces: Requirements and Responses*. Washington, D.C.: The Brookings Institution, 1982.

Davis, Jacquelyn K. *Soviet Theater Strategy*. Washington, D.C.: U.S. Strategic Institute, 1978.

Deane, Michael J. *Strategic Defense in Soviet Strategy*.

Washington, D.C.: Advanced International Studies Institute, 1980.

Despres, John, Lilita Dzirkals, and Barton Whaley. *Timely Lessons of History: The Manchurian Model for Soviet Strategy.* RAND Report R-1825-NA. Santa Monica, Cal: RAND Corporation, 1976.

Dinerstein, H. S. *War and the Soviet Union.* New York: Praeger, 1962 (Reprint by Greenwood Press, 1976).

Douglass, Joseph D., Jr. *Soviet Military Strategy in Europe.* New York: Pergamon Press, 1980.

———. *The Soviet Theater Nuclear Offensive.* Studies in Communist Affairs, Vol. 1. Washington, D.C.: U.S. Government Printing Office, 1976.

Douglass, Joseph D., Jr., and Amoretta M. Hoeber. *Conventional War and Escalation: The Soviet View.* New York: Crane, Russak & Co., 1981.

———, eds. *Selected Readings from Military Thought, 1963-1973.* Studies in Communist Affairs, Vol. 5, Parts I and II. Washington, D.C.: U.S. Government Printing Office, 1982.

———. *Soviet Strategy for Nuclear War.* Stanford, Cal: Hoover Institution, 1979.

Dziak, John J. *Soviet Perceptions of Military Power: The Interaction of Theory and Practice.* New York: Crane, Russak & Co., 1981.

Dzirkals, Lilita I. *"Lightning War" in Manchuria: Soviet Military Analysis of the 1945 Far East Campaign.* RAND Paper P-5589. Santa Monica, Cal: RAND Corporation, 1976.

Garthoff, Raymond L. *How Russia Makes War: Soviet Military Doctrine.* London: George Allen and Unwin, 1954.

———. *Soviet Military Policy: A Historical Analysis.* New York: Praeger, 1966.

Gouré, Leon, et al. *The Role of Nuclear Forces in Current Soviet Strategy.* Coral Gables, Fla: Center for Advanced International Studies, 1974.

Ground Zero. *What About the Russians and Nuclear War?* New York: Pocket Books, 1983.

Hasselkorn, Avigdor. *The Evolution of Soviet Security Strategy, 1956-1975.* New York: Crane, Russak & Co., 1978.

Jacobs, Walter. *Frunze: The Soviet Clausewitz, 1885-1925.* The Hague: Martinus Nijhoff, 1969.

Jukes, Geoffrey. *The Development of Soviet Strategic Thinking Since 1945.* Canberra: Australian National University Press, 1972.

Lambeth, Benjamin S. *Has Soviet Nuclear Strategy Changed?* RAND Paper P-7181. Santa Monica, Cal: RAND Corporation, 1985.

———. *How to Think About Soviet Military Doctrine.* RAND Paper P-5939. Santa Monica, Cal: RAND Corporation, 1978.

———. *Risk and Uncertainty in Soviet Deliberation About War.* RAND Report R-2687-AF. Santa Monica, Cal: RAND Corporation, 1980.

———. *Soviet Strategic Conduct and the Prospects for Stability.* RAND Report R-2579-AF. Santa Monica, Cal: RAND Corporation, 1980.

Lee, William T., and Richard F. Starr. *Soviet Military Policy Since World War II.* Stanford, Cal: Hoover Institute Press, 1986.

Leebaert, Derek, ed. *Soviet Military Thinking.* Boston: Allen & Unwin, 1981.

Leites, Nathan. *Soviet Style in War.* New York: Crane, Russak and Co., 1982.

Luttwak, Edward. *The Grand Strategy of the Soviet Union.* New York: St. Martin's Press, 1983.

Miller, Mark E. *Soviet Strategic Power and Doctrine.* Washington, D.C.: Advanced International Studies Institute, 1982.

Monks, Alfred L. *Soviet Military Doctrine: 1960 to the Present.* New York: Irvington, 1984.

Pipes, Richard, ed. *Soviet Strategy in Europe.* New York: Crane, Russak and Co., 1976.

Scott, Harriet Fast. *Soviet Military Doctrine.* Menlo Park, Cal: Stanford Research Institute, 1971.

———. *Soviet Military Dotrine: Its Continuity, 1960-1970.* Menlo Park, Cal: Stanford Research Institute, 1971.

———. *Soviet Military Doctrine: Its Formulation and Dissemination.* Menlo Park, Cal: Stanford Research Institute, 1971.

Scott, Harriet Fast, and William F. Scott. *The Soviet Art of War: Doctrine, Strategy, and Tactics.* Boulder, Colo: Westview Press, 1982.

Scott, William F. *Soviet Sources of Military Doctrine and Strategy.* New York: Crane Russak and Co., 1975.

Sejna, Jan. *We Will Bury You.* London: Sidgwick and Jackson, 1982.

Semmel, Bernard. *Marxism and the Science of War.* New York: Oxford University Press, 1981.

Snyder, Jack L. *The Soviet Strategic Culture: Implications for Limited Nuclear Options.* RAND Report R-2154-AF. Santa Monica, Cal: RAND Corporation, 1977.

Sokolovskiy, V.D. (Harriet Fast Scott, ed.), *Soviet Military Strategy.* 3rd ed. New York: Crane Russak & Co., 1975.

Vigor, P. H. *Soviet Blitzkrieg Theory.* New York: St. Martin's Press, 1983.

———. *The Soviet View of War, Peace and Neutrality.* London: Routledge and Kegan Paul, 1975.

GROUND FORCES

Bonds, Ray. *An Illustrated Guide to the Weapons of the Modern Soviet Ground Forces.* New York: Arco Publishing, 1981.

Baxter, William P. *Soviet Airland Battle Tactics.* Novato, Ca: Presidio Press, 1986.

Bellamy, Chris. *Red God of War: Soviet Artillery and Rocket Forces.* New York: Brassey's Defense Publishers, 1986.

Erickson, John, Lynn Hansen, and William Schneider. *Soviet Ground Forces: An Operational Assessment.* Boulder, Colo: Westview Press, 1985.

Garder, Michael. *History of the Soviet Army.* New York: Praeger, 1966.

Glanz, David M. *The Soviet Airborne Experience.* Combat Studies Institute Research Survey No. 4. Fort Leavenworth, Kans: U.S. Army Command and General Staff College, 1984.

Isby, David. *Weapons and Tactics of the Soviet Army.* New York: Jane's Publishing, 1981.

Kipp, Jacob W., et al. *Historical Analysis of the Use of Mobile Forces by Russia and the USSR.* Occcasional Paper No. 10. College Station, Tex: Center for Strategic Technology, Texas A & M University, 1985.

Liddell Hart, Basil Henry. *The Red Army.* New York: Harcourt Brace, 1956.

Lototskiy, V. K. *The Soviet Army*. Moscow: Progress Publishers, 1971.

Mackintosh, Malcolm. *Juggernaut: A History of the Soviet Armed Forces*. New York: Macmillan, 1967.

O'Ballance, Edgar. *The Red Army, A Short History*. New York: Praeger, 1964.

Record, Jeffrey. *Sizing Up the Soviet Army*. Washington, D.C.: The Brookings Institution, 1975.

Simpkin, Richard. *Red Armour*. London: Brassey's Publishers, 1984.

Suvorov, Viktor. *The Liberators: My Life in the Soviet Army*. New York: W. W. Norton, 1981.

———. *Inside the Soviet Army*. New York: Macmillan Publishing Co., 1982.

Understanding Soviet Military Developments. U.S. Army Pamphlet. Washington, D.C.: U.S. Government Printing Office, 1978.

AIR FORCES

Barron, John. *MIG Pilot: The Final Escape of Lieutenant Belenko*. New York: Readers Digest Press, 1980.

Berman, Robert P. *Soviet Air Power in Transition*. Washington, D.C.: The Brookings Institution, 1975.

Boyd, Alexander. *The Soviet Air Force Since 1918*. New York: Stein and Day, 1977.

Epstein, Joshua M. *Measuring Military Power: The Soviet Air Threat to Europe*. Princeton, NJ: Princeton University Press, 1984.

Gunston, Bill. *An Illustrated Guide to the Modern Soviet Air Force*. New York: Arco Publishing, 1982.

Gunston, Bill, and Bill Sweetman. *Soviet Air Power*. New York: Crescent Books, 1978.

Hardesty, Von. *Red Phoenix: The Rise of Soviet Air Power*. Washington, D.C.: Smithsonian Institution Press, 1982.

Higham, Robin, and Jacob W. Kipp. *Soviet Aviation and Air Power*. Boulder, Colo: Westview Press, 1977.

Jackson, Robert: *Red Falcons: The Soviet Air Force in Action, 1919–1969*. New York: International Publications Service, 1970.

Kilmarx, Robert A. *A History of Soviet Air Power*. New York: Praeger, 1962.

Lambeth, Benjamin S. *Moscow's Lessons from the 1982 Lebanon Air War*. RAND Report R-3000-AF. Santa Monica, Cal: RAND Corporation, 1984.

———. *Sizing Up the Soviet Air Force: A Review*. RAND Paper P-7205. Santa Monica, Cal: RAND Corporation, 1986.

Lee, Asher, ed. *The Soviet Air and Rocket Forces*. New York: Praeger, 1959.

Mason, R. A., and John W. R. Taylor. *Aircraft, Strategy and Operations of the Soviet Air Force*. New York: Jane's Publishing, 1986.

Miller, Russell. *The Soviet Air Force at War*. The Epic of Flight Series. Alexandria, Va: Time-Life Books, 1983.

Murphy, Paul., ed. *The Soviet Air Forces*. Jefferson, N.C.: McFarland & Co., 1984.

Peterson, Phillip A. *Soviet Air Power and the Pursuit of New Military Options*. Washington, D.C.: U.S. Government Printing Office, 1979.

Smith, Myron J. *The Soviet Air and Strategic Rocket Forces, 1939–1980*. Santa Barbara, Cal: ABC-Clio, 1981.

Soviet Aerospace Handbook. U.S. Air Force Pamphlet 200-21. Washington, D.C.: U.S. Government Printing Office, 1978.

The Soviet Air Force in World War II: The Official History. Originally published by the Minister of Defense of the USSR. Translated by Leland Fetzer and edited by Ray Wagner. Garden City, NY: Doubleday, 1973.

Sweetman, Bill. *The Presidio Concise Guide to Soviet Military Aircraft*. Novato, Ca: Presidio Press, 1981.

Whiting, Kenneth R. *Soviet Air Power*. Boulder, Colo: Westview Press, 1986.

NAVAL FORCES

Bathhurt, Robert R. *Understanding the Soviet Navy: A Handbook*. Newport, RI: Naval War College Press, 1979.

Breyer, Siegfried. *Guide to the Soviet Navy*. Translated by M.W. Henley, Annapolis, Md: Naval Institute Press, 1970.

Dismukes, Bradford, ed. *Soviet Naval Diplomacy*. New York: Pergamon, 1979.

Gorshkov, Sergei G. *Red Star Rising at Sea*. Annapolis, Md: Naval Institute Press, 1979.

———. *The Sea Power of the State*. Annapolis, Md: Naval Institute Press, 1979.

Hansen, Lynn. *Soviet Navy Spetsnaz Operations on the Northern Flanks: Implications for the Defense of Western Europe*. College Station, Tex: Center for Strategic Technology, Texas A & M University, 1984.

Herrick, Robert Waring. *Soviet Naval Strategy*. Annapolis, Md: Naval Institute Press, 1968.

Kime, Steve F. *A Soviet Navy for the Nuclear Age*. Washington, D.C.: National Defense University, 1980.

Kipp, Jacob W. *Naval Art and the Prism of Contemporaneity: Soviet Naval Officers and the Lessons of the Falklands Conflict*. Stratech Paper Series SS83-2. College Station, Tex: Center for Strategic Technology, Texas A & M Univesity, 1984.

Lovett, Christopher C. *Soviet Naval Aviation: Continuity and Change*. Occasional Paper No. 7. College Station, Tex: Center for Strategic Technology, Texas A & M University, 1984.

McGruther, Kenneth R. *The Evolving Soviet Navy*. Newport, R.I.: Naval War College Press, 1978.

MccGwire, Michael, ed. *Soviet Naval Developments: Capability and Context*. Halifax, N.S.: Centre for Foreign Policy Studies, Department of Political Science, Dalhousie, 1973.

———, ed. *Soviet Naval Policy: Objectives and Constraints*. New York: Praeger, 1975.

Morris, Eric. *The Russian Navy: Myth and Reality*. Briarcliff Manor, N.Y.: Stein and Day, 1977.

Murphy, Paul J., ed. *Naval Power in Soviet Policy*. Studies in Communist Affairs, Vol. 2. Washington, D.C.: U.S. Government Printing Office, 1978.

Ranft, Bryan. *The Sea in Soviet Strategy*. Annapolis, Md: Naval Institute Press, 1983.

Tritten, James J. *Soviet Naval Forces and Nuclear Warfare*. Boulder, Colo: Westview Press, 1986.

Understanding Soviet Naval Developments, 5th ed. U.S. Navy Pamphlet (NAVSOP-3560). Washington, D.C.: U.S. Government Printing Office, 1985.

Volgyes, Ivan. *Political Socialization in the Soviet Naval Forces: A Study*. College Station Paper No. 7. College Station, Tex: Center for Strategic Technology, Texas A & M University, 1984.

Watson, Bruce W. *Soviet Navy at Sea: Soviet Naval Operations on the High Seas, 1956–1980*. Boulder, Colo: Westview Press, 1982.

Watson, Bruce W., and Peter M. Dunn, eds. *The Future of the Soviet Navy: An Assessment to the Year 2000*. Boulder, Colo: Westview Press, 1986.

Watson, Bruce W., and Susan M. Watson, eds. *The Soviet Navy, Strengths and Liabilities*. Boulder, Colo: Westview Press, 1986.

Wegener, Edward. *The Soviet Naval Offensive*. Annapolis, Md: Naval Institute Press, 1975.

INTELLIGENCE AND SECURITY FORCES

Barron, John. *KGB: The Secret Works of Soviet Secret Agents*. New York: Readers Digest Press, 1974.

———. *KGB Today: The Hidden Hand*. New York: The Readers Digest, 1983.

Bittman, Ladislav. *The Deception Game*. New York: Ballantine Books, 1972.

———. *The KGB and Soviet Disinformation: An Insider's View*. New York: Pergamon-Brassey's International Defense Publishers, 1985.

Freemantle, Brian. *KGB: Inside the World's Largest Intelligence Network*. New York: Holt Rinehart and Winston, 1982.

Fuller, William C., Jr. *The Internal Troops of the MVD SSSR*. College Station Paper No. 6. College Station, Tex: Center for Strategic Technology, Texas A & M University, 1984.

Godson, Roy, and Richard H. Shultz. *Dezinformatsia: Active Measures in Soviet Strategy*. New York: Pergamon Press, 1984.

Hingley, Ronald. *The Russian Secret Police*. New York: Simon and Schuster, 1970.

Richelson, Jeffrey T. *Sword and Shield: Soviet Intelligence and Security Services*. Boulder, Colo: Westview Press, 1985.

Rositzke, Harry. *The KGB: The Eyes of Russia*. Garden City, N.Y.: Doubleday and Co., 1981.

Suvorov, Victor. *Inside Soviet Military Intelligence*. New York: Macmillan, 1984.

The Federal Republic of Germany and the German Democratic Republic

Jeffrey A. Larsen and Jay L. Lorenzen

Christianity has occasionally calmed the brutal German lust for battle, but it cannot destroy that savage ecstasy . . .
—HEINRICH HEINE

The German soul is opposed to the pacifist ideal of civilization, for is not peace an element of civil corruption?
—THOMAS MANN

German foreign policy means above all maintaining our freedom and strengthening the peace in Europe and in the whole world. To us an active policy for peace is a political necessity and an ethical obligation.
—HELMUT KOHL, 1983

Many in Europe over the past century have had reason to dwell on the German predilection for, and success in, all things military. The situation may have changed as a result of World War II, out of which emerged two distinct German states within the boundaries of the old German nation. The following bibliographic essay attempts to give the reader some recommended sources for further study of the two Germanys and their defense policies. By examining these books and articles, the student of German foreign and defense policy will be better able to decide whether the traditional views of German militarism are still valid in today's much changed and more complex international system, or whether Germany has, as Kohl's remarks suggest, had a major change in its approach to the use of military force as a result of two devastating wars.

These essays are organized into four areas: first, a general overview of key books, articles, and anthologies that address German foreign and defense policy from a broad perspective. Second, the essays turn to relations of the two Germanys with the other actors in their respective alliances and to constraints imposed upon them within the international system. We then focus on domestic concerns within each German state: budgetary impacts on the military, political opposition to defense policies, and the concern over a declining population on manning issues. Finally, we turn to certain issues that could be considered purely military in nature, such as strategies, weapons procurement, arms sales, arms control, and the Strategic Defense Initiative.

The Federal Republic of Germany

The Federal Republic of Germany pillars the Atlantic Alliance's commitment to a European defense, both in its geopolitical situation and in its military charge. A plethora of individual works and anthologies address the FRG's central role in NATO defense arrangements. Additionally, German foreign and defense policies are almost monthly fare in periodicals dedicated to security issues. On occasion, a particularly salient treatment of the defense policy of the FRG appears in these periodicals. We hope to highlight many of the single works dedicated to German defense policy, to direct our readers to key security-oriented periodicals, and to review briefly certain articles deemed helpful.

Certainly the best overall treatment of West German defense policy is the White Paper (Weissbuch) published every two or three years by the FRG Verteidigungsministerium (1985 being the most recent edition). General anthologies of value include *The Foreign Policies of West Germany, France, and Britain* edited by Wolfram F. Hanrieder and Fraeme P. Auton (Englewood Cliffs, N.J.: Prentice-Hall, 1980), *The German Army and NATO Strategy* by the National Defense University, and Wolfram Hanrieder's *West German Foreign Policy, 1949-1979* (Boulder Colo.: Westview Press, 1980). In addition, see "The Security Policy of the Federal Republic of Germany," by Jugen Degner, in *Parameters* (Summer 1985), "European Security and the German Question" by Ulrich Albrecht in *World Policy Journal* (Spring 1984), and Franz Josef Strauss's "Manifesto of a German Atlanticist" in *Strategic Review* (Summer 1982). Former Ambassador Arthur F. Burns examined U.S.-FRG relations in his 1986 Elihu Root Lecture, published as *The United States and Germany: A Vital Partnership* (Council on Foreign Relations, 1986). This topic is covered further by Stephan G. Thomas and Peter Corterier in two chapters entitled "Two Views From West Germany" in *Reagan's Leadership and the Atlantic Alliance: Views From Europe and America*, ed. by Walter Goldstein (New York: Pergamon-Brassey's, 1986). Finally, a new history of Germany's relations with the Atlantic alliance for the past 40 years is John A. Reed, Jr., *Germany and NATO* (Washington, D.C.: National Defense University Press, 1987).

Next, let us examine the constraints and exigencies of the international system on German foreign affairs. One of the best articles on this topic, which examines the history of NATO's 1979 dual-track INF decision in Germany, is by David Yost and Thomas Glad, "West German Party Politics and Theater Nuclear Modernization Since 1977," *Armed Forces and Society* (Summer 1982). In "Public Policy and Security Policy in the Federal Republic of Germany," *Orbis* (Winter 1985), Peter Schmidt analyzes German attitudes towards NATO, the East-West conflict, the use of force, and FRG relations with the United States and the USSR, and then compares these attitudes with similar studies on other major NATO member states. This concern over internal German attitudes and their potential effect on the NATO alliance is reflected in Jonathan Dean's "How to Lose Germany," *Foreign Policy* (Summer 1984). Other valuable articles include Lothar Ruhle, "German Security Policy: Position, Problems, Prospects," *International Security Review* (Summer 1980); "Defense of Germany and the German Defense Contribution," a RAND Corporation pamphlet by Horst Mendershausen; "West German Views on Defense," by Chadwell in the March 1981 issue of *National Defense*; and Peter Bender's "West Germany's Requirements for Security," in *AEI Foreign Policy and Defense Review* 3, no. 4 (1983). German language books that cover many of these same issues include *Die Steitkräfte der NATO auf dem Territorium der BRD*, by Wolfgang Weber, published by Militarverlag, 1984; and *Sicherheit—zu welchem Preis? die Zukunft der westlichen Allianz*, Wolf-Dieter Eberwein and Catherine M. Kelleher, eds., published by Olzog-Studienbuch, 1983. The fact that Germany feels and reacts to these external pressures is evident in publication of

The German Contribution to the Common Defense (Bonn: Federal Press and Information Office, 1986), a pamphlet arguing that Germany is pulling its share of the burden for NATO.

Domestic politics naturally play a role in the formation of Germany's defense policy. James A. Linger examines the growth and role of the German military in "The Emergence of the Bundeswehr as a Pressure Group," *Armed Forces and Society* (Summer 1979) while Ralf Zoll, in the same edition, tackles public opinion in "Public Opinion and Security Policy: The West German Experience." The Bundeswehr's role in society is also examined in two other articles: the first, in the same edition of *Armed Forces and Society*, is "From Scharnhorst to Schmidt: The System of Education and Training in the German Bundeswehr," by Hans Eberhard Radbruch; the second is "The Bundeswehr and German Society," by Joe Gray Taylor, Jr. in *Parameters* (September 1983). Pierre Hassner attempts to understand and explain the changing domestic priorities of the FRG—especially the growth of leftist peace groups—in "The Shifting Foundation," *Foreign Policy* (Fall 1982). "Europe after INF," by Paolo Stoppa-Liebl and Walter Laqueur, also looks at the rise of pacifist tendencies in West Europe and the FRG, in *Washington Quarterly* (Spring 1985). Werner Kaltefleiter addresses public opinion and political party platforms in "German Division," *Policy Review* (Fall 1981). The renewed Eastern European emphasis in FRG foreign policy is seen in two Winter 1984/85 *Foreign Affairs* articles: "The German Question Transformed," by Richard Lowenthal, and "The New Deutschlandpolitik," by Walther L. Kiep. The fundamental security issues at play in West Germany today are covered in an article in *Armed Forces and Society* in Spring 1984, by Wayne Thompson and Peter Wittig: "The West German Defense Policy Consensus: Stable or Eroding?" as well as in "Germany's Security Policy Options from the Elite Perspective," *Air University Review* (March–April 1983). "Debate over German Defense Issues," by Roger Morgan in *AEI Foreign Policy and Defense Review* 4, nos. 3 and 4 (1983), is another source of information on this issue. Peter von Oertzen, (VSA-Verlag, 1984) addresses domestic influences on security policy in *Für einen neuen Reformismus*. Finally, two articles that look strictly at defense spending are "The Expenditure and Revenue Effect of Defense Spending in the FRG," *Policy Sciences* (Amsterdam) (March 1984), and "The Relationship between Defense Spending and Inflation," by Harvey Starr, Francis Hoole, Jeffrey Hart, and John Freeman, *Conflict Resolution* (March 1984).

There are also numerous good articles on what one could consider strictly "military" topics. For instance, NATO strategy and tactics are covered in John Mearsheimer, "Maneuver, Mobile Defense, and the NATO Central Front," *International Security* (Winter 1981–82), wherein he criticizes forward defense as attrition warfare that could be overcome, although with difficulty, through maneuver warfare. Gary L. Guertner, in a Spring 1982 *Orbis* article entitled "Nuclear War in Suburbia," examines NATO strategy in light of the urbanization of Western Germany, claiming that tactical nuclear weapons are self-deterring and should be redressed by enhanced conventional defenses. Samuel Huntingdon picks up this idea in "Conventional Deterrence and Conventional Retaliation in Europe," *Inter-*

national Security, Winter 1983/84, by proposing corrections to NATO's lack of a credible conventional deterrent strategy. The actual force deployments are considered nicely in "NATO's Central Front," a survey in *The Economist*, 30 August 1986. Arms transfers by West Germany are addressed by Frederic S. Pearson in "Of Leopards and Cheetahs: West Germany's Role as a Mid-Sized Arms Supplier," *Orbis* (Spring 1985), and in his "Necessary Evil: Perspectives on West German Arms Transfer Policies," *Armed Forces and Society* (Summer 1986). "West German Perspectives on Nuclear Armament and Arms Control," self-evident in its theme, was written by Gale A. Mattox in *The Annals of the American Academy* (Summer 1983).

German attitudes on strategic defense are found in several articles and books. The formal relations are seen in "Federal Republic of Germany–United States: Agreements on the Transfer of Technology and the Strategic Defense Initiative," *International Legal Materials* (July 1986). General European elite opinion is reflected in *Krieg der Sterne: Ein amerikanischer Traum für Europa*, edited by Andreas Orth (Edition Freitag, 1985). Christoph Bluth examines the opportunities and dangers for the FRG in "SDI: The Challenge to West Germany," *International Affairs* (Spring 1986) while Manfred Hamm looks at the SPD's strategic defense plank in "Strategic Defense and the West German Social Democrats," *Strategic Review* (Spring 1986).

The German Democratic Republic

The available articles, books, and journals dedicated to East Germany's defense and security policy are far fewer than for West Germany, at least in English. A couple of good books on GDR policy that have appeared in recent years are by David Childs, *The GDR: Moscow's German Ally* (London: Allen & Unwin, 1983); *Policymaking in the GDR*, edited by Klaus von Beyme and Hartmut Zimmermann (New York: St. Martin's Press, 1984); and *GDR Foreign Policy*, edited by Eberhard Schulz, Hans-Adolf Jacobsen, Gert Leptin, and Ulrich Scheuner (New York: M. E. Sharpe, 1982). The von Beyme and Zimmermann book, it

should be noted, also has an 80-page bibliography. All three of these books examine the three major issues for East Germany: the GDR government's struggle for legitimacy and the effects of that struggle in the 1970s and 1980s; the search for a national identity of its own; and its relations with the USSR.

Journal articles worthy of mention include Otto Fischer's official East German outlook in "The Foreign Policy of the GDR," *International Affairs* (March 1981). Ronald D. Asmus compares the two Germanys and their relations in the early 1980s in "East and West Germany: Continuity and Change," in *World Today*, April 1984. "Concepts of East German Defence Doctrine," by Stephen R. Bowers in *Army Quarterly and Defense Journal* (October 1978), offers a somewhat dated, but comprehensive, look at the GDR's armed forces and their role, while Maj. Jeff McCausland addresses the same issue in "The East German Army—Spear Point or Weakness?" *Defense Analysis* 2, no. 2 (1986). McCausland's paper provides an overview of the East German army, its size, capabilities, and organization, as well as the question of interoperability with Soviet forces in the Warsaw Pact. Melvin Croan looks at East Germany's "out of area" concerns in "A New Afrika Corps?" *Washington Quarterly* (Winter 1980), analyzing GDR military and security assistance packages to African states.

In the case of East German defense policy, there is more material available to the reader who can handle German. "Wandlandung der kommunistischen Militärdoktrin," by Walter Rehm, was published in *Dtl Arch* 18, no. 11 (1985), and examines East German and Eastern European military theory. There is a section on military policy in Siegmar Quilitzsch et al., *Die DDR in der Welt des Sozialismus* (Staatsverlag, 1985). An official history of the East German army, including current training and relations with the WTO, is *Armee für Frieden und Sozialismus: Geschichte der Nationalen Volksarmee der DDR*, a 744-page tome (Militärverlag, 1985). The same publishing house also printed Erich Honecker's 1982 volume, *Dem Frieden unsere Tat: ausgewählte Reden und Aufsatze zur Militär- und Sicherheitspolitik der SED (Sozialistischen Einheitspartei Deutschlands)*.

France

Frank L. Rosa

France plays a unique global role, adopting an independent nuclear posture, pursuing an activist policy in defense of its former colonies in Africa, and assuming an Atlanticist stance by working in concert with other Western European countries and North America on joint military, economic, and political issues. It was France that first suggested the concept of the annual Economic Summit as a response to the energy crisis of the early 1970s. France takes a European stance in advancing the economic and diplomatic interests of Europe against incursions from either the United States or the Soviet Union—and sometimes even the British.

Global Role

As a nuclear power, France demands and expects respect. It pursues an independent nuclear stance, traditionally arguing that its missiles are pointed both East and West, as is also the case with Great Britain and the United States. France is faced with several security dilemmas. What is the proper role for nuclear forces in defense of the homeland? How can a nuclear deterrence strategy—especially that of a small nuclear power—advance the national interest? What is the correct balance between conventional and nuclear forces?

What are the costs to the strategic environment, if any, of the use of conventional forces?

An understanding of events leading up to and following France's withdrawal from NATO's integrated military structure provides the needed perspective for the study of French defense policy. Such a history is provided in Robert E. Osgood, *NATO: The Entangling Alliance* (Chicago: University of Chicago Press, 1962); Bernard Burrows and Christopher Irwin, *The Security of Western Europe* (London: C. Knight, 1972); and Alfred Grosser, *The Western Alliance: European-American Relations Since 1945* (New York: Random House, Vintage Books, 1982). A thorough review of the French withdrawal decision is found in Henry Kissinger, *Troubled Partnership* (New York: McGraw-Hill, 1965) and Kenneth Hunt, "NATO without France," *Adelphi Papers*, no. 32 (London: International Institute for Strategic Studies, 1966).

By withdrawing from NATO's integrated military structure and creating its own *force de frappe*, France was compelled to develop an independent strategy. Wolf Mendl, *Deterrence and Persuasion* (New York: Praeger, 1970) and Wilfrid Kohl, *French Nuclear Diplomacy* (Princeton, N.J.: Princeton University Press, 1971) examine the early development of French strategy. A later assessment of the international purpose of the French nuclear forces is addressed in "France's Defense Policy," *Military Review* (February 1977): 26–36. This anonymous article is an excerpt from a military report approved by the French Parliament in June 1976. The report states the reason for the existence of a nuclear force in France and for French participation in the Atlantic Pact.

Pierre M. Gallois, "French Defense Planning: The Future in the Past," *International Security* (Fall 1976): 15–31, offers a basic review of the development of defense policies under President Charles de Gaulle. While the purpose of the nuclear forces and strategies was to protect the autonomy of France, Gallois argues, just the opposite may be true. These strategies could be detrimental to the independence of the country. The same argument is advanced by Robin F. Laird, "French Forces in the 1980s and the 1990s," *Comparative Strategy* (1984): 387–412. Laird states that defense modernization in France is forcing the need for greater cooperation with the Western alliance. The increasing capabilities of French forces also make France a more important target for the Soviet Union.

The election of François Mitterrand as president of France brought a socialist government to power, but did little to change the direction of French defense policy. This is the argument advanced by Saint Brides, "Foreign Policy of Socialist France," *Orbis* (Spring 1982): 35–47. The Socialists continued French support for: (1) NATO's rearmament—especially theater forces; (2) global balance between the superpowers; and (3) France's independent nuclear force. The same observation is made by Peter J. Berger, "The Course of French Defense Policy," *Parameters* (September 1982): 19–26. Berger compared the Socialist Party's opposition position and its government position. Faced with the reality of power, the party modified its defense position to the more traditional posture.

The different defense positions of the major French political parties are discussed by Pierre Dabezies, "French Political Parties and Defense Policy: Divergences and Consensus," *Armed Forces and Society* (Winter 1982): 239–56. Dabezies argues that there is a basic consensus over maintaining a nuclear deterrent force.

While there is agreement on the maintenance of a nuclear force, there remain serious questions over the strategies and uses of such a force. In "French Security Policy: Decisions and Dilemmas," *Armed Forces and Society* (Winter 1982): 185–221, Edward A. Kolodziej reviews some of the basic problems facing French decision makers. These include Soviet military expansionism, the threat of increasing international violence, and the increasing military capability—conventional and nuclear—needed to deal with these threats. Marc Geneste, on the other hand, addresses the public debate over an acceptable nuclear strategy for France's independent nuclear force. In "Deterrence through Terror or Deterrence through Defense: The Emerging Nuclear Debate," *Armed Forces and Society* (Winter 1982): 223–38, Geneste reviews the two schools of thought in France: (1) deterrence through terror based on the doctrine of massive retaliation and (2) deterrence through defense.

The territorial scope of French security interests is a further concern. Robin F. Laird explores this issue in "The French Strategic Dilemma," *Orbis* (Summer 1984): 307–28. The dilemma, according to Laird, is that France's nuclear force exists for the defense of France's own national interests; at the same time, there is a greater awareness that French security is tied directly to that of West Germany. The international nature of the strategic environment is forcing changes in the French outlook.

Atlanticist Role

With a socialist government in France, a reorientation is taking place. This is the argument proposed by Robert S. Rudney, "Mitterrand's New Atlanticism: Evolving French Attitudes toward NATO," *Orbis* (Spring 1984): 83–101. Rudney sees France cooperating more with NATO and the United States on military matters. The reason for this shift is examined more thoroughly in A. W. De Porte, "France's New Realism," *Foreign Affairs* (Fall 1984): 144–65. Concern about the Soviet threat and the possibility of a power imbalance in Europe are uppermost in Mitterrand's mind. Unlike Rudney, DePorte argues that cooperation is taking place in European diplomatic arenas. France still possesses an independent military policy and there are major policy differences with the United States over Third World issues.

Does greater cooperation between the two sides of the Atlantic bode well for NATO? During the de Gaulle era, France believed that there were major shortcomings in NATO policies. NATO defense strategy was too inflexible. The range of geographic responsibility was too extended, and the likely theater of conflict between the two superpowers appeared restricted to the destruction of Europe. As previously suggested, the strategic concepts that France has developed since de Gaulle have limited France's ability to maintain autonomy. In "Does NATO Have a Future? A European View," *Washington Quarterly* (Summer 1982): 40–52, Pierre Lellouche presents a pessimistic view. He argues that "there is no basis for genuine defense cooperation because Germany does not want it, England prefers its special relationship with the U.S., and France will neither rejoin NATO nor go along with any plans for Germany's reunification." Lellouche is pointing to the lack of political will within the alliance to tackle the tough issues.

The issues are tough because of increasing public protests over NATO defense policies. There is a political polarization in Europe over significant issue areas according to Gregory Flynn and Hans Rattinger, eds., *The Public and Atlantic Defense* (New York: Rowman & Allanheld, 1985). The policies and actions of the United States are at the heart of the disturbances, leading some to suggest that Europe should take a more active role in its own defense.

European Role

A more politically united Europe, some would argue, would present a greater challenge to the superpowers' hegemony on that continent, permitting the European nations control over their own destinies. This political unity would also permit the Europeans to play a more active role in world affairs. On the other hand, there are those political analysts who argue that such a united, decisive Europe cannot be created. Jean-François Revel, *How Democracies Perish* (New York: Harper & Row, 1983), argues that the political will is missing in Europe; there is an absence of leadership. Nevertheless, President de Gaulle and his successors have envisioned a greater role on the European continent for France.

While there are issues that tend to be divisive, there are others that hold out the possibility of a political and economic renaissance in Europe. Greater political and economic integration make the need for military integration more likely. According to Alex Gliksman, "Under the Nuclear Gun: Three Keys to Europe's Bombs," the key to Europe's security rests on the ability of this region to cooperate on nuclear issues. Gliksman calls for new procedures for controlling nuclear weapons. Three keys would be provided for each system. The Europeans would hold two keys and the United States one. While it would take two keys to launch, the United States would not have veto control. The U.S. key would be identical to one held by a European state. This would override any American reluctance to act.

Helmut Schmidt, *Grand Strategy for the West* (New Haven: Yale University Press, 1985), is more concerned with French inaction than with American inaction. The defense of Europe requires France and French leadership. The West Germans would accept French command of a unified NATO structure. The commitment of France to the defense of Europe, at the boundaries of Western Europe rather than of France, would be a deterrent to any potential aggressor.

The dawning recognition within France of the inability to maintain a completely autonomous decision-making process for its nuclear force may move France into a greater partnership with the other European powers. This is dictated by the reality of the nuclear age and by the dire consequences of failing to do so.

The United Kingdom

Chris L. Jefferies

Periodical Sources

BRITISH

Premier among several British organizations that do research on British defense policy is the Royal United Services Institute for Defence Studies (RUSI) (Whitehall, London SWIA 2ET). Established by royal charter, its purpose is "the study of British Defence and Overseas Policy and . . . the promotion and advancement of the science and literature of the three services." The institute publishes a quarterly journal (*Journal of the Royal United Services Institute for Defence Studies*) and the reports of occasional seminars it sponsors on various subjects relating to British defense, and edits the annual *RUSI and Brassey's Defence Yearbook* (formerly *Brassey's Annual: The Armed Forces Yearbook*). This volume reports significant events of the past year in defense and international relations, as well as weapons development and technology.

The Centre for Defence Studies at the University of Aberdeen, Scotland, is active in both research and pub-

lishing in the field of British defense policy, particularly its economic aspects, and is known for its Aberdeen Studies in Defence Economics (ASIDES) series. These papers are published to make available results of the center's current research. In 1982 the center broadened its research to include more diverse aspects of defense policy, including defense policy in general, and began publishing a new series of occasional papers, entitled CENTREPIECES, reporting its broadened efforts. Copies of both series are available at libraries with defense policy collections, or can be obtained for a nominal fee by writing the Secretary, Centre for Defence Studies, University of Aberdeen, Edward Wright Building, Dunbar Street, Aberdeen AB9274, Scotland.

The International Institute for Strategic Studies (IISS) (23 Tavistock Street, London WC2E 7NQ) has long published defense policy papers. Its well-known Adelphi Papers, monographs exploring "the social and economic sources and political and moral implications of the use and existence of armed forces," also examine on occasion issues of British defense policy and the broader strategic issues that affect them. See also the IISS's periodical *Survival* and the annual *Military Balance* and *Strategic Survey*.

Sources of information frequently underestimated, but which must not be overlooked, are the official publications of the British government. Although they may not be as widely available in the United States as scholarly publications, they are available at major university libraries, through interlibrary loan programs, or through the British Embassy in Washington. These publications provide authoritative information on current defense policy and related expenditures in annual and supplemental statements commonly known as White Papers. (They are entitled "Statement on the Defence Estimates.") Additional sources are the reports of the Defence and External Affairs Subcommittee of the House of Commons Select Committee on Expenditure, although these are not too widely available in the United States.

There are, finally, a large number of defense-related periodicals published in the United Kingdom, some of which circulate in the United States. Just a few that can be of use are *International Affairs*, *Survival*, *Contemporary Review*, *Army Quarterly*, *World Today*, *Navy International*, *Strategic Review*, *International Security Review*, and *Defence and Foreign Affairs Policy*.

AMERICAN

In the United States there are several institutions that occasionally address British defense policy. The Inter-University Seminar on Armed Forces and Society (University of Chicago, Box 46, 1126 East 59th Street, Chicago IL 60637) publishes *Armed Forces and Society*, a quarterly journal exploring civil-military relations, military institutions, arms control, and conflict management. The periodic and continuing Sage Research Series on War, Revolution, and Peacekeeping provides an additional source. The Carnegie Endowment for International Peace (11 Dupont Circle N.W., Washington, D.C. 20036) publishes *Foreign Policy* on a quarterly basis; the Foreign Policy Research Institute (3508 Market Street, Philadelphia, PA 19104) publishes *Orbis: A Journal of World Affairs*, also a quarterly; and the Council on Foreign Relations (58 East 68th Street, New York, NY 10021) publishes its *Foreign Affairs* five times annually. Reviewing the indexes in any of these periodicals will identify British defense policy articles. Of these institutions, the Inter-University Seminar appears to publish most frequently on British defense policy issues.

Periodically addressing the more esoteric military-related British defense issues are official U.S. armed forces journals such as the *Naval War College Review*, *Parameters* (U.S. Army), and *Air University Review*. A recently rejuvenated periodical, *Armed Forces Journal International* (formerly the *Army and Navy Journal*) has often published articles relating to European and NATO strategies and policies, including British defense policy.

Sources by Theme

Discussion and debate of British defense policy encompasses four broad themes which are, in turn, reflected in the literature: First, the history of British de-

fense since World War II; second, Britain's "world" versus its "European" role (that is, "out-of-area" role versus its role in NATO); third, a nuclear versus a non-nuclear defense policy; and fourth, Britain's defense institutions, processes, and priorities. While these themes intersect and overlap at various points, a review of representative literature organized accordingly should prove helpful.

Several wide-ranging, eclectic studies cover this broad spectrum of British defense issues. One of the most useful, edited by John Baylis, is *Alternative Approaches to British Defence Policy* (New York: St. Martin's Press, 1983). Ten analysts address economic constraints and political preferences, the impact of the Falklands experience on policy, defense priorities, alternative strategies, and non-nuclear defense, also providing an outline of the wide-ranging debates over unilateral disarmament, nuclear weapons, and defense versus social programs. Baylis also edited an earlier work, *British Defence Policy in a Changing World* (London: Croom Helm, 1977) that the student of British defense will still find helpful. This volume addresses the military as an instrument of policy, Anglo-American relations, Britain in NATO, Britain's nuclear policy, defense, and other national priorities, and British public opinion and defense. A similar approach to defense policy, though more conceptual, is included in a later study by Dan Smith, *The Defence of the Realm in the 1980s* (London: Croom Helm, 1980).

HISTORY

An understanding of contemporary British defense policy requires, at a minimum, the study of its most recent history. Since the end of World War II, British policy has undergone many important changes as the country has retreated from being a world empire and begun to develop a "European" perspective on defense issues. Even today this transition is reflected in policy debates and deliberations.

Representative of many sources providing an understanding of the historical forces shaping today's British defense policy is C. H. Bartlett, *The Long Retreat* (London: Macmillan, 1972). Bartlett addresses the turbulent period from 1945 to 1970 in a general analysis of the period's defense policy. Phillip Darby, *British Defence Policy East of Suez, 1947–1968* (London: Oxford University Press, 1973), focuses on the "retreat from empire." A comprehensive and useful series of analytical essays on the period 1945 to 1976 is *British Defense Policy in a Changing World*, edited by John Baylis (London: Croom Helm, 1977).

In addition to the books listed above, there are several monographs and articles that give a more condensed account of the period since 1945. John Baylis's article, "British Defense Policy," in *Contemporary Strategy*, edited by John Baylis et al. (New York: Holmes and Meier, 1975 and updated in 1987), is largely an historical account focusing on the adjustments caused by the devolution of empire. He focuses on the efforts to balance commitments and capabilities, conventional and nuclear forces, total and limited war, and service autonomy and centralization. David Greenwood and David Hazel's study *The Evolution of Britain's Defence Priorities, 1957–1976*, ASIDES no. 9 (Aberdeen: Centre for Defence Studies, 1977) traces the major changes in Britain's defense effort since 1957, emphasizes the changing strategic perspectives, and analyzes trends in military manpower and defense budgets. In *British Defense: Policy and Process*, ACIS Working Paper no. 13 (Los Angeles: Center for Arms Control and International Security, UCLA, 1978), Arthur Cyr analyzes the period from an American perspective, identifying the economic problems (of which the withdrawal from empire is a reflection) and the resulting adjustments in strategic doctrine and world role. In brief form, an informative article by P. M. Kennedy in the *RUSI Journal* (December 1977), entitled "British Defense Policy, Part II: An Historian's View," summarizes the political, social, and economic constraints and influences on British defense policy. Finally, Franklin Johnson, *Defense by Ministry*, (New York: Holmes & Meier, 1980), an historical treatment of the evolution of the British Ministry of Defence since World War II, highlights several efforts at reform and the pressures and influences to which the ministry is subject. His work provides useful insight into the origins of recent and ongoing debates on the organization of the ministry. A short summary of the most recent effort at reform is an article by Michael Chichester, "Britain's Defence Organization: The New Look," *Navy International*, June 1985.

A WORLD OR EUROPEAN ROLE?

One of the longest-lasting post–World War II themes, and one of the most difficult to reconcile in British policy, is Britain's defense policy orientation: Should the United Kingdom maintain a "world" defense strategy and posture, or limit itself to the defense of the homeland, the North Atlantic, and Northern Europe? Continuing worldwide Commonwealth ties and access to energy and other natural resources provide strong incentives for a worldwide orientation. Yet the immediacy of European defense issues pulls strongly toward a European focus. Limited resources appear to preclude both. Military action in the Falklands has only served to sharpen the debate.

Michael Carver, former chief of the United Kingdom Defence Staff, addresses this issue in "Britain's Defense Effort," an article in *RUSI and Brassey's Defence Yearbook, 1977–78* (London: Westview Press, 1977). He highlights the pull between demands of warfare on the Continent and war at sea or abroad, the importance and role of NATO commitments, and the declining budget resources available to provide defense needs.

Michael Chichester and John Wilkinson in *The Uncertain Ally* (Aldershot, Eng.: Gower Publishing, 1982) attempt to reconcile the issue. They argue that since the USSR is now a global rather than continental power, threatening Western access to natural resources, European nations, including Britain, must assist the United States in its task of global peacekeeping by increasing their contributions to European defense and being prepared to assist "out of area." The book also reviews British defense policies and problems from 1960 to 1980, outlines a proposed realignment of maritime and air force structures, and addresses the issue of defense resources and acquisitions management. A short article by Gartley, "Can the UK Afford a RDF?" (*Journal of the Royal United Services Institute for Defence Studies*, March 1982) addresses the "out of area" aspect of the issue. On the British campaign against Argentina in the Falklands, see Marilyn B. Yokota's *Bibliography on the Falklands War*, Rand Paper P-7084, (Santa Monica, Calif.: RAND Corporation, August 1985).

James Bellini and Geoffry Pattie, in *A New World Role for the Medium Power* (London: Royal United Services Institute, 1977), argue that a new phase of the international system is beginning in which quality arms and policy ingenuity will be more important than power alone, thus allowing sophisticated medium powers (read the United Kingdom) to recover much of the influence lost during the period of massive deterrence.

A NUCLEAR OR CONVENTIONAL DEFENSE?

The most hotly contested defense issue in recent years concerns Britain's nuclear force and its role in NATO nuclear policy and strategy. Peter Foot, in *The Protestors*, CENTREPIECES, no. 4 (Spring 1983), examines the major arguments opposed to Britain's current nuclear policy and assesses the significance of various viewpoints and their likely impact upon the management of Britain's defense during this decade.

Reviewing a wide range of non-nuclear defense policies is *Defence Without the Bomb* (New York: Taylor & Francis, 1983), a work reporting the recommendations of the Alternate Defence Commission in response to the question, "If Britain does renounce nuclear weapons, what defence policy should it adopt?" The participants do not espouse complete disarmament, but argue that Britain should renounce the use or deployment on its territory of nuclear weapons.

In contrast to the Alternate Defence Commission's views is Peter Malone, who argues in *The British Nuclear Deterrent* (London: Croom Helm, 1984) that the case for operationally independent British nuclear force has never been stronger. He explores the British nuclear, technical, and political legacy; the American connection; doctrinal questions; the Trident decision, the costs and consequences; and the role of Britain in the Atlantic Alliance with its independent deterrent. An interesting series of three articles entitled "The Future of the British Deterrent" was published in the April, May, and June 1983 issues of *Navy International*.

DEFENSE INSTITUTIONS, PROCESSES, AND PRIORITIES

A significant amount of British defense policy literature focuses on the more inward, or domestic, nature of defense: its institutions and their organization; defense policy processes; and the relative priority of defense among competing national priorities.

David Greenwood's *Some Economic Constraints on Force Structure and Doctrine* (Aberdeen: Centre for Defense Studies, 1977) argues that fiscal constraints in the form of reduced budget allocations have forced Britain to reevaluate its defense role and policy. Another monograph from the Centre for Defence Studies at Aberdeen is David Hazel and Phil Williams, *British Defence Effort: Foundations and Alternatives*, ASIDES, no. 11 (1978). It deals with the sequential relations between defense doctrine and policy actions in an analytical framework of four parts: national security *aspirations* based upon societal values; the operational *goals* required to fulfill these aspirations; the national defense *posture* prescribing the roles and missions of the armed forces to achieve goals; and, finally, *provision* in terms of money, matériel, and manpower to allow the fulfillment of roles and missions. Using this analytical framework, the authors examine alternative defense provision, force posture, policy, and aspirations following the pattern established by Washington, D.C.'s Brookings Institution in its annual *Setting National Priorities*.

A dated, but still useful, source contrasting the U.S. and UK defense processes is Richard Neustadt's "London and Washington: Misperceptions between Allies," in *Alliance Politics* (New York: Columbia University Press, 1970). It focuses on several key differences in the decision-making processes of the United States and Great Britain that are still typical of the two systems. The contrast between the processes provides a good understanding of the British system.

A more recent source is an article by John Baylis entitled "Defence Decision-making in Britain and the Determinants of Defence Policy," *RUSI Journal*, March 1975. Baylis identifies several forces affecting the defense decision-making process and the policies themselves: personal characteristics of the decision makers, the machinery of decision making, the role of interest groups and public opinion, and economic and international determinants.

G. H. Green, "British Policy for Defence Procurement," *RUSI Journal*, September 1976, an article with a narrower perspective, summarizes the procurement process and the factors influencing it. Of particular note is his focus on the role of defense industry in British defense policy (a counterpart British "military-industrial complex?"); economic factors and overseas markets; and the issue of transatlantic versus European cooperation in joint research and development and production of weapons systems. Although Green's article was written over a decade age, the question of defense exports remains sensitive, and the issue of cooperative defense research and production continues to be widely debated in NATO fora.

Not to be underrated are sources that address the defense budget and the budget process. Two works are most useful from this perspective. The first is a comparative study by Richard Burt, *Defense Budgeting: The British and American Cases*, Adelphi Papers, no. 112 (London: IISS, 1974–75), in which he reviews the American process and the characteristics unique to it, and then, using that as a basis of comparison, does the same for the British process. He addresses the institutional frameworks, the mechanics of the budgeting process, and, finally, the perspective of the bureaucracy on budgeting. For students with a basic understanding of parliamentary and presidential systems, this article will be of great benefit.

The second study is by Michael Hobkirk, entitled *The Politics of Defense Budgeting* (Washington, D.C.: National Defense University, 1983). Hobkirk, a retired undersecretary in the Ministry of Defence, provides a contrast between the resource allocation processes of the United Kingdom and the United States.

David Greenwood's *Reshaping Britain's Defences* (ASIDES, no. 19, Summer 1981) was written in response to the Thatcher government's efforts to increase defense resources by 3 percent in real terms for the following four years. Greenwood argues that to attempt to do so would result in overstretching defense capabilities, resulting in inadequacies and waste, and presents his own alternatives.

Addressing the issue of public perceptions and defense policy is David Capitanchik, *The Changing Attitude To Defence in Britain* (CENTREPIECES, no. 2, Summer 1982). The author reviews competing domestic and defense policies of the 1960s and 1970s, and outlines the problem of resource allocation and public sentiment. He concludes that although great support existed for the Falklands action, popular support is divided over basic issues of national security, and the public is no longer content to leave defense to the government alone.

Finally, the related issue of civil-military relations, while not a predominant theme in British defense policy, is nonetheless a subject that can increase understanding of the societal constraints on policy. In "British Forces and Internal Security" (*Brassey's Annual*, 1974), D. N. Barclay reviews the role British troops have played since the nineteenth century in maintaining internal order and security, noting that there is still a role for internal security today and in the future—particularly in Northern Ireland. John C. M. Baynes, "British Military Ideology," in *Comparative Defense Policy*, ed. Frank B. Horton III et al. (Baltimore: Johns Hopkins University Press, 1974), studies the military officer in British society by examining the social strata from which officers are drawn, their political indoctrination, the military's role in British society, allies and enemies, and domestic politics. A third source, "British Armed Forces and Politics," *Armed Forces and Society* (August 1977), by Adam Roberts, Oxford University, directly addresses the issue of civil-military relations. He does so from the viewpoint of British military involvement in politics and in domestic disturbances.

Author's Note

While revising and updating this essay for the second edition of *The Defense Policies of Nations*, I was struck by the continuing relevance of many of the sources I included in the first edition, and thus the remarkable constancy of British defense policy despite a change in government, a minor war, and evolutionary change in the Ministry of Defence organization. This thought is well summarized by a commentator (whose name I overlooked) who observed: "The current government faces the same perennial resource allocation problems that have largely determined the pattern of Britain's defence dispositions since World War II." The more things change, the more they stay the same.

This essay is by no means exhaustive, but it does present at least a representative cross-section of readings dealing with the major themes and issues of British defense policy. If the reader is inclined to go further, most of the sources listed above also have bibliographic references providing additional sources. See in particular the notes at the end of David Greenwood's chapter in this volume.

China

Richard J. Latham

A sizeable literature has appeared in the 1980s that focuses on the national security affairs of the People's Republic of China (PRC). In great measure the scholarly enterprise that led to this research is a result of rapprochement with the United States. By the mid 1970s China was increasingly involved in the international system. In December 1978 the Chinese Communist Party (CCP) began a series of domestic political, economic, and social reforms that included a firm commitment to a more open interaction with the global community. In shifting from the ideologically charged Maoist policy of autarky and self-reliance, the Chinese became increasingly familiar with Western ideas, practices, scientific research, and industrial technology. With defense constituting one of China's "four modernization" goals, military exchanges with the West increased. These exchanges, in turn, resulted in greater Chinese awareness of Western national security policies. Research and policy "think tanks" were founded in China; researchers and policy analysts began writing articles about defense matters for the first time since the early 1960s. There was also a resurgence of interest among western researchers. With the exception of a flurry of earlier works about nuclear policy, the Sino-Soviet conflict, and the dominance of the military in domestic politics during the Cultural Revolution, there were relatively few substantive works prior to the late 1970s. The 1980s brought new research opportunities for researchers.

This essay aims to achieve four objectives. First, it identifies the major works of the field. Not every article is listed, but the bibliography does contain the important literature that defines the field of research. Second, the essay identifies the central scholars in the field. This is not a matter of vanity, and I do not mean to suggest that occasional writers do not make important contributions. The intent is to help students of Chinese defense policy recognize the preeminent scholars in the field. Third, the essay identifies the major subject or issue areas of the field. This will be helpful to students, who often invest considerable time in researching intriguing subjects about which little material exists in print.

A final objective is the identification of primary resource materials. Most of these are printed in Chinese or involve gleaning data from translated materials. These are the materials from which Western scholars obtain material for their "secondary" publishing activities.

GENERAL DEFENSE POLICY WORKS

The two most widely cited books dealing with the People's Liberation Army (PLA) by individual authors are Jencks (1982) and Nelsen (1981). The Defense Intelligence Agency's *Handbook of the Chinese People's Lib-*

eration Army (1976, 1984) is also an important reference book. Ray Bonds, *The Chinese War Machine* (1979) is largely a pictorial book, but provides useful descriptive information about weaponry. Edited books have permitted the timely publication of specialized research: Godwin (1983), Segal and Tow (1984), Lovejoy and Watson (1986), and Latham (1987). Segal's *Defending China* (1985) is more historical than contemporary. Important earlier books on the PLA that are now dated include Gittings (1967), Frazer (1967), Griffith (1967), and Whitson (1973).

FOREIGN AND NATIONAL SECURITY POLICIES

When China became a visible participant in the international system in the late 1970s, Chinese foreign policy also became an active area of scholarly research. Important general works included Barnett (1977), Cooper (1980), Harding (1984a, 1980), Heaton (1980a), Hsiung and Kim (1980), Hsuen (1977 and 1982), Kim (1984), Lee (1983), Pillsbury (1975a), and Yahuda (1980). The most influential writer is Jonathan D. Pollack, a RAND Corporation analyst (1984b, 1983, 1981c, 1980a, 1979). Pollack has contributed importantly to an understanding of Chinese foreign policy and strategy in a global context. Still other authors have focused more specifically on the security dimension of China's foreign relations: Godwin (1984), Gregor (1984, 1983), Gurtov and Hwang (1980), Segal (1981a) and Sutter (1986).

STRATEGY, DOCTRINE, AND POLICY

The guerrilla warfare that communist forces waged in the 1930s and 1940s, coupled with Mao Zedong's (1963) and Lin Biao's (1965) canonization of that style, have left an indelible imprint on Chinese defense policy (Griffith/1966, 1978; Johnson/1973). Research by Jencks (1987, 1984), Joffe and Segal (1985), Roberts (1983) and Woodward (1985) explore Chinese efforts to modernize their forces under the rubric of "people's war under modern conditions." Allen S. Whiting's *The Chinese Calculus of Deterrence* (1975) remains an important book in the field. Pollack has been the most prolific writer on Chinese military strategy and strategic thought (1984b, 1981c, 1981d, 1980a, 1979b).

PLA doctrine and tactics have been the subject of publications by Paul Godwin (1978a, 1977), formerly on the faculty of the U.S. Air Force's Air University and now a member of the National Defense University faculty, John W. Lewis (1980), and Ralph Powell (1968). Defense policy issues have been addressed by Harding (1974), Harris (1979), Johnston (1986), Pollack (1981a), and Shambaugh (1987). David Shambaugh examines the new phenomenon of policy inputs from Chinese research institutes and think tanks. Other aspects of Chinese defense strategy, doctrine, policy, military culture and values are discussed in Boorman (1972), Boylan (1982), Chan (1978), Garrett and Glaser (1984), Gurtov and Hwang (1980), Pillsbury (1980/1981), and Whiting (1972).

REGIONAL SECURITY POLICY

Published research on Chinese national security policy focuses principally on the Soviet Union, the shift from confrontation to consultation in U.S.-China relations, Taiwan, and Vietnam. To a lesser extent, writers have examined China's security relations with the two Koreas, Japan, Southeast Asia, India, and Pakistan.

With the Sino-Soviet rift in 1958–59, China's principal benefactor in the modernization of its guerrilla army became China's primary threat. Subsequent border clashes with the USSR along China's northern border further resulted in considerable Western analysis in the 1970s (see Liberthal/1978, Pillsbury/1975a). In recent years Sino-Soviet relations have again been a popular issue among scholars, as the Chinese have found themselves being courted by both the United States and the Soviet Union in a "triangular relationship." These works have included Adelman (1979), Daniel and Jencks (1983), Hiramatsu (1983), Pollack (1982, 1981, 1981b), Segal (1983), Whiting (1984), Wong-Fraser (1981b), and Zagoria (1983).

Security relations between the United States and China have also been extensively analyzed. The notion of playing the China or America "card" has given way to a more subtle exploration of areas of common agreement and discussion of fundamental differences. While both the United States and China once shared considerable concern about the Soviet threat, in recent years the Chinese have deemphasized the "common enemy" concept to steer a more centrist course between the two superpowers. Recent works that deal with various aspects of U.S.-China relations include Bullard (1983), Chang (1984), CRS (1981), Gass (1984), Gregor and Chang (1984), Levin and Pollack (1984), Pillsbury (1975, 1975a), Pollack (1984), Sino-U.S. (1982), Solomon (1981), Stuart and Tow (1982, 1981), Sutter (1983, 1981), Tow (1976), and Whiting (1982).

Taiwan and Vietnam also are the subjects of much analytical research. In recent years both Taiwan and the PRC have reduced the level of confrontation across the Taiwan Strait. Security relations between the United States and Taiwan continue to be a thorny policy issue in U.S.-China relations. At the heart of the issue is the kind of assistance the United States gives to Taiwan in the form of military sales and technology cooperation to maintain Taiwan's defensive force posture. Research on this subject includes Dowen (1979), Gregor (1985), Gregor and Chang (1984a), Lasater (1982), Linder and Gregor (1980), Snyder and Gregor (1981), Snyder, Gregor and Chang (1980), Whiting (1983), and Wolff and Simon (1982). The Sino-Vietnam War of 1979 and subsequent border clashes have been addressed by Jencks (1979), and Linder and Gregor (1981). The Sino-Vietnamese confrontation is described by the Chinese as being linked to the larger issue of Vietnamese hegemony on the Indochina peninsula, particularly Kampuchea (Cambodia).

FORCE STRUCTURE

The composition of the PLA force structure has not changed appreciably since the early 1960s. Conse-

quently, there has been little need to engage in much more than "bean counting" at the margins. Useful resources are Bonds (1979), DIA (1984), and Jencks (1982). The best yearly source of order-of-battle data is the *Military Balance*, published by the International Institute for Strategic Studies, London. Information regarding new weapons systems and modifications is frequently found in periodicals such as *Conmilit* (Hong Kong), *Asian Defense Review* (Malaysia), *Hongkong Zhishi* (Aviation Knowledge, Beijing), *Hongkong Zazhi* (Aviation Magazine, Beijing), *Wugi Zhishi* (Ordnance Knowledge, Beijing), and *Jiefangjun Huabao* (Liberation Army Pictorial, Beijing).

China's strategic forces (missiles and nuclear weapons) are the subject of a small group of writers such as Gelber (1973), Halperin (1965), Hsieh (1962), Pollack (1977, 1972), Richeson (1973), Segal (1981), Sutter (1983), Tow (1976), Treverton (1980), Wang (1983), and Wong-Fraser (1981). Relatively little has been written in recent years since there have been few changes in China's strategic force structure. The implications of the Reagan administration's Strategic Defense Initiative (SDI) for China's minimum deterrent nuclear force have prompted considerable interest among Chinese writers (Johnston 1986).

CIVIL-MILITARY RELATIONS

A consistently popular topic in Chinese national security studies has been civil-military relations. There have been important theoretical works by Albright (1980), Colton (1979), and Herspring and Volgyes (1978) about civil-military relations in general. Chinese civil-military relations have their roots in regional warlordism (Pye, 1971). The dominant role that the PLA played in domestic affairs during the Cultural Revolution (1966–72) gave rise to an extensive literature that included works by Chang (1972), Gittings (1970), Joffe (1975, 1973, 1971, 1965), Parrish (1973), and Jain (1976). Subsequent research on civil-military relations has focused on the diminution of the military's domestic political influence and the PLA's efforts to rebuild favorable relations with the civilian population. Major writers in this area include Dreyer (1982), Godwin (1984), Johnston (1984), Joffe (1983), Latham (1983), Nethercut (1982), and Segal (1981a).

The role of military elites in determining defense policy and garnering appropriations is related to a larger study of Chinese political elites (see Bullard, 1979; Nathan, 1973; Pye, 1980). Earlier approaches included Ting's (1979, 1975) emphasis on military factions while Whitson (1972, 1969, 1968) stressed field army affiliations. Monte Bullard (1985), a former U.S. army attache in Beijing and Hong Kong, has argued that more attention should be given to elite roles as the PLA becomes increasingly regularized and accustomed to operating in permanent military oganizations.

MILITARY MODERNIZATION

Apart from strategy, policy and doctrine, the subject area that has attracted the most attention has been military modernization. Defense modernization comes last on Deng Xiaoping's list of "four modernizations" (i.e., agriculture, industry, science and technology, and defense). Consequently, there is an inherent tension between the external threat that demands "more defense" and domestic programs than currently are given priority consideration. Nearly all writers at least implicitly draw attention to the efforts of the military modernizers to develop a force structure that adequately meets external threats while concurrently trying to achieve that objective without larger defense allocations. Important works on this subject include Baum (1980), Bok (1984), Dreyer (1987, 1984, 1984a, 1982a), Godwin (1981, 1987, 1977), Frankenstein (1987), Fraser (1979), L. Liu (1979), Jencks (1982a), Joffe and Segal (1985), Luttwak (1979), Pollack (1980b, 1979a), Pye (1980a), Robinson (1982), Romance (1980), Shambaugh (1979, 1979a), Segal (1982), Stuart and Tow (1981), Wolfgang (1984), and Woodward (1985).

Several issues are related to the modernization of the PLA. One has been professionalization (frequently called "army-building" in Chinese parlance) and military education and training. Published works in this area include Godwin (1977), Heaton (1978, 1980, 1980b), Joffe (1983), Joffe and Segal (1978), Latham (1983), and Yu (1985).

A second area has involved China's defense industries. On the one hand, they have sought critical modernizing technology transfers from the West to improve their own armed forces. On the other hand, domestic economic reforms have prompted a "civilianization" of the defense industries and an aggressive sale of arms, particularly in the Third world, to put China's defense industries on a profitable basis. Examples of this research are IISS (1980), Chu (1984), CRS (1981), Jencks (1980), Latham (1987, 1986, 1986a, 1984), Mershon (1981), Pollack (1985, 1985a), Shambaugh (1983), Stuart and Tow (1982a, 1981), and Sutter (1981).

Third, defense modernization is closely linked to the acquisition of Western military technology. This has been a controversial area in China as well as among Western governments. The Chinese have sought state-of-the-art military technology that in many cases is not even transferred among Western allies for commercial reasons. Chinese leaders frequently criticize COCOM countries for trying to impede China's military modernization by prohibiting the sale of certain technologies. Concurrently, the Chinese acknowledge that they have serious problems absorbing the technology that is available. Western industrial countries are anxious to sell equipment rather than technology, since they fear the Chinese will become competitors in foreign arms sales. Major works in this area are Deshingkar (1983), Gelb (1979), Gelber (1979), Orleans (1981), Shambaugh (1979a), Simon (1984, 1982), and Suttmeier (1980).

PRIMARY RESEARCH SOURCES

There is a variety of primary research sources, but many are in the Chinese language. The most authoritative Chinese publications include the following: People's Daily (Renmin Ribao, Beijing), Guangming Daily (Guangming Ribao, Beijing), Liberation Army Daily (Jiefangjun Bao, Beijing), and Red Flag (Honggi, Beijing). Editorials are among the best indicators of policy shifts, especially the 1 July (anniversary of the Chinese Communist Party), 1 August (anniversary of the People's Liberation Army), 1 October (anniversary of the People's Republic of China) and 1 January (New Year) editorials, which are frequently used to announce important policies. The Beijing Review, formerly Peking Review, is an English-language tabloid that frequently publishes important policy decisions and documents.

In recent years China has resumed publishing academic and professional journals. Technically they are not "primary" sources, but their official and semi-official status makes them reliable indicators of officially approved or tolerated perspectives. These publications include International Studies (Guoji Wenti Yanjiu, Beijing), International Affairs Study Journal (Guoji Guanxi Xueyan Xuebao, Beijing), Contemporary International Relations (Xiandai Guoji Guanxi, Beijing), Materials on International Studies (Guoji Wenti Ziliao, Shanghai), International Strategic Studies (Guoji Zhanlue Yanjiu, Beijing), International Studies (Guoji Wenti Yanjiu, Beijing), Economic Management (Jingji Guanli, Beijing), Enterprise Management (Qiyue Guanli, Beijing), Outlook (Liaowang, Beijing), Fortnightly (Banyue Tan, Beijing), World Affairs (Shijie Zhishi, Beijing), Modernization (Xiandaihua, Beijing), Aviation Knowledge (Hangkong Zhishi, Beijing), Aviation Magazine (Hangkong Zazhi, Beijing), Aerospace Knowledge (Hangtian Zhishi, Beijing), Ordnance Knowledge (Wugi Zhishi, Beijing), and Historical Studies (Lishi Yanjiu, Beijing). Several Chinese language periodicals are published in Hong Kong and Taiwan such as Contending (Zhengming, Hong Kong), The Eighties, formerly The Seventies (Bashi Niandai, Hong Kong), Conmilit (Xandai Junshi or Hong Kong), Communist Chinese Studies (Chungkung Yenchiu, Taipei), Issues and Studies (in English, Taipei), National Defense Digest (Kuofang Yits'ui, Taipei), and Problems and Research (Went'i yu Yenchiu, Taipei). Asian English language periodicals include Hong Kong's weekly Far Eastern Economic Review and Asian Defence Journal (monthly, Kuala Lumpur, Malaysia).

Many of the important articles from Chinese-language sources are available in English translation. The Foreign Broadcast Information Service (FBIS), a U.S. government organization, publishes the Daily Report: China, which is a daily transcription and translation of Chinese radio broadcasts and publications. The Joint Publications Research Service (JPRS), also a U.S. government organization and associated with FBIS, publishes a series of translations from published Chinese language sources. For researchers who do not have access to original Chinese sources, these are extremely valuable translations: China Report: Red Flag, China Report: Political, Sociological and Military Affairs, China Report: Economic Affairs, China Report: Agriculture, and China Report: Science and Technology. An abbreviated source of translated material can be found in the British Broadcasting Corporation's Summary of World Broadcasts/Far East.

A number of English language academic journals frequently publish articles on Chinese defense policy, including China Quarterly, Asian Survey, Journal of Asian Studies, Journal of Northeast Asian Studies, Modern China, Australian Journal of Chinese Affairs, Pacific Affairs, Current History, and Problems of Communism. The Association of Asian Studies, publisher of the Journal of Asian Studies, also publishes an annual, exhaustive Bibliography of Asian Studies. Unfortunately, it is running several years behind. Each issue of China Quarterly contains a particularly useful, but often overlooked, "Quarterly Chronicle and Documentation" section. Taipei's Issues and Studies frequently contains translations of covertly obtained classified documents from China.

PROSPECTS

In the first edition of *The Defense Policies of Nations* the bibliographic essay was largely an examination of a small body of literature that emphasized the paucity of defense-related information. That situation has changed radically. In recent years the literature on Chinese defense policy has been enriched not only by an increasingly sophisticated Western scholarship, but also by a growing number of Chinese "defense intellectuals," research organizations, and publications. Our understanding of Chinese national security matters is still thin compared to what we understand about defense policy in Western states and even the Soviet Union. Students of Chinese defense policy are, however, developing a more sharply defined sense of community (Jencks, 1986; Latham, 1985), and that community increasingly includes Chinese scholars. In 1986 there was an unprecedented exchange of research fellows and lecturers between the U.S. National Defense University and the PLA's National Defense University. Western academics and military officers have visited and addressed meetings of defense policy scholars, analysts, and military officers in China, as their Chinese counterparts have done in Western countries. Although the doors of libraries, archives, and think tanks have hardly been thrown open, there are at least encouraging signs that the study of Chinese defense policy will move beyond macro-level speculation.

Bibliography

Adelman, Jonathan R. (1979). "The Soviet and Chinese Armies: Their Post–Civil War Roles." *Survey*, 24 (Winter), 57–81.

———. (1978) "The Formative Influence of Civil Wars: Social Roles of the Soviet and Chinese Armies." *Armed Forces and Society*, Vol. 5, 93–116.

Albright, David (1980). "A Comparative Conceptualization of Civil-Military Relations." *World Politics* (July).

Barnett, A. Doak (1985). *The Making of Foreign Policy in China: Structure and Process*, Boulder, CO: Westview Press.

———. (1977). *China and the Major Powers in East Asia*, Washington, D.C.: The Brookings Institution.

Baum, Richard E. (ed.) (1980). *China's Four Modernizations*, Boulder, CO: Westview Press.

Bok, Georges Tan Eng (1984). *La Modernization de la Défense Chinoise et ses Principales Limites, 1977–1983*, Paris: Fondation pour les Etudes de Défense Nationale.

———. (1984a). "Strategic Doctrine." In Gerald Segal and William Tow (eds.), *Chinese Defence Policy*, Urbana and Chicago: University of Illinois Press, 3–17.

———. (1983). "China's Military Doctrine and Stategy." Paper delivered at the Conference on Chinese Defense issues. Garmisch, FRG, May 3–6, 1983.

———. (1980). "La strategie nucleaire chinoise." *Strategique* (Fall), 25–62.

———. (1979). "Système militaire et système politique en Chine communiste." *Strategique* (Spring), 15–57.

———. (1978). "La modernisation de la défense chinoise et ses limites." *Défense national* (May), 69–84.

Bonds, Ray (1979). *The Chinese War Machine*, London: Salamander Books Ltd.

Boorman Scott A. (1972). "Deception in Chinese Strategy." In William W. Whitson (ed.), *The Military and Political Power in China in the 1970s*, New York: Praeger.

Boylan, Edward S. (1982). "The Chinese Cultural Style of Warfare." *Comparative Strategy*, 3, 341–364.

Bullard, Monte R. (1985). *China's Political-Military Evolution: The Party and the Military in the PRC: 1960–1984*, Boulder, CO: Westview Press.

———. (1983). "The U.S.–China Defense Relationship." *Paramaters*, 13 (March), 43–50.

———. (1979). "People's Republic of China Elite Studies: A Review of the Literature." *Asian Survey*, 19 (August), 789–800.

Chan, Steve (1978). "Chinese Conflict Calculus and Behavior: Assessment from a Perspective of Conflict Management." *World Politics*, 30 (April), 391–410.

Chang, Parris H. (1984). "U.S.–China Relations: From Hostility to Euphoria to Realism." *The Annals*, 476 (November), 156–170.

———. (1972). "The Changing Pattern of Military Participation in Chinese Politics." *Orbis*, 16 (Fall).

Chen, K. C. (ed.) (1979). *China and the Three Worlds: A Foreign Policy Reader*, White Plains, NY: M. E. Sharpe, Inc.

Cheng, Chester J. (ed.) (1966). *The Politics of the Chinese Red Army*, Stanford, CA: Stanford University Press.

Chu, Wellington (1984). "Increased Military Sales to China." *Journal of International Affairs*, Vol. 39.

Clough, Ralph N., et al. (1975). *The United States, China, and Arms Control*, Washington, D.C.: The Brookings Institution.

Colton, Timothy (1979). *Commissars, Commanders and Civilian Authority*, Cambridge, MA: Harvard University Press.

Cooper, John E. (1980). *China's Global Role*, Stanford, CA: Hoover Institution Press.

Congressional Research Service (CRS) (1981). *The Implications of U.S.-China Military Cooperation*, Washington, D.C.: United States Government Printing Office. (A workshop sponsored by the Committee on Foreign Relations, U.S. Senate and Congressional Research Service, Library of Congress.)

Daniel, Donald C. and Harlan W. Jencks (1983). "Soviet Military Confrontation with China: Options for the USSR, the PRC, and the United States." *Conflict*, Vol. 5, 57–87.

Defense Intelligence Agency (DIA) (1985). *A Selective Annotated Bibliography on the Chinese People's Liberation Army*, Washington, D.C.: Defense Intelligence Agency. DDB-2600-4737-85. Vols. 1 and 11 (July), Vol. III (October).

———. (1984). *Handbook of the Chinese People's Liberation Army*, Washington, D.C.: Defense Intelligence Agency. DDB-2680-32-84. Supersedes *Handbook of the Chinese Armed Forces* (1976).

Deshingkar, Giri (1983). "Military Technology and the Quest for Self-reliance in India and China." *International Social Science Journal*, 35, 99–121, 3–17.

Downen, Robert L. (1979). *The Taiwan Pawn in the China Game: Congress to the Rescue*, Washington, D.C.: Georgetown University.

Dreyer, June Teufel (1987). "The Streamlining and Reorganization of the Chinese People's Liberation Army." In Richard J. Latham (ed.), *Chinese National*

Security and the Second Revolution, Boulder, CO: Lynne Rienner Publishers.

———. (1984). "China's Military in the 1980's." *Current History*, 83 (September), 269–278.

———. (1984a). "China's Military Modernization." *Orbis*, 27 (Winter), 1011–1026.

———. (1982). "The Chinese Militia: Citizen-Soldiers and Civil-Military Relations in the People's Republic of China." *Armed Forces and Society*, 9 (Fall), 63–82.

———. (1982a). *China's Military Power in the 1980's*, Washington, D.C.: China Council of the Asia Society.

Fingar, Thomas (1980). "Domestic Policy and the Quest for Independence." In Thomas Fingar and the Stanford Journal of International Studies (eds.). *China's Quest for Independence: Policy Evolution in the 1970's*, Boulder, CO: Westview Press, pp. 25–92.

Frankenstein, John (1987). "A Historical Perspective on Chinese Military Modernization." In Richard J. Latham (ed.). *Chinese National Security and the Second Revolution*, Boulder, CO: Lynne Rienner Publishers.

Fraser, Angus M. (1979). "Military Modernization in China." *Problems of Communism*, 28 (September–December), 34–49.

———. (1967). *The People's Liberation Army*, London: Oxford University Press.

Garrett, Bannin N., and Bonnie S. Glaser (1984). *War and Peace: The Views from Moscow and Beijing*, Berkeley, CA: Institute of International Studies.

Gass, Henry B. (1984). *Sino-American Security Relations: Expectations and Realities*, Washington, D.C.: National Defense University Press.

Gelb, Leslie H. (1979). "U.S. Defence Technology, Policy Transfers, and Asian Security." In Richard H. Soloman (ed.), *Asian Security in the 1980s*, Santa Monica, CA: RAND Corporation.

Gelber, Harry G. (1979). *Technology, Defense and External Relations in China*, Boulder, CO: Westview Press.

———. (1973). *Nuclear Weapons and China Policy*, Adelphi Paper No. 99, London: International Institute for Strategic Studies.

Gelman, Harry (1983). "Soviet Policy Towards China." *Survey*, 27 (Autumn–Winter), 165–174, 247–272.

George, Alexander (1967). *The Chinese Communist Army in Action: The Korean War and Its Aftermath*, New York: Columbia University Press.

Gittings, John (1970). "Army-Party Relations in the Context of the Cultural Revolution." In John Wilson Lewis (ed.). *Party Leadership and Revolutionary Power in China*, London: Cambridge University Press.

———. (1967). *The Role of the Chinese Army*, London: Oxford University Press.

Godwin, Paul H. B. (1984). "Soldiers and Statesmen in Conflict: Chinese Defense and Foreign Policies in the 1980s." In Samuel S. Kim (ed.), *China and the World: Chinese Foreign Policy in the Post-Mao Era*, Boulder, CO: Westview Press.

———. (1983). *The Chinese Defense Establishment: Continuity and Change in the 1980s*, Boulder, CO: Westview Press.

———. (1981). "China's Defense Modernization." *Air University Review*, 33 (November/December), 3–19.

———. (1979). "China and the Second World: The Search for Defense Technology." *Contemporary China*, 2 (Fall), 3–9.

———. (1978a). *The Chinese Tactical Air Forces and Strategic Weapons Program: Development, Doctrine, and Strategy*, Maxwell AFB, AL: Air University Documentary Research Study.

———. (1978b). "China's Defense Dilemma: The Modernization Crisis of 1976 and 1977." *Contemporary China*, 2 (Fall), 63–85.

———. (1977). *Doctrine, Strategy, and Ethics: The Modernization of the Chinese People's Liberation Army*, Maxwell AFB, AL: Air University.

Gregor, A. James (1985). "Modernization of the Air Force of the PRC and the Military Balance in the Taiwan Strait. *Issues and Studies*, 21 (October), 58–74.

———. (1984). "Western Security and the Military Potential of the PRC." *Parameters*, Vol. 14, 35–48.

———. (1983). "The People's Republic of China as a Western Security Asset." *Air University Review*, 34 (July–August), 12–23.

Gregor, A. James and Maria Hsia Chang (1984). *The Iron Triangle: A U.S. Security Policy for Northeast Asia*, Stanford, CA: Hoover Institution Press.

———. (1984a). *The Taiwan Relations Act*, Glen Falls, NY: U.S. Committee on Asia-Pacific Peace and Stability.

Griffith, Samuel B. (1967). *The Chinese People's Liberation Army*, New York: McGraw-Hill Book Company.

———. (1978). *Mao Zedong on Guerrilla Warfare*, Garden City, NY: Anchor Press/Doubleday.

———. (1966). *Pekingarfare*, Garden City, NY: Anchor Press/Doubleday.

———. (1966). *Peking and People's Wars*, London: Pall Mall Press.

Gurtov, Melvin and Byong-Moo Hwang (1980). *China Under Threat: The Politics of Strategy and Diplomacy*, Baltimore: Johns Hopkins University Press.

Halperin, Morton (1965). *China and the Bomb*, New York: Fred Praeger.

Harding, Harry (1984). "Competing Models of the Chinese Communist Policy Process: Toward a Sorting and Evaluation." *Issues and Studies*, 20 (February), 13–36.

———. (1984a). *China's Foreign Relations in the 1980s*, New Haven, CT: Yale University Press.

———. (1980). "The Domestic Politics of China's Global Posture, 1973–78." In Thomas Fingar and the Stanford Journal of International Studies (eds.). *China's Quest for Independence: Policy Evolution in the 1970's*, Boulder, CO: Westview Press, 93–146.

———. (1974). "The Evolution of Chinese Military Policy." In Frank B. Horton et al. (eds.), *Comparative Defense Policy*, Baltimore: Johns Hopkins University Press, 216–232.

Harris, Jack H. (1979). "Enduring Chinese Dimensions in Peking's Military Policy and Doctrine." *Issues and Studies*, 15 (July), 77–88.

———. (1979a). "Politics of National Security in China." *Problems of Communism*, 28 (March–April) 64–66.

Heaton, William R., Jr. (1987). "New Trends in China's Professional Military Education and Training." In Richard J. Latham (ed.), *Chinese National Security and the Second Revolution*, Boulder, CO: Lynne Rienner Publishers.

———. (1980). "Professional Military Education in China: A Visit to the Military Academy of the People's Liberation Army." *China Quarterly*, 81 (March), 122–128.

———. (1980a). *A United Front Against Hegemonism: Chinese Foreign Policy into the 1980's*, Washington, D.C.: National Defense University.

———. (1980b). "Professional Military Education in China: A Visit to the Military Academy of the People's Liberation Army." *China Quarterly*, 81 (March), 122–128.

Herspring, Dale and Ivan Volgyes (eds.) (1978). *Civil-Military Relations in Communist Systems*, Boulder, CO: Westview Press.

Hiramatsu, Shingeo (1983). "A Chinese Prespective on Sino-Soviet Relations." *Journal of Northeast Asian Studies*, 2 (September), 60–62.

Hsieh, Alice L. (1962). *Communist China's Strategy in the Nuclear Era*, Englewood Cliffs, NJ: Prentice-Hall.

Hsiung, James C. and Samuel S. Kim (eds.) (1980). *China in the Global Community*, New York: Praeger.

Hsueh, Chun-tu (ed.) (1982). *China's Foreign Relations: New Perspectives*, New York: Praeger.

———. (1977). *Dimensions of China's Foreign Relations*, New York: Praeger Publishers.

Huang, Chen-hsia (1968). *Mao's Generals*, Hong Kong: Research Institute of Contemporary History (in Chinese).

International Institute for Strategic Studies (IISS) (1980). "China's Defence Industries." *Strategic Survey 1979*, London: International Institute for Strategic Studies.

Jain, Jagdish P. (1976). *After Mao What? Army, Party and Group Rivalries in China*, Boulder, CO: Westview Press.

Jencks, Harlan W. (1978). "PRC Defense Strategy as Reflected in Military Reform." In Richard J. Latham (ed.), *Chinese National Security and the Second Revolution*, Boulder, CO: Lynne Rienner Publishers.

———. (1986). "The Current State of Chinese Military Studies: A Personal View." Paper presented at the Asian Studies on the Pacific Coast Conference, 28–30 June 1985. University of Oregon, Eugene.

———. (1985). "Lessons of a 'Lesson': China-Vietnam, 1979." In Robert E. Harkavy and Stephanie E. Newman (eds.), *The Lessons of Recent Wars in the Third World*, Lexington, MA: D.C. Heath.

———. (1984). " 'People's War under Modern Conditions': Wishful Thinking, National Suicide, or Effective Deterrent?" *China Quarterly*, 98 (June), 305–319.

———. (1982). *From Muskets to Missiles: Politics and Professionalism in the Chinese Army, 1945–1981*, Boulder, CO: Westview Press.

———. (1982a). "Defending China in 1982." *Current History*, 81 (September).

———. (1980). "The Chinese Military-Industrial Complex and Defense Modernization." *Asian Survey*, (October).

———. (1979). "China's 'Punitive' War on Vietnam: A Military Assessment." *Asian Survey*, 19 (August), 801–815.

Joffe, Ellis (1983). "Party and Military in China: Professionalism in Command?" *Problems of Communism*, 82 (September–October), 48–63.

———. (1975). "China's Military: The PLA in Internal Politics." *Problems of Communism*, 24 (November/December).

———. (1973). "The Chinese Army after the Cultural Revolution." *China Quarterly*, 55 (July/September).

———. (1971). *Party and Army*, Cambridge, MA: East Asian Research Center, Harvard University.

———. (1965). *Party and Army, Professionalism and Political Control in the Chinese Officer Corps, 1949–1964*, Cambridge, MA: Harvard University Press.

Joffe, Ellis and Gerald Segal (1985). "The PLA Under Modern Conditions." *Survival*, 27 (July/August), 146–157.

———. (1978). "The Chinese Army and Professionalism." *Problems of Communism*, 27 (November/December), 1–19.

Johnson, U. Alexis, George R. Packard, and Alfred D. Wilhelm, Jr. (1984). *China Policy for the Next Decade*, Boston, MA: Oelgeschlager, Gunn and Hain, Publishers.

Johnson, Chalmers (1973). *Autopsy on People's Wars*, Berkeley, CA: University of California Press.

Johnston, Alastair L. (1986). *China and Arms Control: Emerging Issues and Interests in the 1980s*, Ottawa: The Canadian Centre for Arms Control and Disarmament.

———. (1984). "Changing Party-Army Relations in China, 1979–1984." *Asian Survey*, 10 (October), 1012–1040.

Kierman, Frank A., Jr. (1974), *Chinese Ways in Warfare*, Cambridge, MA: Harvard University Press.

Kihl, Young Whan and Lawrence E. Grinter (1986). *Asian-Pacific Security: Emerging Challenges and Responses*, Boulder, CO: Lynne Rienner Publishers.

Kim, Samuel S. (1984). *China and the World: Chinese Foreign Policy in the Post-Mao Era*, Boulder, CO: Westview Press.

———. (1979). *China, the United Nations and World Order*, Princeton, NJ: Princeton University Press.

Lary, Diana (1985). *Warlord Soldiers: Chinese Common Soldiers, 1911–1935*, New York: Cambridge University Press.

Lasater Martin L. (1982). *The Security of Taiwan: Unraveling the Dilemma*, Washington, D.C.: Georgetown University.

Latham, Richard J. (ed.) (1978). *Chinese National Security and the Second Revolution*, Boulder, CO: Lynne Rienner Publishers.

———. (1986). "The Implications of the Post-Mao Reforms on the Chinese Defense Industries." In Douglas Lovejoy and Bruce Watson (eds.), *Chinese Defense Policy in Review*, Boulder, CO: Westview Press.

———. (1986a). "The Implications of Military Industrialization in the PRC." In James E. Katz (ed.), *Sowing the Serpents' Teeth: The Implications of Third World Military Industrialization*, Lexington, MA: Lexington Books.

———. (1985). "Summary of Discussions at the Conference of PRC National Security Affairs: An Assessment of Analytical Trends." Washington, D.C.: Defense Intelligence College.

———. (1984). "People's Republic of China: The Restructuring of Defense-Industrial Policies." In James E. Katz (ed.), *Arms Production in Developing Countries: An Analysis of Decision Making*, Lexington, MA: Lexington Books.

———. (1983). "The Rectification of 'Work Style'

Command and Management Problems in the PLA."
In Paul Godwin (ed.). *The Chinese Defense Establishment: Continuity and Change in the 1980s*, Boulder, CO: Westview Press, 89–120.

Lee, Edmund (1983), "Beijing's Balancing Act." *Foreign Policy*, 51 (Summer), 27–63.

Leng, Shao-chuan (1984). "China's Nuclear Policy: An Overall View." University of Maryland (Occasional Papers, No. 1).

Levin, Norman D. and Jonathan D. Pollack (1984). *Managing the Strategic Triangle: Summary of a Workshop Discussion*, Santa Monica, CA: RAND Corporation.

———. (1984a). "Beijing and the Superpowers." *Problems of Communism*, 33 (November/December).

Lewis, John Wilson (1980). "China's Military Doctrines and Force Posture." In Thomas Fingar and the Stanford Journal of International Studies (eds.). *China's Quest for Independece: Policy Evolution in the 1970's*, Boulder, CO: Westview Press, 147–197.

Liberthal, Kenneth G. (1978). *Sino-Soviet Conflict in the 1970's: Its Evolution and Implications for the Strategic Triangle*, Santa Monica, CA: RAND Corporation.

Lin Piao (1965). *Long Live the Victory of the People's War*, Beijing: Foreign Languages Press.

Linder, James B. and A. James Gregor (1981). "The Chinese Communist Air Force in the 'Punitive' War Against Vietnam." *Air University Review*, 32 (September/October), 67–77.

———. (1980). "Taiwan's Troubled Security Outlook." *Strategic Review*, 9 (Fall), 48–55.

Liu, Alan P. L. (1979). "The 'Gang of Four' and the Chinese People's Liberation Army." *Asian Survey*, 19 (September), 817–837.

Liu, Leo Yueh-yun (1979). "The Modernization of the Chinese Military." *Current History*, 79 (September), 9–40.

Lovejoy, Charles D., Jr., and Bruce W. Watson (eds.) (1986). *China's Military Reforms*, Boulder, CO: Westview Press.

Luttwak, Edward N. (1979). "Military Modernization in the People's Republic of China: Problems and Prospects." *The Journal of Strategic Studies*.

Mao Zedong (1963). *Selected Military Writings of Mao Tsetung*, Beijing: Foreign Languages Press.

McMillen, Donald Hugh (ed.) (1984). *Asian Perspectives on International Security*, New York: St. Martin's Press.

Mershon Center Quarterly Report (1981). *U.S. Military Sales and Technology Transfers to China: The Policy Implications*, Columbus, OH: Ohio State University Press.

Mirsky, Jonathan (1981). "China's 1979 Invasion of Vietnam: A View from the Infantry." *Journal of the Royal United Services Institute for Defence Studies*, 136 (January).

Muller, David G., Jr. (1983). *China as a Maritime Power*, Boulder CO: Westview Press.

———. (1983a). "China's SSBN in Perspective." *U.S. Naval Institute Proceedings*, 109 (March), 125–127.

Natham, Andrew J. (1973). "A Factional Model for CCP Politics." *China Quarterly*, 53 (January–March), 34–66.

Nelsen, Harvey W. (1981). *The Chinese Military System: An Organizational Study of the Chinese Peo-*

ple's Liberation Army, 2nd edition, revised. Boulder, CO: Westview Press.

Nethercut, Richard D. (1982). "Deng and the Gun: Party-Military Relations in the People's Republic of China." *Asian Survey*, 8 (August), 691–705.

Orleans, Leo (ed.) (1981). *Science in Contemporary China*, Stanford, CA: Stanford University Press.

Parrish, William (1973). "Factions in Chinese Military Politics." *China Quarterly*, 56 (October/December), 667–699.

Pillsbury, Michael (1980/81). "Strategic Acupuncture." *Foreign Policy*, 41 (Winter), 44–61.

———. (1975). "U.S.-Chinese Military Ties." *Foreign Policy*, 20 (Fall), 50–64.

———. (1975a). *Chinese Views of the Soviet-American Strategic Balance: Salt on the Dragon*, Santa Monica, CA: RAND Corporation.

Pollack, Jonathan D. (1985). *The R & D Process and Technological Innovation in the Chinese Industrial System*, Santa Monica, CA: RAND Corporation.

———. (1985a). *The Chinese Electronics Industry in Transition*, Santa Monica, CA: RAND Corporation.

———. (1984). *The Lessons of Coalition Politics: Sino-American Security Relations*, Santa Monica, CA: RAND Corporation.

———. (1984a). *China's Role in Pacific Basin Security*, Santa Monica, CA: RAND Corporation; also *Survival*, (July/August), 164–173.

———. (1984b). *China and the Global Strategic Balance*, Santa Monica, CA: RAND Corporation; also in Harry Harding (ed.), *China's Foreign Relations in the 1980's*, New Haven, CT: Yale University Press, 146–176.

———. (1983). *China in the Evolving International System*, Santa Monica, CA: RAND Corporation.

———. (1982). *The Sino-Soviet Rivalry and Chinese Security Debate*, Santa Monica, CA: RAND Corporation.

———. (1981). "Chinese Global Strategy and Soviet Power." *Problems of Communism*, 30 (January/February), 54–69.

———. (1981a). *Strategy and Policy in Chinese Security Debates*, Santa Monica, CA: RAND Corporation.

———. (1981b). *The Sino-Soviet Conflict in the 1980s: Its Dynamics and Policy Implications*, Santa Monica, CA: RAND Corporation.

———. (1981c). *Security, Strategy and the Logic of Chinese Foreign Policy*, Berkeley, CA: University of California Institute of East Asian Studies, Policy Studies Monograph.

———. (1981d). "The Evolution of Chinese Strategic Thought." In Robert O'Neill and D. M. Horner (eds.), *New Directions in Strategic Thinking*, London: George Allen & Unwin, 137–152.

———. (1980). "China as a Military Power." In Onkar Marwah and Jonathan D. Pollack (eds.). *Military Power and Policy in Asian States*, Boulder, CO: Westview Press, 43–99.

———. (1980a). *Security, Strategy, and the Logic of Chinese Foreign Policy*, Berkeley, CA: University of California Institute of East Asian Studies, Policy Studies Monograph.

———. (1980b). "Modernization of National Defense." In Richard E. Baum (ed.), *China's Four Modernizations*, Boulder, CO: Westview Press.

———. (1979). "The People's Republic of China in a Proliferated World." In J. K. King (ed.), *International Political Effects of the Spread of Nuclear Weapons*, Washington, D.C.: U.S. Government Printing Office.

———. (1979a). *Defense Modernization in the People's Republic of China*, Santa Monica, CA: RAND Corporation.

———. (1979b). "The Logic of Chinese Military Strategy." *Bulletin of the Atomic Scientists*, 34 (January), 23–24.

———. (1977). "China as a Nuclear Power." In W. Overholt (ed.), *Asia's Nuclear Future*, Boulder, CO: Westview Press.

———. (1972). "Chinese Attitudes Toward Nuclear Weapons, 1964–9." *China Quarterly*, 50 (April/June), 244–271.

Powell, Ralph L. (1968). "Maoist Military Doctrines." *Asian Survey*, 8 (April), 239–262.

Pye, Lucian (1980). *The Dynamics of Factions and Consensus in Chinese Politics: A Model and Some Proposition*, Santa Monica, CA: RAND Corporation.

———. (1980a). "Dilemmas for America in China's Modernization." *International Security*, (Spring).

———. (1971). *Warlord Politics*, New York: Praeger.

Quester, George H. (1984). "America and the Chinese: The Need for Continuing Ambiguity." *Crossroads*, No. 13, 35–53.

Richeson, Alfred K. (1973). "Evolution of Chinese Nuclear Strategy." *Military Review*, 53 (January), 13–30.

Roberts, Thomas C. (1983). *The Chinese People's Militia and the Doctrine of People's War*, Washington, D.C.: National Defense University Press.

Robinson, Thomas W. (1982). "Chinese Military Modernization in the 1980s." *China Quarterly*, 90 (June), 231–252.

Romance, Francis J. (1980). "Modernization of China's Armed Forces." *Asian Survey*, 20 (March), 298–310.

Shambaugh, David L. (1987). "China's National Security Research Community." In Richard J. Latham (ed.), *Chinese National Security and the Second Revolution*, Boulder, CO: Lynne Rienner Publishers.

———. (1983). "China's Defense Industries: Indigenous and Foreign Procurement." In Paul H. B. Godwin (ed.), *The Chinese Defense Establishment: Continuity and Change in the 1980s*, Boulder, CO: Westview Press, 43–89.

———. (1979). "China's Quest for Military Modernization." *Asian Affairs* (May/June), 305–307.

———. (1979a). "Military Modernization and the Politics of Technology Transfer." *Contemporary China*, 3 (Fall), 4–5.

Segal, Gerald (1985). *Defending China*, Oxford: Oxford University Press.

———. (1983). "The Soviet 'Threat' at China's Gates." *Conflict Studies*, No. 143 (London: Institute for the Study of Conflict).

———. (1982). "China's Security Debate." *Survival*, 24 (March/April), 68–77.

———. (1981). "China's Nuclear Posture for the 1980s." *Survival*, 23 (January/February), 11–18.

———. (1981a). "The PLA and Chinese Foreign Policy Decision-Making." *International Affairs*, 57 (Summer), 449–466.

Segal, Gerald and William T. Tow (eds.) (1984). *Chinese Defense Policy*, Urbana and Chicago, IL: University of Illinois Press.

Simon, Denis Fred (1984). "The Role or Science and Technology in China's Foreign Relations." In Samuel S. Kim (ed.), *China and the World: Chinese Foreign Policy in the Post-Mao Era*, Boulder, CO: Westview Press, 293–318.

———. (1982). "China's Capacity to Assimilate Foreign Technology: An Assessment." In U.S. Congress, Joint Economic Committee. *China Under the Four Modernizations*, Washington, D.C.: Government Printing Office.

"Sino–U.S. Joint Communique (August 17, 1982)." (1982). *Beijing Review* (23 August), p. 14.

Snyder, Edwin K. and A. James Gregor (1981). "The Military Balance in the Taiwan Strait." *Journal of Strategic Studies*, 4 (September), 306–317.

Snyder, Edwin K., A. James Gregor, and Maria Hsia Chang (1980). *The Taiwan Relations Act and the Defense of the Republic of China*, Berkeley: Institute of International Studies.

Solomon, Richard H. (1981). *The China Factor: Sino-American Relations and the Global Scene*, Englewood Cliffs, NJ: Prentice-Hall.

———. (ed.) (1979). *Asian Security in the 1980s: Problems and Policies for a Time of Transition*, Santa Monica, CA: RAND Corporation.

Stuart, Douglas T. and William T. Tow (eds.) (1982). *China, the Soviet Union and the West: Strategic and Political Dimensions in the 1980s*, Boulder, CO: Westview Press.

———. (1982a). "Chinese Military Modernization: The Western Arms Connection." *China Quarterly*, 90 (June), 253–270.

———. (1981). "China's Military Turns to the West." *International Affairs*, 57 (Spring), 291–294.

Sun Tzu (1963). *Art of War*, Oxford: Oxford University Press.

Suttmeier, Richard P. (1980). *Science, Technology and China's Drive for Modernization*, Stanford, CA: Hoover Institution Press.

Sutter, Robert G. (1986). "China: Coping with the Evolving Strategic Environment." In Young Whan Kihl and Lawrence E. Grinter (eds.), *Asian-Pacific Security: Emerging Challenges and Responses*, Boulder, CO: Lynne Rienner Publishers.

———. (1983). *Chinese Nuclear Weapons and American Interests—Conflicting Policy Choices*, Washington, D.C.: Congressional Research Service.

———. (1981). *Increased U.S. Military Sales to China: Arguments and Alternatives*, Washington, D.C.: Congressional Research Service.

Swanson, Bruce (1982). *Eighth Voyage of the Dragon: A History of China's Quest for Seapower*, Annapolis, MD: Naval Institute Press.

Ting, William Pang-yu (1979). "Coalitional Behavior among the Chinese Military Elite: A Nonrecursive, Simultaneous Equations, and Multiplicative Causal Model." *American Political Science Review*, 73 (June), 478–493.

———. (1975). "A Longitudinal Study of Chinese Military Factionalism." *Asian Survey*, 15, 896–910.

Tow, William T. (1983). "Sino-Japanese Security Cooperation: Evolution and Prospects." *Pacific Affairs*, 56 (Spring), 51–83.

———. (1976). "China's Nuclear Strategy and U.S.

Reactions in 'Post-Détente' Era." *Military Review*, 56 (June), 80–90.

Tretiak, Daniel (1981). "Who Makes Chinese Foreign Policy Today." *The Australian Journal of Chinese Affairs*, 56 (June), 80–90.

———. (1980). "China's Vietnam War and its Consequences." *China Quarterly*, 80 (December), 740–767.

Treverton, Gregory (1980). "China's Nuclear Forces and the Stability of Soviet-American Deterrence." *The Future of Strategic Deterrence*, Part I, Adelphi Papers, 160 (Autumn), 38–44.

Wang, Robert (1984). "China's Evolving Strategic Doctrine." *Asian Survey*, 24 (October), 1040–1055.

Wang, Shan-nan (1983). *Chinese Development of Nuclear Science*, Taipei, Taiwan: Kuang Lu Publishing Company.

Whiting, Allen S. (1984). "Sino-Soviet Relations: What Next?" *The Annals*, 476 (November), 142–155.

———. (1983). "PRC-Taiwan Relations, 1983–93." *SAIS Review*, 3 (Winter–Spring) 131–146.

———. (1982). "Sino-American Relations: The Decade Ahead." *Orbis* (Fall), 697–720.

———. (1975). *The Chinese Calculus of Deterrence*, Ann Arbor, MI: University of Michigan Press.

———. (1972). "The Use of Force in Foreign Policy by the People's Republic of China." *Annals*, 402 (July), 55–65.

Whitson, William W. (1973). *The Chinese High Command: A History of Communist Military Politics, 1927–1971*, New York: Praeger.

———. (1972). "Domestic Constraints on Alternative Chinese Military Policies and Strategies in the 1970's." *Annals*, 402 (July), 40–51.

———. (1972a) (ed.). *The Military and Political Power in China in the 1970s*, New York: Praeger.

———. (1969). "Field Army in Chinese Politics." *China Quarterly*, 37 (January/March), 1–23.

———. (1968). "The Concept of Military Generation: The Chinese Communist Case." *Asian Survey*, 8 (November), 921–947.

Wolff, Lester L. and David L. Simon (eds.) (1982). *The Legislative History of the Taiwan Relations Act*, Jamaica, NY: American Association of Chinese Studies.

Wolfgang, Marvin E. (1984). "China in Transition." *The Annals*, 476 (November).

Wong-Fraser, Agatha S. Y. (1981). "China's Nuclear Deterrent." *Current History*, 8 (September), 245–249, 275–276.

———. (1981a). *China's Attitudes Towards Arms control and Disarmament*, London: Macmillan.

———. (1981b). *Sino-Soviet Conflict in the Persian Gulf: A Case Study*, Washington, D.C.: University Press of America.

Woodard, Dennis (1985). "The PLA: A People's Army under Modern Conditions?" In Graham Young (ed.), *China: Dilemmas of Modernization*, Dover, New Hampshire: Longwood Publishing Group.

Yahuda, Michael (1980). *China's Foreign Policy After Mao*, New York: St. Martin's Press.

Yang Shangkun (1984). "Building Chinese-Style Modernized Armed Forces." *Honggi* (Red Flag), 15 (August).

Yu, Yu-lin (1985). "Politics in Teng Hsiao-p'ing's Army-Building Strategy (1977–1984)." *Issues and Studies*, 21 (October), 34–57.

Zagoria, Donald S. (1983). "The Moscow-Beijing Detente." *Foreign Affairs*, 61 (Spring), 853–873.

Zhang Aiping (1983). "Several Questions Concerning Modernization of National Defense." *Honggi* (Red Flag), 5 (March), 21–24. In FBIS. *Daily Report*, 17 March 1983, pp. K2–K7.

Japan and the Koreas

Thomas A. Drohan

Combining Japan, South Korea, and North Korea in this bibliographic essay is an attempt to draw on the complementary sources regarding these nations, whose fates are so interrelated, while at the same time offering a differentiated structure that may help readers focus somewhat on the individual countries. The intent of this modest essay is to describe some examples of the most recent English-language literature in an organized fashion rather than to provide an inclusive catalog of the defense and defense-related writings about each nation. The aim is not only to describe specific examples of work in subject areas, but also to suggest journals and other sources likely to be of value for further research. First, studies at a regional level of analysis, which cover both Japan and the Koreas, are surveyed. This literature typically analyzes the international environment in its treatment of Japan and the Koreas. Next, Japan-specific works are described within the

confines of six major areas or subheadings where the majority of current materials have been found to exist (defense policy, security interests, security issues, constraints on Japan's defense, nuclear weapons policy, Japan–U.S. relations). We then turn to the Korean peninsula, describing sources applicable to both the Republic of Korea (ROK) and the Democratic People's Republic of Korea (DPRK) under two broad headings (integrative works, security issues). South Korea is treated next, using six subheadings to describe the literature (broad studies, leadership, civil-military relations, politics and the economy, military posture, and foreign relations). Finally, sources concerning the defense policy of North Korea are similarly segmented into six subheadings (broad studies, leadership, communist movement, politics and the economy, military posture, and foreign relations).

There is, of course, substantial overlap among studies grouped within each nation's subheading, but such general segmentation will, it may be hoped, prove useful to researchers of subject areas. The essay concludes with suggested sources for keeping current with events in each country.

Regional Sources

An excellent survey of the defense and foreign policies of Japan and the Koreas, as well as of China, the United States, the USSR, and other countries, is contained in *Asian Security, 1984*, edited by Masataka Kosaka and published by Tokyo's Research Institute for Peace and Security. Another cross-sectional work is Donald J. Senese, "The Defense of East Asia," *Journal of Social Political and Economic Studies* (1982), which discusses Japanese defense initiatives and regional actors' perceptions of them, as well as the Korean balance of power. Various perceptions of threats throughout the region are stressed in *Threats to Security in East Asia-Pacific*, edited by Charles E. Morrison (1983). Naotoshi Sakonjo, "Security in Northeast Asia," *Journal of Northeast Asian Studies* (1983), describes the regional activities of the United States, USSR, Japan, and the Koreas. Kensuke Ebata's "Air Forces of the Far East" (1985) is a regularly appearing feature in *Asian Defense Journal*, a publication that provides regular assessments of the military balance and naval forces in Asia.

One Japanese perspective of regional security is provided by Hideaki Kase, "Northeast Asian Security: A View from Japan," *Comparative Strategy* 1 (1978). Japanese security concerns are integrated with South Korean interests in Edward A. Olsen, "Japan–South Korea Security Ties," *Air University Review* (May–June 1981). See also his "Security in Northeast Asia: A Trilateral Alternative," *Naval War College Review* (1985). A Korean perspective is Tong Chin Rhee's "The Military-Strategic Factors in U.S.-Korea Policy in the Changing Political Environment in East-Asia," *Korea and World Affairs* (Winter 1983), which explains, from a Korean perspective, U.S. options in Korea in terms of global constraints on the United States. This article provides a nice counterweight to those that stress only regional problems and concerns. C. I. Eugene Kim focuses on U.S. relations with South Korea in a regional analysis, "The United States and the Security of Northeast Asia," in *Korea and World Affairs* (Spring 1984). U.S. relations with both Japan and South Korea are discussed in a report issued by the U.S. House of Representatives Committee on Foreign Affairs, "United States Relations with Japan and Korea: Security Issues," which was the result of a staff study mission in August 1981.

Japan

In spite of its economic prowess and an interest in the peace and security of East Asia, Japan's security interests and defense policies have been constrained by political, cultural and psychological factors both within and outside Japan. Within Japan, the defense budget is a focal point of constant debate, competing with popular social programs against an historical memory of twentieth century Japanese military imperialism and the dropping of two atomic weapons on Japan. The military role in foreign policy is constrained constitutionally by Article IX and by governmental policies. Yet Japan's global economy and its expansion of ties with nations in the Middle East, Africa, and Latin America, coupled with a growing Soviet regional capability and U.S. concerns, have evoked calls for Japan to reassess its regional role and responsibilities. It is within this general context that Japanese national security policy has developed. Consequently, most of the literature dealing with Japan's defense policy has emphasized its political and economic aspects, offering the researcher a broad interpretation of "national security."

DEFENSE POLICY

An extensive scholarly work is Franklin B. Weinstein, ed., *U.S.-Japan Relations and the Security of East Asia: The Next Decade* (Boulder, Colo.: Westview Press, 1978), which includes Japanese perceptions of U.S. security policy as well as outlooks on Northeast Asian security. The most authoritative source is the Japanese Defense Agency's annual White Paper on defense, which is translated into English by Japan Times, Ltd. and marketed as *Defense of Japan*. It contains both general overviews and details of such areas as the international military environment, fundamental concepts of defense policy, current defense issues and capabilities, the domestic environment, new technologies, and Japan–U.S. defense cooperation. James H. Buck's "Japan's Defense Policy" in *Armed Forces and Society* (Fall 1981) gives an historical background and survey of domestic issues, and posits future directions defense policy may take. For a critical view of the 1986–1990 Japanese defense plan, see Kiyofuku Chuma's "The 1986–90 Defense Plan: Does It Go Too Far?" in *Japan Quarterly* (January–March 1986), which addresses the defense buildup program in light of domestic antimilitarism, U.S. political pressure, and global security concerns. Larry A. Niksch emphasizes the constraining nature of the government's realistic security alternatives in "Japanese Defense Policy: Suzuki's Shrinking Options," *Journal of Northeast Asian Studies* (June 1982).

Articles focusing on the activities and role of the Japan self-defense forces (JSDF) many times reflect a perceived need for an expanded defensive role. John F. O'Connell in "The Role of the Self-Defense Forces in Japan's Sea Lane Defense," *Journal of Northeast Asian Studies* (1984) discusses air defense, mining operations, transport defense, and possible Soviet threats to those missions. Tomohisa Sakanaka explains the need for an expansion of the JSDF due to military threats and current force weaknesses in the context of a national consensus on defense policy in "Military Threats and Japan's Defense Capability," *Asian Survey* (July 1980). An inside view to the JSDF military education system is provided by Edward J. Drea in "Officer Education in Japan," *Military Review* (September 1980).

The Challenge of China and Japan: Politics and Development in East Asia (New York: Praeger, 1985), a comparative study edited by Susan L. Shirk, includes differences in national defense policy making between Japan and China, while Jon Woronoff focuses on Japanese defense industry in "Japan's Defense Industry Is Small but Sophisticated," *Asian Business* (1984) and "Measuring Japanese Military Threat," *Oriental Economist* (1984). Another article on defense industry is Kazuo Tomiyama's "Revival and Growth of Japan's Defense Industry," *Japanese Economic Studies* (Summer 1981).

Pieces on national security strategy typically stem from noted changes in Japan's security environment. Mike Mochizuki, "Japan's Search for Strategy," *International Security* (Winter 1983–84), outlines Japan's postwar strategy, its new policy environment, and existing factional debates on defense, while stressing that the key to strategic thinking must be the external environment. Hisahiko Okazaki, former director-general for foreign relations for the Japan Defense Agency, calls for serious strategic thinking in response to external environment changes and suggests elements of such a strategy in "Japanese Security Policy: A Time for Strategy," *International Security* (Fall 1982). Makoto Mamoi in "Strategic Environments and U.S. Security Policy in Northeast Asia in the 1980s: A Japanese Perception," in *Northeast Asian Security after Vietnam*, ed. Martin Weinstein (Champaign: University of Illinois Press, 1982), describes strategic options the Japanese have, based on Soviet and U.S. military balance.

SECURITY INTERESTS

Works dealing with what Japan's security interests are and why such interests are deemed vital necessarily stress Japan's vibrant, yet vulnerable, economy. An analysis of Japanese national security interests and economic relations is Edward Olsen's *U.S.-Japan Strategic Reciprocity: A Neo-Internationalist View* (Stanford, Calif.: Hoover Institution Press, 1985). The sufficiency and security of strategic supplies of minerals are discussed by W. C. J. van Rensburg, *Strategic Minerals*, vol. 1 (which includes like treatment of the United States and Western Europe). *Japan's Foreign Relations: A Global Search for Economic Security*, edited by Robert S. Ozaki and Walter Arnold, is an excellent compilation of papers that is part of a Westview special studies series on East Asia. Raw material difficulties are highlighted in Nobutoshi Akao, ed., *Japan's Economic Security: Resources as a Factor in Foreign Policy* (New York: St. Martin's Press, 1983). "Seeking the Establishment of Economic Security of Japan" is summarized in the *Journal of Japanese Trade and Industry* (January–February 1983).

The defense of the western Pacific sea lanes and their importance to Japan's security interests are discussed in Taketsugu Tsurutani, "Japan's Security, Defense Responsibilities and Capabilities," *Orbis*. The author also lists some of the JSDF's deficiencies, which he feels need to be corrected. A primary threat to Japan's security interests, the Soviet Union, is analyzed in the context of U.S.-Japan relations in Tetsuya Kataoka, "Japan's Northern Threat," *Problems of Communism* (March–April 1984). Given this growing Soviet regional military presence and capability, some have argued that Japan's security interests would be best served in the future by a Western Pacific Treaty Organization (WEPTO). A Japanese role in such a collective security apparatus to maintain regional peace and security is proposed by Yatsuhiro Nakagawa in "The WEPTO Option: Japan's New Role in East Asia/Pacific Collective Security" (August 1984).

SECURITY ISSUES

While most articles on Japanese security entail a variety of issues, it may be useful to identify some examples of recurring issues. Coverage of security and related economic issues discussed in a meeting between President Reagan and Prime Minister Nakasone may be found in the *Weekly Compilation of Presidential Documents*, 21 April 1986. Alan Murray also frames a few security issues in "Trade, Defense Issues Fray U.S.-Japan Ties," *Congressional Quarterly Weekly Report*, 27 November 1982.

An outstanding review of the defense debate is Tracy Dahlby's "Defense without Militarism," *Far Eastern Economic Review* (May 1981). An interview with Michael Nacht focuses on the rearmament issue in "Japanese Rearmament: Treading the Narrow Path," *Harvard International Review* (April 1984). Pros and cons of rearmament in terms of political and economic considerations are found in an article by Theodore N. Roy, "The Japanese Phoenix," *International Journal of World Peace* (April–June, 1985). Robert W. Barnett addresses Japan's constitutional dilemma regarding rearmament in "In Defense of Japan: Can Toyko Keep Faith with a 'No War' Constitution and Avoid Charges of a 'Free Ride'?" in *Worldview* (March 1984). A thoughtful case for measured rearmament based on the changing security environment, defense capabilities to protect national security interests, and logical options is Masashi Nishihara, "Expanding Japan's Credible Defense Role," *International Security* (Winter 1983–84). An American business perspective of Japanese rearmament, which includes perceived dangers of sharing U.S. technology, can be found in "Rearming Japan: Special Report," *Business Week* (March 1983).

Emphasis on various opinions of different publics in Japan is given by Allen Whiting in "Prospects for Japanese Defense Policy," *Asian Survey* (November 1982). Use of public opinion polls on specific defense issues and coverage of Japanese elite and press reviews enhance the value of this article. Karl Eikenburg describes increased support for defense spending and maintains this public attitude will continue to grow in "The Japanese Defense Debate: A Growing Consensus" (June 1982).

CONSTRAINTS ON JAPAN'S DEFENSE

A paramount constraint on defense policy in Japan is, of course, the government's decision-making process itself. An outstanding work on this is "Government Decisionmaking in Japan: Implications for the United States," a report submitted to the United States House of Representatives Committee on Foreign Affairs, Subcommittee on Asian and Pacific Affairs (1982:Y4F.76/1:G74/2). Constraints such as the relatively low standing of the Defense Agency in the government vis-à-vis other competing agencies and opposition from the Ministry of Finance are noted. Of particular interest and value to those concerned with defense policy are the interview and prepared statement in this report by John Endicott of the National Defense University on the defense decision-making process in the Japanese government.

Tetsuya Kataoka's "Japan's Defense Non-Buildup: What Went Wrong?" in *International Journal of World Peace* (April–June 1985) argues that Japan's cultural aloofness combined with U.S. mistrust of Japan is inhibiting Japan's defense initiatives. *The U.S.-Japan Alliance: Sharing the Burden of Defense* (National Defense University Press, 1983) by Robert F. Reed emphasizes various legal, political, attitudinal and budgetary constraints on Japan's contribution to its defense. Tomohisa Sakanaka gives a Japanese perspective in an editorial in the *Wall Street Journal* (11 January 1982) entitled "Japanese Defense Constraints." He argues that rapid increases in defense spending would be accompanied by severe social and political frictions unless a significant change in the external environment occurred to justify such increases.

NUCLEAR WEAPONS POLICY

Much of the recent literature still centers around the three non-nuclear principles Japan has upheld since 1958—that Japan will neither possess nuclear weapons, produce nuclear weapons nor permit their entry into Japan. For an argument in favor of preserving these principles, see Kamo Takehiko's "The Risk of Nuclear War and Japanese Militarization" in *Japan Quarterly* (April–June 1982). Tsuneo Akaha in "Japan's Three Nonnuclear Principles: A Coming Demise?" *Peace and Change* (Spring 1985) investigates the amount of domestic support for a non-nuclear defense policy, as well as how the Soviet buildup and U.S. responses could weaken the national nonnuclear consensus. An earlier article by the same author, "Japan's Nonnuclear Policy," in *Asian Survey* (August 1984) examines the defense debate over Japan's nonnuclear policy. Daniel I. Okimoto's "Chrysanthemum without the Sword: Japan's Nonnuclear Policy," in *Northeast Asian Security After Vietnam*, ed. Martin Weinstein, also contains excellent coverage of this topic. Toyoda Toshiyuki also examines attitudes toward nuclear issues, considering the arms race, military-industrial complex, and Soviet and American military policies in "The Decreasing Credibility of Nuclear Deterrence" in *Japan Quarterly* (1984).

JAPAN–U.S. RELATIONS

A top collection that assesses and offers predictions of security relations between Japan and the United States is *Comprehensive Security: Japanese and U.S. Perspectives* (Northeast Asia–United States Forum on International Policy, Stanford University, 1981). This is a compilation of papers from a conference of thirty Japanese and American specialists, co-chaired by Kiichi Saeki, chairman of the Nomura Research Institute, and John K. Emmerson, who serves as chairman of the Forum's U.S.–Japan relations program. Especially useful in studying U.S.–Japan relations are Kiichi Saeki's "U.S.–Japan Cooperation in Developing the Security Environment of the 1980s: A Japanese View," John Emmerson's "Prospects for U.S.–Japan Cooperation in Developing the Security Environment of the 1980s: An American View," and William Perry's "The Unique Role of Technology in U.S.–Japan Relations of the 80s." Also examining the two countries' security relations is the previously mentioned *Northeast Asian Security After Vietnam*, ed. Martin E. Weinstein. Several of the contributors in this valuable study incorporate U.S.–Japan relations in their broader articles on regional security.

A Japanese response to President Reagan's Strategic Defense Initiative is contained in Shoju Takase's "What 'Star Wars' Means to Japan," *Japan Quarterly* (1985). Takesugu Tsurutani, in "Old Habits, New Times," *International Security* (Fall 1982), lists three dangers to the alliance which he believes have quietly worsened—Japan's ambiguousness regarding the alliance's pur-

pose, the post-Vietnam American proclivity to change policy abruptly, and the public volatility in Japan on security issues.

Defense debates in particular are treated by John E. Endicott in "U.S.–Japan Defense Cooperation in the 1990s" in *Journal of Northeast Asian Studies* (1984). The alliance's role in regional security is discussed by James V. Young in "A Realistic Approach to the U.S.–Japan Alliance," *Military Review* (May, 1985). David B. H. Denoon, in "Japan and the U.S.—The Security Agenda," *Current History* (November 1983), describes the principal security debate between Japan and the United States and concludes with three alternatives for their defense relations—the most likely one of gradually expanding JSDF capabilities within the framework of the alliance; adopting a more neutral Japanese strategy perhaps within a weaker alliance; or pursuing an autonomous "Gaullist" stance, which would require a real self-defense capability.

The Korean Peninsula

One may find annual coverage of the events on the Korean peninsula, under the subtitle of "East Asia," in recurring articles in *Foreign Affairs* which analyze both South and North Korean developments. *Asian Survey* also carries articles in its January editions each year, with perspectives from authors of varied backgrounds. Robert A. Scalapino's "Current Dynamics of the Korean Peninsula" in *Problems of Communism* (November–December 1981) analyzes military and internal factors and relations between the South and the North as well as with other major powers. Two RAND Corporation studies evaluate relative South and North Korean capabilities to compete militarily in the future. Former U.S. Ambassador to Korea Richard L. Sneider compiled political and social strengths and weaknesses of both Koreas in "The Political and Social Capabilities of North and South Korea for the Long-Term Military Competition" (R-3271-NA, January, 1985). A later report analyzes political-social capabilities as well as technological and economic capabilities of both countries in an overall evaluation of South and North potential for the future: "The Changing Balance: South and North Korean Capabilities for Long-Term Military Competition," by Charles Wolf, Jr., Donald P. Henry, K. C. Yeh, James H. Hayes, John Schenk and Richard L. Sneider (R-3305, December 1985). Two other works which generally cover South and North Korea, with some emphasis on South Korea, are Fuji Kamiya's "The Korean Peninsula After Park Chung Hee," *Asian Survey* (July 1980) and Bae-ho Hahn's "Korea-Japan Relations in the 1970s," *Asian Survey* (November 1980).

Perhaps the best volume on the Korean security problem is the book edited by Franklin B. Weinstein and Fuji Kamiya, *The Security of Korea* (Boulder, Colo: Westview Press, 1980). A combined effort of varying specialists, the book gives U.S. and Japanese perspectives of how to avoid peninsular conflict. For information regarding the peninsula's military balance, the International Institute for Strategic Studies in London provides the annual, authoritative account *The Military Balance*. Lee Young Ho's "Military Balance and Peace for the Korean Peninsula," *Asian Survey* (August 1981), argues that the current military balance deters conflict given existing mutual distrust, but only integration can stop the peninsula arms race. This article contains several useful endnotes for those interested in the military balance in general as well as the conflicting estimates of North Korean military strength during the U.S. troop withdrawal debates. A more recent analysis is Larry A. Niksch's "The Military Balance on the Korean Peninsula," *Korean and World Affairs* (Summer 1986).

Byung-joon Anh provides a broad view of peninsula security in his "The Security Situation on the Korean Peninsula in Global Perspective," *The Journal of Asiatic Studies* (Seoul: September 1981), which surveys security issues and U.S.–ROK agreements. Tong Whan Park addresses the security dilemma and shows how two models of the peninsula arms race fail to account for South-North competition in "The Korean Arms Race: Implications in the International Politics of Northeast Asia," *Asian Survey* (June 1980). Geostrategic issues of the peninsula as they relate to Northeast Asia are analyzed in Kook Chin Kim's "The Pivotal Security Linkage Between the Korean Peninsula and Northeast Asia: A Korean View," *Korea and World Affairs* (Fall 1985).

For viewpoints and discussion regarding the recurring issue of reunification, see Hak-joon Kim's book, *The Unification Policy of South and North: A Comparative Study* (Seoul: Seoul National University Press, 1977), and K. Hwang's book, *The Neutralized Unification of Korea in Perspective* (New York: Praeger, 1980). Various articles in *Congressional Quarterly Weekly Report* in the 1977–1978 time frame also discuss the reunification issue, as does Thomas H. Hoivik's "Korea: Is Peaceful Reunification Possible?" *Washington Quarterly* (Winter 1984). In the spring of 1982, *Korea and World Affairs* devoted the entire edition to the issue of reunification, featuring articles by nine scholars. In *Korea and World Affairs* (Fall 1983) Byung Chul Koh evaluates the impact of external forces as obstacles to reunification in his article, "Reunification Strategies of China and North Korea: A Comparative Assessment."

South Korea

South Korea has been largely able to maintain its spectacular economic growth while devoting one-third of its annual budgetary outlays to national defense in the face of ominous threats from North Korea. The 1954 Mutual Defense Treaty with the United States remains a key ingredient to deterring another attack from the north. Recently, though, some have noted the ROK's expanded trade network with other nations not only designed to promote economic growth but also providing future insurance due to a perceived less-than-unwavering U.S. security commitment. Internally, the Fifth Republic headed by President Chun Doo-Hwan took some liberalizing steps toward more democratic rule. But these measures always have been softened by the persistent external and internal threats from the north. Accordingly, internal information regarding defense in this type of an environment is scarce.

BROAD STUDIES

A thoroughly extensive work on many aspects of South Korea is the Council on East Asian Studies of Harvard University's series, "Studies in the Modernization of the Republic of Korea." This work has extensive volumes on areas such as education, entrepreneurs, the foreign sector, rural development, urbanization, and modernization, which in effect describe the political and economic environment in which Republic of Korea (ROK) defense policy operates. *Asian Survey's* annual articles on South Korea typically review internal developments and external factors of change. These issues which underlie stability are surveyed in Chang-yoon Choi's "Korea: Security and Strategic Issues," *Asian Survey* (November 1980). The possibility of an ROK role in a regional security arrangement is discussed by Larry A. Niksch in "South Korea in Broader Pacific Defense," *Journal of Northwest Asian Studies* (March 1983).

LEADERSHIP

For a well-documented review of South Korean (and North Korean) leaders, see Dae-Sook Suh and Chae-Jin Lee's *Political Leadership in Korea* (University of Washington Press, 1976). Leadership values are stressed in C. I. Eugene Kim's "The Value Congruity Between ROK Civilian and Former Military Party Elites," *Asian Survey* (August 1978), while business elites are discussed in Kyong-Dong Kim's "Political Factors in the Formation of the Entrepreneurial Elite in South Korea," *Asian Survey* (May 1976). *Asian Survey* occasionally features articles concerning such aspects of leadership as political legitimacy and military rule.

CIVIL-MILITARY RELATIONS

While civil-military relations are treated in large works that survey many areas of Korea, such as the country studies compiled by American University, two articles specifically about civil-military relations are C.I. Eugene Kim's "Civil-Military Relations in the Two Koreas," *Armed Forces and Society* (Fall 1984) and Jong-Chun Baek's "The Role of the Republic of Korea Armed Forces in National Development."

POLITICS AND THE ECONOMY

In addition to *Asian Survey's* annual recount of politics in South Korea, *Current History* is a valuable source. Edward Baker's "Politics in South Korea," *Current History* (April 1982) is a critical view of President Chun Doo-Hwan's military government to that date. *Orbis* also provides similar information. Edward Olsen's "'Korea, Inc.': The Political Impact of Park Chung Hee's Economic Miracle," *Orbis* (Spring 1980) describes political and economic aspects of the ROK's growth and prospects for the future. *Asian Affairs* featured Sung-joo Han's "The Emerging Political Process in Korea" (November–December, 1980). For a discussion of ROK political problems as they purportedly stem from military rule, see Roger Benjamin's "The Political Economy of Korea," *Asian Survey* (November 1982). An earlier work edited by Edward Reynolds Wright is his book, *Korean Politics in Transition*, which includes an article by John P. Lovell entitled, "The Military and Politics in Postwar Korea" (Seattle: University of Washington Press, 1975). An excellent essay on several studies of Korean politics is Young Whan Kihl's "Korean Politics in the 1980s," *Problems of Communism* (September–October 1981). Quality works on the politico-economic environment of national security policy can be found in Department of Defense-distributed

Technical Reports. Two such reports, distributed by the Defense Logistics Agency's Defense Technical Information Center, are Thomas W. Robinson's "South Korean Political Development in the 1980s," and P.W. Kuznet's "The South Korean Model of Political and Economic Development: Economic Aspects." Both reports were prepared for the Department of State. A comparative discussion of the ROK and North Korean economies and the implications for peninsula stability is found in Kihwan Kim's "Korea's Economy: Reforms, Prospects, and Implications for the Balance of Power on the Peninsula," *Korea and World Affairs* (Fall 1983).

MILITARY POSTURE

While nearly all sources regarding Korea mention military capabilities, a few articles deal specifically with it. Michael Underdown's "South Korean Defense Capability," in *Australian Outlook* (August 1981) is one example. Donald R. Cotter and N. F. Wikner have a piece in *Strategic Review* (Spring 1982) entitled, "Korea: Force Imbalances and Remedies," which uses statistics of military capability to argue for the necessity of the American military ground presence in the ROK.

An interesting account of military capability intelligence estimates is the Investigations Subcommittee of the House Committee on Armed Services' "Report on Impact of Intelligence of Reassessment on Withdrawal of U.S. Troops From Korea" (7 September 1979).

FOREIGN RELATIONS

Much of the literature about the ROK's foreign policy centers around ROK–U.S., ROK–North Korea, and ROK–Japan relations. However, an excellent examination of the ROK's overall foreign policy as it relates to a changed regional environment is Edward A. Olsen's "The Evolution of the ROK's Foreign Policy," *Washington Quarterly* (Winter 1984). Youngnok Koo provides a comparative discussion of ROK and U.S. views and interests in "Future Perspectives of South Korea's Foreign Relations," *Asian Survey* (November 1980).

ROK–U.S. relations typically are discussed in light of the Mutual Defense Treaty. Sung joo Han discusses the treaty's viability in "South Korea and the United States: The Alliance Survives," *Asian Survey* (November 1980). Yong Kyun Kim offers an appraisal of the feasibility of a Pacific-NATO agreement in "The Mutual Defense Treaty of 1953 with the United States," *Journal of East Asian Affairs* (Fall–Winter 1982). In the same issue, Tae-Hwan Kwok provides a ROK perspective of U.S. interests and changing regional policies in the Korean peninsula in "U.S.–Korea Security Relations." A National Defense University monograph, *U.S.–ROK Combined Operations: A Korean Perspective* by Taek-Hyung Rhee (Washington, D.C.: NDU Press, 1986), details some noted shortcomings in U.S.–ROK combined military operations doctrine. The impact of the People's Republic of China on U.S.–Korean relations is analyzed by Jonathan Pollack in "U.S.–Korean Relations: The China Factor," *Journal of Northeast Asian Studies* (Fall 1983). Tong Chin Rhee explains U.S.–Korea relations in terms of its global context, rather than solely regional problems, in "The Military-Strategic Factors in U.S.–Korea Policy in the Changing Political Environment in East-Asia," *Korea and World Affairs* (Winter 1983). In its December 1982

issue, *Korea Journal* featured "100 Years of Korean-American Relations" by several contributors. Especially useful are Andrew Nahm's "Studies on United States-Korean Relations in the English Language: A Bibliographical Survey," and Yong-su Pae's "A Bibliography on Korean-American Relations." Two articles in the September 1983 issue of *Journal of Northeast Asian Studies* are of note here—Sung Joo Han's "South Korea's Policy Towards the United States" and Soong Hoom Kil's "South Korean Policy Toward Japan." Both reflect a South Korean concern that on the one hand an increasingly powerful Japan is desirable for peninsular security, but on the other hand may encourage the U.S. to decrease its regional presence.

ROK–Japan relations as they relate to security are also discussed in Edward Olsen's "Japan–South Korea Security Ties," *Air University Review* (May–June 1981). A Korean assessment of ROK–Japan relations is Bae-ho Hahn's "Korea–Japan Relations in the 1970s," *Asian Survey* (November 1980), which traces its evolution since the post–World War II era. A recent assessment of the current warm relations between the ROK and Japan is provided by Evelyn Colbert in "Japan and the Republic of Korea: Yesterday, Today, and Tomorrow," *Asian Survey* (March 1986).

Much of the useful information about South-North Korean relations focuses on the reunification issue, such as Thomas Hoivik's article in *Washington Quarterly* (Winter 1984), "Korea: Is Peaceful Reunification Still Possible?" A study of the unification policies of both Koreas can be found in Hak-joon Kim's *The Unification Policy of South and North Korea 1948–1976: A Comparative Study* (Seoul: National University Press, 1977). For coverage of the foreign policy-making apparatus of both South and North Korea, see Byung Chul Koh's *The Foreign Policy Systems of North and South Korea* (Berkeley and Los Angeles: University of California Press, 1984).

North Korea

North Korea's highly centralized government and extremely closed society explain the relative paucity of sources for the researcher. Currently, North Korea is a nation devoting roughly 20% of its GNP to defense in the face of its foreign debt crisis, growing South Korean military and economic might, and a looming internal political power vacuum. Other than the formal institutional power structure and the central figure of Kim Il Sung, little is certain regarding the nature of decision making in this insular state. Thanks to some determined research exhibited in several recent works, however, our knowledge of North Korean defense-related policies has increased.

BROAD STUDIES

Robert A. Scalapino and Jun-yop Kim's book, *North Korea Today: Strategic and Domestic Issues* (Berkeley: Institute of East Asian Studies, 1983), is the work of seventeen writer/scholars and is an excellent compilation of much of what little is known about North Korea today. Its broad scope and diversity of perspectives are particularly strong in the areas of foreign relations and the economy. Another comprehensive study is Tai Sung An's *North Korea: A Political Handbook* (Wilmington:

Scholarly Resources, Inc., 1983). This valuable source is an objective description and analysis that emphasizes the North Korean political system and contains an extensive bibliography. American University's Country Study on the Democratic People's Republic of Korea (DPRK) is another broad work where topical information and sources can be found.

LEADERSHIP

In addition to the broad studies mentioned above, there are others that include political elites in the DPRK. One view is contained in Ilpyong Kim's *Communist Politics in North Korea* (New York: Praeger, 1975). This book portrays Kim Il Sung's efforts to modernize industry in the DPRK in a favorable light. Another viewpoint can be found in the work done by Sukryul Yu, *Power Structure of North Korea* (Seoul: Korea Press Institute). Young Hwan Kihl has done some comparative analysis that is notably strong in the leadership dimension in his *Politics and Policies in Divided Korea* (Boulder, Colo.: Westview Press, 1984). His article in *Current History* (April 1982), "North Korea: A Reevaluation" discusses political succession. Also discussing the leadership's succession issue is Suk-Ryul Yu in "Political Succession in North Korea," *Korea and World Affairs* (Winter 1982). For a very well-documented history of both North and South Korean political elites, see Dae-sook Suh and Chong-sik Lee's *Political Leadership in Korea* (Seattle: University of Washington Press, 1976). In this book, the writers point out a trend toward functional compartmentalization. For viewpoints by North Korean leaders themselves, see *The Korean Conundrum: A Conversation With Kim Il Sung*, a report by U.S. Representative Stephen Solarz to the U.S. House Committee on Foreign Affairs (August, 1981). For updated listings on who the elites in North Korea are, see the CIA's Directorate of Intelligence's "Directory of Officials of the Democratic People's Republic of Korea: A Reference Aid."

COMMUNIST MOVEMENT

Dae-sook Suh's two initial works on communism in North Korea have provided a solid foundation for later studies. *The Korean Communist Movement 1918–1948* (Princeton, 1967) is a remarkable record of the early days of the movement and its old party leaders. This study is complemented by the same author's *Documents of Korean Communism 1918–1948* (Princeton, 1970), a compilation of related material. A more recent book is Chong-sik Lee's *Korean Worker's Party: A Short History* (Stanford, Calif.: Hoover Institution Press, 1978). The same author pulished "Evolution of the Korean Workers' Party and the Rise of Kim Chong-Il" in *Asian Survey* (May 1982). Robert D. Scalapino and Chong-sik Lee's *Communism in Korea* (Berkeley, 1972), is broad in scope and contains a rich bibliography in English, Korean, and Japanese materials. South Korean journals such as *Vantage Point* provide perspectives on North Korea's communist ideology in articles such as Haen Son Kim's "Functions of North Korea's Juche Ideology With Special Reference to Unification Policy" (June, 1984). This article explains the ideology's integrative functions such as political socialization, legitimacy maintenance and regime loyalty. *Washington Quarterly* and *Asian Profile* contain similar subject articles on occasion.

POLITICS AND THE ECONOMY

Some treatment of North Korean politics is included in Gregory Henderson's widely researched and documented account of Korean political processes, *Korea: Politics of the Vortex*. Other works mentioned in other subject areas also provide analyses of North Korean politics, such as Young Whan Kihl's *Politics and Policies in Divided Korea* and Il Pyong Kim's *Communist Politics in North Korea*. Also see Foreign Broadcast Information Service (FBIS) analysis report, "The North Korean Party Congress: Goals and Policies for the 1980s," dated 5 December 1980.

For elite perceptions and political system capabilities as they affect North Korean economic and military capabilities, see a RAND study by Norman D. Levin, "Management and Decisionmaking in the North Korean Economy" (R-1805, Fall 1982). This study focuses on the question, how will North Korea's general style of decision making and management of its economy impact on its ability to sustain high military expenditures? Jong-chul Ahn discusses the primacy of political considerations and how these party politics undermine military professionalism and promote factionalism in "Political Control Over the Military by North Korean Workers' Party," *Vantage Point* (April 1983).

A valuable study of political life in North Korea in general is Tai Sung An's book, *North Korea in Transition: From Dictatorship to Dynasty* (Westport: Greenwood Press, 1983), while an impact of North Korean political struggles on foreign relations can be found in Se Hee Yoo's "The Influence of Factional Struggles in North Korea on Its Relations with China and the Soviet Union," *Chinese Affairs* 1, No. 1.

MILITARY POSTURE

An excellent concise review of the origins, development and structure of ground forces is Mark L. Urban's "The North Korean People's Army: Anatomy of a Giant," *International Defense Review* (July 1983). For a rare study of North Korean military doctrine as it relates to political behavior, see Yong Soon Kim's "North Korean Military Doctrine and Its Policy Implications in North Korean Foreign Policy," *Korea Observer* (Spring 1981). In this work, the author describes contributing factors to the formation of military doctrine, societal structures and capabilities related to the doctrine, and the doctrine's strategic implications for relations with other nations. For a South Korean government perspective on the implications of the doubling North Korean military capabilities since the 1960s, see Young Choi's "The North Korean Military Buildup and Its Impact on North Korean Military Strategy in the 1980s," *Asian Survey* (March 1985). The same author has an earlier work focusing on military strategy, "Military Strategy of North Korea," in *On North Korean Military Affairs* (Seoul: Institute of North Korean Studies, 1978). The ROK government's National Unification Board provides information on the North Korean military posture, such as Lee Byung-joo's "An Analysis of North Korean Military Strength and Our Countermeasures, Particularly on Military Strategy and War Potentials" (Seoul: Policy Planning Office of the NVB, December 1976).

FOREIGN RELATIONS

Two previously mentioned books, Scalapino and Kim's *North Korea Today, Strategic and Domestic Is-*

sues and Koh's *The Foreign Policy Systems of North and South Korea*, focus on North Korean foreign relations. North Korea–China and North Korea–Soviet relations are covered in Young Whan Kihl's "North Korea: A Reevaluation," *Current History* (April 1982). Jae Kyu Park describes North Korean relations with these two powers in terms of striving for equidistance and avoiding alienating either one, in "North Korea's Political and Economic Relations With China and the Soviet Union," *Comparative Strategy* (1984). Park proposes that if recent trends toward increasing relations with western countries continue, this could enhance the liklihood of unification due to decreasing North Korean dependence (economic and military) on China and the Soviet Union. Another article discussing North Korean relations with these two powers is Hak-joon Kim's "North Korea's Foreign Relations Amidst Sino-Soviet Conflict," *Vantage Point* (April 1984). For a study of relations as indicated by foreign trade, see an analysis done by Hong Yoon Lee for Seoul's Institute for International Economic Research, "North Korea's Foreign Trade During the 1970s and Its Prospects For the 1980s" (July 1981). Finally, Young C. Kim addresses objectives of DPRK foreign policy in terms of what motivates these objectives and how the objectives might change in "North Korean Foreign Policy," *Problems of Communism* (January–February 1985).

Keeping Current

For the English-language reader, staying informed of major developments in Japan and the Koreas is reasonably easy, as a fair array of primary sources exists, with the notable exception of North Korean viewpoints. The *Japan Times*, *Japan Weekly*, and *Japan Quarterly* are useful for following events in that country, and South Korea's *Korea Herald* and *Korea Times* provide a timely ROK perspective on events. North Korea's *Rodong Sinmum*, *Minju Chosen* and *Kulloja* provide editorials; the Joint Publications Research Service *Korean Affairs Report* provides translation of some DPRK sources.

For the Japan–Korea region, FBIS's *Daily Report*, Asia and the Pacific version, provides daily summaries of events. Other journals such as *Far Eastern Economic Review* provide weekly accounts of significant occurrences.

The Middle East

Mary Payrow-Olia

Any essay purporting to describe the defense policies of Middle Eastern nations faces a number of difficulties: the complex diversity of the area; polemical tirades substituting for unbiased data; the multilingual nature of the articles written on the subject; and the dearth of information on particular countries. This essay does not pretend to address these problems as a definitive treatise on regional or country-specific defense policies. Rather, it seeks to acquaint the reader with an overview of some of the existing literature. In order to ensure the widest possible use, all non-English language sources are excluded. Prior to 1980, most of the literature addressed the role of the military in society. Since then, a few books and articles have considered the security environment, strategy, doctrine, policy-making processes and procedures, and force structures of the region.

The military plays a pivotal role in Middle Eastern defense and security policies. A good place to start is *The Middle East Military Balance, 1984*, ed. Mark Heller et al. (Tel Aviv: Jaffee Center for Strategic Studies, Tel Aviv University, 1984). This compendium covers strategic developments in the Middle East, regional forces, and the military balance among states. The data on twenty-one Middle Eastern countries include arms transfers, defense expenditures, comparisons of the quality and quantity of arms, the organization of armed forces, the military's role in its respective political system, deployment and employment of troops and matériel, doctrine and tactics, theater maps, and a glossary of military acronyms. This work also projects future regional trends and the outcome of a future conventional conflict. *Defense Planning in Less-Industrialized States: The Middle East and South Asia*, ed. Stephanie G. Neuman (Lexington, Mass.: Lexington Books, 1984) is a good companion text. Defense policies are considered by several contributors. One third of *Security Policies of Developing Countries*, ed. Edward A. Kolodziej and Robert E. Harkavy (Lexington, Mass.: Lexington Books, 1982) covers Pakistan, Egypt, Israel, Iraq, Iran, and Syria. The book's framework focuses on each state's assumptions about the international system and threats from it: military doctrines, force levels, and weapons systems; and the impact of domestic political factors on defense policies. *Gulf Security into the 1980's: Perceptual and Strategic Dimensions*, ed. Robert G. Darius et al. (Stanford, Calif.: Hoover Institution Press, 1984) offers a broad, regional perspective. Some chapters cover the link between Afghanistan, Khomeini's foreign policy, and the security concerns of the Gulf Cooperation Council. A drawback to this book is that it fails to address the impact of the Arab-Israeli conflict on Gulf security concerns. *Regional Security in the Middle East*, ed. Charles Tripp, is a collection of six articles. The best two articles are Adeed Dawisha, "Saudi Arabia's Search for Security," which argues that the crux of Saudi Arabia's security dilemma hinges on its dependence upon the United States and the perceived need to be part of a pan-Arab consensus, and Andrew Duncan, "The Military Threat to Israel," which outlines a shift in the Israeli military's perspective from survival to security after 1967.

Another good collection is *International Security in*

Southwest Asia, ed. Hafeez Milik (New York: Praeger, 1984), which includes "Saudi Arabian Foreign Policy toward the Gulf Security" by Ali E.H. Dessouki. Anthony H. Cordesman, *The Gulf and the Search for Strategic Stability: Saudi Arabia, the Military Balance in the Gulf and Trends in the Arab-Israeli Military Balance* (Boulder, Colo.: Westview Press, 1984) focuses on the impact of estimates of comparative firepower, nationalistic ferment, and religious zeal upon regional peace and conflict. Cordesman also considers how Gulf states view a close military partnership with the United States in light of their security concerns. Abdul-Monem M. Al-Mashat, *National Security in the Third World* (Boulder, Colo.: Westview Press, 1985), argues that national security must be redefined for Middle Eastern and other developing societies.

The impact of regional conflict upon defense policies has also been addressed. Noteworthy in this area are three recent texts. *New Technology and Military Power: General Purpose Military Forces for the 1980's and Beyond*, Seymour J. Deitchman (Boulder, Colo.: Westview Press, 1979) uses Middle East wars to illustrate the impact of new technologies on weapons, tactics, and strategies for conventional forces. Two companion texts contain documents that reflect the declared policies of Middle Eastern states involved in the Arab-Israeli conflict: *Documents on the Israeli-Palestinian Conflict, 1967-1983*, ed. Yehuda Lukas (New York: Cambridge University Press, 1984), which contains peace initiatives and basic policy statements of the PLO, the Arab League and Israel; and *The Israeli-Arab Reader: A Documentary History of the Middle East*, ed. Walter Laqueur and Barry Rubin (New York: Penguin Books, 4th ed., 1984), which documents both sides' justifications and war aims for the military engagements of 1967, 1973, and 1982. *The Arab-Israeli Conflict: Perspectives*, ed. Alvin Rubinstein (New York: Praeger, 1984) is a collection of six essays. Two of the best are Haim Shaked's essay on continuity and change in the causes of escalation and relaxation in the conflict; and Aaron David Miller's essay on "The Palestinian Dimension," which describes the internal and external pressures on the Palestinian community. The military perspective of the PLO is covered in Y. Sayigh, "Palestinian Military Performance in the 1982 War," *Journal of Palestinian Studies* 12 (1983): 3-24. Different aspects of the Israeli incursion into Lebanon and its impact on regional defense policies are considered in Augustus Norton, "Making Enemies in South Lebanon: Harakat Amal, the IDF, and South Lebanon," *Middle East Insight* 3 (January-February 1984): 13-20; and Richard Gabriel, *Operation Peace for Galilee: The Israeli-PLO War in Lebanon* (New York: Hill & Wang, 1984). *Modern Weapons and Third World Powers*, Rodney W. Jones and Steven A. Hildreth (Boulder, Colo.: Westview Press, 1984) assesses the regional goals, ambitions, security perceptions, and defense policies of Middle Eastern states and other Third World countries. Analyses of combat effectiveness, conflict management, and defense performance are also included. *The Regionalization of Warfare: The Falkland/Malvinas Islands, Lebanon, and the Iran-Iraq Conflict*, ed. James Brown and William B. Snyder (New Brunswick, N.J.: Transaction Books, 1985), considers the impact of public opinion upon defense policies, the correlation between technol-

ogy and training, and the necessity for military professionalism and coordination of policies. Mark A. Heller, *The Iran-Iraq War: Implications of Third Parties* (Tel Aviv University, 1984) considers the security and political interests of Arab Gulf states regarding the Iran-Iraq conflict. Another useful book to round out the impact of conflict on regional defense policies is *Middle East Military Guerrilla Balance*, ed. Mark A. Heller et al. (Boulder, Colo.: Westview Press, 1983). A good overview of personalities and political struggles that influenced the Arab-Israeli conflict can be found in Chaim Herzog, *The Arab-Israeli Wars: War and Peace in the Middle East from the War of Independence through Lebanon* (New York: Random House, 1982). Herzog does a fairly good job of describing the various campaigns since 1948, but fails miserably with the Israeli incursion into Lebanon. The October 1973 war sparked a flurry of literature that provides useful insights into the defense policy process of the region. Some of these are John W. Amos II, *Arab-Israeli Military and Political Relations: Arab Perceptions and the Politics of Escalation* (New York: Pergamon, 1979); Nadav Safran, *Israel: The Embattled Ally* (Cambridge: Harvard University Press, 1978); and Trevor N. Dupuy, *Elusive Victory* (New York: Harper & Row, 1978).

Defense policies also have been influenced to a degree by the ongoing peace process in the region. Several studies provide helpful insights: Anthony Cordesman, "Peace in the Middle East: The Value of Small Victories," *Middle East Journal* 38 (Summer 1984): 515-20; N. Tahboub, "Jordan's Role in the Middle East Peace: An Analytical Note," *Journal of South Asia and Middle East Studies* 7 (1984): 58-62; N. Hussein, "Peace Efforts: Principles versus Practices," *American-Arab Affairs* 8 (Spring 1984): 1-17; A. Alireza, "An Arab View of the Peace Process," *American-Arab Affairs* 4 (Spring 1983): 70-76; Adeed Dawisha, "Comprehensive Peace in the Middle East and the Comprehension of Arab Politics," *Middle East Journal* 37 (Winter 1983): 43-53; Daniel Amit, "Strategies for Struggle, Strategies for Peace," *Journal of Palestine Studies* 12 (1983): 23-30; and H. Waller, "Israel and the Peace Process," *Current History* 82 (January 1983): 10-14.

A growing number of sources, some of them disappointing, consider the strategic nuclear policies of the region. Taysu Nashif, *Nuclear Warfare in the Middle East: Dimension and Responsibilities* (Princeton, N.J.: Kingston Press, 1983) is little more than an anti-Israeli polemic. Paul F. Power, "Preventing Nuclear Conflict in the Middle East: The Free Zone Strategy," *Middle East Journal* 37 (Autumn 1983): 617-35, offers very little new in describing Israel's strategic policy as maintaining superior conventional forces while retaining an undisclosed nuclear bomb option. Three rather good sources on the subject remain Steven Rosen, "A Stable System of Nuclear Deterrence in the Arab-Israeli Conflict," *American Political Science Review* 71 (December 1971): 1367-83; Robert Pranger and Dale Tahtinen, *Nuclear Threat in the Middle East* (Washington, D.C.: American Enterprise Institute, 1975); and Steve Weisman and Herbert Krosney, *The Islamic Bomb* (New York: Times Books, 1981). Good background sources are Roger Pajak, *Nuclear Proliferation in the Middle East*, Monograph 82-1 (Washington, D.C.: National Defense University Press, 1982); Rodney W. Jones, *Nu-*

clear Proliferation: Islam, the Bomb, and South Asia (Beverly Hills, Calif.: Sage, 1981); Lewis A. Dunn, "Persian Gulf Nuclearization," in *The Security of the Persian Golf*, Hassein Amirsadeghi ed. (New York: St. Martin's Press, 1981); and Paul Jabbar, *A Nuclear Middle East: Infrastructure, Likely Military Postures, and Prospects for Strategic Stability* (Berkeley and Los Angeles: University of California Press, 1977). A good source is *Small Nuclear Forces and U.S. Security Policy: Threats and Potential Conflicts in the Middle East and South Asia*, ed. Rodney W. Jones (Lexington, Mass.: Lexington Books, 1984). Especially noteworthy in this volume is Robert E. Hunter, "Small Nuclear Forces in the Middle East: The Years 2000–2010," which considers possible future technologies, strategic planning, and outcomes of nuclear conflict.

Another influence on regional defense policies is the role of external forces. A brief sample of the literature in this area would include *The Global Politics of Arms Sales*, Andrew J. Pierre (Princeton: Princeton University Press, 1982), which has a 70-page section on Middle East arms recipients and argues that arms transfer policies contribute to the destabilization of the region. Robert W. Stookey, *The Arabian Peninsula: Zone of Ferment* (Stanford, Calif.: Hoover Institution Press, 1984) argues that Arab Gulf states actively seek arms from Western sources in order to maintain domestic order and regional stability. Alexander Bennet, "Arms Transfer as an Instrument of Soviet Policy in the Middle East," *Middle East Journal* 39 (Autumn 1985): 745–74, discusses the policies of recipients of Soviet arms and attempts to categorize supplier-client relationships in the region. The impact of external influences on regional defense policies can be seen in two representative articles: Robert G. Lawrence, "Arab Perceptions of U.S. Security Policy in Southwest Asia," *American Arab Affairs* 5 (Summer 1983): 27–38; and Rashid Khalidi, "Arab Views of the Soviet Role in the Middle East," *Middle East Journal* 39 (Autumn 1985): 716–32. The role of the U.N. is addressed in Istvan Pogany, *The Security Council and the Arab-Israeli Conflict* (New York: St. Martin's Press, 1984). Nathan Pelcots, *Peacekeeping on Arab-Israeli Fronts: Lessons from the Sinai and Lebanon* (Boulder, Colo.: Westview Press, 1984) compares the advantages and disadvantages of non-U.N. forces with U.N. peacekeeping forces.

A large part of the literature focuses on the role of the military in society. J. C. Hurewitz, *Middle East Politics: The Military Dimensions* (Boulder, Colo.: Westview Press, 1984) considers the impact of military intervention on particular political systems and societies. Past contributions include Amos Perlmutter, *Political Roles and Military Rulers* (Totowa, N.J.: Frank Cass, 1981); id., "The Arab Military Elite," *World Politics* 22 (January 1970): 269–300; Eliezer Beeri, *Army Officers in Arab Politics and Society* (New York: Praeger, 1970); James A. Bill, "Military Modernization in the Middle East," *Comparative Politics* 2 (October 1969): 41–62; Manfred Halpern, "Middle Eastern Armies and the New Middle Class," in *The Role of Military in Underdeveloped Countries*, ed. John Johnson (Princeton: Princeton University Press, 1962); Majid Khadduri, "Army Officer: His Role in Middle Eastern Politics," in *Social Forces in the Middle East*, ed. S. N. Fisher (Ithaca, N.Y.: Cornell University Press, 1955);

Dankwart A. Rustow, "Military in Middle Eastern Society and Politics," in *Political Development and Social Change*, ed. Jason L. Finkle and Richard W. Gable (New York: Wiley, 1966); Faud Il Khuri and Gerald Obermyer, "The Social Bases for Military Intervention in the Middle East," in *Political-Military Systems: Comparative Perspective*, ed. Catherine McArdle Kelleher (Beverly Hills, Calif.: Sage, 1974); and S. N. Fisher, *The Military in the Middle East: Problems in Society and Government* (Columbus: Ohio State University Press, 1963). Gabriel Ben-Dor has written several articles on military intervention in Middle Eastern societies: "The Politics of Threat: Military Intervention in the Middle East," in *World Perspectives in the Sociology of the Military*, ed. George A. Kourvetaris and Betty A. Bebratz (New Brunswick, N.J.: Transaction Books, 1977); "Military Regimes in the Arab World: Prospects and Patterns of Civilization," *Armed Forces and Society* 1 (May 1975): 317–27; "The National Security Policy of Egypt," in *Security Policies of Developing Countries*, ed. Kolodziej and Harkavy; and "State, Society and Military Elites in the Middle East," in *Hierarchy and Stratification in the Middle East* (New York: Social Science Research Council, 1982). A survey of differing explanations of military intervention is considered in William Thompson's "Toward Explaining Arab Military Coups," *Journal of Political and Military Sociology* 2 (Fall 1974): 237–50. Other good articles include John B. Glubb, "The Role of the Army in the Traditional Arab State," in *Modernization of the Arab World*, ed. J. H. Thompson and R. D. Reischauer (Princeton, N.J.: Van Nostrand, 1966); Ayad Al-Qazzaz, "Political Order, Stability and Officers: A Comparative Study of Iraq, Syria and Egypt from Independence till June 1967," *Middle East Forum* 45 (Summer 1969): 31–51; William I. Zartman, "Military Elements in Regional Unrest," in *Soviet-American Rivalry in the Middle East*, ed. J. C. Hurewitz (New York: Praeger, 1972); the chapter entitled "Violence and the Military" in James A. Bill and Carl Leiden, *Politics in the Middle East* (Boston: Little, Brown, 1984); and George M. Haddad, *Revolutions and Military Rule in the Middle East*, 3 vols. (New York: Robert Speller & Sons, 1965–73). *The Foreign Policies of Arab States*, ed. Bahgat Korany and Ali E. H. Dessouki (Boulder, Colo.: Westview Press; Cairo: American University in Cairo, 1984) analyzes Syria, Saudi Arabia, Iraq, Egypt, Algeria, and the PLO in terms of domestic environment, foreign policy orientation, and the decision-making process. Finally, a recent article by Anthony H. Cordesman, "The Middle East and the Cost of the Politics Force," *Middle East Journal* 40 (Winter 1986): 5–15, argues that the primary danger of modernization in the region is not Westernization but militarization. The spiraling arms buildup in the Middle East is characterized as squandering "a priceless and unrenewable patrimony." On the Arab-Israeli conflict, Cordesman contends:

The true military confrontation is now limited to Israel and Syria, and it is a confrontation that neither side can win. Israel can maintain its military security but only at a crippling social and economic cost. Syria can buy the shell of military parity with Israel, but not the training, technology, or sustaining capability to make that parity real. It can help drive a mutual arms race, and possibly help trigger another war, but never "win" any significant goal.

After examining Egypt, Israel, Jordan, and Syria, he reaches the conclusion that: "The U.S. can buy temporary security for its friends in the region through arms transfers, but only peace can bring an end to massive new arms transfers and aid packages. At the same time, the nations in the region can only use arms to make their situation marginally worse, but never significantly better."

Overall, the preponderance of the literature is still geared to the impact of militarization upon society rather than upon doctrine, strategy, or structures of defense policy making. When examining the literature on specific countries, it is apparent that there is proportionally more literature available on Israel than on any other Middle Eastern country. The reader may wish to consult the works of the Foreign Area Studies Series of American University, which publishes a series of area handbooks on individual Middle Eastern states that include a section on national defense.

Israel

Zui Lanir, ed., *Israeli Security Planning in the 1980s: Its Politics and Economics* (New York: Praeger, 1984) considers the widening gap between Israel's military requirements and the capacity of its economy to provide resources while Arab countries continue increasing their military spending. This book also analyzes the impact of the Israeli Defense Forces upon foreign and defense policy making. Efraim Inbar, *Israeli Strategic Thought in the Post-1973 Period* (Jerusalem: Israel Research Institute of Contemporary Society, 1982) not only traces the shifts in Israeli strategy since the 1973 war, but also includes in an appendix Ariel Sharon's statements regarding the extension of Israeli strategic and security interests to Turkey, Pakistan, Iran, the Gulf, and Africa. A critique of Israeli policy in Lebanon is found in *Israel's Lebanon Policy: Where To*, ed. Joseph Alper (Tel Aviv: Jaffee Center for Strategic Studies, Tel Aviv University, 1984). Amos Perlmutter has written extensively on the Israeli military, its policies, and its role in society. His "Unilateral Withdrawal: Israel's Security Option," *Foreign Affairs* 64 (Fall 1985): 141-53, provides a brief overview of security policy shifts between policy based upon some form of political autonomy for Palestinians and stable eastern borders. Perlmutter has also written two books on the developing role of the military in the Israeli foreign and defense policymaking process: *Military and Politics in Israel: Nation Building and Role Expansion* (New York: Praeger, 1969) and *Politics and the Military in Israel, 1967-1977* (London: Cass, 1978). Ben Halpern focuses on the transition from underground military units to a state-controlled army and on how this transition has affected policy in "The Role of the Military in Israel" in *Role of the Military in Underdeveloped Countries*, ed. Johnson. Edward Luttwak and Dan Horowitz, *The Israeli Army* (New York: Harper & Row, 1975), consider various military influences upon Israeli defense policy. Different aspects of Israeli security doctrines and policies are considered in Yoav Ben Horin and Barry Posen, *Israel's Strategic Doctrine* (Santa Monica, Calif.: RAND Corporation, 1981); Efraim Inbar, "Israel's New

Military Doctrine," *Strategic Studies* 7 (1984): 84-100; Aharon Yariv and R. Lieber, "Personal Whim or Strategic Imperative? The Israeli Invasion of Lebanon," *International Security* 8 (1983): 117-42; a two-part series by A. Shalev, "Security Dangers from the East," *Jerusalem Quarterly* 27 (1983): 15-26; and "Security Dangers for the East (2)," *Jerusalem Quarterly* 30 (Winter 1984): 132-44; and Aharon Yariv, "Strategic Depth," *Jerusalem Quarterly* 17 (Fall 1980): 3-12. Excellent background sources on the doctrinal content and processes of the Israeli defense policy community include Michael Handel, *Israel's Political-Military Doctrine* (Cambridge: Harvard University Press, 1975) and Michael Brecher, *Decisions in Israel's Foreign Policy* (New Haven: Yale University Press, 1975).

Geostrategic influences upon Israel and controversies over the role they play in defense policies are explored in Moshe Dayan, "Israel's Border and Security Problems," *Foreign Affairs* 33 (January 1955): 250-67; Merrill A. McPeak, "Israel: Borders and Security," *Foreign Affairs* 54 (April 1976): 426-43; and Yigal Allon, "Israel: The Case for Defensible Borders," *Foreign Affairs* 55 (October 1976): 38-53. The complexity of geostrategic position and Israeli defense policy is illustrated by Israel Tall, who argues in "Israel's Defense Doctrine: Background and Dynamics," *Military Review* 58 (March 1978): 23-37, that the increased territory acquired during the 1967 war resulted in confused defense planning and weakened Israel's security. Mark Heller considers the increased territory in a different light. For an examination of proposals for creation of a Palestinian state and their implications for Israel's military security, its international political standing, and its economic well-being, see Heller's *Palestinian State: The Implications for Israel* (Cambridge: Harvard University Press, 1983).

The significance of security, the American relationship, and the allocation of resources within Israel are addressed in a number of articles: Duncan Clarke and Alan S. Cohen, "The United States, Israel and the Lavi Fighter," *Middle East Journal* 40 (Winter 1986): 16-32; M. Hameed, "The Impact and Implications of the U.S.-Israeli Strategic Cooperation Agreement," *American-Arab Affairs* 8 (1984): 13-19; Y. Somekh, "Supply of F-16 Aircraft and Mobile Hawk Missiles to Jordan: The Military Ramifications for Israel," *Middle East Review* 15 (1982-83): 53-58; and Efraim Inbar, "The American Arms Transfer to Israel," *Middle East Review* 15 (1982-83): 40-52.

The Arab-Israeli wars have also influenced the development of Israeli defense policy. Useful studies in this area include Avi Shalaim and Raymond Tanter, "Decision Process, Choice and Consequences: Israel's Deep Penetration Bombing in Egypt, 1970," *World Politics* 30 (July 1978): 483-516; Dan Horowitz, "Flexible Responsiveness and Military Strategy: The Case of the Israeli Army," *Policy Sciences* 1 (Summer 1970): 191-205; Abraham Wagner *Crisis Decision-Making: Israel's Experiences in 1967 and 1973* (New York: Praeger, 1974); Michael Handel, "The Yom Kippur War and the Inevitability of Surprise," *International Studies Quarterly* 21 (September 1977): 461-502; Avi Shalaim, "Failures in National Intelligence Estimates: The Case of the Yom Kippur War," *World Politics* 28 (April 1976): 348-80; Abraham Wagner, *The Impact of the 1973 October War on Israeli Policy* (Washington, D.C.: American Institute for Research, 1975); and Janice

Gross Stein, "'Intelligence' and 'Stupidity' Recondiered: Estimation and Decision in Isael, 1973," *Journal of Strategic Studies* 3 (September 1980): 147–77. Four recent works are noteworthy. Ze'ev Schiff and Ehud Ya'ari are investigative journalists who describe the ability of former Defense Minister Ariel Sharon to connive or bully his way through policy, and they castigate a cabinet that ignored Sharon's propensity to act first and seek approval later in *Israel's Lebanon War*, trans. Ina Friedman (New York: Simon & Schuster, 1984). Along the same vein, Moshe Lissak, ed., *Israeli Society and Its Defense Establishment: The Social and Political Impact of a Protracted Violent Conflict* (Totowa, N.J.: Frank Cass, 1984) contends that Israeli social and political mechanisms no longer constrain the autonomy of its military, and conversely that the routinization of conflict has led to increased partisan political influence over critical segments of the military. Ruevan Gal, "Israeli Military Commitment," *Armed Forces and Society* 11 (Summer 1985): 553–564, considers the case of Colonel Eli Geva, an IDF armored brigade commander who requested to be relieved of his command in the midst of the Israeli incursion into Lebanon. It explores the demands of obedience and discipline and contrasts them with the requirements of conscience and commitment. William Darryl Henderson, *Cohesion: The Human Element in Combat* (Washington, D.C.: National Defense University Press, 1985), compares the Israeli Army with the armies of North Vietnam, the Soviet Union, and the United States. He concludes that the qualitative edge belongs to armies with good leadership and cohesive forces.

Excellent sources on Israeli nuclear policies include Shai Feldman, *Israeli Nuclear Deterrence: A Strategy for 1980s* (New York: Columbia University Press, 1982), which considers both Arab and Israeli views of Israeli nuclear weapons, and George H. Quester, "Nuclear Weapons and Israel," *Middle East Journal* 37 (Autumn 1983): 547–64, which traces the evolution of Israeli nuclear policies. Other noteworthy contributions are Robert Harkavy, *Spectre of a Middle Eastern Holocaust: The Strategic and Diplomatic Implications of the Israeli Nuclear Weapons Program* (Denver: University of Denver Press, 1977); Robert Pranger and Dale Tahtinen, *Nuclear Threat in the Middle East* (Washington, D.C.: American Enterprise Institute, 1975); Yair Evron, "Israel and the Atom: The Uses and Misuses of Ambiguity, 1957–1967," *Orbis* 17 (Winter 1974): 1326–43; Lawrence Freedman, "Israeli Nuclear Policy," *Survival* 17 (May 1975): 114–20; and Alan Dowth, "Nuclear Proliferation: The Israeli Case," *International Studies Quarterly* (March 1978): 22–23.

Other Middle Eastern countries are not covered as well as Israel. Consequently the information that follows is, at best, fragmentary.

Lebanon

A few articles address different militias and the army in Lebanon. *The Emergence of a New Lebanon: Fantasy and Reality*, ed. Edward Azar (New York: Praeger, 1984), contains two noteworthy articles: R. D. McLaurin, "Lebanon and Its Army: Past, Present and Future" and Lewis Snider, "The Lebanese Forces: Wartime Origins and Political Significance." Snider also has addressed the structure and doctrine of the Lebanese forces, the functions they perform, and their relationship to the army and the government in "The Lebanese Forces: Their Origins and Role in Lebanon's Politics," *Middle East Journal* 38 (Winter 1984): 1–33. The impact of violent conflict during the past decade upon society, the army, the government, and the militias have been covered by a wide range of sources, including Walid Khalidi, *Conflict and Violence in Lebanon* (Cambridge: Harvard University Center for International Affairs, 1979); Halim Barakat, *Lebanon in Strife* (Austin: University of Texas Press, 1977); John Bullock, *Death of a Country: The Civil War in Lebanon* (London: Weidenfeld & Nicolson, 1977); and Fouad Ajami, "Lebanon and Its Inheritors," *Foreign Affairs* 63 (Spring 1985): 778–99.

Syria

Ajami's "Lebanon and Its Inheritors" includes a brief discussion of Syria's security policies regarding Lebanese factions. R. D. McLaurin et al., *Foreign Policy Making in the Middle East: Domestic Influences on Policy in Egypt, Iraq, Israel and Syria* (New York: Praeger, 1977), consider Syrian political and military objectives. Other useful sources include Amos Perlmutter, "From Obscurity to Rule: The Syrian Army and the Ba'ath Party," *Western Political Quarterly* 22 (December 1969): 827–45; Adeed Dawisha, "Syria under Assad, 1970–1978: The Centres of Power," *Government and Opposition* 13 (Summer 1978); and Moshe Ma'oz, "Alawi Military Officers in Syrian Politics, 1966–1974," *Military and State in Modern Asia*, ed. Harold Schiffrin (Jerusalem: Academic Press, 1976).

Iraq

Information on Iraqi defense policy is sparse. There is a brief survey on Iraqi defense policy in W. Seth Carus, "Military Policy in Iraq," in *Defense Planning in Less Industrialized States*, ed. Neuman. Christine Moss Helms, "The Iraqi Dilemma: Political Objectives versus Military Strategy," *American Arab Affairs* 5 (Summer 1983): 76–85, suggests that the Ba'ath Party has purposely constrained military strategy in the Iran-Iraq War. On the other hand, Uriel Dann, "The Iraqi Officer Corps as a Factor for Stability: An Orthodox Approach," in *Military and the State in Modern Asia*, argues that the military acts as a moderating, stabilizing force in domestic politics. McLaurin, *Foreign Policy Making*, has a brief section on Iraqi military policy. Claudia Wright traces the growth of Iraqi military and economic power up to 1979 in "Iraq: New Power in the Middle East," *Arab-American Affairs* 5 (Summer 1983): 76–85. Mohammad Farbush, *The Role of the Military in Politics: A Case Study of Iraq to 1941* (London: Routledge & Kegan Paul, 1982), and E. Koury, "The Impact of the Geopolitical Situation of Iraq upon the Gulf Cooperation Council," *Middle East Insight* 2 (January–February 1983): 28–35, provide useful insights and background material. Jed Snyder's "The Road to Osiraq: Baghdad's Quest for the 'Bomb'" in *Middle East Journal* 37 (Autumn 1983): 565–93 discusses Iraqi nuclear policies and programs and their political-military implications before and after the Israeli raid.

Jordan

Relatively few sources exist regarding Jordanian defense policy. Two good starting points are P. J. Vatikiotis, *Politics and the Military in Jordan* (New York: Praeger, 1967), and Sayed Ali El-Edroos, *The Hashemite Arab Army, 1908–1979* (Amman: The Publishing Committee, 1982). Anthony Cordesman, *Jordanian Arms and the Middle East Balance* (Washington, D.C.: Middle East Institute, 1983) lists individual state's weapons and provides a comparison of the region's weaponry. His charts, graphs, and tables nicely illustrate the text. Cordesman outlines Jordan's unique and extremely vulnerable position given the steady decline in Jordan's forces and military expenditures relative to those of Israel, Syria, and Egypt.

Saudi Arabia and Other Gulf States

The best discussion of the defense policies and structures of Saudi Arabia and other Gulf states is to be found in Anthony Cordesman, *The Gulf and the Search for Strategic Stability: Saudi Arabia, the Military Balance in the Gulf, and Trends in the Arab Israeli Military Balance* (Boulder, Colo.: Westview Press, 1984). Half of the book explores the many facets of Saudi military capability and defense policy; the rest covers the defense communities and policies of the Yemens, Kuwait, Bahrain, Qatar, the United Arab Emirates, Iran, and Iraq. Maps and graphs enrich the text. Other good sources include John Thomas Cummings, Hossein G. Askari, and Michael Skinner, "Military Expenditures and Manpower Requirements in the Arabian Peninsula," *Arab Studies Quarterly* 2 (Winter 1980); Dale Tahtinen, *National Security Challenges to Saudi Arabia* (Washington, D.C.: American Enterprise Institute, 1978); and two articles by Adeed Dawisha, "Internal Values and External Threats: The Making of Saudi Policy," *Orbis* 23 (Spring 1979) and *Saudi Arabia's Search for Security,* Adelphi Papers, no. 158 (London: International Institute for Strategic Studies, 1979–80). Nadav Safran traces Saudi foreign relations and security policies from the founding of the modern kingdom by Ibn Saud to the present in *Saudi Arabia: The Ceaselesss Quest for Security* (Cambridge: Harvard University Press, 1985).

Iran

In addition to the chapters on Iran in Cordesman's, *The Gulf and the Search for Strategic Stability*, two other sources consider postrevolutionary Iran's military forces and doctrines: R. Perron, "The Iranian Islamic Revolutionary Guard Corps," *Middle East Insight* 4 (1985): 35–39; and Willliam Hichman, *Ravaged and Reborn: The Iranian Army, 1982* (Washington, D.C.: Brookings Institution, 1983). Elaine Sciolino traces the emergence of a battle-tested army and a revolutionary militia in Iran since the Revolution in "Iran's Durable Revolution," *Foreign Affairs* 61 (Spring 1983): 803–920. A bit on strategy can be found in Charles G. MacDonald, "Iran's Strategic Interests and the Law of the Sea," *Middle East Journal* (Summer 1980): 302–23.

Egypt

Kolodziej and Harkavy's *Security Policies of Developing Countries* has a wonderful chapter on Egypt's military doctrine, force structure, weapons systems, and the impact of domestic influences on defense policies. Good companion articles are Dessouki's "Egypt and Gulf Security," in *International Security in Southwest Asia* and K. Shikkaki, "The Nuclearization Debates: The Cases of Israel and Egypt," *Journal of Palestine Studies* 14 (1985): 77–91. Discussions of Egyptian national security concerns can be found in Korany and Dessouki, *The Foreign Policies of Arab States* and McLaurin et al., *Foreign Policy Making*. The evolving role of the Egyptian military is considered in Charles Holley, "Egypt's 'Other' Armed Forces," *Middle East Journal* 46 (August 1978): 28–30; Eliezer Berri, "Changing Role of the Military in Egyptian Politics," in *Military and the State in Modern Asia*; and P. J. Vatikiotis, *The Egyptian Army in Politics: Pattern for New Nations*? (Bloomington: Indiana University Press, 1961). The role of the military in society is covered in Anouar Abdel-Malek, *Egypt: Military Society*, trans. Charles Lam Markmann (New York: Vintage Books, 1968); and Amos Perlmutter, *Egypt: The Praetorian State* (New Brunswick, N.J.: Transaction Books, 1974).

This essay has tried to present an overview of available English-language sources on regional and country-specific defense policies in the Middle East. There is a definite requirement for increased scholarly research on the defense policies and defense decision-making processes of Islamic states in the region.

Latin America

Marion David Tunstall

The Western student generally approaches the subject of defense policy with certain preconceived notions of the way things military are. The military is to be externally oriented, subordinate to civilian authorities, and competent in a limited, technical field. In the United States the image is that of the citizen soldier, and since colonial days there has been a mistrust of large standing professional armies. Military subordination has been possible, in part, because of these attitudes and also because of a political evolution that has emphasized compromise, accommodation, and consensus over conflict, with the notable exception of the Civil War. It has also been possible because the geographic position of the United States long kept it largely isolated, focusing the attention of its small military forces on securing the territory of its expanding frontiers. Many scholars have noted the traditional mistrust of the military and the popular image of military officers as inflexible, hierarchical, and disciplined, rather than as broadly capable decision makers. Professionalism also implies a separation of the military from the political currents that swirl about it.

These are the "oughts," perceptions that persist today, even though the military and defense establishment has become the largest standing bureaucracy in the U.S. government. Some critics suggest that technical competence in the profession of arms is declining as military members become more involved in management and the bureaucratic struggle for support and dollars, a process that produces fewer heroes. Nevertheless, whatever the reality, it is still these oughts that provide the lenses through which most North Americans examine the militaries of other nations. Too frequently, North Americans impose their own notions of professionals and professionalism in questioning why Latin American militaries are not more like the admittedly often less-than-accurate image of the U.S. military.

U.S. studies of Latin American militaries or defense policies generally begin with a few basic understandings. First, the military—long a prominent actor and part of the original triumvirate that included the Church and the oligarchs—still retains special rights and privileges in the political system. Second, Latin American militaries began as personal or party armies and did not begin the conversion to national militaries until the victory of one warring faction set the course of national development. Third, professionalization (in the sense of the development of technical skills and of institutionally distinct structures) began for the most part in the late nineteenth and early twentieth centuries under the tutelage of European advisers. This tended to give the military a coherence and disciplinary advantage in relation to many other national institutions, further enhancing the status it has enjoyed as wielder of the coercive force of the nation. Fourth, violence remains a part of the political systems of Latin America, and the military has continued to be involved in a political process characterized by a lack of agreement on the fundamental rules of the game and on the rights of certain actors to play a part.[1] Invited or self-proclaimed, the Latin American military came to consider itself the conservator of the state. Finally, for most Latin American states, significant external challenges largely vanished with the resolution of the border struggles of the late nineteenth and early twentieth centuries, thus turning the attention of the military increasingly inward, reinforcing its political involvement. In general, U.S. studies of Latin American defense policies remain dominated by an internal, civil-military focus, with external defense matters receiving much less attention. Yet all agree with Abraham Lowenthal that "the armed forces are central to what happens in Latin American politics and are likely to remain so."[2]

I make no claim to comprehensiveness in the pages that follow. I have endeavored to select key themes and works I find useful in explaining the evolution of the literature on Latin American militaries and defense policies. This review acknowledges the difficulty of capturing the multidirectional flow of these studies and, with the exception of a few major works, does not attempt to provide coverage of each individual military or country. It also does not consider the military in Cuba and the Caribbean. With regard to the specifics of the Malvinas/Falklands conflict, moreover, the reader is referred to the *Bibliography of the 1982 Falklands War* by Marilyn B. Yakota. I acknowledge, and have benefited from, the efforts of those who have previously and expertly embarked on a similar undertaking: L. N. McAlister, R. C. Rankin, A. F. Lowenthal, and S. J. Fitch.

Studies of Latin American militaries and defense abound, but the serious scholar would do well to begin with writings that appeared around 1960. It was at this point that underlying arguments that have influenced research over the past four decades first took coherent form in debates over the proper role of the military and the best modes of studying the military institution in Latin America. Though studies of the military were legion prior to 1960, few demonstrated the rigor of those that followed. Edwin Lieuwen's bibliographic note in

The author would like to thank Susan Whitson, Betty Fogler, Sharon Johnson, and the reference staff of the Air Force Academy Library and Mrs. Bailey and the staff of the Interamerican Defense College Library for their invaluable assistance during the preparation of this article. A special thanks is also due to Kay McGrew for her patience and special assistance in the final preparation of this study. The views expressed here are those of the author and do not necessarily reflect those of any agency of the U.S. government.

Arms and Politics in Latin America offers a useful synopsis of much of the literature available from 1900 to 1960. These earlier studies were largely historical and descriptive, and dealt with a hodge-podge of subjects and concerns, failing to penetrate very deeply the forces and institutions that the militaries of the region constituted.

How, then, is one to explain the development of the scholarship of the 1960s? In his 1966 review of literature, L. N. McAlister attributes the development to the Cuban revolution, which turned more scholastic attention to the region; to the fact that U.S. policy, concerned with regional penetration, looked to development as a means to overcome systemic invitations to violence and to the military to help provide stability and security; and, finally, to systems analysis and theoretical studies of the military such as Samuel Finer's *The Man on Horseback*, Samuel Huntington's *Soldier and State*, and Morris Janowitz's *The Military in the Political Development of New Nations*. (McAlister, 1966)

Initial efforts at greater rigor did not break completely with the characteristics of previous scholarship. Much of the literature prior to 1960 was prone to ethnocentrism in the application of U.S. standards of military professionalism and democracy. The U.S. model was applied to judge political involvement by the military as an aberration, and intervention as a violation of the institutional role of the military. "Militarism," as it was called, was seen as selfish and reactionary, and the military was not seen as a "normal" political actor. Much of the literature reflected an evaluation (akin to the stages of modernization and development theory offered by W. W. Rostow) that the problems of Latin America were those of systemic immaturity. These problems would be overcome as the systems modernized and progressed with civilian "middle-class" forces wresting control from dominant elites and establishing the conditions for true democracy. Such studies did not limit the "blame" to Latin America, but also directed a critical eye to the role of the United States and other powers. In his 1959 *Twilight of the Tyrants*, Tad Szulc could conclude: "The pattern of events in the late 1950s suggests unmistakably that the republics of the South so recently emancipated from regimes of force have finally crossed the great divide of their political distances and taken the road toward constitutional order and stability." (p. 4)

Lieuwen's previously mentioned work, his *Generals versus Presidents*, and John J. Johnson's *The Military and Society in Latin America* are representative of the literature that bridges the 1960 divide. Historically oriented (and written in a period in which the earlier optimism of Szulc and others had been shattered by the return of military governments to power), all three books attempted to explain the politically involved military as an "objective fact of life." Though Lieuwen asserted that his books were not a rant against militarism, both reflected the "oughts" of the earlier literature. Indeed, he and Johnson examined the institution of the military and its patterns of recruitment and socialization, noting the appearance of younger, more progressive officers.[3] Lieuwen concluded on an essentially normative and optimistic note: "Yet despite its recent setbacks, democracy still has the overwhelming support of Latin America's people." (Lieuwen, 1964: p. 134)

In a study that followed his 1962 edited volume on *The Role of the Military in Underdeveloped Countries*, Johnson offered a revisionist critique that questioned Lieuwen and saw militarism and intervention, not as the disease, but as the symptom of the inability of civilian leaders and institutions to garner the support necessary to create and maintain stable, organized governments that can make decisions and implement them while keeping control of the military. (Johnson, 1964) Thus, in this view, military intervention is a symptom of a systemic disorder, and the military is to be compared with civilian politicians. As often as not, it is the civilian leaders who demonstrate weakness and inability to govern, hence contributing to an environment that "pulls" the military into political action. Violence is employed as much by others as it is by the military, and the military may actually perform positive functions of unification[4] within a less than "ordered" system. Thus, Johnson offered a different perspective than Lieuwen. He viewed the military as an effective agent of development and began to move away from the more descriptive tendencies of the earlier literature and toward explanations offered in such works as L. N. McAlister's "Changing Concepts of the Role of the Military in Latin America."

Efforts thus were taken to analyze social origins, recruitment, socialization, and the development of the military as an institution, describing relations between the military and other institutions and actors within Latin American political systems. Typologies and classifications began to emerge to suggest the likelihood and frequency of military actions (Wyckoff, 1960) and to define civil-military relations. Thus, the military began to be seen not as a political interloper, but as a key actor that can play many distinct roles. (Germani and Silvert, 1976)

Earlier assumptions about automatic democratization by the middle classes were also questioned during this period. One key analysis in this regard is José Nun's "A Latin American Phenomenon: The Middle Class Coup" (1965). Nun disabuses his readers of the notion that one can assume either a unified middle "class" or a middle-class-based military intervention that would result necessarily in progressive development, a view that places him at odds with both Lieuwen and Johnson. More appropriately, the Latin American middle "class" should be called a sector, as it has lacked a unifying social or ideological stance and thus may find itself at a disadvantage in dealing with the more unified laboring and upper-class elements. Lacking unity, and thus the means to protect itself, the middle sector is less a positive force and tends in Nun's view to be resistant to change. The military, increasingly composed of middle-sector officers, acts in a way that reflects the concerns and frustrations of this growing sector.

Nun's explanations are rejected by other scholars such as Luigi Einaudi (*The Peruvian Military: A Summary Political Analysis*), who argues against the "determinism" of Nun and asserts that a broader perspective on the military inclusive of institutional influences and needs, education, isolation, and other factors must be considered in explaining intervention. A stronger refutation based on the argument that the officer is motivated by institutional norms and military allegiance or situations rather than class is found in the work of Carlos Astiz ("The Argentine Armed Forces: Their

Role and Political Involvement") and José Minguens ("The New Latin American Military Coup"). In his work, Minguens foreshadows the "technocratic/institutional" thesis that would come into prominence in the mid 1970s. Additionally, the argument is made that the middle-sector origins of many Latin American officers should not be assumed as equating with a socially based decision for intervention. Indeed, too many other factors must be taken into account.

McAlister notes another phenomenon—the focus on the developmental possibilities of the military. In a move away from the assumption that military action is inevitably regressive, some literature of the early to mid 1960s emphasized the infrastructure-building role or the national unification role of the military. This literature reflected the developing "civic action" orientation and counterinsurgency thrust of the U.S. military programs for the region. Even here, some attention was given to the possible dangers of further involving the military in things political and the possibility of frustrating encounters with problems whose origins could not be handled by building a new school or bridge. Further, there was the danger of the possible rise of what was then called "Nasserism"—the view that military dictatorship offers the only hope for rapid modernization—a prescient view. (Barber and Ronning, 1966)

Toward the end of the period of McAlister's analysis, another trend that was to carry forward developed. The general works characterizing the earlier period began to give way to more detailed and careful case studies. The first generation of these emerged in the early pages of the *Journal of Inter-American Studies* and covered countries such as Argentina and Colombia. Full-length work came in such studies as R. E. Gilmore's *Caudillismo and Militarism in Venezuela, 1810–1910* and L. North's *Civil Military Relations in Argentina, Chile, and Peru*. Not all of the literature of the late 1960s to early 1970s was oriented toward case studies. Indeed, some of the most influential works of the period attempted to generalize on the broader subject of military intervention.

Among the more significant of these efforts are Martin Needler's "Political Development and Military Intervention in Latin America" and Robert D. Putnam's "Toward Explaining Military Intervention in Latin American Politics." Noting the existence of contradictory theories about the relation of military coups to political development, Needler sets himself the task of relating the frequency of coups to social conditions and of discussing the internal workings of the military during and before a coup. His overall theme is that military seizure of power impedes the process of political development and social mobilization. While Needler's linkage of overthrow to worsening economic conditions and his methodology have come under some blistering criticism, his conclusions on internal dynamics have been more favorably received. Needler argues that the military may be hesitant, drawn in by civilian pressure and appeal; that factions within the military may be strengthened in relation to their external connections; and, most important, that coalition building in support of a coup continues until the decisive "swing-man" adds the weight of prestige or critical opposition, frequently becoming the leader of the new government (as was the case with General Castelo Branco in Brazil). Finally,

Needler notes that this very process leads to problems within the military after the government is established. Turning to policy prescription, Needler argues that the United States may sway the military by weighing in to dissuade the less than committed swing-man.

Putnam's 1967 article remains a standard against which quantitative studies of Latin American military behavior are measured. Collecting data from the previous decade, he attempted to evaluate the various, often contradictory, propositions regarding the supposed causes of military intervention. Putnam used four major operational categories: socioeconomic development, political development, institutional characteristics, and foreign influences. Testing propositions against them, he found little explanatory utility in either the level of political development indicators or those for foreign influence. On the other hand, he found that higher levels of social mobilization tend to inhibit military intervention because active political participation complicates the chances for success. At the same time, traditions of military intervention may also legitimize and promote further intervention. Though he did not escape problems of data reliability, Putnam's efforts were accepted by many in the period because they tended to affirm assumptions about a relation between development and a decline in intervention. He proposed a military intervention index, ranking countries on a scale from zero to three, with zero being those in which the military was essentially an apolitical pressure group and three being those in which the military ruled. Interestingly, J. Mark Ruhl's application of Putnam's procedures to the 1969–78 period resulted in the finding that "every one of the moderately strong relationships Putnam discovered in the earlier test era practically disappeared." (Ruhl, 1982: p. 579) Ruhl explained the finding in terms of the literature on bureaucratic authoritarianism (which had become the dominant academic focus in the mid 1970s) and in terms of difficulties in cross-sectional, aggregate data studies.

Drawing on the earlier efforts and noting the concerns of authors like Putnam and Needler, several key figures produced the classics of the late 1960s and early 1970s, most notably Lieuwen's *Mexican Militarism: The Political Rise and Fall of the Revolutionary Army, 1919–1940*; R. A. Potash's *The Army and Politics in Argentina, 1928–1945*; Alfred Stepan's *The Military in Politics: Changing Patterns in Brazil*; R. Clinton's "The Modernizing Military: The Case of Peru"; Victor Villanueva's *El CAEM: La revolución de la fuerza armada*; Luigi Einaudi and Alfred Stepan's *Latin American Institutional Development: Changing Military Perspectives in Peru and Brazil*; and David Ronfeldt's *The Mexican Army and Political Order since 1940*.

Clinton, Potash, Stepan and the others continued research that delved deeply into Latin American military institutions, beginning to bridge the gap between purely historical and political analyses. Using information previously unavailable or overlooked, they provided a detailed examination of changes wrought in these militaries over the years, as well as a much more precise evaluation of factors within the military and their linkages and relationships with civilian authorities. This literature revealed much more about the recruitment, social origins, training, and processes of institutionalization and professionalization of regional military establishments. The focus of these studies was to understand the military first and then to place it within the society; the problem remained in the development of some means of comparative analysis or general theorizing.

Clinton, Stepan, and Einaudi offered another key development in the literature on Latin American militaries—the concept of "new professionalism" and its relation to a new doctrine of national security that called for a larger role for the military in society. In its expanding educational programs, the military came to focus on development as key to security, and hence core to its mission of national defense. In Peru this meant "guided" socioeconomic change to obtain security, as in the Velasco Alvorado government of 1968, while in Brazil, greater concern with security also resulted in "guided" development. Under the "new professionalism" concept, the military was to become more, not less, involved—offsetting the hopes of the "democratic gradualist" and signaling, at least in Brazil, a yielding of the historical military role of moderator for the new role of governor. Stepan and Potash also depicted a military riven by political diversity, but drawn together by institutional factors and the situation in which it finds itself—one lacking in confidence about the competency of civil leadership.

The resurgence of military intervention in the mid 1960s and early 1970s differed from earlier periods in that the military seized and held power as an institution. As George Philip notes, writers in this period began to take for granted a political order with some form of coherent authoritarianism as the norm or logical consequence of the system. (Philip, 1980) There was a search for an explanation as to why the modernizing states of Latin America were subject to military intervention, a development that flew in the face of expectations that advances would lead to democracy. Authors like Frederick Pike and Thomas Stritch (1974), Howard J. Wiarda (1973), Claudio Veliz (1968), and Philippe Schmitter (1974) examined the cultural influences on Latin American political and economic development and criticized the assumptions and omissions of the developmentalists, noting that Latin American corporatism was simply an ill fit for many developmental frameworks. The traditional Latin American system was defined as hierarchical, corporative, elitist, and authoritarian, modified but not destroyed by the challenges of the twentieth century. Thus centralization, government control, general versus individual will, and top-down change were the standards of the system, and administration was more vital than politics. The literature began to refer to Latin American political systems as "living museums"—incorporating the new without abandoning the old.

Evaluations of the military regimes of Latin America led in the late 1960s to a wider reexamination of the assumptions of developmentalists (e.g., see Samuel P. Huntington, *Political Order in Changing Societies*). This general review of developmentalism resulted for Latin America in the concept of "bureaucratic authoritarianism" that reflected, yet rejected, both the developmentalist and dependency approaches. The effort was to focus on the development of states that industrialize late and in the midst of a dependency on foreign capital, technology, and management. The father of this new school of thought, which helped to explain de-

velopments in Brazil, Argentina, and Peru, and later in Chile and Uruguay, was the Argentine political scientist Guillermo O'Donnell.

In his *Modernization and Bureaucratic Authoritarianism: Studies in South American Politics*, O'Donnell bows to the ground-breaking efforts of many of the writings already mentioned above, laying out the assertions that have provided the focus for much of the intellectual debate on Latin American development and the military since. He challenges both the developmentalists and their nemeses, the dependency theorists, who explain the problems of Latin America in terms of Prebisch's center-periphery and imperialist-capitalist designs. In his view, class intransigence and domestic economic conditions necessitate orthodox economic practices and creation of a favorable investment environment, which can be implemented only by a technocratic-military coalition that exercises the control and discipline not being provided by the inefficient civilian political structure.

Focusing on regime, coalition, and policies, O'Donnell develops concepts of exclusionary and inclusionary regimes and a typology of traditional, populist, and bureaucratic authoritarians. Though O'Donnell defines bureaucratic authoritarians as essentially exclusionary and nondemocratic, later writers have noted many structural similarities between bureaucratic authoritarian reforms in exclusionary Brazil and the "revolutionary" inclusionary Peruvian junta (see Stepan's *The State and Society: Peruvian Comparative Perspective*). The efforts of O'Donnell and others to move beyond "cultural" explanations are an attempt to deal with military governments that displace (or attempt to displace) the old politics with a new, disciplined, rapid, militarily and technocratically generated path to development.

As previously noted, the orientation, education, and coherence that encouraged such thinking had been developed in the expanding concepts of professionalism and national security originating in the centers of military higher education. Thus "moderating" militaries became more confident and, in their thinking, more capable of governing. Political restrictions, or "guided democracy," would be necessary to ensure the promise of economic development and modernization. These were seen as enduring, not transitory, regimes. The general thrust of this literature is captured well in J. Malloy's *Authoritarianism and Corporatism in Latin America* and D. Collier's *The New Authoritarianism in Latin America*, which contains an excellent bibliography.

O'Donnell's model captured the attention of many Latin Americanists and became the straw man of the late 1970s and early 1980s. When details of the evolution of military regimes challenged some of the assumptions of bureaucratic authoritarianism, O'Donnell was criticized for having overgeneralized the specific cases of Brazil and Argentina. In "Three Mistaken Theses regarding the Connection between Industrialization and Authoritarian Regimes," José Serra termed Brazil the "paradigmatic case" (p. 102), yet raised questions about the model. O'Donnell came under deeper examination in Collier (1979) and Remmer and Merkx (1982; the same issue of the *Latin American Research Review* carried O'Donnell's rejoinder), and the whole model was given a blistering review in Needler (1986). Needler dismissed bureaucratic authoritarianism as a passing fancy of the mid 1970s that ignored the case of Venezuela. Moreover, in *Generals in Retreat*, Philip O'Brien and Paul Cammach stated that bureaucratic authoritarianism is "in danger of being abandoned; it has already been emasculated."[5]

As the military as an institution continued to govern in much of Latin America, academic attention turned naturally to the consequences of military rule and comparison with the civilian governments of the region, as well as comparisons between military regimes. Philippe C. Schmitter (1973) focused on the political function of direct military rule, the policy consequences of internal military intervention and external military aid, and the likely impact of both on regional and global political systems. (p. vii) Of direct concern was the relation of external assistance, particularly that of the United States, to the military's ability to increase its relative command over national economic resources and decision making. With more capability in its "political" capacity, the military becomes even less willing to relinquish control. The book also raised questions of the potential problems caused by asymmetric military capabilities and a decaying U.S. hegemony. Schmitter found that higher defense spending and a corresponding decrease in social welfare spending accompanied military regimes, particularly intermittent ones, and that this regime type also affected extractive ability, relative burden sharing, reinvestment, and social benefits. Acknowledging the need for more data and analysis, Schmitter set the focus for the next decade. Most of the efforts that followed Schmitter's were case studies of particular regimes. As before, comparative analyses tended to be rather sparse.

One partial compendium of the "consequences" articles is in part 6 of Loveman and Davies (1978). Robert Wesson (1982) also examines military rule, with a bow to John J. Johnson's assumption about reasons for military intervention and an acknowledgement of the much improved qualifications and ability of the military to rule. Wesson's collection also includes some analysis of states that were not under military rule and asks why.

Of necessity, some focus was given to explaining different types of military regimes, i.e., contrasting Peru with Brazil, but attention was also directed at comparisons within a given type. Articles compared the earlier period of Brazilian military rule with later ones and examined the implementation of the Peruvian military's reforms. Individual case studies of military rule abound and are to be found in the pages of regional journals, as well as in Collier (1979), Handelmann and Saunders (1981), Linz and Stepan (1978), Hayes (1975), Lowenthal (1975), Middlebrook and Palmer (1975), and others. It remains a topic of concern (for example, see Grindle, 1987).

A subset of the military literature that predates (but is also coincident with) that of military rule is writing on the evolution of national security doctrine. Stepan relates the development and expansion of the definition of national security within the Brazilian Escuela Superior de Guerra. (1971: 178–83) National security and national development had become inextricably linked, and the military's role grew to encompass concerns not only with territory and resources, but also with popular unity, the nature of the government, industrial capacity, and national morale.

Stepan further develops the concept of "new professionalism" in his article in Lowenthal (1976). Using nationalism and patriotism as sources of appeal and justification, many militaries of the region have sought to organize and control almost all aspects of society, strengthening or creating the capacity they feel they need to sustain the drive to the national security objective of development. As it has evolved, the doctrine has assumed a broader ideological bent and has turned not only to building the state, but also to defeating those who would impede the effort, including "subversives" serving "internal" enemies. Arrigada (1980), Calvo (1979), Varas (1985: ch. 2), and Comblin (1979) give good synopses of the development of this concept of national security.

A useful, if little known, general contribution to the study of the role of Latin American militaries was completed in 1972 by the Center for Advanced International Studies of the University of Miami. Under the direction of Clyde C. Wooten, a staff including several military officers and such notables as McAlister, Suchlicki, and Maingot completed *The Political and Socio-Economic Role of the Military in Latin America*; it has four appendices covering twelve countries. Proceeding from this series of twelve descriptive and uneven studies of militaries and civil-military relations, the work attempted to "provide a wider perspective of the military as a functional institution and a more definitive comparative framework for defining the U.S. long term interest and policy objectives with respect to Latin America." (p. 9) Though the conclusions offered little that is not in keeping with the literature of the time, the effort did present a coherent, easily accessible study.

Don Etchison began his study on *The United States and Militarism in Central America* by quoting Luis Hankes' conclusion that Central America caught the world's attention because of volcanos, imminent communist takeover, or an archaeological discovery. Indeed, in the literature from 1960 on, Central America had largely been ignored. Etchison's descriptive review of the Central American militaries and of their relations with the United States filled a gap, but few heeded the call for more work in this area. One exception was Richard Millet's *Guardians of the Dynasty*, a study of Somoza's National Guard. However, few were attracted by the relatively virgin ground of the military in Central America. Ron Seckinger, "The Central American Militaries: A Survey of the Literature," revealed an embarrassing lack of information on the military in an area that had already captured a predominant share of U.S. foreign policy attention.

Steven Ropp, *Panamanian Politics: From Guarded Nation to National Guard*, fills another gap, but the void is still tremendous. Clearly, the Central American militaries are smaller, and, in relative terms, less professionalized and institutionalized. They have been given more to the cliquish behavior and *caudillismo* that characterized the earlier period of South American military development. Yet, in keeping with Johnson's 1964 study, they still can be said to be more organized and coherent than many of their civilian institutional counterparts.

In 1976 Abraham Lowenthal published what has been considered the standard compendium of writing on Latin American militaries and their political role, *Armies and Politics in Latin America*, which brought together the key theoretical articles from Germani and Silvert to Nun, Putnam, and Schmitter and combined them with a useful collection of case studies reflecting the ongoing debates in the field. Lowenthal's was an effort to facilitate teaching and learning, to stimulate further inquiry, to encourage theorizing, and to point the way to much-needed research and greater coherence in the field.

In the conclusion of his introductory essay, Lowenthal suggests a research requirement to study the relation between the level of organization, coherence, and strength of the military and civilian sectors and the extent of military dominance within the system. As Samuel Fitch, coeditor of the updated version of *Armies and Politics*, indicates, Lowenthal's efforts have had direct utility in much of the work that has followed, such as explaining the ability of the PRI to institutionalize its rule over the army in Mexico, the late turn of Chile to bureaucratic authoritarianism, and the distinctive forms of military regimes in Central America. (p. 36) Unfortunately, many of Lowenthal's research suggestions remain unfulfilled. There continues to be a need for comparative research, for more field research, and for an analysis of those cases in which the military does not intervene.

With the demise of military governments in Ecuador (1979) and Peru (1980) and signs that the Brazilian military's "abertura" was serious, a new trend emerged in the literature, that of explaining the military's withdrawal from government. Here, Needler's concepts of coalition politics within the military (1966), Stepan and Potash's studies of factions within the military, and the work of many case studies began to be examined in terms of what Needler (1980) has called the second phase of military regimes.

Needler describes a two-step internal coup process that removes the original conspirators and replaces them with a group pledged to or open to reconstitutionalization. (p. 621) The reasons for such an internal coup, he argues, are not unlike those that motivate the original takeover: a deteriorating economy, a political crisis, threats to the institutional survival of the military, and so on. Such coalitions usually include civilian coconspirators who may have been partners in the first effort.

In a volume on the political dilemmas of military regimes, George Philip notes that "at one level, military regimes almost always fail . . . in that they are either overthrown or are forced to make a disorderly retreat from power. . . . Their ability to relinquish power under the right circumstances, even if this is done in a disorganized way, may be as important to maintaining the underlying social continuity as the intial seizure of power." (Philip, 1985) In the same volume, an attempt is made to develop a comparative framework that includes chapters on Argentina by Guillermo Makin and Central America by James Dunkerley. Key to military government are the problem of legitimacy, workable organizations, the creation of institutional media for exercising control, and the ability to maintain internal unity and retain the support of technocratic or bureaucratic allies.

As Clapman and Philip suggest, the military is usually good for the short term, but conflicts quickly emerge involving continued rule, military values, and preservation of governmental structures. Clapman and Philip offer a useful analysis of regime types and patterns of regime succession, which may be applied to ongoing studies of military withdrawal from governmental office. In *The Military in South American Politics*,

Philip adds a more detailed examination of the internal politics of the military and offers an interesting perspective on the competition that pits activist minorities against each other. Stanley Hilton (1987) tackles the interesting and academically novel consideration of changing strategic perceptions and the effect they have on the concept of mission and the return to civilian government.

Another work that considers the withdrawal of the military from power is O'Brien and Cammack (1985). The book takes as its point of departure a review of O'Donnell's bureaucratic authoritarianism and the assertion that the military does not have a "special vocation to govern, particularly in times of deep political and economic crisis." (p. vii) The editors' preference for the dependency explanation also is evident in the case studies of Argentina and Chile, although those on Brazil and Uruguay are generally less disposed to use dependency rhetoric.

Another series of articles is found in the useful special edition of *Government and Opposition* 19 (Spring 1984) on the transition from military to civilian government. Claude Welch's work (1987) contributes to the comparative study of the factors that contribute to "successful" military disengagement from politics in Africa and Latin America. The Latin American focus is on Bolivia, Colombia, and Peru.

Fitch's review in the updated *Armies and Politics in Latin America* calls attention to *Transitions from Authoritarian Rule* by Guillermo O'Donnell, Philippe Schmitter, and Lawrence Whitehead. Though the conclusions do not appear to differ greatly from those offered earlier by Needler, the articles do add detail and depth to the understanding of the process by which the military negotiates its withdrawal from power and of the conflicts that emerge within the military over the proper role it should play.

Equally important, the revised edition of *Armies and Politics* cited above contains four excellent articles on "democratization and extrication from military rule." These alone make the revised version a must, but its value is greatly magnified by the many new articles on the Mexican and Central American militaries and on the consequences of military power. This edition succeeds in capturing the essence of the existing literature and debates, as did its predecessor. Regrettably, though understandably, it does not retain some of the classic studies found in the first offering.

Finally, one must note the publication of Robert Wesson, ed., *The Latin American Military Institution*. A study of nine militaries, this is unique for its focus on the ranks, education, and career paths and for the unusual attention it gives to the subject of ideology and doctrine. Though it has suffered in the process of compilation, it is an invaluable source of information on subjects rarely addressed in the literature. Recognizing the strength and coherence of the military and its institutional advantages, it attempts to explain the divergent experiences of Latin American states, and hence to determine the distinguishing factors that explain the role of the military.

U.S. Assistance and Role

The reader of this review will note that relations between the United States and militaries in the region have received passing notice only. U.S.-Latin American military relations since 1960 are the subject of another, equally comprehensive, literature review and will not be attempted here. Instead, this portion of the review will attempt to relate a few major themes evident in the material reviewed above. As has been indicated, the writings labeled here as traditional view the military as a somewhat alien institution. The traditionalist use of *intervention* reflects a perception of the military as outside of the "normal" set of political participants. Though they acknowledge the relative strength of the military, the traditionalists argue that the militaries of Latin America have few real missions, thus revealing a Western concept of military professionalism that expects an externally oriented and subordinate military.

With little real external threat from neighbors and no significant capability to defend the hemisphere in Cold War terms, the Latin American militaries became more inwardly oriented. Yet they continued to absorb an "excessive" share of national budgets. A similar argument had been made against military assistance by Dean Acheson in 1947 (Corbett, 1972). Events of the late 1950s convinced Lieuwen and others that the United States had to share the blame for the continuation of Latin American militarism and alienation of democratic forces. These writers were not persuaded by the argument that U.S. military assistance was merely a cost-effective means of ensuring U.S. access to resources and effecting an economy-of-force approach to the region. Indeed, Lieuwen's *Arms and Politics in Latin America* emerged from a 1959 study that suggested elimination of all military aid within a few years. (Corbett, p. vii) As the focus of U.S. policy turned from continental defense to counterinsurgency following Castro's successful revolution in Cuba, Lieuwen continued to voice his opposition to U.S. military assistance.

Following John J. Johnson, many rejected Western political norms and assumptions for evaluating Latin American militaries. While Johnson was not "pro-military," he acknowledged that the military could play a positive developmental role in society. It could be as a symbol of national unity, could forestall violent radical change, and, utilizing its organizational and technical skills, could contribute directly to development through civic action programs oriented to rural areas and involving part-time efforts. (pp. 263–64)

Not surprisingly, Johnson did not equate U.S. assistance with increased intervention by the military, but did suggest a number of areas in which U.S. assistance could help develop the public service role of the military. (p. 265) Still, if "militarism" was to be overcome, it would have to be done within the constraints of Latin American societies, not because of U.S. policy. The United States did not create the conditions favorable to military involvement in politics and neither could it end them. Thus, Johnson and those who followed his thinking rejected the assertions of Lieuwen. They did this, however, without accepting the equally facile argument that U.S. assistance and training had professionalized the militaries of the region, recreating them in the U.S. image of subordination to civil authorities and with an external orientation. (Center for Advanced International Studies, 1972: p. v and Jenkins and Sereseres, 1977)

As counterinsurgency became the predominant focus of U.S. military assistance programs in the region, the U.S. began a parting of ways with its Latin American allies. To be sure, Latin American militaries were concerned with counterinsurgency, internal security, and stability, but not to the exclusion of more advanced military hardware to satisfy their perception of strength through modernity and their perceived requirements for external defense. This, in part, led to the arms races of the 1960s and 1970s, which Varas chronicled and analyzed in his *Militarization and the Arms Race*. To a certain extent, military elements resisted the U.S. emphasis on counterinsurgency, considering its focus on civic action as diversionary (Glick, 1965), but as Willard F. Barber and C. Neale Ronning argued (1966), the United States continued to emphasize the importance of the counterinsurgency mission and found many willing converts. Though Barber and Ronning agreed that the short-term effects of inhibiting insurgency and yielding a favorable image for the military were useful, they were dubious of the long-term benefits. Their concern was with the "quick fix" aspect of a doctrine that in their view ignored the deeper causes of insurgencies and potentially strengthened a military orientation toward greater involvement in things political.

The debate continued through the 1960s and 1970s, down to the present, with emotionalism often the rule. The United States remained the dominant force and supplier in the region; it continued to provide Latin American militaries with the training and equipment it deemed necessary to meet the perceived threat. A continental defense orientation was supplanted by counterinsurgency, which stressed security and development and assumed declining military costs. (Varas, 1985: pp. 40–45; this source also has a good bibliography) The U.S. change in emphasis was consistent with an inward orientation of the Latin militaries.

The argument, then, is that U.S. policies did not create, but did reinforce, military tendencies to increased involvement. Later executive and congressional policies, institutional rivalries before and after Vietnam, and Latin American perceptions of decreased U.S. flexibility and reliability on the one hand, and growing local "needs" on the other, contributed to a relative decline in U.S. dominance of the Latin arms and training market.

While policy proponents and opponents continued their debates, academics also focused on the subject. John Powell concluded (1965) that the higher proportion of U.S. military assistance would only enhance the ability of better equipped and trained Latin American militaries to intervene in politics. Charles Wolf (1965) and Philippe Schmitter (1973) generally found little statistical evidence to support the thesis that U.S. military assistance was associated with higher frequencies of restrictive regimes. Wolf's admonition against easy assertions was echoed by Elizabeth Hyman (1972: 407–08): "Outside the Caribbean the evidence that foreign countries exerted lasting influence through assistance . . . is far less convincing. . . . The more weakly organized forces of Latin America remain as little able to provide a channel for foreign influence to form and to advance effectively and consistently their own corporate view. . . . The 'professional' forces . . . are by now generally rather resistant to influences from abroad." Critics like Miles Wolpin (1972) remained unconvinced, arguing that U.S. military assistance and training were designed to create dependence, to foment a pro-U.S. orientation, and to develop a hostility to revolution through an elaborate form of bribery.

The more useful academic literature on military assistance moves toward an institutional focus and away from being either pro or con with respect to U.S. policy issues or to the propensity by local militaries to intervene in domestic politics. Though largely descriptive, Etchison's *The United States and Militarism in Central America* gives significant attention to the relation of U.S. military assistance to the development of the Central American militaries. Jenkins and Sereseres conclude their 1977 study of Guatemala with the argument that the important impact of U.S. military assistance was in its contribution to the development of a "more consistent and institutionalized pattern of political behavior. . . . As a result, the political power once wielded by ambitious individual officers has been replaced by a politically more powerful military institution." (p. 588) These studies argue that U.S. military assistance is but one factor among many that have contributed to increased military involvement in politics. (Heller, 1978)

J. S. Fitch has proven to be one of the more productive and penetrating authors on the subject of the impact of U.S. military assistance. His "U.S. Military Aid to Latin America" (1979) captures the essence of the debate that had been raging since the 1960s and assumed such great importance in the years of President Carter's linkage of human rights performance to arms sales and assistance. (Fitch, 1984) Acknowledging the difficulty of acquiring hard data, Fitch reviews the arguments of the radicals and the proponents of aid and observes that "the attitudinal impact of U.S. training and assistance is limited but by no means inconsequential" (p. 369) and that the impact of MAP (i.e., the military assistance program) "is to increase the level of professionalization." (p. 72) This latter element becomes particularly important when the higher level of technical skills, managerial capability, and more broadly based training increase the military's "confidence in itself as an alternative source of national leadership." (p. 376) In his most significant conclusion, Fitch argues that "MAP thus facilitates an expansion of the military role in politics and the institutionalization of the coup d'état as an integral part of the political process" (p. 361), a finding that echoes, in part, those of Jenkins and Sereseres. Clearly, the debate has not ended, but resounds throughout the literature that has emerged around Central America.

External Defense and Latin American Militaries

The long period of quiescence in Latin American interstate conflict extending from the 1932 Chaco war to the 1982 Malvinas/Falklands conflict reaffirmed the academic orientation and bias toward the study of the "political role" of Latin American militaries. Little attention was paid to continued strains between states, and hence to the orientation of the militaries to the external defense role. While many U.S. traditionalists viewed the regional militaries as performing no useful function and argued for their drastic reduction or even abolition, other scholars explained Latin American militaries as useful appendages to U.S. hemispheric or global policy, arguing that they played an essential role in stabilizing the area, turning back revolutionary challenges and, most important, that they allowed the United States to concentrate more of its resources on other, less secure, fronts.

The assumption of the "appendage" scholars became particularly important in regard to U.S. involvement in Vietnam. Policy critics argued that Vietnam contributed further to a "blindness" developed in the Cold War era to regime types. In their view, the United States helped to professionalize the military, but also helped to inculcate an ideology that made the identification of internal enemies as part of the "global struggle" against communism easier. U.S. hubris, confidence in the deterrent posed by its geographic proximity, the demands of other involvements, and détente (relaxation of tensions between the two superpowers) led to a period of relative U.S. neglect of Latin America in the late 1960s and into the 1970s. This coincided with a growing Latin resistance, sometimes radical, to U.S. programs and "interference." Arms sales were the primary U.S. connection, yet they were subject to the vagaries of U.S. domestic politics and changing policies in different administrations, leaving the United States, in the Latin view, an unreliable supplier. U.S. attention was redirected toward the region, however, by the dramatic events in Nicaragua. The U.S. found itself confronted with aggressive arms sales competitors and with many militaries of the region at least rhetorically committed to a more independent role, a position reinforced later by impressions of what appeared to be a pro-British (anti-Argentine) U.S. policy in the Malvinas/Falklands conflict. Although arms sales predominance may have been lost, the United States nevertheless retained a strong political influence in the region. (Varas, 1985: 44).

In analyzing national security concerns, many Latin American militaries, but particularly those of Argentina, Brazil, Chile, and Peru, have turned to a rich heritage in geopolitics. (Child, 1979) Geopolitical orientation is less prevalent in Central America and, as Child comments, has usually been condemned in Mexico. As defined by Child (1985), the term implies a mix of "classical and power politics approaches and is linked to national security doctrine and to the Latin American military's sometimes strongly felt need to justify its existence by making a contribution to national development plans and strategies." (p. 20) In this context, the geopolitical analyst considers the state to be an organic whole, with a heart, peripheral elements, borders, and communications system. The state includes the relations between the society, its territorial wealth and resources, and its place in the international environment. (Varas, 1985:16). Geopolitics is not just a military art, it is to be practiced and used to guide the development and progress of the state. It is understood that the needs of one state place it in conflict with others in competition for position and dominance, a fact reflected in the thinking of Chilean Augusto Pinochet, in his *Geopolítico*. A state derives its power from the ability effectively to manage and exploit its own territory and capacity in pursuit of its national goals. Military power and internal order are key elements of this capacity.

Geopolitical implications for Latin American defense policies are numerous. Neighbors will be seen to be in competition for control of vital sea or land areas, resources are to be coveted, and the state that is internally incomplete or weak will be perceived to be vulnerable to enemy encroachment. In Brazil, geopoliticians have argued for opening the frontier, settling and developing it to remove any temptation to outsiders and to strengthen security. (Kelly, 1874) Geopolitical thought of the ABC countries (Argentina, Brazil, and Chile) has also emphasized the importance of maintaining access to the sea and protecting vital sea lanes, particularly the choke points at which they are most vulnerable. In this context, the Antarctic and South Atlantic are of particular importance, as is the Caribbean Basin for the northern states. (Morris, 1986)

Key to the geopolitical approach is the effort to maintain a favorable balance of power while searching for the greatest status for one's own country. As has been clearly indicated in the Argentine journal *Estratégia*, this may place one Latin state in direct conflict with another; hence, Argentina's consuming concern with Brazil and Brazilian expansion, both in the region and in the world. (Child, 1979: 96) Thus, as Jack Child indicates in his 1985 study: "Conflict may arise over territory, border, resources, ideology, influence and migration and many now perceived as less important may become vital." In this context, a specific area of concern for Argentina and Brazil is their nuclear competition.

Of significant concern to geopolitical thinkers is the status of relations with the United States. As a global power, the United States is seen as inevitably drawn to securing its own vital interests, lines of communication, resources, and alliances. In its quest for allies to help realize U.S. geopolitical objectives, the United States selects key regional actors and partners. Latins see themselves as sharing a common strategic interest in strengthening the region and securing it from extra-hemispheric threats. Many geopolitical writings recognize the importance of Latin America to the United States and to the global balance, and hence attribute a greater significance to regional state capabilities or the lack thereof. Yet they also recognize that Latin America is part of the Third World and, as a consequence, may be in conflict with the developed North over issues of economic injustice and dependency that have an impact on the global status and strength of states in the region. A part of both the Third and, because of inter-American ties, the First worlds, Latin America is seen as the "bridge" between the worlds.

As Child notes in his *Geopolitics in South America*, relations with the United States, while a major preoccupation, have not always been viewed favorably. The inter-American alliance has suffered both the weathering of neglect and the blows of direct policy assault—a reference to the Carter administration and congressionally mandated limitations on arms sales and training. While many railed against what they saw as U.S. fickleness, others flatly rejected the conditional assistance. Though primarily felt by Argentina, the U.S. position on the Malvinas/Falklands conflict led many Latin American states and militaries to question U.S. reliability and the significance of the alliance. Child quotes a Latin American military officer: "The U.S. was going to achieve what the liberator Simon Bolivar had not been able to—the unification of Latin America" against the United States. (p. 10) Long resented, U.S. dominance became even more chaffing. While the United States has continued to play a dominant external role, there also has appeared to be a greater sense of independence among the Latin American states.

Many Latin analysts argue, however, that the United States will work to preserve its geopolitical margins, engaging in regional alliances and continuing to subordinate Latin America to its strategic requirements. While reflecting strategic necessity for the United States, these alliances have an equally significant impact on the regional balance. Argentina has been particularly concerned with U.S.–Brazilian relations and with the impact this has on the balance between the two "major actors" of the Southern cone. Argentines like Guglianelli frequently condemn Brazil's relations with the United States as an extension of the arm of imperialism, and have called on Brazil to back away if it desires a more favorable balance. (Caviedes, 1984) From a Brazilian perspective, Argentina has been seen as politically unstable, haughty, undisciplined, organizationally weak, and headstrong. In part, Argentine concern with these characteristics has given rise to a fixation on the apparently boundless, successful, expansive power to the north. (Selcher, 1985) Though Selcher makes a strong case that it has been toned down in the wake of the return of civilian governments, this deeply embedded "zero-sum" geopolitical thinking persists. Other states like Uruguay, caught in the giants' shadows, strive to assert their separate identities.

Geopolitical thought is also consistent with a strong political role for the military. Extreme emphasis is placed on the efficiency and solidarity of the state in turning domestic resources to external strength. Internal vulnerabilities are to be closed off lest they be temptations to neighboring competitors. Thus, Brazilian authors have repeatedly emphasized the necessity of settling and exploiting the Amazon and of achieving greater economic development to enhance the strength of Brazil. Ultimately, security demands the efficient functioning of the state as an organic whole, and the internal "health" of the organism cannot be allowed to fail. In this brand of geopolitical thinking, the healthy organism is characterized by discipline and an elevation and strengthening of the people and territory toward the unified goal of state security.

Discipline and development become the tonic for the state that has not reached its full power potential. Defense against aggression includes maintaining capabilities against both external and internal enemies, and the state must constantly be attuned to dangers that would sap its capabilities. As Child points out, a combination of the U.S.-modeled national security focus with the geopolitical orientation of many Latin militaries has resulted in a security concept extending far beyond internal defense and development concerns. (Child, 1979: 67)

The national security doctrine developed in Brazil's senior level war college was to be applied by the state military and security apparatus. Education, elimination, or control of internal enemies and a disciplined, controlled, primarily growth-oriented development combined to yield the regime O'Donnell defined as bureaucratic authoritarian. (Varas, 1985: 20–23 and Child, 1985: 70–72) The military inevitably became involved on all four of the major fronts: defense, and internal, international, and economic affairs. In turn, national security became the legitimizing ideology.

It is important to note that not all geopolitical analyses have such a bellicose tone or impact. In *Geosur*, Quagliolli de Bellis of Uruguay has long advocated the geopolitical integration of the region—a pooling of resources and efforts to enhance the status of the whole area. Child also points to the positive effects of geopolitics in terms of its advocacy of national utilization of resources, planned development, opening up of remote areas, and an orientation to reexamine national goals and interests. (Child, 1985: 173) Though *Geosur's* integrationist aspirations have found echoes of support from time to time, the competitive aspect of state relations remains the dominant theme and may yet give rise to conflict.

It is the question of potential conflict that occupies Selcher in "Brazilian-Argentine Relations in the 1980's." In a well-written, persuasive article, Selcher traces a decline in geopolitical policy dominance in Argentine-Brazilian relations dating to 1976. It is his argument that mutual confidence has been developed, supplemented by institutional mechanisms that have moderated traditional suspicions. Selcher sees these developments as promising, though incipient, and cites as examples the resolution of the Itaipu Dam controversy, Brazil's support of Argentina during the Malvinas/Falklands conflict, and Brazil's present concern to couch its Amazonian development in unthreatening terms. Equally, resolution of the Beagle Channel issue has also somewhat relieved Argentina's anxiety regarding Chile. Whether the new problem solving exchanges that Selcher details will overcome the long-standing influence of geopolitical analysis remains to be seen, but Selcher is optimistic.

Present Directions

Through nearly three decades the literature on Latin American militaries has taken many turns. Nevertheless, many of the questions posed in the 1950s remain the focus of today's literature. Chester Brown (1983) raises the question of the justification of military spending and the nature of the external threat. Henry A. Dietz and Karl Schmidt (1984) provide a rebuttal to Brown, offering a careful analysis of the realities of arms spending and the distinction between cost effectiveness and image that affects perspectives on "reasonable levels." Linda Reif (1984) grapples with the issue of why militaries oust civilians and the institutional factors, capabilities, and decision-making aspects of the process. Merilee S. Grindle (1987) examines the issue of defense spending and the nature of the regime and the influence of the military. Literature on demilitarization abounds and is represented by the works of O'Donnell, Schmitter, and Whitehead (1986) and Handy (1986).

Still, many areas remain under- or un-researched, and many of the items of Lowenthal's 1976 research agenda have not received attention. As Fitch notes in *Armies and Politics in Latin America* (1986: 39-41), case studies continue to dominate and the area of comparative analysis is woefully neglected. Though some effort has begun to compare regimes, more needs to be done to explain the "differences," to include explanations such as those attempted by Ronfeldt (1984) as to why the Mexican situation has not resulted in a military coup. Equally, more research could now be initiated to compare the military's behavior over time within the same country. Hilton ties directly into the research fo-

cus on military thought suggested in John Markoff and Silvio Baretta (1986).

In spite of the increased policy focus on Central America, the militaries of that region still have received little serious, academic attention. Steve Ropp's *Panamanian Politics: From Guarded Nation to National Guard* helps to fill a void on Panama, but other countries remain largely ignored. Data collection and field research are as problematic as they were when McAlister penned his ground-breaking review, and the drive to become more sophisticated and complete demands more accurate information by those who research in the region. The militaries of Latin America warrant much more attention from scholars. Unquestionably, policy could profit from a deeper, more informed academic base.

General Research

The quest for information on Latin American militaries should begin in any one of a number of excellent reference works. Perhaps the most useful of the general works are the *Hispanic American Periodicals Index* (HAPI) and the *Handbook of Latin American Studies*. HAPI provides easily accessed information on recent articles and research and has a useful section on journal addresses. A helpful addition is the separate HAPI *Thesaurus and Name Authority*. *The Handbook for Latin American Studies* is also a major source of information, covering not only periodical literature but also recent book publications. Though HAPI may be a bit easier to use, an initial review of both will provide an excellent start to research. *Indexed Journals: A Guide to Latin American Studies* and *A Bibliography of Latin American Bibliographies* are helpful for the researcher less certain of exactly what source of general information to use or the student in search of a bibliography or index for a specific subfield.

Current Military Literature, a recent and more specific index, offers some helpful coverage on Latin American militaries, but should not be relied on as the primary source of information. Of general works, the *International Political Science Abstracts* is excellent in its coverage of international materials and the *Public Affairs Information Service Bulletin* is also useful for finding works in English. Finally, one may consult the *Social Sciences Index* or any one of the other general reference works. Any of these will provide the student of Latin American militaries with a means of accessing information, though the work required and the rewards obtained are varied.

Specific Journals

Articles on Latin American militaries or defense policies are not limited to regional journals, but cross many disciplinary and research lines. The list that follows includes those journals that since 1960 frequently have carried articles on some major aspect of Latin American military studies or have been the focus for the exposition of the ideas that have shaped the literature in this important subfield.

ENGLISH-LANGUAGE JOURNALS

American Political Science Review; 1527 New Hampshire Avenue, NW; Washington, D.C. 20036

Armed Forces and Society; Seven Locks Press; P.O. Box 37; Cabin John, MD 20818

Canadian Journal of Latin American and Caribbean Studies; c/o Department of History, University of Toronto; Messessauga, Ontario L5L1C6 Canada

Canadian Journal of Political Science; University of Toronto Press; Journals Department; 5210 Dufferin Street; Downsview, Ontario M3H5T8 Canada

Caribbean Review; Florida International University; Miami, FL 33199

Comparative Political Studies; Sage Publications, Inc.; 275 S. Beverly Drive; Beverly Hills, CA 90212

Comparative Politics; 49 Sheridan Avenue; Albany, NY 12210

Current History; Current History, Inc.; 4225 Main Street; Philadelphia, PA 19127

Defense Latin America; Whitton Press, Ltd.; Park House Street; Maidenhead, Berkshire LS5 1QS, England

Government and Opposition; Houghton Street; Aldwych, London WL2 2AE, England

Hispanic American Historical Review; Duke University Press; P.O. Box 6697; College Station; Durham, NC 27708

InterAmerican Economic Affairs; P.O. Box 181; Washington, D.C. 20044

International Affairs (UK); Butterworth Publishers; 80 Montvale Avenue; Stoneham, MA 02180

Journal of Development Studies; 11 Gainsborough Road; London, E11 1RS England

Journal of Interamerican Studies and World Affairs; P.O. Box 248134; University of Miami; Coral Gables, FL 33124

Journal of Latin American Studies; Cambridge University Press; Cambridge, CB2 2RU England

Journal of Political and Military Sociology; Transaction Periodicals Consortium; Rutgers University; New Brunswick, NJ 08903

Latin American Perspectives; P.O. Box 5703; Riverside, CA 92517

Latin American Research Review; University of New Mexico; Albuquerque, NM 87131

North/South: Canadian Journal of Latin American Studies; Canadian Association of Latin American Studies; Tabaret Hall, Room 354; University of Ottawa; Ottawa, Ontario KIN-6N5 Canada

Orbis; Foreign Policy Research Institute; 3508 Market Street, Suite 350; Philadelphia, PA 19104

Parameters; U.S. Army War College; Carlisle Barracks, PA 17013

Political Science Quarterly; Academy of Political Sciences; 2852 Broadway; New York, NY 10025-7885

Political Studies; Butterworth Scientific, Ltd; P.O. Box 63; Westbury House, Bury Street; Guildford, GU2 5BH, England

Western Political Quarterly; University of Utah; 258 Orson Spencer Hall; Salt Lake City, UT 84112

World Politics; Princeton University Press; 3175 Princeton Pike; Lawrenceville, NJ 08648

Universities Field Staff International Reports; 620 Union Drive; Indianapolis, IN 46202 (formerly *American Universities*)

LATIN AMERICAN JOURNALS

Many of these are not readily available in the United States or are available only in limited numbers. They are difficult to acquire and maintain. The list that follows is focused primarily on military journals, but includes several political science journals that frequently carry articles on the military. This list does not include journals specifically or primarily technical in concern.

Argentina

Estratégia; Instituto Argentino de Estudios Estratégicos y de las Relaciones Internacionales; Alsena 500, 1087 Buenos Aires, RA; Guglialmelli's journal of geopolitics and strategy.

Estratégia Nacional; Cuadernos de Estratégia; Maipu 889, 2ndo A; 1068 Buenos Aires, RA; Focus on strategy and foreign policy issues.

Geopolítica; Instituto de Estudios Geopolíticos; Libertad 94, 6°L; Corrientes 194 1P; Buenos Aires, RA; Geopolitics, particularly Southern Cone.

Revista Argentina de Estudios Estratégicos; Viamonte 494, 3er Piso Of11; 1035 Buenos Aires, RA; Geopolitics, nuclear matters, Antarctic, Argentine foreign policy, domestic politics.

Revista Argentina de Estudios Internacionales; Centro de Estudios Internacionales Argentinos; Defensa 251-1°B; 1065 Buenos Aires, RA; International relations and law; geopolitics.

Revista de La Escuela de Defensa Nacional; Maipu 262; 1084 Capital Federal, RA; Military and political articles, strategy, balance of power, education and national defense, planning.

Revista de La Escuela de Guerra Naval; Av Libertador No 807; 11429 Buenos Aires, RA; Naval strategy, law of the sea, deterrence, planning.

Revista de La Escuela Superior de Guerra; Luis M. Campos 480; 1426 Buenos Aires, RA; Faculty of ESG on inter-American strategy, armaments. Includes a review of classics on strategy and considers government military relations.

Revista Militar; Círculo Militar; Santa Fé 750; Buenos Aires, RA; Short articles, some on theory, formerly *Revista de Círculo Militar*.

Bolivia

Revista de La Escuela Superior de Guerra; Editorial Carlos Canelas; Cochabamba, Bolivia; Military, general.

Brazil

A Defesa Nacional; Palacio Duque de Caxias; Praca Duque de Caxias 25; 10455 Rio de Janeiro, RJ, Brazil; Geopolitics, strategy, military and government, science and technology, economics.

Defesa Latina; Editora Aero Ltda; Av Joao Pedro Cardoso; 225 Sales 3E5; Sao Paulo, CEP 04355, Brazil; General military strategy, formerly *Brasil Defesa*.

Politica e Estrategia: Revista Trimestral de Política Internacional e Assuntos Militares; Centro de Estudos Estratégicos; Alameda Eduardo Prado; 705-01218-Sao Paulo, Brazil; Military and government, military rule and power, internal and external defense articles from the United States.

Relacoes Internacionais; Asa Norte 70.910; Brasilia, D. F. Brazil; International politics, foreign relations, political theory.

Revista Brasileira Estudos Políticos; Universidade de Minas Gerais; Belo Horizonte, CP 1.301, Minas Gerais Brazil; General political science, political history, constitutional issues.

Revista da Escola Superior de Guerra; Divisao de Documentacao; Rua da Silva, #14; Beneficia CEP 10911; Rio de Janeiro, Brazil; Strategy, broad military subjects, technology, development.

Revista de Ciencia Política; Praia de Botafogo, 190 Sala 1.113; Caixa Postal 9.052-20.000; Rio de Janeiro, Brazil; Occasional articles on military and security matters.

Revista do Clube Militar; Clube Militar; Av Rio Branco 2519; Rio de Janeiro, CEP 20040, Brazil; Broad military subjects, economic development, cultural and institutional concerns.

Revista Do Exercito Brasileiro; Palacio Duque de Caxias; Praca Duque de Caxias; No 25, CEP 20455, Rio de Janeiro, Brazil; Professional focus and institutional news, sections on doctrine and officer education. Formerly *Revista Militar Brasileira*.

Revista Maritima Brasileira; Ministerio de Marinha; Servicio de Documentacao; Geral da Marinha; Rua Dom Manuel 15, Centro 20010; Rio de Janeiro, RJ, Brazil; Naval strategy and history, general military and security, science and technology and international reprints. Note: there is also another *Revista Maritime Brasileira*, published by the Escola de Guerra Naval, Ave Pasteur No 480, Praia Vermelha, Rio de Janeiro CEP 22.290, Brazil.

Seguranca e Desenvolvimento: Revista da Associacao Dos Diplomaclos da Escola Superior de Guerra; Edificio do Ministerio da Fazenda; Av Presidente Antonio Carlos 375; Groupas 1201, 02, 03, 05; Rio de Janeiro, RJ, Brazil; Geopolitics, political, military, with internal focus too.

Chile

Estudios Internacionales: Revista del Instituto de Estudios Internacionales de la Universidad de Chile; Avenida Condell 249; Casella 1487, Sur 21; Santiago, 9, Chile; International relations, debt, general foreign poicy, with articles on national and regional security and integration.

Memorial Del Ejército de Chile; Estado Mayor Ejército de Chile; Correro 21; Santiago, Chile; Historically focused, but has carried several articles on current topics, i.e., intelligence, human rights, and general military concerns.

Política y Geostratégia; Academia Nacional de Estudios Políticos y Estratégicos; Eliodoro Yanez 2760; Santiago, Chile; Geopolitics and strategy, general military, articles on Marxism.

Revista de Ciencia Política; Av Libertador Bernardo O'Higgins; 340, Of 14; Casella 114-D; Santiago, Chile; Occasional articles on military and security matters.

Revista de Marina; Armada de Chile; Correro Naval; Valparaiso, Chile; Shorter articles; historical but includes materials on geopolitics and hemispheric security along with international reprints.

Colombia

Revista de Las Fuerzas Armadas; Escuela Superior de Guerra; Fuerzas Militares de Colombia; Avenida 81, No 45a-40, 4403; Bogotá, D.E., Colombia; General military with some history, intelligence, economics focus.

Fuerzas Armadas; Oficina de Relaciones Públicas; Ministerio de Guerra; Bogotá, Colombia; more general, though with some articles on strategy/doctrine.

Ecuador

Revista Geográfica; Instituto Geográfico Militar; Departamento Geográfico; Quito, Ecuador.

Guatemala

Revista Militar; Centro de Estudios Militares (CEM); Lavanida Zona 17; Ciudad de Guatemala, Guatemala; National security, internal and external, development, revolutionary theory.

Honduras

Revista Centroamericano de Economía; Universidad Nacional Autónoma de Honduras; Tegucigalpa, Honduras; Occasional article on military/militarism.

Mexico

Estados Unidos: Perspectiva Latinoamericana; Centro de Investigación y Docencia Económica; Apartado Postal 41-553; México 10 DF; Occasional articles on military/U.S. military.

Foro Internacional; El Colegio de México; Camino al Ajusco 20; Pedregal de Sta Teresa, 10740; México, DF; Foreign affairs, transfers, U.S. and Soviet policy in Latin America, and international reprints.

Relaciones Internacionales; Facultad de Ciencias Políticas y Sociales; Universidad Nacional Autónoma de México; Apdo 70-266, 04510 México, DF, México; Occasional articles on military.

Revista Del Ejército; Secretaria de la Defensa Nacional; Estado Mayor del Ejército; Mexico City, Mexico; Military professionalism, doctrine, analysis, and history.

Revista Méxicana de Ciencias Políticas y Sociales; Facultad de Ciencias Políticas y Sociales; Instituto Matías Romero de Estudios Diplomáticos; Secretaria de Relaciones Exteriores; Mexico City, Mexico; Occasional articles on military matters.

Paraguay

Boletín Naval; Armada Nacional; Asunción, Paraguay; General naval.

Revista del Ejército y Armada; Centro Militar y Naval; Asunción, Paraguay; General military, doctrine.

Revista Paraguaya de Sociología; Eligio Ayala Número 973; Casella de Correro 2157; Asunción, Paraguay; Occasional articles on the military in Paraguay and area.

Peru

Defensa Nacional; Centro de Altos Estudios Militares (CAEM); Avenida Escuela Militar; SIN Chorrillos, Lima, Peru; Journal of the military theoreticians of Peru; focus is on internal/external defense, development, planning, military and government.

Estudios Geopolíticos y Estratégicos; Avenida Arequipa 310; Lima, 1, Peru; Geopolitics and strategy, Peru and region.

Revista de Marina del Peru; Escuela Naval de Peru; Callao, Peru; Naval history, strategy, and international reviews.

Revista Militar del Peru; Ministerio de Guerra; Avd Bolívar; Lima, Peru; Strategy, political-military, and professional.

Uruguay

Ejército República Oriental del Uruguay; Comando General del Ejército; Departmento de Relaciones Públicas del Estado Mayor de Ejército; Avd Garibaldi 2313; Montevideo, República Oriental del Uruguay; Military strategy and doctrine, geopolitics, development and international reprints.

Geopolítica; Instituto Uruguayo de Estudios Geopolíticos; Casilla de Correros 5039; Soriano 1585-10-6; Montevideo, Uruguay; Geopolitics with focus on the Southern Cone.

Geosur; Asociación Sudamericana de Estudios Geopolíticos y Internacionales; Casella de Correro 5006; Montevideo, Uruguay; Quagliotti de Bellis' journal. Geopolitical focus on "integrated" Latin America.

Revista Militar y Naval; Ministerio de Defensa Nacional; Montevideo, Uruguay; General military, institutional and professional news.

Venezuela

Gaceta Internacional; Apartado 62156; Caracas, 1060-A, Venezuela; Geopolitics, strategy, the inter-American system, foreign policy, relations with the United States.

Mundo Nuevo: Revista de Estudios Latinoamericanos; Apdo 172 71; Caracas, 1015-A, Venezuela; International relations, economics, occasional military subjects.

Revista del Ejército; Comandancia General del Ejército; Caracas, Venezuela; Strategy, history, economics, professional development, international reprints.

Revista de la Armada; Armada 1020-10068-06; Caracas, Venezuela; Geopolitics, strategy, politics, economics.

Revista de Las Fuerzas Armadas de Venezuela; Ministerio de la Defensa; El Ministerio; Caracas, Venezuela; Professional development strategy. Formerly *Fuerzas Armadas de Venezuela*.

Conclusions

Much of the literature of geopolitics develops the perspectives that militaries and nations have of themselves in terms of the international environment, power, capabilities, and threats, both external and internal. This must be supplemented by the literature on foreign policy and diplomacy to be considered complete. Both the geopolitical and the military assistance literatures consider the issues of linkages and interdependencies, with the latter having a decidedly evaluative tone.

Latin American defense writings abound with references to historical experience, and many of the evaluations of the military in politics are based on the persistence of certain forms of behavior within both military and civilian institutions. Though this review has not focused directly on capability studies, many of the works cited refer to military or academic views of the requirements for (and expenses, both political and economic, of) military capability. Certainly, the geopolitical analysts address the issues of capabilities as central to their competitive view of the world, encompassing domestic determinants as well as the key issues of unity, efficiency, and national effectiveness. Geopolitics informs military thinking about weapons and training needs for external defense. Finally, much of the case study literature is replete with analysis of the significance of factionalism—particulary as it applies to the decision to launch a coup or the problems of preserving unity once the military becomes governor.

Far less information is readily available on the intricacies of the defense decision-making process. Latin American militaries remain an elusive target for current research, and much of the field work is based on interviews with retirees or graduates of various military training programs in the United States. Though this remains an impediment, there is a useful literature base for analysis of the import of fragmentation, both civilian and military, and of the relative importance of various actors. The issues of hardware acquisition, armaments industries, military sufficiency, and logistics capabilities have been the focus of many recent articles, including introspective pieces by both Argentinians and Brazilians in the aftermath of the Malvinas/Falklands conflict. Many of the military journals of the region address themselves to the problems of sustaining and maintaining their forces.

Of all of the matters addressed in the organizing framework for the country studies printed in this volume, the issue of civil-military relations has received the greatest amount of attention from the U.S. academic community. Indeed, from Lieuwen to today, it has been the major fixation. Studies have been both objective and evaluative and have attempted to explain the persistent presence of the military in the politics of the region. It has been a rich field, and much remains to be done to explain both why militaries seize (or are invited to take) power or, conversely, avoid doing so.

Arms control has also been a matter of debate for some time. From the earliest U.S. arguments that there was no threat, and hence no need for arms, to the present-day examinations of arms races both in terms of acquisition and industrialization, the question of how much is enough has persisted. Too often, the literature has answered the question from a given scholar's personal perspective rather than in terms of the threats and requirements perceived by the militaries. Very useful studies have been conducted of relative return and civilian versus military spending, but much more remains to be done. Varas' *Militarization and the International Arms Race in Latin America* (1985) is an excellent summary and analysis of the status of these studies and of the problems of arms control in the region.

Little actual fighting has been required of Latin American militaries. Nevertheless, their study remains important. In this regard, recall Lowenthal's opening line in his 1976 *Armies and Politics in Latin America*: "The armed forces are central to what has happened in Latin American politics and are likely to remain so." (p. 3)

Notes

1. See Gary Wynia, *The Politics of Latin American Development* (London: Cambridge University Press, 1984), chap. 2.

2. Abraham F. Lowenthal, ed., *Armies and Politics in Latin America* (New York: Holmes & Meier, 1976), p. 3.

3. For one of the earlier efforts to develop a typology of the officer corps, see Victor Alba, *El militarismo: Ensayo sobre un fenómeno político-social* (Mexico City: Universidad Nacional Autónomo, 1959).

4. Morris Janowitz, *The Military in the Political Development of New Nations* (Chicago: University of Chicago Press, 1964).

5. Philip O'Brien and Paul Cammach, *Generals in Retreat: The Politics of Conformity in Latin America* (Oxford: Oxford University Press, 1985), p. 14.

Bibliography

Alba, Victor. *El militarismo: Ensayos sobre un fenómeno político-social*. Mexico City: Universidad Nacional Autónoma de México, 1959.

Arrigada Herrera, Genario. "National Security Doctrine in Latin America." *Peace and Change* 6, nos. 1–2 (1980): 49–60.

Astiz, Carlos. "The Argentine Armed Forces: Their Role and Political Involvement." *Western Political Quarterly* 22, no. 4 (1969): 862–78.

Barber, Willard F., and Ronning, C. Neale. *Internal Security and Military Power: Counterinsurgency and Civic Action in Latin America*. Columbus: Ohio State University, 1966.

Brown, Chester. "Latin American Arms: For What? The Experience of the Period 1971–1980." *Inter American Economic Affairs* 37, no. 1 (1983): 61–66.

Calvo, Roberto. "The Church and the Doctrine of National Security." *Journal of Interamerican Studies* 21, no. 1 (1979): 69–88.

Caviedes, Cesar. *The Southern Cone: Realities of the Authoritarian State in South America*. Totowa, N.J.: Rowman & Allanheld, 1984.

Center for Advanced International Studies, University of Miami. *The Political and Socio-Economic Role of the Military in Latin America*. Coral Gables, Fla: University of Miami Press, 1972.

Child, Jack. "Geopolitical Thinking in Latin America." *Latin American Research Review* 14, no. 2 (1979): 89–111.

———. *Geopolitics and Conflict in Latin America: Quarrels Among Neighbors*. New York: Praeger, 1985.

Clinton, Richard. "The Modernizing Military: The Case of Peru." *Inter American Economic Affairs*. 24, no. 4 (1971): 43–66.

Collier, David, ed. *The New Authoritarianism in Latin America*. Princeton: Princeton University Press, 1979.

Comblin, José. *The Church and the National Security State*. Maryknoll, N.Y.: Orbis Books, 1979.

Corbett, Charles D. *The Latin American Military as a Socio-Political Force*. Coral Gables, Fla: University of Miami, 1972.

Crahan, Margaret. *Human Rights and Basic Needs in the Americas*. Washington, D.C.: Georgetown University Press, 1982.

Dietz, Henry A., and Schmidt, Karl. "Militarization in Latin America: For What? and Why?" *Inter American Economic Affairs* 38, no. 1 (1984): 44–64.

Einaudi, Luigi. *The Peruvian Military: A Summary Political Analysis*. Santa Monica, Calif.: RAND Corporation, 1969.

Einaudi, Luigi, and Stepan, Alfred C. *Latin American Institutional Development: Changing Military Perspectives in Peru and Brazil*. Santa Monica, Calif.: RAND Corporation, 1971.

Etchison, Don. *The United States and Militarism in Central America*. New York: Praeger, 1975.

Finer, Samuel E. *The Man on Horseback: The Role of the Military in Politics*. London: Pall Mall Press, 1962.

Fitch, J. Samuel. "U.S. Military Aid to Latin America." *Armed Forces and Society* 5, no. 3 (1979): 360–86.

———. "Human Rights and the US Military Training Program: Alternatives for Latin America." *Human Rights Quarterly* 3, no. 4 (1984): 65–80.

Germani, Gino, and Silvert, Kalman. "Politics, Social Structure, and Military Intervention in Latin America." In *Armies and Politics in Latin America*, edited by Abraham F. Lowenthal. New York: Holmes & Meier, 1976.

Gilmore, Robert L. *Caudillismo and Militarism in Venezuela, 1810–1910*. Athens: Ohio University Press, 1964.

Glick, Edward. *The Feasibility of Arms Control and Disarmament in Latin America*. Santa Monica, Calif.: System Development Corporation, 1963.

———. *The Nonmilitary Use of the Latin American Military: A More Realistic Approach to Arms Control and Economic Development*. Santa Monica, Calif.: System Development Corporation, 1965.

Grindle, Merilee S. "Civil-Military Relations and Budgetary Politics in Latin America." *Armed Forces and Society* 13, no. 2 (1987): 255–75.

Handelmann, Howard, and Saunders, Thomas, eds. *Military Government and the Movement toward Democracy in South America*. Bloomington: Indiana University Press, 1981.

Handy, Jim. "Resurgent Democracy and the Guatemalan Military." *Journal of Latin American Studies* 18, no. 2 (1986): 383–408.

Hayes, Margaret Daly. "Policy Consequences of Military Participation in Politics: An Analysis of Trade-offs in Brazilian Federal Expenditures." In *Comparative Public Policy: Issues, Theories and Methods*, edited by Craig Liske et al. Beverly Hills, Calif.: Sage Publications, 1975.

Heller, Claude. "La asistencia militar norteamericana a America Latina: Una perspectiva política." *Estados Unidos: Perspectiva Latinoamericana* (Mexico) 4, no. 2 (1978): 136–68.

Hilton, Stanley. "The Brazilian Military: Changing Strategic Perceptions and the Question of Mission." *Armed Forces and Society* 13, no. 3 (1987): 329–51.

Hovey, Harold. *United States Military Assistance*. New York: Praeger, 1965.

Huntington, Samuel P. *The Soldier and State: The Theory and Politics of Civil-Military Relations*. Cambridge: Harvard University Press, 1959.

———. *Political Order in Changing Societies*. New Haven: Yale University Press, 1968.

Hyman, Elizabeth. "Soldiers in Politics: New Insights on Latin American Armed Forces." *Political Science Quarterly* 83, no. 3 (1972): 401–18.

Imaz, José. *Los que mandan*. Buenos Aires: Editorial Universitaria de Buenos Aires, 1964.

Janowitz, Morris. *The Military in the Political Development of New Nations*. Chicago: University of Chicago Press, 1964.

Jenkins, Brian, and Sereseres, Caesar. "U.S. Military Assistance and the Guatemalan Armed Forces." *Armed Forces and Society* 3, no. 4 (1977), 575–94.

Johnson, John J., ed. *The Role of the Military in Underdeveloped Countries*. Princeton: Princeton University Press, 1962.

———. *The Military and Society in Latin America*. Stanford: Stanford University Press, 1964.

Kelly, Philip L. "Geopolitical Themes in the Writings of General Carlos de Meira Mattos of Brazil." *Journal of Latin American Studies* 16, no.2 (1984): 439–61.

Lieuwen, Edwin. *Arms and Politics in Latin America*. New York: Praeger, 1961.

———. *Generals versus Presidents: Neomilitarism in Latin America*. London: Pall Mall Press, 1964.

———. *Mexican Militarism: The Political Rise and Fall of the Revolutionary Army, 1910–1940*. Albuquerque: University of New Mexico Press, 1968.

Linz, Juan, and Stepan, Alfred C., eds. *The Breakdown of Democratic Regimes*. Baltimore: Johns Hopkins University Press, 1978.

Loveman, Brian, and Davies, Thomas, eds. *The Politics of Antipolitics*. Lincoln: University of Nebraska Press, 1978.

Lowenthal, Abraham F., ed. *The Peruvian Experiment: Continuity and Change under Military Rule*. Princeton: Princeton University Press, 1975.

———, ed. *Armies and Politics in Latin America*. New York: Holmes & Meier, 1976.

Lowenthal, Abraham F., and Fitch, J. Samuel, eds. *Armies and Politics in Latin America*. New York: Holmes & Meier, 1986.

Markoff, John, and Duncan Baretta, Silvio. "What We Don't Know about Coups: Observations on Recent South American Politics." *Armed Forces and Society* 12, no. 2 (1986): 28–53.

McAlister, L. N. "Changing Concepts of the Role of the Military in Latin America." *Annals of the American Academy* 360 (July 1965): 85–98.

———. "Recent Research and Writings on the Role of the Military in Latin America." *Latin American Research Review* 2, no. 1 (1966): 5–37.

Middlebrook, Kevin, and Palmer, David. *Military Government and Political Development: Lessons from Peru*. Beverly Hills, Calif.: Sage Publications, 1975.

Miguens, José. "The New Latin American Military Coup." *Studies in Comparative International Development* 6, no. 1 (1970–71): 3–15.

Millett, Richard. *Guardians of the Dynasty*. Maryknoll, N.Y.: Orbis Books, 1977.

Morris, Michael. "Maritime Politics in Latin America." *Political Geography Quarterly* 5, no. 1 (1986): 43–55.

Needler, Martin. "Political Development and Military Intervention in Latin America." *American Political Science Review* 60, no. 3 (1966): 616–26.

———. "The Military Withdrawal from Power in South America." *Armed Forces and Society* 6, no. 4 (1980): 614–24.

———. "The Military and Politics in Latin America." *Journal of Interamerican Studies and World Affairs* 28, no. 3 (1986), 141–47.

North, Lisa. *Civil Military Relations in Argentina, Chile, and Peru*. Berkeley and Los Angeles: University of California Press, 1966.

Nun, José. "The Middle Class Coup." In *The Politics of Conformity in Latin America*, edited by Claudio Veliz, pp. 66–118. Oxford, Oxford University Press, 1967.

O'Brien, Philip, and Cammack, Paul. *Generals in Retreat: The Crisis of Military Rule in Latin America*. Dover, N.H.: Manchester University Press, 1985.

O'Donnell, Guillermo. *Modernization and Bureaucratic Authoritarianism: Studies in South American Politics*. Berkeley and Los Angeles: University of California Press, 1973.

———. "Reply to Remmer and Merkx." *Latin American Research Review* 17, no. 2 (1982): 41–50.

O'Donnell, Guillermo; Schmitter, Philippe; and Whitehead, Lawrence; eds. *Transitions from Authoritarian Rule*. Baltimore: Johns Hopkins University Press, 1986.

Philip, George. "The Military Institution Revisited: Some Notes on Corporatism and Military Rule in Latin America." *Journal of Latin American Studies* 12, no. 2 (1980): 421–36.

———. *The Military in South American Politics*. London: Croom Helm, 1985.

———. "Military Institutionalization and Political Engagement." In *The Political Dilemmas of Military Regimes*, edited by G. Philip and C. Clapman. Totowa, N.J.: Barnes & Noble, 1985.

Philip, George, and Clapman, C., eds. *The Political Dilemmas of Military Regimes*. Totowa, N.J.: Barnes & Noble, 1985.

Pike, Frederick, and Stritch, Thomas. *The New Corporatism: Social Political Structures in the Iberian World*. South Bend, Ind.: University of Notre Dame Press, 1974.

Pinochet, Augusto. *Geopolítico*. Santiago, Chile: Editorial Andres Bello, 1974.

Potash, Robert A. *The Army and Politics in Argentina, 1928–1945*. Stanford: Stanford University Press, 1969.

———. *The Army and Politics in Argentina, 1945–1962: Peron to Frondizi*. Stanford: Stanford University Press, 1980.

Powell, John. "Military Assistance and Militarism in Latin America." *Western Political Quarterly* 18 (June 1965): 382–93.

Putnam, Robert D. "Toward Explaining Military Intervention in Latin American Politics." *World Politics* 20, no. 1 (1967): 63–110.

Reif, Linda. "Seizing Control: Latin American Military Motives, Capabilities and Risks." *Armed Forces and Society* 10, no. 4 (1984): 563–582.

Remmer, Karen, and Merkx, Gilbert. "Bureaucratic Authoritarianism Revisited." *Latin American Research Review* 17, no. 2 (1982): 3–40.

Ronfeldt, David. *The Mexican Army and Political Order since 1940*. Santa Monica, Calif.: RAND Corporation, 1973.

Ronfeldt, David, et al. *The Modern Mexican Military: A Reassessment*. San Diego: Center for Mexican Studies, University of California, 1984.

Ropp, Steven. *Panamanian Politics: From Guarded Nation to National Guard*. Stanford: Hoover Institution Press, 1982.

Ruhl, J. Mark. "Social Mobilization, Military Tradition, and Current Patterns of Civil-Military Relations in Latin America." *Western Political Quarterly* 35, no. 4 (1982): 574–86.

Schmitter, Philippe C., ed. *Military Rule in Latin America: Function, Consequences, and Perspectives*. Beverly Hills, Calif.: Sage Publications, 1973.

———. "Still the Century of Corporatism." In *The New Corporatism: Social Political Structures in the Iberian World*. Edited by Frederick Pike and Thomas Stritch. South Bend, Ind.: University of Notre Dame Press, 1974.

Seckinger, Ron. "The Central American Militaries: A Survey of the Literature." *Latin American Research Review* 16, no. 2 (1981): 228–46.

Selcher, Wayne A. "Brazilian-Argentine Relations in the 1980s: From Wary Rivalry to Friendly Competition." *Journal of Interamerican Studies and World Affairs* 27, no. 2 (1985): 25–53.

Serra, José. "Three Mistaken Theses regarding the Connection between Industrialization and Authoritarian Regimes." In *The New Authoritarianism in Latin America*, edited by David Collier. Princeton: Princeton University Press, 1979.

Stepan, Alfred. *The Military in Politics: Changing Patterns in Brazil*. Princeton: Princeton University Press, 1971.

Szulc, Tad. *Twilight of the Tyrants*. New York: Holt, 1959.

Varas, Augusto. *Militarization and the International Arms Race in Latin America*. Boulder, Colo: Westview Press, 1985.

Veliz, Claudio. "Centralism and Nationalism in Latin America." *Foreign Affairs* 47, no. 1 (1968): 68–83.

Villanueva, Victor. *El CAEM: La revolución de la fuerza armada*. Lima: Instituto de Estudios Peruanos, 1972.

Welch, Claude E. *No Farewell to Arms? Military Disengagement from Politics in Africa and Latin America*. Boulder, Colo: Westview Press, 1987.

Wesson, Robert, ed. *New Military Politics in Latin America*. New York: Praeger, 1982.

———. *The Latin American Military Institution*. New York: Praeger, 1986.

Wiarda, Howard. "Toward a Framework for the Study of Political Change in the Iberic-Latin Tradition." *World Politics* 25, no. 2 (1973): 206–35.

Wolf, Charles. "The Political Effects of Military Programs: Some Indications for Latin America." *Orbis* 8 (Winter 1965): 871–93.

Wolpin, Miles. *Military Aid and Counterrevolution in the Third World*. Lexington, Mass: Lexington Books, 1972.

Wyckoff, Theodore. "The Role of the Military in Latin American Politics." *Western Political Quarterly* 13 (September 1960): 745–63.

Wynia, Gary. *The Politics of Latin American Development*. New York: Cambridge University Press, 1984.

Yokota, Marilyn B. *Bibliography on the 1982 Falklands War*. Santa Monica, Calif.: RAND Corporation, 1985.

Mexico

Harold Colson

Credit for the first important study of the military in modern Mexico goes to "The Mexican Army" by Virginia Prewett. Writing in the April 1941 issue of *Foreign Affairs*, Prewett adeptly portrayed an institution that had just emerged from three decades of revolutionary upheaval with a new set of organizational structures, institutional roles, political outlooks, and technical capabilities. Despite such an auspicious start, the literature on Mexican military affairs is only now beginning to mature, for very little pertinent research was published in the twenty years immediately following the end of World War II. Indeed, the second major English-language work on the Mexican military did not appear until 1958. Since the late 1960s, however, numerous researchers have begun to explore aspects of the changing politico-military situation in modern Mexico. Just as concerns about political stability and regional security informed much of the initial research, so have questions of domestic hardship and external turmoil helped generate the new cycle of interest regarding Mexican defense matters. Not surprisingly, therefore, the existing scholarship was recently enriched by the publication of *The Modern Mexican Military: A Reassessment*, edited by David Ronfeldt (San Diego: Center for U.S.–Mexican Studies, University of California, 1984). Born during a March 1984 research workshop attended by some thirty-four civilian and military investigators from the United States and Mexico, this anthology contains such articles as Edwin Lieuwen's "Depoliticization of the Mexican Revolutionary Army, 1915–1940," Stephen J. Wager's "Basic Characteristics of the Modern Mexican Military," Alden M. Cunningham's "Mexico's National Security in the 1980s–1990s," Edward J. Williams' "The Mexican Military and Foreign Policy: The Evolution of Influence," and Caesar Sereseres's "The Mexican Army Looks South." Although these and other recent studies have made significant contributions to our understanding of contemporary Mexican security affairs, many fundamental issues still remain unresolved. This essay is thus intended to help guide interested researchers to the leading primary and secondary sources for the study of the topic.

HISTORIES

All of the basic histories of the modern Mexican military are written in Spanish. The most scholarly work is Jorge Alberto Lozoya's *El ejército mexicano* (Mexico City: Colegio de México, 1984). First published in 1970, this vital study is now in its third edition. Lozoya combines a helpful account of key historical developments with a perceptive discussion of current institutional roles. The Secretaría de la Defensa Nacional published its own *El ejército méxicano* in 1979. Written by five high-ranking Mexican officers, this lavishly illustrated tome surveys the evolution of military power in Mexico from Aztec times to the contemporary era. Another introductory work is Gloria Fuentes, *El ejército méxicano* (Mexico City: Editorial Grijalbo, 1983). Medardo Cordova Torres examines the origins of the Mexican air force in *Historia de la iniciación de la fuerza aérea méxicana* (Mexico City: Secretaria de la Defensa Nacional, 1961–62). Several books deal with the military history of the Revolution of 1910, but no major studies probe the institutional development of the armed forces in the years since World War II. This gap is due in large part to the fact that the relevant military archives have long been closed to outside researchers. The Mexican services do publish valuable reports on numerous military topics, but these official works are usually difficult to locate in the United States.

CIVIL-MILITARY RELATIONS

The political role of the modern Mexican military has attracted a relatively large amount of scholarly attention. Ever since Edwin Lieuwen published his pioneering "Curbing Militarism in Mexico" in the *New Mexico Historical Review* (October 1958), a growing number of academic and professional investigators have sought to describe the evolving nature of civil-military relations in twentieth-century Mexico. Among the earliest major studies were Darrina D. Turner's "The Changing Political Role of the Mexican Army, 1934–1940" (M.A. thesis, University of Florida, 1960), Norman M. Smith's "The Role of the Armed Forces in Contemporary Mexican Politics" (M.A. thesis, University of Florida, 1966), and Franklin D. Margiotta's "The Mexican Military: A Case Study in Nonintervention" (M.A. thesis, Georgetown University, 1968). Lieuwen followed his initial article with *Mexican Militarism: The Political Rise and Fall of the Revolutionary Army, 1910–1940* (Albuquerque: University of New Mexico Press, 1968). Lyle N. McAlister's chapter on Mexico in *The Military in Latin American Sociopolitical Evolution: Four Case Studies* (Washington, D.C.: American University Center for Research in Social Systems, 1970) was written nearly two decades ago, but it is still cited by many researchers. Another important government-sponsored report was *The Political and Socio-Economic Role of the Military in Latin America* (Coral Gables, Fla.: Center for Advanced International Studies, University of Miami, 1972). Appendix 3 of this four-volume set contains a lengthy section on Mexico. Karl M. Schmitt's "The Role of the Military in Contemporary Mexico" appeared in *The Caribbean: Mexico Today*, edited by A. Curtis Wilgus (Gainesville: University of Florida Press, 1964). Other early articles included Frederick C. Turner, "Mexico: Las causas de la limitación militar," *Aportes*, no. 6 (October 1967) and Carlos A. Biebrich Torres, "Papel del ejército en la vida democrática," *Pensamiento Político* 8 (December 1971).

The factual and conceptual foundations for the study of civil-military relations in Mexico were established during the 1960s, but the field did not begin to peak until the following decade. First published in 1973, David Ronfeldt's *The Mexican Army and Political Order since 1940* (Santa Monica, Calif.: RAND Corporation) was revised and expanded in 1975. This highly influential work heralded a significant flurry of activity on the

political role of the modern Mexican military, for a number of other major studies of the topic were released around the same time. Margiotta updated his early research through a series of works that culminated with "Civilian Control and the Mexican Military: Changing Patterns of Political Influence," *Civilian Control of the Military: Theory and Cases from Developing Countries*, edited by Claude E. Welch, Jr. (Albany: State University of New York Press, 1976). Gordon C. Schloming's "Civil-Military Relations in Mexico, 1910–1940: A Case Study" (Ph.D. diss., Columbia University, 1974) helped place the Mexican experience in comparative historical and political perspective. Guillermo Boils provided the first comprehensive account of political activity by the Mexican armed forces with *Los militares y la política en México, 1915–1974* (Mexico City: Ediciones El Caballito, 1975), while Francisco Javier Aguilar Oceguera examined an important phase in the depoliticization process with a thesis titled "El papel de los militares en la etapa cardenista" (Universidad Nacional Autónoma de México, 1973). The late 1970s witnessed the appearance of such articles as Randall G. Hansis, "The Political Strategy of Military Reform: Alvaro Obregón and Revolutionary Mexico, 1920–1924," *The Americas* 36 (October 1979) and José Luis Piñeyro Piñeyro, "The Mexican Army and the State: Historical and Political Perspective," *Revue Internationale de Sociologie* 14 (April–August 1978). Alicia Hernández Chávez devoted a substantial part of *La mécanica cardenista* (Mexico City: Colegio de México, 1979) to a discussion of civil-military relations during the 1930s.

Although current studies of the Mexican armed forces tend to emphasize national security and force-modernization issues, a few notable works on civil-military relations have appeared in recent years. William S. Ackroyd's "Civil-Military Relations in Mexico: The Role of the Modern Mexican Military" (Ph.D. diss., University of Arizona, 1987) is the newest major study. Edward J. Williams surveys the contemporary scene in "The Evolution of the Mexican Military and Its Implications for Civil-Military Relations," *Mexico's Political Stability: The Next Five Years*, edited by Roderic A. Camp (Boulder, Colo.: Westview Press, 1986). Two intriguing Defense Intelligence Agency reports, *Civilian Control of the Mexican Military* (1984) and *Political Role and Attitudes of the Mexican Armed Forces* (1985), still carry security classifications. Piñeyro offers another noteworthy addition to the Mexican literature with *Ejército y sociedad en México: Pasado y presente* (Puebla: Universidad Autónoma de Puebla, 1985). Harold Colson identifies these and many other relevant secondary studies in "Military and Politics in Twentieth-Century Mexico: A Bibliography," *South Eastern Latin Americanist* 31 (1987).

NATIONAL SECURITY AND DEFENSE COOPERATION

A number of works provide basic information on contemporary Mexican security affairs. Adrian J. English's *Armed Forces of Latin America: Their Histories, Development, Present Strength and Military Potential* (London: Jane's, 1984) contains a helpful chapter on Mexico. Stephen J. Wager discusses the personnel systems, foreign influences, interservice relations, doctrinal orientations, and political activities of the Mexican armed forces in *The Latin American Military Institu-*

tion, edited by Robert Wesson (New York: Praeger, 1986). Phyllis Greene Walker offers an overview of current national defense matters in *Mexico: A Country Study*, edited by James D. Rudolph (Washington, D.C.: Government Printing Office, 1985). Command organization, force structure, and security policy are among the key topics covered by Walker. Vicente Ernesto Pérez Mendoza highlights civil functions in "The Role of the Armed Forces in the Mexican Economy in the 1980s" (M.S. thesis, Naval Postgraduate School, 1981). David Ronfeldt makes another important contribution with *The Modern Mexican Military: Implications for Mexico's Stability and Security* (Santa Monica, Calif.: RAND Corporation, 1985). A slightly reduced version of this report appears in *Armies and Politics in Latin America*, edited by Abraham Lowenthal and J. Samuel Fitch (New York: Holmes & Meier, 1986). General articles on Mexican national security affairs include Alden M. Cunningham, "Mexico's National Security," *Parameters* 14 (Winter 1984) and Olga Pellicer, "National Security in Mexico: Traditional Notions and New Preoccupations," in *U.S.-Mexico Relations: Economic and Social Aspects*, edited by Clark Reynolds and Carlos Tello (Stanford: Stanford University Press, 1983). Sergio Aguayo's "Mexican National Security and Central America" appears in *Contadora and the Diplomacy of Peace in Central America*, edited by Bruce M. Bagley (Boulder, Colo.: Westview Press, 1987). Thomas H. Moorer and Georges A. Fauriol devote a portion of *Caribbean Basin Security* (New York: Praeger, 1984) to a discussion of Mexican security issues. While attending the Army War College, Hugh Scruggs prepared an essay titled "National Security Policy: Mexico." Researchers may obtain this 1986 report from the National Technical Information Service.

Very few studies examine defense cooperation between Mexico and the United States. Donald F. Harrison treats one major episode in "United States-Mexican Military Collaboration during World War II" (Ph.D. diss., Georgetown University, 1976). More recent developments are featured in a thesis by José Luis Piñeyro Piñeyro titled "El profesional ejército méxico y la asistencia militar de Estados Unidos, 1965–1975" (Colegio de México, 1976). Boils, *Los militares y la política*, and Wager, "Basic Characteristics of the Modern Mexican Military," also provide some discussion of U.S. military influences.

FORCE MODERNIZATION

The recent campaign to upgrade and strengthen the Mexican armed forces has generated a growing body of literature. One standard account is Edward J. Williams, "Mexico's Modern Military: Implications for the Region," *Caribbean Review* 10 (Fall 1981). Otmar Kauck presents "Las fuerzas armadas de México ganan influencia y importancia" and "El nuevo ejército méxicano" in *Tecnología Militar* no. 2 (1981). Michael J. Dziedzic treats a specific aspect of the modernization effort in "The Essence of Decision in a Hegemonic Regime: The Case of Mexico's Acquisition of a Supersonic Fighter" (Ph.D. diss., University of Texas, 1986). Stephen J. Wager delivered "The Modernization of the Mexican Military and Its Significance for Mexico's Central American Policy" during the Military Policy Symposium on Mexico, the United States, and Central American Revolutionary Change held by the Army War

College in November 1982. A copy of this unpublished paper is retained at the Army War College Library. Mexican perspectives on the modernization program are reflected in Otto Granados Roldán, "Regreso a las armas," *Nexos*, no. 50 (February 1982) and Héctor Aguilar Camín, "Regreso a las armas," *Unomasuno*, 2 March 1981. Many other relevant articles have appeared in leading U.S. newspapers. Representative works include Christopher Dickey's "Modernization Could Lead Mexican Military into Politics," *Washington Post*, 23 September 1982, and Alan Riding's "Mexican Army, Parading Pride, Raises Concern," *New York Times*, 5 October 1980. *Status of the Mexican Ground Forces* (Washington, D.C.: Central Intelligence Agency, 1984) is a classified report on current force structure.

FOREIGN POLICY

Growing tensions in the Caribbean basin have helped reinvigorate the study of Mexican foreign policy. Two introductory works on regional diplomacy are Anthony T. Bryan's "Mexico and the Caribbean: New Ventures into the Region," *Caribbean Review* 10 (Summer 1981) and Thomas G. Sanders' *Mexican Policy in Central America* (Hanover, N.H.: Universities Field Staff International, 1982). Edward J. Williams offers such pertinent articles as "Mexico's Central American Policy: Apologies, Motivations, and Principles," *Bulletin of Latin American Research* 2 (October 1982) and "Mexico's Central American Policy: Revolutionary and Prudential Dimensions," in *Colossus Challenged: The Struggle for Caribbean Influence*, edited by H. Michael Erisman and John D. Martz (Boulder, Colo.: Westview Press, 1982). Williams deals more extensively with defense issues in "Mexico's Central American Policy: National Security Considerations," *Rift and Revolution: The Central American Imbroglio*, edited by Howard J. Wiarda (Washington, D.C.: American Enterprise Institute, 1984). Bruce M. Bagley followed "Mexico in the 1980s: A New Regional Power," *Current History* 80 (November 1981) with "Mexican Foreign Policy: The Decline of a Regional Power," *Current History* 82 (December 1983). Bagley has also produced "Mexico in Central America: The Limits of Regional Power," in *Political Change in Central America: Internal and External Dimensions*, edited by Wolf Grabendorff, Heinrich-W. Krumwiede, and Jorg Todt (Boulder, Colo.: Westview Press, 1984). *The Future of Central America: Policy Choices for the U.S. and Mexico*, edited by Richard R. Fagen and Olga Pellicer (Stanford: Stanford University Press, 1983) contains Pellicer's "Mexico in Central America: The Difficult Exercise of Regional Power," Mario Ojeda's "Mexican Policy toward Central America in the Context of U.S.-Mexico Relations," and Adolfo Aguilar Zinser's "Mexico and the Guatemala Crisis." Other articles on Mexican policy regarding Central America include René Herrera Zuñiga and Mario Ojeda, "Mexican Foreign Policy and Central America" in *Central America: International Dimensions of the Crisis*, edited by Richard E. Reinberg (New York: Holmes & Meier, 1982) and John F. McShane, "Emerging Regional Power: Mexico's Role in the Caribbean Basin" in *Latin American Foreign Policies: Global and Regional Dimensions*, edited by Elizabeth G. Ferris and Jennie K. Lincoln (Boulder, Colo.: Westview Press, 1981). Herrera and Ojeda provide a lengthier discussion of the topic with *La política de México hacia Centroamérica, 1979–1982* (Mexico City: Colegio de México, 1983). Ojeda has also edited *Las relaciones de México con los paises de América Central* (Mexico City: Colegio de México, 1985). Two general articles on contemporary Mexican diplomacy are Elizabeth G. Ferris, "Mexico's Foreign Policies: A Study in Contradictions" in *Dynamics of Latin American Foreign Policies: Challenges for the 1980s*, edited by Jennie K. Lincoln and Elizabeth G. Ferris (Boulder, Colo.: Westview Press, 1984), and Olga Pellicer, "Veinte años de política exterior méxicana, 1960–1980," *Foro Internacional* 21 (October–December 1980). Pellicer has also edited *La política exterior de México: desafíos en los ochenta* (Mexico City: Centro de Investigación y Docencia Económicas, 1983). Mario Ojeda's *Alcances y límites de la política exterior de México* (Mexico City: Colegio de México, 1976) remains a standard treatment of Mexican foreign relations in the years since World War II.

SOURCE MATERIALS

A variety of publications furnish ongoing coverage of Mexican defense affairs. The *Memorias* of the Secretaría de la Defensa Nacional and the Secretaría de Marina are key government ministry reports. National security issues also receive some attention in the annual *Informe de Gobierno* delivered by the Mexican president. Published by the Secretaría de la Defensa Nacional, the monthly *Revista del Ejército y Fuerza Aérea Méxicanos* is the official journal of the Mexican army and air force. The corresponding navy journal is the bimonthly *Revista* of the Secretaría de Marina. Good sources of current politico-military news are the daily newspaper *Excélsior* and the weekly magazine *Proceso*, both of which are published in Mexico City. The respected quarterly journal *Foro Internacional* (Mexico City: Colegio de México) frequently examines contemporary Mexican foreign policy issues. Scanning *Carta de Política Exterior Méxicana* (Mexico City: Centro de Investigación y Docencia Económicas), *Informe Relaciones México–Estados Unidos* (Mexico City: Editorial Nueva Imagen), *Relaciones Internacionales* (Mexico City: Universidad Nacional Autónoma de México), and *Revista Méxicana de Política Exterior* (Mexico City: Instituto Matías Romero de Estudios Diplomáticos, Secretaría de Relaciones Exteriores) will also yield relevant articles. *Defensa Latino Americana* (Redhill: Whitton Press), *International Defense Review* (Geneva: Interavia), *Jane's Defence Weekly* (London: Jane's), *Revista Aérea* (New York: Strato Publishing), and *Tecnología Militar* (McLean, Va.: Monch Publishing Group) occasionally discuss current developments in Mexican defense policy. Translations of selected Mexican media broadcasts and print resources are contained in *Daily Report: Latin America* (Washington, D.C.: Foreign Broadcast Information Service) and *Latin America Report* (Arlington, Va.: Joint Publications Research Service). Microfiche versions of FBIS and JPRS reports are available in many academic and research libraries across the United States.

English-language newspapers and newsletters occasionally deal with Mexican security affairs. The *New York Times*, *Washington Post*, and the *Miami Herald* are among the U.S. leaders in Mexican coverage. Important British sources include *Latin America Weekly Report* and *Latin America Regional Reports: Mexico & Central America*, both of which are published in London by Latin American Newsletters. One convenient tool for keeping up with international press coverage of Mexico and the rest of Latin America is *ISLA*, a monthly publication that reprints pertinent articles from nine major newpapers in the United States and Great Britain. *ISLA* is published in Oakland, California, by Information Services on Latin America.

Scholarly and professional journals from several countries have recently published articles on Mexican defense affairs. Works such as Štefica Deren-Antoljak's "Uloga armije u društveno-ekonomskon i političkom preobražaju Meksika," *Politička Misao* 16 (1979) and Volker G. Lehr's "Das mexikanische Militar: Ein lateinamerikanischer Sonderfall," *Verfassung und Recht in Übersee* 13 (1980) reflect the growing interest in the Mexican military. Unfortunately, many more years will pass before the study of Mexican national defense advances to the point that major articles on the subject frequently appear in a core set of leading international journals. Owing to the interdisciplinary nature of the topic, relevant contributions appear in military science periodicals as frequently as they do in political science works, a fact that complicates the bibliographic research process. Because the number of possible outlets for new studies is so large, investigators must consult a variety of indexing sources in order to be reasonably confident of identifying all recent articles. Among the most useful indexes are *Hispanic American Periodicals Index* (Los Angeles: UCLA Latin American Center), *PAIS Bulletin* (New York: Public Affairs Information Service), *PAIS Foreign Language Index* (New York: Public Affairs Information Service), *Historical Abstracts* (Santa Barbara, Calif.: ABC-Clio), *International Political Science Abstracts* (Paris: International Political Science Association), *Sociological Abstracts* (San Diego: Sociological Abstracts), *Air University Library Index to Military Periodicals* (Maxwell Air Force Base, Ala.: Air University Library), and *Current Military Literature* (Oxford: Military Press). *Información Sistemática* (Mexico City: Información Sistemática) provides access to Mexican newspaper literature.

Federal government technical reports constitute another important category of materials. Numerous war colleges, intelligence agencies, and research institutes regularly produce unclassified studies on foreign military forces and international defense affairs. Descriptions of available reports appear in *Government Reports Announcements & Index* (Springfield, Va.: National Technical Information Service) and *Monthly Catalog of United States Government Publications* (Washington, D.C.: Superintendent of Documents). Neither *GRA&I* nor *Monthly Catalog* lists classified studies, but the public catalogs of some federal research libraries do contain unclassified descriptions of many such works.

Two good annual compilations of data about the size and composition of the Mexican armed forces are *The Military Balance* (London: International Institute for Strategic Studies) and *Defense & Foreign Affairs Handbook* (Washington, D.C.: Perth Corporation). Federal researchers also have access to the classified *Ground Order of Battle: Mexico* published by the Defense Intelligence Agency.

Glossary

The glossary of terms that follows is an updated version of glossaries published in the first edition of *The Defense Policies of Nations* (1982) and the fourth edition of *American Defense Policy* (1977), edited by John E. Endicott and Roy W. Stafford, Jr.; both volumes were published by the Johns Hopkins University Press. The glossary is by no means intended as a comprehensive list of all terms and concepts relevant to the comparative study of defense policy. It is hoped, however, that it will be helpful to the general reader.

ABC WEAPONS: Atomic, biological, and chemical weapons. Procurement of any ABC weapons often stirs public controversy in democratic nations. The Geneva Protocol of 1925 prohibits the use of poison gas and bacteriological weapons in warfare.

ACCIDENTAL ATTACK: An unintended attack that occurs without deliberate national design as a direct result of a random event, such as a mechanical failure, a simple human error, or an unauthorized action by a subordinate.

ACTIVE AIR DEFENSE: Direct defensive action taken to destroy attacking enemy aircraft or missiles, or to nullify or reduce the effectiveness of such attack. It includes such measures as the use of aircraft, interceptor missiles, air defense artillery, nonair defense weapons in an air defense role, and electronic countermeasures.

ACTIVE DEFENSE: The employment of limited offensive action and counterattacks to deny a contested area or position to the enemy. See also Passive Defense.

AEROSPACE: Of, or pertaining to, the earth's envelope of atmosphere and the space above it; two separate entities considered as a single realm for activity in launching, guidance, and control of vehicles that will travel in both entities.

AFRIKANERS: South Africa's dominant "white tribe," largely of German, Huguenot French, and Dutch descent.

AIRBORNE COMMAND POST: A suitably equipped aircraft used by the commander for the control of his forces.

AIRBORNE EARLY WARNING: The detection of enemy air or surface units by radar or other equipment carried in an airborne vehicle and the transmission of a warning to friendly units.

AIR-BREATHING MISSILE: A missile with an engine requiring the intake of air for combustion of its fuel, as in a ramjet or turbojet. To be contrasted with the rocket missile, which carries its own oxidizer and can operate beyond the atmosphere. See also Cruise Missile.

AIR DEFENSE FORCES OF THE USSR (PVO STRANY): One of five independent arms of the Soviet military services, the Air Defense Forces have historically received funding sufficient to deploy air defenses greater than those of any Western country. The forces include surface-to-air missiles (SAMs), antiballistic missiles (ABMs), and jet interceptors.

AIR-LAUNCHED CRUISE MISSILE (ALCM): A cruise missile launched from an aircraft. The long-range (1,000–2,000 miles) U.S. ALCM can be loaded internally or externally on the B-1. The Hound Dog, a turbojet-propelled missile designed to be equipped with a nuclear warhead and carried externally on the B-52, is an example of a mid-range cruise missile. The Kangaroo is a Soviet ALCM. See also Sea-launched Cruise Missile.

AIRMOBILE FORCES OPERATION: Ground combat units using assigned and/or attached fixed and rotary-wing aircraft under their control to maneuver rapidly within given areas of operation; the employment of such forces in combat.

AIR STRIKE: An attack on specific objectives by fighter, bomber, or attack aircraft on an offensive or defensive mission. May consist of several air organizations under a single command in the air.

AIR SUPERIORITY: Dominance in the air to a degree that permits friendly land, sea, and air forces to operate at specific times and places without prohibitive interference by enemy air forces.

AIR-TO-AIR MISSILE: A missile launched from an airborne carrier at an airborne target.

AIR-TO-SURFACE MISSILE: A missile launched from an airborne carrier at a surface target.

ALLIANCE: A coalition of states pursuing security or other goals.

ANTIBALLISTIC MISSILE (ABM): A defensive missile designed to intercept and destroy a strategic offensive ballistic missile or its payload. This term is used interchangeably with "ballistic missile defense interceptor missile." See also Interceptor Missile.

ANTIBALLISTIC MISSILE (ABM) SYSTEM: A system to counter strategic ballistic missiles or their elements in flight trajectory, currently consisting of: (1) ABM interceptor missiles, which are interceptor missiles constructed and deployed for an ABM role, or of a type tested in an ABM mode; (2) ABM launchers, which are launchers constructed for launching ABM interceptor missiles; and (3) ABM radars, which are designed and deployed for an ABM role, or of a type tested in an ABM mode.

ANTISUBMARINE WARFARE (ASW): All measures to reduce or nullify the effectiveness of hostile submarines; specifically concerns operations to detect, locate, track, and destroy submarines used for strategic nuclear and conventional purposes.

ANZUS TREATY: A security treaty concluded in 1951 among Australia, New Zealand, and the United States. The treaty declared that an attack upon any of the members would constitute a common danger and that each would respond to it according to its constitutional processes.

ARMS CONTROL: A concept that refers to (1) any plan, arrangement, or process, resting upon explicit or implicit international agreement, governing any aspect of the following: the numbers, types, and performance characteristics of weapons systems (including the command and control, logistics support arrangements, and any related intelligence-gathering mechanisms); the numerical strength, organization, equipment, deployment, or employment of the armed forces retained by the parties (it encompasses "disarmament"); (2) on some occasions, those measures taken for the purpose of reducing instability in the military environment. See also Arms Limitation; Disarmament; General and Complete Disarmament; Strategic Arms Limitation Talks (SALT); Strategic Arms Reduction Talks (START).

ARMS CONTROL AND DISARMAMENT AGENCY (ACDA): This U.S. agency was created in 1961. The director of ACDA is the president and the secretary of state on arms control and disarmament matters, and, under the direction of the secretary of state, has primary responsibility within the government for such matters. He is responsible for the executive direction and coordination of all activities of the agency and its relations with other government agencies and the Congress.

ARMS LIMITATION: An agreement to restrict quantitative holdings of, or qualitative improvements in, specific armaments or weapons systems. See also Arms Control; Disarmament; Strategic Arms Limitation Talks.

ARMS RACE: Competition between two or more countries or coalitions of countries that results in the cumulative proliferation or accretion of weapons; an increase in the destructive power of weapons possessed by those parties; and/or the buildup of their armed forces, incited by convictions that national security objectives demand quantitative superiority, qualitative superiority, or both.

ARMS STABILITY: A strategic force relation in which neither side perceives the necessity for undertaking major new arms programs in order to avoid being placed at a disadvantage. See also Strategic Stability.

ARMY CORPS: A tactical unit larger than a division and smaller than a field army. A corps usually consists of two or more divisions, together with auxiliary arms and services. See also Field Army.

ASEAN: Association of South East Asian Nations.

ASSURED DESTRUCTION CAPABILITY: A highly reliable ability to inflict unacceptable damage on any aggressor or combination of aggressors at any time during the course of a nuclear exchange, even after absorbing a surprise first strike. See also First Strike; Mutual Assured Destruction; Unacceptable Damage.

ATB: Advanced Technology Bomber; a bomber that has a greatly reduced radar signature providing an enhanced penetration capability against projected enemy air defenses.

ATTACK CARRIER: An aircraft carrier designed to accommodate high-performance fighter/attack aircraft whose primary purpose is to project offensive striking power against targets ashore and afloat.

ATTACK SUBMARINE: A submarine designed primarily to destroy enemy merchant shipping and naval vessels, including other submarines. See also Submarine.

B-1 BOMBER: Built by Rockwell International, this swing-wing, supersonic, U.S. strategic bomber can deliver conventional or nuclear ordnance at low altitudes and high speeds. Its Terrain Following Radar (TFR) allows the plane to fly at altitudes lower than could normally be flown, which enables it to evade detection until the last possible moment. It has a very small radar cross-section or "signature," which also helps avoid detection. It is an interim bomber to replace the Boeing B-52 while waiting for development of the Advanced Technology Bomber (ATB). See also Advanced Technology Bomber (ATB).

BALANCE OF POWER: A system of power alignments in which peace and security may be maintained through an equilibrium of power between (or among) rival powers or blocs. In this condition, states enter into alliances with friendly states to protect or enhance their power positions. Critics argue that the balance of power may lead as easily to war as to peace, citing World Wars I and II as examples.

BALANCE OF TERROR: A term describing a state of unstable equilibrium or of mutual deterrence between nuclear powers based not on the balance of power (the whole spectrum of power) between them, but on their possession of weapons that allow either side to deal a mortal blow to the other even while it is absorbing a mortal blow from the other.

BALLISTIC MISSILE: Any missile that does not rely upon aerodynamic surfaces to produce lift and consequently follows a ballistic trajectory (i.e., that resulting when a body is acted upon only by gravity and aerodynamic drag) when thrust is terminated. See also Intercontinental Ballistic Missile (ICBM).

BALLISTIC MISSILE DEFENSE (BMD) SYSTEM: A system designed to destroy offensive strategic ballistic missiles or their warheads before they reach their targets. See also Antiballistic Missile (ABM) System.

BALLISTIC MISSILE EARLY WARNING SYSTEM (BMEWS): An electronic system for providing detection and early warning of attack by enemy ICBMs.

BARGAINING CHIP: Any military force, weapons system, or other resource, present or projected, that a country expresses willingness to downgrade or discard in return for concessions by a particular rival.

BIOLOGICAL OPERATIONS (WARFARE): Employment of biological agents to produce casualties in man or animals and damage to plants or matériel; or defense against such employment. See also CBR Weapons; Defoliant Operations.

BIPOLAR: A world power distribution or structure as may be characterized in the present period by the predominance of the United States and the USSR.

BLUE WATER: Oceangoing; high seas naval capability beyond a nation's immediate coastal area.

BOMBERS: Military aircraft designed to deliver nuclear or non-nuclear weapons against targets on the ground. Generally, bombers such as the Soviet Bison, Bear, and Blackjack and the U.S. B-52 and B-1 have been considered heavy bombers; Soviet Badgers and Blinders and the U.S. FB-111 have been considered medium bombers; and Soviet Beagles have been considered light bombers. See also Long-Range Bomber Aircraft; Medium Bomber.

BOERS: See Afrikaners; the name derives from the Afrikaans word for farmer, *boer* (plural *boere*), and came to be applied to those original white inhabitants of the Cape who trekked into the interior in the 1830s to escape British rule, ultimately founding the Transvaal and Orange Free State republics.

BRD: Federal Republic of Germany; see FRG; BRD is the abbreviation in German: *Bundesrepublik Deutschland*; West Germany

BREZHNEV DOCTRINE: The Soviet policy of maintaining friendly communist regimes in power in neighboring states, using force when necessary. The invasions of Czechoslovakia in 1968 and Afghanistan in 1979 demonstrated the doctrine in action.

BRIGADE: A unit, often part of a division, to which are attached groups and/or battalions and smaller units tailored to meet anticipated requirements. See also Division.

BRINKMANSHIP: Conduct in a crisis intended to prevail over an adversary by showing greater willingness to approach the brink of disaster. The term is attributed to Thomas C. Schelling in his book *Strategy of Conflict* (New York: Oxford University Press, 1963), p. 200.

BRUSHFIRE WAR: A local war that can flare up suddenly and either subside prior to great power intervention or escalate to greater magnitude.

BUNDESWEHR: West German armed forces.

BURDEN SHARING: See Cost Sharing.

BUS: The part of a MIRVed missile's payload that carries the reentry vehicles (RVs) and has a guidance package, fuel, and thrust devices for modifying the ballistic flight path so that the RVs can be dispensed sequentially toward different targets. See also Multiple Independently Targetable Reentry Vehicles (MIRV); Reentry Vehicles (RV).

CAPABILITY: The potential for executing a specified course of action. A capability may or may not be accompanied by an intention to carry out a particular course of action. Capabilities are conditioned by many variables, including the balance of military forces, time, space, terrain, and weather.

CAPITALIST ENCIRCLEMENT: A Soviet term referring to the ring of capitalist nations surrounding the USSR that, in the Soviet view, pose a security problem.

CARTER DOCTRINE: Usually refers to a commitment by President Carter to use force, if necessary, to assure continuation of the flow of oil from the Persian Gulf.

CATALYTIC ATTACK: An attack designed to bring about a war between major powers through the disguised machinations of a third power.

CBM: Confidence Building Measures. See also CSBM. Notification of troop movements, mutual observation of military exercises, and related activities designed to improve the degree of trust and confidence between adversaries.

CBR (CHEMICAL, BIOLOGICAL, AND RADIOLOGICAL OPERATIONS): A collective term used to refer to chemical, biological, and radiological operations. See also NBC.

CBR WEAPON: Abbreviated term for chemical, biological, and radiological agents of warfare. Also referred to as "special weapons." See also Biological Operations.

CDE: Conference on Disarmament in Europe, a part of the CSCE process.

CDU: Christian Democratic Union, a political party in West Germany generally considered to be right of center or center-right on the West German political spectrum.

CENTRAL STRATEGIC FORCES: Term usually refers to U.S. and Soviet ICBMs, SLBMs, and long-range bombers or cruise missile carriers.

CIRCULAR ERROR PROBABLE (CEP): A measure of weapons system accuracy used as a factor in determining probable damage to targets. CEP is defined as the radius of a circle within which a warhead has a 0.5 probability of falling.

CIVIL DEFENSE: Passive measures designed to minimize the effects of enemy action on all aspects of civilian life, particularly to protect the population base. This includes emergency steps to repair or restore vital utilities and facilities. See also Passive Defense.

CIVIL RESERVE AIR FLEET (CRAF): U.S. commercial aircraft and crews allocated in an emergency for exclusive military use in international and domestic service.

CLOSE-AIR SUPPORT: Air strikes against targets near enough to ground combat units that detailed coordination between participating air and ground elements is required.

CMEA: See Council for Mutual Economic Assistance.

COLD LAUNCH: The technique of ejecting a missile from a silo before full ignition of the main engine, sometimes called "pop-up." All current U.S. submarine-launched ballistic missiles (SLBMs) are ejected in this manner. The Soviet Union has recently been testing intercontinental ballistic missile (ICBM) launches using the cold-launch technique. Since full ignition of the main engine occurs only after the missile has cleared the silo, the requirement for extensive shielding of the missile in the silo at launch from its own exhaust gases is reduced, thus making it possible for the silo to accommodate a larger missile. Moreover, the cold-launch technique leaves the missile silo essentially undamaged and available for reloading. The 1972 Interim Agreement, an outcome of the Strategic Arms Limitation Talks (SALT), did not restrict the number of missiles each site could have but did restrict the number of launchers. See also Rapid Reload Capacity; Sea/Submarine Launched Ballistic Missiles; Strategic Arms Limitation Talks.

COLD WAR: A state of tension between adversaries in which measures short of sustained combat by regular forces are used to achieve national objectives. These measures may include political, economic, technological, sociological, paramilitary, and small-scale military efforts. The term *Cold War* is commonly used to characterize relations between the United States and the USSR from the latter 1940s to the late 1960s. See also Conflict Spectrum; National Objectives.

COLLATERAL CASUALTIES AND DAMAGE: Physical harm done to persons and property collocated with, or adjacent to, targets. Collateral effects may be welcome or unwanted, depending on circumstances.

COLOURED: Racially mixed population of Khoikhoi (Hottentot), European, Cape Malay, and African heredity in South Africa.

COMBAT POWER: A compilation of capabilities related to a specific military balance between countries or coalitions. Ingredients include numbers and types of forces; technological attributes of weapons and equipment; discipline; morale; pride; confidence; hardiness; elan; loyalty; training; combat experience; command/control arrangements; staying power; and leadership. Combat power is illusory unless accompanied by the national will to use it as required. See also National Will.

COMBINED ARMS CONCEPT: Consistent with Soviet warfighting doctrine, different air, naval, and ground-force units are orchestrated in coordinated attacks, working together and not at cross-purposes. See Joint Force.

COMECON: See Council for Mutual Economic Assistance (CMEA).

COMINFORM (COMMUNIST INFORMATION BUREAU): Stalin established the Cominform in September 1947 as a successor to the Comintern (Communist International) to help integrate and consolidate the communist countries under Soviet control. Nine Communist parties originally joined: those of the USSR, Poland, Czechoslovakia, Bulgaria, Hungary, Romania, France, Italy, and Yugoslavia. The organization soon encountered difficulties; Yugoslavia was expelled, and in 1956 the bureau ceased to exist.

COMMAND AND CONTROL COMMUNICATIONS AND INTELLIGENCE (C³I): A comprehensive concept that refers to an arrangement of facilities, equipment, personnel, and procedures used to obtain, process, and distribute information needed by decision makers to plan, direct, and control military operations.

COMPELLENCE: The process of influencing another party, through one instrument or a variety of instruments, either to cease some specified action or to embark on a course that would not otherwise have been taken. Compellence is positive in nature; deterrence is negative. For further information on compellence, see Thomas C. Schelling, *Arms and Influence* (New Haven: Yale University Press, 1966). See also Deterrence.

CONDENSATION TRAIL: A visible cloud streak, usually brilliantly white in color, that trails behind a missile or other vehicle in flight under certain conditions. Also called a vapor trail or contrail.

CONFERENCE ON SECURITY AND COOPERATION IN EUROPE (CSCE): The conference that led to the signing of the Helsinki Agreements of 1975 and subsequent follow-up conferences of the same name. See also Helsinki Agreements.

CONFLICT SPECTRUM: A continuum of hostilities that ranges from subcrisis maneuvering in Cold War situations to the most violent form of general war. See also Cold War; Spectrum of War.

CONTAINMENT: Measures to discourage or prevent the expansion of enemy territorial holdings or influence. Specifically, a U.S. policy directed against communist expansion. Containment became an official part of U.S. policy with the enunciation of the Truman Doctrine on 12 March 1947. Immediately thereafter, in July 1947, strong support for the policy of containment was set forth in the now famous article, signed "X" and written by George F. Kennan, entitled "The Sources of Soviet Conduct" (*Foreign Affairs*, July 1947).

CONTINGENCY PLANS AND OPERATIONS: Preparation for major events that can reasonably be anticipated and that probably would have a detrimental effect on national security—actions in case such events occur.

CONTRAIL: See Condensation Trail.

CONTROLLED COUNTERFORCE WAR: War in which one or both sides concentrate on reducing enemy strategic retaliatory forces and take special precautions to minimize collateral casualties and damage. See also Collateral Casualties and Damage; Counterforce.

CONTROLLED RESPONSE: The selection from a wide variety of feasible options of the one that will provide the specific military response most advantageous under the circumstances. Responding to a military attack with military action matched to the circumstances in a manner designed to avoid all-out nuclear war.

CONVENTIONAL WEAPONS: Nonnuclear weapons. Excludes all biological weapons, and generally excludes chemical weapons except for existing smoke, incendiary, and riot-control agents.

CORDON SANITAIRE: A territorial buffer between two opposing forces or states.

CORRELATION OF FORCES: A term that in Soviet usage refers to the overall balance of economic, military, scientific, and sociopolitical capabilities between two states or coalitions of states. For a related, but different, concept, see Military Balance.

COST-EFFECTIVENESS: A condition that matches ends with means in ways that create maximum capabilities at minimum expense—in colloquial terms, getting the most for your money.

COST SHARING: An attempt by NATO members to distribute defense costs among themselves fairly. The concept is in response to the perception that some states have been paying more than their "fair" share of NATO's defense expenditures. Also referred to as "burden sharing." See Three-Percent Guideline.

COUNCIL OF MUTUAL ECONOMIC ASSISTANCE (CMEA): CMEA (sometimes referred to as COMECON) was formed in January 1949 in response to the Marshall Plan and is the economic counterpart of the Warsaw Pact. Its stated objective is to promote the economic development of all members and it has, in practice, led to greater division of labor, coordination of five-year plans, and trade and economic ties that as a whole have tended to benefit the USSR. Members include the Soviet Union, Poland, Czechoslovakia, Romania, Hungary, Bulgaria, and East Germany.

COUNTERFORCE: The employment of strategic air and missile forces to destroy, or render impotent, military capabilities of an enemy force. Bombers and their bases, ballistic missile submarines, ICBM silos, ABM and air defense installations, command and control centers, and nuclear stockpiles are typical counterforce targets. See also Counterforce; First Strike.

COUNTERINSURGENCY (COIN): Those military, paramilitary, political, economic, psychological, and civic actions taken by a government to defeat subversive insurgency.

COUNTERVAILING STRATEGY: Secretary of Defense Harold Brown committed the United States to a countervailing strategy during the Carter administration. This strategy requires forces capable of responding to any attack such that the enemy could not hope to gain any rational objective; any enemy gain would entail offsetting losses. Specifically, forces must be able to: (1) survive a surprise attack, (2) be deployed in a controlled manner by national command authorities, (3) penetrate enemy defenses, and (4) destroy their assigned targets.

COUNTERVALUE: A strategic concept that calls for the destruction or neutralization of selected enemy population centers, industries, resources, and institutions that constitute the fabric of society. See also Counterforce.

COUPLING (STRATEGIC): The linking of U.S. forces (particularly central strategic forces such as ICBMs, heavy bombers, and SLBMs) to the defense of allies as part of extended deterrence.

CREDIBILITY: Clear evidence that capabilities and intentions are sufficient to support purported policies. See also National Will.

CRISIS STABILITY: The ability of a government to manage a nuclear crisis in a rational and unhurried manner, thereby avoiding rash decisions.

CROSS-TARGETING: Attack planning that assigns a number of warheads carried by different delivery vehicles to a specific target with the goal of increasing the probability of target destruction.

CRUISE MISSILE: A pilotless aircraft, propelled by an air-breathing engine, that operates entirely within the earth's atmosphere. Thrust continues throughout its flight. Inflight guidance and control can be remote or on-board equipment. Conventional and nuclear warheads are available. See also Air-launched Cruise Missile and Sea-launched Cruise Missile.

CRUISER: A large, long-endurance surface warship armed for independent offensive operations against surface ships and land targets. Also acts as an escort to protect aircraft carriers, merchantmen, and other ships against surface or air attack. May have antisubmarine capability. Its own aircraft-handling capability is usually restricted to one or two float planes, helicopters, or other *STOL* (short takeoff and landing) types.

CSBM: Confidence and Security Building Measures. See also CBM.

CSCE: See Conference on Security and Cooperation in Europe.

CSU: Christian Social Union, the leading political party in the West German state of Bavaria; right-of-center party usually aligned with the CDU.

CULTURAL REVOLUTION: The People's Republic of China underwent a period of political violence and turmoil from 1966 to 1969 known as the Cultural Revolution. Mao Zedong initiated the revolution by forming the Red Guards to eliminate opposition to his policies. The guards' zeal became excessive and the People's Liberation Army assumed an enlarged role in the political system to help restore order.

DAMAGE LIMITATION: Active or passive efforts to restrict the level or geographic extent of devastation during war. Includes counterforce actions of all kinds, as well as civil defense measures. See also Active Defense; Civil Defense; Counterforce; Passive Defense.

D-DAY: The unnamed day on which a particular operation commences or is to commence. An operation may be the commencement of hostilities; the date of a major military effort; the execution date of an operation (as distinguished from the date the order to execute is issued); the date the operations phase is implemented, either by land assault, air strike, naval bombardment, parachute assault, or amphibious assault. The highest command headquarters responsible for coordinating the planning will specify the exact meaning of D-Day within the aforementioned definition. The term *D-Day* is often used historically to refer to allied landings at Normandy in France on 6 June 1944. (See also H-Hour; K-Day; M-Day.)

DDR: German Democratic Republic or East Germany; see GDR; DDR is the abbreviation in German: *Deutsche Demokratische Republik*.

DÉFENSE (DE) TOUS AZIMUTS: The use of defense forces geared to meet threats from any direction, usually used in reference to French refusal under de Gaulle to specify either superpower as the primary security threat. It was popularized as France's military policy under de Gaulle.

DEFENSE IN DEPTH: Protective measures in successive positions along axes of enemy advance, as opposed to a single line of resistance. Designed to absorb and progressively weaken enemy penetrations or attack, prevent initial observations of the whole position by the enemy, and allow the commander to maneuver his reserve.

DEFENSE PLANNING COMMITTEE (DPC): The Defense Planning Committee of NATO was formed in 1966 after France left the integrated military organization. The fourteen-nation committee deals with issues related to alliance-integrated military planning and other matters in which France does not participate.

DEFOLIANT OPERATIONS: The employment of defoliating agents on vegetated areas in support of military operations. See also Biological Operations.

DEPRESSED TRAJECTORY: The trajectory of a ballistic missile fired at an angle to the ground significantly lower than the angle of a minimum energy trajectory. See also Minimum Energy Trajectory.

DESTROYER: A medium-sized warship configured to escort and protect other ships against air, submarine, and surface attacks. May also be used for independent offensive operations against enemy ships or land targets. Some carry one or two helicopters.

DÉTENTE: Lessening of tensions in international relations. May be achieved formally or informally.

DETERRENCE: (1) Steps taken to prevent opponents from initiating armed actions and to inhibit escalation if combat occurs. Threats of force predominate. (2) The prevention of opponents from action by fear of the consequences. Deterrence is a state of mind brought about by the existence of a credible threat of unacceptable counteraction. See also Compellence; Credibility; Deterrence by Denial; Finite Deterrence; Graduated Deterrence; Intrawar Deterrence; Maximum Deterrence; Minimum Deterrence; Type I, Type II, and Type III Deterrence.

DETERRENCE BY DENIAL: Deterring another power from first strike by convincing the opponent that no military benefit could be gained by striking first. This basically counterforce posture requires deployment of damage-limiting and disarming forces. Often associated with the Soviet approach to deterrence.

DIRECT APPROACH: Any grand strategy in which the use of force predominates; any military strategy that depends primarily on physical pressure, as opposed to deterrence, surprise, or maneuver. Direct assaults on fortified positions would be an example of the direct approach. See also Grand Strategy; Indirect Approach; Strategy.

DISARMAMENT: The reduction of a military establishment at some level set by international agreement. See also Arms Control; General and Complete Disarmament.

DIVISION: (1) A tactical unit or formation as follows: (a) a major administrative and tactical unit or formation that combines in itself the necessary arms and services required for sustained combat (larger than a regiment or brigade and smaller than a corps); (b) a number of naval ships of smaller type grouped together for operational and administrative command, or a tactical unit of a naval aircraft squadron, consisting of two or more sections; (c) an air division is an air combat organization normally consisting of two or more wings with appropriate service units. The combat wings of an air division will normally contain units of similar type. (2) The organizational part of a headquarters that handles military matters of a particular nature, such as personnel, intelligence, plans and training, or supply and evacuation. (3) A number of personnel of a ship's complement grouped together for operational and administrative command.

DIVISION EQUIVALENT: Separate brigades, regiments, and comparable combat forces whose aggregate capabilities approximate those of a division, except for staying power. See also Division.

DOCTRINE: Fundamental principles by which the military forces or elements thereof guide their actions in support of national objectives. It is authorative but requires judgment in application. See also National Objectives; Principles of War.

DOSAAF: Russian acronym referring in the USSR to the "voluntary" society for the support of the army, navy, and the air force.

DUAL CAPABLE: Refers to weapons systems capable of using either nuclear warheads or "conventional" (non-nuclear) ordnance.

DUAL-CAPABLE SYSTEM: Those systems capable of delivering either conventional or nuclear weapons. Certain artillery pieces, short-range missiles, and tactical aircraft are dual-capable delivery systems.

DUAL-TRACK DECISION: The decision made by NATO in 1979 to pursue two courses simultaneously concerning intermediate-range nuclear forces in Europe (INF)—modernizing nuclear forces (developing for deployment of both Pershing IIs and GLCMs) *and*, at the same time, seeking an arms control agreement with the USSR relating INF systems. See also Two-Track Decision.

ECONOMIC WARFARE: The offensive or defensive use of trade, foreign aid programs, financial transactions, and other factors that influence the production, distribution, and consumption of goods and services. Seeks to achieve national security objectives by augmenting friendly capabilities and diminishing or neutralizing enemy capabilities and potential. See also Sanctions.

ELECTRONIC COUNTERCOUNTERMEASURES (ECCM): Electronic warfare involving actions taken to retain effective use of the electromagnetic spectrum despite the enemy's use of electronic countermeasures. See Electronic Countermeasures.

ELECTRONIC COUNTERMEASURES (ECM): Electronic warfare (EW) involving actions taken to prevent or reduce an enemy's effective use of equipment and tactics employing (or affected by) electromagnetic radiation and to exploit the enemy's use of such radiation. ECM may be further classified as follows: (1) Passive ECM (sometimes called Electronic Support Measures or ESM), i.e., ECM without active transmissions by the searcher such as intercept search for enemy electronic emissions and tactical evasion (measures taken to impede detection and tracking by the enemy); (2) Active ECM: ECM involving active emissions that may be detected by an enemy, such as jamming (the deliberate radiating or reradiating of electronic signals in order to obliterate or obscure signals the enemy is attempting to receive) or deception (the deliberate radiating or reradiating of signals received by his electronic equipment).

ENHANCED RADIATION WEAPONS (ERW): Refers to nuclear weapons that maximize initial radiation while minimizing blast effects; intended for use against tank or troop concentrations.

EQUIVALENT MEGATONNAGE (EMT): A measure used to compare the destructive potential of differing combinations of nuclear warhead yields. EMT calculations are useful in estimating the effects of small numbers of high-yield warheads in contrast to larger numbers of smaller-yield warheads against the same targets. EMT is computed from the expression: $EMT = NY^x$, where $N =$ number of actual warheads of yield Y; $Y =$ yield of the actual warheads, in megatons; and $x =$ scaling factor. Scaling factors vary with the size and characteristics of the target base and the number of targets attacked. See also Countervalue; Soft Target.

ERETZ ISRAEL: The common Hebrew name that roughly corresponds geographically to Palestine under the British mandate boundaries. The term also refers to the idea of a "greater Israel" that would include such territories as Judea and Samaria on the

West Bank as well as other areas that were part of biblical Israel.

ESCALATION: (1) Intensification or broadening of a conflict through the use of more powerful weapons, larger numbers of forces, or the geographic spread of the conflict. (2) An increase, deliberate or unpremeditated, in the scope or intensity of a conflict.

ESCALATION LADDER: Successive levels of intensity in the conflict spectrum, with nuclear warfare options as the uppermost rungs. See also Conflict Spectrum.

ESSENTIAL EQUIVALENCE: A force structure standard that demands capabilities approximately equal in overall effectiveness to those of particular opponents, but does not insist on numerical equality in all cases. See also Nuclear Parity; Parity.

EUROGROUP: The Eurogroup was established in 1968 by ten Western European members of NATO. Its objective is to coordinate and improve the Western European military contribution to the alliance through greater overall cooperation in defense matters.

EUROPEAN ECONOMIC COMMUNITY (EEC): An association established in 1958 with the purpose of promoting the economic welfare of members by abolishing trade barriers among signatories and adopting common import duties on items from other countries. Also known as the Common Market.

EUROSTRATEGIC WEAPONS: Term usually refers to nuclear weapons deployed by the USSR and designed for use against Western Europe (e.g., the SS-20 IRBM).

EXEMPLARY ATTACK: The isolated engagement of a military target or civilian population center, designed primarily for psychological effect. It demonstrates a capability. The atomic attacks on Hiroshima and Nagasaki were exemplary. See also Symbolic Attack.

EXTENDED DETERRENCE: (1) The deterrent power of a country or coalition of countries projected to protect allies, neutrals, or its own forces on foreign soil. (2) Extension of the deterrent value of the U.S. strategic nuclear forces to protect other allied countries (e.g., NATO and Japan) from aggression. See also Deterrence.

FAIL-SAFE: A plan that prevents a manned nuclear weapons delivery vehicle from proceeding on a mission against the enemy in contradiction of ultimate decisions or orders, by arrangements that require it, when transmission of orders fails, to return to its base (RTB).

FDP: Free Democratic Party; West Germany's centrist party that has added its small margin of seats to forming coalition governments with either to CDU and CSU or SPD. See CDU, CSU, SPD.

FEDAYEEN: So-called "men of sacrifice"—Arab guerrillas opposed to Zionism (the creation of a religious state in Israel).

FIELD ARMY: Administrative and tactical organization composed of a headquarters, certain organic army troops, service support troops, a variable number of corps, and a variable number of divisions. See also Division.

FINITE DETERRENCE: Deterrent power predicated on objective capabilities sufficient to satisfy precisely calculable needs under any conceivable circumstances. Cities are targeted. See also Deterrence.

FIREBREAK: A psychological barrier that inhibits escalation from one type of warfare to another, as from conventional to nuclear combat. See also Threshold.

FIRST STRIKE: The first offensive move of a war. As applied to general nuclear war, it implies the ability to eliminate effective retaliation by the opposition. See also Counterforce; Second Strike.

FIRST-STRIKE CAPABILITY: A military capability sufficient to eliminate effective retaliation by initiating an attack against the opponent's forces. It usually involves targeting nuclear weapons in a counterforce mode.

FIRST USE: The initial employment of specific military measures, such as nuclear weapons, during the conduct of war. A belligerent could execute a second strike in response to aggression, yet be the first to employ nuclear weapons. See also First Strike; Second Strike.

FISSION: The splitting of an atomic nucleus of certain heavy elements, such as uranium and plutonium, by bombardment with neutrons, resulting in the release of substantial quantities of energy. See also Fusion; Thermonuclear.

FLEET BALLISTIC MISSILE SUBMARINE (SSBN): A nuclear-powered submarine designed to deliver ballistic missile attacks against assigned targets from either a submerged or surfaced position. See also Ballistic Missile; Sea/Submarine-launched Ballistic Missile.

FLEXIBLE RESPONSE: (1) A strategy prescribing forces able to respond to a threat at any point along the conflict spectrum. Robert McNamara adopted flexible response as the U.S. strategy in the early 1960s as a replacement for massive retaliation, which was commonly preceived to be an almost immediate resort to nuclear weapons in response to communist aggression. NATO adopted a flexible response strategy in 1967 in its document MC 14/3. (2) A strategy predicated on meeting aggression at an appropriate level or place with the capability of escalating the level of conflict if required or desired. See also Maxwell D. Taylor, *The Uncertain Trumpet* (New York: Harper and Row, 1960), a book that set the tone for this change in U.S. defense strategy.

FLIGHT: (1) In U.S. Navy and Marine Corps usage, a specified group of aircraft usually engaged in a common mission. (2) The basic tactical unit in the U.S. Air Force, consisting of four or more aircraft in two or more elements. (3) A single aircraft airborne on a nonoperational mission.

FORCE DE DISSUASION: The name commonly given to France's nuclear weapons, which are intended to provide the country with minimum deterrence.

FORCE DE FRAPPE: A label applied to France's nuclear forces, as they would become a striking force should their deterrent power fail.

FORWARD-BASED SYSTEM (FBS): A term introduced by the USSR to refer to those U.S. nuclear systems based in third countries or on aircraft carriers and capable of delivering a nuclear strike against the territory of the USSR.

FORWARD DEFENSE: (1) The NATO strategy that dictates resistance to a Warsaw Pact invasion at the point of penetration, as opposed to an orderly retreat to more defensible lines. This strategy has been particularly espoused by West Germany, as it is German territory that would be lost by any falling back. (2) A strategic concept that calls for containing or repulsing military aggression as close to the original line of contact as possible to protect important areas.

FORWARD EDGE OF THE BATTLE AREA (FEBA): The foremost limits of a series of areas in which ground combat units are deployed, excluding the areas in which the covering or screening forces are operating, designated to coordinate fire support, the positioning of forces, or the maneuver of units.

FREE ROCKET: A missile with a completely self-contained propellant package that is neither guided nor controlled in flight.

FRELIMO: Mozambique Liberation Front (in power); see also RENAMO.

FRENCH COMMUNITY: With the advent of France's Fifth Republic in 1958, a new constitutional arrangement established the French Community to preside over the country's overseas territories. These territories were given the choice of independence or autonomous status in the community. Initially only Guinea chose independence, but within three years several others made the same decision. In the past two decades the formal community has largely given way to a series of bilateral agreements between France and its former possessions.

FRG: Federal Republic of Germany (West Germany); see also BRD.

FRIGATE: A medium to small surface warship armed as an escort against surface attack and either air or submarine attack. May be capable of embarking and handling one or two helicopters.

FRONTAL AVIATION: The primary mission of Frontal Aviation (USSR) has traditionally been to provide air support—air defense, ground assault, reconnaissance, and electronic warfare—to ground forces. This mission has been broadened of late to encompass air strikes against theater nuclear reserves and tactical air forces.

FRONT LINE STATES: Those states on the "front line" in the struggle against South Africa—Angola, Botswana, Mozambique, Tanzania, Zimbabwe, and Zambia.

FUSION: The process, accompanied by the release of tremendous amounts of energy, whereby the nuclei of light elements combine to form the nucleus of heavier elements. See also Fission; Thermonuclear.

FY: Fiscal year; in the United States government a given fiscal year begins on 1 October and ends the following 30 September.

GANG OF FOUR: Four members of the Politburo of the People's Republic of China (Jiang Qing, Wang Hungwen, Chang Ch'un-Ch'ia, and Yao Wen-yuan) helped spearhead the radical thrust of the Cultural Revolution and were subsequently labeled the Gang of Four. Vying for political power following Mao's death, the Gang of Four was purged by a more moderate faction.

GAO: Government Accounting Office (United States).

GDP: Gross domestic product.

GDR: German Democratic Republic (East Germany); see also DDR.

GENERAL AND COMPLETE DISARMAMENT (GCD): An extreme form of arms control that would reduce armed forces and armaments to levels sufficient only for domestic security. See also Arms Control; Disarmament.

GENERAL PURPOSE FORCES: All combat forces not designed primarily to accomplish strategic nuclear missions. See also Strategic Defense; Strategic Mobility; Strategic Offense.

GENERAL STAFF: A group of officers in the headquarters of divisions (or larger units or for the armed forces as a whole) that helps its commanders in planning, coordinating, and supervising operations.

GENERAL WAR: Armed conflict between major powers in which the total resources of the belligerents are employed. See also Limited War.

GLASNOST: Term refers to Soviet General Secretary Mikhail Gorbachev's program of openness and reform.

GOLAN HEIGHTS: A 714-square-mile area in the southwestern corner of Syria with a long history of conflict in the Arab–Israeli dispute. Israel has been loath to relinquish the region since capturing it in the 1967 Middle East War, for it had long been used by guerrillas to shell nearby Israeli settlements.

GOSPLAN: The Soviet State Planning Committee, which is responsible for the coordination and guidance of all economic planning in the USSR.

GRADUATED DETERRENCE: A range of deterrent power that affords credible capabilities to inhibit aggression across all, or a considerable portion, of the conflict spectrum. See also Conflict Spectrum; Deterrence.

GRADUATED RESPONSE: The incremental application of national power in ways that allow the opposition to accommodate one step at a time. Sometimes called "piecemealing." See also Flexible Response.

GRAND STRATEGY: The art and science of employing national power under all circumstances to exert desired types and degrees of control over the opposition by applying force, the threat of force, indirect pressures, diplomacy, subterfuge, and other imaginative means to attain national security objectives. See also National Objectives; Strategy.

GREENS: Small political party in FRG; concerns include antinuclear and pro-environmental issues.

GROUND FIRE: Small arms ground-to-air fire directed against aircraft.

GROUND-LAUNCHED CRUISE MISSILE (GLCM): A cruise missile launched from a ground platform. See also Cruise Missile.

GROUND ZERO (GZ): The point on the surface of the earth at, or vertically below or above, the center of a planned or actual nuclear detonation.

GUERRILLA WARFARE: Military and paramilitary operations conducted in enemy-held or hostile territory by irregular, predominantly indigenous forces. See also Unconventional Warfare; Counterinsurgency.

HALF-LIFE: The time required for the activity of a given radioactive element or isotope to decay to half of its initial radioactivity. The half-life is a characteristic property of each radioactive element and is independent of quantity or condition. The effective half-life of a given isotope is the time in which the quantity in the body will decrease to half as a result of both radioactive decay and biological elimination.

HALLSTEIN DOCTRINE: Policy in Adenauer Germany that withdrew diplomatic relations from states recognizing the GDR.

HARDENED SITE: A site constructed to withstand the blasts and associated effects of a nuclear attack and likely to be protected against a chemical, biological, or radiological attack. See also Hard Target.

HARD TARGET: A point or area protected to some significant degree against the blast, heat, and radiation effects of nuclear explosions of particular yields. See also Overpressure; Soft Targets.

HEAVY TANK: Tanks weighing more than sixty tons are generally designated as "heavies," although the United States no longer uses heavy, medium, and light as classifications.

HELSINKI AGREEMENTS: Signed on 1 August 1975, the Helsinki Agreements were the final act of the thirty-five-nation Conference on Security and Cooperation in Europe. The four sections of the agreement on East-West relations included measures on economic cooperation, humanitarian issues, and increased human contacts among nations, and plans for a follow-up conference. The Western nations viewed the agreements on human rights as a major victory, but in exchange they, in effect, endorsed the post–World War II boundaries in Europe.

H-HOUR: The specific hour on D-Day at which a particular operation commences. See also D-Day.

HI-LOW MIX: Mingling high-cost, high-performance items with relatively low-cost, low-performance items in any given weapons system to achieve the best balance between quantity and quality in ways that maximize capabilities and minimize expenses. Term can also refer to tactic of combining attacks by aircraft at different altitudes.

HLG: High-level working group in NATO dealing in particular with arms control negotiations.

IAF: Refers to Israeli Air Force.

ICBM: See Intercontinental Ballistic Missile.

IDF: See Israel Defense Forces.

IDFN: Israel Defense Forces Navy.

IEPG: See Independent European Program Group.

IMEMO: Institute for the World Economy and International Affairs (USSR).

INCIDENTS: Brief clashes or other military disturbances generally of a transitory nature and not involving protracted hostilities.

INDEPENDENT EUROPEAN PROGRAM GROUP (IEPG): An independent forum for European cooperation in defense equipment in which France can participate. Membership includes Belgium, Denmark, France, West Germany, Italy, Greece, Luxembourg, the Netherlands, Norway, Portugal, Turkey, and the United Kingdom.

INDIAN OCEAN ZONE OF PEACE (IOZP): An Indian proposal that would exclude extraregional powers from the Indian Ocean.

INDIRECT APPROACH: Any grand strategy that emphasizes political, economic, social, and psychological pressures instead of direct military force; any military strategy that seeks to throw the enemy off balance before engaging main forces—doing the unexpected in space, time and direction. See also Direct Approach; Grand Strategy; Strategy.

INERTIAL GUIDANCE SYSTEM: A guidance system designed to direct a missile to a predetermined point on the earth's surface by measuring acceleration. The path of the missile is controlled during powered flight on the basis of acceleration measurements made by instruments wholly within the missile and independent of outside information. The system is

thus immune from jamming, atmospheric conditions in the launch area, and other forms of interference.

INF: Intermediate-Range Nuclear Forces. Nuclear weapons systems with a range of 500–5,500 km. These forces include short-range INF (SRINF), with ranges of 500–1,000 km, and long-range INF (LRINF), with ranges of 1,000–5,500 km. See Dual-track Decision.

INFRASTRUCTURE: A term generally applicable to all fixed and permanent installations, fabrications, or facilities for the support and control of military forces.

INF TREATY: Ratified in 1988, this treaty provides for the elimination, over a three-year period, of all American and Soviet missiles of intermediate range (500–5500 km). The treaty eliminates over 400 U.S. and 1,400 Soviet INF warheads. The INF treaty is unique in that it contains extensive on-site verification clauses. It does not, however, apply to short-range nuclear systems (with ranges of less than 500 km) or to aircraft of intermediate range. See INF.

INNERE FÜHRUNG: Concept in West German democratic society of "inner leadership"—the citizen-in-uniform idea that makes the military a part of the society it is to defend, not divorced or isolated from it.

INTELLIGENCE: The product resulting from the collection, evaluation, analysis, integration, and interpretation of all information concerning one or more aspects of foreign countries or areas, which is immediately or potentially significant to the development and execution of plans, policies, and operations.

INTELLIGENCE ESTIMATE: An appraisal of the elements of intelligence relating to a specific situation or condition with a view to determining the courses of action open to the enemy or potential enemy and the probable order of their adoption.

INTERCEPTOR AIRCRAFT: A manned aircraft capable of identifying and engaging other aircraft. See also Interceptor Missile.

INTERCEPTOR MISSILE: A missile designed to counter enemy offensive missiles, reentry vehicles, or aircraft. See also Antiballistic Missile (ABM); Interceptor Aircraft; Reentry Vehicle (RV).

INTERCONTINENTAL BALLISTIC MISSILE (ICBM): A land-based, rocket-propelled vehicle capable of delivering a warhead to intercontinental ranges (ranges in excess of about 3,000 nautical miles). An ICBM consists of a booster stage, one or more sustainer propulsion stages, a reentry vehicle or vehicles, possibly including penetration aids, and, in the case of a MIRVed missile, a bus. See also Ballistic Missile; Bus; Inertial Guidance System; INF; Intermediate-Range Ballistic Missile (IRBM); Medium-Range Ballistic Missile (MRBM); Modern Large Ballistic Missile; Older Heavy Ballistic Missile Launcher; Reentry Vehicle; Short-Range Ballistic Missile (SRBM).

INTERDICT (INTERDICTION): To prevent or hinder, by any means, enemy use of an area or route.

INTERMEDIATE-RANGE BALLISTIC MISSILE (IRBM): A ballistic missile with a range capability from about 1,500 to 3,000 nautical miles. See also INF and Intercontinental Ballistic Missile (ICBM).

INTEROPERABILITY: The ability of the armed forces of

different nations to operate each other's equipment and to interchange the components of such equipment. See also Standardization.

INTRAWAR DETERRENCE: Deterrent power exercised during the conduct of a war to inhibit escalation by the enemy or to limit damage. See also Deterrence.

ISRAEL DEFENSE FORCES (IDF): The armed forces of Israel, consisting of an army, air force, and navy. See also IAF and IDFN.

JCS: U.S. Joint Chiefs of Staff.

JOINT FORCE: In American usage, a general term applied to a force composed of significant elements of the U.S. Army, Navy, Marine Corps, and Air Force, or two or more of these services, operating under a single commander authorized to exercise unified command or operational control over such joint forces. See Combined Arms.

JSDF: Japanese Self-Defense Forces.

JUST WAR: In the classic sense, conflict conducted by competent authorities with irreproachable motives to defend rights, rectify wrongs, or punish transgressors. Just war today connotes actions by a state to defend its own territory or the sovereignty of other nations beset by aggressors. In its conduct, a just war is one subject to moral limits.

K-DAY: The basic date for the introduction of a convoy system or any particular convoy lane. See also D-Day.

KGB: Committee for State Security (Komitet Gosudarstvennoye Bezopasnosti). The predominant state and internal security police organization of the USSR.

KILOTON: The equivalent explosive power of 1,000 tons of trinitrotoluene (TNT), used as a measure of yield for nuclear weapons.

KILOTON WEAPON: A nuclear weapon, the yield of which is measured in terms of thousands of tons of trinitrotoluene (TNT) explosive equivalents, producing yields from 1 to 999 kilotons. See also Megaton Weapons, TNT Equivalent.

KOMSOMOL: Young Communist League (USSR).

LAUNCHER: A structural device designed to support and hold a missile in position for firing. See also Cold Launch; Transporter-Erector-Launcher (TEL).

LAUNCH-ON-WARNING: A doctrine calling for the launch of ballistic missiles when a missile attack against them is detected and before the attacking warheads reach their targets.

LDP: Liberal Democratic Party (Japan).

LEAD TIME: The amount of time between the start of research and development on a weapons system and its operational deployment.

LIGHT TANK: Tanks weighing less than 40 tons are generally designated as "light," although the United States no longer uses heavy, medium, and light as classifications. See also Heavy Tank, Medium Tank.

LIMITED WAR: (1) Armed conflict short of general war, exclusive of incidents, involving the overt engagement of the military forces of two or more nations. (2) Armed encounters, exclusive of incidents, in which one or more major powers or their proxies voluntarily exercise various types and degrees of restraint to prevent unmanageable escalation. Objectives, forces, weapons, targets, and geographic areas all can be limited. See also Escalation; General War; Graduated Response; Incidents; Proxy War.

LOGISTICS: The science of planning and carrying out the movement and maintenance of forces. In its most comprehensive sense, those aspects of military operations that deal with (a) design and development, acquisition, storage, movement, distribution, maintenance, evacuation, and disposition of matériel; (b) movement, evacuation, and hospitalization of personnel; (c) acquisition or construction, maintenance, operations, and disposition of facilities; and (d) acquisition or furnishing of services.

LONG-RANGE BOMBER AIRCRAFT: A bomber designed for a tactical operating radius over 2,500 nautical miles at design gross weight and design bomb load. See also Bomber; Medium Bomber.

MAIN POLITICAL ADMINISTRATION (MPA): The department of the Central Committee of the Communist Party of the Soviet Union whose responsibility it is to maintain firm Party control of the military.

MAJOR NATO COMMANDERS: Major NATO commanders are Supreme Allied Commander Atlantic, Supreme Allied Commander Europe, Allied Commander-in-Chief, Channel.

MANEUVERABLE REENTRY VEHICLE (MaRV): A ballistic reentry vehicle equipped with its own navigation and control systems capable of adjusting its trajectory during reentry into the atmosphere. The advantages of MaRV are twofold. First, the on-board guidance and control systems give some types of MaRVs greater ultimate potential for accuracy due to their ability to make course corrections in the terminal reentry phase. Such accuracy may be essential if the intent is to strike key targets while avoiding or minimizing collateral damage. Second, the MaRV has a high degree of maneuverability and thus the inherent ability to evade terminal ABM defense interceptor missiles. See also Ballistic Missile; Collateral Casualties and Damage; Counterforce; Inertial Guidance System.

MANHATTAN PROJECT: A term referring to the collective research and development efforts that led to the successful detonation of the atomic bombs over Japan in August 1945. The actual research and development took place at numerous sites in the United States and Canada with the help of scientists of several nationalities.

MASSIVE RETALIATION: The act of countering aggression of any type with tremendous destructive power; particularly, a crushing nuclear response to any provocation deemed serious enough to warrant military action. The doctrine was first set forth by Secretary of State John Foster Dulles in an address delivered by him on 12 January 1954. This doctrine, seen by many as essentially a cost-cutting measure, was part of the Eisenhower administration's "New Look" approach to defense. See also Brinkmanship.

MAXIMUM DETERRENCE: Diversified, survivable deterrent power of such quality and magnitude that it affords optimum capabilities to inhibit aggression across the entire conflict spectrum. See also Deterrence; Minimum Deterrence.

MC 14/3: NATO plan outlining alliance strategy agreed upon in 1967; "MC 14/3" reflects the Military Committee's numbering system for such documents.

M-DAY: The term used to designate the day on which mobilization is to begin. See also D-Day.

MEDIUM BOMBER: (1) A multi-engine aircraft that lacks intercontinental range without in-flight refueling but

is suitable for strategic bombing on one-way intercontinental missions, even lacking tanker support.
(2) A bomber designed for a tactical operating radius
of under 1,000 nautical miles at design gross weight
and design bomb load. See also Bombers; Long-
Range Bomber Aircraft.

MEDIUM-RANGE BALLISTIC MISSILE (MRBM): A ballistic
missile with a range capability from about 600 to
1,500 nautical miles. See also Ballistic Missile; Intercontinental Ballistic Missile (ICBM).

MEDIUM TANK: Tanks weighing between 40 and 60 tons
are generally designated as "medium," although the
United States no longer uses heavy, medium, and
light as classifications. See also Heavy Tank; Light
Tank.

MEGATON: The equivalent explosive power of one million tons of trinitrotoluene (TNT), used as a measure
of yield for nuclear weapons.

MEGATON WEAPONS: A nuclear weapon, the yield of
which is measured in terms of millions of tons of
trinitrotoluene (TNT) explosive equivalents. See also
Kiloton Weapon; TNT Equivalent.

MERCHANT MARINE: All nonmilitary vessels of a nation,
publicly and privately owned, together with crews,
that engage in domestic or international trade and
commerce.

MIDGETMAN: Nickname for a small, mobile, single-
warhead ICBM under development in the United
States.

MIG: The name "MiG" stands for Mikoyan and
Gurevich, noted Soviet aircraft designers, and refers
to a type of Soviet tactical aircraft.

MILITARY ASSISTANCE ADVISORY GROUP (MAAG): A
joint service group, normally under the military commander of a unified command and representing the
secretary of defense, that primarily administers U.S.
military assistance planning and programming in the
host country. See also Joint Force; Unified Command.

MILITARY ASSISTANCE PROGRAM (MAP): The U.S. program for providing military assistance under the Foreign Assistance Act of 1961, as amended, distinct
from economic aid and other programs authorized
by the act; includes the furnishing of defense articles
and defense services through grant aid or military
sales to eligible allies specified by Congress.

MILITARY BALANCE: The comparative combat power of
two competing countries or coalitions. See also Combat Power. For a related, but more inclusive, concept
used in the USSR, see Correlation of Forces.

MILITARY DOCTRINE: Fundamental principles by which
the military forces guide their actions in support of
national objectives. It is authoritative but requires
judgment in application.

MILITARY INTERVENTION: The deliberate act of a nation or group of nations to introduce its military
forces into the course of an existing controversy.

MILITARY NECESSITY: The principle whereby a belligerent has the right to apply any measures required to
bring about the successful conclusion of a military
operation and not forbidden by the laws of war.

MILITARY STRATEGY: The art and science of employing
military power under all circumstances to attain national security objectives by applying force or the
threat of force. See also National Objectives; National Security; Strategy; Tactics.

MINIMUM DETERRENCE: Deterrent power predicated
on the belief that countries possessing even few nuclear weapons are automatically guaranteed immunity from rational attack, since the penalty for aggression presumably would be intolerable. See also
Deterrence.

MINIMUM ENERGY TRAJECTORY: The missile flight path
that reaches a given range with the least expenditure
of propellant energy. See also Depressed Trajectory.

MINUTEMAN III: Designated the LGM-30G, this missile
has a 76,000 pound launch weight, carries a one
megaton thermonuclear warhead, and has an 8,000-
mile range. It is a three-stage, solid-propellant, ballistic missile and is guided to its target by an all-iner-
tial guidance and control system. With its improved
third stage and postboost vehicle, the Minuteman III
can deliver multiple independently targetable reentry
vehicles (MIRVs) and their penetration aids to multiple targets. See also Ballistic Missile; Hardened Site;
Hard Target; Intercontinental Ballistic Missile
(ICBM); Mobile Missile.

MISSILE EXPERIMENTAL (MX): The MX, named "Peace-
keeper" to reflect its deterrence role, has been added
to the U.S. ICBM force as a complement to the Minuteman. See Peacekeeper.

MITI: Ministry of International Trade and Industry (Japan).

MOBILE MISSILE: Any ballistic or cruise missile
mounted on and fired from a movable platform,
such as a truck, train, ground effects machine, ship,
or aircraft. See also Minuteman III.

MOBILIZATION: (1) The act of preparing for war or
other emergency through assembling and organizing
national resources. (2) The process by which the
armed forces or part of them are brought to a state of
readiness for war or other national emergency. This
includes assembling and organizing personnel, supplies, and matériel for active service.

MOBILIZATION BASE: The total of all resources available, or that can be made available, to meet foreseeable wartime needs. Such resources include the manpower and material resources and services required
for the support of essential military, civilian, and survival activities, as well as the elements affecting their
state of readiness, such as (but not limited to) the following: manning levels, state of training, modernization of equipment, mobilization of material reserves
and facilities, continuity of government, civil defense
plans and preparedness measures, psychological preparedness of the people, international agreements,
planning with industry, dispersion, and standby legislation and controls. See also Combat Power.

MOD: Ministry of Defense

MODERN LARGE BALLISTIC MISSILE (MLBM): A term in
the SALT negotiations referring to an intercontinental ballistic missile (ICBM) of a type deployed since
1964 and having a volume significantly greater than
the largest light ICBM operational in 1972 (the Soviet SS-11). The U.S. has no MLBMs. The Soviet
SS-9 and the SS-18 are examples of MLBMs. See
also Ballistic Missile; Intercontinental Ballistic Missile (ICBM); Older Heavy Ballistic Missile Launcher.

MOSSAD: The oldest of Israel's intelligence agencies.

MRBM: See Medium-Range Ballistic Missile.

MULTIPLE INDEPENDENTLY TARGETABLE REENTRY VE-
HICLE (MIRV): A reentry vehicle carried by a delivery

system that can place one or more reentry vehicles independently over each of several separate targets. See also Bus; Reentry Vehicle (RV).

MULTIPLE REENTRY VEHICLE (MRV): The reentry vehicle of a delivery system that places more than one reentry vehicle over an individual target. See also Reentry Vehicle (RV).

MULTIPOLAR: Distribution of power among several states or blocs of states in the international community, as opposed to the two-way power division of a bipolar world.

MUTUAL AND BALANCED FORCE REDUCTIONS (MBFR): A form of arms control in which opposing powers concurrently reduce the capabilities of their overall military establishments or selected elements thereof. Personnel strengths and numbers or types of weapons have been the most common considerations. Substantive MBFR talks between the NATO and Warsaw Pact countries began in Vienna, Austria, in October 1973. The official name for the MBFR talks regarding force reductions in Central Europe is Mutual Reduction of Forces and Armaments and Associated Measures in Central Europe. Lack of progress in MBFR has been followed by efforts within the CSCE framework. See also Mutual Force Reductions (MFR); CSCE; CDE; and Arms Control.

MUTUALLY ASSURED DESTRUCTION (MAD): Sometimes referred to as Mutual, Assured Destruction; a condition in which an assured destruction capability is possessed by opposing sides—a force posture on both sides that includes enough survivable, second-strike or retaliatory forces. See also Assured Destruction; Unacceptable Damage.

MUTUAL FORCE REDUCTIONS (MFR): The original name (and one preferred by the East) for the Mutual and Balanced Force Reduction (MBFR) talks between NATO and the Warsaw Pact countries. The word "balanced" was included by the NATO countries seeking to reduce the asymmetry in force levels.

MUTUAL SECURITY TREATY (MST): Japan and the United States signed the Mutual Security Treaty in 1952 to ensure the defense of the Japanese island chain. In return for the right to maintain bases on Japanese territory, the United States assumed primary responsibility for the country's defense.

MVD: Ministry of Internal Affairs (USSR).

NATIONAL COMMAND AUTHORITIES (NCA): The president and the secretary of defense or their duly deputized alternates.

NATIONAL INTELLIGENCE ESTIMATE (NIE): A strategic estimate of capabilities, vulnerabilities, and probable courses of action of foreign nations that is produced at the national level as a composite of the views of the intelligence community. It can be formulated on a current topic or situation in a particular country at the direction of the director of central intelligence (DCI) and represents the pooled judgment of the U.S. intelligence community in policy making at the highest levels of government.

NATIONAL INTERESTS: A highly generalized concept of elements that constitute a state's compelling needs, including self-preservation, independence, national integrity, military security, and economic well-being.

NATIONAL OBJECTIVES: The fundamental aims, goals, or purposes of a nation toward which policies are directed and energies are applied. These may be short, mid, or long-range in nature.

NATIONAL POLICY: A broad course of action or guiding statements adopted by a government to help meet national objectives.

NATIONAL POWER: The sum total of any nation's capabilities or potential derived from available political, economic, military, geographic, social, scientific, and technological resources. Leadership and national will are the unifying factors. See also Combat Power; National Will.

NATIONAL SECURITY: The protection of a nation from all types of external aggression, espionage, hostile reconnaissance, sabotage, subversion, annoyance, and other inimical influences.

NATIONAL SECURITY COUNCIL (NSC): The primary functions of the NSC, created by the National Security Act of 1947, include policy coordination, advice, planning, and crisis management. While serving as the focal point for ideas and initiatives within the national security community, the council's nature and role vary greatly with the personality and desires of the president it serves.

NATIONAL STRATEGY: The art and science of developing and applying the political, economic, psychological, and military power of a nation during peace and war to meet national objectives.

NATIONAL TECHNICAL MEANS (NTM) OF VERIFICATION: Techniques under national control for monitoring compliance with the provisions of an agreement, e.g., reconnaissance via satellite overflight.

NATIONAL WILL: The temper and morale of the people, as they influence a nation's ability to satisfy national security interests or attain national security objectives. See also Combat Power; National Objectives; National Power; National Security.

NATO: See North Atlantic Treaty Organization.

NBC: Nuclear, biological, and chemical weapons.

NEUTRALITY: In international law, the attitude of impartiality, during periods of war, adopted by third states toward belligerents and recognized by the belligerents, which creates rights and duties between the impartial states and the belligerents. In a UN enforcement action, the rules of neutrality apply to impartial members of the United Nations except insofar as they are excluded by the obligation of such under the United Nations Charter. See also Nonalignment.

NEUTRON BOMB: See Enhanced Radiation Weapon.

NEW LOOK: See Massive Retaliation.

NIXON DOCTRINE: Pronounced by President Richard Nixon in 1970, the Nixon Doctrine pledged to U.S. allies that in deterring nuclear warfare primary reliance would remain with American forces, but that at the local warfare level the primary defense burden would fall on the country threatened. The Nixon Doctrine (also known as the Guam Doctrine) reflected domestic pressures to reduce defense spending and overseas commitments.

NNA: Neutral and nonaligned states.

NOMENKLATURA: Ruling elite jobs that are designated by the Communist Party (USSR).

NONALIGNMENT: The political attitude of a state that does not associate or identify itself with the political ideology or objective espoused by other states, groups of states, or international causes, or with the foreign policies stemming therefrom. It does not preclude involvement, but expresses the attitude of no precommitment to a particular state (or bloc) or policy before a situation arises. See also Neutrality.

NONCENTRAL SYSTEM: A U.S. term for nuclear weapons systems other than central systems; generally tactical systems with an alliance or regional orientation.

NONPROLIFERATION TREATY (NPT): The treaty to prohibit the spread of nuclear weapons or the technology to build them to states that do not possess this capability. See Arms Control.

NORTH ATLANTIC TREATY ORGANIZATION (NATO): A regional organization formed in 1949 by the North Atlantic Treaty. Its primary mission is to deter and defend the North Atlantic area against aggression by Warsaw Pact nations. Current membership includes Belgium, the United Kingdom, Denmark, West Germany, Greece, Iceland, Italy, Luxembourg, the Netherlands, Norway, Portugal, Turkey, Canada, France, Spain, and the United States.

NTH COUNTRY: A reference to additions to the group of powers possessing nuclear weapons—the next country of a series to acquire nuclear capabilities.

NUCLEAR CLUB: A slang term referring to countries that have developed their own nuclear weapons capability.

NUCLEAR DELIVERY SYSTEM: A nuclear weapon, together with its means of propulsion and associated installations. Includes carriers such as aircraft, ships, rockets, and motor vehicles.

NUCLEAR-FREE ZONES: Areas in which the production and stationing of nuclear weapons are prohibited. The Treaty for the Prohibition of Nuclear Weapons in Latin America, for example, came into force in 1968.

NUCLEAR PARITY: A condition at a given point in time when opposing forces possess nuclear offensive and defensive systems approximately equal in overall combat effectiveness. See also Essential Equivalence; Parity.

NUCLEAR PROLIFERATION: See Proliferation of Nuclear Weapons.

NUCLEAR THRESHOLD: The psychological line between conventional and nuclear warfare. The difficulty of crossing this threshold varies directly with a state's reluctance to use nuclear weapons.

NUCLEAR UMBRELLA: The protection that the United States offers to friendly nations with its deterrent forces. This protection against aggression is provided by linking the security of another country to use of U.S. nuclear weapons.

NUCLEAR YIELD: The energy released in the detonation of a nuclear weapon, measured in terms of the kilotons or megatons of trinitrotoluene (TNT) required to produce the same energy release. Yields are categorized as: very low—less than 1 kiloton; low—1 to 10 kilotons; medium—over 10 kilotons to 50 kilotons; high—over 50 kilotons to 500 kilotons; and very high—over 500 kilotons. See also Kiloton Weapon; Megaton Weapon; TNT Equivalent.

NVA: Nationale Volksarmee (National People's Army, GDR).

OAS: Organization of American States.

OECD: Organization for Economic Cooperation and Development.

OFFICE OF MANAGEMENT AND BUDGET (OMB): The agency in the Executive Office of the President having primary responsibility for efficient and economical conduct of government operations and for budget preparation and administration.

OLDER HEAVY BALLISTIC MISSILE LAUNCHER: A term in the SALT negotiations referring to a ballistic missile launcher for an ICBM of a type deployed before 1964 that has a volume significantly greater than the largest light ICBM operational in 1972. The U.S. Titan II and Soviet SS-7 and SS-8 launchers are examples. See also Modern Large Ballistic Missile (MLBM).

OMB: See Office of Management and Budget.

OPERATIONS RESEARCH: The analytical study of military problems, undertaken to provide responsible commanders and staff agencies with a scientific basis for decision on actions to improve military operations. See also Systems Analysis.

ORDER OF BATTLE: The identification, strength, command structure, and disposition of the personnel, units, and equipment of any military force.

OSD: Office of the U.S. Secretary of Defense.

OSTPOLITIK: FRG policy of détente and expanded relations with the East.

OVERKILL: Destructive capabilities in excess of those that should logically be adequate to destroy specified targets and/or attain specific security objectives.

OVERPRESSURE: The pressure resulting from the blast wave of an explosion. It is referred to as "positive" when it exceeds atmospheric pressure and "negative" during the passage of the wave when resulting pressures are less than atmospheric pressure. See also Hardened Site; Hard Target.

OVER-THE-HORIZON: A radar system that makes use of the atmospheric reflection and refraction phenomena to extend its range of detection beyond line-of-sight. Over-the-horizon radars may be either forward-scatter or back-scatter systems.

PALESTINE LIBERATION ORGANIZATION (PLO): The PLO was established to represent the Palestinian Arabs. The organization has served as a base for much anti-Israeli guerrilla activity. Its role in the settlement of Middle East problems is an issue of contention, with Israel refusing to recognize it as the legitimate representative of Palestinian Arabs.

PARAMILITARY FORCES: Forces or groups of any country that are distinct from its regular armed forces but resembling them in organization, equipment, training, or mission.

PARITY: A force-structure standard that demands that capabilities or specific forces and weapons systems be approximately equal in effectiveness to enemy counterparts. See also Essential Equivalence; Nuclear Parity.

PASSIVE AIR DEFENSE: All measures, other than active defense, taken to minimize the effects of hostile air action. These include the use of cover, concealment, camouflage, deception, dispersion, and protective construction, e.g., missile site hardening. See also Active Air Defense; Hardened Site; Hard Target.

PASSIVE DEFENSE: All measures, other than the use of armed force, taken to minimize the effects of hostile action. These include the use of cover, concealment, dispersion, protective construction, mobility, and subterfuge. See also Active Defense; Civil Defense.

PAUSE: In the defense of Western Europe, a moment of reflection imposed on any aggressor before the defense resorts to nuclear weapons, i.e., one function of NATO's conventional troop strength is to make such pause possible.

PAYLOAD: The weapon or cargo capacity of any aircraft or missile system, expressed variously in pounds, numbers of bombs, air-to-air and air-to-surface missiles, CW canisters, guns, sensors, ECM packets, etc.; and in terms of missile warhead yields (kilotons, megatons). See also Throw Weight.

PD (PRESIDENTIAL DECISION): A document associated with the Carter administration.

PEACEKEEPER: Also known as Missile X, or the MX missile, it is the latest-generation operational U.S. ICBM. it carries ten warheads and has significant hard target killing capabilities. See also Missile Experimental.

PENETRATION AIDS ("PEN" AIDS): Techniques and/or devices employed by offensive aerospace weapon systems to increase the probability of penetration of enemy defenses.

PEOPLE'S WAR: As defined under Mao in the People's Republic of China, People's War involves defending the country with armed infantry forces, guerrilla units, and a large popular militia. The requirements of minimum deterrence guide deployment of nuclear weapons. The sectors of Chinese society advocating People's War envision a significant political role for the armed forces and constitute one pole in a continuing struggle over what military doctrine to follow. See also People's War Under Modern Conditions.

PEOPLE'S WAR UNDER MODERN CONDITIONS: This concept implied a shift in doctrinal emphasis (versus People's War) for the armed forces of the People's Republic of China. Conventional defense is stressed more than reliance on militia forces, and the armed forces' political role is relatively reduced.

PERESTROIKA: Restructuring (USSR).

PERMISSIVE ACTION LINK (PAL): A device included in, or attached to, a nuclear weapons system to preclude arming and launching until the insertion of a prescribed discrete code or combination. It may include equipment and cabling external to the weapon or weapons system to activate components within the weapon or weapon system.

PLA (PEOPLE'S LIBERATION ARMY): The formal designation of the armed forces of the People's Republic of China.

PLUTON: A French land-mobile tactical nuclear weapon with a maximum range of 120 km and a warhead of 15 or 25 kilotons. It is to be succeeded by a new version known as "Hades."

POLARIS: An underwater/surface-launched, surface-to-surface, solid propellant ballistic missile with inertial guidance and nuclear warhead. Designated as UGM-27. See also Ballistic Missile; Inertial Guidance System; Sea/Submarine-launched Ballistic Missile (SLBM).

POLITBURO: The highest Soviet policy-making body, with ten to fifteen full members. Although the Politburo's operation is cloaked in secrecy, it is known that military influence in the body varies with the changing composition of its membership.

POLITICAL CONSULTATIVE COMMITTEE: A Soviet-dominated, high-level Warsaw Pact committee composed of the Communist party first secretaries, heads of government, and defense and foreign ministers from each member. The committee ostensibly serves as the pact's policy-formulation organ.

POSEIDON: The Poseidon submarine-launched ballistic missile, which gave MIRV capability to the U.S. SLBM arsenal.

POWER: See National Power.

PPBS (PLANNING, PROGRAMMING, AND BUDGETING SYSTEM): A resource management process used by the U.S. Department of Defense to provide military capabilities to meet defined national security objectives.

PRC: People's Republic of China.

PRECAUTIONARY LAUNCH: The launching of nuclear-loaded aircraft under imminent nuclear attack so as to preclude their destruction.

PREEMPTIVE ATTACK: An attack initiated on the basis of incontrovertible evidence that an enemy attack is imminent. See also Preventive War.

PRESIDENTIAL REVIEW MEMORANDUM (PRM): Under the Carter administration, Presidential Review Memoranda functioned within the National Security System. They defined a particular security-related problem, set a deadline, and assigned the study to one of two NSC committees—the Policy Review Committee or the Special Coordinating Committee. The responsible committee investigated the issue and made a recommendation to the President on any action to be taken.

PREVENTIVE WAR: A war initiated in the belief that military conflict, while not imminent, is inevitable, and that to delay would involve greater risk. See also Preemptive Attack.

PRINCIPLES OF WAR: A collection of abstract considerations that have been distilled from historical experience and that, applied to specific circumstances with acumen, assist strategists and tacticians in selecting suitable courses of action.

PROLIFERATION OF NUCLEAR WEAPONS: The acquisition of national nuclear capabilities by states not previously possessing them, either by the dissemination by nuclear powers of weapons or information necessary for their manufacture or by the development of domestic nuclear weapons programs. See also Nth Country; Nuclear Club.

PROPAGANDA: Any form of communication in support of national objectives designed to influence the opinions, emotions, attitudes, or behavior of any group in order to benefit the sponsor, either directly or indirectly.

PROPORTIONAL DETERRENCE: Medium powers can obtain proportional deterrence by deploying enough nuclear striking power to inflict unacceptable damage—damage that would outweigh any gain anticipated by the attacker—on any aggressor. Proportional deterrence is the foundation of France's *force de dissuasion*, as it theoretically protects France from superpower aggression even with a far smaller nuclear force.

PROTOCOL OF 1974: In conjunction with the ABM treaty of SALT I, the 1974 protocol limits the United States and the USSR to one ABM site each, with a maximum of 100 ABM launchers deployed.

PROXY WAR: A form of limited war in which great powers avoid a direct confrontation by furthering their national security interests and objectives through conflicts between their respective representatives or associates sometimes referred to as "clients." See also Limited War.

PSYCHOLOGICAL WARFARE: The planned use of propaganda and other psychological actions having the primary purpose of influencing the opinions, emotions, attitudes, and behavior of hostile foreign groups in such a way as to support the achievement of national objectives. See also National Objectives; Propaganda.

PVO-STRANY: See Air Defense Forces of the USSR.

PYRRHIC VICTORY: The attainment of national security objectives at a cost so high in proportion to gains that national interests suffer. See also National Interests; National Security.

RADIUS OF ACTION: The maximum distance a ship, aircraft, or vehicle can travel away from its base along a given course with normal combat load and return without refueling, allowing for all safety and operation factors. See also Long-Range Bomber Aircraft; Medium Bomber.

RAPID DEPLOYMENT FORCE (RDF): A U.S. troop force originally proposed for the United States by President Carter with the capability of rapid deployment anywhere in the world, but particularly in response to threats to oil supply lines in the Persian Gulf. See also Carter Doctrine.

RAPID RELOAD CAPACITY: The ability of a strategic nuclear delivery system to conduct multiple strikes. This characteristic presently is confined to aircraft, but landmobile missiles and hard-site ICBMs have the potential. Submarines conceivably could be replenished at sea, but a significantly greater time lag would occur. See also Cold Launch.

R AND D: Research and Development.

REAGAN DOCTRINE: Usually refers to the commitment by the Reagan administration to support anti-communist movements (e.g., support for the "Contras" in Nicaragua).

REENTRY VEHICLE (RV): That portion of a ballistic missile designed to carry a nuclear warhead and to reenter the earth's atmosphere in the terminal portion of the missile's trajectory. See also Maneuverable Reentry Vehicle (MaRV); Multiple Independently Targetable Reentry Vehicle (MIRV); Multiple Reentry Vehicle (MRV).

RENAMO: Mozambique National Resistance Movement—supported by South Africa. See also FRELIMO.

RESERVE COMPONENT: Armed forces not in active service. U.S. reserve components include the Army National Guard and Army Reserve; the Naval Reserve; the Marine Corps Reserve; the Air National Guard, and the Air Force Reserve.

RESIDUAL FORCES: Unexpended portions of remaining forces in a military operation that have immediate combat potential and have been deliberately withheld from battle.

REVOLUTIONARY WAR: Efforts to seize political power, destroying existing systems of government and social structures in the process.

RODINA: Motherland (USSR).

SALT: See Strategic Arms Limitation Talks.

SANCTIONS: An economic warfare tool, usually adopted by several states acting in concert, to compel a country or coalition of countries to cease undesirable practices or otherwise bow to the wielder's will. See also Compellence; Economic Warfare.

SCC: See Standing Consultative Commission.

SCG: Special Consultative Group in NATO that meets on matters relating to allied nuclear forces.

SDF: Self-Defense Forces (Japan).

SEA CONTROL: The employment of naval forces, supplemented by land and aerospace forces as appropriate, to destroy enemy naval forces, suppress enemy oceangoing commerce, protect vital shipping lanes, and establish local superiority in areas of naval operations.

SEA-LAUNCHED CRUISE MISSILE (SLCM): A cruise missile capable of being launched from a submerged or surfaced submarine or from a surface ship. See also Air-launched Cruise Missile (ALCM); Cruise Missile; Sea-launched Ballistic Missile (SLBM).

SEA/SUBMARINE-LAUNCHED BALLISTIC MISSILE (SLBM): A ballistic missile carried in and launched from a submarine (also called fleet ballistic missiles, or FBM). SLBMs, along with strategic bombers and ICBMs, comprise the basic "triad" structure of the U.S. strategic deterrent force. Excluded in this category are cruise missiles, which, although carried by and launched from submarines, do not fly a ballistic trajectory. Polaris, Poseidon, and Trident are examples of U.S. and the SS-N-6, SS-N-8, SS-N-20, and SS-N-23 are examples of Soviet SLBMs that have been deployed. See also Ballistic Missile; Cruise Missile; Fleet Ballistic Missile Submarine (SSBN); Polaris; Sea-launched Cruise Missile (SLCM).

SECOND STRIKE: The first counterblow of a war, generally associated with nuclear operations.

SECOND-STRIKE CAPABILITY: The ability to survive a first strike with sufficient resources to deliver an effective counterblow—generally associated with nuclear weapons. See also Assured Destruction; First Strike; Mutually Assured Destruction; Unacceptable Damage.

SED: The Communist Party in East Germany.

SENSORS: Devices used to detect objects or environmental conditions. Examples are radar and optical systems used in missile and aircraft warning/tracking/engagement systems, seismographs used in detection of underground nuclear tests, and devices used to detect long-range emissions from nuclear tests that vent to the atmosphere.

SHAPE: Supreme Headquarters, Allied Powers Europe, NATO's military headquarters near Mons, Belgium.

SHORT-RANGE BALLISTIC MISSILE (SRBM): A ballistic missile with a range up to about 600 nautical miles. The Lance is an example of a U.S. SRBM that is currently deployed. See also Ballistic Missile; Intercontinental Ballistic Missile (ICBM).

SHOW OF FORCE: The purposeful exhibition of armed might before an enemy or potential enemy, usually in a crisis situation, to reinforce deterrent demands. See also Symbolic Attack.

SINO-SOVIET PACT OF 1950: The result of determined bargaining between Mao Zedong and Josef Stalin, the Sino-Soviet Pact of 1950 committed each country to thirty years of mutual security and friendship. In it the USSR also pledged to provide China with $300 million in economic aid and to return Manchurian rail and port facilities it had acquired in 1945.

SIOP: Single Integrated Operations Plan. This plan is the overall coordinating plan for carrying out U.S. strategic doctrine and operations.

SLBM (SEA-LAUNCHED BALLISTIC MISSILE): A ballistic missile carried in and launched from a submarine.

SLCM (SEA-LAUNCHED CRUISE MISSILE): A cruise missile carried by and launched from a surface ship or submarine.

SNDV: Strategic Nuclear Delivery Vehicle.

SOFT TARGET: A target not protected against the blast, heat, and radiation produced by nuclear explosions. There are many degrees of softness. Some missiles and aircraft, for example, are built in ways that ward off certain effects, but they are "soft" in comparison with shelters and silos. See also Hardened Site; Hard Targets; Overpressure.

SORTIE (AIR): An operational flight by one aircraft. See also Flight.

SPD: Social Democratic Party, a left-of-center party in the FRG. See also CDU, CSU, FDP, Greens.

SPECIAL FORCES: See U.S. Army Special Forces.

SPECIFIED COMMAND: A top-echelon U.S. combatant organization with regional or functional responsibilities, which normally is composed of forces under direction of one military service. It has a broad, continuing mission and is established by the president, through the secretary of defense, with the advice and assistance of the Joint Chiefs of Staff. See also Unified Command.

SPECTRUM OF WAR: A term that encompasses the full range of conflict—cold, limited, and general war. See also Cold War; Conflict Spectrum; General War; Limited War.

SPETSNAZ: Special Forces (USSR).

SQUADRON: An organization consisting of two or more divisions of ships or two or more (navy) divisions or flights of aircraft. It is normally, but not necessarily, composed of ships or aircraft of the same type. Also the basic administration unit of the U.S. Army, Navy, Marine Corps, and Air Force. An air force squadron is a component of a wing. See also Flight.

SRBM: See Short-Range Ballistic Missile.

SRF: Strategic Rocket Forces (USSR).

SSBN (STRATEGIC SUBMARINE, BALLISTIC, NUCLEAR): A nuclear-powered submarine equipped to carry and launch ballistic missiles.

SSOD: Special Session on Disarmament in the United Nations.

STANDARDIZATION: The adoption of like or similar military equipment, ammunition, supplies, and operational, logistical, and administrative procedures among countries of an alliance. See also Interoperability.

STANDING CONSULTATIVE COMMISSION (SCC): A permanent U.S.–Soviet commission established in accordance with the provisions of the ABM treaty. Its purpose is "to promote the objectives and implementation of the provisions" of the treaty and subsequent agreements in which SCC jurisdiction is specified. The SCC was established in December 1972 and has since met regularly. See also Antiballistic Missile System (ABM); Strategic Arms Limitations Talks (SALT).

START: Strategic Arms Reduction Talks. Talks between the superpowers aimed not just at limits or caps on numbers of deployed offensive systems (as under SALT), but rather at verifiable *reductions* in the arsenals of strategic nuclear weapons of both superpowers.

STRAIT OF TIRAN: A vital choke point between the Sinai Peninsula and Saudi Arabia that controls Israeli access to the Red Sea. Closure of the Strait of Tiran by President Gamal Abdel Nasser in the spring of 1967 helped bring on the 1967 Middle East War.

STRATEGIC: Relates to a nation's military, economic, and political power and its ability to control the course of military and political events.

STRATEGIC ADVANTAGE: The overall relative relations of opponents that enable one nation or group of nations effectively to control the course of a military or political situation.

STRATEGIC AIRLIFT: Transport aircraft, both military and civilian, used to move armed forces, equipment, and supplies expeditiously over long distances, especially intercontinentally. See also Civil Reserve Air Fleet (CRAF); Military Airlift Command (MAC).

STRATEGIC AIR WARFARE: Air combat and supporting operations designed to effect the progressive destruction and disintegration of the enemy's war-making capacity through the systematic application of force to a selected series of vital targets to a point where he no longer retains the ability or the will to wage war. Vital targets may include key manufacturing systems, sources of raw material, critical material, stockpiles, power systems, transportation systems, communication facilities, concentrations of uncommitted elements of enemy armed forces, key agricultural areas, and other such target systems. See also Counterforce; Countervalue; Residual Forces.

STRATEGIC ARMS LIMITATION TALKS (SALT): The Strategic Arms Limitation Talks between the United States and the USSR were begun in 1969. SALT I, concluded in 1972, encompassed the Treaty on the Limitation of Antiballistic Missile Systems and the Interim Agreement on Certain Measures with Respect to the Limitations of Strategic Offensive Arms. The agreement essentially froze the number of ballistic launchers, operational or under construction, at existing levels. The protocol of 1974 to the treaty on the limitation of ABM systems restricts each side to a single ABM site with a maximum of 100 launchers deployed. The SALT II negotiations began in November 1972 and resulted in a 1979 agreement on limits relating to development, testing, and deployment of weapons systems categorized as strategic offense, but the proposed treaty was never ratified.

STRATEGIC BALANCE: See Military Balance and Correlation of Forces.

STRATEGIC DEFENSE: The strategy and forces designed primarily to protect a nation, its outposts, and possibly its allies from the hazards of general war. It features defense against missiles, both land and sea-launched, and long-range bombers. See also Strategic Offense.

STRATEGIC DELIVERY VEHICLE: A vehicle capable of delivering a strategic nuclear weapon. Manned bombers, sea-launched ballistic missiles, and land-based ballistic missiles are examples of strategic delivery vehicles currently deployed by the world's nuclear powers. Also referred to as the Strategic Nuclear Delivery Vehicle, or SNDV.

STRATEGIC MOBILITY: The ability to shift personnel,

equipment, and supplies effectively and expeditiously between theaters of operation. See also Strategic Airlift.

STRATEGIC OFFENSE: The strategy and forces designed primarily to destroy the enemy's war-making capacity during general war or to so degrade it that the opposition collapses. See also Counterforce; General War; Strategic Defense.

STRATEGIC RESERVE: Uncommitted forces of a country or coalition of countries that are intended to support national security interests and objectives, as required. See also National Interests; National Objectives; Residual Forces.

STRATEGIC RETALIATORY (CONCEPTS AND FORCES): Second-strike strategies and forces designed primarily to destroy the enemy's war-making capacity during general war or to so degrade it that the opposition collapses. See also Combat Power; General War; Second Strike; Second-Strike Capability; Strategic Offense.

STRATEGIC SIGNAL: An act, attitude, or communication that conveys threats or promises intended to influence enemy decisions.

STRATEGIC STABILITY: Strategic stability encompasses both crisis stability and arms stability and refers to relations in which neither side has an incentive to initiate the use of strategic nuclear forces in a crisis or perceives the necessity to undertake major new arms programs to avoid being placed at a strategic disadvantage. See also Arms Stability; Crisis Stability.

STRATEGY: The art and science of developing and using political, economic, psychological, and military force as necessary during peace and war to afford the maximum support to policies, in order to increase the probabilities and favorable consequences of victory and to lessen the chances of defeat. See also Direct Approach; Grand Strategy; Indirect Approach; Military Strategy; National Strategy; Tactics.

SUBMARINE (SSBM, SSB, SSN, SS, SSG, SSGN): A warship designed for operations under the surface of the seas. Nuclear-powered submarines are given the letter designation N. U.S. nuclear-powered submarines that carry SLBMs are known as SSBNs. Soviet SSBNs include the H, Y, C, D, and T classes. Attack submarines, designated SS or SSN, are used to attack enemy surface ships and submarines. Submarines designed for launching cruise missiles are designated SSGN or SSG, and include the Soviet J, W, E, C, and O class submarines. The Soviet long-range, diesel-powered ballistic missile submarines (Golf class) are designated SSB. The Soviet Union has deployed all of the above types of submarines. See also Ballistic Missile; Fleet Ballistic Missile Submarine (SSBN); Polaris; Sea/submarine-launched Ballistic Missile (SLBM); Sea/submarine-launched Cruise Missile (SLCM).

SUBVERSION: Action designed to undermine the military, economic, psychological, morale, or political strength of a regime. See also Propaganda; Unconventional War.

SUFFICIENCY: A force structure standard that demands capabilities adequate to attain desired ends without undue waste. Superiority thus is essential in some circumstances; parity or "essential equivalence" suffices under less demanding conditions; and inferiority, qualitative as well as quantitative, is sometimes

deemed acceptable as in forces designed for "proportional deterrence." See also Essential Equivalence; Parity.

SURFACE-TO-AIR MISSILE (SAM): Surface-launched missile designed to operate against a target above the earth's surface.

SURFACE-TO-SURFACE MISSILE (SSM): A surface-launched missile designed to operate against a target on the earth's surface.

SURVEILLANCE: The systematic observation of aerospace, surface, or subsurface areas, places, persons, or things by visual, aural, electronic, photographic, or other means. See also National Technical Means of Verification.

SURVIVABILITY: The ability of armed forces and civilian communities to withstand attack and still function effectively. It is derived mainly from passive and active defenses. See also Active Defense; Passive Defense.

SYMBOLIC ATTACK: A specialized form of exemplary attack that deliberately avoids casualties or damage, but nevertheless communicates a message to the enemy. A display of nuclear fire power near a great city just outside the radius of destruction would serve symbolic purposes. See also Exemplary Attack; Strategic Signal.

SYSTEMS ANALYSIS: An interdisciplinary technique used by strategic planners. It isolates and examines relevant facts, logical propositions, and assumptions in ways that highlight alternatives, so that decision makers can apply judgment sagaciously and relations between ends and means can be optimized. See also Operations Research.

TACIT ARMS CONTROL AGREEMENT: An arms control course of action in which two or more nations participate without any formal agreement having been made. See also Arms Control.

TACTICAL: A term referring to battlefield operations in general.

TACTICAL NUCLEAR DELIVERY VEHICLE (TNDV): Nuclear delivery vehicles designed to be employed against enemy targets in a limited conflict. Usually relating to vehicles of shorter range than those necessary for the conduct of strategic operations. See also Strategic Delivery Vehicle.

TACTICAL NUCLEAR WEAPONS: Nuclear weapons usually with a range of less than 100 km. Examples include nuclear warheads delivered by artillery pieces and the French Pluton short-range missile.

TACTICAL NUCLEAR WEAPON (TNW) FORCES OR OPERATIONS: Nuclear combat power expressly designed for deterrent, offensive, and defensive purposes that contributes to the accomplishments of localized military missions; the threatened or actual application of such power. May be employed in general as well as limited wars. See also General War; Limited War; Strategic Defense; Strategic Offense.

TACTICS: The detailed methods used to carry out strategic designs. Military tactics involve the employment of units in combat, including the arrangement and maneuvering of units in relation to each other and to the enemy. See also Military Strategy; Strategy.

TALIONIC ATTACK: A "tit-for-tat" exchange. The punishment inflicted by defenders corresponds in kind and degree to the injuries they received, as in "an eye for an eye" approach.

TANK, MAIN BATTLE: A tracked vehicle providing heavy armor protection and serving as the principal assault weapon of armored and infantry troops. See also Heavy Tank; Light Tank; Medium Tank.

TARGET ACQUISITION SYSTEM: A system that detects, identifies, and locates a target in enough detail to allow effective use of weapons.

TARGET LIST: The list of targets maintained and promulgated by the senior echelon of command; it identifies those targets to be engaged by supporting arms, as distinct from a list that may be maintained by any echelon as confirmed, suspect, or possible targets for informational and planning purposes.

TARGET OF OPPORTUNITY: A target visible to a surface or air sensor or observer that is within range of available weapons and against which fire has not been scheduled or requested.

TERMINAL GUIDANCE SYSTEM: A system that directs a missile between midcourse and its arrival in the vicinity of the target. The purpose of such systems is to achieve greater accuracy.

THEATER: In American usage, the geographical area outside the continental United States for which a commander of a unified or specified command has been assigned military responsibility. See also Specified Command; Unified Command.

THEATER NUCLEAR WEAPONS (TNW): Nuclear weapons below the strategic level deployed for use within a particular geographic area such as Europe.

THERMONUCLEAR: An adjective referring to the process (or processes) in which very high temperatures are used to bring about the fusion of light nuclei, with accompanying liberation of energy. See also Fission; Fusion; Thermonuclear Weapon.

THERMONUCLEAR WEAPON: A weapon in which very high temperatures are used to bring about the fusion of light nuclei such as those of hydrogen isotopes (e.g., deuterium and tritium) with the accompanying release of energy. The high temperatures required are obtained by means of fission. See also Fission; Fusion.

THINK TANK: A private company specializing in defense-related research and analysis.

THREE-PERCENT GUIDELINE: In response to the growing strength of Warsaw Pact forces, the NATO countries pledged themselves in 1977 to an annual growth rate in defense spending of 3 percent (real growth). Meeting this guideline proved to be problematic. See also Cost Sharing.

THRESHOLD: An intangible and adjustable line between levels and types of conflicts, such as the separation between nuclear and non-nuclear warfare. The greater the reluctance to use nuclear weapons, the higher the threshold. See also Firebreak.

THROW WEIGHT: Ballistic missile throw weight is the maximum useful weight that has been flight-tested on the boost stages of the missile. The useful weight includes weight of the reentry vehicles (RVs), penetration ("Pen") aids, dispensing and release mechanisms, reentry shrouds, covers, buses, and propulsion devices with their propellants (but not the final boost stages) which are present at the end of the boost phase.

TIME-SENSITIVE TARGET: Any counterforce target that is vulnerable only if it can be struck before it is launched (as with bombers and missiles) or rede-ployed (as with ground combat troops and ships). See also Counterforce.

TITAN: A liquid-propellant, two-stage, rocket-powered intercontinental ballistic missile equipped with a nuclear warhead. No longer in service as an ICBM, it has also been used as a space booster.

TNT EQUIVALENT: A measure of the energy released from the detonation of a nuclear weapon, or from the explosion of a given quantity of fissionable of fusionable material, in terms of the amount of trinitrotoluene (TNT) that would release the same amount of energy when exploded. See also Kiloton Weapon; Megaton Weapon; Yield.

TOOTH-TO-TAIL RATIO: The proportion of combat forces to administrative or logistics support in a nation's armed forces and in specific military organizations such as divisions, air wings, and fleets. See also Division; Wing.

TRANSPORT AIRCRAFT: Aircraft designed primarily for carrying personnel or cargo.

TRANSPORTER-ERECTOR-LAUNCHER (TEL): A surface vehicle in which land-mobile ballistic missiles can be moved into position, prepared for launch, and fired.

TREATY OF FRIENDSHIP, COOPERATION, AND MUTUAL ASSISTANCE (TFCMA): Bilateral treaties that the USSR has signed with East Germany, Finland, and a number of other states.

TRIAD: In U.S. usage, a term commonly used to refer to the basic structure of the U.S. strategic deterrent force. It is comprised of land-based ICBMs, the strategic bomber force, and the Polaris/Poseidon/Trident submarine fleet. The U.S. triad of forces evolved from an allocation of national resources and priorities in order to meet certain strategic objectives, the most important of which was the capability to deter nuclear conflict. Each element of the triad relies on somewhat different means for survival; hence, an enemy's potential for a successful first-strike attack is severely complicated. Bombers rely on warning, fast reaction, and ground or airborne dispersal for survival. The ICBMs are placed in individual hardened silos for survivability. SLBMs depend on the uncertainty of location of the submarine to enhance survivability. In NATO usage, "triad" also refers to the three-part mix of central-strategic nuclear (ICBMs, SLBMs, and bombers), theater nuclear, and conventional forces. See also Bomber; Deterrence; Hardened Site; Intercontinental Ballistic Missile (ICBM); Sea/Submarine-launched Ballistic Missile (SLBM).

TRIDENT: A general descriptive term for the sea-based strategic weapons system consisting of the highly survivable nuclear-powered Trident submarine, long-range Trident ballistic missiles, and the integrated refit facilities required to support the submarine and missile subsystems, as well as associated personnel.

TRIPWIRE: A largely symbolic force positioned on an ally's soil to advertise commitment to a particular country or coalition of countries. Attacks against the token force would trigger a massive response. U.S. forces in Europe have been said to have been serving a "tripwire" function.

TRIPWIRE CONCEPT: Ground forces located near the border of a powerful potential invader can serve as a tripwire. Insufficient to repel the aggressor themselves, their engagement in a significant conflict would trigger large-scale escalation, usually entailing the use of nuclear weapons. As such, they serve a deterrent function. U.S. troops in West Germany and French infantry divisions along the Franco-German border are both known by this term.

TROMPE L'OEIL: A visual deception.

TUBE ARTILLERY: Howitzers and guns, as opposed to rockets and guided missiles. May be towed or self-propelled.

TURNAROUND TIME: The length of time necessary for servicing of an aircraft between operational missions.

TVD: Soviet theater of military operations.

TWO-MAN RULE (CONTROL): A system designed to prohibit access by an individual to nuclear weapons and certain designated components by requiring the presence at all times of at least two authorized persons, each capable of detecting incorrect or unauthorized procedures with respect to the task to be performed.

TWO-TRACK DECISION: See Dual-Track Decision.

TWO-WAY STREET: NATO objective that arms trade over the Atlantic be two-way, not just the U.S. selling to NATO allies.

TYPE I DETERRENCE: Deterrent power that inhibits direct attacks against the wielder's homeland. See also Deterrence; Type II Deterrence; Type III Deterrence.

TYPE II DETERRENCE: Deterrent power that inhibits serious infractions, short of attacks, against the wielder's homeland, such as aggression against friends or allies. See also Deterrence; Type I Deterrence; Type III Deterrence.

TYPE III DETERRENCE: Deterrent power that inhibits aggressive adventurism by making limited provocations appear unprofitable. See also Deterrence; Type I Deterrence; Type II Deterrence.

UNACCEPTABLE DAMAGE: Degrees of destruction anticipated from an enemy second strike that are sufficient to deter a nuclear power from launching a first strike. The degree of damage that will deter a first strike is a function, in part, of national value preferences and economic considerations and is therefore difficult or impossible to predict. See also Assured Destruction; First Strike; Mutually Assured Destruction; National Will; Second Strike.

UNCONVENTIONAL WARFARE: A broad spectrum of military and paramilitary operations conducted in enemy-held, enemy denied, or politically sensitive territory. Unconventional warfare includes but is not limited to, the interrelated fields of guerrilla warfare, evasion and escape, subversion, sabotage, direct action missions, and other operations of a low visibility, cover, or clandestine nature. These interrelated aspects of unconventional warfare may be prosecuted singly or collectively, but predominantly by indigenous personnel, usually supported and directed in varying degrees by an external source or sources during all conditions of war or peace. See also Conflict Spectrum; Guerrilla Warfare; Spectrum of War; Subversion.

UNIFIED COMMAND: In the U.S., a top-echelon combatant organization with regional or functional responsibilities, normally composed of forces from two or more military services. It has a broad, continuing mission and is established by the president, through the secretary of defense, with advice and assistance from the Joint Chiefs of Staff (JCS). See also Specified Command; Theater.

U.S. ARMY SPECIAL FORCES: Military personnel with cross-training in basic and specialized military skills organized into small, multiple-purpose detachments to train, organize, supply, direct, and control indigenous forces in guerrilla warfare and counterinsurgency operations and to conduct unconventional warfare operations. See also Counterinsurgency; Guerrilla Warfare; Unconventional Warfare.

U.S. COUNTRY TEAM: The senior in-country U.S. coordinating and supervising body, headed by the chief of the U.S. diplomatic mission—usually the ambassador—and composed of the senior member of each U.S. department or agency represented.

VERIFICATION: In arms control, any action, including inspection, detection, and identification, taken to ascertain compliance with agreed measures. See also Arms Control; National Technical Means of Verification.

VLADIVOSTOCK ACCORDS: President Gerald Ford and First Secretary Leonid Brezhnev met in Vladivostock in 1974 to discuss further limitations of strategic offensive arms. They agreed on four basic elements to be contained in a SALT II treaty: the new treaty would last through 1985; each side would be limited to 2,400 total nuclear delivery vehicles; each side would be limited to 1,320 MIRVed systems; and forward-based systems (such as U.S. nuclear-capable fighters in Europe) were not to be discussed. See also Strategic Arms Limitations Talks.

VLF: Very low frequency.

V/STOL: Vertical/short take-off and landing.

WAR-FIGHTING/WINNING DOCTRINE: This doctrine prescribes forces equipped to conduct and win a conflict at any level, to include the use of nuclear weapons. Such forces may be used for deterrence purposes by posing a credible challenge to any would-be attacker. Alternatively, should deterrence fail, they can be used for the warfighting purposes for which they were designed. War-fighting doctrine is usually associated with the USSR; however, the United States has also dealt with the possibility of having to fight at least limited nuclear war-fighting engagements.

WAR GAME: A simulation, by whatever means, of a military operation involving two or more opposing forces, using rules, data, and procedures designed to depict an actual or assumed real-life situation.

WARHEAD: That part of a missile, projectile, torpedo, rocket, or other munition that contains either a nuclear or thermonuclear system, high-explosive system, chemical or biological agent, or inert materials intended to inflict damage.

WAR POWERS ACT OF 1972: Initiated in response to dissatisfaction with presidential authority to conduct the Vietnam War, the War Powers Act attempts to reduce the president's authority to deploy armed forces abroad. Specifically, if the president commits American forces to battle on foreign soil, he must report his reasons to Congress within forty-eight hours and obtain congressional approval of the commitment within sixty days; otherwise, the commitment is to be halted. Some have questioned the constitutionality of these provisions because they infringe substantially on presidential prerogatives as commander-in-chief of the armed forces.

WARSAW PACT (WARSAW TREATY ORGANIZATION OR WTO): An East European military alliance that is committed to the defense of the member states' territory. The signatories are Bulgaria, Czechoslovakia, the German Democratic Republic (East Germany), Hungary, Poland, Romania, and the Soviet Union.

WEAPONS OF MASS DESTRUCTION: In arms control usage, weapons that are capable of a high order of destruction or of being used in such a manner as to destroy large numbers of people. These can be nuclear, chemical, biological, and radiological weapons. The term excludes the means of transporting or propelling the weapon where such means is a separable and divisible part of the weapon. See also Arms Control; CBR Weapon.

WEHRMACHT: German armed forces in World War II.

WEST BANK: A U.N. Resolution of 1947 set aside 2,270 square miles west of the Jordan River for the establishment of an independent Arab state. Jordan subsequently gained control of the area by the Israel–Jordan Armistice Agreement of 1949. Israel captured the West Bank in 1967, an acquisition making Israel far more defensible. Israeli control of the West Bank remains in dispute.

WEU: Western European Union.

WILL: See National Will.

WING: (1) In the U.S. Air Force, a unit composed normally of one primary mission group and the necessary supporting organization, i.e., organizations designed to render supply, maintenance, hospi- talization, and other services required by the primary mission groups. Two examples are a tactical air wing and a bomber wing. Primary missions groups may be functional, such as combat, training, transport, or service. (2) A fleet air wing is the basic organizational administrative unit for naval land and tender-based aviation. Such wings are mobile units to which aircraft squadrons and tenders are assigned for administrative control. See also Division.

YIELD: The force of a nuclear explosion expressed in terms of the number of tons of TNT that would have to be exploded to produce the same energy. See also Nuclear Yield; TNT Equivalent.

ZAHAL: Acronym for Zvah Haganah Le Israel—the Israel Defense Forces (IDF). The terms Zahal and IDF are often used interchangeably.

ZERO-BASED BUDGETING (ZBB): With the goal of matching expenditures to objectives, ZBB forces organizations to justify their total spending program for each new budget period. President Jimmy Carter implemented ZBB for the national government, and some state and local units also have used it. Different degrees of success have been reported.

ZERO-SUM GAME: A term expressing a relative situation in which there can only be one winner; one's gain is the other's equal and corresponding loss.

ZULU TIME: Greenwich mean time.

Index

Aaron, David, 51
Abu Nidal, 443
Acheson, Dean, 264
Achille Lauro, 297
Adelman, Kenneth, 372
Adenauer, Konrad, 143, 146, 149, 150, 154, 162, 163, 171
Advanced Technology Fighter (ATF), 303
Aeritalia, 303
Afghanistan, 80, 333, 641; Soviet invasion of, 68, 81, 87, 93, 122, 124, 130, 195, 524, 542, 603, 668; Soviet withdrawal from, 30, 69
Africa, 186, 495, 519n.129; France and, 213, 248, 252; Soviet Union and, 478, 481, 484, 485, 512
African National Congress (ANC), 483-84, 486, 492, 494, 496, 501, 503, 515n.26, 518n.117
Afrikaners, 476, 479, 480-81, 488, 496, 505, 512, 514n.4
Agriculture: Canada, 314; Italy, 292; Soviet Union, 91, 92
Aguilar Zinser, Adolfo, 578n.160
Ahn Byung-Joon, 412
Air forces: Canada, 327-28, 330; China, 368, 370; East Germany, 196; Egypt, 447, 449, 450, 471n.46, 474n.119; France, 211-12, 240, 241, 243-46; India, 523, 527-28, 530-31, 534, 535, 540, 541-42, 543, 543n.29, 545n.101; Israel, 445-46, 447-48, 451-52, 453, 454, 455-56, 459, 464, 470n.28, 472nn.75, 76, 474-75n.124; Italy, 294, 295, 303, 305; Japan, 389, 390, 393, 397, 399; Mexico, 559, 560, 562, 563, 564, 568, 569-70, 571-72, 577n.124; NATO, 272; North Korea, 405, 410; South Africa, 490-91, 509, 511; South Korea, 405, 409, 410, 416; Soviet Union, 30, 31, 116, 117, 119-20, 122-23, 124, 204n.61; U.K., 261, 267-68, 269, 282-84, 285; U.S., 28, 29, 64, 65, 326-27, 328, 350, 609, 685
Air Industries Association of Canada, 341
Akhromeyev, Sergei F., 85, 86, 87, 101, 104, 112, 127
Albonetti, Achille, 296
Alekseyev, N.N., 136n.150

Alexander, Arthur J., 232
Al Fatah, 440
Algeria, 186
Aliboni, Roberto, 300
Alisky, Marvin, 572
Allen, Richard, 49-50
Allende Gossens, Salvador, 69, 550
Alliances, 12, 17: Canada and, 312-13; French Union, 213; Mexico and, 573; Soviet Union and, 18-19, 79-80, 607; U.S. and, 18-19, 35-39, 57, 603. *See also* NATO; Warsaw Pact
Allied Command Europe Mobile Land Force (AMF[L]), 325, 331-32
Allison, Graham, 56, 592
Allon, Yigal, 463, 470n.19
Amalric, Jacques, 213
Anderson, Jack, 416
Andropov, Yuri, 76, 89, 190
Anglo-American Industrial Corporation, Ltd., 482
Angola, 186, 478, 482, 483, 484, 492, 496; South African invasion of, 485, 491, 493-94, 495, 501, 503; Soviet Union and, 31, 80, 125, 128-29
Antia, S.N., 538
Antiballistic missiles (ABM), 666; Canadian, 312, 331; Soviet, 30, 119, 120; U.S., 604-5
Antiballistic missile (ABM) Treaty (1972), 56, 57, 67, 68, 120, 126, 328, 329
Antimilitarism, 169
Antinuclear movement, 156
Antisatellite (ASAT) system: Soviet, 30; U.S., 56
Antisubmarine warfare (ASW), 97, 118-19; India, 526, 543n.26; Italy, 295, 303; Soviet, 120-21
ANZUS (U.S. treaty with Australia and New Zealand), 36, 38-39
Apartheid, 476, 478, 480-81, 483, 493, 496-97, 514n.4, 515n.13, 588
Apel, Hans, 163, 172
Arab League, 434
Arabs: armed forces, 442, 466-67, 472n.81, 473n.98; and Israel, 434-37, 439, 448-49, 456, 464-65, 469n.2, 586, 643-44; in Israel, 431-32, 440, 470n.19, 474n.117

Programming and Problem Solving with C++

Second Edition

Programming and Problem Solving with C++

Second Edition

Nell Dale
University of Texas, Austin

Chip Weems
University of Massachusetts, Amherst

Mark Headington
University of Wisconsin—La Crosse

JONES AND BARTLETT PUBLISHERS
Sudbury, Massachusetts
BOSTON   TORONTO   LONDON   SINGAPORE

World Headquarters
Jones and Bartlett Publishers
40 Tall Pine Drive
Sudbury, MA 01776
978-443-5000
info@jbpub.com
www.jbpub.com

Jones and Bartlett Publishers Canada
2100 Bloor St. West
Suite 6-272
Toronto, ON M6S 5A5
CANADA

Jones and Bartlett Publishers International
Barb House, Barb Mews
London W6 7PA
UK

CHIEF EXECUTIVE OFFICER: Clayton Jones
CHIEF OPERATING OFFICER: Don Jones, Jr.
PUBLISHER: Tom Walker
V.P., SALES AND MARKETING: Tom Manning
V.P., COLLEGE EDITORIAL DIRECTOR: Brian L. McKean
V.P., DIRECTOR OF INTERACTIVE TECHNOLOGY: Mike Campbell
V.P., MANAGING EDITOR: Judith H. Hauck
MARKETING DIRECTOR: Rich Pirozzi
MARKETING MANAGER: Jennifer M. Jacobson
DIRECTOR OF DESIGN AND PRODUCTION: Anne Spencer
SENIOR ACQUISITIONS EDITOR: J. Michael Stranz
PRODUCTION EDITOR: Rebecca S. Marks
DIRECTOR OF MANUFACTURING AND INVENTORY CONTROL: Therese Bräuer
COVER DESIGN: Anne Spencer
TEXT DESIGN: George McLean
COMPOSITION: PageMasters & Company
PRINTING AND BINDING: Courier Companies
COVER PRINTING: Courier Companies

Library of Congress Cataloging-in-Publication Data
Dale, Nell B.
   Programming and problem solving in C++ / Nell Dale, Chip Weems,
and Mark Headington.--2nd ed.
      p.   cm.
   ISBN 0–7637–1063–6
   1. C++ (Computer program language)   I. Weems, Chip.
II. Headington, Mark R.   III. Title.
QA76.73C153D34   1999
005.13'3—dc21   99-25436
                                                  CIP

ISBN: 0-7637-1063-6

Printed in the United States of America
03 02 01 00 99   10 9 8 7 6 5 4 3 2

Cover image © James Archambeault.

*To you, and to all of our other students for whom it
was begun and without whom it would
never have been completed.*

N.D.   C.W.   M.H.

*To the memory of my parents, Rog and Anne, who
fostered in me a lifelong love of reading and learning.*

M.H.

Programming and Problem Solving with C++, Second Edition *Program Disk*

Jones and Bartlett Publishers offers free to students and instructors a program disk with all the complete programs found in *Programming and Problem Solving with C++*, Second Edition. The program disk is available through the Jones and Bartlett World Wide Web site on the Internet.*

Download Instructions

1. Connect to the Jones and Bartlett student diskette home page (www.jbpub.com/disks).
2. Choose *Programming and Problem Solving with C++*, Second Edition.
3. Follow the instructions for downloading and saving the *Programming and Problem Solving with C++*, Second Edition data disk.
4. If you need assistance downloading a Jones and Bartlett student diskette, please send email to: help@jbpub.com.

---

* Downloading the *Programming and Problem Solving with C++*, Second Edition program disk via the Jones and Bartlett home page requires access to the Internet and a World Wide Web browser, such as Netscape Navigator or Microsoft Internet Explorer. Instructors at schools without Internet access may call 1-800-832-0034 and request a copy of the program disk. Jones and Bartlett grants adopters of *Programming and Problem Solving with C++*, Second Edition the right to duplicate copies of the program disk or to store the files on any stand-alone computer or network.

Contents

17 Recursion 1013

Preface

Shortly after its introduction in 1996, the first edition of *Programming and Problem Solving with C++* became one of the best-selling computer science textbooks in the United States. Although this second edition incorporates numerous changes, including reorganization of chapter material, one thing has not changed: our commitment to the student. As always, our efforts are directed toward making the sometimes difficult concepts of computer science more accessible to all students.

The first edition and the Pascal and Ada versions of this book have been widely accepted as model textbooks for the ACM-recommended curriculum for CS1 and the Advanced Placement AP exam in computer science. The content and organization have been guided by the ACM-recommended curriculum for CS1 (October 1984) and the following knowledge units from the ACM/IEEE Computing Curricula 1991 recommendations for a C101 course: AL1–AL4, AL6, NU1, PL3–PL5, and SE1–SE5.

This edition of *Programming and Problem Solving with C++* continues to reflect our experience that topics once considered too advanced can be taught in the first course. For example, we address metalanguages explicitly as the formal means of specifying programming language syntax. We introduce Big-*O* notation early and use it to compare algorithms in later chapters. We discuss modular design in terms of abstract steps, concrete steps, functional equivalence, and functional cohesion. Preconditions and postconditions are used in the context of the algorithm walk-through, in the development of testing strategies, and as interface documentation for user-written functions. The discussion of function interface design includes encapsulation, control abstraction, and communication complexity. Data abstraction and abstract data types (ADTs) are explained in conjunction with the C++ class mechanism, forming a natural lead-in to object-oriented programming.

Changes in the Second Edition

The second edition incorporates the following changes:

- *Conformance to ISO/ANSI standard C++.* ISO/ANSI standard C++ (officially approved in July 1998) is used throughout the book, including relevant portions of the new C++ standard library. However, readers with pre–standard C++ compilers are also supported. A new appendix discusses how to modify the textbook's programs to compile and run successfully with an earlier compiler.

- *An earlier introduction to classes, data abstraction, and object-oriented concepts.* Chapters 11–19 of the first edition have been reorganized into the following Chapters 11–17:

  11 Structured Types, Data Abstraction, and Classes
  12 Arrays
  13 Array-Based Lists
  14 Object-Oriented Software Development
  15 Pointers, Dynamic Data, and Reference Types
  16 Linked Structures
  17 Recursion

  The visible changes are the deletion of two chapters ("Records" and "Multidimensional Arrays"), whose contents have been merged into Chapters 11 and 12, respectively, and the movement of the chapter "Structured Types, Data Abstraction, and Classes" (Chapter 15 in the first edition) to become Chapter 11. With this reorganization, the concept of the C++ class as both a structuring mechanism and a tool for abstraction now comes earlier in the book.

  Introducing classes before arrays has several benefits. In their first exposure to composite types, many students find it easier to comprehend accessing a component by name rather than by position. Chapter 12 on arrays can now rather easily introduce the idea of an array of class objects or an array of structs. Also, Chapter 13, which deals with the list as an ADT, can now be handled in a better way, namely, encapsulating both the data representation (an array) and the length variable within a class, rather than the first edition's approach of using two loosely coupled variables (an array and a separate length variable) to represent the list. Finally, with three chapters' worth of exposure to classes and objects, students reading Chapter 14 can focus on the more difficult aspects of the chapter: inheritance, composition, and dynamic binding.

  A natural result of this reorganization is that the chapter "Object-Oriented Software Development" comes earlier in the sequence: Chapter 14 rather than the first edition's Chapter 16.

- *Attention to length.* In response to feedback from our users and reviewers about the length of the first edition, we have made the following changes:
  - Presentations of certain topics have been streamlined or moved elsewhere. (For example, the material on loop invariants has been moved to the *Instructor's Guide.*)
  - The number of case studies has been reduced substantially. Whereas the first edition presented two or three case studies per chapter, most chapters now have one case study.
  - The first edition's two chapters on one-dimensional arrays and multidimensional arrays have been combined into a single chapter.

- The first edition's appendix containing all syntax templates in one location has been moved to the publisher's Web site.

C++ and Object-Oriented Programming

Some educators reject the C++ language as too permissive and too conducive to writing cryptic, unreadable programs. Our experience does not support this view, *provided that the use of language features is modeled appropriately*. That C++ permits a terse, compact programming style cannot be labeled simply as "good" or "bad." Almost any programming language can be used to write in a style that is too terse and clever to be easily understood. C++ may indeed be used in this manner more often than are other languages, but we have found that with careful instruction in software engineering and a programming style that is straightforward, disciplined, and free of intricate language features, students can learn to use C++ to produce clear, readable code.

It must be emphasized that although we use C++ as a vehicle for teaching computer science concepts, the book is not a language manual and does not attempt to cover all of C++. Certain language features—templates, exceptions, operator overloading, default arguments, and mechanisms for advanced forms of inheritance, to name a few—are omitted in an effort not to overwhelm the beginning student with too much too fast.

Currently, there are diverse opinions about when to introduce the topic of object-oriented programming (OOP). Some educators advocate an immersion in OOP from the very beginning, whereas others (for whom this book is intended) favor a more heterogeneous approach in which both functional decomposition and object-oriented design are presented as design tools. The chapter organization of *Programming and Problem Solving with C++* reflects a transitional approach to OOP. Although we provide an early preview of object-oriented design in Chapter 4, we delay a focused discussion until Chapter 14. The sequence of topics in Chapters 1 through 13 mirrors our belief that OOP is best understood after a firm grounding in algorithm design, control abstraction, and data abstraction with classes. As one reviewer of the first edition, who was originally critical of the delayed introduction to OOP, stated in a subsequent review, "The logical flow of the chapters is excellent. In the earlier review, I commented on the late introduction to OOP. I now (having nearly completed teaching a CS1 with C++) believe that is a good strategy."

Synopsis

Chapter 1 is designed to create a comfortable rapport between students and the subject. The basics of hardware and software are presented, and problem-solving techniques are discussed and reinforced in a Problem-Solving Case Study. We have added a section on ethics to round out this introduction.

Chapters 2 and 3 have been revised as follows. Chapter 2, instead of overwhelming the student right away with the various numeric types available in C++, concentrates on two types only: char and string. (The string type is the ISO/ANSI string class provided by the standard library.) With fewer data types to keep track of, students can focus on overall program structure and get an earlier start on creating and running a simple program. Chapter 3 then begins with a discussion of the C++ numeric types and proceeds as in the first edition, with material on arithmetic expressions, function calls, and output. Unlike many books that detail *all* of the C++ data types and *all* of the C++ operators at once, these two chapters focus only on the int, float, char, and string types and the basic arithmetic operators. Details of the other data types and the more elaborate C++ operators are postponed until Chapter 10.

The functional decomposition and object-oriented design methodologies are a major focus of Chapter 4, and the discussion is written with a healthy degree of formalism. This early in the book, the treatment of object-oriented design is necessarily more superficial than that of functional decomposition. However, students gain the perspective that there are two—not one—design methodologies in widespread use and that each serves a specific purpose. Chapter 4 also covers input and file I/O. The early introduction of files permits the assignment of programming problems that require the use of sample data files.

Students learn to recognize functions in Chapters 1 and 2, and they learn to use standard library functions in Chapter 3. Chapter 4 reinforces the basic concepts of function calls, argument passing, and function libraries. Chapter 4 also relates functions to the implementation of modular designs and begins the discussion of interface design that is essential to writing proper functions.

Chapter 5 begins with Boolean data, but its main purpose is to introduce the concept of flow of control. Selection, using If-Then and If-Then-Else structures, is used to demonstrate the distinction between physical ordering of statements and logical ordering. We also develop the concept of nested control structures. Chapter 5 concludes with a lengthy Testing and Debugging section that expands on the modular design discussion by introducing preconditions and postconditions. The algorithm walk-through and code walk-through are introduced as means of preventing errors, and the execution trace is used to find errors that made it into the code. We also cover data validation and testing strategies extensively in this section.

Chapter 6 is devoted to loop control strategies and looping operations using the syntax of the While statement. Rather than introducing multiple syntactical structures, our approach is to teach the concepts of looping using only the While statement. However, because many instructors have told us that they prefer to show students the syntax for all of C++'s looping statements at once, the discussion of For and Do-While statements in Chapter 9 can be covered optionally after Chapter 6.

By Chapter 7, the students are already comfortable with breaking problems into modules and using library functions, and they are receptive to the idea of writing their own functions. Chapter 7 focuses on passing arguments by value and covers flow of control in function calls, arguments and parameters, local variables, and interface design. The last topic includes preconditions and postconditions in the interface documentation, control abstraction, encapsulation, and physical versus conceptual hiding of an implementation. Chapter 8 expands the discussion to include reference parameters, scope and lifetime, stubs and drivers, and more on interface design, including side effects.

Chapter 9 covers the remaining "ice cream and cake" control structures in C++ (Switch, Do-While, and For), along with the Break and Continue statements. Chapter 9 forms a natural ending point for the first quarter of a two-quarter introductory course sequence.

Chapter 10 begins a transition between the control structures orientation of the first half of the book and the abstract data type orientation of the second half. We examine the built-in simple data types in terms of the set of values represented by each type and the allowable operations on those values. We introduce more C++ operators and discuss the problems of floating-point representation and precision at length. User-defined simple types, user-written header files, and type coercion are among the other topics covered in this chapter.

We begin Chapter 11 with a discussion of simple versus structured data types. We introduce the record (`struct` in C++) as a heterogeneous data structure, describe the syntax for accessing its components, and demonstrate how to combine record types into a hierarchical record structure. From this base, we make a transition to the concept of data abstraction and give a precise definition to the notion of an ADT, emphasizing the separation of specification from implementation. The C++ class mechanism is introduced as a programming language representation of an ADT. The concepts of encapsulation, information hiding, and public and private class members are stressed. We describe the separate compilation of program files, and students learn the technique of placing a class's declaration and implementation into two separate files: the specification (`.h`) file and the implementation file.

In Chapter 12, the array is introduced as a homogeneous data structure whose components are accessed by position rather than by name. One-dimensional arrays are examined in depth, including arrays of structs and arrays of class objects. Material on multidimensional arrays, formerly a separate chapter in the first edition, has been moved to this chapter to complete the discussion.

Chapter 13 integrates the material from Chapters 11 and 12 by defining the list as an ADT. Because we have already introduced classes and arrays, we can clearly differentiate the concepts of array and list from the beginning. The array is a built-in, fixed-size data structure. The list is a user-defined, variable-size structure represented as a length and an array of items, bound together in a class object. The elements in the list are those elements in the array from position 0 through position *length* − 1. In this chapter, we design C++ classes for unsorted and sorted list ADTs, and we code the list algorithms as class member functions. We use Big-*O* notation to compare the various searching and sorting algorithms developed for these ADTs. Finally, we examine C strings in order to give students some insight into how a higher-level abstraction (a string as a list of characters) might be implemented in terms of a lower-level abstraction (a null-terminated `char` array).

Chapter 14 extends the concepts of data abstraction and C++ classes to an exploration of object-oriented software development. Object-oriented design, introduced briefly in Chapter 4, is revisited in greater depth. Students learn to distinguish between inheritance and composition relationships during the design phase, and C++'s derived classes are used to implement inheritance. This chapter also introduces C++ virtual functions, which support polymorphism in the form of run-time binding of operations to objects.

Chapter 15 examines pointer and reference types. We present pointers as a way of making programs more efficient and of allowing the run-time allocation of program data. The coverage of dynamic data structures continues in Chapter 16, in which we present linked lists, linked-list algorithms, and alternative representations of linked lists.

Chapter 17 covers recursion. There is no consensus as to the best place to introduce this subject. We believe that it is better to wait until at least the second semester to cover this topic. However, we have included recursion for those instructors who have requested it. Although Chapter 17 is the last chapter, we divide the examples into two parts: those that require only simple data types and those that require structured data types. Instructors can cover the first part after Chapter 8. The second part contains examples from simple arrays to dynamic linked lists. These examples could be used individually after the appropriate chapter (for example, simple arrays after Chapter 12) or as a unit after Chapter 16.

Additional Features

Web Links Special Web icons found in the Special Sections (see below) prompt students to visit the text's companion Web site located at `www.jbpub.com/dale` for additional information about selected topics. These Web Links give students instant access to real-world applications of material presented in the text. The Web Links are updated on a regular basis to ensure that students receive the most recent information available on the Internet.

Special Sections   Five kinds of features are set off from the main text. Theoretical Foundations sections present material related to the fundamental theory behind various branches of computer science. Software Engineering Tips discuss methods of making programs more reliable, robust, or efficient. Matters of Style address stylistic issues in the coding of programs. Background Information sections explore side issues that enhance the student's general knowledge of computer science. May We Introduce sections contain biographies of computing pioneers such as Blaise Pascal, Ada Lovelace, and Grace Murray Hopper. Web Links appear in most of these Special Sections prompting students to visit the companion Web site at www.jbpub.com/dale for expanded material.

Goals   Each chapter begins with a list of learning objectives for the student. These goals are reinforced and tested in the end-of-chapter exercises.

Problem-Solving Case Studies   Problem solving is best demonstrated through case studies. In each case study, we present a problem and use problem-solving techniques to develop a manual solution. Next, we expand the solution to an algorithm, using functional decomposition, object-oriented design, or both; then we code the algorithm in C++. We show sample test data and output and follow up with a discussion of what is involved in thoroughly testing the program.

Testing and Debugging   Following the case studies in each chapter, this section considers in depth the implications of the chapter material with regard to thorough testing of programs. The section concludes with a list of testing and debugging hints.

Quick Checks   At the end of each chapter are questions that test the student's recall of major points associated with the chapter goals. Upon reading each question, the student immediately should know the answer, which he or she can then verify by glancing at the answers at the end of the section. The page number on which the concept is discussed appears at the end of each question so that the student can review the material in the event of an incorrect response.

Exam Preparation Exercises   These questions help the student prepare for tests. The questions usually have objective answers and are designed to be answerable with a few minutes of work. Answers to selected questions are given in the back of the book, and the remaining questions are answered in the *Instructor's Guide.*

Programming Warm-up Exercises   This section provides the student with experience in writing C++ code fragments. The student can practice the syntactic constructs in each chapter without the burden of writing a complete program. Solutions to selected questions from each chapter appear in the back of the book; the remaining solutions may be found in the *Instructor's Guide.*

Programming Problems These exercises, drawn from a wide range of disciplines, require the student to design solutions and write complete programs.

Case Study Follow-Up These questions require the student to analyze or modify the case studies in the chapter. The exercises afford experience in reading and understanding the documentation and code for existing programs.

Supplements

Instructor's Guide and Test Bank The *Instructor's Guide* features chapter-by-chapter teaching notes, answers to the balance of the exercises, and a compilation of exam questions with answers. The *Instructor's Guide* is available to adopters on request from Jones and Bartlett.

Instructor's ToolKit CD-ROM Also available to adopters upon request from the publisher is a powerful teaching tool entitled "Instructor's ToolKit." This CD-ROM contains an electronic version of the *Instructor's Guide,* a computerized test bank, PowerPoint lecture presentations containing over 900 slides, and the complete programs from the text (see below).

Programs The programs contain the source code for all of the complete programs that are found within the textbook. They are available on the Instructor's ToolKit CD-ROM and also as a free download for instructors and students from the publisher's Web site: www.jbpub.com/disks. The programs from all the case studies, plus several programs that appear in the chapter bodies, are included. Fragments or snippets of program code are not included nor are the solutions to the chapter-ending "Programming Problems." These program files can be viewed or edited using any standard text editor, but in order to compile and run the programs, a C++ compiler must be used.

Companion Web Site This Web site features integrated Web Links from the textbook, the complete programs from the text, and Appendix D entitled "Using this Book with a Prestandard Version of C++," which describes the changes needed to allow the programs in the textbook to run successfully with a prestandard compiler. The Web site also includes the syntax templates in one location. These appeared as an appendix in the last edition.

A Laboratory Course in C++, Second Edition Written by Nell Dale, this lab manual follows the organization of the second edition of the text. The lab manual is designed to allow the instructor maximum flexibility and may be used in both open and closed laboratory settings. Each chapter contains three types of activities: Prelab, Inlab and Postlab. Each lesson is broken into exercises that thoroughly demonstrate the concept covered in the chapter. A disk that contains the programs, program shells (partial programs), and data files accompanies the lab manual.

Student Lecture Notebook Designed from the PowerPoint presentations developed for this text, the Student Lecture Notebook is an invaluable tool for learning. The notebook is designed to encourage students to focus their energies on listening to the lecture as they fill in additional details. The skeletal outline concept helps students organize their notes and readily recognize the important concepts in each chapter.

About the Cover

The broken and scrambled cover image was created from a unique aspect of the 40-room Centre Family Dwelling, a building in The Shaker Village of Pleasant Hill, Kentucky. Built to accommodate 100 celibate inhabitants, Centre Family Dwelling boasts two entranceways, dual stairways, and a wide common passageway on each floor that separates brothers' and sisters' apartments.

Completed in 1834, the massive building's exterior is hand-hewn Kentucky River Limestone which was quarried from the nearby Kentucky Palisades. In the hallways, the floors are covered in quarter-sawed white oak.

Centre Family Dwelling's high ceilings and vast windows are exceptional features for architecture of the time. These unusual characteristics reflect a concern for proper ventilation and lighting, embracing small, high interior windows and transoms to permit light into intimate spaces.

Acknowledgments

We would like to thank the many individuals who have helped us in the preparation of this second edition. We are indebted to the members of the faculties of the Computer Science Departments at the University of Texas at Austin, the University of Massachusetts at Amherst, and the University of Wisconsin–La Crosse.

We extend special thanks to Jeff Brumfield for developing the syntax template metalanguage and allowing us to use it in the text.

For their many helpful suggestions, we thank the lecturers, teaching assistants, consultants, and student proctors who run the courses for which this book was written, and the students themselves.

We are grateful to the following people who took the time to review our manuscript: J. Ken Collier, Northern Arizona State; Lee Cornell, Mankato State University; Charles Dierbach, Towsen State University; Judy Etchison, Collin County Community College; David Galles, University of San Francisco; Susan Gauch, University of Kansas; Wagar Haque, University of Northern British Columbia; Ilga Higbee, Black Hawk College; Jeanine Ingber, University of New Mexico; Paula Jech, Pennsylvania State University; Hikyoo Koh, Lamar University; I. Stephen Leach, Florida State University; Joseph Marti, College of the Canyons; Kenrick Mock, Oregon State University; Viera Proulx, Northeastern University; Howard Pyron, University of Missouri-Rolla; Dennis Ray, Old Dominion University; Sujan Sarkar, Santa Rosa Junior College; Lynn Stauffer, Sonoma State University; Greg Steuben, Rensselaer Polytechnic Institute.

We also thank Karen Jolie and PageMasters & Company along with the many people at Jones and Bartlett who contributed so much, especially Tom Walker, Rebecca Marks, Jennifer Jacobson, Anne Spencer, J. Michael Stranz, W. Scott Smith, and Mike DeFronzo.

Anyone who has ever written a book—or is related to someone who has—can appreciate the amount of time involved in such a project. To our families—all the Dale clan and the extended Dale family (too numerous to name); to Lisa, Charlie, and Abby; to Anne, Brady, and Kari—thanks for your tremendous support and indulgence.

N. D.
C. W.
M. H.

Overview of Programming and Problem Solving

- To understand what a computer program is.
- To be able to list the basic stages involved in writing a computer program.
- To understand what an algorithm is.
- To learn what a high-level programming language is.
- To be able to describe what a compiler is and what it does.
- To understand the compilation and execution processes.
- To learn the history of the C++ programming language.
- To learn what the major components of a computer are and how they work together.
- To be able to distinguish between hardware and software.
- To learn about some of the basic ethical issues confronting computing professionals.
- To be able to choose an appropriate problem-solving method for developing an algorithmic solution to a problem.

Overview of Programming

---

com•put•er \kəm-'pyüt-ər   *n, often attrib* (1646): one that computes; *specif*: a
programmable electronic device that can store, retrieve, and process data*

What a brief definition for something that has, in just a few decades,
changed the way of life in industrialized societies! Computers touch all
areas of our lives: paying bills, driving cars, using the telephone, shopping.
In fact, it would be easier to list those areas of our lives that are not
affected by computers.

It is sad that a device that does so much good is so often maligned and
feared. How many times have you heard someone say, "I'm sorry, our computer fouled things up" or "I just don't understand computers; they're too
complicated for me"? The very fact that you are reading this book, however, means that you are ready to set aside prejudice and learn about computers. But be forewarned: This book is not just about computers in the
abstract. This is a text to teach you how to program computers.

What Is Programming?

Much of human behavior and thought is characterized by logical sequences.
Since infancy, you have been learning how to act, how to do things. And
you have learned to expect certain behavior from other people.

A lot of what you do every day you do automatically. Fortunately, it is
not necessary for you to consciously think of every step involved in a
process as simple as turning a page by hand:

1. Lift hand.
2. Move hand to right side of book.
3. Grasp top right corner of page.
4. Move hand from right to left until page is positioned so that you can
    read what is on the other side.
5. Let go of page.

Think how many neurons must fire and how many muscles must respond,
all in a certain order or sequence, to move your arm and hand. Yet you do
it unconsciously.

Much of what you do unconsciously you once had to learn. Watch how
a baby concentrates on putting one foot before the other while learning to
walk. Then watch a group of three-year-olds playing tag.

---

* By permission. From *Merriam-Webster's Collegiate Dictionary*, Tenth Edition. © 1994 by
Merriam-Webster Inc.

On a broader scale, mathematics never could have been developed without logical sequences of steps for solving problems and proving theorems. Mass production never would have worked without operations taking place in a certain order. Our whole civilization is based on the order of things and actions.

We create order, both consciously and unconsciously, through a process we call **programming**. This book is concerned with the programming of one of our tools, the **computer**.

Programming   Planning or scheduling the performance of a task or an event.

Computer   A programmable device that can store, retrieve, and process data.

Computer programming   The process of planning a sequence of steps for a computer to follow.

Just as a concert program lists the order in which the players perform pieces, a **computer program** lists the sequence of steps the computer performs. From now on, when we use the words *programming* and *program*, we mean *computer programming* and *computer program*.

Computer program   A sequence of instructions to be performed by a computer.

The computer allows us to do tasks more efficiently, quickly, and accurately than we could by hand—if we could do them by hand at all. In order to use this powerful tool, we must specify what we want done and the order in which we want it done. We do this through programming.

How Do We Write a Program?

A computer is not intelligent. It cannot analyze a problem and come up with a solution. A human (the *programmer*) must analyze the problem, develop a sequence of instructions for solving the problem, and then communicate it to the computer. What's the advantage of using a computer if it can't solve problems? Once we have written the solution as a sequence of instructions for the computer, the computer can repeat the solution very quickly and consistently, again and again. The computer frees people from repetitive and boring tasks.

To write a sequence of instructions for a computer to follow, we must go through a two-phase process: *problem solving* and *implementation* (see Figure 1-1).

Problem-Solving Phase

1. *Analysis and specification.*   Understand (define) the problem and what the solution must do.
2. *General solution (algorithm).*   Develop a logical sequence of steps that solves the problem.
3. *Verify.*   Follow the steps exactly to see if the solution really does solve the problem.

Implementation Phase

1. *Concrete solution (program).*   Translate the algorithm into a programming language.
2. *Test.*   Have the computer follow the instructions. Then manually check the results. If you find errors, analyze the program and the algorithm to determine the source of the errors, and then make corrections.

Once a program has been written, it enters a third phase: *maintenance*.

Maintenance Phase

1. *Use.*   Use the program.
2. *Maintain.*   Modify the program to meet changing requirements or to correct any errors that show up in using it.

The programmer begins the programming process by analyzing the problem and developing a general solution called an **algorithm.** Understanding and analyzing a problem take up much more time than Figure 1-1 implies. They are the heart of the programming process.

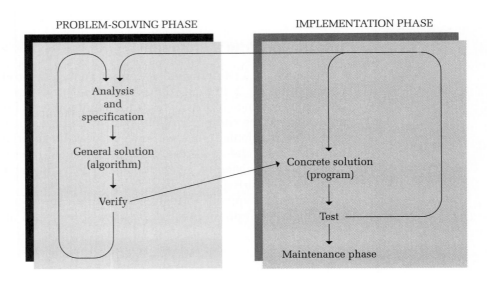

FIGURE 1-1
Programming
Process

Algorithm   A step-by-step procedure for solving a problem in a finite amount of time.

If our definitions of a computer program and an algorithm look similar, it is because all programs are algorithms. A program is simply an algorithm that has been written for a computer.

An algorithm is a verbal or written description of a logical sequence of actions. We use algorithms every day. Recipes, instructions, and directions are all examples of algorithms that are not programs.

When you start your car, you follow a step-by-step procedure. The algorithm might look something like this:

1. Insert the key.
2. Make sure the transmission is in Park (or Neutral).
3. Depress the gas pedal.
4. Turn the key to the start position.
5. If the engine starts within six seconds, release the key to the ignition position.
6. If the engine doesn't start in six seconds, release the key and gas pedal, wait ten seconds, and repeat steps 3 through 6, but not more than five times.
7. If the car doesn't start, call the garage.

Without the phrase "but not more than five times" in step 6, you could be trying to start the car forever. Why? Because if something is wrong with the car, repeating steps 3 through 6 over and over again will not start it. This kind of never-ending situation is called an *infinite loop*. If we leave the phrase "but not more than five times" out of step 6, the procedure does not fit our definition of an algorithm. An algorithm must terminate in a finite amount of time for all possible conditions.

Suppose a programmer needs an algorithm to determine an employee's weekly wages. The algorithm reflects what would be done by hand:

1. Look up the employee's pay rate.
2. Determine the number of hours worked during the week.
3. If the number of hours worked is less than or equal to 40, multiply the number of hours by the pay rate to calculate regular wages.
4. If the number of hours worked is greater than 40, multiply 40 by the pay rate to calculate regular wages, and then multiply the difference between the number of hours worked and 40 by $1\frac{1}{2}$ times the pay rate to calculate overtime wages.
5. Add the regular wages to the overtime wages (if any) to determine total wages for the week.

The steps the computer follows are often the same steps you would use to do the calculations by hand.

After developing a general solution, the programmer tests the algorithm, walking through each step mentally or manually. If the algorithm doesn't work, the programmer repeats the problem-solving process, analyzing the problem again and coming up with another algorithm. Often the second algorithm is just a variation of the first. When the programmer is satisfied with the algorithm, he or she translates it into a **programming language.** We use the C++ programming language in this book.

Programming language   A set of rules, symbols, and special words used to construct a computer program.

A programming language is a simplified form of English (with math symbols) that adheres to a strict set of grammatical rules. English is far too complicated a language for today's computers to follow. Programming languages, because they limit vocabulary and grammar, are much simpler.

Although a programming language is simple in form, it is not always easy to use. Try giving someone directions to the nearest airport using a vocabulary of no more than 45 words, and you'll begin to see the problem. Programming forces you to write very simple, exact instructions.

FIGURE 1-2

Differences in
Implementation

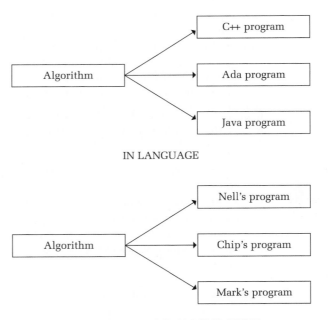

IN LANGUAGE

IN PERSONAL PROGRAMMING STYLE

Translating an algorithm into a programming language is called *coding* the algorithm. The product of that translation—the program—is tested by running (*executing*) it on the computer. If the program fails to produce the desired results, the programmer must *debug* it—that is, determine what is wrong and then modify the program, or even the algorithm, to fix it. The combination of coding and testing an algorithm is called *implementation*.

There is no single way to implement an algorithm. For example, an algorithm can be translated into more than one programming language. Each translation produces a different implementation. Even when two people translate an algorithm into the same programming language, they are likely to come up with different implementations (see Figure 1-2). Why? Because every programming language allows the programmer some flexibility in how an algorithm is translated. Given this flexibility, people adopt their own styles in writing programs, just as they do in writing short stories or essays. Once you have some programming experience, you develop a style of your own. Throughout this book, we offer tips on good programming style.

Some people try to speed up the programming process by going directly from the problem definition to coding the program (see Figure 1-3). A shortcut here is very tempting and at first seems to save a lot of time. However, for many reasons that will become obvious to you as you read this book, this kind of shortcut actually takes *more* time and effort. Developing a general solution before you write a program helps you manage the problem, keep your thoughts straight, and avoid mistakes. If you don't take the time at the beginning to think out and polish your algorithm, you'll spend a lot of extra time debugging and revising your program. So think first and code later! The sooner you start coding, the longer it takes to write a program that works.

Once a program has been put into use, it is often necessary to modify it. Modification may involve fixing an error that is discovered during the use of the program or changing the program in response to changes in the user's requirements. Each time the program is modified, it is necessary to repeat the problem-solving and implementation phases for those aspects of

FIGURE 1-3

Programming
Shortcut?

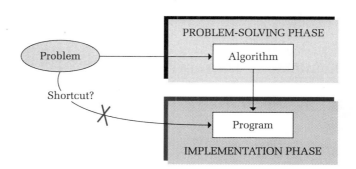

the program that change. This phase of the programming process is known as maintenance and actually accounts for the majority of the effort expended on most programs. For example, a program that is implemented in a few months may need to be maintained over a period of many years. Thus, it is a cost-effective investment of time to develop the initial problem solution and program implementation carefully. Together, the problem-solving, implementation, and maintenance phases constitute the program's *life cycle.*

In addition to solving the problem, implementing the algorithm, and maintaining the program, **documentation** is an important part of the programming process. Documentation includes written explanations of the problem being solved and the organization of the solution, comments embedded within the program itself, and user manuals that describe how to use the program. Most programs are worked on by many different people over a long period of time. Each of those people must be able to read and understand your code.

Documentation   The written text and comments that make a program easier for others to understand, use, and modify.

After you write a program, you must give the computer the information or data necessary to solve the problem. **Information** is any knowledge that can be communicated, including abstract ideas and concepts such as "the earth is round." **Data** is information in a form the computer can use—for example, the numbers and letters making up the formulas that relate the earth's radius to its volume and surface area. But data is not restricted to numbers and letters. These days, computers also process data that represents sound (to be played through speakers), graphic images (to be displayed on a computer screen or printer), video (to be played on a VCR), and so forth.

Information   Any knowledge that can be communicated.

Data   Information in a form a computer can use.

THEORETICAL FOUNDATIONS

Binary Representation of Data

In a computer, data is represented electronically by pulses of electricity. Electric circuits, in their simplest form, are either on or off. Usually a circuit that is on is represented by the number 1; a circuit that is off is represented by the number 0. Any kind of data can be represented by combinations of enough 1s and 0s. We simply have to choose which combination represents each piece of data we are using. For example, we could arbitrarily choose the pattern 1101000110 to represent the name *C++*.

Data represented by 1s and 0s is in *binary form*. The binary (base-2) number system uses only 1s and 0s to represent numbers. (The decimal [base-10] number system uses the digits 0 through 9.) The word *bit* (short for **b**inary dig**it**) often is used to refer to a single 1 or 0. The pattern 1101000110 thus has 10 bits. A binary number with 10 bits can represent 2^{10} (1024) different patterns. A *byte* is a group of 8 bits; it can represent 2^8 (256) patterns. Inside the computer, each character (such as the letter *A*, the letter *g*, or a question mark) is usually represented by a byte. Four bits, or half of a byte, is called a *nibble* or *nybble*—a name that originally was proposed with tongue in cheek but now is standard terminology. Groups of 16, 32, and 64 bits are generally referred to as *words* (although the terms *short word* and *long word* are sometimes used to refer to 16-bit and 64-bit groups, respectively).

The process of assigning bit patterns to pieces of data is called *coding*—the same name we give to the process of translating an algorithm into a programming language. The names are the same because the only language that the first computers recognized was binary in form. Thus, in the early days of computers, programming meant translating both data and algorithms into patterns of 1s and 0s.

Binary coding schemes are still used inside the computer to represent both the instructions that it follows and the data that it uses. For example, 16 bits can represent the decimal integers from 0 to $2^{16} - 1$ (65,535). Characters also can be represented by bit combinations. In one coding scheme, 01001101 represents *M* and 01101101 represents *m*. More complicated coding schemes are necessary to represent negative numbers, real numbers, numbers in scientific notation, sound, graphics, and video. In Chapter 10, we examine in detail the representation of numbers and characters in the computer.

The patterns of bits that represent data vary from one computer to another. Even on the same computer, different programming languages can use different binary representations for the same data. A single programming language may even use the same pattern of bits to represent different things in different contexts. (People do this too. The word formed by the four letters *tack* has different meanings depending on whether you are talking about upholstery, sailing, sewing, paint, or horseback riding.) The point is that patterns of bits by themselves are meaningless. It is the way in which the patterns are used that gives them their meaning.

Fortunately, we no longer have to work with binary coding schemes. Today the process of coding is usually just a matter of writing down the data in letters, numbers, and symbols. The computer automatically converts these letters, numbers, and symbols into binary form. Still, as you work with computers, you will continually run into numbers that are related to powers of 2—numbers such as 256, 32,768, and 65,536—reminders that the binary number system is lurking somewhere nearby.

What Is a Programming Language?

In the computer, all data, whatever its form, is stored and used in binary codes, strings of 1s and 0s. Instructions and data are stored together in the computer's memory using these binary codes. If you were to look at the binary codes representing instructions and data in memory, you could not tell the difference between them; they are distinguished only by the manner in which the computer uses them. It is thus possible for the computer to process its own instructions as a form of data.

When computers were first developed, the only programming language available was the primitive instruction set built into each machine, the **machine language,** or *machine code.*

Machine language   The language, made up of binary-coded instructions, that is used directly by the computer.

Even though most computers perform the same kinds of operations, their designers choose different sets of binary codes for each instruction. So the machine code for one computer is not the same as for another.

When programmers used machine language for programming, they had to enter the binary codes for the various instructions, a tedious process that was prone to error. Moreover, their programs were difficult to read and modify. In time, **assembly languages** were developed to make the programmer's job easier.

Assembly language   A low-level programming language in which a mnemonic is used to represent each of the machine language instructions for a particular computer.

Instructions in an assembly language are in an easy-to-remember form called a *mnemonic* (pronounced ni-MON-ik). Typical instructions for addition and subtraction might look like this:

Assembly Language	**Machine Language**
ADD	100101
SUB	010011

Although assembly language is easier for humans to work with, the computer cannot directly execute the instructions. One of the fundamental discoveries in computer science is that, because a computer can process its own instructions as a form of data, it is possible to write a program to translate the assembly language instructions into machine code. Such a program is called an **assembler**.

Assembler   A program that translates an assembly language program into machine code.

Assembly language is a step in the right direction, but it still forces programmers to think in terms of individual machine instructions. Eventually, computer scientists developed high-level programming languages. These languages are easier to use than assembly languages or machine code because they are closer to English and other natural languages (see Figure 1-4).

FIGURE 1-4

Levels of Abstraction

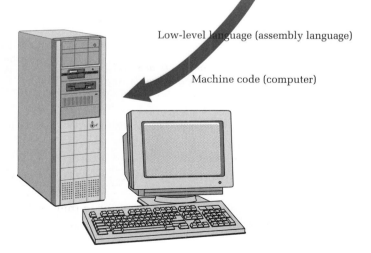

Human thought

Natural language (English, French, German, etc.)

High-level language (C++, FORTRAN, COBOL, etc.)

Low-level language (assembly language)

Machine code (computer)

A program called a **compiler** translates programs written in certain high-level languages (C++, Pascal, FORTRAN, COBOL, Modula-2, and Ada, for example) into machine language. If you write a program in a high-level language, you can run it on any computer that has the appropriate compiler. This is possible because most high-level languages are *standardized*, which means that an official description of the language exists.

Compiler   A program that translates a high-level language into machine code.

A program in a high-level language is called a **source program.** To the compiler, a source program is just input data. It translates the source program into a machine language program called an **object program** (see Figure 1-5). Some compilers also output a *listing*—a copy of the program with error messages and other information inserted.

Source program   A program written in a high-level programming language.
Object program   The machine language version of a source program.

A benefit of standardized high-level languages is that they allow you to write *portable* (or *machine-independent*) code. As Figure 1-5 emphasizes,

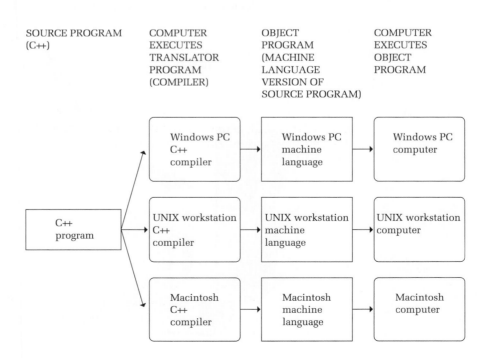

FIGURE 1-5

High-Level Programming Languages Allow Programs to Be Compiled on Different Systems

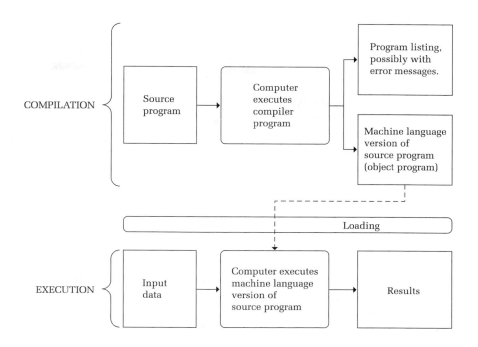

FIGURE 1-6

Compilation and
Execution

a single C++ program can be used on different machines, whereas a program written in assembly language or machine language is not portable from one computer to another. Because each computer has its own machine language, a machine language program written for computer A will not run on computer B.

It is important to understand that *compilation* and *execution* are two distinct processes. During compilation, the computer runs the compiler program. During execution, the object program is loaded into the computer's memory unit, replacing the compiler program. The computer then runs the object program, doing whatever the program instructs it to do (see Figure 1-6).

BACKGROUND INFORMATION

Compilers and Interpreters

Some programming languages—LISP, Prolog, and many versions of BASIC, for example—are translated by an *interpreter* rather than a compiler. An interpreter translates *and executes* each instruction in the source program, one at a time. In contrast, a compiler translates the entire source program into machine language, after which execution of the object program takes place.

The Java language uses both a compiler and an interpreter. First, a Java program is compiled, not into a particular computer's machine language, but into an intermediate code called bytecode. Next, a program called the Java Virtual Machine (JVM) takes the bytecode program and interprets it (translates a bytecode instruction into machine language and executes it, translates the next one and executes it, and so on). Thus, a Java program compiled into bytecode is portable to many different computers, as long as each computer has its own specific JVM that can translate bytecode into the computer's machine language

---

The instructions in a programming language reflect the operations a computer can perform:

- A computer can transfer data from one place to another.
- A computer can input data from an input device (a keyboard or mouse, for example) and output data to an output device (a screen, for example).
- A computer can store data into and retrieve data from its memory and secondary storage (parts of a computer that we discuss in the next section).
- A computer can compare two data values for equality or inequality.
- A computer can perform arithmetic operations (addition and subtraction, for example) very quickly.

Programming languages require that we use certain *control structures* to express algorithms as programs. There are four basic ways of structuring statements (instructions) in most programming languages: sequentially, conditionally, repetitively, and with subprograms (see Figure 1-7). A *sequence* is a series of statements that are executed one after another. *Selection*, the conditional control structure, executes different statements depending on certain conditions. The repetitive control structure, the *loop*, repeats statements while certain conditions are met. The *subprogram* allows us to structure a program by breaking it into smaller units. Each of these ways of structuring statements controls the order in which the computer executes the statements, which is why they are called control structures.

Imagine you're driving a car. Going down a straight stretch of road is like following a sequence of instructions. When you come to a fork in the road, you must decide which way to go and then take one or the other branch of the fork. This is what the computer does when it encounters a selection control structure (sometimes called a *branch* or *decision*) in a program. Sometimes you have to go around the block several times to find a place to park. The computer does the same sort of thing when it encounters a loop in a program.

A subprogram is a process that consists of multiple steps. Every day, for example, you follow a procedure to get from home to work. It makes sense, then, for someone to give you directions to a meeting by saying, "Go

FIGURE 1-7
Basic Structures of Programming Languages

SEQUENCE

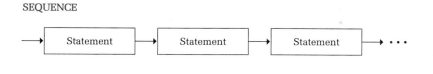

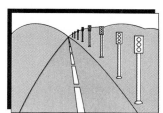

SELECTION (also called *branch* or *decision*)

IF condition THEN statement1 ELSE statement2

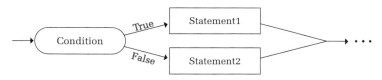

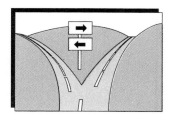

LOOP (also called *repetition* or *iteration*)

WHILE condition DO statement1

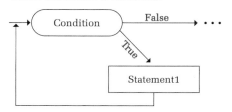

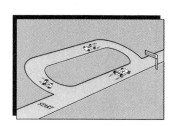

SUBPROGRAM (also called *procedure, function, method,* or *subroutine*)

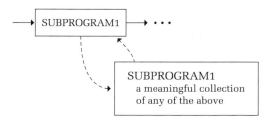

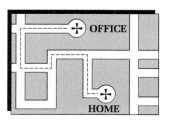

Figure 1-8

Basic Components
of a Computer

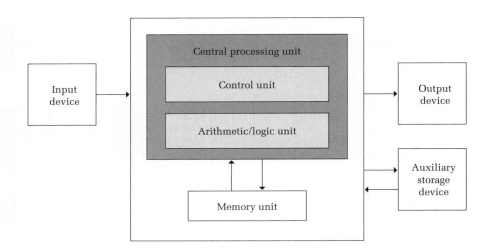

to the office, then go four blocks west" without specifying all the steps you have to take to get to the office. Subprograms allow us to write parts of our programs separately and then assemble them into final form. They can greatly simplify the task of writing large programs.

What Is a Computer?

You can learn a programming language, how to write programs, and how to run (execute) these programs without knowing much about computers. But if you know something about the parts of a computer, you can better understand the effect of each instruction in a programming language.

Most computers have six basic components: the memory unit, the arithmetic/logic unit, the control unit, input devices, output devices, and auxiliary storage devices. Figure 1-8 is a stylized diagram of the basic components of a computer.

The **memory unit** is an ordered sequence of storage cells, each capable of holding a piece of data. Each memory cell has a distinct address to which we refer in order to store data into it or retrieve data from it. These storage cells are called *memory cells*, or *memory locations*.* The memory unit holds data (input data or the product of computation) and instructions (programs), as shown in Figure 1-9.

Memory unit   Internal data storage in a computer.

---

* The memory unit is also referred to as RAM, an acronym for **r**andom **a**ccess **m**emory (so called because we can access any location at random).

FIGURE 1-9

Memory

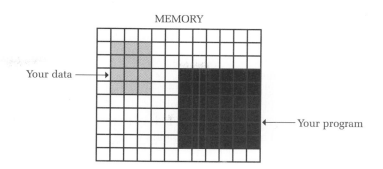

The part of the computer that follows instructions is called the **central processing unit (CPU).** The CPU usually has two components. The **arithmetic/logic unit (ALU)** performs arithmetic operations (addition, subtraction, multiplication, and division) and logical operations (comparing two values). The **control unit** controls the actions of the other components so that program instructions are executed in the correct order.

Central processing unit (CPU) The part of the computer that executes the instructions (program) stored in memory; made up of the arithmetic/logic unit and the control unit.

Arithmetic/logic unit (ALU) The component of the central processing unit that performs arithmetic and logical operations.

Control unit The component of the central processing unit that controls the actions of the other components so that instructions (the program) are executed in the correct sequence.

For us to use computers, there must be some way of getting data into and out of them. **Input/output (I/O) devices** accept data to be processed (input) and present data values that have been processed (output). A keyboard is a common input device. Another is a *mouse*, a pointing device. A video display is a common output device, as are printers and liquid crystal display (LCD) screens. Some devices, such as a connection to a computer network, are used for both input and output.

Input/output (I/O) devices The parts of the computer that accept data to be processed (input) and present the results of that processing (output).

For the most part, computers simply move and combine data in memory. The many types of computers differ primarily in the size of their memories, the speed with which data can be recalled, the efficiency with which data can be moved or combined, and limitations on I/O devices.

When a program is executing, the computer proceeds through a series of steps, the *fetch-execute cycle:*

1. The control unit retrieves (*fetches*) the next coded instruction from memory.
2. The instruction is translated into control signals.
3. The control signals tell the appropriate unit (arithmetic/logic unit, memory, I/O device) to perform (execute) the instruction.
4. The sequence repeats from step 1.

Computers can have a wide variety of **peripheral devices** attached to them. An **auxiliary storage device,** or *secondary storage device*, holds coded data for the computer until we actually want to use the data. Instead of inputting data every time, we can input it once and have the computer store it onto an auxiliary storage device. Whenever we need to use the data, we tell the computer to transfer the data from the auxiliary storage device to its memory. An auxiliary storage device therefore serves as both an input and an output device. Typical auxiliary storage devices are disk drives and magnetic tape drives. A *disk drive* is a cross between a compact disc player and a tape recorder. It uses a thin disk made out of magnetic material. A read/write head (similar to the record/playback head in a tape recorder) travels across the spinning disk, retrieving or recording data. A *magnetic tape drive* is like a tape recorder and is most often used to *back up* (make a copy of) the data on a disk in case the disk is ever damaged.

Other examples of peripheral devices include the following:

- Scanners, which "read" visual images on paper and convert them into binary data
- CD-ROM (compact disc–read-only memory) drives, which read (but cannot write) data stored on removable compact discs
- CD-R (compact disc–recordable) drives, which can write to a particular CD once only but can read from it many times
- CD-RW (compact disc–rewritable) drives, which can both write to and read from a particular CD many times
- DVD-ROM (digital video disc [or digital versatile disc]–read-only memory) drives, which use CDs with far greater storage capacity than conventional CDs
- Modems (modulator/demodulators), which convert back and forth between binary data and signals that can be sent over conventional telephone lines
- Audio sound cards and speakers
- Voice synthesizers
- Digital cameras

Together, all of these physical components are known as **hardware.** The programs that allow the hardware to operate are called **software.** Hardware usually is fixed in design; software is easily changed. In fact, the ease with which software can be manipulated is what makes the computer such a versatile, powerful tool.

Peripheral device   An input, output, or auxiliary storage device attached to a computer.

Auxiliary storage device   A device that stores data in encoded form outside the computer's main memory.

Hardware   The physical components of a computer.

Software   Computer programs; the set of all programs available on a computer.

---

*B*ACKGROUND INFORMATION

PCs, Workstations, and Mainframes

There are many different sizes and kinds of computers. *Mainframes* are very large (they can fill a room!) and very fast. A typical mainframe computer consists of several cabinets full of electronic components. Inside those cabinets are the memory, the central processing unit, and input/output units. It's easy to spot the various peripheral devices: Separate cabinets contain the disk drives and tape drives. Other units are obviously printers and terminals (monitors with keyboards). It is common to be able to connect hundreds of terminals to a single mainframe. For example, all of the cash registers in a chain of department stores might be linked to a single mainframe.

At the other end of the spectrum are *personal computers (PCs)*. These are small enough to fit comfortably on top of a desk. Because of their size, it can be difficult to spot the individual parts inside personal computers. Many PCs are just a single box with a screen, a keyboard, and a mouse. You have to open up the case to see the central processing unit, which is usually just an electronic component called an *integrated circuit* or *chip*.

Some personal computers have tape drives, but most operate only with disk drives, CD-ROM drives, and printers. The CD-ROM and disk drives for personal computers typically hold much less data than disks used with mainframes. Similarly, the printers that are attached to personal computers typically are much slower than those used with mainframes.

Laptop or *notebook* computers are PCs that have been reduced to the size of a large notebook and operate on batteries so that they are portable. They typically consist of two parts that are connected by a hinge at the back of the case. The upper part holds a flat, liquid crystal display (LCD) screen, and the lower part has the keyboard, pointing device, processor, memory, and disk drives.

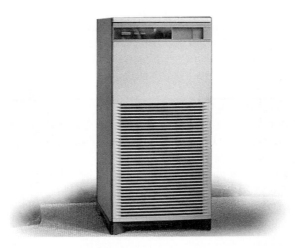

Mainframe Computer

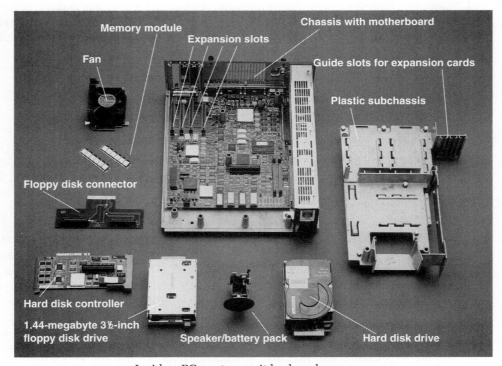

Inside a PC, system unit broken down

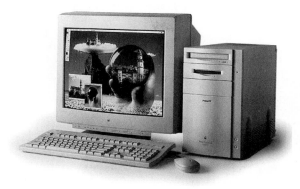

Personal Computer, Macintosh

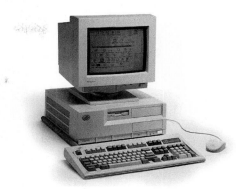

Personal Computer, IBM

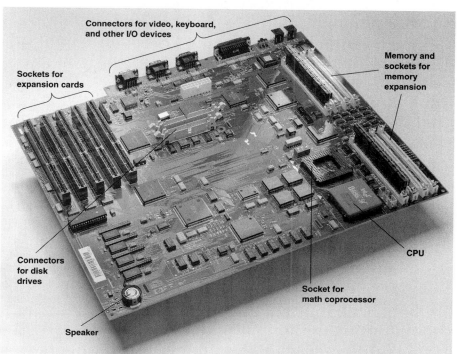

Inside a PC, close-up of a system board

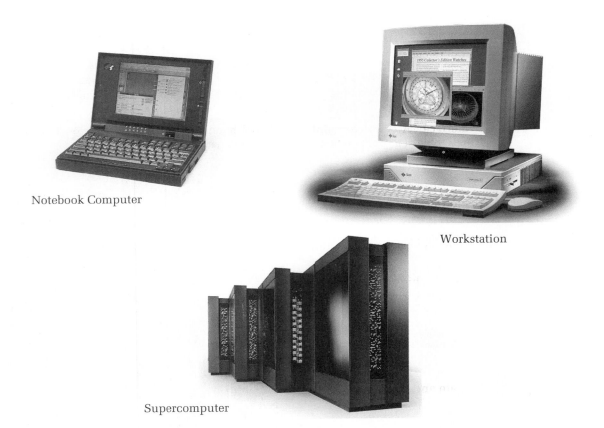

Notebook Computer

Workstation

Supercomputer

Between mainframes and personal computers are *workstations.* These intermediate-sized computer systems are usually less expensive than mainframes and more powerful than personal computers. Workstations are often set up for use primarily by one person at a time. A workstation may also be configured to act like a small mainframe, in which case it is called a *server.* A typical workstation looks very much like a PC. In fact, as PCs have grown more powerful and workstations have become more compact, the distinction between them has begun to fade.

One last type of computer that we should mention is the *supercomputer,* the most powerful class of computer in existence. Supercomputers typically are designed to perform scientific and engineering calculations on immense sets of data with great speed. They are very expensive and thus are not in widespread use.

In addition to the programs that we write or purchase, there are programs in the computer that are designed to simplify the user/computer **interface,** making it easier for us to use the machine. The interface between user and computer is a set of I/O devices—for example, a keyboard, mouse, and screen—that allow the user to communicate with the computer. We work with the keyboard, mouse, and screen on our side of the interface boundary; wires attached to these devices carry the electronic pulses that the computer works with on its side of the interface boundary. At the boundary itself is a mechanism that translates information for the two sides.

Interface A connecting link at a shared boundary that allows independent systems to meet and act on or communicate with each other.

When we communicate directly with the computer, we are using an **interactive system.** Interactive systems allow direct entry of programs and data and provide immediate feedback to the user. In contrast, *batch systems* require that all data be entered before a program is run and provide feedback only after a program has been executed. In this text we focus on interactive systems, although in Chapter 4 we discuss file-oriented programs, which share certain similarities with batch systems.

The set of programs that simplify the user/computer interface and improve the efficiency of processing is called *system software*. It includes the compiler as well as the operating system and the editor (see Figure 1-10). The **operating system** manages all of the computer's resources. It can input programs, call the compiler, execute object programs, and carry out any other system commands. The **editor** is an interactive program used to create and modify source programs or data.

Interactive system A system that allows direct communication between user and computer.

Operating system A set of programs that manages all of the computer's resources.

Editor An interactive program used to create and modify source programs or data.

Although solitary (*stand-alone*) computers are often used in private homes and small businesses, it is very common for many computers to be connected together, forming a *network*. A *local area network* (*LAN*) is one in which the computers are connected by wires and must be reasonably close together, as in a single office building. In a *wide area network* (*WAN*) or *long-haul network*, the computers can be far apart geographically and communicate through phone lines, fiber optic cable, and other media. The most well-known long-haul network is the Internet, which was originally devised as a means for universities, businesses, and government agencies to exchange research information. The Internet exploded in popularity with the establishment of the World Wide Web, a system of linked Internet computers that support specially formatted documents (*Web pages*) that contain text, graphics, audio, and video.

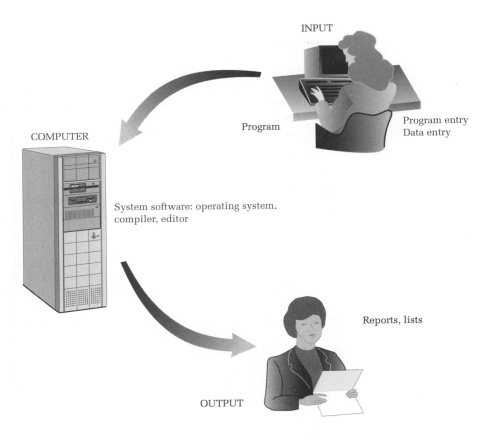

FIGURE 1-10

User/Computer
Interface

INPUT

Program

Program entry
Data entry

COMPUTER

System software: operating system,
compiler, editor

Reports, lists

OUTPUT

*B*ACKGROUND INFORMATION

The Origins of C++

In the late 1960s and early 1970s, Dennis Ritchie created the C programming language
at AT&T Bell Labs. At the time, a group of people within Bell Labs were designing the
UNIX operating system. Initially, UNIX was written in assembly language, as was the
custom for almost all system software in those days. To escape the difficulties of programming in assembly language, Ritchie invented C as a system programming language. C combines the low-level features of an assembly language with the ease of
use and portability of a high-level language. UNIX was reprogrammed so that approximately 90 percent was written in C, and the remainder in assembly language.

   People often wonder where the cryptic name C came from. In the 1960s a programming language named BCPL (Basic Combined Programming Language) had a
small but loyal following, primarily in Europe. From BCPL, another language arose with

its name abbreviated to B. For his language, Dennis Ritchie adopted features from the B language and decided that the successor to B naturally should be named C. So the progression was from BCPL to B to C.

In 1985 Bjarne Stroustrup, also of Bell Labs, invented the C++ programming language. To the C language he added features for data abstraction and object-oriented programming (topics we discuss later in this book). Instead of naming the language D, the Bell Labs group in a humorous vein named it C++. As we see later, ++ signifies the increment operation in the C and C++ languages. Given a variable x, the expression x++ means to increment (add one to) the current value of x. Therefore, the name C++ suggests an enhanced ("incremented") version of the C language.

In the years since Dr. Stroustrup invented C++, the language began to evolve in slightly different ways in different C++ compilers. Although the fundamental features of C++ were nearly the same in all companies' compilers, one company might add a new language feature, whereas another would not. As a result, C++ programs were not always portable from one compiler to the next. The programming community agreed that the language needed to be standardized, and a joint committee of the International Standards Organization (ISO) and the American National Standards Institute (ANSI) began the long process of creating a C++ language standard. After several years of discussion and debate, the ISO/ANSI language standard for C++ was officially approved in mid-1998. Most of the current C++ compilers support the ISO/ANSI standard (hereafter called *standard C++*). To assist you if you are using a pre–standard compiler, throughout the book we point out discrepancies between older language features and new ones that may affect how you write your programs.

Although C originally was intended as a system programming language, both C and C++ are widely used today in business, industry, and personal computing. C++ is powerful and versatile, embodying a wide range of programming concepts. In this book you will learn a substantial portion of the language, but C++ incorporates sophisticated features that go well beyond the scope of an introductory programming course.

Ethics and Responsibilities in the Computing Profession

Every profession operates with a set of ethics that help to define the responsibilities of people who practice the profession. For example, medical professionals have an ethical responsibility to keep information about their patients confidential. Engineers have an ethical responsibility to their employers to protect proprietary information, but they also have a responsibility to protect the public and the environment from harm that may result from their work. Writers are ethically bound not to plagiarize the work of others, and so on.

The computer presents us with a vast new range of capabilities that can affect people and the environment in dramatic ways. It thus challenges society with many new ethical issues. Some of our existing ethical practices apply to the computer, whereas other situations require new ethical rules. In some cases, there may not be established guidelines, but it is up to you to decide what is ethical. In this section we examine some common situations encountered in the computing profession that raise particular ethical issues.

A professional in the computing industry, like any other professional, has knowledge that enables him or her to do certain things that others cannot do. Knowing how to access computers, how to program them, and how to manipulate data gives the computer professional the ability to create new products, solve important problems, and help people to manage their interactions with the ever more complex world in which we all live. Knowledge of computers can be a powerful means to effect positive change.

Knowledge also can be used in unethical ways. A computer can be programmed to trigger a terrorist's bomb, to sabotage a competitor's production line, or to steal money. Although these blatant examples make an extreme point and are unethical in any context, there are more subtle examples that are unique to computers.

Software Piracy

Computer software is easy to copy. But just like books, software is usually copyrighted. It is illegal to copy software without the permission of its creator. Such copying is called **software piracy.**

Software piracy   The unauthorized copying of software for either personal use or use by others.

Copyright laws exist to protect the creators of software (and books and art) so that they can make a profit from the effort and money spent developing the software. A major software package can cost millions of dollars to develop, and this cost (along with the cost of producing the package, shipping it, supporting customers, and allowing for retailer markup) is reflected in the purchase price. If people make unauthorized copies of the software, then the company loses those sales and either has to raise its prices to compensate or spend less money to develop improved versions of the software—in either case, a desirable piece of software becomes harder to obtain.

Software pirates sometimes rationalize their software theft with the excuse that they're just making one copy for their own use. It's not that they're selling a bunch of bootleg copies, after all. But if thousands of people do the same, then it adds up to millions of dollars in lost revenue for the company, which leads to higher prices for everyone.

Computing professionals have an ethical obligation to not engage in software piracy and to try to stop it from occurring. You should never copy software without permission. If someone asks you for a copy of a piece of software, you should refuse to supply it. If someone says that he or she just wants to "borrow" the software to "try it out," tell that person that he or she is welcome to try it out on your machine (or at a retailer's shop) but not to make a copy.

This rule isn't restricted to duplicating copyrighted software; it includes plagiarism of all or part of code that belongs to anyone else. If someone gives you permission to copy some of his or her code, then, just like any responsible writer, you should acknowledge that person with a citation in the code.

Privacy of Data

The computer enables the compilation of databases containing useful information about people, companies, geographic regions, and so on. These databases allow employers to issue payroll checks, banks to cash a customer's check at any branch, the government to collect taxes, and mass merchandisers to send out junk mail. Even though we may not care for every use of databases, they generally have positive benefits. However, they also can be used in negative ways.

For example, a car thief who gains access to the state motor vehicle registry could print out a shopping list of valuable car models together with their owners' addresses. An industrial spy might steal customer data from a company database and sell it to a competitor. Although these are obviously illegal acts, computer professionals face other situations that are not so obvious.

Suppose your job includes managing the company payroll database. In that database are the names and salaries of the employees in the company. You might be tempted to poke around in the database to see how your salary compares with your associates; however, this act is unethical and an invasion of your associates' right to privacy, because this information is confidential. Any information about a person that is not clearly public should be considered confidential. An example of public information is a phone number listed in a telephone directory. Private information includes any data that has been provided with an understanding that it will be used only for a specific purpose (such as the data on a credit card application).

A computing professional has a responsibility to avoid taking advantage of special access that he or she may have to confidential data. The professional also has a responsibility to guard that data from unauthorized access. Guarding data can involve such simple things as shredding old printouts, keeping backup copies in a locked cabinet, and not using passwords that are easy to guess (such as a name or word) as well as more complex measures such as *encryption* (keeping data stored in a secret coded form).

Use of Computer Resources

If you've ever bought a computer, you know that it costs money. A personal computer can be relatively inexpensive, but it is still a major purchase. Larger computers can cost millions of dollars. Operating a PC may cost a few dollars a month for electricity and an occasional outlay for paper, disks, and repairs. Larger computers can cost tens of thousands of dollars per month to operate. Regardless of the type of computer, whoever owns it has to pay these costs. They do so because the computer is a resource that justifies its expense.

The computer is an unusual resource because it is valuable only when a program is running. Thus, the computer's time is really the valuable resource. There is no significant physical difference between a computer that is working and one that is sitting idle. By contrast, a car is in motion when it is working. Thus, unauthorized use of a computer is different from unauthorized use of a car. If one person uses another's car without permission, that individual must take possession of it physically—that is, steal it. If someone uses a computer without permission, the computer isn't physically stolen, but just as in the case of car theft, the owner is being deprived of a resource that he or she is paying for.

For some people, theft of computer resources is a game—like joyriding in a car. The thief really doesn't want the resources, just the challenge of breaking through a computer's security system and seeing how far he or she can get without being caught. Success gives a thrilling boost to this sort of person's ego. Many computer thieves think that their actions are acceptable if they do no harm, but whenever real work is displaced from the computer by such activities, then harm is clearly being done. If nothing else, the thief is trespassing in the computer owner's property. By analogy, consider that even though no physical harm may be done by someone who breaks into your bedroom and takes a nap while you are away, such an action is certainly disturbing to you because it poses a threat of potential physical harm. In this case, and in the case of breaking into a computer, mental harm can be done.

Other thieves can be malicious. Like a joyrider who purposely crashes a stolen car, these people destroy or corrupt data to cause harm. They may feel a sense of power from being able to hurt others with impunity. Sometimes these people leave behind programs that act as time bombs, to cause harm long after they have gone. Another kind of program that may be left is a virus—a program that replicates itself, often with the goal of spreading to other computers. Viruses can be benign, causing no other harm than to use up some resources. Others can be destructive and cause widespread damage to data. Incidents have occurred in which viruses have cost millions of dollars in lost computer time and data.

Virus A computer program that replicates itself, often with the goal of spreading to other computers without authorization, and possibly with the intent of doing harm.

Computing professionals have an ethical responsibility never to use computer resources without permission, which includes activities such as doing personal work on an employer's computer. We also have a responsibility to help guard resources to which we have access—by using unguessable passwords and keeping them secret, by watching for signs of unusual computer use, by writing programs that do not provide loopholes in a computer's security system, and so on.

Software Engineering

Humans have come to depend greatly on computers in many aspects of their lives. That reliance is fostered by the perception that computers function reliably; that is, they work correctly most of the time. However, the reliability of a computer depends on the care that is taken in writing its software.

Errors in a program can have serious consequences, as the following examples of real incidents involving software errors illustrate. An error in the control software of the F-18 jet fighter caused it to flip upside down the first time it flew across the equator. A rocket launch went out of control and had to be blown up because there was a comma typed in place of a period in its control software. A radiation therapy machine killed several patients because a software error caused the machine to operate at full power when the operator typed certain commands too quickly.

Even when the software is used in less critical situations, errors can have significant effects. Examples of such errors include the following:

- An error in your word processor that causes your term paper to be lost just hours before it is due
- An error in a statistical program that causes a scientist to draw a wrong conclusion and publish a paper that must later be retracted
- An error in a tax preparation program that produces an incorrect return, leading to a fine

Programmers thus have a responsibility to develop software that is free from errors. The process that is used to develop correct software is known as **software engineering.**

Software engineering The application of traditional engineering methodologies and techniques to the development of software.

Software engineering has many aspects. The software life cycle described at the beginning of this chapter outlines the stages in the development of software. Different techniques are used at each of these stages. We address many of the techniques in this text. In Chapter 4 we introduce methodologies for developing correct algorithms. We discuss strategies for testing and validating programs in every chapter. We use a modern programming language that enables us to write readable, well-organized programs, and so on. Some aspects of software engineering, such as the development of a formal, mathematical specification for a program, are beyond the scope of this text.

Problem-Solving Techniques

You solve problems every day, often unaware of the process you are going through. In a learning environment, you usually are given most of the information you need: a clear statement of the problem, the necessary input, and the required output. In real life, the process is not always so simple. You often have to define the problem yourself and then decide what information you have to work with and what the results should be.

After you understand and analyze a problem, you must come up with a solution—an algorithm. Earlier we defined an algorithm as a step-by-step procedure for solving a problem in a finite amount of time. Although you work with algorithms all the time, most of your experience with them is in the context of *following* them. You follow a recipe, play a game, assemble a toy, take medicine. In the problem-solving phase of computer programming, you will be *designing* algorithms, not following them. This means you must be conscious of the strategies you use to solve problems in order to apply them to programming problems.

Ask Questions

If you are given a task orally, you ask questions—When? Why? Where?—until you understand exactly what you have to do. If your instructions are written, you might put question marks in the margin, underline a word or a sentence, or in some other way indicate that the task is not clear. Your questions may be answered by a later paragraph, or you might have to discuss them with the person who gave you the task.

These are some of the questions you might ask in the context of programming:

- What do I have to work with—that is, what is my data?
- What do the data items look like?
- How much data is there?

- How will I know when I have processed all the data?
- What should my output look like?
- How many times is the process going to be repeated?
- What special error conditions might come up?

Look for Things That Are Familiar

Never reinvent the wheel. If a solution exists, use it. If you've solved the same or a similar problem before, just repeat your solution. People are good at recognizing similar situations. We don't have to learn how to go to the store to buy milk, then to buy eggs, and then to buy candy. We know that going to the store is always the same; only what we buy is different.

In programming, certain problems occur again and again in different guises. A good programmer immediately recognizes a subtask he or she has solved before and plugs in the solution. For example, finding the daily high and low temperatures is really the same problem as finding the highest and lowest grades on a test. You want the largest and smallest values in a set of numbers (see Figure 1-11).

Solve by Analogy

Often a problem reminds you of a similar problem you have seen before. You may find solving the problem at hand easier if you remember how you

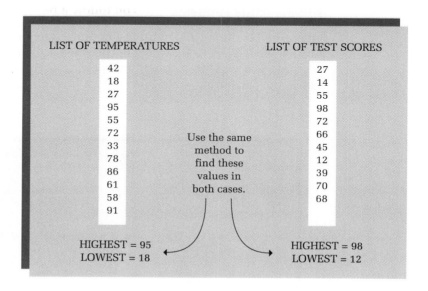

FIGURE 1-11

Look for Things That Are Familiar

FIGURE 1-12

Analogy

A library catalog system can give insight into how to organize a parts inventory.

solved the other problem. In other words, draw an analogy between the two problems. For example, a solution to a perspective projection problem from an art class might help you figure out how to compute the distance to a landmark when you are on a cross-country hike. As you work your way through the new problem, you come across things that are different than they were in the old problem, but usually these are just details that you can deal with one at a time.

Analogy is really just a broader application of the strategy of looking for things that are familiar. When you are trying to find an algorithm for solving a problem, don't limit yourself to computer-oriented solutions. Step back and try to get a larger view of the problem. Don't worry if your analogy doesn't match perfectly—the only reason for using an analogy is that it gives you a place to start (see Figure 1-12). The best programmers are people who have broad experience solving all kinds of problems.

Means-Ends Analysis

Often the beginning state and the ending state are given; the problem is to define a set of actions that can be used to get from one to the other. Suppose you want to go from Boston, Massachusetts, to Austin, Texas. You know the beginning state (you are in Boston) and the ending state (you

FIGURE 1-13

Means-Ends
Analysis

Start: Boston **Goal:** Austin	**Means:** *Fly,* walk, hitchhike, bike, drive, sail, bus
Start: Boston **Goal:** Austin	**Revised Means:** Fly to Chicago and then Austin; *fly to Newark and then Austin:* fly to Atlanta and then Austin
Start: Boston **Intermediate Goal:** Newark **Goal:** Austin	**Means to Intermediate Goal:** *Commuter flight,* walk, hitchhike, bike, drive, sail, bus
Solution: Take commuter flight to Newark and then catch cheap flight to Austin	

want to be in Austin). The problem is how to get from one to the other. In this example, you have lots of choices. You can fly, walk, hitchhike, ride a bike, or whatever. The method you choose depends on your circumstances. If you're in a hurry, you'll probably decide to fly.

Once you've narrowed down the set of actions, you have to work out the details. It may help to establish intermediate goals that are easier to meet than the overall goal. Let's say there is a really cheap, direct flight to Austin out of Newark, New Jersey. You might decide to divide the trip into legs: Boston to Newark and then Newark to Austin. Your intermediate goal is to get from Boston to Newark. Now you only have to examine the means of meeting that intermediate goal (see Figure 1-13).

The overall strategy of means-ends analysis is to define the ends and then to analyze your means of getting between them. The process translates easily to computer programming. You begin by writing down what the input is and what the output should be. Then you consider the actions a computer can perform and choose a sequence of actions that can transform the data into the results.

Divide and Conquer

We often break up large problems into smaller units that are easier to handle. Cleaning the whole house may seem overwhelming; cleaning the rooms one at a time seems much more manageable. The same principle applies to programming. We break up a large problem into smaller pieces that we can solve individually (see Figure 1-14). In fact, the functional

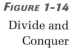

FIGURE 1-14

Divide and Conquer

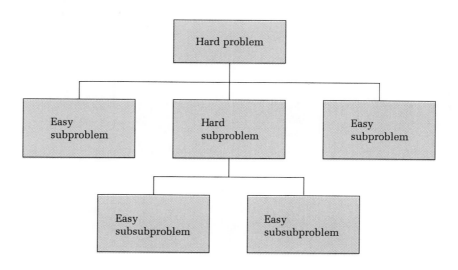

decomposition and object-oriented methodologies, which we describe in Chapter 4, are based on the principle of divide and conquer.

The Building-Block Approach

Another way of attacking a large problem is to see if any solutions for smaller pieces of the problem exist. It may be possible to put some of these solutions together end to end to solve most of the big problem. This strategy is just a combination of the look-for-familiar-things and divide-and-conquer approaches. You look at the big problem and see that it can be divided into smaller problems for which solutions already exist. Solving the big problem is just a matter of putting the existing solutions together, like mortaring together blocks to form a wall (see Figure 1-15).

Merging Solutions

Another way to combine existing solutions is to merge them on a step-by-step basis. For example, to compute the average of a list of values, we must both sum and count the values. If we already have separate solutions for summing values and for counting values, we can combine them. But if we first do the summing and then do the counting, we have to read the list twice. We can save steps if we merge these two solutions: Read a value and then add it to the running total and add 1 to our count before going on to the next value. Whenever the solutions to subproblems duplicate steps, think about merging them instead of joining them end to end.

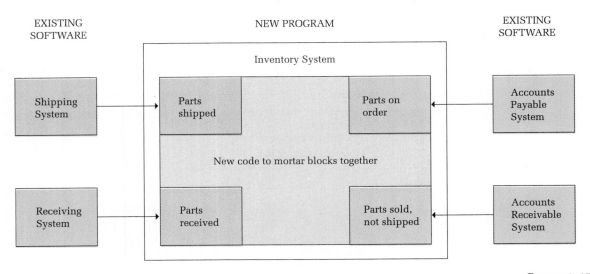

FIGURE 1-15
Building-Block Approach

FIGURE 1-16

Mental Block

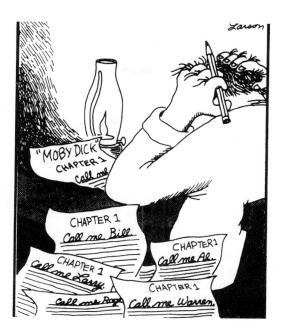

Mental Blocks: The Fear of Starting

Writers are all too familiar with the experience of staring at a blank page, not knowing where to begin. Programmers have the same difficulty when they first tackle a big problem. They look at the problem and it seems overwhelming (see Figure 1-16).

Remember that you always have a way to begin solving any problem: Write it down on paper in your own words so that you understand it. Once you paraphrase the problem, you can focus on each of the subparts individually instead of trying to tackle the entire problem at once. This process gives you a clearer picture of the overall problem. It helps you see pieces of the problem that look familiar or that are analogous to other problems you have solved, and it pinpoints areas where something is unclear, where you need more information.

As you write down a problem, you tend to group things together into small, understandable chunks, which may be natural places to split the problem up—to divide and conquer. Your description of the problem may collect all of the information about data and results into one place for easy reference. Then you can see the beginning and ending states necessary for means-ends analysis.

Most mental blocks are caused by not really understanding the problem. Rewriting the problem in your own words is a good way to focus on the subparts of the problem, one at a time, and to understand what is required for a solution.

Algorithmic Problem Solving

Coming up with a step-by-step procedure for solving a particular problem is not always a cut-and-dried process. In fact, it is usually a trial-and-error process requiring several attempts and refinements. We test each attempt to see if it really solves the problem. If it does, fine. If it doesn't, we try again. Solving any nontrivial problem typically requires a combination of the techniques we've described.

Remember that the computer can only do certain things (see p. 14). Your primary concern, then, is how to make the computer transform, manipulate, calculate, or process the input data to produce the desired output. If you keep in mind the allowable instructions in your programming language, you won't design an algorithm that is difficult or impossible to code.

In the case study that follows, we develop a program for calculating employees' weekly wages. It typifies the thought processes involved in writing an algorithm and coding it as a program, and it shows you what a complete C++ program looks like.

PROBLEM-SOLVING CASE STUDY

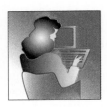

An Algorithm for a Company Payroll

Problem: A small company needs an interactive program (the payroll clerk will input the data) to figure its weekly payroll. The input data and each employee's wages should be saved in a secondary storage file, and the total wages for the week should be displayed on the screen so that the payroll clerk can transfer the appropriate amount into the payroll account.

Discussion: At first glance, this seems like a simple problem. But if you think about how you would do it by hand, you see that you need to ask questions about the specifics of the process. What employee data is input? How are wages computed? In what file should the results be stored? How does the clerk indicate that all of the data has been entered?

- The data for each employee includes an employee identification number, the employee's hourly pay rate, and the hours worked that week.
- Wages equal the employee's pay rate times the number of hours worked, up to 40 hours. If an employee worked more than 40 hours, wages equal the employee's pay rate times 40 hours, plus $1\frac{1}{2}$ times the employee's regular pay rate times the number of hours worked above 40.
- The results should be stored in a file called payFile.

<u>*PROBLEM-SOLVING CASE STUDY cont'd.*</u>

■ There is no employee number 0, so the clerk can indicate the end of the data by entering a 0 when asked for an employee number.

Let's apply the *divide-and-conquer* approach to this problem. There are three obvious steps in almost any problem of this type:

1. Get the data.
2. Compute the results.
3. Output the results.

First we need to get the data. (By *get*, we mean *read* or *input* the data.) We need three pieces of data for each employee: employee identification number, hourly pay rate, and number of hours worked. So that the clerk will know when to enter each value, we must have the computer output a message that indicates when it is ready to accept each of the values (this is called a *prompting message*, or a *prompt*). Therefore, to input the data, we take these steps:

Prompt the user for the employee number (put a message on the screen)
Read the employee number
Prompt the user for the employee's hourly pay rate
Read the pay rate
Prompt the user for the number of hours worked
Read the number of hours worked

The next step is to compute the wages. Let's apply *means-ends analysis*. Our starting point is the set of data values that was input; our desired ending, the payroll for the week. The means at our disposal are the basic operations that the computer can perform, which include calculation and control structures. Let's begin by working backward from the end.

We know that there are two formulas for computing wages: one for regular hours and one for overtime. If there is no overtime, wages are simply the pay rate times the number of hours worked. If the number of hours worked is greater than 40, however, wages are 40 times the pay rate, plus the number of overtime hours times $1^1/_2$ times the pay rate. The number of overtime hours is computed by subtracting 40 from the total number of hours worked. Here are the two formulas:

wages = hours worked × pay rate
wages = (40.0 × pay rate) + (hours worked − 40.0) × 1.5 × pay rate

We now have the means to compute wages for each case. Our intermediate goal is to execute the correct formula given the input data. We must decide which formula to use and employ a branching control structure to make the computer execute the appropriate formula. The decision that controls the branching structure is simply whether more than 40 hours have been worked. We now have the means to get from our starting point to the desired end. To figure the wages, then, we take the following steps:

If hours worked is greater than 40.0, then
    wages = (40.0 × pay rate) + (hours worked – 40.0) × 1.5 × pay rate
otherwise
    wages = hours worked × pay rate

The last step, outputting the results, is simply a matter of directing the computer to write the employee number, the pay rate, the number of hours worked, and the wages into `payFile`:

Write the employee number, pay rate, hours worked, and wages into payFile

There are two things we've overlooked. First, we must repeat this process for each employee, and second, we must compute the total wages for the week. Let's use the *building-block approach* to combine our three main steps (getting the data, computing the wages, and outputting the results) with a structure that repeats the steps for each employee as long as the employee number is not 0. When the employee number is 0, this structure should skip to the end of the algorithm. Next we should insert a step just after the wages are computed that adds them to a running total.

Finally, we must take care of a couple of housekeeping chores. Before we start processing, we must prepare the output file to receive the results and set the running total to zero. At the end of the algorithm, we must tell the computer to stop processing.

What follows is the complete algorithm. Calculating the wages is written as a separate subalgorithm that is defined below the main algorithm. Notice that the algorithm is simply a very precise description of the same steps you would follow to do this process by hand.

Main Algorithm

Prepare to write a list of the employees' wages (open file payFile)
Set the total payroll to zero
Prompt the user for the employee number (put a message on the screen)
Read the employee number
As long as the employee number is not 0, repeat the following steps:
    Prompt the user for the employee's hourly pay rate
    Read the pay rate
    Prompt the user for the number of hours worked
    Read the number of hours worked

Perform the subalgorithm for calculating pay (below)
Add the employee's wages to the total payroll
Write the employee number, pay rate, hours worked, and wages onto the list (file payFile)
Prompt the user for the employee number
Read the employee number
When an employee number equal to 0 is read, continue with the following steps:
Write the total company payroll on the screen
Stop

Subalgorithm for Calculating Pay

If hours worked is greater than 40.0, then
wages = (40.0 × pay rate) + (hours worked − 40.0) × 1.5 × pay rate
otherwise
wages = hours worked × pay rate

Before we implement this algorithm, we should test it. Case Study Follow-Up Exercise 2 asks you to carry out this test.

What follows is the C++ program for this algorithm. It's here to give you an idea of what you'll be learning. If you've had no previous exposure to programming, you probably won't understand most of the program. Don't worry; you will soon. In fact, throughout this book as we introduce new constructs, we refer you back to the Payroll program. One more thing: The remarks following the symbols // are called comments. They are here to help you understand the program; the compiler ignores them. Words enclosed by the symbols /* and */ also are comments and are ignored by the compiler.

```cpp
//*****************************************************************
// Payroll program
// This program computes each employee's wages and
// the total company payroll
//*****************************************************************
#include <iostream>
#include <fstream>      // For file I/O

using namespace std;

void CalcPay( float, float, float& );

const float MAX_HOURS = 40.0;    // Maximum normal work hours
const float OVERTIME = 1.5;      // Overtime pay rate factor

int main()
{
```

```
    float    payRate;      // Employee's pay rate
    float    hours;        // Hours worked
    float    wages;        // Wages earned
    float    total;        // Total company payroll
    int      empNum;       // Employee ID number
    ofstream payFile;      // Company payroll file

    payFile.open("payfile.dat");           // Open the output file
    total = 0.0;                           // Initialize total
    cout << "Enter employee number: ";     // Prompt
    cin >> empNum;                         // Read employee ID no.
    while (empNum != 0)                    // While employee number
    {                                      //   isn't zero
        cout << "Enter pay rate: ";        // Prompt
        cin >> payRate;                    // Read hourly pay rate
        cout << "Enter hours worked: ";    // Prompt
        cin >> hours;                      // Read hours worked
        CalcPay(payRate, hours, wages);    // Compute wages
        total = total + wages;             // Add wages to total
        payFile << empNum << payRate       // Put results into file
               << hours << wages;
        cout << "Enter employee number: "; // Prompt
        cin >> empNum;                     // Read ID number
    }
    cout << "Total payroll is "            // Print total payroll
        << total << endl;                  //    on screen
    return 0;                              // Indicate successful
}                                          //    completion


//******************************************************************

void CalcPay( /* in */  float  payRate,      // Employee's pay rate
              /* in */  float  hours,        // Hours worked
              /* out */ float& wages )       // Wages earned

// CalcPay computes wages from the employee's pay rate
// and the hours worked, taking overtime into account

{
    if (hours > MAX_HOURS)                    // Is there overtime?
        wages = (MAX_HOURS * payRate) +       // Yes
               (hours - MAX_HOURS) * payRate * OVERTIME;
    else
        wages = hours * payRate;              // No
}
```

Summary

We think nothing of turning on the television and sitting down to watch it. It's a communication tool we use to enhance our lives. Computers are becoming as common as televisions, just a normal part of our lives. And like televisions, computers are based on complex principles but are designed for easy use.

Computers are dumb; they must be told what to do. A true computer error is extremely rare (usually due to a component malfunction or an electrical fault). Because we tell the computer what to do, most errors in computer-generated output are really human errors.

Computer programming is the process of planning a sequence of steps for a computer to follow. It involves a problem-solving phase and an implementation phase. After analyzing a problem, we develop and test a general solution (algorithm). This general solution becomes a concrete solution—our program—when we write it in a high-level programming language. The sequence of instructions that makes up our program is then compiled into machine code, the language the computer uses. After correcting any errors ("bugs") that show up during testing, our program is ready to use.

Once we begin to use the program, it enters the maintenance phase. Maintenance involves correcting any errors discovered while the program is being used and changing the program to reflect changes in the user's requirements.

Data and instructions are represented as binary numbers (numbers consisting of just 1s and 0s) in electronic computers. The process of converting data and instructions into a form usable by the computer is called coding.

A programming language reflects the range of operations a computer can perform. The basic control structures in a programming language—sequence, selection, loop, and subprogram—are based on these fundamental operations. In this text, you will learn to write programs in the high-level programming language called C++.

Computers are composed of six basic parts: the memory unit, the arithmetic/logic unit, the control unit, input and output devices, and auxiliary storage devices. The arithmetic/logic unit and control unit together are called the central processing unit. The physical parts of the computer are called hardware. The programs that are executed by the computer are called software.

System software is a set of programs designed to simplify the user/computer interface. It includes the compiler, the operating system, and the editor.

Computing professionals are guided by a set of ethics, as are members of other professions. Among the responsibilities that we have are copying software only with permission and including attribution to other programmers when we make use of their code, guarding the privacy of confidential data, using computer resources only with permission, and carefully engineering our programs so that they work correctly.

We've said that problem solving is an integral part of the programming process. Although you may have little experience programming computers, you have lots of experience solving problems. The key is to stop and think about the strategies you use to solve problems, and then to use those strategies to devise workable algorithms. Among those strategies are asking questions, looking for things that are familiar, solving by analogy, applying means-ends analysis, dividing the problem into subproblems, using existing solutions to small problems to solve a larger problem, merging solutions, and paraphrasing the problem in order to overcome a mental block.

The computer is widely used today in science, engineering, business, government, medicine, consumer goods, and the arts. Learning to program in C++ can help you use this powerful tool effectively.

Quick Check

The Quick Check is intended to help you decide if you've met the goals set forth at the beginning of each chapter. If you understand the material in the chapter, the answer to each question should be fairly obvious. After reading a question, check your response against the answers listed at the end of the Quick Check. If you don't know an answer or don't understand the answer that's provided, turn to the page(s) listed at the end of the question to review the material.

1. What is a computer program? (p. 3)
2. What are the three phases in a program's life cycle? (p. 4)
3. Is an algorithm the same as a program? (p. 5)
4. What is a programming language? (p. 6)
5. What are the advantages of using a high-level programming language? (p. 11)
6. What does a compiler do? (p. 12)
7. What part does the object program play in the compilation and execution processes? (p. 12)
8. Name the four basic ways of structuring statements in C++ and other languages. (p. 15)
9. What are the six basic components of a computer? (p. 16)
10. What is the difference between hardware and software? (p. 19)
11. In what regard is theft of computer time like stealing a car? How are the two crimes different? (p. 28)
12. What is the divide-and-conquer approach? (p. 33)

Answers **1.** A computer program is a sequence of instructions performed by a computer. **2.** The three phases of a program's life cycle are problem solving, implementation, and maintenance. **3.** No. All programs are algorithms, but not all algorithms are programs. **4.** A set of rules, symbols, and special words used to construct a program. **5.** A high-level programming language is easier to use than an assembly language or a machine language. Also, programs written in a high-level language can be run on many different computers. **6.** The compiler translates a program written in a high-level language into machine language. **7.** The object program is the machine language version of a program. It is created by a compiler. The object program is what is loaded into the computer's memory and executed. **8.** Sequence, selection, loop, and subprogram.   **9.** The basic components of a computer are the memory unit, arithmetic/logic unit, control unit, input and output devices, and auxiliary storage devices. **10.** Hardware is the physical components of the computer; software is the collection of programs that run on the computer.   **11.** Both crimes deprive the owner of access to a resource. A physical object is taken in a car theft, whereas time is the thing being stolen from the computer owner.   **12.** The divide-and-conquer approach is a problem-solving technique that breaks a large problem into smaller, simpler subproblems.

Exam Preparation Exercises

1. Explain why the following series of steps is not an algorithm, then rewrite the series so it is.

   Shampooing
   (1) Rinse.
   (2) Lather.
   (3) Repeat.

2. Describe the input and output files used by a compiler.
3. In the following recipe for chocolate pound cake, identify the steps that are branches (selection) and loops, and the steps that are references to subalgorithms outside the algorithm.

   Preheat the oven to 350 degrees
   Line the bottom of a 9-inch tube pan with wax paper
   Sift $2^3/_4$ c flour, $^3/_4$ t cream of tartar, $^1/_2$ t baking soda, $1^1/_2$ t salt, and $1^3/_4$ c sugar
       into a large bowl
   Add 1 c shortening to the bowl
   If using butter, margarine, or lard, then
       add $^2/_3$ c milk to the bowl,
   else
       (for other shortenings) add 1 c minus 2 T of milk to the bowl
   Add 1 t vanilla to the mixture in the bowl
   If mixing with a spoon, then
       see the instructions in the introduction to the chapter on cakes,
   else
       (for electric mixers) beat the contents of the bowl for 2 minutes at medium
       speed, scraping the bowl and beaters as needed
   Add 3 eggs plus 1 extra egg yolk to the bowl
   Melt 3 squares of unsweetened chocolate and add to the mixture in the bowl
   Beat the mixture for 1 minute at medium speed
   Pour the batter into the tube pan
   Put the pan into the oven and bake for 1 hour and 10 minutes
   Perform the test for doneness described in the introduction to the chapter on
       cakes
   Repeat the test once each minute until the cake is done
   Remove the pan from the oven and allow the cake to cool for 2 hours
   Follow the instructions for removing the cake from the pan, given in the
       introduction to the chapter on cakes
   Sprinkle powdered sugar over the cracks on top of the cake just before serving

4. Put a check next to each item below that is a peripheral device.
    _____ a. Disk drive
    _____ b. Arithmetic/logic unit
    _____ c. Magnetic tape drive
    _____ d. Printer
    _____ e. CD-ROM drive
    _____ f. Memory
    _____ g. Auxiliary storage device
    _____ h. Control unit
    _____ i. LCD screen
    _____ j. Mouse
5. Next to each item below, indicate whether it is hardware (H) or software (S).
    _____ a. Disk drive
    _____ b. Memory
    _____ c. Compiler
    _____ d. Arithmetic/logic unit
    _____ e. Editor
    _____ f. Operating system
    _____ g. Object program
    _____ h. Mouse
    _____ i. Central processing unit
6. Means-ends analysis is a problem-solving strategy.
    a. What are three things you must know in order to apply means-ends analysis to a problem?
    b. What is one way of combining this technique with the divide-and-conquer strategy?
7. Show how you would use the divide-and-conquer approach to solve the problem of finding a job.

Programming Warm-up Exercises

1. Write an algorithm for driving from where you live to the nearest airport that has regularly scheduled flights. Restrict yourself to a vocabulary of 74 words plus numbers and place names. You must select the appropriate set of words for this task. An example of a vocabulary is given in Appendix A, the list of reserved words (words with special meaning) in the C++ programming language. Notice that there are just 74 words in that list. The purpose of this exercise is to give you practice writing simple, exact instructions with an equally small vocabulary.
2. Write an algorithm for making a peanut butter and jelly sandwich, using a vocabulary of just 74 words (you choose the words). Assume that all ingredients are in the refrigerator and that the necessary tools are in a drawer under the kitchen counter. The instructions must be very simple and exact because the person making the sandwich has no knowledge of food preparation and takes every word literally.
3. In Exercise 1 above, identify the sequential, conditional, repetitive, and subprogram steps.

Case Study Follow-Up

1. Using Figure 1-14 as a guide, construct a divide-and-conquer diagram of the Problem-Solving Case Study, "An Algorithm for a Company Payroll."
2. Use the following data set to test the payroll algorithm presented on pages 38–39. Follow each step of the algorithm just as it is written, as if you were a computer. Then check your results by hand to be sure that the algorithm is correct.

ID Number	Pay Rate	Hours Worked
327	8.30	48
201	6.60	40
29	12.50	40
166	9.25	51
254	7.00	32
0		

3. In the Company Payroll case study, we used means-ends analysis to develop the subalgorithm for calculating pay. What are the *ends* in the analysis? That is, what information did we start with and what information did we want to end up with?
4. In the Payroll program, certain remarks are preceded by the symbols //. What are these remarks called, and what does the compiler do with them? What is their purpose?

2

C++ Syntax and Semantics, and the Program Development Process

- To understand how a C++ program is composed of one or more subprograms (functions).
- To be able to read syntax templates in order to understand the formal rules governing C++ programs.
- To be able to create and recognize legal C++ identifiers.
- To be able to declare named constants and variables of type `char` and `string`.
- To be able to distinguish reserved words in C++ from user-defined identifiers.
- To be able to assign values to variables.
- To be able to construct simple string expressions made up of constants, variables, and the concatenation operator.
- To be able to construct a statement that writes to an output stream.
- To be able to determine what is printed by a given output statement.
- To be able to use comments to clarify your programs.
- To be able to construct simple C++ programs.
- To learn the steps involved in entering and running a program.

The Elements of C++ Programs

Programmers develop solutions to problems using a programming language. In this chapter, we start looking at the rules and symbols that make up the C++ programming language. We also review the steps required to create a program and make it work on a computer.

C++ Program Structure

In Chapter 1, we talked about the four basic structures for expressing actions in a programming language: sequence, selection, loop, and subprogram. We said that subprograms allow us to write parts of our program separately and then assemble them into final form. In C++, all subprograms are referred to as **functions,** and a C++ program is a collection of one or more functions.

Each function performs some particular task, and collectively they all cooperate to solve the entire problem.

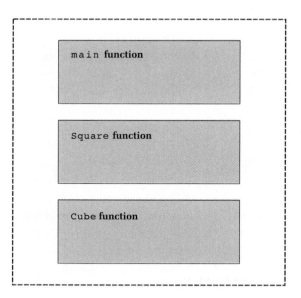

Function   A subprogram in C++.

Every C++ program must have a function named `main`. Execution of the program always begins with the `main` function. You can think of `main` as the master and the other functions as the servants. When `main` wants the function `Square` to perform a task, `main` *calls* (or *invokes*) `Square`. When the `Square` function completes execution of its statements, it obediently returns control to the master, `main`, so the master can continue executing.

Let's look at an example of a C++ program with three functions: `main`, `Square`, and `Cube`. Don't be too concerned with the details in the program—just observe its overall look and structure.

```
#include <iostream>

using namespace std;

int Square( int );
int Cube( int );

int main()
{
    cout << "The square of 27 is " << Square(27) << endl;
    cout << "and the cube of 27 is " << Cube(27) << endl;
    return 0;
}

int Square( int n )
{
    return n * n;
}

int Cube( int n )
{
    return n * n * n;
}
```

In each of the three functions, the left brace ({) and right brace (}) mark the beginning and end of the statements to be executed. Statements appearing between the braces are known as the *body* of the function.

Execution of a program always begins with the first statement of the `main` function. In our program, the first statement is

```
cout << "The square of 27 is " << Square(27) << endl;
```

This is an output statement that causes information to be printed on the computer's display screen. You will learn how to construct output statements like this later in the chapter. Briefly, this statement prints two items. The first is the message

```
The square of 27 is
```

The second to be printed is the value obtained by calling (invoking) the Square function, with the value 27 as the number to be squared. As the servant, the Square function performs its task of squaring the number and sending the computed result (729) back to its *caller*, the main function. Now main can continue executing by printing the value 729 and proceeding to its next statement.

In a similar fashion, the second statement in main prints the message

```
and the cube of 27 is
```

and then invokes the Cube function and prints the result, 19683. The complete output produced by executing this program is, therefore,

```
The square of 27 is 729
and the cube of 27 is 19683
```

Both Square and Cube are examples of *value-returning functions*. A value-returning function returns a single value to its caller. The word int at the beginning of the first line of the Square function

```
int Square( int n )
```

states that the function returns an integer value.

Now look at the main function again. You'll see that the first line of the function is

```
int main()
```

The word int indicates that main is a value-returning function that should return an integer value. And it does. After printing the square and cube of 27, main executes the statement

```
return 0;
```

to return the value 0 to its caller. But who calls the main function? The answer is: the computer's operating system.

When you work with C++ programs, the operating system is considered to be the caller of the main function. The operating system expects main to return a value when main finishes executing. By convention, a return value of 0 means everything went OK. A return value of anything else (typically 1, 2, ...) means something went wrong. Later in this book we look at situations in which you might want to return a value other than 0 from main. For the time being, we always conclude the execution of main by returning the value 0.

We have looked only briefly at the overall picture of what a C++ program looks like—a collection of one or more functions, including `main`. We have also mentioned what is special about the `main` function—it is a required function, execution begins there, and it returns a value to the operating system. Now it's time to begin looking at the details of the C++ language.

Syntax and Semantics

A programming language is a set of rules, symbols, and special words used to construct a program. There are rules for both **syntax** (grammar) and **semantics** (meaning).

Syntax   The formal rules governing how valid instructions are written in a programming language.

Semantics   The set of rules that determines the meaning of instructions written in a programming language.

Syntax is a formal set of rules that defines exactly what combinations of letters, numbers, and symbols can be used in a programming language. There is no room for ambiguity in the syntax of a programming language because the computer can't think; it doesn't "know what we mean." To avoid ambiguity, syntax rules themselves must be written in a very simple, precise, formal language called a **metalanguage.**

Metalanguage   A language that is used to write the syntax rules for another language.

Learning to read a metalanguage is like learning to read the notations used in the rules of a sport. Once you understand the notations, you can read the rule book. It's true that many people learn a sport simply by watching others play, but what they learn is usually just enough to allow them to take part in casual games. You could learn C++ by following the examples in this book, but a serious programmer, like a serious athlete, must take the time to read and understand the rules.

Syntax rules are the blueprints we use to build instructions in a program. They allow us to take the elements of a programming language—the basic building blocks of the language—and assemble them into *constructs*, syntactically correct structures. If our program violates any of the rules of the language—by misspelling a crucial word or leaving out an important comma, for instance—the program is said to have *syntax errors* and cannot compile correctly until we fix them.

THEORETICAL FOUNDATIONS

Metalanguages

Metalanguage is the word *language* with the prefix *meta-*, which means "beyond" or "more comprehensive." A metalanguage is a language that goes beyond a normal language by allowing us to speak precisely about that language. It is a language for talking about languagesOne of the oldest computer-oriented metalanguages is *Backus-Naur Form* (*BNF*), which is named for John Backus and Peter Naur, who developed it in 1960. BNF syntax definitions are written out using letters, numbers, and special symbols. For example, an *identifier* (a name for something in a program) in C++ must be at least one letter or underscore (_), which may or may not be followed by additional letters, underscores, or digits. The BNF definition of an identifier in C++ is

<Identifier> ::= <Nondigit> | <Nondigit> <NondigitOrDigitSequence>
<NondigitOrDigitSequence> ::= <NondigitOrDigit> | <NondigitOrDigit> <NondigitOrDigitSequence>
<NondigitOrDigit> ::= <Nondigit> | <Digit>
<Nondigit> ::= _ | A | B | C | D | E | F | G | H | I | J | K | L | M | N | O | P | Q | R | S | T | U | V | W | X | Y | Z |
        a | b | c | d | e | f | g | h | i | j | k | l | m | n | o | p | q | r | s | t | u | v | w | x | y | z
<Digit> ::= 0 | 1 | 2 | 3 | 4 | 5 | 6 | 7 | 8 | 9

where the symbol ::= is read "is defined as," the symbol | means "or," the symbols < and > are used to enclose words called *nonterminal symbols* (symbols that still need to be defined), and everything else is called a *terminal symbol.*

The first line of the definition reads as follows: "An identifier is defined as either a nondigit or a nondigit followed by a nondigit-or-digit sequence." This line contains nonterminal symbols that must be defined. In the second line, the nonterminal symbol NondigitOrDigitSequence is defined as either a NondigitOrDigit or a NondigitOrDigit followed by another NondigitOrDigitSequence. The self-reference in the definition is a roundabout way of saying that a NondigitOrDigitSequence can be a series of one or more nondigits or digits. The third line defines NondigitOrDigit to be either a Nondigit or a Digit. In the fourth and last lines, we finally encounter terminal symbols, which define Nondigit to be an underscore or any upper- or lowercase letter and Digit as any one of the numeric symbols 0 through 9.

BNF is an extremely simple language, but that simplicity leads to syntax definitions that can be long and difficult to read. An alternative metalanguage, the *syntax diagram*, is easier to follow. It uses arrows to indicate how symbols can be combined. The syntax diagrams that define an identifier in C++ appear on the next page.

To read the diagrams, start at the left and follow the arrows. When you come to a branch, take any one of the branch paths. Symbols in boldface are terminal symbols, and words not in boldface are nonterminal symbols.

The first diagram shows that an identifier consists of a nondigit followed, optionally, by any number of nondigits or digits. The second diagram defines the nonterminal symbol Nondigit to be an underscore or any one of the alphabetic characters. The third diagram defines Digit to be one of the numeric characters. Here, we have eliminated the BNF nonterminal symbols NondigitOrDigitSequence and NondigitOrDigit by using arrows in the first syntax diagram to allow a sequence of consecutive nondigits or digits.

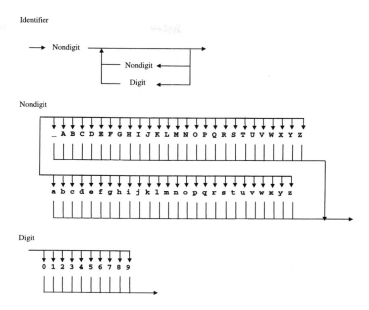

Syntax diagrams are easier to interpret than BNF definitions, but they still can be difficult to read. In this text, we introduce another metalanguage, called a *syntax template*. Syntax templates show at a glance the form a C++ construct takes.

One final note: Metalanguages only show how to write instructions that the compiler can translate. They do not define what those instructions do (their semantics). Formal languages for defining the semantics of a programming language exist, but they are beyond the scope of this text. Throughout this book, we describe the semantics of C++ in English.

Syntax Templates

In this book, we write the syntax rules for C++ using a metalanguage called a *syntax template*. A syntax template is a generic example of the C++ construct being defined. Graphic conventions show which portions are optional and which can be repeated. A boldface word or symbol is a literal word or symbol in the C++ language. A nonboldface word can be replaced by another template. A curly brace is used to indicate a list of items, from which one item can be chosen.

Let's look at an example. This template defines an identifier in C++:

Identifier

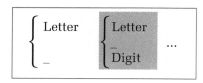

The shading indicates a part of the definition that is optional. The three dots (. . .) mean that the preceding symbol or shaded block can be repeated. Thus, an identifier in C++ must begin with a letter or underscore and is optionally followed by one or more letters, underscores, or digits.

Remember that a word not in boldface type can be replaced with another template. These are the templates for Letter and Digit:

Letter   **Digit**

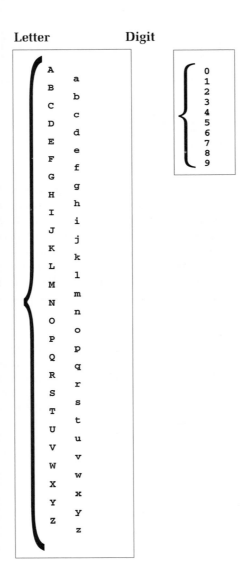

In these templates, the braces again indicate lists of items from which any one item can be chosen. So a letter can be any one of the upper- or lower-case letters, and a digit can be any of the numeric characters 0 through 9.

Now let's look at the syntax template for the C++ `main` function:

MainFunction

```
int main()
{
    Statement
       ⋮
}
```

The `main` function begins with the word `int`, followed by the word `main` and then left and right parentheses. This first line of the function is the *heading*. After the heading, the left brace signals the start of the statements in the function (its body). The shading and the three dots indicate that the function body consists of zero or more statements. (In this diagram we have placed the three dots vertically to suggest that statements usually are arranged vertically, one above the next.) Finally, the right brace indicates the end of the function.

In principle, the syntax template allows the function body to have no statements at all. In practice, however, the body should include a Return statement because the word `int` in the function heading states that `main` returns an integer value. Thus, the shortest C++ program is

```
int main()
{
    return 0;
}
```

As you might guess, this program does absolutely nothing useful when executed!

As we introduce C++ language constructs throughout the book, we use syntax templates to display the proper syntax. At the publisher's Web site, you will find these syntax templates gathered into one central location.*

When you finish this chapter, you should know enough about the syntax and semantics of statements in C++ to write simple programs. But before we can talk about writing statements, we must look at how names are written in C++ and at some of the elements of a program.

---

* The publisher's Web site is `www.jbpub.com/dale`

Naming Program Elements: Identifiers

As we noted in our discussion of metalanguages, **identifiers** are used in C++ to name things—things such as subprograms and places in the computer's memory. Identifiers are made up of letters (A–Z, a–z), digits (0–9), and the underscore character (_), but must begin with a letter or underscore.

Identifier   A name associated with a function or data object and used to refer to that function or data object.

Remember that an identifier *must* start with a letter or underscore:

Identifier

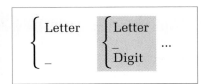

(Identifiers beginning with an underscore have special meanings in some C++ systems, so it is best to begin an identifier with a letter.)
Here are some examples of valid identifiers:

```
sum_of_squares  J9  box_22A  GetData  Bin3D4  count
```

And here are some examples of invalid identifiers and the reasons why they are invalid:

Invalid Identifier	Explanation
40Hours	Identifiers cannot begin with a digit.
Get Data	Blanks are not allowed in identifiers.
box-22	The hyphen (–) is a math symbol (minus) in C++.
cost_in_$	Special symbols such as $ are not allowed.
int	The word int is predefined in the C++ language.

The last identifier in the table, int, is an example of a **reserved word**. Reserved words are words that have specific uses in C++; you cannot use them as programmer-defined identifiers. Appendix A lists all of the reserved words in C++.

Reserved word   A word that has special meaning in C++; it cannot be used as a programmer-defined identifier.

The Payroll program in Chapter 1 uses the programmer-defined identifiers listed below. (Most of the other identifiers in the program are C++ reserved words.) Notice that we chose the names to convey how the identifiers are used.

Identifier	*How It Is Used*
MAX_HOURS	Maximum normal work hours
OVERTIME	Overtime pay rate factor
payRate	An employee's hourly pay rate
hours	The number of hours an employee worked
wages	An employee's weekly wages
total	The sum of weekly wages for all employees (total company payroll)
empNum	An employee's identification number
payFile	The output file (where the employee's number, pay rate, hours, and wages are written)
CalcPay	A function for computing an employee's wages

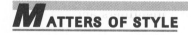

ATTERS OF STYLE

Using Meaningful, Readable Identifiers

The names we use to refer to things in our programs are totally meaningless to the computer. The computer behaves in the same way whether we call the value 3.14159265 pi or cake, as long as we always call it the same thing. However, it is much easier for somebody to figure out how a program works if the names we choose for elements actually tell something about them. Whenever you have to make up a name for something in a program, try to pick one that is meaningful to a person reading the program.

C++ is a *case-sensitive* language. Uppercase letters are different from lowercase letters. The identifiers

PRINTTOPPORTION   printtopportion   pRiNtToPpOrTiOn   PrintTopPortion

are four distinct names and are not interchangeable in any way. As you can see, the last of these forms is the easiest to read. In this book, we use combinations of uppercase letters, lowercase letters, and underscores in identifiers. We explain our conventions for choosing between uppercase and lowercase as we proceed through this chapter.

Now that we've seen how to write identifiers, we look at some of the things that C++ allows us to name.

Data and Data Types

A computer program operates on data (stored internally in memory, stored externally on disk or tape, or input from a device such as a keyboard, scanner, or electrical sensor) and produces output. In C++, each piece of data must be of a specific **data type.** The data type determines how the data is represented in the computer and the kinds of processing the computer can perform on it.

Data type   A specific set of data values, along with a set of operations on those values.

Some types of data are used so frequently that C++ defines them for us. Examples of these *standard* (or *built-in*) *types* are `int` (for working with integer numbers), `float` (for working with real numbers having decimal points), and `char` (for working with character data).

Additionally, C++ allows programmers to define their own data types—*programmer-defined* (or *user-defined*) *types.* Beginning in Chapter 10, we show you how to define your own data types.

In this chapter, we focus on two data types—one for representing data consisting of a single character, the other for representing strings of characters. In the next chapter, we examine the numeric types (such as `int` and `float`) in detail.

*B*ACKGROUND INFORMATION

Data Storage

Where does a program get the data it needs to operate? Data is stored in the computer's memory. Remember that memory is divided into a large number of separate locations or cells, each of which can hold a piece of data. Each memory location has a unique address we refer to when we store or retrieve data. We can visualize memory as a set of post office boxes, with the box numbers as the addresses used to designate particular locations.

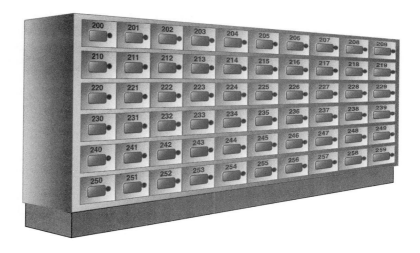

Of course, the actual address of each location in memory is a binary number in a machine language code. In C++ we use identifiers to name memory locations; the compiler then translates them into binary for us. This is one of the advantages of a high-level programming language: It frees us from having to keep track of the numeric addresses of the memory locations in which our data and instructions are stored.

The char *Data Type* The built-in type `char` describes data consisting of one alphanumeric character—a letter, a digit, or a special symbol:

```
'A'    'a'    '8'    '2'    '+'    '-'    '$'    '?'    '*'    ' '
```

Each machine uses a particular *character set*, the set of alphanumeric characters it can represent. (See Appendix E for some sample character sets.) Notice that each character is enclosed in single quotes (apostrophes). The C++ compiler needs the quotes to differentiate, say, between the character data '8' and the integer value 8 because the two are stored differently inside the machine. Notice also that the blank, ' ', is a valid character.*

---

* Most programming languages use ASCII (the American Standard Code for Information Interchange) to represent the English alphabet and other symbols. Each ASCII character is stored in a single byte of memory.

A newly developed character set called Unicode includes the larger alphabets of many international human languages. A single Unicode character occupies two bytes of memory. C++ provides the data type `wchar_t` (for "wide character") to accommodate larger character sets such as Unicode. In C++, the notation L'*something*' denotes a value of type `wchar_t`, where the *something* depends on the particular wide character being used. We do not examine wide characters any further in this book.

You wouldn't want to add the character 'A' to the character 'B' or subtract the character '3' from the character '8', but you might want to compare character values. Each character set has a *collating sequence*, a predefined ordering of all the characters. Although this sequence varies from one character set to another, 'A' always compares less than 'B', 'B' less than 'C', and so forth. And '1' compares less than '2', '2' less than '3', and so on. None of the identifiers in the Payroll program is of type `char`.

The `string` *Data Type*   Whereas a value of type `char` is limited to a single character, a *string* is a sequence of characters, such as a word, name, or sentence, enclosed in double quotes. For example, the following are strings in C++:

```
"Problem Solving"    "C++"    "Programming and "    "   "    " .  "
```

A string must be typed entirely on one line. For example, the string

```
"This string is invalid because it
is typed on more than one line."
```

is not valid because it is split across two lines. In this situation, the C++ compiler issues an error message at the first line. The message may say something like "UNTERMINATED STRING," depending on the particular compiler.

The quotes are not considered to be part of the string but are simply there to distinguish the string from other parts of a C++ program. For example, `"amount"` (in double quotes) is the character string made up of the letters *a, m, o, u, n,* and *t* in that order. On the other hand, `amount` (without the quotes) is an identifier, perhaps the name of a place in memory. The symbols `"12345"` represent a string made up of the characters *1, 2, 3, 4,* and *5* in that order. If we write `12345` without the quotes, it is an integer quantity that can be used in calculations.

A string containing no characters is called the *null string* (or *empty string*). We write the null string using two double quotes with nothing (not even spaces) between them:

```
""
```

The null string is not equivalent to a string of spaces; it is a special string that contains no characters.

To work with string data, this book uses a data type named `string`. This data type is not part of the C++ language (that is, it is not a built-in type). Rather, `string` is a programmer-defined type that is supplied by the C++ *standard library*, a large collection of prewritten functions and data types that any C++ programmer can use. Operations on `string` data include comparing the values of strings, searching a string for a particular character, and joining one string to another. We look at some of these operations later in this chapter and cover additional operations in subsequent chapters. None of the identifiers in the Payroll program is of type `string`, although string values are used directly in several places in the program.

Naming Elements: Declarations

Identifiers can be used to name both constants and variables. In other words, an identifier can be the name of a memory location whose contents are not allowed to change or it can be the name of a memory location whose contents can change.

How do we tell the computer what an identifier represents? By using a **declaration,** a statement that associates a name (an identifier) with a description of an element in a C++ program (just as a dictionary definition associates a name with a description of the thing being named). In a declaration, we name an identifier and what it represents. For example, the Payroll program uses the declaration

```
int empNum;
```

to announce that `empNum` is the name of a variable whose contents are of type `int`. When we declare a variable, the compiler picks a location in memory to be associated with the identifier. We don't have to know the actual address of the memory location because the computer automatically keeps track of it for us.

Declaration A statement that associates an identifier with a data object, a function, or a data type so that the programmer can refer to that item by name.

Suppose that when we mailed a letter, we only had to put a person's name on it and the post office would look up the address. Of course, everybody in the world would need a different name; otherwise, the post office wouldn't be able to figure out whose address was whose. The same is true in C++. Each identifier can represent just one thing (except under special circumstances, which we talk about in Chapters 7 and 8). Every identifier you use in a program must be different from all others.

Constants and variables are collectively called *data objects*. Both data objects and the actual instructions in a program are stored in various memory locations. You have seen that a group of instructions—a function—can be given a name. A name also can be associated with a programmer-defined data type.

In C++, you must declare every identifier before it is used. This allows the compiler to verify that the use of the identifier is consistent with what it was declared to be. If you declare an identifier to be a constant and later try to change its value, the compiler detects this inconsistency and issues an error message.

There is a different form of declaration statement for each kind of data object, function, or data type in C++. The forms of declarations for variables and constants are introduced here; others are covered in later chapters.

Variables   A program operates on data. Data is stored in memory. While a program is executing, different values may be stored in the same memory location at different times. This kind of memory location is called a **variable,** and its content is the *variable value*. The symbolic name that we associate with a memory location is the *variable name* or *variable identifier* (see Figure 2-1). In practice, we often refer to the variable name more briefly as the *variable.*

Variable   A location in memory, referenced by an identifier, that contains a data value that can be changed.

Declaring a variable means specifying both its name and its data type. This tells the compiler to associate a name with a memory location whose contents are of a specific type (for example, char or string). The following statement declares myChar to be a variable of type char:

```
char myChar;
```

In C++, a variable can contain a data value only of the type specified in its declaration. Because of the above declaration, the variable myChar can contain *only* a char value. If the C++ compiler comes across an instruction that tries to store a float value into myChar, it generates extra instructions to convert the float value to the proper type. In Chapter 3, we examine how such type conversions take place.

Here's the syntax template for a variable declaration:

VariableDeclaration

DataType Identifier   , Identifier   . . . ;

where DataType is the name of a data type such as char or string. Notice that a variable declaration always ends with a semicolon.

Figure 2-1
Variable

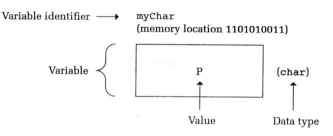

From the syntax template, you can see that it is possible to declare several variables in one statement:

```
char letter, middleInitial, ch;
```

Here, all three variables are declared to be `char` variables. Our preference, though, is to declare each variable with a separate statement:

```
char letter;
char middleInitial;
char ch;
```

With this form it is easier, when modifying a program, to add new variables to the list or delete ones you no longer want.

Declaring each variable with a separate statement also allows you to attach comments to the right of each declaration, as we do in the Payroll program:

```
float payRate;      // Employee's pay rate
float hours;        // Hours worked
float wages;        // Wages earned
float total;        // Total company payroll
int   empNum;       // Employee ID number
```

These declarations tell the compiler to reserve memory space for four `float` variables—payRate, hours, wages, and total—and one `int` variable, empNum. The comments explain to someone reading the program what each variable represents.

Now that we've seen how to declare variables in C++, let's look at how to declare constants.

Constants All single characters (enclosed in single quotes) and strings (enclosed in double quotes) are constants.

```
'A'    '@'    "Howdy boys"    "Please enter an employee number:"
```

In C++ as in mathematics, a constant is something whose value never changes. When we use the actual value of a constant in a program, we are using a **literal value** (or *literal*).

Literal value   Any constant value written in a program.

An alternative to the literal constant is the **named constant** (or **symbolic constant**), which is introduced in a declaration statement. A named constant is just another way of representing a literal value. Instead of using the literal value in an instruction, we give it a name in a declaration statement, then use that name in the instruction. For example, we can write an instruction that prints the title of this book using the literal string "Programming and Problem Solving with C++". Or we can declare a named constant called BOOK_TITLE that equals the same string and then use the constant name in the instruction. That is, we can use either

"Programming and Problem Solving with C++"

or

BOOK_TITLE

in the instruction.

Named constant (symbolic constant)   A location in memory, referenced by an identifier, that contains a data value that cannot be changed.

Using the literal value of a constant may seem easier than giving it a name and then referring to it by that name. But, in fact, named constants make a program easier to read because they make the meaning of literal constants clearer. Named constants also make it easier to change a program later on.

This is the syntax template for a constant declaration:

ConstantDeclaration

```
const DataType  Identifier = LiteralValue ;
```

Notice that the reserved word `const` begins the declaration, and an equal sign (=) appears between the identifier and the literal value.

The following are examples of constant declarations:

```
const string STARS = "********";
const char   BLANK = ' ';
const string BOOK_TITLE = "Programming and Problem Solving with C++";
const string MESSAGE = "Error condition";
```

As we have done above, many C++ programmers capitalize the entire identifier of a named constant and separate the English words with an underscore. The idea is to let the reader quickly distinguish between variable names and constant names when they appear in the middle of a program.

It's a good idea to add comments to constant declarations as well as variable declarations. In the Payroll program, we describe in comments what each constant represents:

```
const float MAX_HOURS = 40.0;    // Maximum normal work hours
const float OVERTIME = 1.5;      // Overtime pay rate factor
```

MATTERS OF STYLE

Capitalization of Identifiers

Programmers often use capitalization as a quick visual clue to what an identifier represents. Different programmers adopt different conventions for using uppercase letters and lowercase letters. Some people use only lowercase letters, separating the English words in an identifier with the underscore character:

```
pay_rate    emp_num  pay_file
```

The conventions we use in this book are as follows:

- For identifiers representing variables, we begin with a lowercase letter and capitalize each successive English word.

  ```
  lengthInYards   middleInitial    hours
  ```

- Names of programmer-written functions and programmer-defined data types (which we examine later in the book) are capitalized in the same manner as variable names except that they begin with capital letters.

  ```
  CalcPay(payRate, hours, wages)    Cube(27)    MyDataType
  ```

Capitalizing the first letter allows a person reading the program to tell at a glance that an identifier represents a function name or data type rather than a variable. However, we cannot use this capitalization convention everywhere. C++ expects every program to have a function named main—all in lowercase letters—so we cannot name it Main. Nor can we use Char for the built-in data type char. C++ reserved words use all lowercase letters, as do most of the identifiers declared in the standard library (such as string).

- For identifiers representing named constants, we capitalize every letter and use underscores to separate the English words.

```
BOOK_TITLE    OVERTIME    MAX_LENGTH
```

This convention, widely used by C++ programmers, is an immediate signal that BOOK_TITLE is a named constant and not a variable, a function, or a data type.

These conventions are only that—conventions. C++ does not require this particular style of capitalizing identifiers. You may wish to capitalize in a different fashion. But whatever system you use, it is essential that you use a consistent style throughout your program. A person reading your program will be confused or misled if you use a random style of capitalization.

Taking Action: Executable Statements

Up to this point, we've looked at ways of declaring data objects in a program. Now we turn our attention to ways of acting, or performing operations, on data.

Assignment   The value of a variable can be set or changed through an **assignment statement.** For example,

```
lastName = "Lincoln";
```

assigns the string value "Lincoln" to the variable lastName (that is, it stores the sequence of characters "Lincoln" into the memory associated with the variable named lastName).

Assignment statement   A statement that stores the value of an expression into a variable.

Here's the syntax template for an assignment statement:

AssignmentStatement

> Variable = Expression ;

The semantics (meaning) of the assignment operator (=) is "store"; the value of the **expression** is *stored* into the variable. Any previous value in the variable is destroyed and replaced by the value of the expression.

Expression An arrangement of identifiers, literals, and operators that can be evaluated to compute a value of a given type.

Only one variable can be on the left-hand side of an assignment statement. An assignment statement is *not* like a math equation ($x + y = z + 4$); the expression (what is on the right-hand side of the assignment operator) is **evaluated,** and the resulting value is stored into the single variable on the left of the assignment operator. A variable keeps its assigned value until another statement stores a new value into it.

Evaluate To compute a new value by performing a specified set of operations on given values.

Given the declarations

```
string firstName;
string middleName;
string lastName;
string title;
char   middleInitial;
char   letter;
```

the following assignment statements are valid:

```
firstName = "Abraham";
middleName = firstName;
middleName = "";
lastName = "Lincoln";
title = "President";
middleInitial = ' ';
letter = middleInitial;
```

However, these assignments are not valid:

Invalid Assignment Statement	Reason
`middleInitial = "A.";`	`middleInitial` is of type `char`; `"A."` is a string.
`letter = firstName;`	`letter` is of type `char`; `firstName` is of type `string`.
`firstName = Thomas;`	`Thomas` is an undeclared identifier.
`"Edison" = lastName;`	Only a variable can appear to the left of `=`.
`lastName = ;`	The expression to the right of `=` is missing.

String Expressions   Although we can't perform arithmetic on strings, the `string` data type provides a special string operation, called *concatenation*, that uses the + operator. The result of concatenating (joining) two strings is a new string containing the characters from both strings. For example, given the statements

```
string bookTitle;
string phrase1;
string phrase2;

phrase1 = "Programming and ";
phrase2 = "Problem Solving";
```

we could write

```
bookTitle = phrase1 + phrase2;
```

This statement retrieves the value of `phrase1` from memory and concatenates the value of `phrase2` to form a new, temporary string containing the characters

```
"Programming and Problem Solving"
```

This temporary string (which is of type `string`) is then assigned to (stored into) `bookTitle`.

The order of the strings in the expression determines how they appear in the resulting string. If we instead write

```
bookTitle = phrase2 + phrase1;
```

then `bookTitle` contains

```
"Problem SolvingProgramming and "
```

Concatenation works with named `string` constants, literal strings, and `char` data as well as with `string` variables. The only restriction is that at least one of the operands of the + operator *must* be a `string` variable or named constant (so you cannot use expressions like `"Hi"` + `"there"` or `'A'` + `'B'`). For example, if we have declared the following constants:

```
const string WORD1 = "rogramming";
const string WORD3 = "Solving";
const string WORD5 = "C++";
```

then we could write the following assignment statement to store the title of this book into the variable `bookTitle`:

```
bookTitle = 'P' + WORD1 + " and Problem " + WORD3 + " with " + WORD5;
```

As a result, `bookTitle` contains the string

```
"Programming and Problem Solving with C++"
```

The preceding example demonstrates how we can combine identifiers, `char` data, and literal strings in a concatenation expression. Of course, if we simply want to assign the complete string to `bookTitle`, we can do so directly:

```
bookTitle = "Programming and Problem Solving with C++";
```

But occasionally we encounter a situation in which we want to add some characters to an existing string value. Suppose that `bookTitle` already contains `"Programming and Problem Solving"` and that we wish to complete the title. We could use a statement of the form

```
bookTitle = bookTitle + " with C++";
```

Such a statement retrieves the value of `bookTitle` from memory, concatenates the string `" with C++"` to form a new string, and then stores the new string back into `bookTitle`. The new string replaces the old value of `bookTitle` (which is destroyed).

Keep in mind that concatenation works only with values of type `string`. Even though an arithmetic plus sign is used for the operation, we cannot concatenate values of numeric data types, such as `int` and `float`, with strings.

If you are using pre–standard C++ (any version of C++ prior to the ISO/ANSI standard) and your standard library does not provide the `string` type, see Section D.1 of Appendix D for a discussion of how to proceed.

Output   Have you ever asked someone, "Do you know what time it is?" only to have the person smile smugly, say, "Yes, I do," and walk away? This situation is like the one that currently exists between you and the computer. You now know enough C++ syntax to tell the computer to assign values to variables and to concatenate strings, but the computer won't give you the results until you tell it to write them out.

In C++ we write out the values of variables and expressions by using a special variable named `cout` (pronounced "see-out") along with the *insertion operator* (<<):

```
cout << "Hello";
```

This statement displays the characters `Hello` on the *standard output device*, usually the video display screen.

The variable `cout` is predefined in C++ systems to denote an *output stream*. You can think of an output stream as an endless sequence of characters going to an output device. In the case of `cout`, the output stream goes to the standard output device.

The insertion operator << (often pronounced as "put to") takes two operands. Its left-hand operand is a stream expression (in the simplest case, just a stream variable such as `cout`). Its right-hand operand is an expression, which could be as simple as a literal string:

```
cout << "The title is ";
cout << bookTitle + ", 2nd Edition";
```

The insertion operator converts its right-hand operand to a sequence of characters and inserts them into (or, more precisely, appends them to) the output stream. Notice how the << points in the direction the data is going—*from* the expression written on the right *to* the output stream on the left.

You can use the << operator several times in a single output statement. Each occurrence appends the next data item to the output stream. For example, we can write the preceding two output statements as

```
cout << "The title is " << bookTitle + ", 2nd Edition";
```

If `bookTitle` contains `"American History"`, both versions produce the same output:

```
The title is American History, 2nd Edition
```

The output statement has the following form:

OutputStatement

```
cout << Expression << Expression ...;
```

The following output statements yield the output shown. These examples assume that the char variable ch contains the value '2', the string variable firstName contains "Marie", and the string variable lastName contains "Curie".

Statement	What Is Printed (□ means blank)
cout << ch;	2
cout << "ch = " << ch;	ch□=□2
cout << firstName + " " + lastName;	Marie□Curie
cout << firstName << lastName;	MarieCurie
cout << firstName << ' ' << lastName;	Marie□Curie
cout << "ERROR MESSAGE";	ERROR□MESSAGE
cout << "Error=" << ch;	Error=2

An output statement prints literal strings exactly as they appear. To let the computer know that you want to print a literal string—not a named constant or variable—you must remember to use double quotes to enclose the string. If you don't put quotes around a string, you'll probably get an error message (such as "UNDECLARED IDENTIFIER") from the C++ compiler. If you want to print a string that includes a double quote, you must type a backslash (\) character and a double quote, with no space between them, in the string. For example, to print the characters

```
Al "Butch" Jones
```

the output statement looks like this:

```
cout << "Al \"Butch\" Jones";
```

To conclude this introductory look at C++ output, we should mention how to terminate an output line. Normally, successive output statements cause the output to continue along the same line of the display screen. The sequence

```
cout << "Hi";
cout << "there";
```

writes the following to the screen, all on the same line:

```
Hithere
```

To print the two words on separate lines, we can do this:

```
cout << "Hi" << endl;
cout << "there" << endl;
```

The output from these statements is

```
Hi
there
```

The identifier endl (meaning "end line") is a special C++ feature called a *manipulator*. We discuss manipulators in the next chapter. For now, the important thing to note is that endl lets you finish an output line and go on to the next line whenever you wish.

Beyond Minimalism: Adding Comments to a Program

All you need to create a working program is the correct combination of declarations and executable statements. The compiler ignores comments, but they are of enormous help to anyone who must read the program. Comments can appear anywhere in a program except in the middle of an identifier, a reserved word, or a literal constant.

   C++ comments come in two forms. The first is any sequence of characters enclosed by the /* */ pair. The compiler ignores anything within the pair. Here's an example:

```
string idNumber;    /* Identification number of the aircraft */
```

   The second, and more common, form begins with two slashes (//) and extends to the end of that line of the program:

```
string idNumber;    // Identification number of the aircraft
```

The compiler ignores anything after the two slashes.

Writing fully commented programs is good programming style. A comment should appear at the beginning of a program to explain what the program does:

```
// This program computes the weight and balance of a Beechcraft
// Starship-1 airplane, given the amount of fuel, number of
// passengers, and weight of luggage in fore and aft storage.
// It assumes that there are two pilots and a standard complement
// of equipment, and that passengers weigh 170 pounds each
```

Another good place for comments is in constant and variable declarations, where the comments explain how each identifier is used. In addition, comments should introduce each major step in a long program and should explain anything that is unusual or difficult to read (for example, a lengthy formula).

It is important to make your comments concise and to arrange them in the program so that they are easy to see and it is clear what they refer to. If comments are too long or crowd the statements in the program, they make the program more difficult to read—just the opposite of what you intended!

Program Construction

We have looked at basic elements of C++ programs: identifiers, declarations, variables, constants, expressions, statements, and comments. Now let's see how to collect these elements into a program. As you saw earlier, C++ programs are made up of functions, one of which must be named `main`. A program also can have declarations that lie outside of any function. The syntax template for a program looks like this:

Program

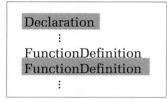

A function definition consists of the function heading and its body, which is delimited by left and right braces:

FunctionDefinition

```
Heading
{
    Statement
      ⋮
}
```

Here's an example of a program with just one function, the `main` function:

```cpp
//******************************************************************
// PrintName program
// This program prints a name in two different formats
//******************************************************************
#include <iostream>
#include <string>

using namespace std;

const string FIRST = "Herman";    // Person's first name
const string LAST = "Smith";      // Person's last name
const char   MIDDLE = 'G';        // Person's middle initial

int main()
{
    string firstLast;    // Name in first-last format
    string lastFirst;    // Name in last-first format

    firstLast = FIRST + " " + LAST;
    cout << "Name in first-last format is " << firstLast << endl;

    lastFirst = LAST + ", " + FIRST + ", ";
    cout << "Name in last-first-initial format is ";
    cout << lastFirst << MIDDLE << '.' << endl;

    return 0;
}
```

The program begins with a comment that explains what the program does. Immediately after the comment, the following lines appear:

```cpp
#include <iostream>
#include <string>

using namespace std;
```

The #include lines instruct the C++ system to insert into our program the contents of the files named iostream and string. The first file contains information that C++ needs in order to output values to a stream such as cout. The second file contains information about the programmer-defined data type string. We discuss the purpose of these #include lines and the using statement a little later in the chapter.

Next comes a declaration section in which we define the constants FIRST, LAST, and MIDDLE. Comments explain how each identifier is used. The rest of the program is the function definition for our main function. The first line is the function heading: the reserved word int, the name of the function, and then opening and closing parentheses. (The parentheses inform the compiler that main is the name of a function, not a variable or named constant.) The body of the function includes the declarations of two variables, firstLast and lastFirst, followed by a list of executable statements. The compiler translates these executable statements into machine language instructions. During the execution phase of the program, these are the instructions that are executed.

Our main function finishes by returning 0 as the function value:

```
return 0;
```

Remember that main returns an integer value to the operating system when it completes execution. This integer value is called the *exit status*. On most computer systems, you return an exit status of 0 to indicate successful completion of the program; otherwise, you return a nonzero value.

Notice how we use spacing in the PrintName program to make it easy for someone to read. We use blank lines to separate statements into related groups, and we indent the entire body of the main function. The compiler doesn't require us to format the program this way; we do so only to make it more readable. We have more to say in the next chapter about formatting a program.

Blocks (Compound Statements)

The body of a function is an example of a *block* (or *compound statement*). This is the syntax template for a block:

Block

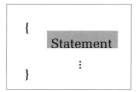

A block is just a sequence of zero or more statements enclosed (delimited) by a { } pair. Now we can redefine a function definition as a heading followed by a block:

FunctionDefinition

```
Heading
Block
```

In later chapters when we learn how to write functions other than `main`, we define the syntax of Heading in detail. In the case of the `main` function, Heading is simply

```
int main()
```

Here is the syntax template for a statement, limited to the C++ statements discussed in this chapter:

Statement

```
⎧ NullStatement
⎪ Declaration
⎨ AssignmentStatement
⎪ OutputStatement
⎩ Block
```

A statement can be empty (the *null statement*). The null statement is just a semicolon (;) and looks like this:

```
;
```

It does absolutely nothing at execution time; execution just proceeds to the next statement. It is not used often.

As the syntax template shows, a statement also can be a declaration, an executable statement, or even a block. The latter means that you can use an entire block wherever a single statement is allowed. In later chapters in which we introduce the syntax for branching and looping structures, this fact is very important.

We use blocks often, especially as parts of other statements. Leaving out a { } pair can dramatically change the meaning as well as the execution of a program. This is why we always indent the statements inside a block—the indentation makes a block easy to spot in a long, complicated program.

Notice in the syntax templates for the block and the statement that there is no mention of semicolons. Yet the PrintName program contains many semicolons. If you look back at the templates for constant declaration, variable declaration, assignment statement, and output statement, you can see that a semicolon is required at the end of each kind of statement. However, the syntax template for the block shows no semicolon after the right brace. The rule for using semicolons in C++, then, is quite simple: Terminate each statement *except* a compound statement (block) with a semicolon.

One more thing about blocks and statements: According to the syntax template for a statement, a declaration is officially considered to be a statement. A declaration, therefore, can appear wherever an executable statement can. In a block, we can mix declarations and executable statements if we wish:

```
{
    char ch;
    ch = 'A';
    cout << ch;
    string str;
    str = "Hello";
    cout << str;
}
```

It's far more common, though, for programmers to group the declarations together before the start of the executable statements:

```
{
    char    ch;
    string str;

    ch = 'A';
    cout << ch;
    str = "Hello";
    cout << str;
}
```

The C++ Preprocessor

Imagine that you are the C++ compiler. You are presented with the following program. You are to check it for syntax errors and, if there are no syntax errors, you are to translate it into machine language code.

```
//***********************************
// This program prints Happy Birthday
//***********************************

int main()
{
    cout << "Happy Birthday" << endl;
    return 0;
}
```

You, the compiler, recognize the identifier `int` as a C++ reserved word and the identifier `main` as the name of a required function. But what about the identifiers `cout` and `endl`? The programmer has not declared them as variables or named constants, and they are not reserved words. You have no choice but to issue an error message and give up.

To fix this program, the first thing we must do is insert a line near the top that says

```
#include <iostream>
```

just as we did in the PrintName program (as well as in the sample program at the beginning of this chapter and the Payroll program of Chapter 1).

The line says to insert the contents of a file named `iostream` into the program. This file contains declarations of `cout`, `endl`, and other items needed to perform stream input and output. The `#include` line is not handled by the C++ compiler but by a program known as the *preprocessor*.

The preprocessor concept is fundamental to C++. The preprocessor is a program that acts as a filter during the compilation phase. Your source program passes through the preprocessor on its way to the compiler (see Figure 2-2).

A line beginning with a pound sign (#) is not considered to be a C++ language statement (and thus is not terminated by a semicolon). It is called a *preprocessor directive*. The preprocessor expands an `#include` directive by physically inserting the contents of the named file into your source program. A file whose name appears in an `#include` directive is called a *header file*. Header files contain constant, variable, data type, and function declarations needed by a program.

FIGURE 2-2
C++ Preprocessor

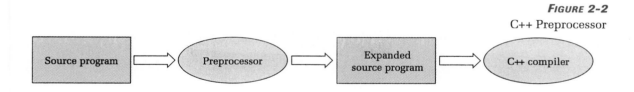

In the directives

```
#include <iostream>
#include <string>
```

the angle brackets **< >** are required. They tell the preprocessor to look for the files in the standard *include directory*—a location in the computer system that contains all the header files that are related to the C++ standard library. The file `iostream` contains declarations of input/output facilities, and the file `string` contains declarations about the `string` data type. In Chapter 3, we make use of standard header files other than `iostream` and `string`.

In the C language and in pre–standard C++, the standard header files end in the suffix `.h` (for example, `iostream.h`), where the *h* suggests "header file." In ISO/ANSI C++, the standard header files no longer use the `.h` suffix.

An Introduction to Namespaces

In our Happy Birthday program, even if we add the preprocessor directive `#include <iostream>`, the program will not compile. The compiler *still* doesn't recognize the identifiers `cout` and `endl`. The problem is that the header file `iostream` (and, in fact, every standard header file) declares all of its identifiers to be in a *namespace* called `std`:

```
namespace std
{
    :          Declarations of variables, data types, and so forth
}
```

An identifier declared within a namespace block can be accessed directly only by statements within that block. To access an identifier that is "hidden" inside a namespace, the programmer has several options. We describe two options here. Chapter 8 describes namespaces in more detail.

The first option is to use a *qualified name* for the identifier. A qualified name consists of the name of the namespace, then the `::` operator (the *scope resolution operator*), and then the desired identifier:

```
std::cout
```

With this approach, our program looks like the following:

```
#include <iostream>

int main()
{
    std::cout << "Happy Birthday" << std::endl;
    return 0;
}
```

Notice that both `cout` and `endl` must be qualified.

The second option is to use a statement called a **using** *directive:*

```
using namespace std;
```

When we place this statement near the top of the program before the `main` function, we make *all* the identifiers in the `std` namespace accessible to our program without having to qualify them:

```
#include <iostream>

using namespace std;

int main()
{
    cout << "Happy Birthday" << endl;
    return 0;
}
```

This second option is the one we used in the PrintName program and the sample program at the beginning of the chapter. In many of the following chapters, we continue to use this method. However, in Chapter 8 we discuss why it is not advisable to use the method in large programs.

If you are using a pre–standard C++ compiler that does not recognize namespaces and the newer header files (`iostream`, `string`, and so forth), you should turn to Section D.2 of Appendix D for a discussion of incompatibilities.

More About Output

We can control both the horizontal and vertical spacing of our output to make it more appealing (and understandable). Let's look first at vertical spacing.

Creating Blank Lines

We control vertical spacing by using the `endl` manipulator in an output statement. You have seen that a sequence of output statements continues to write characters across the current line until an `endl` terminates the line. Here are some examples:

Statements Output Produced*

```
cout << "Hi there, ";
cout << "Lois Lane. " << endl;        Hi there, Lois Lane.
cout << "Have you seen ";
cout << "Clark Kent?" << endl;        Have you seen Clark Kent?

cout << "Hi there, " << endl;         Hi there,
cout << "Lois Lane. " << endl;        Lois Lane.
cout << "Have you seen " << endl;     Have you seen
cout << "Clark Kent?" << endl;        Clark Kent?

cout << "Hi there, " << endl;         Hi there,
cout << "Lois Lane. ";
cout << "Have you seen " << endl;     Lois Lane. Have you seen
cout << "Clark Kent?" << endl;        Clark Kent?
```

*The output lines are shown next to the output statement that ends each of them. There are no blank lines in the actual output from these statements.

What do you think the following statements print out?

```
cout << "Hi there, " << endl;
cout << endl;
cout << "Lois Lane." << endl;
```

The first output statement causes the words *Hi there,* to be printed; the `endl` causes the screen cursor to go to the next line. The next statement prints nothing but goes on to the next line. The third statement prints the words *Lois Lane.* and terminates the line. The resulting output is the three lines

```
Hi there,

Lois Lane.
```

Whenever you use an `endl` immediately after another `endl`, a blank line is produced. As you might guess, three consecutive uses of `endl` produce two blank lines, four consecutive uses produce three blank lines, and so forth.

Note that we have a great deal of flexibility in how we write an output statement in a C++ program. We could combine the three preceding statements into two statements:

```
cout << "Hi there, " << endl << endl;
cout << "Lois Lane." << endl;
```

In fact, we could do it all in one statement. One possibility is

```
cout << "Hi there, " << endl << endl << "Lois Lane." << endl;
```

Here's another:

```
cout << "Hi there, " << endl << endl
    << "Lois Lane." << endl;
```

The last example shows that you can spread a single C++ statement onto more than one line of the program. The compiler treats the semicolon, not the physical end of a line, as the end of a statement.

Inserting Blanks Within a Line

To control the horizontal spacing of the output, one technique is to send extra blank characters to the output stream. (Remember that the blank character, generated by pressing the spacebar on a keyboard, is a perfectly valid character in C++.)

For example, to produce this output:

```
*   *   *   *   *   *   *   *   *

*   *   *   *   *   *   *   *   *   *

*   *   *   *   *   *   *   *   *
```

you would use these statements:

```
cout << "  *   *   *   *   *   *   *   *   *" << endl << endl;
cout << "*   *   *   *   *   *   *   *   *" << endl << endl;
cout << "  *   *   *   *   *   *   *   *   *" << endl;
```

All of the blanks and asterisks are enclosed in double quotes, so they print literally as they are written in the program. The extra `endl` manipulators give you the blank lines between the rows of asterisks.

If you want blanks to be printed, you *must* enclose them in quotes. The statement

```
cout << '*' <<                              '*';
```

produces the output

```
**
```

Despite all of the blanks we included in the output statement, the asterisks print side by side because the blanks are not enclosed by quotes.

▰ *Program Entry, Correction, and Execution*

Once you have a program on paper, you must enter it on the keyboard. In this section, we examine the program entry process in general. You should consult the manual for your specific computer to learn the details.

Entering a Program

The first step in entering a program is to get the computer's attention. With a personal computer, this usually means turning it on if it is not already running. Workstations connected to a network are usually left running all the time. You must *log on* to such a machine to get its attention. This means entering a user name and a password. The password system protects information that you've stored in the computer from being tampered with or destroyed by someone else.

Once the computer is ready to accept your commands, you tell it that you want to enter a program by having it run the editor. The editor is a program that allows you to create and modify programs by entering information into an area of the computer's secondary storage called a **file.**

File   A named area in secondary storage that is used to hold a collection of data; the collection of data itself.

A file in a computer system is like a file folder in a filing cabinet. It is a collection of data that has a name associated with it. You usually choose the name for the file when you create it with the editor. From that point on, you refer to the file by the name you've given it.

There are so many different types of editors, each with different features, that we can't begin to describe them all here. But we can describe some of their general characteristics.

The basic unit of information in an editor is a display screen full of characters. The editor lets you change anything that you see on the screen. When you create a new file, the editor clears the screen to show you that the file is empty. Then you enter your program, using the mouse and keyboard to go back and make corrections as necessary. Figure 2-3 shows an example of an editor's display screen.

Compiling and Running a Program

Once your program is stored in a file, you compile it by issuing a command to run the C++ compiler. The compiler translates the program, then stores the machine language version into a file. The compiler may display a window with messages indicating errors in the program. Some systems

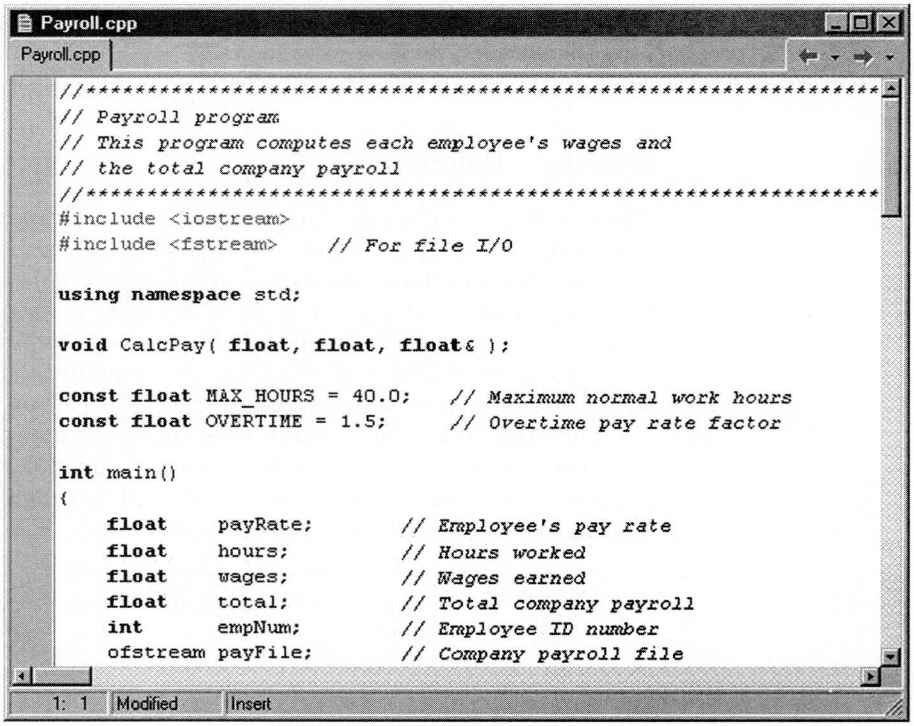

FIGURE 2-3
Display Screen for
an Editor

```
┌─────────────────────────────────────────────────────────────────┐
│ 🗎 Payroll.cpp                                          _ □ ✕     │
├─────────────────────────────────────────────────────────────────┤
│ Payroll.cpp │                                         ← ▾  → ▾    │
├─────────────────────────────────────────────────────────────────┤
│ //*********************************************************** ▲    │
│ // Payroll program                                                │
│ // This program computes each employee's wages and               │
│ // the total company payroll                                      │
│ //***********************************************************      │
│ #include <iostream>                                               │
│ #include <fstream>      // For file I/O                           │
│                                                                   │
│ using namespace std;                                              │
│                                                                   │
│ void CalcPay( float, float, float& );                            │
│                                                                   │
│ const float MAX_HOURS = 40.0;    // Maximum normal work hours     │
│ const float OVERTIME = 1.5;      // Overtime pay rate factor      │
│                                                                   │
│ int main()                                                        │
│ {                                                                 │
│     float    payRate;        // Employee's pay rate               │
│     float    hours;          // Hours worked                      │
│     float    wages;          // Wages earned                      │
│     float    total;          // Total company payroll             │
│     int      empNum;         // Employee ID number                │
│     ofstream payFile;        // Company payroll file          ▼   │
│ ◄ ▬▬▬                                                        ►    │
├─────────────────────────────────────────────────────────────────┤
│  1: 1   Modified    Insert                                        │
└─────────────────────────────────────────────────────────────────┘
```

let you click on an error message to automatically position the cursor in the editor window at the point where the error was detected.

If the compiler finds errors in your program (syntax errors), you have to determine their cause, go back to the editor and fix them, and then run the compiler again. Once your program compiles without errors, you can run (execute) it.

Some systems automatically run a program when it compiles successfully. On other systems, you have to issue a separate command to run the program. Still other systems require that you specify an extra step called *linking* between compiling and running a program. Whatever series of commands your system uses, the result is the same: Your program is loaded into memory and executed by the computer.

Even though a program runs, it still may have errors in its design. The computer does exactly what you tell it to do, even if that's not what you wanted it to do. If your program doesn't do what it should (a *logic error*), you have to go back to the algorithm and fix it, and then go to the editor and fix the program. Finally, you compile and run the program again. This *debugging* process is repeated until the program does what it is supposed to do (see Figure 2-4).

FIGURE 2-4
Debugging Process

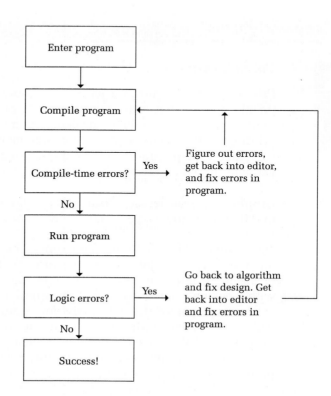

Finishing Up

On a workstation, once you finish working on your program you have to *log off* by issuing a command with the mouse or keyboard. This frees up the workstation so that someone else can use it. It also prevents someone from walking up after you leave and tampering with your files.

On a personal computer, when you're done working you save your files and quit the editor. Turning off the power wipes out what's in the computer's memory, but your files are stored safely on disk. It is a wise precaution to periodically back up (make a copy of) your program files onto a removable diskette. When a disk in a computer suffers a hardware failure, it is often impossible to retrieve your files. With a backup copy on a diskette, you can restore your files to the disk once it is repaired.

Be sure to read the manual for your particular system and editor before you enter your first program. Don't panic if you have trouble at first—almost everyone does. It becomes much easier with practice. That's why it's a good idea to first go through the process with a program such as PrintName, where mistakes don't matter—unlike a class programming assignment!

PROBLEM-SOLVING CASE STUDY

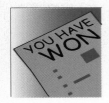

Contest Letter

Problem: You've taken a job with a company that is running a promotional contest. They want you to write a program to print a personalized form letter for each of the contestants. As a first effort, they want to get the printing of the letter straight for just one name. Later on, they plan to have you extend the program to read a mailing list file, so the output should use variables in which the name appears in the letter.

Output: A form letter with a name inserted at the appropriate points so that it appears to be a personal letter.

Discussion: The marketing department for the company has written the letter already. Your job is to write a program that prints it out. The majority of the letter must be entered verbatim into a series of output statements, with a person's name inserted at the appropriate places.

In some places the letter calls for printing the full name, in others it uses a title (such as Mr. or Mrs.), and in others it uses just the first name. Because you plan to eventually use a data file that provides each name in four parts (title, first name, middle initial, last name), you decide that this preliminary program should start with a set of named `string` constants containing the four parts of a name. The program can then use concatenation expressions to form `string` variables in the different formats required by the letter. In that way, all the name strings can be created before the output statements are executed.

The form letter requires the name in four formats: the full name with the title, the last name preceded by the title, the first name alone, and the first and last names without the title or middle initial. Here is the algorithmic solution:

Define Constants

```
TITLE = "Dr."
FIRST_NAME = "Margaret"
MIDDLE_INITIAL = "H"
LAST_NAME = "Sklaznick"
```

Create First Name with Blank

```
Set first = FIRST_NAME + " "
```

Create Full Name

```
Set fullName = TITLE + " " + first + MIDDLE_INITIAL
Set fullName = fullName + ". " + LAST_NAME
```

Create First and Last Name

```
Set firstLast = first + LAST_NAME
```

Create Title and Last Name

```
Set titleLast = TITLE + " " + LAST_NAME
```

Print the Form Letter

Series of output statements containing the text of the letter with the names inserted in the appropriate places

PROBLEM-SOLVING CASE STUDY cont'd.

From the algorithm we can create tables of constants and variables that help us write the declarations in the program.

Constants

Name	Value	Description
TITLE	"Dr."	Salutary title for the name
FIRST_NAME	"Margaret"	First name of addressee
MIDDLE_INITIAL	"H"	Middle initial of addressee
LAST_NAME	"Sklaznick"	Last name of addressee

Variables

Name	Data Type	Description
first	string	Holds the first name plus a blank
fullName	string	Complete name, including title
firstLast	string	First name and last name
titleLast	string	Title followed by the last name

Now we're ready to write the program. Let's call it FormLetter. We can take the declarations from the tables and create the executable statements from the algorithm and the draft of the letter. We also include comments as necessary.

(The following program is written in ISO/ANSI standard C++. If you are working with pre–standard C++, see the alternate version of the program in the PRE_STD directory of the program disk, available at the publisher's Web site, www.jbpub.com/disks.)

```
//****************************************************************
// FormLetter program
// This program prints a form letter for a promotional contest.
// It uses the four parts of a name to build name strings in four
// different formats to be used in personalizing the letter
//****************************************************************
#include <iostream>
#include <string>

using namespace std;
```

<u>*PROBLEM-SOLVING CASE STUDY* cont'd.</u>

```cpp
const string TITLE = "Dr.";                  // Salutary title
const string FIRST_NAME = "Margaret";        // First name of addressee
const string MIDDLE_INITIAL = "H";           // Middle initial
const string LAST_NAME = "Sklaznick";        // Last name of addressee

int main()
{
    string first;        // Holds the first name plus a blank
    string fullName;     // Complete name, including title
    string firstLast;    // First name and last name
    string titleLast;    // Title followed by the last name

    // Create first name with blank

    first = FIRST_NAME + " ";

    // Create full name

    fullName = TITLE + " " + first + MIDDLE_INITIAL;
    fullName = fullName + ". " + LAST_NAME;

    // Create first and last name

    firstLast = first + LAST_NAME;

    // Create title and last name

    titleLast = TITLE + " " + LAST_NAME;

    // Print the form letter

    cout << fullName << " is a GRAND PRIZE WINNER!!!!!!" << endl
         << endl;
    cout << "Dear " << titleLast << "," << endl << endl;
    cout << "Yes it's true! " << firstLast << " has won our"
         << endl;
    cout << "GRAND PRIZE -- your choice of a 42-INCH* COLOR"
         << endl;
    cout << "TELEVISION or a FREE WEEKEND IN NEW YORK CITY.**"
         << endl;
    cout << "All that you have to do to collect your prize is"
         << endl;
    cout << "attend one of our fun-filled all-day presentations"
         << endl;
    cout << "on the benefits of owning a timeshare condominium"
         << endl;
```

```
        cout << "trailer at the Happy Acres Mobile Campground in"
             << endl;
        cout << "beautiful Panhard, Texas! Now " << first << "I realize"
             << endl;
        cout << "that the three-hour drive from the nearest airport"
             << endl;
        cout << "to Panhard may seem daunting at first, but isn't"
             << endl;
        cout << "it worth a little extra effort to receive such a"
             << endl;
        cout << "FABULOUS PRIZE? So why wait? Give us a call right"
             << endl;
        cout << "now to schedule your visit and collect your" << endl;
        cout << "GRAND PRIZE!" << endl << endl;
        cout << "Most Sincerely," << endl << endl;
        cout << "Argyle M. Sneeze" << endl << endl << endl << endl;
        cout << "* Measured around the circumference of the packing"
             << endl;
        cout << "crate. ** Includes air fare and hotel accommodations."
             << endl;
        cout << "Departure from Nome, Alaska; surcharge applies to"
             << endl;
        cout << "other departure airports. Accommodations within"
             << endl;
        cout << "driving distance of New York City at the Cheap-O-Tel"
             << endl;
        cout << "in Plattsburgh, NY." << endl;
        return 0;
}
```

The output from the program is

```
Dr. Margaret H. Sklaznick is a GRAND PRIZE WINNER!!!!!!

Dear Dr. Sklaznick,

Yes it's true! Margaret Sklaznick has won our
GRAND PRIZE -- your choice of a 42-INCH* COLOR
TELEVISION or a FREE WEEKEND IN NEW YORK CITY.**
All that you have to do to collect your prize is
attend one of our fun-filled all-day presentations
on the benefits of owning a timeshare condominium
trailer at the Happy Acres Mobile Campground in
beautiful Panhard, Texas! Now Margaret I realize
that the three-hour drive from the nearest airport
to Panhard may seem daunting at first, but isn't
it worth a little extra effort to receive such a
FABULOUS PRIZE? So why wait? Give us a call right
now to schedule your visit and collect your
```

PROBLEM-SOLVING CASE STUDY cont'd.

GRAND PRIZE!

Most Sincerely,

Argyle M. Sneeze

* Measured around the circumference of the packing crate. ** Includes air fare and hotel accommodations. Departure from Nome, Alaska; surcharge applies to other departure airports. Accommodations within driving distance of New York City at the Cheap-O-Tel in Plattsburgh, NY.

Testing and Debugging

1. Every identifier that isn't a C++ reserved word must be declared. If you use a name that hasn't been declared—either by your own declaration statements or by including a header file—you get an error message.
2. If you try to declare an identifier that is the same as a reserved word in C++, you get an error message from the compiler. See Appendix A for a list of reserved words.
3. C++ is a case-sensitive language. Two identifiers that are capitalized differently are treated as two different identifiers. The word `main` and all C++ reserved words use only lowercase letters.
4. To use identifiers from the standard library, such as `cout` and `string`, you must either (a) give a qualified name such as `std::cout` or (b) put a `using` directive near the top of your program:

   `using namespace std;`

5. Check for mismatched quotes in `char` and string literals. Each `char` literal begins and ends with an apostrophe (single quote). Each string literal begins and ends with a double quote.
6. Be sure to use only the apostrophe (') to enclose `char` literals. Most keyboards also have a reverse apostrophe (`), which is easily confused with the apostrophe. If you use the reverse apostrophe, the compiler issues an error message.
7. To use a double quote within a literal string, use the two symbols \" in a row. If you use just a double quote, it ends the string, and the compiler then sees the remainder of the string as an error.

8. In an assignment statement, be sure that the identifier to the left of = is a variable and not a named constant.

9. In assigning a value to a `string` variable, the expression to the right of = must be a `string` expression, a literal string, or a `char`.

10. In a concatenation expression, at least one of the two operands of + must be of type `string`. For example, the operands cannot both be literal strings or `char` values.*

11. Make sure your statements end in semicolons (except compound statements, which do not have a semicolon after the right brace).

Summary

The syntax (grammar) of the C++ language is defined by a metalanguage. In this text, we use a form of metalanguage called syntax templates. We describe the semantics (meaning) of C++ statements in English.

Identifiers are used in C++ to name things. Some identifiers, called reserved words, have predefined meanings in the language; others are created by the programmer. The identifiers you invent are restricted to those *not* reserved by the C++ language. Reserved words are listed in Appendix A.

Identifiers are associated with memory locations by declarations. A declaration may give a name to a location whose value does not change (a constant) or to one whose value can change (a variable). Every constant and variable has an associated data type. C++ provides many built-in data types, the most common of which are `int`, `float`, and `char`. Additionally, C++ permits programmer-defined types such as the `string` type from the standard library.

The assignment operator is used to change the value of a variable by assigning it the value of an expression. At execution time, the expression is evaluated and the result is stored into the variable. With the `string` type, the plus sign (+) is an operator that concatenates two strings. A string expression can concatenate any number of strings to form a new `string` value.

Program output is accomplished by means of the output stream variable `cout`, along with the insertion operator (<<). Each insertion operation sends output data to the standard output device. When an `endl` manipulator appears instead of a data item, the computer terminates the current output line and goes on to the next line.

Output should be clear, understandable, and neatly arranged. Messages in the output should describe the significance of values. Blank lines (produced by successive uses of the `endl` manipulator) and blank spaces within lines help to organize the output and improve its appearance.

---

* The invalid concatenation expression "Hi" + "there" results in a syntax error message such as "INVALID POINTER ADDITION." This can be confusing, especially because the topic of pointers is not covered until much later in this book.

A C++ program is a collection of one or more function definitions (and optionally some declarations outside of any function). One of the functions *must* be named `main`. Execution of a program always begins with the `main` function. Collectively, the functions all cooperate to produce the desired results.

Quick Check

1. Every C++ program consists of at least how many functions? (p. 51)
2. Use the following syntax template to decide whether your last name is a valid C++ identifier. (pp. 53–55)

Identifier

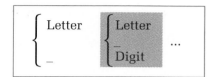

3. Write a C++ constant declaration that gives the name ZED to the value 'z'. (pp. 64–65)
4. Which of the following words are reserved words in C++? (*Hint:* Look in Appendix A.)

       const   pi   float   integer   sqrt

   (pp. 56–57)
5. Declare a `char` variable named `letter` and a `string` variable named `street`. (pp. 62–63)
6. Assign the value `"Elm"` to the `string` variable `street`. (pp. 67–68)
7. Write an output statement to print out the title of this book (*Programming and Problem Solving with C++*). (pp. 70–72)
8. What does the following code segment print out?

   ```
   string str;

   str = "Abraham";
   cout << "The answer is " << str + "Lincoln" << endl;
   ```

   (pp. 68–72)
9. The following program code is incorrect. Rewrite it, using correct syntax for the comment.

   ```
   string address;   / Employee's street address,
                     / including apartment
   ```

   (pp. 72–73)

10. Fill in the blanks in this program.

```
#include _____

#include _____

using _____

const string TITLE = "Mr";    // First part of salutary title

int _____()

____

    string guest1;    // First guest

    string guest2;    // Second guest

    guest1 ____ TITLE + ". Jones";

    guest2 ____ TITLE + "s. Smith";

    _____ << "The guests in attendance were" _____ endl;

    _____ << guest1 << " and ";

    _____ << guest2 _____ endl;

    return _____;
```

_____

(pp. 73–80)
11. Show precisely the output produced by running the program in Question 10 above.
12. If you want to print the word *Hello* on one line and then print a blank line, how many consecutive endl manipulators should you insert after the output of "Hello"? (pp. 81–82)

Answers   1. A program must have at least one function—the main function.   2. Unless your last name is hyphenated, it probably is a valid C++ identifier.
3. const char ZED = 'Z';   4. const, float
5. char letter;
   string street;
6. street = "Elm";
7. cout << "Programming and Problem Solving with C++" << endl;
8. The answer is AbrahamLincoln
9. string address;   // Employee's street address,
                      // including apartment

   or

   string address;   /* Employee's street address, */
                      /* including apartment   */

```
10.#include <iostream>
   #include <string>

   using namespace std;

   const string TITLE = "Mr";      // First part of salutary title

   int main()
   {
       string guest1;      // First guest
       string guest2;      // Second guest

       guest1 = TITLE + ". Jones";
       guest2 = TITLE + "s. Smith";
       cout << "The guests in attendance were" << endl;
       cout << guest1 << " and ";
       cout << guest2 << endl;
       return 0;
   }
```
11. The guests in attendance were
    Mr. Jones and Mrs. Smith
12. Two consecutive endl manipulators are necessary.

Exam Preparation Exercises

1. Mark the following identifiers either valid or invalid.

	Valid	Invalid
a. item#1	_____	_____
b. data	_____	_____
c. y	_____	_____
d. 3Set	_____	_____
e. PAY_DAY	_____	_____
f. bin-2	_____	_____
g. num5	_____	_____
h. Sq Ft	_____	_____

2. Given these four syntax templates:

Dwit	**Twitnit**	**Twit**	**Nit**
Twitnit . . .	Twit . . . Nit . . .	$\begin{cases} X \\ Y \\ Z \end{cases}$	$\begin{cases} 1 \\ 2 \\ 3 \end{cases}$

mark the following "Dwits" either valid or invalid.

	Valid	Invalid
a. XYZ	_____	_____
b. 123	_____	_____
c. X1	_____	_____
d. 23Y	_____	_____
e. XY12	_____	_____
f. Y2Y	_____	_____
g. ZY2	_____	_____
h. XY23X1	_____	_____

3. Match each of the following terms with the correct definition (1 through 15) given below. There is only one correct definition for each term.

_____ a. program	_____ g. variable
_____ b. algorithm	_____ h. constant
_____ c. compiler	_____ i. memory
_____ d. identifier	_____ j. syntax
_____ e. compilation phase	_____ k. semantics
_____ f. execution phase	_____ l. block

(1) A symbolic name made up of letters, digits, and underscores but not beginning with a digit

(2) A place in memory where a data value that cannot be changed is stored

(3) A program that takes a program written in a high-level language and translates it into machine code

(4) An input device

(5) The time spent planning a program

(6) Grammar rules

(7) A sequence of statements enclosed by braces

(8) Meaning

(9) A program that translates assembly language instructions into machine code

(10) When the machine code version of a program is being run

(11) A place in memory where a data value that can be changed is stored

(12) When a program in a high-level language is converted into machine code

(13) A part of the computer that can hold both program and data

(14) A step-by-step procedure for solving a problem in a finite amount of time

(15) A sequence of instructions that enables a computer to perform a particular task

4. Which of the following are reserved words and which are programmer-defined identifiers?

	Reserved	Programmer-Defined
a. char	_____	_____
b. sort	_____	_____
c. INT	_____	_____
d. long	_____	_____
e. Float	_____	_____

5. Reserved words can be used as variable names. (True or False?)

6. In a C++ program consisting of just one function, that function can be named either main or Main. (True or False?)

7. If s1 and s2 are `string` variables containing `"blue"` and `"bird"`, respectively, what output does each of the following statements produce?

    a. `cout << "s1 = " << s1 << "s2 = " << s2 << endl;`
    b. `cout << "Result:" << s1 + s2 << endl;`
    c. `cout << "Result:   " << s1 + s2 << endl;`
    d. `cout << "Result:   " << s1 << ' ' << s2 << endl;`

8. Show precisely what is output by the following statement.

    ```
    cout << "A rolling" << endl
         << "stone" << endl << endl
         << "gathers" << endl
         << endl << endl << endl << "no"
         << "moss" << endl;
    ```

9. How many characters can be stored into a variable of type `char`?
10. How many characters are in the null string?
11. A variable of type `string` can be assigned to a variable of type `char`. (True or False?)
12. A literal string can be assigned to a variable of type `string`. (True or False?)
13. What is the difference between the literal string `"computer"` and the identifier `computer`?
14. What is output by the following code segment? (All variables are of type `string`.)

    ```
    street = "Elm St.";
    address = "1425B";
    city = "Amaryllis";
    state = "Iowa";
    firstLine = address + ' ' + street;
    cout << firstLine << endl;
    cout << city;
    cout << ", " << state << endl;
    ```

15. Identify the syntax errors in the following program.

    ```
    // This program is full of errors
    #include <iostream

    constant string FIRST : Martin";
    constant string MID : "Luther;
    constant string LAST : King

    int main
    {
        string name;
        character initial;

        name = Martin + Luther + King;
        initial = MID;
        LAST = "King Jr.";
        count << 'Name = ' << name << endl;
    ```

```
cout << mid
cout << endl;
```

Programming Warm-up Exercises

1. Write an output statement that prints your name.
2. Write three consecutive output statements that print the following three lines:

    ```
    The moon
    is
    blue.
    ```

3. Write declaration statements to declare three variables of type `string` and two variables of type `char`. The `string` variables should be named `make`, `model`, and `color`. The `char` variables should be named `plateType` and `classification`.
4. Write a series of output statements that print out the values in the variables declared in Exercise 3. The values should each appear on a separate line, with a blank line between the `string` and `char` values. Each value should be preceded by an identifying message on the same line.
5. Change the PrintName program (page 74) so that it also prints the name in the format

    First-name Middle-initial. Last-name

    Make `MIDDLE` a `string` constant rather than a `char` constant. Define a new `string` variable to hold the name in the new format and assign it the string using the existing named constants, any literal strings that are needed for punctuation and spacing, and concatenation operations. Print the string, labeled appropriately.
6. Write C++ output statements that produce exactly the following output.

    a. ```
        Four score
        and seven years ago
        ```
    b.  ```
        Four score
        and seven
        years ago
        ```
    c. ```
        Four score
        and

        seven
        years ago
        ```
    d.  ```
        Four
            score
                and
        seven
            years
                ago
        ```

7. Enter and run the following program. Be sure to type it exactly as it appears here.

```
//*************************************************************
// HelloWorld program
// This program prints two simple messages
//*************************************************************
#include <iostream>
#include <string>

using namespace std;

const string MSG1 = "Hello world.";

int main()
{
    string msg2;

    cout << MSG1 << endl;
    msg2 = MSG1 + " " + MSG1 + " " + MSG1;
    cout << msg2 << endl;
    return 0;
}
```

Programming Problems

1. Write a C++ program that prints your initials in large block letters, each letter made up of the same character it represents. The letters should be a minimum of seven printed lines high and should appear all in a row. For example, if your initials were DOW, your program should print out

```
DDDDDDD              OOOOO         W         W
D      D            O     O        W         W
D      D           O       O       W         W
D      D           O       O       W    W    W
D      D           O       O       W   W W   W
D      D            O     O        W  W   W  W
DDDDDDD              OOOOO          WW     WW
```

    Be sure to include appropriate comments in your program, choose meaningful identifiers, and use indentation as we do in the programs in this chapter.

2. Write a program that simulates the child's game "My Grandmother's Trunk." In this game, the players sit in a circle, and the first player names something that goes in the trunk: "In my grandmother's trunk, I packed a pencil." The next player restates the sentence and adds something new to the trunk: "In my grandmother's trunk, I packed a pencil and a red ball." Each player in turn adds something to the trunk, attempting to keep track of all the items that are already there.

    Your program should simulate just five turns in the game. Starting with the null string, simulate each player's turn by concatenating a new word or phrase to the existing string, and print the result on a new line. The output should be formatted as follows:

```
In my grandmother's trunk, I packed
a flower.
In my grandmother's trunk, I packed
a flower and a shirt.
In my grandmother's trunk, I packed
a flower and a shirt and a cup.
In my grandmother's trunk, I packed
a flower and a shirt and a cup and a blue marble.
In my grandmother's trunk, I packed
a flower and a shirt and a cup and a blue marble and a ball.
```

3. Write a program that prints its own grading form. The program should output the name and number of the class, the name and number of the programming assignment, your name and student number, and labeled spaces for scores reflecting correctness, quality of style, late deduction, and overall score. An example of such a form is the following:

```
CS-101 Introduction to Programming and Problem Solving

Programming Assignment 1

Sally A. Student
ID Number 431023877

Grade Summary:

    Program Correctness:
    Quality of Style:
    Late Deduction:
    Overall Score:
    Comments:
```

Case Study Follow-Up

1. Change the FormLetter program so that the name of the town is Wormwood, Massachusetts, instead of Panhard, Texas.
2. In the FormLetter program, explain what takes place in each of the two statements that assign values to the string variable fullName.
3. For obvious reasons, the president of the company wants more space inserted between the signature and the footnotes describing the prizes. How would you accomplish this?
4. Change the FormLetter program so that your name is printed in the appropriate places in the letter. (*Hint:* You need to change only four lines in the program.)

3

Numeric Types, Expressions, and Output

GOALS

- To be able to declare named constants and variables of type `int` and `float`.
- To be able to construct simple arithmetic expressions.
- To be able to evaluate simple arithmetic expressions.
- To be able to construct and evaluate expressions that include multiple arithmetic operations.
- To understand implicit type coercion and explicit type conversion.
- To be able to call (invoke) a value-returning function.
- To be able to recognize and understand the purpose of function arguments.
- To be able to use C++ library functions in expressions.
- To be able to call (invoke) a void function (one that does not return a function value).
- To be able to use C++ manipulators to format the output.
- To learn and be able to use additional operations associated with the `string` type.
- To be able to format the statements in a program in a clear and readable fashion.

In Chapter 2, we examined enough C++ syntax to be able to construct simple programs using assignment and output. We focused on the `char` and `string` types and saw how to construct expressions using the concatenation operator. In this chapter we continue to write programs that use assignment and output, but we concentrate on additional built-in data types: `int` and `float`. These numeric types are supported by numerous operators that allow us to construct complex arithmetic expressions. We show how to make expressions even more powerful by using *library functions*—prewritten functions that are part of every C++ system and are available for use by any program.

We also return to the subject of formatting the output. In particular, we consider the special features that C++ provides for formatting numbers in the output. We finish by looking at some additional operations on `string` data.

Overview of C++ Data Types

The C++ built-in data types are organized into simple types, structured types, and address types (see Figure 3-1). Do not feel overwhelmed by the quantity of data types shown in this figure. Our purpose is simply to give you an overall picture of what is available in C++. This chapter concentrates on the integral and floating types. Details of the other types come later in the book. First we look at the integral types (those used primarily to represent integers), and then we consider the floating types (used to represent real numbers containing decimal points).

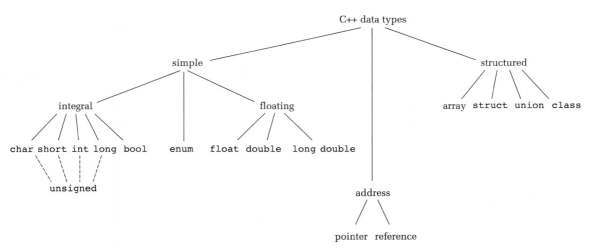

FIGURE 3-1
C++ Data Types

Numeric Data Types

You already are familiar with the basic concepts of integer and real numbers in math. However, as used on a computer, the corresponding data types have certain limitations, which we now consider.

Integral Types

The data types `char`, `short`, `int`, and `long` are known as integral types (or integer types) because they refer to integer values—whole numbers with no fractional part. (We postpone talking about the remaining integral type, `bool`, until Chapter 5.)

In C++, the simplest form of integer value is a sequence of one or more digits:

```
22   16   1   498   0   4600
```

Commas are not allowed.

In most cases, a minus sign preceding an integer value makes the integer negative:

```
-378   -912
```

The exception is when you explicitly add the reserved word `unsigned` to the data type name:

```
unsigned int
```

An `unsigned` integer value is assumed to be only positive or zero. The `unsigned` types are used primarily in specialized situations. With a few exceptions later in this chapter, we rarely use `unsigned` in this book.

The data types `char`, `short`, `int`, and `long` are intended to represent different sizes of integers, from smaller (fewer bits) to larger (more bits). The sizes are machine dependent (that is, they may vary from machine to machine). For one particular machine, we might picture the sizes this way:

char memory cell

short memory cell

int memory cell

long memory cell

On another machine, the size of an int might be the same as the size of a long. In general, the more bits there are in the memory cell, the larger the integer value that can be stored.

Although we used the char type in Chapter 2 to store character data such as 'A', there are reasons why C++ classifies char as an integral type. Chapter 10 discusses the reasons.

int is by far the most common data type for manipulating integer data. In the Payroll program, the identifier for the employee number, empNum, is of data type int. You nearly always use int for manipulating integer values, but sometimes you have to use long if your program requires values larger than the maximum int value. (On some personal computers, the range of int values is from −32768 through +32767. More commonly, ints range from −2147483648 through +2147483647.) If your program tries to compute a value larger than your machine's maximum value, the result is *integer overflow*. Some machines give you an error message when overflow occurs, but others don't. We talk more about overflow in later chapters.

One caution about integer values in C++: A literal constant beginning with a zero is taken to be an octal (base-8) number instead of a decimal (base-10) number. If you write

```
015
```

the C++ compiler takes this to mean the decimal number 13. If you aren't familiar with the octal number system, don't worry about why an octal 15 is the same as a decimal 13. The important thing to remember is not to start a decimal integer constant with a zero (unless you simply want the number 0, which is the same in both octal and decimal). In Chapter 10, we discuss the various integral types in more detail.

Floating-Point Types

Floating-point types (or floating types), the second major category of simple types in C++, are used to represent real numbers. Floating-point numbers have an integer part and a fractional part, with a decimal point in between. Either the integer part or the fractional part, but not both, may be missing. Here are some examples:

```
18.0   127.54   0.57   4.   193145.8523   .8
```

Starting 0.57 with a zero does not make it an octal number. It is only with integer values that a leading zero indicates an octal number.

Just as the integral types in C++ come in different sizes (char, short, int, and long), so do the floating-point types. In increasing order of size, the floating-point types are float, double (meaning double precision), and `long double`. Again, the exact sizes are machine dependent. Each larger size potentially gives us a wider range of values and more precision (the number of significant digits in the number), but at the expense of more memory space to hold the number.

Floating-point values also can have an exponent, as in scientific notation. (In scientific notation, a number is written as a value multiplied by 10 to some power.) Instead of writing 3.504×10^{12}, in C++ we write `3.504E12`. The `E` means exponent of base 10. The number preceding the letter `E` doesn't need to include a decimal point. Here are some examples of floating-point numbers in scientific notation:

```
1.74536E-12    3.652442E4    7E20
```

Most programs don't need the `double` and `long double` types. The `float` type usually provides sufficient precision and range of values for floating-point numbers. Even personal computers provide `float` values with a precision of six or seven significant digits and a maximum value of about `3.4E+38`. In the Payroll program, the identifiers MAX_HOURS, OVER-TIME, payRate, hours, wages, and total are all of type `float` because they are identifiers for data items that may have fractional parts.

We talk more about floating-point numbers in Chapter 10. But there is one more thing you should know about them now. Computers cannot always represent floating-point numbers exactly. You learned in Chapter 1 that the computer stores all data in binary (base-2) form. Many floating-point values can only be approximated in the binary number system. Don't be surprised if your program prints out the number 4.8 as 4.7999998. In most cases, slight inaccuracies in the rightmost fractional digits are to be expected and are not the result of programmer error.

Declarations for Numeric Types

Just as with the types `char` and `string`, we can declare named constants and variables of type `int` and `float`. Such declarations use the same syntax as before, except that the literals and the names of the data types are different.

Named Constant Declarations

In the case of named constant declarations, the literal values in the declarations are numeric instead of being characters in single or double quotes. For example, here are some constant declarations that define values of type `int` and `float`. For comparison, declarations of `char` and `string` values are included.

```
const float  PI = 3.14159;
const float  E = 2.71828;
const int    MAX_SCORE = 100;
const int    MIN_SCORE = -100;
const char   LETTER = 'W';
const string NAME = "Elizabeth";
```

Although character and string literals are put in quotes, literal integers and floating-point numbers are not, because there is no chance of confusing them with identifiers. Why? Because identifiers must start with a letter or underscore, and numbers must start with a digit or sign.

SOFTWARE ENGINEERING TIP

Using Named Constants Instead of Literals

It's a good idea to use named constants instead of literals. In addition to making your program more readable, named constants can make your program easier to modify. Suppose you wrote a program last year to compute taxes. In several places you used the literal 0.05, which was the sales tax rate at the time. Now the rate has gone up to 0.06. To change your program, you must locate every literal 0.05 and change it to 0.06. And if 0.05 is used for some other reason—to compute deductions, for example—you need to look at each place where it is used, figure out what it is used for, and then decide whether to change it.

The process is much simpler if you use a named constant. Instead of using a literal constant, suppose you had declared a named constant, TAX_RATE, with a value of 0.05. To change your program, you would simply change the declaration, setting TAX_RATE equal to 0.06. This one modification changes all of the tax rate computations without affecting the other places where 0.05 is used.

C++ allows us to declare constants with different names but the same value. If a value has different meanings in different parts of a program, it makes sense to declare and use a constant with an appropriate name for each meaning.

Named constants also are reliable; they protect us from mistakes. If you mistype the name PI as PO, the C++ compiler tells you that the name PO has not been declared. On the other hand, even though we recognize that the number 3.14149 is a mistyped version of pi (3.14159), the number is perfectly acceptable to the compiler. It won't warn us that anything is wrong.

Variable Declarations

We declare numeric variables the same way in which we declare char and string variables, except that we use the names of numeric types. The following are valid variable declarations:

```
int     studentCount;    // Number of students
int     sumOfScores;     // Sum of their scores
float   average;         // Average of the scores
char    grade;           // Student's letter grade
string stuName;          // Student's name
```

Given the declarations

```
int    num;
int    alpha;
float rate;
char   ch;
```

the following are appropriate assignment statements:

Variable	Expression
alpha =	2856;
rate =	0.36;
ch =	'B';
num =	alpha;

In each of these assignment statements, the data type of the expression matches the data type of the variable to which it is assigned. Later in the chapter we see what happens if the data types do not match.

Simple Arithmetic Expressions

Now that we have looked at declaration and assignment, we consider how to calculate with values of numeric types. Calculations are performed with expressions. We first look at simple expressions that involve at most one operator so that we may examine each operator in detail. Then, we move on to compound expressions that combine multiple operations.

Arithmetic Operators

Expressions are made up of constants, variables, and operators. The following are all valid expressions:

```
alpha + 2    rate - 6.0    4 - alpha    rate    alpha * num
```

The operators allowed in an expression depend on the data types of the constants and variables in the expression. The *arithmetic operators* are

+ Unary plus
– Unary minus
+ Addition
– Subtraction
* Multiplication
/ { Floating-point division (floating-point result)
   { Integer division (no fractional part)
% Modulus (remainder from integer division)

The first two operators are **unary operators**—they take just one operand. The remaining five are **binary operators**, taking two operands. Unary plus and minus are used as follows:

```
-54    +259.65    -rate
```

Programmers rarely use the unary plus. Without any sign, a numeric constant is assumed to be positive anyway.

Unary operator   An operator that has just one operand.
Binary operator   An operator that has two operands.

You may not be familiar with integer division and modulus (%). Let's look at them more closely. Note that % is used only with integers. When you divide one integer by another, you get an integer quotient and a remainder. Integer division gives only the integer quotient, and % gives only the remainder. (If either operand is negative, the sign of the remainder may vary from one C++ compiler to another.)

$$
\begin{array}{ll}
\dfrac{3}{2\overline{)6}} \quad \leftarrow 6\ /\ 2 & \dfrac{3}{2\overline{)7}} \quad \leftarrow 7\ /\ 2 \\
\dfrac{6}{0} \quad \leftarrow 6\ \%\ 2 & \dfrac{6}{1} \quad \leftarrow 7\ \%\ 2
\end{array}
$$

In contrast, floating-point division yields a floating-point result. The expression

```
7.0 / 2.0
```

yields the value 3.5.

Here are some expressions using arithmetic operators and their values:

Expression	Value
3 + 6	9
3.4 - 6.1	−2.7
2 * 3	6
8 / 2	4
8.0 / 2.0	4.0
8 / 8	1
8 / 9	0
8 / 7	1
8 % 8	0
8 % 9	8
8 % 7	1
0 % 7	0
5 % 2.3	error (both operands must be integers)

Be careful with division and modulus. The expressions `7.0 / 0.0`, `7 / 0`, and `7 % 0` all produce errors. The computer cannot divide by zero.

Because variables are allowed in expressions, the following are valid assignments:

```
alpha = num + 6;
alpha = num / 2;
num = alpha * 2;
num = 6 % alpha;
alpha = alpha + 1;
num = num + alpha;
```

As we saw with assignment statements involving `string` expressions, the same variable can appear on both sides of the assignment operator. In the case of

```
num = num + alpha;
```

the value in `num` and the value in `alpha` are added together, and then the sum of the two values is stored back into `num`, replacing the previous value stored there. This example shows the difference between mathematical equality and assignment. The mathematical equality

$$num = num + alpha$$

is true only when *alpha* equals 0. The assignment statement

```
num = num + alpha;
```

is valid for *any* value of `alpha`.

Here's a simple program that uses arithmetic expressions:

```
//*******************************************************************
// FreezeBoil program
// This program computes the midpoint between
// the freezing and boiling points of water
//*******************************************************************
#include <iostream>

using namespace std;

const float FREEZE_PT = 32.0;    // Freezing point of water
const float BOIL_PT = 212.0;     // Boiling point of water

int main()
{
    float avgTemp;                 // Holds the result of averaging
                                   //    FREEZE_PT and BOIL_PT

    cout << "Water freezes at " << FREEZE_PT << endl;
    cout << " and boils at " << BOIL_PT << " degrees." << endl;

    avgTemp = FREEZE_PT + BOIL_PT;
    avgTemp = avgTemp / 2.0;

    cout << "Halfway between is ";
    cout << avgTemp << " degrees." << endl;

    return 0;
}
```

The program begins with a comment that explains what the program does. Next comes a declaration section where we define the constants `FREEZE_PT` and `BOIL_PT`. The body of the `main` function includes a declaration of the variable `avgTemp` and then a sequence of executable statements. These statements print a message, add `FREEZE_PT` and `BOIL_PT`, divide the sum by 2, and finally print the result.

Increment and Decrement Operators

In addition to the arithmetic operators, C++ provides *increment* and *decrement operators*:

```
.++        Increment
--         Decrement
```

These are unary operators that take a single variable name as an operand. For integer and floating-point operands, the effect is to add 1 to (or subtract 1 from) the operand. If `num` currently contains the value 8, the statement

```
num++;
```

causes `num` to contain 9. You can achieve the same effect by writing the assignment statement

```
num = num + 1;
```

but C++ programmers typically prefer the increment operator. (Recall from Chapter 1 how the C++ language got its name: C++ is an enhanced ["incremented"] version of the C language.)

The ++ and -- operators can be either *prefix operators*

```
++num;
```

or *postfix operators*

```
num++;
```

Both of these statements behave in exactly the same way; they add 1 to whatever is in `num`. The choice between the two is a matter of personal preference.

C++ allows the use of ++ and -- in the middle of a larger expression:

```
alpha = num++ * 3;
```

In this case, the postfix form of ++ does *not* give the same result as the prefix form. In Chapter 10, we explain the ++ and -- operators in detail. In the meantime, you should use them only to increment or decrement a variable as a separate, stand-alone statement:

IncrementStatement

```
{ Variable ++  ;
{ ++ Variable ;
```

DecrementStatement

```
{ Variable --  ;
{ -- Variable ;
```

Compound Arithmetic Expressions

The expressions we've used so far have contained at most a single arithmetic operator. We also have been careful not to mix integer and floating-point values in the same expression. Now we look at more complicated expressions—ones that are composed of several operators and ones that contain mixed data types.

Precedence Rules

Arithmetic expressions can be made up of many constants, variables, operators, and parentheses. In what order are the operations performed? For example, in the assignment statement

```
avgTemp = FREEZE_PT + BOIL_PT / 2.0;
```

is `FREEZE_PT + BOIL_PT` calculated first or is `BOIL_PT / 2.0` calculated first?

The basic arithmetic operators (unary +, unary –, + for addition, – for subtraction, * for multiplication, / for division, and % for modulus) are ordered the same way mathematical operators are, according to *precedence rules:*

Highest precedence level:	Unary + Unary –
Middle level:	* / %
Lowest level:	+ –

Because division has higher precedence than addition, the expression in the example above is implicitly parenthesized as

```
FREEZE_PT + (BOIL_PT / 2.0)
```

That is, we first divide `BOIL_PT` by 2.0 and then add `FREEZE_PT` to the result.

You can change the order of evaluation by using parentheses. In the statement

```
avgTemp = (FREEZE_PT + BOIL_PT) / 2.0;
```

`FREEZE_PT` and `BOIL_PT` are added first, and then their sum is divided by 2.0. We evaluate subexpressions in parentheses first and then follow the precedence of the operators.

When an arithmetic expression has several binary operators with the same precedence, their *grouping order* (or *associativity*) is from left to right. The expression

```
int1 - int2 + int3
```

means (int1 – int2) + int3, not int1 – (int2 + int3). As another example, we would use the expression

```
(float1 + float2) / float1 * 3.0
```

to evaluate the expression in parentheses first, then divide the sum by float1, and multiply the result by 3.0. Below are some more examples.

Expression	Value
10 / 2 * 3	15
10 % 3 - 4 / 2	−1
5.0 * 2.0 / 4.0 * 2.0	5.0
5.0 * 2.0 / (4.0 * 2.0)	1.25
5.0 + 2.0 / (4.0 * 2.0)	5.25

In C++, all unary operators (such as unary + and unary –) have right-to-left associativity. Though this fact may seem strange at first, it turns out to be the natural grouping order. For example, – + x means – (+ x) rather than the meaningless (– +) x.

Type Coercion and Type Casting

Integer values and floating-point values are stored differently inside a computer's memory. The pattern of bits that represents the constant 2 does not look at all like the pattern of bits representing the constant 2.0. (In Chapter 10, we examine why floating-point numbers need a special representation inside the computer.) What happens if we mix integer and floating-point values together in an assignment statement or an arithmetic expression? Let's look first at assignment statements.

Assignment Statements If you make the declarations

```
int   someInt;
float someFloat;
```

then someInt can hold *only* integer values, and someFloat can hold *only* floating-point values. The assignment statement

```
someFloat = 12;
```

may seem to store the integer value 12 into `someFloat`, but this is not true. The computer refuses to store anything other than a `float` value into `someFloat`. The compiler inserts extra machine language instructions that first convert 12 into 12.0 and then store 12.0 into `someFloat`. This implicit (automatic) conversion of a value from one data type to another is known as **type coercion.**

The statement

```
someInt = 4.8;
```

also causes type coercion. When a floating-point value is assigned to an `int` variable, the fractional part is truncated (cut off). As a result, `someInt` is assigned the value 4.

With both of the assignment statements above, the program would be less confusing for someone to read if we avoided mixing data types:

```
someFloat = 12.0;
someInt = 4;
```

More often, it is not just constants but entire expressions that are involved in type coercion. Both of the assignments

```
someFloat = 3 * someInt + 2;
someInt = 5.2 / someFloat - anotherFloat;
```

lead to type coercion. Storing the result of an `int` expression into a `float` variable generally doesn't cause loss of information; a whole number such as 24 can be represented in floating-point form as 24.0. However, storing the result of a floating-point expression into an `int` variable can cause loss of information because the fractional part is truncated. It is easy to overlook the assignment of a floating-point expression to an `int` variable when we try to discover why our program is producing the wrong answers.

To make our programs as clear (and error free) as possible, we can use explicit **type casting** (or **type conversion**). A C++ *cast operation* consists of a data type name and then, within parentheses, the expression to be converted:

```
someFloat = float(3 * someInt + 2);
someInt = int(5.2 / someFloat - anotherFloat);
```

Type coercion   The implicit (automatic) conversion of a value from one data type to another.

Type casting   The explicit conversion of a value from one data type to another; also called type conversion.

Both of the statements

```
someInt = someFloat + 8.2;
someInt = int(someFloat + 8.2);
```

produce identical results. The only difference is in clarity. With the cast operation, it is perfectly clear to the programmer and to others reading the program that the mixing of types is intentional, not an oversight. Countless errors have resulted from unintentional mixing of types.

Note that there is a nice way to round off rather than truncate a floating-point value before storing it into an int variable. Here is the way to do it:

```
someInt = int(someFloat + 0.5);
```

With pencil and paper, see for yourself what gets stored into someInt when someFloat contains 4.7. Now try it again, assuming someFloat contains 4.2. (This technique of rounding by adding 0.5 assumes that someFloat is a positive number.)

Arithmetic Expressions So far we have been talking about mixing data types across the assignment operator (=). It's also possible to mix data types within an expression:

```
someInt * someFloat
4.8 + someInt - 3
```

Such expressions are called **mixed type** (or **mixed mode**) **expressions**.

Mixed type expression An expression that contains operands of different data types; also called mixed mode expression.

Whenever an integer value and a floating-point value are joined by an operator, implicit type coercion occurs as follows.

1. The integer value is temporarily coerced to a floating-point value.
2. The operation is performed.
3. The result is a floating-point value.

Let's examine how the machine evaluates the expression 4.8 + someInt - 3, where someInt contains the value 2. First, the operands of the + operator have mixed types, so the value of someInt is coerced to 2.0. (This conversion is only temporary; it does not affect the value that is stored in someInt.) The addition takes place, yielding a value of 6.8. Next, the subtraction (-) operator joins a floating-point value (6.8) and an integer value (3). The value 3 is coerced to 3.0, the subtraction takes place, and the result is the floating-point value 3.8.

Just as with assignment statements, you can use explicit type casts within expressions to lessen the risk of errors. Writing expressions such as

```
float(someInt) * someFloat
4.8 + float(someInt - 3)
```

makes it clear what your intentions are.

Explicit type casts are not only valuable for program clarity, but also are mandatory in some cases for correct programming. Given the declarations

```
int    sum;
int    count;
float average;
```

suppose that `sum` and `count` currently contain 60 and 80, respectively. If `sum` represents the sum of a group of integer values and `count` represents the number of values, let's find the average value:

```
average = sum / count;      // Wrong
```

Unfortunately, this statement stores the value 0.0 into `average`. Here's why. The expression to the right of the assignment operator is not a mixed type expression. Both operands of the / operator are of type `int`, so integer division is performed. 60 divided by 80 yields the integer value 0. Next, the machine implicitly coerces 0 to the value 0.0 before storing it into `average`. The way to find the average correctly, as well as clearly, is this:

```
average = float(sum) / float(count);
```

This statement gives us floating-point division instead of integer division. As a result, the value 0.75 is stored into `average`.

As a final remark about type coercion and type conversion, you may have noticed that we have concentrated only on the `int` and `float` types. It is also possible to stir `char` values, `short` values, and `double` values into the pot. The results can be confusing and unexpected. In Chapter 10, we return to the topic with a more detailed discussion. In the meantime, you should avoid mixing values of these types within an expression.

MAY WE INTRODUCE

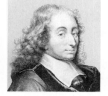

Blaise Pascal

One of the great historical figures in the world of computing was the French mathematician and religious philosopher Blaise Pascal (1623–1662), the inventor of one of the earliest known mechanical calculators.

Pascal's father, Etienne, was a noble in the French court, a tax collector, and a mathematician. Pascal's mother died when Pascal was 3 years old. Five years later, the family moved to Paris and Etienne took over the education of the children. Pascal quickly showed a talent for mathematics. When he was only 17, he published a mathematical essay that earned the jealous envy of René Descartes, one of the founders of modern geometry. (Pascal's work actually had been completed before he was 16.) It was based on a theorem, which he called the *hexagrammum mysticum*, or mystic hexagram, that described the inscription of hexagons in conic sections (parabolas, hyperbolas, and ellipses). In addition to the theorem (now called Pascal's theorem), his essay included over 400 corollaries.

When Pascal was about 20, he constructed a mechanical calculator that performed addition and subtraction of eight-digit numbers. That calculator required the user to dial in the numbers to be added or subtracted; the sum or difference then appeared in a set of windows. It is believed that his motivation for building this machine was to aid his father in collecting taxes. The earliest version of the machine does indeed split the numbers into six decimal digits and two fractional digits, as would be used for calculating sums of money. The machine was hailed by his contemporaries as a great advance in mathematics, and Pascal built several more in different forms. It achieved such popularity that many fake, nonfunctional copies were built by others and displayed as novelties. Several of Pascal's calculators still exist in various museums.

Pascal's box, as it is called, was long believed to be the first mechanical calculator. However, in 1950 a letter from Wilhelm Shickard to Johannes Kepler written in 1624 was discovered. This letter described an even more sophisticated calculator built by Shickard 20 years prior to Pascal's box. Unfortunately, the machine was destroyed in a fire and never rebuilt.

During his twenties, Pascal solved several difficult problems related to the cycloid curve, indirectly contributing to the development of differential calculus. Working with Pierre de Fermat, he laid the foundation of the calculus of probabilities and combinatorial analysis. One of the results of this work came to be known as Pascal's triangle, which simplifies the calculation of the coefficients of the expansion of $(X + Y)^N$, where N is a positive integer.

Pascal also published a treatise on air pressure and conducted experiments that showed that barometric pressure decreases with altitude, helping to confirm theories that had been proposed by Galileo and Torricelli. His work on fluid dynamics forms a significant part of the foundation of that field. Among the most famous of his contributions is Pascal's law, which states that pressure applied to a fluid in a closed vessel is transmitted uniformly throughout the fluid.

When Pascal was 23, his father became ill, and the family was visited by two disciples of Jansenism, a reform movement in the Catholic Church that had begun six years earlier. The family converted, and five years later one of his sisters entered a convent. Initially, Pascal was not so taken with the new movement, but by the time he was 31, his sister had persuaded him to abandon the world and devote himself to religion.

His religious works are considered no less brilliant than his mathematical and scientific writings. Some consider *Provincial Letters*, his series of 18 essays on various aspects of religion, as the beginning of modern French prose.

Pascal returned briefly to mathematics when he was 35, but a year later his health, which had always been poor, took a turn for the worse. Unable to perform his usual work, he devoted himself to helping the less fortunate. Three years later, he died while staying with his sister, having given his own house to a poor family.

Function Calls and Library Functions

Value-Returning Functions

At the beginning of Chapter 2, we showed a program consisting of three functions: `main`, `Square`, and `Cube`. Here is a portion of the program:

```cpp
int main()
{
    cout << "The square of 27 is " << Square(27) << endl;
    cout << "and the cube of 27 is " << Cube(27) << endl;
    return 0;
}

int Square( int n )
{
    return n * n;
}

int Cube( int n )
{
    return n * n * n;
}
```

We said that all three functions are value-returning functions. `Square` returns to its caller a value—the square of the number sent to it. `Cube` returns a value—the cube of the number sent to it. And `main` returns to the operating system a value—the program's exit status.

Let's focus for a moment on the Cube function. The main function contains a statement

```
cout << " and the cube of 27 is " << Cube(27) << endl;
```

In this statement, the master (main) causes the servant (Cube) to compute the cube of 27 and give the result back to main. The sequence of symbols

```
Cube(27)
```

is a **function call** or **function invocation.** The computer temporarily puts the main function on hold and starts the Cube function running. When Cube has finished doing its work, the computer goes back to main and picks up where it left off.

Function call (function invocation)   The mechanism that transfers control to a function.

In the above function call, the number 27 is known as an *argument* (or *actual parameter*). Arguments make it possible for the same function to work on many different values. For example, we can write statements like these:

```
cout << Cube(4);
cout << Cube(16);
```

Here's the syntax template for a function call:

FunctionCall

FunctionName (ArgumentList)

The **argument list** is a way for functions to communicate with each other. Some functions, like Square and Cube, have a single argument in the argument list. Other functions, like main, have no arguments in the list. And some functions have two, three, or more arguments in the argument list, separated by commas.

Argument list   A mechanism by which functions communicate with each other.

Value-returning functions are used in expressions in much the same way that variables and constants are. The value computed by a function simply takes its place in the expression. For example, the statement

```
someInt = Cube(2) * 10;
```

stores the value 80 into `someInt`. First the `Cube` function is executed to compute the cube of 2, which is 8. The value 8—now available for use in the rest of the expression—is multiplied by 10. Note that a function call has higher precedence than multiplication, which makes sense if you consider that the function result must be available before the multiplication takes place.

Here are several facts about value-returning functions:

- The function call is used within an expression; it does not appear as a separate statement.
- The function computes a value (*result*) that is then available for use in the expression.
- The function returns exactly one result—no more, no less.

The `Cube` function expects to be given (or *passed*) an argument of type `int`. What happens if the caller passes a `float` argument? The answer is that the compiler applies implicit type coercion. The function call `Cube(6.9)` computes the cube of 6, not 6.9.

Although we have been using literal constants as arguments to `Cube`, the argument could just as easily be a variable or named constant. In fact, the argument to a value-returning function can be any expression of the appropriate type. In the statement

```
alpha = Cube(int1 * int1 + int2 * int2);
```

the expression in the argument list is evaluated first, and only its result is passed to the function. For example, if `int1` contains 3 and `int2` contains 5, the above function call passes 34 as the argument to `Cube`.

An expression in a function's argument list can even include calls to functions. For example, we could use the `Square` function to rewrite the above assignment statement as follows:

```
alpha = Cube(Square(int1) + Square(int2));
```

Library Functions

Certain computations, such as taking square roots or finding the absolute value of a number, are very common in programs. It would be an enormous waste of time if every programmer had to start from scratch and create functions to perform these tasks. To help make the programmer's life easier, every C++ system includes a standard library—a large collection of prewritten functions, data types, and other items that any C++ programmer may use. Here is a very small sample of some standard library functions:

Header File*	Function	Argument Type(s)	Result Type	Result (Value Returned)
<cstdlib>	abs(i)	int	int	Absolute value of i
<cmath>	cos(x)	float	float	Cosine of x (x is in radians)
<cmath>	fabs(x)	float	float	Absolute value of x
<cstdlib>	labs(j)	long	long	Absolute value of j
<cmath>	pow(x, y)	float	float	x raised to the power y (if x = 0.0, y must be positive; if x ≤ 0.0, y must be a whole number)
<cmath>	sin(x)	float	float	Sine of x (x is in radians)
<cmath>	sqrt(x)	float	float	Square root of x (x ≥ 0.0)

* The names of these header files are not the same as in pre–standard C++. If you are working with pre–standard C++, see Section D.2 of Appendix D.

Technically, the entries in the table marked `float` should all say `double`. These library functions perform their work using double-precision floating-point values. But because of type coercion, the functions work just as you would like them to when you pass `float` values to them.

Using a library function is easy. First, you place an `#include` directive near the top of your program, specifying the appropriate header file. This directive ensures that the C++ preprocessor inserts declarations into your program that give the compiler some information about the function. Then, whenever you want to use the function, you just make a function call.* Here's an example:

```
#include <iostream>
#include <cmath>        // For sqrt() and fabs()

using namespace std;
    ⋮
float alpha;
float beta;
    ⋮
alpha = sqrt(7.3 + fabs(beta));
```

* Some systems require you to specify a particular compiler option if you use the math functions. For example, with some versions of UNIX, you must add the option –lm when compiling your program.

Remember from Chapter 2 that all identifiers in the standard library are in the namespace `std`. If we omit the `using` directive from the above code, we must use qualified names for the library functions (`std::sqrt`, `std::fabs`, and so forth).

The C++ standard library provides dozens of functions for you to use. Appendix C lists a much larger selection than we have presented here. You should glance briefly at this appendix now, keeping in mind that much of the terminology and C++ language notation will make sense only after you have read further into the book.

Void Functions

In this chapter, the only kind of function that we have looked at is the value-returning function. C++ provides another kind of function as well. If you look at the Payroll program in Chapter 1, you see that the function definition for `CalcPay` begins with the word `void` instead of a data type like `int` or `float`:

```
void CalcPay( ... )
{
     ⋮
}
```

`CalcPay` is an example of a function that doesn't return a function value to its caller. Instead, it just performs some action and then quits. We refer to a function like this as a *non-value-returning function,* a *void-returning function,* or, most briefly, a **void function.** In many programming languages, a void function is known as a **procedure.**

Void functions are invoked differently from value-returning functions. With a value-returning function, the function call appears in an expression. With a void function, the function call is a separate, stand-alone statement. In the Payroll program, `main` calls the `CalcPay` function like this:

```
CalcPay(payRate, hours, wages);
```

From the caller's perspective, a call to a void function has the flavor of a command or built-in instruction:

```
DoThis(x, y, z);
DoThat();
```

In contrast, a call to a value-returning function doesn't look like a command; it looks like a value in an expression:

```
y = 4.7 + Cube(x);
```

Value-returning function A function that returns a single value to its caller and is invoked from within an expression.

Void function (procedure) A function that does not return a function value to its caller and is invoked as a separate statement.

For the next few chapters, we won't be writing our own functions (except main). Instead, we'll be concentrating on how to use existing functions, including functions for performing stream input and output. Some of these functions are value-returning functions; others are void functions. Again, we emphasize the difference in how you invoke these two kinds of functions: A call to a value-returning function occurs in an expression, whereas a call to a void function occurs as a separate statement.

Formatting the Output

To format a program's output means to control how it appears visually on the screen or on a printer. In Chapter 2, we considered two kinds of output formatting: creating extra blank lines by using the endl manipulator and inserting blanks within a line by putting extra blanks into literal strings. In this section, we examine how to format the output values themselves.

Integers and Strings

By default, consecutive integer and string values are output with no spaces between them. If the variables i, j, and k contain the values 15, 2, and 6, respectively, the statement

```
cout << "Results: " << i << j << k;
```

outputs the stream of characters

```
Results: 1526
```

Without spacing between the numbers, this output is difficult to interpret.

To separate the output values, you could print a single blank (as a char constant) between the numbers:

```
cout << "Results: " << i << ' ' << j << ' ' << k;
```

This statement produces the output

```
Results: 15 2 6
```

If you want even more spacing between items, you can use literal strings containing blanks, as we discussed in Chapter 2:

```
cout << "Results: " << i << "    " << j << "    " << k;
```

Here, the resulting output is

```
Results: 15    2    6
```

Another way to control the horizontal spacing of the output is to use *manipulators*. For some time now, we have been using the endl manipulator to terminate an output line. In C++, a manipulator is a rather curious thing that behaves like a function but travels in the disguise of a data object. Like a function, a manipulator causes some action to occur. But like a data object, a manipulator can appear in the midst of a series of insertion operations:

```
cout << someInt << endl << someFloat;
```

Manipulators are used *only* in input and output statements.

Here's a revised syntax template for the output statement, showing that not only arithmetic and string expressions but also manipulators are allowed:

OutputStatement

```
cout << ExpressionOrManipulator << ExpressionOrManipulator ...;
```

The C++ standard library supplies many manipulators, but for now we look at only five of them: endl, setw, fixed, showpoint, and setprecision. The endl, fixed, and showpoint manipulators come "for free" when we #include the header file iostream to perform I/O. The other two manipulators, setw and setprecision, require that we also #include the header file iomanip:

```
#include <iostream>
#include <iomanip>

using namespace std;
   ⋮
cout << setw(5) << someInt;
```

The manipulator `setw`—meaning "set width"—lets us control how many character positions the next data item should occupy when it is output. (`setw` is only for formatting numbers and strings, not `char` data.) The argument to `setw` is an integer expression called the *fieldwidth specification;* the group of character positions is called the *field*. The next data item to be output is printed *right-justified* (filled with blanks on the left to fill up the field).

Let's look at an example. Assuming two `int` variables have been assigned values as follows:

```
ans = 33;
num = 7132;
```

then the following output statements produce the output shown to their right.

Statement	Output (□ *means blank*)

1. `cout << setw(4) << ans`
`      << setw(5) << num`
`      << setw(4) << "Hi";`
	□□33□7132□□Hi
	  4 5 4

2. `cout << setw(2) << ans`
`      << setw(4) << num`
`      << setw(2) << "Hi";`
	337132Hi
	 2 4 2

3. `cout << setw(6) << ans`
`      << setw(3) << "Hi"`
`      << setw(5) << num;`
	□□□□33□Hi□7132
	   6 3 5

4. `cout << setw(7) << "Hi"` `      << setw(4) << num;`	□□□□□Hi7132 7 4
5. `cout << setw(1) << ans` `      << setw(5) << num;`	33□7132 ↑ 5 Field automatically expands to fit the two-digit value

---

In (1), each value is specified to occupy enough positions so that there is at least one space separating them. In (2), the values all run together because the fieldwidth specified for each value is just large enough to hold the value. This output obviously is not very readable. It's better to make the fieldwidth larger than the minimum size required so that some space is left between values. In (3), there are extra blanks for readability; in (4), there are not. In (5), the fieldwidth is not large enough for the value in ans, so it automatically expands to make room for all of the digits.

Setting the fieldwidth is a one-time action. It holds only for the very next item to be output. After this output, the fieldwidth resets to 0, meaning "extend the field to exactly as many positions as are needed." In the statement

```
cout << "Hi" << setw(5) << ans << num;
```

the fieldwidth resets to 0 after ans is output. As a result, we get the output

```
Hi    337132
```

Floating-Point Numbers

You can specify a fieldwidth for floating-point values just as for integer values. But you must remember to allow for the decimal point when you specify the number of character positions. The value 4.85 requires four output positions, not three. If x contains the value 4.85, the statement

```
cout << setw(4) << x << endl
     << setw(6) << x << endl
     << setw(3) << x << endl;
```

produces the output

```
4.85
  4.85
4.85
```

In the third line, a fieldwidth of 3 isn't sufficient, so the field automatically expands to accommodate the number.

There are several other issues related to output of floating-point numbers. First, large floating-point values are printed in scientific (E) notation. The value 123456789.5 may print on some systems as

```
1.23457E+08
```

You can use the manipulator named `fixed` to force all subsequent floating-point output to appear in decimal form rather than scientific notation:

```
cout << fixed << 3.8 * x;
```

Second, if the number is a whole number, C++ doesn't print a decimal point. The value 95.0 prints as

```
95
```

To force decimal points to be displayed in subsequent floating-point output, even for whole numbers, you can use the manipulator `showpoint`:

```
cout << showpoint << floatVar;
```

(If you are using a pre–standard version of C++, the `fixed` and `showpoint` manipulators may not be available. See Section D.3 of Appendix D for an alternative way of achieving the same results.)

Third, you often would like to control the number of *decimal places* (digits to the right of the decimal point) that are displayed. If your program is supposed to print the 5% sales tax on a certain amount, the statement

```
cout << "Tax is $" << price * 0.05;
```

may output

```
Tax is $17.7435
```

Here, you clearly would prefer to display the result to two decimal places. To do so, use the `setprecision` manipulator as follows:

```
cout << fixed << setprecision(2) << "Tax is $" << price * 0.05;
```

Provided that `fixed` has already been specified, the argument to `setprecision` specifies the desired number of decimal places. Unlike `setw`, which applies only to the very next item printed, the value sent to `setprecision` remains in effect for all subsequent output (until you change it with another call to `setprecision`). Here are some examples of using `setprecision` in conjunction with `setw`:

Value of x	Statement	Output (□ means blank)
	`cout << fixed;`	
310.0	`cout << setw(10)`	
	`        << setprecision(2) << x;`	□□□□310.00
310.0	`cout << setw(10)`	
	`        << setprecision(5) << x;`	□310.00000
310.0	`cout << setw(7)`	
	`        << setprecision(5) << x;`	310.00000 (expands to nine positions)
4.827	`cout << setw(6)`	
	`        << setprecision(2) << x;`	□□4.83 (last displayed digit is rounded off)
4.827	`cout << setw(6)`	
	`        << setprecision(1) << x;`	□□□4.8 (last displayed digit is rounded off)

Again, the total number of print positions is expanded if the fieldwidth specified by `setw` is too narrow. However, the number of positions for fractional digits is controlled entirely by the argument to `setprecision`.

The following table summarizes the manipulators we have discussed in this section. Manipulators without arguments are available through the header file `iostream`. Those with arguments require the header file `iomanip`.

Header File	Manipulator	Argument Type	Effect
`<iostream>`	`endl`	None	Terminates the current output line
`<iostream>`	`showpoint`	None	Forces display of decimal point in floating-point output
`<iostream>`	`fixed`	None	Suppresses scientific notation in floating-point output
`<iomanip>`	`setw(n)`	int	Sets fieldwidth to n*
`<iomanip>`	`setprecision(n)`	int	Sets floating-point precision to n digits

*`setw` is only for numbers and strings, not `char` data. Also, `setw` applies only to the very next output item, after which the fieldwidth is reset to 0 (meaning "use only as many positions as are needed").

MATTERS OF STYLE

Program Formatting

As far as the compiler is concerned, C++ statements are *free format:* They can appear anywhere on a line, more than one can appear on a single line, and one statement can span several lines. The compiler only needs blanks (or comments or new lines) to separate important symbols, and it needs semicolons to terminate statements. However, it is extremely important that your programs be readable, both for your sake and for the sake of anyone else who has to examine them.

When you write an outline for an English paper, you follow certain rules of indentation to make it readable. These same kinds of rules can make your programs easier to read. It is much easier to spot a mistake in a neatly formatted program than in a messy one. Thus, you should keep your program neatly formatted while you are working on it. If you've gotten lazy and let your program become messy while making a series of changes, take the time to straighten it up. Often the source of an error becomes obvious during the process of formatting the code.

Take a look at the following program for computing the cost per square foot of a house. Although it compiles and runs correctly, it does not conform to any formatting standards.

```cpp
// HouseCost program
// This program computes the cost per square foot of
    // living space for a house, given the dimensions of
// the house, the number of stories, the size of the
// nonliving space, and the total cost less land
#include <iostream>
#include <iomanip>// For setw() and setprecision()
using namespace
std;
const float WIDTH = 30.0; // Width of the house
    const float LENGTH = 40.0; // Length of the house
const float STORIES = 2.5; // Number of full stories
const float NON_LIVING_SPACE = 825.0;// Garage, closets, etc.

const float PRICE = 150000.0; // Selling price less land
int main() { float grossFootage;// Total square footage
    float livingFootage;         // Living area
float costPerFoot;      // Cost/foot of living area
    cout << fixed << showpoint;   // Set up floating-pt.
//   output format

grossFootage = LENGTH * WIDTH * STORIES; livingFootage =
grossFootage - NON_LIVING_SPACE; costPerFoot = PRICE /
livingFootage; cout << "Cost per square foot is "
<< setw(6) << setprecision(2) << costPerFoot << endl;
return 0; }
```

Now look at the same program with proper formatting:

```
//*****************************************************************
// HouseCost program
// This program computes the cost per square foot of
// living space for a house, given the dimensions of
// the house, the number of stories, the size of the
// nonliving space, and the total cost less land
//*****************************************************************
#include <iostream>
#include <iomanip>       // For setw() and setprecision()

using namespace std;

const float WIDTH = 30.0;                // Width of the house
const float LENGTH = 40.0;               // Length of the house
const float STORIES = 2.5;               // Number of full stories
const float NON_LIVING_SPACE = 825.0;    // Garage, closets, etc.
const float PRICE = 150000.0;            // Selling price less land

int main()
{
    float grossFootage;      // Total square footage
    float livingFootage;     // Living area
    float costPerFoot;       // Cost/foot of living area

    cout << fixed << showpoint;              // Set up floating-pt.
                                             //   output format

    grossFootage = LENGTH * WIDTH * STORIES;
    livingFootage = grossFootage - NON_LIVING_SPACE;
    costPerFoot = PRICE / livingFootage;

    cout << "Cost per square foot is "
         << setw(6) << setprecision(2) << costPerFoot << endl;
    return 0;
}
```

Need we say more?

Appendix F talks about programming style. Use it as a guide when you are writing programs.

Additional string *Operations*

Now that we have introduced numeric types and function calls, we can take advantage of additional features of the string data type. In this section, we introduce four functions that operate on strings: length, size, find, and substr.

The length and size Functions

The length function, when applied to a string variable, returns an unsigned integer value that equals the number of characters currently in the string. If myName is a string variable, a call to the length function looks like this:

```
myName.length()
```

You specify the name of a string variable (here, myName), then a dot (period), and then the function name and argument list. The length function requires no arguments to be passed to it, but you still must use parentheses to signify an empty argument list. Also, length is a value-returning function, so the function call must appear within an expression:

```
string firstName;
string fullName;

firstName = "Alexandra";
cout << firstName.length() << endl;        // Prints 9
fullName = firstName + " Jones";
cout << fullName.length() << endl;         // Prints 15
```

Perhaps you are wondering about the syntax in a function call like

```
firstName.length()
```

This expression uses a C++ notation called *dot notation*. There is a dot (period) between the variable name firstName and the function name length. Certain programmer-defined data types, such as string, have functions that are tightly associated with them, and dot notation is required in the function calls. If you forget to use dot notation, writing the function call as

```
length()
```

you get a compile-time error message, something like "UNDECLARED IDENTIFIER." The compiler thinks you are trying to call an ordinary function named length, not the length function associated with the string type. In Chapter 4, we discuss the meaning behind dot notation.

Some people refer to the length of a string as its *size*. To accommodate both terms, the string type provides a function named size. Both firstName.size() and firstName.length() return the same value.

We said that the length function returns an unsigned integer value. If we want to save the result into a variable len, as in

```
len = firstName.length();
```

then what should we declare the data type of len to be? To keep us from having to guess whether unsigned int or unsigned long is correct for the particular compiler we're working with, the string type defines a data type size_type for us to use:

```
string firstName;
string::size_type len;

firstName = "Alexandra";
len = firstName.length();
```

Notice that we must use the qualified name string::size_type (just as we do with identifiers in namespaces) because the definition of size_type is otherwise hidden inside the definition of the string type.

Before leaving the length and size functions, we should make a remark about capitalization of identifiers. In the guidelines given in Chapter 2, we said that in this book we begin the names of programmer-defined functions and data types with uppercase letters. We follow this convention when we write our own functions and data types in later chapters. However, we have no control over the capitalization of items supplied by the C++ standard library. Identifiers in the standard library generally use all-lowercase letters.

The **find** Function

The find function searches a string to find the first occurrence of a particular substring and returns an unsigned integer value (of type string:: size_type) giving the result of the search. The substring, passed as an argument to the function, can be a literal string or a string expression. If str1 and str2 are of type string, the following are valid function calls:

```
str1.find("the")        str1.find(str2)        str1.find(str2 + "abc")
```

In each case above, str1 is searched to see if the specified substring can be found within it. If so, the function returns the position in str1 where the match begins. (Positions are numbered starting at 0, so the first character in a string is in position 0, the second is in position 1, and so on.) For a successful search, the match must be exact, including identical capitalization. If the substring could not be found, the function returns the special value string::npos, a named constant meaning "not a position within the string." (string::npos is the largest possible value of type string::size_type, a number like 4294967295 on many machines. This value is suitable for "not a valid position" because the string operations do not let any string become this long.)

Given the code segment

```
string phrase;
string::size_type position;

phrase = "The dog and the cat";
```

the statement

```
position = phrase.find("the");
```

assigns to position the value 12, whereas the statement

```
position = phrase.find("rat");
```

assigns to position the value string::npos, because there was no match.

The argument to the find function can also be a char value. In this case, find searches for the first occurrence of that character within the string and returns its position (or string::npos, if the character was not found). For example, the code segment

```
string theString;

theString = "Abracadabra";
cout << theString.find('a');
```

outputs the value 3, which is the position of the first occurrence of a lower-case *a* in theString.

Below are some more examples of calls to the find function, assuming the following code segment has been executed:

```
string str1;
string str2;

str1 = "Programming and Problem Solving";
str2 = "gram";
```

Function Call	*Value Returned by Function*
str1.find("and")	12
str1.find("Programming")	0
str2.find("and")	string::npos
str1.find("Pro")	0
str1.find("ro" + str2)	1
str1.find("Pr" + str2)	string::npos
str1.find(' ')	11

Notice in the fourth example that there are two copies of the substring "Pro" in str1, but find returns only the position of the first copy. Also notice that the copies can be either separate words or parts of words— find merely tries to match the sequence of characters given in the argument list. The final example demonstrates that the argument can be as simple as a single character, even a single blank.

The substr Function

The substr function returns a particular substring of a string. Assuming myString is of type string, here is a sample function call:

```
myString.substr(5, 20)
```

The first argument is an unsigned integer that specifies a position within the string, and the second is an unsigned integer that specifies the length of the desired substring. The function returns the piece of the string that starts with the specified position and continues for the number of characters given by the second argument. Note that substr doesn't change myString; it returns a new, temporary string value that is a copy of a portion of the string. Below are some examples, assuming the statement

```
myString = "Programming and Problem Solving";
```

has been executed.

Function Call	*String Contained in Value Returned by Function*
myString.substr(0, 7)	"Program"
myString.substr(7, 8)	"ming and"
myString.substr(10, 0)	""
myString.substr(24, 40)	"Solving"
myString.substr(40, 24)	None. Program terminates with an execution error message.

In the third example, specifying a length of 0 produces the null string as the result. The fourth example shows what happens if the second argument specifies more characters than are present after the starting position: substr returns the characters from the starting position to the end of the string. The last example illustrates that the first argument, the position, must not be beyond the end of the string.

Because substr returns a value of type string, you can use it with the concatenation operator (+) to copy pieces of strings and join them together to form new strings. The find and length functions can be useful in determining the location and end of a piece of a string to be passed to substr as arguments.

Here is a code segment that uses several of the string operations:

```
string fullName;
string name;
string::size_type startPos;

fullName = "Jonathan Alexander Peterson";
startPos = fullName.find("Peterson");
name = "Mr. " + fullName.substr(startPos, 8);
cout << name << endl;
```

This code outputs Mr. Peterson when it is executed. First it stores a string into the variable fullName, and then it uses find to locate the start of the name Peterson within the string. Next, it builds a new string by concatenating the literal "Mr. " with the characters Peterson, which are copied from the original string. Last, it prints out the new string. As we see in later chapters, string operations are an important aspect of many computer programs.

The following table summarizes the string operations we have looked at in this chapter.

Function Call (s is of type string)	Argument Type(s)	Result Type	Result (Value Returned)
s.length() s.size()	None	string::size_type	Number of characters in the string
s.find(arg)	string, literal string, or char	string::size_type	Starting position in s where arg was found. If not found, result is string::npos
s.substr(pos,len)	string::size_type	string	Substring of at most len characters, starting at position pos of s. If len is too large, it means "to the end" of string s. If pos is too large, execution of the program is terminated.*

*Technically, if pos is too large, the program generates what is called an out-of-range *exception*—a topic we do not discuss at this time. Unless we write additional program code to deal explicitly with this out-of-range exception, the program simply terminates with a message such as "ABNORMAL PROGRAM TERMINATION."

SOFTWARE ENGINEERING TIP

Understanding Before Changing

When you are in the middle of getting a program to run and you come across an error, it's tempting to start changing parts of the program to try to make it work. *Don't!* You'll nearly always make things worse. It's essential that you understand what is causing the error and that you carefully think through the solution. The only thing you should try is running the program with different data to determine the pattern of the unexpected behavior.

There is no magic trick—inserting an extra semicolon or right brace, for example— that can automatically fix a program. If the compiler tells you that a semicolon or a right brace is missing, you need to examine the program in light of the syntax rules and determine precisely what the problem is. Perhaps you accidentally typed a colon instead of a semicolon. Or maybe there's an extra left brace.

If the source of a problem isn't immediately obvious, a good rule of thumb is to leave the computer and go somewhere where you can quietly look over a printed copy of the program. Studies show that people who do all of their debugging away from the computer actually get their programs to work in less time *and in the end produce better programs* than those who continue to work on the machine—more proof that there is still no mechanical substitute for human thought.*

---

*Basili, V. R., and Selby, R. W., "Comparing the Effectiveness of Software Testing Strategies," *IEEE Trans. on Software Engineering* SE-13, no. 12 (1987): 1278–1296.

PROBLEM-SOLVING CASE STUDY

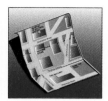

Map Measurements

Problem: You're spending a day in the city. You plan to visit the natural history museum, a record store, a gallery, and a bookshop, and then go to a concert. You have a tourist map that shows where these places are located. You want to determine how far apart they are and how far you'll walk during the entire day. Then you can decide when it would be better to take a taxi. According to the map's legend, one inch on the map equals one quarter of a mile on the ground.

Output: The distance between each of the places and the total distance, rounded to the nearest tenth of a mile. The values on which the calculations are based should also be printed for verification purposes.

Discussion: You can measure the distances between two points on the map with a ruler. The program must output miles, so you need to multiply the number of inches by 0.25. You then write down the figure, rounded to the nearest tenth of a mile. When you've done this for each pair of places, you add the distances to get the total mileage. This is essentially the algorithm we use in the program.

The only tricky part is how to round a value to the nearest tenth of a mile. In this chapter, we showed how to round a floating-point value to the nearest integer by adding 0.5 and using a type cast to truncate the result:

```
int(floatValue + 0.5)
```

To round to the nearest tenth, we first multiply the value by 10, round the result to the nearest integer, and then divide by 10 again. For example, if `floatValue` contains 5.162, then

```
float(int(floatValue * 10.0 + 0.5)) / 10.0
```

gives 5.2 as its result.

Let's treat all of the quantities as named constants so that it is easier to change the program later. From measuring the map, you know that the distance from the museum to the record store is 1.5 inches, from the record store to the gallery is 2.3 inches, from the gallery to the bookshop is 5.9 inches, and from the bookshop to the concert is 4.0 inches. Here is the algorithmic solution:

Define Constants

```
DISTANCE1 = 1.5
DISTANCE2 = 2.3
DISTANCE3 = 5.9
DISTANCE4 = 4.0
SCALE = 0.25
```

Initialize the Total Miles

```
Set totMiles = 0.0
```

Compute Miles for Each Distance on the Map

```
Set miles = float(int(DISTANCE1 * SCALE * 10.0 + 0.5)) / 10.0
Print DISTANCE1, miles
Add miles to totMiles
Set miles = float(int(DISTANCE2 * SCALE * 10.0 + 0.5)) / 10.0
Print DISTANCE2, miles
Add miles to totMiles
Set miles = float(int(DISTANCE3 * SCALE * 10.0 + 0.5)) / 10.0
Print DISTANCE3, miles
Add miles to totMiles
Set miles = float(int(DISTANCE4 * SCALE * 10.0 + 0.5)) / 10.0
Print DISTANCE4, miles
Add miles to totMiles
```

Print the Total Miles

```
Print a blank line
Print totMiles
```

From the algorithm we can create tables of constants and variables that help us write the declarations in the program.

PROBLEM-SOLVING CASE STUDY *cont'd.*

Constants

Name	Value	Description
DISTANCE1	1.5	Measurement for first distance
DISTANCE2	2.3	Measurement for second distance
DISTANCE3	5.9	Measurement for third distance
DISTANCE4	4.0	Measurement for fourth distance
SCALE	0.25	Scale factor of map

Variables

Name	Data Type	Description
totMiles	float	Total of rounded mileages
miles	float	An individual rounded mileage

Now we're ready to write the program. Let's call it Walk. We take the declarations from the tables and create the executable statements from the algorithm. We have labeled the output with explanatory messages and formatted the values to one decimal place. We've also added comments where needed.

(The following program is written in ISO/ANSI standard C++. If you are working with pre–standard C++, see the alternate version of the program in the PRE_STD directory of the program disk, available at the publisher's Web site, www.jbpub.com/disks.)

```
//*****************************************************************
// Walk program
// This program computes the mileage (rounded to tenths of a mile)
// for each of four distances between points in a city, given
// the measurements on a map with a scale of one inch equal to
// one quarter of a mile
//*****************************************************************
#include <iostream>
#include <iomanip>     // For setprecision()

using namespace std;

const float DISTANCE1 = 1.5;    // Measurement for first distance
const float DISTANCE2 = 2.3;    // Measurement for second distance
const float DISTANCE3 = 5.9;    // Measurement for third distance
const float DISTANCE4 = 4.0;    // Measurement for fourth distance
const float SCALE = 0.25;       // Map scale (miles per inch)
```

```
int main()
{
    float totMiles;         // Total of rounded mileages
    float miles;            // An individual rounded mileage

    cout << fixed << showpoint              // Set up floating-pt.
        << setprecision(1);                 //    output format

    // Initialize the total miles

    totMiles = 0.0;

    // Compute miles for each distance on the map

    miles = float(int(DISTANCE1 * SCALE * 10.0 + 0.5)) / 10.0;
    cout << "For a measurement of " << DISTANCE1
        << " the first distance is " << miles << " mile(s) long."
        << endl;
    totMiles = totMiles + miles;

    miles = float(int(DISTANCE2 * SCALE * 10.0 + 0.5)) / 10.0;
    cout << "For a measurement of " << DISTANCE2
        << " the second distance is " << miles << " mile(s) long."
        << endl;
    totMiles = totMiles + miles;

    miles = float(int(DISTANCE3 * SCALE * 10.0 + 0.5)) / 10.0;
    cout << "For a measurement of " << DISTANCE3
        << " the third distance is " << miles << " mile(s) long."
        << endl;
    totMiles = totMiles + miles;

    miles = float(int(DISTANCE4 * SCALE * 10.0 + 0.5)) / 10.0;
    cout << "For a measurement of " << DISTANCE4
        << " the fourth distance is " << miles << " mile(s) long."
        << endl;
    totMiles = totMiles + miles;

    // Print the total miles

    cout << endl;
    cout << "Total mileage for the day is " << totMiles << " miles."
        << endl;
    return 0;
}
```

The output from the program is

```
For a measurement of 1.5 the first distance is 0.4 mile(s) long.
For a measurement of 2.3 the second distance is 0.6 mile(s) long.
For a measurement of 5.9 the third distance is 1.5 mile(s) long.
For a measurement of 4.0 the fourth distance is 1.0 mile(s) long.

Total mileage for the day is 3.5 miles.
```

Testing and Debugging

1. An `int` constant other than 0 should not start with a zero. If it starts with a zero, it is an octal (base-8) number.
2. Watch out for integer division. The expression `47 / 100` yields 0, the integer quotient. This is one of the major sources of wrong output in C++ programs.
3. When using the `/` and `%` operators, remember that division by zero is not allowed.
4. Double-check every expression according to the precedence rules to be sure that the operations are performed in the desired order.
5. Avoid mixing integer and floating-point values in expressions. If you must mix them, consider using explicit type casts to reduce the chance of mistakes.
6. For each assignment statement, check that the expression result has the same data type as the variable to the left of the assignment operator (=). If not, consider using an explicit type cast for clarity and safety. And remember that storing a floating-point value into an `int` variable truncates the fractional part.
7. For every library function you use in your program, be sure to `#include` the appropriate header file.
8. Examine each call to a library function to see that you have the right number of arguments and that the data types of the arguments are correct.
9. With the `string` type, positions of characters within a string are numbered starting at 0, not 1.
10. If the cause of an error in a program is not obvious, leave the computer and study a printed listing. Change your program only after you understand the source of the error.

Summary

C++ provides several built-in numeric data types, of which the most commonly used are `int` and `float`. The integral types are based on the mathematical integers, but the computer limits the range of integer values that can be represented. The floating-point types are based on the mathematical notion of real numbers. As with integers, the computer limits the range of floating-point numbers that can be represented. Also, it limits the number of digits of precision in floating-point values. We can write literals of type `float` in several forms, including scientific (E) notation.

Much of the computation of a program is performed in arithmetic expressions. Expressions can contain more than one operator. The order in which the operations are performed is determined by precedence rules. In arithmetic expressions, multiplication, division, and modulus are performed first, then addition and subtraction. Multiple binary (two-operand) operations of the same precedence are grouped from left to right. You can use parentheses to override the precedence rules.

Expressions may include function calls. C++ supports two kinds of functions: value-returning functions and void functions. A value-returning function is called by writing its name and argument list as part of an expression. A void function is called by writing its name and argument list as a complete C++ statement.

The C++ standard library is an integral part of every C++ system. The library contains many prewritten data types, functions, and other items that any programmer can use. These items are accessed by using `#include` directives to the C++ preprocessor, which inserts the appropriate header files into the program.

In output statements, the `setw`, `showpoint`, `fixed`, and `setprecision` manipulators control the appearance of values in the output. These manipulators do *not* affect the values actually stored in memory, only their appearance when displayed on the output device.

Not only should the output produced by a program be easy to read, but the format of the program itself should be clear and readable. C++ is a free-format language. A consistent style that uses indentation, blank lines, and spaces within lines helps you (and other programmers) understand and work with your programs.

Quick Check

1. Write a C++ constant declaration that gives the name PI to the value 3.14159. (pp. 105–106)
2. Declare an `int` variable named `count` and a `float` variable named `sum`. (pp. 106–107)

3. You want to divide 9 by 5.
   a. How do you write the expression if you want the result to be the floating-point value 1.8?
   b. How do you write it if you want only the integer quotient?
      (pp. 107–110)
4. What is the value of the following C++ expression?

   `5 % 2`

   (pp. 108–110)
5. What is the result of evaluating the expression

   `(1 + 2 * 2) / 2 + 1`

   (pp. 112–113)
6. How would you write the following formula as a C++ expression that produces a floating-point value as a result? (pp. 112–113)

$$\frac{9}{5}c + 32$$

7. Add type casts to the following statements to make the type conversions clear and explicit. Your answers should produce the same results as the original statements. (pp. 113–116)
   a. `someFloat = 5 + someInt;`
   b. `someInt = 2.5 * someInt / someFloat;`
8. You want to compute the square roots and absolute values of some floating-point numbers.
   a. Which C++ library functions would you use? (pp. 120–122)
   b. Which header file(s) must you #include in order to use these functions?
9. Which part of the following function call is its argument list? (p. 119)

   `Square(someInt + 1)`

10. In the statement

    `alpha = 4 * Beta(gamma, delta) + 3;`

    would you conclude that Beta is a value-returning function or a void function? (pp. 120–123)
11. In the statement

    `Display(gamma, delta);`

    would you conclude that Display is a value-returning function or a void function? (pp. 120–123)
12. Assume the float variable pay contains the value 327.66101. Using the fixed, setw, and setprecision manipulators, what output statement would you use to print pay in dollars and cents with three leading blanks? (pp. 124–128)
13. If the string variable str contains the string "Now is the time", what is output by the following statement? (pp. 131–136)

    `cout << str.length() << ' ' << str.substr(1, 2) << endl;`

14. Reformat the following program to make it clear and readable. (pp. 129–130)

```
//*************************************************************
                 // SumProd program
  // This program computes the sum and product of two integers
//*************************************************************
#include <iostream>
using namespace std;
const int INT1=20;const int INT2=8;int main() { cout <<
"The sum of " << INT1 << " and "
<< INT2 << " is " << INT1+INT2 << endl;cout
<< "Their product is " << INT1*INT2 << endl;return 0; }
```

15. What should you do if a program fails to run correctly and the reason for the error is not immediately obvious? (p. 136)

Answers 1. `const float PI = 3.14159;`
2. `int    count;`
    `float sum;`
3. a. `9.0 / 5.0` b. `9 / 5` **4.** The value is 1. **5.** The result is 3. **6.** `9.0 / 5.0 * c +`
`32.0` **7.** a. `someFloat = float(5 + someInt);` b. `someInt = int(2.5 *`
`float(someInt) / someFloat);` **8.** a. `sqrt` and `fabs` b. `math` **9.** `someInt + 1` **10.**
A value-returning function **11.** A void function **12.** `cout << fixed << setw(9) <<`
`setprecision(2) << pay;` **13.** 15 ow
14.
```
//*************************************************************
  // SumProd program
  // This program computes the sum and product of two integers
//*************************************************************
#include <iostream>

using namespace std;

const int INT1 = 20;
const int INT2 = 8;

int main()
{
    cout << "The sum of " << INT1 << " and " << INT2
         << " is " << INT1 + INT2 << endl;
    cout << "Their product is " << INT1 * INT2 << endl;
    return 0;
}
```
15. Get a fresh printout of the program, leave the computer, and study the program until you understand the cause of the problem. Then correct the algorithm and the program as necessary before you go back to the computer and make any changes in the program file.

Exam Preparation Exercises

1. Mark the following constructs either valid or invalid. Assume all variables are of type int.

	Valid	Invalid
a. x * y = c;	_____	_____
b. y = con;	_____	_____
c. const int x : 10;	_____	_____
d. int x;	_____	_____
e. a = b % c;	_____	_____

2. If alpha and beta are int variables with alpha containing 4 and beta containing 9, what value is stored into alpha in each of the following? Answer each part independently of the others.
   a. alpha = 3 * beta;
   b. alpha = alpha + beta;
   c. alpha++;
   d. alpha = alpha / beta;
   e. alpha--;
   f. alpha = alpha + alpha;
   g. alpha = beta % 6;

3. Compute the value of each legal expression. Indicate whether the value is an integer or a floating-point value. If the expression is not legal, explain why.

	Integer	Floating Point
a. 10.0 / 3.0 + 5 * 2	_____	_____
b. 10 % 3 + 5 % 2	_____	_____
c. 10 / 3 + 5 / 2	_____	_____
d. 12.5 + (2.5 / (6.2 / 3.1))	_____	_____
e. -4 * (-5 + 6)	_____	_____
f. 13 % 5 / 3	_____	_____
g. (10.0 / 3.0 % 2) / 3	_____	_____

4. What value is stored into the int variable result in each of the following?
   a. result = 15 % 4;
   b. result = 7 / 3 + 2;
   c. result = 2 + 7 * 5;
   d. result = 45 / 8 * 4 + 2;
   e. result = 17 + (21 % 6) * 2;
   f. result = int(4.5 + 2.6 * 0.5);

5. If a and b are int variables with a containing 5 and b containing 2, what output does each of the following statements produce?
   a. cout << "a = " << a << "b = " << b << endl;
   b. cout << "Sum:" << a + b << endl;
   c. cout << "Sum: " << a + b << endl;
   d. cout << a / b << " feet" << endl;

6. What does the following program print?

   ```
   #include <iostream>

   using namespace std;

   const int LBS = 10;
   ```

```
int main()
{
    int   price;
    int   cost;
    char ch;

    price = 30;
    cost = price * LBS;
    ch = 'A';
    cout << "Cost is " << endl;
    cout << cost << endl;
    cout << "Price is " << price << "Cost is " << cost << endl;
    cout << "Grade " << ch << " costs " << endl;
    cout << cost << endl;
    return 0;
}
```

7. Translate the following C++ code into algebraic notation. (All variables are float variables.)

```
y = -b + sqrt(b * b - 4.0 * a * c);
```

8. Given the following program fragment:

```
int   i;
int   j;
float z;

i = 4;
j = 17;
z = 2.6;
```

determine the value of each expression below. If the result is a floating-point value, include a decimal point in your answer.

a. i / float(j)
b. 1.0 / i + 2
c. z * j
d. i + j % i
e. (1 / 2) * i
f. 2 * i + j - i
g. j / 2
h. 2 * 3 - 1 % 3
i. i % j / i
j. int(z + 0.5)

9. To use each of the following statements, a C++ program must #include which header file(s)?

a. cout << x;
b. int1 = abs(int2);
c. y = sqrt(7.6 + x);

d. `cout << y << endl;`
e. `cout << setw(5) << someInt;`

10. Evaluate the following expressions. If the result is a floating-point number, include a decimal point in your answer.

    a. `fabs(-9.1)`
    b. `sqrt(49.0)`
    c. `3 * int(7.8) + 3`
    d. `pow(4.0, 2.0)`
    e. `sqrt(float(3 * 3 + 4 * 4))`
    f. `sqrt(fabs(-4.0) + sqrt(25.0))`

11. Show precisely the output of the following C++ program. Use a □ to indicate each blank.

```
#include <iostream>
#include <iomanip>      // For setw()

using namespace std;

int main()
{
    char   ch;
    int    n;
    float  y;

    ch = 'A';
    cout << ch;
    ch = 'B';
    cout << ch << endl;
    n = 413;
    y = 21.8;
    cout << setw(5) << n << " is the value of n" << endl;
    cout << setw(7) << y << " is the value of y" << endl;
    return 0;
}
```

12. Given that x is a `float` variable containing 14.3827, show the output of each statement below. Use a □ to indicate each blank. (Assume that `cout << fixed` has already executed.)

    a. `cout << "x is" << setw(5) << setprecision(2) << x;`
    b. `cout << "x is" << setw(8) << setprecision(2) << x;`
    c. `cout << "x is" << setw(0) << setprecision(2) << x;`
    d. `cout << "x is" << setw(7) << setprecision(3) << x;`

13. Given the statements

```
string heading;
string str;

heading = "Exam Preparation Exercises";
```

what is the output of each code segment below?

```
a. cout << heading.length();
b. cout << heading.substr(6, 10);
c. cout << heading.find("Ex");
d. str = heading.substr(2, 24);
   cout << str.find("Ex");
e. str = heading.substr(heading.find("Ex") + 2, 24);
   cout << str.find("Ex");
f. str = heading.substr(heading.find("Ex") + 2,
                        heading.length() - heading.find("Ex") + 2);
   cout << str.find("Ex");
```

14. Formatting a program incorrectly causes an error. (True or False?)

Programming Warm-up Exercises

1. Change the program in Exam Preparation Exercise 6 so that it prints the cost for 15 pounds.

2. Write an assignment statement to calculate the sum of the numbers from 1 through n using Gauss's formula:
$$sum = \frac{n(n+1)}{2}$$

   Store the result into the int variable sum.

3. Given the declarations

```
int    i;
int    j;
float x;
float y;
```

   write a valid C++ expression for each of the following algebraic expressions.

   a. $\dfrac{x}{y} - 3$ e. $\dfrac{i}{j}$ (the floating-point result)

   b. $(x + y)(x - y)$ f. $\dfrac{i}{j}$ (the integer quotient)

   c. $\dfrac{1}{x + y}$ g. $\dfrac{\dfrac{x+y}{3} - \dfrac{x-y}{5}}{4x}$

   d. $\dfrac{1}{x} + y$

4. Given the declarations

```
int    i;
long   n;
float x;
float y;
```

   write a valid C++ expression for each of the following algebraic expressions. Use calls to library functions wherever they are useful.

a. $|i|$ (absolute value)   e. $\dfrac{x^3}{y}$

b. $|n|$ f. $\sqrt{x^6 + y^5}$

c. $|x + y|$ g. $(x + \sqrt{y})^7$

d. $|x| + |y|$

5. Write expressions to compute both solutions for the quadratic formula. The formula is

$$\frac{-b \pm \sqrt{b^2 - 4ac}}{2a}$$

The ± means "plus or minus" and indicates that there are two solutions to the equation: one in which the result of the square root is added to $-b$ and one in which the result is subtracted from $-b$. Assume all variables are float variables.

6. Enter the following program into your computer and run it. In the initial comments, replace the items within parentheses with your own information. (Omit the parentheses.)

```
//**********************************
// Programming Assignment (assignment number)
// (your name)
// (date program was run)
// (description of the problem)
//**********************************
#include <iostream>

using namespace std;

const float DEBT = 300.0;      // Original value owed
const float PMT = 22.4;        // Payment
const float INT_RATE = 0.02;   // Interest rate

int main()
{
    float charge;       // Interest times debt
    float reduc;        // Amount debt is reduced
    float remaining;    // Remaining balance

    charge = INT_RATE * DEBT;
    reduc = PMT - charge;
    remaining = DEBT - reduc;
    cout << "Payment: " << PMT
         << " Charge: " << charge
         << " Balance owed: " << remaining << endl;
    return 0;
}
```

7. Enter the following program into your computer and run it. Add comments, using the pattern shown in Exercise 6 above. (Notice how hard it is to tell what the program does without the comments.)

```cpp
#include <iostream>

using namespace std;

const int TOT_COST = 1376;
const int POUNDS = 10;
const int OUNCES = 12;

int main()
{
    int    totOz;
    float  uCost;

    totOz = 16 * POUNDS;
    totOz = totOz + OUNCES;
    uCost = TOT_COST / totOz;
    cout << "Cost per unit: " << uCost << endl;
    return 0;
}
```

8. Complete the following C++ program. The program should find and output the perimeter and area of a rectangle, given the length and the width. Be sure to label the output. And don't forget to use comments.

```cpp
//***********************************************
// Rectangle program
// This program finds the perimeter and the area
// of a rectangle, given the length and width
//***********************************************
#include <iostream>

using namespace std;

int main()
{
    float length;        // Length of the rectangle
    float width;         // Width of the rectangle
    float perimeter;     // Perimeter of the rectangle
    float area;          // Area of the rectangle

    length = 10.7;
    width = 5.2;
```

9. Write an expression whose result is the position of the first occurrence of the characters "res" in a string variable named sentence. If the variable contains the first sentence of this question, then what is the result? (Look at the sentence carefully!)

10. Write a sequence of C++ statements to output the positions of the second and third occurrences of the characters "res" in the `string` variable named sentence. You may assume that there are always at least three occurrences in the variable. (*Hint:* Use the `substr` function to create a new string whose contents are the portion of sentence following an occurrence of "res".)

Programming Problems

1. C++ systems provide a header file `climits`, which contains declarations of constants related to the specific compiler and machine on which you are working. Two of these constants are `INT_MAX` and `INT_MIN`, the largest and smallest int values for your particular computer. Write a program to print out the values of `INT_MAX` and `INT_MIN`. The output should identify which value is `INT_MAX` and which value is `INT_MIN`. Be sure to include appropriate comments in your program, and use indentation as we do in the programs in this chapter.

2. Write a program that outputs three lines, labeled as follows:

   ```
   7 / 4 using integer division equals   <result>
   7 / 4 using floating-point division equals   <result>
   7 modulo 4 equals   <result>
   ```

   where <result> stands for the result computed by your program. Use named constants for 7 and 4 everywhere in your program (including the output statements) to make the program easy to modify. Be sure to include appropriate comments in your program, choose meaningful identifiers, and use indentation as we do in the programs in this chapter.

3. Write a C++ program that converts a Celsius temperature to its Fahrenheit equivalent. The formula is

   $$Fahrenheit = \frac{9}{5} \, Celsius + 32$$

   Make the Celsius temperature a named constant so that its value can be changed easily. The program should print both the value of the Celsius temperature and its Fahrenheit equivalent, with appropriate identifying messages. Be sure to include appropriate comments in your program, choose meaningful identifiers, and use indentation as we do in the programs in this chapter.

4. Write a program to calculate the diameter, the circumference, and the area of a circle with a radius of 6.75. Assign the radius to a `float` variable, and then output the radius with an appropriate message. Declare a named constant PI with the value 3.14159. The program should output the diameter, the circumference, and the area, each on a separate line, with identifying labels. Print each value to five decimal places within a total fieldwidth of 10. Be sure to include appropriate comments in your program, choose meaningful identifiers, and use indentation as we do in the programs in this chapter.

5. You have bought a car, taking out a loan with an annual interest rate of 9%. You will make 36 monthly payments of $165.25 each. You want to keep track of the remaining balance you owe after each monthly payment. The formula for the remaining balance is

$$bal_k = pmt\left[\frac{1 - (1 + i)^{k-n}}{i}\right]$$

where

bal_k	=	balance remaining after the kth payment
k	=	payment number (1, 2, 3, ...)
pmt	=	amount of the monthly payment
i	=	interest rate per month (annual rate ÷ 12)
n	=	total number of payments to be made

Write a program to calculate and print the balance remaining after the first, second, and third monthly car payments. Before printing these three results, the program should output the values on which the calculations are based (monthly payment, interest rate, and total number of payments). Label all output with identifying messages, and print all money amounts to two decimal places. Be sure to include appropriate comments in your program, choose meaningful identifiers, and use indentation as we do in the programs in this chapter.

Case Study Follow-Up

1. What is the advantage of using named constants instead of literal constants in the Walk program?
2. Modify the Walk program to include a round-off factor so that the rounding of `miles` can be modified easily. Currently, the program uses a literal constant (10.0) in several places to round `miles` to the nearest tenth, requiring us to make multiple changes if we want a different round-off factor.
3. Should the round-off factor in Question 2 be a constant or a variable? Explain.
4. In the Walk program, a particular pattern of statements is repeated four times with small variations. Identify the repeating pattern. Next, circle those parts of the statements that vary with each repetition. Having done this, now modify the Walk program to work with a fifth distance measurement.

4

Program Input and the Software Design Process

GOALS

- To be able to construct input statements to read values into a program.
- To be able to determine the contents of variables assigned values by input statements.
- To be able to write appropriate prompting messages for interactive programs.
- To know when noninteractive input/output is appropriate and how it differs from interactive input/output.
- To be able to write programs that use data files for input and output.
- To understand the basic principles of object-oriented design.
- To be able to apply the functional decomposition methodology to solve a simple problem.
- To be able to take a functional decomposition and code it in C++, using self-documenting code.

A program needs data on which to operate. We have been writing all of the data values in the program itself, in literal and named constants. If this were the only way we could enter data, we would have to rewrite a program each time we wanted to apply it to a different set of values. In this chapter, we look at ways of entering data into a program while it is running.

Once we know how to input data, process the data, and output the results, we can begin to think about designing more complicated programs. We have talked about general problem-solving strategies and writing simple programs. For a simple problem, it's easy to choose a strategy, write the algorithm, and code the program. But as problems become more complex, we have to use a more organized approach. In the second part of this chapter, we look at two general methodologies for developing software: object-oriented design and functional decomposition.

Getting Data into Programs

One of the biggest advantages of computers is that a program can be used with many different sets of data. To do so, we must keep the data separate from the program until the program is executed. Then instructions in the program copy values from the data set into variables in the program. After storing these values into the variables, the program can perform calculations with them (see Figure 4-1).

FIGURE 4-1
Separating the
Data from the
Program

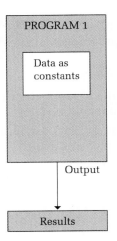

This program must
be changed to work
with different data
values.

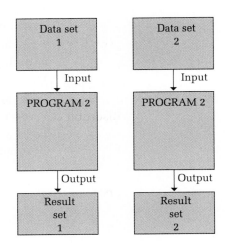

This program inputs its data
from outside, so it can work
with different data sets without
being changed.

The process of placing values from an outside data set into variables in a program is called *input*. In widely used terminology, the computer is said to *read* outside data into the variables. The data for the program can come from an input device or from a file on an auxiliary storage device. We look at file input later in this chapter; here we consider the *standard input device*, the keyboard.

Input Streams and the Extraction Operator (>>)

The concept of a stream is fundamental to input and output in C++. As we stated in Chapter 3, you can think of an output stream as an endless sequence of characters going from your program to an output device. Likewise, think of an *input stream* as an endless sequence of characters coming into your program from an input device.

To use stream I/O, you must use the preprocessor directive

```
#include <iostream>
```

The header file `iostream` contains, among other things, the definitions of two data types: `istream` and `ostream`. These are data types representing input streams and output streams, respectively. The header file also contains declarations that look like this:

```
istream cin;
ostream cout;
```

The first declaration says that `cin` (pronounced "see-in") is a variable of type `istream`. The second says that `cout` (pronounced "see-out") is a variable of type `ostream`. Furthermore, `cin` is associated with the standard input device (the keyboard), and `cout` is associated with the standard output device (usually the display screen).

As you have already seen, you can output values to `cout` by using the insertion operator (<<), which is sometimes pronounced "put to":

```
cout << 3 * price;
```

In a similar fashion, you can input data from `cin` by using the *extraction operator* (>>), sometimes pronounced "get from":

```
cin >> cost;
```

When the computer executes this statement, it inputs the next number you type on the keyboard (425, for example) and stores it into the variable `cost`.

The extraction operator >> takes two operands. Its left-hand operand is a stream expression (in the simplest case, just the variable `cin`). Its right-hand operand is a variable into which we store the input data. For the time being, we assume the variable is of a simple type (`char`, `int`, `float`, and so forth). Later in the chapter we discuss the input of string data.

You can use the `>>` operator several times in a single input statement. Each occurrence extracts (inputs) the next data item from the input stream. For example, there is no difference between the statement

```
cin >> length >> width;
```

and the pair of statements

```
cin >> length;
cin >> width;
```

Using a sequence of extractions in one statement is a convenience for the programmer.

When you are new to C++, you may get the extraction operator (`>>`) and the insertion operator (`<<`) reversed. Here is an easy way to remember which one is which: Always begin the statement with either `cin` or `cout`, and use the operator that points in the direction in which the data is going. The statement

```
cout << someInt;
```

sends data from the variable `someInt` *to* the output stream. The statement

```
cin >> someInt;
```

sends data from the input stream *to* the variable `someInt`.

Here's the syntax template for an input statement:

InputStatement

```
cin >> Variable  >> Variable ...;
```

Unlike the items specified in an output statement, which can be constants, variables, or complicated expressions, the items specified in an input statement can *only* be variable names. Why? Because an input statement indicates where input data values should be stored. Only variable names refer to memory locations where we can store values while a program is running.

When you enter input data at the keyboard, you must be sure that each data value is appropriate for the data type of the variable in the input statement.

Data Type of Variable in an >> Operation	Valid Input Data
`char`	A single printable character other than a blank
`int`	An `int` literal constant, optionally preceded by a sign
`float`	An `int` or `float` literal constant (possibly in scientific, E, notation), optionally preceded by a sign

Notice that when you input a number into a `float` variable, the input value doesn't have to have a decimal point. The integer value is automatically coerced to a `float` value. Any other mismatches, such as trying to input a `float` value into an `int` variable or a `char` value into a `float` variable, can lead to unexpected and sometimes serious results. Later in this chapter we discuss what might happen.

When looking for the next input value in the stream, the >> operator skips any leading *whitespace characters*. Whitespace characters are blanks and certain nonprintable characters such as the character that marks the end of a line. (We talk about this end-of-line character in the next section.) After skipping any whitespace characters, the >> operator proceeds to extract the desired data value from the input stream. If this data value is a `char` value, input stops as soon as a single character is input. If the data value is `int` or `float`, input of the number stops at the first character that is inappropriate for the data type, such as a whitespace character. Here are some examples, where i, j, and k are `int` variables, ch is a `char` variable, and x is a `float` variable:

Statement	Data	Contents After Input
1. `cin >> i;`	32	i = 32
2. `cin >> i >> j;`	4 60	i = 4, j = 60
3. `cin >> i >> ch >> x;`	25 A 16.9	i = 25, ch = 'A', x = 16.9
4. `cin >> i >> ch >> x;`	25	
	A	
	16.9	i = 25, ch = 'A', x = 16.9
5. `cin >> i >> ch >> x;`	25A16.9	i = 25, ch = 'A', x = 16.9
6. `cin >> i >> j >> x;`	12 8	i = 12, j = 8 (Computer waits for a third number)
7. `cin >> i >> x;`	46 32.4 15	i = 46, x = 32.4 (15 is held for later input)

Examples (1) and (2) are straightforward examples of integer input. Example (3) shows that you do not use quotes around character data values when they are input (quotes around character constants are needed in a program, though, to distinguish them from identifiers). Example (4) demonstrates how the process of skipping whitespace characters includes going on to the next line of input if necessary. Example (5) shows that the first character encountered that is inappropriate for a numeric data type ends the number. Input for the variable i stops at the input character A, after which the A is stored into ch, and then input for x stops at the end of the input line. Example (6) shows that if you are at the keyboard and haven't entered enough values to satisfy the input statement, the computer waits (and waits and waits. . .) for more data. Example (7) shows that if more values are entered than there are variables in the input statement, the extra values remain waiting in the input stream until they can be read by the next input statement. If there are extra values left when the program ends, the computer disregards them.

The Reading Marker and the Newline Character

To help explain stream input in more detail, we introduce the concept of the *reading marker*. The reading marker works like a bookmark, but instead of marking a place in a book, it keeps track of the point in the input stream where the computer should continue reading. The reading marker indicates the next character waiting to be read. The extraction operator >> leaves the reading marker on the character following the last piece of data that was input.

Each input line has an invisible end-of-line character (the *newline character*) that tells the computer where one line ends and the next begins. To find the next input value, the >> operator crosses line boundaries (newline characters) if it has to.

Where does the newline character come from? What is it? The answer to the first question is easy. When you are working at a keyboard, you generate a newline character yourself each time you hit the Return or Enter key. Your program also generates a newline character when it uses the endl manipulator in an output statement. The endl manipulator outputs a newline, telling the screen cursor to go to the next line. The answer to the second question varies from computer system to computer system. The newline character is a nonprintable control character that the system recognizes as meaning the end of a line, whether it's an input line or an output line.

In a C++ program, you can refer directly to the newline character by using the two symbols \n, a backslash and an n with no space between them. Although \n consists of two symbols, it refers to a single character—the newline character. Just as you can store the letter *A* into a char variable ch like this:

```
ch = 'A';
```

so you can store the newline character into a variable:

```
ch = '\n';
```

You also can put the newline character into a string, just as you can any printable character:

```
cout << "Hello\n";
```

This last statement has exactly the same effect as the statement

```
cout << "Hello" << endl;
```

But back to our discussion of input. Let's look at some examples using the reading marker and the newline character. In the following table, i is an int variable, ch is a char variable, and x is a float variable. The input statements produce the results shown. The part of the input stream printed in color is what has been extracted by input statements. The reading marker, denoted by the shaded block, indicates the next character waiting to be read. The \n denotes the newline character produced by striking the Return or Enter key.

Statements	Contents After Input	Marker Position in the Input Stream
1.		25 A 16.9\n
cin >> i;	i = 25	25 A 16.9\n
cin >> ch;	ch = 'A'	25 A 16.9\n
cin >> x;	x = 16.9	25 A 16.9 \n
2.		25\n
		A\n
		16.9\n
cin >> i;	i = 25	25 \n
		A\n
		16.9\n
cin >> ch;	ch = 'A'	25\n
		A \n
		16.9\n
cin >> x;	x = 16.9	25\n
		A\n
		16.9 \n

Statements	Contents After Input	Marker Position in the Input Stream
3.		25A16.9\n
cin >> i;	i = 25	25A16.9\n
cin >> ch;	ch = 'A'	25A16.9\n
cin >> x;	x = 16.9	25A16.9\n

Reading Character Data with the get Function

As we have discussed, the >> operator skips any leading whitespace characters (such as blanks and newline characters) while looking for the next data value in the input stream. Suppose that ch1 and ch2 are char variables and the program executes the statement

cin >> ch1 >> ch2;

If the input stream consists of

R 1

then the extraction operator stores 'R' into ch1, skips the blank, and stores '1' into ch2. (Note that the char value '1' is not the same as the int value 1. The two are stored completely differently in a computer's memory. The extraction operator interprets the same data in different ways, depending on the data type of the variable that's being filled.)

What if we had wanted to input *three* characters from the input line: the *R*, the blank, and the 1? With the extraction operator, it's not possible. Whitespace characters such as blanks are skipped over.

The istream data type provides a second way in which to read character data, in addition to the >> operator. You can use the get function, which inputs the very next character in the input stream without skipping any whitespace characters. A function call looks like this:

cin.get(someChar);

The get function is associated with the istream data type, and you must use dot notation to make a function call. (Recall that we used dot notation in Chapter 3 to invoke certain functions associated with the string type. Later in this chapter we explain the reason for dot notation.) To use the get function, you give the name of an istream variable (here, cin), then a dot (period), and then the function name and argument list. Notice that the call to get uses the syntax for calling a void function, not a value-returning function. The function call is a complete statement; it is not part of a larger expression.

The effect of the above function call is to input the next character waiting in the stream—even if it is a whitespace character like a blank—and store it into the variable `someChar`. The argument to the `get` function *must* be a variable, not a constant or arbitrary expression; we must tell the function where we want it to store the input character.

Using the `get` function, we now can input all three characters of the input line

```
R 1
```

We can use three consecutive calls to the `get` function:

```
cin.get(ch1);
cin.get(ch2);
cin.get(ch3);
```

or we can do it this way:

```
cin >> ch1;
cin.get(ch2);
cin >> ch3;
```

The first version is probably a bit clearer for someone to read and understand.

Here are some more examples of character input using both the `>>` operator and the `get` function. `ch1`, `ch2`, and `ch3` are all `char` variables. As before, `\n` denotes the newline character.

Statements	Contents After Input	Marker Position in the Input Stream
1.		A B\n CD\n
`cin >> ch1;`	ch1 = 'A'	A█B\n CD\n
`cin >> ch2;`	ch2 = 'B'	A B\n CD\n
`cin >> ch3;`	ch3 = 'C'	A B\n C█\n
2.		A B\n CD\n
`cin.get(ch1);`	ch1 = 'A'	A█B\n CD\n
`cin.get(ch2);`	ch2 = ' '	A B\n CD\n
`cin.get(ch3);`	ch3 = 'B'	A B\n CD\n

Statements	Contents After Input	Marker Position in the Input Stream
3.		A B\n CD\n
cin >> ch1;	ch1 = 'A'	A B\n CD\n
cin >> ch2;	ch2 = 'B'	A B\n CD\n
cin.get(ch3);	ch3 = '\n'	A B\n CD\n

THEORETICAL FOUNDATIONS

More About Functions and Arguments

When your main function tells the computer to go off and follow the instructions in another function, SomeFunc, the main function is *calling* SomeFunc. In the call to SomeFunc, the arguments in the argument list are *passed* to the function. When SomeFunc finishes, the computer *returns* to the main function.

With some functions you have seen, like sqrt and abs, you can pass constants, variables, and arbitrary expressions to the function. The get function for reading character data, however, accepts only a variable as an argument. The get function stores a value into its argument when it returns, and only variables can have values stored into them while a program is running. Even though get is called as a void function—not a value-returning function—it *returns* or *passes back* a value through its argument list. The point to remember is that you can use arguments both to send data into a function and to get results back out.

Skipping Characters with the ignore Function

Most of us have a specialized tool lying in a kitchen drawer or in a toolbox. It gathers dust and cobwebs because we almost never use it. But when we suddenly need it, we're glad we have it. The ignore function associated with the istream type is like this specialized tool. You rarely have occasion to use ignore; but when you need it, you're glad it's available.

The ignore function is used to skip (read and discard) characters in the input stream. It is a function with two arguments, called like this:

```
cin.ignore(200, '\n');
```

The first argument is an `int` expression; the second, a `char` value. This particular function call tells the computer to skip the next 200 input characters *or* to skip characters until a newline character is read, whichever comes first.

Here are some examples that use a `char` variable `ch` and three `int` variables, `i`, `j`, and `k`:

Statements	Contents After Input	Marker Position in the Input Stream
1.		957 34 1235\n 128 96\n
`cin >> i >> j;`	i = 957, j = 34	957 34 1235\n 128 96\n
`cin.ignore(100, '\n');`		957 34 1235\n 128 96\n
`cin >> k;`	k = 128	957 34 1235\n 128 96\n
2.		A 22 B 16 C 19\n
`cin >> ch;`	ch = 'A'	A 22 B 16 C 19\n
`cin.ignore(100, 'B');`		A 22 B 16 C 19\n
`cin >> i;`	i = 16	A 22 B 16 C 19\n
3.		ABCDEF\n
`cin.ignore(2, '\n');`		ABCDEF\n
`cin >> ch;`	ch = 'C'	ABCDEF\n

Example (1) shows the most common use of the `ignore` function, which is to skip the rest of the data on the current input line. Example (2) demonstrates the use of a character other than '\n' as the second argument. We skip over all input characters until a *B* has been found, then read the next input number into `i`. In both (1) and (2), we are focusing on the second argument to the `ignore` function, and we arbitrarily choose any large number, such as 100, for the first argument. In (3), we change our focus and concentrate on the first argument. Our intention is to skip the next two input characters on the current line.

Reading String Data

To input a character string into a `string` variable, we have two options. The first is to use the extraction operator (`>>`). When reading input characters into a `string` variable, the `>>` operator skips any leading whitespace characters such as blanks and newlines. It then reads successive characters into the variable, stopping at the first *trailing* whitespace character (which is not consumed, but remains as the first character waiting in the input stream). For example, assume we have the following code:

```
string firstName;
string lastName;

cin >> firstName >> lastName;
```

If the input stream initially looks like this (where □ denotes a blank):

□□Mary□Smith□□□18

then our input statement stores the four characters Mary into firstName, stores the five characters Smith into lastName, and leaves the input stream as

□□□18

Although the >> operator is widely used for string input, it has a potential drawback: it cannot be used to input a string that has blanks within it. (Remember that it stops reading as soon as it encounters a whitespace character.) This fact leads us to the second option for performing string input: the getline function. A call to this function looks like this:

```
getline(cin, myString);
```

The function call, which does not use dot notation, requires two arguments. The first is an input stream variable (here, cin) and the second is a string variable. The getline function does not skip leading whitespace characters and continues until it reaches the newline character '\n'. That is, getline reads and stores an entire input line, embedded blanks and all. Note that with getline, the newline character *is* consumed (but is not stored into the string variable). Given the code segment

```
string inputStr;

getline(cin, inputStr);
```

and the input line

□□Mary□Smith□□□18

the result of the call to getline is that all 17 characters on the input line (including blanks) are stored into inputStr, and the reading marker is positioned at the beginning of the next input line.

The following table summarizes the differences between the >> operator and the getline function when reading string data into string variables.

Statement	*Skips Leading Whitespace?*	*Stops Reading When?*
`cin >> inputStr;`	Yes	When a trailing whitespace character is encountered (which is *not* consumed)
`getline(cin, inputStr);`	No	When '\n' is encountered (which *is* consumed)

Interactive Input/Output

In Chapter 1, we defined an interactive program as one in which the user communicates directly with the computer. Many of the programs that we write are interactive. There is a certain "etiquette" involved in writing interactive programs that has to do with instructions for the user to follow.

To get data into an interactive program, we begin with *input prompts*, printed messages that explain what the user should enter. Without these messages, the user has no idea what data values to type. In many cases, a program also should print out all of the data values typed in so that the user can verify that they were entered correctly. Printing out the input values is called *echo printing*. Here's a program segment showing the proper use of prompts:

```
cout << "Enter the part number:" << endl;            // Prompt
cin >> partNumber;
cout << "Enter the quantity of this part ordered:"    // Prompt
     << endl;
cin >> quantity;
cout << "Enter the unit price for this part:"         // Prompt
     << endl;
cin >> unitPrice;
totalPrice = quantity * unitPrice;
cout << "Part " << partNumber                         // Echo print
     << ", quantity " << quantity
     << ", at $ " << setprecision(2) << unitPrice
     << " each" << endl;
cout << "totals $ " << totalPrice << endl;
```

And here's the output, with the user's input shown in color:

```
Enter the part number:
4671
Enter the quantity of this part ordered:
10
```

```
Enter the unit price for this part:
27.25
Part 4671, quantity 10, at $ 27.25 each
totals $ 272.50
```

The amount of information you should put into your prompts depends on who is going to be using a program. If you are writing a program for people who are not familiar with computers, your messages should be more detailed. For example, "Type a four-digit part number, then press the key marked Enter." If the program is going to be used frequently by the same people, you might shorten the prompts: "Enter PN" and "Enter Qty." If the program is for very experienced users, you can prompt for several values at once and have them type all of the values on one input line:

```
Enter PN, Qty, Unit Price:
4176 10 27.25
```

In programs that use large amounts of data, this method saves the user keystrokes and time. However, it also makes it easier for the user to enter values in the wrong order. In such situations, echo printing the data is especially important.

Whether a program should echo print its input or not also depends on how experienced the users are and on the task the program is to perform. If the users are experienced and the prompts are clear, as in the first example, then echo printing is probably not required. If the users are novices or multiple values can be input at once, echo printing should be used. If the program inputs a large quantity of data and the users are experienced, rather than echo print the data, it may be stored in a separate file that can be checked after all of the data is input. We discuss how to store data into a file later in this chapter.

Prompts are not the only way in which programs interact with users. It can be helpful to have a program print out some general instructions at the beginning ("Press Enter after typing each data value. Enter a negative number when done."). When data is not entered in the correct form, a message that indicates the problem should be printed. For users who haven't worked much with computers, it's important that these messages be informative and "friendly." The message

```
ILLEGAL DATA VALUES!!!!!!!
```

is likely to upset an inexperienced user. Moreover, it doesn't offer any constructive information. A much better message would be

```
That is not a valid part number.
Part numbers must be no more than four digits long.
Please reenter the number in its proper form:
```

In Chapter 5, we introduce the statements that allow us to test for erroneous data.

Noninteractive Input/Output

Although we tend to use examples of interactive I/O in this text, many programs are written using noninteractive I/O. A common example of noninteractive I/O on large computer systems is batch processing (see Chapter 1). Remember that in batch processing, the user and the computer do not interact while the program is running. This method is most effective when a program is going to input or output large amounts of data. An example of batch processing is a program that inputs a file containing semester grades for thousands of students and prints grade reports to be mailed out.

When a program must read in many data values, the usual practice is to prepare them ahead of time, storing them into a disk file. This allows the user to go back and make changes or corrections to the data as necessary before running the program. When a program is designed to print lots of data, the output can be sent directly to a high-speed printer or another disk file. After the program has been run, the user can examine the data at leisure. In the next section, we discuss input and output with disk files.

Programs designed for noninteractive I/O do not print prompting messages for input. It is a good idea, however, to echo print each data value that is read. Echo printing allows the person reading the output to verify that the input values were prepared correctly. Because noninteractive programs tend to print large amounts of data, their output often is in the form of a table—columns with descriptive headings.

Most C++ programs are written for interactive use. But the flexibility of the language allows you to write noninteractive programs as well. The biggest difference is in the input/output requirements. Noninteractive programs are generally more rigid about the organization and format of the input and output data.

File Input and Output

In everything we've done so far, we've assumed that the input to our programs comes from the keyboard and that the output from our programs goes to the screen. We look now at input/output to and from files.

Files

Earlier we defined a file as a named area in secondary storage that holds a collection of information (for example, the program code we have typed into the editor). The information in a file usually is stored on an auxiliary storage device, such as a disk. Our programs can read data from a file in the same way they read data from the keyboard, and they can write output to a disk file in the same way they write output to the screen.

Why would we want a program to read data from a file instead of the keyboard? If a program is going to read a large quantity of data, it is easier to enter the data into a file with an editor than to enter it while the program is running. With the editor, we can go back and correct mistakes. Also, we do not have to enter the data all at once; we can take a break and come back later. And if we want to rerun the program, having the data stored in a file allows us to do so without retyping the data.

Why would we want the output from a program to be written to a disk file? The contents of a file can be displayed on a screen or printed. This gives us the option of looking at the output over and over again without having to rerun the program. Also, the output stored in a file can be read into another program as input. For example, the Payroll program writes its output to a file named `payFile`. We can take `payFile` and read it into another program, perhaps one that prints out paychecks.

Using Files

If we want a program to use file I/O, we have to do four things:

1. Request the preprocessor to include the header file `fstream`.
2. Use declaration statements to declare the file streams we are going to use.
3. Prepare each file for reading or writing by using a function named `open`.
4. Specify the name of the file stream in each input or output statement.

***Including the Header File* `fstream`**   Suppose we want the Walk program (p. 139) to read data from a file and to write its output to a file. The first thing we must do is use the preprocessor directive

```
#include <fstream>
```

Through the header file `fstream`, the C++ standard library defines two data types, `ifstream` and `ofstream` (standing for *input file stream* and *output file stream*). Consistent with the general idea of streams in C++, the `ifstream` data type represents a stream of characters coming from an input file, and `ofstream` represents a stream of characters going to an output file.

All of the istream operations you have learned about—the extraction operator (>>), the get function, and the ignore function—are also valid for the ifstream type. And all of the ostream operations, such as the insertion operator (<<) and the endl, setw, and setprecision manipulators, apply also to the ofstream type. To these basic operations, the ifstream and ofstream types add some more operations designed specifically for file I/O.

Declaring File Streams   In a program, you declare stream variables the same way that you declare any variable—you specify the data type and then the variable name:

```
int       someInt;
float     someFloat;
ifstream  inFile;
ofstream  outFile;
```

(You don't have to declare the stream variables cin and cout. The header file iostream already does this for you.)

For our Walk program, let's name the input and output file streams inData and outData. We declare them like this:

```
ifstream inData;      // Holds map distances in inches
ofstream outData;     // Holds walking distances in miles
```

Note that the ifstream type is for input files only, and the ofstream type is for output files only. With these data types, you cannot read from and write to the same file.

Opening Files   The third thing we have to do is prepare each file for reading or writing, an act called *opening a file*. Opening a file causes the computer's operating system to perform certain actions that allow us to proceed with file I/O.

In our example, we want to read from the file stream inData and write to the file stream outData. We open the relevant files by using these statements:

```
inData.open("walk.dat");
outData.open("results.dat");
```

Both of these statements are function calls (notice the telltale arguments—the mark of a function). In each function call, the argument is a literal string enclosed by quotes. The first statement is a call to a function named open, which is associated with the ifstream data type. The second is a call to another function (also named open) associated with the ofstream data type. As we have seen earlier, we use dot notation (as in inData.open) to call certain library functions that are tightly associated with data types.

Exactly what does an open function do? First, it associates a stream variable used in your program with a physical file on disk. Our first function call creates a connection between the stream variable inData and the actual disk file, named walk.dat. (Names of file streams must be identifiers; they are variables in your program. But some computer systems do not use this syntax for file names on disk. For example, many systems allow or even require a dot within a file name.) Similarly, the second function call associates the stream variable outData with the disk file results.dat. Associating a program's name for a file (outData) with the actual name for the file (results.dat) is much the same as associating a program's name for the standard output device (cout) with the actual device (the screen).

The next thing the open function does depends on whether the file is an input file or an output file. With an input file, the open function sets the file's reading marker to the first piece of data in the file. (Each input file has its own reading marker.)

With an output file, the open function checks to see whether the file already exists. If the file doesn't exist, open creates a new, empty file for you. If the file already exists, open erases the old contents of the file. Then the writing marker is set at the beginning of the empty file (see Figure 4-2). As output proceeds, each successive output operation advances the writing marker to add data to the end of the file.

FIGURE 4-2
The Effect of
Opening a File

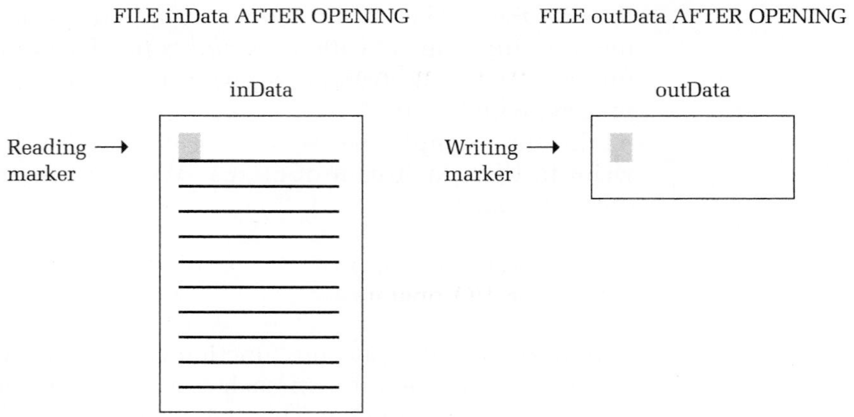

FILE inData AFTER OPENING   FILE outData AFTER OPENING

inData   outData

Reading →   Writing →
marker   marker

Because the reason for opening files is to *prepare* the files for reading or writing, you must open the files before using any input or output statements that refer to the files. In a program, it's a good idea to open files right away to be sure that the files are prepared before the program attempts any file I/O.

```
    ⋮

int main()
{

    ⋮   } Declarations

    // Open the files

    inData.open("walk.dat");
    outData.open("results.dat");
      ⋮
}
```

Specifying File Streams in Input/Output Statements   There is just one more thing we have to do in order to use files. As we said earlier, all `istream` operations are also valid for the `ifstream` type, and all `ostream` operations are valid for the `ofstream` type. So, to read from or write to a file, all we need to do in our input and output statements is substitute the appropriate file stream variable for `cin` or `cout`. In our Walk program, we would use a statement like

```
inData >> distance1 >> distance2 >> distance3 >> distance4 >> scale;
```

to instruct the computer to read data from the file `inData` instead of from `cin`. Similarly, all of the output statements that write to the file `outData` would specify `outData`, not `cout`, as the destination:

```
outData << "Total mileage for the day is " << totMiles << " miles."
        << endl;
```

What is nice about C++ stream I/O is that we have a uniform syntax for performing I/O operations, regardless of whether we're working with the keyboard and screen, with files, or with other I/O devices.

An Example Program Using Files

The reworked Walk program is shown below. Now it reads its input from the file inData and writes its output to the file outData. Compare this program with the original version on page 139 and notice that the named constants have disappeared because the data is now input at execution time. Notice also that to set up the floating-point output format, the fixed, showpoint, and setprecision manipulators are applied to the outData stream variable, not to cout.

```cpp
//******************************************************************
// Walk program
// This program computes the mileage (rounded to tenths of a mile)
// for each of four distances between points in a city, given
// the measurements on a map with a scale whose value is also
// input
//******************************************************************
#include <iostream>
#include <iomanip>      // For setprecision()
#include <fstream>      // For file I/O

using namespace std;

int main()
{
    float    distance1;        // Measurement for first distance
    float    distance2;        // Measurement for second distance
    float    distance3;        // Measurement for third distance
    float    distance4;        // Measurement for fourth distance
    float    scale;            // Map scale (miles per inch)
    float    totMiles;         // Total of rounded mileages
    float    miles;            // An individual rounded mileage
    ifstream inData;           // Holds map distances in inches
    ofstream outData;          // Holds walking distances in miles

    outData << fixed << showpoint         // Set up floating-pt.
            << setprecision(1);           //    output format

    // Open the files

    inData.open("walk.dat");
    outData.open("results.dat");

    // Get data

    inData >> distance1 >> distance2 >> distance3 >> distance4
           >> scale;
```

```
// Initialize the total miles

totMiles = 0.0;

// Compute miles for each distance on the map

miles = float(int(distance1 * scale * 10.0 + 0.5)) / 10.0;
outData << "For a measurement of " << distance1
        << " the first distance is " << miles
        << " mile(s) long." << endl;
totMiles = totMiles + miles;

miles = float(int(distance2 * scale * 10.0 + 0.5)) / 10.0;
outData << "For a measurement of " << distance2
        << " the second distance is " << miles
        << " mile(s) long." << endl;
totMiles = totMiles + miles;

miles = float(int(distance3 * scale * 10.0 + 0.5)) / 10.0;
outData << "For a measurement of " << distance3
        << " the third distance is " << miles
        << " mile(s) long." << endl;
totMiles = totMiles + miles;

miles = float(int(distance4 * scale * 10.0 + 0.5)) / 10.0;
outData << "For a measurement of " << distance4
        << " the fourth distance is " << miles
        << " mile(s) long." << endl;
totMiles = totMiles + miles;

// Print the total miles

outData << endl;
outData << "Total mileage for the day is " << totMiles
        << " miles." << endl;
return 0;
}
```

Before running the program, you would use the editor to create and save a file walk.dat to serve as input. The contents of the file might look like this:

```
1.5 2.3 5.9 4.0 0.25
```

In writing the new Walk program, what happens if you mistakenly specify cout instead of outData in one of the output statements? Nothing disastrous; the output of that one statement merely goes to the screen instead of the output file. And what if, by mistake, you specify cin instead of `inData` in the input statement? The consequences are not as pleasant. When you run the program, the computer will appear to go dead (to *hang*). Here's the reason: Execution reaches the input statement and the computer waits for you to enter the data from the keyboard. But you don't know that the computer is waiting. There's no message on the screen prompting you for input, and you are assuming (wrongly) that the program is getting its input from a data file. So the computer waits, and you wait, and the computer waits, and you wait. Every programmer at one time or another has had the experience of thinking the computer has hung, when, in fact, it is working just fine, silently waiting for keyboard input.

Run-Time Input of File Names

Until now, our examples of opening a file for input have included code similar to the following:

```
ifstream inFile;

inFile.open("datafile.dat");
   ⋮
```

The `open` function associated with the `ifstream` data type requires an argument that specifies the name of the actual data file on disk. By using a literal string, as in the example above, the file name is fixed at compile time. Therefore, the program works only for this one particular disk file.

We often want to make a program more flexible by allowing the file name to be determined at *run time*. A common technique is to prompt the user for the name of the file, read the user's response into a variable, and pass the variable as an argument to the `open` function. In principle, the following code should accomplish what we want. Unfortunately, the compiler does not allow it.

```
ifstream inFile;
string   fileName;

cout << "Enter the input file name: ";
cin >> fileName;
inFile.open(fileName);                // Compile-time error
```

The problem is that the `open` function does not expect an argument of type `string`. Instead, it expects a *C string*. A C string (so named because it originated in the C language, the forerunner of C++) is a limited form of string whose properties we discuss much later in the book. A literal string, such as `"datafile.dat"`, happens to be a C string and thus is acceptable as an argument to the `open` function.

To make the above code work correctly, we need to convert a `string` variable to a C string. The `string` data type provides a value-returning function named `c_str` that is applied to a `string` variable as follows:

```
fileName.c_str()
```

This function returns the C string that is equivalent to the one contained in the `fileName` variable. (The original string contained in `fileName` is not changed by the function call.) The primary purpose of the `c_str` function is to allow programmers to call library functions that expect C strings, not `string` strings, as arguments.

Using the `c_str` function, we can code the run-time input of a file name as follows:

```
ifstream inFile;
string   fileName;

cout << "Enter the input file name: ";
cin >> fileName;
inFile.open(fileName.c_str());
```

Input Failure

When a program inputs data from the keyboard or an input file, things can go wrong. Let's suppose that we're executing a program. It prompts us to enter an integer value, but we absentmindedly type some letters of the alphabet. The input operation fails because of the invalid data. In C++ terminology, the `cin` stream has entered the *fail state*. Once a stream has entered the fail state, any further I/O operations using that stream are considered to be null operations—that is, they have no effect at all. Unfortunately for us, *the computer does not halt the program or give any error message*. The computer just continues executing the program, silently ignoring each additional attempt to use that stream.

Invalid data is the most common reason for input failure. When your program inputs an `int` value, it is expecting to find only digits in the input stream, possibly preceded by a plus or minus sign. If there is a decimal point somewhere within the digits, does the input operation fail? Not necessarily; it depends on where the reading marker is. Let's look at an example.

Assume that a program has `int` variables `i`, `j`, and `k`, whose contents are currently 10, 20, and 30, respectively. The program now executes the following two statements:

```
cin >> i >> j >> k;
cout << "i: " << i << "  j: " << j << "  k: " << k;
```

If we type these characters for the input data:

```
1234.56 7 89
```

then the program produces this output:

```
i: 1234   j: 20   k: 30
```

Let's see why.

Remember that when reading int or float data, the extraction operator >> stops reading at the first character that is inappropriate for the data type (whitespace or otherwise). In our example, the input operation for i succeeds. The computer extracts the first four characters from the input stream and stores the integer value 1234 into i. The reading marker is now on the decimal point:

```
1234.56 7 89
```

The next input operation (for j) fails; an int value cannot begin with a decimal point. The cin stream is now in the fail state, and the current value of j (20) remains unchanged. The third input operation (for k) is ignored, as are all the rest of the statements in our program that read from cin.

Another way to make a stream enter the fail state is to try to open an input file that doesn't exist. Suppose that you have a data file on your disk named myfile.dat. In your program you have the following statements:

```
ifstream inFile;

inFile.open("myfil.dat");
inFile >> i >> j >> k;
```

In the call to the open function, you misspelled the name of your disk file. At run time, the attempt to open the file fails, so the stream inFile enters the fail state. The next three input operations (for i, j, and k) are null operations. Without issuing any error message, the program proceeds to use the (unknown) contents of i, j, and k in calculations. The results of these calculations are certain to be puzzling.

The point of this discussion is not to make you nervous about I/O but to make you aware. The Testing and Debugging section at the end of this chapter offers suggestions for avoiding input failure, and Chapters 5 and 6 introduce program statements that let you test the state of a stream.

Software Design Methodologies

Over the last two chapters and the first part of this one, we have introduced elements of the C++ language that let us input data, perform calculations, and output results. The programs we wrote were short and straightforward because the problems to be solved were simple. We are ready to write programs for more complicated problems, but first we need to step back and look at the overall process of programming.

As you learned in Chapter 1, the programming process consists of a problem-solving phase and an implementation phase. The problem-solving phase includes *analysis* (analyzing and understanding the problem to be solved) and *design* (designing a solution to the problem). Given a complex problem—one that results in a 10,000-line program, for example—it's simply not reasonable to skip the design process and go directly to writing C++ code. What we need is a systematic way of designing a solution to a problem, no matter how complicated the problem is.

In the remainder of this chapter, we describe two important methodologies for designing solutions to more complex problems: *functional decomposition* and *object-oriented design*. These methodologies help you create solutions that can be easily implemented as C++ programs. The resulting programs are readable, understandable, and easy to debug and modify.

One software design methodology that is in widespread use is known as **object-oriented design (OOD)**. C++ evolved from the C language primarily to facilitate the use of the OOD methodology. In the next two sections, we present the essential concepts of OOD; we expand our treatment of the approach later in the book. OOD is often used in conjunction with the other methodology that we discuss in this chapter, **functional decomposition.**

Object-oriented design A technique for developing software in which the solution is expressed in terms of objects—self-contained entities composed of data and operations on that data.

Functional decomposition A technique for developing software in which the problem is divided into more easily handled subproblems, the solutions of which create a solution to the overall problem.

OOD focuses on entities (*objects*) consisting of data and operations on the data. In OOD, we solve a problem by identifying the components that make up a solution and identifying how those components interact with each other through operations on the data that they contain. The result is a design for a set of objects that can be assembled to form a solution to a problem. In contrast, functional decomposition views the solution to a problem as a task to be accomplished. It focuses on the sequence of operations that are required to complete the task. When the problem requires a sequence of steps that is long or complex, we divide it into subproblems that are easier to solve.

The choice of which methodology we use depends on the problem at hand. For example, a large problem might involve several sequential phases of processing, such as gathering data and verifying its correctness with noninteractive processing, analyzing the data interactively, and printing reports noninteractively at the conclusion of the analysis. This process has a natural functional decomposition. Each of the phases, however, may best be solved by a set of objects that represent the data and the operations that can be applied to it. Some of the individual operations may be sufficiently complex that they require further decomposition, either into a sequence of operations or into another set of objects.

If you look at a problem and see that it is natural to think about it in terms of a collection of component parts, then you should use OOD to solve it. For example, a banking problem may require a `checkingAccount` object with associated operations `OpenAccount`, `WriteCheck`, `MakeDeposit`, and `IsOverdrawn`. The `checkingAccount` object consists of not only data (the account number and current balance, for example) but also these operations, all bound together into one unit.

On the other hand, if you find that it is natural to think of the solution to the problem as a series of steps, then you should use functional decomposition. For example, when computing some statistical measures on a large set of real numbers, it is natural to decompose the problem into a sequence of steps that read a value, perform calculations, and then repeat the sequence. The C++ language and the standard library supply all of the operations that we need, and we simply write a sequence of those operations to solve the problem.

What Are Objects?

Let's take a closer look at what objects are and how they work before we examine OOD further. We said earlier that an object is a collection of data together with associated operations. Several programming languages, called *object-oriented programming languages,* have been created specifically to support OOD. Examples are C++, Java, Smalltalk, CLOS, Eiffel, and Object-Pascal. In these languages, a *class* is a programmer-defined data type from which objects are created. Although we did not say it at the time, we have been using classes and objects to perform input and output in C++. `cin` is an object of a data type (class) named `istream`, and `cout` is an object of a class `ostream`. As we explained earlier, the header file `iostream` defines the classes `istream` and `ostream` and also declares `cin` and `cout` to be objects of those classes:

```
istream cin;
ostream cout;
```

Similarly, the header file `fstream` defines classes `ifstream` and `ofstream`, from which you can declare your own input file stream and output file stream objects.

Another example you have seen already is `string`—a programmer-defined class from which you create objects by using declarations such as

```
string lastName;
```

In Figure 4-3, we picture the `cin` and `lastName` objects as entities that have a private part and a public part. The private part includes data and functions that the user cannot access and doesn't need to know about in order to use the object. The public part, shown as ovals in the side of the object, represents the object's *interface*. The interface consists of operations that are available to programmers wishing to use the object. In C++, public operations are written as functions and are known as *member functions*. Except for operations using symbols such as << and >>, a member function is invoked by giving the name of the class object, then a dot, and then the function name and argument list:

```
cin.ignore(100, '\n');
cin.get(someChar);
cin >> someInt;
len = lastName.length();
pos = lastName.find('A');
```

Object-Oriented Design

The first step in OOD is to identify the major objects in the problem, together with their associated operations. The final problem solution is ultimately expressed in terms of these objects and operations.

OOD leads to programs that are collections of objects. Each object is responsible for one part of the entire solution, and the objects communicate by accessing each other's member functions. There are many libraries of prewritten classes, including the C++ standard library, public libraries (called *freeware* or *shareware*), libraries that are sold commercially, and libraries that are developed by companies for their own use. In many cases, it is possible to browse through a library, choose classes you need for a problem, and assemble them to form a substantial portion of your program. Putting existing pieces together in this fashion is an excellent example of the building-block approach we discussed in Chapter 1.

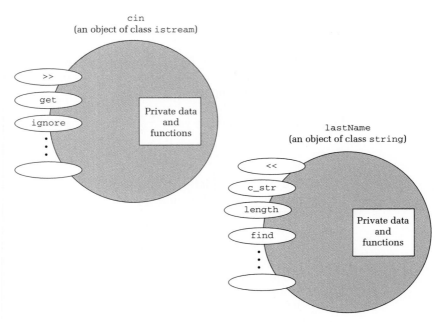

FIGURE 4-3
Objects and Their
Operations

When there isn't a suitable class available in a library, it is necessary to define a new class. We see how this is done in Chapter 11. The design of a new class begins with the specification of its interface. We must decide what operations are needed on the outside of the class to make its objects useful. Once the interface is defined, we can design the implementation of the class, including all of its private members.

One of the goals in designing an interface is to make it flexible so the new class can be used in unforeseen circumstances. For example, we may provide a member function that converts the value of an object into a string, even though we don't need this capability in our program. When the time comes to debug the program, it may be very useful to display values of this type as strings.

Useful features are often absent from an interface, sometimes due to lack of foresight and sometimes for the purpose of simplifying the design. It is quite common to discover a class in a library that is almost right for your purpose but is missing some key feature. OOD addresses this situation with a concept called *inheritance,* which allows you to adapt an existing class to meet your particular needs. You can use inheritance to add features to a class (or restrict the use of existing features) without having to inspect and modify its source code. Inheritance is considered such an integral part of object-oriented programming that a separate term, *object-based programming*, is used to describe programming with objects but not inheritance.

In Chapter 14, we see how to define classes that inherit members from existing classes. Together, OOD, class libraries, and inheritance can dramatically reduce the time and effort required to design, implement, and maintain large software systems.

To summarize the OOD process: We identify the major components of a problem solution and how they interact. We then look in the available libraries for classes that correspond to the components. When we find a class that is almost right, we can use inheritance to adapt it. When we can't find a class that corresponds to a component, we must design a new class. Our design specifies the interface for the class, and we then implement the interface with public and private members as necessary. OOD isn't always used in isolation. Functional decomposition may be used in designing member functions within a class or in coordinating the interactions of objects.

In this section, we have presented only an introduction to OOD. A more complete discussion requires knowledge of topics that we explore in Chapters 5 through 10: flow of control, programmer-written functions, and more about data types. In Chapters 11 through 13, we learn how to write our own classes, and we return to OOD in Chapter 14. Until then, our programs are relatively small, so we use object-based programming and functional decomposition to arrive at our problem solutions.

Functional Decomposition

The second design technique we use is functional decomposition (it's also called *structured design*, *top-down design*, *stepwise refinement*, and *modular programming*). In functional decomposition, we work from the abstract (a list of the major steps in our solution) to the particular (algorithmic steps that can be translated directly into C++ code). You can also think of this as working from a high-level solution, leaving the details of implementation unspecified, down to a fully detailed solution.

The easiest way to solve a problem is to give it to someone else and say, "Solve this problem." This is the most abstract level of a problem solution: a single-statement solution that encompasses the entire problem without specifying any of the details of implementation. It's at this point that we programmers are called in. Our job is to turn the abstract solution into a concrete solution, a program.

If the solution clearly involves a series of major steps, we break it down (decompose it) into pieces. In the process, we move to a lower level of abstraction—that is, some of the implementation details (but not too many) are now specified. Each of the major steps becomes an independent subproblem that we can work on separately. In a very large project, one person (the *chief architect* or *team leader*) formulates the subproblems and then gives them to other members of the programming team, saying, "Solve this problem." In the case of a small project, we give the subproblems to ourselves. Then we choose one subproblem at a time to solve. We may break the chosen subproblem into another series of steps that, in turn, become smaller subproblems. Or we may identify components that are naturally represented as objects. The process continues until each subproblem cannot be divided further or has an obvious solution.

Why do we work this way? Why not simply write out all of the details? Because it is much easier to focus on one problem at a time. For example, suppose you are working on part of a program to output certain values and discover that you need a complex formula to calculate an appropriate fieldwidth for printing one of the values. Calculating fieldwidths is not the purpose of this part of the program. If you shift your focus to the calculation, you are likely to forget some detail of the overall output process. What you do is write down an abstract step—"Calculate the fieldwidth required"—and go on with the problem at hand. Once you've written the major steps, you can go back to solving the step that does the calculation.

By subdividing the problem, you create a hierarchical structure called a *tree structure*. Each level of the tree is a complete solution to the problem that is less abstract (more detailed) than the level above it. Figure 4-4 shows a generic solution tree for a problem. Steps that are shaded have enough implementation details to be translated directly into C++ statements. These are **concrete steps.** Those that are not shaded are **abstract steps;** they reappear as subproblems in the next level down. Each box in the figure represents a **module.** Modules are the basic building blocks in a functional decomposition. The diagram in Figure 4-4 is also called a *module structure chart.*

Concrete step   A step for which the implementation details are fully specified.

Abstract step   A step for which some implementation details remain unspecified.

Module   A self-contained collection of steps that solves a problem or subproblem; can contain both concrete and abstract steps.

Like OOD, functional decomposition uses the divide-and-conquer approach to problem solving. Both techniques break up large problems into smaller units that are easier to handle. The difference is that in OOD the units are objects, whereas the units in functional decomposition are modules representing algorithms.

Modules

A module begins life as an abstract step in the next-higher level of the solution tree. It is completed when it solves a given subproblem—that is, when

FIGURE 4-4
Hierarchical Solution Tree

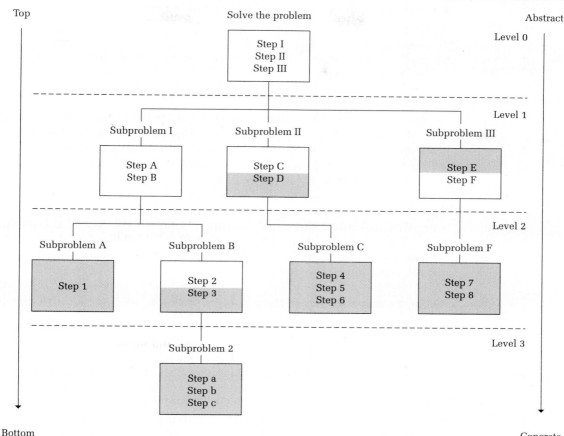

it specifies a series of steps that does the same thing as the higher-level abstract step. At this stage, a module is **functionally equivalent** to the abstract step. (Don't confuse our use of *function* with C++ functions. Here we use the term to refer to the specific role that the module or step plays in an algorithmic solution.)

Functional equivalence A property of a module that performs exactly the same operation as the abstract step it defines. A pair of modules are also functionally equivalent to each other when they perform exactly the same operation.

In a properly written module, the only steps that directly address the given subproblem are concrete steps; abstract steps are used for significant new subproblems. This is called **functional cohesion.**

Functional cohesion A property of a module in which all concrete steps are directed toward solving just one problem, and any significant subproblems are written as abstract steps.

The idea behind functional cohesion is that each module should do just one thing and do it well. Functional cohesion is not a well-defined property; there is no quantitative measure of cohesion. It is a product of the human need to organize things into neat chunks that are easy to understand and remember. Knowing which details to make concrete and which to leave abstract is a matter of experience, circumstance, and personal style. For example, you might decide to include a fieldwidth calculation in a printing module if there isn't so much detail in the rest of the module that it becomes confusing. On the other hand, if the calculation is performed several times, it makes sense to write it as a separate module and just refer to it each time you need it.

Writing Cohesive Modules Here's one approach to writing modules that are cohesive:

1. Think about how you would solve the subproblem by hand.
2. Begin writing down the major steps.
3. If a step is simple enough that you can see how to implement it directly in C++, it is at the concrete level; it doesn't need any further refinement.
4. If you have to think about implementing a step as a series of smaller steps or as several C++ statements, it is still at an abstract level.
5. If you are trying to write a series of steps and start to feel overwhelmed by details, you probably are bypassing one or more levels of abstraction. Stand back and look for pieces that you can write as more abstract steps.

We could call this the "procrastinator's technique." If a step is cumbersome or difficult, put it off to a lower level; don't think about it today, think about it tomorrow. Of course, tomorrow does come, but the whole process can be applied again to the subproblem. A trouble spot often seems much simpler when you can focus on it. And eventually the whole problem is broken up into manageable units.

As you work your way down the solution tree, you make a series of design decisions. If a decision proves awkward or wrong (and many times it does!), you can backtrack (go back up the tree to a higher-level module) and try something else. You don't have to scrap your whole design—only the small part you are working on. There may be many intermediate steps and trial solutions before you reach a final design.

Pseudocode   You'll find it easier to implement a design if you write the steps in pseudocode. *Pseudocode* is a mixture of English statements and C++-like control structures that can be translated easily into C++. (We've been using pseudocode in the algorithms in the Problem-Solving Case Studies.) When a concrete step is written in pseudocode, it should be possible to rewrite it directly as a C++ statement in a program.

Implementing the Design

The product of functional decomposition is a hierarchical solution to a problem with multiple levels of abstraction. Figure 4-5 shows a functional decomposition for the Walk program of Chapter 3. This kind of solution forms the basis for the implementation phase of programming.

How do we translate a functional decomposition into a C++ program? If you look closely at Figure 4-5, you can see that the concrete steps (those that are shaded) can be assembled into a complete algorithm for solving the problem. The order in which they are assembled is determined by their position in the tree. We start at the top of the tree, at level 0, with the first step, "Initialize the total miles." Because it is abstract, we must go to the next level, level 1. There we find a single concrete step that corresponds to this step; this step becomes the first part of our algorithm. Because the conversion process is now concrete, we can go back to level 0 and go on to the next step, computing the miles for each distance. We find that this step is abstract, but when we look at level 1, we see that it is broken into a series of abstract steps that are further expanded at level 2. Going through each of the abstract steps at level 1, we incorporate the corresponding concrete steps from level 2 into our algorithm. The last step at level 0 is abstract, so level 1 contains the corresponding concrete steps. Here's the resulting algorithm:

```
DISTANCE1 = 1.5
DISTANCE2 = 2.3
DISTANCE3 = 5.9
DISTANCE4 = 4.0
SCALE = 0.25
Set totMiles = 0.0
Set miles = float(int(DISTANCE1 * SCALE * 10.0 + 0.5)) / 10.0
Print DISTANCE1, miles
Add miles to totMiles
Set miles = float(int(DISTANCE2 * SCALE * 10.0 + 0.5)) / 10.0
Print DISTANCE2, miles
Add miles to totMiles
```

FIGURE 4-5
Solution Tree for
Walk Program

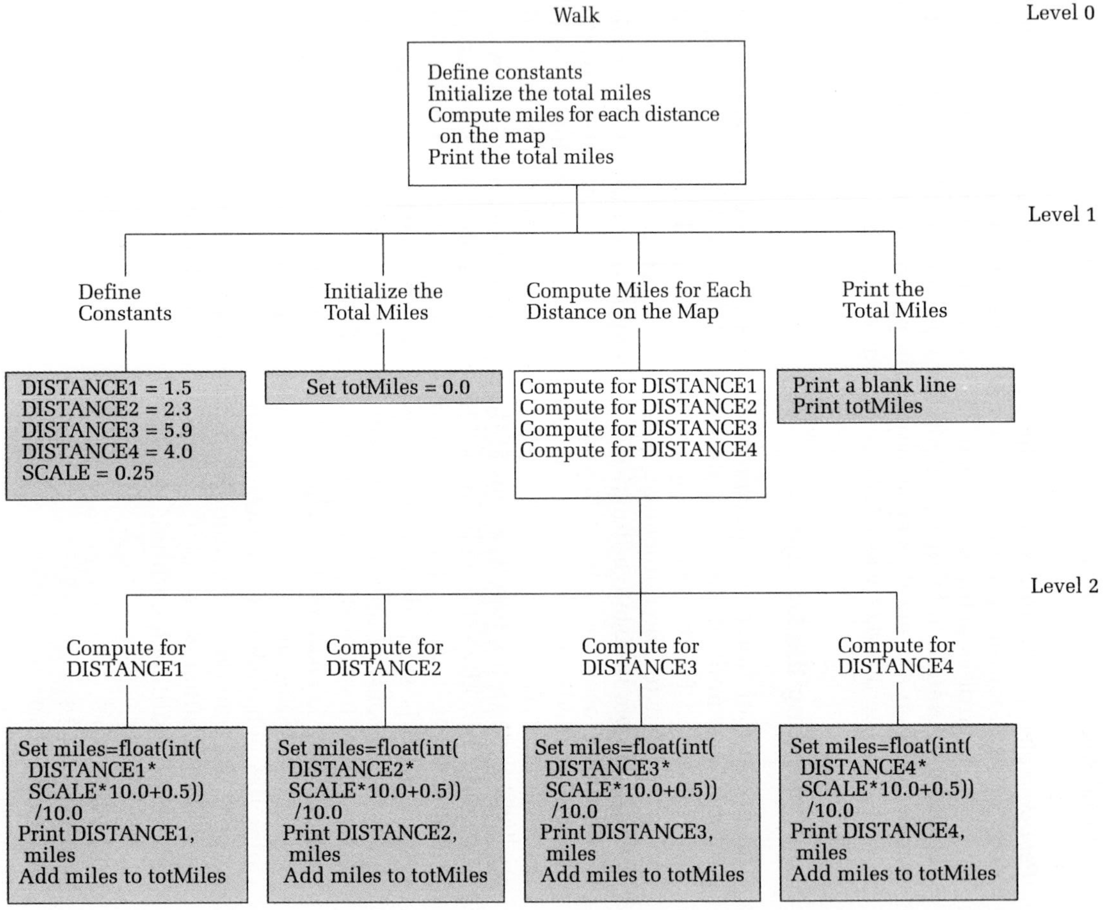

```
Set miles = float(int(DISTANCE3 * SCALE * 10.0 + 0.5)) / 10.0
Print DISTANCE3, miles
Add miles to totMiles
Set miles = float(int(DISTANCE4 * SCALE * 10.0 + 0.5)) / 10.0
Print DISTANCE4, miles
Add miles to totMiles
Print a blank line
Print totMiles
```

From this algorithm we can construct a table of the constants and variables required, and then write the declarations and executable statements of the program.

In practice, you write your design not as a tree diagram but as a series of modules grouped by levels of abstraction, as we've done below.

Main Module   **Level 0**

```
Define constants
Initialize the total miles
Compute miles for each distance on the map
Print the total miles
```

Define Constants   **Level 1**

```
DISTANCE1 = 1.5
DISTANCE2 = 2.3
DISTANCE3 = 5.9
DISTANCE4 = 4.0
SCALE = 0.25
```

Initialize the Total Miles

```
Set totMiles = 0.0
```

Compute Miles for Each Distance on the Map

```
Compute for DISTANCE1
Compute for DISTANCE2
Compute for DISTANCE3
Compute for DISTANCE4
```

Print the Total Miles

```
Print a blank line
Print totMiles
```

Compute for DISTANCE1   Level 2

```
Set miles = float(int(DISTANCE1 * SCALE * 10.0 + 0.5)) / 10.0
Print DISTANCE1, miles
Add miles to totMiles
```

Compute for DISTANCE2

```
Set miles = float(int(DISTANCE2 * SCALE * 10.0 + 0.5)) / 10.0
Print DISTANCE2, miles
Add miles to totMiles
```

Compute for DISTANCE3

```
Set miles = float(int(DISTANCE3 * SCALE * 10.0 + 0.5)) / 10.0
Print DISTANCE3, miles
Add miles to totMiles
```

Compute for DISTANCE4

Set miles = float(int(DISTANCE4 * SCALE * 10.0 + 0.5)) / 10.0
Print DISTANCE4, miles
Add miles to totMiles

If you look at the C++ program for Walk, you can see that it closely resembles this solution. You can also see that the names of the modules have been paraphrased as comments in the code.

The type of implementation that we've introduced here is called *flat* or *inline implementation*. We are flattening the two-dimensional, hierarchical structure of the solution by writing all of the steps as one long sequence. This kind of implementation is adequate when a solution is short and has only a few levels of abstraction. The programs it produces are clear and easy to understand, assuming appropriate comments and good style.

Longer programs, with more levels of abstraction, are difficult to work with as flat implementations. In Chapter 7, you'll see that it is preferable to implement a hierarchical solution by using a *hierarchical implementation*. There we implement many of the modules by writing them as separate C++ functions, and the abstract steps in the design are replaced with calls to those functions.

One of the advantages of implementing modules as functions is that they can be called from different places in a program. For example, if a problem requires that the volume of a cylinder be computed in several places, we could write a single function to perform the calculation and simply call it in each place. This gives us a *semihierarchical implementation*. The implementation does not preserve a pure hierarchy because abstract steps at various levels of the solution tree share one implementation of a module (see Figure 4-6). A shared module actually falls outside the hierarchy because it doesn't really belong at any one level.

Another advantage of implementing modules as functions is that you can pick them up and use them in other programs. Over time, you will build a library of your own functions to complement those that are supplied by the C++ standard library.

We postpone a detailed discussion of hierarchical implementations until Chapter 7. For now, our programs remain short enough for flat implementations to suffice. Chapters 5 and 6 examine topics such as flow of control, preconditions and postconditions, interface design, side effects, and others you'll need in order to develop hierarchical implementations.

From now on, we use the following outline for the functional decompositions in our case studies, and we recommend that you adopt a similar outline in solving your own programming problems:

Problem statement
Input description
Output description
Discussion
Assumptions (if any)
Main module
Remaining modules by levels
Module structure chart

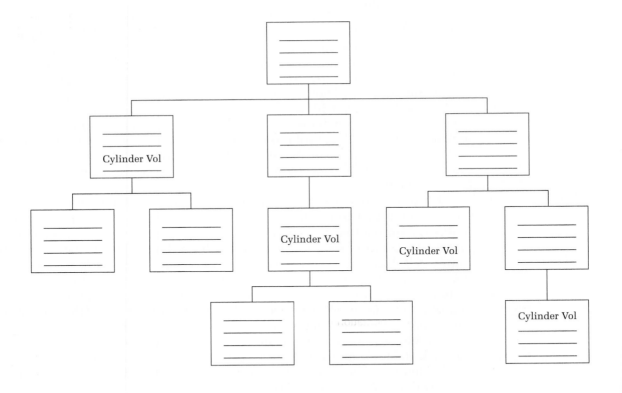

Cylinder Vol

Set volume = $\pi r^2 h$

FIGURE 4-6
A Semihierarchical Module Structure Chart with a Shared Module

In some of our case studies, the outline is reorganized, with the input and output descriptions following the discussion. In later chapters, we also expand the outline with additional sections. Don't think of this outline as a rigid prescription—it is more like a list of things to do. We want to be sure to do everything on the list, but the individual circumstances of each problem guide the order in which we do them.

A Perspective on Design

We have looked at two design methodologies, object-oriented design and functional decomposition. Until we learn about additional C++ language features that support OOD, we use functional decomposition (and object-based programming) in the next several chapters to come up with our problem solutions.

An important perspective to keep in mind is that functional decomposition and OOD are not separate, disjoint techniques. OOD decomposes a problem into objects. Objects not only contain data but also have associated operations. The operations on objects require algorithms. Sometimes the algorithms are complicated and must be decomposed into subalgorithms by using functional decomposition. Experienced programmers are familiar with both methodologies and know when to use one or the other, or a combination of the two.

Remember that the problem-solving phase of the programming process takes time. If you spend the bulk of your time analyzing and designing a solution, then coding and implementing the program take relatively little time.

Software Engineering Tip

Documentation

As you create your functional decomposition or object-oriented design, you are developing documentation for your program. *Documentation* includes the written problem specifications, design, development history, and actual code of a program.

Good documentation helps other programmers read and understand a program and is invaluable when software is being debugged and modified (maintained). If you haven't looked at your program for six months and need to change it, you'll be happy that you documented it well. Of course, if someone else has to use and modify your program, documentation is indispensable.

Documentation is both external and internal to the program. External documentation includes the specifications, the development history, and the design documents. Internal documentation includes the program format and **self-documenting code**—

meaningful identifiers and comments. You can use the pseudocode from the design process as comments in your programs.

This kind of documentation may be sufficient for someone reading or maintaining your programs. However, if a program is going to be used by people who are not programmers, you must provide a user's manual as well.

Be sure to keep documentation up-to-date. Indicate any changes you make in a program in all of the pertinent documentation. Use self-documenting code to make your programs more readable.

Self-documenting code Program code containing meaningful identifiers as well as judiciously used clarifying comments.

Now let's look at a case study that demonstrates functional decomposition.

*P*ROBLEM-SOLVING CASE STUDY

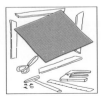

Stretching a Canvas

Problem: You are taking an art class in which you are learning to make your own painting canvas by stretching the cloth over a wooden frame and stapling it to the back of the frame. For a given size of painting, you must determine how much wood to buy for the frame, how large a piece of canvas to purchase, and the cost of the materials.

Input: Four floating-point numbers: the length and width of the painting, the cost per inch of the wood, and the cost per square foot of the canvas.

Output: Prompting messages, the input data (echo print), the length of wood to buy, the dimensions of the canvas, the cost of the wood, the cost of the canvas, and the total cost of the materials.

Discussion: The length of the wood is twice the sum of the length and width of the painting. The cost of the wood is simply its length times its cost per inch.

PROBLEM-SOLVING CASE STUDY cont'd.

According to the art instructor, the dimensions of the canvas are the length and width of the painting, each with 5 inches added (for the part that wraps around to the back of the frame). The area of the canvas in square inches is its length times its width. However, we are given the cost for a square foot of the canvas. Thus, we must divide the area of the canvas by the number of square inches in a square foot (144) before multiplying by the cost.

Assumptions: The input values are positive (checking for erroneous data is not done).

Main Module   **Level 0**

Get length and width
Get wood cost
Get canvas cost
Compute dimensions and costs
Print dimensions and costs

Get Length and Width   **Level 1**

Print "Enter length and width of painting:"
Read length, width

Get Wood Cost

Print "Enter cost per inch of the framing wood in dollars:"
Read woodCost

PROBLEM-SOLVING CASE STUDY cont'd.

Get Canvas Cost

> Print "Enter cost per square foot of canvas in dollars:"
> Read canvasCost

Compute Dimensions and Costs

> Set lengthOfWood = (length + width) * 2
> Set canvasWidth = width + 5
> Set canvasLength = length + 5
> Set canvasAreaInches = canvasWidth * canvasLength
> Set canvasAreaFeet = canvasAreaInches / 144.0
> Set totWoodCost = lengthOfWood * woodCost
> Set totCanvasCost = canvasAreaFeet * canvasCost
> Set totCost = totWoodCost + totCanvasCost

Print Dimensions and Costs

> Print "For a painting", length, "in. long and", width, "in. wide,"
> Print "you need to buy", lengthOfWood, "in. of wood, and"
> Print "the canvas must be", canvasLength, "in. long and",
> canvasWidth, "in. wide."
>
> Print "Given a wood cost of $", woodCost, "per in."
> Print "and a canvas cost of $", canvasCost, "per sq. ft.,"
> Print "the wood will cost $", totWoodCost, ','
> Print "the canvas will cost $", totCanvasCost, ','
> Print "and the total cost of materials will be $", totCost, '.'

Module Structure Chart:

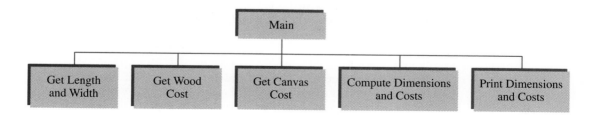

Variables

Name	Data Type	Description
length	float	Length of painting in inches
width	float	Width of painting in inches
woodCost	float	Cost of wood per inch in dollars
canvasCost	float	Cost of canvas per square foot
lengthOfWood	float	Amount of wood to buy
canvasWidth	float	Width of canvas to buy
canvasLength	float	Length of canvas to buy
canvasAreaInches	float	Area of canvas in square inches
canvasAreaFeet	float	Area of canvas in square feet
totCanvasCost	float	Total cost of canvas being bought
totWoodCost	float	Total cost of wood being bought
totCost	float	Total cost of materials

Constants

Name	Value	Description
SQ_IN_PER_SQ_FT	144.0	Number of square inches in one square foot

Here is the complete program. Notice how we've used the module names as comments to help distinguish the modules from one another in our flat implementation.

PROBLEM-SOLVING CASE STUDY cont'd.

(The following program is written in ISO/ANSI standard C++. If you are working with pre–standard C++, see the alternate version of the program in the PRE_STD directory of the program disk, available at the publisher's Web site, www.jbpub.com/disks.)

```cpp
//*****************************************************************
// Canvas program
// This program computes the dimensions and costs of materials
// to build a painting canvas of given dimensions. The user is
// asked to enter the length and width of the painting and the
// costs of the wood (per inch) and canvas (per square foot)
//*****************************************************************
#include <iostream>
#include <iomanip>     // For setprecision()

using namespace std;

const float SQ_IN_PER_SQ_FT = 144.0;    // Square inches per
                                        //   square foot
int main()
{
    float length;              // Length of painting in inches
    float width;               // Width of painting in inches
    float woodCost;            // Cost of wood per inch in dollars
    float canvasCost;          // Cost of canvas per square foot
    float lengthOfWood;        // Amount of wood to buy
    float canvasWidth;         // Width of canvas to buy
    float canvasLength;        // Length of canvas to buy
    float canvasAreaInches;    // Area of canvas in square inches
    float canvasAreaFeet;      // Area of canvas in square feet
    float totCanvasCost;       // Total cost of canvas being bought
    float totWoodCost;         // Total cost of wood being bought
    float totCost;             // Total cost of materials

    cout << fixed << showpoint;              // Set up floating-pt.
                                             //   output format

    // Get length and width

    cout << "Enter length and width of painting:" << endl;
    cin >> length >> width;

    // Get wood cost

    cout << "Enter cost per inch of the framing wood in dollars:"
         << endl;
    cin >> woodCost;
```

PROBLEM-SOLVING CASE STUDY cont'd.

```
// Get canvas cost

cout << "Enter cost per square foot of canvas in dollars:"
     << endl;
cin >> canvasCost;

// Compute dimensions and costs

lengthOfWood = (length + width) * 2;
canvasWidth = width + 5;
canvasLength = length + 5;
canvasAreaInches = canvasWidth * canvasLength;
canvasAreaFeet = canvasAreaInches / SQ_IN_PER_SQ_FT;
totWoodCost = lengthOfWood * woodCost;
totCanvasCost = canvasAreaFeet * canvasCost;
totCost = totWoodCost + totCanvasCost;

// Print dimensions and costs

cout << endl << setprecision(1);
cout << "For a painting " << length << " in. long and "
     << width << " in. wide," << endl;
cout << "you need to buy " << lengthOfWood << " in. of wood,"
     << " and" << endl;
cout << "the canvas must be " << canvasLength << " in. long"
     << " and " << canvasWidth << " in. wide." << endl;

cout << endl << setprecision(2);
cout << "Given a wood cost of $" << woodCost << " per in."
     << endl;
cout << "and a canvas cost of $" << canvasCost
     << " per sq. ft.," << endl;
cout << "the wood will cost $" << totWoodCost << ',' << endl;
cout << "the canvas will cost $" << totCanvasCost << ','
     << endl;
cout << "and the total cost of materials will be $" << totCost
     << '.' << endl;
return 0;
}
```

This is an interactive program. The data values are input while the program is executing. If the user enters this data:

```
24.0 36.0 0.08 2.80
```

then the dialogue with the user looks like this:

```
Enter length and width of painting:
24.0 36.0
Enter cost per inch of the framing wood in dollars:
0.08
Enter cost per square foot of canvas in dollars:
2.80

For a painting 24.0 in. long and 36.0 in. wide,
you need to buy 120.0 in. of wood, and
the canvas must be 29.0 in. long and 41.0 in. wide.

Given a wood cost of $0.08 per in.
and a canvas cost of $2.80 per sq. ft.,
the wood will cost $9.60,
the canvas will cost $23.12,
and the total cost of materials will be $32.72.
```

*B*ACKGROUND INFORMATION

Programming on Many Scales

To help you put the topics in this book into context, we describe in broad terms the way programming in its many forms is done in "the real world." Obviously, we can't cover every possibility, but we'll try to give you a flavor of the state of the art.

Programming projects range in size from the small scale, in which a student or computer hobbyist writes a short program to try out something new, to large-scale multicompany programming projects involving hundreds of people. Between these two extremes are efforts of many other sizes. There are people who use programming in their professions, even though it isn't their primary job. For example, a scientist might write a special-purpose program to analyze data from a particular experiment.

Even among professional programmers, there are many specialized programming areas. An individual might have a specialty in business data processing, in writing compilers or developing word processors (a specialty known as "tool making"), in research and development support, in graphical display development, in writing entertainment software, or in one of many other areas. However, one person can produce only fairly small programs (a few tens of thousands of lines of code at best). Work of this kind is called *programming in the small*.

A larger application, such as the development of a new operating system, might require hundreds of thousands or even millions of lines of code. Such large-scale projects require teams of programmers, many of them specialists, who must be organized in some manner or they waste valuable time just trying to communicate with one another.

Usually, a hierarchical organization is set up along the lines of the module structure chart. One person, the *chief architect* or *project director*, determines the basic structure of the program and then delegates the responsibility of implementing the major components. These components may be modules produced by a functional decomposition, or they might be classes and objects resulting from an object-oriented design. In smaller projects, the components may be delegated directly to programmers. In larger projects, the components may be given to team leaders, who divide them into subcomponents that are then delegated to individual programmers or groups of programmers. At each stage, the person in charge must have the knowledge and experience necessary to define the next-lower level of the hierarchy and to estimate the resources necessary to implement it. This sort of organization is called *programming in the large*.

Programming languages and software tools can help a great deal in supporting programming in the large. For example, if a programming language lets programmers develop, compile, and test parts of a program independently before they are put together, then it enables several people to work on the program simultaneously. Of course, it is hard to appreciate the complexity of programming in the large when you are writing a small program for a class assignment. However, the experience you gain in this course will be valuable as you begin to develop larger programs.

The following is a classic example of what happens when a large program is developed without careful organization and proper language support. In the 1960s, IBM developed a major new operating system called OS/360, which was one of the first true examples of programming in the large. After the operating system was written, more than 1000 significant errors were found. Despite years of trying to fix these errors, the programmers never did get the number of errors below 1000, and sometimes the "fixes" produced far more errors than they eliminated.

What led to this situation? Hindsight analysis showed that the code was badly organized and that different pieces were so interrelated that nobody could keep it all straight. A seemingly simple change in one part of the code caused several other parts of the system to fail. Eventually, at great expense, an entirely new system was created using better organization and tools.

In those early days of computing, everyone expected occasional errors to occur, and it was still possible to get useful work done with a faulty operating system. Today, however, computers are used more and more in critical applications such as medical equipment and aircraft control systems, where errors can prove fatal. Many of these applications depend on large-scale programming. If you were stepping onto a modern jetliner right now, you might well pause and wonder, "Just what sort of language and tools did they use when they wrote the programs for this thing?" Fortunately, most large software development efforts today use a combination of good methodology, appropriate language, and extensive organizational tools—an approach known as *software engineering*.

Testing and Debugging

An important part of implementing a program is testing it (checking the results). By now you should realize that there is nothing magical about the computer. It is infallible only if the person writing the instructions and entering the data is infallible. Don't trust it to give you the correct answers until you've verified enough of them by hand to convince yourself that the program is working.

From here on, these Testing and Debugging sections offer tips on how to test your programs and what to do if a program doesn't work the way you expect it to work. But don't wait until you've found a bug to read the Testing and Debugging sections. It's much easier to prevent bugs than to fix them.

When testing programs that input data values from a file, it's possible for input operations to fail. And when input fails in C++, the computer doesn't issue a warning message or terminate the program. The program simply continues executing, ignoring any further input operations on that file. The two most common reasons for input failure are invalid data and the *end-of-file error*.

An end-of-file error occurs when the program has read all of the input data available in the file and needs more data to fill the variables in its input statements. It might be that the data file simply was not prepared properly. Perhaps it contains fewer data items than the program requires. Or perhaps the format of the input data is wrong. Leaving out whitespace between numeric values is guaranteed to cause trouble. For example, we may want a data file to contain three integer values—25, 16, and 42. Look what happens with this data:

```
2516   42
```

and this code:

```
inFile >> i >> j >> k;
```

The first two input operations use up the data in the file, leaving the third with no data to read. The stream `inFile` enters the fail state, so k isn't assigned a new value and the computer quietly continues executing at the next statement in the program.

If the data file is prepared correctly and there is still an end-of-file error, the problem is in the program logic. For some reason, the program is attempting too many input operations. It could be a simple oversight such as specifying too many variables in a particular input statement. It could be a misuse of the `ignore` function, causing values to be skipped inadvertently. Or it could be a serious flaw in the algorithm. You should check all of these possibilities.

The other major source of input failure, invalid data, has several possible causes. The most common is an error in the preparation or entry of the data. Numeric and character data mixed inappropriately in the input can cause the input stream to fail if it is supposed to read a numeric value but the reading marker is positioned at a character that isn't allowed in the number. Another cause is using the wrong variable name (which happens to be of the wrong data type) in an input statement. Declaring a variable to be of the wrong data type is a variation on the problem. Last, leaving out a variable (or including an extra one) in an input statement can cause the reading marker to end up positioned on the wrong type of data.

Another oversight, one that doesn't cause input failure but causes programmer frustration, is to use `cin` or `cout` in an I/O statement when you meant to specify a file stream. If you mistakenly use `cin` instead of an input file stream, the program stops and waits for input from the keyboard. If you mistakenly use `cout` instead of an output file stream, you get unexpected output on the screen.

By giving you a framework that can help you organize and keep track of the details involved in designing and implementing a program, functional decomposition (and, later, object-oriented design) should help you avoid many of these errors in the first place.

In later chapters, you'll see that you can test modules separately. If you make sure that each module works by itself, your program should work when you put all the modules together. Testing modules separately is less work than trying to test an entire program. In a smaller section of code, it's less likely that multiple errors will combine to produce behavior that is difficult to analyze.

Testing and Debugging Hints

1. Input and output statements always begin with the name of a stream object, and the >> and << operators point in the direction in which the data is going. The statement

```
cout << n;
```

sends data *to* the output stream `cout`, and the statement

```
cin >> n;
```

sends data *to* the variable n.

2. When a program inputs from or outputs to a file, be sure each I/O statement from or to the file uses the name of the file stream, not `cin` or `cout`.

3. The `open` function associated with an `ifstream` or `ofstream` object requires a C string as an argument. The argument cannot be a `string` object. At this point in the book, the argument can only be (a) a literal string or (b) the C string returned by the function call `myString.c_str()`, where `myString` is of type `string`.

4. When you open a data file for input, make sure that the argument to the `open` function supplies the correct name of the file as it exists on disk.

5. When reading a character string into a `string` object, the `>>` operator stops at, *but does not consume,* the first trailing whitespace character.

6. Be sure that each input statement specifies the correct number of variables and that each of those variables is of the correct data type.

7. If your input data is mixed (character and numeric values), be sure to deal with intervening blanks.

8. Echo print the input data to verify that each value is where it belongs and is in the proper format. (This is crucial, because an input failure in C++ doesn't produce an error message or terminate the program.)

Summary

Programs operate on data. If data and programs are kept separate, the data is available to use with other programs, and the same program can be run with different sets of input data.

The extraction operator (`>>`) inputs data from the keyboard or a file, storing the data into the variable specified as its right-hand operand. The extraction operator skips any leading whitespace characters to find the next data value in the input stream. The `get` function does not skip leading whitespace characters; it inputs the very next character and stores it into the `char` variable specified in its argument list. Both the `>>` operator and the `get` function leave the reading marker positioned at the next character to be read. The next input operation begins reading at the point indicated by the marker.

The newline character (denoted by `\n` in a C++ program) marks the end of a data line. You create a newline character each time you press the Return or Enter key. Your program generates a newline each time you use the `endl` manipulator or explicitly output the `\n` character. Newline is a control character; it does not print. It controls the movement of the screen cursor or the position of a line on a printer.

Interactive programs prompt the user for each data entry and directly inform the user of results and errors. Designing interactive dialogue is an exercise in the art of communication.

Noninteractive input/output allows data to be prepared before a program is run and allows the program to run again with the same data in the event that a problem crops up during processing.

Data files often are used for noninteractive processing and to permit the output from one program to be used as input to another program. To use these files, you must do four things: (1) include the header file `fstream`, (2) declare the file streams along with your other variable declarations, (3) prepare the files for reading or writing by calling the `open` function, and (4) specify the name of the file stream in each input or output statement that uses it.

Object-oriented design and functional decomposition are methodologies for tackling nontrivial programming problems. Object-oriented design produces a problem solution by focusing on objects and their associated operations. The first step is to identify the major objects in the problem and choose appropriate operations on those objects. An object is an instance of a data type called a class. During object-oriented design, classes can be designed from scratch, obtained from class libraries and used as is, or customized from existing classes by using the technique of inheritance. The result of the design process is a program consisting of self-contained objects that manage their own data and communicate by invoking each other's operations.

Functional decomposition begins with an abstract solution that then is divided into major steps. Each step becomes a subproblem that is analyzed and subdivided further. A concrete step is one that can be translated directly into C++; those steps that need more refining are abstract steps. A module is a collection of concrete and abstract steps that solves a subproblem. Programs can be built out of modules using a flat implementation, a hierarchical implementation, or a semihierarchical implementation.

Careful attention to program design, program formatting, and documentation produces highly structured and readable programs.

Quick Check

1. Write a C++ statement that inputs values from the standard input stream into two `float` variables, x and y. (pp. 155–158)
2. Your program is reading from the standard input stream. The next three characters waiting in the stream are a blank, a blank, and the letter *A*. Indicate what character is stored into the `char` variable ch by each of the following statements. (Assume the same initial stream contents for each.)

   a. `cin >> ch;`
   b. `cin.get(ch);`

   (pp. 158–162)
3. An input line contains a person's first, middle, and last names, separated by spaces. To read the entire name into a single `string` variable, which is appropriate: the >> operator or the `getline` function? (pp. 163–165)

4. Input prompts should acknowledge the user's experience.
   a. What sort of message would you have a program print to prompt a novice user to input a Social Security number?
   b. How would you change the wording of the prompting message for an experienced user? (pp. 165–166)
5. If a program is going to input 1000 numbers, is interactive input appropriate? (p. 167)
6. What four things must you remember to do in order to use data files in a C++ program? (pp. 168–171)
7. How many levels of abstraction are there in a functional decomposition before you reach the point at which you can begin coding a program? (pp. 181–191)
8. When is a flat implementation of a functional decomposition appropriate? (pp. 185–191)
9. Modules are the building blocks of functional decomposition. What are the building blocks of object-oriented design? (pp. 177–182)

Answers **1.** cin >> x >> y; **2.** a. 'A' b. ' ' (a blank) **3.** The getline function **4.** a. Please type a nine-digit Social Security number, then press the key marked Enter. b. Enter SSN. **5.** No. Batch input is more appropriate for programs that input large amounts of data. **6.** (1) Include the header file fstream. (2) Declare the file streams along with your other variable declarations. (3) Call the open function to prepare each file for reading or writing. (4) Specify the name of the file stream in each I/O statement that uses it. **7.** There is no fixed number of levels of abstraction. You keep refining the solution through as many levels as necessary until the steps are all concrete. **8.** A flat implementation is appropriate when a design is short and has just one or two levels of abstraction. **9.** The building blocks are objects, each of which has associated operations.

Exam Preparation Exercises

1. What is the main advantage of having a program input its data rather than writing all the data values as constants in the program?
2. Given these two lines of data:

```
17 13
7 3 24 6
```

and this input statement:

```
cin >> int1 >> int2 >> int3;
```

   a. What is the value of each variable after the statement is executed?
   b. What happens to any leftover data values in the input stream?
3. The newline character signals the end of a line.
   a. How do you generate a newline character when typing input data at the keyboard?
   b. How do you generate a newline character in a program's output?
4. When reading char data from an input stream, what is the difference between using the >> operator and using the get function?
5. Integer values can be read from the input data into float variables. (True or False?)

6. You may use either spaces or newlines to separate numeric data values being entered into a C++ program. (True or False?)
7. Consider this input data:

```
14  21  64
19  67  91
73  89  27
23  96  47
```

What are the values of the int variables a, b, c, and d after the following program segment is executed?

```
cin >> a;
cin.ignore(200, '\n');
cin >> b >> c;
cin.ignore(200, '\n');
cin >> d;
```

8. Given the input data

```
123W 56
```

what is printed by the output statement when the following code segment is executed?

```
int1 = 98;
int2 = 147;
cin >> int1 >> int2;
cout << int1 << ' ' << int2;
```

9. Given the input data

```
11 12.35 ABC
```

what is the value of each variable after the following statements are executed? Assume that i is of type int, x is of type float, and ch1 is of type char.
a. cin >> i >> x >> ch1 >> ch1;
b. cin >> ch1 >> i >> x;

10. Consider the input data

```
40 Tall Pine Drive
Sudbury, MA 01776
```

and the program code

```
string address;

cin >> address;
```

After the code is executed,
a. what string is contained in address?
b. where is the reading marker positioned?

11. Answer Exercise 10 again, replacing the input statement with

```
getline(cin, address);
```

12. Define the following terms as they apply to interactive input/output.
    a. Input prompt
    b. Echo printing
13. Correct the following program so that it reads a value from the file stream inData and writes it to the file stream outData.

```
#include <iostream>

using namespace std;

int main()
{
    int      n;
    ifstream inData;

    outData.open("results.dat");
    cin >> n;
    outData << n << endl;
    return 0;
}
```

14. Use your corrected version of the program in Exercise 13 to answer the following questions.
    a. If the file stream inData initially contains the value 144, what does it contain after the program is executed?
    b. If the file stream outData is initially empty, what are its contents after the program is executed?
15. List three characteristics of programs that are designed using a highly organized methodology such as functional decomposition or object-oriented design.
16. The get and ignore functions are member functions of the istream class. (True or False?)
17. The find and substr functions are member functions of the string class. (True or False?)
18. The getline function is a member function of the string class. (True or False?)

Programming Warm-up Exercises

1. Your program has three char variables: ch1, ch2, and ch3. Given the input data

    A B C\n

    write the input statement(s) required to store the *A* into ch1, the *B* into ch2, and the *C* into ch3. Note that each pair of input characters is separated by two blanks.
2. Change your answer to Exercise 1 so that the *A* is stored into ch1 and the next two blanks are stored into ch2 and ch3.

3. Write a single input statement that reads the input lines

```
10.25    7.625\n
8.5\n
1.0\n
```

and stores the four values into the float variables length1, height1, length2, and height2.

4. Write a series of statements that input the first letter of each of the following names into the char variables chr1, chr2, and chr3.

```
Peter\n
Kitty\n
Kathy\n
```

5. Write a set of variable declarations and a series of input statements to read the following lines of data into variables of the appropriate type. You can make up the variable names. Notice that the values are separated from one another by a single blank and that there are no blanks to the left of the first character on each line.

```
A 100 2.78 g 14\n
207.98 w q 23.4 92\n
R 42 L 27 R 63\n
```

6. Write a program segment that reads nine integer values from a file and writes them to the screen, three numbers per output line. The file is organized one value to a line.

7. Write a code segment for an interactive program to input values for a person's age, height, and weight and the initials of his or her first and last names. The numeric values are all integers. Assume that the person using the program is a novice user. How would you rewrite the code for an experienced user?

8. Fill in the blanks in the following program, which should read four values from the file stream dataIn and output them to the file stream resultsOut.

```
#include _____
#include _____
using _____
int main()
{
    int             val1;
    int             val2;
    int             val3;
    int             val4;
    _____     dataIn;
    ofstream        _____;
    _____ ("myinput.dat");
    _____ ("myoutput.dat");
    _____ >> val1 >> val2 >> val3 >> val4;
    _____ << val1 << val2 << val3 << val4 << endl;
    return 0;
}
```

9. Modify the program in Exercise 8 so that the name of the input file is prompted for and read in from the user at run time instead of being specified as a literal string.
10. Use functional decomposition to write an algorithm for starting the engine of an automobile with a manual transmission.
11. Use functional decomposition to write an algorithm for logging on to your computer system and entering and running a program. The algorithm should be simple enough for a novice user to follow.
12 The quadratic formula is

$$x = \frac{-b \pm \sqrt{b^2 - 4ac}}{2a}$$

Use functional decomposition to write an algorithm to read the three coefficients of a quadratic polynomial from a file (inQuad) and write the two floating-point solutions to another file (outQuad). Assume that the discriminant (the portion of the formula inside the square root) is nonnegative. You may use the standard library function sqrt. (Express your solution as pseudocode, not as a C++ program.)

Programming Problems

1. Write a functional decomposition and a C++ program to read an invoice number, quantity ordered, and unit price (all integers) and compute the total price. The program should write out the invoice number, quantity, unit price, and total price with identifying phrases. Format your program with consistent indentation, and use appropriate comments and meaningful identifiers. Write the program to be run interactively, with informative prompts for each data value.
2 How tall is a rainbow? Because of the way in which light is refracted by water droplets, the angle between the level of your eye and the top of a rainbow is always the same. If you know the distance to the rainbow, you can multiply it by the tangent of that angle to find the height of the rainbow. The magic angle is 42.3333333 degrees. The C++ standard library works in radians, however, so you have to convert the angle to radians with this formula:

$$radians = degrees \times \frac{\pi}{180}$$

where π equals 3.14159265.

Through the header file `cmath`, the C++ standard library provides a tangent function named `tan`. This is a value-returning function that takes a floating-point argument and returns a floating-point result:

```
x = tan(someAngle);
```

If you multiply the tangent by the distance to the rainbow, you get the height of the rainbow.

Write a functional decomposition and a C++ program to read a single floating-point value—the distance to the rainbow—and compute the height of the rainbow. The program should print the distance to the rainbow and its height, with phrases that identify which number is which. Display the floating-point values to four decimal places. Format your program with consistent indentation, and use appropriate comments and meaningful identifiers. Write the program so that it prompts the user for the input value.

3. Sometimes you can see a second, fainter rainbow outside a bright rainbow. This second rainbow has a magic angle of 52.25 degrees. Modify the program in Problem 2 so that it prints the height of the main rainbow, the height of the secondary rainbow, and the distance to the main rainbow, with a phrase identifying each of the numbers.

4. Write a program that reads a person's name in the format First Middle Last and then prints each of the names on a separate line. Following the last name, the program should print the initials for the name. For example, given the input `James Tiberius Kirk`, the program should output

```
James
Tiberius
Kirk
JTK
```

Assume that the first name begins in the first position on a line (there are no leading blanks) and that the names are separated from each other by a single blank.

Case Study Follow-Up

1. In the Canvas problem, look at the module structure chart and identify each level 1 module as an input module, a computational module, or an output module.

2. Redraw the module structure chart for the Canvas program so that level 1 contains modules named Get Data, Compute Values, and Print Results. Decide whether each of the level 1 modules in the original module structure chart corresponds directly to one of the three new modules or if it fits best as a level 2 module under one of the three. In the latter case, add the level 2 modules to the new module structure chart in the appropriate places.

3. Modify the Canvas program so that it reads the input data from a file rather than the keyboard. At run time, prompt the user for the name of the file containing the data.

5

Conditions, Logical Expressions, and Selection Control Structures

GOALS

- To be able to construct a simple logical (Boolean) expression to evaluate a given condition.
- To be able to construct a complex logical expression to evaluate a given condition.
- To be able to construct an If-Then-Else statement to perform a specific task.
- To be able to construct an If-Then statement to perform a specific task.
- To be able to construct a set of nested If statements to perform a specific task.
- To be able to determine the precondition and postcondition for a module and to use them to perform an algorithm walk-through.
- To be able to trace the execution of a C++ program.
- To be able to test and debug a C++ program.

So far, the statements in our programs have been executed in their physical order. The first statement is executed, then the second, and so on until all of the statements have been executed. But what if we want the computer to execute the statements in some other order? Suppose we want to check the validity of input data and then perform a calculation *or* print an error message, not both. To do so, we must be able to ask a question and then, based on the answer, choose one or another course of action.

The If statement allows us to execute statements in an order that is different from their physical order. We can ask a question with it and do one thing if the answer is yes (true) or another if the answer is no (false). In the first part of this chapter, we deal with asking questions; in the second part, we deal with the If statement itself.

Flow of Control

The order in which statements are executed in a program is called the **flow of control.** In a sense, the computer is under the control of one statement at a time. When a statement has been executed, control is turned over to the next statement (like a baton being passed in a relay race).

Flow of control   The order in which the computer executes statements in a program.

Flow of control is normally sequential (see Figure 5-1). That is, when one statement is finished executing, control passes to the next statement in the program. When we want the flow of control to be nonsequential, we

FIGURE 5-1
Sequential Control

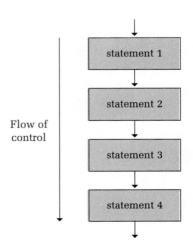

Flow of
control

use **control structures,** special statements that transfer control to a statement other than the one that physically comes next. Control structures are so important that we focus on them in the remainder of this chapter and in the next four chapters.

Control structure A statement used to alter the normally sequential flow of control.

Selection

We use a selection (or branching) control structure when we want the computer to choose between alternative actions. We make an assertion, a claim that is either true or false. If the assertion is true, the computer executes one statement. If it is false, it executes another (see Figure 5-2). The computer's ability to solve practical problems is a product of its ability to make decisions and execute different sequences of instructions.

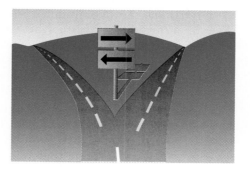

The Payroll program in Chapter 1 shows the selection process at work. The computer must decide whether or not a worker has earned overtime pay. It does this by testing the assertion that the person has worked more

FIGURE 5-2
Selection
(Branching)
Control Structure

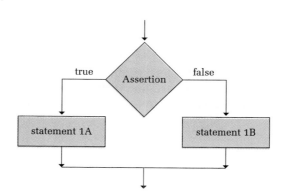

than 40 hours. If the assertion is true, the computer follows the instructions for computing overtime pay. If the assertion is false, the computer simply computes the regular pay. Before we examine selection control structures in C++, let's look closely at how we get the computer to make decisions.

Conditions and Logical Expressions

To ask a question in C++, we don't phrase it as a question; we state it as an assertion. If the assertion we make is true, the answer to the question is yes. If the statement is not true, the answer to the question is no. For example, if we want to ask, "Are we having spinach for dinner tonight?" we would say, "We are having spinach for dinner tonight." If the assertion is true, the answer to the question is yes. If not, the answer is no.

So, asking questions in C++ means making an assertion that is either true or false. The computer *evaluates* the assertion, checking it against some internal condition (the values stored in certain variables, for instance) to see whether it is true or false.

The `bool` Data Type

In C++, the `bool` data type is a built-in type consisting of just two values, the constants `true` and `false`. The reserved word `bool` is short for Boolean (pronounced 'BOOL-ē-un).* Boolean data is used for testing conditions in a program so that the computer can make decisions (with a selection control structure).

We declare variables of type `bool` the same way we declare variables of other types, that is, by writing the name of the data type and then an identifier:

```
bool dataOK;     // True if the input data is valid
bool done;       // True if the process is done
bool taxable;    // True if the item has sales tax
```

Each variable of type `bool` can contain one of two values: `true` or `false`. It's important to understand right from the beginning that `true` and `false` are not variable names and they are not strings. They are special constants in C++ and, in fact, are reserved words.

---

* The word *Boolean* is a tribute to George Boole, a nineteenth-century English mathematician who described a system of logic using variables with just two values, True and False. (See the May We Introduce box on page 224)

BACKGROUND INFORMATION

Before the bool *Type*

The C language does not have a `bool` data type, and prior to the ISO/ANSI C++ language standard, neither did C++. In C and pre–standard C++, the value 0 represents *false*, and any nonzero value represents *true*. In these languages, it is customary to use the `int` type to represent Boolean data:

```
int dataOK;
    ⋮
dataOK = 1;    // Store "true" into dataOK
    ⋮
dataOK = 0;    // Store "false" into dataOK
```

To make the code more self-documenting, many C and pre–standard C++ programmers prefer to define their own Boolean data type by using a *Typedef statement*. This statement allows you to introduce a new name for an existing data type:

```
typedef int bool;
```

All this statement does is tell the compiler to substitute the word `int` for every occurrence of the word `bool` in the rest of the program. Thus, when the compiler encounters a statement such as

```
bool dataOK;
```

it translates the statement into

```
int dataOK;
```

With the Typedef statement and declarations of two named constants, `true` and `false`, the code at the beginning of this discussion becomes the following:

```
typedef int bool;
const int true = 1;
const int false = 0;
    ⋮
bool dataOK;
    ⋮
dataOK = true;
    ⋮
dataOK = false;
```

With standard C++, none of this is necessary because `bool` is a built-in type. If you are working with pre-standard C++, see Section D.4 of Appendix D for more information about defining your own `bool` type so that you can work with the programs in this book.

Logical Expressions

In programming languages, assertions take the form of *logical expressions* (also called *Boolean expressions*). Just as an arithmetic expression is made up of numeric values and operations, a logical expression is made up of logical values and operations. Every logical expression has one of two values: true or false.

Here are some examples of logical expressions:

- A Boolean variable or constant
- An expression followed by a relational operator followed by an expression
- A logical expression followed by a logical operator followed by a logical expression

Let's look at each of these in detail.

Boolean Variables and Constants As we have seen, a Boolean variable is a variable declared to be of type `bool`, and it can contain either the value `true` or the value `false`. For example, if `dataOK` is a Boolean variable, then

```
dataOK = true;
```

is a valid assignment statement.

Relational Operators Another way of assigning a value to a Boolean variable is to set it equal to the result of comparing two expressions with a *relational operator*. Relational operators test a relationship between two values.

Let's look at an example. In the following program fragment, `lessThan` is a Boolean variable and `i` and `j` are `int` variables:

```
cin >> i >> j;
lessThan = (i < j);   // Compare i and j with the "less than"
                      // relational operator, and assign the
                      // truth value to lessThan
```

By comparing two values, we assert that a relationship (like "less than") exists between them. If the relationship does exist, the assertion is true; if not, it is false. These are the relationships we can test for in C++:

Operator Relationship Tested

==	Equal to
!=	Not equal to
>	Greater than
<	Less than
>=	Greater than or equal to
<=	Less than or equal to

An expression followed by a relational operator followed by an expression is called a *relational expression.* The result of a relational expression is of type bool. For example, if x is 5 and y is 10, the following expressions all have the value true:

```
x != y
y > x
x < y
y >= x
x <= y
```

If x is the character 'M' and y is 'R', the values of the expressions are still true because the relational operator <, used with letters, means "comes before in the alphabet," or, more properly, "comes before in the collating sequence of the character set." For example, in the widely used ASCII character set, all of the uppercase letters are in alphabetical order, as are the lowercase letters, but all of the uppercase letters come before the lowercase letters. So

```
'M' < 'R'
```

and

```
'm' < 'r'
```

have the value true, but

```
'm' < 'R'
```

has the value false.

Of course, we have to be careful about the data types of things we compare. The safest approach is to always compare ints with ints, floats with floats, chars with chars, and so on. If you mix data types in a comparison, implicit type coercion takes place just as in arithmetic expressions. If an int value and a float value are compared, the computer temporarily coerces the int value to its float equivalent before making the comparison. As with arithmetic expressions, it's wise to use explicit type casting to make your intentions known:

```
someFloat >= float(someInt)
```

If you compare a bool value with a numeric value (probably by mistake), the value false is temporarily coerced to the number 0, and true is coerced to 1. Therefore, if boolVar is a bool variable, the expression

```
boolVar < 5
```

yields true because 0 and 1 both are less than 5.

Until you learn more about the char type in Chapter 10, be careful to compare char values only with other char values. For example, the comparisons

```
'0' < '9'
```

and

```
0 < 9
```

are appropriate, but

```
'0' < 9
```

generates an implicit type coercion and a result that probably isn't what you expect.

We can use relational operators not only to compare variables or constants, but also to compare the values of arithmetic expressions. In the following table, we compare the results of adding 3 to x and multiplying y by 10 for different values of x and y.

Value of x	Value of y	Expression	Result
12	2	x + 3 <= y * 10	true
20	2	x + 3 <= y * 10	false
7	1	x + 3 != y * 10	false
17	2	x + 3 == y * 10	true
100	5	x + 3 > y * 10	true

Caution: It's easy to confuse the assignment operator (=) and the == relational operator. These two operators have very different effects in a program. Some people pronounce the relational operator as "equals-equals" to remind themselves of the difference.

Comparing Strings   Recall from Chapter 4 that string is a class—a programmer-defined type from which you declare variables that are more commonly called objects. Contained within each string object is a character string. The string class is designed such that you can compare these strings using the relational operators. Syntactically, the operands of a relational operator can either be two string objects, as in

myString < yourString

or a string object and a C string:

myString >= "Johnson"

However, the operands cannot both be C strings.

Comparison of strings follows the collating sequence of the machine's character set (ASCII, for instance). When the computer tests a relationship between two strings, it begins with the first character of each, compares them according to the collating sequence, and if they are the same repeats the comparison with the next character in each string. The character-by-character test proceeds until either a mismatch is found or the final characters have been compared and are equal. If all their characters are equal, then the two strings are equal. If a mismatch is found, then the string with the character that comes before the other is the "lesser" string.

For example, given the statements

string word1;
string word2;

```
word1 = "Tremendous";
word2 = "Small";
```

the relational expressions in the following table have the indicated values.

Expression	Value	Reason
word1 == word2	false	They are unequal in the first character.
word1 > word2	true	'T' comes after 'S' in the collating sequence.
word1 < "Tremble"	false	Fifth characters don't match, and 'b' comes before 'e'.
word2 == "Small"	true	They are equal.
"cat" < "dog"	Unpredictable	The operands cannot both be C strings.*

*The expression is syntactically legal in C++ but results in a *pointer* comparison, not a string comparison. Pointers are not discussed until Chapter 15.

In most cases, the ordering of strings corresponds to alphabetical ordering. But when strings have mixed-case letters, we can get nonalphabetical results. For example, in a phone book we expect to see Macauley before MacPherson, but the ASCII collating sequence places all uppercase letters before the lowercase letters, so the string "MacPherson" compares as less than "Macauley". To compare strings for strict alphabetical ordering, all the characters must be in the same case. In a later chapter we show an algorithm for changing the case of a string.

If two strings with different lengths are compared and the comparison is equal up to the end of the shorter string, then the shorter string compares as less than the longer string. For example, if word2 contains "Small", the expression

```
word2 < "Smaller"
```

yields true, because the strings are equal up to their fifth character position (the end of the string on the left), and the string on the right is longer.

Logical Operators   In mathematics, the *logical* (or *Boolean*) *operators* AND, OR, and NOT take logical expressions as operands. C++ uses special symbols for the logical operators: && (for AND), || (for OR), and ! (for NOT). By combining relational operators with logical operators, we can make more complex assertions. For example, suppose we want to determine whether a final score is greater than 90 *and* a midterm score is greater than 70. In C++, we would write the expression this way:

```
finalScore > 90 && midtermScore > 70
```

The AND operation (`&&`) requires both relationships to be true in order for the overall result to be true. If either or both of the relationships are false, the entire result is false.

The OR operation (`||`) takes two logical expressions and combines them. If *either* or *both* are true, the result is true. Both values must be false for the result to be false. Now we can determine whether the midterm grade is an A *or* the final grade is an A. If either the midterm grade or the final grade equals A, the assertion is true. In C++, we write the expression like this:

```
midtermGrade == 'A' || finalGrade == 'A'
```

The `&&` and `||` operators always appear between two expressions; they are binary (two-operand) operators. The NOT operator (`!`) is a unary (one-operand) operator. It precedes a single logical expression and gives its opposite as the result. If (`grade == 'A'`) is false, then `!` (`grade == 'A'`) is true. NOT gives us a convenient way of reversing the meaning of an assertion. For example,

```
!(hours > 40)
```

is the equivalent of

```
hours <= 40
```

In some contexts, the first form is clearer; in others, the second makes more sense.

The following pairs of expressions are equivalent:

Expression	Equivalent Expression
`!(a == b)`	`a != b`
`!(a == b || a == c)`	`a != b && a != c`
`!(a == b && c > d)`	`a != b || c <= d`

Take a close look at these expressions to be sure you understand why they are equivalent. Try evaluating them with some values for a, b, c, and d. Notice the pattern: The expression on the left is just the one to its right with `!` added and the relational and logical operators reversed (for example, `==` instead of `!=` and `||` instead of `&&`). Remember this pattern. It allows you to rewrite expressions in the simplest form.*

---

* In Boolean algebra, the pattern is formalized by a theorem called *DeMorgan's law*.

Logical operators can be applied to the results of comparisons. They also can be applied directly to variables of type `bool`. For example, instead of writing

```
isElector = (age >= 18 && district == 23);
```

to assign a value to the Boolean variable `isElector`, we could use two intermediate Boolean variables, `isVoter` and `isConstituent`:

```
isVoter = (age >= 18);
isConstituent = (district == 23);
isElector = isVoter && isConstituent;
```

The two tables below summarize the results of applying `&&` and `||` to a pair of logical expressions (represented here by Boolean variables x and y).

Value of x	*Value of* y	*Value of* x `&&` y
true	true	true
true	false	false
false	true	false
false	false	false

Value of x	*Value of* y	*Value of* x `||` y
true	true	true
true	false	true
false	true	true
false	false	false

The following table summarizes the results of applying the `!` operator to a logical expression (represented by Boolean variable x).

Value of x	*Value of* !x
true	false
false	true

Technically, the C++ operators !, &&, and || are not required to have logical expressions as operands. Their operands can be of any simple data type, even floating-point types. If an operand is not of type `bool`, its value is temporarily coerced to type `bool` as follows: A 0 value is coerced to `false`, and any nonzero value is coerced to `true`. As an example, you sometimes encounter C++ code that looks like this:

```
float height;
bool   badData;
   :
cin >> height;
badData = !height;
```

The assignment statement says to set `badData` to `true` if the coerced value of `height` is `false`. That is, the statement really is saying, "Set `badData` to `true` if `height` equals 0.0." Although this assignment statement works correctly according to the C++ language, many programmers find the following statement to be more readable:

```
badData = (height == 0.0);
```

Throughout this text we apply the logical operators *only* to logical expressions, not to arithmetic expressions.

Caution: It's easy to confuse the logical operators && and || with two other C++ operators, & and |. We don't discuss the & and | operators here, but we'll tell you that they are used for manipulating individual bits within a memory cell—a role quite different from that of the logical operators. If you accidentally use & instead of &&, or | instead of ||, you won't get an error message from the compiler, but your program probably will compute wrong answers. Some programmers pronounce && as "and-and" and || as "or-or" to avoid making mistakes.

Short-Circuit Evaluation   Consider the logical expression

```
i == 1 && j > 2
```

Some programming languages use *full evaluation* of logical expressions. With full evaluation, the computer first evaluates both subexpressions (both i == 1 and j > 2) before applying the && operator to produce the final result.

In contrast, C++ uses **short-circuit (or conditional) evaluation** of logical expressions. Evaluation proceeds from left to right, and the computer stops evaluating subexpressions as soon as possible—that is, as soon as it knows the truth value of the entire expression. How can the computer know if a lengthy logical expression yields `true` or `false` if it doesn't examine all the subexpressions? Let's look first at the AND operation.

An AND operation yields the value `true` only if both of its operands are `true`. In the expression above, suppose that the value of i happens to be 95. The first subexpression yields `false`, so it isn't necessary even to look at the second subexpression. The computer stops evaluation and produces the final result of `false`.

Short-circuit (conditional) evaluation   Evaluation of a logical expression in left-to-right order with evaluation stopping as soon as the final truth value can be determined.

With the OR operation, the left-to-right evaluation stops as soon as a subexpression yielding `true` is found. Remember that an OR produces a result of `true` if either one or both of its operands are `true`. Given this expression:

```
c <= d || e == f
```

if the first subexpression is `true`, evaluation stops and the entire result is `true`. The computer doesn't waste time with an unnecessary evaluation of the second subexpression.

*M*AY WE INTRODUCE

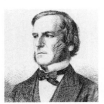

George Boole

Boolean algebra is named for its inventor, English mathematician George Boole, born in 1815. His father, a tradesman, began teaching him mathematics at an early age. But Boole initially was more interested in classical literature, languages, and religion— interests he maintained throughout his life. By the time he was 20, he had taught himself French, German, and Italian. He was well versed in the writings of Aristotle, Spinoza, Cicero, and Dante, and wrote several philosophical papers himself.

At 16, to help support his family, he took a position as a teaching assistant in a private school. His work there and a second teaching job left him little time to study. A few years later, he opened a school and began to learn higher mathematics on his own. In spite of his lack of formal training, his first scholarly paper was published in the *Cambridge Mathematical Journal* when he was just 24. Boole went on to publish over 50 papers and several major works before he died in 1864, at the peak of his career.

Boole's *The Mathematical Analysis of Logic* was published in 1847. It would eventually form the basis for the development of digital computers. In the book, Boole set forth the formal axioms of logic (much like the axioms of geometry) on which the field of symbolic logic is built.

Boole drew on the symbols and operations of algebra in creating his system of logic. He associated the value 1 with the universal set (the set representing everything in the universe) and the value 0 with the empty set, and restricted his system to these two quantities. He then defined operations that are analogous to subtraction, addition, and multiplication. Variables in the system have symbolic values. For example, if a Boolean variable *P* represents the set of all plants, then the expression 1 − *P* refers to the set of all things that are not plants. We can simplify the expression by using −*P* to mean "*not* plants." (0 − *P* is simply 0 because we can't remove elements from the empty set.) The subtraction operator in Boole's system corresponds to the ! (NOT) operator in C++. In a C++ program, we might set the value of the Boolean variable plant to true when the name of a plant is entered, whereas !plant is true when the name of anything else is input.

The expression 0 + *P* is the same as *P*. However, 0 + *P* + *F*, where *F* is the set of all foods, is the set of all things that are either plants or foods. So the addition operator in Boole's algebra is the same as the C++ || (OR) operator.

The analogy can be carried to multiplication: 0 × *P* is 0, and 1 × *P* is *P*. But what is *P* × *F*? It is the set of things that are both plants and foods. In Boole's system, the multiplication operator is the same as the && (AND) operator.

In 1854, Boole published *An Investigation of the Laws of Thought, on Which Are Founded the Mathematical Theories of Logic and Probabilities*. In the book, he described theorems built on his axioms of logic and extended the algebra to show how probabilities could be computed in a logical system. Five years later, Boole published *Treatise on Differential Equations*, then *Treatise on the Calculus of Finite Differences*. The latter is one of the cornerstones of numerical analysis, which deals with the accuracy of computations. (In Chapter 10, we examine the important role numerical analysis plays in computer programming.)

Boole received little recognition and few honors for his work. Given the importance of Boolean algebra in modern technology, it is hard to believe that his system of logic was not taken seriously until the early twentieth century. George Boole was truly one of the founders of computer science.

Precedence of Operators

In Chapter 3, we discussed the rules of precedence, the rules that govern the evaluation of complex arithmetic expressions. C++'s rules of precedence also govern relational and logical operators. Here's a list showing the order of precedence for the arithmetic, relational, and logical operators (with the assignment operator thrown in as well):

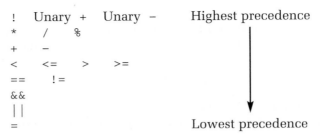

```
!    Unary +   Unary -        Highest precedence
*    /    %
+    -
<    <=    >    >=
==    !=
&&
||
=                              Lowest precedence
```

Operators on the same line in the list have the same precedence. If an expression contains several operators with the same precedence, most of the operators group (or *associate*) from left to right. For example, the expression

```
a / b * c
```

means (a / b) * c, not a / (b * c). However, the unary operators (!, unary +, unary -) group from right to left. Although you'd never have occasion to use this expression:

```
!!badData
```

the meaning of it is !(!badData) rather than the meaningless (!!)badData. Appendix B, "Precedence of Operators," lists the order of precedence for all operators in C++. In skimming the appendix, you can see that a few of the operators associate from right to left (for the same reason we just described for the ! operator).

Parentheses are used to override the order of evaluation in an expression. If you're not sure whether parentheses are necessary, use them anyway. The compiler disregards unnecessary parentheses. So if they clarify an expression, use them. Some programmers like to include extra parentheses when assigning a relational expression to a Boolean variable:

```
dataInvalid = (inputVal == 0);
```

The parentheses are not needed; the assignment operator has the lowest precedence of all the operators we've just listed. So we could write the statement as

```
dataInvalid = inputVal == 0;
```

but some people find the parenthesized version more readable.

One final comment about parentheses: C++, like other programming languages, requires that parentheses always be used in pairs. Whenever you write a complicated expression, take a minute to go through and pair up all of the opening parentheses with their closing counterparts.

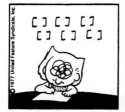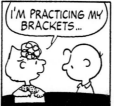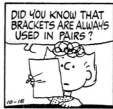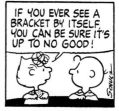

PEANUTS reprinted by permission of United Features Syndicate, Inc.

SOFTWARE ENGINEERING TIP

Changing English Statements into Logical Expressions

In most cases, you can write a logical expression directly from an English statement or mathematical term in an algorithm. But you have to watch out for some tricky situations. Remember our sample logical expression:

```
midtermGrade == 'A' || finalGrade == 'A'
```

In English, you would be tempted to write this expression: "Midterm grade or final grade equals A." In C++, you can't write the expression as you would in English. That is,

```
midtermGrade || finalGrade == 'A'
```

won't work because the || operator is connecting a char value (midtermGrade) and a logical expression (finalGrade == 'A'). The two operands of || should be logical expressions. (Note that this expression is wrong in terms of logic, but it isn't "wrong" to the C++ compiler. Recall that the || operator may legally connect two expressions of any data type, so this example won't generate a syntax error message. The program will run, but it won't work the way you intended.)

A variation of this mistake is to express the English assertion "*i* equals either 3 or 4" as

```
i == 3 || 4
```

Again, the syntax is correct but the semantics are not. This expression always evaluates to true. The first subexpression, i == 3, may be true or false. But the second subexpression, 4, is nonzero and therefore is coerced to the value true. Thus, the || operation causes the entire expression to be true. We repeat: Use the || operator (and the && operator) only to connect two logical expressions. Here's what we want:

```
i == 3 || i == 4
```

In math books, you might see a notation like this:

$$12 < y < 24$$

which means "*y* is between 12 and 24." This expression is legal in C++ but gives an unexpected result. First, the relation $12 < y$ is evaluated, giving the result `true` or `false`. The computer then coerces this result to 1 or 0 in order to compare it with the number 24. Because both 1 and 0 are less than 24, the result is always `true`. To write this expression correctly in C++, you must use the `&&` operator as follows:

```
12 < y && y < 24
```

Relational Operators with Floating-Point Types

So far, we've talked only about comparing `int`, `char`, and `string` values. Here we look at `float` values.

Do not compare floating-point numbers for equality. Because small errors in the rightmost decimal places are likely to arise when calculations are performed on floating-point numbers, two `float` values rarely are exactly equal. For example, consider the following code that uses two `float` variables named `oneThird` and `x`:

```
oneThird = 1.0 / 3.0;
x = oneThird + oneThird + oneThird;
```

We would expect `x` to contain the value 1.0, but it probably doesn't. The first assignment statement stores an *approximation* of 1/3 into `oneThird`, perhaps 0.333333. The second statement stores a value like 0.999999 into `x`. If we now ask the computer to compare `x` with 1.0, the comparison yields `false`.

Instead of testing floating-point numbers for equality, we test for *near* equality. To do so, we compute the difference between the two numbers and test to see if the result is less than some maximum allowable difference. For example, we often use comparisons like this:

```
fabs(r - s) < 0.00001
```

where `fabs` is the floating-point absolute value function from the C++ standard library. The expression `fabs(r - s)` computes the absolute value of the difference between two `float` variables `r` and `s`. If the difference is less than 0.00001, the two numbers are close enough to call them equal. We discuss this problem with floating-point accuracy in more detail in Chapter 10.

The If Statement

Now that we've seen how to write logical expressions, let's use them to alter the normal flow of control in a program. The *If statement* is the fundamental control structure that allows branches in the flow of control. With it, we can ask a question and choose a course of action: *If* a certain condition exists, *then* perform one action, *else* perform a different action.

At run time, the computer performs just one of the two actions, depending on the result of the condition being tested. Yet we must include the code for *both* actions in the program. Why? Because, depending on the circumstances, the computer can choose to execute *either* of them. The If statement gives us a way of including both actions in a program and gives the computer a way of deciding which action to take.

The If-Then-Else Form

In C++, the If statement comes in two forms: the *If-Then-Else* form and the *If-Then* form. Let's look first at the If-Then-Else. Here is its syntax template:

IfStatement (the If-Then-Else form)

```
if ( Expression )
    Statement1A
else
    Statement1B
```

The expression in parentheses can be of any simple data type. Almost without exception, this will be a logical (Boolean) expression; if not, its value is implicitly coerced to type `bool`. At run time, the computer evaluates the expression. If the value is `true`, the computer executes Statement1A. If the value of the expression is `false`, Statement1B is executed. Statement1A often is called the *then-clause;* Statement1B, the *else-clause*. Figure 5-3 illustrates the flow of control of the If-Then-Else. In the figure, Statement2 is the next statement in the program after the entire If statement.

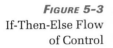

FIGURE 5-3

If-Then-Else Flow
of Control

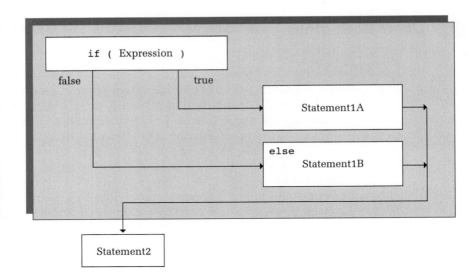

Notice that a C++ If statement uses the reserved words `if` and `else` but does not include the word *then*. Still, we use the term *If-Then-Else* because it corresponds to how we say things in English: "*If* something is true, *then* do this, *else* do that."

The code fragment below shows how to write an If statement in a program. Observe the indentation of the then-clause and the else-clause, which makes the statement easier to read. And notice the placement of the statement following the If statement.

```
if (hours <= 40.0)
    pay = rate * hours;
else
    pay = rate * (40.0 + (hours - 40.0) * 1.5);
cout << pay;
```

In terms of instructions to the computer, the above code fragment says, "If `hours` is less than or equal to 40.0, compute the regular pay and then go on to execute the output statement. But if `hours` is greater than 40, compute the regular pay and the overtime pay, and then go on to execute the output statement." Figure 5-4 shows the flow of control of this If statement.

If-Then-Else often is used to check the validity of input. For example, before we ask the computer to divide by a data value, we should be sure that the value is not zero. (Even computers can't divide something by zero. If you try, most computers halt the execution of your program.) If the divisor is zero, our program should print out an error message. Here's the code:

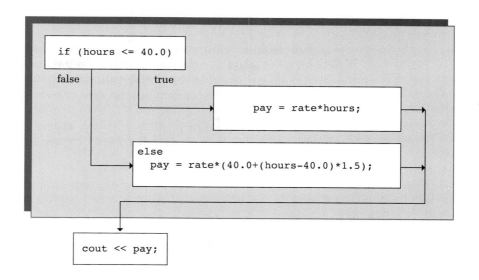

FIGURE 5-4
Flow of Control for
Calculating Pay

```
if (divisor != 0)
    result = dividend / divisor;
else
    cout << "Division by zero is not allowed." << endl;
```

As another example of an If-Then-Else, suppose we want to determine where in a string variable the first occurrence (if any) of the letter *A* is located. Recall from Chapter 3 that the string class has a member function named find, which returns the position where the item was found (or the named constant string::npos if the item wasn't found). The following code outputs the result of the search:

```
string myString;
string::size_type pos;
        ⋮
pos = myString.find('A');
if (pos == string::npos)
    cout << "No 'A' was found" << endl;
else
    cout << "An 'A' was found in position " << pos << endl;
```

Before we look any further at If statements, take another look at the syntax template for the If-Then-Else. According to the template, there is no semicolon at the end of an If statement. In all of the program fragments above—the worker's pay, division-by-zero, and string search examples—there seems to be a semicolon at the end of each If statement. However, the semicolons belong to the statements in the else-clauses in those examples; assignment statements end in semicolons, as do output statements. The If statement doesn't have its own semicolon at the end.

Blocks (Compound Statements)

In our division-by-zero example, suppose that when the divisor is equal to zero we want to do *two* things: print the error message *and* set the variable named `result` equal to a special value like 9999. We would need two statements in the same branch, but the syntax template seems to limit us to one.

What we really want to do is turn the else-clause into a *sequence* of statements. This is easy. Remember from Chapter 2 that the compiler treats the block (compound statement)

```
{
    ⋮
}
```

like a single statement. If you put a { } pair around the sequence of statements you want in a branch of the If statement, the sequence of statements becomes a single block. For example:

```
if (divisor != 0)
    result = dividend / divisor;
else
{
    cout << "Division by zero is not allowed." << endl;
    result = 9999;
}
```

If the value of `divisor` is 0, the computer both prints the error message and sets the value of `result` to 9999 before continuing with whatever statement follows the If statement.

Blocks can be used in both branches of an If-Then-Else. For example:

```
if (divisor != 0)
{
    result = dividend / divisor;
    cout << "Division performed." << endl;
}
else
{
    cout << "Division by zero is not allowed." << endl;
    result = 9999;
}
```

When you use blocks in an If statement, there's a rule of C++ syntax to remember: *Never use a semicolon after the right brace of a block.* Semicolons are used only to terminate simple statements such as assignment statements, input statements, and output statements. If you look at the examples above, you won't see a semicolon after the right brace that signals the end of each block.

MATTERS OF STYLE

Braces and Blocks

C++ programmers use different styles when it comes to locating the left brace of a block. The style we use puts the left and right braces directly below the words `if` and `else`, each brace on its own line:

```
if (n >= 2)
{
    alpha = 5;
    beta = 8;
}
else
{
    alpha = 23;
    beta = 12;
}
```

Another popular style is to place the left braces at the end of the `if` line and the `else` line; the right braces still line up directly below the words `if` and `else`. This way of formatting the If statement originated with programmers using the C language, the predecessor of C++.

```
if (n >= 2) {
    alpha = 5;
    beta = 8;
}
else {
    alpha = 23;
    beta = 12;
}
```

It makes no difference to the C++ compiler which style you use (and there are other styles as well). It's a matter of personal preference. Whichever style you use, though, you should always use the same style throughout a program. Inconsistency can confuse the person reading your program and give the impression of carelessness.

The If-Then Form

Sometimes you run into a situation where you want to say, "*If* a certain condition exists, *then* perform some action; otherwise, don't do anything." In other words, you want the computer to skip a sequence of instructions if a certain condition isn't met. You could do this by leaving the else branch empty, using only the null statement:

```
if (a <= b)
    c = 20;
else
    ;
```

Better yet, you can simply leave off the else part. The resulting statement is the If-Then form of the If statement. This is its syntax template:

IfStatement (the If-Then form)

```
if ( Expression )
    Statement
```

Here's an example of an If-Then. Notice the indentation and the placement of the statement that follows the If-Then.

```
if (age < 18)
    cout << "Not an eligible ";
cout << "voter." << endl;
```

This statement means that if age is less than 18, first print "Not an eligible " and then print "voter." If age is not less than 18, skip the first output statement and go directly to print "voter." Figure 5-5 shows the flow of control for an If-Then.

Like the two branches in an If-Then-Else, the one branch in an If-Then can be a block. For example, let's say you are writing a program to compute income taxes. One of the lines on the tax form reads "Subtract line 23 from line 17 and enter result on line 24; if result is less than zero, enter zero and check box 24A." You can use an If-Then to do this in C++:

```
result = line17 - line23;
if (result < 0.0)
{
    cout << "Check box 24A" << endl;
    result = 0.0;
}
line24 = result;
```

FIGURE 5-5

If-Then Flow of
Control

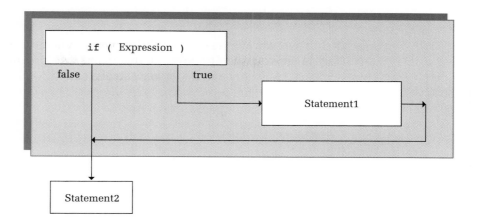

This code does exactly what the tax form says it should. It computes the result of subtracting line 23 from line 17. Then it looks to see if `result` is less than 0. If it is, the fragment prints a message telling the user to check box 24A and then sets `result` to 0. Finally, the calculated result (or 0, if the result is less than 0) is stored into a variable named `line24`.

What happens if we leave out the left and right braces in the code fragment above? Let's look at it:

```
result = line17 - line23;              // Incorrect version
if (result < 0.0)
    cout << "Check box 24A" << endl;
    result = 0.0;
line24 = result;
```

Despite the way we have indented the code, the compiler takes the then-clause to be a single statement—the output statement. If `result` is less than 0, the computer executes the output statement, then sets `result` to 0, and then stores `result` into `line24`. So far, so good. But if `result` is initially greater than or equal to 0, the computer skips the then-clause and proceeds to the statement following the If statement—the assignment statement that sets `result` to 0. The unhappy outcome is that `result` ends up as 0 no matter what its initial value was! The moral here is not to rely on indentation alone; you can't fool the compiler. If you want a compound statement for a then- or else-clause, you must include the left and right braces.

A Common Mistake

Earlier we warned against confusing the = operator and the == operator. Here is an example of a mistake that every C++ programmer is guaranteed to make at least once in his or her career:

```
cin >> n;
if (n = 3)                      // Wrong
    cout << "n equals 3";
else
    cout << "n doesn't equal 3";
```

This code segment *always* prints out

```
n equals 3
```

no matter what was input for n.

Here is the reason: We've used the wrong operator in the If test. The expression n = 3 is not a logical expression; it's called an *assignment expression*. (If an assignment is written as a separate statement ending with a semicolon, it's an assignment *statement*.) An assignment expression has a *value* (above, it's 3) and a *side effect* (storing 3 into n). In the If statement of our example, the computer finds the value of the tested expression to be 3. Because 3 is a nonzero value and thus is coerced to true, the then-clause is executed, no matter what the value of n is. Worse yet, the side effect of the assignment expression is to store 3 into n, destroying what was there.

Our intention is not to focus on assignment expressions; we discuss their use later in the book. What's important now is that you see the effect of using = when you meant to use ==. The program compiles correctly but runs incorrectly. When debugging a faulty program, always look at your If statements to see whether you've made this particular mistake.

Nested If Statements

There are no restrictions on what the statements in an If can be. Therefore, an If within an If is OK. In fact, an If within an If within an If is legal. The only limitation here is that people cannot follow a structure that is too involved, and readability is one of the marks of a good program.

When we place an If within an If, we are creating a *nested control structure*. Control structures nest much like mixing bowls do, with smaller ones tucked inside larger ones. Here's an example, written in pseudocode:

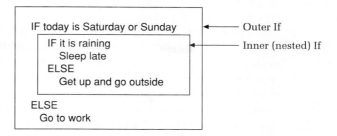

In general, any problem that involves a *multiway branch* (more than two alternative courses of action) can be coded using nested If statements. For example, to print out the name of a month given its number, we could use a sequence of If statements (unnested):

```
if (month == 1)
    cout << "January";
if (month == 2)
    cout << "February";
if (month == 3)
    cout << "March";
    ⋮
if (month == 12)
    cout << "December";
```

But the equivalent nested If structure,

```
if (month == 1)
    cout << "January";
else
    if (month == 2)              // Nested If
        cout << "February";
    else
        if (month == 3)              // Nested If
            cout << "March";
        else
            if (month == 4)              // Nested If
                ⋮
```

is more efficient because it makes fewer comparisons. The first version—the sequence of independent If statements—always tests every condition (all 12 of them), even if the first one is satisfied. In contrast, the nested If solution skips all remaining comparisons after one alternative has been selected. As fast as modern computers are, many applications require so much computation that inefficient algorithms can waste hours of computer time. Always be on the lookout for ways to make your programs more efficient, as long as doing so doesn't make them difficult for other programmers to understand. It's usually better to sacrifice a little efficiency for the sake of readability.

In the last example, notice how the indentation of the then- and else-clauses causes the statements to move continually the right. Instead, we can use a special indentation style with deeply nested If-Then-Else statements to indicate that the complex structure is just choosing one of a set of alternatives. This general multiway branch is known as an *If-Then-Else-If* control structure:

```
if (month == 1)
    cout << "January";
else if (month == 2)         // Nested If
    cout << "February";
else if (month == 3)         // Nested If
    cout << "March";
else if (month == 4)         // Nested If
    ⋮
else
    cout << "December";
```

This style prevents the indentation from marching continuously to the right. But, more important, it visually conveys the idea that we are using a 12-way branch based on the variable `month`.

It's important to note one difference between the sequence of If statements and the nested If: More than one alternative can be taken by the sequence of Ifs, but the nested If can select only one. To see why this is important, consider the analogy of filling out a questionnaire. Some questions are like a sequence of If statements, asking you to circle all the items in a list that apply to you (such as all your hobbies). Other questions ask you to circle only one item in a list (your age group, for example) and are thus like a nested If structure. Both kinds of questions occur in programming problems. Being able to recognize which type of question is being asked permits you to immediately select the appropriate control structure.

Another particularly helpful use of the nested If is when you want to select from a series of consecutive ranges of values. For example, suppose that we want to print out an appropriate activity for the outdoor temperature, given the following table.

Activity	Temperature
Swimming	Temperature > 85
Tennis	$70 < \text{temperature} \leq 85$
Golf	$32 < \text{temperature} \leq 70$
Skiing	$0 < \text{temperature} \leq 32$
Dancing	Temperature ≤ 0

At first glance, you may be tempted to write a separate If statement for each range of temperatures. On closer examination, however, it is clear that these If conditions are interdependent. That is, if one of the statements is executed, none of the others should be executed. We really are selecting one alternative from a set of possibilities—just the sort of situation in which we can use a nested If structure as a multiway branch. The only difference between this problem and our earlier example of printing the month name from its number is that we must check ranges of numbers in the If expressions of the branches.

When the ranges are consecutive, we can take advantage of that fact to make our code more efficient. We arrange the branches in consecutive order by range. Then, if a particular branch has been reached, we know that the preceding ranges have been eliminated from consideration. Thus, the If expressions must compare the temperature to only the lowest value of each range.

```
cout << "The recommended activity is ";
if (temperature > 85)
    cout << "swimming." << endl;
else if (temperature > 70)
    cout << "tennis." << endl;
else if (temperature > 32)
    cout << "golf." << endl;
else if (temperature > 0)
    cout << "skiing." << endl;
else
    cout << "dancing." << endl;
```

To see how this If-Then-Else-If structure works, consider the branch that tests for `temperature` greater than 70. If it has been reached, we know that `temperature` must be less than or equal to 85 because that condition causes this particular `else` branch to be taken. Thus, we only need to test whether `temperature` is above the bottom of this range (> 70). If that test fails, then we enter the next else-clause knowing that `temperature` must be less than or equal to 70. Each successive branch checks the bottom of its range until we reach the final `else`, which takes care of all the remaining possibilities.

Note that if the ranges aren't consecutive, then we must test the data value against both the highest and lowest value of each range. We still use an If-Then-Else-If because that is the best structure for selecting a single branch from multiple possibilities, and we may arrange the ranges in consecutive order to make them easier for a human reader to follow. But there is no way to reduce the number of comparisons when there are gaps between the ranges.

The Dangling `else`

When If statements are nested, you may find yourself confused about the `if-else` pairings. That is, to which `if` does an `else` belong? For example, suppose that if a student's average is below 60, we want to print "Failing"; if it is at least 60 but less than 70, we want to print "Passing but marginal"; and if it is 70 or greater, we don't want to print anything.

We code this information with an If-Then-Else nested within an If-Then:

```
if (average < 70.0)
    if (average < 60.0)
        cout << "Failing";
    else
        cout << "Passing but marginal";
```

How do we know to which `if` the `else` belongs? Here is the rule that the C++ compiler follows: In the absence of braces, an `else` is always paired with the closest preceding `if` that doesn't already have an `else` paired with it. We indented the code to reflect this pairing.

Suppose we write the fragment like this:

```
if (average >= 60.0)        // Incorrect version
    if (average < 70.0)
        cout << "Passing but marginal";
else
    cout << "Failing";
```

Here we want the `else` branch attached to the outer If statement, not the inner, so we indent the code as you see it. But indentation does not affect the execution of the code. Even though the `else` aligns with the first `if`, the compiler pairs it with the second `if`. An `else` that follows a nested If-Then is called a *dangling else*. It doesn't logically belong with the nested If but is attached to it by the compiler.

To attach the `else` to the first `if`, not the second, you can turn the outer then-clause into a block:

```
if (average >= 60.0)        // Correct version
{
    if (average < 70.0)
        cout << "Passing but marginal";
}
else
    cout << "Failing";
```

The { } pair indicates that the inner If statement is complete, so the `else` must belong to the outer `if`.

Testing the State of an I/O Stream

In Chapter 4, we talked about the concept of input and output streams in C++. We introduced the classes `istream`, `ostream`, `ifstream`, and `ofstream`. We said that any of the following can cause an input stream to enter the fail state:

- Invalid input data
- An attempt to read beyond the end of a file
- An attempt to open a nonexistent file for input

C++ provides a way to check whether a stream is in the fail state. In a logical expression, you simply use the name of the stream object (such as `cin`) as if it were a Boolean variable:

```
if (cin)
    ⋮

if ( !inFile )
    ⋮
```

When you do this, you are said to be **testing the state of the stream.** The result of the test is either `true` (meaning the last I/O operation on that stream succeeded) or `false` (meaning the last I/O operation failed).

Conceptually, you want to think of a stream object in a logical expression as being a Boolean variable with a value `true` (the stream state is OK) or `false` (the state isn't OK).

Notice in the second If statement above that we typed spaces around the expression `!inFile`. The spaces are not required by C++ but are there for readability. Without the spaces, it is harder to see the exclamation mark: `if (!inFile)`.

Testing the state of a stream   The act of using a C++ stream object in a logical expression as if it were a Boolean variable; the result is `true` if the last I/O operation on that stream succeeded, and `false` otherwise.

In an If statement, the way you phrase the logical expression depends on what you want the then-clause to do. The statement

```
if (inFile)
    ⋮
```

executes the then-clause if the last I/O operation on `inFile` succeeded. The statement

```
if ( !inFile )
    ⋮
```

executes the then-clause if `inFile` is in the fail state. (And remember that once a stream is in the fail state, it remains so. Any further I/O operations on that stream are null operations.)

Here's an example that shows how to check whether an input file was opened successfully:

```
#include <iostream>
#include <fstream>      // For file I/O

using namespace std;

int main()
{
    int       height;
    int       width;
    ifstream inFile;

    inFile.open("mydata.dat");            // Attempt to open input file
    if ( !inFile )                        // Was it opened?
    {
        cout << "Can't open the input file.";   // No--print message
        return 1;                               // Terminate program
    }
    inFile >> height >> width;
    ⋮
    return 0;
}
```

In this program, we begin by attempting to open the disk file `mydata.dat` for input. Immediately, we check to see whether the attempt succeeded. If it was successful, the value of the expression !inFile in the If statement is false and the then-clause is skipped. The program proceeds to read data from the file and then, presumably, to perform some computations. It concludes by executing the statement

```
return 0;
```

With this statement, the main function returns control to the computer's operating system. Recall that the function value returned by main is known as the exit status. The value 0 signifies normal completion of the program. Any other value (typically 1, 2, 3, ...) means that something went wrong.

Let's trace through the program again, assuming we weren't able to open the input file. Upon return from the open function, the stream inFile is in the fail state. In the If statement, the value of the expression !inFile is true. Thus, the then-clause is executed. The program prints an error message to the user and then terminates, returning an exit status of 1 to inform the operating system of an abnormal termination of the program. (Our choice of the value 1 for the exit status is purely arbitrary. System programmers sometimes use several different values in a program to signal different reasons for program termination. But most people just use the value 1.)

Whenever you open a data file for input, be sure to test the stream state before proceeding. If you forget to, and the computer cannot open the file, your program quietly continues executing and ignores any input operations on the file.

*P*ROBLEM-SOLVING CASE STUDY

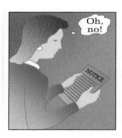

Warning Notices

Problem: Many universities send warning notices to freshmen who are in danger of failing a class. Your program should calculate the average of three test grades and print out a student's ID number, average, and whether or not the student is passing. Passing is a 60-point average or better. If the student is passing with less than a 70 average, the program should indicate that he or she is marginal.

Input: Student ID number (of type long) followed by three test grades (of type int). On some personal computers, the maximum int value is 32767. The student ID number is of type long (meaning long integer) to accommodate larger values such as nine-digit Social Security numbers.

Output:

A prompt for input

The input values (echo print)

Student ID number, average grade, passing/failing message, marginal indication, and error message if any of the test scores are negative

Discussion: To calculate the average, we have to read in the three test scores, add them, and divide by 3.

To print the appropriate message, we have to determine whether or not the average is below 60. If it is at least 60, we have to determine if it is less than 70.

If you were doing this by hand, you probably would notice if a test grade was negative and question it. If the semantics of your data imply that the values should be nonnegative, then your program should test to be sure they are. We test to make sure each grade is nonnegative, using a Boolean variable to report the result of the test. Here is the main module for our algorithm.

Main Module   **Level 0**

```
Get data
Test data
IF data OK
     Calculate average
     Print message indicating status
ELSE
     Print "Invalid Data: Score(s) less than zero."
```

Which of these steps require(s) expansion? *Get data*, *Test data*, and *Print message indicating status* all require multiple statements in order to solve their particular subproblem. On the other hand, we can translate *Print "Invalid Data:..."* directly into a C++ output statement. What about the step *Calculate average*? We can write it as a single C++ statement, but there's another level of detail that we must fill in—the actual formula to be used. Because the formula is at a lower level of detail than the rest of the main module, we chose to expand *Calculate average* as a level 1 module.

PROBLEM-SOLVING CASE STUDY *cont'd.*

Get Data

```
Prompt for input
Read studentID, test1, test2, test3
Print studentID, test1, test2, test3
```

Test Data

```
IF test1 < 0 OR test2 < 0 OR test3 < 0
        Set dataOK = false
ELSE
        Set dataOK = true
```

Calculate Average

```
Set average = (test1 + test2 + test3) / 3.0
```

Print Message Indicating Status

```
Print average
IF average >= 60.0
        Print "Passing"
        IF average < 70.0
                Print " but marginal"
        Print '.'
ELSE
        Print "Failing."
```

<u>*PROBLEM-SOLVING CASE STUDY cont'd.*</u>

Module Structure Chart:

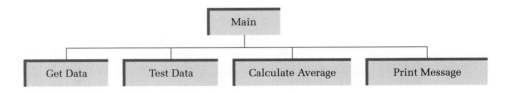

Variables

Name	Data Type	Description
average	float	Average of three test scores
studentID	long	Student's identification number
test1	int	Score for first test
test2	int	Score for second test
test3	int	Score for third test
dataOK	bool	True if data is correct

To save space, from here on we omit the list of constants and variables from the Problem-Solving Case Studies. But we recommend that you continue writing those lists as you design your own algorithms. The lists save you a lot of work when you are writing the declarations for your programs. Here is the program that implements our design.

(The following program is written in ISO/ANSI standard C++. If you are working with pre–standard C++, see the alternate version of the program in the PRE_STD directory of the program disk, available at the publisher's Web site, www.jbpub.com/disks.)

```
//****************************************************************
// Notices program
// This program determines (1) a student's average based on three
// test scores and (2) the student's passing/failing status
//****************************************************************
#include <iostream>
#include <iomanip>     // For setprecision()

using namespace std;
```

PROBLEM-SOLVING CASE STUDY cont'd.

```cpp
int main()
{
    float average;          // Average of three test scores
    long  studentID;        // Student's identification number
    int   test1;            // Score for first test
    int   test2;            // Score for second test
    int   test3;            // Score for third test
    bool  dataOK;           // True if data is correct

    cout << fixed << showpoint;              // Set up floating-pt.
                                             //    output format
    // Get data

    cout << "Enter a Student ID number and three test scores:"
         << endl;
    cin >> studentID >> test1 >> test2 >> test3;
    cout << "Student number: " << studentID << "  Test Scores: "
         << test1 << ", " << test2 << ", " << test3 << endl;

    // Test data

    if (test1 < 0 || test2 < 0 || test3 < 0)
        dataOK = false;
    else
        dataOK = true;

    if (dataOK)
    {
        // Calculate average

        average = float(test1 + test2 + test3) / 3.0;

        // Print message

        cout << "Average score is "
             << setprecision(2) << average << "--";
        if (average >= 60.0)
        {
            cout << "Passing";                // Student is passing
            if (average < 70.0)
                cout << " but marginal";      // But marginal
            cout << '.' << endl;
        }
        else                                  // Student is failing
            cout << "Failing." << endl;
    }
```

```
    else                                    // Invalid data
        cout << "Invalid Data:  Score(s) less than zero." << endl;

    return 0;
}
```

Here's a sample run of the program. Again, the input is in color.

```
Enter a Student ID number and three test scores:
9483681   73   62   68
Student Number: 9483681   Test Scores: 73, 62, 68
Average score is 67.67--Passing but marginal.
```

And here's a sample run with invalid data:

```
Enter a Student ID number and three test scores:
9483681   73   -10   62
Student Number: 9483681   Test Scores: 73, -10, 62
Invalid Data:  Score(s) less than zero.
```

In this program, we use a nested If structure that's easy to understand although somewhat inefficient. We assign a value to dataOK in one statement before testing it in the next. We could reduce the code by saying

```
dataOK = ! (test1 < 0 || test2 < 0 || test3 < 0);
```

Using DeMorgan's law, we also could write this statement as

```
dataOK = (test1 >= 0 && test2 >= 0 && test3 >= 0);
```

In fact, we could reduce the code even more by eliminating the variable dataOK and using

```
if (test1 >= 0 && test2 >= 0 && test3 >= 0)
    ⋮
```

in place of

```
if (dataOK)
    ⋮
```

To convince yourself that these three variations work, try them by hand with some test data.

If all of these statements do the same thing, how do you choose which one to use? If your goal is efficiency, the final variation—the compound condition in the main If statement—is best. If you are trying to express as clearly as possible what your code is doing, the longer form shown in the program may be best. The other variations lie somewhere in between. (However, some people would find the compound condition in the main If statement to be not only the most efficient but also the clearest to understand.) There are no absolute rules to follow here, but the general guideline is to strive for clarity, even if you must sacrifice a little efficiency.

Testing and Debugging

In Chapter 1, we discussed the problem-solving and implementation phases of computer programming. Testing is an integral part of both phases. Here we test both phases of the process used to develop the Notices program. Testing in the problem-solving phase is done after the solution is developed but before it is implemented. In the implementation phase, we test after the algorithm is translated into a program, and again after the program has compiled successfully. The compilation itself constitutes another stage of testing that is performed automatically.

Testing in the Problem-Solving Phase: The Algorithm Walk-Through

Determining Preconditions and Postconditions To test during the problem-solving phase, we do a *walk-through* of the algorithm. For each module in the functional decomposition, we establish an assertion called a precondition and another called a postcondition. A **precondition** is an assertion that must be true before a module is executed in order for the module to execute correctly. A **postcondition** is an assertion that should be true after the module has executed, if it has done its job correctly. To test a module, we "walk through" the algorithmic steps to confirm that they produce the required postcondition, given the stated precondition.

Precondition   An assertion that must be true before a module begins executing.

Postcondition   An assertion that should be true after a module has executed.

Our algorithm has five modules: the main module, Get Data, Test Data, Calculate Average, and Print Message Indicating Status. Usually there is no precondition for a main module. Our main module's postcondition is that it outputs the correct results, given the correct input. More specifically, the postcondition for the main module is

- the computer has input four integer values into `studentID`, `test1`, `test2`, and `test3`.
- the input values have been echo printed.
- if the input is invalid, an error message has been printed; otherwise, the average of the last three input values has been printed, along with the message "Passing" if the average is greater than or equal to 70.0, "Passing but marginal." if the average is less than 70.0 and greater than or equal to 60.0, or "Failing." if the average is less than 60.0.

Because Get Data is the first module executed in the algorithm and because it does not assume anything about the contents of the variables it is about to manipulate, it has no precondition. Its postcondition is that it has input four integer values into `studentID`, `test1`, `test2`, and `test3`.

The precondition for module Test Data is that `test1`, `test2`, and `test3` have been assigned meaningful values. Its postcondition is that `dataOK` contains `true` if the values in `test1`, `test2`, and `test3` are non-negative; otherwise, `dataOK` contains `false`.

The precondition for module Calculate Average is that `test1`, `test2`, and `test3` contain meaningful values. Its postcondition is that the variable named `average` contains the mean (the average) of `test1`, `test2`, and `test3`.

The precondition for module Print Message Indicating Status is that `average` contains the mean of the values in `test1`, `test2`, and `test3`. Its postcondition is that the value in `average` has been printed, along with the message "Passing" if the average is greater than or equal to 70.0, "Passing but marginal." if the average is less than 70.0 and greater than or equal to 60.0, or "Failing." if the average is less than 60.0.

Below we summarize the module preconditions and postconditions in tabular form. In the table, we use *AND* with its usual meaning in an assertion—the logical AND operation. Also, a phrase like "`someVariable` is assigned" is an abbreviated way of asserting that `someVariable` has already been assigned a meaningful value.

Module	Precondition	Postcondition
Main	—	Four integer values have been input AND The input values have been echo printed AND If the input is invalid, an error message has been printed; otherwise, the average of the last three input values has been printed, along with a message indicating the student's status
Get Data	—	`studentID`, `test1`, `test2`, and `test3` have been input
Test Data	`test1`, `test2`, and `test3` are assigned	`dataOK` contains `true` if `test1`, `test2`, and `test3` are nonnegative; otherwise, `dataOK` contains `false`
Calculate Average	`test1`, `test2`, and `test3` are assigned	`average` contains the average of `test1`, `test2`, and `test3`
Print Message Indicating Status	`average` contains the average of `test1`, `test2`, and `test3`	The value of `average` has been printed, along with a message indicating the student's status

Performing the Algorithm Walk-Through Now that we've established the preconditions and postconditions, we walk through the main module. At this point, we are concerned only with the steps in the main module, so for now we assume that each lower-level module executes correctly. At each step, we must determine the current conditions. If the step is a reference to another module, we must verify that the precondition of that module is met by the current conditions.

B.C. by johnny hart

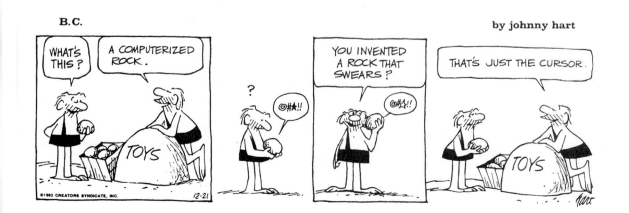

We begin with the first statement in the main module. Get Data does not have a precondition, and we assume that Get Data satisfies its postcondition that it correctly inputs four integer values into `studentID`, `test1`, `test2`, and `test3`.

The precondition for module Test Data is that `test1`, `test2`, and `test3` are assigned values. This must be the case if Get Data's postcondition is true. Again, because we are concerned only with the step at level 0, we assume that Test Data satisfies its postcondition that `dataOK` contains `true` or `false`, depending on the input values.

Next, the If statement checks to see if `dataOK` is `true`. If it is, the algorithm performs the then-clause. Assuming that Calculate Average correctly calculates the mean of `test1`, `test2`, and `test3` and that Print Message Indicating Status prints the average and the appropriate message (remember, we're assuming that the lower-level modules are correct for now), then the If statement's then-clause is correct. If the value in `dataOK` is `false`, the algorithm performs the else-clause and prints an error message.

We now have verified that the main (level 0) module is correct, assuming the level 1 modules are correct. The next step is to examine each module at level 1 and answer this question: If the level 2 modules (if any) are assumed to be correct, does this level 1 module do what it is supposed to do? We simply repeat the walk-through process for each module, starting with its particular precondition. In this example, there are no level 2 modules, so the level 1 modules must be complete.

Get Data correctly reads in four values—`studentID`, `test1`, `test2`, and `test3`—thereby satisfying its postcondition. (The next refinement is to code this instruction in C++. Whether it is coded correctly or not is *not* an issue in this phase; we deal with the code when we perform testing in the implementation phase.)

Test Data checks to see if all three of the variables contain nonnegative scores. The If condition correctly uses OR operators to combine the relational expressions so that if any of them are `true`, the then-clause is executed. It thus assigns `false` to `dataOK` if any of the numbers are negative; otherwise, it assigns `true`. The module therefore satisfies its postcondition.

Calculate Average sums the three test scores, divides the sum by 3.0, and assigns the result to `average`. The required postcondition therefore is true.

Print Message Indicating Status outputs the value in `average`. It then tests whether `average` is greater than or equal to 60.0. If so, "Passing" is printed and it then tests whether `average` is less than 70.0. If so, the words "but marginal" are added after "Passing". On the other hand, if `average` is less than 60.0, the message "Failing." is printed. Thus the module satisfies its postcondition.

Once we've completed the algorithm walk-through, we have to correct any discrepancies and repeat the process. When we know that the modules do what they are supposed to do, we start translating the algorithm into our programming language.

A standard postcondition for any program is that the user has been notified of invalid data. You should *validate* every input value for which any restrictions apply. A data-validation If statement tests an input value and outputs an error message if the value is not acceptable. (We validated the data when we tested for negative scores in the Notices program.) The best place to validate data is immediately after it is input. To satisfy the data-validation postcondition, the Warning Notices algorithm also should test the input values to ensure that they aren't too large.

For example, if the maximum score on a test is 100, then module Test Data should check for values in `test1`, `test2`, and `test3` that are greater than 100. The printing of the error message also should be modified to indicate the particular error condition that occurred. It would be best if it also specified the score that is invalid. Such a change makes it clear that Test Data should be the module to print the error messages. If Test Data prints the error message, then the If-Then-Else in the main module can be rewritten as an If-Then.

Testing in the Implementation Phase

Now that we've talked about testing in the problem-solving phase, we turn to testing in the implementation phase. In this phase, you need to test at several points.

Code Walk-Through After the code is written, you should go over it line by line to be sure that you've faithfully reproduced the algorithm—a process known as a *code walk-through*. In a team programming situation, you ask other team members to walk through the algorithm and code with you, to double-check the design and code.

Execution Trace You also should take some actual values and hand-calculate what the output should be by doing an *execution trace* (or *hand trace*). When the program is executed, you can use these same values as input and check the results.

The computer is a very literal device—it does exactly what we tell it to do, which may or may not be what we want it to do. We try to make sure that a program does what we want by tracing the execution of the statements.

We use a nonsense program below to demonstrate the technique. We keep track of the values of the program variables on the right-hand side. Variables with undefined values are indicated with a dash. When a variable is assigned a value, that value is listed in the appropriate column.

	Value of		
Statement	a	b	c
`const int x = 5;`			
`int main()`			
`{`			
`    int a, b, c;`	—	—	—
`    b = 1;`	—	1	—
`    c = x + b;`	—	1	6
`    a = x + 4;`	9	1	6
`    a = c;`	6	1	6
`    b = c;`	6	6	6
`    a = a + b + c;`	18	6	6
`    c = c % x;`	18	6	1
`    c = c * a;`	18	6	18
`    a = a % b;`	0	6	18
`    cout << a << b`			
`         << c;`	0	6	18
`    return 0;`	0	6	18
`}`			

Now that you've seen how the technique works, let's apply it to the Notices program. We list only the executable statement portion here. The input values are 6483, 73, 62, and 60. (The table is on page 255.)

The then-clause of the first If statement is not executed for this input data, so we do not fill in any of the variable columns to its right. The same situation occurs with the else-clauses in the other If statements. The test data causes only the then-clauses to be executed. We always create columns for all of the variables, even if we know that some will stay empty. Why? Because it's possible that later we'll encounter an erroneous reference to an empty variable; having a column for the variable reminds us to check for just such an error.

Statement	Value of					
	test1	test2	test3	average	dataOK	studentID
`cout << "Enter a Student ID number and three "`						
`    << "test scores:" << endl;`	—	—	—	—	—	—
`cin >> studentID >> test1 >> test2 >> test3;`	73	62	60	—	—	6483
`cout << "Student number: " << studentID`						
`    << " Test Scores: " << test1 << ", "`						
`    << test2 << ", " << test3 << endl;`	73	62	60	—	—	6483
`if (test1 < 0 || test2 < 0 || test3 < 0)`	73	62	60	—	—	6483
`    dataOK = false;`						
`else`						
`    dataOK = true;`	73	62	60	—	true	6483
`if (dataOK)`	73	62	60	—	true	6483
`{`						
`    average = float(test1 + test2 + test3) /`						
`              3.0;`	73	62	60	67.67	true	6483
`    cout << "Average score is "`						
`         << setprecision(2) << average << "--";`	73	62	60	67.67	true	6483
`    if (average >= 60.0)`	73	62	60	67.67	true	6483
`    {`						
`        cout << "Passing";`	73	62	60	67.67	true	6483
`        if (average < 70.0)`	73	62	60	67.67	true	6483
`            cout << " but marginal";`	73	62	60	67.67	true	6483
`        cout << '.' << endl;`	73	62	60	67.67	true	6483
`    }`						
`    else`						
`        cout << "Failing." << endl;`						
`}`						
`else`						
`    cout << "Invalid Data: Score(s) less "`						
`         << "than zero." << endl;`						
`return 0;`	73	62	60	67.67	true	6483

When a program contains branches, it's a good idea to retrace its execution with different input data so that each branch is traced at least once. In the next section, we describe how to develop data sets that test each of a program's branches.

Testing Selection Control Structures   To test a program with branches, we need to execute each branch at least once and verify the results. For example, in the Notices program there are four If-Then-Else statements (see Figure 5-6). We need a series of data sets to test the different branches. For example, the following sets of input values for `test1`, `test2`, and `test3` cause all of the branches to be executed:

	test1	test2	test3
Set 1	100	100	100
Set 2	60	60	63
Set 3	50	50	50
Set 4	−50	50	50

Figure 5-7 shows the flow of control through the branching structure of the Notices program for each of these data sets. Set 1 is valid and gives an average of 100, which is passing and not marginal. Set 2 is valid and gives an average of 61, which is passing but marginal. Set 3 is valid and gives an average of 50, which is failing. Set 4 has an invalid test grade, which generates an error message.

Every branch in the program is executed at least once through this series of test runs; eliminating any of the test data sets would leave at least one branch untested. This series of data sets provides what is called *minimum complete coverage* of the program's branching structure. Whenever you test a program with branches in it, you should design a series of tests that covers all of the branches. It may help to draw diagrams like those in Figure 5-7 so that you can see which branches are being executed.

FIGURE 5-6
Branching
Structure for
Notices Program

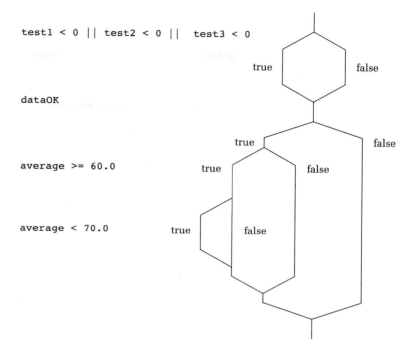

```
test1 < 0 || test2 < 0 || test3 < 0
```

```
dataOK
```

```
average >= 60.0
```

```
average < 70.0
```

FIGURE 5-7
Flow of Control
Through Notices
Program for Each
of Four Data Sets

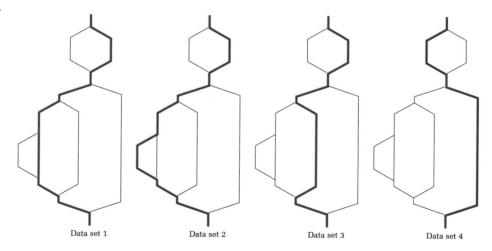

Data set 1   Data set 2   Data set 3   Data set 4

Because an action in one branch of a program often affects processing in a later branch, it is critical to test as many *combinations of branches*, or paths, through a program as possible. By doing so, we can be sure that there are no interdependencies that could cause problems. Of course, some combinations of branches may be impossible to follow. For example, if the else is taken in the first branch of the Notices program, the else in the second branch cannot be taken. Shouldn't we try all possible paths? Yes, in theory we should. However, the number of paths in even a small program can be very large.

The approach to testing that we've used here is called *code coverage* because the test data is designed by looking at the code of the program. Code coverage is also called *white box* (or *clear box*) *testing* because we are allowed to see the program code while designing the tests. Another approach to testing, *data coverage*, attempts to test as many allowable data values as possible without regard to the program code. Because we need not see the code in this form of testing, it is also called *black box testing*— we would design the same set of tests even if the code were hidden in a black box. Complete data coverage is as impractical as complete code coverage for many programs. For example, the Notices program reads four integer values and thus has approximately $(2 * \text{INT\_MAX})^4$ possible inputs. (INT_MAX and INT_MIN are constants declared in the header file climits. They represent the largest and smallest possible int values, respectively, on your particular computer and C++ compiler.)

Often, testing is a combination of these two strategies. Instead of trying every possible data value (data coverage), we examine the code (code coverage) and look for ranges of values for which processing is identical. Then we test the values at the boundaries and, sometimes, a value in the middle of each range. For example, a simple condition such as

```
alpha < 0
```

divides the integers into two ranges:

1. INT_MIN through −1
2. 0 through INT_MAX

Thus, we should test the four values INT_MIN, −1, 0, and INT_MAX. A compound condition such as

```
alpha >= 0 && alpha <= 100
```

divides the integers into three ranges:

1. INT_MIN through −1
2. 0 through 100
3. 101 through INT_MAX

Thus, we have six values to test. In addition, to verify that the relational operators are correct, we should test for values of 1 (> 0) and 99 (< 100).

Conditional branches are only one factor in developing a testing strategy. We consider more of these factors in later chapters.

The Test Plan

We've discussed strategies and techniques for testing programs, but how do you approach the testing of a specific program? You do it by designing and implementing a **test plan**—a document that specifies the test cases that should be tried, the reason for each test case, and the expected output. **Implementing a test plan** involves running the program using the data specified by the test cases in the plan and checking and recording the results.

Test plan A document that specifies how a program is to be tested.

Test plan implementation Using the test cases specified in a test plan to verify that a program outputs the predicted results.

The test plan should be developed together with the functional decomposition. As you create each module, write out its precondition and postcondition and note the test data required to verify them. Consider code coverage and data coverage to see if you've left out tests for any aspects of the program (if you've forgotten something, it probably also indicates that a precondition or postcondition is incomplete).

The following table shows a partial test plan for the Notices program. It has eight test cases. The first test case is just to check that the program echo prints its input properly. The next three cases test the different paths through the program for valid data. Three more test cases check that each of the scores is appropriately validated by separately entering an invalid score for each. The last test case checks the boundary where a score is considered valid—when it is 0. We could further expand this test plan to check the valid data boundary separately for each score by providing three test cases in which one score in each case is 0. We also could test the boundary conditions of the different paths for valid data. That is, we could check that averages of exactly 60 and 70, and slightly higher and slightly lower, produce the desired output. Case Study Follow-Up Exercise 1 asks you to complete this test plan and implement it.

Test Plan for Notices Program

Reason for Test Case	Input Values	Expected Output	Observed Output
Echo-print check	9999, 100, 100, 100	Student Number: 9999 Test Scores: 100, 100, 100	

Note to implementor: Once echo printing has been checked, it is omitted from the expected output column in subsequent test cases, but still appears in the program's output.

Passing scores	9999, 80, 70, 90	Average score is 80.00-- Passing.	
Passing but marginal scores	9999, 55, 65, 75	Average score is 65.00-- Passing but marginal.	
Failing scores	9999, 30, 40, 50	Average score is 40.00-- Failing.	
Invalid data, Test 1	9999, −1, 20, 30	Invalid Data: Score(s) less than zero.	
Invalid data, Test 2	9999, 10, −1, 30	Invalid Data: Score(s) less than zero.	
Invalid data, Test 3	9999, 10, 20, −1	Invalid Data: Score(s) less than zero.	
Boundary of valid data	9999, 0, 0, 0	Average score is 0.00-- Failing.	

Implementing a test plan does not guarantee that a program is completely correct. It means only that a careful, systematic test of the program has not demonstrated any bugs. The situation shown in Figure 5-8 is analogous to trying to test a program without a plan—depending only on luck, you may completely miss the fact that a program contains numerous errors. Developing and implementing a written test plan, on the other hand, casts a wide net that is much more likely to find errors.

Tests Performed Automatically During Compilation and Execution

Once a program is coded and test data has been prepared, it is ready for compiling. The compiler has two responsibilities: to report any errors and (if there are no errors) to translate the program into object code.

Errors can be syntactic or semantic. The compiler finds syntactic errors. For example, the compiler warns you when reserved words are misspelled, identifiers are undeclared, semicolons are missing, and operand types are mismatched. But it won't find all of your typing errors. If you type > instead of < , you won't get an error message; instead, you get erroneous results when you test the program. It's up to you to design a test plan and carefully check the code to detect errors of this type.

FIGURE 5-8

When You Test a
Program Without a
Plan, You Never
Know What You
Might Be Missing

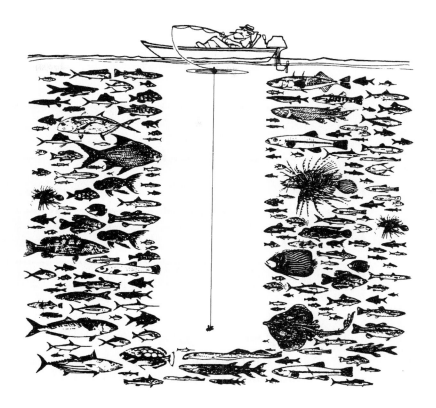

Semantic errors (also called *logic errors*) are mistakes that give you the wrong answer. They are more difficult to locate than syntactic errors and usually surface when a program is executing. C++ detects only the most obvious semantic errors—those that result in an invalid operation (dividing by zero, for example). Although semantic errors sometimes are caused by typing errors, they are more often a product of a faulty algorithm design. The lack of checking for test scores over 100 that we found in the algorithm walk-through for the Warning Notices problem is a typical semantic error.

By walking through the algorithm and the code, tracing the execution of the program, and developing a thorough test strategy, you should be able to avoid, or at least quickly locate, semantic errors in your programs.

Figure 5-9 illustrates the testing process we've been discussing. The figure shows where syntax and semantic errors occur and in which phase they can be corrected.

Figure 5-9
Testing Process

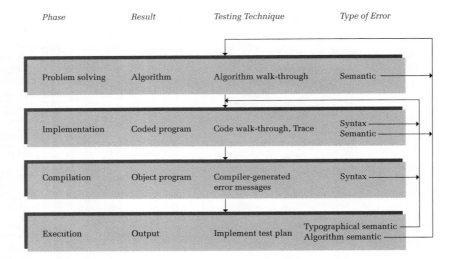

Phase	Result	Testing Technique	Type of Error
Problem solving	Algorithm	Algorithm walk-through	Semantic
Implementation	Coded program	Code walk-through, Trace	Syntax / Semantic
Compilation	Object program	Compiler-generated error messages	Syntax
Execution	Output	Implement test plan	Typographical semantic / Algorithm semantic

Testing and Debugging Hints

1. C++ has three pairs of operators that are similar in appearance but very different in effect: == and =, && and &, and | | and |. Double-check all of your logical expressions to be sure you're using the "equals-equals," "and-and," and "or-or" operators.

2. If you use extra parentheses for clarity, be sure that the opening and closing parentheses match up. To verify that parentheses are properly paired, start with the innermost pair and draw a line connecting them. Do the same for the others, working your way out to the outermost pair. For example,

```
if ( ( (total/scores) > 50) && ( (total/(scores - 1) ) < 100 ) )
```

Here is a quick way to tell whether you have an equal number of opening and closing parentheses. The scheme uses a single number (the "magic number"), whose value initially is 0. Scan the expression from left to right. At each opening parenthesis, add 1 to the magic number; at each closing parenthesis, subtract 1. At the final closing parenthesis, the magic number should be 0. For example,

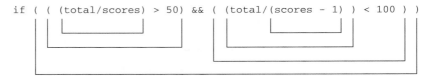

```
if ((( total/scores) > 50) && ((total/(scores - 1)) < 100))
   0   123              2   1   23       4            32     10
```

3. Don't use =< to mean "less than or equal to"; only the symbol <= works. Likewise, => is invalid for "greater than or equal to"; you must use >= for this operation.

4. In an If statement, remember to use a { } pair if the then-clause or else-clause is a sequence of statements. And be sure not to put a semicolon after the right brace.

5. Echo print all input data. By doing so, you know that your input values are what they are supposed to be.

6. Test for bad data. If a data value must be positive, use an If statement to test the value. If the value is negative or 0, an error message should be printed; otherwise, processing should continue. For example, module Test Data in the Notices program could be rewritten to test for scores greater than 100 as follows (this change also requires that we remove the else branch in the main module):

```
dataOK = true;
if (test1 < 0 || test2 < 0 || test3 < 0)
{
    cout << "Invalid Data:   Score(s) less than zero."
<< endl;
    dataOK = false;
}
if (test1 > 100 || test2 > 100 || test3 > 100)
{
    cout << "Invalid Data:   Score(s) greater than
100." << endl;
    dataOK = false;
}
```

These If statements test the limits of reasonable scores, and the rest of the program continues only if the data values are reasonable.

7. Take some sample values and try them by hand as we did for the Notices program. (There's more on this method in Chapter 6.)

8. If your program reads data from an input file, it should verify that the file was opened successfully. Immediately after the call to the open function, an If statement should test the state of the file stream.

9. If your program produces an answer that does not agree with a value you've calculated by hand, try these suggestions:

   a. Redo your arithmetic.

   b. Recheck your input data.

   c. Carefully go over the section of code that does the calculation. If you're in doubt about the order in which the operations are performed, insert clarifying parentheses.

   d. Check for integer overflow. The value of an int variable may have exceeded INT_MAX in the middle of a calculation. Some systems give an error message when this happens, but most do not.

   e. Check the conditions in branching statements to be sure that the correct branch is taken under all circumstances.

Summary

Using logical expressions is a way of asking questions while a program is running. The program evaluates each logical expression, producing the value `true` if the expression is true or the value `false` if the expression is not true.

The If statement allows you to take different paths through a program based on the value of a logical expression. The If-Then-Else is used to choose between two courses of action; the If-Then is used to choose whether or not to take a particular course of action. The branches of an If-Then or If-Then-Else can be any statement, simple or compound. They can even be other If statements.

The algorithm walk-through requires us to define a precondition and a postcondition for each module in an algorithm. Then we need to verify that those assertions are true at the beginning and end of each module. By testing our design in the problem-solving phase, we can eliminate errors that can be more difficult to detect in the implementation phase.

An execution trace is a way of finding program errors once we've entered the implementation phase. It's a good idea to trace a program before you run it, so that you have some sample results against which to check the program's output. A written test plan is an essential part of any program development effort.

Quick Check

1. Write a C++ expression that compares the variable `letter` to the constant 'Z' and yields `true` if `letter` is less than 'Z'. (pp. 214–220)
2. Write a C++ expression that yields `true` if `letter` is between 'A' and 'Z' inclusive. (pp. 214–224)
3. What form of the If statement would you use to make a C++ program print out "Is an uppercase letter" if the value in `letter` is between 'A' and 'Z' inclusive, and print out "Is not an uppercase letter" if the value in `letter` is outside that range? (pp. 229–231)
4. What form of the If statement would you use to make a C++ program print out "Is a digit" only if the value in the variable `someChar` is between '0' and '9' inclusive? (pp. 234–236)
5. On a telephone, each of the digits 2 through 9 has a segment of the alphabet associated with it. What kind of control structure would you use to decide which segment a given letter falls into and to print out the corresponding digit? (pp. 236–240)
6. What is one postcondition that every program should have? (pp. 249–253)
7. In what phase of the program development process should you carry out an execution trace? (pp. 253–256)

8.   You've written a program that prints out the corresponding digit on a phone, given a letter of the alphabet. Everything seems to work right except that you can't get the digit '5' to print out; you keep getting the digit '6'. What steps would you take to find and fix this bug? (pp. 256–259)

9.   How do we satisfy the postcondition that the user has been notified of invalid data values? (pp. 249–253)

Answers   **1.** `letter < 'Z'`   **2.** `letter >= 'A' && letter <= 'Z'`   **3.** The If-Then-Else form   **4.** The If-Then form   **5.** A nested If statement   **6.** The user has been notified of invalid data values.   **7.** The implementation phase   **8.** Carefully review the section of code that should print out '5'. Check the branching condition and the output statement there. Try some sample values by hand.   **9.** The program must validate every input for which any restrictions apply and print an error message if the data violates any of the restrictions.

Exam Preparation Exercises

1.   Given these values for the Boolean variables x, y, and z:

      `x = true, y = false, z = true`

      evaluate the following logical expressions. In the blank next to each expression, write a T if the result is `true` or an F if the result is `false`.

      _____   a. `x && y || x && z`
      _____   b. `(x || !y) && (!x || z)`
      _____   c. `x || y && z`
      _____   d. `!(x || y) && z`

2.   Given these values for variables i, j, p, and q:

      $i = 10$, $j = 19$, p = true, q = false

      add parentheses (if necessary) to the expressions below so that they evaluate to true.

      a. `i == j || p`
      b. `i >= j || i <= j && p`
      c. `!p || p`
      d. `!q && q`

3.   Given these values for the int variables i, j, m, and n:

      $i = 6$, $j = 7$, $m = 11$, $n = 11$

      what is the output of the following code?

```
cout << "Madam";
if (i < j)
    if (m != n)
        cout << "How";
    else
        cout << "Now";
cout << "I'm";
if (i >= m)
    cout << "Cow";
else
    cout << "Adam";
```

4. Given the int variables x, y, and z, where x contains 3, y contains 7, and z contains 6, what is the output from each of the following code fragments?

```
a. if (x <= 3)
       cout << x + y << endl;
   cout << x + y << endl;
b. if (x != -1)
       cout << "The value of x is " << x << endl;
   else
       cout << "The value of y is " << y << endl;
c. if (x != -1)
   {
       cout << x << endl;
       cout << y << endl;
       cout << z << endl;
   }
   else
       cout << "y" << endl;
       cout << "z" << endl;
```

5. Given this code fragment:

```
if (height >= minHeight)
    if (weight >= minWeight)
        cout << "Eligible to serve." << endl;
    else
        cout << "Too light to serve." << endl;
else
    if (weight >= minWeight)
        cout << "Too short to serve." << endl;
    else
        cout << "Too short and too light to serve." << endl;
```

a. What is the output when height exceeds minHeight and weight exceeds minWeight?

b. What is the output when height is less than minHeight and weight is less than minWeight?

6. Match each logical expression in the left column with the logical expression in the right column that tests for the same condition.

_____	a. x < y && y < z	(1) !(x != y) && y == z
_____	b. x > y && y >= z	(2) !(x <= y || y < z)
_____	c. x != y || y == z	(3) (y < z || y == z) || x == y
_____	d. x == y || y <= z	(4) !(x >= y) && !(y >= z)
_____	e. x == y && y == z	(5) !(x == y && y != z)

7. The following expressions make sense but are invalid according to C++'s rules of syntax. Rewrite them so that they are valid logical expressions. (All the variables are of type int.)

    a. x < y <= z

    b. x, y, and z are greater than 0

    c. x is equal to neither y nor z

    d. x is equal to y and z

8. Given these values for the Boolean variables x, y, and z:

    x = true, y = true, z = false

    indicate whether each expression is true (T) or false (F).

    _____ a. !(y || z) || x

    _____ b. z && x && y

    _____ c. ! y || (z || !x)

    _____ d. z || (x && (y || z))

    _____ e. x || x && z

9. For each of the following problems, decide which is more appropriate, an If-Then-Else or an If-Then. Explain your answers.

    a. Students who are candidates for admission to a college submit their SAT scores. If a student's score is equal to or above a certain value, print a letter of acceptance for the student. Otherwise, print a rejection notice.

    b. For employees who work more than 40 hours a week, calculate overtime pay and add it to their regular pay.

    c. In solving a quadratic equation, whenever the value of the discriminant (the quantity under the square root sign) is negative, print out a message noting that the roots are complex (imaginary) numbers.

    d. In a computer-controlled sawmill, if a cross section of a log is greater than certain dimensions, adjust the saw to cut 4-inch by 8-inch beams; otherwise, adjust the saw to cut 2-inch by 4-inch studs.

10. What causes the error message "UNEXPECTED ELSE" when this code fragment is compiled?

```
if (mileage < 24.0)
{
    cout << "Gas ";
    cout << "guzzler.";
};
else
    cout << "Fuel efficient.";
```

11. The following code fragment is supposed to print "Type AB" when Boolean variables typeA and typeB are both true, and print "Type O" when both variables are false. Instead it prints "Type O" whenever just one of the variables is false. Insert a { } pair to make the code segment work the way it should.

```
if (typeA || typeB)
    if (typeA && typeB)
        cout << "Type AB";
else
    cout << "Type O";
```

12. The nested If structure below has five possible branches depending on the values read into char variables ch1, ch2, and ch3. To test the structure, you need five sets of data, each set using a different branch. Create the five test data sets.

```
cin >> ch1 >> ch2 >> ch3;
if (ch1 == ch2)
    if (ch2 == ch3)
        cout << "All initials are the same." << endl;
    else
        cout << "First two are the same." << endl;
else if (ch2 == ch3)
    cout << "Last two are the same." << endl;
else if (ch1 == ch3)
    cout << "First and last are the same." << endl;
else
    cout << "All initials are different." << endl;
```

a. Test data set 1:   ch1 = _____   ch2 = _____   ch3 = _____
b. Test data set 2:   ch1 = _____   ch2 = _____   ch3 = _____
c. Test data set 3:   ch1 = _____   ch2 = _____   ch3 = _____
d. Test data set 4:   ch1 = _____   ch2 = _____   ch3 = _____
e. Test data set 5:   ch1 = _____   ch2 = _____   ch3 = _____

13. If x and y are Boolean variables, do the following two expressions test the same condition?

```
x != y
(x || y) && !(x && y)
```

14. The following If condition is made up of three relational expressions:

```
if (i >= 10 && i <= 20 && i != 16)
    j = 4;
```

If i contains the value 25 when this If statement is executed, which relational expression(s) does the computer evaluate? (Remember that C++ uses short-circuit evaluation.)

Programming Warm-up Exercises

1. Declare eligible to be a Boolean variable, and assign it the value true.
2. Write a statement that sets the Boolean variable available to true if numberOrdered is less than or equal to numberOnHand minus numberReserved.
3. Write a statement containing a logical expression that assigns true to the Boolean variable isCandidate if satScore is greater than or equal to 1100, gpa is not less than 2.5, and age is greater than 15. Otherwise, isCandidate should be false.
4. Given the declarations

```
bool leftPage;
int  pageNumber:
```

write a statement that sets leftPage to true if pageNumber is even. (*Hint:* Consider what the remainders are when you divide different integers by 2.)

5. Write an If statement (or a series of If statements) that assigns to the variable biggest the greatest value contained in variables i, j, and k. Assume the three values are distinct.

6. Rewrite the following sequence of If-Thens as a single If-Then-Else.

```cpp
if (year % 4 == 0)
    cout << year << " is a leap year." << endl;
if (year % 4 != 0)
{
    year = year + 4 - year % 4;
    cout << year << " is the next leap year." << endl;
}
```

7. Simplify the following program segment, taking out unnecessary comparisons. Assume that age is an int variable.

```cpp
if (age > 64)
    cout << "Senior voter";
if (age < 18)
    cout << "Under age";
if (age >= 18 && age < 65)
    cout << "Regular voter";
```

8. The following program fragment is supposed to print out the values 25, 60, and 8, in that order. Instead, it prints out 50, 60, and 4. Why?

```cpp
length = 25;
width = 60;
if (length = 50)
    height = 4;
else
    height = 8;
cout << length << ' ' << width << ' ' << height << endl;
```

9. The following C++ program segment is almost unreadable because of the inconsistent indentation and the random placement of left and right braces. Fix the indentation and align the braces properly.

```cpp
// This is a nonsense program
if (a > 0)
if (a < 20)
        {
    cout << "A is in range." << endl;
b = 5;
    }
        else
                {
cout << "A is too large." << endl;
    b = 3;
}
    else
cout << "A is too small." << endl;
        cout << "All done." << endl;
```

10. Given the `float` variables x1, x2, y1, y2, and m, write a program segment to find the slope of a line through the two points (x1, y1) and (x2, y2). Use the formula

$$m = \frac{y1 - y2}{x1 - x2}$$

to determine the slope of the line. If x1 equals x2, the line is vertical and the slope is undefined. The segment should write the slope with an appropriate label. If the slope is undefined, it should write the message "Slope undefined."

11. Given the `float` variables a, b, c, root1, root2, and discriminant, write a program segment to determine whether the roots of a quadratic polynomial are real or complex (imaginary). If the roots are real, find them and assign them to root1 and root2. If they are complex, write the message "No real roots."

   The formula for the solution to the quadratic equation is

$$\frac{-b \pm \sqrt{b^2 - 4ac}}{2a}$$

The ± means "plus or minus" and indicates that there are two solutions to the equation: one in which the result of the square root is added to −b and one in which the result is subtracted from −b. The roots are real if the discriminant (the quantity under the square root sign) is not negative.

12. The following program reads data from an input file without checking to see if the file was opened successfully. Insert statements that print an error message and terminate the program if the file cannot be opened.

```cpp
#include <iostream>
#include <fstream>      // For file I/O

using namespace std;

int main()
{
    int      m;
    int      n;
    ifstream info;

    info.open("indata.dat");
    info >> m >> n;
    cout << "The sum of " << m << " and " << n
         << " is " << m + n << endl;
    return 0;
}
```

Programming Problems

1. Using functional decomposition, write a C++ program that inputs a single letter and prints out the corresponding digit on the telephone. The letters and digits on a telephone are grouped this way:

   2 = ABC   4 = GHI   6 = MNO   8 = TUV

   3 = DEF   5 = JKL   7 = PRS   9 = WXY

   No digit corresponds to either Q or Z. For these two letters, your program should print a message indicating that they are not used on a telephone.

   The program might operate like this:

   ```
   Enter a single letter, and I will tell you what the corresponding
   digit is on the telephone.
   R
   The digit 7 corresponds to the letter R on the telephone.
   ```

   Here's another example:

   ```
   Enter a single letter, and I will tell you what the corresponding
   digit is on the telephone.
   Q
   There is no digit on the telephone that corresponds to Q.
   ```

   Your program should print a message indicating that there is no matching digit for any nonalphabetic character the user enters. Also, the program should recognize only uppercase letters. Include the lowercase letters with the invalid characters.

   Prompt the user with an informative message for the input value, as shown above. The program should echo-print the input letter as part of the output.

   Use proper indentation, appropriate comments, and meaningful identifiers throughout the program.

2. People who deal with historical dates use a number called the *Julian day* to calculate the number of days between two events. The Julian day is the number of days that have elapsed since January 1, 4713 B.C. For example, the Julian day for October 16, 1956, is 2435763. There are formulas for computing the Julian day from a given date and vice versa.

   One very simple formula computes the day of the week from a given Julian day:

   $$\textit{day of the week} = (\textit{Julian day} + 1) \, \% \, 7$$

   where % is the C++ modulus operator. This formula gives a result of 0 for Sunday, 1 for Monday, and so on up to 6 for Saturday. For Julian day 2435763, the result is 2 (a Tuesday). Your job is to write a C++ program that inputs a Julian day, computes the day of the week using the formula, and then prints out the name of the day that corresponds to that number. If the maximum `int` value on your machine is small (32767, for instance), use the `long` data type instead of `int`. Be sure to echo-print the input data and to use proper indentation and comments.

Your output might look like this:

```
Enter a Julian day number:
2451545
Julian day number 2451545 is a Saturday.
```

3. You can compute the date for any Easter Sunday from 1982 to 2048 as follows (all variables are of type int):

```
a is year % 19
b is year % 4
c is year % 7
d is (19 * a + 24) % 30
e is (2 * b + 4 * c + 6 * d + 5) % 7
Easter Sunday is March (22 + d + e)*
```

Write a program that inputs the year and outputs the date (month and day) of Easter Sunday for that year. Echo-print the input as part of the output. For example:

```
Enter the year (for example, 1999):
1985
Easter is Sunday, April 7, in 1985.
```

4. The algorithm for computing the date of Easter can be extended easily to work with any year from 1900 to 2099. There are four years—1954, 1981, 2049, and 2076—for which the algorithm gives a date that is seven days later than it should be. Modify the program for Problem 3 to check for these years and subtract 7 from the day of the month. This correction does not cause the month to change. Be sure to change the documentation for the program to reflect its broadened capabilities.

5. Write a C++ program that calculates and prints the diameter, the circumference, or the area of a circle, given the radius. The program inputs two data items. The first is a character—'D' (for diameter), 'C' (for circumference), or 'A' (for area)—to indicate the calculation needed. The next data value is a floating-point number indicating the radius of the particular circle.

   The program should echo-print the input data. The output should be labeled appropriately and formatted to two decimal places. For example, if the input is

```
A 6.75
```

your program should print something like this:

```
The area of a circle with radius 6.75 is 143.14.
```

Here are the formulas you need:

Diameter = $2r$
Circumference = $2\pi r$
Area of a circle = πr^2

where r is the radius. Use 3.14159265 for π.

---

* Notice that this formula can give a date in April.

6. The factorial of a number n is $n * (n-1) * (n-2) * \ldots * 2 * 1$. Stirling's formula approximates the factorial for large values of n:

$$\frac{n^n \sqrt{2\pi n}}{e^n}$$

where $\pi = 3.14159265$ and $e = 2.718282$.

Write a C++ program that inputs an integer value (but stores it into a float variable n), calculates the factorial of n using Stirling's formula, assigns the (rounded) result to a long integer variable, and then prints the result appropriately labeled.

Depending on the value of n, you should obtain one of these results:

- A numerical result.
- If n equals 0, the factorial is defined to be 1.
- If n is less than 0, the factorial is undefined.
- If n is too large, the result exceeds LONG_MAX.

(LONG_MAX is a constant declared in the header file climits. It gives the maximum long value for your particular machine and C++ compiler.)

Because Stirling's formula is used to calculate the factorial of very large numbers, the factorial approaches LONG_MAX quickly. If the factorial exceeds LONG_MAX, it causes an arithmetic overflow in the computer, in which case the program either stops running or continues with a strange-looking integer result, perhaps negative. Before you write the program, then, you first must write a small program that lets you determine, by trial and error, the largest value of n for which your computer system can compute a factorial using Stirling's formula. After you've determined this value, you can write the program using nested Ifs that print different messages depending on the value of n. If n is within the acceptable range for your computer system, output the number and the result with an appropriate message. If n is 0, write the message, "The number is 0. The factorial is 1." If the number is less than 0, write "The number is less than 0. The factorial is undefined." If the number is greater than the largest value of n for which your computer system can compute a factorial, write "The number is too large."

Suggestion: Don't compute Stirling's formula directly. The values of n^n and e^n can be huge, even in floating-point form. Take the natural logarithm of the formula and manipulate it algebraically to work with more reasonable floating-point values. If r is the result of these intermediate calculations, the final result is e^r. Make use of the standard library functions log and exp, available through the header file cmath. These functions, described in Appendix C, compute the natural logarithm and natural exponentiation, respectively.

Case Study Follow-Up

1. a. Complete the test plan for the Notices program that was begun in the Testing and Debugging section on page 259. That section describes the remaining tests to be written.

    b. Implement the complete test plan and record the observed output.

2. Could the data validation test in the Notices program be changed to the following?

    ```
    dataOK = (test1 + test2 + test3) >= 0;
    ```

    Explain.

3. Modify the Notices program so that it prints "Passing with high marks." if the value in average is above 90.0.

4. If the Notices program is modified to input and average four scores, what changes (if any) to the control structures are required?

5. Change the Notices program so that it checks each of the test scores individually and prints error messages indicating which of the scores is invalid and why.

6. Rewrite the preconditions and postconditions for the modules in the Warning Notices algorithm to reflect the changes to the design of the Notices program requested in Case Study Follow-Up Exercise 4.

7. Write a test plan that achieves complete code coverage for the Notices program as modified in Case Study Follow-Up Exercise 4.

CHAPTER

6

Looping

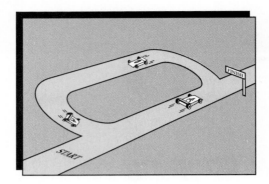

In Chapter 5, we said that the flow of control in a program can differ from the physical order of the statements. The *physical order* is the order in which the statements appear in a program; the order in which we want the statements to be executed is called the *logical order*.

The If statement is one way of making the logical order different from the physical order. Looping control structures are another. A **loop** executes the same statement (simple or compound) over and over, as long as a condition or set of conditions is satisfied.

Loop   A control structure that causes a statement or group of statements to be executed repeatedly.

In this chapter, we discuss different kinds of loops and how they are constructed using the While statement. We also discuss *nested loops* (loops that contain other loops) and introduce a notation for comparing the amount of work done by different algorithms.

The While Statement

The While statement, like the If statement, tests a condition. Here is the syntax template for the While statement:

WhileStatement

```
while ( Expression )
    Statement
```

and this is an example of one:

```
while (inputVal != 25)
    cin >> inputVal;
```

The While statement is a looping control structure. The statement to be executed each time through the loop is called the *body* of the loop. In the example above, the body of the loop is the input statement that reads in a value for `inputVal`. This While statement says to execute the body repeatedly as long as the input value does not equal 25. The While statement is completed (hence, the loop stops) when `inputVal` equals 25. The effect of this loop, then, is to consume and ignore all the values in the input stream until the number 25 is read.

Just like the condition in an If statement, the condition in a While statement can be an expression of any simple data type. Nearly always, it is a logical (Boolean) expression; if not, its value is implicitly coerced to type `bool` (recall that a zero value is coerced to `false`, and any nonzero value is coerced to `true`). The While statement says, "If the value of the expression is `true`, execute the body and then go back and test the expression again. If the expression's value is `false`, skip the body." The loop body is thus executed over and over as long as the expression is `true` when it is tested. When the expression is `false`, the program skips the body and execution continues at the statement immediately following the loop. Of course, if the expression is `false` to begin with, the body is not even executed. Figure 6-1 shows the flow of control of the While statement, where Statement1 is the body of the loop and Statement2 is the statement following the loop.

The body of a loop can be a compound statement (block), which allows us to execute any group of statements repeatedly. Most often we use While loops in the following form:

```
while (Expression)
{
    ⋮
}
```

In this structure, if the expression is `true`, the entire sequence of statements in the block is executed, and then the expression is checked again. If it is still `true`, the statements are executed again. The cycle continues until the expression becomes `false`.

Although in some ways the If and While statements are alike, there are fundamental differences between them (see Figure 6-2). In the If structure, Statement1 is either skipped or executed exactly once. In the While structure, Statement1 can be skipped, executed once, or executed over and over.

FIGURE 6-1
While Statement
Flow of Control

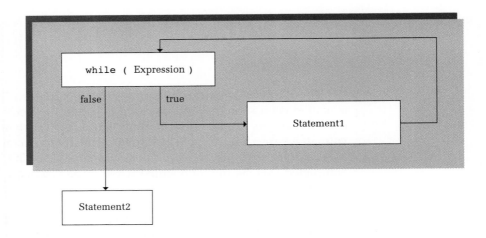

The If is used to *choose* a course of action; the While is used to *repeat* a course of action.

Phases of Loop Execution

The body of a loop is executed in several phases:

- The moment that the flow of control reaches the first statement inside the loop body is the **loop entry.**
- Each time the body of a loop is executed, a pass is made through the loop. This pass is called an **iteration.**
- Before each iteration, control is transferred to the **loop test** at the beginning of the loop.
- When the last iteration is complete and the flow of control has passed to the first statement following the loop, the program has **exited the loop.** The condition that causes a loop to be exited is the **termination condition.** In the case of a While loop, the termination condition is that the While expression becomes false.

FIGURE 6-2
A Comparison of If and While

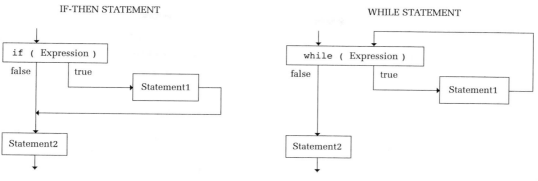

IF-THEN STATEMENT

WHILE STATEMENT

Loop entry   The point at which the flow of control reaches the first statement inside a loop.

Iteration   An individual pass through, or repetition of, the body of a loop.

Loop test   The point at which the While expression is evaluated and the decision is made either to begin a new iteration or skip to the statement immediately following the loop.

Loop exit   The point at which the repetition of the loop body ends and control passes to the first statement following the loop.

Termination condition   The condition that causes a loop to be exited.

Notice that the loop exit occurs only at one point: when the loop test is performed. Even though the termination condition may become satisfied midway through the execution of the loop, the current iteration is completed before the computer checks the While expression again.

The concept of looping is fundamental to programming. In this chapter, we spend some time looking at typical kinds of loops and ways of implementing them with the While statement. These looping situations come up again and again when you are analyzing problems and designing algorithms.

Loops Using the While Statement

In solving problems, you will come across two major types of loops: **count-controlled loops,** which repeat a specified number of times, and **event-controlled loops,** which repeat until something happens within the loop.

Count-controlled loop   A loop that executes a specified number of times.

Event-controlled loop   A loop that terminates when something happens inside the loop body to signal that the loop should be exited.

If you are making an angel food cake and the recipe reads "Beat the mixture 300 strokes," you are executing a count-controlled loop. If you are making a pie crust and the recipe reads "Cut with a pastry blender until the mixture resembles coarse meal," you are executing an event-controlled loop; you don't know ahead of time the exact number of loop iterations.

Count-Controlled Loops

A count-controlled loop uses a variable we call the *loop control variable* in the loop test. Before we enter a count-controlled loop, we have to *initialize* (set the initial value of) the loop control variable and then test it. Then, as part of each iteration of the loop, we must *increment* (increase by 1) the loop control variable. Here's an example:

```
loopCount = 1;                      // Initialization
while (loopCount <= 10)             // Test
{
    .
    .                               // Repeated actions
    .
    loopCount = loopCount + 1;      // Incrementation
}
```

Here `loopCount` is the loop control variable. It is set to 1 before loop entry. The While statement tests the expression

```
loopCount <= 10
```

and executes the loop body as long as the expression is `true`. The dots inside the compound statement represent a sequence of statements to be repeated. The last statement in the loop body increments `loopCount` by adding 1 to it.

Look at the statement in which we increment the loop control variable. Notice its form:

```
variable = variable + 1;
```

This statement adds 1 to the current value of the variable, and the result replaces the old value. Variables that are used this way are called *counters*. In our example, loopCount is incremented with each iteration of the loop—we use it to count the iterations. The loop control variable of a count-controlled loop is always a counter.

We've encountered another way of incrementing a variable in C++. The incrementation operator (++) increments the variable that is its operand. The statement

```
loopCount++;
```

has precisely the same effect as the assignment statement

```
loopCount = loopCount + 1;
```

From here on, we typically use the ++ operator, as do most C++ programmers.

When designing loops, it is the programmer's responsibility to see that the condition to be tested is set correctly (initialized) before the While statement begins. The programmer also must make sure that the condition changes within the loop so that it eventually becomes false; otherwise, the loop is never exited.

```
loopCount = 1;                    ←Variable loopCount must be initialized
while (loopCount <= 10)
{
      ⋮
    loopCount++;                  ←loopCount must be incremented
}
```

A loop that never exits is called an *infinite loop* because, in theory, the loop executes forever. In the code above, omitting the incrementation of loopCount at the bottom of the loop leads to an infinite loop; the While expression is always true because the value of loopCount is forever 1. If your program goes on running for much longer than you expect it to, chances are that you've created an infinite loop. You may have to issue an operating system command to stop the program.

How many times does the loop in our example execute—9 or 10? To determine this, we have to look at the initial value of the loop control variable and then at the test to see what its final value is. Here we've initialized loopCount to 1, and the test indicates that the loop body is executed for each value of loopCount up through 10. If loopCount starts out at 1 and runs up to 10, the loop body is executed 10 times. If we want the loop to execute 11 times, we have to either initialize `loopCount` to 0 or change the test to

```
loopCount <= 11
```

Event-Controlled Loops

There are several kinds of event-controlled loops: sentinel-controlled, end-of-file-controlled, and flag-controlled. In all of these loops, the termination condition depends on some event occurring while the loop body is executing.

Sentinel-Controlled Loops   Loops often are used to read in and process long lists of data. Each time the loop body is executed, a new piece of data is read and processed. Often a special data value, called a *sentinel* or *trailer value*, is used to signal the program that there is no more data to be processed. Looping continues as long as the data value read is *not* the sentinel; the loop stops when the program recognizes the sentinel. In other words, reading the sentinel value is the event that controls the looping process.

A sentinel value must be something that never shows up in the normal input to a program. For example, if a program reads calendar dates, we could use February 31 as a sentinel value:

```
// This code is incorrect:

while ( !(month == 2 && day == 31) )
{
    cin >> month >> day;              // Get a date
     ⋮                                // Process it
}
```

There is a problem in the loop in the example above. The values of `month` and `day` are not defined before the first pass through the loop. Somehow we have to initialize these variables. We could assign them arbitrary values, but then we would run the risk that the first values input are the sentinel values, which would then be processed as data. Also, it's inefficient to initialize variables with values that are never used.

We can solve the problem by reading the first set of data values *before* entering the loop. This is called a *priming read*. (The idea is similar to priming a pump by pouring a bucket of water into the mechanism before starting it.) Let's add the priming read to the loop:

```
// This is still incorrect:

cin >> month >> day;                        // Get a date--priming read
while ( !(month == 2 && day == 31) )
{
    cin >> month >> day;                    // Get a date
       ⋮                                    // Process it
}
```

With the priming read, if the first values input are the sentinel values, then the loop correctly does not process them. We've solved one problem, but now there is a problem when the first values input are valid data. Notice that the first thing the program does inside the loop is to get a date, destroying the values obtained by the priming read. Thus, the first date in the data list is never processed. Given the priming read, the *first* thing that the loop body should do is process the data that's already been read. But then at what point do we read the next data set? We do this *last* in the loop. In this way, the While condition is applied to the next data set before it gets processed. Here's how it looks:

```
// This version is correct:

cin >> month >> day;                        // Get a date--priming read
while ( !(month == 2 && day == 31) )
{
       ⋮                                    // Process it
    cin >> month >> day;                    // Get the next date
}
```

This segment works fine. The first data set is read in; if it is not the sentinel, it gets processed. At the end of the loop, the next data set is read in, and we go back to the beginning of the loop. If the new data set is not the sentinel, it gets processed just like the first. When the sentinel value is read, the While expression becomes `false` and the loop exits (*without* processing the sentinel).

Many times the problem dictates the value of the sentinel. For example, if the problem does not allow data values of 0, then the sentinel value should be 0. Sometimes a combination of values is invalid. The combination of February and 31 as a date is such a case. Sometimes a range of values (negative numbers, for example) is the sentinel. And when you process char data one line of input at a time, the newline character (`'\n'`) often serves as the sentinel. Here's a code segment that reads and prints all of the characters on an input line (`inChar` is of type `char`):

```
cin.get(inChar);                    // Get first character
while (inChar != '\n')
{
    cout << inChar;                 // Echo it
    cin.get(inChar);               // Get next character
}
```

(Notice that for this particular task we use the get function, not the >> operator, to input a character. Remember that the >> operator skips white-space characters—including blanks and newlines—to find the next data value in the input stream. In this example, we want to input *every* character, even a blank and especially the newline character.)

When you are choosing a value to use as a sentinel, what happens if there aren't any invalid data values? Then you may have to input an extra value in each iteration, a value whose only purpose is to signal the end of the data. For example, look at this code segment:

```
cin >> dataValue >> sentinel;       // Get first data value
while (sentinel == 1)
{
        ⋮                           // Process it
    cin >> dataValue >> sentinel;   // Get next data value
}
```

The second value on each line of the following data set is used to indicate whether or not there is more data. In this data set, when the sentinel value is 0, there is no more data; when it is 1, there is more data.

Data values	Sentinel values
10	1
0	1
−5	1
8	1
−1	1
47	0

What happens if you forget to enter the sentinel value? In an interactive program, the loop executes again, prompting for input. At that point, you can enter the sentinel value, but your program logic may be wrong if you already entered what you thought was the sentinel value. If the input to the program is from a file, once all the data has been read from the file, the loop body is executed again. However, there isn't any data left—because the computer has reached the end of the file—so the file stream enters the fail state. In the next section, we describe a way to use the end-of-file situation as an alternative to using a sentinel.

Before we go on, we mention an issue that is related not to the design of loops but to C++ language usage. In Chapter 5, we talked about the common mistake of using the assignment operator (=) instead of the relational operator (==) in an If condition. This same mistake can happen when you write While statements. See what happens when we use the wrong operator in the previous example:

```
cin >> dataValue >> sentinel;
while (sentinel = 1)                    // Whoops
{
    ⋮
    cin >> dataValue >> sentinel;
}
```

This mistake creates an infinite loop. The While expression is now an assignment expression, not a relational expression. The expression's value is 1 (interpreted in the loop test as `true` because it's nonzero), and its side effect is to store the value 1 into `sentinel`, replacing the value that was just input into the variable. Because the While expression is always `true`, the loop never stops.

End-of-File-Controlled Loops You already have learned that an input stream (such as `cin` or an input file stream) goes into the fail state (a) if it encounters unacceptable input data, (b) if the program tries to open a nonexistent input file, or (c) if the program tries to read past the end of an input file. Let's look at the third of these three possibilities.

After a program has read the last piece of data from an input file, the computer is at the end of the file (EOF, for short). At this moment, the stream state is all right. But if we try to input even one more data value, the stream goes into the fail state. We can use this fact to our advantage. To write a loop that inputs an unknown number of data items, we can use the failure of the input stream as a form of sentinel.

In Chapter 5, we described how to test the state of an I/O stream. In a logical expression, we use the name of the stream as though it were a Boolean variable:

```
if (inFile)
    ⋮
```

In a test like this, the result is `true` if the most recent I/O operation succeeded, or `false` if it failed. In a While statement, testing the state of a stream works the same way. Suppose we have a data file containing integer values. If `inData` is the name of the file stream in our program, here's a loop that reads and echoes all of the data values in the file:

```
inData >> intVal;                    // Get first value
while (inData)                       // While the input succeeded...
{
    cout << intVal << endl;          // Echo it
    inData >> intVal;                // Get next value
}
```

Let's trace this code, assuming there are three values in the file: 10, 20, and 30. The priming read inputs the value 10. The While condition is true because the input succeeded. Therefore, the computer executes the loop body. First the body prints out the value 10, and then it inputs the second data value, 20. Looping back to the loop test, the expression inData is true because the input succeeded. The body executes again, printing the value 20 and reading the value 30 from the file. Looping back to the test, the expression is true. Even though we are at the end of the file, the stream state is still OK—the previous input operation succeeded. The body executes a third time, printing the value 30 and executing the input statement. This time, the input statement fails; we're trying to read beyond the end of the file. The stream inData enters the fail state. Looping back to the loop test, the value of the expression is false and we exit the loop.

When we write EOF-controlled loops like the one above, we are expecting that the end of the file is the reason for stream failure. But keep in mind that *any* input error causes stream failure. The above loop terminates, for example, if input fails because of invalid characters in the input data. This fact emphasizes again the importance of echo printing. It helps us verify that all the data was read correctly before the EOF was encountered.

EOF-controlled loops are similar to sentinel-controlled loops in that the program doesn't know in advance how many data items are to be input. In the case of sentinel-controlled loops, the program reads until it encounters the sentinel value. With EOF-controlled loops, it reads until it reaches the end of the file.

Is it possible to use an EOF-controlled loop when we read from the standard input device (via the cin stream) instead of a data file? On many systems, yes. With the UNIX operating system, you can type Ctrl-D (that is, you hold down the Ctrl key and tap the D key) to signify end-of-file during interactive input. With the MS-DOS operating system, the end-of-file keystrokes are Ctrl-Z. Other systems use similar keystrokes. Here's a program segment that tests for EOF on the cin stream in UNIX:

```
cout << "Enter an integer (or Ctrl-D to quit): ";
cin >> someInt;
while (cin)
{
    cout << someInt << " doubled is " << 2 * someInt << endl;
    cout << "Next number (or Ctrl-D to quit): ";
    cin >> someInt;
}
```

Flag-Controlled Loops A *flag* is a Boolean variable that is used to control the logical flow of a program. We can set a Boolean variable to `true` before a While loop; then, when we want to stop executing the loop, we reset it to `false`. That is, we can use the Boolean variable to record whether or not the event that controls the process has occurred. For example, the following code segment reads and sums values until the input value is negative. (`nonNegative` is the Boolean flag; all of the other variables are of type `int`.)

```
sum = 0;
nonNegative = true;                   // Initialize flag
while (nonNegative)
{
    cin >> number;
    if (number < 0)                   // Test input value
        nonNegative = false;          // Set flag if event occurred
    else
        sum = sum + number;
}
```

Notice that we can code sentinel-controlled loops with flags. In fact, this code uses a negative value as a sentinel.

You do not have to initialize flags to `true`; you can initialize them to `false`. If you do, you must use the NOT operator (`!`) in the While expression and reset the flag to `true` when the event occurs. Compare the code segment above with the one below; both perform the same task. (Assume that `negative` is a Boolean variable.)

```
sum = 0;
negative = false;                     // Initialize flag
while ( !negative )
{
    cin >> number;
    if (number < 0)                   // Test input value
        negative = true;              // Set flag if event occurred
    else
        sum = sum + number;
}
```

As one more example, look at the While statement in the Payroll program at the end of Chapter 1. This is a sentinel-controlled loop because an employee number (empNum) with a value of 0 is used to stop the loop. We could have used a flag instead, as follows. (moreData is a Boolean variable.)

```
cin >> empNum;
moreData = (empNum != 0);              // true if empNum != 0
while (moreData)
{
     ⋮
    cin >> empNum;                      // Get the next employee number
    moreData = (empNum != 0);           // Update the flag accordingly
}
```

Looping Subtasks

We have been looking at ways to use loops to affect the flow of control in programs. But looping by itself does nothing. The loop body must perform a task in order for the loop to accomplish something. In this section, we look at three tasks—counting, summing, and keeping track of a previous value—that often are used in loops.

Counting A common task in a loop is to keep track of the number of times the loop has been executed. For example, the following program fragment reads and counts input characters until it comes to a period. (inChar is of type char; count is of type int.) The loop in this example has a counter variable, but the loop is not a count-controlled loop because the variable is not being used as a loop control variable.

```
count = 0;                             // Initialize counter
cin.get(inChar);                       // Read the first character
while (inChar != '.')
{
    count++;                           // Increment counter
    cin.get(inChar);                   // Get the next character
}
```

The loop continues until a period is read. After the loop is finished, count contains one less than the number of characters read. That is, it counts the number of characters up to, but not including, the sentinel value (the period). Notice that if a period is the first character, the loop body is not entered and count contains a 0, as it should. We use a priming read here because the loop is sentinel-controlled.

The counter variable in this example is called an **iteration counter** because its value equals the number of iterations through the loop.

Iteration counter   A counter variable that is incremented with each iteration of a loop.

According to our definition, the loop control variable of a count-controlled loop is an iteration counter. However, as you've just seen, not all iteration counters are loop control variables.

Summing   Another common looping task is to sum a set of data values. Notice in the following example that the summing operation is written the same way, regardless of how the loop is controlled.

```
sum = 0;                            // Initialize the sum
count = 1;
while (count <= 10)
{
    cin >> number;                  // Input a value
    sum = sum + number;             // Add the value to sum
    count++;
}
```

We initialize sum to 0 before the loop starts so that the first time the loop body executes, the statement

```
sum = sum + number;
```

adds the current value of sum (0) to number to form the new value of sum. After the entire code fragment has executed, sum contains the total of the ten values read, count contains 11, and number contains the last value read.

Here count is being incremented in each iteration. For each new value of count, there is a new value for number. Does this mean we could decrement count by 1 and inspect the previous value of number? No. Once a new value has been read into number, the previous value is gone forever unless we've saved it in another variable. You'll see how to do that in the next section.

Let's look at another example. We want to count and sum the first ten odd numbers in a data set. We need to test each number to see if it is even or odd. (We can use the modulus operator to find out. If number % 2 equals 1, number is odd; otherwise, it's even.) If the input value is even, we do nothing. If it is odd, we increment the counter and add the value to our sum. We use a flag to control the loop because this is not a normal count-controlled loop. In the following code segment, all variables are of type int except the Boolean flag, lessThanTen.

```
count = 0;                        // Initialize event counter
sum = 0;                          // Initialize sum
lessThanTen = true;              // Initialize loop control flag
while (lessThanTen)
{
    cin >> number;               // Get the next value
    if (number % 2 == 1)         // Is the value odd?
    {
        count++;                 // Yes--Increment counter
        sum = sum + number;      // Add value to sum
        lessThanTen = (count < 10);  // Update loop control flag
    }
}
```

In this example, there is no relationship between the value of the counter variable and the number of times the loop is executed. We could have written the While expression this way:

```
while (count < 10)
```

but this might mislead a reader into thinking that the loop is count-controlled in the normal way. So, instead, we control the loop with the flag lessThanTen to emphasize that count is incremented only when an odd number is read. The counter in this example is an **event counter;** it is initialized to 0 and incremented only when a certain event occurs. The counter in the previous example was an *iteration counter;* it was initialized to 1 and incremented during each iteration of the loop.

Event counter   A variable that is incremented each time a particular event occurs.

Keeping Track of a Previous Value   Sometimes we want to remember the previous value of a variable. Suppose we want to write a program that counts the number of not-equal operators (!=) in a file that contains a C++ program. We can do so by simply counting the number of times an exclamation mark (!) followed by an equal sign (=) appears in the input. One way in which to do this is to read the input file one character at a time, keeping track of the two most recent characters, the current value and the previous value. In each iteration of the loop, a new current value is read and the old current value becomes the previous value. When EOF is reached, the loop is finished. Here's a program that counts not-equal operators in this way:

```cpp
//******************************************************************
// NotEqualCount program
// This program counts the occurrences of "!=" in a data file
//******************************************************************
#include <iostream>
#include <fstream>      // For file I/O

using namespace std;

int main()
{
    int      count;        // Number of != operators
    char     prevChar;     // Last character read
    char     currChar;     // Character read in this loop iteration
    ifstream inFile;       // Data file

    inFile.open("myfile.dat");              // Attempt to open input file
    if ( !inFile )                          // Was it opened?
    {
        cout << "** Can't open input file **"  // No--print message
            << endl;
        return 1;                              // Terminate program
    }
    count = 0;                  // Initialize counter
    inFile.get(prevChar);       // Initialize previous value
    inFile.get(currChar);       // Initialize current value
    while (inFile)              // While previous input succeeded...
    {
        if (currChar == '=' &&  // Test for event
            prevChar == '!')
            count++;               // Increment counter
        prevChar = currChar;    // Replace previous value
                                //    with current value
        inFile.get(currChar);   // Get next value
    }
    cout << count << " != operators were found." << endl;
    return 0;
}
```

Study this loop carefully. It's going to come in handy. There are many problems in which you must keep track of the last value read in addition to the current value.

How to Design Loops

It's one thing to understand how a loop works when you look at it and something else again to design a loop that solves a given problem. In this section, we look at how to design loops. We can divide the design process into two tasks: designing the control flow and designing the processing that takes place in the loop. We can in turn break each task into three phases: the task itself, initialization, and update. It's also important to specify the state of the program when it exits the loop, because a loop that leaves variables and files in a mess is not well designed.

There are seven different points to consider in designing a loop:

1. What is the condition that ends the loop?
2. How should the condition be initialized?
3. How should the condition be updated?
4. What is the process being repeated?
5. How should the process be initialized?
6. How should the process be updated?
7. What is the state of the program on exiting the loop?

We use these questions as a checklist. The first three help us design the parts of the loop that control its execution. The next three help us design the processing within the loop. The last question reminds us to make sure that the loop exits in an appropriate manner.

Designing the Flow of Control

The most important step in loop design is deciding what should make the loop stop. If the termination condition isn't well thought out, there's the potential for infinite loops and other mistakes. So here is our first question:

-   What is the condition that ends the loop?

This question usually can be answered through a close examination of the problem statement. The following table lists some examples.

Key Phrase in Problem Statement	Termination Condition
"Sum 365 temperatures"	The loop ends when a counter reaches 365 (count-controlled loop).
"Process all the data in the file"	The loop ends when EOF occurs (EOF-controlled loop).
"Process until ten odd integers have been read"	The loop ends when ten odd numbers have been input (event counter).
"The end of the data is indicated by a negative test score"	The loop ends when a negative input value is encountered (sentinel-controlled loop).

Now we need statements that make sure the loop gets started correctly and statements that allow the loop to reach the termination condition. So we have to ask the next two questions:

- How should the condition be initialized?
- How should the condition be updated?

The answers to these questions depend on the type of termination condition.

Count-Controlled Loops If the loop is count-controlled, we initialize the condition by giving the loop control variable an initial value. For count-controlled loops in which the loop control variable is also an iteration counter, the initial value is usually 1. If the process requires the counter to run through a specific range of values, the initial value should be the lowest value in that range.

The condition is updated by increasing the value of the counter by 1 for each iteration. (Occasionally, you may come across a problem that requires a counter to count from some value *down* to a lower value. In this case, the initial value is the greater value, and the counter is decremented by 1 for each iteration.) So, for count-controlled loops that use an iteration counter, these are the answers to the questions:

- Initialize the iteration counter to 1.
- Increment the iteration counter at the end of each iteration.

If the loop is controlled by a variable that is counting an event within the loop, the control variable usually is initialized to 0 and is incremented each time the event occurs. For count-controlled loops that use an event counter, these are the answers to the questions:

- Initialize the event counter to 0.
- Increment the event counter each time the event occurs.

Sentinel-Controlled Loops In sentinel-controlled loops, a priming read may be the only initialization necessary. If the source of input is a file rather than the keyboard, it also may be necessary to open the file in preparation for reading. To update the condition, a new value is read at the end of each iteration. So, for sentinel-controlled loops, we answer our questions this way:

- Open the file, if necessary, and input a value before entering the loop (priming read).
- Input a new value for processing at the end of each iteration.

EOF-Controlled Loops EOF-controlled loops require the same initialization as sentinel-controlled loops. You must open the file, if necessary, and perform a priming read. Updating the loop condition happens implicitly; the stream state is updated to reflect success or failure every time a value is input. However, if the loop doesn't read any data, it can never reach EOF, so updating the loop condition means the loop must keep reading data.

Flag-Controlled Loops In flag-controlled loops, the Boolean flag variable must be initialized to `true` or `false` and then updated when the condition changes.

- Initialize the flag variable to `true` or `false`, as appropriate.
- Update the flag variable as soon as the condition changes.

In a flag-controlled loop, the flag variable essentially remains unchanged until it is time for the loop to end. Then the code detects some condition within the process being repeated that changes the value of the flag (through an assignment statement). Because the update depends on what the process does, at times we have to design the process before we can decide how to update the condition.

Designing the Process Within the Loop

Once we've determined the looping structure itself, we can fill in the details of the process. In designing the process, we first must decide what we want a single iteration to do. Assume for a moment that the process is going to execute only once. What tasks must the process perform?

- What is the process being repeated?

To answer this question, we have to take another look at the problem statement. The definition of the problem may require the process to sum up data values or to keep a count of data values that satisfy some test. For example:

Count the number of integers in the file howMany.

This statement tells us that the process to be repeated is a counting operation.

Here's another example:

Read a stock price for each business day in a week and compute the average price.

In this case, part of the process involves reading a data value. We have to conclude from our knowledge of how an average is computed that the process also involves summing the data values.

In addition to counting and summing, another common loop process is reading data, performing a calculation, and writing out the result. Many other operations can appear in looping processes. We've mentioned only the simplest here; we look at some other processes later on.

After we've determined the operations to be performed if the process is executed only once, we design the parts of the process that are necessary for it to be repeated correctly. We often have to add some steps to take into account the fact that the loop executes more than once. This part of the design typically involves initializing certain variables before the loop and then reinitializing or updating them before each subsequent iteration.

- How should the process be initialized?
- How should the process be updated?

For example, if the process within a loop requires that several different counts and sums be performed, each must have its own statements to initialize variables, increment counting variables, or add values to sums. Just deal with each counting or summing operation by itself—that is, first write the initialization statement, and then write the incrementing or summing statement. After you've done this for one operation, you go on to the next.

The Loop Exit

When the termination condition occurs and the flow of control passes to the statement following the loop, the variables used in the loop still contain values. And if the cin stream has been used, the reading marker has been left at some position in the stream. Or maybe an output file has new contents. If these variables or files are used later in the program, the loop must leave them in an appropriate state. So, the final step in designing a loop is answering this question:

- What is the state of the program on exiting the loop?

Now we have to consider the consequences of our design and double-check its validity. For example, suppose we've used an event counter and that later processing depends on the number of events. It's important to be sure (with an algorithm walk-through) that the value left in the counter is the exact number of events—that it is not off by 1.

Look at this code segment:

```
commaCount = 1;              // This code is incorrect
cin.get(inChar);
while (inChar != '\n')
{
    if (inChar == ',')
        commaCount++;
    cin.get(inChar);
}
cout << commaCount << endl;
```

This loop reads characters from an input line and counts the number of commas on the line. However, when the loop terminates, `commaCount` equals the actual number of commas plus 1 because the loop initializes the event counter to 1 before any events take place. By determining the state of `commaCount` at loop exit, we've detected a flaw in the initialization. `commaCount` should be initialized to 0.

Designing correct loops depends as much on experience as it does on the application of design methodology. At this point, you may want to read through the Problem-Solving Case Study at the end of the chapter to see how the loop design process is applied to a real problem.

Nested Logic

In Chapter 5, we described nested If statements. It's also possible to nest While statements. Both While and If statements contain statements and are, themselves, statements. So the body of a While statement or the branch of an If statement can contain other While and If statements. By nesting, we can create complex control structures.

Suppose we want to extend our code for counting commas on one line, repeating it for all the lines in a file. We put an EOF-controlled loop around it:

```
cin.get(inChar);              // Initialize outer loop
while (cin)                   // Outer loop test
{
    commaCount = 0;           // Initialize inner loop
                              //   (Priming read is taken care of
                              //    by outer loop's priming read)
```

```
    while (inChar != '\n')        // Inner loop test
    {
        if (inChar == ',')
            commaCount++;
        cin.get(inChar);          // Update inner termination condition
    }
    cout << commaCount << endl;
    cin.get(inChar);              // Update outer termination condition
}
```

In this code, notice that we have omitted the priming read for the inner loop. The priming read for the outer loop has already "primed the pump." It would be a mistake to include another priming read just before the inner loop; the character read by the outer priming read would be destroyed before we could test it.

Let's examine the general pattern of a simple nested loop. The dots represent places where the processing and update may take place in the outer loop.

```
Initialize outer loop

while ( Outer loop condition )

{
        ⋮
    ┌──────────────────────────────────────────┐
    │ Initialize inner loop                      │
    │                                            │
    │ while ( Inner loop condition )             │
    │                                            │
    │ {                                          │
    │   Inner loop processing and update         │
    │ }                                          │
    └──────────────────────────────────────────┘

        ⋮
}
```

Notice that each loop has its own initialization, test, and update. It's possible for an outer loop to do no processing other than to execute the inner loop repeatedly. On the other hand, the inner loop might be just a small part of the processing done by the outer loop; there could be many statements preceding or following the inner loop.

Let's look at another example. For nested count-controlled loops, the pattern looks like this (where outCount is the counter for the outer loop, inCount is the counter for the inner loop, and limit1 and limit2 are the number of times each loop should be executed):

```
outCount = 1;                           // Initialize outer loop counter
while (outCount <= limit1)
{
    ⋮
    inCount = 1;                        // Initialize inner loop counter
    while (inCount <= limit2)
    {
        ⋮
        inCount++;                      // Increment inner loop counter
    }
    ⋮
    outCount++;                         // Increment outer loop counter
}
```

Here, both the inner and outer loops are count-controlled loops, but the pattern can be used with any combination of loops.

The following program fragment shows a count-controlled loop nested within an EOF-controlled loop. The outer loop inputs an integer value telling how many asterisks to print out across a row of the screen. (We use the numbers to the right of the code to trace the execution of the program.)

```
cin >> starCount;                       1
while (cin)                             2
{
    loopCount = 1;                      3
    while (loopCount <= starCount)      4
    {
        cout << '*';                    5
        loopCount++;                    6
    }
    cout << endl;                       7
    cin >> starCount;                   8
}
cout << "Goodbye" << endl;              9
```

To see how this code works, let's trace its execution with these data values (<EOF> denotes the end-of-file keystrokes pressed by the user):

```
3
1
<EOF>
```

We'll keep track of the variables starCount and loopCount, as well as the logical expressions. To do this, we've numbered each line (except those containing only a left or right brace). As we trace the program, we indicate the first execution of line 3 by 3.1, the second by 3.2, and so on.

Table 6-1 Code Trace

| | Variables | | | Logical Expressions | |
Statement	starCount	loopCount	cin	loopCount <= starCount	Output
1.1	3	—	—	—	—
2.1	3	—	T	—	—
3.1	3	1	—	—	—
4.1	3	1	—	T	—
5.1	3	1	—	—	*
6.1	3	2	—	—	—
4.2	3	2	—	T	—
5.2	3	2	—	—	*
6.2	3	3	—	—	—
4.3	3	3	—	T	—
5.3	3	3	—	—	*
6.3	3	4	—	—	—
4.4	3	4	—	F	—
7.1	3	4	—	—	\n (newline)
8.1	1	4	—	—	—
2.2	1	4	T	—	—
3.2	1	1	—	—	—
4.5	1	1	—	T	—
5.4	1	1	—	—	*
6.4	1	2	—	—	—
4.6	1	2	—	F	—
7.2	1	2	—	—	\n (newline)
8.2	1	2	—	—	—
	(null operation)				
2.3	1	2	F	—	—
9.1	1	2	—	—	Goodbye

Here's a sample run of the program. The user's input is in color. Again, the symbol <EOF> denotes the end-of-file keystrokes pressed by the user (the symbol would not appear on the screen).

```
3
***
1
*
<EOF>
Goodbye
```

Because `starCount` and `loopCount` are variables, their values remain the same until they are explicitly changed, as indicated by the repeating values in Table 6-1. The values of the logical expressions `cin` and `loopCount <= starCount` exist only when the test is made. We indicate this fact with dashes in those columns at all other times.

Designing Nested Loops

To design a nested loop, we begin with the outer loop. The process being repeated includes the nested loop as one of its steps. Because that step is more complex than a single statement, our functional decomposition methodology tells us to make it a separate module. We can come back to it later and design the nested loop just as we would any other loop.

For example, here's the design process for the preceding code segment:

1. *What is the condition that ends the loop?* EOF is reached in the input.
2. *How should the condition be initialized?* A priming read should be performed before the loop starts.
3. *How should the condition be updated?* An input statement should occur at the end of each iteration.
4. *What is the process being repeated?* Using the value of the current input integer, the code should print that many asterisks across one output line.
5. *How should the process be initialized?* No initialization is necessary.
6. *How should the process be updated?* A sequence of asterisks is output and then a newline character is output. There are no counter variables or sums to update.
7. *What is the state of the program on exiting the loop?* The `cin` stream is in the fail state (because the program tried to read past EOF), `starCount` contains the last integer read from the input stream, and the rows of asterisks have been printed along with a concluding message.

From the answers to these questions, we can write this much of the algorithm:

```
Read starCount
WHILE NOT EOF
    Print starCount asterisks
    Output newline
    Read starCount
Print "Goodbye"
```

After designing the outer loop, it's obvious that the process in its body (printing a sequence of asterisks) is a complex step that requires us to design an inner loop. So we repeat the methodology for the corresponding lower-level module:

1. *What is the condition that ends the loop?* An iteration counter exceeds the value of starCount.
2. *How should the condition be initialized?* The iteration counter should be initialized to 1.
3. *How should the condition be updated?* The iteration counter is incremented at the end of each iteration.
4. *What is the process being repeated?* The code should print a single asterisk on the standard output device.
5. *How should the process be initialized?* No initialization is needed.
6. *How should the process be updated?* No update is needed.
7. *What is the state of the program on exiting the loop?* A single row of asterisks has been printed, the writing marker is at the end of the current output line, and loopCount contains a value one greater than the current value of starCount.

Now we can write the algorithm:

```
Read starCount
WHILE NOT EOF
      Set loopCount = 1
      WHILE loopCount <= starCount
            Print ' * '
            Increment loopCount
      Output newline
      Read starCount
Print "Goodbye"
```

Of course, nested loops themselves can contain nested loops (called *doubly nested loops*), which can contain nested loops (*triply nested loops*), and so on. You can use this design process for any number of levels of nesting. The trick is to defer details by using the functional decomposition methodology—that is, focus on the outermost loop first and treat each new level of nested loop as a module within the loop that contains it.

It's also possible for the process within a loop to include more than one loop. For example, here's an algorithm that reads and prints people's names from a file, omitting the middle name in the output:

        Read and print first name (ends with a comma)
        WHILE NOT EOF
                Read and discard characters from middle name (ends with a comma)
                Read and print last name (ends at newline)
                Output newline
                Read and print first name (ends with a comma)

The steps for reading the first name, middle name, and last name require us to design three separate loops. All of these loops are sentinel-controlled.

This kind of complex control structure would be difficult to read if written out in full. There are simply too many variables, conditions, and steps to remember at one time. In the next two chapters, we examine the control structure that allows us to break programs down into more manageable chunks—the subprogram.

THEORETICAL FOUNDATIONS

Analysis of Algorithms

If you were given the choice of cleaning a room with a toothbrush or a broom, you probably would choose the broom. Using a broom sounds like less work than using a toothbrush. True, if the room were in a dollhouse, it might be easier to use the toothbrush, but in general a broom is the faster way to clean. If you were given the choice of adding numbers together with a pencil and paper or a calculator, you would probably choose the calculator because it is usually less work. If you were given the choice of walking or driving to a meeting, you would probably choose to drive; it sounds like less work.

What do these examples have in common? What do they have to do with computer science? In each of the situations mentioned, one of the choices seems to involve significantly less work. Precisely measuring the amount of work is difficult in each case because there are unknowns. How large is the room? How many numbers are there? How far away is the meeting? In each case, the unknown information is related to the size of the problem. If the problem is especially small (for example, adding 2 plus 2), our original estimate of which approach to take (using the calculator) might be wrong. However, our intuition is usually correct, because most problems are reasonably large.

In computer science, we need a way of measuring the amount of work done by an algorithm relative to the size of a problem, because there is usually more than one algorithm that solves any given problem. We often must choose the most efficient algorithm—the algorithm that does the least work for a problem of a given size.

The amount of work involved in executing an algorithm relative to the size of the problem is called the **complexity** of the algorithm. We would like to be able to look at an algorithm and determine its complexity. Then we could take two algorithms that perform the same task and determine which completes the task faster (requires less work).

Complexity   A measure of the effort expended by the computer in performing a computation, relative to the size of the computation.

How do we measure the amount of work required to execute an algorithm? We use the total number of *steps* executed as a measure of work. One statement, such as an assignment, may require only one step; another, such as a loop, may require many steps. We define a step as any operation roughly equivalent in complexity to a comparison, an I/O operation, or an assignment.

Given an algorithm with just a sequence of simple statements (no branches or loops), the number of steps performed is directly related to the number of statements. When we introduce branches, however, we make it possible to skip some statements in the algorithm. Branches allow us to subtract steps without physically removing them from the algorithm because only one branch is executed at a time. But because we usually want to express work in terms of the worst-case scenario, we use the number of steps in the longest branch.

Now consider the effect of a loop. If a loop repeats a sequence of 15 simple statements 10 times, it performs 150 steps. Loops allow us to multiply the work done in an algorithm without physically adding statements.

Now that we have a measure for the work done in an algorithm, we can compare algorithms. For example, if algorithm A always executes 3124 steps and algorithm B always does the same task in 1321 steps, then we can say that algorithm B is more efficient—that is, it takes fewer steps to accomplish the same task.

If an algorithm, from run to run, always takes the same number of steps or fewer, we say that it executes in an amount of time bounded by a constant. Such algorithms are referred to as having *constant-time* complexity. Be careful: Constant time doesn't mean small; it means that the amount of work done does not exceed some amount from one run to another.

If a loop executes a fixed number of times, the work done is greater than the physical number of statements but still is constant. What happens if the number of loop iterations can change from one run to the next? Suppose a data file contains N data values to be processed in a loop. If the loop reads and processes one value during each iteration, then the loop executes N iterations. The amount of work done thus depends on a variable, the number of data values. The variable N determines the size of the problem in this example.

If we have a loop that executes N times, the number of steps to be executed is some factor times N. The factor is the number of steps performed within a single iteration of the loop. Specifically, the work done by an algorithm with a data-dependent loop is given by the expression

Steps performed
by the loop

$$\overbrace{S_1 \times N} + \underline{S_0}$$

Steps performed
outside the loop

where S_1 is the number of steps in the loop body (a constant for a given simple loop), N is the number of iterations (a variable representing the size of the problem), and S_0 is the number of steps outside the loop. Mathematicians call expressions of this form *linear;* hence, algorithms such as this are said to have *linear-time* complexity. Notice that if N grows very large, the term $S_1 \times N$ dominates the execution time. That is, S_0 becomes an insignificant part of the total execution time. For example, if S_0 and S_1 are each 20 steps, and N is 1,000,000, then the total number of steps is 20,000,020. The 20 steps contributed by S_0 are a tiny fraction of the total.

What about a data-dependent loop that contains a nested loop? The number of steps in the inner loop, S_2, and the number of iterations performed by the inner loop, L, must be multiplied by the number of iterations in the outer loop:

Steps performed　　　Steps performed　　　Steps performed outside
by the nested loop　　by the outer loop　　　the outer loop

$$\overbrace{(S_2 \times L \times N)} \quad + \quad \overbrace{(S_1 \times N)} \quad + \quad \overbrace{S_0}$$

By itself, the inner loop performs $S_2 \times L$ steps, but because it is repeated N times by the outer loop, it accounts for a total of $S_2 \times L \times N$ steps. If L is a constant, then the algorithm still executes in linear time.

Now, suppose that for each of the N outer loop iterations, the inner loop performs N steps ($L = N$). Here the formula for the total steps is

$$(S_2 \times N \times N) + (S_1 \times N) + S_0$$

or

$$(S_2 \times N^2) + (S_1 \times N) + S_0$$

Because N^2 grows much faster than N (for large values of N), the inner loop term $(S_2 \times N^2)$ accounts for the majority of steps executed and of the work done. The corresponding execution time is thus essentially proportional to N^2. Mathematicians call this type of formula *quadratic*. If we have a doubly nested loop in which each loop depends on N, then the expression is

$$(S_3 \times N^3) + (S_2 \times N^2) + (S_1 \times N) + S_0$$

and the work and time are proportional to N^3 whenever N is reasonably large. Such a formula is called *cubic*.

The following table shows the number of steps required for each increase in the exponent of N, where N is a size factor for the problem, such as the number of input values.

N	N^0 *(Constant)*	N^1 *(Linear)*	N^2 *(Quadratic)*	N^3 *(Cubic)*
1	1	1	1	1
10	1	10	100	1,000
100	1	100	10,000	1,000,000
1,000	1	1,000	1,000,000	1,000,000,000
10,000	1	10,000	100,000,000	1,000,000,000,000

As you can see, each time the exponent increases by 1, the number of steps is multiplied by an additional order of magnitude (factor of 10). That is, if N is made 10 times greater, the work involved in an N^2 algorithm increases by a factor of 100, and the work involved in an N^3 algorithm increases by a factor of 1000. To put this in more concrete terms, an algorithm with a doubly nested loop in which each loop depends on the number of data values takes 1000 steps for 10 input values and 1 trillion steps for 10,000 values. On a computer that executes 10 million instructions per second, the latter case would take more than a day to run.

The table also shows that the steps outside of the innermost loop account for an insignificant portion of the total number of steps as N gets bigger. Because the innermost loop dominates the total time, we classify the complexity of an algorithm according to the highest order of N that appears in its complexity expression, called the *order of magnitude*, or simply the *order*, of that expression. So we talk about algorithms having "order N squared complexity" (or cubed or so on) or we describe them with what is called *Big-O notation*. We express the complexity by putting the highest-order term in parentheses with a capital O in front. For example, $O(1)$ is constant time, $O(N)$ is linear time, $O(N^2)$ is quadratic time, and $O(N^3)$ is cubic time.

Determining the complexities of different algorithms allows us to compare the work they require without having to program and execute them. For example, if you had an $O(N^2)$ algorithm and a linear algorithm that performed the same task, you probably would choose the linear algorithm. We say *probably* because an $O(N^2)$ algorithm actually may execute fewer steps than an $O(N)$ algorithm for small values of N. Remember that if the size factor N is small, the constants and lower-order terms in the complexity expression may be significant.

Let's look at an example. Suppose that algorithm A is $O(N^2)$ and that algorithm B is $O(N)$. For large values of N, we would normally choose algorithm B because it requires less work than A. But suppose that in algorithm B, $S_0 = 1000$ and $S_1 = 1000$. If $N = 1$, then algorithm B takes 2000 steps to execute. Now suppose that for algorithm A, $S_0 = 10$, $S_1 = 10$, and $S_2 = 10$. If $N = 1$, then algorithm A takes only 30 steps. Here is a table that compares the number of steps taken by these two algorithms for different values of N.

N	Algorithm A	Algorithm B
1	30	2000
2	70	3000
3	130	4000
10	1110	11,000
20	4210	21,000
30	9310	31,000
50	25,510	51,000
100	101,010	101,000
1,000	10,010,010	1,001,000
10,000	1,000,100,010	10,001,000

From this table we can see that the $O(N^2)$ algorithm A is actually faster than the $O(N)$ algorithm B, up to the point that N equals 100. Beyond that point, algorithm B becomes more efficient. Thus, if we know that N is always less than 100 in a particular problem, we would choose algorithm A. For example, if the size factor N is the number of test scores on an exam and the class size is limited to 30 students, algorithm A would be more efficient. On the other hand, if N is the number of scores at a university with 25,000 students, we would choose algorithm B.

Constant, linear, quadratic, and cubic expressions are all examples of *polynomial* expressions. Algorithms whose complexity is characterized by such expressions are therefore said to execute in *polynomial time* and form a broad class of algorithms that encompasses everything we've discussed so far.

In addition to polynomial-time algorithms, we encounter a logarithmic-time algorithm in Chapter 13. There are also factorial ($O(N!)$), exponential ($O(N^N)$), and hyperexponential ($O(N^{N^N})$) classes of algorithms, which can require vast amounts of time to execute and are beyond the scope of this book. For now, the important point to remember is that different algorithms that solve the same problem can vary significantly in the amount of work they do.

PROBLEM-SOLVING CASE STUDY

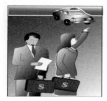

Average Income by Gender

Problem: You've been hired by a law firm that is working on a sex discrimination case. Your firm has obtained a file of incomes, incFile, that contains the salaries for every employee in the company being sued. Each salary amount is preceded by 'F' for female or 'M' for male. As a first pass in the analysis of this data, you've been asked to compute the average income for females and the average income for males.

Input: A file, incFile, of floating-point salary amounts, with one amount per line. Each amount is preceded by a character ('F' for female, 'M' for male). This code is the first character on each input line and is followed by a blank, which separates the code from the amount.

Output:

All the input data (echo print)
The number of females and their average income
The number of males and their average income

Discussion: The problem breaks down into three main steps. First, we have to process the data, counting and summing the salary amounts for each sex. Next, we compute the averages. Finally, we have to print the calculated results.

The first step is the most difficult. It involves a loop with several subtasks. We use our checklist of questions to develop these subtasks in detail.

1. *What is the condition that ends the loop?* The termination condition is EOF on the file incFile. It leads to the following loop test (in pseudocode).

       WHILE NOT EOF on incFile

2. *How should the condition be initialized?* We must open the file for input, and a priming read must take place.
3. *How should the condition be updated?* We must input a new data line with a gender code and amount at the end of each iteration. Here's the resulting algorithm:

       Open incFile for input (and verify the attempt)
       Read sex and amount from incFile
       WHILE NOT EOF on incFile
         : (Process being repeated)
         Read sex and amount from incFile

4. *What is the process being repeated?* From our knowledge of how to compute an average, we know that we have to count the number of amounts and divide this number into the sum of the amounts. Because we have to do this separately for females and males, the process consists of four parts: counting the females and summing their incomes, and then counting the males and summing their incomes. We develop each of these in turn.

5. *How should the process be initialized?* femaleCount and femaleSum should be set to zero. maleCount and maleSum also should be set to zero.

6. *How should the process be updated?* When a female income is input, femaleCount is incremented and the income is added to femaleSum. Otherwise, an income is assumed to be for a male, so maleCount is incremented and the amount is added to maleSum.

7. *What is the state of the program on exiting the loop?* The file stream incFile is in the fail state, femaleCount contains the number of input values preceded by 'F', femaleSum contains the sum of the values preceded by 'F', maleCount contains the number of values not preceded by 'F', and maleSum holds the sum of those values.

From the description of how the process is updated, we can see that the loop must contain an If-Then-Else structure, with one branch for female incomes and the other for male incomes. Each branch must increment the correct event counter and add the income amount to the correct total. After the loop has exited, we have enough information to compute and print the averages, dividing each total by the corresponding count.

Assumptions: There is at least one male and one female among all the data sets. The only gender codes in the file are 'M' and 'F'—any other codes are counted as 'M'. (This last assumption invalidates the results if there are any illegal codes in the data. Case Study Follow-Up Exercise 1 asks you to change the program as necessary to address this problem.)

Now we're ready to write the complete algorithm:

Main Module   **Level 0**

Separately count females and males, and sum incomes
Compute average incomes
Output results

PROBLEM-SOLVING CASE STUDY cont'd.

Separately Count Females and Males, and Sum Incomes   Level 1

> Initialize ending condition
> Initialize process
> WHILE NOT EOF on incFile
>   Update process
>   Update ending condition

Compute Average Incomes

> Set femaleAverage = femaleSum / femaleCount
> Set maleAverage = maleSum / maleCount

Output Results

> Print femaleCount and femaleAverage
> Print maleCount and maleAverage

Initialize Ending Condition   Level 2

> Open incFile for input (and verify the attempt)
> Read sex and amount from incFile

Initialize Process

> Set femaleCount = 0
> Set femaleSum = 0.0
> Set maleCount = 0
> Set maleSum = 0.0

PROBLEM-SOLVING CASE STUDY cont'd.

Update Process

```
Echo print sex and amount
IF sex is 'F'
        Increment femaleCount
        Add amount to femaleSum
ELSE
        Increment maleCount
        Add amount to maleSum
```

Update Ending Condition

```
Read sex and amount from incFile
```

Module Structure Chart:

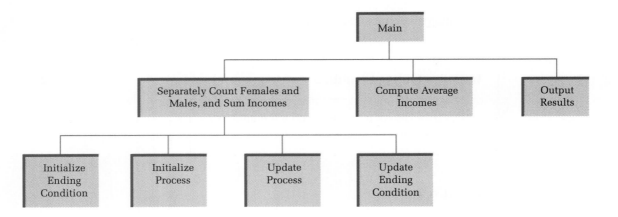

PROBLEM-SOLVING CASE STUDY cont'd.

(The following program is written in ISO/ANSI standard C++. If you are working with pre–standard C++, see the alternate version of the program in the PRE_STD directory of the program disk, available at the publisher's Web site, www.jbpub.com/disks.)

```cpp
//****************************************************************
// Incomes program
// This program reads a file of income amounts classified by
// gender and computes the average income for each gender
//****************************************************************
#include <iostream>
#include <iomanip>     // For setprecision()
#include <fstream>     // For file I/O
#include <string>      // For string type

using namespace std;

int main()
{
    char     sex;           // Coded 'F' = female, 'M' = male
    int      femaleCount;   // Number of female income amounts
    int      maleCount;     // Number of male income amounts
    float    amount;        // Amount of income for a person
    float    femaleSum;     // Total of female income amounts
    float    maleSum;       // Total of male income amounts
    float    femaleAverage; // Average female income
    float    maleAverage;   // Average male income
    ifstream incFile;       // File of income amounts
    string   fileName;      // External name of file

    cout << fixed << showpoint          // Set up floating-pt.
         << setprecision(2);            //    output format

    // Separately count females and males, and sum incomes

    // Initialize ending condition

    cout << "Name of the income data file: ";
    cin >> fileName;
    incFile.open(fileName.c_str());     // Open input file
    if ( !incFile )                     //    and verify attempt
    {
        cout << "** Can't open input file **" << endl;
        return 1;
    }
    incFile >> sex >> amount;           // Perform priming read
```

PROBLEM-SOLVING CASE STUDY   cont'd.

```
// Initialize process

femaleCount = 0;
femaleSum = 0.0;
maleCount = 0;
maleSum = 0.0;

while (incFile)
{
    // Update process

    cout << "Sex: " << sex << " Amount: " << amount << endl;
    if (sex == 'F')
    {
        femaleCount++;
        femaleSum = femaleSum + amount;
    }
    else
    {
        maleCount++;
        maleSum = maleSum + amount;
    }

    // Update ending condition

    incFile >> sex >> amount;
}

// Compute average incomes

femaleAverage = femaleSum / float(femaleCount);
maleAverage = maleSum / float(maleCount);

// Output results

cout << "For " << femaleCount << " females, the average "
    << "income is " << femaleAverage << endl;
cout << "For " << maleCount << " males, the average "
    << "income is " << maleAverage << endl;
return 0;
}
```

Testing: With an EOF-controlled loop, the obvious test cases are a file with data and an empty file. We should test input values of both 'F' and 'M' for the gender, and try some typical data (so we can compare the results with our hand-calculated values) and some atypical data (to see how the process behaves). An atypical data set for testing a counting operation is an empty file, which should result in a count of zero. Any other result for the count indicates an error. For a summing operation, atypical data might include negative or zero values.

The Incomes program is not designed to handle empty files or negative income values. An empty file causes both `femaleCount` and `maleCount` to equal zero at the end of the loop. Although this is correct, the statements that compute average income cause the program to crash because they divide by zero. A negative income would be treated like any other value, even though it is probably a mistake.

To correct these problems, we should insert If statements to test for the error conditions at the appropriate points in the program. When an error is detected, the program should print an error message instead of carrying out the usual computation. This prevents a crash and allows the program to keep running. We call a program that can recover from erroneous input and keep running a *robust program*.

Testing and Debugging

Loop-Testing Strategy

Even if a loop has been properly designed and verified, it is still important to test it rigorously because the chance of an error creeping in during the implementation phase is always present. Because loops allow us to input many data sets in one run, and because each iteration may be affected by preceding ones, the test data for a looping program is usually more extensive than for a program with just sequential or branching statements. To test a loop thoroughly, we must check for the proper execution of both a single iteration and multiple iterations.

Remember that a loop has seven parts (corresponding to the seven questions in our checklist). A test strategy must test each part. Although all seven parts aren't implemented separately in every loop, the checklist reminds us that some loop operations serve multiple purposes, each of which should be tested. For example, the incrementing statement in a count-controlled loop may be updating both the process and the ending condition, so it's important to verify that it performs both actions properly with respect to the rest of the loop.

To test a loop, we try to devise data sets that could cause the variables to go out of range or leave the files in improper states that violate either the loop postcondition (an assertion that must be true immediately after loop exit) or the postcondition of the module containing the loop.

It's also good practice to test a loop for four special cases: (1) when the loop is skipped entirely, (2) when the loop body is executed just once, (3) when the loop executes some normal number of times, and (4) when the loop fails to exit.

Statements following a loop often depend on its processing. If a loop can be skipped, those statements may not execute correctly. If it's possible to execute a single iteration of a loop, the results can show whether the body performs correctly in the absence of the effects of previous iterations, which can be very helpful when you're trying to isolate the source of an error. Obviously, it's important to test a loop under normal conditions, with a wide variety of inputs. If possible, you should test the loop with real data in addition to mock data sets. Count-controlled loops should be tested to be sure they execute exactly the right number of times. And finally, if there is any chance that a loop might never exit, your test data should try to make that happen.

Testing a program can be as challenging as writing it. To test a program, you need to step back, take a fresh look at what you've written, and then attack it in every way possible to make it fail. This isn't always easy to do, but it's necessary if your programs are going to be reliable. (A *reliable program* is one that works consistently and without errors regardless of whether the input data is valid or invalid.)

Test Plans Involving Loops

In Chapter 5, we introduced formal test plans and discussed the testing of branches. Those guidelines still apply to programs with loops, but here we provide some additional guidelines that are specific to loops.

Unfortunately, when a loop is embedded in a larger program, it sometimes is difficult to control and observe the conditions under which the loop executes using test data and output alone. In come cases we must use indirect tests. For example, if a loop reads floating-point values from a file and prints their average without echo printing them, you cannot tell directly that the loop processes all the data—if the data values in the file are all the same, then the average appears correct as long as even one of them is processed. You must construct the input file so that the average is a unique value that can be arrived at only by processing all the data.

To simplify our testing of such loops, we would like to observe the values of the variables associated with the loop at the start of each iteration. How can we observe the values of variables while a program is running? Two common techniques are the use of the system's *debugger* program and the use of extra output statements designed solely for debugging purposes. We discuss these techniques in the next section, Testing and Debugging Hints.

Now let's look at some test cases that are specific to the different types of loops that we've seen in this chapter.

Count-Controlled Loops When a loop is count-controlled, you should include a test case that specifies the output for all the iterations. It may help to add an extra column to the test plan that lists the iteration number. If the loop reads data and outputs a result, then each input value should produce a different output to make it easier to spot errors. For example, in a loop that is supposed to read and print 100 data values, it is easier to tell that the loop executes the correct number of iterations when the values are 1, 2, 3, ..., 100 than if they are all the same.

If the program inputs the iteration count for the loop, you need to test the cases in which an invalid count, such as a negative number, is input (an error message should be output and the loop should be skipped), a count of 0 is input (the loop should be skipped), a count of 1 is input (the loop should execute once), and some typical number of iterations is input (the loop should execute the specified number of times).

Event-Controlled Loops In an event-controlled loop, you should test the situation in which the event occurs before the loop, in the first iteration, and in a typical number of iterations. For example, if the event is that EOF occurs, then try an empty file, a file with one data set, and another with several data sets. If your testing involves reading from test files, you should attach printed copies of the files to the test plan and identify each in some way so that the plan can refer to them. It also helps to identify where each iteration begins in the Input and Expected Output columns of the test plan.

When the event is the input of a sentinel value, you need the following test cases: the sentinel is the only data set, the sentinel follows one data set, and the sentinel follows a typical number of data sets. Given that sentinel-controlled loops involve a priming read, it is especially important to verify that the first and last data sets are processed properly.

Testing and Debugging Hints

1. Plan your test data carefully to test all sections of a program.
2. Beware of infinite loops, in which the expression in the While statement never becomes `false`. The symptom: the program doesn't stop. If you are on a system that monitors the execution time of a program, you may see a message such as "TIME LIMIT EXCEEDED."

   If you have created an infinite loop, check your logic and the syntax of your loops. Be sure there's no semicolon immediately after the right parenthesis of the While condition:

```
while (Expression);          // Wrong
   Statement
```

This semicolon causes an infinite loop in most cases; the compiler thinks the loop body is the null statement (the do-nothing statement composed only of a semicolon). In a count-controlled loop, make sure the loop control variable is incremented within the loop. In a flag-controlled loop, make sure the flag eventually changes.

And, as always, watch for the = versus == problem in While conditions as well as in If conditions. The line

```
while (someVar = 5)      // Wrong (should be ==)
```

produces an infinite loop. The value of the assignment (not relational) expression is always 5, which is interpreted as true.

3. Check the loop termination condition carefully and be sure that something in the loop causes it to be met. Watch closely for values that cause one iteration too many or too few (the "off-by-1" syndrome).

4. Remember to use the get function rather than the >> operator in loops that are controlled by detection of a newline character.

5. Perform an algorithm walk-through to verify that all of the appropriate preconditions and postconditions occur in the right places.

6. Trace the execution of the loop by hand with a code walk-through. Simulate the first few passes and the last few passes very carefully to see how the loop really behaves.

7. Use a *debugger* if your system provides one. A debugger is a program that runs your program in "slow motion," allowing you to execute one instruction at a time and to examine the contents of variables as they change. If you haven't already done so, check to see if a debugger is available on your system.

8. If all else fails, use *debug output statements*—output statements inserted into a program to help debug it. They output messages that indicate the flow of execution in the program or report the values of variables at certain points in the program.

   For example, if you want to know the value of variable beta at a certain point in a program, you could insert this statement:

```
cout << "beta = " << beta << endl;
```

If this output statement is in a loop, you will get as many values of beta output as there are iterations of the body of the loop.

After you have debugged your program, you can remove the debug output statements or just precede them with // so that they'll be treated as comments. (This practice is referred to as *commenting out* a piece of code.) You can remove the double slashes if you need to use the statements again.

9. An ounce of prevention is worth a pound of debugging. Use the checklist questions to design your loop correctly at the outset. It may seem like extra work, but it pays off in the long run.

Summary

The While statement is a looping construct that allows the program to repeat a statement as long as the value of an expression is `true`. When the value of the expression becomes `false`, the body of the loop is skipped and execution continues with the first statement following the loop.

With the While statement, you can construct several types of loops that you will use again and again. These types of loops fall into two categories: count-controlled loops and event-controlled loops.

In a count-controlled loop, the loop body is repeated a specified number of times. You initialize a counter variable right before the While statement. This variable is the loop control variable. The control variable is tested against the limit in the While expression. The last statement in the loop body increments the control variable.

Event-controlled loops continue executing until something inside the body signals that the looping process should stop. Event-controlled loops include those that test for a sentinel value in the data, for end-of-file, or for a change in a flag variable.

Sentinel-controlled loops are input loops that use a special data value as a signal to stop reading. EOF-controlled loops are loops that continue to input (and process) data values until there is no more data. To implement them with a While statement, you must test the state of the input stream by using the name of the stream object as if it were a Boolean variable. The test yields `false` when there are no more data values. A flag is a variable that is set in one part of the program and tested in another. In a flag-controlled loop, you must set the flag before the loop begins, test it in the While expression, and change it somewhere in the body of the loop.

Counting is a looping operation that keeps track of how many times a loop is repeated or how many times some event occurs. This count can be used in computations or to control the loop. A counter is a variable that is used for counting. It may be the loop control variable in a count-controlled loop, an iteration counter in a counting loop, or an event counter that counts the number of times a particular condition occurs in a loop.

Summing is a looping operation that keeps a running total of certain values. It is like counting in that the variable that holds the sum is initialized outside the loop. The summing operation, however, adds up unknown values; the counting operation adds a constant (1) to the counter each time.

When you design a loop, there are seven points to consider: how the termination condition is initialized, tested, and updated; how the process in the loop is initialized, performed, and updated; and the state of the program upon exiting the loop. By answering the checklist questions, you can bring each of these points into focus.

To design a nested loop structure, begin with the outermost loop. When you get to where the inner loop must appear, make it a separate module and come back to its design later.

The process of testing a loop is based on the answers to the checklist questions and the patterns the loop might encounter (for example, executing a single iteration, multiple iterations, an infinite number of iterations, or no iterations at all).

Quick Check

1. Write the first line of a While statement that loops until the value of the Boolean variable done becomes true. (pp. 276–279)
2. What are the four parts of a count-controlled loop? (pp. 280–282)
3. Should you use a priming read with an EOF-controlled loop? (pp. 285–287)
4. How is a flag variable used to control a loop? (pp. 287–288)
5. What is the difference between a counting operation in a loop and a summing operation in a loop? (pp. 288–291)
6. What is the difference between a loop control variable and an event counter? (pp. 288–291)
7. What kind of loop would you use in a program that reads the closing price of a stock for each day of the week? (pp. 292–296)
8. How would you extend the loop in Question 7 to make it read prices for 52 weeks? (pp. 296–302)
9. How would you test a program that is supposed to count the number of females and the number of males in a data set? (Assume that females are coded with 'F' in the data; males, with 'M'.) (pp. 313–315)

Answers **1.** while (!done) **2.** The process being repeated, plus initializing, testing, and incrementing the loop control variable **3.** Yes **4.** The flag is set outside the loop. The While expression checks the flag, and an If inside the loop resets the flag when the termination condition occurs. **5.** A counting operation increments by a fixed value with each iteration of the loop; a summing operation adds unknown values to the total. **6.** A loop control variable controls the loop; an event counter simply counts certain events during execution of the loop. **7.** Because there are five days in a business week, you would use a count-controlled loop that runs from 1 to 5. **8.** Nest the original loop inside a count-controlled loop that runs from 1 to 52. **9.** Run the program with data sets that have a different number of females and males, only females, only males, illegal values (other characters), and an empty input file.

Exam Preparation Exercises

1. In one or two sentences, explain the difference between loops and branches.
2. What does the following loop print out? (number is of type int.)

```
number = 1;
while (number < 11)
{
    number++;
    cout << number << endl;
}
```

3. By rearranging the order of the statements (don't change the way they are written), make the loop in Exercise 2 print the numbers from 1 through 10.

4. When the following code is executed, how many iterations of the loop are performed?

```
number = 2;
done = false;
while ( !done )
{
    number = number * 2;
    if (number > 64)
        done = true;
}
```

5. What is the output of this nested loop structure?

```
i = 4;
while (i >= 1)
{
    j = 2;
    while (j >= 1)
    {
        cout << j << ' ';
        j--;
    }
    cout << i << endl;
    i--;
}
```

6. The following code segment is supposed to write out the even numbers between 1 and 15. (n is an int variable.) It has two flaws in it.

```
n = 2;
while (n != 15)
{
    n = n + 2;
    cout << n << ' ';
}
```

a. What is the output of the code as written?
b. Correct the code so that it works as intended.

7. The following code segment is supposed to copy one line from the standard input device to the standard output device.

```
cin.get(inChar);
while (inChar != '\n')
{
    cin.get(inChar);
    cout << inChar;
}
```

a. What is the output if the input line consists of the characters ABCDE?
b. Rewrite the code so that it works properly.

8. Does the following program segment need any priming reads? If not, explain why. If so, add the input statement(s) in the proper place. (`letter` is of type `char`.)

```
while (cin)
{
    while (letter != '\n')
    {
        cout << letter;
        cin.get(letter);
    }
    cout << endl;
    cout << "Another line read..." << endl;
    cin.get(letter);
}
```

9. What sentinel value would you choose for a program that reads telephone numbers as integers?

10. Consider this program:

```
#include <iostream>

using namespace std;

const int LIMIT = 8;

int main()
{
    int   sum;
    int   i;
    int   number;
    bool finished;

    sum = 0;
    i = 1;
    finished = false;
    while (i <= LIMIT && !finished)
    {
        cin >> number;
        if (number > 0)
            sum = sum + number;
        else if (number == 0)
            finished = true;
        i++;
    }
    cout << "End of test. " << sum << ' ' << number << endl;
    return 0;
}
```

and these data values:

```
5   6   -3   7   -4   0   5   8   9
```

a. What are the contents of sum and number after exit from the loop?
b. Do the data values fully test the program? Explain your answer.
11. Here is a simple count-controlled loop:

```
count = 1;
while (count < 20)
    count++;
```

a. List three ways of changing the loop so that it executes 20 times instead of 19.
b. Which of those changes makes the value of count range from 1 through 21?
12. What is the output of the following program segment? (All variables are of type int.)

```
i = 1;
while (i <= 5)
{
    sum = 0;
    j = 1;
    while (j <= i)
    {
        sum = sum + j;
        j++;
    }
    cout << sum << ' ';
    i++;
}
```

Programming Warm-up Exercises

1. Write a program segment that sets a Boolean variable dangerous to true and stops reading data if pressure (a float variable being read in) exceeds 510.0. Use dangerous as a flag to control the loop.
2. Write a program segment that counts the number of times the integer 28 occurs in a file of 100 integers.
3. Write a nested loop code segment that produces this output:

```
1
1 2
1 2 3
1 2 3 4
```

4. Write a program segment that reads a file of student scores for a class (any size) and finds the class average.
5. Write a program segment that reads in integers and then counts and prints out the number of positive integers and the number of negative integers. If a value is 0, it should not be counted. The process should continue until end-of-file occurs.
6. Write a program segment that adds up the even integers from 16 through 26, inclusive.
7. Write a program segment that prints out the sequence of all the hour and minute combinations in a day, starting with 1:00 A.M. and ending with 12:59 A.M.

8. Rewrite the code segment for Exercise 7 so that it prints the times in ten-minute intervals, arranged as a table with six columns and 24 rows.

9. Write a code segment that inputs one line of data containing an unknown number of character strings that are separated by spaces. The final value on the line is the sentinel string End. The segment should output the number of strings on the input line (excluding End), the number of strings that contained at least one letter *e*, and the percentage of strings that contained at least one *e*. (*Hint*: To determine if *e* occurs in a string, use the find function of the string class.)

10. Extend the code segment of Exercise 9 so that it processes all the lines in a data file inFile and prints the three pieces of information for each input line.

11. Modify the code segment of Exercise 10 so that it also keeps a count of the total number of strings in the file and the total number of strings containing at least one *e*. (Again, do not count the sentinel string on each line.) When EOF is reached, print the three pieces of information for the entire file.

Programming Problems

1. Write a functional decomposition and a C++ program that inputs an integer and a character. The output should be a diamond composed of the character and extending the width specified by the integer. For example, if the integer is 11 and the character is an asterisk (*), the diamond would look like this:

```
          *
         ***
        *****
       *******
      *********
     ***********
      *********
       *******
        *****
         ***
          *
```

If the input integer is an even number, it should be increased to the next odd number. Use meaningful variable names, proper indentation, appropriate comments, and good prompting messages.

2. Write a functional decomposition and a C++ program that inputs an integer larger than 1 and calculates the sum of the squares from 1 to that integer. For example, if the integer equals 4, the sum of the squares is 30 (1 + 4 + 9 + 16). The output should be the value of the integer and the sum, properly labeled. The program should repeat this process for several input values. A negative input value signals the end of the data.

3. You are putting together some music tapes for a party. You've arranged a list of songs in the order in which you want to play them. However, you would like to minimize the empty tape left at the end of each side of a cassette (the cassette plays for 45 minutes on a side). So you want to figure out the total time for a group of songs and see how well they fit. Write a functional decomposition and a C++ program to help you do this. The program should input a reference number and a time for each song until it encounters a reference number of

0. The times should each be entered as minutes and seconds (two integer values). For example, if song number 4 takes 7 minutes and 42 seconds to play, the data entered for that song would be

```
4   7   42
```

The program should echo print the data for each song and the current running time total. The last data entry (reference number 0) should not be added to the total time. After all the data has been read, the program should print a message indicating the time remaining on the tape.

If you are writing this program to read data from a file, the output should be in the form of a table with columns and headings. For example,

Song Number	Song Minutes	Time Seconds	Total Minutes	Time Seconds
1	5	10	5	10
2	7	42	12	52
5	4	19	17	11
3	4	33	21	44
4	10	27	32	11
6	8	55	41	6
0	0	1	41	6

```
There are 3 minutes and 54 seconds of tape left.
```

If you are using interactive input, your output should have prompting messages interspersed with the results. For example,

```
Enter the song number:
1
Enter the number of minutes:
5
Enter the number of seconds:
10
Song number 1, 5 minutes and 10 seconds
Total time is 5 minutes and 10 seconds.
For the next song,
Enter the song number:
   ⋮
```

Use meaningful variable names, proper indentation, and appropriate comments. If you're writing an interactive program, use good prompting messages. The program should discard any invalid data sets (negative numbers, for example) and print an error message indicating that the data set has been discarded and what was wrong with it.

4. Using functional decomposition, write a program that prints out the approximate number of words in a file of text. For our purposes, this is the same as the number of gaps following words. A *gap* is defined as one or more spaces in a row, so a sequence of spaces counts as just one gap. The newline character also counts as a gap. Anything other than a space or newline is considered to be part of a word. For example, there are 13 words in this sentence, according to our definition. The program should echo print the data.

Solve this problem with two different programs:

a. Use a `string` object into which you input each word as a string. This approach is quite straightforward.

b. Assume the `string` class does not exist, and input the data one character at a time. This approach is more complicated. (*Hint*: Only count a space as a gap if the previous character read is something other than a space.)

Use meaningful variable names, proper indentation, and appropriate comments. Thoroughly test the programs with your own data sets.

Case Study Follow-Up

1. Change the Incomes program so that it does the following:

   a. Prints an error message when a negative income value is input and then goes on processing any remaining data. The erroneous data should not be included in any of the calculations. Thoroughly test the modified program with your own data sets.

   b. Does not crash when there are no males in the input file or no females (or the file is empty). Instead, it should print an appropriate error message. Test the revised program with your own data sets.

   c. Rejects data sets that are coded with a letter other than 'F' or 'M' and prints an error message before continuing to process the remaining data. The program also should print a message indicating the number of erroneous data sets encountered in the file.

2. Develop a thorough set of test data for the Incomes program as modified in Exercise 1.

3. Modify the Incomes program so that it reports the highest and lowest incomes for each gender.

4. Develop a thorough set of test data for the Incomes program as modified in Exercise 3.

7

Functions

- To be able to write a program that uses functions to reflect the structure of your functional decomposition.
- To be able to write a module of your own design as a void function.
- To be able to define a void function to do a specified task.
- To be able to distinguish between value and reference parameters.
- To be able to use arguments and parameters correctly.
- To be able to do the following tasks, given a functional decomposition of a problem:

  Determine what the parameter list should be for each module.

  Determine which parameters should be reference parameters and which should be value parameters.

  Code the program correctly.

- To be able to define and use local variables correctly.
- To be able to write a program that uses multiple calls to a single function.

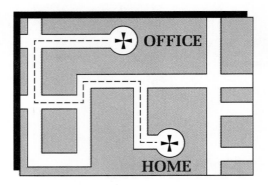

You have been using C++ functions since we introduced standard library routines such as sqrt and abs in Chapter 3. By now, you should be quite comfortable with the idea of calling these subprograms to perform a task. So far, we have not considered how the programmer can create his or her own functions other than main. That is the topic of this chapter and the next.

You might wonder why we waited until now to look at user-defined subprograms. The reason, and the major purpose for using subprograms, is that we write our own value-returning functions and void functions to help organize and simplify larger programs. Until now, our programs have been relatively small and simple, so we didn't need to write subprograms. Now that we've covered the basic control structures, we are ready to introduce subprograms so that we can begin writing larger and more complex programs.

Functional Decomposition with Void Functions

As a brief refresher, let's review the two kinds of subprograms that the C++ language works with: value-returning functions and void functions. A value-returning function receives some data through its argument list, computes a single function value, and returns this function value to the calling code. The caller invokes (calls) a value-returning function by using its name and argument list in an expression:

```
y = 3.8 * sqrt(x);
```

In contrast, a void function (*procedure*, in some languages) does not return a function value. Nor is it called from within an expression. Instead, the function call appears as a complete, stand-alone statement. An example is the get function associated with the istream and ifstream classes:

```
cin.get(inputChar);
```

In this chapter, we concentrate exclusively on creating our own void functions. In Chapter 8, we examine how to write value-returning functions.

From the early chapters on, you have been designing your programs as collections of modules. Many of these modules are naturally implemented as *user-defined void functions*. We now look at how to turn the modules in your algorithms into user-defined void functions.

When to Use Functions

In general, you can code any module as a function, although some are so simple that this really is unnecessary. In designing a program, then, we frequently need to decide which modules should be implemented as functions. The decision should be based on whether the overall program is easier to understand as a result. Other factors can affect this decision, but for now this is the simplest heuristic (strategy) to use.

If a module is a single line only, it is usually best to write it directly in the program. Turning it into a function only complicates the overall program, which defeats the purpose of using subprograms. On the other hand, if a module is many lines long, it is easier to understand the program if the module is turned into a function.

Keep in mind that whether you choose to code a module as a function or not affects only the readability of the program and may make it more or less convenient to change the program later. Your choice does not affect the correct functioning of the program.

Writing Modules as Void Functions

It is quite simple to turn a module into a void function in C++. Basically, a void function looks like the `main` function except that the function heading uses `void` rather than `int` as the data type of the function. Additionally, the body of a void function does not contain a statement like

```
return 0;
```

as does `main`. A void function does not return a function value to its caller.

Let's look at a program using void functions. A friend of yours is returning from a long trip, and you want to write a program that prints the following message:

```
* * * * * * * * * * * * * *
* * * * * * * * * * * * * *
 Welcome Home!
* * * * * * * * * * * * * *
* * * * * * * * * * * * * *
* * * * * * * * * * * * * *
* * * * * * * * * * * * * *
```

Here is a design for the program.

Main   **Level 0**

Print two lines of asterisks
Print "Welcome Home!"
Print four lines of asterisks

Print 2 Lines   **Level 1**

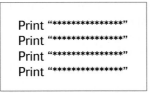

Print "**************"
Print "**************"

Print 4 Lines

Print "**************"
Print "**************"
Print "**************"
Print "**************"

If we write the two first-level modules as void functions, the main function is simply

```
int main()
{
    Print2Lines();
    cout << "Welcome Home!" << endl;
    Print4Lines();
    return 0;
}
```

Notice how similar this code is to the main module of our functional decomposition. It contains two function calls—one to a function named Print2Lines and another to a function named Print4Lines. Both of these functions have empty argument lists.

The following code should look familiar to you, but look carefully at the function heading.

```
void Print2Lines()                          // Function heading
{
    cout << "***************" << endl;
    cout << "***************" << endl;
}
```

This segment is a *function definition*. A function definition is the code that extends from the function heading to the end of the block that is the body of the function. The function heading begins with the word `void`, signaling the compiler that this is not a value-returning function. The body of the function executes some ordinary statements and does *not* finish with a `return` statement to return a function value.

Now look again at the function heading. Just like any other identifier in C++, the name of a function cannot include blanks, even though our paper-and-pencil module names do. Following the function name is an empty argument list—that is, there is nothing between the parentheses. Later we see what goes inside the parentheses if a function uses arguments. Now let's put `main` and the other two functions together to form a complete program.

```
//******************************************************************
// Welcome program
// This program prints a "Welcome Home" message
//******************************************************************
#include <iostream>

using namespace std;

void Print2Lines();                         // Function prototypes
void Print4Lines();

int main()
{
    Print2Lines();                          // Function call
    cout << " Welcome Home!" << endl;
    Print4Lines();                          // Function call
    return 0;
}


//******************************************************************

void Print2Lines()                          // Function heading

// This function prints two lines of asterisks
```

```
{
    cout << "***************" << endl;
    cout << "***************" << endl;
}


//******************************************************************

void Print4Lines()                              // Function heading

// This function prints four lines of asterisks

{
    cout << "***************" << endl;
    cout << "***************" << endl;
    cout << "***************" << endl;
    cout << "***************" << endl;
}
```

C++ function definitions can appear in any order. We could have chosen to place the main function last instead of first, but C++ programmers typically put main first and any supporting functions after it.

In the Welcome program, the two statements just before the main function are called *function prototypes*. These declarations are necessary because of the C++ rule requiring you to declare an identifier before you can use it. Our main function uses the identifiers Print2Lines and Print4Lines, but the definitions of those functions don't appear until later. We must supply the function prototypes to inform the compiler in advance that Print2Lines and Print4Lines are the names of functions, that they do not return function values, and that they have no arguments. We say more about function prototypes later in the chapter.

Because the Welcome program is so simple to begin with, it may seem more complicated with its modules written as functions. However, it is clear that it much more closely resembles our functional decomposition. This is especially true of the main function. If you handed this code to someone, the person could look at the main function (which, as we said, usually appears first) and tell you immediately what the program does—it prints two lines of something, prints "Welcome Home!", and prints four lines of something. If you asked the person to be more specific, he or she could then look up the details in the other function definitions. The person is able to begin with a top-level view of the program and then study the lower-level modules as necessary, without having to read the entire program or look at a module structure chart. As our programs grow to include many modules nested several levels deep, the ability to read a program in the same manner as a functional decomposition aids greatly in the development and debugging process.

MAY WE INTRODUCE

Charles Babbage

The British mathematician Charles Babbage (1791–1871) is generally credited with designing the world's first computer. Unlike today's electronic computers, however, Babbage's machine was mechanical. It was made of gears and levers, the predominant technology of the 1820s and 1830s.

Babbage actually designed two different machines. The first, called the Difference Engine, was to be used in computing mathematical tables. For example, the Difference Engine could produce a table of squares:

x	x^2
1	1
2	4
3	9
4	16
⋮	⋮

It was essentially a complex calculator that could not be programmed. Babbage's Difference Engine was designed to improve the accuracy of the computation of tables, not the speed. At that time, all tables were produced by hand, a tedious and error-prone job. Because much of science and engineering depended on accurate table information, an error could have serious consequences. Even though the Difference Engine could perform the calculations only a little faster than a human could, it did so without error. In fact, one of its most important features was that it would stamp its output directly onto copper plates, which could then be placed into a printing press, thereby avoiding even typographical errors.

By 1833, the project to build the Difference Engine had run into financial trouble. The engineer whom Babbage had hired to do the construction was dishonest and had drawn the project out as long as possible so as to extract more money from Babbage's sponsors in the British government. Eventually the sponsors became tired of waiting for the machine and withdrew their support. At about the same time, Babbage lost interest in the project because he had developed the idea for a much more powerful machine, which he called the Analytical Engine—a truly programmable computer.

The idea for the Analytical Engine came to Babbage as he toured Europe to survey the best technology of the time in preparation for constructing the Difference Engine. One of the technologies that he saw was the Jacquard automatic loom, in which a series of paper cards with punched holes was fed through the machine to produce a woven cloth pattern. The pattern of holes constituted a program for the loom and made it possible to weave patterns of arbitrary complexity automatically. In fact, its inventor even had a detailed portrait of himself woven by one of his machines.

Babbage realized that this sort of device could be used to control the operation of a computing machine. Instead of calculating just one type of formula, such a machine could be programmed to perform arbitrarily complex computations, including the manipulation of algebraic symbols. As his associate, Ada Lovelace (the world's first computer programmer), elegantly put it, "We may say most aptly that the Analytical Engine weaves algebraical patterns." It is clear that Babbage and Lovelace fully understood the power of a programmable computer and even contemplated the notion that someday such machines could achieve artificial thought.

Unfortunately, Babbage never completed construction of either of his machines. Some historians believe that he never finished them because the technology of the period could not support such complex machinery. But most feel that Babbage's failure was his own doing. He was both brilliant and somewhat eccentric (it is known that he was afraid of Italian organ grinders, for example). As a consequence, he had a tendency to abandon projects in midstream so that he could concentrate on newer and better ideas. He always believed that his new approaches would enable him to complete a machine in less time than his old ideas would.

When he died, Babbage had many pieces of computing machines and partial drawings of designs, but none of the plans were complete enough to produce a single working computer. After his death, his ideas were dismissed and his inventions ignored. Only after modern computers were developed did historians recognize the true importance of his contributions. Babbage recognized the potential of the computer an entire century before one was fully developed. Today, we can only imagine how different the world would be if he had succeeded in constructing his Analytical Engine.

An Overview of User-Defined Functions

Now that we've seen an example of how a program is written with functions, let's look briefly and informally at some of the more important points of function construction and use.

Flow of Control in Function Calls

We said that C++ function definitions can be arranged in any order, although main usually appears first. During compilation, the functions are translated in the order in which they physically appear. When the program is executed, however, control begins at the first statement in the main function, and the program proceeds in logical sequence. When a function call is encountered, logical control is passed to the first statement in that function's body. The statements in the function are executed in logical order. After the last one is executed, control returns to the point immediately following the function call. Because function calls alter the logical order of execution, functions are considered control structures. Figure 7-1 illustrates this physical versus logical ordering of functions. In the figure, functions A, B, and C are written in the physical order A, B, C but are executed in the order C, B, A.

In the Welcome program, execution begins with the first executable statement in the `main` function (the call to `Print2Lines`). When `Print2Lines` is called, control passes to its first statement and subsequent statements in its body. After the last statement in `Print2Lines` has executed, control returns to the `main` function at the point following the call (the output statement that prints "Welcome Home!").

Function Parameters

Looking at the Welcome program, you can see that `Print2Lines` and `Print4Lines` are very similar functions. They differ only in the number of lines that they print. Do we really need two different functions in this program? Maybe we should write only one function that prints *any* number of lines, where the "any number of lines" is passed as an argument by the caller (`main`). Here is a second version of the program, which uses only one function to do the printing. We call it NewWelcome.

FIGURE 7-1

Physical Versus
Logical Order of
Functions

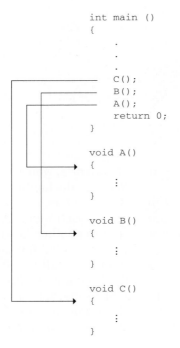

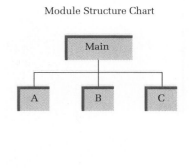

Module Structure Chart

```
//*****************************************************************
// NewWelcome program
// This program prints a "Welcome Home" message
//*****************************************************************
#include <iostream>

using namespace std;

void PrintLines( int );                      // Function prototype

int main()
{
    PrintLines(2);
    cout << " Welcome Home!" << endl;
    PrintLines(4);
    return 0;
}


//*****************************************************************

void PrintLines( int numLines )

// This function prints lines of asterisks, where
// numLines specifies how many lines to print

{
    int count;        // Loop control variable

    count = 1;
    while (count <= numLines)
    {
        cout << "**************" << endl;
        count++;
    }
}
```

In the function heading of PrintLines, you see some code between the parentheses that looks like a variable declaration. This is a *parameter declaration*. As you learned in earlier chapters, arguments represent a way for two functions to communicate with each other. Arguments enable the calling function to input (pass) values to another function to use in its processing and—in some cases—to allow the called function to output (return) results to the caller. The items listed in the call to a function are the **arguments.** The variables declared in the function heading are the **parameters.** (Some programmers use the pair of terms *actual argument* and *formal argument* instead of *argument* and *parameter.* Others use the term *actual parameter* in place of *argument*, and *formal parameter* in place of *parame-*

ter.) Notice that the `main` function in the code above is a *parameterless* function.

Parameter   A variable declared in a function heading; also called *formal argument* or *formal parameter.*

Argument   A variable or expression listed in a call to a function; also called *actual argument* or *actual parameter.*

In the NewWelcome program, the arguments in the two function calls are the constants 2 and 4, and the parameter in the `PrintLines` function is named `numLines`. The `main` function first calls `PrintLines` with an argument of 2. When control is turned over to `PrintLines`, the parameter `numLines` is initialized to 2. Within `PrintLines`, the count-controlled loop executes twice and the function returns. The second time `PrintLines` is called, the parameter `numLines` is initialized to the value of the argument, 4. The loop executes four times, after which the function returns.

Although there is no benefit in doing so, we could write the `main` function this way:

```
int main()
{
    int lineCount;

    lineCount = 2;
    PrintLines(lineCount);
    cout << " Welcome Home!" << endl;
    lineCount = 4;
    PrintLines(lineCount);
    return 0;
}
```

In this version, the argument in each call to `PrintLines` is a variable rather than a constant. Each time `main` calls `PrintLines`, a copy of the argument's value is passed to the function to initialize the parameter `numLines`. This version shows that when you pass a variable as an argument, the argument and the parameter can have different names.

The NewWelcome program brings up a second major reason for using functions—namely, a function can be called from many places in the `main` function (or from other functions). Use of multiple calls can save a great deal of effort in coding many problem solutions. If a task must be done in more than one place in a program, we can avoid repetitive coding by writing it as a function and then calling it wherever we need it. Another example that illustrates this use of functions appears in the Problem-Solving Case Study at the end of this chapter.

If more than one argument is passed to a function, the arguments and parameters are matched by their relative positions in the two lists. For example, if you want `PrintLines` to print lines consisting of any selected character, not only asterisks, you might rewrite the function so that its heading is

```
void PrintLines( int   numLines,
                 char whichChar )
```

and a call to the function might look like this:

```
PrintLines(3, '#');
```

The first argument, 3, is matched with `numLines` because `numLines` is the first parameter. Likewise, the second argument, '#', is matched with the second parameter, `whichChar`.

Syntax and Semantics of Void Functions

Function Call (Invocation)

To call (or invoke) a void function, we use its name as a statement, with the arguments in parentheses following the name. A **function call** in a program results in the execution of the body of the called function. This is the syntax template of a function call to a void function:

FunctionCall (to a void function)

```
FunctionName ( ArgumentList );
```

Function call (to a void function)   A statement that transfers control to a void function. In C++, this statement is the name of the function, followed by a list of arguments.

According to the syntax template for a function call, the argument list is optional. A function is not required to have arguments. However, as the syntax template also shows, the parentheses are required even if the argument list is empty.

If there are two or more arguments in the argument list, you must separate them with commas. Here is the syntax template for ArgumentList:

ArgumentList

Expression , Expression . . .

When a function call is executed, the arguments are passed to the parameters according to their positions, left to right, and control is then transferred to the first executable statement in the function body. When the last statement in the function has executed, control returns to the point from which the function was called.

Function Declarations and Definitions

In C++, you must declare every identifier before it can be used. In the case of functions, a function's declaration must physically precede any function call.

A function declaration announces to the compiler the name of the function, the data type of the function's return value (either `void` or a data type like `int` or `float`), and the data types of the parameters it uses. The NewWelcome program shows a total of three function declarations. The first declaration (the statement labeled "Function prototype") does not include the body of the function. The remaining two declarations—for `main` and `PrintLines`—include bodies for the functions.

In C++ terminology, a function declaration that omits the body is called a **function prototype,** and a declaration that does include the body is a **function definition.** We can use a Venn diagram to picture the fact that all definitions are declarations, but not all declarations are definitions:

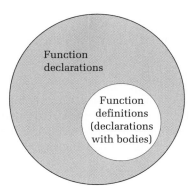

Function prototype   A function declaration without the body of the function.

Function definition   A function declaration that includes the body of the function.

Whether we are talking about functions or variables, the general idea in C++ is that a declaration becomes a definition if it also allocates memory space for the item. (There are exceptions to this rule of thumb, but we don't concern ourselves with them now.) For example, a function prototype is merely a declaration—that is, it specifies the properties of a function: its name, its data type, and the data types of its parameters. But a function definition does more; it causes the compiler to allocate memory for the instructions in the body of the function. (Technically, all of the variable declarations we've used so far have been variable *definitions* as well as declarations—they allocate memory for the variable. In Chapter 8, we see examples of variable declarations that aren't variable definitions.)

The rule throughout C++ is that you can declare an item as many times as you wish, but you can define it only once. In the NewWelcome program, we could include many function prototypes for `PrintLines` (though we'd have no reason to), but only one function definition is allowed.

Function Prototypes   We have said that the definition of the `main` function usually appears first in a program, followed by the definitions of all other functions. To satisfy the requirement that identifiers be declared before they are used, C++ programmers typically place all function prototypes near the top of the program, before the definition of `main`.

A function prototype (known as a *forward declaration* in some languages) specifies in advance the data type of the function value to be returned (or the word `void`) and the data types of the parameters. A prototype for a void function has the following form:

FunctionPrototype (for a void function)

```
void FunctionName ( ParameterList );
```

As you can see in the syntax template, no body is included for the function, and a semicolon terminates the declaration. The parameter list is optional, to allow for parameterless functions. If the parameter list is present, it has the following form:

ParameterList (in a function prototype)

DataType **&** VariableName **,** DataType **&** VariableName . . .

The ampersand (&) attached to the name of a data type is optional and has a special significance that we cover later in the chapter.

In a function prototype, the parameter list must specify the data types of the parameters, but their names are optional. You could write either

```
void DoSomething( int, float );
```

or

```
void DoSomething( int velocity, float angle );
```

Sometimes it's useful for documentation purposes to supply names for the parameters, but the compiler ignores them.

Function Definitions You learned in Chapter 2 that a function definition consists of two parts: the function heading and the function body, which is syntactically a block (compound statement). Here's the syntax template for a function definition, specifically, for a void function:

FunctionDefinition (for a void function)

```
void FunctionName ( ParameterList )
{
      Statement
          ⋮
}
```

Notice that the function heading does *not* end in a semicolon the way a function prototype does. It is a common syntax error to put a semicolon at the end of the line.

The syntax of the parameter list differs slightly from that of a function prototype in that you *must* specify the names of all the parameters. Also, it's our style preference (but not a language requirement) to declare each parameter on a separate line:

ParameterList (in a function definition)

```
DataType & VariableName ,
DataType & VariableName
    ⋮
```

Local Variables

Because a function body is a block, any function—not only the `main` function—can include variable declarations within its body. These variables are called **local variables** because they are accessible only within the block in which they are declared. As far as the calling code is concerned, they don't exist. If you tried to print the contents of a local variable from another function, a compile-time error such as "UNDECLARED IDENTIFIER" would occur. You saw an example of a local variable in the NewWelcome program—the `count` variable declared within the `PrintLines` function.

Local variable   A variable declared within a block and not accessible outside of that block.

In contrast to local variables, variables declared outside of all the functions in a program are called *global variables*. We return to the topic of global variables in Chapter 8.

Local variables occupy memory space only while the function is executing. At the moment the function is called, memory space is created for its local variables. When the function returns, its local variables are destroyed.* Therefore, every time the function is called, its local variables start out with their values undefined. Because every call to a function is independent of every other call to that same function, you must initialize the local variables within the function itself. And because local variables are destroyed when the function returns, you cannot use them to store values between calls to the function.

The following code segment illustrates each of the parts of the function declaration and calling mechanism that we have discussed.

```
#include <iostream>

using namespace std;

void TryThis( int, int, float );     // Function prototype
```

---
* We'll see an exception to this rule in the next chapter.

```
void TryThis( int, int, float );        // Function prototype

int main()                              // Function definition
{
    int    int1;                        // Variables local to main
    int    int2;
    float someFloat;
    ⋮
    TryThis(int1, int2, someFloat);     // Function call with three
                                        //   arguments
    ⋮
}

void TryThis( int    param1,            // Function definition with
              int    param2,            //   three parameters
              float param3 )

{
    int    i;                           // Variables local to TryThis
    float x;
    ⋮
}
```

The Return Statement

The `main` function uses the statement

```
return 0;
```

to return the value 0 (or 1 or some other value) to its caller, the operating system. Every value-returning function must return its function value this way.

A void function does not return a function value. Control returns from the function when it "falls off" the end of the body—that is, after the final statement has executed. As you saw in the NewWelcome program, the `PrintLines` function simply prints some lines of asterisks and then returns.

Alternatively, there is a second form of the Return statement. It looks like this:

```
return;
```

This statement is valid *only* for void functions. It can appear anywhere in the body of the function; it causes control to exit the function immediately and return to the caller. Here's an example:

```
void SomeFunc( int n )
{
    if (n > 50)
    {
        cout << "The value is out of range.";
        return;
    }
    n = 412 * n;
    cout << n;
}
```

In this (nonsense) example, there are two ways for control to exit the function. At function entry, the value of n is tested. If it is greater than 50, the function prints a message and returns immediately without executing any more statements. If n is less than or equal to 50, the If statement's then-clause is skipped and control proceeds to the assignment statement. After the last statement, control returns to the caller.

Another way of writing the above function is to use an If-Then-Else structure:

```
void SomeFunc( int n )
{
    if (n > 50)
        cout << "The value is out of range.";
    else
    {
        n = 412 * n;
        cout << n;
    }
}
```

If you asked different programmers about these two versions of the function, you would get differing opinions. Some prefer the first version, saying that it is most straightforward to use Return statements whenever it logically makes sense to do so. Others insist on the *single-entry, single-exit* approach in the second version. With this philosophy, control enters a function at one point only (the first executable statement) and exits at one point only (the end of the body). They argue that multiple exits from a function make the program logic hard to follow and difficult to debug. Other programmers take a position somewhere between these two philosophies, allowing occasional use of the Return statement when the logic is clear. Our advice is to use `return` sparingly; overuse can lead to confusing code.

MATTERS OF STYLE

Naming Void Functions

When you choose a name for a void function, keep in mind how calls to it will look. A call is written as a statement; therefore, it should sound like a command or an instruction to the computer. For this reason, it is a good idea to choose a name that is an imperative verb or has an imperative verb as part of it. (In English, an imperative verb is one representing a command: *Listen! Look! Do something!*) For example, the statement

```
Lines(3);
```

has no verb to suggest that it's a command. Adding the verb *Print* makes the name sound like an action:

```
PrintLines(3);
```

When you are picking a name for a void function, write down sample calls with different names until you come up with one that sounds like a command to the computer.

Header Files

From the very beginning, we have been using `#include` directives that request the C++ preprocessor to insert the contents of header files into our programs:

```
#include <iostream>
#include <cmath>      // For sqrt() and fabs()
#include <fstream>    // For file I/O
#include <climits>    // For INT_MAX and INT_MIN
```

Exactly what do these header files contain?

It turns out that there is nothing magical about header files. Their contents are nothing more than a series of C++ declarations. There are declarations of items such as named constants (`INT_MAX`, `INT_MIN`), classes (`istream`, `ostream`, `string`), and objects (`cin`, `cout`). But most of the items in a header file are function prototypes.

Suppose that your program needs to use the library function `sqrt` in a statement like this:

```
y = sqrt(x);
```

Every identifier must be declared before it can be used. If you forget to #include the header file cmath, the compiler gives you an "UNDE-CLARED IDENTIFIER" error message. The file cmath contains function prototypes for sqrt and other math-oriented library functions. With this header file included in your program, the compiler not only knows that the identifier sqrt is the name of a function but it also can verify that your function call is correct with respect to the number of arguments and their data types.

Header files save you the trouble of writing all of the library function prototypes yourself at the beginning of your program. With just one line—the #include directive—you cause the preprocessor to go out and find the header file and insert the prototypes into your program. In later chapters, we see how to create our own header files that contain declarations specific to our programs.

Parameters

When a function is executed, it uses the arguments given to it in the function call. How is this done? The answer to this question depends on the nature of the parameters. C++ supports two kinds of parameters: **value parameters** and **reference parameters.** With a value parameter, which is declared without an ampersand (&) at the end of the data type name, the function receives a copy of the argument's value. With a reference parameter, which is declared by adding an ampersand to the data type name, the function receives the location (memory address) of the caller's argument. Before we examine in detail the difference between these two kinds of parameters, let's look at an example of a function heading with a mixture of reference and value parameter declarations.

```
void Example( int&   param1,      // A reference parameter
              int    param2,      // A value parameter
              float  param3 )     // Another value parameter
```

With simple data types—int, char, float, and so on—a value parameter is the default (assumed) kind of parameter. In other words, if you don't do anything special (add an ampersand), a parameter is assumed to be a value parameter. To specify a reference parameter, you have to go out of your way to do something extra (attach an ampersand).

Value parameter   A parameter that receives a copy of the value of the corresponding argument.

Reference parameter   A parameter that receives the location (memory address) of the caller's argument.

Let's look at both kinds of parameters, starting with value parameters.

Value Parameters

In the NewWelcome program, the `PrintLines` function heading is

```
void PrintLines( int numLines )
```

The parameter `numLines` is a value parameter because its data type name doesn't end in `&`. If the function is called using an argument `lineCount`,

```
PrintLines(lineCount);
```

then the parameter `numLines` receives a copy of the value of `lineCount`. At this moment, there are two copies of the data—one in the argument `lineCount` and one in the parameter `numLines`. If a statement inside the `PrintLines` function were to change the value of `numLines`, this change would not affect the argument `lineCount` (remember, there are two copies of the data). Using value parameters thus helps us avoid unintentional changes to arguments.

Because value parameters are passed copies of their arguments, anything that has a value may be passed to a value parameter. This includes constants, variables, and even arbitrarily complicated expressions. (The expression is simply evaluated and a copy of the result is sent to the corresponding value parameter.) For the `PrintLines` function, the following function calls are all valid:

```
PrintLines(3);
PrintLines(lineCount);
PrintLines(2 * abs(10 - someInt));
```

There must be the same number of arguments in a function call as there are parameters in the function heading.* Also, each argument should have the same data type as the parameter in the same position. Notice how each parameter in the following example is matched to the argument in the same position (the data type of each argument below is what you would assume from its name):

Function heading: `void ShowMatch(float num1, int num2, char letter)`

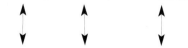

Function call: `ShowMatch(floatVariable, intVariable, charVariable);`

---

* This statement is not the whole truth. C++ has a special language feature—*default parameters*—that lets you call a function with fewer arguments than parameters. We do not cover default parameters in this book.

If the matched items are not of the same data type, implicit type coercion takes place. For example, if a parameter is of type int, an argument that is a float expression is coerced to an int value before it is passed to the function. As usual in C++, you can avoid unintended type coercion by using an explicit type cast or, better yet, by not mixing data types at all.

As we have stressed, a value parameter receives a copy of the argument, and therefore the caller's argument cannot be accessed directly or changed. When a function returns, the contents of its value parameters are destroyed, along with the contents of its local variables. The difference between value parameters and local variables is that the values of local variables are undefined when a function starts to execute, whereas value parameters are automatically initialized to the values of the corresponding arguments.

Because the contents of value parameters are destroyed when the function returns, they cannot be used to return information to the calling code. What if we *do* want to return information by modifying the caller's arguments? We must use the second kind of parameter available in C++: reference parameters. Let's look at these now.

Reference Parameters

A reference parameter is one that you declare by attaching an ampersand to the name of its data type. It is called a reference parameter because the called function can refer to the corresponding argument directly. Specifically, the function is allowed to inspect *and modify* the caller's argument.

When a function is invoked using a reference parameter, it is the *location* (memory address) of the argument, not its value, that is passed to the function. There is only one copy of the information, and it is used by both the caller and the called function. When a function is called, the argument and the parameter become synonyms for the same location in memory. Whatever value is left by the called function in this location is the value that the caller will find there. Therefore, you must be careful when using a reference parameter because any change made to it affects the argument in the calling code. Let's look at an example.

In Chapter 5, we wrote an If-Then-Else-If structure that prints an appropriate activity for a given outdoor temperature. Suppose we want a program that reads in a temperature from the user and prints the recommended activity. Here is its design.

Main   **Level 0**

```
Get temperature
Print activity
```

Get Temperature   **Level 1**

```
Prompt user for temperature
Read temperature
Echo print temperature
```

Print Activity

```
Print "The recommended activity is"
IF temperature > 85
      Print "swimming."
ELSE IF temperature > 70
      Print "tennis."
ELSE IF temperature > 32
      Print "golf."
ELSE IF temperature > 0
      Print "skiing."
ELSE
      Print "dancing."
```

Let's write the two level 1 modules as void functions, `GetTemp` and `PrintActivity`, so that the `main` function looks like the main module of our functional decomposition. Here is the resulting program.

```
//*******************************************************************
// Activity program
// This program outputs an appropriate activity
// for a given temperature
//*******************************************************************
#include <iostream>

using namespace std;

void GetTemp( int& );                    // Function prototypes
```

```
void PrintActivity( int );

int main()
{
    int temperature;     // The outside temperature

    GetTemp(temperature);                    // Function call
    PrintActivity(temperature);              // Function call
    return 0;
}

//****************************************************************

void GetTemp( int& temp )                    // Reference parameter

// This function prompts for a temperature to be entered,
// reads the input value into temp, and echo prints it

{
    cout << "Enter the outside temperature:" << endl;
    cin >> temp;
    cout << "The current temperature is " << temp << endl;
}

//****************************************************************

void PrintActivity( int temp )               // Value parameter

// Given the value of temp, this function prints a message
// indicating an appropriate activity

{
    cout << "The recommended activity is ";
    if (temp > 85)
        cout << "swimming." << endl;
    else if (temp > 70)
        cout << "tennis." << endl;
    else if (temp > 32)
        cout << "golf." << endl;
    else if (temp > 0)
        cout << "skiing." << endl;
    else
        cout << "dancing." << endl;
}
```

In the Activity program, the arguments in the two function calls are both named temperature. The parameter in GetTemp is a reference parameter named temp. The parameter in PrintActivity is a value parameter, also named temp.

The main function tells GetTemp where to leave the temperature by giving it the location of the variable temperature when it makes the function call. We *must* use a reference parameter here so that GetTemp knows where to deposit the result. In a sense, the parameter temp is just a convenient placeholder in the function definition. When GetTemp is called with temperature as its argument, all the references to temp inside the function actually are made to temperature. If the function were to be called again with a different variable as an argument, all the references to temp would actually refer to that other variable until the function returned control to main.

In contrast, PrintActivity's parameter is a value parameter. When PrintActivity is called, main sends a copy of the value of temperature for the function to work with. It's appropriate to use a value parameter in this case because PrintActivity is not supposed to modify the argument temperature.

Because arguments and parameters can have different names, we can call a function at different times with different arguments. Suppose we wanted to change the Activity program to print an activity for both the indoor and outdoor temperatures. We could declare integer variables in the main function named indoorTemp and outdoorTemp, then write the body of main as follows:

```
GetTemp(indoorTemp);
PrintActivity(indoorTemp);
GetTemp(outdoorTemp);
PrintActivity(outdoorTemp)
return 0;
```

In GetTemp and PrintActivity, the parameters would receive values from, or pass values to, either indoorTemp or outdoorTemp.

The following table summarizes the usage of arguments and parameters.

Item	Usage
Argument	Appears in a function *call*. The corresponding parameter may be either a reference or a value parameter.
Value parameter	Appears in a function *heading*. Receives a *copy* of the value of the corresponding argument.
Reference parameter	Appears in a function *heading*. Receives the *address* of the corresponding argument.

An Analogy

Before we talk more about parameter passing, let's look at an analogy from daily life. You're at the local discount catalog showroom to buy a Father's Day present. To place your order, you fill out an order form. The form has places to write in the quantity of each item and its catalog number, and places where the order clerk will fill in the prices. You write down what you want and hand the form to the clerk. You wait for the clerk to check whether the items are available and calculate the cost. He returns the form, and you see that the items are in stock and the price is $48.50. You pay the clerk and go on about your business.

This illustrates how function calls work. The clerk is like a void function. You, acting as the `main` function, ask him to do some work for you. You give him some information: the item numbers and quantities. These are his input parameters. You wait until he returns some information to you: the availability of the items and their prices. These are the clerk's output parameters. The clerk does this task all day long with different input values. Each order activates the same process. The shopper waits until the clerk returns information based on the specific input.

The order form is analogous to the arguments of a function call. The spaces on the form represent variables in the `main` function. When you hand the form to the clerk, some of the places contain information and some are empty. The clerk holds the form while doing his job so he can write information in the blank spaces. These blank spaces correspond to reference parameters; you expect the clerk to return results to you in the spaces.

When the `main` function calls another function, reference parameters allow the called function to access and change the variables in the argument list. When the called function finishes, `main` continues, making use of whatever new information the called function left in the variables.

The parameter list is like the set of shorthand or slang terms the clerk uses to describe the spaces on the order form. For example, he may think in terms of "units," "codes," and "receipts." These are his terms (parameters) for what the order form calls "quantity," "catalog number," and "price" (the arguments). But he doesn't waste time reading the names on the form every time; he knows that the first item is the units (quantity), the second is the code (catalog number), and so on. In other words, he looks only at the position of each space on the form. This is how arguments are matched to parameters—by their relative positions in the two lists.

Matching Arguments with Parameters

Earlier we said that with reference parameters, the argument and the parameter become synonyms for the same memory location. When a function returns control to its caller, the link between the argument and the parameter is broken. They are synonymous only during a particular call to the function. The only evidence that a matchup between the two ever occurred is that the contents of the argument may have changed (see Figure 7-2).

Only a variable can be passed as an argument to a reference parameter because a function can assign a new value to the argument. (In contrast, remember that an arbitrarily complicated expression can be passed to a value parameter.) Suppose that we have a function with the following heading:

```
void DoThis( float val,      // Value parameter
             int&  count )   // Reference parameter
```

Then the following function calls are all valid.

```
DoThis(someFloat, someInt);
DoThis(9.83, intCounter);
DoThis(4.9 * sqrt(y), myInt);
```

When flow of control is in the main function,
temperature can be accessed as shown by the arrow.

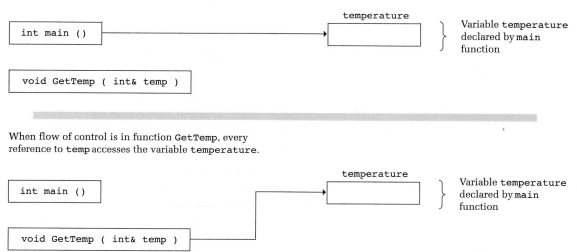

FIGURE 7-2
Using a Reference Parameter to Access an Argument

In the `DoThis` function, the first parameter is a value parameter, so any expression is allowed as the argument. The second parameter is a reference parameter, so the argument *must* be a variable name. The statement

```
DoThis(y, 3);
```

generates a compile-time error because the second argument isn't a variable name. Earlier we said the syntax template for an argument list is

ArgumentList

Expression , Expression ...

But you must keep in mind that Expression is restricted to a variable name if the corresponding parameter is a reference parameter.

There is another important difference between value and reference parameters when it comes to matching arguments with parameters. With value parameters, we said that implicit type coercion occurs if the matched items have different data types (the value of the argument is coerced, if possible, to the data type of the parameter). In contrast, with reference parameters, the matched items *must* have exactly the same data type.

The following table summarizes the appropriate forms of arguments.

Parameter	*Argument*
Value parameter	A variable, constant, or arbitrary expression (type coercion may take place)
Reference parameter	A variable *only*, of exactly the same data type as the parameter

Finally, it is the programmer's responsibility to make sure that the argument list and parameter list match up semantically as well as syntactically. For example, suppose we had written the indoor/outdoor modification to the Activity program as follows.

```
int main()
{
    ⋮
    GetTemp(indoorTemp);
    PrintActivity(indoorTemp);
```

```
GetTemp(outdoorTemp);
PrintActivity(indoorTemp)     // Wrong argument
return 0;
}
```

The argument list in the last function call matches the corresponding parameter list in its number and type of arguments, so no syntax error would be signaled. However, the output would be erroneous because the argument is the wrong temperature value. Similarly, if a function has two parameters of the same data type, you must be careful that the arguments are in the right order. If they are in the wrong order, no syntax error will result, but the answers will be wrong.

THEORETICAL FOUNDATIONS

Argument-Passing Mechanisms

There are three major ways of passing arguments to and from subprograms. C++ supports only two of these mechanisms; however, it's useful to know about all three in case you have occasion to use them in another language.

C++ reference parameters employ a mechanism called a *pass by address* or *pass by location*. A memory address is passed to the function. Another name for this is a *pass by reference* because the function can refer directly to the caller's variable that is specified in the argument list.

C++ value parameters are an example of a *pass by value*. The function receives a copy of the value of the caller's argument. Passing by value can be less efficient than passing by address because the value of an argument may occupy many memory locations (as we see in Chapter 11), whereas an address usually occupies only a single location. For the simple data types `int`, `char`, `bool`, and `float`, the efficiency of either mechanism is about the same.

A third method of passing arguments is called a *pass by name*. The argument is passed to the function as a character string that must be interpreted by special run-time support software (called a *thunk*) supplied by the compiler. For example, if the name of a variable is passed to a function, the run-time interpreter looks up the name of the argument in a table of declarations to find the address of the variable. Passing by name can have unexpected results. If an argument has the same spelling as a local variable in the function, the function will refer to the local version of the variable instead of the variable in the calling code.

Some versions of the pass by name allow an expression or even a code segment to be passed to a function. Each time the function refers to the parameter, an interpreter performs the action specified by the parameter. An interpreter is similar to a compiler and nearly as complex. Thus, a pass by name is the least efficient of the three argument-passing mechanisms. Passing by name is supported by the ALGOL and LISP programming languages, but not by C++.

There are two different ways of matching arguments with parameters, although C++ supports only one of them. Most programming languages, C++ among them, match arguments and parameters by their relative positions in the argument and parameter lists. This is called *positional matching*, *relative matching*, or *implicit matching*. A few languages, such as Ada, also support *explicit* or *named matching*. In explicit matching, the argument list specifies the name of the parameter to be associated with each argument. Explicit matching allows arguments to be written in any order in the function call. The real advantage is that each call documents precisely which values are being passed to which parameters.

Designing Functions

We've looked at some examples of functions and defined the syntax of function prototypes and function definitions. But how do we design functions? First, we need to be more specific about what functions do. We've said that they allow us to organize our programs more like our functional decompositions, but what really is the advantage of doing that?

The body of a function is like any other segment of code, except that it is contained in a separate block within the program. Isolating a segment of code in a separate block means that its implementation details can be "hidden" from view. As long as you know how to call a function and what its purpose is, you can use it without looking at the code inside the function body. For example, you don't know how the code for a library function like sqrt is written (its implementation is hidden from view), yet you still can use it effectively.

The specification of what a function does and how it is invoked defines its **interface** (see Figure 7-3). By hiding a module implementation, or **encapsulating** the module, we can make changes to it without changing the main function, as long as the interface remains the same. For example, you might rewrite the body of a function using a more efficient algorithm.

Interface   A connecting link at a shared boundary that permits independent systems to meet and act on or communicate with each other. Also, the formal description of the purpose of a subprogram and the mechanism for communicating with it.

Encapsulation   Hiding a module implementation in a separate block with a formally specified interface.

FIGURE 7-3
Function Interface
(Visible) and
Implementation
(Hidden)

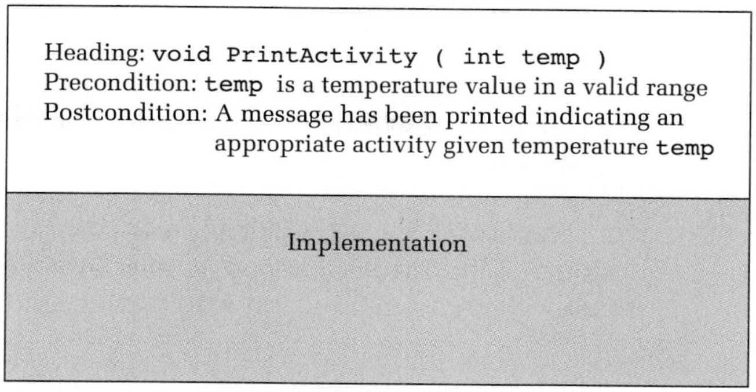

Heading: `void PrintActivity ( int temp )`
Precondition: `temp` is a temperature value in a valid range
Postcondition: A message has been printed indicating an
appropriate activity given temperature `temp`

Implementation

Encapsulation is what we do in the functional decomposition process when we postpone the solution of a difficult subproblem. We write down its purpose, its precondition and postcondition, and what information it takes and returns, and then we write the rest of our design as if the subproblem had already been solved. We could hand this interface specification to someone else, and that person could develop a function for us that solves the subproblem. We needn't be concerned about how it works, as long as it conforms to the interface specification. Interfaces and encapsulation are the basis for *team programming,* in which a group of programmers work together to solve a large problem.

Thus, designing a function can (and should) be divided into two tasks: designing the interface and designing the implementation. We already know how to design an implementation—it is a segment of code that corresponds to an algorithm. To design the interface, we focus on the *what,* not the *how.* We must define the behavior of the function (what it does) and the mechanism for communicating with it.

You already know how to specify formally the behavior of a function. Because a function corresponds to a module, its behavior is defined by the precondition and postcondition of the module. All that remains is to define the mechanism for communicating with the function. To do so, make a list of the following items:

1. *Incoming values* that the function receives from the caller.
2. *Outgoing values* that the function produces and returns to the caller.
3. *Incoming/outgoing values*—values the caller has that the function changes (receives and returns).

Now decide which identifiers inside the module match the values in this list. These identifiers become the variables in the parameter list for the function. Then the parameters are declared in the function heading. All other variables that the function needs are local and must be declared within the body of the function. This process is repeated for all the modules at each level.

Let's look more closely at designing the interface. First we examine function preconditions and postconditions. After that, we consider in more detail the notion of incoming, outgoing, and incoming/outgoing parameters.

Writing Assertions as Program Comments

We have been writing module preconditions and postconditions as informal, English-language assertions. From now on, we include preconditions and postconditions as comments to document the interfaces of C++ functions. Here's an example:

```
void PrintAverage( float sum,
                   int   count )

// Precondition:
//      sum is assigned  &&  count > 0
// Postcondition:
//      The average sum/count has been output on one line

{
    cout << "Average is " << sum / float(count) << endl;
}
```

The precondition is an assertion describing everything that the function requires to be true at the moment the caller invokes the function. The postcondition describes the state of the program at the moment the function finishes executing.

You can think of the precondition and postcondition as a contract. The contract states that if the precondition is true at function entry, then the postcondition must be true at function exit. The *caller* is responsible for ensuring the precondition, and the *function code* must ensure the postcondition. If the caller fails to satisfy its part of the contract (the precondition), the contract is off; the function cannot guarantee that the postcondition will be true.

Above, the precondition warns the caller to make sure that sum has been assigned a meaningful value and to be sure that count is positive. If this precondition is true, the function guarantees it will satisfy the postcondition. If count isn't positive when PrintAverage is invoked, the effect of the function is undefined. (For example, if count equals 0, the postcondition surely isn't satisfied—the program crashes!)

Sometimes the caller doesn't need to satisfy any precondition before calling a function. In this case, the precondition can be written as the value `true` or simply omitted. In the following example, no precondition is necessary:

```
void Get2Ints( int& int1,
               int& int2 )

// Postcondition:
//     User has been prompted to enter two integers
//  && int1 == first input value
//  && int2 == second input value

{
    cout << "Please enter two integers: ";
    cin >> int1 >> int2;
}
```

In assertions written as C++ comments, we use either `&&` or AND to denote the logical AND operator, either `||` or OR to denote a logical OR, either `!` or NOT to denote a logical NOT, and `==` to denote "equals." (Notice that we do *not* use = to denote "equals." Even when we write program comments, we want to keep C++'s == operator distinct from the assignment operator.)

There is one final notation we use when we express assertions as program comments. Preconditions implicitly refer to values of variables at the moment the function is invoked. Postconditions implicitly refer to values at the moment the function returns. But sometimes you need to write a postcondition that refers to parameter values that existed at the moment the function was invoked. To signify "at the time of entry to the function," we attach the symbol `@entry` to the end of the variable name. Below is an example of the use of this notation. The `Swap` function exchanges, or swaps, the contents of its two parameters.

```
void Swap( int& firstInt,
           int& secondInt )

// Precondition:
//     firstInt and secondInt are assigned
// Postcondition:
//     firstInt == secondInt@entry
//  && secondInt == firstInt@entry

{
    int temporaryInt;
```

```
        temporaryInt = firstInt;
        firstInt = secondInt;
        secondInt = temporaryInt;
}
```

*M*ATTERS OF STYLE

Function Preconditions and Postconditions

Preconditions and postconditions, when well written, are a concise but accurate description of the behavior of a function. A person reading your program should be able to see at a glance how to use the function by looking only at its interface (the function heading and the precondition and postcondition). The reader should never have to look into the code of the function body to understand the purpose of the function or how to use it.

A function interface describes *what* the function does, not the details of *how* it does it. For this reason, the postcondition should mention (by name) each outgoing parameter and its value but should not mention any local variables. Local variables are implementation details; they are irrelevant to the function's interface.

Documenting the Direction of Data Flow

Another helpful piece of documentation in a function interface is the direction of **data flow** for each parameter in the parameter list. Data flow is the flow of information between the function and its caller. We said earlier that each parameter can be classified as an *incoming* parameter, an *outgoing* parameter, or an *incoming/outgoing* parameter. (Some programmers refer to these as *input* parameters, *output* parameters, and *input/output* parameters.)

Data flow   The flow of information from the calling code to a function and from the function back to the calling code.

For an incoming parameter, the direction of data flow is one-way—into the function. The function inspects and uses the current value of the parameter but does not modify it. In the function heading, we attach the comment

```
/* in */
```

to the declaration of the parameter. (Remember that C++ comments come in two forms. The first, which we use most often, starts with two slashes and extends to the end of the line. The second form encloses a comment between /* and */ and allows us to embed a comment within a line of code.) Here is the `PrintAverage` function with comments added to the parameter declarations:

```
void PrintAverage( /* in */ float sum,
                   /* in */ int   count )

// Precondition:
//      sum is assigned  &&  count > 0
// Postcondition:
//      The average sum/count has been output on one line

{
    cout << "Average is " << sum / float(count) << endl;
}
```

Passing by value is appropriate for each parameter that is incoming only. As you can see in the function body, `PrintAverage` does not modify the values of the parameters `sum` and `count`. It merely uses their current values. The direction of data flow is one-way—into the function.

The data flow for an outgoing parameter is one-way—out of the function. The function produces a new value for the parameter without using the old value in any way. The comment /* out */ identifies an outgoing parameter. Here we've added comments to the `Get2Ints` function heading:

```
void Get2Ints( /* out */ int& int1,
               /* out */ int& int2 )
```

Passing by reference must be used for an outgoing parameter. If you look back at the body of `Get2Ints`, you'll see that the function stores new values into the two variables (by means of the input statement), replacing whatever values they originally contained.

Finally, the data flow for an incoming/outgoing parameter is two-way—into and out of the function. The function uses the old value and also produces a new value for the parameter. We use /* inout */ to document this two-way direction of data flow. Here is an example of a function that uses two parameters, one of them incoming only and the other one incoming/outgoing:

```
void Calc( /* in */      int  alpha,
           /* inout */ int& beta  )

// Precondition:
//    alpha and beta are assigned
// Postcondition
//    beta == beta@entry * 7 - alpha

{
    beta = beta * 7 - alpha;
}
```

This function first inspects the incoming value of beta so that it can evaluate the expression to the right of the equal sign. Then it stores a new value into beta by using the assignment operation. The data flow for beta is therefore considered a two-way flow of information. A pass by value is appropriate for alpha (it's incoming only), but a pass by reference is required for beta (it's an incoming/outgoing parameter).

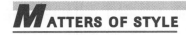ATTERS OF STYLE

Formatting Function Headings

From here on, we follow a specific style when coding our function headings. Comments appear next to the parameters to explain how each parameter is used. Also, embedded comments indicate which of the three data flow categories each parameter belongs to (In, Out, or Inout).

```
void Print( /* in */      float val,     // Value to be printed
            /* inout */ int&  count )   // Number of lines printed
                                          //   so far
```

Notice that the first parameter above is a value parameter. The second is a reference parameter, presumably because the function changes the value of the counter.

We use comments in the form of rows of asterisks (or dashes or some other character) before and after a function to make the function stand out from the surrounding code. Each function also has its own block of introductory comments, just like those at the start of a program, as well as its precondition and postcondition.

It's important to put as much care into documenting each function as you would into the documentation at the beginning of a program.

The following table summarizes the correspondence between a parameter's data flow and the appropriate argument-passing mechanism.

Data Flow for a Parameter	Argument-Passing Mechanism
Incoming	Pass by value
Outgoing	Pass by reference
Incoming/outgoing	Pass by reference

There are exceptions to the guidelines in this table. C++ requires that I/O stream objects be passed by reference because of the way streams and files are implemented. We encounter another exception in Chapter 12.

SOFTWARE ENGINEERING TIP

Conceptual Versus Physical Hiding of a Function Implementation

In many programming languages, the encapsulation of an implementation is purely conceptual. If you want to know how a function is implemented, you simply look at the function body. C++, however, permits function implementations to be written and stored separately from the `main` function.

Larger C++ programs are usually split up and stored into separate files on a disk. One file might contain just the source code for the `main` function; another file, the source code for one or two functions invoked by `main`; and so on. This organization is called a *multifile program*. To translate the source code into object code, the compiler is invoked for each file independently of the others, possibly at different times. A program called the *linker* then collects all the resulting object code into a single executable program.

When you write a program that invokes a function located in another file, it isn't necessary for that function's source code to be available. All that's required is for you to include a function prototype so that the compiler can check the syntax of the call to the function. After the compiler is done, the linker finds the object code for that function and links it with your `main` function's object code. We do this kind of thing all the time when we invoke library functions. C++ systems supply only the object code, not the source code, for library functions like `sqrt`. The source code for their implementations are physically hidden from view.

One advantage of physical hiding is that it helps the programmer avoid the temptation to take advantage of any unusual features of a function's implementation. For example, suppose we want to change the Activity program to read temperatures and output activities repeatedly. Knowing that the `GetTemp` function doesn't perform range checking on the input value, we might be tempted to use –1000 as a sentinel for the loop:

```
int main()
{
    int temperature;

    GetTemp(temperature);
    while (temperature != -1000)
    {
        PrintActivity(temperature);
        GetTemp(temperature);
    }
    return 0;
}
```

This code works fine for now, but later another programmer decides to improve GetTemp so that it checks for a valid temperature range (as it should):

```
void GetTemp( /* out */ int& temp )

// This function prompts for a temperature to be entered, reads
// the input value, checks to be sure it is in a valid temperature
// range, and echo prints it

// Postcondition:
//     User has been prompted for a temperature value (temp)
//  && Error messages and additional prompts have been printed
//     in response to invalid data
//  && IF no valid data was encountered before EOF
//         Value of temp is undefined
//     ELSE
//         -50 <= temp <= 130  &&  temp has been printed

{
    cout << "Enter the outside temperature (-50 through 130): ";
    cin >> temp;
    while (cin &&                          // While not EOF and
           (temp < -50 || temp > 130))     //   temp is invalid...
    {
        cout << "Temperature must be"
             << " -50 through 130." << endl;
        cout << "Enter the outside temperature: ";
        cin >> temp;
    }
    if (cin)                               // If not EOF...
        cout << "The current temperature is "
             << temp << endl;
}
```

Unfortunately, this improvement causes the `main` function to be stuck in an infinite loop because `GetTemp` won't let us enter the sentinel value –1000. If the original implementation of `GetTemp` had been physically hidden, we would not have relied on the knowledge that it does not perform error checking. Instead, we would have written the `main` function in a way that is unaffected by the improvement to `GetTemp`:

```
int main()
{
    int temperature;

    GetTemp(temperature);
    while (cin)                      // While not EOF...
    {
        PrintActivity(temperature);
        GetTemp(temperature);
    }
    return 0;
}
```

Later in the book, you learn how to write multifile programs and hide implementations physically. In the meantime, conscientiously avoid writing code that depends on the internal workings of a function.

PROBLEM-SOLVING CASE STUDY

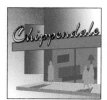

Comparison of Furniture-Store Sales

Problem: A new regional sales manager for the Chippendale Furniture Stores has just come into town. She wants to see a monthly, department-by-department comparison, in the form of bar graphs, of the two Chippendale stores in town. The daily sales for each department are kept in each store's accounting files. Data on each store is stored in the following form:

Department ID number
Number of business days for the department
Daily sales for day 1
Daily sales for day 2
    ⋮
Daily sales for last day in period
Department ID number
Number of business days for the department
Daily sales for day 1
    ⋮

PROBLEM-SOLVING CASE STUDY cont'd.

The bar graph is to be printed in the following form:

```
Bar Graph Comparing Departments of Store #1 and Store #2

Store  Sales in 1,000s of dollars
   #   0         5        10        15        20        25
       |.........|.........|.........|.........|.........|

       Dept 1030
   1   **********************
       Dept 1030
   2   ******************************************

       Dept 1210
   1   *************************************************
       Dept 1210
   2   ****************************************

       Dept 2040
   1   **********************************************
       Dept 2040
   2   ******************************
```

As you can see from the bar graph, each star represents $500 in sales. No stars are printed if a department's sales are less than or equal to $250.

Input: Two data files (store1 and store2), each containing the following values for each department:

Department ID number (int)
Number of business days (int)
Daily sales (several float values)

Output: A bar graph showing total sales for each department.

Discussion: Reading the input data from both files is straightforward. To make the program flexible, we'll prompt the user for the names of the disk files, read the names as strings, and associate the strings with file stream objects (let's call them store1 and store2). We need to read a department ID number, the number of business days, and the daily sales for that department. After processing each department, we can read the data for the next department, continuing until we run out of departments (EOF is encountered). Because the reading process is the same for both store1 and store2, we can use one function for reading both files. All we have to do is pass the appropriate file stream as an argument to the function. We

PROBLEM-SOLVING CASE STUDY cont'd.

want total sales for each department, so this function has to sum the daily sales for a department as they are read. A function can be used to print the output heading. Another function can be used to print out each department's sales for the month in graphic form.

There are three loops in this program: one in the `main` function (to read and process the file data), one in the function that gets the data for one department (to read all the daily sales amounts), and one in the function that prints the bar graph (to print the stars in the graph). The loop for the `main` function tests for EOF on *both* `store1` and `store2`. One graph for each store must be printed for each iteration of this loop.

The loop for the `GetData` function requires an iteration counter that ranges from 1 through the number of days for the department. Also, a summing operation is needed to total the sales for the period.

At first glance, it might seem that the loop for the `PrintData` function is like any other counting loop, but let's look at how we would do this process by hand. Suppose we want to print a bar for the value 1850. We first make sure the number is greater than 250, then print a star and subtract 500 from the original value. We check again to see if the new value is greater than 250, then print a star and subtract 500. This process repeats until the resulting value is less than or equal to 250. Thus, the loop requires a counter that is decremented by 500 for each iteration, with a termination value of 250 or less. A star is printed for each iteration of the loop.

Function `PrintHeading` does not receive any values from `main`, nor does it return any. Thus, its parameter list is empty.

Function `GetData` receives the file stream object from `main` and returns it, modified, after having read some values. The function also returns to `main` the values of the department ID and its sales for the month. Thus, `GetData` has three parameters: the file stream object (with data flow Inout), department ID (data flow Out), and department sales (data flow Out).

Function `PrintData` must receive the department ID, store number, and department sales from the `main` function to print the bar graph for an input record. Therefore, the function has those three items as its parameters, all with data flow In.

We include one more function named `OpenForInput`. This function receives a file stream object, prompts the user for the name of the associated disk file, and attempts to open the file. The function returns the file stream object to its caller, either successfully opened or in the fail state (if the file could not be opened). The single parameter to this function—the file stream object—therefore has data flow Inout.

PROBLEM-SOLVING CASE STUDY *cont'd.*

Assumptions: Each file is in order by department ID. Both stores have the same departments.

Main   **Level 0**

```
Open data files for input
IF either file could not be opened
        Terminate program
Print heading
Get data for a Store 1 department
Get data for a Store 2 department
WHILE NOT EOF on file store1 AND NOT EOF on file store2
        Print data for the Store 1 department
        Print data for the Store 2 department
        Get data for a Store 1 department
        Get data for a Store 2 department
```

Open for Input (Inout: someFile)   **Level 1**

```
Prompt user for name of disk file
Read fileName
Associate fileName with stream someFile,
        and try to open it
IF file could not be opened
        Print error message
```

Print Heading (No parameters)

```
Print chart title
Print heading
Print bar graph scale
```

Get Data (Inout: dataFile; Out: deptID, deptSales)

```
Read deptID from dataFile
IF EOF on dataFile
        Return
Read numDays from dataFile
Set deptSales = 0.0
Set day (loop control variable) = 1
WHILE day <= numDays
        Read sale from dataFile
        Add sale to deptSales
        Increment day
```

Print Data (In: deptID, storeNum, deptSales)

```
Print deptID
Print storeNum
WHILE deptSales > 250.0
        Print a '*'
        Subtract 500.0 from deptSales
Terminate current output line
```

To develop this functional decomposition, we had to make several passes through the design process, and several mistakes had to be fixed to arrive at the design you see here. Don't get discouraged if you don't have a perfect functional decomposition on the first try every time.

Module Structure Chart: Because we are expressing our modules as C++ functions, the module structure chart now includes the names of parameters and uses arrows to show the direction of data flow.

PROBLEM-SOLVING CASE STUDY cont'd.

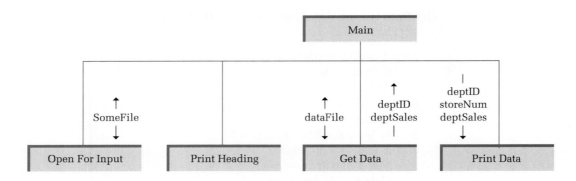

(The following program is written in ISO/ANSI standard C++. If you are working with pre–standard C++, see the alternate version of the program in the PRE_STD directory of the program disk, available at the publisher's Web site, www.jbpub.com/disks.)

```
//******************************************************************
// Graph program
// This program generates bar graphs of monthly sales
// by department for two Chippendale furniture stores, permitting
// department-by-department comparison of sales
//******************************************************************
#include <iostream>
#include <iomanip>      // For setw()
#include <fstream>      // For file I/O
#include <string>       // For string type

using namespace std;

void GetData( ifstream&, int&, float& );
void OpenForInput( ifstream& );
void PrintData( int, int, float );
void PrintHeading();

int main()
{
    int      deptID1;      // Department ID number for Store 1
    int      deptID2;      // Department ID number for Store 2
    float    sales1;       // Department sales for Store 1
    float    sales2;       // Department sales for Store 2
```

PROBLEM-SOLVING CASE STUDY cont'd.

```cpp
    ifstream store1;        // Accounting file for Store 1
    ifstream store2;        // Accounting file for Store 2

    cout << "For Store 1," << endl;
    OpenForInput(store1);
    cout << "For Store 2," << endl;
    OpenForInput(store2);
    if ( !store1 || !store2 )              // Make sure files
        return 1;                          //    were opened

    PrintHeading();

    GetData(store1, deptID1, sales1);      // Priming reads
    GetData(store2, deptID2, sales2);
    while (store1 && store2)               // While not EOF...
    {
        cout << endl;
        PrintData(deptID1, 1, sales1);     // Process Store 1
        PrintData(deptID2, 2, sales2);     // Process Store 2
        GetData(store1, deptID1, sales1);
        GetData(store2, deptID2, sales2);
    }
    return 0;
}


//******************************************************************

void OpenForInput( /* inout */ ifstream& someFile )     // File to be
                                                        // opened
// Prompts the user for the name of an input file
// and attempts to open the file

// Postcondition:
//      The user has been prompted for a file name
//   && IF the file could not be opened
//          An error message has been printed
// Note:
//      Upon return from this function, the caller must test
//      the stream state to see if the file was successfully opened

{
    string fileName;     // User-specified file name

    cout << "Input file name: ";
    cin >> fileName;
```

PROBLEM-SOLVING CASE STUDY *cont'd.*

```cpp
        someFile.open(fileName.c_str());
        if ( !someFile )
            cout << "** Can't open " << fileName << " **" << endl;
}


//****************************************************************

void PrintHeading()

// Prints the title for the bar chart, a heading, and the numeric
// scale for the chart.  The scale uses one mark per $500

// Postcondition:
//     The heading for the bar chart has been printed

{
    cout
        << "Bar Graph Comparing Departments of Store #1 and Store #2"
        << endl << endl
        << "Store  Sales in 1,000s of dollars" << endl
        << " #     0        5        10       15       20       25"
        << endl
        << "        |.........|.........|.........|.........|.........|"
        << endl;
}


//****************************************************************

void GetData( /* inout */ ifstream& dataFile,    // Input file
              /* out */    int&       deptID,     // Department number
              /* out */    float&     deptSales ) // Department's
                                                  //   monthly sales

// Takes an input accounting file as a parameter, reads the
// department ID number and number of days of sales from that file,
// then reads one sales figure for each of those days, computing a
// total sales figure for the month.  This figure is returned in
// deptSales.  (If input of the department ID fails due to
// end-of-file, deptID and deptSales are undefined.)

// Precondition:
//     dataFile has been successfully opened
//  && For each department, the file contains a department ID,
//     number of days, and one sales figure for each day
// Postcondition:
//     IF input of deptID failed due to end-of-file
//         deptID and deptSales are undefined
```

PROBLEM-SOLVING CASE STUDY cont'd.

```
//      ELSE
//          The data file reading marker has advanced past one
//          department's data
//      && deptID == department ID number as read from the file
//      && deptSales == sum of the sales values for the department

{
    int    numDays;   // Number of business days in the month
    int    day;       // Loop control variable for reading daily sales
    float  sale;      // One day's sales for the department

    dataFile >> deptID;
    if ( !dataFile )            // Check for EOF
        return;                 // If so, exit the function

    dataFile >> numDays;
    deptSales = 0.0;
    day = 1;                    // Initialize loop control variable
    while (day <= numDays)
    {
        dataFile >> sale;
        deptSales = deptSales + sale;
        day++;                  // Update loop control variable
    }
}


//****************************************************************

void PrintData( /* in */ int    deptID,      // Department ID number
                /* in */ int    storeNum,    // Store number
                /* in */ float  deptSales )  // Total sales for the
                                             //    department

// Prints the department ID number, the store number, and a
// bar graph of the sales for the department.  The bar graph
// is printed at a scale of one mark per $500

// Precondition:
//     deptID contains a valid department number
//   && storeNum contains a valid store number
//   && 0.0 <= deptSales <= 25000.0
// Postcondition:
//     A line of the bar chart has been printed with one * for
//     each $500 in sales, with remainders over $250 rounded up
//   && No stars have been printed for sales <= $250

{
```

```
cout << setw(12) << "Dept " << deptID << endl;
cout << setw(3) << storeNum << "      ";
while (deptSales > 250.0)
{
    cout << '*' ;                          // Print '*' for each $500
    deptSales = deptSales - 500.0;         // Update loop control
}                                          //   variable
cout << endl;
}
```

Testing: We should test this program with data files that contain the same number of data sets for both stores and with data files that contain different numbers of data sets for both stores. The case in which one or both of the files are empty also should be tested. The test data should include a set that generates a monthly sales figure of $0.00 and one that generates more than $25,000 in sales. We also should test the program to see what it does with negative days, negative sales, and mismatched department IDs. This series of tests would reveal that for this program to work correctly for the furniture-store employees who are to use it, we should add several checks for invalid data.

The `main` function of the Graph program not only reflects our functional decomposition but also contains multiple calls to `OpenForInput`, `GetData`, and `PrintData`. The resulting program is shorter and more readable than one in which the code for each function is physically duplicated.

Testing and Debugging

The parameters declared by a function and the arguments that are passed to the function by the caller must satisfy the interface to the function. Errors that occur with the use of functions often are due to an incorrect use of the interface between the calling code and the called function.

One source of errors is mismatched argument lists and parameter lists. The C++ compiler ensures that the lists have the same number of items and that they are compatible in type. It's the programmer's responsibility, however, to verify that each argument list contains the correct items. This is a matter of comparing the parameter declarations to the argument list in every call to the function. This job is much easier if the function heading gives each parameter a distinct name and describes its purpose in a comment. You can avoid mistakes in writing an argument list by using descriptive variable names in the calling code to suggest exactly what information is being passed to the function.

Another source of error is the failure to ensure that the precondition for a function is met before it is called. For example, if a function assumes that the input file is not at EOF when it is called, then the calling code must ensure that this is true before making the call to the function. If a function behaves incorrectly, review its precondition, then trace the program execution up to the point of the call to verify the precondition. You can waste a lot of time trying to locate an error in a correct function when the error is really in the part of the program prior to the call.

If the arguments match the parameters and the precondition is correctly established, then the source of the error is most likely in the function itself. Trace the function to verify that it transforms the precondition into the proper postcondition. Check that all local variables are initialized properly. Parameters that are supposed to return data to the caller must be declared as reference parameters (with an & symbol attached to the data type name).

An important technique for debugging a function is to use your system's debugger program, if one is available, to step through the execution of the function. If a debugger is not available, you can insert debug output statements to print the values of the arguments immediately before and after calls to the function. It also may help to print the values of all local variables at the end of the function. This information provides a snapshot of the function (a picture of its status at a particular moment in time) at its two most critical points, which is useful in verifying hand traces.

To test a function thoroughly, you must arrange the incoming values so that the precondition is pushed to its limits; then the postcondition must be verified. For example, if a function requires a parameter to be within a certain range, try calling the function with values in the middle of that range and at its extremes.

Testing a function also involves trying to arrange the data to *violate* its precondition. If the precondition can be violated, then errors may crop up that appear to be in the function being tested, when they are really in the main function or another function. For example, function PrintData in the Graph program assumes that a department's sales do not exceed $25,000. If a figure of $250,000 is entered by mistake, the main function does not check this number before the call, and the function tries to print a row of 500 stars. When this happens, you might assume that PrintData has gone haywire, but it's the main function's fault for not checking the validity of the data. (The program should perform this test in function GetData.) Thus, a side effect of one function can multiply and give the appearance of errors elsewhere in a program. We take a closer look at the concept of side effects in the next chapter.

The `assert` *Library Function*

We have discussed how function preconditions and postconditions are useful for debugging (by checking that the precondition of each function is true prior to a function call, and by verifying that each function correctly transforms the precondition into the postcondition) and for testing (by pushing the precondition to its limits and even violating it). To state the preconditions and postconditions for our functions, we've been writing the assertions as program comments:

```
// Precondition:
//     studentCount > 0
```

All comments, of course, are ignored by the compiler. They are not executable statements; they are for humans to examine.

On the other hand, the C++ standard library gives us a way in which to write *executable assertions*. Through the header file `cassert`, the library provides a void function named `assert`. This function takes a logical (Boolean) expression as an argument and halts the program if the expression is false. Here's an example:

```
#include <cassert>
   ⋮
assert(studentCount > 0);
average = sumOfScores / studentCount;
```

The argument to the `assert` function must be a valid C++ logical expression. If its value is `true`, nothing happens; execution continues on to the next statement. If its value is `false`, execution of the program terminates immediately with a message stating (a) the assertion as it appears in the argument list, (b) the name of the file containing the program source code, and (c) the line number in the program. In the example above, if the value of `studentCount` is less than or equal to 0, the program halts after printing a message like this:

```
Assertion failed: studentCount > 0, file myprog.cpp, line 48
```

(This message is potentially confusing. It doesn't mean that `studentCount` *is* greater than 0. In fact, it's just the opposite. The message tells you that the assertion `studentCount > 0` is *false*.)

Executable assertions have a profound advantage over assertions expressed as comments: the effect of a false assertion is highly visible (the program terminates with an error message). The `assert` function is therefore valuable in software testing. A program under development might be filled with calls to the `assert` function to help identify where errors are occurring. If an assertion is false, the error message gives the precise line number of the failed assertion.

Additionally, there is a way to "remove" the assertions without really removing them. If you use the preprocessor directive #define NDEBUG before including the header file cassert, like this:

```
#define NDEBUG
#include <cassert>
    ⋮
```

then all calls to the assert function are ignored when you run the program. (NDEBUG stands for "No debug," and a #define directive is a preprocessor feature that we don't discuss right now.) After program testing and debugging, programmers often like to "turn off" debugging statements yet leave them physically present in the source code in case they might need the statements later. Inserting the line #define NDEBUG turns off assertion checking without having to remove the assertions.

As useful as the assert function is, it has two limitations. First, the argument to the function must be expressed as a C++ logical expression. We can turn the comment

```
//   0.0 <= deptSales <= 25000.0
```

into an executable assertion with the statement

```
assert(0.0 <= deptSales && deptSales <= 25000.0);
```

But there is no easy way to turn the comment

```
//   For each department, the file contains a department ID,
//   number of days, and one sales figure for each day
```

into a C++ logical expression.

The second limitation is that the assert function is appropriate only for testing a program that is under development. A production program (one that has been completed and released to the public) must be robust and must furnish helpful error messages to the user of the program. You can imagine how baffled a user would be if the program suddenly quit and displayed an error message such as

```
Assertion failed: sysRes <= resCount, file newproj.cpp, line 298
```

Despite these limitations, you should consider using the assert function as a regular tool for testing and debugging your programs.

Testing and Debugging Hints

1. Follow documentation guidelines carefully when writing functions (see Appendix F). As your programs become more complex and therefore prone to errors, it becomes increasingly important to adhere to documentation and formatting standards. Even if the function name seems to reflect the process being done, describe that process in comments. Include comments stating the function precondition (if any) and postcondition to make the function interface complete. Use comments to explain the purposes of all parameters and local variables whose roles are not obvious.

2. Provide a function prototype near the top of your program for each function you've written. Make sure that the prototype and its corresponding function heading are an *exact* match (except for the absence of parameter names in the prototype).

3. Be sure to put a semicolon at the end of a function prototype. But do *not* put a semicolon at the end of the function heading in a function definition. Because function prototypes look so much like function headings, it's common to get one of them wrong.

4. Be sure the parameter list gives the data type of each parameter.

5. Use value parameters unless a result is to be returned through a parameter. Reference parameters can change the contents of the caller's argument; value parameters cannot.

6. In a parameter list, be sure the data type of each reference parameter ends with an ampersand (&). Without the ampersand, the parameter is a value parameter.

7. Make sure that the argument list of every function call matches the parameter list in number and order of items, and be very careful with their data types. The compiler will trap any mismatch in the number of arguments. But if there is a mismatch in data types, there may be no compile-time error. Specifically, with a pass by value, a type mismatch can lead to implicit type coercion rather than a compile-time error.

8. Remember that an argument matching a reference parameter *must* be a variable, whereas an argument matching a value parameter can be any expression that supplies a value of the same data type (except as noted in hint 7).

9. Become familiar with *all* the tools available to you when you're trying to locate the sources of errors—the algorithm walk-through, hand tracing, the system's debugger program, the `assert` function, and debug output statements.

Summary

C++ allows us to write programs in modules expressed as functions. The structure of a program, therefore, can parallel its functional decomposition even when the program is complicated. To make your `main` function look exactly like level 0 of your functional decomposition, simply write each lower-level module as a function. The `main` function then executes these other functions in logical sequence.

Functions communicate by means of two lists: the parameter list (which specifies the data type of each identifier) in the function heading, and the argument list in the calling code. The items in these lists must agree in number and position, and they should agree in data type.

Part of the functional decomposition process involves determining what data must be received by a lower-level module and what information must be returned from it. The names of these data items, together with the precondition and postcondition of a module, define its interface. The names of the data items become the parameter list, and the module name becomes the name of the function. With void functions, a call to the function is accomplished by writing the function's name as a statement, enclosing the appropriate arguments in parentheses.

C++ has two kinds of parameters: reference and value. Reference parameters have data types ending in `&` in the parameter list, whereas value parameters do not. Parameters that return values from a function must be reference parameters. All others should be value parameters. This minimizes the risk of errors, because only a copy of the value of an argument is passed to a value parameter, and thus the argument is protected from change.

In addition to the variables declared in its parameter list, a function may have local variables declared within it. These variables are accessible only within the block in which they are declared. Local variables must be initialized each time the function containing them is called because their values are destroyed when the function returns.

You may call functions from more than one place in a program. The positional matching mechanism allows the use of different variables as arguments to the same function. Multiple calls to a function, from different places and with different arguments, can simplify greatly the coding of many complex programs.

Quick Check

1. If a design has one level 0 module and three level 1 modules, how many C++ functions is the program likely to have? (pp. 326–330)
2. Does a C++ function have to be declared before it can be used in a function call? (p. 330)
3. What is the difference between a function declaration and a function definition in C++? (pp. 337–340)
4. Given the function heading

```
void QuickCheck( int    size,
                 float& length,
                 char   initial )
```

indicate which parameters are value parameters and which are reference parameters. (p. 344)

5. a. What would a call to the QuickCheck function look like if the arguments were the variables radius (a float), number (an int), and letter (a char)? (pp. 336–337)

    b. How is the matchup between these arguments and the parameters made? What information is actually passed from the calling code to the QuickCheck function, given these arguments? (pp. 344–353)

    c. Which of these arguments is (are) protected from being changed by the QuickCheck function? (pp. 344–353)

6. Where in a function are local variables declared, and what are their initial values equal to? (pp. 340–341)

7. You are designing a program and you need a void function that reads any number of floating-point values and returns their average. The number of values to be read is in an integer variable named dataPoints, declared in the calling code.

    a. How many parameters should there be in the parameter list, and what should their data type(s) be? (pp. 354–356)

    b. Which parameter(s) should be passed by reference and which should be passed by value? (pp. 354–361)

8. Describe one way in which you can use a function to simplify the coding of an algorithm. (pp. 335–336)

Answers **1.** Four (including main) **2.** Yes **3.** A definition is a declaration that includes the function body. **4.** length is a reference parameter; size and initial are value parameters. **5.** a. QuickCheck(number, radius, letter); b. The matchup is done on the basis of the variables' positions in each list. Copies of the values of size and initial are passed to the function; the location (memory address) of length is passed to the function. c. size and initial are protected from change because only copies of their values are sent to the function. **6.** In the block that forms the body of the function. Their initial values are undefined. **7.** a. There should be two parameters: an int containing the number of values to be read and a float containing the computed average. b. The int should be a value parameter; the float should be a reference parameter. **8.** The coding may be simplified if the function is called from more than one place in the program.

Exam Preparation Exercises

1. Define the following terms:

function call	parameter
argument list	argument
parameterless function	local variable

2. Identify the following items in the program fragment shown below.

function prototype	function definition
function heading	parameters
arguments	function call
local variables	function body

```
void Test( int, int, int );

int main()
{
    int a;
    int b;
    int c;
    ⋮
    Test(a, c, b);
    Test(b, a, c);
    ⋮
}

void Test( int d,
           int e,
           int f )
{
    int g;
    int h;
    ⋮
}
```

3. For the program in Exercise 2, fill in the blanks below with variable names to show the matching that takes place between the arguments and parameters in each of the two calls to the Test function.

First Call to Test		*Second Call to* Test	
Parameter	*Argument*	*Parameter*	*Argument*
1. _____	_____	1. _____	_____
2. _____	_____	2. _____	_____
3. _____	_____	3. _____	_____

4. What is the output of the following program?

```
#include <iostream>

using namespace std;

void Print( int, int );

int main()
{
    int n;

    n = 3;
    Print(5, n);
    Print(n, n);
    Print(n * n, 12);
    return 0;
}
```

(continued on next page)

```
void Print( int a,
            int b )
{
    int c;

    c = 2 * a + b;
    cout << a << ' ' << b << ' ' << c << endl;
}
```

5. Using a reference parameter (passing by reference), the called function can obtain the initial value of an argument as well as change the value of the argument. (True or False?)

6. Using a value parameter, the value of a variable can be passed to a function and used for computation there without any modification of the caller's argument. (True or False?)

7. Given the declarations

```
const int ANGLE = 90;

char letter;
int  number;
```

indicate whether each of the following arguments would be valid using a pass by value, a pass by reference, or both.

a. `letter`
b. `ANGLE`
c. `number`
d. `number + 3`
e. `23`
f. `ANGLE * number`
g. `abs(number)`

8. A variable named `widgets` is stored in memory location 13571. When the statements

```
widgets = 23;
Drop(widgets);
```

are executed, what information is passed to the parameter in the `Drop` function? (Assume the parameter is a reference parameter.)

9. Assume that, in Exercise 8, the parameter within the `Drop` function is named `clunkers`. After the function body performs the assignment

```
clunkers = 77;
```

what is the value in `widgets`? in `clunkers`?

10. Using the data values

    3 2 4

    show what is printed by the following program.

```
#include <iostream>

using namespace std;

void Test( int&, int&, int& );

int main()
{
    int a;
    int b;
    int c;

    Test(a, b, c);
    b = b + 10;
    cout << "The answers are " << b << ' ' << c << ' ' << a;
    return 0;
}

void Test( int& z,
           int& x,
           int& a )
{
    cin >> z >> x >> a;
    a = z * x + a;
}
```

11. The program below has a function named Change. Fill in the values of all variables before and after the function is called. Then fill in the values of all variables after the return to the main function. (If any value is undefined, write *U* instead of a number.)

```
#include <iostream>

using namespace std;

void Change( int, int& );

int main()
{
    int a;
    int b;
```

```
        a = 10;
        b = 7;
        Change(a, b);
        cout << a << ' ' << b << endl;
        return 0;
    }

    void Change( int   x,
                 int& y )
    {
        int b;

        b = x;
        y = y + b;
        x = y;
    }
```

Variables in `main` just before `Change` is called:

a _____

b _____

Variables in `Change` at the moment control enters the function:

x _____

y _____

b _____

Variables in `main` after return from `Change`:

a _____

b _____

12. Show the output of the following program.

```
#include <iostream>

using namespace std;

void Test( int&, int );

int main()
{
    int d;
    int e;

    d = 12;
    e = 14;
    Test(d, e);
    cout << "In the main function after the first call, "
         << "the variables equal " << d << ' ' << e << endl;
    d = 15;
    e = 18;
    Test(e, d);
    cout << "In the main function after the second call, "
         << "the variables equal " << d << ' ' << e << endl;
    return 0;
}
```

```
void Test( int& s,
           int  t )
{
    s = 3;
    s = s + 2;
    t = 4 * s;
    cout << "In function Test, the variables equal "
        << s << ' ' << t << endl;
}
```

13. Number the marked statements in the following program to show the order in which they are executed (the logical order of execution).

```
#include <iostream>

using namespace std;

void DoThis( int&, int& );

int main()
{
    int number1;
    int number2;

_____    cout << "Exercise ";
_____    DoThis(number1, number2);
_____    cout << number1 << ' ' << number2 << endl;
              return 0;
}

void DoThis( int& value1,
             int& value2 )
{
    int value3;

_____    cin >> value3 >> value1;
_____    value2 = value1 + 10;
}
```

14. If the program in Exercise 13 were run with the data values 10 and 15, what would be the values of the following variables just before execution of the Return statement in the main function?

number1 _____ number2 _____ value3 _____

Programming Warm-up Exercises

1. Write the function heading for a void function named PrintMax that accepts a pair of integers and prints out the greater of the two. Document the data flow of each parameter with /* in */, /* out */, or /* inout */.

2. Write the heading for a void function that corresponds to the following list.

   Rocket Simulation Module

Incoming	thrust (floating point)
Incoming/Outgoing	weight (floating point)
Incoming	timeStep (integer)
Incoming	totalTime (integer)
Outgoing	velocity (floating point)
Outgoing	outOfFuel (Boolean)

3. Write a void function that reads in a specified number of `float` values and returns their average. A call to this function might look like

   ```
   GetMeanOf(5, mean);
   ```

   where the first argument specifies the number of values to be read, and the second argument contains the result. Document the data flow of each parameter with /* in */, /* out */, or /* inout */.

4. Given the function heading

   ```
   void Halve( /* inout */ int& firstNumber,
               /* inout */ int& secondNumber )
   ```

   write the body of the function so that when it returns, the original values in firstNumber and secondNumber are halved.

5. Add comments to the preceding Halve function that state the function precondition and postcondition.

6. a. Write a single void function to replace the repeated pattern of statements you identified in Case Study Follow-Up Exercise 4 of Chapter 3. Document the data flow of the parameters with /* in */, /* out */, or /* inout */. Include comments giving the function precondition and postcondition.
   b. Show the function calls with arguments.

7. a. Write a void function that reads in data values of type int (heartRate) until a normal heart rate (from 60 through 80) is read or EOF occurs. The function has one parameter, named normal, that contains true if a normal heart rate was read or false if EOF occurred.
   b. Write a statement that invokes your function. You may use the same variable name for the argument and the parameter.

8. Consider the following function definition.

   ```
   void Rotate( /* inout */ int& firstValue,
                /* inout */ int& secondValue,
                /* inout */ int& thirdValue  )
   {
       int temp;

       temp = firstValue;
       firstValue = secondValue;
       secondValue = thirdValue;
       thirdValue = temp;
   }
   ```

   a. Add comments to the function that tell a reader what the function does and what is the purpose of each parameter and local variable.

b. Write a program that reads three values into variables, echo prints them, calls the Rotate function with the three variables as arguments, and then prints the arguments after the function returns.

9. Modify the function in Exercise 8 to perform the same sort of operation on four values. Modify the program you wrote for part b of Exercise 8 to work with the new version of this function.

10. Write a void function named CountUpper that counts the number of uppercase letters on one line of input. The function should return this number to the calling code in a parameter named upCount.

11. Write a void function named AddTime that has three parameters: hours, minutes, and elapsedTime. elapsedTime is an integer number of minutes to be added to the starting time passed in through hours and minutes. The resulting new time is returned through hours and minutes. Here is an example, assuming that the arguments are also named hours, minutes, and elapsedTime:

Before Call	*After Call*
to AddTime	*to AddTime*
hours = 12	hours = 16
minutes = 44	minutes = 2
elapsedTime = 198	elapsedTime = 198

12. Write a void function named GetNonBlank that returns the first nonblank character it encounters in the standard input stream. In your function, use the cin.get function to read each character. (This GetNonBlank function is just for practice. It's unnecessary because you could use the >> operator, which skips leading blanks, to accomplish the same result.)

13. Write a void function named SkipToBlank that skips all characters in the standard input stream until a blank is encountered. In your function, use the cin.get function to read each character. (This function is just for practice. There's already a library function, cin.ignore, that allows you to do the same thing.)

14. Modify the function in Exercise 13 so that it returns a count of the number of characters that were skipped.

Programming Problems

1. Using functions, rewrite the program developed for Programming Problem 4 in Chapter 6. The program is to determine the number of words encountered in the input stream. For the sake of simplicity, we define a word to be any sequence of characters except whitespace characters (such as blanks and newlines). Words can be separated by any number of whitespace characters. A word can be any length, from a single character to an entire line of characters. If you are writing the program to read data from a file, then it should echo print the input. For an interactive implementation, you do not need to echo print for this program.

For example, for the following data, the program would indicate that 26 words were entered.

```
This isn't exactly an example of g00d english, but it
does demonstrate that a w0rd is just a se@uence of
characters          with0u+ any blank$.   #####   .......
```

As with Programming Problem 4 in Chapter 6, solve this problem with two different programs:

a. Use a `string` object into which you input each word as a string.

b. Assume the `string` class does not exist, and input the data one character at a time. (*Hint:* Consider turning the `SkipToBlank` function of Programming Warm-up Exercise 13 into a `SkipToWhitespace` function.)

Now that your programs are becoming more complex, it is even more important for you to use proper indentation and style, meaningful identifiers, and appropriate comments.

2. Write a C++ program that reads characters representing binary (base-2) numbers from a data file and translates them to decimal (base-10) numbers. The binary and decimal numbers should be output in two columns with appropriate headings. Here is a sample of the output:

```
Binary Number    Decimal Equivalent
     1                    1
    10                    2
    11                    3
 10000                   16
 10101                   21
```

There is only one binary number per input line, but an arbitrary number of blanks can precede the number. The program must read the binary numbers one character at a time. As each character is read, the program multiplies the total decimal value by 2 and adds either 1 or 0, depending on the input character. The program should check for bad data; if it encounters anything except a 0 or a 1, it should output the message "Bad digit on input."

As always, use appropriate comments, proper documentation and coding style, and meaningful identifiers throughout this program. You must decide which of your design modules should be coded as functions to make the program easier to understand.

3. Develop a functional decomposition and write a C++ program to print a calendar for one year, given the year and the day of the week that January 1 falls on. It may help to think of this task as printing 12 calendars, one for each month, given the day of the week on which a month starts and the number of days in the month. Each successive month starts on the day of the week that follows the last day of the preceding month. Days of the week should be numbered 0 through 6 for Sunday through Saturday. Years that are divisible by 4 are leap years. (Determining leap years actually is more complicated than this, but for this program it will suffice.) Here is a sample run for an interactive program:

```
What year do you want a calendar for?
2002
What day of the week does January 1 fall on?
(Enter 0 for Sunday, 1 for Monday, etc.)
2
```

2002

```
                January
         S   M   T   W   T   F   S
         --------------------
                 1   2   3   4   5
         6   7   8   9  10  11  12
        13  14  15  16  17  18  19
        20  21  22  23  24  25  26
        27  28  29  30  31

               February
         S   M   T   W   T   F   S
         --------------------
                             1   2
         3   4   5   6   7   8   9
        10  11  12  13  14  15  16
        17  18  19  20  21  22  23
        24  25  26  27  28


                  .

                  .

                  .


               December
         S   M   T   W   T   F   S
         --------------------
         1   2   3   4   5   6   7
         8   9  10  11  12  13  14
        15  16  17  18  19  20  21
        22  23  24  25  26  27  28
        29  30  31
```

When writing your program, be sure to use proper indentation and style, meaningful identifiers, and appropriate comments.

4. Write a functional decomposition and a C++ program with functions to help you balance your checking account. The program should let you enter the initial balance for the month, followed by a series of transactions. For each transaction entered, the program should echo print the transaction data, the current balance for the account, and the total service charges. Service charges are $0.10 for a deposit and $0.15 for a check. If the balance drops below $500.00 at any point during the month, a service charge of $5.00 is assessed for the month. If the balance drops below $50.00, the program should print a warning message. If the balance becomes negative, an additional service charge of $10.00 should be assessed for each check until the balance becomes positive again.

A transaction takes the form of a letter, followed by a blank and a float number. If the letter is a *C*, then the number is the amount of a check. If the letter is a *D*, then the number is the amount of a deposit. The last transaction consists of the letter *E*, with no number following it. A sample run might look like this:

```
Enter the beginning balance:
879.46
Enter a transaction:
C 400.00
Transaction: Check in amount of $400.00
Current balance: $479.46
Service charge: Check - $0.15
Service charge: Below $500 - $5.00
Total service charges: $5.15
Enter a transaction:
D 100.0
Transaction: Deposit in amount of $100.00
Current balance: $579.46
Service charge: Deposit - $0.10
Total service charges: $5.25
Enter a transaction:
E
Transaction: End
Current balance: $579.46
Total service charges: $5.25
Final balance: $574.21
```

As usual, your program should use proper style and indentation, meaningful identifiers, and appropriate comments. Also, be sure to check for data errors such as invalid transaction codes or negative amounts.

5. In this problem, you are to design and implement a Roman numeral calculator. The subtractive Roman numeral notation commonly in use today (such as IV, meaning 4) was used only rarely during the time of the Roman Republic and Empire. For ease of calculation, the Romans most frequently used a purely additive notation in which a number was simply the sum of its digits (4 equals IIII, in this notation). Each number starts with the digit of highest value and ends with the digit of smallest value. This is the notation we use in this problem.

   Your program inputs two Roman numbers and an arithmetic operator and prints out the result of the operation, also as a Roman number. The values of the Roman digits are as follows:

I	1
V	5
X	10
L	50
C	100
D	500
M	1000

   Thus, the number MDCCCCLXXXXVIIII represents 1999. The arithmetic operators that your program should recognize in the input are +, − , *, and /. These should perform the C++ operations of integer addition, subtraction, multiplication, and division.

One way of approaching this problem is to convert the Roman numbers into decimal integers, perform the required operation, and then convert the result back into a Roman number for printing. The following is a sample run of the program:

```
Enter the first number:
MCCXXVI
The first number is 1226
Enter the second number:
LXVIIII
The second number is 69
Enter the desired arithmetic operation:
+
The sum of MCCXXVI and LXVIIII is MCCLXXXXV (1295)
```

Your program should use proper style and indentation, appropriate comments, and meaningful identifiers. It also should check for errors in the input, such as illegal digits or arithmetic operators, and take appropriate actions when these are found. The program also might check to ensure that the numbers are in purely additive form—that is, digits are followed only by digits of the same or lower value.

6. Develop a functional decomposition and write a program to produce a bar chart of gourmet-popcorn production for a cooperative farm group on a farm-by-farm basis. The input to the program is a series of data sets, one per line, with each set representing the production for one farm. The output is a bar chart that identifies each farm and displays its production in pints of corn per acre.

    Each data set consists of the name of a farm, followed by a comma and one or more spaces, a `float` number representing acres planted, one or more spaces, and an `int` number representing pint jars of popcorn produced.

    The output is a single line for each farm, with the name of the farm starting in the first position on a line and the bar chart starting in position 30. Each mark in the bar chart represents 250 jars of popcorn per acre. The production goal for the year is 5000 jars per acre. A vertical bar should appear in the chart for farms with lower production, and a special mark is used for farms with production greater than or equal to 5000 jars per acre. For example, given the input file

```
Orville's Acres,     114.8   43801
Hoffman's Hills,     77.2    36229
Jiffy Quick Farm,    89.4    24812
Jolly Good Plantation,   183.2   104570
Organically Grown Inc.,  45.5    14683
```

the output would be

```
                        Pop CoOp
        Farm Name                     Production in
                                      Thousands of
                                      Pint Jars per Acre
                                       1   2   3   4   5   6
                                      ---|---|---|---|---|---
        Orville's Acres               ***************     |
        Hoffman's Hills               ******************* |
        Jiffy Quick Farm              ***********         |
        Jolly Good Plantation         ********************#***
        Organically Grown Inc.        *************       |
```

This problem should decompose neatly into several functions. You should write your program in proper programming style with appropriate comments. It should handle data errors (such as a farm name longer than 29 characters) without crashing.

Case Study Follow-Up

1. Write a separate function for the Graph program that creates a bar of asterisks in a string object, given a sales figure.
2. Rewrite the existing PrintData function so that it calls the function you wrote for Exercise 1.
3. Modify the Graph program to print an error message when a negative value is input for the number of days in a department's month.
4. Rewrite the Graph program to check for sales greater than $25,000. It should print a bar of asterisks out to the $25,000 mark and then print an exclamation point (!) at the end of the bar.
5. Write a program, to be run prior to the Graph program, that compares the two data files. The program should signal an error if it finds mismatched department ID numbers or if the files contain different numbers of departments.

8

Scope, Lifetime, and More on Functions

- To be able to do the following tasks, given a C++ program composed of several functions:

  Determine whether a variable is being referenced globally.

  Determine which variables are local variables.

  Determine which variables are accessible within a given block.

- To be able to determine the lifetime of each variable in a program.

- To understand and be able to avoid unwanted side effects.

- To know when to use a value-returning function.

- To be able to design and code a value-returning function for a specific task.

- To be able to invoke a value-returning function properly.

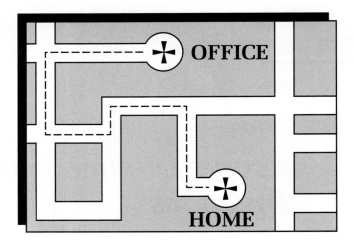

As programs get larger and more complicated, the number of identifiers in a program increases. We invent function names, variable names, constant identifiers, and so on. Some of these identifiers we declare inside blocks. Other identifiers—function names, for example—we declare outside of any block. This chapter examines the C++ rules by which a function may access identifiers that are declared outside its own block. Using these rules, we return to the discussion of interface design that we began in Chapter 7.

Finally, we look at the second kind of subprogram provided by C++: the *value-returning function*. Unlike void functions, which return results (if any) through the parameter list, a value-returning function returns a single result—the function value—to the expression from which it was called. In this chapter, you learn how to write user-defined value-returning functions.

Scope of Identifiers

As we saw in Chapter 7, local variables are those declared inside a block, such as the body of a function. Recall that local variables cannot be accessed outside the block that contains them. The same access rule applies to declarations of named constants: Local constants may be accessed only in the block in which they are declared.

Any block, not only a function body, can contain variable and constant declarations. For example, this If statement contains a block that declares a local variable n:

```
if (alpha > 3)
{
    int n;

    cin >> n;
    beta = beta + n;
}
```

As with any local variable, n cannot be accessed by any statement outside the block containing its declaration.

If we listed all the places from which an identifier could be accessed legally, we would describe that identifier's **scope of visibility** or **scope of access,** often just called its **scope.**

Scope   The region of program code where it is legal to reference (use) an identifier.

C++ defines several categories of scope for any identifier. We begin by describing three of these categories.

1. *Class scope.*   This term refers to the data type called a *class*, which we introduced briefly in Chapter 4. We postpone a detailed discussion of class scope until Chapter 11.
2. *Local scope.*   The scope of an identifier declared inside a block extends from the point of declaration to the end of that block. Also, the scope of a function parameter (formal parameter) extends from the point of declaration to the end of the block that is the body of the function.
3. *Global scope.*   The scope of an identifier declared outside all functions and classes extends from the point of declaration to the end of the entire file containing the program code.

C++ function names have global scope. (There is an exception to this rule, which we discuss in Chapter 11 when we examine C++ classes.) Once a function name has been declared, the function can be invoked by any other function in the rest of the program. In C++, there is no such thing as a local function—that is, you cannot nest a function definition inside another function definition.

Global variables and constants are those declared outside all functions. In the following code fragment, gamma is a global variable and can be accessed directly by statements in main and SomeFunc.

```
int gamma;     // Global variable

int main()
{
    gamma = 3;
      ⋮
}

void SomeFunc()
{
    gamma = 5;
      ⋮
}
```

When a function declares a local identifier with the same name as a global identifier, the local identifier takes precedence within the function. This principle is called **name precedence** or **name hiding**.

Name precedence   The precedence that a local identifier in a function has over a global identifier with the same name in any references that the function makes to that identifier; also called *name hiding*.

Here's an example that uses both local and global declarations:

```
#include <iostream>

using namespace std;

void SomeFunc( float );

const int a = 17;    // A global constant
int b;               // A global variable
int c;               // Another global variable

int main()
{
    b = 4;                     // Assignment to global b
    c = 6;                     // Assignment to global c
    SomeFunc(42.8);
    return 0;
}

void SomeFunc( float c )      // Prevents access to global c
{
    float b;                  // Prevents access to global b
```

```
    b = 2.3;                    // Assignment to local b
    cout << "a = " << a;        // Output global a (17)
    cout << " b = " << b;       // Output local b (2.3)
    cout << " c = " << c;       // Output local c (42.8)
}
```

In this example, function SomeFunc accesses global constant a but declares its own local variable b and parameter c. Thus, the output would be

```
a = 17 b = 2.3 c = 42.8
```

Local variable b takes precedence over global variable b, effectively hiding global b from the statements in function SomeFunc. Parameter c also blocks access to global variable c from within the function. Function parameters act just like local variables in this respect; that is, parameters have local scope.

Scope Rules

When you write C++ programs, you rarely declare global variables. There are negative aspects to using global variables, which we discuss later. But when a situation crops up in which you have a compelling need for global variables, it pays to know how C++ handles these declarations. The rules for accessing identifiers that aren't declared locally are called **scope rules.**

Scope rules   The rules that determine where in the program an identifier may be accessed, given the point where that identifier is declared.

In addition to local and global access, the C++ scope rules define what happens when blocks are nested within other blocks. Anything declared in a block that contains a nested block is **nonlocal** to the inner block. (Global identifiers are nonlocal with respect to all blocks in the program.) If a block accesses any identifier declared outside its own block, it is a *nonlocal access.*

Nonlocal identifier   With respect to a given block, any identifier declared outside that block.

Here are the detailed scope rules, excluding class scope and certain language features we have not yet discussed:

1. A function name has global scope. Function definitions cannot be nested within function definitions.
2. The scope of a function parameter is identical to the scope of a local variable declared in the outermost block of the function body.
3. The scope of a global variable or constant extends from its declaration to the end of the file, except as noted in rule 5.
4. The scope of a local variable or constant extends from its declaration to the end of the block in which it is declared. This scope includes any nested blocks, except as noted in rule 5.
5. The scope of an identifier does not include any nested block that contains a locally declared identifier with the same name (local identifiers have name precedence).

Here is a sample program that demonstrates C++ scope rules. To simplify the example, only the declarations and headings are spelled out. Note how the While-loop body labeled Block3, located within function `Block2`, contains its own local variable declarations.

```
// ScopeRules program

#include <iostream>

using namespace std;

void Block1( int, char& );
void Block2();

int  a1;          // One global variable
char a2;          // Another global variable

int main()
{
    ⋮
}

//***************************************************************

void Block1( int   a1,         // Prevents access to global a1
             char& b2 )        // Has same scope as c1 and d2
{
    int c1;       // A variable local to Block1
    int d2;       // Another variable local to Block1
      ⋮
}

//***************************************************************
```

```
void Block2()
{
    int a1;        // Prevents access to global a1
    int b2;        // Local to Block2; no conflict with b2 in Block1

    while (...)
    {              // Block3
        int c1;    // Local to Block3; no conflict with c1 in Block1
        int b2;    // Prevents nonlocal access to b2 in Block2; no
                   //   conflict with b2 in Block1

        ⋮
    }
}
```

Let's look at the ScopeRules program in terms of the blocks it defines and see just what these rules mean. Figure 8-1 shows the headings and declarations in the ScopeRules program with the scopes of visibility indicated by boxes.

Anything inside a box can refer to anything in a larger surrounding box, but outside-in references aren't allowed. Thus, a statement in Block3 could access any identifier declared in Block2 or any global variable. A statement in Block3 could not access identifiers declared in Block1 because it would have to enter the Block1 box from outside.

Notice that the parameters for a function are inside the function's box, but the function name itself is outside. If the name of the function were inside the box, no function could call another function. This demonstrates merely that function names are globally accessible.

Imagine the boxes in Figure 8-1 as rooms with walls made of two-way mirrors, with the reflective side facing out and the see-through side facing in. If you stood in the room for Block3, you would be able to see out through all the surrounding rooms to the declarations of the global variables (and anything between). You would not be able to see into any other rooms (such as Block1), however, because their mirrored outer surfaces would block your view. Because of this analogy, the term *visible* is often used in describing a scope of access. For example, variable a2 is visible throughout the program, meaning that it can be accessed from anywhere in the program.

Figure 8-1 does not tell the whole story; it represents only scope rules 1 through 4. We also must keep rule 5 in mind. Variable a1 is declared in three different places in the ScopeRules program. Because of name precedence, Block2 and Block3 access the a1 declared in Block2 rather than the global a1. Similarly, the scope of the variable b2 declared in Block2 does *not* include the "hole" created by Block3, because Block3 declares its own variable b2.

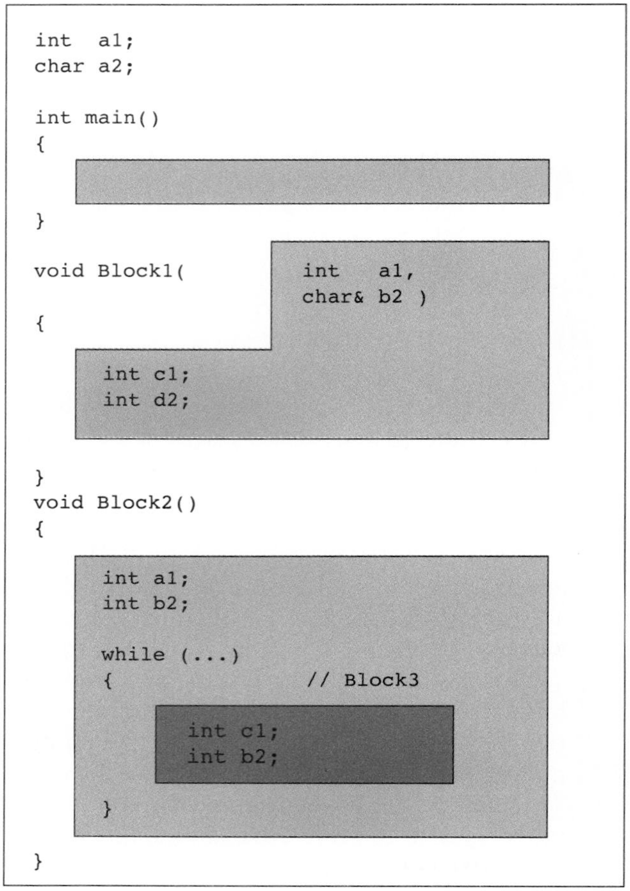

FIGURE 8-1

Scope Diagram
for ScopeRules
Program

```
int   a1;
char a2;

int main()
{



}
void Block1(        int    a1,
                    char& b2 )

{
       int c1;
       int d2;



}
void Block2()
{
       int a1;
       int b2;

       while (...)
       {                    // Block3
              int c1;
              int b2;

       }

}
```

Name precedence is implemented by the compiler as follows. When an expression refers to an identifier, the compiler first checks the local declarations. If the identifier isn't local, the compiler works its way outward through each level of nesting until it finds an identifier with the same name. There it stops. If there is an identifier with the same name declared at a level even further out, it is never reached. If the compiler reaches the global declarations (including identifiers inserted by #include directives) and still can't find the identifier, an error message such as "UNDECLARED IDENTIFIER" is issued.

Such a message most likely indicates a misspelling or an incorrect capitalization, or it could mean that the identifier was not declared before the reference to it or was not declared at all. It may also indicate, however, that the blocks are nested so that the identifier's scope doesn't include the reference.

Variable Declarations and Definitions

In Chapter 7, you learned that C++ terminology distinguishes between a function declaration and a function definition. A function prototype is a declaration only—that is, it doesn't cause memory space to be reserved for the function. In contrast, a function declaration that includes the body is called a function definition. The compiler reserves memory for the instructions in the function body.

C++ applies the same terminology to variable declarations. A variable declaration becomes a variable definition if it also reserves memory for the variable. All of the variable declarations we have used from the beginning have been variable definitions. What would a variable declaration look like if it were *not* also a definition?

In the previous chapter, we talked about the concept of a multifile program, a program that physically occupies several files containing individual pieces of the program. C++ has a reserved word `extern` that lets you reference a global variable located in another file. A "normal" declaration such as

```
int someInt;
```

causes the compiler to reserve a memory location for `someInt`. On the other hand, the declaration

```
extern int someInt;
```

is known as an *external declaration.* It states that `someInt` is a global variable located in another file and that no storage should be reserved for it here. System header files such as `iostream` contain external declarations so that user programs can access important variables defined in system files. For example, `iostream` includes declarations like these:

```
extern istream cin;
extern ostream cout;
```

These declarations allow you to reference `cin` and `cout` as global variables in your program, but the variable definitions are located in another file supplied by the C++ system.

In C++ terminology, the statement

```
extern int someInt;
```

is a declaration but not a definition of `someInt`. It associates a variable name with a data type so that the compiler can perform type checking. But the statement

```
int someInt;
```

is both a declaration and a definition of someInt. It is a definition because it reserves memory for someInt. In C++, you can declare a variable or a function many times, but there can be only one definition.

Except in situations in which it's important to distinguish between declarations and definitions of variables, we'll continue to use the more general phrase *variable declaration* instead of the more specific *variable definition*.

Namespaces

For some time, we have been including the following using directive in our programs:

```
using namespace std;
```

What exactly is a namespace? As a general concept, *namespace* is another word for *scope*. However, as a specific C++ language feature, a namespace is a mechanism by which the programmer can create a named scope. For example, the standard header file cstdlib contains function prototypes for several library functions, one of which is the absolute value function, abs. The declarations are contained within a *namespace definition* as follows:

```
// In header file cstdlib:

namespace std
{
    ⋮
    int abs( int );
    ⋮
}
```

A namespace definition consists of the word namespace, then an identifier of the programmer's choice, and then the *namespace body* between braces. Identifiers declared within the namespace body are said to have *namespace scope*. Such identifiers cannot be accessed outside the body except by using one of three methods.

The first method, introduced in Chapter 2, is to use a qualified name: the name of the namespace, followed by the scope resolution operator (::), followed by the desired identifier. Here is an example:

```
#include <cstdlib>

int main()
{
    int alpha;
    int beta;
    ⋮
    alpha = std::abs(beta);    // A qualified name
    ⋮
}
```

The general idea is to inform the compiler that we are referring to the `abs` declared in the `std` namespace, not some other `abs` (such as a global function named `abs` that we might have written ourselves).

The second method is to use a statement called a *using declaration* as follows:

```
#include <cstdlib>

int main()
{
    int alpha;
    int beta;
    using std::abs;    // A using declaration
    ⋮
    alpha = abs(beta);
    ⋮
}
```

This `using` declaration allows the identifier `abs` to be used throughout the body of `main` as a synonym for the longer `std::abs`.

The third method—one with which we are familiar—is to use a `using` directive (not be confused with a `using` declaration).

```
#include <cstdlib>

int main()
{
    int alpha;
    int beta;
    using namespace std;    // A using directive
    ⋮
```

```
        alpha = abs(beta);
          ⋮
}
```

With a `using` directive, *all* identifiers from the specified namespace are accessible, but only in the scope in which the `using` directive appears. Above, the `using` directive is in local scope (it's within a block), so identifiers from the `std` namespace are accessible only within `main`. On the other hand, if we put the `using` directive outside all functions (as we have been doing), like this:

```
#include <cstdlib>

using namespace std;

int main()
{
   ⋮
}
```

then the `using` directive is in global scope; consequently, identifiers from the `std` namespace are accessible globally.

Placing a `using` directive in global scope can be a convenience. For example, all of the functions we write can refer to identifiers such as `abs`, `cin`, and `cout` without our having to insert a `using` directive locally in each function. However, global `using` directives are considered a bad idea when creating large, multifile programs. Programmers often make use of several libraries, not just the C++ standard library, when developing complex software. Two or more libraries may, just by coincidence, use the same identifier for completely different purposes. If global `using` directives are employed, *name clashes* (multiple definitions of the same identifier) can occur because all the identifiers have been brought into global scope. (C++ programmers refer to this as "polluting the global namespace.") Over the next several chapters, we continue to use global `using` directives for the `std` namespace because our programs are relatively small and therefore name clashes aren't likely.

Given the concept of namespace scope, we refine our description of C++ scope categories as follows.

1. *Class scope.* This term refers to the data type called a *class*. We postpone a detailed discussion of class scope until Chapter 11.
2. *Local scope.* The scope of an identifier declared inside a block extends from the point of declaration to the end of that block. Also, the scope of a function parameter (formal parameter) extends from the point of declaration to the end of the block that is the body of the function.

3. *Namespace scope.* The scope of an identifier declared in a namespace definition extends from the point of declaration to the end of the namespace body, *and* its scope includes the scope of a `using` directive specifying that namespace.
4. *Global* (or *global namespace*) *scope.* The scope of an identifier declared outside all namespaces, functions, and classes extends from the point of declaration to the end of the entire file containing the program code.

Note that these are general descriptions of scope categories and not scope rules. The descriptions do not account for name hiding (the redefinition of an identifier within a nested block).

Lifetime of a Variable

A concept related to but separate from the scope of a variable is its **lifetime**—the period of time during program execution when an identifier actually has memory allocated to it. We have said that storage for local variables is created (allocated) at the moment control enters a function. Then the variables are "alive" while the function is executing, and finally the storage is destroyed (deallocated) when the function exits. In contrast, the lifetime of a global variable is the same as the lifetime of the entire program. Memory is allocated only once, when the program begins executing, and is deallocated only when the entire program terminates. Observe that scope is a *compile-time* issue, but lifetime is a *run-time* issue.

Lifetime The period of time during program execution when an identifier has memory allocated to it.

In C++, an **automatic variable** is one whose storage is allocated at block entry and deallocated at block exit. A **static variable** is one whose storage remains allocated for the duration of the entire program. All global variables are static variables. By default, variables declared within a block are automatic variables. However, you can use the reserved word `static` when you declare a local variable. If you do so, the variable is a static variable and its lifetime persists from function call to function call:

```
void SomeFunc()
{
    float   someFloat;      // Destroyed when function exits
    static int someInt;     // Retains its value from call to call
      ⋮
}
```

It is usually better to declare a local variable as `static` than to use a global variable. Like a global variable, its memory remains allocated throughout the lifetime of the entire program. But unlike a global variable, its local scope prevents other functions in the program from tinkering with it.

Automatic variable   A variable for which memory is allocated and deallocated when control enters and exits the block in which it is declared.

Static variable   A variable for which memory remains allocated throughout the execution of the entire program.

Initializations in Declarations

One of the most common things we do in programs is first declare a variable and then, in a separate statement, assign an initial value to the variable. Here's a typical example:

```
int sum;

sum = 0;
```

C++ allows you to combine these two statements into one. The result is known as an *initialization in a declaration.* Here we initialize `sum` in its declaration:

```
int sum = 0;
```

In a declaration, the expression that specifies the initial value is called an *initializer.* Above, the initializer is the constant 0. Implicit type coercion takes place if the data type of the initializer is different from the data type of the variable.

An automatic variable is initialized to the specified value each time control enters the block:

```
void SomeFunc( int someParam )
{
    int i = 0;                  // Initialized each time
    int n = 2 * someParam + 3;  // Initialized each time
     ⋮
}
```

In contrast, initialization of a static variable (either a global variable or a local variable explicitly declared `static`) occurs once only, the first time control reaches its declaration. Here's an example in which two local static variables are initialized only once (the first time the function is called):

```
void AnotherFunc( int param )
{
    static char ch = 'A';        // Initialized once only
    static int  m  = param + 1;  // Initialized once only
     ⋮
}
```

Although an initialization gives a variable an initial value, it is perfectly acceptable to reassign it another value during program execution.

There are differing opinions about initializing a variable in its declaration. Some programmers never do it, preferring to keep an initialization close to the executable statements that depend on that variable. For example,

```
int loopCount;
     ⋮
loopCount = 1;
while (loopCount <= 20)
{
     ⋮
}
```

Other programmers maintain that one of the most frequent causes of program errors is forgetting to initialize variables before using their contents; initializing each variable in its declaration eliminates these errors. As with any controversial topic, most programmers seem to take a position somewhere between these two extremes.

Interface Design

We return now to the issue of interface design, which we first discussed in Chapter 7. Recall that the data flow through a function interface can take three forms: incoming only, outgoing only, and incoming/outgoing. Any item that can be classified as purely incoming should be coded as a value parameter. Items in the remaining two categories (outgoing and incoming/outgoing) must be reference parameters; the only way the function can deposit results into the caller's arguments is to have the addresses of those arguments. For emphasis, we repeat the following table from Chapter 7.

Data Flow for a Parameter	Argument-Passing Mechanism
Incoming	Pass by value
Outgoing	Pass by reference
Incoming/outgoing	Pass by reference

As we said in the last chapter, there are exceptions to the guidelines in this table. C++ requires that I/O stream objects be passed by reference because of the way streams and files are implemented. We encounter another exception in Chapter 12.

Sometimes it is tempting to skip the interface design step when writing a function, letting it communicate with other functions by referencing global variables. Don't! Without the interface design step, you would actually be creating a poorly structured and undocumented interface. Except in well-justified circumstances, the use of global variables is a poor programming practice that can lead to program errors. These errors are extremely hard to locate and usually take the form of unwanted side effects.

Side Effects

Suppose you made a call to the `sqrt` library function in your program:

```
y = sqrt(x);
```

You expect the call to `sqrt` to do one thing only: compute the square root of the variable x. You'd be surprised if `sqrt` also changed the value of your variable x because `sqrt`, by definition, does not make such changes. This would be an example of an unexpected and unwanted **side effect.**

Side effect   Any effect of one function on another that is not a part of the explicitly defined interface between them.

Side effects are sometimes caused by a combination of reference parameters and careless coding in a function. Perhaps an assignment statement in the function stores a temporary result into one of the reference parameters, accidentally changing the value of an argument back in the calling code. As we mentioned before, using value parameters avoids this type of side effect by preventing the change from reaching the argument.

Side effects also can occur when a function accesses a global variable. An error in the function might cause the value of a global variable to be changed in an unexpected way, causing an error in other functions that access that variable.

The symptoms of a side-effect error are misleading because the trouble shows up in one part of the program when it really is caused by something in another part. To avoid such errors, the only external effect that a function should have is to transfer information through the well-structured interface of the parameter list (see Figure 8-2). If functions access nonlocal variables *only* through their parameter lists, and if all incoming-only parameters are value parameters, then each function is essentially isolated from other parts of the program and side effects cannot occur.

When a function is free of side effects, we can treat it as an independent module and reuse it in other programs. It is hazardous or impossible to reuse functions with side effects.

Here is a short example of a program that runs but produces incorrect results because of global variables and side effects.

```
//********************************************************************
// Trouble program
// This is an example of poor program design, which
// causes an error when the program is executed
//********************************************************************
#include <iostream>

using namespace std;

void CountChars();

int   count;          // Supposed to count input lines, but does it?
char ch;              // Holds one input character

int main()
{
    count = 0;
    cin.get(ch);
    while (cin)
    {
        count++;
        CountChars();
        cin.get(ch);
    }
    cout << count << " lines of input processed." << endl;
    return 0;
}


//********************************************************************

void CountChars()

// Counts the number of characters on one input line
// and prints the count
// Note: main() has already read the first character on a line
```

```
{
    count = 0;                                      // Side effect
    while (ch != '\n')
    {
        count++;                                    // Side effect
        cin.get(ch);
    }
    cout << count << " characters on this line." << endl;
}
```

The Trouble program is supposed to count and print the number of characters on each line of input. After the last line has been processed, it should print the number of lines. Strangely enough, each time the program is run, it reports that the number of lines of input is the same as the number of characters in the last line of input. This is because the CountChars function accesses the global variable count and uses it to store the number of characters on each input line.

There is no reason for count to be a global variable. If a local variable count is declared in main and another local variable count is declared in CountChars, the program works correctly. There is no conflict between the two variables because each is visible only inside its own block.

The Trouble program also demonstrates one common exception to the rule of not accessing global variables. Technically, cin and cout are global objects declared in the header file iostream. The CountChars function reads and writes directly to these streams. To be absolutely correct, cin and cout should be passed as arguments to the function. However, cin

FIGURE 8-2
Side Effects

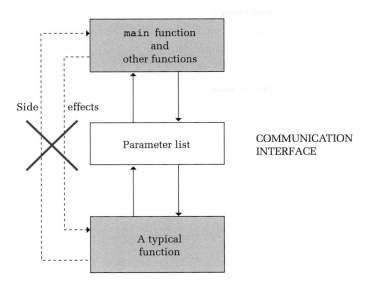

and `cout` are fundamental I/O facilities supplied by the standard library, and it is conventional for C++ functions to access them directly.

Global Constants

Contrary to what you might think, it is acceptable to reference named constants globally. Because the values of global constants cannot be changed while the program is running, no side effects can occur.

There are two advantages to referencing constants globally: ease of change, and consistency. If you need to change the value of a constant, it's easier to change only one global declaration than to change a local declaration in every function. By declaring a constant in only one place, we also ensure that all parts of the program use exactly the same value.

This is not to say that you should declare *all* constants globally. If a constant is needed in only one function, then it makes sense to declare it locally within that function.

At this point, you may want to turn to the first Problem-Solving Case Study at the end of this chapter. This case study further illustrates the interface design process and the use of value and reference parameters.

MAY WE INTRODUCE

Ada Lovelace

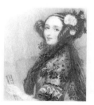

On December 10, 1815 (the same year in which George Boole was born), a daughter— Augusta Ada Byron—was born to Anna Isabella (Annabella) Byron and George Gordon, Lord Byron. In England at that time, Byron's fame derived not only from his poetry but also from his wild, scandalous behavior. The marriage was strained from the beginning, and Annabella left Byron shortly after Ada's birth. By April of 1816, the two had signed separation papers. Byron left England, never to return. Throughout the rest of his life, he regretted being unable to see his daughter. At one point, he wrote of her:

I see thee not. I hear thee not.
But none can be so wrapt in thee.

Before he died in Greece at age 36, he exclaimed, "Oh my poor dear child! My dear Ada! My God, could I but have seen her!"

Meanwhile, Annabella, who would eventually become a baroness in her own right, and who was educated as both a mathematician and a poet, carried on with Ada's upbringing and education. Annabella gave Ada her first instruction in mathematics, but it soon became clear that Ada was gifted in the subject and should receive more extensive tutoring. Ada received further training from Augustus DeMorgan, famous today for one of the basic theorems of Boolean algebra, the logical foundation for modern computers. By age 8, Ada had also demonstrated an interest in mechanical devices and was building detailed model boats.

When she was 18, Ada visited the Mechanics Institute to hear Dr. Dionysius Lardner's lectures on the Difference Engine, a mechanical calculating machine being built by Charles Babbage. She became so interested in the device that she arranged to be introduced to Babbage. It was said that, upon seeing Babbage's machine, Ada was the only person in the room to understand immediately how it worked and to recognize its significance. Ada and Charles Babbage became lifelong friends. She worked with him, helping to document his designs, translating writings about his work, and developing programs for his machines. In fact, today Ada is recognized as the first computer programmer in history, and the modern Ada programming language is named in her honor.

When Babbage designed his Analytical Engine, Ada foresaw that it could go beyond arithmetic computations and become a general manipulator of symbols, and that it would thus have far-reaching capabilities. She even suggested that such a device could eventually be programmed with rules of harmony and composition so that it could produce "scientific" music. In effect, Ada foresaw the field of artificial intelligence more than 150 years ago.

In 1842, Babbage gave a series of lectures in Turin, Italy, on his Analytical Engine. One of the attendees was Luigi Menabrea, who was so impressed that he wrote an account of Babbage's lectures. At age 27, Ada decided to translate the account into English with the intent of adding a few of her own notes about the machine. In the end, her notes were twice as long as the original material, and the document, "The Sketch of the Analytical Engine," became the definitive work on the subject.

It is obvious from Ada's letters that her "notes" were entirely her own and that Babbage was sometimes making unsolicited editorial changes. At one point, Ada wrote to him,

> I am much annoyed at your having altered my Note. You know I am always willing to make any required alterations myself, but that I cannot endure another person to meddle with my sentences.

Ada gained the title Countess of Lovelace when she married Lord William Lovelace. The couple had three children, whose upbringing was left to Ada's mother while Ada pursued her work in mathematics. Her husband was supportive of her work, but for a woman of that day, such behavior was considered almost as scandalous as some of her father's exploits.

Ada Lovelace died of cancer in 1852, just one year before a working Difference Engine was built in Sweden from one of Babbage's designs. Like her father, Ada lived only to age 36, and even though they led very different lives, she had undoubtedly admired him and taken inspiration from his unconventional, rebellious nature. In the end, Ada asked to be buried beside him at the family's estate.

Value-Returning Functions

In Chapter 7 and the first part of this chapter, we have been writing our own void functions. We now look at the second kind of subprogram in C++, the value-returning function. You already know several value-returning functions supplied by the C++ standard library: sqrt, abs, fabs, and others. From the caller's perspective, the main difference between void functions and value-returning functions is the way in which they are called. A call to a void function is a complete statement; a call to a value-returning function is part of an expression.

From a design perspective, value-returning functions are used when there is only one result returned by a function and that result is to be used directly in an expression. For example, suppose we are writing a program that calculates a prorated refund of tuition for students who withdraw in the middle of a semester. The amount to be refunded is the total tuition times the remaining fraction of the semester (the number of days remaining divided by the total number of days in the semester). The people who use the program want to be able to enter the dates on which the semester begins and ends and the date of withdrawal, and they want the program to calculate the fraction of the semester that remains.

Because each semester at this particular school begins and ends within one calendar year, we can calculate the number of days in a period by determining the day number of each date and subtracting the starting day number from the ending day number. The day number is the number associated with each day of the year if you count sequentially from January 1. December 31 has the day number 365, except in leap years, when it is 366. For example, if a semester begins on 1/3/01 and ends on 5/17/01, the calculation is as follows.

> The day number of 1/3/01 is 3
> The day number of 5/17/01 is 137
> The length of the semester is 137 − 3 + 1 = 135

We add 1 to the difference of the days because we count the first day as part of the period.

The algorithm for calculating the day number for a date is complicated by leap years and by months of different lengths. We could code this algorithm as a void function named ComputeDay. The refund could then be computed by the following code segment.

```
ComputeDay(startMonth, startDay, startYear, start);
ComputeDay(lastMonth, lastDay, lastYear, last);
ComputeDay(withdrawMonth, withdrawDay, withdrawYear, withdraw);
fraction = float(last - withdraw + 1) / float(last - start + 1);
refund = tuition * fraction;
```

The first three arguments to `ComputeDay` are received by the function, and the last one is returned to the caller. Because `ComputeDay` returns only one value, we can write it as a value-returning function instead of a void function. Let's look at how the calling code would be written if we had a value-returning function named `Day` that returned the day number of a date in a given year.

```
start = Day(startMonth, startDay, startYear);
last = Day(lastMonth, lastDay, lastYear);
withdraw = Day(withdrawMonth, withdrawDay, withdrawYear);
fraction = float(last - withdraw + 1) / float(last - start + 1);
refund = tuition * fraction;
```

The second version of the code segment is much more intuitive. Because `Day` is a value-returning function, you know immediately that all its parameters receive values and that it returns just one value (the day number for a date).

Let's look at the function definition for `Day`. Don't worry about how `Day` works; for now, you should concentrate on its syntax and structure.

```
int Day( /* in */ int month,          // Month number, 1 - 12
         /* in */ int dayOfMonth,      // Day of month, 1 - 31
         /* in */ int year       )     // Year. For example, 2001

// This function computes the day number within a year, given
// the date. It accounts correctly for leap years. The
// calculation is based on the fact that months average 30 days
// in length. Thus, (month - 1) * 30 is roughly the number of
// days in the year at the start of any month. A correction
// factor is used to account for cases where the average is
// incorrect and for leap years. The day of the month is then
// added to produce the day number

// Precondition:
//      1 <= month <= 12
//   && dayOfMonth is in valid range for the month
//   && year is assigned
// Postcondition:
//      Function value == day number in the range 1 - 365
//                   (or 1 - 366 for a leap year)

{
    int correction = 0;   // Correction factor to account for leap
                          //   year and months of different lengths

    // Test for leap year
```

```
if (year % 4 == 0 && (year % 100 != 0 || year % 400 == 0))
    if (month >= 3)              // If date is after February 29
        correction = 1;          //    then add one for leap year

// Correct for different-length months

if (month == 3)
    correction = correction - 1;
else if (month == 2 || month == 6 || month == 7)
    correction = correction + 1;
else if (month == 8)
    correction = correction + 2;
else if (month == 9 || month == 10)
    correction = correction + 3;
else if (month == 11 || month == 12)
    correction = correction + 4;
return (month - 1) * 30 + correction + dayOfMonth;
}
```

The first thing to note is that the function definition looks like a void function, except for the fact that the heading begins with the data type int instead of the word void. The second thing to observe is the Return statement at the end, which includes an integer expression between the word return and the semicolon.

A value-returning function returns one value, not through a parameter but by means of a Return statement. The data type at the beginning of the heading declares the type of value that the function returns. This data type is called the *function type,* although a more precise term is **function value type** (or *function return type* or *function result type*).

Function value type   The data type of the result value returned by a function.

The last statement in the Day function evaluates the expression

```
(month - 1) * 30 + correction + dayOfMonth
```

and returns the result as the function value (see Figure 8-3).

You now have seen two forms of the Return statement. The form

```
return;
```

is valid *only* in void functions. It causes control to exit the function immediately and return to the caller. The second form is

```
return Expression;
```

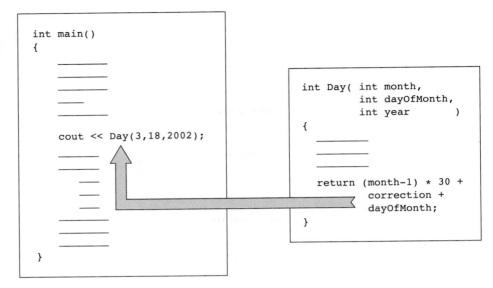

Figure 8-3

Returning a
Function Value to
the Expression
That Called the
Function

This form is valid *only* in a value-returning function. It returns control to the caller, sending back the value of Expression as the function value. (If the data type of Expression is different from the declared function type, its value is coerced to the correct type.)

In Chapter 7, we presented a syntax template for the function definition of a void function. We now update the syntax template to cover both void functions and value-returning functions:

FunctionDefinition

```
DataType FunctionName ( ParameterList )
    {
        Statement
            ⋮
    }
```

If DataType is the word `void`, the function is a void function; otherwise, it is a value-returning function. Notice from the shading in the syntax template that DataType is optional. If you omit the data type of a function, `int` is assumed. We mention this point only because you sometimes encounter programs where DataType is missing from the function heading. Many programmers do not consider this practice to be good programming style.

The parameter list for a value-returning function has exactly the same form as for a void function: a list of parameter declarations, separated by commas. Also, a function prototype for a value-returning function looks just like the prototype for a void function except that it begins with a data type instead of `void`.

Let's look at two more examples of value-returning functions. The C++ standard library provides a power function, `pow`, that raises a floating-point number to a floating-point power. The library does not supply a power function for `int` values, so let's build one of our own. The function receives two integers, x and n (where $n \geq 0$), and computes x^n. We use a simple approach, multiplying repeatedly by x. Because the number of iterations is known in advance, a count-controlled loop is appropriate. The loop counts down to 0 from the initial value of n. For each iteration of the loop, x is multiplied by the previous product.

```
int Power( /* in */ int x,       // Base number
           /* in */ int n )      // Power to raise base to

// This function computes x to the n power

// Precondition:
//      x is assigned  &&  n >= 0  &&  (x to the n) <= INT_MAX
// Postcondition:
//      Function value == x to the n power

{
    int result;      // Holds intermediate powers of x

    result = 1;
    while (n > 0)
    {
        result = result * x;
        n--;
    }
    return result;
}
```

Notice the notation we use in the postcondition of a value-returning function. Because a value-returning function returns a single value, it is most concise if you simply state what that value equals. Except in complicated examples, the postcondition looks like this:

```
// Postcondition
//      Function value == ...
```

Another function that is used frequently in calculating probabilities is the factorial. For example, 5 factorial (written 5! in mathematical notation) is $5 \times 4 \times 3 \times 2 \times 1$. Zero factorial, by definition, equals 1. This function has one integer parameter. As with the `Power` function, we use repeated multiplication, but we decrement the multiplier on each iteration.

```
int Factorial( /* in */ int n )    // Number whose factorial is
                                   //    to be computed
// This function computes n!

// Precondition:
//     n >= 0  &&  n! <= INT_MAX
// Postcondition:
//     Function value == n!

{
    int result;      // Holds partial products

    result = 1;
    while (n > 0)
    {
        result = result * n;
        n--;
    }
    return result;
}
```

A call to the `Factorial` function might look like this:

```
combinations = Factorial(n) / (Factorial(m) * Factorial(n - m));
```

Boolean Functions

Value-returning functions are not restricted to returning numerical results. We can also use them, for example, to evaluate a condition and return a Boolean result. Boolean functions can be useful when a branch or loop depends on some complex condition. Rather than code the condition directly into the If or While statement, we can call a Boolean function to form the controlling expression.

Suppose we are writing a program that works with triangles. The program reads three angles as floating-point numbers. Before performing any calculations on those angles, however, we want to check that they really form a triangle by adding the angles to confirm that their sum equals 180 degrees. We can write a value-returning function that takes the three angles as parameters and returns a Boolean result. Such a function would look like this (recall from Chapter 5 that you should test floating-point numbers only for near equality):

```cpp
#include <cmath>    // For fabs()
 ⋮
bool IsTriangle( /* in */ float angle1,    // First angle
                 /* in */ float angle2,    // Second angle
                 /* in */ float angle3 )   // Third angle

// This function checks to see if its three incoming values
// add up to 180 degrees, forming a valid triangle

// Precondition:
//     angle1, angle2, and angle3 are assigned
// Postcondition:
//     Function value == true, if (angle1 + angle2 + angle3) is
//                                 within 0.00000001 of 180.0 degrees
//                          == false, otherwise

{
    return (fabs(angle1 + angle2 + angle3 - 180.0) < 0.00000001);
}
```

The following program fragment shows how the `IsTriangle` function might be called:

```cpp
cin >> angleA >> angleB >> angleC;
if (IsTriangle(angleA, angleB, angleC))              // Function call
    cout << "The three angles form a valid triangle.";
else
    cout << "Those angles do not form a triangle.";
```

The If statement is much easier to understand with the function than it would be if the entire condition were coded directly. When a conditional test is at all complicated, a Boolean function is in order.

The C++ standard library provides a number of helpful functions that let you test the contents of `char` variables. To use them, you `#include` the header file `cctype`. Here are some of the available functions; Appendix C contains a more complete list.

Header File	Function	Function Type	Function Value
<cctype>	isalpha(ch)	int	Nonzero, if ch is a letter ('A'–'Z', 'a'–'z'); 0, otherwise
<cctype>	isalnum(ch)	int	Nonzero, if ch is a letter or a digit ('A'–'Z', 'a'–'z', '0'–'9'); 0, otherwise
<cctype>	isdigit(ch)	int	Nonzero, if ch is a digit ('0'–'9'); 0, otherwise
<cctype>	islower(ch)	int	Nonzero, if ch is a lowercase letter ('a'–'z'); 0, otherwise
<cctype>	isspace(ch)	int	Nonzero, if ch is a whitespace character (blank, newline, tab, carriage return, form feed); 0, otherwise
<cctype>	isupper(ch)	int	Nonzero, if ch is an uppercase letter ('A'–'Z'); 0, otherwise

Although they return int values, the "is..." functions behave like Boolean functions. They return an int value that is nonzero (coerced to true in an If or While condition) or 0 (coerced to false in an If or While condition). These functions are convenient to use and make programs more readable. For example, the test

```
if (isalnum(inputChar))
```

is easier to read and less prone to error than if you coded the test the long way:

```
if (inputChar >= 'A' && inputChar <= 'Z' ||
    inputChar >= 'a' && inputChar <= 'z' ||
    inputChar >= '0' && inputChar <= '9'     )
```

In fact, this complicated logical expression doesn't work correctly on some machines. We'll see why when we examine character data in Chapter 10.

MATTERS OF STYLE

Naming Value-Returning Functions

In Chapter 7, we said that it's good style to use imperative verbs when naming void functions. The reason is that a call to a void function is a complete statement and should look like a command to the computer:

```
PrintResults(a, b, c);
DoThis(x);
DoThat();
```

This naming scheme, however, doesn't work well with value-returning functions. A statement such as

```
z = 6.7 * ComputeMaximum(d, e, f);
```

sounds awkward when you read it aloud: "Set z equal to 6.7 times the *compute maximum* of d, e, and f."

With a value-returning function, the function call represents a value within an expression. Things that represent values, such as variables and value-returning functions, are best given names that are nouns or, occasionally, adjectives. See how much better this statement sounds when you pronounce it out loud:

```
z = 6.7 * Maximum(d, e, f);
```

You would read this as "Set z equal to 6.7 times the *maximum* of d, e, and f." Other names that suggest values rather than actions are SquareRoot, Cube, Factorial, StudentCount, SumOfSquares, and SocialSecurityNum. As you see, they are all nouns or noun phrases.

Boolean value-returning functions (and variables) are often named using adjectives or phrases beginning with *Is*. Here are a few examples:

```
while (Valid(m, n))
if (Odd(n))
if (IsTriangle(s1, s2, s3))
```

When you are choosing a name for a value-returning function, try to stick with nouns or adjectives so that the name suggests a value, not a command to the computer.

Interface Design and Side Effects

The interface to a value-returning function is designed in much the same way as the interface to a void function. We simply write down a list of what the function needs and what it must return. Because value-returning functions return only one value, there is only one item labeled "outgoing" in the list: the function return value. Everything else in the list is labeled "incoming," and there aren't any "incoming/outgoing" parameters.

Returning more than one value from a value-returning function (by modifying the caller's arguments) is a side effect and should be avoided. If your interface design calls for multiple values to be returned, then you should use a void function instead of a value-returning function.

A rule of thumb is never to use reference parameters in the parameter list of a value-returning function, but to use value parameters exclusively. Let's look at an example that demonstrates the importance of this rule. Suppose we define the following function:

```
int SideEffect( int& n )
{
    int result = n * n;

    n++;                    // Side effect
    return result;
}
```

This function returns the square of its incoming value, but it also increments the caller's argument before returning. Now suppose we call this function with the following statement:

```
y = x + SideEffect(x);
```

If x is originally 2, what value is stored into y? The answer depends on the order in which your compiler generates code to evaluate the expression. If the compiled code first calls the function, then the answer is 7. If it accesses x first in preparation for adding it to the function result, the answer is 6. This uncertainty is precisely why reference parameters shouldn't be used with value-returning functions. A function that causes an unpredictable result has no place in a well-written program.

An exception is the case in which an I/O stream object is passed to a value-returning function. Remember that C++ allows a stream object to be passed only to a reference parameter. Within a value-returning function, the only operation that should be performed is testing the state of the stream (for EOF or I/O errors). A value-returning function should not perform input or output operations. Such operations are considered to be side effects of the function. (We should point out that not everyone agrees with this point of view. Some programmers feel that performing I/O within a value-returning function is perfectly acceptable. You will find strong opinions on both sides of this issue.)

There is another advantage to using only value parameters in a value-returning function definition: You can use constants and expressions as arguments. For example, we can call the `IsTriangle` function using literals and other expressions:

```
if (IsTriangle(30.0, 60.0, 30.0 + 60.0))
    cout << "A 30-60-90 angle combination forms a triangle.";
else
    cout << "Something is wrong.";
```

When to Use Value-Returning Functions

There aren't any formal rules for determining when to use a void function and when to use a value-returning function, but here are some guidelines:

1. If the module must return more than one value or modify any of the caller's arguments, do not use a value-returning function.
2. If the module must perform I/O, do not use a value-returning function. (This guideline is not universally agreed upon.)
3. If there is only one value returned from the module and it is a Boolean value, a value-returning function is appropriate.
4. If there is only one value returned and that value is to be used immediately in an expression, a value-returning function is appropriate.
5. When in doubt, use a void function. You can recode any value-returning function as a void function by adding an extra outgoing parameter to carry back the computed result.
6. If both a void function and a value-returning function are acceptable, use the one you feel more comfortable implementing.

Value-returning functions were included in C++ to provide a way of simulating the mathematical concept of a function. The C++ standard library supplies a set of commonly used mathematical functions through the header file `cmath`. A list of these appears in Appendix C.

*B*ACKGROUND INFORMATION

Ignoring a Function Value

A peculiarity of the C++ language is that it lets you ignore the value returned by a value-returning function. For example, you could write the following statement in your program without any complaint from the compiler:

```
sqrt(x);
```

When this statement is executed, the value returned by `sqrt` is promptly discarded. This function call has absolutely no effect except to waste the computer's time by calculating a value that is never used.

Clearly, the above call to `sqrt` is a mistake. No programmer would write that statement intentionally. But C++ programmers occasionally write value-returning functions in a way that allows the caller to ignore the function value. Here is a specific example from the C++ standard library.

The library provides a function named `remove`, the purpose of which is to delete a disk file from the system. It takes a single argument—a C string specifying the name of the file—and it returns a function value. This function value is an integer notifying you of the status: 0 if the operation succeeded, and nonzero if it failed. Here is how you might call the `remove` function:

```
status = remove("junkfile.dat");
if (status != 0)
    PrintErrorMsg();
```

On the other hand, if you assume that the system always succeeds at deleting a file, you can ignore the returned status by calling `remove` as though it were a void function:

```
remove("junkfile.dat");
```

The `remove` function is sort of a hybrid between a void function and a value-returning function. Conceptually, it is a void function; its principal purpose is to delete a file, not to compute a value to be returned. Literally, however, it's a value-returning function. It does return a function value—the status of the operation (which you can choose to ignore).

In this book, we don't write hybrid functions. We prefer to keep the concept of a void function distinct from a value-returning function. But there are two reasons why every C++ programmer should know about the topic of ignoring a function value. First, if you accidentally call a value-returning function as if it were a void function, the compiler won't prevent you from making the mistake. Second, you sometimes encounter this style of coding in other people's programs and in the C++ standard library. Several of the library functions are technically value-returning functions, but the function value is used merely to return something of secondary importance such as a status value.

PROBLEM-SOLVING CASE STUDY

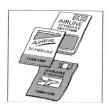

Reformat Dates

Problem: You work for a company that publishes the schedules for international airlines. The firm must print three versions of the schedules because of the different formats for dates used around the world. Your job is to write a program that takes dates written in American format (mm/dd/yyyy) from file stream `dataIn` and converts them to British format (dd/mm/yyyy) and International Standards Organization (ISO) format (yyyy-mm-dd). The output should be a table written to file stream `dataOut` that contains the dates lined up in three columns as follows:

```
American Format        British Format          ISO Format

  mm/dd/yyyy             dd/mm/yyyy            yyyy-mm-dd
  mm/dd/yyyy             dd/mm/yyyy            yyyy-mm-dd
```

There is one small problem. Although the dates are in American format, one per line, embedded blanks can occur anywhere in the line. For example, the input file may look like this:

```
10/11/1935
1 1     / 2 3         / 1 9   2 6
              5/2/2004
05    /28                      /1965
7/   3/    19  56
```

Given this input, the output (written to file stream `dataOut`) would be

```
    American Format        British Format          ISO Format

      10/11/1935             11/10/1935            1935-10-11
      11/23/1926             23/11/1926            1926-11-23
      05/02/2004             02/05/2004            2004-05-02
      05/28/1965             28/05/1965            1965-05-28
      07/03/1956             03/07/1956            1956-07-03
```

Input: A data file (stream `dataIn`) containing dates, one per line, in American format, mm/dd/yyyy (may include embedded blanks).

The number of input lines is unknown. The program should continue to process input lines until EOF occurs.

Output: A file (stream `dataOut`) containing a table with each date in the following formats:

PROBLEM-SOLVING CASE STUDY *cont'd.*

mm/dd/yyyy   dd/mm/yyyy   yyyy-mm-dd

See the preceding sample output for the formatting of the table.

Discussion: It is easy for a human to scan the input line, skipping over the embedded blanks and the slash (/) to pick up each number. We also easily identify a one-character number. The key to this problem is making explicit what our eyes do implicitly.

First, we know that we cannot read values as int data because the digits may have blanks between them, and the terminating character may be a slash, a blank, or, in the case of the year, the newline character ('\n'). Therefore, we must read everything as char data.

We recognize the first character in the month because it is the first nonblank character on a line. If the next character is a digit, then we have the complete month, and we can skip over blanks and the slash. If the next character is not a digit, we must skip over blanks until we find a digit or a slash. If we find a slash, we know that the month is a one-digit month, and we must insert a leading zero. Once we have both characters of the month, we can store them into a string.

The same algorithm works for finding the day. The algorithm for finding the year is easier. Assuming that four digits are always present, we simply input four characters, skipping blanks along the way. Let's convert these observations into a functional decomposition.

Assumptions: Each line in dataIn contains a valid date in American format.

Main   **Level 0**

```
Open the input and output files
IF either file could not be opened
        Terminate program
Write headings
Get month
WHILE NOT EOF on dataIn
        Get day
        Get year
        Write date in American format
        Write date in British format
        Write date in ISO format
        Get month
```

PROBLEM-SOLVING CASE STUDY cont'd.

Writing the headings can be done in a single C++ output statement, so we can code it directly in the `main` function instead of creating a separate module.

Open for Input (Inout: someFile)   **Level 1**

> We can reuse the Open for Input module from the Graph program in Chapter 7

Open for Output (Inout: someFile)

> We can modify the Open for Input module so that it opens an output file

Get Month (Inout: dataIn; Out: twoChars)

The parameter `twoChars` is a string variable that holds both digit characters of the month.

> Read firstChar from dataIn, skipping leading whitespace chars
> IF EOF on dataIn
>   Return
> Read secondChar from dataIn, skipping leading whitespace chars
> IF secondChar is '/'
>   Set secondChar = firstChar
>   Set firstChar = '0'
> ELSE
>   Read dummy from dataIn, skipping leading whitespace chars
> Set twoChars = firstChar
> Concatenate secondChar to twoChars

The else-clause uses a variable named dummy to move the reading marker past the slash if there is a two-digit month.

We must remember to test both one-digit and two-digit numbers, with the digits together and separated. We also must test digits at the beginning of the line and immediately before and after the slash.

Get Day (Inout: dataIn; Out: twoChars)

Because the reading marker is left pointing to the character immediately to the right of the slash, the Get Day module is identical to the Get Month module.

Get Year (Inout: dataIn; Out: year)

The outgoing parameter year is a string variable that holds the four digit characters of the month.

```
Set year = ""      (the null string)
Set loopCount = 1
WHILE loopCount ≤ 4
        Read digitChar from dataIn, skipping leading whitespace chars
        Concatenate digitChar to year
        Increment loopCount
```

The algorithm begins by storing the null string into year. Then, using a count-controlled loop, we input exactly four characters, concatenating each one to the end of year as we go.

Write Date in American Format (Inout: dataOut; In: month, day, year)

```
Write month, '/', day, '/', year to dataOut
```

PROBLEM-SOLVING CASE STUDY cont'd.

Write Date in British Format (Inout: dataOut; In: month, day, year)

Write day, '/', month, '/', year to dataOut

Write Date in ISO Format (Inout: dataOut; In: month, day, year)

Write year, '–', month, '–', day to dataOut

As we noted during the design phase, modules Get Month and Get Day are identical. We can replace them with a single module, Get Two Digits. We also can combine modules Write Date in American Format, Write Date in British Format, and Write Date in ISO Format into one module named Write. Here is the resulting module structure chart. The chart emphasizes the importance of interface design. The arrows indicate which identifiers are received or returned by each module.

Module Structure Chart:

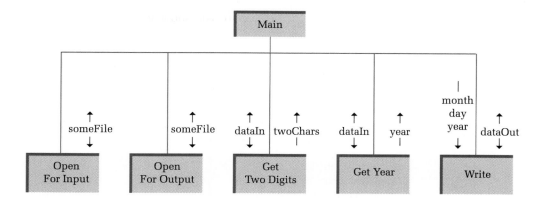

PROBLEM-SOLVING CASE STUDY cont'd.

Here is the program that corresponds to our design. We have omitted the precondition and postcondition from the comments at the beginning of each function. Case Study Follow-Up Exercise 1 asks you to fill them in.

(The following program is written in ISO/ANSI standard C++. If you are working with pre–standard C++, see the alternate version of the program in the PRE_STD directory of the program disk, available at the publisher's Web site, www.jbpub.com/disks.)

```cpp
//****************************************************************
// ConvertDates program
// This program reads dates in American form from an input file and
// writes them to an output file in American, British, and ISO form.
// No data validation is done on the input file
//****************************************************************
#include <iostream>
#include <iomanip>     // For setw()
#include <fstream>     // For file I/O
#include <string>      // For string type

using namespace std;

void Get2Digits( ifstream&, string& );
void GetYear( ifstream&, string& );
void OpenForInput( ifstream& );
void OpenForOutput( ofstream& );
void Write( ofstream&, string, string, string );

int main()
{
    string    month;      // Both digits of month
    string    day;        // Both digits of day
    string    year;       // Four digits of year
    ifstream dataIn;      // Input file of dates
    ofstream dataOut;     // Output file of dates

    OpenForInput(dataIn);
    OpenForOutput(dataOut);
    if ( !dataIn || !dataOut )           // Make sure files
        return 1;                        //   were opened

    dataOut << setw(20) << "American Format"    // Write headings
            << setw(20) << "British Format"
            << setw(20) << "ISO Format" << endl << endl;

    Get2Digits(dataIn, month);                  // Priming read
    while (dataIn)                              // While not EOF...
    {
```

```
            Get2Digits(dataIn, day);
            GetYear(dataIn, year);
            Write(dataOut, month, day, year);
            Get2Digits(dataIn, month);
        }
        return 0;
}


//****************************************************************

void OpenForInput( /* inout */ ifstream& someFile )    // File to be
                                                       // opened
// Prompts the user for the name of an input file
// and attempts to open the file

// Postcondition: Exercise
//
// Note:
//     Upon return from this function, the caller must test
//     the stream state to see if the file was successfully opened

{
    string fileName;    // User-specified file name

    cout << "Input file name: ";
    cin >> fileName;

    someFile.open(fileName.c_str());
    if ( !someFile )
        cout << "** Can't open " << fileName << " **" << endl;
}


//****************************************************************

void OpenForOutput( /* inout */ ofstream& someFile )   // File to be
                                                       // opened
// Prompts the user for the name of an output file
// and attempts to open the file

// Postcondition: Exercise
//
// Note:
//     Upon return from this function, the caller must test
//     the stream state to see if the file was successfully opened

{
    string fileName;    // User-specified file name
```

PROBLEM-SOLVING CASE STUDY cont'd.

```cpp
    cout << "Output file name: ";
    cin >> fileName;

    someFile.open(fileName.c_str());
    if ( !someFile )
        cout << "** Can't open " << fileName << " **" << endl;
}

//*****************************************************************

void Get2Digits( /* inout */ ifstream& dataIn,       // Input file
                 /* out */    string&   twoChars )   // Two digits

// Reads characters up to a slash from dataIn and returns two
// digit characters in the string twoChars.  If only one digit
// is found before the slash, a leading '0' is inserted.
// (If input fails due to end-of-file, twoChars is undefined.)

// Precondition:  Exercise
// Postcondition: Exercise

{
    char firstChar;     // First character of a two-digit value
    char secondChar;    // Second character of value
    char dummy;         // To consume the slash, if necessary

    dataIn >> firstChar;
    if ( !dataIn )                  // Check for EOF
        return;                     // If so, exit the function

    dataIn >> secondChar;
    if (secondChar == '/')
    {
        secondChar = firstChar;
        firstChar = '0';
    }
    else
        dataIn >> dummy;            // Consume the slash

    twoChars = firstChar;
    twoChars = twoChars + secondChar;
}

//*****************************************************************

void GetYear( /* inout */ ifstream& dataIn,      // Input file
              /* out */    string&   year   )    // Four digits
                                                 //   of year
```

PROBLEM-SOLVING CASE STUDY *cont'd.*

```
// Reads characters from dataIn and returns four digit characters
// in the year string

// Precondition:  Exercise
// Postcondition: Exercise

{
    char digitChar;     // One digit of the year
    int  loopCount;     // Loop control variable

    year = "";
    loopCount = 1;
    while (loopCount <= 4)
    {
        dataIn >> digitChar;
        year = year + digitChar;
        loopCount++;
    }
}


//*******************************************************************

void Write( /* inout */ ofstream& dataOut,     // Output file
            /* in */    string    month,       // Month string
            /* in */    string    day,         // Day string
            /* in */    string    year    )    // Year string

// Writes the date represented by month, day, and year to file
// dataOut in American, British, and ISO form

// Precondition:  Exercise
// Postcondition: Exercise

{
    dataOut << setw(9) << month << '/' << day << '/' << year;
    dataOut << setw(13) << day << '/' << month << '/' << year;
    dataOut << setw(16) << year << '-' << month
            << '-' << day << endl;
}
```

The Write function in this program contains only three statements in the body (and could have been written as a single, long output statement). We could just as easily have written these statements directly in the main function in place of the call to the function.

We don't mean to imply that you should never write a function with as few as one, two, or three statements. In some cases, decomposition of a problem makes a small function quite appropriate. When deciding whether to code a module directly in the next-higher level or as a function, ask yourself the following question: Which way will make the overall program easier to read, understand, and modify later? With experience, you will develop your own set of guidelines for making this decision. For example, if a two-line module is to be called from several places in the program, you should code it as a function. If it is called from only one place, it may be better to code it directly at the next-higher level, unless doing so would contribute to making the calling function too long.

Testing: The ConvertDates program allows a great deal of variation in the formatting of its input. Such flexibility makes it necessary to test the program with many combinations of input. The test data should include digits, slashes, and blanks in every valid arrangement and in some arrangements that are invalid.

Blanks can appear in a date in 11 places: between each pair of the 10 characters, before the first character, and after the last. At a minimum, we should test with a data set containing 11 dates in which a single blank appears in each of these positions. To be thorough, we should test all possible combinations of a blank or no blank in these positions. There are 2^{11} (or 2048) such combinations.

In theory, we also should test for combinations with single or multiple blanks in each position. If we check only for combinations of none, one, or two blanks in each position, then there are 3^{11} (or 177,147) such combinations. Creating such a comprehensive test data set by hand would be both difficult and time-consuming. However, we could write a program to generate it. Such programs, called *test generators,* often provide the simplest way of testing a program with a large test data set.

We actually can test the ConvertDates program with far fewer than 177,147 combinations of blanks, because we know that the >> operator is used to skip all blanks preceding a character. Thus, once we have verified that >> works correctly in one place in a date, it isn't necessary to test it for every combination of blanks in other places. In addition to testing for correctly skipping blanks, we must test that the program properly handles months and days with one or two digits. We should try a date in which the month and day are each a single digit, and another date in which they both have two digits.

Here is a sample test data file for the ConvertDates program:

```
10/23/1999
10/23/200 1
```

```
10/23/ 2002
10/23 /2003
10/2 3/2004
10/ 23/2005
10 /23/2006
1 0/23/2007
 10/23/2008
  1  0  /  2  3  /  2  0  0  9
1/2/1946
  1  /  2  /  1 946
```

For this data, here is the output from the program:

American Format	British Format	ISO Format
10/23/1999	23/10/1999	1999-10-23
10/23/2001	23/10/2001	2001-10-23
10/23/2002	23/10/2002	2002-10-23
10/23/2003	23/10/2003	2003-10-23
10/23/2004	23/10/2004	2004-10-23
10/23/2005	23/10/2005	2005-10-23
10/23/2006	23/10/2006	2006-10-23
10/23/2007	23/10/2007	2007-10-23
10/23/2008	23/10/2008	2008-10-23
10/23/2009	23/10/2009	2009-10-23
01/02/1946	02/01/1946	1946-01-02
01/02/1946	02/01/1946	1946-01-02

The ConvertDates program is actually too flexible in how it allows dates to be entered. For instance, a "digit" can be any nonblank character. Because slashes appear in the correct places, an input sequence such as

```
#$ / () / A@
```

is treated as a valid date. On the other hand, a seemingly valid date such as

```
12-27-65
```

is not recognized because dashes aren't valid separators. Furthermore, ConvertDates does not handle erroneous dates gracefully. If part of a date is missing, for example, the program may end up reading the remainder of the input file incorrectly. Case Study Follow-Up Exercise 2 asks you to add data validation to the ConvertDates program.

SOFTWARE ENGINEERING TIP

Control Abstraction, Functional Cohesion, and Communication Complexity

The ConvertDates program contains two different While loops. The control structure for this program has the potential to be fairly complex. Yet if you look at the individual modules, the most complicated control structure is a While loop without any If or While statements nested within it.

The complexity of a program is hidden by reducing each of the major control structures to an abstract action performed by a function call. In the ConvertDates program, for example, finding the year is an abstract action that appears as a call to `GetYear`. The logical properties of the action are separated from its implementation (a While loop). This aspect of a design is called **control abstraction**.

Control abstraction   The separation of the logical properties of an action from its implementation.

Control abstraction can serve as a guideline for deciding which modules to code as functions and which to code directly. If a module contains a control structure, it is a good candidate for being implemented as a function. On the other hand, the `Write` function lacks control abstraction. Its body is a sequence of three statements, which could just as well be located in the `main` function. But even if a module does not contain a control structure, you still want to consider other factors. Is it lengthy, or is it called from more than one place? If so, you should use a function.

Somewhat related to control abstraction is the concept of **functional cohesion,** which states that a module should perform exactly one abstract action.

Functional cohesion   The principle that a module should perform exactly one abstract action.

If you can state the action that a module performs in one sentence with no conjunctions (*and*s), then it is highly cohesive. A module that has more than one primary purpose lacks cohesion. Apart from `main`, all the functions in the ConvertDates program have good cohesion.

A module that only partially fulfills a purpose also lacks cohesion. Such a module should be combined with whatever other modules are directly related to it. For example, it would make no sense to have a separate function that prints the first digit of a date because printing a date is one abstract action.

A third and related aspect of a module's design is its **communication complexity**, the amount of data that passes through a module's interface—for example, the number of arguments. A module's communication complexity is often an indicator of its cohesiveness. Usually, if a module requires a large number of arguments, it either is trying to accomplish too much or is only partially fulfilling a purpose. You should step back and see if there is an alternative way of dividing up the problem so that a minimal amount of data is communicated between modules. The modules in ConvertDates have low communication complexity.

Communication complexity   A measure of the quantity of data passing through a module's interface.

PROBLEM-SOLVING CASE STUDY

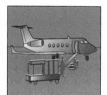

Starship Weight and Balance

Problem: The company you work for has just upgraded its fleet of corporate aircraft by adding the Beechcraft Starship-1. As with any airplane, it is essential that the pilot know the total weight of the loaded plane at takeoff and its center of gravity. If the plane weighs too much, it won't be able to lift off. If its center of gravity is outside the limits established for the plane, it might be impossible to control. Either situation can lead to a crash. You have been asked to write a program that determines the weight and center of gravity of this new plane, based on the number of crew members and passengers as well as the weight of the baggage, closet contents, and fuel.

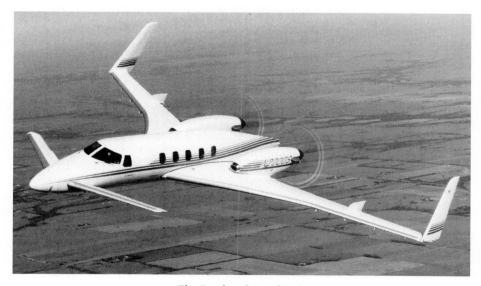

The Beechcraft Starship-1

PROBLEM-SOLVING CASE STUDY cont'd.

Input: Number of crew members, number of passengers, weight of closet contents, baggage weight, fuel in gallons.

Output: Total weight, center of gravity.

Discussion: As with most real-world problems, the basic solution is simple but is complicated by special cases. We use value-returning functions to hide the complexity so that the main function remains simple.

The total weight is basically the sum of the empty weight of the airplane plus the weight of each of the following: crew members, passengers, baggage, contents of the storage closet, and fuel. We use the standard average weight of a person, 170 pounds, to compute the total weight of the people. The weight of the baggage and the contents of the closet are given. Fuel weighs 6.7 pounds per gallon. Thus, the total weight is

$$totalWeight = emptyWeight + (crew + passengers) \times 170 + baggage + closet + fuel \times 6.7$$

To compute the center of gravity, each weight is multiplied by its distance from the front of the airplane, and the products—called *moment arms* or simply *moments*—are then summed and divided by the total weight (see Figure 8-4). The formula is thus

$$centerOfGravity = (emptyMoment + crewMoment + passengerMoment +$$
$$cargoMoment + fuelMoment) / totalWeight$$

The Starship-1 manual gives the distance from the front of the plane to the crew's seats, closet, baggage compartment, and fuel tanks. There are four rows of passenger seats, so this calculation depends on where the individual passengers sit. We have to make some assumptions about how passengers arrange themselves. Each row has two seats. The most popular seats are in row 2 because they are near the entrance and face forward. Once row 2 is filled, passengers usually take seats in row 1, facing their traveling companions. Row 3 is usually the next to fill up, even though it faces backward, because row 4 is a fold-down bench seat that is less comfortable than the armchairs in the forward rows. The following table gives the distance from the nose of the plane to each of the "loading stations."

PROBLEM-SOLVING CASE STUDY cont'd.

FIGURE 8-4
A Passenger
Moment Arm

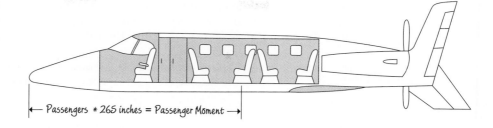

Loading Station	Distance from Nose (inches)
Crew seats	143
Row 1 seats	219
Row 2 seats	265
Row 3 seats	295
Row 4 seats	341
Closet	182
Baggage	386

The distance for the fuel varies because there are several tanks, and the tanks are in different places. As fuel is added to the plane, it automatically flows into the different tanks so that the center of gravity changes as the tanks are filled. There are four formulas for computing the distance from the nose to the "center" of the fuel tanks, depending on how much fuel is being loaded into the plane. The following table lists these distance formulas.

Gallons of Fuel (G)	Distance (D) Formula
0–59	$D = 314.6 \times G$
60–360	$D = 305.8 + (\,-0.01233 \times (G - 60\,))$
361–520	$D = 303.0 + (\;\;0.12500 \times (G - 361\,))$
521–565	$D = 323.0 + (\,-0.04444 \times (G - 521\,))$

We define one value-returning function for each of the different moments, and we name these functions `CrewMoment`, `PassengerMoment`, `CargoMoment`, and `FuelMoment`. The center of gravity is then computed with the formula we gave earlier and the following arguments:

$$centerOfGravity \ = \ (CrewMoment(crew) + PassengerMoment(passengers) +$$
$$CargoMoment(closet, baggage) + FuelMoment(fuel) +$$
$$emptyMoment) \ / \ totalWeight$$

The empty weight of the Starship is 9887 pounds, and its empty center of gravity is 319 inches from the front of the airplane. Thus, the empty moment is 3,153,953 inch-pounds.

We now have enough information to write the algorithm to solve this problem. In addition to printing the results, we'll also print a warning message that states the assumptions of the program and tells the pilot to double-check the results by hand if the weight or center of gravity is near the allowable limits.

Main   **Level 0**

```
Get data
Set totalWt =
      EMPTY_WEIGHT + (passengers + crew) * 170 +
      baggage + closet + fuel * 6.7
Set centerOfGravity =
      (CrewMoment(crew) + PassengerMoment(passengers) +
      CargoMoment(closet, baggage) + FuelMoment(fuel) +
      EMPTY_MOMENT) / totalWt
Print totalWt, centerOfGravity
Print warning
```

Get Data (Out: crew, passengers, closet, baggage, fuel)   **Level 1**

```
Prompt for number of crew, number of passengers,
      weight in closet and baggage compartments,
      and gallons of fuel
Read crew, passengers, closet, baggage, fuel
Echo print the input
```

PROBLEM-SOLVING CASE STUDY cont'd.

Crew Moment (In: crew)

Out: Function value

```
Return crew * 170 * 143
```

Passenger Moment (In: passengers)

Out: Function value

```
Set moment = 0.0
IF passengers > 6
      Add (passengers – 6) * 170 * 341 to moment
      Set passengers = 6
IF passengers > 4
      Add (passengers – 4) * 170 * 295 to moment
      Set passengers = 4
IF passengers > 2
      Add (passengers – 2) * 170 * 219 to moment
      Set passengers = 2
IF passengers > 0
      Add passengers * 170 * 265 to moment
Return moment
```

Cargo Moment (In: closet, baggage)

Out: Function value

```
Return closet * 182 + baggage * 386
```

Fuel Moment (In: fuel)

Out: Function value

```
Set fuelWt = fuel * 6.7
IF fuel < 60
      Set fuelDistance = fuel * 314.6
ELSE IF fuel < 361
      Set fuelDistance = 305.8 + (−0.01233 * (fuel − 60))
ELSE IF fuel < 521
      Set fuelDistance = 303.0 + ( 0.12500 * (fuel − 361))
ELSE
      Set fuelDistance = 323.0 + (−0.04444 * (fuel − 521))
Return fuelDistance * fuelWt
```

Print Warning (No parameters)

Print a warning message about the assumptions of
the program and when to double-check the results

Module Structure Chart: In the following chart, you'll see a new notation. The box corresponding to each value-returning function has an
upward arrow originating at its right side. This arrow signifies the function
value that is returned.

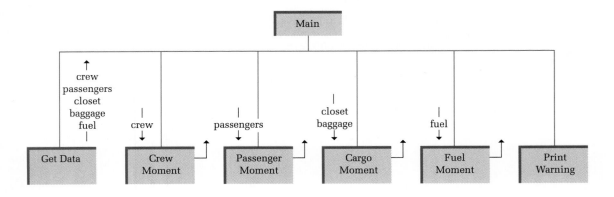

PROBLEM-SOLVING CASE STUDY *cont'd.*

(The following program is written in ISO/ANSI standard C++. If you are working with pre–standard C++, see the alternate version of the program in the PRE_STD directory of the program disk, available at the publisher's Web site, www.jbpub.com/disks.)

```
//******************************************************************
// Starship program
// This program computes the total weight and center of gravity
// of a Beechcraft Starship-1, given the number of crew members
// and passengers, weight of closet and baggage compartment cargo,
// and gallons of fuel loaded.  It assumes that each person
// weighs 170 pounds, and that the fuel weighs 6.7 pounds per
// gallon.  Thus, the output is approximate and should be hand-
// checked if the Starship is loaded near its limits
//******************************************************************
#include <iostream>
#include <iomanip>      // For setw() and setprecision()

using namespace std;

const float PERSON_WT = 170.0;          // Average person weighs
                                        //    170 lbs.
const float LBS_PER_GAL = 6.7;          // Jet-A weighs 6.7 lbs.
                                        //    per gal.
const float EMPTY_WEIGHT = 9887.0;      // Standard empty weight
const float EMPTY_MOMENT = 3153953.0;   // Standard empty moment

float CargoMoment( int, int );
float CrewMoment( int );
float FuelMoment( int );
void  GetData( int&, int&, int&, int&, int& );
float PassengerMoment( int );
void  PrintWarning();

int main()
{
    int   crew;              // Number of crew on board (1 or 2)
    int   passengers;        // Number of passengers (0 through 8)
    int   closet;            // Weight in closet (160 lbs. maximum)
    int   baggage;           // Weight of baggage (525 lbs. max.)
    int   fuel;              // Gallons of fuel (10 through 565 gals.)
    float totalWt;           // Total weight of the loaded Starship
    float centerOfGravity;   // Center of gravity of loaded Starship
```

PROBLEM-SOLVING CASE STUDY cont'd.

```cpp
    cout << fixed << showpoint            // Set up floating-pt.
         << setprecision(2);              //    output format

    GetData(crew, passengers, closet, baggage, fuel);

    totalWt =
        EMPTY_WEIGHT + float(passengers + crew) * PERSON_WT +
        float(baggage + closet) + float(fuel) * LBS_PER_GAL;
    centerOfGravity =
        (CrewMoment(crew) + PassengerMoment(passengers) +
        CargoMoment(closet, baggage) + FuelMoment(fuel) +
        EMPTY_MOMENT) / totalWt;

    cout << "Total weight is " << totalWt << " pounds." << endl;
    cout << "Center of gravity is " << centerOfGravity
         << " inches from the front of the plane." << endl;
    PrintWarning();
    return 0;
}


//**************************************************************

void GetData( /* out */ int& crew,         // Number of crew members
              /* out */ int& passengers,   // Number of passengers
              /* out */ int& closet,       // Weight of closet cargo
              /* out */ int& baggage,      // Weight of baggage
              /* out */ int& fuel       )  // Gallons of fuel

// Prompts for the input of crew, passengers, closet, baggage, and
// fuel values and returns the five values after echo printing them

// Postcondition:
//      All parameters (crew, passengers, closet, baggage, and fuel)
//      have been prompted for, input, and echo printed

{
    cout << "Enter the number of crew members." << endl;
    cin >> crew;
    cout << "Enter the number of passengers." << endl;
    cin >> passengers;
    cout << "Enter the weight, in pounds, of cargo in the" << endl
         << " closet, rounded up to the nearest whole number."
         << endl;
    cin >> closet;
    cout << "Enter the weight, in pounds, of cargo in the" << endl
         << " aft baggage compartment, rounded up to the" << endl
         << " nearest whole number." << endl;
```

PROBLEM-SOLVING CASE STUDY cont'd.

```
        cin >> baggage;
        cout << "Enter the number of U.S. gallons of fuel" << endl
            << " loaded, rounded up to the nearest whole number."
            << endl;
        cin >> fuel;
        cout << endl;
        cout << "Starship loading data as entered:" << endl
            << "    Crew:          " << setw(6) << crew << endl
            << "    Passengers:    " << setw(6) << passengers << endl
            << "    Closet weight: " << setw(6) << closet << " pounds"
            << endl
            << "    Baggage weight:" << setw(6) << baggage << " pounds"
            << endl
            << "    Fuel:          " << setw(6) << fuel << " gallons"
            << endl << endl;
}


//******************************************************************

float CrewMoment( /* in */ int crew )    // Number of crew members

// Computes the crew moment arm in inch-pounds from the number of
// crew members.  Global constant PERSON_WT is used as the weight
// of each crew member

// Precondition:
//    crew == 1  OR  crew == 2
// Postcondition:
//    Function value == Crew moment arm, based on the crew parameter

{
    const float CREW_DISTANCE = 143.0;  // Distance to crew seats
                                        //    from front

    return float(crew) * PERSON_WT * CREW_DISTANCE;
}

//******************************************************************

float PassengerMoment( /* in */ int passengers )    // Number of
                                                    //    passengers

// Computes the passenger moment arm in inch-pounds from the number
// of passengers.  Global constant PERSON_WT is used as the weight
// of each passenger.  It is assumed that the first two passengers
// sit in row 2, the second two in row 1, the next two in row 3,
// and remaining passengers sit in row 4
```

```
// Precondition:
//      0 <= passengers <= 8
// Postcondition:
//      Function value == Passenger moment arm, based on the
//                          passengers parameter

{
    const float ROW1_DIST = 219.0;   // Distance to row 1 seats
                                     //    from front
    const float ROW2_DIST = 265.0;   // Distance to row 2 seats
    const float ROW3_DIST = 295.0;   // Distance to row 3 seats
    const float ROW4_DIST = 341.0;   // Distance to row 4 seats

    float moment = 0.0;              // Running total of moment as
                                     //    rows are added

    if (passengers > 6)                      // For passengers 7 and 8
    {
        moment = moment +
                float(passengers - 6) * PERSON_WT * ROW4_DIST;
        passengers = 6;                      // 6 remain
    }
    if (passengers > 4)                      // For passengers 5 and 6
    {
        moment = moment +
                float(passengers - 4) * PERSON_WT * ROW3_DIST;
        passengers = 4;                      // 4 remain
    }
    if (passengers > 2)                      // For passengers 3 and 4
    {
        moment = moment +
                float(passengers - 2) * PERSON_WT * ROW1_DIST;
        passengers = 2;                      // 2 remain
    }
    if (passengers > 0)                      // For passengers 1 and 2
        moment = moment +
                float(passengers) * PERSON_WT * ROW2_DIST;
    return moment;
}

//********************************************************************

float CargoMoment( /* in */ int closet,     // Weight in closet
                   /* in */ int baggage )    // Weight of baggage

// Computes the total moment arm for cargo loaded into the
// front closet and aft baggage compartment

// Precondition:
```

PROBLEM-SOLVING CASE STUDY *cont'd.*

```
//      0 <= closet <= 160  &&  0 <= baggage <= 525
// Postcondition:
//      Function value == Cargo moment arm, based on the closet and
//                         baggage parameters

{
    const float CLOSET_DIST = 182.0;     // Distance from front
                                         //    to closet
    const float BAGGAGE_DIST = 386.0;    // Distance from front
                                         //    to bagg. comp.

    return float(closet) * CLOSET_DIST +
           float(baggage) * BAGGAGE_DIST;
}


//******************************************************************

float FuelMoment( /* in */ int fuel )    // Fuel in gallons

// Computes the moment arm for fuel on board.  There are four
// different formulas for this calculation, depending on
// the amount of fuel, due to fuel tank layout.
// This function uses the global constant LBS_PER_GAL
// to compute the weight of the fuel

// Precondition:
//     10 <= fuel <= 565
// Postcondition:
//     Function value == Fuel moment arm, based on the
//                        fuel parameter

{
    float fuelWt;          // Weight of fuel in pounds
    float fuelDistance;    // Distance from front of plane

    fuelWt = float(fuel) * LBS_PER_GAL;
    if (fuel < 60)
        fuelDistance = float(fuel) * 314.6;
    else if (fuel < 361)
        fuelDistance = 305.8 + (-0.01233 * float(fuel - 60));
    else if (fuel < 521)
        fuelDistance = 303.0 + ( 0.12500 * float(fuel - 361));
    else
        fuelDistance = 323.0 + (-0.04444 * float(fuel - 521));
    return fuelDistance * fuelWt;
}


//******************************************************************
```

PROBLEM-SOLVING CASE STUDY cont'd.

```
void PrintWarning()

// Warns the user of assumptions made by the program
// and when to double-check the program's results

// Postcondition:
//      An informational warning message has been printed

{
    cout << endl
         << "Notice:  This program assumes that passengers" << endl
         << "  fill the seat rows in order 2, 1, 3, 4, and" << endl
         << "  that each passenger and crew member weighs " 
         << PERSON_WT << " pounds." << endl
         << "  It also assumes that Jet-A fuel weighs "
         << LBS_PER_GAL << " pounds" << endl
         << "  per U.S. gallon.  The center of gravity" << endl
         << "  calculations for fuel are approximate.  If" << endl
         << "  the aircraft is loaded near its limits, the" << endl
         << "  pilot's operating handbook should be used" << endl
         << "  to compute weight and center of gravity" << endl
         << "  with more accuracy." << endl;
}
```

Testing: Because someone could use the output of this program to make decisions that could result in property damage, injury, or death, it is essential to test the program thoroughly. In particular, it should be checked for maximum and minimum input values in different combinations. In addition, a wide range of test cases should be tried and verified against results calculated by hand. If possible, the program's output should be checked against sample calculations done by experienced pilots for actual flights.

Notice that the main function neglects to guarantee any of the function preconditions before calling the functions. If this program were actually to be used by pilots, it should have data validation checks added in the GetData function.

Testing and Debugging

One of the advantages of a modular design is that you can test it long before the code has been written for all of the modules. If we test each module individually, then we can assemble the modules into a complete program with much greater confidence that the program is correct. In this section, we introduce a technique for testing a module separately.

Stubs and Drivers

Suppose you were given the code for a module and your job was to test it. How would you test a single module by itself? First of all, it must be called by something (unless it is the `main` function). Second, it may have calls to other modules that aren't available to you. To test the module, you must fill in these missing links.

When a module contains calls to other modules, we can write dummy functions called **stubs** to satisfy those calls. A stub usually consists of an output statement that prints a message such as "Function such-and-such just got called." Even though the stub is a dummy, it allows us to determine whether the function is called at the right time by the `main` function or another function.

Stub A dummy function that assists in testing part of a program. A stub has the same name and interface as a function that actually would be called by the part of the program being tested, but it is usually much simpler.

A stub can also be used to print the set of values that are passed to it; this tells us whether or not the module being tested is supplying the correct information. Sometimes a stub assigns new values to its reference parameters to simulate data being read or results being computed in order to give the calling module something to keep working on. Because we can choose the values that are returned by the stub, we have better control over the conditions of the test run.

Here is a stub that simulates the `GetYear` function in the ConvertDates program by returning an arbitrarily chosen string.

```
void GetYear( /* inout */ ifstream& dataIn,      // Input file
              /* out */    string&   year )       // Four digits
                                                   //   of year

// Stub for GetYear function in the ConvertDates program

{
    cout << "GetYear was called here. Returning \"1948\"." << endl;
    year = "1948";
}
```

This stub is simpler than the function it simulates, which is typical because the object of using a stub is to provide a simple, predictable environment for testing a module.

In addition to supplying a stub for each call within the module, you must provide a dummy program—a **driver**—to call the module itself. A driver program contains the bare minimum of code required to call the module being tested.

Driver   A simple `main` function that is used to call a function being tested. The use of a driver permits direct control of the testing process.

By surrounding a module with a driver and stubs, you gain complete control of the conditions under which it executes. This allows you to test different situations and combinations that may reveal errors. For example, the following program is a driver for the `FuelMoment` function in the Starship program. Because `FuelMoment` doesn't call any other functions, no stubs are necessary.

```
//*****************************************************************
// FuelMomentDriver program
// This program provides an environment for testing the
// FuelMoment function in isolation from the Starship program
//*****************************************************************
#include <iostream>

using namespace std;

const float LBS_PER_GAL = 6.7;

float FuelMoment( int );

int main()
{
    int testVal;     // Test value for fuel in gallons

    cout << "Fuel moment for gallons from 10 through 565"
         << " in steps of 15:" << endl;
    testVal = 10;
    while (testVal <= 565)
    {
        cout << FuelMoment(testVal) << endl;
        testVal = testVal + 15;
    }
    return 0;
}

//*****************************************************************

float FuelMoment( /* in */ int Fuel )    // Fuel in gallons
```

```
{
    float fuelWt;            // Weight of fuel in pounds
    float fuelDistance;      // Distance from front of plane

    fuelWt = float(fuel) * LBS_PER_GAL;
    if (fuel < 60)
        fuelDistance = float(fuel) * 314.6;
    else if (fuel < 361)
        fuelDistance = 305.8 + (-0.01233 * float(fuel - 60));
    else if (fuel < 521)
        fuelDistance = 303.0 + ( 0.12500 * float(fuel - 361));
    else
        fuelDistance = 323.0 + (-0.04444 * float(fuel - 521));
    return fuelDistance * fuelWt;
}
```

Stubs and drivers are important tools in team programming. The programmers develop the overall design and the interfaces between the modules. Each programmer then designs and codes one or more of the modules and uses drivers and stubs to test the code. When all of the modules have been coded and tested, they are assembled into what should be a working program.

For team programming to succeed, it is essential that all of the module interfaces be defined explicitly and that the coded modules adhere strictly to the specifications for those interfaces. Obviously, global variable references must be carefully avoided in a team-programming situation because it is impossible for each person to know how the rest of the team is using every variable.

Testing and Debugging Hints

1. Make sure that variables used as arguments to a function are declared in the block where the function call is made.
2. Carefully define the precondition, postcondition, and parameter list to eliminate side effects. Variables used only in a function should be declared as local variables. *Do not* use global variables in your programs. (Exception: It is acceptable to reference cin and cout globally.)
3. If the compiler displays a message such as "UNDECLARED IDENTI-FIER," check that the identifier isn't misspelled (and that it is, in fact, declared), that the identifier is declared before it is referenced, and that the scope of the identifier includes the reference to it.
4. If you intend to use a local name that is the same as a nonlocal name, a misspelling in the local declaration will wreak havoc. The C++ compiler won't complain, but will cause every reference to the local name to go to the nonlocal name instead.

5. Remember that the same identifier cannot be used in both the parameter list and the outermost local declarations of a function.

6. With a value-returning function, be sure the function heading and prototype begin with the correct data type for the function return value.

7. With a value-returning function, don't forget to use a statement

    ```
    return Expression;
    ```

    to return the function value. Make sure the expression is of the correct type, or implicit type coercion will occur.

8. Remember that a call to a value-returning function is part of an expression, whereas a call to a void function is a separate statement. (C++ softens this distinction, however, by letting you call a value-returning function as if it were a void function, ignoring the return value. Be careful here.)

9. In general, don't use reference parameters in the parameter list of a value-returning function. A reference parameter must be used, however, when an I/O stream object is passed as a parameter.

10. If necessary, use your system's debugger (or use debug output statements) to indicate when a function is called and if it is executing correctly. The values of the arguments can be displayed immediately before the call to the function (to show the incoming values) and immediately after (to show the outgoing values). You also may want to display the values of local variables in the function itself to indicate what happens each time it is called.

Summary

The scope of an identifier refers to the parts of the program in which it is visible. C++ function names have global scope, as do the names of variables and constants that are declared outside all functions and namespaces. Variables and constants declared within a block have local scope; they are not visible outside the block. The parameters of a function have the same scope as local variables declared in the outermost block of the function.

With rare exceptions, it is not considered good practice to declare global variables and reference them directly from within a function. All communication between the modules of a program should be through the argument and parameter lists (and via the function value sent back by a value-returning function). The use of global constants, on the other hand, is considered to be an acceptable programming practice because it adds consistency and makes a program easier to change while avoiding the pitfalls of side effects. Well-designed and well-documented functions that are free of side effects can often be reused in other programs. Many programmers keep a library of functions that they use repeatedly.

The lifetime of a variable is the period of time during program execution when memory is allocated to it. Global variables have static lifetime (memory remains allocated for the duration of the program's execution). By default, local variables have automatic lifetime (memory is allocated and deallocated at block entry and block exit). A local variable may be given static lifetime by using the word `static` in its declaration. This variable has the lifetime of a global variable but the scope of a local variable.

C++ allows a variable to be initialized in its declaration. For a static variable, the initialization occurs once only—when control first reaches its declaration. An automatic variable is initialized each time control reaches the declaration.

C++ provides two kinds of subprograms, void functions and value-returning functions, for us to use. A value-returning function is called from within an expression and returns a single result that is used in the evaluation of the expression. For the function value to be returned, the last statement executed by the function must be a Return statement containing an expression of the appropriate data type.

All the scope rules, as well as the rules about reference and value parameters, apply to both void functions and value-returning functions. It is considered poor programming practice, however, to use reference parameters in a value-returning function definition. Doing so increases the potential for unintended side effects. (An exception is when I/O stream objects are passed as parameters. Other exceptions are noted in later chapters.)

We can use stubs and drivers to test functions in isolation from the rest of a program. They are particularly useful in the context of team-programming projects.

Quick Check

1. a. How can you tell if a variable that is referenced inside a function is local or global? (pp. 392–398)
   b. Where are local variables declared? (pp. 392–398)
   c. When does the scope of an identifier declared in block A exclude a block nested within block A? (pp. 392–398)
2. A program consists of two functions, main and DoCalc. A variable x is declared outside both functions. DoCalc declares two variables, a and b, within its body; b is declared as static. In what function(s) are each of a, b, and x visible, and what is the lifetime of each variable? (pp. 392–398, 403–404)
3. Why should you use value parameters whenever possible? Why should you avoid the use of global variables? (pp. 405–409, 420–421)
4. For each of the following, decide whether a value-returning function or a void function is the most appropriate implementation. (pp. 411–421)
   a. Selecting the larger of two values for further processing in an expression.
   b. Printing a paycheck.
   c. Computing the area of a hexagon.

    d. Testing whether an incoming value is valid and returning `true` if it is.

    e. Computing the two roots of a quadratic equation.

5.   What would the heading for a value-returning function named `Min` look like if it had two `float` parameters, `num1` and `num2`, and returned a `float` result? (pp. 411–421)

6.   What would a call to `Min` look like if the arguments were a variable named `deductions` and the literal `2000.0`? (pp. 411–421)

Answers   **1.** a. If the variable is not declared in either the body of the function or its parameter list, then the reference is global. b. Local variables are declared within a block (compound statement). c. When the nested block declares an identifier with the same name.   **2.** x is visible to both functions, but a and b are visible only within DoCalc. x and b are static variables; once memory is allocated to them, they are "alive" until the program terminates. a is an automatic variable; it is "alive" only while DoCalc is executing.   **3.** Both using value parameters and avoiding global variables will minimize side effects. Also, passing by value allows the arguments to be arbitrary expressions.   **4.** a. Value-returning function b. Void function c. Value-returning function d. Value-returning function e. Void function

5. `float Min( float num1,`
                `float num2 )`

6. `smaller = Min(deductions, 2000.0);`

Exam Preparation Exercises

1.   If a function contains a locally declared variable with the same name as a global variable, no confusion results because references to variables in functions are first interpreted as references to local variables. (True or False?)

2.   Variables declared at the beginning of a block are accessible to all remaining statements in that block, including those in nested blocks (assuming the nested blocks don't declare local variables with the same names). (True or False?)

3.   Define the following terms.

    local variable   scope
    global variable side effects
    lifetime   name precedence (name hiding)

4.   What is the output of the following C++ program? (This program is an example of poor interface design practices.)

```
#include <iostream>

using namespace std;

void DoGlobal();
void DoLocal();
void DoReference( int& );
void DoValue( int );

int x;

int main()
{
    x = 15;
```

```
        DoReference(x);
        cout << "x = " << x << " after the call to DoReference."
             << endl;
        x = 16;
        DoValue(x);
        cout << "x = " << x << " after the call to DoValue."
             << endl;
        x = 17;
        DoLocal();
        cout << "x = " << x << " after the call to DoLocal."
             << endl;
        x = 18;
        DoGlobal();
        cout << "x = " << x << " after the call to DoGlobal."
             << endl;
        return 0;
}

void DoReference( int& a )
{
    a = 3;
}

void DoValue( int b )
{
    b = 4;
}

void DoLocal()
{
    int x;

    x = 5;
}

void DoGlobal()
{
    x = 7;
}
```

5. What is the output of the following program?

```
#include <iostream>

using namespace std;

void Test();

int main()
{
```

```
        Test();
        Test();
        Test();
        return 0;
    }

    void Test()
    {
        int i = 0;
        static int j = 0;

        i++;
        j++;
        cout << i << ' ' << j << endl;
    }
```

6. The following function calculates the sum of the integers from 1 through n. However, it has an unintended side effect. What is it?

```
    void SumInts( int& n,
                  int& sum )
    {
        sum = 0;
        while (n >= 1)
        {
            sum = sum + n;
            n = n - 1;
        }
    }
```

7. Given the function heading

```
    bool HighTaxBracket( int inc,
                         int ded )
```

is the following statement a legal call to the function if income and deductions are of type int?

```
    if (HighTaxBracket(income, deductions))
        cout << "Upper Class";
```

8. The statement

```
    Power(k, l, m);
```

is a call to the void function whose definition follows. Rewrite the function as a value-returning function, then write a function call that assigns the function value to the variable m.

```
    void Power( float  base,
                int    exponent,
                float& answer  )
    {
        int i;
```

```
      answer = 1.0;
      i = 1;
      while (i <= exponent)
      {
          answer = answer * base;
          i++;
      }
  }
```

9. You are given the following `Test` function and a C++ program in which the variables a, b, c, and `result` are declared to be of type `float`. In the calling code, a = −5.0, b = 0.1, and c = 16.2. What is the value of `result` when each of the following calls returns?

```
float Test( float x,
            float y,
            float z )
{
    if (x > y || y > z)
        return 0.5;
    else
        return -0.5;
}
```

    a. result = Test(5.2, 5.3, 5.6);
    b. result = Test(fabs(a), b, c);

10. What is wrong with each of the following C++ function definitions?
    a. void Test1(int m,
                   int n)

```
    {
        return 3 * m + n;
    }
```

    b. float Test2(int   i,
                     float x)

```
    {
        i = i + 7;
        x = 4.8 + float(i);
    }
```

11. Explain why it is risky to use a reference parameter as a parameter of a value-returning function.

Programming Warm-up Exercises

1. The following program is written with very poor style. For one thing, global variables are used in place of arguments. Rewrite it without global variables, using good programming style.

```
#include <iostream>
using namespace std;
void MashGlobals();
```

```
int a, b, c;
int main()
{
cin >> a >> b >> c;
MashGlobals();
cout << "a=" << a << ' ' << "b=" << b << ' '
<< "c=" << c << endl;
return 0;
}
void MashGlobals()
{
int temp;
temp = a + b;
a = b + c;
b = temp;
}
```

2. Write the heading for a value-returning function Epsilon that receives two float parameters named high and low and returns a float result.

3. Write the heading for a value-returning function named NearlyEqual that receives three float parameters—num1, num2, and difference—and returns a Boolean result.

4. Given the heading you wrote in Exercise 3, write the body of the function. The function returns true if the absolute value of the difference between num1 and num2 is less than the value in difference and returns false otherwise.

5. Write a value-returning function named CompassHeading that returns the sum of its four float parameters: trueCourse, windCorrAngle, variance, and deviation.

6. Write a value-returning function named FracPart that receives a floating-point number and returns the fractional part of that number. Use a single parameter named x. For example, if the incoming value of x is 16.753, the function return value is 0.753.

7. Write a value-returning function named Circumf that finds the circumference of a circle given the radius. The formula for calculating the circumference of a circle is π multiplied by twice the radius. Use 3.14159 for π.

8. Given the function heading

```
float Hypotenuse( float side1,
                  float side2 )
```

write the body of the function to return the length of the hypotenuse of a right triangle. The parameters represent the lengths of the other two sides. The formula for the hypotenuse is

$$\sqrt{side1^2 + side2^2}$$

9. Write a value-returning function named FifthPow that returns the fifth power of its float parameter.

10. Write a value-returning function named Min that returns the smallest of its three integer parameters.

11. The following If conditions work correctly on most, but not all, machines. Rewrite them using the "is..." functions from the C++ standard library (header file cctype).

    a. `if (inChar >= '0' && inChar <= '9')`
       `DoSomething();`

    b. `if (inChar >= 'A' && inChar <= 'Z' ||`
       `    inChar >= 'a' && inChar <= 'z'  )`
       `DoSomething();`

    c. `if (inChar >= 'A' && inChar <= 'Z' ||`
       `    inChar >= '0' && inChar <= '9'  )`
       `DoSomething();`

    d. `if (inChar < 'a' || inChar > 'z')`
       `DoSomething();`

12. Write a Boolean value-returning function IsPrime that receives an integer parameter n, tests it to see if it is a prime number, and returns true if it is. (A prime number is an integer greater than or equal to 2 whose only divisors are 1 and the number itself.) A call to this function might look like this:

```
if (IsPrime(n))
    cout << n << " is a prime number.";
```

(*Hint:* If n is not a prime number, it is exactly divisible by an integer in the range 2 through $\sqrt{n}$.)

13. Write a value-returning function named Postage that returns the cost of mailing a package, given the weight of the package in pounds and ounces and the cost per ounce.

Programming Problems

1. If a principal amount P, for which the interest is compounded Q times per year, is placed in a savings account, then the amount of money in the account (the balance) after N years is given by the following formula, where I is the annual interest rate as a floating-point number:

$$balance = P \times \left(1 + \frac{I}{Q}\right)^{N \times Q}$$

   Write a C++ program that inputs the values for P, I, Q, and N and outputs the balance for each year up through year N. Use a value-returning function to compute the balance. Your program should prompt the user appropriately, label the output values, and have good style.

2. Euclid's algorithm is a method for finding the greatest common divisor (GCD) of two positive integers. It states that for any two positive integers M and N such that $M \leq N$, the GCD is calculated as follows:

    a. Divide N by M.

    b. If the remainder $R = 0$, then the GCD = M.

    c. If $R > 0$, then M becomes N, and R becomes M, and repeat from step (a) until $R = 0$.

Write a program that uses a value-returning function to find the GCD of two numbers. The main function reads pairs of numbers from a file stream named dataFile. For each pair read in, the two numbers and the GCD should be labeled properly and written to a file stream named gcdList.

3. The distance to the landing point of a projectile, launched at an angle angle (in radians) with an initial velocity of velocity (in feet per second), ignoring air resistance, is given by the formula

$$distance = \frac{velocity^2 \times \sin (2 \ x \ angle)}{32.2}$$

Write a C++ program that implements a game in which the user first enters the distance to a target. The user then enters the angle and velocity for launching a projectile. If the projectile comes within 0.1% of the distance to the target, the user wins the game. If the projectile doesn't come close enough, the user is told how far off the projectile is and is allowed to try again. If there isn't a winning input after five tries, then the user loses the game.

To simplify input for the user, your program should allow the angle to be input in degrees. The formula for converting degrees to radians is

$$radians = \frac{degrees \times 3.14159265}{180.0}$$

Each of the formulas in this problem should be implemented as a C++ value-returning function. Your program should prompt the user for input appropriately, label the output values, and have proper programming style.

4. Write a program that computes the number of days between two dates. One way of doing this is to have the program compute the Julian day number for each date and subtract one from the other. The Julian day number is the number of days that have elapsed since noon on January 1, 4713 B.C. The following algorithm can be used to calculate the Julian day number.

Given year (an integer, such as 2001), month (an integer from 1 through 12), and day (an integer from 1 through 31), if month is 1 or 2, then subtract 1 from year and add 12 to month.

If the date comes from the Gregorian calendar (later than October 15, 1582), then compute an intermediate result with the following formula (otherwise, let intRes1 equal 0):

$$intRes1 = 2 - year \ / \ 100 + year \ / \ 400 \quad (integer \ division)$$

Compute a second intermediate result with the formula

$$intRes2 = int(365.25 \times year)$$

Compute a third intermediate result with the formula

$$intRes3 = int(30.6001 \times (month + 1))$$

Finally, the Julian day number is computed with the formula

$$julianDay = intRes1 + intRes2 + intRes3 + day + 1720994.5$$

Your program should make appropriate use of value-returning functions in solving this problem. These formulas require nine significant digits; you may have to use the integer type `long` and the floating-point type `double`. Your program should prompt appropriately for input (the two dates) if it is to be run interactively. Use proper style with appropriate comments.

Case Study Follow-Up

1. Supply the missing precondition and postcondition in the comments at the beginning of each function in the ConvertDates program.
2. Add data validation to the ConvertDates program as follows.
    a. Have the program check the input characters and print an error message if any of the "digits" are not numeric characters ('0' through '9'). This validation test should be written as a separate function.
    b. Have the program check the date to be sure that it is valid. `month` should be in the range 01 through 12, and `day` should be in the appropriate range for the particular month. (For example, reject a date of 06/31/99 because June has only 30 days.) Remember that February can have either 28 or 29 days, depending on the year. This validation test should be written as a separate function.
3. Modify the ConvertDates program so that it can input the dates with digits separated by either slashes (/) or dashes (–).
4. In the Starship program, the `main` function neglects to guarantee any of the function preconditions before calling the functions. Modify the `GetData` function to validate the input data. When control returns from `GetData`, the `main` function should be able to assume that all the data values are within the proper ranges.

9

Additional Control Structures

GOALS

- To be able to write a Switch statement for a multiway branching problem.
- To be able to write a Do-While statement and contrast it with a While statement.
- To be able to write a For statement as an alternative to a While statement.
- To understand the purpose of the Break and Continue statements.
- To be able to choose the most appropriate looping statement for a given problem.

In the preceding chapters, we introduced C++ statements for sequence, selection, loop, and subprogram structures. In some cases, we introduced more than one way of implementing these structures. For example, selection may be implemented by an If-Then structure or an If-Then-Else structure. The If-Then is sufficient to implement any selection structure, but C++ provides the If-Then-Else for convenience because the two-way branch is frequently used in programming.

This chapter introduces five new statements that are also nonessential to, but nonetheless convenient for, programming. One, the Switch statement, makes it easier to write selection structures that have many branches. Two new looping statements, For and Do-While, make it easier to program certain types of loops. The other two statements, Break and Continue, are control statements that are used as part of larger looping and selection structures.

The Switch Statement

The Switch statement is a selection control structure that allows us to list any number of branches. In other words, it is a control structure for multi-way branches. A Switch is similar to nested If statements. The value of the **switch expression**—an expression whose value is matched with a label attached to a branch—determines which one of the branches is executed. For example, look at the following statement:

```
switch (letter)
{
    case 'X'  : Statement1;
            break;
    case 'L'  :
    case 'M'  : Statement2;
            break;
    case 'S'  : Statement3;
            break;
    default   : Statement4;
}
Statement5;
```

In this example, `letter` is the switch expression. The statement means "If `letter` is 'X', execute Statement1 and break out of the Switch statement, continuing with Statement5. If `letter` is 'L' or 'M', execute Statement2 and continue with Statement5. If `letter` is 'S', execute Statement3 and continue with Statement5. If `letter` is none of the characters mentioned, execute Statement4 and continue with Statement5." The Break statement causes an immediate exit from the Switch statement. We'll see shortly what happens if we omit the Break statements.

Switch expression The expression whose value determines which switch label is selected. It cannot be a floating-point or string expression.

The syntax template for the Switch statement is

SwitchStatement

```
switch ( IntegralOrEnumExpression )
{
    SwitchLabel ...  Statement
            ⋮
}
```

IntegralOrEnumExpression is an expression of integral type—char, short, int, long, bool—or of enum type (we discuss enum in the next chapter). The optional SwitchLabel in front of a statement is either a *case label* or a *default label:*

SwitchLabel

```
⎧  case ConstantExpression :
⎨
⎩  default :
```

In a case label, ConstantExpression is an integral or enum expression whose operands must be literal or named constants. The following are examples of constant integral expressions (where CLASS_SIZE is a named constant of type int):

```
3
CLASS_SIZE
'A'
2 * CLASS_SIZE + 1
```

The data type of ConstantExpression is coerced, if necessary, to match the type of the switch expression.

In our opening example that tests the value of `letter`, the following are the case labels:

```
case 'X' :
case 'L' :
case 'M' :
case 'S' :
```

As that example shows, a single statement may be preceded by more than one case label. Each case value may appear only once in a given Switch statement. If a value appears more than once, a syntax error results. Also, there can be only one default label in a Switch statement.

The flow of control through a Switch statement goes like this. First, the switch expression is evaluated. If this value matches one of the values in a case label, control branches to the statement following that case label. From there, control proceeds sequentially until either a Break statement or the end of the Switch statement is encountered. If the value of the switch expression doesn't match any case value, then one of two things happens. If there is a default label, control branches to the statement following that label. If there is no default label, all statements within the Switch are skipped and control simply proceeds to the statement following the entire Switch statement.

The following Switch statement prints an appropriate comment based on a student's grade (`grade` is of type `char`):

```
switch (grade)
{
    case 'A' :
    case 'B' : cout << "Good Work";
               break;
    case 'C' : cout << "Average Work";
               break;
    case 'D' :
    case 'F' : cout << "Poor Work";
               numberInTrouble++;
               break;                    // Unnecessary, but a good habit
}
```

Notice that the final Break statement is unnecessary. But programmers often include it anyway. One reason is that it's easier to insert another case label at the end if a Break statement is already present.

If `grade` does not contain one of the specified characters, none of the statements within the Switch is executed. Unless a precondition of the Switch statement is that `grade` is definitely one of 'A', 'B', 'C', 'D', or 'F', it would be wise to include a default label to account for an invalid grade:

```
switch (grade)
{
    case 'A' :
    case 'B' : cout << "Good Work";
               break;
    case 'C' : cout << "Average Work";
               break;
    case 'D' :
    case 'F' : cout << "Poor Work";
               numberInTrouble++;
               break;
    default  : cout << grade << " is not a valid letter grade.";
               break;
}
```

A Switch statement with a Break statement after each case alternative behaves exactly like an If-Then-Else-If control structure. For example, our Switch statement is equivalent to the following code:

```
if (grade == 'A' || grade == 'B')
    cout << "Good Work";
else if (grade == 'C')
    cout << "Average Work";
else if (grade == 'D' || grade == 'F')
{
    cout << "Poor Work";
    numberInTrouble++;
}
else
    cout << grade << " is not a valid letter grade.";
```

Is either of these two versions better than the other? There is no absolute answer to this question. For this particular example, our opinion is that the Switch statement is easier to understand because of its two-dimensional, table-like form. But some may find the If-Then-Else-If version easier to read. When implementing a multiway branching structure, our advice is to write down both a Switch and an If-Then-Else-If and then compare them for readability. Keep in mind that C++ provides the Switch statement as a matter of convenience. Don't feel obligated to use a Switch statement for every multiway branch.

Finally, we said we would look at what happens if you omit the Break statements inside a Switch statement. Let's rewrite our letter grade example without the Break statements:

```
switch (grade)      // Wrong version
{
    case 'A' :
    case 'B' : cout << "Good Work";
    case 'C' : cout << "Average Work";
    case 'D' :
    case 'F' : cout << "Poor Work";
               numberInTrouble++;
    default  : cout << grade << " is not a valid letter grade.";
}
```

If `grade` happens to be 'H', control branches to the statement at the default label and the output is

```
H is not a valid letter grade.
```

Unfortunately, this case alternative is the only one that works correctly. If `grade` is 'A', the resulting output is this:

```
Good WorkAverage WorkPoor WorkA is not a valid letter grade.
```

Remember that after a branch is taken to a specific case label, control proceeds sequentially until either a Break statement or the end of the Switch statement is encountered. Forgetting a Break statement in a case alternative is a very common source of errors in C++ programs.

*M*AY WE INTRODUCE

Admiral Grace Murray Hopper

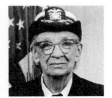

From 1943 until her death on New Year's Day in 1992, Admiral Grace Murray Hopper was intimately involved with computing. In 1991, she was awarded the National Medal of Technology "for her pioneering accomplishments in the development of computer programming languages that simplified computer technology and opened the door to a significantly larger universe of users."

Admiral Hopper was born Grace Brewster Murray in New York City on December 9, 1906. She attended Vassar and received a Ph.D. in mathematics from Yale. For the next ten years, she taught mathematics at Vassar.

In 1943, Admiral Hopper joined the U.S. Navy and was assigned to the Bureau of Ordnance Computation Project at Harvard University as a programmer on the Mark I. After the war, she remained at Harvard as a faculty member and continued work on the Navy's Mark II and Mark III computers. In 1949, she joined Eckert-Mauchly Computer Corporation and worked on the UNIVAC I. It was there that she made a legendary contribution to computing: She discovered the first computer "bug"—a moth caught in the hardware.

Admiral Hopper had a working compiler in 1952, at a time when the conventional wisdom was that computers could do only arithmetic. Although not on the committee that designed the computer language COBOL, she was active in its design, implementation, and use. COBOL (which stands for Common Business-Oriented Language) was developed in the early 1960s and is still widely used in business data processing.

Admiral Hopper retired from the Navy in 1966, only to be recalled within a year to full-time active duty. Her mission was to oversee the Navy's efforts to maintain uniformity in programming languages. It has been said that just as Admiral Hyman Rickover was the father of the nuclear navy, Rear Admiral Hopper was the mother of computerized data automation in the Navy. She served with the Naval Data Automation Command until she retired again in 1986 with the rank of rear admiral. At the time of her death, she was a senior consultant at Digital Equipment Corporation.

During her lifetime, Admiral Hopper received honorary degrees from more than 40 colleges and universities. She was honored by her peers on several occasions, including the first Computer Sciences Man of the Year award given by the Data Processing Management Association, and the Contributions to Computer Science Education Award given by the Special Interest Group for Computer Science Education of the ACM (Association for Computing Machinery).

Admiral Hopper loved young people and enjoyed giving talks on college and university campuses. She often handed out colored wires, which she called nanoseconds because they were cut to a length of about one foot—the distance that light travels in a nanosecond (billionth of a second). Her advice to the young was, "You manage things, you lead people. We went overboard on management and forgot about leadership."

When asked which of her many accomplishments she was most proud of, she answered, "All the young people I have trained over the years."

The Do-While Statement

The Do-While statement is a looping control structure in which the loop condition is tested at the end (bottom) of the loop. This format guarantees that the loop body executes at least once. The syntax template for the Do-While is this:

DoWhileStatement

```
do
      Statement
while ( Expression ) ;
```

As usual in C++, Statement is either a single statement or a block. Also, note that the Do-While ends with a semicolon.

The Do-While statement

```
do
{
    Statement1;
    Statement2;
      ⋮
    StatementN;
} while (Expression);
```

means "Execute the statements between `do` and `while` as long as Expression still has the value `true` at the end of the loop."

Let's compare a While loop and a Do-While loop that do the same task: They find the first period in a file of data. Assume that there is at least one period in the file.

While Solution

```
dataFile >> inputChar;
while (inputChar != '.')
    dataFile >> inputChar;
```

Do-While Solution

```
do
    dataFile >> inputChar;
while (inputChar != '.');
```

The While solution requires a priming read so that `inputChar` has a value before the loop is entered. This isn't required for the Do-While solution because the input statement within the loop is executed before the loop condition is evaluated.

Let's look at another example. Suppose a program needs to read a person's age interactively. The program requires that the age be positive. The following loops ensure that the input value is positive before the program proceeds any further.

While Solution

```
cout << "Enter your age: ";
cin >> age;
while (age <= 0)
{
    cout << "Your age must be positive." << endl;
    cout << "Enter your age: ";
    cin >> age;
}
```

Do-While Solution

```
do
{
    cout << "Enter your age: ";
    cin >> age;
    if (age <= 0)
        cout << "Your age must be positive." << endl;
} while (age <= 0);
```

Notice that the Do-While solution does not require the prompt and input steps to appear twice—once before the loop and once within it—but it does test the input value twice.

We can also use the Do-While to implement a count-controlled loop *if* we know in advance that the loop body should always execute at least once. Below are two versions of a loop to sum the integers from 1 through n.

While Solution

```
sum = 0;
counter = 1;
while (counter <= n)
{
    sum = sum + counter;
    counter++;
}
```

Do-While Solution

```
sum = 0;
counter = 1;
do
{
    sum = sum + counter;
    counter++;
} while (counter <= n);
```

If n is a positive number, both of these versions are equivalent. But if n is 0 or negative, the two loops give different results. In the While version, the final value of sum is 0 because the loop body is never entered. In the Do-While version, the final value of sum is 1 because the body executes once and *then* the loop test is made.

Because the While statement tests the condition before executing the body of the loop, it is called a *pretest loop.* The Do-While statement does

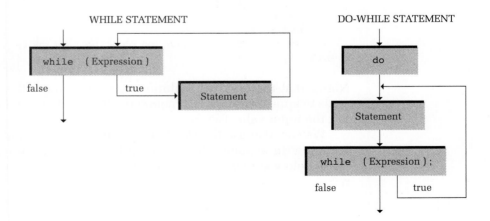

Figure 9-1
Flow of Control:
While and
Do-While

the opposite and thus is known as a *posttest loop.* Figure 9-1 compares the flow of control in the While and Do-While loops.

After we look at two other new looping constructs, we offer some guidelines for determining when to use each type of loop.

The For Statement

The For statement is designed to simplify the writing of count-controlled loops. The following statement prints out the integers from 1 through n:

```
for (count = 1; count <= n; count++)
    cout << count << endl;
```

This For statement means "Initialize the loop control variable `count` to 1. While `count` is less than or equal to n, execute the output statement and increment `count` by 1. Stop the loop after `count` has been incremented to n + 1."

In C++, a For statement is merely a compact notation for a While loop. In fact, the compiler essentially translates a For statement into an equivalent While loop as follows:

```
for (  count = 1  ;  count <= n  ;  count++  )
        cout << count << endl;


        count = 1;
        while (count <= n)
        {
            cout << count << endl;
            count++;
        }
```

The syntax template for a For statement is

ForStatement

for (InitStatement Expression1 ; Expression2)
Statement

Expression1 is the While condition. InitStatement can be one of the following: the null statement (just a semicolon), a declaration statement (which
always ends in a semicolon), or an expression statement (an expression
ending in a semicolon). Therefore, there is always a semicolon before
Expression1. (This semicolon isn't shown in the syntax template because
InitStatement always ends with its own semicolon.)

Most often, a For statement is written such that InitStatement initializes a loop control variable and Expression2 increments or decrements the
loop control variable. Here are two loops that execute the same number of
times (50):

```
for (loopCount = 1; loopCount <= 50; loopCount++)
    ⋮

for (loopCount = 50; loopCount >= 1; loopCount--)
    ⋮
```

Just like While loops, Do-While and For loops may be nested. For
example, the nested For structure

```
for (lastNum = 1; lastNum <= 7; lastNum++)
{
    for (numToPrint = 1; numToPrint <= lastNum; numToPrint++)
        cout << numToPrint;
    cout << endl;
}
```

prints the following triangle of numbers.

```
1
12
123
1234
12345
123456
1234567
```

Although For statements are used primarily for count-controlled loops, C++ allows you to write *any* While loop by using a For statement. To use For loops intelligently, you should know the following facts.

1. In the syntax template, InitStatement can be the null statement, and Expression2 is optional. If Expression2 is omitted, there is no statement for the compiler to insert at the bottom of the loop. As a result, you could write the While loop

    ```
    while (inputVal != 999)
        cin >> inputVal;
    ```

    as the equivalent For loop

    ```
    for ( ; inputVal != 999; )
        cin >> inputVal;
    ```

2. According to the syntax template, Expression1—the While condition—is optional. If you omit it, the expression `true` is assumed. The loop

    ```
    for ( ; ; )
        cout "Hi" << endl;
    ```

    is equivalent to the While loop

    ```
    while (true)
        cout << "Hi" << endl;
    ```

    Both of these are infinite loops that print "Hi" endlessly.

3. The initializing statement, InitStatement, can be a declaration with initialization:

    ```
    for (int i = 1; i <= 20; i++)
        cout << "Hi" << endl;
    ```

    Here, the variable `i` has local scope, even though there are no braces creating a block. The scope of `i` extends only to the end of the For statement. Like any local variable, `i` is inaccessible outside its scope (that is, outside the For statement). Because `i` is local to the For statement, it's possible to write code like this:

    ```
    for (int i = 1; i <= 20; i++)
        cout << "Hi" << endl;
    for (int i = 1; i <= 100; i++)
        cout << "Ed" << endl;
    ```

This code does *not* generate a compile-time error (such as "MULTIPLY DEFINED IDENTIFIER"). We have declared two distinct variables named i, each of which is local to its own For statement.*

As you have seen by now, the For statement in C++ is a very flexible structure. Its use can range from a simple count-controlled loop to a general-purpose, "anything goes" While loop. Some programmers squeeze a lot of work into the heading (the first line) of a For statement. For example, the program fragment

```
cin >> ch;
while (ch != '.')
    cin >> ch;
```

can be compressed into the following For loop:

```
for (cin >> ch; ch != '.'; cin >> ch)
    ;
```

Because all the work is done in the For heading, there is nothing for the loop body to do. The body is simply the null statement.

With For statements, our advice is to keep things simple. The trickier the code is, the harder it will be for another person (or you!) to understand your code and track down errors. In this book, we use For loops for count-controlled loops only.

The Break and Continue Statements

The Break statement, which we introduced with the Switch statement, is also used with loops. A Break statement causes an immediate exit from the innermost Switch, While, Do-While, or For statement in which it appears. Notice the word *innermost*. If break is in a loop that is nested inside another loop, control exits the inner loop but not the outer.

One of the more common ways of using break with loops is to set up an infinite loop and use If tests to exit the loop. Suppose we want to input ten pairs of integers, performing data validation and computing the square root of the sum of each pair. For data validation, assume that the first number of each pair must be less than 100 and the second must be greater than 50. Also, after each input, we want to test the state of the stream for EOF. Here's a loop using Break statements to accomplish the task:

---

* In versions of C++ prior to the ISO/ANSI language standard, i would not be local to the body of the loop. Its scope would extend to the end of the block surrounding the For statement. In other words, it would be as if i had been declared outside the loop. If you are using an older version of C++ and your compiler tells you something like "MULTIPLY DEFINED IDENTIFIER" in code similar to the pair of For statements above, simply choose a different variable name in the second For loop.

```
loopCount = 1;
while (true)
{
    cin >> num1;
    if ( !cin || num1 >= 100)
        break;
    cin >> num2;
    if ( !cin || num2 <= 50)
        break;
    cout << sqrt(float(num1 + num2)) << endl;
    loopCount++;
    if (loopCount > 10)
        break;
}
```

Note that we could have used a For loop to count from 1 to 10, breaking out of it as necessary. However, this loop is both count-controlled and event-controlled, so we prefer to use a While loop.

The above loop contains three distinct exit points. Some people vigorously oppose this style of programming, as it violates the single-entry, single-exit philosophy we discussed with multiple returns from a function. Is there any advantage to using an infinite loop in conjunction with break? To answer this question, let's rewrite the loop without using Break statements. The loop must terminate when num1 is invalid or num2 is invalid or loopCount exceeds 10. We'll use Boolean flags to signal invalid data in the While condition:

```
num1Valid = true;
num2Valid = true;
loopCount = 1;
while (num1Valid && num2Valid && loopCount <= 10)
{
    cin >> num1;
    if ( !cin || num1 >= 100)
        num1Valid = false;
    else
    {
        cin >> num2;
        if ( !cin || num2 <= 50)
            num2Valid = false;
        else
        {
            cout << sqrt(float(num1 + num2)) << endl;
            loopCount++;
        }
    }
}
```

One could argue that the first version is easier to follow and understand than this second version. The primary task of the loop body—computing the square root of the sum of the numbers—is more prominent in the first version. In the second version, the computation is obscured by being buried within nested Ifs. The second version also has a more complicated control flow.

The disadvantage of using `break` with loops is that it can become a crutch for those who are too impatient to think carefully about loop design. It's easy to overuse (and abuse) the technique. Here's an example, printing the integers 1 through 5:

```
i = 1;
while (true)
{
    cout << i;
    if (i == 5)
        break;
    i++;
}
```

There is no real justification for setting up the loop this way. Conceptually, it is a pure count-controlled loop, and a simple For loop does the job:

```
for (i = 1; i <= 5; i++)
    cout << i;
```

The For loop is easier to understand and is less prone to error.

A good rule of thumb is: Use `break` within loops only as a last resort. Specifically, use it only to avoid baffling combinations of multiple Boolean flags and nested Ifs.

Another statement that alters the flow of control in a C++ program is the Continue statement. This statement, valid only in loops, terminates the current loop iteration (but not the entire loop). It causes an immediate branch to the bottom of the loop—skipping the rest of the statements in the loop body—in preparation for the next iteration. Here is an example of a reading loop in which we want to process only the positive numbers in an input file:

```
for (dataCount = 1; dataCount <= 500; dataCount++)
{
    dataFile >> inputVal;
    if (inputVal <= 0)
        continue;
    cout << inputVal;
        ⋮
}
```

If `inputVal` is less than or equal to 0, control branches to the bottom of the loop. Then, as with any For loop, the computer increments `dataCount` and performs the loop test before going on to the next iteration.

The Continue statement is not used often, but we present it for completeness (and because you may run across it in other people's programs). Its primary purpose is to avoid obscuring the main process of the loop by indenting the process within an If statement. For example, the above code would be written without a Continue statement as follows:

```
for (dataCount = 1; dataCount <= 500; dataCount++)
{
    dataFile >> inputVal;
    if (inputVal > 0)
    {
        cout << inputVal;
         ⋮
    }
}
```

Be sure to note the difference between `continue` and `break`. The Continue statement means "Abandon the current iteration of the loop, and go on to the next iteration." The Break statement means "Exit the entire loop immediately."

Guidelines for Choosing a Looping Statement

Here are some guidelines to help you decide when to use each of the three looping statements (While, Do-While, and For).

1. If the loop is a simple count-controlled loop, the For statement is a natural. Concentrating the three loop control actions—initialize, test, and increment/decrement—into one location (the heading of the For statement) reduces the chances of forgetting to include one of them.
2. If the loop is an event-controlled loop whose body should execute at least once, a Do-While statement is appropriate.
3. If the loop is an event-controlled loop and nothing is known about the first execution, use a While (or perhaps a For) statement.
4. When in doubt, use a While statement.
5. An infinite loop with Break statements sometimes clarifies the code but more often reflects an undisciplined loop design. Use it only after careful consideration of While, Do-While, and For.

P ROBLEM-SOLVING CASE STUDY

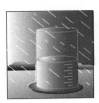

Monthly Rainfall Averages

Problem: Meteorologists have recorded monthly rainfall amounts at several sites throughout a region of the country. You have been asked to write an interactive program that lets the user enter one year's rainfall amounts at a particular site and prints out the average of the 12 values. After the data for a site is processed, the program asks whether the user would like to repeat the process for another recording site. A user response of 'y' means yes, and 'n' means no. The program must trap erroneous input data (negative values for rainfall amounts and invalid responses to the "Do you wish to continue?" prompt).

Input: For each recording site, 12 floating-point rainfall amounts. For each "Do you wish to continue?" prompt, either a 'y' or an 'n'.

Output: For each recording site, the floating-point average of the 12 rainfall amounts, displayed to two decimal places.

Discussion: A solution to this problem requires several looping structures. At the topmost level of the design, we need a loop to process the data from all the sites. Each iteration must process one site's data, then ask the user whether to continue with another recording site. The program does not know in advance how many recording sites there are, so the loop cannot be a count-controlled loop. Although we can make any of For, While, or Do-While work correctly, we'll use a Do-While under the assumption that the user definitely wants to process at least one site's data. Therefore, we can set up the loop so that it processes the data from a recording site and then, at the *bottom* of the loop, decides whether to iterate again.

Another loop is required to input 12 monthly rainfall amounts and form their sum. Using the summing technique we are familiar with by now, we initialize the sum to 0 before starting the loop, and each loop iteration reads another number and adds it to the accumulating sum. A For loop is appropriate for this task, because we know that exactly 12 iterations must occur.

We'll need two more loops to perform data validation—one loop to ensure that a rainfall amount is nonnegative and another to verify that the user types only 'y' or 'n' when prompted to continue. As we saw earlier in the chapter, Do-While loops are well suited to this kind of data validation. We want the loop body to execute at least once, reading an input value and testing for valid data. As long as the user keeps entering invalid data, the loop continues. Control exits the loop only when the user finally gets it right.

PROBLEM-SOLVING CASE STUDY *cont'd.*

      Assumptions: The user processes data for at least one site.

Main

Level 0

```
DO
        Get 12 rainfall amounts and sum them
        Print sum / 12
        Prompt user to continue
        Get yes or no response ('y' or 'n')
WHILE response is 'y'
```

Get 12 Amounts (Out: sum)

Level 1

```
Set sum = 0
FOR count going from 1 through 12
        Prompt user for a rainfall amount
        Get and verify one rainfall amount
        Add amount to sum
```

Get Yes or No (Out: response)

```
DO
        Read response
        IF response isn't 'y' or 'n'
                Print error message
WHILE response isn't 'y' or 'n'
```

PROBLEM-SOLVING CASE STUDY cont'd.

Get One Amount (Out: amount)   **Level 2**

```
DO
        Read amount
        IF amount < 0.0
                Print error message
WHILE amount < 0.0
```

Module Structure Chart:

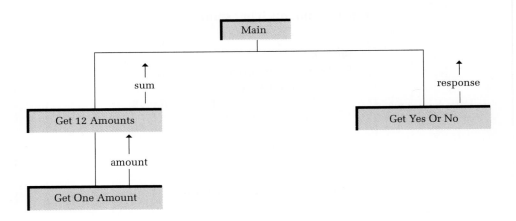

(The following program is written in ISO/ANSI standard C++. If you are working with pre–standard C++, see the alternate version of the program in the PRE_STD directory of the program disk, available at the publisher's Web site, www.jbpub.com/disks.)

PROBLEM-SOLVING CASE STUDY *cont'd.*

```
//**********************************************************************
// Rainfall program
// This program inputs 12 monthly rainfall amounts from a
// recording site and computes the average monthly rainfall.
// This process is repeated for as many recording sites as
// the user wishes.
//**********************************************************************
#include <iostream>
#include <iomanip>      // For setprecision()

using namespace std;

void Get12Amounts( float& );
void GetOneAmount( float& );
void GetYesOrNo( char& );

int main()
{
    float sum;            // Sum of 12 rainfall amounts
    char  response;       // User response ('y' or 'n')

    cout << fixed << showpoint              // Set up floating-pt.
         << setprecision(2);                //   output format

    do
    {
        Get12Amounts(sum);
        cout << endl << "Average rainfall is " << sum / 12.0
             << " inches" << endl << endl;
        cout << "Do you have another recording site? (y or n) ";
        GetYesOrNo(response);
    } while (response == 'y');
    return 0;
}


//**********************************************************************

void Get12Amounts( /* out */ float& sum )    // Sum of 12 rainfall
                                             // amounts

// Inputs 12 monthly rainfall amounts, verifying that
// each is nonnegative, and returns their sum

// Postcondition:
//      12 rainfall amounts have been read and verified to be
//      nonnegative
//   && sum == sum of the 12 input values
```

PROBLEM-SOLVING CASE STUDY cont'd.

```cpp
{
    int   count;        // Loop control variable
    float amount;       // Rainfall amount for one month

    sum = 0;
    for (count = 1; count <= 12; count++)
    {
        cout << "Enter rainfall amount " << count << ": ";
        GetOneAmount(amount);
        sum = sum + amount;
    }
}

//****************************************************************

void GetYesOrNo( /* out */ char& response )    // User response char

// Inputs a character from the user and, if necessary,
// repeatedly prints an error message and inputs another
// character if the character isn't 'y' or 'n'

// Postcondition:
//      response has been input (repeatedly, if necessary, along
//      with output of an error message)
//   && response == 'y' or 'n'

{
    do
    {
        cin >> response;
        if (response != 'y' && response != 'n')
            cout << "Please type y or n: ";
    } while (response != 'y' && response != 'n');
}

//****************************************************************

void GetOneAmount( /* out */ float& amount )    // Rainfall amount
                                                // for one month

// Inputs one month's rainfall amount and, if necessary,
// repeatedly prints an error message and inputs another
// value if the value is negative
```

PROBLEM-SOLVING CASE STUDY cont'd.

```
// Postcondition:
//      amount has been input (repeatedly, if necessary, along
//      with output of an error message)
//   && amount >= 0.0

{
    do
    {
        cin >> amount;
        if (amount < 0.0)
            cout << "Amount cannot be negative. Enter again: ";
    } while (amount < 0.0);
}
```

Testing: We should test two separate aspects of the Rainfall program. First, we should verify that the program works correctly given valid input data. Supplying arbitrary rainfall amounts of 0 or greater, we must confirm that the program correctly adds up the values and divides by 12 to produce the average. Also, we should make sure that the program behaves correctly whether we type 'y' or 'n' when prompted to continue.

The second aspect to test is the data validation code that we included in the program. When prompted for a rainfall amount, we should type negative numbers repeatedly to verify that an error message is printed and that we cannot escape the Do-While loop until we eventually type a nonnegative number. Similarly, when prompted to type 'y' or 'n' to process another recording site, we must press several incorrect keys to exercise the loop in the GetYesOrNo function. Here's a sample run showing the testing of the data validation code:

```
Enter rainfall amount 1: 0
Enter rainfall amount 2: 0
Enter rainfall amount 3: 0
Enter rainfall amount 4: 3.4
Enter rainfall amount 5: 9.6
Enter rainfall amount 6: 1.2
Enter rainfall amount 7: -3.4
Amount cannot be negative. Enter again: -9
Amount cannot be negative. Enter again: -4.2
Amount cannot be negative. Enter again: 1.3
Enter rainfall amount 8: 0
Enter rainfall amount 9: 0
Enter rainfall amount 10: 0
Enter rainfall amount 11: 0
Enter rainfall amount 12: 0
```

PROBLEM-SOLVING CASE STUDY cont'd.

```
Average rainfall is 1.29 inches

Do you have another recording site? (y or n) d
Please type y or n: q
Please type y or n: Y
Please type y or n: n
```

Testing and Debugging

The same testing techniques we used with While loops apply to Do-While and For loops. There are, however, a few additional considerations with these loops.

The body of a Do-While loop always executes at least once. Thus, you should try data sets that show the result of executing a Do-While loop the minimal number of times.

With a data-dependent For loop, it is important to test for proper results when the loop executes zero times. This occurs when the starting value is greater than the ending value (or less than the ending value if the loop control variable is being decremented).

When a program contains a Switch statement, you should test it with enough different data sets to ensure that each branch is selected and executed correctly. You should also test the program with a switch expression whose value is not in any of the case labels.

Testing and Debugging Hints

1. In a Switch statement, make sure there is a Break statement at the end of each case alternative. Otherwise, control "falls through" to the code in the next case alternative.
2. Case labels in a Switch statement are made up of values, not variables. They may, however, include named constants and expressions involving only constants.
3. A switch expression cannot be a floating-point or string expression, and case constants cannot be floating-point or string constants.
4. If there is a possibility that the value of the switch expression might not match one of the case constants, you should provide a default alternative.
5. Double-check long Switch statements to make sure that you haven't omitted any branches.
6. The Do-While loop is a posttest loop. If there is a possibility that the loop body should be skipped entirely, use a While statement or a For statement.

7. The For statement heading (the first line) always has three pieces within the parentheses. Most often, the first piece initializes a loop control variable, the second piece tests the variable, and the third piece increments or decrements the variable. The three pieces must be separated by semicolons. Any of the pieces can be omitted, but the semicolons still must be present.

8. With nested control structures, the Break statement can exit only one level of nesting—the innermost Switch or loop in which the `break` is located.

Summary

The Switch statement is a multiway selection statement. It allows the program to choose among a set of branches. A Switch containing Break statements can always be simulated by an If-Then-Else-If structure. If a Switch can be used, however, it often makes the code easier to read and understand. A Switch statement cannot be used with floating-point or string values in the case labels.

The Do-While is a general-purpose looping statement. It is like the While loop except that its test occurs at the end of the loop, guaranteeing at least one execution of the loop body. As with a While loop, a Do-While continues as long as the loop condition is `true`. A Do-While is convenient for loops that test input values and repeat if the input is not correct.

The For statement is also a general-purpose looping statement, but its most common use is to implement count-controlled loops. The initialization, testing, and incrementation (or decrementation) of the loop control variable are centralized in one location, the first line of the For statement.

The For, Do-While, and Switch statements are the ice cream and cake of C++. We can live without them if we absolutely must, but they are very nice to have.

Quick Check

1. Given a switch expression that is the `int` variable `nameVal`, write a Switch statement that prints your first name if `nameVal = 1`, your middle name if `nameVal = 2`, and your last name if `nameVal = 3`. (pp. 462–466])

2. How would you change the answer to Question 1 so that it prints an error message if the value is not 1, 2, or 3? (pp. 462–466)

3. What is the primary difference between a While loop and a Do-While loop? (pp. 468–471)

4. A certain problem requires a count-controlled loop that starts at 10 and counts down to 1. Write the heading (the first line) of a For statement that controls this loop. (pp. 471–474)

5. Within a loop, how does a Continue statement differ from a Break statement? (pp. 474–477)

6. What C++ looping statement would you choose for a loop that is both count-controlled and event-controlled and whose body might not execute even once? (p. 477)

Answers

1. ```
switch (nameVal)
{
    case 1 : cout << "Mary";
             break;
    case 2 : cout << "Lynn";
             break;
    case 3 : cout << "Smith";
             break;   // Not required
}
```

2. ```
switch (nameVal)
{
    case 1   : cout << "Mary";
               break;
    case 2   : cout << "Lynn";
               break;
    case 3   : cout << "Smith";
               break;
    default  : cout << "Invalid name value.";
               break;   // Not required
}
```

3. The body of a Do-While always executes at least once; the body of a While may not execute at all. 4. `for (count = 10; count >= 1; count--)` 5. A Continue statement terminates the current iteration and goes on to the next iteration (if possible). A Break statement causes an immediate loop exit. 6. A While (or perhaps a For) statement

Exam Preparation Exercises

1. Define the following terms:
   switch expression
   pretest loop
   posttest loop
2. A switch expression may be an expression that results in a value of type int, float, bool, or char. (True or False?)
3. The values in case labels may appear in any order, but duplicate case labels are not allowed within a given Switch statement. (True or False?)
4. All possible values for the switch expression must be included among the case labels for a given Switch statement. (True or False?)
5. Rewrite the following code fragment using a Switch statement.

   ```
   if (n == 3)
       alpha++;
   else if (n == 7)
       beta++;
   else if (n == 10)
       gamma++;
   ```

6. What is printed by the following code fragment if n equals 3? (Be careful here.)

```
switch (n + 1)
{
    case 2  : cout << "Bill";
    case 4  : cout << "Mary";
    case 7  : cout << "Joe";
    case 9  : cout << "Anne";
    default : cout << "Whoops!";
}
```

7. If a While loop whose condition is delta <= alpha is converted into a Do-While loop, the loop condition of the Do-While loop is delta > alpha. (True or False?)

8. A Do-While statement always ends in a semicolon. (True or False?)

9. What is printed by the following program fragment, assuming the input value is 0? (All variables are of type int.)

```
cin >> n;
i = 1;
do
{
    cout << i;
    i++;
} while (i <= n);
```

10. What is printed by the following program fragment, assuming the input value is 0? (All variables are of type int.)

```
cin >> n;
for (i = 1; i <= n; i++)
    cout << i;
```

11. What is printed by the following program fragment? (All variables are of type int.)

```
for (i = 4; i >= 1; i--)
{
    for (j = i; j >= 1; j--)
        cout << j << ' ';
    cout << i << endl;
}
```

12. What is printed by the following program fragment? (All variables are of type int.)

```
for (row = 1; row <= 10; row++)
{
    for (col = 1; col <= 10 - row; col++)
        cout << '*';
    for (col = 1; col <= 2*row - 1; col++)
        cout << ' ';
    for (col = 1; col <= 10 - row; col++)
```

```
        cout << '*';
    cout << endl;
}
```

13. A Break statement located inside a Switch statement that is within a While loop causes control to exit the loop immediately. (True or False?)

Programming Warm-up Exercises

1. Write a Switch statement that does the following:
    If the value of grade is
       'A', add 4 to sum
       'B', add 3 to sum
       'C', add 2 to sum
       'D', add 1 to sum
       'F', print "Student is on probation"

2. Modify the code for Exercise 1 so that an error message is printed if grade does not equal one of the five possible grades.

3. Rewrite the Day function of Chapter 8 (pages 412–413), replacing the If-Then-Else-If structure with a Switch statement.

4. Write a program segment that reads and sums until it has summed ten data values or until a negative value is read, whichever comes first. Use a Do-While loop for your solution.

5. Rewrite the following code segment using a Do-While loop instead of a While loop.

```
cout << "Enter 1, 2, or 3: ";
cin >> response;
while (response < 1 || response > 3)
{
    cout << "Enter 1, 2, or 3: ";
    cin >> response;
}
```

6. Rewrite the following code segment using a While loop.

```
cin >> ch;
if (cin)
    do
    {
        cout << ch;
        cin >> ch;
    } while (cin);
```

7. Rewrite the following code segment using a For loop.

```
sum = 0;
count = 1;
while (count <= 1000)
{
    sum = sum + count;
    count++;
}
```

8. Rewrite the following For loop as a While loop.

```
for (m = 93; m >= 5; m--)
    cout << m << ' ' << m * m << endl;
```

9. Rewrite the following For loop using a Do-While loop.

```
for (k = 9; k <= 21; k++)
    cout << k << ' ' << 3 * k << endl;
```

10. Write a value-returning function that accepts two int parameters, base and exponent, and returns the value of base raised to the exponent power. Use a For loop in your solution.

11. Make the logic of the following loop easier to understand by using an infinite loop with Break statements.

```
sum = 0;
count = 1;
do
{
    cin >> int1;
    if ( !cin || int1 <= 0)
        cout << "Invalid first integer.";
    else
    {
        cin >> int2;
        if ( !cin || int2 > int1)
            cout << "Invalid second integer.";
        else
        {
            cin >> int3;
            if ( !cin || int3 == 0)
                cout << "Invalid third integer.";
            else
            {
                sum = sum + (int1 + int2) / int3;
                count++;
            }
        }
    }
} while (cin && int1 > 0 && int2 <= int1 && int3 != 0 &&
        count <= 100);
```

Programming Problems

1. Develop a functional decomposition and write a C++ program that inputs a two-letter abbreviation for one of the 50 states and prints out the full name of the state. If the abbreviation isn't valid, the program should print an error message and ask for an abbreviation again. The names of the 50 states and their abbreviations are given in the following table.

State	Abbreviation	State	Abbreviation
Alabama	AL	Montana	MT
Alaska	AK	Nebraska	NE
Arizona	AZ	Nevada	NV
Arkansas	AR	New Hampshire	NH
California	CA	New Jersey	NJ
Colorado	CO	New Mexico	NM
Connecticut	CT	New York	NY
Delaware	DE	North Carolina	NC
Florida	FL	North Dakota	ND
Georgia	GA	Ohio	OH
Hawaii	HI	Oklahoma	OK
Idaho	ID	Oregon	OR
Illinois	IL	Pennsylvania	PA
Indiana	IN	Rhode Island	RI
Iowa	IA	South Carolina	SC
Kansas	KS	South Dakota	SD
Kentucky	KY	Tennessee	TN
Louisiana	LA	Texas	TX
Maine	ME	Utah	UT
Maryland	MD	Vermont	VT
Massachusetts	MA	Virginia	VA
Michigan	MI	Washington	WA
Minnesota	MN	West Virginia	WV
Mississippi	MS	Wisconsin	WI
Missouri	MO	Wyoming	WY

(*Hint:* Use nested Switch statements, where the outer statement uses the first letter of the abbreviation as its switch expression.)

2. Write a functional decomposition and a C++ program that reads a date in numeric form and prints it in English. For example:

```
Enter a date in the form mm dd yyyy.
10   27   1942
October twenty-seventh, nineteen hundred forty-two.
```

Here is another example:

```
Enter a date in the form mm dd yyyy.
12   10   2010
December tenth, two thousand ten.
```

The program should print an error message for any invalid date, such as 2 29 1883 (1883 wasn't a leap year).

3. Write a C++ program that reads full names from an input file and writes the initials for the names to an output file stream named `initials`. For example, the input

```
John James Henry
```

should produce the output

```
JJH
```

The names are stored in the input file first name first, then middle name, then last name, separated by an arbitrary number of blanks. There is only one name per line. The first name or the middle name could be just an initial, or there may not be a middle name.

4. Write a functional decomposition and a C++ program that converts letters of the alphabet into their corresponding digits on the telephone. The program should let the user enter letters repeatedly until a 'Q' or a 'Z' is entered. (Q and Z are the two letters that are not on the telephone.) An error message should be printed for any nonalphabetic character that is entered.

The letters and digits on the telephone have the following correspondence.

ABC	=	2	DEF	=	3	GHI	=	4
JKL	=	5	MNO	=	6	PRS	=	7
TUV	=	8	WXY	=	9			

Here is an example:

```
Enter a letter: P
The letter P corresponds to 7 on the telephone.
Enter a letter: A
The letter A corresponds to 2 on the telephone.
Enter a letter: D
The letter D corresponds to 3 on the telephone.
Enter a letter: 2
Invalid letter. Enter Q or Z to quit.
Enter a letter: Z
Quit.
```

Case Study Follow-Up

1. Rewrite the GetYesOrNo and GetOneAmount functions in the Rainfall program, replacing the Do-While loops with While loops.
2. Rewrite the Get12Amounts function in the Rainfall program, replacing the For loop with a Do-While loop.
3. Rewrite the Get12Amounts function in the Rainfall program, replacing the For loop with a While loop.
4. In the GetYesOrNo function of the Rainfall program, is it possible to replace the If statement with a Switch statement? If so, is it advisable to do so?
5. In the GetOneAmount function of the Rainfall program, is it possible to replace the If statement with a Switch statement? If so, is it advisable to do so?

10

Simple Data Types: Built-In and User-Defined

GOALS

- To be able to identify all of the simple data types provided by the C++ language.
- To become familiar with specialized C++ operators and expressions.
- To be able to distinguish between external and internal representations of character data.
- To understand how floating-point numbers are represented in the computer.
- To understand how the limited numeric precision of the computer can affect calculations.
- To be able to select the most appropriate simple data type for a given variable.
- To be able to declare and use an enumeration type.
- To be able to use the For and Switch statements with user-defined enumeration types.
- To be able to distinguish a named user-defined type from an anonymous user-defined type.
- To be able to create a user-written header file.
- To understand the concepts of type promotion and type demotion.

This chapter represents a transition point in your study of computer science and C++ programming. So far, we have emphasized simple variables, control structures, and named processes (functions). After this chapter, the focus shifts to ways to structure (organize) data and to the algorithms necessary to process data in these structured forms. In order to make this transition, we must examine the concept of data type in greater detail.

Until now, we have worked primarily with the data types `int`, `char`, `bool`, and `float`. These four data types are adequate for solving a wide variety of problems. But certain programs need other kinds of data. In this chapter, we take a closer look at all of the simple data types that are part of the C++ language. As part of this look, we discuss the limitations of the computer in doing calculations. We examine how these limitations can cause numerical errors and how to avoid such errors.

There are times when even the built-in data types cannot adequately represent all the data in a program. C++ has several mechanisms for creating *user-defined* data types; that is, we can define new data types ourselves. This chapter introduces one of these mechanisms, the enumeration type. In subsequent chapters, we introduce additional user-defined data types.

Built-In Simple Types

In Chapter 2, we defined a data type as a specific set of data values (which we call the *domain*) along with a set of operations on those values. For the `int` type, the domain is the set of whole numbers from `INT_MIN` through `INT_MAX`, and the allowable operations we have seen so far are +, −, *, /, %, ++, --, and the relational and logical operations. The domain of the `float` type is the set of all real numbers that a particular computer is capable of representing, and the operations are the same as those for the `int` type except that modulus (%) is excluded. For the `bool` type, the domain is the set consisting of the two values `true` and `false`, and the allowable operations are the logical (!, &&, ||) and relational operations. The `char` type, though used primarily to manipulate character data, is classified as an integral type because it uses integers in memory to stand for characters. Later in the chapter we see how this works.

The `int`, `char`, `bool`, and `float` types have a property in common. The domain of each type is made up of indivisible, or atomic, data values. Data types with this property are called **simple** (or **atomic**) **data types.** When we say that a value is atomic, we mean that it has no component parts that can be accessed individually. For example, a single character of type `char` is atomic, but the string "Good Morning" is not (it is composed of 12 individual characters).

Simple (atomic) data type   A data type in which each value is atomic (indivisible).

Another way of describing a simple type is to say that only one value can be associated with a variable of that type. In contrast, a *structured type* is one in which an entire collection of values is associated with a single variable of that type. For example, a string object represents a collection of characters that are given a single name. Beginning in Chapter 11, we look at structured types.

Figure 10-1 displays the simple types that are built into the C++ language. This figure is a portion of the complete diagram of C++ data types that you saw in Figure 3-1.

In this figure, one of the types—enum—is not actually a single data type in the sense that int and float are data types. Instead, it is a mechanism with which we can define our own simple data types. We look at enum later in the chapter.

The integral types char, short, int, and long represent nothing more than integers of different sizes. Similarly, the floating-point types float, double, and long double simply refer to floating-point numbers of different sizes. What do we mean by *sizes*?

In C++, sizes are measured in multiples of the size of a char. By definition, the size of a char is 1. On most—but not all—computers, the 1 means one byte. (Recall from Chapter 1 that a byte is a group of eight consecutive bits [1s or 0s].)

Let's use the notation *sizeof* (SomeType) to denote the size of a value of type SomeType. Then, by definition, *sizeof* (char) = 1. Other than char, the sizes of data objects in C++ are machine dependent. On one machine, it might be the case that

FIGURE 10-1
C++ Simple Types

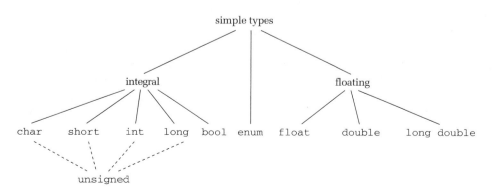

sizeof (char) = 1
sizeof (short) = 2
sizeof (int) = 4
sizeof (long) = 8

On another machine, the sizes might be as follows:

sizeof (char) = 1
sizeof (short) = 2
sizeof (int) = 2
sizeof (long) = 4

Despite these variations, the C++ language guarantees that the following statements are true:

- $1 = sizeof$ (char) $\leq sizeof$ (short) $\leq sizeof$ (int) $\leq sizeof$ (long).
- $1 \leq sizeof$ (bool) $\leq sizeof$ (long).
- $sizeof$ (float) $\leq sizeof$ (double) $\leq sizeof$ (long double).
- A char is at least 8 bits.
- A short is at least 16 bits.
- A long is at least 32 bits.

For numeric data, the size of a data object determines its **range of values.** Let's look in more detail at the sizes, ranges of values, and literal constants for each of the built-in types.

Range of values   The interval within which values of a numeric type must fall, specified in terms of the largest and smallest allowable values.

Integral Types

Before looking at how the sizes of integral types affect their possible values, we remind you that the reserved word unsigned may precede the name of certain integral types—unsigned char, unsigned short, unsigned int, unsigned long. Values of these types are nonnegative integers with values from 0 through some machine-dependent maximum value. Although we rarely use unsigned types in this book, we include them in this discussion for thoroughness.

Ranges of Values   The following table displays sample ranges of values for the char, short, int, and long data types and their unsigned variations.

Type	Size in Bytes*	Minimum Value*	Maximum Value*
char	1	−128	127
unsigned char	1	0	255
short	2	−32,768	32,767
unsigned short	2	0	65,535
int	2	−32,768	32,767
unsigned int	2	0	65,535
long	4	−2,147,483,648	2,147,483,647
unsigned long	4	0	4,294,967,295

* These values are for one particular machine. Your machine's values may be different.

C++ systems provide the header file `climits`, from which you can determine the maximum and minimum values for your machine. This header file defines the constants CHAR_MAX and CHAR_MIN, SHRT_MAX and SHRT_MIN, INT_MAX and INT_MIN, and LONG_MAX and LONG_MIN. The unsigned types have a minimum value of 0 and maximum values defined by UCHAR_MAX, USHRT_MAX, UINT_MAX, and ULONG_MAX. To find out the values specific to your computer, you could print them out like this:

```
#include <climits>
using namespace std;
    ⋮
cout << "Max. long = " << LONG_MAX << endl;
cout << "Min. long = " << LONG_MIN << endl;
    ⋮
```

Literal Constants In C++, the valid `bool` constants are `true` and `false`. Integer constants can be specified in three different number bases: decimal (base 10), octal (base 8), and hexadecimal (base 16). Just as the decimal number system has ten digits—0 through 9—the octal system has eight digits—0 through 7. The hexadecimal system has digits 0, 1, 2, 3, 4, 5, 6, 7, 8, 9, A, B, C, D, E, and F, which correspond to the decimal values 0 through 15. Octal and hexadecimal values are used in system software (compilers, linkers, and operating systems, for example) to refer directly to individual bits in a memory cell and to control hardware devices. These manipulations of low-level objects in a computer are the subject of more advanced study and are outside the scope of this book.

The following table shows examples of integer constants in C++. Notice that an L or a U (either uppercase or lowercase) can be added to the end of a constant to signify `long` or `unsigned`, respectively.

Constant	Type	Remarks
1658	int	Decimal (base-10) integer.
03172	int	Octal (base-8) integer. Begins with 0 (zero). Decimal equivalent is 1658.
0x67A	int	Hexadecimal (base-16) integer. Begins with 0 (zero), then either x or X. Decimal equivalent is 1658.
65535U	unsigned int	Unsigned constants end in U or u.
421L	long	Explicit long constant. Ends in L or l.
53100	long	Implicit long constant, assuming the machine's maximum int is, say, 32767.
389123487UL	unsigned long	Unsigned long constants end in UL or LU in any combination of uppercase and lowercase letters.

Notice that this table presents only numeric constants for the integral types. We discuss char constants later in a separate section.

Here is the syntax template for an integer constant:

IntegerConstant

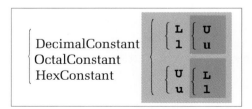

DecimalConstant is a nonzero digit followed, optionally, by a sequence of decimal digits:

DecimalConstant

NonzeroDigit DigitSeq

NonzeroDigit, DigitSeq, and Digit are defined as follows:

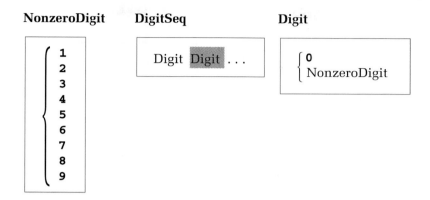

NonzeroDigit   **DigitSeq**   **Digit**

The second form of integer constant, OctalConstant, has the following syntax:

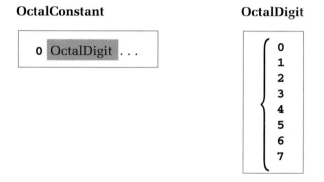

OctalConstant   **OctalDigit**

Finally, HexConstant is defined as

HexConstant   **HexDigit**

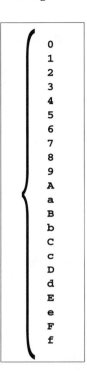

Floating-Point Types

Ranges of Values   Below is a table that gives sample ranges of values for the three floating-point types, float, double, and long double. In this table we show, for each type, the maximum positive value and the minimum positive value (a tiny fraction that is very close to 0). Negative numbers have the same range but the opposite sign. Ranges of values are expressed in exponential (scientific) notation, where 3.4E+38 means 3.4×10^{38}.

Type	Size in Bytes*	Minimum Positive Value*	Maximum Positive Value*
float	4	3.4E−38	3.4E+38
double	8	1.7E−308	1.7E+308
long double	10	3.4E−4932	1.1E+4932

*These values are for one particular machine. Your machine's values may be different.

The standard header file `cfloat` defines the constants `FLT_MAX` and `FLT_MIN`, `DBL_MAX` and `DBL_MIN`, and `LDBL_MAX` and `LDBL_MIN`. To determine the ranges of values for your machine, you could write a short program that prints out these constants.

Literal Constants When you use a floating-point constant such as 5.8 in a C++ program, its type is assumed to be `double` (double precision). If you store the value into a `float` variable, the computer coerces its type from `double` to `float` (single precision). If you insist on a constant being of type `float` rather than `double`, you can append an `F` or an `f` at the end of the constant. Similarly, a suffix of `L` or `l` signifies a `long double` constant. Here are some examples of floating-point constants in C++:

Constant	Type	Remarks
6.83	double	By default, floating-point constants are of type double.
6.83F	float	Explicit float constants end in F or f.
6.83L	long double	Explicit long double constants end in L or l.
4.35E-9	double	Exponential notation, meaning 4.35×10^{-9}.

Here's the syntax template for a floating-point constant in C++:

FloatingPtConstant

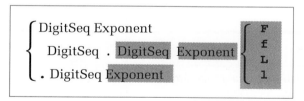

DigitSeq is the same as defined in the section on integer constants—a sequence of decimal (base-10) digits. The form of Exponent is the following:

Exponent

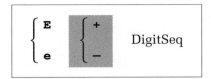

Additional C++ Operators

C++ has a rich, sometimes bewildering, variety of operators that allow you to manipulate values of the simple data types. Operators you have learned about so far include the assignment operator (=), the arithmetic operators (+, -, *, /, %), the increment and decrement operators (++, --), the relational operators (==, !=, <, <=, >, >=), and the logical operators (!, &&, ||). In certain cases, a pair of parentheses is also considered to be an operator—namely, the function call operator,

```
ComputeSum(x, y);
```

and the type cast operator,

```
y = float(someInt);
```

C++ also has many specialized operators that are seldom found in other programming languages. Here is a table of these additional operators. As you inspect the table, don't panic—a quick scan will do.

Operator	Remarks
Combined assignment operators	
+= Add and assign	
-= Subtract and assign	
*= Multiply and assign	
/= Divide and assign	
Increment and decrement operators	
++ Pre-increment	Example: ++someVar
++ Post-increment	Example: someVar++
-- Pre-decrement	Example: --someVar
-- Post-decrement	Example: --someVar

Operator	Remarks
Bitwise operators	Integer operands only
`<<` Left shift	
`>>` Right shift	
`&` Bitwise AND	
`|` Bitwise OR	
`^` Bitwise EXCLUSIVE OR	
`~` Complement (invert all bits)	
More combined assignment operators	Integer operands only
`%=` Modulus and assign	
`<<=` Shift left and assign	
`>>=` Shift right and assign	
`&=` Bitwise AND and assign	
`|=` Bitwise OR and assign	
`^=` Bitwise EXCLUSIVE OR and assign	
Other operators	
`()` Cast	
`sizeof` Size of operand in bytes	Form: `sizeof` Expr or `sizeof`(Type)
`?:` Conditional operator	Form: Expr1 `?` Expr2 `:` Expr3

The operators in this table, along with those you already know, comprise most—but not all—of the C++ operators. We introduce a few more operators in later chapters as the need arises.

Assignment Operators and Assignment Expressions

C++ has several assignment operators. The equal sign (=) is the basic assignment operator. When combined with its two operands, it forms an **assignment expression** (*not* an assignment statement). Every assignment expression has a *value* and a *side effect*, namely, that the value is stored into the object denoted by the left-hand side. For example, the expression

```
delta = 2 * 12
```

has the value 24 and the side effect of storing this value into `delta`.

In C++, any expression becomes an **expression statement** when it is terminated by a semicolon. All three of the following are valid C++ statements, although the first two have no effect whatsoever at run time:

```
23;
2 * (alpha + beta);
delta = 2 * 12;
```

The third expression statement *is* useful because of its side effect of storing 24 into `delta`.

Assignment expression   A C++ expression with (1) a value and (2) the side effect of storing the expression value into a memory location.

Expression statement   A statement formed by appending a semicolon to an expression.

Because an assignment is an expression, not a statement, you can use it anywhere an expression is allowed. Here is a statement that stores the value 20 into `firstInt`, the value 30 into `secondInt`, and the value 35 into `thirdInt`:

```
thirdInt = (secondInt = (firstInt = 20) + 10) + 5;
```

Some C++ programmers use this style of coding, but others find it hard to read and error-prone.

In Chapter 5, we cautioned against the mistake of using the = operator in place of the == operator:

```
if (alpha = 12)   // Wrong
   ⋮
else
   ⋮
```

The condition in the If statement is an assignment expression, not a relational expression. The value of the expression is 12 (interpreted in the If condition as `true`), so the else-clause is never executed. Worse yet, the side effect of the assignment expression is to store 12 into `alpha`, destroying its previous contents.

In addition to the = operator, C++ has several combined assignment operators (+=, *=, and the others listed in our table of operators). These operators have the following semantics:

Statement	Equivalent Statement
`i += 5;`	`i = i + 5;`
`pivotPoint *= n + 3;`	`pivotPoint = pivotPoint * (n + 3);`

The combined assignment operators are another example of "ice cream and cake." They are sometimes convenient for writing a line of code more compactly, but you can do just fine without them.

Increment and Decrement Operators

The increment and decrement operators (++ and --) operate only on variables, not on constants or arbitrary expressions. Suppose a variable someInt contains the value 3. The expression ++someInt denotes preincrementation. The side effect of incrementing someInt occurs first, so the resulting value of the expression is 4. In contrast, the expression someInt++ denotes post-incrementation. The value of the expression is 3, and *then* the side effect of incrementing someInt takes place. The following code illustrates the difference between pre- and post-incrementation:

```
int1 = 14;
int2 = ++int1;
// Assert: int1 == 15  &&  int2 == 15

int1 = 14;
int2 = int1++;
// Assert: int1 == 15  &&  int2 == 14
```

Using side effects in the middle of larger expressions is always a bit dangerous. It's easy to make semantic errors, and the code may be confusing to read. Look at this example:

```
a = (b = c++) * --d / (e += f++);
```

Some people make a game of seeing how much they can do in the fewest keystrokes possible. But they should remember that serious software development requires writing code that other programmers can read and understand. Overuse of side effects hinders this goal. By far the most common use of ++ and -- is to do the incrementation or decrementation as a separate expression statement:

```
count++;
```

Here, the value of the expression is unused, but we get the desired side effect of incrementing count. In this example, it doesn't matter whether you use pre-incrementation or post-incrementation. The choice is up to you.

Bitwise Operators

The bitwise operators listed in the operator table (<<, >>, &, |, and so forth) are used for manipulating individual bits within a memory cell. This book does not explore the use of these operators; the topic of bit-level operations is most often covered in a course on computer organization and assembly language programming. However, we point out two things about the bit-wise operators.

First, the built-in operators << and >> are the left shift and right shift operators, respectively. Their purpose is to take the bits within a memory cell and shift them to the left or right. Of course, we have been using these operators all along, but in an entirely different context—program input and output. The header file `iostream` uses an advanced C++ technique called *operator overloading* to give additional meanings to these two operators. An overloaded operator is one that has multiple meanings, depending on the data types of its operands. When looking at the << operator, the compiler determines by context whether a left shift operation or an output operation is desired. Specifically, if the first (left-hand) operand denotes an output stream, then it is an output operation. If the first operand is an integer variable, it is a left shift operation.

Second, we repeat our caution from Chapter 5: Do not confuse the && and || operators with the & and | operators. The statement

```
if (i == 3 & j == 4)    // Wrong
    k = 20;
```

is syntactically correct because & is a valid operator (the bitwise AND operator). The program containing this statement compiles correctly but executes incorrectly. Although we do not examine what the bitwise AND and OR operators do, just be careful to use the relational operators && and || in your logical expressions.

The Cast Operation

You have seen that C++ is very liberal about letting the programmer mix data types in expressions, in assignment operations, in argument passing, and in returning a function value. However, implicit type coercion takes place when values of different data types are mixed together. Instead of relying on implicit type coercion in a statement such as

```
intVar = floatVar;
```

we have recommended using an explicit type cast to show that the type conversion is intentional:

```
intVar = int(floatVar);
```

In C++, the cast operation comes in two forms:

```
intVar = int(floatVar);      // Functional notation
intVar = (int) floatVar;     // Prefix notation. Parentheses required
```

The first form is called functional notation because it looks like a function call. It isn't really a function call (there is no user-defined or predefined subprogram named `int`), but it has the syntax and visual appearance of a function call. The second form, prefix notation, doesn't look like any familiar language feature in C++. In this notation, the parentheses surround the name of the data type, not the expression being converted. Prefix notation is the only form available in the C language; C++ added the functional notation.

Although most C++ programmers use the functional notation for the cast operation, there is one restriction on its use. The data type name must be a single identifier. If the type name consists of more than one identifier, you *must* use prefix notation. For example,

```
myVar = unsigned int(someFloat);    // No
myVar = (unsigned int) someFloat;   // Yes
```

The `sizeof` Operator

The `sizeof` operator is a unary operator that yields the size, in bytes, of its operand. The operand can be a variable name, as in

```
sizeof someInt
```

or the operand can be the name of a data type, enclosed in parentheses:

```
sizeof(float)
```

You could find out the sizes of various data types on your machine by using code like this:

```
cout << "Size of a short is " << sizeof(short) << endl;
cout << "Size of an int is " << sizeof(int) << endl;
cout << "Size of a long is " << sizeof(long) << endl;
```

The `?:` Operator

The last operator in our operator table is the `?:` operator, sometimes called the conditional operator. It is a ternary (three-operand) operator with the following syntax:

ConditionalExpression

> Expression1 **?** Expression2 **:** Expression3

Here's how it works. First, the computer evaluates Expression1. If the value is `true`, then the value of the entire expression is Expression2; otherwise, the value of the entire expression is Expression3. (Only one of Expression2 and Expression3 is evaluated.) A classic example of its use is to set a variable `max` equal to the larger of two variables `a` and `b`. Using an If statement, we would do it this way:

```
if (a > b)
    max = a;
else
    max = b;
```

With the `?:` operator, we can use the following assignment statement:

```
max = (a > b) ? a : b;
```

Here is another example. The absolute value of a number x is defined as

$$|x| = \begin{cases} x, & \text{if } x \geq 0 \\ -x, & \text{if } x < 0 \end{cases}$$

To compute the absolute value of a variable `x` and store it into `y`, you could use the `?:` operator as follows:

```
y = (x >= 0) ? x : -x;
```

In both the `max` and the absolute value examples, we used parentheses around the expression being tested. These parentheses are unnecessary because, as we'll see shortly, the conditional operator has very low precedence. But it is customary to include the parentheses for clarity.

Operator Precedence

Below is a summary of operator precedence for the C++ operators we have encountered so far, excluding the bitwise operators. (Appendix B contains the complete list.) In the table, the operators are grouped by precedence level, and a horizontal line separates each precedence level from the next-lower level.

Operator	**Precedence (highest to lowest)** Associativity	Remarks
()	Left to right	Function call and function-style cast
++ --	Right to left	++ and -- as postfix operators
++ -- ! Unary + Unary –	Right to left	++ and -- as prefix operators
(cast) sizeof	Right to left	
* / %	Left to right	
+ –	Left to right	
< <= > >=	Left to right	
== !=	Left to right	
&&	Left to right	
||	Left to right	
?:	Right to left	
= += -= *= /=	Right to left	

The column labeled *Associativity* describes grouping order. Within a precedence level, most operators group from left to right. For example,

```
a - b + c
```

means

```
(a - b) + c
```

and not

```
a - (b + c)
```

Certain operators, though, group from right to left—specifically, the unary operators, the assignment operators, and the ?: operator. Look at the assignment operators, for example. The expression

```
sum = count = 0
```

means

```
sum = (count = 0)
```

This associativity makes sense because the assignment operation is naturally a right-to-left operation.

A word of caution: Although operator precedence and associativity dictate the *grouping* of operators with their operands, C++ does not define the *order* in which subexpressions are evaluated. Therefore, using side effects in expressions requires extra care. For example, if i currently contains 5, the statement

```
j = ++i + i;
```

stores either 11 or 12 into j, depending on the particular compiler being used. Let's see why. There are three operators in the expression statement above: =, ++, and +. The ++ operator has the highest precedence, so it operates just on i, not the expression i + i. The addition operator has higher precedence than the assignment operator, giving implicit parentheses as follows:

```
j = (++i + i);
```

So far, so good. But now we ask this question: In the addition operation, is the left operand or the right operand evaluated first? The C++ language doesn't dictate the order. If a compiler generates code to evaluate the left operand first, the result is 6 + 6, or 12. Another compiler might generate code to evaluate the right operand first, yielding 6 + 5, or 11. To be assured of left-to-right evaluation in this example, you should force the ordering with two separate statements:

```
++i;
j = i + i;
```

The moral here is that if you use multiple side effects in expressions, you increase the risk of unexpected or inconsistent results. For the newcomer to C++, it's better to avoid unnecessary side effects altogether.

___ *Working with Character Data*

We have been using `char` variables to store character data, such as the character 'A' or 'e' or '+':

```
char someChar;
    ⋮
someChar = 'A';
```

However, because `char` is defined to be an integral type and `sizeof(char)` equals 1, we also can use a `char` variable to store a small (usually one-byte) integer constant. For example,

```
char counter;
    ⋮
counter = 3;
```

On computers with a very limited amount of memory space, programmers sometimes use the `char` type to save memory when they are working with small integers.

A natural question to ask is, How does the computer know the difference between integer data and character data when the data is sitting in a memory cell? The answer is, The computer *can't* tell the difference! To explain this surprising fact, we must look more closely at how character data is stored in a computer.

Character Sets

Each computer uses a particular character set, the set of all possible characters with which it is capable of working. Two character sets widely in use today are the ASCII character set and the EBCDIC character set. ASCII is used by the vast majority of all computers, whereas EBCDIC is found primarily on IBM mainframe computers. ASCII consists of 128 different characters, and EBCDIC has 256 characters. Appendix E shows the characters that are available in these two character sets.

A more recently developed character set called *Unicode* allows many more distinct characters than either ASCII or EBCDIC. Unicode was invented primarily to accommodate the larger alphabets and symbols of various international human languages. In C++, the data type `wchar_t` rather than `char` is used for Unicode characters. In fact, `wchar_t` can be used for other, possibly infrequently used, "wide character" sets in addition to Unicode. In this book, we do not examine Unicode or the `wchar_t` type. We continue to focus our attention on the `char` type and the ASCII and EBCDIC character sets.

Whichever character set is being used, each character has an **external representation**—the way it looks on an I/O device like a printer—and an **internal representation**—the way it is stored inside the computer's memory unit. If you use the `char` constant 'A' in a C++ program, its external representation is the letter *A*. That is, if you print it out you see an *A*, as you would expect. Its internal representation, though, is an integer value. The 128 ASCII characters have internal representations 0 through 127; the EBCDIC characters, 0 through 255. For example, the ASCII table in Appendix E shows that the character 'A' has internal representation 65, and the character 'b' has internal representation 98.

External representation   The printable (character) form of a data value.

Internal representation   The form in which a data value is stored inside the memory unit.

Let's look again at the statement

```
someChar = 'A';
```

Assuming our machine uses the ASCII character set, the compiler translates the constant 'A' into the integer 65. We could also have written the statement as

```
someChar = 65;
```

Both statements have exactly the same effect—that of storing 65 into `someChar`. However, the second version is *not* recommended. It is not as understandable as the first version, and it is nonportable (the program won't work correctly on a machine that uses EBCDIC, which uses a different internal representation—193—for 'A').

Earlier we mentioned that the computer cannot tell the difference between character and integer data in memory. Both are stored internally as integers. However, when we perform I/O operations, the computer does the right thing—it uses the external representation that corresponds to the data type of the expression being printed. Look at this code segment, for example:

```
// This example assumes use of the ASCII character set
int  someInt = 97;
char someChar = 97;

cout << someInt << endl;
cout << someChar << endl;
```

When these statements are executed, the output is

```
97
a
```

When the << operator outputs someInt, it prints the sequence of characters 9 and 7. To output someChar, it prints the single character a. Even though both variables contain the value 97 internally, the data type of each variable determines how it is printed.

What do you think is output by the following sequence of statements?

```
char ch = 'D';

ch++;
cout << ch;
```

If you answered E, you are right. The first statement declares ch and initializes it to the integer value 68 (assuming ASCII). The next statement increments ch to 69, and then its external representation (the letter *E*) is printed. Extending this idea of incrementing a char variable, we could print the letters *A* through *G* as follows:

```
char ch;

for (ch = 'A'; ch <= 'G'; ch++)
    cout << ch;
```

This code initializes ch to 'A' (65 in ASCII). Each time through the loop, the external representation of ch is printed. On the final loop iteration, the *G* is printed and ch is incremented to 'H' (72 in ASCII). The loop test is then false, so the loop terminates.

C++ char Constants

In C++, char constants come in two different forms. The first form, which we have been using regularly, is a single printable character enclosed by apostrophes (single quotes):

```
'A'   '8'   ')'   '+'
```

Notice that we said *printable* character. Character sets include both printable characters and *control characters* (or *nonprintable characters*). Control characters are not meant to be printed but are used to control the screen, printer, and other hardware devices. If you look at the ASCII character table, you see that the printable characters are those with integer values 32–126. The remaining characters (with values 0–31 and 127) are nonprintable control characters. In the EBCDIC character set, the control characters are those with values 0–63 and 250–255 (and some that are intermingled with the printable characters). One control character you already know about is the newline character, which causes the screen cursor to advance to the next line.

To accommodate control characters, C++ provides a second form of `char` constant: the *escape sequence*. An escape sequence is one or more characters preceded by a backslash (\). You are familiar with the escape sequence \n, which represents the newline character. Here is the complete description of the two forms of `char` constant in C++:

1. A single printable character—except an apostrophe (') or backslash (\)—enclosed by apostrophes.
2. One of the following escape sequences, enclosed by apostrophes:

\n	Newline (Line feed in ASCII)
\t	Horizontal tab
\v	Vertical tab
\b	Backspace
\r	Carriage return
\f	Form feed
\a	Alert (a bell or beep)
\\	Backslash
\'	Single quote (apostrophe)
\"	Double quote (quotation mark)
\0	Null character (all 0 bits)
\ddd	Octal equivalent (one, two, or three octal digits specifying the integer value of the desired character)
\xddd	Hexadecimal equivalent (one or more hexadecimal digits specifying the integer value of the desired character)

Even though an escape sequence is written as two or more characters, each escape sequence represents a single character in the character set. The alert character (\a) is the same as what is called the BEL character in ASCII and EBCDIC. To ring the bell (well, these days, beep the beeper) on your computer, you can output the alert character like this:

```
cout << '\a';
```

In the list of escape sequences above, the entries labeled *Octal equivalent* and *Hexadecimal equivalent* let you refer to any character in your machine's character set by specifying its integer value in either octal or hexadecimal form.

Note that you can use an escape sequence within a string just as you can use any printable character within a string. The statement

```
cout << "\aWhoops!\n";
```

beeps the beeper, displays Whoops!, and terminates the output line. The statement

```
cout << "She said \"Hi\"";
```

outputs She said "Hi" and does not terminate the output line.

Programming Techniques

What kinds of things can we do with character data in a program? The possibilities are endless and depend, of course, on the particular problem we are solving. But several techniques are so widely used that it's worth taking a look at them.

Comparing Characters In previous chapters, you have seen examples of comparing characters for equality. We have used tests such as

```
if (ch == 'a')
```

and

```
while (inputChar != '\n')
```

Characters can also be compared by using <, <=, >, and >=. For example, if the variable firstLetter contains the first letter of a person's last name, we can test to see if the last name starts with *A* through *H* by using this test:

```
if (firstLetter >= 'A' && firstLetter <= 'H')
```

On one level of thought, a test like this is reasonable if you think of < as meaning "comes before" in the character set and > as meaning "comes after." On another level, the test makes even more sense when you consider that the underlying representation of a character is an integer number. The machine literally compares the two integer values using the mathematical meaning of less than or greater than.

When you write a logical expression to check whether a character lies within a certain range of values, you sometimes have to keep in mind the character set your machine uses. In Chapter 8, we hinted that a test like

```
if (ch >= 'a' && ch <= 'z')
```

works correctly on some machines but not on others. In ASCII, this If test behaves correctly because the lowercase letters occupy 26 consecutive positions in the character set. In EBCDIC, however, there is a gap between the lowercase letters *i* and *j* that includes nonprintable characters, and there is another gap between *r* and *s*. (There are similar gaps between the uppercase letters *I* and *J* and between *R* and *S*.) If your machine uses EBCDIC, you must rephrase the If test to be sure you include *only* the desired characters. A better approach, though, is to take advantage of the "is..." functions supplied by the standard library through the header file cctype. If you replace the above If test with this one:

```
if (islower(ch))
```

then your program is more portable; the test works correctly on any machine, regardless of its character set. It's a good idea to become well acquainted with these character-testing library functions (Appendix C). They can save you time and help you to write more portable programs.

Converting Digit Characters to Integers Suppose you want to convert a digit that is read in character form to its numeric equivalent. Because the digit characters '0' through '9' are consecutive in both the ASCII and EBCDIC character sets, subtracting '0' from any digit in character form gives the digit in numeric form:

```
'0' - '0' = 0
'1' - '0' = 1
'2' - '0' = 2
   ⋮
```

For example, in ASCII, '0' has internal representation 48 and '2' has internal representation 50. Therefore, the expression

```
'2' - '0'
```

equals $50 - 48$ and evaluates to 2.

Why would you want to do this? Recall that when the extraction operator (>>) reads data into an int variable, the input stream fails if an invalid character is encountered. (And once the stream has failed, no further input will succeed). Suppose you're writing a program that prompts an inexperienced user to enter a number from 1 through 5. If the input variable is of type int and the user accidentally types a letter of the alphabet, the program is in trouble. To defend against this possibility, you might read the user's response as a character and convert it to a number, performing error checking along the way. Here's a code segment that demonstrates the technique:

```
#include <cctype>    // For isdigit()
using namespace std;
   ⋮
void GetResponse( /* out */ int& response )
```

```
// Postcondition:
//      User has been prompted to enter a digit from 1
//      through 5 (repeatedly, and with error messages,
//      if data is invalid)
//  && 1 <= response <= 5

{
    char inChar;
    bool badData = false;

    do
    {
        cout << "Enter a number from 1 through 5: ";
        cin >> inChar;
        if ( !isdigit(inChar) )
            badData = true;                   // It's not a digit
        else
        {
            response = int(inChar - '0');
            if (response < 1 || response > 5)
                badData = true;               // It's a digit, but
        }                                     // it's out of range
        if (badData)
            cout << "Please try again." << endl;
    } while (badData);
}
```

Converting to Lowercase and Uppercase   When working with character
data, you sometimes find that you need to convert a lowercase letter to
uppercase, or vice versa. Fortunately, the programming technique required
to do these conversions is easy—a simple call to a library function is all it
takes. Through the header file cctype, the standard library provides not
only the "is..." functions we have discussed, but also two value-returning
functions named toupper and tolower. Here are their descriptions:

Header File	Function	Function Type	Function Value
<cctype>	toupper(ch)	char*	Uppercase equivalent of ch, if ch is a lowercase letter; ch, otherwise
<cctype>	tolower(ch)	char	Lowercase equivalent of ch, if ch is an uppercase letter; ch, otherwise

*Technically, both the argument and the return value are of type int. But conceptu-
ally, the functions operate on character data.

Notice that the value returned by each function is just the original character if the condition is not met. For example, `tolower('M')` returns the character 'm', whereas `tolower('+')` returns '+'.

A common use of these two functions is to let the user respond to certain input prompts by using either uppercase or lowercase letters. For example, if you want to allow either *Y* or *y* for a "Yes" response from the user, and either *N* or *n* for "No," you might do this:

```
#include <cctype>      // For toupper()
using namespace std;
    ⋮
cout << "Enter Y or N: ";
cin >> inputChar;
if (toupper(inputChar) == 'Y')
{
    ⋮
}
else if (toupper(inputChar) == 'N')
{
    ⋮
}
else
    PrintErrorMsg();
```

Below is a function named `Lower`, which is our implementation of the `tolower` function. (You wouldn't actually want to waste time by writing this function because `tolower` is already available to you.) This function returns the lowercase equivalent of an uppercase letter. In ASCII, each lowercase letter is exactly 32 positions beyond the corresponding uppercase letter. And in EBCDIC, the lowercase letters are 64 positions *before* their corresponding uppercase letters. To make our `Lower` function work on both ASCII-based and EBCDIC-based machines, we define a constant DIS-TANCE to have the value

```
'a' - 'A'
```

In ASCII, the value of this expression is 32. In EBCDIC, the value is −64.

```
#include <cctype>      // For isupper()
using namespace std;
  ⋮
char Lower( /* in */ char ch )

// Postcondition:
//      Function value == lowercase equivalent of ch, if ch is
//                        an uppercase letter
//                     == ch, otherwise

{
```

```
        const int DISTANCE = 'a' - 'A';   // Fixed distance between
                                          // uppercase and lowercase
                                          // letters
        if (isupper(ch))
            return ch + DISTANCE;
        else
            return ch;
    }
```

Accessing Characters Within a String   In the last section, we gave the outline of a code segment that prompts the user for a "Yes" or "No" response. The code accepted a response of 'Y' or 'N' in uppercase or lowercase letters. If a problem requires the user to type the entire word *Yes* or *No* in any combination of uppercase and lowercase letters, the code becomes more complicated. Reading the user's response as a string into a `string` object named `inputStr`, we would need a lengthy If-Then-Else-If structure to compare `inputStr` to "yes", "Yes", "yEs", "yeS", and so on.

As an alternative, let's inspect only the first character of the input string, comparing it with 'Y', 'y', 'N', or 'n', and then ignore the rest of the string. The `string` class allows you to access an individual character in a string by giving its position number in square brackets:

StringObject [Position]

Within a string, the first character is at position 0, the second is at position 1, and so forth. Therefore, the value of Position must be greater than or equal to 0 and less than or equal to the string length minus 1. For example, if `inputStr` is a `string` object and `ch` is a `char` variable, the statement

```
ch = inputStr[2];
```

accesses the character at position 2 of the string (the third character) and copies it into `ch`.

Now we can sketch out the code for reading a "Yes" or "No" response, checking only the first letter of that response.

```
string inputStr;
    ⋮
cout << "Enter Yes or No: ";
cin >> inputStr;
if (toupper(inputStr[0]) == 'Y')
```

```
{
    ⋮
}
else if (toupper(inputStr[0]) == 'N')
{
    ⋮
}
else
    PrintErrorMsg();
```

More on Floating-Point Numbers

We have used floating-point numbers off and on since we introduced them in Chapter 2, but we have not examined them in depth. Floating-point numbers have special properties when used on the computer. Thus far, we've almost ignored these properties, but now it's time to consider them in detail.

Representation of Floating-Point Numbers

Let's assume we have a computer in which each memory location is the same size and is divided into a sign plus five decimal digits. When a variable or constant is defined, the location assigned to it consists of five digits and a sign. When an `int` variable or constant is defined, the interpretation of the number stored in that place is straightforward. When a `float` variable or constant is defined, the number stored there has both a whole number part and a fractional part, so it must be coded to represent both parts.

Let's see what such coded numbers might look like. The range of whole numbers we can represent with five digits is −99,999 through +99,999:

−99999 through +99999

| + | 9 | 9 | 9 | 9 | 9 | Largest positive number |

| + | 0 | 0 | 0 | 0 | 0 | Zero |

| − | 9 | 9 | 9 | 9 | 9 | Largest negative number |

Our **precision** (the number of digits we can represent) is five digits, and each number within that range can be represented exactly.

What happens if we allow one of those digits (the leftmost one, for example) to represent an exponent?

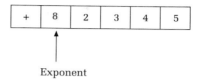

Exponent

Then +82345 represents the number $+2345 \times 10^8$. The range of numbers we now can represent is much larger:

-9999×10^9 through 9999×10^9

or

$-9,999,000,000,000$ through $+9,999,000,000,000$

However, our precision is now only four digits; that is, only four-digit numbers can be represented exactly in our system. What happens to numbers with more digits? The four leftmost digits are represented correctly, and the rightmost digits, or least significant digits, are lost (assumed to be 0). Figure 10-2 shows what happens. Note that 1,000,000 can be repre-

NUMBER	POWER OF TEN NOTATION	CODED REPRESENTATION						VALUE
		Sign	Exp					
+99,999	$+9999 \times 10^1$	+	1	9	9	9	9	+99,990
		Sign	Exp					
−999,999	-9999×10^2	−	2	9	9	9	9	−999,900
		Sign	Exp					
+1,000,000	-1000×10^3	+	3	1	0	0	0	+1,000,000
		Sign	Exp					
−4,932,416	-4932×10^3	−	3	4	9	3	2	−4,932,000

FIGURE 10-2   Coding Using Positive Exponents

Figure 10-3 Coding Using Positive and Negative Exponents

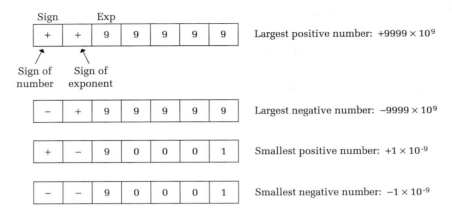

Largest positive number: $+9999 \times 10^9$

Largest negative number: -9999×10^9

Smallest positive number: $+1 \times 10^{-9}$

Smallest negative number: -1×10^{-9}

sented exactly but −4,932,416 cannot, because our coding scheme limits us to four **significant digits.**

To extend our coding scheme to represent floating-point numbers, we must be able to represent negative exponents. Examples are

$$7394 \times 10^{-2} = 73.94$$

and

$$22 \times 10^{-4} = .0022$$

Because our scheme does not include a sign for the exponent, let's change it slightly. The existing sign becomes the sign of the exponent, and we add a sign to the far left to represent the sign of the number itself (see Figure 10-3).

All the numbers between -9999×10^9 and 9999×10^9 can now be represented accurately to four digits. Adding negative exponents to our scheme allows us to represent fractional numbers as small as 1×10^{-9}.

Figure 10-4 shows how we would encode some floating-point numbers. Note that our precision is still only four digits. The numbers 0.1032, −5.406, and 1,000,000 can be represented exactly. The number 476.0321, however, with seven significant digits, is represented as 476.0; the *321* cannot be represented. (We should point out that some computers perform *rounding* rather than simple truncation when discarding excess digits. Using our assumption of four significant digits, such a machine would store 476.0321 as 476.0 but would store 476.0823 as 476.1. We continue our discussion assuming simple truncation rather than rounding.)

Figure 10-4 Coding of Some Floating-Point Numbers

NUMBER	POWER OF TEN NOTATION	CODED REPRESENTATION Sign		Exp					VALUE
0.1032	$+1032 \times 10^{-4}$	+	–	4	1	0	3	2	0.1032
–5.4060	-5406×10^{-3}	–	–	3	5	4	0	6	–5.406
–0.003	-3000×10^{-6}	–	–	6	3	0	0	0	–0.0030
476.0321	$+4760 \times 10^{-1}$	+	–	1	4	7	6	0	476.0
1,000,000	$+1000 \times 10^{3}$	+	+	3	1	0	0	0	1,000,000

Arithmetic with Floating-Point Numbers

When we use integer arithmetic, our results are exact. Floating-point arithmetic, however, is seldom exact. To understand why, let's add three floating-point numbers *x*, *y*, and *z* using our coding scheme.

First, we add *x* to *y* and then we add *z* to the result. Next, we perform the operations in a different order, adding *y* to *z*, and then adding *x* to that result. The associative law of arithmetic says that the two answers should be the same—but are they? Let's use the following values for *x*, *y*, and *z*:

$$x = -1324 \times 10^3 \qquad y = 1325 \times 10^3 \qquad z = 5424 \times 10^0$$

Here is the result of adding *z* to the sum of *x* and *y*:

$$\begin{array}{lll} (x) & -1324 \times 10^3 & \\ (y) & \underline{1325 \times 10^3} & \\ & 1 \times 10^3 & = 1000 \times 10^0 \\ & & \\ (x+y) & 1000 \times 10^0 & \\ (z) & \underline{5424 \times 10^0} & \\ & 6424 \times 10^0 & \leftarrow (x+y)+z \end{array}$$

Now here is the result of adding x to the sum of y and z:

(y)	1325000×10^0	
(z)	5424×10^0	
	1330424×10^0	$= 1330 \times 10^3$ (truncated to four digits)

(y + z)	1330×10^3	
(x)	-1324×10^3	
	6×10^3	$= 6000 \times 10^0 \leftarrow x + (y + z)$

These two answers are the same in the thousands place but are different thereafter. The error behind this discrepancy is called **representational error.**

Because of representational errors, it is unwise to use a floating-point variable as a loop control variable. Because precision may be lost in calculations involving floating-point numbers, it is difficult to predict when (or even *if*) a loop control variable of type `float` (or `double` or `long double`) will equal the termination value. A count-controlled loop with a floating-point control variable can behave unpredictably.

Also because of representational errors, you should never compare floating-point numbers for exact equality. Rarely are two floating-point numbers exactly equal, and thus you should compare them only for near equality. If the difference between the two numbers is less than some acceptable small value, you can consider them equal for the purposes of the given problem.

Implementation of Floating-Point Numbers in the Computer

Let's formally define some of the terms we used informally in the previous sections.

Significant digits   Those digits from the first nonzero digit on the left to the last nonzero digit on the right (plus any 0 digits that are exact).

Precision   The maximum number of significant digits.

Representational error   Arithmetic error that occurs when the precision of the true result of an arithmetic operation is greater than the precision of the machine.

More on Floating-Point Numbers

All computers limit the precision of floating-point numbers, although modern machines use binary rather than decimal arithmetic. In our representation, we used only 5 digits to simplify the examples, and some computers really are limited to only 4 or 5 digits of precision. A more typical system might provide 6 significant digits for `float` values, 15 digits for `double` values, and 19 for the `long double` type. We have shown only a single-digit exponent, but most systems allow 2 digits for the `float` type and up to 4-digit exponents for type `long double`.

When you declare a floating-point variable, part of the memory location is assumed to contain the exponent, and the number itself (called the *mantissa*) is assumed to be in the balance of the location. The system is called floating-point representation because the number of significant digits is fixed, and the decimal point conceptually is allowed to float (move to different positions as necessary). In our coding scheme, every number is stored as four digits, with the leftmost digit being nonzero and the exponent adjusted accordingly. Numbers in this form are said to be *normalized*. The number 1,000,000 is stored as

+	+	3	1	0	0	0

and 0.1032 is stored as

+	−	4	1	0	3	2

Normalization provides the maximum precision possible.

Model Numbers Any real number that can be represented exactly as a floating-point number in the computer is called a *model number*. A real number whose value cannot be represented exactly is approximated by the model number closest to it. In our system with four digits of precision, 0.3021 is a model number. The values 0.3021409, 0.3021222, and 0.30209999999 are examples of real numbers that are represented in the computer by the same model number. The following table shows all of the model numbers for an even simpler floating-point system that has one digit in the mantissa and an exponent that can be −1, 0, or 1.

0.1×10^{-1}	0.1×10^{0}	$0.1 \times 10^{+1}$
0.2×10^{-1}	0.2×10^{0}	$0.2 \times 10^{+1}$
0.3×10^{-1}	0.3×10^{0}	$0.3 \times 10^{+1}$
0.4×10^{-1}	0.4×10^{0}	$0.4 \times 10^{+1}$
0.5×10^{-1}	0.5×10^{0}	$0.5 \times 10^{+1}$
0.6×10^{-1}	0.6×10^{0}	$0.6 \times 10^{+1}$
0.7×10^{-1}	0.7×10^{0}	$0.7 \times 10^{+1}$
0.8×10^{-1}	0.8×10^{0}	$0.8 \times 10^{+1}$
0.9×10^{-1}	0.9×10^{0}	$0.9 \times 10^{+1}$

The difference between a real number and the model number that represents it is a form of representational error called *rounding error.* We can measure rounding error in two ways. The *absolute error* is the difference between the real number and the model number. For example, the absolute error in representing 0.3021409 by the model number 0.3021 is 0.0000409. The *relative error* is the absolute error divided by the real number and sometimes is stated as a percentage. For example, 0.0000409 divided by 0.3021409 is 0.000135, or 0.0135%.

The maximum absolute error depends on the *model interval*—the difference between two adjacent model numbers. In our example, the interval between 0.3021 and 0.3022 is 0.0001. The maximum absolute error in this system, for this interval, is less than 0.0001. Adding digits of precision makes the model interval (and thus the maximum absolute error) smaller.

The model interval is not a fixed number; it varies with the exponent. To see why the interval varies, consider that the interval between 3021.0 and 3022.0 is 1.0, which is 10^4 times larger than the interval between 0.3021 and 0.3022. This makes sense, because 3021.0 is simply 0.3021 times 10^4. Thus, a change in the exponent of the model numbers adjacent to the interval has an equivalent effect on the size of the interval. In practical terms, this means that we give up significant digits in the fractional part in order to represent numbers with large integer parts. Figure 10-5 illustrates this by graphing all of the model numbers listed in the preceding table.

We also can use relative and absolute error to measure the rounding error resulting from calculations. For example, suppose we multiply 1.0005 by 1000. The correct result is 1000.5, but because of rounding error, our four-digit computer produces 1000.0 as its result. The absolute error of the computed result is 0.5, and the relative error is 0.05%. Now suppose we multiply 100,050.0 by 1000. The correct result is 100,050,000, but the computer produces 100,000,000 as its result. If we look at the relative error, it is still a modest 0.05%, but the absolute error has grown to 50,000. Notice that this example is another case of changing the size of the model interval.

FIGURE 10-5
A Graphical
Representation of
Model Numbers

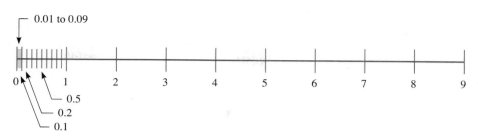

Whether it is more important to consider the absolute error or the relative error depends on the situation. It is unacceptable for an audit of a company to discover a $50,000 accounting error; the fact that the relative error is only 0.05% is not important. On the other hand, a 0.05% relative error is acceptable in representing prehistoric dates because the error in measurement techniques increases with age. That is, if we are talking about a date roughly 10,000 years ago, an absolute error of 5 years is acceptable; if the date is 100,000,000 years ago, then an absolute error of 50,000 years is equally acceptable.

Comparing Floating-Point Numbers We have cautioned against comparing floating-point numbers for exact equality. Our exploration of representational errors in this chapter reveals why calculations may not produce the expected results even though it appears that they should. In Chapter 5, we wrote an expression that compares two floating-point variables r and s for near equality using the floating-point absolute value function fabs:

```
fabs(r - s) < 0.00001
```

From our discussion of model numbers, you now can recognize that the constant 0.00001 in this expression represents a maximum absolute error. We can generalize this expression as

```
fabs(r - s) < ERROR_TERM
```

where ERROR_TERM is a value that must be determined for each programming problem.

What if we want to compare floating-point numbers with a relative error measure? We must multiply the error term by the value in the problem that the error is relative to. For example, if we want to test whether r and s are "equal" within 0.05% of s, we write the following expression:

```
fabs(r - s) < 0.0005 * s
```

Keep in mind that the choice of the acceptable error and whether it should be absolute or relative depends on the problem being solved. The error terms we have shown in our example expressions are completely arbitrary and may not be appropriate for most problems. In solving a problem that involves the comparison of floating-point numbers, you typically want an error term that is as small as possible. Sometimes the choice is specified in the problem description or is reasonably obvious. Some cases require careful analysis of both the mathematics of the problem and the representational limits of the particular computer. Such analyses are the domain of a branch of mathematics called *numerical analysis* and are beyond the scope of this text.

Underflow and Overflow   In addition to representational errors, there are two other problems to watch out for in floating-point arithmetic: *underflow* and *overflow*.

Underflow is the condition that arises when the value of a calculation is too small to be represented. Going back to our decimal representation, let's look at a calculation involving small numbers:

$$\begin{array}{r} 4210 \times 10^{-8} \\ \times\, 2000 \times 10^{-8} \\ \hline 8420000 \times 10^{-16} \quad = 8420 \times 10^{-13} \end{array}$$

This value cannot be represented in our scheme because the exponent −13 is too small. Our minimum is −9. One way to resolve the problem is to set the result of the calculation to 0.0. Obviously, any answer depending on this calculation will not be exact.

Overflow is a more serious problem because there is no logical recourse when it occurs. For example, the result of the calculation

$$\begin{array}{r} 9999 \times 10^{9} \\ \times\, 1000 \times 10^{9} \\ \hline 9999000 \times 10^{18} \quad = 9999 \times 10^{21} \end{array}$$

cannot be stored, so what should we do? To be consistent with our response to underflow, we could set the result to 9999×10^{9} (the maximum representable value in this case). Yet this seems intuitively wrong. The alternative is to stop with an error message.

C++ does not define what should happen in the case of overflow or underflow. Different implementations of C++ solve the problem in different ways. You might try to cause an overflow with your system and see what happens. Some systems may print a run-time error message such as

"FLOATING POINT OVERFLOW." On other systems, you may get the largest number that can be represented.

Although we are discussing problems with floating-point numbers, integer numbers also can overflow both negatively and positively. Most implementations of C++ ignore integer overflow. To see how your system handles the situation, you should try adding 1 to INT_MAX and −1 to INT_MIN. On most systems, adding 1 to INT_MAX sets the result to INT_MIN, a negative number.

Sometimes you can avoid overflow by arranging computations carefully. Suppose you want to know how many different five-card poker hands can be dealt from a deck of cards. What we are looking for is the number of *combinations* of 52 cards taken 5 at a time. The standard mathematical formula for the number of combinations of n things taken r at a time is

$$\frac{n!}{r!\,(n-r)!}$$

We could use the Factorial function we wrote in Chapter 8 and write this formula in an assignment statement:

```
hands = Factorial(52) / (Factorial(5) * Factorial(47));
```

The only problem is that 52! is a very large number (approximately 8.0658×10^{67}). And 47! is also large (approximately 2.5862×10^{59}). Both of these numbers are well beyond the capacity of most systems to represent exactly as integers (52! requires 68 digits of precision). Even though they can be represented on many machines as floating-point numbers, most of the precision is still lost. By rearranging the calculations, however, we can achieve an exact result on any system with 9 or more digits of precision. How? Consider that most of the multiplications in computing 52! are canceled when the product is divided by 47!

$$\frac{52!}{5! \times 47!} = \frac{52 \times 51 \times 50 \times 49 \times 48 \times 47 \times 46 \times 45 \times 44 \times \ldots}{(5 \times 4 \times 3 \times 2 \times 1) \times (47 \times 46 \times 45 \times 44 \times \ldots)}$$

So, we really only have to compute

```
hands = 52 * 51 * 50 * 49 * 48 / Factorial(5);
```

which means the numerator is 311,875,200 and the denominator is 120. On a system with 9 or more digits of precision, we get an exact answer: 2,598,960 poker hands.

Cancellation Error   Another type of error that can happen with floating-point numbers is called *cancellation error*, a form of representational error that occurs when numbers of widely differing magnitudes are added or subtracted. Let's look at an example:

$$(1 + 0.00001234 - 1) = 0.00001234$$

The laws of arithmetic say this equation should be true. But is it true if the computer does the arithmetic?

$$
\begin{array}{r}
100000000 \times 10^{-8} \\
+ \quad 1234 \times 10^{-8} \\
\hline
100001234 \times 10^{-8}
\end{array}
$$

To four digits, the sum is 1000×10^{-3}. Now the computer subtracts 1:

$$
\begin{array}{r}
1000 \times 10^{-3} \\
-1000 \times 10^{-3} \\
\hline
0
\end{array}
$$

The result is 0, not .00001234.

Sometimes you can avoid adding two floating-point numbers that are drastically different in size by carefully arranging the calculations. Suppose a problem requires many small floating-point numbers to be added to a large floating-point number. The result is more accurate if the program first sums the smaller numbers to obtain a larger number and then adds the sum to the large number.

At this point, you may want to turn to the first Problem-Solving Case Study at the end of the chapter. This case study involves floating-point computations, and it addresses some of the issues you have learned about in this section.

---

*B*ACKGROUND INFORMATION

Practical Implications of Limited Precision

A discussion of representational, overflow, underflow, and cancellation errors may seem purely academic. In fact, these errors have serious practical implications in many problems. We close this section with three examples illustrating how limited precision can have costly or even disastrous effects.

During the Mercury space program, several of the spacecraft splashed down a considerable distance from their computed landing points. This delayed the recovery of the spacecraft and the astronaut, putting both in some danger. Eventually, the problem was traced to an imprecise representation of the Earth's rotation period in the program that calculated the landing point.

As part of the construction of a hydroelectric dam, a long set of high-tension cables had to be constructed to link the dam to the nearest power distribution point. The cables were to be several miles long, and each one was to be a continuous unit. (Because of the high power output from the dam, shorter cables couldn't be spliced together.) The cables were constructed at great expense and strung between the two points. It turned out that they were too short, however, so another set had to be manufactured. The problem was traced to errors of precision in calculating the length of the catenary curve (the curve that a cable forms when hanging between two points).

An audit of a bank turned up a mysterious account with a large amount of money in it. The account was traced to an unscrupulous programmer who had used limited precision to his advantage. The bank computed interest on its accounts to a precision of a tenth of a cent. The tenths of cents were not added to the customers' accounts, so the programmer had the extra tenths for all the accounts summed and deposited into an account in his name. Because the bank had thousands of accounts, these tiny amounts added up to a large amount of money. And because the rest of the bank's programs did not use as much precision in their calculations, the scheme went undetected for many months.

The moral of this discussion is twofold: (1) The results of floating-point calculations are often imprecise, and these errors can have serious consequences; and (2) if you are working with extremely large numbers or extremely small numbers, you need more information than this book provides and should consult a numerical analysis text.

SOFTWARE ENGINEERING TIP

Choosing a Numeric Data Type

A first encounter with all the numeric data types of C++ may leave you feeling overwhelmed. To help in choosing an alternative, you may even feel tempted to toss a coin. You should resist this temptation, because each data type exists for a reason. Here are some guidelines:

1. In general, int is preferable.

    As a rule, you should use floating-point types *only* when absolutely necessary—that is, when you definitely need fractional values. Not only is floating-point arithmetic subject to representational errors, it also is significantly slower than integer arithmetic on most computers.

    For ordinary integer data, use int instead of char or short. It's easy to make overflow errors with these smaller data types. (For character data, though, the char type is appropriate.)

2. Use `long` only if the range of `int` values on your machine is too restrictive.
   Compared to `int`, the `long` type requires more memory space and execution time.

3. Use `double` and `long double` only if you need enormously large or small numbers, or if your machine's `float` values do not carry enough digits of precision.
   The cost of using `double` and `long double` is increased memory space and execution time.

4. Avoid the `unsigned` forms of integral types.
   These types are primarily for manipulating bits within a memory cell, a topic this book does not cover. You might think that declaring a variable as `unsigned` prevents you from accidentally storing a negative number into the variable. However, the C++ compiler does *not* prevent you from doing so. Later in this chapter, we explain why.

By following these guidelines, you'll find that the simple types you use most often are `int` and `float`, along with `char` for character data and `bool` for Boolean data. Only rarely do you need the longer and shorter variations of these fundamental types.

User-Defined Simple Types

The concept of a data type is fundamental to all of the widely used programming languages. One of the strengths of the C++ language is that it allows programmers to create new data types, tailored to meet the needs of a particular program. Much of the remainder of this book is about user-defined data types. In this section, we examine how to create our own simple types.

The Typedef Statement

The *Typedef statement* allows you to introduce a new name for an existing type. Its syntax template is

TypedefStatement

> **typedef** ExistingTypeName NewTypeName ;

Before the `bool` data type was part of the C++ language, many programmers used code like the following to simulate a Boolean type:

```
typedef int Boolean;
const int TRUE = 1;
const int FALSE = 0;
   ⋮
Boolean dataOK;
   ⋮
dataOK = TRUE;
```

In this code, the Typedef statement causes the compiler to substitute the word `int` for every occurrence of the word `Boolean` in the rest of the program.

The Typedef statement provides a very limited way of defining our own data types. In fact, Typedef does not create a new data type at all: It merely creates an additional name for an existing data type. As far as the compiler is concerned, the domain and operations of the above `Boolean` type are identical to the domain and operations of the `int` type.

Despite the fact that Typedef cannot truly create a new data type, it is a valuable tool for writing self-documenting programs. Before `bool` was a built-in type, program code that used the identifiers `Boolean`, `TRUE`, and `FALSE` was more descriptive than code that used `int`, 1, and 0 for Boolean operations.

Names of user-defined types obey the same scope rules that apply to identifiers in general. Most types like `Boolean` above are defined globally, although it is reasonable to define a new type within a subprogram if that is the only place it is used. The guidelines that determine where a named constant should be defined apply also to data types.

Enumeration Types

C++ allows the user to define a new simple type by listing (enumerating) the literal values that make up the domain of the type. These literal values must be *identifiers*, not numbers. The identifiers are separated by commas, and the list is enclosed in braces. Data types defined in this way are called **enumeration types.** Here's an example:

```
enum Days {SUN, MON, TUE, WED, THU, FRI, SAT};
```

This declaration creates a new data type named `Days`. Whereas Typedef merely creates a synonym for an existing type, an enumeration type like `Days` is truly a new type and is distinct from any existing type.

The values in the Days type—SUN, MON, TUE, and so forth—are called **enumerators.** The enumerators are *ordered*, in the sense that SUN < MON < TUE ... < FRI < SAT. Applying relational operators to enumerators is like applying them to characters: The relation that is tested is whether an enumerator "comes before" or "comes after" in the ordering of the data type.

Enumeration type   A user-defined data type whose domain is an ordered set of literal values expressed as identifiers.

Enumerator   One of the values in the domain of an enumeration type.

Earlier we saw that the internal representation of a char constant is a nonnegative integer. The 128 ASCII characters are represented in memory as the integers 0 through 127. Values in an enumeration type are also represented internally as integers. By default, the first enumerator has the integer value 0, the second has the value 1, and so forth. Our declaration of the Days enumeration type is similar to the following set of declarations:

```
typedef int Days;
const int SUN = 0;
const int MON = 1;
const int TUE = 2;
   ⋮
const int SAT = 6;
```

If there is some reason that you want different internal representations for the enumerators, you can specify them explicitly like this:

```
enum Days {SUN = 4, MON = 18, TUE = 9, ... };
```

There is rarely any reason to assign specific values to enumerators. With the Days type, we are interested in the days of the week, not in the way the machine stores them internally. We do not discuss this feature any further, although you may occasionally see it in C++ programs.

Notice the style we use to capitalize enumerators. Because enumerators are, in essence, named constants, we capitalize the entire identifier. This is purely a style choice. Many C++ programmers use both uppercase and lowercase letters when they invent names for the enumerators.

Here is the syntax template for the declaration of an enumeration type. It is a simplified version; later in the chapter we expand it.

EnumDeclaration

> **enum** Name **{** Enumerator **,** Enumerator **. . . }** **;**

Each enumerator has the following form:

Enumerator

> Identifier = ConstIntExpression

where the optional ConstIntExpression is an integer expression composed only of literal or named constants.

The identifiers used as enumerators must follow the rules for any C++ identifier. For example,

```
enum Vowel {'A', 'E', 'I', 'O', 'U'};     // Error
```

is not legal because the items are not identifiers. The declaration

```
enum Places {1st, 2nd, 3rd};     // Error
```

is not legal because identifiers cannot begin with digits. In the declarations

```
enum Starch {CORN, RICE, POTATO, BEAN};
enum Grain {WHEAT, CORN, RYE, BARLEY, SORGHUM};     // Error
```

type `Starch` and type `Grain` are legal individually, but together they are not. Identifiers in the same scope must be unique. `CORN` cannot be defined twice.

Suppose you are writing a program for a veterinary clinic. The program must keep track of different kinds of animals. The following enumeration type might be used for this purpose.

Type identifier   Literal values in the domain

```
enum Animals {RODENT, CAT, DOG, BIRD, REPTILE, HORSE, BOVINE, SHEEP};
```

```
Animals inPatient;        Creation of two variables of type Animals
Animals outPatient;
```

`RODENT` is a literal, one of the values in the data type `Animals`. Be sure you understand that `RODENT` is not a variable name. Instead, `RODENT` is one of the values that can be stored into the variables `inPatient` and `outPatient`. Let's look at the kinds of operations we might want to perform on variables of enumeration types.

Assignment   The assignment statement

```
inPatient = DOG;
```

does not assign to `inPatient` the character string "DOG", nor the contents of a variable named `DOG`. It assigns the *value* `DOG`, which is one of the values in the domain of the data type `Animals`.

Assignment is a valid operation, as long as the value being stored is of type `Animals`. Both of the statements

```
inPatient = DOG;
outPatient = inPatient;
```

are acceptable. Each expression on the right-hand side is of type `Animals`—`DOG` is a literal of type `Animals`, and `inPatient` is a variable of type `Animals`. Although we know that the underlying representation of `DOG` is the integer 2, the compiler prevents us from using this assignment:

```
inPatient = 2;    // Not allowed
```

Here is the precise rule:

Implicit type coercion is defined from an enumeration type to an integral type but not from an integral type to an enumeration type.

Applying this rule to the statements

```
someInt = DOG;    // Valid
inPatient = 2;    // Error
```

we see that the first statement stores 2 into `someInt` (because of implicit type coercion), but the second produces a compile-time error. The restriction against storing an integer value into a variable of type `Animals` is to keep you from accidentally storing an out-of-range value:

```
inPatient = 65;    // Error
```

Incrementation Suppose that you want to "increment" the value in `inPatient` so that it becomes the next value in the domain:

```
inPatient = inPatient + 1;    // Error
```

This statement is illegal for the following reason. The right-hand side is OK because implicit type coercion lets you add `inPatient` to 1; the result is an `int` value. But the assignment operation is not valid because you can't store an `int` value into `inPatient`. The statement

```
inPatient++;    // Error
```

is also invalid because the compiler considers it to have the same semantics as the assignment statement above. However, you can escape the type coercion rule by using an *explicit* type conversion—a type cast—as follows:

```
inPatient = Animals(inPatient + 1);    // Correct
```

When you use the type cast, the compiler assumes that you know what you are doing and allows it.

Incrementing a variable of enumeration type is very useful in loops. Sometimes we need a loop that processes all the values in the domain of the type. We might try the following For loop:

```
Animals patient;

for (patient=RODENT; patient <= SHEEP; patient++)   // Error
    ⋮
```

However, as we explained above, the compiler will complain about the expression `patient++`. To increment `patient`, we must use an assignment expression and a type cast:

```
for (patient=RODENT; patient <= SHEEP; patient=Animals(patient + 1))
    ⋮
```

The only caution here is that when control exits the loop, the value of patient is 1 *greater than* the largest value in the domain (SHEEP). If you want to use patient outside the loop, you must reassign it a value that is within the appropriate range for the Animals type.

Comparison   The most common operation performed on values of enumeration types is comparison. When you compare two values, their ordering is determined by the order in which you listed the enumerators in the type declaration. For instance, the expression

```
inPatient <= BIRD
```

has the value true if inPatient contains the value RODENT, CAT, DOG, or BIRD.

You can also use values of an enumeration type in a Switch statement. Because RODENT, CAT, and so on are literals, they can appear in case labels:

```
switch (inPatient)
{
    case RODENT  :
    case CAT     :
    case DOG     :
    case BIRD    : cout << "Cage ward";
                     break;
    case REPTILE : cout << "Terrarium ward";
                     break;
    case HORSE   :
    case BOVINE  :
    case SHEEP   : cout << "Barn";
}
```

Input and Output   Stream I/O is defined only for the basic built-in types (int, float, and so on), not for user-defined enumeration types. Values of enumeration types must be input or output indirectly.

To input values, one strategy is to read a string that spells one of the constants in the enumeration type. The idea is to input the string and translate it to one of the literals in the enumeration type by looking only at as many letters as are necessary to determine what it is.

For example, the veterinary clinic program could read the kind of animal as a string, then assign one of the values of type Animals to that patient. *Cat, dog, horse,* and *sheep* can be determined by their first letter. *Bovine, bird, rodent,* and *reptile* cannot be determined until the second letter is examined. The following program fragment reads in a string representing an animal name and converts it to one of the values in type Animals.

```
#include <cctype>      // For toupper()
#include <string>      // For string type
    ⋮
string animalName;
    ⋮
cin >> animalName;
switch (toupper(animalName[0]))
{
    case 'R' : if (toupper(animalName[1]) == 'O')
                   inPatient = RODENT;
               else
                   inPatient = REPTILE;
               break;
    case 'C' : inPatient = CAT;
               break;
    case 'D' : inPatient = DOG;
               break;
    case 'B' : if (toupper(animalName[1]) == 'I')
                   inPatient = BIRD;
               else
                   inPatient = BOVINE;
               break;
    case 'H' : inPatient = HORSE;
               break;
    default  : inPatient = SHEEP;
}
```

Enumeration type values cannot be printed directly either. Printing is done by using a Switch statement that prints a character string corresponding to the value.

```
switch (inPatient)
{
    case RODENT  : cout << "Rodent";
                   break;
    case CAT     : cout << "Cat";
                   break;
    case DOG     : cout << "Dog";
                   break;
    case BIRD    : cout << "Bird";
                   break;
    case REPTILE : cout << "Reptile";
                   break;
    case HORSE   : cout << "Horse";
                   break;
    case BOVINE  : cout << "Bovine";
                   break;
    case SHEEP   : cout << "Sheep";
}
```

You might ask, Why not use just a pair of letters or an integer number as a code to represent each animal in a program? The answer is that we use enumeration types to make our programs more readable; they are another way to make the code more self-documenting.

Returning a Function Value We have been using value-returning functions to compute and return values of built-in types such as int, float, and char:

```
int Factorial( int );
float CargoMoment( int );
```

C++ allows a function return value to be of *any* data type—built-in or user-defined—except an array (a data type we examine in later chapters).

In the last section, we wrote a Switch statement to convert an input string into a value of type Animals. Let's write a value-returning function that performs this task. Notice how the function heading declares the data type of the return value to be Animals.

```
Animals StrToAnimal( /* in */ string str )
{
    switch (toupper(str[0]))
    {
        case 'R' : if (toupper(str[1]) == 'O')
                       return RODENT;
                   else
                       return REPTILE;
        case 'C' : return CAT;
        case 'D' : return DOG;
        case 'B' : if (toupper(str[1]) == 'I')
                       return BIRD;
                   else
                       return BOVINE;
        case 'H' : return HORSE;
        default  :  return SHEEP;
    }
}
```

In this function, why didn't we include a Break statement after each case alternative? Because when one of the alternatives executes a Return statement, control immediately exits the function. It's not possible for control to "fall through" to the next alternative.

Here is a sample of code that calls the StrToAnimal function:

```
enum Animals {RODENT, CAT, DOG, BIRD, REPTILE, HORSE, BOVINE, SHEEP};

Animals StrToAnimal( string );
  ⋮
int main()
{
    Animals inPatient;
    Animals outPatient;
    string  inputStr;
      ⋮
    cin >> inputStr;
    inPatient = StrToAnimal(inputStr);
      ⋮
    cin >> inputStr;
    outPatient = StrToAnimal(inputStr);
      ⋮
}
```

Named and Anonymous Data Types

The enumeration types we have looked at, `Animals` and `Days`, are called **named types** because their declarations included names for the types. Variables of these new data types are declared separately using the type identifiers `Animals` and `Days`.

Named type A user-defined type whose declaration includes a type identifier that gives a name to the type.

C++ also lets us introduce a new type directly in a variable declaration. Instead of the declarations

```
enum CoinType {NICKEL, DIME, QUARTER, HALF_DOLLAR};
enum StatusType {OK, OUT_OF_STOCK, BACK_ORDERED};

CoinType   change;
StatusType status;
```

we could write

```
enum {NICKEL, DIME, QUARTER, HALF_DOLLAR} change;
enum {OK, OUT_OF_STOCK, BACK_ORDERED} status;
```

A new type declared in a variable declaration is called an **anonymous type** because it does not have a name—that is, it does not have a type identifier associated with it.

Anonymous type   A type that does not have an associated type identifier.

If we can create a data type in a variable declaration, why bother with a separate type declaration that creates a named type? Named types, like named constants, make a program more readable, more understandable, and easier to modify. Also, declaring a type and declaring a variable of that type are two distinct concepts; it is best to keep them separate.

We now give a more complete syntax template for an enumeration type declaration. This template shows that the type name is optional (yielding an anonymous type) and that a list of variables may optionally be included in the declaration.

EnumDeclaration

enum Name **{** Enumerator **,** Enumerator ... **}** VariableName **,** VariableName ... **;**

User-Written Header Files

As you create your own user-defined data types, you often find that a data type can be useful in more than one program. For example, you may be working on several programs that need an enumeration type consisting of the names of the 12 months of the year. Instead of typing the statement

```
enum Months
{
    JANUARY, FEBRUARY, MARCH, APRIL, MAY, JUNE,
    JULY, AUGUST, SEPTEMBER, OCTOBER, NOVEMBER, DECEMBER
};
```

at the beginning of every program that uses the Months type, you can put this statement into a separate file named, say, months.h. Then you use months.h just as you use system-supplied header files such as iostream and cmath. By using an #include directive, you ask the C++ preprocessor to insert the contents of the file physically into your program. (Although many C++ systems use the filename extension .h [or no extension at all] to denote header files, other systems use extensions such as .hpp or .hxx.)

When you enclose the name of a header file in angle brackets, as in

```
#include <iostream>
```

the preprocessor looks for the file in the standard *include directory,* a directory that contains all the header files supplied by the C++ system. On the other hand, you can enclose the name of a header file in double quotes, like this:

```
#include "months.h"
```

In this case, the preprocessor looks for the file in the programmer's current directory. This mechanism allows us to write our own header files that contain type declarations and constant declarations. We can use a simple #include directive instead of retyping the declarations in every program that needs them (see Figure 10-6.)

More on Type Coercion

As you have learned over the course of several chapters, C++ performs implicit type coercion whenever values of different data types are used in the following:

1. Arithmetic and relational expressions
2. Assignment operations
3. Argument passing
4. Return of the function value from a value-returning function

For item 1—mixed type expressions—the C++ compiler follows one set of rules for type coercion. For items 2, 3, and 4, the compiler follows a second set of rules. Let's examine each of these two rules.

FIGURE 10-6
Including
Header Files

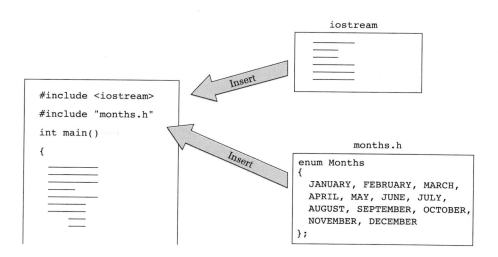

Type Coercion in Arithmetic and Relational Expressions

Suppose that an arithmetic expression consists of one operator and two operands—for example, `3.4*sum` or `var1/var2`. If the two operands are of different data types, then one of them is temporarily **promoted** (or **widened**) to match the data type of the other. To understand exactly what promotion means, let's look at the rule for type coercion in an arithmetic expression.*

Step 1:   Each `char`, `short`, `bool`, or enumeration value is promoted (widened) to `int`. If both operands are now `int`, the result is an `int` expression.

Step 2:   If step 1 still leaves a mixed type expression, the following precedence of types is used:

$$\text{lowest} \longrightarrow \text{highest}$$

`int, unsigned int, long, unsigned long, float, double, long double`

The value of the operand of "lower" type is promoted to that of the "higher" type, and the result is an expression of that type.

A simple example is the expression `someFloat+2`. This expression has no `char`, `short`, `bool`, or enumeration values in it, so step 1 still leaves a mixed type expression. In step 2, `int` is a "lower" type than `float`, so the value 2 is coerced temporarily to the `float` value, say, 2.0. Then the addition takes place, and the type of the entire expression is `float`.

This description of type coercion also holds for relational expressions such as

`someInt <= someFloat`

The value of `someInt` is temporarily coerced to floating-point representation before the comparison takes place. The only difference between arithmetic expressions and relational expressions is that the resulting type of a relational expression is always `bool`—the value `true` or `false`.

Promotion (widening)   The conversion of a value from a "lower" type to a "higher" type according to a programming language's precedence of data types.

---

* The rule we give for type coercion is a simplified version of the rule found in the C++ language definition. The complete rule has more to say about unsigned types, which we rarely use in this book.

Here is a table that describes the result of promoting a value from one simple type to another in C++:

From	To	Result of Promotion
double	long double	Same value, occupying more memory space
float	double	Same value, occupying more memory space
Integral type	Floating-point type	Floating-point equivalent of the integer value; fractional part is zero
Integral type	Its unsigned counterpart	Same value, if original number is nonnegative; a radically different positive number, if original number is negative
Signed integral type	Longer signed integral type	Same value, occupying more memory space
unsigned integral type	Longer integral type (either signed or unsigned)	Same nonnegative value, occupying more memory space

NOTE: The result of promoting a char to an int is compiler dependent. Some compilers treat char as unsigned char, so promotion always yields a nonnegative integer. With other compilers, char means signed char, so promotion of a negative value yields a negative integer.

The note at the bottom of the table suggests a potential problem if you are trying to write a portable C++ program. If you use the char type only to store character data, there is no problem. C++ guarantees that each character in a machine's character set (such as ASCII) is represented as a nonnegative value. Using character data, promotion from char to int gives the same result on any machine with any compiler.

But if you try to save memory by using the char type for manipulating small signed integers, then promotion of these values to the int type can produce different results on different machines! That is, one machine may promote negative char values to negative int values, whereas the same program on another machine might promote negative char values to *positive* int values. The moral is this: Unless you are squeezed to the limit for memory space, do not use char to manipulate small signed numbers. Use char only to store character data.

Type Coercion in Assignments, Argument Passing, and Return of a Function Value

In general, promotion of a value from one type to another does not cause loss of information. Think of promotion as moving your baseball cards from a small shoe box to a larger shoe box. All of the cards still fit into the new box and there is room to spare. On the other hand, **demotion** (or **narrowing**) of data values can potentially cause loss of information. Demotion is like moving a shoe box full of baseball cards into a smaller box—something has to be thrown out.

Demotion (narrowing)   The conversion of a value from a "higher" type to a "lower" type according to a programming language's precedence of data types. Demotion may cause loss of information.

Consider an assignment operation

$$v = e$$

where v is a variable and e is an expression. Regarding the data types of v and e, there are three possibilities:

1. If the types of v and e are the same, no type coercion is necessary.
2. If the type of v is "higher" than that of e (using the type precedence we explained with promotion), then the value of e is promoted to v's type before being stored into v.
3. If the type of v is "lower" than that of e, the value of e is demoted to v's type before being stored into v.

Demotion, which you can think of as shrinking a value, may cause loss of information:

- Demotion from a longer integral type to a shorter integral type (such as `long` to `int`) results in discarding the leftmost (most significant) bits in the binary number representation. The result may be a drastically different number.
- Demotion from a floating-point type to an integral type causes truncation of the fractional part (and an undefined result if the whole-number part will not fit into the destination variable). The result of truncating a negative number is machine dependent.
- Demotion from a longer floating-point type to a shorter floating-point type (such as `double` to `float`) may result in a loss of digits of precision.

Our description of type coercion in an assignment operation also holds for argument passing (the mapping of arguments onto parameters) and for returning a function value with a Return statement. For example, assume that `INT_MAX` on your machine is 32767 and that you have the following function:

```
void DoSomething( int n )
{
    ⋮
}
```

If the function is called with the statement

```
DoSomething(50000);
```

then the value 50000 (which is implicitly of type `long` because it is larger than `INT_MAX`) is demoted to a completely different, smaller value that fits into an `int` location. In a similar fashion, execution of the function

```
int SomeFunc( float x )
{
    ⋮
    return 70000;
}
```

causes demotion of the value 70000 to a smaller `int` value because `int` is the declared type of the function return value.

One interesting consequence of implicit type coercion is the futility of declaring a variable to be `unsigned`, hoping that the compiler will prevent you from making a mistake like this:

```
unsignedVar = -5;
```

The compiler does not complain at all. It generates code to coerce the `int` value to an `unsigned int` value. If you now print out the value of `unsignedVar`, you'll see a strange-looking positive integer. As we have pointed out before, `unsigned` types are most appropriate for advanced techniques that manipulate individual bits within memory cells. It's best to avoid using `unsigned` for ordinary numeric computations.

*P*ROBLEM-SOLVING CASE STUDY

Finding the Area Under a Curve

Problem: Find the area under the curve of the function X^3 over an interval specified by the user. In other words, given a pair of floating-point numbers, find the area under the graph of X^3 between those two numbers (see Figure 10-7).

Input: Two floating-point numbers specifying the interval over which to find the area, and an integer number of intervals to use in approximating the area.

FIGURE 10-7

Area Under Graph
of X^3 Between 0
and 3

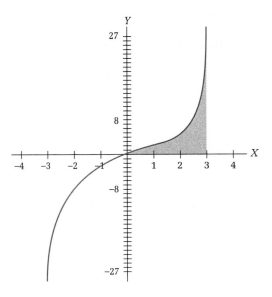

Output: The input data (echo print) and the value calculated for the area over the given interval.

Discussion: Our approach is to compute an approximation to this area. If the area under the curve is divided into equal, narrow, rectangular strips, the sum of the areas of these rectangles is close to the actual area under the curve (see Figure 10-8). The narrower the rectangles, the more accurate the approximation should be.

We can use a value-returning function to compute the area of each rectangle. The user enters the low and high values for X, as well as the number of rectangles into which the area should be subdivided (`divisions`). The width of a rectangle is then

```
(high - low) / divisions
```

The height of a rectangle equals the value of X^3 when X is at the horizontal midpoint of the rectangle. The area of a rectangle equals its height times its width. Because the leftmost rectangle has its midpoint at

```
(low + width/2.0)
```

its area equals the following (see Figure 10-9):

PROBLEM-SOLVING CASE STUDY cont'd.

FIGURE 10-8
Approximation
of Area Under a
Curve

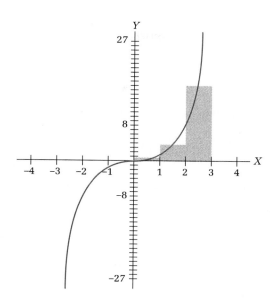

FIGURE 10-9
Area of the Left-
most Rectangle

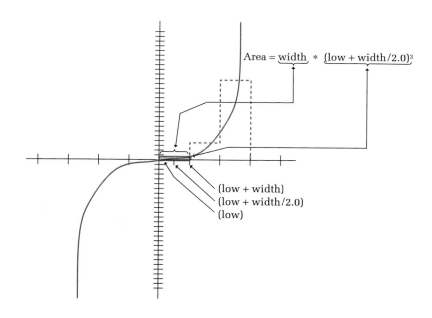

Area = width * (low + width/2.0)³

(low + width)
(low + width/2.0)
(low)

`(low + width/2.0)`^{3} `* width`

The second rectangle has its left edge at the point where X equals

`low + width`

and its area equals the following (see Figure 10-10):

`(low + width + width/2.0)`^{3} `* width`

The left edge of each rectangle is at a point that is `width` greater than the left edge of the rectangle to its left. Thus, we can step through the rectangles by using a count-controlled loop with the number of iterations equal to the value of `divisions`. This loop contains a second counter (not the loop control variable) starting at `low` and counting by steps of `width` up to (`high` − `width`). Two counters are necessary because the second counter must be of type `float`, and it is poor programming technique to have a loop control variable be a `float` variable. For each iteration of this loop, we compute the area of the corresponding rectangle and add this value to the total area under the curve.

We want a value-returning function to compute the area of a rectangle, given the position of its left edge and its width. Let's also make X^3 a separate function named `Funct`, so we can substitute other mathematical func-

FIGURE 10-10
Area of the
Second
Rectangle

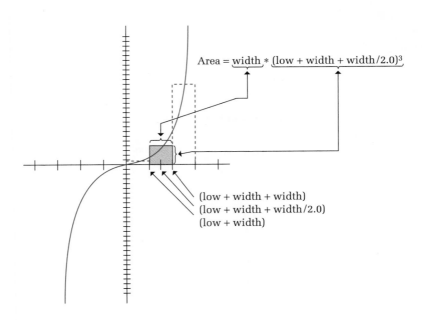

Area = $\dfrac{\text{width}}{} * \underline{(\text{low} + \text{width} + \text{width}/2.0)^3}$

(low + width + width)
(low + width + width/2.0)
(low + width)

tions in its place without changing the rest of the design. Our program can then be converted quickly to find the area under the curve of any single-variable function.

Here is our design:

Main   **Level 0**

```
Get data
Set width = (high − low) / divisions
Set area = 0.0
Set leftEdge = low
FOR count going from 1 through divisions
    Set area = area + RectArea(leftEdge, width)
    Set leftEdge = leftEdge + width
Print area
```

RectArea (In: leftEdge, width)   **Level 1**

    Out: Function value

```
Return  Funct(leftEdge + width/2.0) * width
```

Get Data (Out: low, high, divisions)

```
Prompt for low and high
Read low, high
Prompt for divisions
Read divisions
Echo print input data
```

Funct (In: x)   **Level 2**

    Out: Function value

```
Return x * x * x
```

PROBLEM-SOLVING CASE STUDY *cont'd.*

Module Structure Chart:

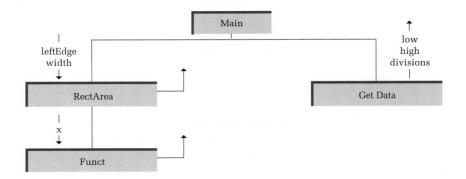

(The following program is written in ISO/ANSI standard C++. If you are working with pre–standard C++, see the alternate version of the program in the PRE_STD directory of the program disk, available at the publisher's Web site, www.jbpub.com/disks.)

```
//******************************************************************
// Area program
// This program finds the area under the curve of a mathematical
// function in a specified interval.  Input consists of two float
// values and one int.  The first two are the low, high values for
// the interval.  The third is the number of slices to be used in
// approximating the area.  As written, this program finds the
// area under the curve of the function x cubed; however, any
// single-variable function may be substituted for the function
// named Funct
//******************************************************************
#include <iostream>
#include <iomanip>       // For setprecision()

using namespace std;

float Funct( float );
void  GetData( float&, float&, int& );
float RectArea( float, float );

int main()
{
    float low;          // Lowest value in the desired interval
    float high;         // Highest value in the desired interval
    float width;        // Computed width of a rectangular slice
    float leftEdge;     // Left edge point in a rectangular slice
    float area;         // Total area under the curve
```

PROBLEM-SOLVING CASE STUDY cont'd.

```
        int    divisions;    // Number of slices to divide the interval by
        int    count;        // Loop control variable

        cout << fixed << showpoint;              // Set up floating-pt.
                                                 //   output format
        GetData(low, high, divisions);
        width = (high - low) / float(divisions);
        area = 0.0;
        leftEdge = low;

        // Calculate and sum areas of slices

        for (count = 1; count <= divisions; count++)
        {
            area = area + RectArea(leftEdge, width);
            leftEdge = leftEdge + width;
        }

        // Print result

        cout << "The result is equal to "
             << setprecision(7) << area << endl;
        return 0;
    }

    //*****************************************************************

    void GetData( /* out */ float& low,       // Bottom of interval
                  /* out */ float& high,      // Top of interval
                  /* out */ int&   divisions ) // Division factor

    // Prompts for the input of low, high, and divisions values
    // and returns the three values after echo printing them

    // Postcondition:
    //     All parameters (low, high, and divisions)
    //     have been prompted for, input, and echo printed
    {
        cout << "Enter low and high values of desired interval"
             << " (floating point)." << endl;
        cin >> low >> high;
        cout << "Enter the number of divisions to be used (integer)."
             << endl;
        cin >> divisions;
        cout << "The area is computed over the interval "
             << setprecision(7) << low << endl
             << "to " << high << " with " << divisions
             << " subdivisions of the interval." << endl;
    }
```

PROBLEM-SOLVING CASE STUDY cont'd.

```
//****************************************************************

float RectArea( /* in */ float leftEdge,    // Left edge point of
                                            //    rectangle
                 /* in */ float width    )  // Width of rectangle

// Computes the area of a rectangle that starts at leftEdge and is
// "width" units wide.  The rectangle's height is given by the value
// computed by Funct at the horizontal midpoint of the rectangle

// Precondition:
//      leftEdge and width are assigned
// Postcondition:
//      Function value == area of specified rectangle

{
    return Funct(leftEdge + width / 2.0) * width;
}

//****************************************************************

float Funct( /* in */ float x )     // Value to be cubed

// Computes x cubed.  You may replace this function with any
// single-variable function

// Precondition:
//      The absolute value of x cubed does not exceed the
//      machine's maximum float value
// Postcondition:
//      Function value == x cubed

{
    return x * x * x;
}
```

Testing: We should test this program with sets of data that include positive, negative, and zero values. It is especially important to try to input values of 0 and 1 for the number of divisions. The results from the program should be compared against values calculated by hand using the same algorithm and against the true value of the area under the curve of X^3, which is given by the formula

$$\frac{1}{4} \times (high^4 - low^4)$$

PROBLEM-SOLVING CASE STUDY cont'd.

(This formula comes from the mathematical topic of calculus. What we have been referring to as the area under the curve in the interval a to b is called the *integral* of the function from a to b.)

Let's consider for a moment the effects of representational error on this program. The user specifies the low and high values of the interval, as well as the number of subdivisions to be used in computing the result. The more subdivisions used, the more accurate the result should be because the rectangles are narrower and thus approximate more closely the shape of the area under the curve. It seems that we can obtain precise results by using a large number of subdivisions. In fact, however, there is a point beyond which an increase in the number of subdivisions *decreases* the precision of the results. If we specify too many subdivisions, the area of an individual rectangle becomes so small that the computer can no longer represent its value accurately. Adding all those inaccurate values produces a total area that has an even greater error.

PROBLEM-SOLVING CASE STUDY

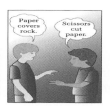

Rock, Paper, Scissors

Problem: Play the children's game Rock, Paper, Scissors. In this game, two people simultaneously choose one of the following: rock, paper, or scissors. Whether a player wins or loses depends not only on that player's choice but also on the opponent's choice. The rules are as follows:

Rock breaks scissors; rock wins.
Paper covers rock; paper wins.
Scissors cut paper; scissors win.
All matching combinations are ties.
The overall winner is the player who wins the most individual games.

Input: A series of letters representing player A's plays (fileA, one letter per line) and a series of letters representing player B's plays (fileB, one letter per line), with each play indicated by 'R' (for Rock), 'P' (for Paper), or 'S' (for Scissors).

Output: For each game, the game number and the player who won that game; at the end, the total number of games won by each player, and the overall winner.

Discussion: We assume that everyone has played this game and understands it. Therefore, our discussion centers on how to simulate the game in a program.

PROBLEM-SOLVING CASE STUDY cont'd.

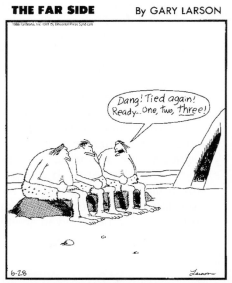

THE FAR SIDE   By GARY LARSON

Before paper and fire

In the algorithm we developed to read in animal names, we used as input a string containing the entire animal name and translated the string into a corresponding literal in an enumeration type. Here, we show an alternative approach. For input, we use a single character to stand for rock, paper, or scissors. We input 'R', 'P', or 'S' and convert the letter to a value of an enumeration type made up of the literals ROCK, PAPER, and SCIS-SORS.

Each player creates a file composed of a series of the letters 'R', 'P', and 'S', representing a series of individual games. A pair of letters is read, one from each file, and converted into the appropriate enumeration type literals. Let's call each literal a play. The plays are compared, and a winner is determined. The number of games won is incremented for the winning player each time. The game is over when there are no more plays (the files are empty).

Assumptions: The game is over when one of the files runs out of plays.

PROBLEM-SOLVING CASE STUDY cont'd.

Main   Level 0

```
Open data files (and verify success)
Get plays
WHILE NOT EOF on fileA AND NOT EOF on fileB
      IF plays are legal
                  Process plays
      ELSE
                  Print an error message
      Get plays
Print big winner
```

Get Plays (Out: playForA, playForB, legal)   Level 1

```
Read charForA (player A's play) from fileA
Read charForB (player B's play) from fileB
IF EOF on fileA OR EOF on fileB
      Return
Set legal =  (charForA is 'R', 'P', or 'S') AND
                  (charForB is 'R', 'P', or 'S')
IF legal
      Set playForA = ConversionValue(charForA)
      Set playForB = ConversionValue(charForB)
```

Process Plays (In: gameNumber, playForA, playForB; Inout: winsForA, winsForB)

```
IF playForA == playForB
      Print gameNumber, " is a tie"
ELSE IF   playForA == PAPER AND playForB == ROCK OR
                  playForA == SCISSORS AND playForB == PAPER OR
                  playForA == ROCK AND playForB == SCISSORS
      Record a win for Player A, incrementing winsForA (the number
            of games won by Player A)
ELSE
      Record a win for Player B, incrementing winsForB
```

Print Big Winner (In: winsForA, winsForB)

```
Print winsForA
Print winsForB
IF winsForA > winsForB
      Print "Player A has won the most games."
ELSE IF winsForB > winsForA
      Print "Player B has won the most games."
ELSE
      Print "Players A and B have tied."
```

ConversionValue (In: someChar)   **Level 2**
   Out: Function value

```
SWITCH someChar
      'R': Return ROCK
      'P': Return PAPER
      'S': Return SCISSORS
```

Record a Win (In: player, gameNumber; Inout: numOfWins)

```
Print message saying which player has won game number gameNumber
Increment numOfWins by 1
```

Now we are ready to code the simulation of the game. We must remember to initialize our counters. We assumed that we knew the game number for each game, yet nowhere have we kept track of the game number. We need to add a counter to our loop in the main module. Here's the revised main module:

PROBLEM-SOLVING CASE STUDY cont'd.

Main

Open data files (and verify success)
Set winsForA and winsForB = 0
Set gameNumber = 0
Get plays
WHILE NOT EOF on fileA AND NOT EOF on fileB
    Increment gameNumber by 1
    IF plays are legal
        Process plays
    ELSE
        Print an error message
    Get plays
Print big winner

Module Structure Chart:

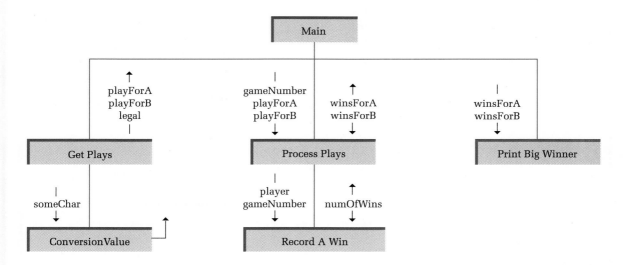

(The following program is written in ISO/ANSI standard C++. If you are working with pre–standard C++, see the alternate version of the program in the PRE_STD directory of the program disk, available at the publisher's Web site, www.jbpub.com/disks.)

PROBLEM-SOLVING CASE STUDY _cont'd._

```cpp
//*****************************************************************
// Game program
// This program simulates the children's game Rock, Paper, and
// Scissors.  Each game consists of inputs from two players,
// coming from fileA and fileB.  A winner is determined for each
// individual game and for the games overall
//*****************************************************************
#include <iostream>
#include <fstream>      // For file I/O

using namespace std;

enum PlayType {ROCK, PAPER, SCISSORS};

PlayType ConversionVal( char );
void GetPlays( ifstream&, ifstream&, PlayType&, PlayType&, bool& );
void PrintBigWinner( int, int );
void ProcessPlays( int, PlayType, PlayType, int&, int& );
void RecordAWin( char, int, int& );

int main()
{
    PlayType playForA;              // Player A's play
    PlayType playForB;              // Player B's play
    int      winsForA = 0;          // Number of games A wins
    int      winsForB = 0;          // Number of games B wins
    int      gameNumber = 0;        // Number of games played
    bool     legal;                 // True if play is legal
    ifstream fileA;                 // Player A's plays
    ifstream fileB;                 // Player B's plays

    // Open the input files

    fileA.open("filea.dat");
    fileB.open("fileb.dat");
    if ( !fileA || !fileB )
    {
        cout << "** Can't open input file(s) **" << endl;
        return 1;
    }

    // Play a series of games and keep track of who wins

    GetPlays(fileA, fileB, playForA, playForB, legal);
    while (fileA && fileB)
    {
        gameNumber++;
```

PROBLEM-SOLVING CASE STUDY cont'd.

```
            if (legal)
                ProcessPlays(gameNumber, playForA, playForB, winsForA,
                            winsForB);
            else
                cout << "Game number " << gameNumber
                    << " contained an illegal play." << endl;
            GetPlays(fileA, fileB, playForA, playForB, legal);
    }

    // Print overall winner

    PrintBigWinner(winsForA, winsForB);

    return 0;
}

//*****************************************************************

void GetPlays( /* inout */ ifstream& fileA,      // Plays for A
               /* inout */ ifstream& fileB,      // Plays for B
               /* out */   PlayType& playForA,   // A's play
               /* out */   PlayType& playForB,   // B's play
               /* out */   bool&     legal    )  // True if plays
                                                 //   are legal

// Reads the players' plays from the data files, converts the plays
// from char form to PlayType form, and reports whether the plays
// are legal.  If end-of-file is encountered on either file, the
// outgoing parameters are undefined.

// Precondition:
//      fileA and fileB have been successfully opened
// Postcondition:
//      IF input from either file failed due to end-of-file
//          playForA, playForB, and legal are undefined
//      ELSE
//          Player A's play has been read from fileA and Player B's
//          play has been read from fileB
//       && IF both plays are legal
//              legal == TRUE
//           && playForA == PlayType equivalent of Player A's play
//                          char
//           && playForB == PlayType equivalent of Player B's play
//                          char
//          ELSE
//              legal == FALSE
//           && playForA and playForB are undefined
```

```
{
    char charForA;      // Player A's input
    char charForB;      // Player B's input

    fileA >> charForA;          // Skip whitespace, including newline
    fileB >> charForB;
    if ( !fileA || !fileB)
        return;

    legal = (charForA=='R' || charForA=='P' || charForA=='S') &&
            (charForB=='R' || charForB=='P' || charForB=='S');
    if (legal)
    {
        playForA = ConversionVal(charForA);
        playForB = ConversionVal(charForB);
    }
}

//******************************************************************

PlayType ConversionVal( /* in */ char someChar )    // Play character

// Converts a character into an associated PlayType value

// Precondition:
//      someChar == 'R' or 'P' or 'S'
// Postcondition:
//      Function value == ROCK, if someChar == 'R'
//                     == PAPER, if someChar == 'P'
//                     == SCISSORS, if someChar == 'S'

{
    switch (someChar)
    {
        case 'R': return ROCK;      // No break needed after
        case 'P': return PAPER;     //    return statement
        case 'S': return SCISSORS;
    }
}

//******************************************************************

void ProcessPlays( /* in */     int      gameNumber,   // Game number
                   /* in */     PlayType playForA,      // A's play
                   /* in */     PlayType playForB,      // B's play
                   /* inout */  int&     winsForA,      // A's wins
                   /* inout */  int&     winsForB  )    // B's wins
```

PROBLEM-SOLVING CASE STUDY cont'd.

```cpp
// Determines whether there is a winning play or a tie.  If there
// is a winner, the number of wins of the winning player is
// incremented.  In all cases, a message is written

// Precondition:
//     All arguments are assigned
// Postcondition:
//     IF Player A won
//         winsForA == winsForA@entry + 1
//     ELSE IF Player B won
//         winsForB == winsForB@entry + 1
//  && A message, including gameNumber, has been written specifying
//     either a tie or a winner

{
    if (playForA == playForB)
        cout << "Game number " << gameNumber << " is a tie."
            << endl;
    else if (playForA == PAPER && playForB == ROCK ||
            playForA == SCISSORS && playForB == PAPER ||
            playForA == ROCK && playForB == SCISSORS)
        RecordAWin('A', gameNumber, winsForA);       // Player A wins
    else
        RecordAWin('B', gameNumber, winsForB);       // Player B wins
}


//****************************************************************

void RecordAWin( /* in */     char player,         // Winning player
                 /* in */     int  gameNumber,     // Game number
                 /* inout */  int& numOfWins  )    // Win count

// Outputs a message telling which player has won the current game
// and updates that player's total

// Precondition:
//     player == 'A' or 'B'
//  && gameNumber and numOfWins are assigned
// Postcondition:
//     A winning message, including player and gameNumber, has
//     been written
//  && numOfWins == numOfWins@entry + 1

{
    cout << "Player " << player << " has won game number "
        << gameNumber << '.' << endl;
    numOfWins++;
}
```

PROBLEM-SOLVING CASE STUDY cont'd.

```
//*****************************************************************
void PrintBigWinner( /* in */ int winsForA,      // A's win count
                     /* in */ int winsForB )     // B's win count

// Prints number of wins for each player and the
// overall winner (or tie)

// Precondition:
//      winsForA and winsForB are assigned
// Postcondition:
//      The values of winsForA and winsForB have been output
//   && A message indicating the overall winner (or a tie) has been
//      output

{
    cout << endl;
    cout << "Player A has won " << winsForA << " games." << endl;
    cout << "Player B has won " << winsForB << " games." << endl;
    if (winsForA > winsForB)
        cout << "Player A has won the most games." << endl;
    else if (winsForB > winsForA)
        cout << "Player B has won the most games." << endl;
    else
        cout << "Players A and B have tied." << endl;
}
```

Testing: We tested the Game program with the following files. They are listed side by side so that you can see the pairs that made up each game. Note that each combination of 'R', 'P', and 'S' is used at least once. In addition, there is an erroneous play character in each file.

fileA	fileB
R	R
S	S
S	S
R	S
R	P
P	P
P	P
R	S
S	T
A	P
P	S
P	R
S	P
R	S

PROBLEM-SOLVING CASE STUDY *cont'd.*

```
R            S
P            P
S            R
```

Given the data in these files, the program produced the following output.

```
Game number 1 is a tie.
Game number 2 is a tie.
Game number 3 is a tie.
Player A has won game number 4.
Player B has won game number 5.
Game number 6 is a tie.
Game number 7 is a tie.
Player A has won game number 8.
Game number 9 contained an illegal play.
Game number 10 contained an illegal play.
Player B has won game number 11.
Player A has won game number 12.
Player A has won game number 13.
Player A has won game number 14.
Player A has won game number 15.
Game number 16 is a tie.
Player B has won game number 17.

Player A has won 6 games.
Player B has won 3 games.
Player A has won the most games.
```

An examination of the output shows it to be correct: Player A did win six games, player B did win three games, and player A won the most games. This one set of test data is not enough to test the program completely, though. It should be run with test data in which player B wins, player A and player B tie, `fileA` is longer than `fileB`, and `fileB` is longer than `fileA`.

Testing and Debugging

Floating-Point Data

When a problem requires the use of floating-point numbers that are extremely large, small, or precise, it is important to keep in mind the limitations of the particular system you are using. When testing a program that performs floating-point calculations, determine the acceptable margin of error beforehand, and then design your test data to try to push the program beyond those limits. Carefully check the accuracy of the computed results.

(Remember that when you hand-calculate the correct results, a pocket calculator may have *less* precision than your computer system.) If the program produces acceptable results when given worst-case data, it probably performs correctly on typical data.

Coping with Input Errors

Several times in this book, we've had our programs test for invalid data and write an error message. Writing an error message is certainly necessary, but it is only the first step. We must also decide what the program should do next. The problem itself and the severity of the error should determine what action is taken in any error condition. The approach taken also depends on whether or not the program is being run interactively.

In a program that reads its data only from an input file, there is no interaction with the person who entered the data. The program, therefore, should try to adjust for the bad data items, if at all possible.

If the invalid data item is not essential, the program can skip it and continue; for example, if a program averaging test grades encounters a negative test score, it could simply skip the negative score. If an educated guess can be made about the probable value of the bad data, it can be set to that value before being processed. In either event, a message should be written stating that an invalid data item was encountered and outlining the steps that were taken. Such messages form an *exception report.*

If the data item is essential and no guess is possible, processing should be terminated. A message should be written to the user with as much information as possible about the invalid data item.

In an interactive environment, the program can prompt the user to supply another value. The program should indicate to the user what is wrong with the original data. Another possibility is to write out a list of actions and ask the user to choose among them.

These suggestions on how to handle bad data assume that the program recognizes bad data values. There are two approaches to error detection: passive and active. Passive error detection leaves it to the system to detect errors. This may seem easier, but the programmer relinquishes control of processing when an error occurs. An example of passive error detection is the system's division-by-zero error.

Active error detection means having the program check for possible errors and determine an appropriate action if an error occurs. An example of active error detection would be to read a value and use an If statement to see if the value is 0 before dividing it into another number.

The Area program in the first Problem-Solving Case Study uses *no* error detection. If the input is typed incorrectly, the program either crashes (if `divisions` is 0) or produces erroneous output (if `high < low`). Case Study Follow-Up Exercise 2 asks you to supply active error detection for these situations.

Testing and Debugging Hints

1. Avoid using unnecessary side effects in expressions. The test

   ```
   if ((x = y) < z)
       ⋮
   ```

   is less clear and more prone to error than the equivalent sequence of statements

   ```
   x = y;
   if (y < z)
       ⋮
   ```

   Also, if you accidentally omit the parentheses around the assignment operation, like this:

   ```
   if (x = y < z)
   ```

   then, according to C++ operator precedence, x is *not* assigned the value of y. It is assigned the value 1 or 0 (the coerced value of the Boolean result of the relational expression y < z).
2. Programs that rely on a particular machine's character set may not run correctly on another machine. Check to see what character-handling functions are supplied by the standard library. Functions such as `tolower`, `toupper`, `isalpha`, and `iscntrl` automatically account for the character set being used.
3. Don't directly compare floating-point values for equality. Instead, check them for near equality. The tolerance for near equality depends on the particular problem you are solving.
4. Use integers if you are dealing with whole numbers only. Any integer can be represented exactly by the computer, as long as it is within the machine's allowable range of values. Also, integer arithmetic is faster than floating-point arithmetic on most machines.
5. Be aware of representational, cancellation, overflow, and underflow errors. If possible, try to arrange calculations in your program to keep floating-point numbers from becoming too large or too small.
6. If your program increases the value of a positive integer and the result suddenly becomes a negative number, you should suspect integer overflow. On most computers, adding 1 to `INT_MAX` yields `INT_MIN`, a negative number.
7. Except when you really need to, avoid mixing data types in expressions, assignment operations, argument passing, and the return of a function value. If you must mix types, explicit type casts can prevent unwelcome surprises caused by implicit type coercion.
8. Consider using enumeration types to make your programs more readable, understandable, and modifiable.
9. Avoid anonymous data typing. Give each user-defined type a name.
10. Enumeration type values cannot be input or output directly.
11. Type demotion can lead to decreased precision or corruption of data.

Summary

A data type is a set of values (the domain) along with the operations that can be applied to those values. Simple data types are data types whose values are atomic (indivisible).

The integral types in C++ are `char`, `short`, `int`, `long`, and `bool`. The most commonly used integral types are `int` and `char`. The `char` type can be used for storing small (usually one-byte) numeric integers or, more often, for storing character data. Character data includes both printable and nonprintable characters. Nonprintable characters—those that control the behavior of hardware devices—are expressed in C++ as escape sequences such as `\n`. Each character is represented internally as a nonnegative integer according to the particular character set (such as ASCII or EBCDIC) that a computer uses.

The floating-point types built into the C++ language are `float`, `double`, and `long double`. Floating-point numbers are represented in the computer with a mantissa and an exponent. This representation permits numbers that are much larger or much smaller than those that can be represented with the integral types. Floating-point representation also allows us to perform calculations on numbers with fractional parts.

However, there are drawbacks to using floating-point numbers in arithmetic calculations. Representational errors, for example, can affect the accuracy of a program's computations. When using floating-point numbers, keep in mind that if two numbers are vastly different from each other in size, adding or subtracting them can produce the wrong answer. Remember, also, that the computer has a limited range of numbers that it can represent. If a program tries to compute a value that is too large or too small, an error message may result when the program executes.

C++ allows the programmer to define additional data types. The Typedef statement is a simple mechanism for renaming an existing type, although the result is not truly a new data type. An enumeration type, created by listing the identifiers that make up the domain, is a new data type that is distinct from any existing type. Values of an enumeration type may be assigned, compared in relational expressions, used as case labels in a Switch statement, passed as arguments, and returned as function values. Enumeration types are extremely useful in the writing of clear, self-documenting programs. In succeeding chapters, we look at language features that let us create even more powerful user-defined types.

Quick Check

1. The C++ simple types are divided into integral types, floating-point types, and enum types. What are the five integral types (ignoring the unsigned variations) and the three floating-point types? (pp. 494–496)
2. What is the difference between an expression and an expression statement in C++? (pp. 503–505)
3. Assume that the following code segment is executed on a machine that uses the ASCII character set. What is the final value of the char variable someChar? Give both its external and internal representations. (pp. 511–513)

```
someChar = 'T';
someChar = someChar + 4;
```

4. Why is it inappropriate to use a variable of a floating-point type as a loop control variable? (pp. 520–531)
5. If a computer has four digits of precision, what would be the result of the following addition operation? (pp. 520–531)

$$400400.000 + 199.9$$

6. When choosing a data type for a variable that stores whole numbers only, why should int be your first choice? (pp. 531–532)
7. Declare an enumeration type named AutoMakes, consisting of the names of five of your favorite car manufacturers. (pp. 533–541)
8. Given the type declaration

```
enum VisibleColors
{
    RED, ORANGE, YELLOW, GREEN, BLUE, INDIGO, VIOLET
};
```

write the first line of a For statement that "counts" from RED through VIOLET. Use a loop control variable named rainbow that is of type VisibleColors. (pp. 533–541)
9. Why is it better to use a named type than an anonymous type? (pp. 541–542)
10. Suppose that many of your programs need an enumeration type named Days and another named Months. If you place the type declarations into a file named calendar.h, what would an #include directive look like that inserts these declarations into a program? (pp. 542–543)
11. In arithmetic and relational expressions, which of the following could occur: type promotion, type demotion, or both? (pp. 543–547)

Answers **1.** The integral types are char, short, int, long, and bool. The floating-point types are float, double, and long double. **2.** An expression becomes an expression statement when it is terminated by a semicolon. **3.** The external representation is the letter X; the internal representation is the integer 88. **4.** Because representational errors can cause the loop termination condition to be evaluated with unpredictable results. **5.** 400500.000 (Actually, 4.005E+5) **6.** Floating-point arithmetic is subject to numerical inaccuracies and is slower than integer arithmetic on most machines. Use of the smaller integral types, char and short, can more easily lead to overflow errors. The long type usually requires more memory than int, and the arithmetic is usually slower. **7.** enum AutoMakes {SAAB, JAGUAR,

CITROEN, CHEVROLET, FORD}; **8.** for (rainbow = RED; rainbow <= VIOLET; rainbow = VisibleColors(rainbow + 1)) **9.** Named types make a program more readable, more understandable, and easier to modify. **10.** #include "calendar.h" **11.** Type promotion

Exam Preparation Exercises

1. Every C++ compiler guarantees that sizeof(int) < sizeof(long). (True or False?)
2. Classify each of the following as either an expression or an expression statement.
   a. sum = 0
   b. sqrt(x)
   c. y = 17;
   d. count++
3. Rewrite each statement as described.
   a. Using the += operator, rewrite the statement

      sumOfSquares = sumOfSquares + x * x;

   b. Using the decrement operator, rewrite the statement

      count = count - 1;

   c. Using a single assignment statement that uses the ?: operator, rewrite the statement

      if (n > 8)
          k = 32;
      else
          k = 15 * n;

4. What is printed by each of the following program fragments? (In both cases, ch is of type char.)
   a. for (ch = 'd'; ch <= 'g'; ch++)
      cout << ch;
   b. ch = 'F';
      cout << ch << ' ' << int(ch);   // Assume ASCII
5. What is printed by the following output statement?

   cout << "Notice that\nthe character \\ is a backslash.\n";

6. If a system supports ten digits of precision for floating-point numbers, what are the results of the following computations?
   a. 1.4E+12 + 100.0
   b. 4.2E−8 + 100.0
   c. 3.2E−5 + 3.2E+5
7. Define the following terms:

   mantissa   significant digits
   exponent   overflow
   representational error

8. Given the type declaration

   ```
   enum Agents {SMITH, JONES, GRANT, WHITE};
   ```

   does the expression JONES > GRANT have the value true or false?
9. Given the following declarations,

   ```
   enum Perfumes {POISON, DIOR_ESSENCE, CHANEL_NO_5, COTY};
   Perfumes sample;
   ```

   indicate whether each statement below is valid or invalid.
   a. sample = POISON;
   b. sample = 3;
   c. sample++;
   d. sample = Perfumes(sample + 1);
10. Using the declarations

    ```
    enum SeasonType {WINTER, SPRING, SUMMER, FALL};
    SeasonType season;
    ```

    indicate whether each statement below is valid or invalid.
    a. cin >> season;
    b. if (season >= SPRING)
         ⋮
    c. for (season = WINTER; season <= SUMMER; season =
                                    SeasonType(season + 1))
         ⋮
11. Given the following program fragment,

    ```
    enum Colors {RED, GREEN, BLUE};

    Colors myColor;
    enum {RED, GREEN, BLUE} yourColor;
    ```

    the data type of myColor is a named type, and the data type of yourColor is an anonymous type. (True or False?)
12. If you have written your own header file named mytypes.h, then the preprocessor directive

    ```
    #include <mytypes.h>
    ```

    is the correct way to insert the contents of the header file into a program. (True or False?)
13. In each of the following situations, indicate whether promotion or demotion occurs. (The names of the variables are meant to suggest their data types.)
    a. Execution of the assignment operation someInt = someFloat
    b. Evaluation of the expression someFloat + someLong
    c. Passing the argument someDouble to the parameter someFloat
    d. Execution of the following statement within an int function:

       ```
       return someShort;
       ```

14. Active error detection leaves error hunting to C++ and the operating system, whereas passive error detection requires the programmer to do the error hunting. (True or False?)

Programming Warm-up Exercises

1. Find out the maximum and minimum values for each of the C++ integral and floating-point types on your machine. These values are declared as named constants in the files `climits` and `cfloat` in the standard include directory.

2. Using a combination of printable characters and escape sequences within *one* literal string, write a single output statement that does the following in the order shown:
   - Prints `Hello`
   - Prints a (horizontal) tab character
   - Prints `There`
   - Prints two blank lines
   - Prints `"Ace"` (including the double quotes)

3. Write a While loop that copies all the characters (including whitespace characters) from an input file stream `inFile` to an output file stream `outFile`, except that every lowercase letter is converted to uppercase. Assume that both files have been opened successfully before the loop begins. The loop should terminate when end-of-file is detected.

4. Given the following declarations

   ```
   int   n;
   char  ch1;
   char  ch2;
   ```

   and given that n contains a two-digit number, translate n into two single characters such that `ch1` holds the higher-order digit, and `ch2` holds the lower-order digit. For example, if n = 59, `ch1` would equal '5', and `ch2` would equal '9'. Then output the two digits as characters in the same order as the original numbers. (*Hint:* Consider how you might use the `/` and `%` operators in your solution.)

5. In a program you are writing, a `float` variable `beta` potentially contains a very large number. Before multiplying `beta` by 100.0, you want the program to test whether it is safe to do so. Write an If statement that tests for a possible overflow *before* multiplying by 100.0. Specifically, if the multiplication would lead to overflow, print a message and don't perform the multiplication; otherwise, go ahead with the multiplication.

6. Declare an enumeration type for the course numbers of computer courses at your school.

7. Declare an enumeration type for the South American countries.

8. Declare an enumeration type for the work days of the week (Monday through Friday).

9. Write a value-returning function that converts the first two letters of a work day into the type declared in Exercise 8.

10. Write a void function that prints a value of the type declared in Exercise 8.

11. Using a loop control variable `today` of the type declared in Exercise 8, write a For loop that prints out all five values in the domain of the type. To print each value, invoke the function of Exercise 10.

12. Below is a function that is supposed to return the ratio of two integers, rounded up or down to the nearest integer.

```
int Ratio( /* in */ int int1,
           /* in */ int int2 )
{
    return float(int1) / float(int2);
}
```

Sometimes this function returns an incorrect result. Describe what the problem is in terms of type promotion or demotion and fix the problem.

Programming Problems

1. Read in the lengths of the sides of a triangle and determine whether the triangle is isosceles (two sides are equal), equilateral (three sides are equal), or scalene (no sides are equal). Use an enumeration type whose enumerators are ISOSCELES, EQUILATERAL, and SCALENE.

   The lengths of the sides of the triangle are to be entered as integer values. For each set of sides, print out the kind of triangle or an error message saying that the three sides do not make a triangle. (For a triangle to exist, any two sides together must be longer than the remaining side.) Continue analyzing triangles until end-of-file occurs.

2. Write a C++ program that reads a single character from 'A' through 'Z' and produces output in the shape of a pyramid composed of the letters up to and including the letter that is input. The top letter in the pyramid should be 'A', and on each level, the next letter in the alphabet should fall between two copies of the letter that was introduced in the level above it. For example, if the input is 'E', the output looks like the following:

   ```
       A
      ABA
     ABCBA
    ABCDCBA
   ABCDEDCBA
   ```

3. Read in a floating-point number character by character, ignoring any characters other than digits and a decimal point. Convert the valid characters into a single floating-point number and print the result. Your algorithm should convert the whole number part to an integer and the fractional part to an integer and combine the two integers as follows:

   $$\text{Set result} = \text{wholePart} + \text{fractionalPart} / (10^{\text{number of digits in fraction}})$$

   For example, 3A4.21P6 would be converted into 34 and 216, and the result would be the value of the sum

   $$34 + \frac{216}{1000}$$

   You may assume that the number has at least one digit on either side of the decimal point.

4. The program that plays Rock, Paper, and Scissors takes its input from two files. Rewrite the program so that it uses interactive input from two players. The main module should be as follows:

```
DO
    Get command
    IF command is CONTINUE
        Play game
    ELSE IF command is PRINT_STATS
        Print statistics
WHILE command isn't STOP
```

command should be a variable of an enumeration type whose enumerators are CONTINUE, PRINT_STATS, and STOP. The statistics to be printed are the current game number, the current number of wins for the first player, and the current number of wins for the second player. The Get Command module should begin by asking if the players want to see the current statistics. If they do not, the first player should be prompted to enter a 'C' to continue or an 'S' to stop. If the first player wishes to continue, ask the second player; command should be CONTINUE if both players enter a 'C', and STOP otherwise. If both players wish to continue, the first player and then the second player should be prompted to enter a play.

Case Study Follow-Up

1. In the Area program, it would be more efficient to go directly from midpoint to midpoint and not use the left edge of a rectangle at all. How would you change the program to use this approach?
2. The following exercises pertain to the Area program.
   a. Why does the program crash if the user enters 0 for divisions?
   b. Add active error detection to the GetData function so that, upon return from the function, it is guaranteed that divisions > 0 and high ≥ low.
3. Enter and repeatedly run the Area program to observe the effect of increasing the number of divisions. On each run, enter 0 for low and 2 for high. Start with one division, then use 10, 100, 1000, 10,000, 100,000, and 1,000,000 divisions on successive runs.
   a. What is the result from each run?
   b. Does the result ever equal the exact answer, 4.0? If so, which run gives the correct answer? If not, which run comes closest? Does it help to use even more divisions?
   c. Approximately how long does the computer take to execute each of the runs? From these times, estimate how long it would take to execute with 100,000,000 divisions.
4. Repeat Exercise 3, using 0 for low and 1000 for high.

5. What is the advantage of converting 'R', 'P', and 'S' into values of an enumeration type in the Rock, Paper, Scissors case study?
6. Modify the Game program so that it prompts the user for the names of the two external files before opening them.
7. Write a comprehensive test plan for the Game program.
8. Implement your test plan for the Game program.

11

Structured Types, Data Abstraction, and Classes

GOALS

- To be able to declare a record (struct) data type, a data structure whose components may be heterogeneous.
- To be able to access a member of a record variable.
- To be able to define a hierarchical record structure.
- To be able to access values stored in a hierarchical record variable.
- To understand the general concept of a C++ union type.
- To understand the difference between specification and implementation of an abstract data type.
- To be able to declare a C++ class type.
- To be able to declare class objects, given the declaration of a class type.
- To be able to write client code that invokes class member functions.
- To be able to implement class member functions.
- To understand how encapsulation and information hiding are enforced by the C++ compiler.
- To be able to organize the code for a C++ class into two files: the specification (.h) file and the implementation file.
- To be able to write a C++ class constructor.

In the last chapter, we examined the concept of a data type and looked at how to define simple data types. In this chapter, we expand the definition of a data type to include structured types, which represent collections of components that are referred to by a single name. We begin with a discussion of structured types in general and then examine two structured types provided by the C++ language: the struct and the union.

Next, we introduce the concept of *data abstraction,* the separation of a data type's logical properties from its implementation. Data abstraction is important because it allows us to create data types not otherwise available in a programming language. Another benefit of data abstraction is the ability to produce *off-the-shelf software*—pieces of software that can be used over and over again in different programs either by the creator of the software or by any programmer wishing to use them.

The primary concept for practicing data abstraction is the *abstract data type.* In this chapter, we examine abstract data types in depth and introduce the C++ language feature designed expressly for creating abstract data types: the *class.* We conclude with two case studies that demonstrate data abstraction, abstract data types, and C++ classes.

Simple Versus Structured Data Types

In Chapter 10, we examined simple, or atomic, data types. A value in a simple type is a single data item; it cannot be broken down into component parts. For example, each int value is a single integer number and cannot be further decomposed. In contrast, a **structured data type** is one in which each value is a *collection* of component items. The entire collection is given a single name, yet each component can still be accessed individually. An example of a structured data type in C++ is the string class, used for creating and manipulating strings. When you declare a variable myString to be of type string, myString does not represent just one atomic data value; it represents an entire collection of characters. But each of the components in the string can be accessed individually (by using an expression such as myString[3], which accesses the char value at position 3).

Structured data type   A data type in which each value is a collection of components and whose organization is characterized by the method used to access individual components. The allowable operations on a structured data type include the storage and retrieval of individual components.

Simple data types, both built-in and user-defined, are the building blocks for structured types. A structured type gathers together a set of com-

FIGURE 11-1
Atomic (Simple)
and Structured
Data Types

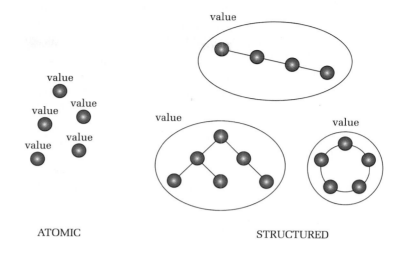

ATOMIC   STRUCTURED

ponent values and usually imposes a specific arrangement on them (see Figure 11-1). The method used to access the individual components of a structured type depends on how the components are arranged. As we discuss various ways of structuring data, we look at the corresponding access mechanisms.

Figure 11-2 shows the structured types available in C++. This figure is a portion of the complete diagram presented in Figure 3-1.

In this chapter, we examine the `struct`, `union`, and `class` types. Array data types are the topic of Chapter 12.

Records (C++ Structs)

In computer science, a **record** is a heterogeneous structured data type. By *heterogeneous*, we mean that the individual components of a record can be of different data types. Each component of a record is called a **field** of the

FIGURE 11-2
C++ Structured
Types

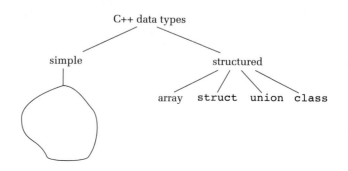

record, and each field is given a name called the *field name*. C++ uses its own terminology with records. A record is called a **structure**, the fields of a record are called **members** of the structure, and each member has a *member name*.

Record (structure, in C++)   A structured data type with a fixed number of components that are accessed by name. The components may be heterogeneous (of different types).

Field (member, in C++)   A component of a record.

In C++, record data types are most commonly declared according to the following syntax:

StructDeclaration

```
struct TypeName
{
      MemberList
};
```

where TypeName is an identifier giving a name to the data type, and MemberList is defined as

MemberList

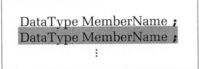

The reserved word `struct` is an abbreviation for *structure*, the C++ term for a record. Because the word *structure* has many other meanings in computer science, we'll use *struct* or *record* to avoid any possible confusion about what we are referring to.

You probably recognize the syntax of a member list as being nearly identical to a series of variable declarations. Be careful: A `struct` declaration is a type declaration, and we still must declare variables of this type for any memory locations to be associated with the member names. As an example, let's use a struct to describe a student in a class. We want to store the first and last names, the overall grade point average prior to this class, the grade on programming assignments, the grade on quizzes, the final exam grade, and the final course grade.

```
// Type declarations

enum GradeType {A, B, C, D, F};

struct StudentRec
{
    string     firstName;
    string     lastName;
    float      gpa;               // Grade point average
    int        programGrade;      // Assume 0..400
    int        quizGrade;         // Assume 0..300
    int        finalExam;         // Assume 0..300
    GradeType  courseGrade;
};


// Variable declarations

StudentRec firstStudent;
StudentRec student;
int        grade;
```

Notice, both in this example and in the syntax template, that a `struct` declaration ends with a semicolon. By now, you have learned not to put a semicolon after the right brace of a compound statement (block). However, the member list in a `struct` declaration is not considered to be a compound statement; the braces are simply required syntax in the declaration. A `struct` declaration, like all C++ declaration statements, must end with a semicolon.

`firstName`, `lastName`, `gpa`, `programGrade`, `quizGrade`, `finalExam`, and `courseGrade` are member names within the `struct` type `StudentRec`. These member names make up the member list. Note that each member name is given a type. Also, member names must be unique within a `struct` type, just as variable names must be unique within a block.

`firstName` and `lastName` are of type `string`. `gpa` is a `float` member. `programGrade`, `quizGrade`, and `finalExam` are `int` members. `courseGrade` is of an enumeration data type made up of the grades A through D and F.

None of these struct members are associated with memory locations until we declare a variable of the `StudentRec` type. `StudentRec` is merely a pattern for a struct (see Figure 11-3). The variables `firstStudent` and `student` are variables of type `StudentRec`.

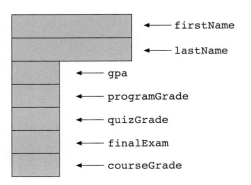

FIGURE 11-3
Pattern for a Struct

Accessing Individual Components

To access an individual member of a struct variable, you give the name of the variable, followed by a dot (period), and then the member name. This expression is called a **member selector**. The syntax template is

MemberSelector

> StructVariable . MemberName

This syntax for selecting individual components of a struct is often called *dot notation*. To access the grade point average of `firstStudent`, we would write

`firstStudent.gpa`

To access the final exam score of `student`, we would write

`student.finalExam`

Member selector   The expression used to access components of a struct variable. It is formed by using the struct variable name and the member name, separated by a dot (period).

The component of a struct accessed by the member selector is treated just like any other variable of the same type. It may be used in an assignment statement, passed as an argument, and so on. Figure 11-4 shows the struct variable `student` with the member selector for each member. In this example, we assume that some processing has already taken place, so values are stored in some of the components.

Let's demonstrate the use of these member selectors. Using our `student` variable, the following code segment reads in a final exam grade; adds up the program grade, the quiz grade, and the final exam grade; and then assigns a letter grade to the result.

```
cin >> student.finalExam;
grade = student.finalExam + student.programGrade +
        student.quizGrade;
if (grade >= 900)
    student.courseGrade = A;
else if (grade >= 800)
    student.courseGrade = B;
else   .
       .
       .
```

Aggregate Operations on Structs

In addition to accessing individual components of a struct variable, we can in some cases use **aggregate operations**. An aggregate operation is one that manipulates the struct as an entire unit.

Aggregate operation   An operation on a data structure as a whole, as opposed to an operation on an individual component of the data structure.

The following table summarizes the aggregate operations that are allowed on struct variables.

FIGURE 11-4
Struct Variable
`student` with
Member Selectors

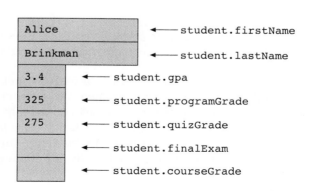

Aggregate Operation	Allowed on Structs?
I/O	No
Assignment	Yes
Arithmetic	No
Comparison	No
Argument passage	Yes, by value or by reference
Return as a function's return value	Yes

According to the table, one struct variable can be assigned to another. However, both variables must be declared to be of the same type. For example, given the declarations

```
StudentRec student;
StudentRec anotherStudent;
```

the statement

```
anotherStudent = student;
```

copies the entire contents of the struct variable `student` to the variable `anotherStudent`, member by member.

On the other hand, aggregate arithmetic operations and comparisons are not allowed (primarily because they wouldn't make sense):

```
student = student * anotherStudent;     // Not allowed
if (student < anotherStudent)           // Not allowed
```

Furthermore, aggregate I/O is not permitted:

```
cin >> student;                         // Not allowed
```

We must input or output a struct variable one member at a time:

```
cin >> student.firstName;
cin >> student.lastName;
    ⋮
```

According to the table, an entire struct can be passed as an argument, either by value or by reference, and a struct can be returned as the value of a value-returning function. Let's define a function that takes a `StudentRec` variable as a parameter.

The task of this function is to determine if a student's grade in a course is consistent with his or her overall grade point average (GPA). We define *consistent* to mean that the course grade corresponds correctly to the rounded GPA. The GPA is calculated on a four-point scale, where A is 4, B is 3, C is 2, D is 1, and F is 0. If the rounded GPA is 4 and the course grade is A, then the function returns `true`. If the rounded GPA is 4 and the course grade is not A, then the function returns `false`. Each of the other grades is tested in the same way.

The `Consistent` function is coded below. The parameter `aStudent`, a struct variable of type `StudentRec`, is passed by value.

```cpp
bool Consistent( /* in */ StudentRec aStudent )

// Precondition:
//      0.0 <= aStudent.gpa <= 4.0
// Postcondition:
//      Function value == true, if the course grade is consistent
//                                with the overall GPA
//                        == false, otherwise

{
    int roundedGPA = int(aStudent.gpa + 0.5);

    switch (roundedGPA)
    {
        case 0: return (aStudent.courseGrade == F);
        case 1: return (aStudent.courseGrade == D);
        case 2: return (aStudent.courseGrade == C);
        case 3: return (aStudent.courseGrade == B);
        case 4: return (aStudent.courseGrade == A);
    }
}
```

More About Struct Declarations

To complete our initial look at C++ structs, we give a more complete syntax template for a `struct` type declaration:

StructDeclaration

```
struct TypeName
{
      MemberList
} VariableList ;
```

As you can see in the syntax template, two items are optional: TypeName (the name of the `struct` type being declared), and VariableList (a list of variable names between the right brace and the semicolon). Our examples thus far have declared a type name but have not included a variable list. The variable list allows you not only to declare a `struct` type but also to declare variables of that type, all in one statement. For example, you could write the declarations

```
struct StudentRec
{
    string firstName;
    string lastName;
        ⋮
};

StudentRec firstStudent;
StudentRec student;
```

more compactly in the form

```
struct StudentRec
{
    string firstName;
    string lastName;
        ⋮
} firstStudent, student;
```

In this book, we avoid combining variable declarations with type declarations, preferring to keep the two notions separate.

If you omit the type name but include the variable list, you create an anonymous type:

```
struct
{
    int   firstMember;
    float secondMember;
} someVar;
```

Here, `someVar` is a variable of an anonymous type. No other variables of that type can be declared because the type has no name. Therefore, `someVar` cannot participate in aggregate operations such as assignment or argument passage. The cautions given in Chapter 10 against anonymous typing of enumeration types apply to `struct` types as well.

Hierarchical Records

We have seen examples in which the components of a record are simple variables and strings. A component of a record can also be another record. Records whose components are themselves records are called **hierarchical records.**

Hierarchical record   A record in which at least one of the components is itself a record.

Let's look at an example in which a hierarchical structure is appropriate. A small machine shop keeps information about each of its machines. There is descriptive information, such as the identification number, a description of the machine, the purchase date, and the cost. Statistical information is also kept, such as the number of down days, the failure rate, and the date of last service. What is a reasonable way of representing all this information? First, let's look at a flat (nonhierarchical) record structure that holds this information.

```
struct MachineRec
{
    int     idNumber;
    string  description;
    float   failRate;
    int     lastServicedMonth;   // Assume 1..12
    int     lastServicedDay;     // Assume 1..31
    int     lastServicedYear;    // Assume 1900..2050
    int     downDays;
    int     purchaseDateMonth;   // Assume 1..12
    int     purchaseDateDay;     // Assume 1..31
    int     purchaseDateYear;    // Assume 1900..2050
    float   cost;
};
```

The `MachineRec` type has 11 members. There is so much detailed information here that it is difficult to quickly get a feeling for what the record represents. Let's see if we can reorganize it into a hierarchical structure that makes more sense. We can divide the information into two groups: information that changes and information that does not. There are also two dates to be kept: date of purchase and date of last service. These observations suggest use of a record describing a date, a record describing the statistical data, and an overall record containing the other two as components. The following type declarations reflect this structure.

```
struct DateType
{
    int month;   // Assume 1..12
    int day;     // Assume 1..31
    int year;    // Assume 1900..2050
};
struct StatisticsType
{
    float     failRate;
    DateType lastServiced;
    int       downDays;
};
struct MachineRec
{
    int            idNumber;
    string         description;
    StatisticsType history;
    DateType       purchaseDate;
    float          cost;
};

MachineRec machine;
```

The contents of a machine record are now much more obvious. Two of the components of the struct type MachineRec are themselves structs: purchaseDate is of struct type DateType, and history is of struct type StatisticsType. One of the components of struct type StatisticsType is a struct of type DateType.

How do we access the components of a hierarchical structure such as this one? We build the accessing expressions (member selectors) for the members of the embedded structs from left to right, beginning with the struct variable name. Here are some expressions and the components they access:

Expression	Component Accessed
machine.purchaseDate	DateType struct variable
machine.purchaseDate.month	month member of a DateType struct variable
machine.purchaseDate.year	year member of a DateType struct variable
machine.history.lastServiced.year	year member of a DateType struct variable contained in a struct of type StatisticsType

Figure 11-5 is a pictorial representation of machine with values. Look carefully at how each component is accessed.

Unions

In Figure 11-2, we presented a diagram showing the four structured types available in C++. We have discussed `struct` types and now look briefly at *union* types.

In C++, a union is defined to be a struct that holds only one of its members at a time during program execution. Here is a declaration of a `union` type and a union variable:

```
union WeightType
{
    long  wtInOunces;
    int   wtInPounds;
    float wtInTons;
};

WeightType weight;
```

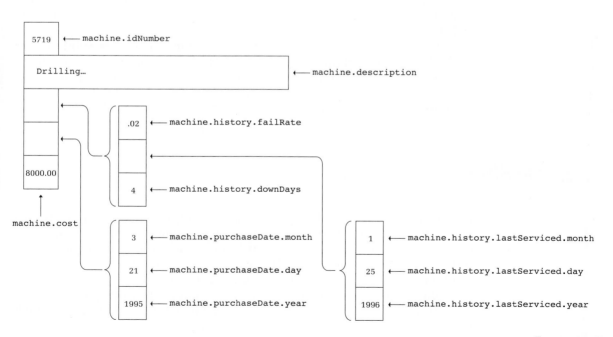

FIGURE 11-5
Hierarchical Records in machine Variable

The syntax for declaring a union type is identical to that of a struct type, except that the word union is substituted for struct.

At run time, the memory space allocated to the variable weight does *not* include room for three distinct components. Instead, weight can contain only one of the following: *either* a long value *or* an int value *or* a float value. The assumption is that the program will never need a weight in ounces, a weight in pounds, and a weight in tons simultaneously while executing. The purpose of a union is to conserve memory by forcing several values to use the same memory space, one at a time. The following code shows how the weight variable might be used.

```
weight.wtInTons = 4.83;
    ⋮
// Weight in tons is no longer needed. Reuse the memory space.

weight.wtInPounds = 35;
    ⋮
```

After the last assignment statement, the previous float value 4.83 is gone, replaced by the int value 35.

It's quite reasonable to argue that a union is not a data structure at all. It does not represent a collection of values; it represents only a single value from among several *potential* values. On the other hand, unions are grouped together with the structured types because of their similarity to structs.

There is much more to be said about unions, including subtle issues related to their declaration and usage. However, these issues are more appropriate in an advanced study of data structures and system programming. We have introduced unions only to present a complete picture of the structured types provided by C++ and to acquaint you with the general idea in case you encounter unions in other C++ programs.

Data Abstraction

As the software we develop becomes more complex, we design algorithms and data structures in parallel. We progress from the logical or abstract data structure envisioned at the top level through the refinement process until we reach the concrete coding in C++. We have illustrated two ways of representing the logical structure of a machine record in a shop inventory. The first used a record in which all the components were defined (made concrete) at the same time. The second used a hierarchical record in which the dates and statistics describing a machine's history were defined in lower-level records.

Let's look again at the two different ways in which we represented our logical data structure.

```
// **************** Version 1 ****************

struct MachineRec
{
    int     idNumber;
    string  description;
    float   failRate;
    int     lastServicedMonth;   // Assume 1..12
    int     lastServicedDay;     // Assume 1..31
    int     lastServicedYear;    // Assume 1900..2050
    int     downDays;
    int     purchaseDateMonth;   // Assume 1..12
    int     purchaseDateDay;     // Assume 1..31
    int     purchaseDateYear;    // Assume 1900..2050
    float   cost;
};


// **************** Version 2 ****************

struct DateType
{
    int month;   // Assume 1..12
    int day;     // Assume 1..31
    int year;    // Assume 1900..2050
};
struct StatisticsType
{
    float     failRate;
    DateType  lastServiced;
    int       downDays;
};
struct MachineRec
{
    int            idNumber;
    string         description;
    StatisticsType history;
    DateType       purchaseDate;
    float          cost;
};
```

Which of these two representations is better? The second one is better for two reasons.

First, it groups elements together logically. The statistics and the dates are entities within themselves. We may want a date or a machine history in another record structure. If we define the dates and statistics only within

MachineRec (as in the first structure), we would have to define them again for every other data structure that needs them, giving us multiple definitions of the same logical entity.

Second, the details of the entities (statistics and dates) are pushed down to a lower level in the second structure. The principle of deferring details to as low a level as possible should be applied to designing data structures as well as to designing algorithms. How a machine history or a date is represented is not relevant to our concept of a machine record, so the details need not be specified until it is time to write the algorithms to manipulate those members.

Pushing the implementation details of a data type to a lower level separates the logical description from the implementation. This concept is analogous to control abstraction, which we discussed in Chapter 8. The separation of the logical properties of a data type from its implementation details is called **data abstraction,** which is a goal of effective programming and the foundation upon which abstract data types are built. (We explore the concept of abstract data types in the next section.)

Data abstraction   The separation of a data type's logical properties from its implementation.

Eventually, all the logical properties must be defined in terms of concrete data types and routines written to manipulate them. If the implementation is properly designed, we can use the same routines to manipulate the structure in a wide variety of applications. For example, if we have a routine to compare dates, we can use that routine to compare dates representing days on which equipment was bought or maintained, or dates representing people's birthdays. The concept of designing a low-level structure and writing routines to manipulate it is the basis for C++ class types, which we examine later in the chapter.

Abstract Data Types

We live in a complex world. Throughout the course of each day, we are constantly bombarded with information, facts, and details. To cope with complexity, the human mind engages in *abstraction*—the act of separating the essential qualities of an idea or object from the details of how it works or is composed.

With abstraction, we focus on the *what,* not the *how.* For example, our understanding of automobiles is largely based on abstraction. Most of us know *what* the engine does (it propels the car), but fewer of us know—or want to know—precisely *how* the engine works internally. Abstraction allows us to discuss, think about, and use automobiles without having to know everything about how they work.

In the world of software design, it is now recognized that abstraction is an absolute necessity for managing immense, complex software projects. In introductory computer science courses, programs are usually small (perhaps 50 to 200 lines of code) and understandable in their entirety by one person. However, large commercial software products composed of hundreds of thousands—even millions—of lines of code cannot be designed, understood, or tested thoroughly without using abstraction in various forms. To manage complexity, software developers regularly use two important abstraction techniques: control abstraction and data abstraction.

In Chapter 8, we defined control abstraction as the separation of the logical properties of an action from its implementation. We engage in control abstraction whenever we write a function that reduces a complicated algorithm to an abstract action performed by a function call. By invoking a library function, as in the expression

```
4.6 + sqrt(x)
```

we depend only on the function's *specification,* a written description of what it does. We can use the function without having to know its *implementation* (the algorithms that accomplish the result). By invoking the sqrt function, our program is less complex because all the details involved in computing square roots are absent.

Abstraction techniques also apply to data. Every data type consists of a set of values (the domain) along with a collection of allowable operations on those values. In the preceding section, we described data abstraction as the separation of a data type's logical properties from its implementation details. Data abstraction comes into play when we need a data type that is not built into the programming language. We can define the new data type as an **abstract data type (ADT)**, concentrating only on its logical properties and deferring the details of its implementation.

Abstract data type A data type whose properties (domain and operations) are specified independently of any particular implementation.

As with control abstraction, an abstract data type has both a specification (the *what*) and an implementation (the *how*). The specification of an ADT describes the characteristics of the data values as well as the behavior of each of the operations on those values. The user of the ADT needs to understand only the specification, not the implementation, in order to use it. Here's a very informal specification of a list ADT:

TYPE
   IntList
DOMAIN
   Each IntList value is a collection of up to 100 separate integer numbers.
OPERATIONS
   Insert an item into the list.
   Delete an item from the list.
   Search the list for an item.
   Return the current length of the list.
   Sort the list into ascending order.
   Print the list.

Notice the complete absence of implementation details. We have not mentioned how the data might actually be stored in a program or how the operations might be implemented. Concealing the implementation details reduces complexity for the user and also shields the user from changes in the implementation.

   Below is the specification of another ADT, one that might be useful for representing time in a program.

TYPE
   TimeType
DOMAIN
   Each TimeType value is a time of day in the form of hours, minutes, and seconds.
OPERATIONS
   Set the time.
   Print the time.
   Increment the time by one second.
   Compare two times for equality.
   Determine if one time is "less than" (comes before) another.

   The specification of an ADT defines abstract data values and abstract operations for the user. Ultimately, of course, the ADT must be implemented in program code. To implement an ADT, the programmer must do two things:

1. Choose a concrete **data representation** of the abstract data, using data types that already exist.
2. Implement each of the allowable operations in terms of program instructions.

Data representation   The concrete form of data used to represent the abstract values of an abstract data type.

To implement the IntList ADT, we could choose a concrete data representation consisting of two items: a 100-element data structure (such as an *array*, the topic of the next chapter) and an `int` variable that keeps track of the current length of the list. To implement the IntList operations, we must create algorithms based on the chosen data representation. In the next two chapters, we discuss in detail the array data structure and its use in implementing list ADTs.

To implement the TimeType ADT, we might use three `int` variables for the data representation—one for the hours, one for the minutes, and one for the seconds. Or we might use three strings as the data representation. The specification of the ADT does not confine us to any particular data representation. As long as we satisfy the specification, we are free to choose among alternative data representations and their associated algorithms. Our choice may be based on time efficiency (the speed at which the algorithms execute), space efficiency (the economical use of memory space), or simplicity and readability of the algorithms. Over time, you will acquire knowledge and experience that help you decide which implementation is best for a particular context.

THEORETICAL FOUNDATIONS

Categories of Abstract Data Type Operations

In general, the basic operations associated with an abstract data type fall into three categories: **constructors, transformers,** and **observers.**

Constructor An operation that creates a new instance (variable) of an ADT.

Transformer An operation that builds a new value of the ADT, given one or more previous values of the type.

An operation that creates a new instance of an ADT (such as a list) is a constructor. Operations that insert an item into a list and delete an item from a list are transformers. An operation that takes one list and appends it to the end of a second list is also a transformer.

Observer An operation that allows us to observe the state of an instance of an ADT without changing it.

A Boolean function that returns `true` if a list is empty and `false` if it contains any components is an example of an observer. A Boolean function that tests to see if a certain value is in the list is another observer.

Some operations are combinations of observers and constructors. An operation that takes two lists and merges them into a (new) third list is both an observer (of the two existing lists) and a constructor (of the third list).

In addition to the three basic categories of ADT operations, a fourth category is sometimes defined: **iterators.**

Iterator   An operation that allows us to process—one at a time—all the components in an instance of an ADT.

An example of an iterator is an operation that returns the first item in a list when it is called initially and returns the next one with each successive call.

C++ Classes

In previous chapters, we have treated data values as passive quantities to be acted upon by functions. In Chapter 10, we viewed Rock, Paper, Scissors game plays as passive data, and we implemented operations as

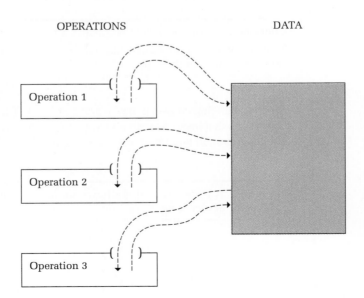

FIGURE 11-6
Data and
Operations as
Separate Entities

OPERATIONS   DATA

Operation 1

Operation 2

Operation 3

functions that took `PlayType` values as parameters. Similarly, earlier in this chapter we treated a student record as a passive quantity, using a struct as the data representation and implementing the operation `Consistent` as a function receiving a struct as a parameter (see Figure 11-6).

This separation of operations and data does not correspond very well with the notion of an abstract data type. After all, an ADT consists of *both* data values and operations on those values. It is preferable to view an ADT as defining an *active* data structure—one that combines both data and operations into a single, cohesive unit (see Figure 11-7). C++ supports this view by providing a built-in structured type known as a **class.**

In Figure 11-2, we listed the four structured types available in the C++ language: the array, the struct, the union, and the class. A class is a structured type provided specifically for representing abstract data types. A class is similar to a struct but is nearly always designed so that its components (**class members**) include not only data but also functions that manipulate that data. Here is a C++ class declaration corresponding to the TimeType ADT that we defined in the previous section:

```
class TimeType
{
public:
    void Set( int, int, int );
    void Increment();
    void Write() const;
    bool Equal( TimeType ) const;
    bool LessThan( TimeType ) const;
private:
    int hrs;
    int mins;
    int secs;
};
```

(For now, you should ignore the word `const` appearing in some of the function prototypes. We explain this use of `const` later in the chapter.)

FIGURE 11-7

Data and Operations Bound into a Single Unit

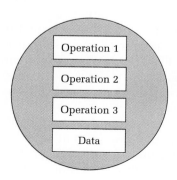

The `TimeType` class has eight members—five member functions (`Set`, `Increment`, `Write`, `Equal`, `LessThan`) and three member variables (`hrs`, `mins`, `secs`). As you might guess, the three member variables form the concrete data representation for the TimeType ADT. The five member functions correspond to the operations we listed for the TimeType ADT: set the time (to the hours, minutes, and seconds passed as arguments to the `Set` function), increment the time by one second, print the time, compare two times for equality, and determine if one time is less than another. Although the `Equal` function compares two `TimeType` variables for equality, its parameter list has only one parameter—a `TimeType` variable. Similarly, the `LessThan` function has only one parameter, even though it compares two times. We'll see the reason later.

Like a `struct` declaration, the declaration of `TimeType` defines a data type but does not create variables of the type. Class variables (more often referred to as **class objects** or **class instances**) are created by using ordinary variable declarations:

```
TimeType startTime;
TimeType endTime;
```

Any software that declares and manipulates `TimeType` objects is called a **client** of the class.

Class   A structured type in a programming language that is used to represent an abstract data type.

Class member   A component of a class. Class members may be either data or functions.

Class object (class instance)   A variable of a `class` type.

Client   Software that declares and manipulates objects of a particular class.

As you look at the preceding declaration of the `TimeType` class, you can see the reserved words `public` and `private`, each followed by a colon. Data and/or functions declared between the words `public` and `private` constitute the public interface; clients can access these class members directly. Class members declared after the word `private` are considered private information and are inaccessible to clients. If client code attempts to access a private item, the compiler signals an error.

Private class members can be accessed only by the class's member functions. In the `TimeType` class, the private variables `hrs`, `mins`, and `secs` can be accessed only by the member functions `Set`, `Increment`, `Write`, `Equal`, and `LessThan`, not by client code. This separation of class members into private and public parts is a hallmark of ADT design. To preserve the properties of an ADT correctly, an instance of the ADT should be manipulated *only* through the operations that form the public interface. We have more to say about this issue later in the chapter.

MATTERS OF STYLE

Declaring Public and Private Class Members

C++ does not require you to declare public and private class members in a fixed order. Several variations are possible.

By default, class members are private; the word `public` must be used to "open up" any members for public access. Therefore, we could write the `TimeType` class declaration as follows:

```
class TimeType
{
    int hrs;
    int mins;
    int secs;
public:
    void Set( int, int, int );
    void Increment();
    void Write() const;
    bool Equal( TimeType ) const;
    bool LessThan( TimeType ) const;
};
```

By default, the variables `hrs`, `mins`, and `secs` are private. The public part extends from the word `public` to the end of the class declaration.

Even with the private part located first, some programmers use the reserved word `private` to be as explicit as possible:

```
class TimeType
{
private:
    int hrs;
    int mins;
    int secs;
public:
    void Set( int, int, int );
    void Increment();
    void Write() const;
    bool Equal( TimeType ) const;
    bool LessThan( TimeType ) const;
};
```

Our preference is to locate the public part first so as to focus attention on the public interface and deemphasize the private data representation:

```
class TimeType
{
public:
    void Set( int, int, int );
    void Increment();
    void Write() const;
    bool Equal( TimeType ) const;
    bool LessThan( TimeType ) const;
private:
    int hrs;
    int mins;
    int secs;
};
```

We use this style throughout the remainder of the book.

Regarding public versus private accessibility, we can now describe more fully the difference between C++ structs and classes. C++ defines a struct to be a class whose members are all, by default, public. In contrast, members of a class are, by default, private. Furthermore, it is most common to use only data, not functions, as members of a struct. Note that you *can* declare struct members to be private and you *can* include member functions in a struct, but then you might as well use a class!

Classes, Class Objects, and Class Members

It is important to restate that a class is a type, not a data object. Like any type, a class is a pattern from which you create (or *instantiate*) many objects of that type. Think of a type as a cookie cutter and objects of that type as the cookies.

The declarations

```
TimeType time1;
TimeType time2;
```

create two objects of the TimeType class: time1 and time2. Each object has its own copies of hrs, mins, and secs, the private data members of the class. At a given moment during program execution, time1's copies of hrs, mins, and secs might contain the values 5, 30, and 10; and time2's copies might contain the values 17, 58, and 2. Figure 11-8 is a visual image of the class objects time1 and time2.

(In truth, the C++ compiler does not waste memory by placing duplicate copies of a member function—say, Increment—into both time1 and time2. The compiler generates just one physical copy of Increment, and any class object executes this one copy of the function. Nevertheless, the diagram in Figure 11-8 is a good mental picture of two different class objects.)

FIGURE 11-8
Conceptual View of Two Class Objects

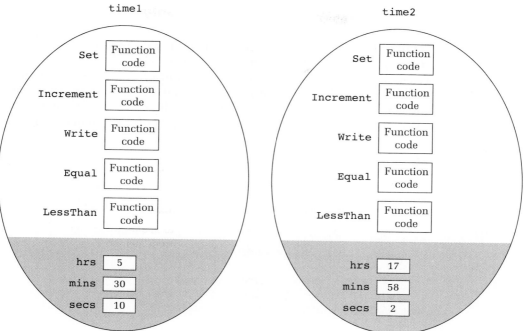

Be sure you are clear about the difference between the terms *class object* and *class member*. Figure 11-8 depicts two objects of the `TimeType` class, and each object has eight members.

Built-in Operations on Class Objects

In many ways, programmer-defined classes are like built-in types. You can declare as many objects of a class as you like. You can pass class objects as arguments to functions and return them as function values. Like any variable, a class object can be automatic (created each time control reaches its declaration and destroyed when control exits its surrounding block) or static (created once when control reaches its declaration and destroyed when the program terminates).

In other ways, C++ treats structs and classes differently from built-in types. Most of the built-in operations do not apply to structs or classes. You cannot use the + operator to add two `TimeType` objects, nor can you use the == operator to compare two `TimeType` objects for equality.

Two built-in operations that are valid for struct and class objects are member selection (.) and assignment (=). As with structs, you select an individual member of a class by using dot notation. That is, you write the name of the class object, then a dot, then the member name. The statement

```
time1.Increment();
```

invokes the `Increment` function for the `time1` object, presumably to add one second to the time stored in `time1`. The other built-in operation, assignment, performs aggregate assignment of one class object to another with the following semantics: If x and y are objects of the same class, then the assignment x = y copies the data members of y into x. Below is a fragment of client code that demonstrates member selection and assignment.

```
TimeType  time1;
TimeType  time2;
int       inputHrs;
int       inputMins;
int       inputSecs;

time1.Set(5, 20, 0);
// Assert: time1 corresponds to 5:20:0

cout << "Enter hours, minutes, seconds: ";
cin >> inputHrs >> inputMins >> inputSecs;
time2.Set(inputHrs, inputMins, inputSecs);

if (time1.LessThan(time2))
    DoSomething();

time2 = time1;                    // Member-by-member assignment
time2.Write();
// Assert: 5:20:0 has been output
```

Earlier we remarked that the `Equal` and `LessThan` functions have only one parameter each, even though they are comparing two `TimeType` objects. In the If statement of the code segment above, we are comparing `time1` and `time2`. Because `LessThan` is a class member function, we invoke it by giving the name of a class object (`time1`), then a dot, then the function name (`LessThan`). Only one item remains unspecified: the class object with which `time1` should be compared (`time2`). Therefore, the `LessThan` function requires only one parameter, not two. Here is another way of explaining it: If a class member function represents a binary (two-operand) operation, the first operand appears to the left of the dot operator, and the second operand is in the parameter list. (To generalize, an *n*-ary operation has *n* − 1 operands in the parameter list. Thus, a unary operation—such as `Write` or `Increment` in the `TimeType` class—has an empty parameter list.)

In addition to member selection and assignment, a few other built-in operators are valid for class objects and structs. These operators are used for manipulating memory addresses, and we defer discussing them until later in the book. For now, think of . and = as the only valid built-in operators.

From the very beginning, you have been working with C++ classes in a particular context: input and output. The standard header file `iostream` contains the declarations of two classes—`istream` and `ostream`—that manage a program's I/O. The C++ standard library declares `cin` and `cout` to be objects of these classes:

```
istream cin;
ostream cout;
```

The `istream` class has many member functions, two of which—the `get` function and the `ignore` function—you have already seen in statements like these:

```
cin.get(someChar);
cin.ignore(200, '\n');
```

As with any C++ class object, we use dot notation to select a particular member function to invoke.

You also have used C++ classes when performing file I/O. The header file `fstream` contains declarations for the `ifstream` and `ofstream` classes. The client code

```
ifstream dataFile;

dataFile.open("input.dat");
```

declares an `ifstream` class object named `dataFile`, then invokes the class member function `open` to try to open a file `input.dat` for input.

We do not examine in detail the `istream`, `ostream`, `ifstream`, and `ofstream` classes and all of their member functions. To study these would be beyond the goals of this book. What is important to recognize is that classes and objects are fundamental to all I/O activity in a C++ program.

Class Scope

We said earlier that member names must be unique within a struct. Additionally, in Chapter 8 we mentioned four kinds of scope in C++: local scope, global scope, namespace scope, and *class scope*. Class scope applies to the member names within structs, unions, and classes. To say that a member name has class scope means that the name is bound to that class (or struct or union). If the same identifier happens to be declared outside the class, the two identifiers are unrelated. Let's look at an example.

The TimeType class has a member function named Write. In the same program, another class (say, SomeClass) could also have a member function named Write. Furthermore, the program might have a global Write function that is completely unrelated to any classes. If the program has statements like

```
TimeType   checkInTime;
SomeClass someObject;
int        n;
  ⋮
checkInTime.Write();
someObject.Write();
Write(n);
```

then the C++ compiler has no trouble distinguishing among the three Write functions. In the first two function calls, the dot notation denotes class member selection. The first statement invokes the Write function of the TimeType class, and the second statement invokes the Write function of the SomeClass class. The final statement does not use dot notation, so the compiler knows that the function being called is the global Write function.

Information Hiding

Conceptually, a class object has an invisible wall around it. This wall, called the **abstraction barrier,** protects private data and functions from being accessed by client code. The barrier also prohibits the class object from directly accessing data and functions outside the object. This barrier is a critical characteristic of classes and abstract data types.

For a class object to share information with the outside world (that is, with clients), there must be a gap in the abstraction barrier. This gap is the public interface—the class members declared to be public. The only way that a client can manipulate the internals of the class object is indirectly—through the operations in the public interface. Engineers have a similar concept called a **black box.** A black box is a module or device whose inner workings are hidden from view. The user of the black box depends only on the written specification of *what* it does, not on *how* it does it. The user connects wires to the interface and assumes that the module works correctly by satisfying the specification (see Figure 11-9).

In software design, the black box concept is referred to as **information hiding.** Information hiding protects the user of a class from having to know all the details of its implementation. Information hiding also assures the

FIGURE 11-9
A Black Box

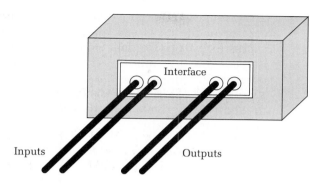

class's implementor that the user cannot directly access any private code or data and compromise the correctness of the implementation.

You have been introduced to encapsulation and information hiding before. In Chapter 7, we discussed the possibility of hiding a function's implementation in a separate file. In this chapter, you'll see how to hide the implementations of class member functions by placing them in files that are separate from the client code.

Abstraction barrier   The invisible wall around a class object that encapsulates implementation details. The wall can be breached only through the public interface.

Black box   An electrical or mechanical device whose inner workings are hidden from view.

Information hiding   The encapsulation and hiding of implementation details to keep the user of an abstraction from depending on or incorrectly manipulating these details.

The creator of a C++ class is free to choose which members are private and which are public. However, making data members public (as in a struct) allows the client to inspect and modify the data directly. Because information hiding is so fundamental to data abstraction, most classes exhibit a typical pattern: The private part contains data, and the public part contains the functions that manipulate the data.

The TimeType class exemplifies this organization. The data members hrs, mins, and secs are private, so the compiler prohibits a client from accessing these members directly. The following client statement therefore results in a compile-time error:

```
TimeType checkInTime;

checkInTime.hrs = 9;     // Prohibited in client code
```

Because only the class's member functions can access the private data, the creator of the class can offer a reliable product, knowing that external access to the private data is impossible. If it is acceptable to let the client *inspect* (but not modify) private data members, a class might provide observer functions. The `TimeType` class has three such functions: `Write`, `Equal`, and `LessThan`. Because these observer functions are not intended to modify the private data, they are declared with the word `const` following the parameter list:

```
void Write() const;
bool Equal( TimeType ) const;
bool LessThan( TimeType ) const;
```

C++ refers to these functions as *const member functions*. Within the body of a `const` member function, a compile-time error occurs if any statement tries to modify a private data member. Although not required by the language, it is good practice to declare as `const` those member functions that do not modify private data.

Specification and Implementation Files

An abstract data type consists of two parts: a specification and an implementation. The specification describes the behavior of the data type without reference to its implementation. The implementation creates an abstraction barrier by hiding the concrete data representation as well as the code for the operations.

The `TimeType` class declaration serves as the specification of `TimeType`. This declaration presents the public interface to the user in the form of function prototypes. To implement the `TimeType` class, we must provide function definitions (declarations with bodies) for all the member functions.

In C++, it is customary (though not required) to package the class declaration and the class implementation into separate files. One file—the *specification file*—is a header (`.h`) file containing only the class declaration. The second file—the *implementation file*—contains the function definitions for the class member functions. Let's look first at the specification file.

The Specification File

Below is the specification file for the `TimeType` class. On our computer system, we have named the file `timetype.h`. The class declaration is the same as we presented earlier, with one important exception: We include function preconditions and postconditions to specify the semantics of the member functions as unambiguously as possible for the user of the class.

```
//****************************************************************
// SPECIFICATION FILE (timetype.h)
// This file gives the specification
// of a TimeType abstract data type
//****************************************************************

class TimeType
{
public:
    void Set( /* in */ int hours,
              /* in */ int minutes,
              /* in */ int seconds );
        // Precondition:
        //     0 <= hours <= 23  &&  0 <= minutes <= 59
        //  && 0 <= seconds <= 59
        // Postcondition:
        //     Time is set according to the incoming parameters
        // NOTE:
        //     This function MUST be called prior to
        //     any of the other member functions

    void Increment();
        // Precondition:
        //     The Set function has been invoked at least once
        // Postcondition:
        //     Time has been advanced by one second, with
        //     23:59:59 wrapping around to 0:0:0

    void Write() const;
        // Precondition:
        //     The Set function has been invoked at least once
        // Postcondition:
        //     Time has been output in the form HH:MM:SS

    bool Equal( /* in */ TimeType otherTime ) const;
        // Precondition:
        //     The Set function has been invoked at least once
        //     for both this time and otherTime
        // Postcondition:
        //     Function value == true, if this time equals otherTime
        //                    == false, otherwise

    bool LessThan( /* in */ TimeType otherTime ) const;
        // Precondition:
        //     The Set function has been invoked at least once
        //     for both this time and otherTime
```

```
//   && This time and otherTime represent times in the
//      same day
// Postcondition:
//      Function value == true, if this time is earlier
//                              in the day than otherTime
//                        == false, otherwise
private:
    int hrs;
    int mins;
    int secs;
};
```

Notice the preconditions for the `Increment`, `Write`, `Equal`, and `LessThan` functions. It is the responsibility of the client to set the time before incrementing, printing, or testing it. If the client fails to set the time, the effect of each of these functions is undefined.

In principle, a specification file should not reveal any implementation details to the user of the class. The file should specify *what* each member function does without disclosing *how* it does it. However, as you can see in the class declaration, there is one implementation detail that is visible to the user: the concrete data representation of our ADT that is listed in the private part. However, the data representation is still considered hidden information in the sense that the compiler prohibits client code from accessing the data directly.

The Implementation File

The specification (`.h`) file for the `TimeType` class contains only the class declaration. The implementation file must provide the function definitions for all the class member functions. In the opening comments of the implementation file below, we document the file name as `timetype.cpp`. Your system may use a different file name suffix for source code files, perhaps `.c`, `.C`, or `.cxx`.

We recommend that you first skim the C++ code below, not being too concerned about the new language features such as prefixing the name of each function with the symbols

```
TimeType::
```

Immediately following the program code, we explain the new features.

```
//*****************************************************************
// IMPLEMENTATION FILE (timetype.cpp)
// This file implements the TimeType member functions
//*****************************************************************
```

```cpp
#include "timetype.h"
#include <iostream>

using namespace std;

// Private members of class:
//      int hrs;
//      int mins;
//      int secs;

//*****************************************************************

void TimeType::Set( /* in */ int hours,
                    /* in */ int minutes,
                    /* in */ int seconds )

// Precondition:
//      0 <= hours <= 23   &&   0 <= minutes <= 59
//   && 0 <= seconds <= 59
// Postcondition:
//      hrs == hours  &&  mins == minutes  &&  secs == seconds
// NOTE:
//      This function MUST be called prior to
//      any of the other member functions

{
    hrs = hours;
    mins = minutes;
    secs = seconds;
}

//*****************************************************************

void TimeType::Increment()

// Precondition:
//      The Set function has been invoked at least once
// Postcondition:
//      Time has been advanced by one second, with
//      23:59:59 wrapping around to 0:0:0

{
    secs++;
    if (secs > 59)
    {
        secs = 0;
        mins++;
        if (mins > 59)
        {
```

```
            mins = 0;
            hrs++;
            if (hrs > 23)
                hrs = 0;
        }
    }
}


//****************************************************************

void TimeType::Write() const

// Precondition:
//      The Set function has been invoked at least once
// Postcondition:
//      Time has been output in the form HH:MM:SS

{
    if (hrs < 10)
        cout << '0';
    cout << hrs << ':';
    if (mins < 10)
        cout << '0';
    cout << mins << ':';
    if (secs < 10)
        cout << '0';
    cout << secs;
}


//****************************************************************

bool TimeType::Equal( /* in */ TimeType otherTime ) const

// Precondition:
//      The Set function has been invoked at least once
//      for both this time and otherTime
// Postcondition:
//      Function value == true, if this time equals otherTime
//                     == false, otherwise

{
    return (hrs == otherTime.hrs && mins == otherTime.mins &&
            secs == otherTime.secs);
}


//****************************************************************
```

```
bool TimeType::LessThan( /* in */ TimeType otherTime ) const

// Precondition:
//      The Set function has been invoked at least once
//      for both this time and otherTime
//   && This time and otherTime represent times in the
//      same day
// Postcondition:
//      Function value == true, if this time is earlier
//                               in the day than otherTime
//                     == false, otherwise

{
    return (hrs < otherTime.hrs ||
            hrs == otherTime.hrs && mins < otherTime.mins ||
            hrs == otherTime.hrs && mins == otherTime.mins
                                 && secs < otherTime.secs);
}
```

This implementation file demonstrates several important points.

1. The file begins with the preprocessor directive

    ```
    #include "timetype.h"
    ```

    Both the implementation file and the client code must #include the specification file. Figure 11-10 pictures this shared access to the specification file. This sharing guarantees that all declarations related to an abstraction are consistent. That is, both client.cpp and timetype.cpp must reference the same declaration of the TimeType class located in timetype.h.

2. Near the top of the implementation file we have included a comment that restates the private members of the TimeType class.

    ```
    // Private members of class:
    //      int hrs;
    //      int mins;
    //      int secs;
    ```

    This comment reminds the reader that any references to these identifiers are references to the private class members.

3. In the heading of each function definition, the name of the member function is prefixed by the class name (TimeType) and the C++ scope resolution operator (::). As we discussed earlier, it is possible for several different classes to have member functions with the same name, say, Write. In addition, there may be a global Write function that is not a member of any class. The scope resolution operator eliminates any uncertainty about which particular function is being defined.

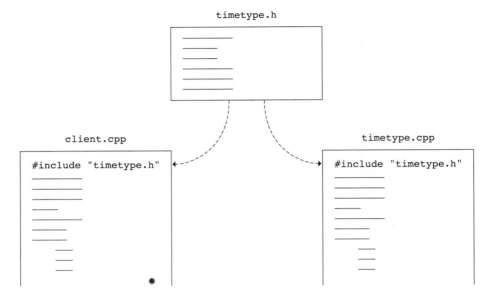

4. Although clients of a class must use the dot operator to refer to class members (for example, `startTime.Write()`), members of a class refer to each other directly without using dot notation. Looking at the bodies of the `Set` and `Increment` functions, you can see that the statements refer directly to the member variables `hrs`, `mins`, and `secs` without using the dot operator.

    An exception to this rule occurs when a member function manipulates two or more class objects. Consider the `Equal` function. Suppose that the client code has two class objects, `startTime` and `endTime`, and uses the statement

    ```
    if (startTime.Equal(endTime))
       ⋮
    ```

    At execution time, the `startTime` object is the object for which the `Equal` function is invoked. In the body of the `Equal` function, the relational expression

    ```
    hrs == otherTime.hrs
    ```

    refers to class members of two different class objects. The unadorned identifier `hrs` refers to the `hrs` member of the class object for which the function is invoked (that is, `startTime`). The expression `otherTime.hrs` refers to the `hrs` member of the class object that is passed as a function argument: `endTime`.

5. `Write`, `Equal`, and `LessThan` are observer functions; they do not modify the private data of the class. Because we have declared these to be `const` member functions, the compiler prevents them from assigning new values to the private data. The use of `const` is both an aid to the user of the class (as a visual signal that this function does not modify any private data) and an aid to the class implementor (as a way of preventing accidental modification of the data). Note that the word `const` must appear in both the function prototype (in the class declaration) and the heading of the function definition.

Compiling and Linking a Multifile Program

Now that we have created a specification file and an implementation file for our `TimeType` class, how do we (or any other programmer) make use of these files in our programs? Let's begin by looking at the notion of *separate compilation* of source code files.

In earlier chapters, we have referred to the concept of a multifile program—a program divided up into several files containing source code. In C++, it is possible to compile each of these files separately and at different times. The compiler translates each source code file into an object code file. Figure 11-11 shows a multifile program consisting of the source code files `myprog.cpp`, `file2.cpp`, and `file3.cpp`. We can compile each of these files independently, yielding object code files `myprog.obj`, `file2.obj`, and `file3.obj`. Although each `.obj` file contains machine language code, it is not yet in executable form. The system's linker program brings the object code together to form an executable program file. (In Figure 11-11, we use the file name suffixes `.cpp`, `.obj`, and `.exe`. Your C++ system may use different file name conventions.)

Files such as `file2.cpp` and `file3.cpp` typically contain function definitions for functions that are called by the code in `myprog.cpp`. An important benefit of separate compilation is that modifying the code in just one file requires recompiling only that file. The new `.obj` file is then relinked with the other existing `.obj` files. Of course, if a modification to one file affects the code in another file—for example, changing a function's interface by altering the number or data types of the function parameters—then the affected files also need to be modified and recompiled.

Returning to our `TimeType` class, let's assume we have used the system's editor to create the `timetype.h` and `timetype.cpp` files. Now we can compile `timetype.cpp` into object code. If we are working at the operating system's command line, we use a command similar to the following:

```
cc -c timetype.cpp
```

FIGURE 11-11

Separate
Compilation and
Linking

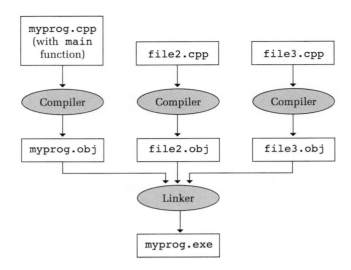

In this example, we assume that cc is the name of a command that invokes either the C++ compiler or the linker or both, depending on various options given on the command line. The command-line option -c means, on many systems, "compile but do not link." In other words, this command produces an object code file, say, timetype.obj, but does not attempt to link this file with any other file.

A programmer wishing to use the TimeType class will write code that #includes the file timetype.h, then declares and uses TimeType objects:

```
#include "timetype.h"
  ⋮
TimeType appointment;

appointment.Set(15, 30, 0);
appointment.Write();
  ⋮
```

If this client code is in a file named diary.cpp, an operating system command like

```
cc diary.cpp timetype.obj
```

compiles the client program into object code, links this object code with timetype.obj, and produces an executable program (see Figure 11-12).

The mechanics of compiling, linking, and executing vary from one computer system to another. Our examples using the cc command assume you are working at the operating system's command line. Many C++ sys-

FIGURE 11-12
Linking with the
TimeType
Implementation
File

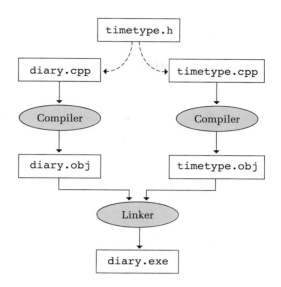

tems provide an *integrated environment*—a program that bundles the editor, the compiler, and the linker into one package. Integrated environments put you back into the editor when a compile-time or link-time error occurs, pinpointing the location of the error. Some integrated environments also manage *project files*. Project files contain information about all the constituent files of a multifile program. With project files, the system automatically recompiles or relinks any files that have become out-of-date because of changes to other files of the program.

Whichever environment you use—the command-line environment or an integrated environment—the overall process is the same: You compile the individual source code files into object code, link the object files into an executable program, then execute the program.

Before leaving the topic of multifile programs, we stress an important point. Referring to Figure 11-12, the files timetype.h and timetype.obj must be available to users of the TimeType class. The user needs to examine timetype.h to see what TimeType objects do and how to use them. The user must also be able to link his or her program with timetype.obj to produce an executable program. But the user does *not* need to see timetype.cpp. The implementation of TimeType should be treated as a black box. The main purpose of abstraction is to simplify the programmer's job by reducing complexity. Users of an abstraction should not have to look at its implementation to learn how to use it, nor should they write programs that depend on implementation details. In the latter case, any changes in the implementation could "break" the user's programs. In Chapter 7, the Software Engineering Tip box entitled "Conceptual Versus Physical Hiding of a Function Implementation" discussed the hazards of writing code that relies on implementation details.

Guaranteed Initialization with Class Constructors

The TimeType class we have been discussing has a weakness. It depends on the client to invoke the Set function before calling any other member function. For example, the Increment function's precondition is

```
// Precondition:
//     The Set function has been invoked at least once
```

If the client fails to invoke the Set function first, this precondition is false and the contract between the client and the function implementation is broken. Because classes nearly always encapsulate data, the creator of a class should not rely on the user to initialize the data. If the user forgets to do so, unpleasant results may occur.

C++ provides a mechanism, called a *class constructor,* to guarantee the initialization of a class object. A constructor is a member function that is implicitly invoked whenever a class object is created.

A constructor function has an unusual name: the name of the class itself. Let's change the TimeType class by adding two class constructors:

```
class TimeType
{
public:
    void Set( int, int, int );
    void Increment();
    void Write() const;
    bool Equal( TimeType ) const;
    bool LessThan( TimeType ) const;
    TimeType( int, int, int );          // Constructor
    TimeType();                         // Constructor
private:
    int hrs;
    int mins;
    int secs;
};
```

This class declaration includes two constructors, differentiated by their parameter lists. The first has three int parameters, which, as we will see, are used to initialize the private data when a class object is created. The second constructor is parameterless and initializes the time to some default value, such as 0:0:0. A parameterless constructor is known in C++ as a *default constructor.*

Constructor declarations are unique in two ways. First, as we have mentioned, the name of the function is the same as the name of the class. Second, the data type of the function is omitted. The reason is that a constructor cannot return a function value. Its purpose is only to initialize a class object's private data.

In the implementation file, the function definitions for the two `TimeType` constructors might look like the following:

```
//****************************************************************

TimeType::TimeType( /* in */ int initHrs,
                    /* in */ int initMins,
                    /* in */ int initSecs )
// Constructor

// Precondition:
//     0 <= initHrs <= 23  &&  0 <= initMins <= 59
// && 0 <= initSecs <= 59
// Postcondition:
//     hrs == initHrs  &&  mins == initMins  &&  secs == initSecs

{
    hrs = initHrs;
    mins = initMins;
    secs = initSecs;
}


//****************************************************************

TimeType::TimeType()

// Default constructor

// Postcondition:
//     hrs == 0  &&  mins == 0  &&  secs == 0

{
    hrs = 0;
    mins = 0;
    secs = 0;
}
```

Invoking a Constructor

Although a constructor is a member of a class, it is never invoked using dot notation. A constructor is automatically invoked whenever a class object is created. The client declaration

```
TimeType lectureTime(10, 30, 0);
```

includes an argument list to the right of the name of the class object being declared. When this declaration is encountered at execution time, the first (parameterized) constructor is automatically invoked, initializing the private data of lectureTime to the time 10:30:0. The client declaration

```
TimeType startTime;
```

has no argument list after the identifier startTime. The default (parameterless) constructor is implicitly invoked, initializing startTime's private data to the time 0:0:0.

Remember that a declaration in C++ is a genuine statement and can appear anywhere among executable statements. Placing declarations among executable statements is extremely useful when creating class objects whose initial values are not known until execution time. Here's an example:

```
cout << "Enter appointment time in hours, minutes, and seconds: ";
cin >> hours >> minutes >> seconds;

TimeType appointmentTime(hours, minutes, seconds);

cout << "The appointment time is ";
appointmentTime.Write();
  ⋮
```

Revised Specification and Implementation Files for `TimeType`

By including constructors for the TimeType class, we are sure that each class object is initialized before any subsequent calls to the class member functions. One of the constructors allows the client code to specify an initial time; the other creates an initial time of 0:0:0 if the client does not specify a time. Because of these constructors, it is *impossible* for a TimeType object to be in an uninitialized state after it is created. As a result, we can delete from the TimeType specification file the warning to call Set before calling any other member functions. Also, we can remove all of the function preconditions that require Set to be called previously. Here is the revised TimeType specification file:

```
//*****************************************************************
// SPECIFICATION FILE (timetype.h)
// This file gives the specification
// of a TimeType abstract data type
//*****************************************************************
```

```cpp
class TimeType
{
public:
    void Set( /* in */ int hours,
              /* in */ int minutes,
              /* in */ int seconds );
        // Precondition:
        //     0 <= hours <= 23  &&  0 <= minutes <= 59
        //  && 0 <= seconds <= 59
        // Postcondition:
        //     Time is set according to the incoming parameters

    void Increment();
        // Postcondition:
        //     Time has been advanced by one second, with
        //     23:59:59 wrapping around to 0:0:0

    void Write() const;
        // Postcondition:
        //     Time has been output in the form HH:MM:SS

    bool Equal( /* in */ TimeType otherTime ) const;
        // Postcondition:
        //     Function value == true, if this time equals otherTime
        //                    == false, otherwise

    bool LessThan( /* in */ TimeType otherTime ) const;
        // Precondition:
        //     This time and otherTime represent times in the
        //     same day
        // Postcondition:
        //     Function value == true, if this time is earlier
        //                              in the day than otherTime
        //                    == false, otherwise

    TimeType( /* in */ int initHrs,
              /* in */ int initMins,
              /* in */ int initSecs );
        // Precondition:
        //     0 <= initHrs <= 23  &&  0 <= initMins <= 59
        //  && 0 <= initSecs <= 59
        // Postcondition:
        //     Class object is constructed
        //  && Time is set according to the incoming parameters

    TimeType();
        // Postcondition:
        //     Class object is constructed  &&  Time is 0:0:0
```

```
private:
    int hrs;
    int mins;
    int secs;
};
```

To save space, we do not include the revised implementation file here. The only changes are as follows:

1. The inclusion of the function definitions for the two class constructors, which we presented earlier.
2. The deletion of all function preconditions stating that the Set function must be invoked previously.

At this point, you may wonder whether we need the Set function at all. After all, both the Set function and the parameterized constructor seem to do the same thing—set the time according to values passed as arguments—and the implementations of the two functions are essentially identical. The difference is that Set can be invoked for an existing class object whenever and as often as we wish, whereas the parameterized constructor is invoked once only—at the moment a class object is created. Therefore, we retain the Set function to provide maximum flexibility to clients of the class.

Guidelines for Using Class Constructors

The class is an essential language feature for creating abstract data types in C++. The class mechanism is a powerful design tool, but along with this power come rules for using classes correctly.

C++ has some very intricate rules about using constructors, many of which relate to language features we have not yet discussed. Below are some guidelines that are pertinent at this point.

1. A constructor cannot return a function value, so the function is declared without a return value type.
2. A class may provide several constructors. When a class object is declared, the compiler chooses the appropriate constructor according to the number and data types of the arguments to the constructor.
3. Arguments to a constructor are passed by placing the argument list immediately after the name of the class object being declared:

    ```
    SomeClass anObject(arg1, arg2);
    ```

4. If a class object is declared without an argument list, as in the statement

    ```
    SomeClass anObject;
    ```

then the effect depends upon what constructors (if any) the class provides.

If the class has no constructors at all, memory is allocated for anObject but its private data members are in an uninitialized state.

If the class does have constructors, then the default (parameterless) constructor is invoked if there is one. If the class has constructors but no default constructor, a syntax error occurs.

Before leaving the topic of constructors, we give you a brief preview of another special member function supported by C++: the *class destructor.* Just as a constructor is implicitly invoked when a class object is created, a destructor is implicitly invoked when a class object is destroyed—for example, when control leaves the block in which a local object is declared. A class destructor is named the same as a constructor except that the first character is a tilde (~):

```cpp
class SomeClass
{
public:
    ⋮
    SomeClass();      // Constructor
    ~SomeClass();     // Destructor
private:
    ⋮
};
```

In the next few chapters, we won't be using destructors; the kinds of classes we'll be writing have no need to perform special actions at the moment a class object is destroyed. In Chapter 15, we explore destructors in detail and describe the situations in which you need to use them.

PROBLEM-SOLVING CASE STUDY

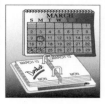

Manipulating Dates

Dates are often necessary pieces of information. In programs, our processing of dates may call for us to compare two dates, print a date, or determine the date a certain number of days in the future. The machine shop example had a date as part of the data. In fact, the machine shop example had two dates: the date of purchase and the date of last service. Each time we needed a date, we defined it again.

Let's stop this duplication of effort and do the job once and for all—let's write the code to support a date as an abstract data type.

The format for this case study needs to be a little different. Because we are developing only one software component—an ADT—and not a complete program, we omit the Input and Output sections. Instead, we include two sections entitled Specification of the ADT and Implementation of the ADT.

Problem: Design and implement an ADT to represent a date. Make the domain and operations general enough to be used in any program that needs to perform these operations on dates. The informal specification of the ADT is given below.

TYPE
  DateType
DOMAIN
  Each DateType value is a single date after the year 1582 A.D. in the form of month, day, and year.
OPERATIONS
  Construct a new DateType instance.
  Set the date.
  Inspect the date's month.
  Inspect the date's day.
  Inspect the date's year.
  Print the date.
  Compare two dates for "before," "equal," or "after."
  Increment the date by one day.

Discussion: We create the DateType ADT in two stages: specification, followed by implementation. The result of the first stage is a C++ specification (.h) file containing the declaration of a DateType class. This file must describe for the user the precise semantics of each ADT operation. The informal specification given above would be unacceptable to the user of the ADT. The descriptions of the operations are too imprecise and ambiguous to be helpful to the user.

The second stage—implementation—requires us to (a) choose a concrete data representation for a date, and (b) implement each of the operations as a C++ function definition. The result is a C++ implementation file containing these function definitions.

Specification of the ADT: The domain of our ADT is the set of all dates after the year 1582 A.D. in the form of a month, a day, and a year. We restrict the year to be after 1582 A.D. in order to simplify the ADT opera-

<u>*PROBLEM-SOLVING CASE STUDY cont'd.*</u>

tions (ten days were skipped in 1582 in switching from the Julian to the Gregorian calendar).

To represent the DateType ADT as program code, we use a C++ class named `DateType`. The ADT operations become public member functions of the class. Let's now specify the operations more carefully.

Construct a new DateType instance: For this operation, we use a C++ default constructor that initializes the date to January 1 of the year 1583. The client code can reset the date at any time using the "Set the date" operation.

Set the date: The client must supply three arguments for this operation: month, day, and year. Although we haven't yet determined a concrete data representation for a date, we must decide what data types the client should use for these arguments. We choose integers, where the month must be in the range 1 through 12, the day must be in the range 1 through the maximum number of days in the month, and the year must be greater than 1582. Notice that these range restrictions will become the precondition for invoking this operation.

Inspect the date's month, inspect the date's day, and inspect the date's year: All three of these operations are observer operations. They give the client access, indirectly, to the private data. In the `DateType` class, we represent these operations as value-returning member functions with the following prototypes:

```
int Month();
int Day();
int Year();
```

Why do we need these observer operations? Why not simply let the data representation of the month, day, and year be public instead of private so that the client can access the values directly? The answer is that the client should be allowed to inspect *but not modify* these values. If the data were public, a client could manipulate the data incorrectly (such as incrementing January 31 to January 32), thereby compromising the correct behavior of the ADT.

Print the date: This operation prints the date on the standard output device in the following form:

```
January 12, 2001
```

Compare two dates: This operation compares two dates and determines whether the first one comes before the second one, they are the same, or the first one comes after the second one. To indicate the result of the comparison, we define an enumeration type with three values:

```
enum RelationType {BEFORE, SAME, AFTER};
```

Then we can code the comparison operation as a class member function that returns a value of type `RelationType`. Here is the function prototype:

```
RelationType ComparedTo( /* in */ DateType otherDate ) const;
```

Because this is a class member function, the date being compared to `otherDate` is the class object for which the member function is invoked. For example, the following client code tests to see whether `date1` comes before `date2`.

```
DateType date1;
DateType date2;
  ⋮
if (date1.ComparedTo(date2) == BEFORE)
    DoSomething();
```

Increment the date by one day: This operation advances the date to the next day. For example, given the date March 31, 2000, this operation changes the date to April 1, 2000.

We are now almost ready to write the C++ specification file for our `DateType` class. However, the class declaration requires us to include the private part—the private variables that are the concrete data representation of the ADT. Choosing a concrete data representation properly belongs in the ADT implementation phase, not the specification phase. But to satisfy the C++ class declaration requirement, we now choose a data representation. The simplest representation for a date is three `int` values—one each for the month, day, and year. Here, then, is the specification file containing the `DateType` class declaration (along with the declaration of the `RelationType` enumeration type).

```
//****************************************************************
// SPECIFICATION FILE (datetype.h)
// This file gives the specification of a DateType abstract data
// type and provides an enumeration type for comparing dates
//****************************************************************
```

PROBLEM-SOLVING CASE STUDY cont'd.

```cpp
enum RelationType {BEFORE, SAME, AFTER};

class DateType
{
public:
    void Set( /* in */ int newMonth,
              /* in */ int newDay,
              /* in */ int newYear  );
        // Precondition:
        //     1 <= newMonth <= 12
        //  && 1 <= newDay <= maximum no. of days in month newMonth
        //  && newYear > 1582
        // Postcondition:
        //     Date is set according to the incoming parameters

    int Month() const;
        // Postcondition:
        //     Function value == this date's month

    int Day() const;
        // Postcondition:
        //     Function value == this date's day

    int Year() const;
        // Postcondition:
        //     Function value == this date's year

    void Print() const;
        // Postcondition:
        //     Date has been output in the form
        //         month day, year
        //     where the name of the month is printed as a string

    RelationType ComparedTo( /* in */ DateType otherDate ) const;
        // Postcondition:
        //     Function value == BEFORE, if this date is
        //                                   before otherDate
        //                    == SAME, if this date equals otherDate
        //                    == AFTER, if this date is
        //                                   after otherDate

    void Increment();
        // Postcondition:
        //     Date has been advanced by one day

    DateType();
        // Postcondition:
```

```
//      New DateType object is constructed with a
//      month, day, and year of 1, 1, and 1583
private:
    int mo;
    int day;
    int yr;
};
```

Implementation of the ADT: We have already chosen a concrete data representation for a date, shown in the specification file as the `int` variables `mo`, `day`, and `yr`. Now we must implement each class member function, placing the function definitions into a C++ implementation file named, say, `datetype.cpp`. As we implement the member functions, we also discuss testing strategies that can help to convince us that the implementations are correct.

The class constructor, `Set`, `Month`, `Day`, *and* `Year` *functions:* The implementations of these functions are so straightforward that no discussion is needed.

The class constructor DateType ( )

```
Set mo = 1
Set day = 1
Set yr = 1583
```

Set (In: newMonth, newDay, newYear)

```
Set mo = newMonth
Set day = newDay
Set yr = newYear
```

Month ( )

Out: Function value

```
Return mo
```

PROBLEM-SOLVING CASE STUDY cont'd.

Day ( )

Out: Function value

┌─────────────────┐
│ Return day   │
└─────────────────┘

Year ( )

Out: Function value

┌─────────────────┐
│ Return yr   │
└─────────────────┘

Testing: The `Month`, `Day`, and `Year` observer functions can be used to verify that the class constructor and `Set` functions work correctly. The code

```
DateType someDate;

cout << someDate.Month() << ' ' << someDate.Day() << ' '
    << someDate.Year() << endl;
```

should print out 1 1 1583. To test the `Set` function, it is sufficient to set a `DateType` object to a few different values (obeying the precondition for the `Set` function), then print out the month, day, and year as above.

The Print function The date is to be printed in the form month, day, comma, and year. We need a blank to separate the month and the day, and a comma followed by a blank to separate the day and the year. Because the month is represented as an integer in the range 1 through 12, we can use a Switch statement to print out the month in word form.

Print ( )

┌──────────────────────────────────┐
│ SWITCH mo   │
│   1: Print "January"   │
│   2: Print "February"   │
│   ⋮   │
│   12: Print "December"   │
│ Print ' ', day, ", ", yr   │
└──────────────────────────────────┘

Testing: In testing the `Print` function, we should print each month at least once. Both the year and the day should be tested at their end points and at several points between.

The `ComparedTo` function: If we were to compare two dates in our heads, we would look first at the years. If the years were different, we would immediately know which date came first. If the years were the same, we would look at the months. If the months were the same, we would have to look at the days. As so often happens, we can use this algorithm directly in our function.

ComparedTo (In: otherDate)

   Out: Function value

IF yr < otherDate.yr
        Return BEFORE
IF yr > otherDate.yr
        Return AFTER

// Years are equal. Compare months
IF mo < otherDate.mo
        Return BEFORE
IF mo > otherDate.mo
        Return AFTER

// Years and months are equal. Compare days
IF day < otherDate.day
        Return BEFORE
IF day > otherDate.day
        Return AFTER

// Years, months, and days are equal
Return SAME

Testing: In testing this function, we should ensure that each path is taken at least once. Case Study Follow-Up Exercises 2 and 3 ask you to design test data for this function and to write a driver that does the testing.

PROBLEM-SOLVING CASE STUDY *cont'd.*

The Increment *function:* The algorithm to increment the date is similar to our earlier algorithm for incrementing a TimeType value by one second. If the current date plus 1 is still within the same month, we are done. If the current date plus 1 is within the next month, then we must increment the month and reset the day to 1. Finally, we must not forget to increment the year when the month changes from December to January.

To determine whether the current date plus 1 is within the current month, we add 1 to the current day and compare this value with the maximum number of days in the current month. In this comparison, we must remember to check for leap year if the month is February.

Increment ( )

```
Increment day by 1
IF day > number of days in month "mo"
        Set day = 1
        Increment mo by 1
        IF mo > 12
                Set mo = 1
                Increment yr by 1
```

We can code the algorithm for finding the number of days in a month as a separate function—an auxiliary ("helper") function that is not a member of the DateType class. The number of days in February might need to be adjusted for leap year, so this function must receive as parameters both a month and a year.

DaysInMonth (In: month, year)

Out: Function value

```
SWITCH month
        1, 3, 5, 7, 8, 10, 12 : Return 31
        4, 6, 9, 11 : Return 30
        2 :    // It's February.  Check for leap year
                IF (year MOD 4 is 0 AND year MOD 100 isn't 0)
                OR year MOD 400 is 0
                        Return 29
        ELSE
                Return 28
```

Testing: To test the `Increment` function, we need to create a driver that calls the function with different values for the date. Values that cause the month to change must be tested, as well as values that cause the year to change. Leap year must be tested, including years with the last two digits 00. Case Study Follow-Up Exercises 4 and 5 ask you to carry out this testing.

Here is the implementation file that contains function definitions for all of the ADT operations:

```
//*****************************************************************
// IMPLEMENTATION FILE (datetype.cpp)
// This file implements the DateType member functions
//*****************************************************************
#include "datetype.h"
#include <iostream>

using namespace std;

// Private members of class:
//      int mo;
//      int day;
//      int yr;

int DaysInMonth( int, int );  // Prototype for auxiliary function

//*****************************************************************

DateType::DateType()

// Constructor

// Postcondition:
//      mo == 1  &&  day == 1  &&  yr == 1583

{
    mo = 1;
    day = 1;
    yr = 1583;
}

//*****************************************************************

void DateType::Set( /* in */ int newMonth,
                    /* in */ int newDay,
                    /* in */ int newYear  )

// Precondition:
//      1 <= newMonth <= 12
```

PROBLEM-SOLVING CASE STUDY cont'd.

```
//    && 1 <= newDay <= maximum no. of days in month newMonth
//    && newYear > 1582
// Postcondition:
//      mo == newMonth  &&  day == newDay  &&  yr == newYear

{
    mo = newMonth;
    day = newDay;
    yr = newYear;
}

//*****************************************************************

int DateType::Month() const

// Postcondition:
//      Function value == mo

{
    return mo;
}

//*****************************************************************

int DateType::Day() const

// Postcondition:
//      Function value == day

{
    return day;
}

//*****************************************************************

int DateType::Year() const

// Postcondition:
//      Function value == yr

{
    return yr;
}

//*****************************************************************
```

PROBLEM-SOLVING CASE STUDY cont'd.

```cpp
void DateType::Print() const

// Postcondition:
//      Date has been output in the form
//          month day, year
//      where the name of the month is printed as a string

{
    switch (mo)
    {
        case 1 : cout << "January";
                break;
        case 2 : cout << "February";
                break;
        case 3 : cout << "March";
                break;
        case 4 : cout << "April";
                break;
        case 5 : cout << "May";
                break;
        case 6 : cout << "June";
                break;
        case 7 : cout << "July";
                break;
        case 8 : cout << "August";
                break;
        case 9 : cout << "September";
                break;
        case 10 : cout << "October";
                break;
        case 11 : cout << "November";
                break;
        case 12 : cout << "December";
    }
    cout << ' ' << day << ", " << yr;
}

//****************************************************************

RelationType DateType::ComparedTo(
                    /* in */ DateType otherDate ) const

// Postcondition:
//      Function value == BEFORE, if this date is
//                              before otherDate
//                      == SAME, if this date equals otherDate
//                      == AFTER, if this date is
//                              after otherDate
```

PROBLEM-SOLVING CASE STUDY *cont'd.*

```
    {
        if (yr < otherDate.yr)              // Compare years
            return BEFORE;
        if (yr > otherDate.yr)
            return AFTER;

        if (mo < otherDate.mo)              // Years are equal. Compare
            return BEFORE;                  //    months
        if (mo > otherDate.mo)
            return AFTER;

        if (day < otherDate.day)            // Years and months are equal.
            return BEFORE;                  //    Compare days
        if (day > otherDate.day)
            return AFTER;

        return SAME;                        // Years, months, and days
    }                                       //    are equal

//*******************************************************************

void DateType::Increment()

// Postcondition:
//      Date has been advanced by one day

{
    day++;
    if (day > DaysInMonth(mo, yr))
    {
        day = 1;
        mo++;
        if (mo > 12)
        {
            mo = 1;
            yr++;
        }
    }
}

//*******************************************************************

int DaysInMonth( /* in */ int month,
                 /* in */ int year  )

// Returns the number of days in month "month", taking
// leap year into account
```

```
// Precondition:
//     1 <= month <= 12  &&  year > 1582
// Postcondition:
//     Function value == number of days in month "month "

{
    switch (month)
    {
        case 1: case 3: case 5: case 7: case 8: case 10: case 12:
            return 31;
        case 4: case 6: case 9: case 11:
            return 30;
        case 2:    // It's February.  Check for leap year
            if ((year % 4 == 0 && year % 100 != 0) ||
                year % 400 == 0)
                return 29;
            else
                return 28;
    }
}
```

A date is a logical entity for which we now have developed an implementation. We have designed, implemented, and tested a date ADT that we (or any programmer) can use whenever we have a date as part of our program data. If we discover in the future that additional operations on a date would be useful, we can implement, test, and add them to our set of date operations.

We have said that data abstraction is an important principle of software design. What we have done here is an example of data abstraction. From now on, when a problem needs a date, we can stop our decomposition at the logical level. We do not need to worry about implementing a date each time.

PROBLEM-SOLVING CASE STUDY

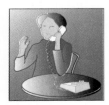

Birthday Calls

Problem: Everyone has at least one friend who always remembers everyone's birthday. Each year when we receive greetings on our birthday from this friend, we promise to do better about remembering others' birthdays. Let's write a program to go through your address book and print the names and phone numbers of all the people who have birthdays within the next two weeks, so you can give them a call. Here, the "address book" is a data file containing information about your friends.

Input: Today's date (from the keyboard); and a list of names, phone numbers, and birth dates (from file `friendFile`). Entries in this file are in the form

```
John Arbuthnot
(493) 384-2938
 1/12/1970

Mary Smith
(123) 123-4567
10/12/1960
```

Output: The names, phone numbers, and birthdays of any friends whose birthdays are within the next two weeks. A sample of the output is

```
John Arbuthnot
(493) 384-2938
January 12, 2001
```

Note that the date printed is the friend's next birthday, not the friend's birth date.

Discussion: As we start our design phase for this problem, we call all the information about one person an *entry*. An entry consists of the following items: first name, last name, phone number, and birth date. To go any further, we must decide how we will represent these items as a C++ data structure. And we must design specific algorithms associated with our data structure.

Two of the items are names—that is, sequences of alphabetic characters. We can represent them as strings. The area code and local phone number could both be integer numbers, but we would like to store the hyphen that is between the third and fourth digits of the local number, because this is how phone numbers are usually printed. Therefore, we make the area code an integer, but we make the local phone number a string. (We assume that an area code is 100 or greater so that we don't have to worry about how to print leading zeros in area codes such as 052. A Case Study Follow-Up exercise asks you to rethink this assumption.) Because a phone number has two components—an area code and a local number—it makes sense to represent it as a struct:

```
struct PhoneType
{
    int    areaCode;
    string number;
};
```

Finally, we represent a birth date as a `DateType` object, where `DateType` is the class we developed in the preceding case study.

Putting this all together, we define the following `struct` type to represent an entry for one person.

```
struct EntryType
{
    string   firstName;
    string   lastName;
    PhoneType phone;
    DateType  birthDate;
};
```

`firstName`, `lastName`, `phone`, and `birthDate` are member names within the `struct` type `EntryType`. The members `firstName` and `lastName` are strings of type `string`, `phone` is a struct of type

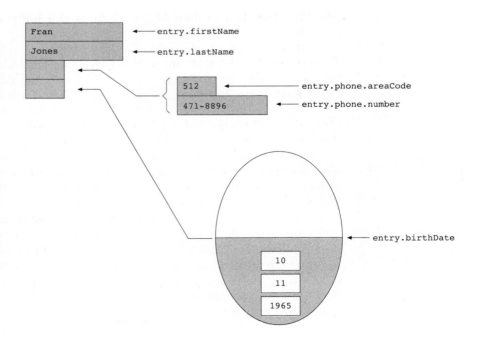

FIGURE 11-13
Struct Variable
entry, of type
EntryType

<u>*PROBLEM-SOLVING CASE STUDY cont'd.*</u>

PhoneType, and birthDate is a class object of type DateType. Notice that EntryType is a hierarchical record type, because the phone member is also a record. A complete entry with values stored in a struct variable named entry is shown in Figure 11-13.

When looking for birthdays, we are interested in month and day only—the year is not important. If we were going through a conventional address book checking for birthdays by hand, we would write down the month and day of the date two weeks away and compare it to the month and day of each friend's birth date.

We can use the same algorithm in our program. Using the DateType class that we developed, the member function Increment can be used to calculate the date two weeks (14 days) from the current date. We can use the class member function ComparedTo to determine whether a friend's birthday lies between the current date and the date two weeks away, inclusive. How do we ignore the year? We set the year of each friend's birth date to the current year for the comparison. However, if the current date plus 14 days is in the next year, and the friend's birthday is in January, then we must set the year to the current year plus 1 for the comparison to work correctly.

Data Structures:

The DateType class, for manipulating dates.

A struct type PhoneType that stores an area code (integer) and a local phone number (string).

A struct type EntryType that stores a first name (string), a last name (string), a telephone number of type PhoneType, and a birth date of type DateType.

PROBLEM-SOLVING CASE STUDY cont'd.

Main   **Level 0**

Open friendFile for input (and verify success)
Get current date into class object currentDate
Set targetDate = currentDate
FOR count going from 1 through 14
    targetDate.Increment()

Get entry
WHILE NOT EOF on friendFile
    IF targetDate.Year() isn't currentDate.Year() AND
                 entry.birthDate.Month() is 1
        Set birthdayYear = targetDate.Year()
    ELSE
        Set birthdayYear = currentDate.Year()
    birthday.Set(entry.birthDate.Month(), entry.birthDate.Day(), birthdayYear)
    IF birthday.ComparedTo(currentDate) ≥ SAME AND
              birthday.ComparedTo(targetDate) ≤ SAME
        Print entry
    Get entry

Get Current Date (Out: currentDate)   **Level 1**

Prompt user for current date
Read month, day, year
currentDate.Set(month, day, year)

PROBLEM-SOLVING CASE STUDY cont'd.

Get Entry (Inout: friendFile; Out: entry)

```
Read entry.firstName from friendFile
IF EOF on friendFile
        Return
Read entry.lastName from friendFile

// Below, dummy is a char variable to consume the '(' and ')'
Read dummy, entry.phone.areaCode,
        dummy, entry.phone.number from friendFile

// Below, dummy consumes the '/' and '/'
Read month, dummy, day, dummy, year from friendFile

entry.birthDate.Set(month, day, year)
```

Print Entry (In: entry, birthday)

```
Print entry.firstName, ' ', entry.lastName
Print '(', entry.phone.areaCode, ')', entry.phone.number
birthday.Print()
```

Because the `DateType` member functions (`Increment`, `ComparedTo`, and so on) already exist, no more decomposition is necessary.

Module Structure Chart:

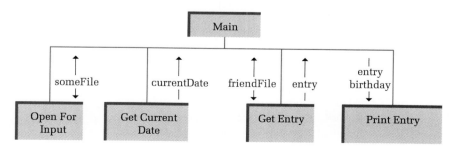

Below is the BirthdayCalls program that implements our design. By using the preexisting `DateType` class, the program is significantly shorter and easier to understand than if it included all the code to manipulate dates. All we have to do is `#include` the header file `datetype.h` to make use of `DateType` class objects. To run the program, we link its object code file with the `DateType` object code file, the place where all the `DateType` implementation details are hidden.

(The following program is written in ISO/ANSI standard C++. If you are working with pre–standard C++, see the alternate version of the program in the PRE_STD directory of the program disk, available at the publisher's Web site, `www.jbpub.com/disks`.)

```cpp
//****************************************************************
// BirthdayCalls program
// A data file contains people's names, phone numbers, and birth
// dates.  This program reads a date from standard input, calculates
// a date two weeks away, and prints the names, phone numbers, and
// birthdays of all those in the file whose birthdays come on or
// before the date two weeks away
//****************************************************************
#include "datetype.h"
#include <iostream>
#include <fstream>      // For file I/O
#include <string>       // For string type

using namespace std;

struct PhoneType
{
    int     areaCode;
    string number;
};
struct EntryType
{
    string    firstName;
    string    lastName;
    PhoneType phone;
    DateType  birthDate;
};

void GetCurrentDate( DateType& );
void GetEntry( ifstream&, EntryType& );
void OpenForInput( ifstream& );
void PrintEntry( EntryType, DateType );
```

PROBLEM-SOLVING CASE STUDY cont'd.

```cpp
int main()
{
    ifstream  friendFile;     // Input file of friends' records
    EntryType entry;          // Current record from friendFile
                              //   being checked
    DateType  currentDate;    // Month, day, and year of current day
    DateType  birthday;       // Date of next birthday
    DateType  targetDate;     // Two weeks from current date
    int       birthdayYear;   // Year of next birthday
    int       count;          // Loop counter

    OpenForInput(friendFile);
    if ( !friendFile )
        return 1;

    GetCurrentDate(currentDate);
    targetDate = currentDate;
    for (count = 1; count <= 14; count++)
        targetDate.Increment();

    GetEntry(friendFile, entry);
    while (friendFile)
    {
        if (targetDate.Year() != currentDate.Year() &&
                entry.birthDate.Month() == 1)
            birthdayYear = targetDate.Year();
        else
            birthdayYear = currentDate.Year();
        birthday.Set(entry.birthDate.Month(), entry.birthDate.Day(),
                    birthdayYear);
        if (birthday.ComparedTo(currentDate) >= SAME &&
                birthday.ComparedTo(targetDate) <= SAME)
            PrintEntry(entry, birthday);
        GetEntry(friendFile, entry);
    }
    return 0;
}


//****************************************************************

void OpenForInput( /* inout */ ifstream& someFile )    // File to be
                                                       // opened
// Prompts the user for the name of an input file
// and attempts to open the file
```

PROBLEM-SOLVING CASE STUDY cont'd.

```
// Postcondition:
//     The user has been prompted for a file name
//  && IF the file could not be opened
//         An error message has been printed
// Note:
//     Upon return from this function, the caller must test
//     the stream state to see if the file was successfully opened

{
    .
    .          (Same as in ConvertDates program of Chapter 8)
    .
}

//****************************************************************

void GetCurrentDate( /* out */ DateType& currentDate )    // Today's
                                                          //    date
// Reads the current date from standard input

// Postcondition:
//     User has been prompted for the current month, day, and year
//  && currentDate is set according to the input values

{
    int month;
    int day;
    int year;

    cout << "Enter current date as three integers, separated by"
         << " spaces: MM DD YYYY" << endl;
    cin >> month >> day >> year;
    currentDate.Set(month, day, year);
}

//****************************************************************

void GetEntry(
    /* inout */ ifstream&  friendFile,    // Input file of records
    /* out */   EntryType& entry        )  // Next record from file

// Reads an entry from file friendFile

// Precondition:
//     friendFile is open for input
// Postcondition:
```

PROBLEM-SOLVING CASE STUDY *cont'd.*

```
//      IF input of the firstName member failed due to end-of-file
//          entry is undefined
//      ELSE
//          All members of entry are filled with the values
//          for one person read from friendFile

{
    char dummy;    // Used to input and ignore certain characters
    int  month;
    int  day;
    int  year;

    friendFile >> entry.firstName;
    if ( !friendFile )
        return;
    friendFile >> entry.lastName;

    friendFile >> dummy                    // Consume '('
               >> entry.phone.areaCode
               >> dummy                    // Consume ')'
               >> entry.phone.number;

    friendFile >> month
               >> dummy                    // Consume '/'
               >> day
               >> dummy                    // Consume '/'
               >> year;
    entry.birthDate.Set(month, day, year);
}


//****************************************************************


void PrintEntry( /* in */ EntryType entry,     // Friend's record
                 /* in */ DateType  birthday )  // Friend's birthday
                                                //    this year
// Prints the name, phone number, and birthday

// Precondition:
//      entry is assigned
// Postcondition:
//      entry.firstName, entry.lastName, entry.phone, and birthday
//      have been printed

{
    cout << entry.firstName << ' ' << entry.lastName << endl;
    cout << '(' << entry.phone.areaCode << ") "
```

```
                  << entry.phone.number << endl;
          birthday.Print();
          cout << endl << endl;
   }
```

Testing: The only portions of this program that need to be checked are the `main` function and the input and output routines. The operations on dates have already been tested thoroughly.

The logic in the `main` function is straightforward. The test data should include birthdays less than two weeks away, exactly two weeks away, and more than two weeks away. The current date should include the cases in which two weeks away is within the same month, within the next month, and within the next year.

Testing and Debugging

Testing and debugging a C++ class amounts to testing and debugging each member function of the class. All of the techniques you have learned about—algorithm walk-throughs, code walk-throughs, hand traces, test drivers, verification of preconditions and postconditions, the system debugger, the `assert` function, and debug outputs—may be brought into play.

Consider how we might test this chapter's `TimeType` class. Here is the class declaration, abbreviated by leaving out the function preconditions and postconditions:

```
class TimeType
{
public:
    void Set( /* in */ int hours,
              /* in */ int minutes,
              /* in */ int seconds );
        // Precondition: ...
        // Postcondition: ...

    void Increment();
        // Postcondition: ...

    void Write() const;
        // Postcondition: ...

    bool Equal( /* in */ TimeType otherTime ) const;
        // Postcondition: ...

    bool LessThan( /* in */ TimeType otherTime ) const;
```

```
        // Precondition: ...
        // Postcondition: ...

    TimeType( /* in */ int initHrs,
              /* in */ int initMins,
              /* in */ int initSecs );
        // Precondition: ...
        // Postcondition: ...

    TimeType();
        // Postcondition: ...
private:
    int hrs;
    int mins;
    int secs;
};
```

To test this class fully, we must test each of the member functions. Let's step through the process of testing just one of them: the `Increment` function.

When we implemented the `Increment` function, we presumably started with a pseudocode algorithm, performed an algorithm walk-through, and translated the pseudocode into the following C++ function:

```
void TimeType::Increment()

// Postcondition:
//      Time has been advanced by one second, with
//      23:59:59 wrapping around to 0:0:0

{
    secs++;
    if (secs > 59)
    {
        secs = 0;
        mins++;
        if (mins > 59)
        {
            mins = 0;
            hrs++;
            if (hrs > 23)
                hrs = 0;
        }
    }
}
```

Now we perform a code walk-through, verifying that the C++ code faithfully matches the pseudocode algorithm. At this point (or earlier, during the algorithm walk-through), we do a hand trace to confirm that the logic is correct.

For the hand trace we should pick values of hrs, mins, and secs that ensure code coverage. To execute every path though the control flow, we need cases in which the following conditions occur:

1. The first If condition is false.
2. The first If condition is true and the second is false.
3. The first If condition is true, the second is true, and the third is false.
4. The first If condition is true, the second is true, and the third is true.

Below is a table displaying values of hrs, mins, and secs that correspond to these four cases. For each case we also write down what we hope will be the values of the variables after executing the algorithm.

	Initial Values				*Expected Results*		
Case	*hrs*	*mins*	*secs*		*hrs*	*mins*	*secs*
1	10	5	30		10	5	31
2	4	6	59		4	7	0
3	13	59	59		14	0	0
4	23	59	59		0	0	0

Using the initial values for each case, a hand trace of the code confirms that the algorithm produces the desired results.

Finally, we write a test driver for the Increment function, just to be sure that our understanding of the algorithm logic is the same as the computer's! Here is a possible test driver:

```
#include <iostream>
#include "timetype.h"

using namespace std;

int main()
{
    TimeType time;
    int      hours;
    int      minutes;
    int      seconds;

    cout << "Enter a time (use hours < 0 to quit): ";
    cin >> hours >> minutes >> seconds;
    while (hours >= 0)
```

```
    {
        time.Set(hours, minutes, seconds);
        time.Increment();
        cout << "Incremented time is ";
        time.Write();
        cout << endl;
        cout << "Enter a time (use hours < 0 to quit): ";
        cin >> hours >> minutes >> seconds;
    }
    return 0;
}
```

The `timetype.cpp` implementation file only needs to contain function definitions for the following member functions: `Set`, `Increment`, `Write`, and the default constructor. The other member functions do not need to be implemented yet. Now we compile the test driver and `timetype.cpp`, link the two object files, and execute the program. For input data, we supply at least the four test cases discussed earlier. The program's output should match the desired results.

Now that we have tested the `Increment` function, we can apply the same steps to the remaining class member functions. We can create a separate test driver for each function, or we can write just one driver that tests all of the functions. The disadvantage of writing just one driver is that devising different combinations of input values to test several functions at once can quickly become complicated.

Before leaving the topic of testing a class, we must emphasize an important point. Even though a class has been tested thoroughly, it is still possible for errors to arise. Let's look at two examples using the `TimeType` class. The first example is the client statement

```
time.Set(24, 0, 0);
```

The second example is the comparison

```
if (time1.LessThan(time2))
    ⋮
```

where the programmer intends `time1` to be 11:00:00 on a Wednesday and `time2` to be 1:20:00 on a Thursday. (The result of the test is `false`, not `true` as the programmer expects.) Do you see the problem? In each example, the client has violated the function precondition. The precondition of `Set` requires the first argument to have a value from 0 through 23. The precondition of `LessThan` requires the two times to be on the same day, not on two different days.

If a class has been well tested and there are errors when client code uses the class, always check the member function preconditions. You can waste many hours trying to debug a class member function when, in fact, the function is correct. The error may lie in the client code.

Testing and Debugging Hints

1. The declarations of `struct` and `class` types must end with semi-colons.
2. Be sure to specify the full member selector when referencing a component of a struct variable or class object.
3. Avoid using anonymous `struct` types.
4. Regarding semicolons, the declarations and definitions of class member functions are treated the same as any C++ function. The member function prototype, located in the class declaration, ends with a semi-colon. The function heading—the part of the function definition preceding the body—does not end with a semicolon.
5. When implementing a class member function, don't forget to prefix the function name with the name of the class and the scope resolution operator (`::`).

```
void TimeType::Increment()
{
    ⋮
}
```

6. For now, the only built-in operations that apply to struct variables and class objects are member selection (`.`) and assignment (`=`). To perform other operations, such as comparing two struct variables or class objects, you must access the components individually (in the case of struct variables) or write class member functions (in the case of class objects).
7. If a class member function inspects but does not modify the private data, it is a good idea to make it a `const` member function.
8. A class member function does not use dot notation to access private members of the class object for which the function is invoked. In contrast, a member function *must* use dot notation to access the private members of a class object that is passed to it as an argument.
9. To avoid errors caused by uninitialized data, it is good practice to always include a class constructor when designing a class.
10. A class constructor is declared without a return value type and cannot return a function value.
11. If a client of a class has errors that seem to be related to the class, start by checking the preconditions of the class member functions. The errors may be in the client, not the class.

Summary

In addition to being able to create user-defined atomic data types, we can create structured data types. In a structured data type, a name is given to an entire group of components. With many structured types, the group can be accessed as a whole, or each individual component can be accessed separately.

The record is a data structure for grouping together heterogeneous data—data items that are of different types. Individual components of a record are accessed by name. In C++, records are referred to as *structures* or as *structs*. We can use a struct variable to refer to the struct as a whole, or we can use a member selector to access any individual member (component) of the struct. Entire structs of the same type may be assigned directly to each other, passed as arguments, or returned as function return values. Comparison of structs, however, must be done member by member. Reading and writing of structs must also be done member by member.

Data abstraction is a powerful technique for reducing the complexity and increasing the reliability of programs. Separating the properties of a data type from the details of its implementation frees the user of the type from having to write code that depends on a particular implementation of the type. This separation also assures the implementor of the type that client code cannot accidentally compromise a correct implementation.

An abstract data type (ADT) is a type whose specification is separate from its implementation. The specification announces the abstract properties of the type. The implementation consists of (a) a concrete data representation and (b) the implementations of the ADT operations. In C++, an ADT can be realized by using the class mechanism. A class is similar to a struct, but the members of a class are not only data but also functions. Class members can be designated as public or private. Most commonly, the private members are the concrete data representation of the ADT, and the public members are the functions corresponding to the ADT operations.

Among the public member functions of a class, the programmer often includes one or more class constructors—functions that are invoked automatically whenever a class object is created.

Separate compilation of program units is central to the separation of specification from implementation. The declaration of a C++ class is typically placed in a specification (.h) file, and the implementations of the class member functions reside in another file: the implementation file. The client code is compiled separately from the class implementation file, and the two resulting object code files are linked together to form an executable file. Through separate compilation, the user of an ADT can treat the ADT as an off-the-shelf component without ever seeing how it is implemented.

Quick Check

1. Write the type declaration for a struct data type named PersonRec with three members: age, height, and weight. All three members are intended to store integer values, with height and weight representing height in inches and weight in pounds, respectively. (pp. 579–586)

2. Assume a variable named now, of type PersonRec, has been declared. Write assignment statements to store into now the data for a 28-year old person measuring 5'6" and weighing 140 pounds. (pp. 579–586)

3. Declare a hierarchical record type named HistoryRec that consists of two members of type PersonRec. The members are named past and present. (pp. 587–589)

4. Assume a variable named history, of type HistoryRec, has been declared. Write assignment statements to store into the past member of history the data for a 15-year-old person measuring 5'0" and weighing 96 pounds. Write the assignment statement that copies the contents of variable now into the present member of history. (pp. 587–589)

5. What is the primary purpose of C++ union types? (pp. 589–590)

6. The specification of an ADT describes only its properties (the domain and allowable operations). To implement the ADT, what two things must a programmer do? (pp. 592–595)

7. Write a C++ class declaration for the following Checkbook ADT. Do not implement the ADT other than to include in the private part a concrete data representation for the current balance. All monetary amounts are to be represented as floating-point numbers.

   TYPE
       Checkbook
   DOMAIN
       Each instance of the Checkbook type is a value representing one customer's current checking account balance.
   OPERATIONS
       Open the checking account, specifying an initial balance.
       Write a check for a specified amount.
       Deposit a specified amount into the checking account.
       Return the current balance.

   (pp. 596–600)

8. Write a segment of client code that declares two Checkbook objects, one for a personal checkbook and one for a business account. (pp. 596–600)

9. For the personal checkbook in Question 8, write a segment of client code that opens the account with an initial balance of $300.00, writes two checks for $50.25 and $150.00, deposits $87.34 into the account, and prints out the resulting balance. (pp. 600–603)

10. Implement the following Checkbook member functions. (pp. 608–613)
    a. Open
    b. WriteCheck
    c. CurrentBalance

11. A compile-time error occurs if a client of Checkbook tries to access the private class members directly. Give an example of such a client statement. (pp. 604–605)

12. In which file—the specification file or the implementation file—would the solution to Question 7 be located? In which file would the solution to Question 10 be located? (pp. 606–613)

13. For the Checkbook class, replace the Open function with two C++ class constructors. One (the default constructor) initializes the account balance to zero. The other initializes the balance to an amount passed as an argument. (pp. 616–621)

    a. Revise the class declaration.

    b. Implement the two class constructors.

Answers

1.
```
struct PersonRec
{
    int age;
    int height;
    int weight;
};
```

2.
```
now.age = 28;
now.height = 66;
now.weight = 140;
```

3.
```
struct HistoryRec
{
    PersonRec past;
    PersonRec present;
};
```

4.
```
history.past.age = 15;
history.past.height = 60;
history.past.weight = 96;
history.present = now;
```

5. The primary purpose is to save memory by forcing different values to share the same memory space, one at a time.   **6.** a. Choose a concrete data representation of the abstract data, using data types that already exist. b. Implement each of the allowable operations in terms of program instructions.

7.
```
class Checkbook
{
public:
    void Open( /* in */ float initBalance );
    void WriteCheck( /* in */ float amount );
    void Deposit( /* in */ float amount );
    float CurrentBalance() const;
private:
    float balance;
};
```

8.
```
Checkbook personalAcct;
Checkbook businessAcct;
```

9.
```
personalAcct.Open(300.0);
personalAcct.WriteCheck(50.25);
personalAcct.WriteCheck(150.0);
personalAcct.Deposit(87.34);
cout << '$' << personalAcct.CurrentBalance() << endl;
```

10. a.
```
void Checkbook::Open( /* in */ float initBalance )
{
    balance = initBalance;
}
```
    b.
```
void Checkbook::WriteCheck( /* in */ float amount )
{
    balance = balance - amount;
}
```
    c.
```
float Checkbook::CurrentBalance() const
{
    return balance;
}
```

11. `personalAcct.balance = 10000.0;`

12. The C++ class declaration of Question 7 would be located in the specification file. The C++ function definitions of Question 10 would be located in the implementation file.

13. a.
```
class Checkbook
{
public:
    void WriteCheck( /* in */ float amount );
    void Deposit( /* in */ float amount );
    float CurrentBalance() const;
    Checkbook();
    Checkbook( /* in */ float initBalance );
private:
    float balance;
};
```
    b.
```
Checkbook::Checkbook()
{
    balance = 0.0;
}
Checkbook::Checkbook( /* in */ float initBalance )
{
    balance = initBalance;
}
```

Exam Preparation Exercises

1. Define the following terms that relate to records (structs in C++):
   record
   member
   member selector
   hierarchical record

2. Declare a `struct` type named `RecType` to contain an integer variable representing a person's number of dependents, a floating-point variable representing the person's salary, and a Boolean variable indicating whether the person has major medical insurance coverage (`true`) or basic company coverage only (`false`).

3. Using the second version of the `MachineRec` type in this chapter (p. 588), the code below is supposed to print a message if a machine has not been serviced within the current year. The code has an error. Correct the error by using a proper member selector in the If statement.

```
DateType     currentDate;
MachineRec machine;
    ⋮
if (machine.lastServiced.year != currentDate.year)
    PrintMsg();
```

4. Given the declarations

```
struct NameType
{
    string first;
    string last;
};
struct AddrType
{
    string city;
    string state;
    long    zipCode;
};
struct PersonType
{
    NameType name;
    AddrType address;
};


PersonType person;
```

write C++ code that stores the following information into person:
Beverly Johnson
2638 Oak Dr.
La Crosse, WI 54601

5. The specification of an abstract data type (ADT) should not mention implementation details. (True or False?)

6. Below are some real-world objects you might want to represent in a program as ADTs. For each, give some abstract operations that might be appropriate. (Ignore the concrete data representation for each object.)
   a. A thesaurus
   b. An automatic dishwasher
   c. A radio-controlled model airplane

7. Consider the following C++ class declaration and client code:

Class Declaration   *Client Code*

```
class SomeClass              SomeClass object1;
{                            SomeClass object2;
public:                      int       m;
    void Func1( int n );
    int  Func2( int n ) const;   object1.Func1(3);
    void Func3();                m = object2.Func2(5);
private:
    int someInt;
};
```

a. List all the identifiers that refer to data types (both built-in and programmer-defined).

b. List all the identifiers that are names of class members.

c. List all the identifiers that are names of class objects.

d. List the names of all member functions that are allowed to inspect the private data.

e. List the names of all member functions that are allowed to modify the private data.

f. In the implementation of `SomeClass`, which one of the following would be the correct function definition for `Func3`?

  i.   `void Func3()`
```
    {
        ⋮
    }
```
  ii. `void SomeClass::Func3()`
```
    {
        ⋮
    }
```
  iii. `SomeClass::void Func3()`
```
    {
        ⋮
    }
```

8. If you do not use the reserved words `public` and `private`, all members of a C++ class are private and all members of a struct are public. (True or False?)

9. Define the following terms:
instantiate
`const` member function
specification file
implementation file

10. To the `TimeType` class we wish to add three observer operations: `CurrentHrs`, `CurrentMins`, and `CurrentSecs`. These operations simply return the current values of the private data to the client. We can amend the class declaration by inserting the following function prototypes into the public part:

```
int CurrentHrs() const;
    // Postcondition:
    //      Function value == hours part of the time of day

int CurrentMins() const;
    // Postcondition:
    //      Function value == minutes part of the time of day

int CurrentSecs() const;
    // Postcondition:
    //      Function value == seconds part of the time of day
```

Write the function definitions for these three functions as they would appear in the implementation file.

11. Answer the following questions about Figure 11-11, which illustrates the process of compiling and linking a multifile program.
   a. If only the file myprog.cpp is modified, which files must be recompiled?
   b. If only the file myprog.cpp is modified, which files must be relinked?
   c. If only the files file2.cpp and file3.cpp are modified, which files must be recompiled? (Assume that the modifications do not affect existing code in myprog.cpp.)
   d. If only the files file2.cpp and file3.cpp are modified, which files must be relinked? (Assume that the modifications do not affect existing code in myprog.cpp.)

12. Define the following terms:
    separate compilation
    C++ class constructor
    default constructor

13. The following class has two constructors among its public member functions:

```
class SomeClass
{
public:
    float Func1() const;
      ⋮
    SomeClass( /* in */ float f );
        // Precondition:
        //      f is assigned
        // Postcondition:
        //      Private data is initialized to f
    SomeClass();
        // Postcondition:
        //      Private data is initialized to 8.6
private:
    float someFloat;
};
```

   Write declarations for the following class objects.
   a. An object obj1, initialized to 0.0.
   b. An object obj2, initialized to 8.6.

14. The C++ compiler will signal a syntax error in the following class declaration. What is the error?

```
class SomeClass
{
public:
    void Func1( int n );
    int  Func2();
    int  SomeClass();
private:
    int privateInt;
};
```

Programming Warm-up Exercises

1. a. Write a `struct` declaration to contain the following information about a student:
    Name (string of characters)
    Social Security number (string of characters)
    Year (freshman, sophomore, junior, senior)
    Grade point average (floating-point number)
    Sex (M, F)

    b. Declare a struct variable of the type in part (a), and write a program segment that prints the information in each member of the variable.

2. a. Declare a `struct` type named `AptType` for an apartment locator service. The following information should be included:
    Landlord (string of characters)
    Address (string of characters)
    Bedrooms (integer)
    Price (floating-point number)

    b. Declare `anApt` to be a variable of type `AptType`.

    c. Write a function to read values into the members of a variable of type `AptType`. (The struct variable should be passed as an argument.) The order in which the data is read is the same as that of the items in the struct.

3. Write a hierarchical C++ `struct` declaration to contain the following information about a student:
    Name (string of characters)
    Student ID number
    Credit hours to date
    Number of courses taken
    Date first enrolled (month and year)
    Year (freshman, sophomore, junior, senior)
    Grade point average
    Each `struct` and enumeration type should have a separate type declaration.

4. You are writing the subscription renewal system for a magazine. For each subscriber, the system is to keep the following information:
    Name (first, last)
    Address (street, city, state, zip code)
    Expiration date (month, year)
    Date renewal notice was sent (month, day, year)
    Number of renewal notices sent so far
    Number of years for which subscription is being renewed (0 for renewal not yet received; otherwise, 1, 2, or 3 years)
    Whether or not the subscriber's name may be included in a mailing list for sale to other companies
    Write a hierarchical record type declaration to represent this information. Each subrecord should be declared separately as a named data type.

5. The `TimeType` class supplies two member functions, `Equal` and `LessThan`, that correspond to the relational operators `==` and `<`. Show how *client code* can simulate the other four relational operators (`!=`, `<=`, `>`, and `>=`) using only the `Equal` and `LessThan` functions. Specifically, express each of the following pseudocode statements in C++, where `time1` and `time2` are objects of type `TimeType`.

a. IF time1 ≠ time2
   Set n = 1
b. IF time1 ≤ time2
   Set n = 5
c. IF time1 > time2
   Set n = 8
d. IF time1 ≥ time2
   Set n = 5

6. In reference to Programming Warm-up Exercise 5, make life easier for the user of the `TimeType` class by adding new member functions `NotEqual`, `LessOrEqual`, `GreaterThan`, and `GreaterOrEqual` to the class.
   a. Show the function specifications (prototypes and preconditions and post-conditions) as they would appear in the new class declaration.
   b. Write the function definitions as they would appear in the implementation file. (*Hint:* Instead of writing the algorithms from scratch, simply have the function bodies invoke the existing functions `Equal` and `LessThan`. And remember: Class members can refer to each other directly without using dot notation.)

7. Enhance the `TimeType` class by adding a new member function `WriteAmPm`. This function prints the time in 12-hour rather than 24-hour form, adding *AM* or *PM* at the end. Show the function specification (prototype and precondition and postcondition) as it would appear in the new class declaration. Then write the function definition as it would appear in the implementation file.

8. Add a member function named `Minus` to the `TimeType` class. This value-returning function yields the difference in seconds between the times represented by two class objects. Show the function specification (prototype and precondition and postcondition) as it would appear in the new class declaration. Then write the function definition as it would appear in the implementation file.

9. a. Design the data sets necessary to thoroughly test the `LessThan` function of the `TimeType` class.
   b. Write a driver and test the `LessThan` function using your test data.

10. a. Design the data sets necessary to thoroughly test the `Write` function of the `TimeType` class.
    b. Write a driver and test the `Write` function using your test data.

11. a. Design the data sets necessary to thoroughly test the `WriteAmPm` function of Programming Warm-Up Exercise 7.
    b. Write a driver and test the `WriteAmPm` function using your test data.

12. Reimplement the `TimeType` class so that the private data representation is a single variable:

```
long secs;
```

This variable represents time as the number of seconds since midnight. *Do not change the public interface in any way.* The user's view is still hours, minutes, and seconds, but the class's view is seconds since midnight.

Notice how this data representation simplifies the `Equal` and `LessThan` functions but makes the other operations more complicated by converting seconds back and forth to hours, minutes, and seconds. Use auxiliary functions, hidden inside the implementation file, to perform these conversions instead of duplicating the algorithms in several places.

Programming Problems

1. The Emerging Manufacturing Company has just installed its first computer and hired you as a junior programmer. Your first program is to read employee pay data and produce two reports: (1) an error and control report, and (2) a report on pay amounts. The second report must contain a line for each employee and a line of totals at the end of the report.

    Input:
    Transaction File
    Set of three job site number/name pairs
    One line for each employee containing ID number, job site number, and number of hours worked

    These data items have been presorted by ID number.

    Master File
    ID number
    Name
    Pay rate per hour
    Number of dependents
    Type of employee (1 is management, 0 is union)
    Job site
    Sex (M, F)

    This file is ordered by ID number.
    NOTE: (1) Union members, unlike management, get time and a half for hours over 40. (2) The tax formula for tax computation is as follows: If number of dependents is 1, tax rate is 15%. Otherwise, the tax rate is the greater of 2.5% and

    $$\left[1 - \left(\frac{No.\ of\ dep.}{No.\ of\ dep.\ +\ 6} \right) \right] \times 15\%$$

    Output:
    Error and Control Report
    Lists the input lines for which there is no corresponding master record, or where the employees' job site numbers do not agree with those in the master file. Continues processing with the next line of data.
    Gives the total number of employee records that were processed correctly during the run.

    Payroll Report (Labeled for Management)
    Contains a line for each employee showing the name, ID number, job site name, gross pay, and net pay.
    Contains a total line showing the total amount of gross pay and total amount of net pay.

2. You have taken a job with the IRS because you want to learn how to save on your income tax. They want you to write a toy tax computing program so that they can get an idea of your programming abilities. The program reads in the names of the members of families and each person's income, and computes the tax that the family owes. You may assume that people with the same last name who appear consecutively in the input are in the same family. The number of deductions that a family can count is equal to the number of people listed in

that family in the input data. Tax is computed as follows:

adjusted income	=	income – (5000 × number of deductions)
tax rate	=	$\begin{cases} \text{adjusted income}/100{,}000 \text{ if income} < 60{,}000 \\ 50\%, \text{ otherwise} \end{cases}$
tax	=	tax rate × adjusted income

There will be no refunds, so you must check for people whose tax would be negative and set it to zero.

Input entries are in the following form:

Last name First name Total income

Sample Data:
```
Jones Ralph 19765.43
Jones Mary 8532.00
Jones Francis 0
Atwell Humphrey 5678.12
Murphy Robert 13432.20
Murphy Ellen 0
Murphy Paddy 0
Murphy Eileen 0
Murphy Conan 0
Murphy Nora 0
```

Input:
The data as described above, with end-of-file indicating the end of the input data.

Output:
A table containing all the families, one family per line, with each line containing the last name of the family, their total income, and their computed tax.

3. A rational number is a number that can be expressed as a fraction whose numerator and denominator are integers. Examples of rational numbers are 0.75 (which is 3/4) and 1.125 (which is 9/8). The value π is not a rational number; it cannot be expressed as the ratio of two integers.

Working with rational numbers on a computer is often a problem. Inaccuracies in floating-point representation can yield imprecise results. For example, the result of the C++ expression

```
1.0 / 3.0 * 3.0
```

is likely to be a value like 0.999999 rather than 1.0.

Design, implement, and test a Rational class that represents a rational number as a pair of integers instead of a single floating-point number. The Rational class should have two class constructors. The first one lets the client specify an initial numerator and denominator. The other—the default constructor—creates the rational number 0, represented as a numerator of 0 and a denominator of 1. The segment of client code

```
Rational num1(1, 3);
Rational num2(3, 1);
Rational result;

cout << "The product of ";
```

```
num1.Write();
cout << " and ";
num2.Write();
cout << " is ";
result = num1.MultipliedBy(num2);
result.Write();
```

would produce the output

```
The product of 1/3 and 3/1 is 1/1
```

At the very least, you should provide the following operations:
- Constructors for explicit as well as default initialization of Rational objects.
- Arithmetic operations that add, subtract, multiply, and divide two Rational objects. These should be implemented as value-returning functions, each returning a Rational object.
- A Boolean operation that compares two Rational objects for equality.
- An output operation that displays the value of a Rational object in the form numerator/denominator.

Include any additional operations that you think would be useful for a rational number class.

4. A complex ("imaginary") number has the form $a + bi$, where i is the square root of -1. Here, a is called the real part and b is called the imaginary part. Alternatively, $a + bi$ can be expressed as the ordered pair of real numbers (a, b).

Arithmetic operations on two complex numbers (a, b) and (c, d) are as follows:

$$(a,b) + (c,d) = (a + c, b + d)$$
$$(a,b) - (c,d) = (a - c, b - d)$$
$$(a,b) \times (c,d) = (a \times c - b \times d, a \times d + b \times c)$$
$$(a,b) \div (c,d) = \left(\frac{a \times c + b \times d}{c^2 + d^2}, \frac{b \times c + a \times d}{c^2 + d^2} \right)$$

Also, the absolute value (or magnitude) of a complex number is defined as

$$| (a,b) | = \sqrt{a^2 + b^2}$$

Design, implement, and test a complex number class that represents the real and imaginary parts as double-precision values (data type double) and provides at least the following operations:
- Constructors for explicit as well as default initialization. The default initial value should be (0.0, 0.0).
- Arithmetic operations that add, subtract, multiply, and divide two complex numbers. These should be implemented as value-returning functions, each returning a class object.
- A complex absolute value operation.
- Two observer operations, RealPart and ImagPart, that return the real and imaginary parts of a complex number.

5. Design, implement, and test a countdown timer class named Timer. This class mimics a real-world timer by counting off seconds, starting from an initial value. When the timer reaches zero, it beeps (by sending the alert character, '\a', to the standard output device). Some appropriate operations might be the following:

   - Create a timer, initializing it to a specified number of seconds.
   - Start the timer.
   - Reset the timer to some value.

   When the Start operation is invoked, it should repeatedly decrement and output the current value of the timer approximately every second. To delay the program for one second, use a For loop whose body does absolutely nothing; that is, its body is the null statement. Experiment with the number of loop iterations to achieve as close to a one-second delay as you can.

   If your C++ system provides functions to clear the screen and to position the cursor anywhere on the screen, you might want to do the following. Begin by clearing the screen. Then, always display the timer value at the same position in the center of the screen. Each output should overwrite the previous value displayed, just like a real-world timer.

Case Study Follow-Up

1. Classify each of the eight member functions of the DateType class as a constructor, a transformer, or an observer operation.
2. Write a test plan for testing the ComparedTo function of the DateType class.
3. Write a driver to implement your test plan for the ComparedTo function.
4. Write a test plan for testing the Increment function of the DateType class.
5. Write a driver to implement your test plan for the Increment function.
6. In the BirthdayCalls program, we represented a person's area code as an int value. Printing an int area code works fine for North American phone numbers, where area codes are greater than 200. But international area codes may start with a zero. Our program would print an area code of 052 as 52. Suggest two ways of accommodating international area codes so that leading zeros are printed.
7. Write a test plan for the BirthdayCalls program.
8. Implement your test plan for the BirthdayCalls program.
9. Modify the BirthdayCalls program as follows. Add an additional date called babyBoomerDate. As the first action in the program, read a value for babyBoomerDate. Keep track of how many friends were born before babyBoomerDate and how many were born on or after that date. Print these two counts at the end of the program.

12

Arrays

GOALS

- To be able to declare a one-dimensional array.
- To be able to perform fundamental operations on a one-dimensional array:

    Assign a value to an array component.

    Access a value stored in an array component.

    Fill an array with data, and process the data in the array.
- To be able to initialize a one-dimensional array in its declaration.
- To be able to pass one-dimensional arrays as arguments to functions.
- To be able to use arrays of records and class objects.
- To be able to apply subarray processing to a given one-dimensional array.
- To be able to declare and use a one-dimensional array with index values that have semantic content.
- To be able to declare a two-dimensional array.
- To be able to perform fundamental operations on a two-dimensional array:

    Access a component of the array.

    Initialize the array.

    Print the values in the array.

    Process the array by rows.

    Process the array by columns.
- To be able to declare a two-dimensional array as a parameter.
- To be able to view a two-dimensional array as an array of arrays.
- To be able to declare and process a multidimensional array.

Data structures play an important role in the design process. The choice of data structure directly affects the design because it determines the algorithms used to process the data. In Chapter 11, we saw how the record (struct) and the class give us the ability to refer to an entire group of components by one name. This simplifies the design of many programs.

In many problems, however, a data structure has so many components that it is difficult to process them if each one must have a unique member name. For example, the IntList abstract data type (ADT) we proposed briefly in Chapter 11 represents a collection of up to 100 integer values. If we used a struct or a class to hold these values, we would need to invent 100 different member names, write 100 different input statements to read values into the members, and write 100 different output statements to display the values—an incredibly tedious task! An *array*—the fourth of the structured data types supported by C++—is a data type that allows us to program operations of this kind with ease.

In this chapter, we examine array data types as provided by the C++ language; in Chapter 13, we show how to combine classes and arrays to implement an ADT such as IntList.

One-Dimensional Arrays

If we wanted to input 1000 integer values and print them in reverse order, we could write a program of this form:

```
//****************************
// ReverseNumbers program
//****************************
#include <iostream>

using namespace std;

int main()
{
    int value0;
    int value1;
    int value2;
      ⋮
    int value999;

    cin >> value0;
    cin >> value1;
    cin >> value2;
      ⋮
    cin >> value999;
```

```
    cout << value999 << endl;
    cout << value998 << endl;
    cout << value997 << endl;
      ⋮
    cout << value0 << endl;
    return 0;
}
```

This program is over 3000 lines long, and we have to use 1000 separate variables. Note that all the variables have the same name except for an appended number that distinguishes them. Wouldn't it be convenient if we could put the number into a counter variable and use For loops to go from 0 through 999, and then from 999 back down to 0? For example, if the counter variable were `number`, we could replace the 2000 original input/output statements with the following four lines of code (we enclose `number` in brackets to set it apart from `value`):

```
for (number = 0; number < 1000; number++)
    cin >> value[number];
for (number = 999; number >= 0; number--)
    cout << value[number] << endl;
```

This code fragment is correct in C++ *if* we declare `value` to be a *one-dimensional array,* which is a collection of variables—all of the same type—in which the first part of each variable name is the same, and the last part is an *index value* enclosed in square brackets. In our example, the value stored in `number` is called the *index*.

The declaration of a one-dimensional array is similar to the declaration of a simple variable (a variable of a simple data type), with one exception: You must also declare the size of the array. To do so, you indicate within brackets the number of components in the array:

```
int value[1000];
```

This declaration creates an array with 1000 components, all of type `int`. The first component has index value 0, the second component has index value 1, and the last component has index value 999.

Here is the complete ReverseNumbers program, using array notation. This is certainly much shorter than our first version of the program.

```
//***************************
// ReverseNumbers program
//***************************
#include <iostream>

using namespace std;
```

```
int main()
{
    int value[1000];
    int number;

    for (number = 0; number < 1000; number++)
        cin >> value[number];
    for (number = 999; number >= 0; number--)
        cout << value[number] << endl;
    return 0;
}
```

As a data structure, an array differs from a struct or class in two fundamental ways:

1. An array is a *homogeneous* data structure (all components are of the same data type), whereas structs and classes are heterogeneous types (their components may be of different types).
2. A component of an array is accessed by its *position* in the structure, whereas a component of a struct or class is accessed by an identifier (the member name).

Let's now define arrays formally and look at the rules for accessing individual components.

Declaring Arrays

A **one-dimensional array** is a structured collection of components (often called *array elements*) that can be accessed individually by specifying the position of a component with a single index value. (Later in the chapter, we introduce multidimensional arrays, which are arrays that have more than one index value.)

One-dimensional array A structured collection of components, all of the same type, that is given a single name. Each component (array element) is accessed by an index that indicates the component's position within the collection.

Here is a syntax template describing the simplest form of a one-dimensional array declaration:

ArrayDeclaration

> DataType ArrayName **[** ConstIntExpression **]** **;**

In the syntax template, DataType describes what is stored in each component of the array. Array components may be of almost any type, but for now we limit our discussion to atomic components. ConstIntExpression is an integer expression composed only of literal or named constants. This expression, which specifies the number of components in the array, must have a value greater than 0. If the value is n, the range of index values is 0 through $n - 1$, not 1 through n. For example, the declarations

```
float angle[4];
int    testScore[10];
```

create the arrays shown in Figure 12-1. The `angle` array has four components, each capable of holding one `float` value. The `testScore` array has a total of ten components, all of type `int`.

Accessing Individual Components

Recall that to access an individual component of a struct or class, we use dot notation—the name of the struct variable or class object, followed by a period, followed by the member name. In contrast, to access an individual array component, we write the array name, followed by an expression enclosed in square brackets. The expression specifies which component to access. The syntax template for accessing an array component is

FIGURE 12-1

`angle` and `testScore` Arrays

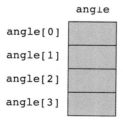
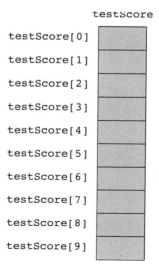

ArrayComponentAccess

ArrayName [IndexExpression]

The index expression may be as simple as a constant or a variable name or as complex as a combination of variables, operators, and function calls. Whatever the form of the expression, it must result in an integer value. Index expressions can be of type `char`, `short`, `int`, `long`, or `bool` because these are all integral types. Additionally, values of enumeration types can be used as index expressions, with an enumeration value implicitly coerced to an integer.

The simplest form of index expression is a constant. Using our `angle` array, the sequence of assignment statements

```
angle[0] = 4.93;
angle[1] = -15.2;
angle[2] = 0.5;
angle[3] = 1.67;
```

fills the array components one at a time (see Figure 12-2).

Each array component—`angle[2]`, for instance—can be treated exactly the same as any simple variable of type `float`. For example, we can do the following to the individual component `angle[2]`:

`angle[2] = 9.6;`	Assign it a value.
`cin >> angle[2];`	Read a value into it.
`cout << angle[2];`	Write its contents.
`y = sqrt(angle[2]);`	Pass it as an argument.
`x = 6.8 * angle[2] + 7.5;`	Use it in an arithmetic expression.

Let's look at index expressions that are more complicated than constants. Suppose we declare a 1000-element array of `int` values with the statement

```
int value[1000];
```

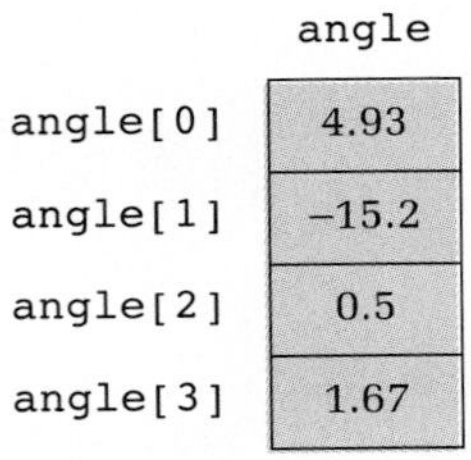

FIGURE 12-2
`angle` Array with
Values

angle

angle[0]	4.93
angle[1]	−15.2
angle[2]	0.5
angle[3]	1.67

and execute the following two statements.

```
value[counter] = 5;
if (value[number+1] % 10 != 0)
   ⋮
```

In the first statement, 5 is stored into an array component. If `counter` is 0, 5 is stored into the first component of the array. If `counter` is 1, 5 is stored into the second place in the array, and so forth.

In the second statement, the expression `number+1` selects an array component. The specific array component accessed is divided by 10 and checked to see if the remainder is nonzero. If `number+1` is 0, we are testing the value in the first component; if `number+1` is 1, we are testing the second place; and so on. Figure 12-3 shows the index expression as a constant, a variable, and a more complex expression.

Note that we have seen the use of square brackets before. In earlier chapters, we said that the `string` class allows you to access an individual character within a string:

```
string aString;

aString = "Hello";
cout << aString[1];     // Prints 'e'
```

FIGURE 12-3

An Index as a Constant, a Variable, and an Arbitrary Expression

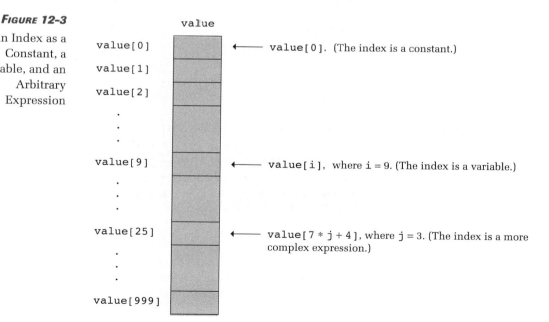

Although `string` is a class, not an array, the `string` class was written using the advanced C++ technique of *operator overloading* to give the `[]` operator another meaning (string component selection) in addition to its standard meaning (array element selection). The result is that a `string` object is similar to an array of characters but has special properties.

Out-of-Bounds Array Indexes

Given the declaration

```
float alpha[100];
```

the valid range of index values is 0 through 99. What happens if we execute the statement

```
alpha[i] = 62.4;
```

when `i` is less than 0 or when `i` is greater than 99? The result is that a memory location outside the array is accessed. C++ does not check for invalid (*out-of-bounds*) array indexes either at compile time or at run time. If `i` happens to be 100 in the statement above, the computer stores 62.4 into the next memory location past the end of the array, destroying whatever value was contained there. It is entirely the programmer's responsibility to make sure that an array index does not step off either end of the array.

Out-of-bounds array index   An index value that, in C++, is either less than 0 or greater than the array size minus 1.

Array-processing algorithms often use For loops to step through the array elements one at a time. Here is a loop to zero out our 100-element `alpha` array (`i` is an `int` variable):

```
for (i = 0; i < 100; i++)
    alpha[i] = 0.0;
```

We could also write the first line as

```
for (i = 0; i <= 99; i++)
```

However, C++ programmers commonly use the first version so that the number in the loop test (100) is the same as the array size. With this pattern, it is important to remember to test for *less-than*, not less-than-or-equal.

Initializing Arrays in Declarations

You learned in Chapter 8 that C++ allows you to initialize a variable in its declaration:

```
int delta = 25;
```

The value 25 is called an initializer. You also can initialize an array in its declaration, using a special syntax for the initializer. You specify a list of initial values for the array elements, separate them with commas, and enclose the list within braces:

```
int age[5] = {23, 10, 16, 37, 12};
```

In this declaration, age[0] is initialized to 23, age[1] is initialized to 10, and so on. There must be at least one initial value between the braces. If you specify too many initial values, you get a syntax error message. If you specify too few, the remaining array elements are initialized to zero.

Arrays follow the same rule as simple variables about the time(s) at which initialization occurs. A static array (one that is either global or declared as static within a block) is initialized once only, when control reaches its declaration. An automatic array (one that is local and not declared as static) is reinitialized each time control reaches its declaration.

An interesting feature of C++ is that you are allowed to omit the size of an array when you initialize it in a declaration:

```
float temperature[] = {0.0, 112.37, 98.6};
```

The compiler figures out the size of the array (here, 3) according to how many initial values are listed. In general, this feature is not particularly useful. In Chapter 13, though, we'll see that it can be convenient for initializing certain kinds of char arrays called C strings.

(Lack of) Aggregate Array Operations

In Chapter 11, we defined an aggregate operation as an operation on a data structure as a whole. Some programming languages allow aggregate operations on arrays, but C++ does not. If x and y are declared as

```
int x[50];
int y[50];
```

there is no aggregate assignment of y to x:

```
x = y;    // Not valid
```

To copy array y into array x, you must do it yourself, element by element:

```
for (index = 0; index < 50; index++)
    x[index] = y[index];
```

Similarly, there is no aggregate comparison of arrays:

```
if (x == y)    // Not valid
```

nor can you perform aggregate I/O of arrays:

```
cout << x;    // Not valid
```

or aggregate arithmetic on arrays:

```
x = x + y;    // Not valid
```

(C++ allows one exception for I/O, which we discuss in Chapter 13. Aggregate I/O is permitted for C strings, which are special kinds of char arrays.) Finally, it's not possible to return an entire array as the value of a value-returning function:

```
return x;    // Not valid
```

The only thing you can do to an array as a whole is to pass it as an argument to a function:

```
DoSomething(x);
```

Passing an array as an argument gives the function access to the entire array. The following table compares arrays, structs, and classes with respect to aggregate operations.

Aggregate Operation	Arrays	Structs and Classes
I/O	No (except C strings)	No
Assignment	No	Yes
Arithmetic	No	No
Comparison	No	No
Argument passage	By reference only	By value or by reference
Return as a function's return value	No	Yes

Later in the chapter, we look in detail at passing arrays as arguments.

Examples of Declaring and Accessing Arrays

We now look in detail at some specific examples of declaring and accessing arrays. Here are some declarations that a program might use to analyze occupancy rates in an apartment building:

```
const int BUILDING_SIZE = 350;   // Number of apartments

int occupants[BUILDING_SIZE];    // occupants[i] is the number of
                                 //    occupants in apartment i
int totalOccupants;              // Total number of occupants
int counter;                     // Loop control and index variable
```

occupants is a 350-element array of integers (see Figure 12-4). occupants[0] = 3 if the first apartment has three occupants; occupants[1] = 5 if the second apartment has five occupants; and so on. If values have been stored into the array, then the following code totals the number of occupants in the building.

```
totalOccupants = 0;
for (counter = 0; counter < BUILDING_SIZE; counter++)
    totalOccupants = totalOccupants + occupants[counter];
```

The first time through the loop, counter is 0. We add the contents of totalOccupants (that is, 0) to the contents of occupants[0], storing the result into totalOccupants. Next, counter becomes 1 and the loop test occurs. The second loop iteration adds the contents of totalOccupants to the contents of occupants[1], storing the result into totalOccupants. Now counter becomes 2 and the loop test is made. Eventually, the loop adds the contents of occupants[349] to the sum and increments counter to 350. At this point, the loop condition is false, and control exits the loop.

Note how we used the named constant BUILDING_SIZE in both the array declaration and the For loop. When constants are used in this manner, changes are easy to make. If the number of apartments changes from 350 to 400, we need to change only one line: the const declaration of BUILDING_SIZE. If we had used the literal value 350 in place of BUILD-ING_SIZE, we would need to update several of the statements in the code above, and probably many more throughout the rest of the program.

FIGURE 12-4
occupants Array

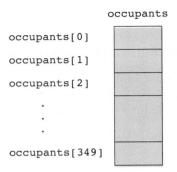

occupants

occupants[0]

occupants[1]

occupants[2]

occupants[349]

Because an array index is an integer value, we access the components by their position in the array—that is, the first, the second, the third, and so on. Using an `int` index is the most common way of thinking about an array. C++, however, provides more flexibility by allowing an index to be of any integral type or enumeration type. (The index expression still must evaluate to an integer in the range from 0 through one less than the array size.) The next example shows an array in which the indexes are values of an enumeration type.

```
enum Drink {ORANGE, COLA, ROOT_BEER, GINGER_ALE, CHERRY, LEMON};

float salesAmt[6];  // Array of 6 floats, to be indexed by Drink type
Drink flavor;       // Variable of the index type
```

`Drink` is an enumeration type in which the enumerators ORANGE, COLA, ..., LEMON have internal representations 0 through 5, respectively. `salesAmt` is a group of six `float` components representing dollar sales figures for each kind of drink (see Figure 12-5). The following code prints the values in the array (see Chapter 10 to review how to increment values of enumeration types in For loops).

FIGURE 12-5
salesAmt Array

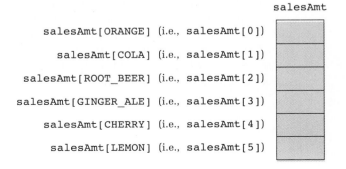

salesAmt

salesAmt[ORANGE] (i.e., salesAmt[0])

salesAmt[COLA] (i.e., salesAmt[1])

salesAmt[ROOT_BEER] (i.e., salesAmt[2])

salesAmt[GINGER_ALE] (i.e., salesAmt[3])

salesAmt[CHERRY] (i.e., salesAmt[4])

salesAmt[LEMON] (i.e., salesAmt[5])

FIGURE 12-6
grade Array with
Values

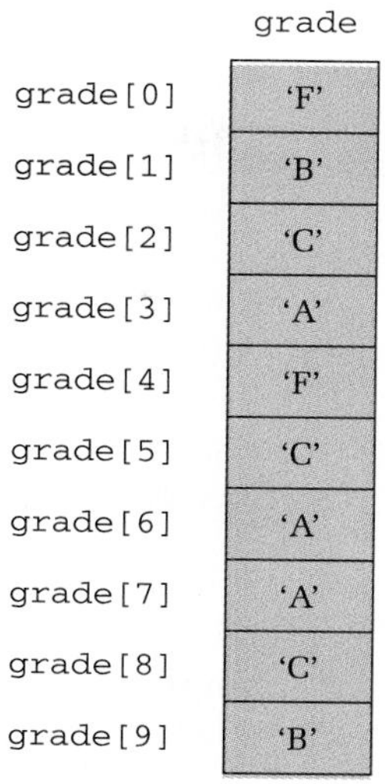

```
for (flavor = ORANGE; flavor <= LEMON; flavor = Drink(flavor + 1))
    cout << salesAmt[flavor] << endl;
```

Here is one last example.

```
const int NUM_STUDENTS = 10;
```

```
char grade[NUM_STUDENTS];   // Array of 10 student letter grades
int  idNumber;              // Student ID number (0 through 9)
```

The grade array is pictured in Figure 12-6. Values are shown in the components, which implies that some processing of the array has already occurred. Following are some simple examples showing how the array might be used.

`cin >> grade[2];`	Reads the next nonwhitespace character from the input stream and stores it into the component in grade indexed by 2.
`grade[3] = 'A';`	Assigns the character 'A' to the component in grade indexed by 3.
`idNumber = 5;`	Assigns 5 to the index variable idNumber.

`grade[idNumber] = 'C';`	Assigns the character 'C' to the component of `grade` indexed by `idNumber` (that is, by 5).

`for (idNumber = 0; idNumber < NUM_STUDENTS;`
`    idNumber++)`
`  cout << grade[idNumber];`
	Loops through the `grade` array, printing each component. For this loop, the output would be FBCAFCAACB.

`for (idNumber = 0; idNumber < NUM_STUDENTS;`
`    idNumber++)`
`  cout << "Student " << idNumber`
`      << " Grade " << grade[idNumber]`
`      << endl;`
	Loops through `grade`, printing each component in a more readable form.

In the last example, `idNumber` is used as the index, but it also has semantic content—it is the student's identification number. The output would be

```
Student 0 Grade F
Student 1 Grade B
   ⋮
Student 9 Grade B
```

Passing Arrays as Arguments

In Chapter 8, we said that if a variable is passed to a function and it is not to be changed by the function, then the variable should be passed by value instead of by reference. We specifically excluded stream variables (such as those representing data files) from this rule and said that there would be one more exception. Arrays are this exception.

By default, C++ simple variables are always passed by value. To pass a simple variable by reference, you must append an ampersand (&) to the data type name in the function's parameter list:

```
int SomeFunc( float param1,     // Pass-by-value
              char& param2 )    // Pass-by-reference
{
    ⋮
}
```

It is impossible to pass a C++ array by value; arrays are *always* passed by reference. Therefore, you never use & when declaring an array as a parameter. When an array is passed as an argument, its **base address**—the memory address of the first element of the array—is sent to the function. The function then knows where the caller's actual array is located and can access any element of the array.

Base address   The memory address of the first element of an array.

Here is a C++ function that will zero out a one-dimensional `float` array of any size:

```
void ZeroOut( /* out */ float arr[],
              /* in */  int   numElements )
{
    int i;

    for (i = 0; i < numElements; i++)
        arr[i] = 0.0;
}
```

In the parameter list, the declaration of `arr` does not include a size within the brackets. If you include a size, the compiler ignores it. The compiler only wants to know that it is a `float` array, not a `float` array of any particular size. Therefore, in the `ZeroOut` function you must include a second parameter—the number of array elements—in order for the For loop to work correctly.

The calling code can invoke the `ZeroOut` function for a `float` array of any size. The following code fragment makes function calls to zero out two arrays of different sizes. Notice how an array parameter is declared in a function prototype.

```
void ZeroOut( float[], int );    // Function prototype
  ⋮
int main()
{
    float velocity[30];
    float refractionAngle[9000];
      ⋮
    ZeroOut(velocity, 30);
    ZeroOut(refractionAngle, 9000);
      ⋮
}
```

With simple variables, passing by value prevents a function from modifying the caller's argument. Although you cannot pass arrays by value in C++, you can still prevent the function from modifying the caller's array.

To do so, you use the reserved word const in the declaration of the parameter. Below is a function that copies one int array into another. The first parameter—the destination array—is expected to be modified, but the second array is not.

```
void Copy( /* out */      int destination[],
           /* in */  const int source[],
           /* in */       int size         )
{
    int i;

    for (i = 0; i < size; i++)
        destination[i] = source[i];

}
```

The word const guarantees that any attempt to modify the source array within the Copy function results in a compile-time error.

Here's a table that summarizes argument passage for simple variables and one-dimensional arrays:

Argument	*Parameter Declaration for a Pass by Value*	*Parameter Declaration for a Pass by Reference*
Simple variable	int cost	int& price
Array	Impossible*	int arr[]

*However, prefixing the array declaration with the word const prevents the function from modifying the parameter.

One final remark about argument passage: It is a common mistake to pass an array *element* to a function when passing the entire array was intended. For example, our ZeroOut function expects the base address of a float array to be sent as the first argument. In the following code fragment, the function call is an error.

```
float velocity[30];
   ⋮
ZeroOut(velocity[30], 30);    // Error
```

First of all, velocity[30] denotes a single array element—one floating-point number—and not an entire array. Furthermore, there is no array element with an index of 30. The indexes for the velocity array run from 0 through 29.

BACKGROUND INFORMATION

C, C++, and Arrays as Arguments

Some programming languages allow arrays to be passed either by value or by reference. Remember that with passing by value, a copy of the argument is sent to the function. When an array is passed by value, the entire array is copied. Not only is extra space required in the function to hold the copy, but the copying itself takes time. Passing by reference requires only that the address of the argument be passed to the function, so when an array is passed by reference, just the address of the first array component is passed. Thus, passing large arrays by reference saves both memory and time.

The C programming language—the direct predecessor of C++—was designed to be a system programming language. System programs, such as compilers, assemblers, linkers, and operating systems, must be both fast and economical with memory space. In the design of the C language, passing arrays by value was judged to be an unnecessary language feature. Serious system programmers never used a pass by value when working with arrays. Therefore, both C and C++ pass arrays only by reference.

Of course, using a reference parameter can lead to inadvertent errors if the values are changed within the function. In early versions of the C language, there was no way to protect the caller's array from being modified by the function.

C++ (and recent versions of C) added the ability to declare an array parameter as const. By declaring the array as const, a compile-time error occurs if the function attempts to modify the array. As a result, C++ supports the efficiency of passing arrays by reference yet also provides the protection (through const) of passing by value.

Whenever your design of a function's interface identifies an array parameter as incoming-only (to be inspected but not modified by the function), declare the array as const to obtain the same protection as passing by value.

Assertions About Arrays

In assertions written as comments, we often need to refer to a range of array elements:

```
// Assert: alpha[i] through alpha[j] have been printed
```

To specify such ranges, it is more convenient to use an abbreviated notation consisting of two dots:

```
// Assert: alpha[i]..alpha[j] have been printed
```

or, more briefly:

```
// Assert: alpha[i..j] have been printed
```

Note that this dot-dot notation is not valid syntax in C++ language statements. We are talking only about comments in a program.

As an example of the use of this notation, here is how we would write the precondition and postcondition for our ZeroOut function:

```
void ZeroOut( /* out */ float arr[],
              /* in */  int   numElements )

// Precondition:
//     numElements is assigned
// Postcondition:
//     arr[0..numElements-1] == 0.0

{
    int i;

    for (i = 0; i < numElements; i++)
        arr[i] = 0.0;
}
```

Using Typedef with Arrays

In Chapter 10, we discussed the Typedef statement as a way of giving an additional name to an existing data type. We said that before bool became a built-in type in C++, programmers often used a Typedef statement such as the following:

```
typedef int Boolean;
```

We can also use Typedef to give a name to an array type. Here's an example:

```
typedef float FloatArr[100];
```

This statement says that the type FloatArr is the same as the type "100-element array of float." (Notice that the array size in brackets comes at the very end of the statement.) We can now declare variables to be of type FloatArr:

```
FloatArr angle;
FloatArr velocity;
```

The compiler essentially translates these declarations into

```
float angle[100];
float velocity[100];
```

In this book, we don't often use Typedefs to give names to one-dimensional array types. However, when we discuss multidimensional arrays later in the chapter, we'll see that the technique can come in handy.

Arrays of Records and Class Objects

Although arrays with atomic components are very common, many applications require a collection of records or class objects. For example, a business needs a list of parts records, and a teacher needs a list of students in a class. Arrays are ideal for these applications. We simply define an array whose components are records or class objects.

Arrays of Records

Let's define a grade book to be a collection of student records as follows:

```
const int MAX_STUDENTS = 150;

enum GradeType {A, B, C, D, F};

struct StudentRec
{
    string      stuName;
    float       gpa;
    int         examScore[4];
    GradeType   courseGrade;
};

StudentRec gradeBook[MAX_STUDENTS];
int         count;
```

This data structure can be visualized as shown in Figure 12-7.

An element of `gradeBook` is selected by an index. For example, `gradeBook[2]` is the third component in the array `gradeBook`. Each component of `gradeBook` is a record of type `StudentRec`. To access the course grade of the third student, we use the following expression:

FIGURE 12-7

gradeBook Array
with Records as
Elements

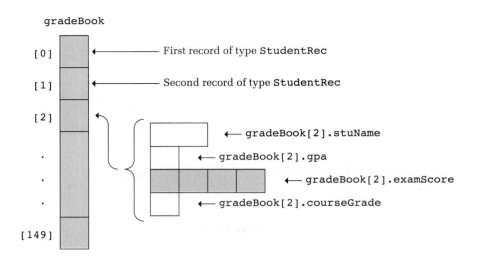

gradeBook

[0] ←——————— First record of type StudentRec

[1] ←——————— Second record of type StudentRec

[2]

gradeBook[2].stuName

gradeBook[2].gpa

gradeBook[2].examScore

gradeBook[2].courseGrade

[149]

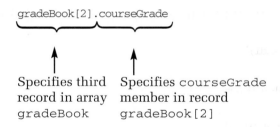

gradeBook[2].courseGrade

Specifies third   Specifies courseGrade
record in array   member in record
gradeBook   gradeBook[2]

The record component gradeBook[2].examScore is an array. We can access the individual elements in this component just as we would access the elements of any other array: We give the name of the array followed by the index, which is enclosed in brackets.

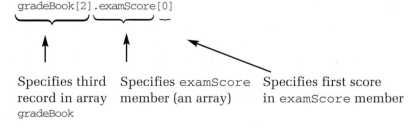

gradeBook[2].examScore[0]

Specifies third   Specifies examScore   Specifies first score
record in array   member (an array)   in examScore member
gradeBook

The following code fragment prints the name of each student in the class:

```
for (count = 0; count < MAX_STUDENTS; count++)
    cout << gradeBook[count].stuName << endl;
```

Arrays of Class Objects

The syntax for declaring and using arrays of class objects is the same as for arrays of structs. Given the TimeType class of Chapter 11, we can maintain a collection of ten appointment times by starting with the declaration

```
TimeType appointment[10];
```

This statement creates a ten-element array named appointment, in which each element is a TimeType object. The following statements set the first two appointment times to 8:45:00 and 10:00:00.

```
appointment[0].Set(8, 45, 0);
appointment[1].Set(10, 0, 0);
```

To output all ten appointment times, we would write

```
for (index = 0; index < 10; index++)
{
    appointment[index].Write();
    cout << endl;
}
```

Recall that the TimeType class has two constructors defined for it. One is the default (parameterless) constructor, which sets the time for a newly created object to 00:00:00. The other is a parameterized constructor with which the client code can specify an initial time when the class object is created. How are constructors handled when you declare an array of class objects? Here is the rule in C++:

If a class has at least one constructor, and an array of class objects is declared:

```
SomeClass arr[50];
```

then one of the constructors *must* be the default (parameterless) constructor. This constructor is invoked for each element of the array.

Therefore, with our declaration of the appointment array

```
TimeType appointment[10];
```

the default constructor is called for all ten array elements, setting each time to an initial value of 00:00:00.

Special Kinds of Array Processing

Two types of array processing occur especially often: using only part of the declared array (a subarray) and using index values that have specific meaning within the problem (indexes with semantic content). We describe both of these methods briefly here and give further examples in the remainder of the chapter.

Subarray Processing

The *size* of an array—the declared number of array components—is established at compile time. We have to declare it to be as big as it would ever need to be. Because the exact number of values to be put into the array often depends on the data itself, however, we may not fill all of the array components with values. The problem is that to avoid processing empty ones, we must keep track of how many components are actually filled.

As values are put into the array, we keep a count of how many components are filled. We then use this count to process only components that have values stored in them. Any remaining places are not processed. For example, if there are 250 students in a class, a program to analyze test grades would set aside 250 locations for the grades. However, some students may be absent on the day of the test. So the number of test grades must be counted, and that number, rather than 250, is used to control the processing of the array.

If the number of data items actually stored in an array is less than its declared size, functions that receive array parameters must also receive the number of data items as a parameter. For example,

```
void Print( /* in */ const char grade[],      // Array for up to
                                                //    250 students
               /* in */         int  numGrades )  // Number of grades
                                                //    actually in array
```

The first case study at the end of this chapter demonstrates the technique of subarray processing.

Indexes with Semantic Content

In some problems, an array index has meaning beyond simple position; that is, the index has *semantic content.* An example is the salesAmt array we showed earlier. This array is indexed by a value of enumeration type Drink. The index of a specific sales amount is the kind of soft drink sold; for example, salesAmt[ROOT_BEER] is the dollar sales figure for root beer.

The next section gives additional examples of indexes with semantic content.

Two-Dimensional Arrays

A one-dimensional array is used to represent items in a list or sequence of values. In many problems, however, the relationships between data items are more complex than a simple list. A **two-dimensional array** is used to represent items in a table with rows and columns, provided each item in the table is of the same data type. Two-dimensional arrays are useful for representing board games, such as chess, tic-tac-toe, or Scrabble, and in computer graphics, where the screen is thought of as a two-dimensional array. A component in a two-dimensional array is accessed by specifying the row and column indexes of the item in the array. This is a familiar task. For example, if you want to find a street on a map, you look up the street name on the back of the map to find the coordinates of the street, usually a letter and a number. The letter specifies a column to look on, and the number specifies a row. You find the street where the row and column meet.

Two-dimensional array   A collection of components, all of the same type, structured in two dimensions. Each component is accessed by a pair of indexes that represent the component's position in each dimension.

Figure 12-8 shows a two-dimensional array with 100 rows and 9 columns. The rows are accessed by an integer ranging from 0 through 99; the columns are accessed by an integer ranging from 0 through 8. Each component is accessed by a row-column pair—for example, 0, 5.

A two-dimensional array is declared in exactly the same way as a one-dimensional array, except that sizes must be specified for two dimensions. Below is the syntax template for declaring an array with more than one dimension, along with an example.

ArrayDeclaration

DataType ArrayName **[** ConstIntExpression **]**   **[** ConstIntExpression **]** . . . **;**

FIGURE 12-8
A Two-
Dimensional
Array

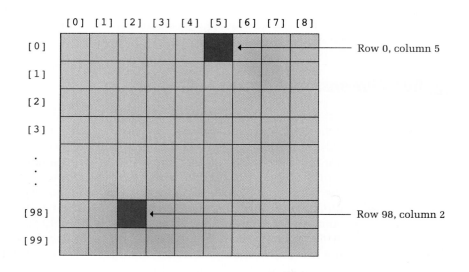

Row 0, column 5

Row 98, column 2

```
const int NUM_ROWS = 100;
const int NUM_COLS = 9;
    ⋮
float alpha[NUM_ROWS][NUM_COLS];
```

First Second
dimension dimension

This example declares `alpha` to be a two-dimensional array, all of whose components are `float` values. The declaration creates the array that is pictured in Figure 12-8.

To access an individual component of the `alpha` array, two expressions (one for each dimension) are used to specify its position. Each expression is in its own pair of brackets next to the name of the array:

```
alpha[0][5] = 36.4;
```

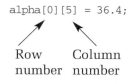

Row   Column
number   number

The syntax template for accessing an array component is

ArrayComponentAccess

ArrayName **[** IndexExpression **]** **[** IndexExpression **]** . . .

As with one-dimensional arrays, each index expression must result in an integer value.

Let's look now at some examples. Here is the declaration of a two-dimensional array with 364 integer components ($52 \times 7 = 364$):

```
int hiTemp[52][7];
```

hiTemp is an array with 52 rows and 7 columns. Each place in the array (each component) can contain any int value. Our intention is that the array contains high temperatures for each day in a year. Each row represents one of the 52 weeks in a year, and each column represents one of the 7 days in a week. (To keep the example simple, we ignore the fact that there are 365—and sometimes 366—days in a year.) The expression hiTemp[2][6] refers to the int value in the third row (row 2) and the seventh column (column 6). Semantically, hiTemp[2][6] is the temperature for the seventh day of the third week. The code fragment shown in Figure 12-9 would print the temperature values for the third week.

Another representation of the same data might be as follows:

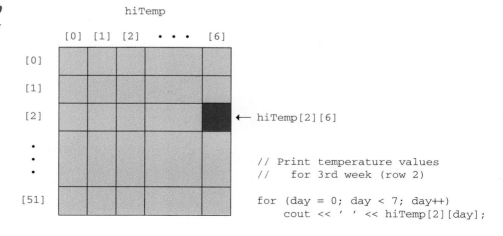

FIGURE 12-9

hiTemp Array

```
// Print temperature values
//    for 3rd week (row 2)

for (day = 0; day < 7; day++)
    cout << ' ' << hiTemp[2][day];
```

```
enum DayType
{
     MONDAY,  TUESDAY,  WEDNESDAY,  THURSDAY,  FRIDAY,  SATURDAY,  SUNDAY
};

int hiTemp[52][7];
```

Here, `hiTemp` is declared the same as before, but we can use an expression of type `DayType` for the column index. `hiTemp[2][SUNDAY]` corresponds to the same component as `hiTemp[2][6]` in the first example. (Recall that enumerators such as MONDAY, TUESDAY, ... are represented internally as the integers 0, 1, 2, ...) If `day` is of type `DayType` and `week` is of type `int`, the code fragment shown in Figure 12-10 sets the entire array to 0. (Notice that by using `DayType`, the temperature values in the array begin with the first Monday of the year, not necessarily with January 1.)

Another way of looking at a two-dimensional array is to see it as a structure in which each component has two features. For example, in the following code,

```
enum Colors {RED, ORANGE, YELLOW, GREEN, BLUE, INDIGO, VIOLET};
enum Makes
{
     FORD,  TOYOTA,  HYUNDAI,  JAGUAR,  CITROEN,  BMW,  FIAT,  SAAB
};
const int NUM_COLORS = 7;
const int NUM_MAKES = 8;
```

FIGURE 12-10

`hiTemp` Array
(Alternate Form)

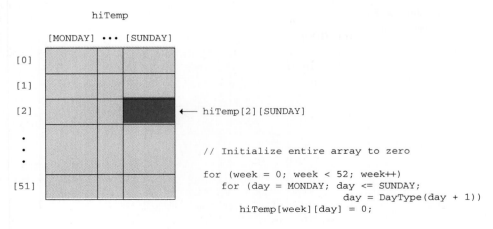

```
// Initialize entire array to zero

for (week = 0; week < 52; week++)
    for (day = MONDAY; day <= SUNDAY;
                       day = DayType(day + 1))
        hiTemp[week][day] = 0;
```

```
float crashRating[NUM_COLORS][NUM_MAKES];    // Array of crash
                                             // likelihoods by color
                                             // and make
      ⋮
crashRating[BLUE][JAGUAR] = 0.83;            // Blue Jaguars have a crash
                                             //    likelihood of 0.83
crashRating[RED][FORD] = 0.19;               // Red Fords have a crash
                                             //    likelihood of 0.19
```

the data structure uses one dimension to represent the color and the other to represent the make of automobile. In other words, both indexes have semantic content—a concept we discussed in the previous section.

Processing Two-Dimensional Arrays

Processing data in a two-dimensional array generally means accessing the array in one of four patterns: randomly, along rows, along columns, or throughout the entire array. Each of these may also involve subarray processing.

The simplest way to access a component is to look directly in a given location. For example, a user enters map coordinates that we use as indexes into an array of street names to access the desired name at those coordinates. This process is referred to as *random access* because the user may enter any set of coordinates at random.

There are many cases in which we might wish to perform an operation on all the elements of a particular row or column in an array. Consider the hiTemp array defined previously, in which the rows represent weeks of the year and the columns represent days of the week. If we wanted the average high temperature for a given week, we would sum the values in that row and divide by 7. If we wanted the average for a given day of the week, we would sum the values in that column and divide by 52. The former case is access by row; the latter case is access by column.

Now suppose that we wish to determine the average for the year. We must access every element in the array, sum them, and divide by 364. In this case, the order of access—by row or by column—is not important. (The same is true when we initialize every element of an array to zero.) This is access throughout the array.

There are times when we must access every array element in a particular order, either by rows or by columns. For example, if we wanted the average for every week, we would run through the entire array, taking each row in turn. However, if we wanted the average for each day of the week, we would run through the array a column at a time.

Let's take a closer look at these patterns of access by considering four common examples of array processing.

1. Sum the rows.
2. Sum the columns.
3. Initialize the array to all zeros (or some special value).
4. Print the array.

First, let's define some constants and variables using general identifiers, such as `row` and `col`, rather than problem-dependent identifiers. Then let's look at each algorithm in terms of generalized two-dimensional array processing.

```
const int NUM_ROWS = 50;
const int NUM_COLS = 50;

int arr[NUM_ROWS][NUM_COLS];    // A two-dimensional array
int row;                        // A row index
int col;                        // A column index
int total;                      // A variable for summing
```

Sum the Rows

Suppose we want to sum row number 3 (the fourth row) in the array and print the result. We can do this easily with a For loop:

```
total = 0;
for (col = 0; col < NUM_COLS; col++)
    total = total + arr[3][col];
cout << "Row sum: " << total << endl;
```

This For loop runs through each column of `arr`, while keeping the row index fixed at 3. Every value in row 3 is added to `total`.

Now suppose we want to sum and print two rows—row 2 and row 3. We can use a nested loop and make the row index a variable:

```
for (row = 2; row < 4; row++)
{
    total = 0;
    for (col = 0; col < NUM_COLS; col++)
        total = total + arr[row][col];
    cout << "Row sum: " << total << endl;
}
```

The outer loop controls the rows, and the inner loop controls the columns. For each value of row, every column is processed; then the outer loop moves to the next row. In the first iteration of the outer loop, row is held at 2 and col goes from 0 through NUM_COLS−1. Therefore, the array is accessed in the following order:

```
arr[2][0]   [2][1]   [2][2]   [2][3] ... [2][NUM_COLS-1]
```

In the second iteration of the outer loop, row is incremented to 3, and the array is accessed as follows:

```
arr[3][0]   [3][1]   [3][2]   [3][3] ... [3][NUM_COLS-1]
```

We can generalize this row processing to run through every row of the array by having the outer loop run from 0 through NUM_ROWS−1. However, if we want to access only part of the array (subarray processing), given variables declared as

```
int rowsFilled;    // Data is in 0..rowsFilled-1
int colsFilled;    // Data is in 0..colsFilled-1
```

then we write the code fragment as follows:

```
for (row = 0; row < rowsFilled; row++)
{
    total = 0;
    for (col = 0; col < colsFilled; col++)
        total = total + arr[row][col];
    cout << "Row sum: " << total << endl;
}
```

Figure 12-11 illustrates subarray processing by row.

Sum the Columns

Suppose we want to sum and print each column. The code to perform this task follows. Again, we have generalized the code to sum only the portion of the array that contains valid data.

```
for (col = 0; col < colsFilled; col++)
{
    total = 0;
    for (row = 0; row < rowsFilled; row++)
        total = total + arr[row][col];
    cout << "Column sum: " << total << endl;
}
```

In this case, the outer loop controls the column, and the inner loop controls the row. All the components in the first column are accessed and summed before the outer loop index changes and the components in the second column are accessed. Figure 12-12 illustrates subarray processing by column.

Initialize the Array

As with one-dimensional arrays, we can initialize a two-dimensional array either by initializing it in its declaration or by using assignment statements. If the array is small, it is simplest to initialize it in its declaration. To initialize a two-row by three-column array to look like this:

```
14    3   -5
 0   46    7
```

FIGURE 12-11
Partial Array
Processing by Row

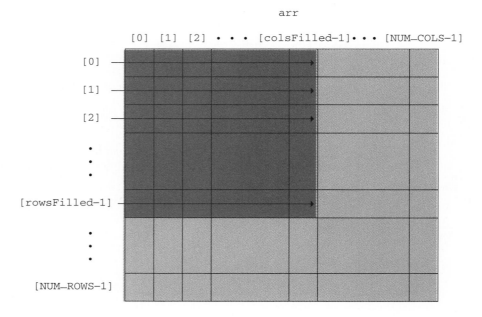

we can use the following declaration.

```
int arr[2][3] =
{
    {14, 3, -5},
    {0, 46, 7}
};
```

In this declaration, the initializer list consists of two items, each of which is itself an initializer list. The first inner initializer list stores 14, 3, and −5 into row 0 of the array; the second stores 0, 46, and 7 into row 1. The use of two initializer lists makes sense if you think of each row of the two-dimensional array as a one-dimensional array of three ints. The first initializer list initializes the first array (the first row), and the second list initializes the second array (the second row). Later in the chapter, we revisit this notion of viewing a two-dimensional array as an array of arrays.

Initializing an array in its declaration is impractical if the array is large. For a 100-row by 100-column array, you don't want to list 10,000 values. If the values are all different, you should store them into a file and input them into the array at run time. If the values are all the same, the usual approach is to use nested For loops and an assignment statement. Here is a general-purpose code segment that zeros out an array with NUM_ROWS rows and NUM_COLS columns:

Figure 12-12
Partial Array
Processing by
Column

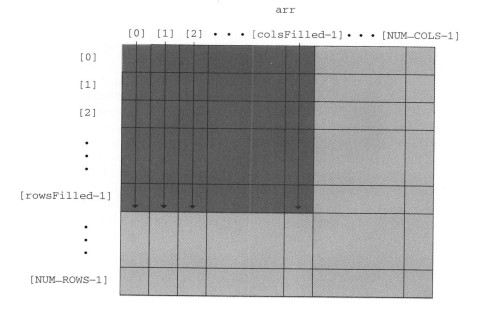

```
for (row = 0; row < NUM_ROWS; row++)
    for (col = 0; col < NUM_COLS; col++)
        arr[row][col] = 0;
```

In this case, we initialized the array a row at a time, but we could just as easily have run through each column instead. The order doesn't matter as long as we access every element.

Print the Array

If we wish to print out an array with one row per line, then we have another case of row processing:

```
#include <iomanip>    // For setw()
    ⋮
for (row = 0; row < NUM_ROWS; row++)
{
    for (col = 0; col < NUM_COLS; col++)
        cout << setw(15) << arr[row][col];
    cout << endl;
}
```

This code fragment prints the values of the array in columns that are 15 characters wide. As a matter of proper style, this fragment should be preceded by code that prints headings over the columns to identify their contents.

There's no rule that we have to print each row on a line. We could turn the array sideways and print each column on one line simply by exchanging the two For loops. When you are printing a two-dimensional array, you must consider which order of presentation makes the most sense and how the array fits on the page. For example, an array with 6 columns and 100 rows would be best printed as 6 columns, 100 lines long.

Almost all processing of data stored in a two-dimensional array involves either processing by row or processing by column. In most of our examples the index type has been int, but the pattern of operation of the loops is the same no matter what types the indexes are.

The looping patterns for row processing and column processing are so useful that we summarize them below. To make them more general, we use minRow for the first row number and minCol for the first column number. Remember that row processing has the row index in the outer loop, and column processing has the column index in the outer loop.

Row Processing

```
for (row = minRow; row < rowsFilled; row++)
    for (col = minCol; col < colsFilled; col++)
        ⋮              // Whatever processing is required
```

Column Processing

```
for (col = minCol; col < colsFilled; col++)
    for (row = minRow; row < rowsFilled; row++)
        ⋮              // Whatever processing is required
```

Passing Two-Dimensional Arrays as Arguments

Earlier in the chapter, we said that when one-dimensional arrays are declared as parameters in a function, the size of the array usually is omitted from the square brackets:

```
void SomeFunc( /* inout */ float alpha[],
               /* in */    int   size   )
{
    ⋮
}
```

If you include a size in the brackets, the compiler ignores it. As you learned, the base address of the caller's argument (the memory address of the first array element) is passed to the function. The function works for an argument of any size. Because the function cannot know the size of the caller's array, we either pass the size as an argument—as in SomeFunc above—or use a named constant if the function always operates on an array of a certain size.

When a two-dimensional array is passed as an argument, again the base address of the caller's array is sent to the function. But you cannot leave off the sizes of both of the array dimensions. You can omit the size of the first dimension (the number of rows) but not the second (the number of columns). Here is the reason.

In the computer's memory, C++ stores two-dimensional arrays in row order. Thinking of memory as one long line of memory cells, the first row of the array is followed by the second row, which is followed by the third, and so on (see Figure 12-13). To locate beta[1][0] in this figure, a function that receives beta's base address must be able to know that there are four elements in each row—that is, that the array consists of four columns. Therefore, the declaration of a parameter must always state the number of columns:

```
void AnotherFunc( /* inout */ int beta[][4] )
{
    ⋮
}
```

Furthermore, the number of columns declared for the parameter must be *exactly* the same as the number of columns in the caller's array. As you can tell from Figure 12-13, if there is any discrepancy in the number of columns, the function will access the wrong array element in memory.

Our AnotherFunc function works for a two-dimensional array of any number of rows, as long as it has exactly four columns. In practice, we seldom write programs that use arrays with a varying number of rows but the same number of columns. To avoid problems with mismatches in argument and parameter sizes, it's practical to use a Typedef statement to define a two-dimensional array type and then declare both the argument and the parameter to be of that type. For example, we might make the declarations

```
const int NUM_ROWS = 10;
const int NUM_COLS = 20;
typedef int ArrayType[NUM_ROWS][NUM_COLS];
```

and then write the following general-purpose function that initializes all elements of an array to a specified value:

```
void Initialize( /* out */ ArrayType arr,      // Array to initialize
                 /* in */   int       initVal) // Initial value

// Initializes each element of arr to initVal

// Precondition:
//      initVal is assigned
// Postcondition:
//      arr[0..NUM_ROWS-1][0..NUM_COLS-1] == initVal
```

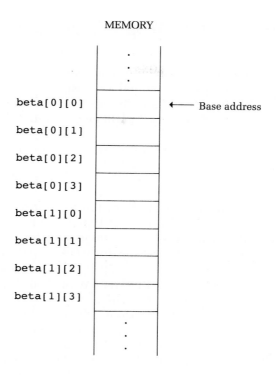

FIGURE 12-13
Memory Layout for
a Two-Row by
Four-Column
Array

```
{
    int row;
    int col;

    for (row = 0; row < NUM_ROWS; row++)
        for (col = 0; col < NUM_COLS; col++)
            arr[row][col] = initVal;
}
```

The calling code could then declare and initialize one or more arrays of type `ArrayType` by making calls to the `Initialize` function. For example,

```
ArrayType delta;
ArrayType gamma;

Initialize(delta, 0);
Initialize(gamma, -1);
  ⋮
```

Another Way of Defining Two-Dimensional Arrays

We hinted earlier that a two-dimensional array can be viewed as an array of arrays. This view is supported by C++ in the sense that the components of a one-dimensional array do not have to be atomic. The components can themselves be structured—structs, class objects, even arrays. For example, our hiTemp array could be declared as follows.

```
typedef int WeekType[7];    // Array type for 7 temperature readings

WeekType hiTemp[52];        // Array of 52 WeekType arrays
```

With this declaration, the 52 components of the hiTemp array are one-dimensional arrays of type WeekType. In other words, hiTemp has two dimensions. We can refer to each row as an entity: hiTemp[2] refers to the array of temperatures for week 2. We can also access each individual component of hiTemp by specifying both indexes: hiTemp[2][0] accesses the temperature on the first day of week 2.

Does it matter which way we declare a two-dimensional array? Not to C++. The choice should be based on readability and understandability. Sometimes the features of the data are shown more clearly if both indexes are specified in a single declaration. At other times, the code is clearer if one dimension is defined first as a one-dimensional array type.

Here is an example of when it is advantageous to define a two-dimensional array as an array of arrays. If the rows have been defined first as a one-dimensional array type, each row can be passed to a function whose parameter is a one-dimensional array of the same type. For example, the following function calculates and returns the maximum value in an array of type WeekType.

```
int Maximum( /* in */ const WeekType data )   // Array to be examined

// Precondition:
//     data[0..6] are assigned
// Postcondition:
//     Function value == maximum value in data[0..6]

{
    int max;        // Temporary max. value
    int index;      // Loop control and index variable
```

```
    max = data[0];
    for (index = 1; index < 7; index++)
        if (data[index] > max)
            max = data[index];
    return max;
}
```

Our two-part declaration of hiTemp permits us to call Maximum using a component of hiTemp as follows.

```
highest = Maximum(hiTemp[20]);
```

Row 20 of hiTemp is passed to Maximum, which treats it like any other one-dimensional array of type WeekType (see Figure 12-14). It makes sense to pass the row as an argument because both it and the function parameter are of the same named type, WeekType.

With hiTemp declared as an array of arrays, we can output the maximum temperature of each week of the year with the following code:

```
cout << " Week  Maximum" << endl
     << "Number Temperature" << endl;
for (week = 0; week < 52; week++)
    cout << setw(6) << week
         << setw(9) << Maximum(hiTemp[week]) << endl;
```

FIGURE 12-14

A One-Dimensional Array of One-Dimensional Arrays

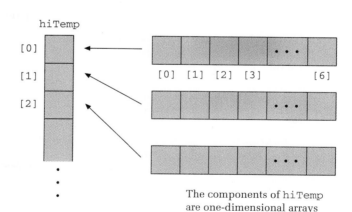

The components of hiTemp are one-dimensional arrays of type WeekType.

Multidimensional Arrays

C++ does not place a limit on the number of dimensions that an array can have. We can generalize our definition of an array to cover all cases.

Array A collection of components, all of the same type, ordered on N dimensions ($N \geq 1$). Each component is accessed by N indexes, each of which represents the component's position within that dimension.

You might have guessed from the syntax templates that you can have as many dimensions as you want. How many should you have in a particular case? Use as many as there are features that describe the components in the array.

Take, for example, a chain of department stores. Monthly sales figures must be kept for each item by store. There are three important pieces of information about each item: the month in which it was sold, the store from which it was purchased, and the item number. We can define an array type to summarize this data as follows:

```
const int NUM_ITEMS = 100;
const int NUM_STORES = 10;

typedef int SalesType[NUM_STORES][12][NUM_ITEMS];

SalesType sales;     // Array of sales figures
int       item;
int       store;
int       month;
int       numberSold;
int       currentMonth;
```

A graphic representation of the `sales` array is shown in Figure 12-15.

The number of components in `sales` is 12,000 (10 × 12 × 100). If sales figures are available only for January through June, then half the array is empty. If we want to process the data in the array, we must use subarray processing. The following program fragment sums and prints the total number of each item sold this year to date by all stores.

FIGURE 12-15
Graphical
Representation of
sales Array

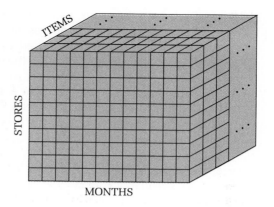

```
for (item = 0; item < NUM_ITEMS; item++)
{
    numberSold = 0;
    for (store = 0; store < NUM_STORES; store++)
        for (month = 0; month <= currentMonth; month++)
            numberSold = numberSold + sales[store][month][item];
    cout << "Item #" << item << " Sales to date = " << numberSold
        << endl;
}
```

Because item controls the outer For loop, we are summing each item's sales by month and store. If we want to find the total sales for each store, we use store to control the outer For loop, summing its sales by month and item with the inner loops.

```
for (store = 0; store < NUM_STORES; store++)
{
    numberSold = 0;
    for (item = 0; item < NUM_ITEMS; item++)
        for (month = 0; month <= currentMonth; month++)
            numberSold = numberSold + sales[store][month][item];
    cout << "Store #" << store << " Sales to date = " << numberSold
        << endl;
}
```

It takes two loops to access each component in a two-dimensional array; it takes three loops to access each component in a three-dimensional array. The task to be accomplished determines which index controls the outer loop, the middle loop, and the inner loop. If we want to calculate monthly sales by store, month controls the outer loop and store controls the middle loop. If we want to calculate monthly sales by item, month controls the outer loop and item controls the middle loop.

If we want to keep track of the departments that sell each item, we can add a fourth dimension.

```
enum Departments {A, B, C, D, E, F, G};
const int NUM_DEPTS = 7;
typedef int SalesType[NUM_STORES][12][NUM_ITEMS][NUM_DEPTS];
```

How would we visualize this new structure? Not very easily! Fortunately, we do not have to visualize a structure in order to use it. If we want the number of sales in store 1 during June for item number 4 in department C, we simply access the array element

```
sales[1][5][4][C]
```

When a multidimensional array is declared as a parameter in a function, C++ requires you to state the sizes of all dimensions except the first. For our four-dimensional version of SalesType, a function heading would look either like this:

```
void DoSomething( /* inout */ int arr[][12][NUM_ITEMS][NUM_DEPTS] )
```

or, better yet, like this:

```
void DoSomething( /* inout */ SalesType arr )
```

The second version is the safest (and the most uncluttered to look at). It ensures that the sizes of all dimensions of the parameter match those of the argument exactly. With the first version, the reason that you must declare the sizes of all but the first dimension is the same as we discussed earlier for two-dimensional arrays. Because arrays are stored linearly in memory (one array element after another), the compiler must use this size information to locate correctly an element that lies within the array.

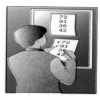

PROBLEM-SOLVING CASE STUDY

Comparison of Two Lists

Problem: You are writing a program for an application that does not tolerate erroneous input data. Therefore, the data values are prepared by entering them twice into one file. The file contains two lists of positive integer numbers, separated by a negative number. These two lists of numbers should be identical; if they are not, then a data entry error has occurred. For example, if the input file contains the sequence of numbers 17, 14, 8, −5, 17, 14, 8, then the two lists of three numbers are identical. However, the sequence 17, 14, 8, −5, 17, 12, 8 shows a data entry error.

You decide to write a separate program to compare the lists and print out any pairs of numbers that are not the same. The exact number of integers in each list is unknown, but each list has no more than 500.

Input: A file (`dataFile`) containing two lists of positive integers. The lists are separated by a negative integer, and both lists have the same number of integers.

Output: A statement that the lists are identical, or a list of the pairs of values that do not match.

Discussion: Because the lists are in the same file, the first list has to be read and stored until the negative number is read. Then the second list can be read and compared with the first list.

If we were checking the lists by hand, we would write the numbers from the first list on a pad of paper, one per line. The line number would correspond to the number's position in the list; that is, the first number would be on the first line, the second number on the second line, and so on. The first number in the second list would then be compared to the number on the first line, the second number to the number on the second line, and so forth.

We use an array named `firstList` to represent the pad of paper. Its declaration looks like this:

```
const int MAX_NUMBER = 500;    // Maximum in each list

int firstList[MAX_NUMBER];     // Holds first list
```

Because the first array component has index 0, we must think of our pad of paper as having its lines numbered from 0, not 1.

Now we can complete the design and program for our problem.

PROBLEM-SOLVING CASE STUDY cont'd.

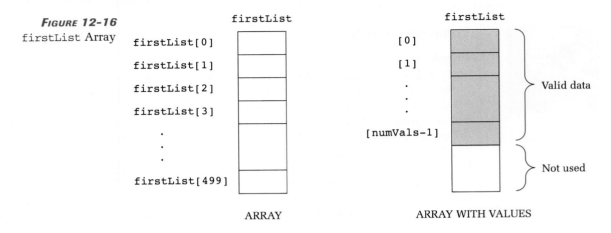

FIGURE 12-16
firstList Array

Assumption: The two lists to be compared have the same number of integers.

Data Structures: A one-dimensional int array (firstList) to hold the first list of numbers. If numVals is the actual number of values in each list, only positions 0 through numVals − 1 of the array will be filled (see Figure 12-16).

Main   **Level 0**

> Open dataFile (and verify success)
> Read first list
> Set allOK = true
> Compare lists, changing allOK if necessary
> IF allOK
>   Print "The two lists are identical"

In the module Read First List, the first input value is stored into firstList[0], the second into firstList[1], the third into firstList[2]. This implies that we need a counter to keep track of which number is being read. When the negative number is encountered, the counter tells us how many of the 500 places set aside were actually needed. We can use this value (call it numVals) to control the reading and comparing loop in the Compare Lists module. This is an example of subarray processing.

Read First List (Inout: dataFile; Out: numVals, firstList)   Level 1

```
Set counter = 0
Read number from dataFile
WHILE number >= 0
        Set firstList[counter] = number
        Increment counter
        Read number from dataFile
Set numVals= counter
```

Compare Lists (In: firstList, numVals; Inout: dataFile, allOK)

```
FOR counter going from 0 through numVals−1
        Read number from second list
        IF numbers not the same
                Set allOK = false
                Print both numbers
```

Numbers Not the Same   Level 2

```
number != firstList[counter]
```

Print Both Numbers

```
Print firstList[counter], number
```

PROBLEM-SOLVING CASE STUDY cont'd.

Because the last two modules are only one line each, we can code them directly in the Compare Lists module.

Module Structure Chart:

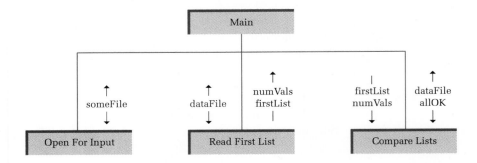

(The following program is written in ISO/ANSI standard C++. If you are working with pre–standard C++, see the alternate version of the program in the PRE_STD directory of the program disk, available at the publisher's Web site, www.jbpub.com/disks.)

```
//****************************************************************
// CheckLists program
// There are two lists of positive integers in a data file,
// separated by a negative integer.  This program compares the two
// lists.  If they are identical, a message is printed.  If not,
// nonmatching pairs are printed.  Assumption: The number of values
// in both lists is the same and is <= 500
//****************************************************************
#include <iostream>
#include <iomanip>      // For setw()
#include <fstream>      // For file I/O
#include <string>       // For string class

using namespace std;

const int MAX_NUMBER = 500;      // Maximum in each list

void CompareLists( const int[], int, ifstream&, bool& );
void OpenForInput( ifstream& );
```

PROBLEM-SOLVING CASE STUDY cont'd.

```
void ReadFirstList( int[], int&, ifstream& );

int main()
{
    int       firstList[MAX_NUMBER];   // Holds first list
    bool      allOK;                   // True if lists are identical
    int       numVals;                 // No. of values in first list
    ifstream dataFile;                 // Input file

    OpenForInput(dataFile);
    if ( !dataFile )
        return 1;

    ReadFirstList(firstList, numVals, dataFile);
    allOK = true;
    CompareLists(firstList, numVals, dataFile, allOK);
    if (allOK)
        cout << "The two lists are identical" << endl;
    return 0;
}

//******************************************************************

void OpenForInput( /* inout */ ifstream& someFile )    // File to be
                                                       // opened
// Prompts the user for the name of an input file
// and attempts to open the file

{
    .
    .         (Same as in ConvertDates program of Chapter 8)
    .
}

//******************************************************************

void ReadFirstList(
            /* out */    int       firstList[],   // Filled first list
            /* out */    int&      numVals,        // Number of values
            /* inout */ ifstream& dataFile    )   // Input file

// Reads the first list from the data file
// and counts the number of values in the list

// Precondition:
//    dataFile has been successfully opened for input
//  && The no. of input values in the first list <= MAX_NUMBER
```

PROBLEM-SOLVING CASE STUDY cont'd.

```
// Postcondition:
//     numVals == number of input values in the first list
//  && firstList[0..numVals-1] contain the input values

{
    int counter;     // Index variable
    int number;      // An input value

    counter = 0;
    dataFile >> number;
    while (number >= 0)
    {
        firstList[counter] = number;
        counter++;
        dataFile >> number;
    }
    numVals = counter;
}

//*******************************************************************

void CompareLists(
    /* in */      const int      firstList[],   // 1st list of numbers
    /* in */            int      numVals,        // Number in 1st list
    /* inout */      ifstream& dataFile,         // Input file
    /* inout */         bool&   allOK        )   // True if lists match

// Reads the second list of numbers
// and compares it to the first list

// Precondition:
//     allOK is assigned
//  && numVals <= MAX_NUMBER
//  && firstList[0..numVals-1] are assigned
//  && The two lists have the same number of values
// Postcondition:
//     Values from the second list have been read from the
//     input file
//  && IF all values in the two lists match
//         allOK == allOK@entry
//     ELSE
//         allOK == false
//        && The positions and contents of mismatches have been
//           printed
```

PROBLEM-SOLVING CASE STUDY *cont'd.*

```
{
    int counter;      // Loop control and index variable
    int number;       // An input value

    for (counter = 0; counter < numVals; counter++)
    {
        dataFile >> number;
        if (number != firstList[counter])
        {
            allOK = false;
            cout << "Position " << counter << ": "
                 << setw(4) << firstList[counter] << " != "
                 << setw(4) << number << endl;
        }
    }
}
```

Testing: The program is run with two sets of data, one in which the two lists are identical and one in which there are errors. The data and the results from each are shown below.

Data Set 1	*Data Set 2*
21	21
32	32
76	76
22	22
21	21
-4	-4
21	21
32	32
76	176
22	12
21	21

Output

The two lists are identical.

Output

Position 2: 76 != 176
Position 3: 22 != 12

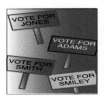

PROBLEM-SOLVING CASE STUDY

City Council Election

Problem: There has just been a hotly contested city council election. In four voting precincts, citizens have cast their ballots for four candidates. Let's do an analysis of the votes for the four candidates by precinct. We want to know how many votes each candidate received in each precinct, how many total votes each candidate received, and how many total votes were cast in each precinct.

Input: An arbitrary number of votes in a file voteFile, with each vote represented as a pair of numbers: a precinct number (1 through 4) and a candidate number (1 through 4); and candidate names, entered from the keyboard (to be used for printing the output).

Output: The following three items, written to a file reportFile: a tabular report showing how many votes each candidate received in each precinct, the total number of votes for each candidate, and the total number of votes in each precinct.

Discussion: The data consists of a pair of numbers for each vote. The first number is the precinct number; the second number is the candidate number.

   If we were doing the analysis by hand, our first task would be to go through the data, counting how many people in each precinct voted for each candidate. We would probably create a table with precincts down the side and candidates across the top. Each vote would be recorded as a hash mark in the appropriate row and column (see Figure 12-17).

   When all of the votes had been recorded, a sum of each column would tell us how many votes each candidate had received. A sum of each row would tell us how many people had voted in each precinct.

   As is so often the case, we can use this by-hand algorithm directly in our program. We can create a two-dimensional array in which each component is a counter for the number of votes for a particular candidate in each

FIGURE 12-17
Vote-Counting
Table

Precinct	Smith	Jones	Adams	Smiley
1	ﬀﬀ ||	||	ﬀﬀ ﬀﬀ ||	ﬀﬀ
2	ﬀﬀ ﬀﬀ	||	ﬀﬀ	|||
3	||	ﬀﬀ |||	ﬀﬀ ﬀﬀ ﬀﬀ	|||
4	ﬀﬀ	ﬀﬀ |||	ﬀﬀ ﬀﬀ	||

PROBLEM-SOLVING CASE STUDY cont'd.

FIGURE 12-18

Data Structures for
Election Program

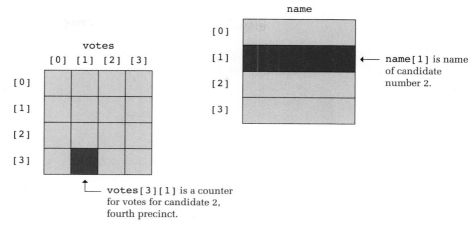

votes[3][1] is a counter
for votes for candidate 2,
fourth precinct.

name[1] is name
of candidate
number 2.

precinct; for example, the value indexed by [2][1] would be the counter
for the votes in precinct 2 for candidate 1. Well, not quite. C++ arrays are
indexed beginning at 0, so the correct array component would be indexed
by [1][0]. When we input a precinct number and candidate number, we
must remember to subtract 1 from each before indexing into the array.
Likewise, we must add 1 to an array index that represents a precinct number or candidate number before printing it out.

Data Structures:

A two-dimensional array named votes, where the rows represent
precincts and the columns represent candidates
A one-dimensional array of strings containing the names of the candidates,
to be used for printing (see Figure 12-18).

In the design that follows, we use the named constants
NUM_PRECINCTS and NUM_CANDIDATES in place of the literal constants 4
and 4.

Main   **Level 0**

```
Open voteFile for input (and verify success)
Open reportFile for output (and verify success)
Get candidate names
Set votes array to 0
Read precinct, candidate from voteFile
WHILE NOT EOF on voteFile
        Increment votes[precinct-1][candidate-1] by 1
        Read precinct, candidate from voteFile
Write report to reportFile
Write totals per candidate to reportFile
Write totals per precinct to reportFile
```

Get Candidate Names (Out: name)   **Level 1**

```
Print  "Enter the names of the candidates, one per line,
                in the order they appear on the ballot."
FOR candidate going from 0 through NUM_CANDIDATES - 1
        Read name[candidate]
```

Note that each candidate's name is stored in the slot in the name array corresponding to his or her candidate number (minus 1). These names are useful when the totals are printed.

Set Votes to Zero (Out: votes)

```
FOR each precinct
        FOR each candidate
                Set votes[precinct][candidate] = 0
```

PROBLEM-SOLVING CASE STUDY cont'd.

Write Report (In: votes, name; Inout: reportFile)

```
// Set up headings
FOR each candidate
        Write name[candidate] to reportFile
Write newline to reportFile
// Print array by row
FOR each precinct
        FOR each candidate
                Write votes[precinct][candidate] to reportFile
        Write newline to reportFile
```

Write Totals per Candidate (In: votes, name; Inout: reportFile)

```
FOR each candidate
        Set total = 0
        // Compute column sum
        FOR each precinct
                Add votes[precinct][candidate] to total
Write "Total votes for", name[candidate], total to reportFile
```

Write Totals per Precinct (In: votes; Inout: reportFile)

```
FOR each precinct
        Set total = 0
        // Compute row sum
        FOR each candidate
                Add votes[precinct][candidate] to total
Write "Total votes for precinct", precinct, ':', total to reportFile
```

Module Structure Chart:

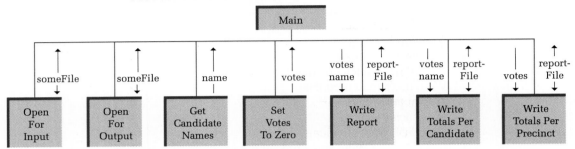

(The following program is written in ISO/ANSI standard C++. If you are working with pre–standard C++, see the alternate version of the program in the PRE_STD directory of the program disk, available at the publisher's Web site, www.jbpub.com/disks.)

```
//****************************************************************
// Election program
// This program reads votes represented by precinct number and
// ballot position from a data file, calculates the sums per
// precinct and per candidate, and writes all totals to an
// output file
//****************************************************************
#include <iostream>
#include <iomanip>     // For setw()
#include <fstream>     // For file I/O
#include <string>      // For string class

using namespace std;

const int NUM_PRECINCTS = 4;
const int NUM_CANDIDATES = 4;

typedef int VoteArray[NUM_PRECINCTS][NUM_CANDIDATES];
                            // 2-dimensional array type
                            //    for votes
```

PROBLEM-SOLVING CASE STUDY cont'd.

```cpp
void GetNames( string[] );
void OpenForInput( ifstream& );
void OpenForOutput( ofstream& );
void WritePerCandidate( const VoteArray, const string[],
                        ofstream& );
void WritePerPrecinct( const VoteArray, ofstream& );
void WriteReport( const VoteArray, const string[], ofstream& );
void ZeroVotes( VoteArray );

int main()
{
    string    name[NUM_CANDIDATES];  // Array of candidate names
    VoteArray votes;             // Totals for precincts vs. candidates
    int       candidate;         // Candidate number input from voteFile
    int       precinct;          // Precinct number input from voteFile
    ifstream  voteFile;          // Input file of precincts, candidates
    ofstream  reportFile;        // Output file receiving summaries

    OpenForInput(voteFile);
    if ( !voteFile )
        return 1;
    OpenForOutput(reportFile);
    if ( !reportFile )
        return 1;

    GetNames(name);
    ZeroVotes(votes);

    // Read and tally votes

    voteFile >> precinct >> candidate;
    while (voteFile)
    {
        votes[precinct-1][candidate-1]++;
        voteFile >> precinct >> candidate;
    }

    // Write results to report file

    WriteReport(votes, name, reportFile);
    WritePerCandidate(votes, name, reportFile);
    WritePerPrecinct(votes, reportFile);
```

```
        return 0;
}

//******************************************************************

void OpenForInput( /* inout */ ifstream& someFile )    // File to be
                                                        // opened
// Prompts the user for the name of an input file
// and attempts to open the file

{
        .
        .       (Same as in ConvertDates program of Chapter 8)
        .
}

//******************************************************************

void OpenForOutput( /* inout */ ofstream& someFile )   // File to be
                                                        // opened
// Prompts the user for the name of an output file
// and attempts to open the file

{
        .
        .       (Same as in ConvertDates program of Chapter 8)
        .
}

//******************************************************************

void GetNames( /* out */ string name[] )    // Array of candidate
                                            //    names
// Reads the candidate names from standard input

// Postcondition:
//      The user has been prompted to enter the candidate names
//   && name[0..NUM_CANDIDATES-1] contain the input names,
//      truncated to 10 characters each

{
    string inputStr;       // An input string
    int    candidate;      // Loop counter
```

PROBLEM-SOLVING CASE STUDY cont'd.

```
          cout << "Enter the names of the candidates, one per line,"
               << endl << "in the order they appear on the ballot."
               << endl;

          for (candidate = 0; candidate < NUM_CANDIDATES; candidate++)
          {
              cin >> inputStr;
              name[candidate] = inputStr.substr(0, 10);
          }
      }


//*****************************************************************

void ZeroVotes( /* out */ VoteArray votes )   // Array of vote totals

// Zeros out the votes array

// Postcondition:
//     All votes[0..NUM_PRECINCTS-1][0..NUM_CANDIDATES-1] == 0

{
    int precinct;       // Loop counter
    int candidate;      // Loop counter

    for (precinct = 0; precinct < NUM_PRECINCTS; precinct++)
        for (candidate = 0; candidate < NUM_CANDIDATES; candidate++)
            votes[precinct][candidate] = 0;
}


//*****************************************************************

void WriteReport(
        /* in */     const VoteArray votes,       // Total votes
        /* in */     const string    name[],      // Candidate names
        /* inout */      ofstream& reportFile )    // Output file

// Writes the vote totals in tabular form to the report file

// Precondition:
//     votes[0..NUM_PRECINCTS-1][0..NUM_CANDIDATES] are assigned
//   && name[0..NUM_CANDIDATES-1] are assigned
// Postcondition:
//     The name array has been output across one line, followed by
//     the votes array, one row per line
```

PROBLEM-SOLVING CASE STUDY cont'd.

```
{
    int precinct;        // Loop counter
    int candidate;       // Loop counter

    // Set up headings

    reportFile << "            ";
    for (candidate = 0; candidate < NUM_CANDIDATES; candidate++)
        reportFile << setw(12) << name[candidate];
    reportFile << endl;

    // Print array by row

    for (precinct = 0; precinct < NUM_PRECINCTS; precinct++)
    {
        reportFile << "Precinct" << setw(4) << precinct + 1;
        for (candidate = 0; candidate < NUM_CANDIDATES; candidate++)
            reportFile << setw(12) << votes[precinct][candidate];
        reportFile << endl;
    }
    reportFile << endl;
}


//*********************************************************************

void WritePerCandidate(
        /* in */      const VoteArray votes,          // Total votes
        /* in */      const string    name[],         // Candidate names
        /* inout */       ofstream& reportFile )      // Output file

// Sums the votes per person and writes the totals to the
// report file

// Precondition:
//     votes[0..NUM_PRECINCTS-1][0..NUM_CANDIDATES] are assigned
//   && name[0..NUM_CANDIDATES-1] are assigned
// Postcondition:
//     For each person i, name[i] has been output,
//     followed by the sum
//     votes[0][i] + votes[1][i] + ... + votes[NUM_PRECINCTS-1][i]
```

PROBLEM-SOLVING CASE STUDY *cont'd.*

```
    {
        int precinct;        // Loop counter
        int candidate;       // Loop counter
        int total;           // Total votes for a candidate

        for (candidate = 0; candidate < NUM_CANDIDATES; candidate++)
        {
            total = 0;

            // Compute column sum

            for (precinct = 0; precinct < NUM_PRECINCTS; precinct++)
                total = total + votes[precinct][candidate];

            reportFile << "Total votes for"
                        << setw(10) << name[candidate] << ":"
                        << setw(3) << total << endl;
        }
        reportFile << endl;
    }


    //*****************************************************************

    void WritePerPrecinct(
                /* in */     const VoteArray votes,      // Total votes
                /* inout */       ofstream& reportFile )  // Output file

    // Sums the votes per precinct and writes the totals to the
    // report file

    // Precondition:
    //      votes[0..NUM_PRECINCTS-1][0..NUM_CANDIDATES] are assigned
    // Postcondition:
    //      For each precinct i, the value i+1 has been output,
    //      followed by the sum
    //      votes[i][0] + votes[i][1] + ... + votes[i][NUM_CANDIDATES-1]

    {
        int precinct;        // Loop counter
        int candidate;       // Loop counter
        int total;           // Total votes for a precinct
```

PROBLEM-SOLVING CASE STUDY *cont'd.*

```
    for (precinct = 0; precinct < NUM_PRECINCTS; precinct++)
    {
        total = 0;

        // Compute row sum

        for (candidate = 0; candidate < NUM_CANDIDATES; candidate++)
            total = total + votes[precinct][candidate];

        reportFile << "Total votes for precinct"
                   << setw(3) << precinct + 1 << ':'
                   << setw(3) << total << endl;
    }
}
```

Testing: This program was executed with the data listed below. (We list the data in three columns to save space.) The names of the candidates entered from the keyboard were Smith, Jones, Adams, and Smiley. In this data set, there is at least one vote for each candidate in each precinct. Case Study Follow-Up Exercise 4 asks you to outline a complete testing strategy for this program.

Input Data

1 1	3 1	3 3
1 1	4 3	4 4
1 2	3 4	4 4
1 2	3 2	4 3
1 3	3 3	4 4
1 4	2 1	4 4
2 2	2 3	4 1
2 2	4 3	4 2
2 3	4 4	2 4
2 1	3 2	4 4

The output, which was written to file reportFile, is shown below.

		Jones	Smith	Adams	Smiley
Precinct	1	2	2	1	1
Precinct	2	2	2	2	1
Precinct	3	1	2	2	1
Precinct	4	1	1	3	6

```
Total votes for      Jones:   6
Total votes for      Smith:   7
Total votes for      Adams:   8
Total votes for     Smiley:   9

Total votes for precinct  1:   6
Total votes for precinct  2:   7
Total votes for precinct  3:   6
Total votes for precinct  4:  11
```

Testing and Debugging

One-Dimensional Arrays

The most common error in processing arrays is an out-of-bounds array index. That is, the program attempts to access a component using an index that is either less than 0 or greater than the array size minus 1. For example, given the declarations

```
char line[100];
int   counter;
```

the following For statement would print the 100 elements of the `line` array and then print a 101st value—the value that resides in memory immediately beyond the end of the array.

```
for (counter = 0; counter <= 100; counter++)
    cout << line[counter];
```

This error is easy to detect, because 101 characters get printed instead of 100. The loop test should be `counter < 100`. But you won't always use a simple For statement when accessing arrays. Suppose we read data into the `line` array in another part of the program. Let's use a While statement that reads to the newline character:

```
counter = 0;
cin.get(ch);
while (ch != '\n')
{
    line[counter] = ch;
    counter++;
    cin.get(ch);
}
```

This code seems reasonable enough, but what if the input line has more than 100 characters? After the hundredth character is read and stored into the array, the loop continues to execute with the array index out of bounds. Characters are stored into memory locations past the end of the array, wiping out other data values (or even machine language instructions in the program!).

The moral is: When processing arrays, give special attention to the design of loop termination conditions. Always ask yourself if the loop could possibly keep running after the last array component has been processed.

Whenever an array index goes out of bounds, the first suspicion should be a loop that fails to terminate properly. The second thing to check is any array access involving an index that is based on input data or a calculation. When an array index is input as data, a data validation check is an absolute necessity.

Complex Structures

As we have demonstrated in many examples in this chapter and the last, it is possible to combine data structures in various ways: structs whose components are structs, structs whose components are arrays, arrays whose components are structs or class objects, arrays whose components are arrays (multidimensional arrays), and so forth. When arrays, structs, and class objects are combined, there can be confusion about precisely where to place the operators for array element selection ([]) and struct or class member selection (.).

To summarize the correct placement of these operators, let's use the StudentRec type we introduced in this chapter:

```
struct StudentRec
{
    string     stuName;
    float      gpa;
    int        examScore[4];
    GradeType  courseGrade;
};
```

If we declare a variable of type StudentRec,

```
StudentRec student;
```

then what is the syntax for selecting the first exam score of the student (that is, for selecting element 0 of the examScore member of student)? The dot operator is a binary (two-operand) operator; its left operand denotes a struct variable, and its right operand is a member name:

StructVariable.MemberName

The `[]` operator is a unary (one-operand) operator; it comes immediately after an expression denoting an array:

Array **[**IndexExpression**]**

Therefore, the expression

`student`

denotes a struct variable, the expression

`student.examScore`

denotes an array, and the expression

`student.examScore[0]`

denotes an integer—the integer located in element 0 of the `student.examScore` array.

With arrays of structs or class objects, again you have to be sure that the `[]` and `.` operators are in the proper positions. Given the declaration

`StudentRec gradeBook[150];`

we can access the `gpa` member of the first element of the `gradeBook` array with the expression

`gradeBook[0].gpa`

The index `[0]` is correctly attached to the identifier `gradeBook` because `gradeBook` is the name of an array. Furthermore, the expression

`gradeBook[0]`

denotes a struct, so the dot operator selects the `gpa` member of this struct.

Multidimensional Arrays

Errors with multidimensional arrays usually fall into two major categories: index expressions that are out of order and index range errors.

Suppose we were to expand the Election program to accommodate ten candidates and four precincts. Let's declare the `votes` array as

```
int votes[4][10];
```

The first dimension represents the precincts, and the second represents the candidates. An example of the first kind of error—incorrect order of the index expressions—would be to print out the votes array as follows.

```
for (precinct = 0; precinct < 4; precinct++)
{
    for (candidate = 0; candidate < 10; candidate++)
        cout << setw(4) << votes[candidate][precinct];
    cout << endl;
}
```

The output statement specifies the array indexes in the wrong order. The loops march through the array with the first index ranging from 0 through 9 (instead of 0 through 3) and the second index ranging from 0 through 3 (instead of 0 through 9). The effect of executing this code may vary from system to system. The program may output the wrong array components and continue executing, or the program may crash with a memory access error.

An example of the second kind of error—an incorrect index range in an otherwise correct loop—can be seen in this code:

```
for (precinct = 0; precinct < 10; precinct++)
{
    for (candidate = 0; candidate < 4; candidate++)
        cout << setw(4) << votes[precinct][candidate];
    cout << endl;
}
```

Here, the output statement correctly uses precinct for the first index and candidate for the second. However, the For statements use incorrect upper limits for the index variables. As with the preceding example, the effect of executing this code is undefined but is certainly wrong. A valuable way to prevent this kind of error is to use named constants instead of the literals 10 and 4. In the case study, we used NUM_PRECINCTS and NUM_CANDIDATES. You are much more likely to spot an error (or to avoid making an error in the first place) if you write something like this:

```
for (precinct = 0; precinct < NUM_PRECINCTS; precinct++)
```

than if you use a literal constant as the upper limit for the index variable.

Testing and Debugging Hints

1. When an individual component of a one-dimensional array is accessed, the index must be within the range 0 through the array size minus 1. Attempting to use an index value outside this range causes your program to access memory locations outside the array.

2. The individual components of an array are themselves variables of the component type. When values are stored into an array, they should either be of the component type or be explicitly converted to the component type; otherwise, implicit type coercion occurs.

3. C++ does not allow aggregate operations on arrays. There is no aggregate assignment, aggregate comparison, aggregate I/O, or aggregate arithmetic. You must write code to do all of these operations, one array element at a time.

4. Omitting the size of a one-dimensional array in its declaration is permitted only in two cases: (1) when an array is declared as a parameter in a function heading and (2) when an array is initialized in its declaration. In all other declarations, you *must* specify the size of the array with a constant integer expression.

5. If an array parameter is incoming-only, declare the parameter as const to prevent the function from modifying the caller's argument accidentally.

6. Don't pass an individual array component as an argument when the function expects to receive the base address of an entire array.

7. The size of an array is fixed at compile time, but the number of values actually stored there is determined at run time. Therefore, an array must be declared to be as large as it could ever be for the particular problem. Subarray processing is used to process only the components that have data in them.

8. When functions perform subarray processing on a one-dimensional array, pass both the array name and the number of data items actually stored in the array.

9. With multidimensional arrays, use the proper number of indexes when referencing an array component, and make sure the indexes are in the correct order.

10. In loops that process multidimensional arrays, double-check the upper and lower bounds on each index variable to be sure they are correct for that dimension of the array.

11. When declaring a multidimensional array as a parameter, you must state the sizes of all but the first dimension. Also, these sizes must agree exactly with the sizes of the caller's argument.

12. To eliminate the chances of the size mismatches referred to in item 11, use a Typedef statement to define a multidimensional array type. Declare both the argument and the parameter to be of this type.

Summary

The one-dimensional array is a homogeneous data structure that gives a name to a sequential group of like components. Each component is accessed by its relative position within the group (rather than by name, as in a struct or class), and each component is a variable of the component type. To access a particular component, we give the name of the array and an index that specifies which component of the group we want. The index can be an expression of any integral type, as long as it evaluates to an integer from 0 through the array size minus 1. Array components can be accessed in random order directly, or they can be accessed sequentially by stepping through the index values one at a time.

Two-dimensional arrays are useful for processing information that is represented naturally in tabular form. Processing data in two-dimensional arrays usually takes one of two forms: processing by row or processing by column. An array of arrays, which is useful if rows of the array must be passed as arguments, is an alternative way of defining a two-dimensional array.

A multidimensional array is a collection of like components that are ordered on more than one dimension. Each component is accessed by a set of indexes, one for each dimension, that represents the component's position on the various dimensions. Each index may be thought of as describing a feature of a given array component.

Quick Check

1. Declare a one-dimensional array named quizAnswer that contains 12 components indexed by the integers 0 through 11. The component type is bool. (pp. 664–667)

2. Given the declarations

    ```
    const int SIZE = 30;

    char firstName[SIZE];
    ```

    a. Write an assignment statement that stores 'A' into the first component of array firstName. (pp. 667–669)
    b. Write an output statement that prints the value of the fourteenth component of array firstName. (pp. 667–669)
    c. Write a For statement that fills array firstName with blanks. (p. 670)

3. Declare a five-element one-dimensional int array named oddNums, and initialize it (in its declaration) to contain the first five odd integers, starting with 1. (p. 671)

4. Give the function heading for a void function named SomeFunc, where
   a. SomeFunc has a single parameter: a one-dimensional float array x that is an Inout parameter.
   b. SomeFunc has a single parameter: a one-dimensional float array x that is an In parameter.
   (pp. 676–678)

5. Given the declaration

   ```
   StudentRec gradeBook[150];
   ```

   where StudentRec is the struct type defined in this chapter, do the following.
   a. Write an assignment statement that records the fact that the tenth student has a grade point average of 3.25.
   b. Write an assignment statement that records the fact that the fourth student scored 78 on the third exam. (pp. 681–683)

6. Given the declarations in Question 2 and the following program fragment, which reads characters into array firstName until a blank is encountered, write a For statement that prints out the portion of the array that is filled with input data. (p. 684)

   ```
   n = 0;
   cin.get(letter);
   while (letter != ' ')
   {
       firstName[n] = letter;
       n++;
       cin.get(letter);
   }
   ```

7. Define an enumeration type for the musical notes A through G (excluding sharps and flats). Then declare a one-dimensional array in which the index values represent musical notes, and the component type is float. Finally, show an example of a For loop that prints out the contents of the array. (p. 684)

8. Declare a two-dimensional array, named plan, with 30 rows and 10 columns. The component type of the array is float. (p. 685–689)

9. a. Assign the value 27.3 to the component in row 13, column 7 of the array plan from Question 8. (pp. 685–689)
   b. Nested For loops can be used to sum the values in each row of array plan. What range of values would the outer For loop count through to do this? (pp. 690–691)
   c. Nested For loops can be used to sum the values in each column of array plan. What range of values would the outer For loop count through to do this? (pp. 691–692)
   d. Write a program fragment that initializes array plan to all zeros. (pp. 692–694)

e. Write a program fragment that prints the contents of array `plan`, one row per line of output. (pp. 694–695)

10. Suppose array `plan` is passed as an argument to a function in which the corresponding parameter is named `someArray`. What would the declaration of `someArray` look like in the parameter list? (pp. 695–697)

11. Given the declarations

```
typedef int OneDimType[100];

OneDimType twoDim[40];
```

rewrite the declaration of `twoDim` without referring to type `OneDimType`. (pp. 698–699)

12. Given the declarations

```
const int SIZE = 10;
typedef char FourDim[SIZE][SIZE][SIZE][SIZE-1];

FourDim quick;
```

a. How many components does array `quick` contain? (pp. 700–702)
b. Write a program fragment that fills array `quick` with blanks. (pp. 700–702)

Answers

1. `bool quizAnswer[12];`
2. a. `firstName[0] = 'A';`
   b. `cout << firstName[13];`
   c. `for (index = 0; index < SIZE; index++)`
      `    firstName[index] = ' ';`
3. `int oddNums[5] = {1, 3, 5, 7, 9};`
4. a. `void SomeFunc( float x[] )`
   b. `void SomeFunc( const float x[] )`
5. a. `gradeBook[9].gpa = 3.25;`
   b. `gradeBook[3].examScore[2] = 78;`
6. `for (index = 0; index < n; index++)`
   `    cout << firstName[index];`
7. `enum NoteType {A, B, C, D, E, F, G};`
   `float noteVal[7];`
   `NoteType index;`
   `for (index = A; index <= G; index = NoteType(index + 1))`
   `    cout << noteVal[index] << endl;`
8. `float plan[30][10];`
9. a. `plan[13][7] = 27.3;`
   b. `for (row = 0; row < 30; row++)`
   c. `for (col = 0; col < 10; col++)`
   d. `for (row = 0; row < 30; row++)`
      `    for (col = 0; col < 10; col++)`
      `        plan[row][col] = 0.0;`

```
e.  for (row = 0; row < 30; row++)
    {
        for (col = 0; col < 10; col++)
            cout << setw(8) << plan[row][col];
        cout << endl;
    }
```
10. Either
```
    float someArray[30][10]
```
or
```
    float someArray[][10]
```
11. `int twoDim[40][100];`
12. a. Nine thousand ($10 \times 10 \times 10 \times 9$)
    b.
```
    for (dim1 = 0; dim1 < SIZE; dim1++)
        for (dim2 = 0; dim2 < SIZE; dim2++)
            for (dim3 = 0; dim3 < SIZE; dim3++)
                for (dim4 = 0; dim4 < SIZE - 1; dim4++)
                    quick[dim1][dim2][dim3][dim4] = ' ';
```

Exam Preparation Exercises

1. Every component in an array must have the same type, and the number of components is fixed at compile time. (True or False?)
2. The components of an array must be of an integral or enumeration type. (True or False?)
3. Declare one-dimensional arrays according to the following descriptions.
   a. A 24-element `float` array
   b. A 500-element `int` array
   c. A 50-element double-precision floating-point array
   d. A 10-element `char` array
4. Write a code fragment to do the following tasks:
   a. Declare a constant named CLASS_SIZE representing the number of students in a class.
   b. Declare a one-dimensional array `quizAvg` of size CLASS_SIZE whose components will contain floating-point quiz score averages.
5. Write a code fragment to do the following tasks:
   a. Declare an enumeration type `BirdType` made up of bird names.
   b. Declare a one-dimensional `int` array `sightings` that is to be indexed by `BirdType`.
6. Given the declarations

```
const int SIZE = 100;

enum Colors
{
    BLUE, GREEN, GOLD, ORANGE, PURPLE, RED, WHITE, BLACK
};
```

```
int      count[8];
Colors cIndex;                      // Index for count array
Colors rainbow[SIZE];
int      rIndex;                    // Index for rainbow array
```

write code fragments to do the following tasks:

a. Set count to all zeros.

b. Set rainbow to all WHITE.

c. Count the number of times GREEN appears in rainbow.

d. Print the value in count indexed by BLUE.

e. Total the values in count.

7. What is the output of the following program? The data for the program is given below it.

```cpp
#include <iostream>

using namespace std;

int main()
{
    int a[100];
    int b[100];
    int j;
    int m;
    int sumA = 0;
    int sumB = 0;
    int sumDiff = 0;

    cin >> m;
    for (j = 0; j < m; j++)
    {
        cin >> a[j] >> b[j];
        sumA = sumA + a[j];
        sumB = sumB + b[j];
        sumDiff = sumDiff + (a[j] - b[j]);
    }
    for (j = m - 1; j >= 0; j--)
        cout << a[j] << ' ' << b[j] << ' '
             << a[j] - b[j] << endl;
    cout << endl;
    cout << sumA << ' ' << sumB << ' ' << sumDiff << endl;
    return 0;
}
```

Data

```
   5
11 15
19 14
 4  2
17  6
 1  3
```

8. A person wrote the following code fragment, intending to print 10 20 30 40.

```
int arr[4] = {10, 20, 30, 40};
int index;

for (index = 1; index <= 4; index++)
    cout << ' ' << arr[index];
```

Instead, the code printed 20 30 40 24835. Explain the reason for this output.

9. Given the declarations

```
int sample[8];
int i;
int k;
```

show the contents of the array sample after the following code segment is executed. Use a question mark to indicate any undefined values in the array.

```
for (k = 0; k < 8; k++)
    sample[k] = 10 - k;
```

10. Using the same declarations given for Exercise 9, show the contents of the array sample after the following code segment is executed.

```
for (i = 0; i < 8; i++)
    if (i <= 3)
        sample[i] = 1;
    else
        sample[i] = -1;
```

11. Using the same declarations given for Exercise 9, show the contents of the array sample after the following code segment is executed.

```
for (k = 0; k < 8; k++)
    if (k % 2 == 0)
        sample[k] = k;
    else
        sample[k] = k + 100;
```

12. What are the two basic differences between a record and an array?
13. If the members of a record are all the same data type, an array data structure could be used instead. (True or False?)
14. For each of the following descriptions of data, determine which general type of data structure (array, record, array of records, or hierarchical record) is appropriate.
    a. A payroll entry with a name, address, and pay rate.
    b. A person's address.
    c. An inventory entry for a part.
    d. A list of addresses.
    e. A list of hourly temperatures.
    f. A list of passengers on an airliner, including names, addresses, fare class, and seat assignment.
    g. A departmental telephone directory with last name and extension number.

15. Given the declarations

```
const int NUM_SCHOOLS = 10;
const int NUM_SPORTS = 3;
enum SportType {FOOTBALL, BASKETBALL, VOLLEYBALL};

int    kidsInSports[NUM_SCHOOLS][NUM_SPORTS];
float costOfSports[NUM_SPORTS][NUM_SCHOOLS];
```

answer the following questions:
a. What is the number of rows in kidsInSports?
b. What is the number of columns in kidsInSports?
c. What is the number of rows in costOfSports?
d. What is the number of columns in costOfSports?
e. How many components does kidsInSports have?
f. How many components does costOfSports have?
g. What kind of processing (row or column) would be needed to total the amount of money spent on each sport?
h. What kind of processing (row or column) would be needed to total the number of children participating in sports at a particular school?

16. Given the following code segments, draw the arrays and their contents after the code is executed. Indicate any undefined values with the letter *U.*
a.
```
int exampleA[4][3];
int i, j;

for (i = 0; i < 4; i++)
    for (j = 0; j < 3; j++)
        exampleA[i][j] = i * j;
```
b.
```
int exampleB[4][3];
int i, j;

for (i = 0; i < 3; i++)
    for (j = 0; j < 3; j++)
        exampleB[i][j] = (i + j) % 3;
```
c.
```
int exampleC[8][2];
int i, j;

exampleC[7][0] = 4;
exampleC[7][1] = 5;
for (i = 0; i < 7; i++)
{
    exampleC[i][0] = 2;
    exampleC[i][1] = 3;
}
```

17. a. Define enumeration types for the following:
TeamType made up of classes (freshman, sophomore, etc.) on your campus
ResultType made up of game results (won, lost, or tied)

b. Using Typedef, declare a two-dimensional integer array type named `Outcome`, intended to be indexed by `TeamType` and `ResultType`.

c. Declare an array variable `standings` to be of type `Outcome`.

d. Give a C++ statement that increases the number of freshman wins by 1.

18. The following code fragment includes a call to a function named `DoSomething`.

```
typedef float ArrType[100][20];

ArrType x;
    :
DoSomething(x);
```

Indicate whether each of the following would be valid or invalid as the function heading for `DoSomething`.

a. `void DoSomething( /* inout */ ArrType arr )`
b. `void DoSomething( /* inout */ float arr[100][20] )`
c. `void DoSomething( /* inout */ float arr[100][] )`
d. `void DoSomething( /* inout */ float arr[][20] )`
e. `void DoSomething( /* inout */ float arr[][] )`
f. `void DoSomething( /* inout */ float arr[][10] )`

19. Declare the two-dimensional array variables described below. Use proper style.

a. An array with five rows and six columns that contains Boolean values.

b. An array, indexed from 0 through 39 and 0 through 199, that contains `float` values.

c. A `char` array with rows indexed by a type

```
enum FruitType {LEMON, PEAR, APPLE, ORANGE};
```

and columns indexed by the integers 0 through 15.

20. A logging operation keeps records of 37 loggers' monthly production for purposes of analysis, using the following array structure:

```
const int NUM_LOGGERS = 37;

int logsCut[NUM_LOGGERS][12];   // Logs cut per logger per month
int monthlyHigh;
int monthlyTotal;
int yearlyTotal;
int high;
int month;
int bestMonth;
int logger;
int bestLogger;
```

a. The following statement assigns the January log total for logger number 7 to `monthlyTotal`. (True or False?)

```
monthlyTotal = logsCut[7][0];
```

b. The following statements compute the yearly total for logger number 11. (True or False?)

```
yearlyTotal = 0;
for (month = 0; month < NUM_LOGGERS; month++)
    yearlyTotal = yearlyTotal + logsCut[month][10];
```

c. The following statements find the best logger (most logs cut) in March. (True or False?)

```
monthlyHigh = 0;
for (logger = 0; logger < NUM_LOGGERS; logger++)
    if (logsCut[logger][2] > monthlyHigh)
    {
        bestLogger = logger;
        monthlyHigh = logsCut[logger][2];
    }
```

d. The following statements find the logger with the highest monthly production and the logger's best month. (True or False?)

```
high = -1;
for (month = 0; month < 12; month++)
    for (logger = 0; logger < NUM_LOGGERS; logger++)
        if (logsCut[logger][month] > high)
        {
            high = logsCut[logger][month];
            bestLogger = logger;
            bestMonth = month;
        }
```

21. Declare the float array variables described below. Use proper style.
    a. A three-dimensional array in which the first dimension is indexed from 0 through 9, the second dimension is indexed by an enumeration type representing the days of the week, and the third dimension is indexed from 0 through 20.
    b. A four-dimensional array in which the first two dimensions are indexed from 0 through 49, and the third and fourth are indexed by any valid ASCII character.

Programming Warm-up Exercises

Use the following declarations in Exercises 1–7. You may declare any other variables that you need.

```
const int NUM_STUDS = 100;   // Number of students

bool failing[NUM_STUDS];
bool passing[NUM_STUDS];
int  grade;
int  score[NUM_STUDS];
```

1. Write a C++ function that initializes all components of failing to false. The failing array is a parameter.

2. Write a C++ function that has `failing` and `score` as parameters. Set the components of `failing` to `true` wherever the corresponding value in `score` is less than 60.

3. Write a C++ function that has `passing` and `score` as parameters. Set the components of `passing` to `true` wherever the corresponding value in `score` is greater than or equal to 60.

4. Write a C++ value-returning function `PassTally` that takes `passing` as a parameter and reports how many components in `passing` are `true`.

5. Write a C++ value-returning function `Error` that takes `passing` and `failing` as parameters. `Error` returns `true` if any corresponding components in `passing` and `failing` are the same.

6. Write a C++ value-returning function that takes `grade` and `score` as parameters. The function reports how many values in `score` are greater than or equal to `grade`.

7. Write a C++ function that takes `score` as a parameter and reverses the order of the components in `score`; that is, `score[0]` goes into `score[NUM_STUDS-1]`, `score[1]` goes into `score[NUM_STUDS-2]`, and so on.

8. Write a program segment to read in a set of part numbers and associated unit costs. Use an array of structs with two members, `number` and `cost`, to represent each pair of input values. Assume the end-of-file condition terminates the input.

9. Below is the specification of a "safe array" class, which halts the program if an array index goes out of bounds. (Recall that C++ does not check for out-of-bounds indexes when you use built-in arrays.)

```
const int MAX_SIZE = 200;

class IntArray
{
public:
    int ValueAt( /* in */ int i ) const;
        // Precondition:
        //     i is assigned
        // Postcondition:
        //     IF i >= 0  &&  i < declared size of array
        //         Function value == value of array element
        //                           at index i
        //     ELSE
        //         Program has halted with error message

    void Store( /* in */ int val,
                /* in */ int i   );
        // Precondition:
        //     val and i are assigned
        // Postcondition:
        //     IF i >= 0  &&  i < declared size of array
        //         val is stored in array element i
        //     ELSE
        //         Program has halted with error message
```

```
            IntArray( /* in */ int arrSize );
               // Precondition:
               //     arrSize is assigned
               // Postcondition:
               //     IF arrSize >= 1  &&  arrSize <= MAX_SIZE
               //         Array created with all array elements == 0
               //     ELSE
               //         Program has halted with error message
        private:
            int arr[MAX_SIZE];
            int size;
        };
```

Implement each member function as it would appear in the implementation file. To halt the program, use the `exit` function supplied by the C++ standard library through the header file `cstdlib` (see Appendix C).

10. Write a C++ value-returning function that returns `true` if all the values in a certain subarray of a two-dimensional array are positive, and returns `false` otherwise. The array (of type `ArrayType`), the number of columns in the subarray, and the number of rows in the subarray should be passed as arguments.

11. Write a C++ function `Copy` that takes a two-dimensional `int` array `data`, defined to be `NUM_ROWS` by `NUM_COLS`, and copies the values into a second array `data2`, defined the same way. `data` and `data2` are of type `TwoDimType`. The constants `NUM_ROWS` and `NUM_COLS` may be accessed globally.

12. Write a C++ function that finds the largest value in a two-dimensional `float` array of 50 rows and 50 columns.

13. Using the declarations in Exam Preparation Exercise 15, write functions, in proper style, to do the following tasks. Only constants may be accessed globally.
    a. Determine which school spent the most money on football.
    b. Determine which sport the last school spent the most money on.
    c. Determine which school had the most students playing basketball.
    d. Determine in which sport the third school had the most students participating.
    e. Determine the total amount spent by all the schools on volleyball.
    f. Determine the total number of students who played any sport. (Assume that each student played only one sport.)
    g. Determine which school had the most students participating in sports.
    h. Determine which was the most popular sport in terms of money spent.
    i. Determine which was the most popular sport in terms of student participation.

14. Given the following declarations

```
const int NUM_DEPTS = 100;
const int NUM_STORES = 10;
const int NUM_MONTHS = 12;

typedef int SalesType[NUM_STORES][NUM_MONTHS][NUM_DEPTS];
```

write a C++ function to initialize an array of type SalesType to 0. The constants NUM_STORES, NUM_MONTHS, and NUM_DEPTS may be accessed globally. The array should be a parameter.

15. Sales figures are kept on items sold by store, by department, and by month. Write a C++ function to calculate and print the total number of items sold during the year by each department in each store. The data is stored in an array of type SalesType as defined in Programming Warm-up Exercise 14. The array containing the data should be a parameter. The constants NUM_STORES, NUM_MONTHS, and NUM_DEPTS may be accessed globally.

16. Write a C++ value-returning function that returns the sum of the elements in a specified row of a two-dimensional array. The array, the number of filled-in columns, and which row is to be totaled should be parameters.

Programming Problems

1. The local baseball team is computerizing its records. You are to write a program that computes batting averages. There are 20 players on the team, identified by the numbers 1 through 20. Their batting records are coded in a file as follows. Each line contains four numbers: the player's identification number and the number of hits, walks, and outs he or she made in a particular game. Here is a sample:

   3   2   1   1

   The example above indicates that during a game, player number 3 was at bat four times and made 2 hits, 1 walk, and 1 out. For each player there are several lines in the file. Each player's batting average is computed by adding the player's total number of hits and dividing by the total number of times at bat. A walk does not count as either a hit or a time at bat when the batting average is being calculated. Your program prints a table showing each player's identification number, batting average, and number of walks. (Be careful: The players' identification numbers are 1 through 20, but C++ array indexes start at 0.)

2 Write a program that calculates the mean and standard deviation of integers stored in a file. The output should be of type float and should be properly labeled and formatted to two decimal places. The formula for calculating the mean of a series of integers is to add all the numbers, then divide by the number of integers. Expressed in mathematical terms, the mean $\overline{X}$ of N numbers X_1, X_2, ... X_N is

$$\overline{X} = \frac{\sum_{i=1}^{N} X_i}{N}$$

To calculate the standard deviation of a series of integers, subtract the mean from each integer (you may get a negative number) and square the result, add all these squared differences, divide by the number of integers minus 1, then take the square root of the result. Expressed in mathematical terms, the standard deviation S is

$$S = \sqrt{\frac{\sum_{i=1}^{N} (X_i - \overline{X})^2}{N - 1}}$$

3. One of the local banks is gearing up for a big advertising campaign and would like to see how long its customers are waiting for service at drive-up windows. Several employees have been asked to keep accurate records for the 24-hour drive-up service. The collected information, which is read from a file, consists of the time the customer arrived in hours, minutes, and seconds; the time the customer actually was served; and the ID number of the teller. Write a program that does the following:
   a. Reads in the wait data.
   b. Computes the wait time in seconds.
   c. Calculates the mean, standard deviation (defined in Programming Problem 2), and range.
   d. Prints a single-page summary showing the values calculated in part c.

   Input
   The first data line contains a title.
   The remaining lines each contain a teller ID, an arrival time, and a service time. The times are broken up into integer hours, minutes, and seconds according to a 24-hour clock.

   Processing
   Calculate the mean and the standard deviation.
   Locate the shortest wait time and the longest wait time for any number of records up to 100.

   Output
   The input data (echo print).
   The title.
   The following values, all properly labeled: number of records, mean, standard deviation, and range (minimum and maximum).

4. Your history professor has so many students in her class that she has trouble determining how well the class does on exams. She has discovered that you are a computer whiz and has asked you to write a program to perform some simple statistical analyses on exam scores. Your program must work for any class size up to 100. Write and test a computer program that does the following:
   a. Reads the test grades from file inData.
   b. Calculates the class mean, standard deviation (defined in Programming Problem 2), and percentage of the test scores falling in the ranges <10, 10–19, 20–29, 30–39, ... , 80–89, and ≥90.
   c. Prints a summary showing the mean and the standard deviation, as well as a histogram showing the percentage distribution of test scores.

   Input
   The first data line contains the number of exams to be analyzed and a title for the report.
   The remaining lines have ten test scores on each line until the last line, and one to ten scores on the last. The scores are all integers.

   Output
   The input data as they are read.
   A report consisting of the title that was read from the data, the number of scores, the mean, the standard deviation (all clearly labeled), and the histogram.

5. The final exam in your psychology class consists of 30 multiple-choice questions. Your instructor says that if you write the program to grade the finals, you won't have to take the exam.

   Input

   The first data line contains the key to the exam. The correct answers are the first 30 characters; they are followed by an integer number that says how many students took the exam (call it n).

   The next n lines contain student answers in the first 30 character positions, followed by the student's name in the next 10 character positions.

   Output

   For each student—the student's name; followed by the number of correct answers; followed by *PASS* if the number correct is 60 percent or better, or *FAIL* otherwise.

6. Write an interactive program that plays tic-tac-toe. Represent the board as a 3×3 character array. Initialize the array to blanks and ask each player in turn to input a position. The first player's position is marked on the board with an *O,* and the second player's position is marked with an *X.* Continue the process until a player wins or the game is a draw. To win, a player must have three marks in a row, in a column, or on a diagonal. A draw occurs when the board is full and no one has won.

   Each player's position should be input as indexes into the tic-tac-toe board—that is, a row number, a space, and a column number. Make the program user-friendly.

   After each game, print out a diagram of the board showing the ending positions. Keep a count of the number of games each player has won and the number of draws. Before the beginning of each game, ask each player if he or she wishes to continue. If either player wishes to quit, print out the statistics and stop.

7. Photos taken in space by the Galileo spacecraft are sent back to earth as a stream of numbers. Each number represents a level of brightness. A large number represents a high brightness level, and a small number represents a low level. Your job is to take a matrix (a two-dimensional array) of the numbers and print it as a picture.

   One approach to generating a picture is to print a dark character (such as a $) when the brightness level is low, and to print a light character (such as a blank or a period) when the level is high. Unfortunately, errors in transmission sometimes occur. Thus, your program should first attempt to find and correct these errors. Assume a value is in error if it differs by more than 1 from each of its four neighboring values. Correct the erroneous value by giving it the average of its neighboring values, rounded to the nearest integer.

   Example:

   ```
         5          The 2 would be regarded as an error and would be given
      4  2  5       a corrected value of 5.
         5
   ```

   Note that values on the corners or boundaries of the matrix have to be processed differently than the values on the interior. Your program should print an image of the uncorrected picture and then an image of the corrected picture.

8. The following diagram represents an island surrounded by water (shaded area).

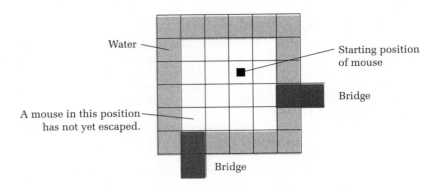

Two bridges lead out of the island. A mouse is placed on the black square. Write a program to make the mouse take a walk across the island. The mouse is allowed to travel one square at a time, either horizontally or vertically. A random number from 1 through 4 should be used to decide which direction the mouse is to take.* The mouse drowns when he hits the water; he escapes when he enters a bridge. You may generate a random number up to 100 times. If the mouse does not find his way by the hundredth try, he will die of starvation. Restart the mouse in a reinitialized array and go back and repeat the whole process. Count the number of times he escapes, drowns, and starves.

Input

First input line—the size of the array, including border of water and bridges (not larger than 20 × 20)

Next *N* input lines—the rows of the two-dimensional array, where the positions containing negative numbers represent the water, the positions in the edge containing a 0 represent the bridges, the position containing a 1 represents the starting position of the mouse, and all other positions contain 0s

Output

A line stating whether the mouse escaped, drowned, or starved

A line showing the mouse's starting position and the position of the two bridges

A map showing the frequency of the mouse's visits to each position

You should print the items above (double spaced between trips) for each trip by the mouse.

---

* Through the header file `cstdlib`, the C++ standard library supplies a value-returning, parameterless function named `rand`. Each time it is called, `rand` returns a random `int` in the range 0 through `RAND_MAX`, a constant defined in `cstdlib` (usually the same as `INT_MAX`). The following statement assigns to `randNum` a random integer in the range 1 through 4:

```
randNum = rand() % 4 + 1;
```

See Appendix C for further details.

9. In competitive diving, each diver makes three dives of varying degrees of difficulty. Nine judges score each dive from 0 through 10 in steps of 0.5. The total score is obtained by discarding the lowest and highest of the judges' scores, adding the remaining scores, and then multiplying the scores by the degree of difficulty. The divers take turns, and when the competition is finished, they are ranked according to score. Write a program to calculate the outcome of a competition, using the following input and output specifications.

Input

Number of divers

Diver's name (ten characters), difficulty (float), and judges' ratings (nine floats)

There is a line of data for each diver for each dive. All the data for Dive 1 are grouped together, then all for Dive 2, then all for Dive 3.

Output

The input data, echo printed in tabular form with appropriate headings—for example, Name, Difficulty, judge's number (1–9)

A table that contains the following information:

Name   Dive 1   Dive 2   Dive 3   Total

where Name is the diver's name; Dive 1, Dive 2, and Dive 3 are the total points received for a single dive, as described above; and Total is the overall total

Case Study Follow-Up

1. In the CheckLists program, the ReadFirstList function declares a parameter firstList. Would it be all right to prefix the declaration of firstList with the word const? Explain.
2. The CheckLists program compares two lists of integers. Exactly what changes would be necessary for the program to compare two lists of float values?
3. Modify the CheckLists program so that it works even if the lists are not the same length or they contain more than 500 values. Print appropriate error messages and stop the comparison.
4. Outline a testing strategy that fully tests the Election program.
5. The Election program is designed for 4 precincts and 4 candidates. Modify the program so that it works for 12 precincts and 3 candidates.

13

Array-Based Lists

Chapter 12 introduced the array, a data structure that is a collection of components of the same type given a single name. In general, a one-dimensional array is a structure used to hold a list of items. In this chapter, we examine algorithms that build and manipulate data stored as a list in a one-dimensional array. These algorithms are implemented as general-purpose functions that can be modified easily to work with many kinds of lists.

We also consider the *C string*, a special kind of built-in one-dimensional array that is used for storing character strings. We conclude with a case study that uses list algorithms developed in this chapter.

The List as an Abstract Data Type

As defined in Chapter 12, a one-dimensional array is a built-in data structure that consists of a fixed number of homogeneous components. One use for an array is to store a list of values. A list may contain fewer values than the number of places reserved in the array. In Chapter 12's Comparison of Two Lists case study, we used a variable numVals to keep track of the number of values currently stored in the array, and we employed subarray processing to prevent processing array components that were not part of the list of values. In Figure 12-16, you can see that the *array* goes from firstList[0] through firstList[499], but the *list* stored in the array goes from firstList[0] through firstList[numVals-1]. The number of places in the array is fixed, but the number of values in the list stored there may vary.

For a moment, let's think of the concept of a list not in terms of arrays but as a separate data type. We can define a **list** as a varying-length, linear collection of homogeneous components. That's quite a mouthful. By *linear* we mean that each component (except the first) has a unique component that comes before it and each component (except the last) has a unique component that comes after it. The **length** of a list—the number of values currently stored in the list—can vary during the execution of the program.

List   A variable-length, linear collection of homogeneous components.

Length   The number of values currently stored in a list.

Like any data type, a list must have associated with it a set of allowable operations. What kinds of operations would we want to define for a list? Here are some possibilities: create a list, add an item to a list, delete an item from a list, print a list, search a list for a particular value, sort a list into alphabetical or numerical order, and so on. When we define a data type formally—by specifying its properties and the operations that preserve those properties—we are creating an abstract data type (ADT). In fact, in Chapter 11 we proposed an ADT named IntList, a data type for a list of up to 100 integer values. At the time, we did not implement this ADT because we did not have at our disposal a suitable concrete data representation. Now that we are familiar with the idea of using a one-dimensional array to represent a list, we can combine C++ classes and arrays to implement list ADTs.

Let's generalize the IntList ADT by (a) allowing the components to be of *any* simple type or of type `string`, (b) replacing the maximum length of 100 with a maximum of MAX_LENGTH, a defined constant, and (c) including a wider variety of allowable operations. Here is the specification of the more general ADT:

TYPE
  List
DOMAIN
  Each instance of type List is a collection of up to MAX_LENGTH components, each of type ItemType.
OPERATIONS
  Create an initially empty list.
  Report whether the list is empty (`true` or `false`).
  Report whether the list is full (`true` or `false`).
  Return the current length of the list.
  Insert an item into the list.
  Delete an item from the list.
  Search for a specified item, returning `true` or `false` according to
    whether the item is present in the list.
  Sort the list into ascending order.
  Print the list.

We can use a C++ class named `List` to represent the List ADT in our programs. For the concrete data representation, we use two items: a one-dimensional array to hold the list items, and an `int` variable that stores the current length of the list. When we compile the `List` class, we need to supply definitions for MAX_LENGTH and `ItemType`:

```
const int MAX_LENGTH = [        ] ;    // Maximum possible number of
                                       //    components needed
typedef [        ] ItemType;           // Type of each component
                                       //    (a simple type or the
                                       //    string class)
```

Here is the specification file for our List ADT. Notice that we use 50 for MAX_LENGTH and `int` for `ItemType`. Notice also that the abstract operation

Create an initially empty list is implemented as the class constructor
List().

```
//*****************************************************************
// SPECIFICATION FILE (list.h)
// This file gives the specification of a list abstract data type.
// The list components are not assumed to be in order by value
//*****************************************************************

const int MAX_LENGTH = 50;      // Maximum possible number of
                                //    components needed
typedef int ItemType;           // Type of each component
                                //    (a simple type or string class)


class List
{
public:
    bool IsEmpty() const;
        // Postcondition:
        //      Function value == true, if list is empty
        //                     == false, otherwise

    bool IsFull() const;
        // Postcondition:
        //      Function value == true, if list is full
        //                     == false, otherwise

    int Length() const;
        // Postcondition:
        //      Function value == length of list

    void Insert( /* in */ ItemType item );
        // Precondition:
        //      NOT IsFull()
        //   && item is assigned
        // Postcondition:
        //      item is in list
        //   && Length() == Length()@entry + 1

    void Delete( /* in */ ItemType item );
        // Precondition:
        //      NOT IsEmpty()
        //   && item is assigned
        // Postcondition:
        //      IF item is in list at entry
        //          First occurrence of item is no longer in list
        //       && Length() == Length()@entry - 1
        //      ELSE
        //          List is unchanged
```

```
      bool IsPresent( /* in */ ItemType item ) const;
          // Precondition:
          //     item is assigned
          // Postcondition:
          //     Function value == true, if item is in list
          //                    == false, otherwise

      void SelSort();
          // Postcondition:
          //     List components are in ascending order of value

      void Print() const;
          // Postcondition:
          //     All components (if any) in list have been output

      List();
          // Constructor
          // Postcondition:
          //     Empty list is created
  private:
      int       length;
      ItemType data[MAX_LENGTH];
  };
```

In Chapter 11, we classified ADT operations as constructors, transformers, observers, and iterators. `IsEmpty`, `IsFull`, `Length`, `IsPresent`, and `Print` are observers. `Insert`, `Delete`, and `SelSort` are transformers. The class constructor is an ADT constructor operation.

The private part of the class declaration shows our data representation of a list: an `int` variable and an array (see Figure 13-1). However, notice that the preconditions and postconditions of the member functions mention nothing about an array. The abstraction is a list, not an array. The user of the class is interested only in manipulating lists of items and does not care how we implement a list. If we change to a different data representation (as we do in Chapter 15), neither the public interface nor the client code needs to be changed.

We now consider how to implement each of the ADT operations, given that the list items are stored in an array. Before we do so, however, we must distinguish between lists whose components must always be kept in alphabetical or numerical order (*sorted lists*) and lists in which the components are not arranged in any particular order (*unsorted lists*). We begin with unsorted lists.

FIGURE 13-1

myList, a Class
Object of
Type List

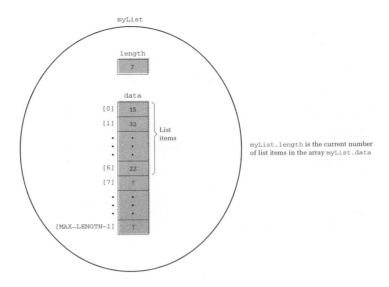

myList.length is the current number
of list items in the array myList.data

Unsorted Lists

Basic Operations

As we discussed in Chapter 11, an ADT is typically implemented in C++ by using a pair of files: the specification file (such as the preceding list.h file) and the implementation file, which contains the implementations of the class member functions. Here is how the implementation file list.cpp starts out:

```
//********************************************************************
// IMPLEMENTATION FILE (list.cpp)
// This file implements the List class member functions
// List representation: a one-dimensional array and a length
//                      variable
//********************************************************************
#include "list.h"
#include <iostream>

using namespace std;

// Private members of class:
//     int      length;          Length of the list
//     ItemType data[MAX_LENGTH];    Array holding the list
```

Let's look now at the implementations of the basic list operations.

Creating an Empty List   As Figure 13-1 shows, the list exists in the array elements data[0] through data[length-1]. To create an empty list, it is sufficient to set the length member to 0. We do not need to store any special values into the `data` array to make the list empty, because only those values in `data[0]` through `data[length-1]` are processed by the list algorithms.

In the `List` class, the appropriate place to initialize the list to be empty is the class constructor:

```
List::List()

// Constructor

// Postcondition:
//       length == 0

{
    length = 0;
}
```

One thing you will notice as we go through the `List` member functions is that the *implementation assertions* (the preconditions and postconditions appearing in the implementation file) are often stated differently from the *abstract assertions* (those located in the specification file). Abstract assertions are written in terms that are meaningful to the user of the ADT; implementation details should not be mentioned. In contrast, implementation assertions can be made more precise by referring directly to variables and algorithms in the implementation code. In the case of the `List` class constructor, the abstract postcondition is simply that an empty list has been created. On the other hand, the implementation postcondition

```
// Postcondition:
//       length == 0
```

is phrased in terms of our private data representation.

The IsEmpty Operation   This operation returns `true` if the list is empty and `false` if the list is not empty. Using our convention that `length` equals 0 if the list is empty, the implementation of this operation is straightforward.

```
bool List::IsEmpty() const

// Reports whether list is empty

// Postcondition:
//       Function value == true, if length == 0
//                      == false, otherwise

{
    return (length == 0);
}
```

The IsFull Operation   The list is full if there is no more room in the array holding the list items—that is, if the list length equals MAX_LENGTH.

```
bool List::IsFull() const

// Reports whether list is full

// Postcondition:
//     Function value == true, if length == MAX_LENGTH
//                    == false, otherwise

{
    return (length == MAX_LENGTH);
}
```

The Length Operation   This operation simply returns to the client the current length of the list.

```
int List::Length() const

// Returns current length of list

// Postcondition:
//     Function value == length

{
    return length;
}
```

The Print Operation   To output the components of the list, we can simply use a For loop that steps through the data array, printing each array element in sequence.

```
void List::Print() const

// Prints the list

// Postcondition:
//     Contents of data[0..length-1] have been output

{
    int index;     // Loop control and index variable

    for (index = 0; index < length; index++)
        cout << data[index] << endl;
}
```

Insertion and Deletion

To devise an algorithm for inserting a new item into the list, we first observe that we are working with an unsorted list and that the values do not have to be maintained in any particular order. Therefore, we can store a new value into the next available position in the array—data[length]—and then increment length. This algorithm brings up a question: Do we need to check that there is room in the list for the new item? We have two choices. The Insert function can test length against MAX_LENGTH and return an error flag if there isn't any room, or we can let the client code make the test before calling Insert (that is, make it a precondition that the list is not full). If you look back at the List class declaration in list.h, you can see that we have chosen the second approach. The client can use the IsFull operation to make sure the precondition is true. If the client fails to satisfy the precondition, the contract between client and function is broken, and the function is not required to satisfy the postcondition.

```
void List::Insert( /* in */ ItemType item )

// Inserts item into the list

// Precondition:
//      length < MAX_LENGTH
//   && item is assigned
// Postcondition:
//      data[length@entry] == item
//   && length == length@entry + 1

{
    data[length] = item;
    length++;
}
```

Deleting a component from a list consists of two parts: finding the component and removing it from the list. Before we can write the algorithm, we must know what to do if the component is not there. *Delete* can mean "Delete, if it's there" or "Delete, it *is* there." According to the List class declaration in list.h, we assume the first meaning; the code for the first definition works for the second as well but is not as efficient. We must start at the beginning of the list and search for the value to be deleted. If we find it, how do we remove it? We take the last value in the list (the one stored in data[length-1]), put it where the item to be deleted is located, and then decrement length. Moving the last item from its original position is appropriate only for an unsorted list because we don't need to preserve the order of the items in the list.

The definition "Delete, if it's there" requires a searching loop with a compound condition. We examine each component in turn and stop looking when we find the item to be deleted or when we have looked at all the items and know that it is not there.

```
void List::Delete( /* in */ ItemType item )

// Deletes item from the list, if it is there

// Precondition:
//     length > 0
//  && item is assigned
// Postcondition:
//     IF item is in data array at entry
//           First occurrence of item is no longer in array
//        && length == length@entry - 1
//     ELSE
//        length and data array are unchanged

{
    int index = 0;     // Index variable

    while (index < length && item != data[index])
        index++;

    if (index < length)
    {                                       // Remove item
        data[index] = data[length-1];
        length--;
    }
}
```

To see how the While loop and the subsequent If statement work, let's look at the two possibilities: Either item is in the list or it is not. If item is in the list, the loop terminates when the expression index < length is true and the expression item != data[index] is false. After the loop exit, the If statement finds the expression index < length to be true and removes the item. On the other hand, if item is not in the list, the loop terminates when the expression index < length is false—that is, when index becomes equal to length. Subsequently, the If condition is false, and the function returns without changing anything.

Sequential Search

In the Delete function, the algorithm we used to search for the item to be deleted is known as a *sequential* or *linear search* in an unsorted list. We use the same algorithm to implement the `IsPresent` function of the `List` class.

```
bool List::IsPresent( /* in */ ItemType item ) const

// Searches the list for item, reporting whether it was found

// Precondition:
//      item is assigned
// Postcondition:
//      Function value == true, if item is in data[0..length-1]
//                     == false, otherwise

{
    int index = 0;     // Index variable

    while (index < length && item != data[index])
        index++;

    return (index < length);
}
```

This algorithm is called a sequential search because we start at the beginning of the list and look at each item in sequence. We stop the search as soon as we find the item we are looking for (or when we reach the end of the list, concluding that the desired item is not present in the list).

We can use this algorithm in any program requiring a list search. In the form shown, it searches a list of `ItemType` components, provided that `ItemType` is an integral type or the `string` class. To use the function with a list of floating-point values, we must modify it so that the While statement tests for near equality rather than exact equality (for the reasons discussed in Chapter 10). In the following statement, we assume that `EPSILON` is defined as a global constant.

```
while (index < length && fabs(item - data[index]) >= EPSILON)
    index++;
```

The sequential search algorithm finds the first occurrence of the searched-for item. How would we modify it to find the last occurrence? We would initialize `index` to `length–1` and decrement `index` each time through the loop, stopping when we found the item we wanted or when `index` became `–1`.

Before we leave this search algorithm, let's introduce a variation that makes the program more efficient, although a little more complex. The While loop contains a compound condition: It stops when it either finds `item` or reaches the end of the list. We can insert a copy of `item` into `data[length]`—that is, into the array component beyond the end of the list—as a sentinel. By doing so, we are guaranteed to find `item` in the list.

FIGURE 13-2
Sequential Search
with Copy of item
in data[length]

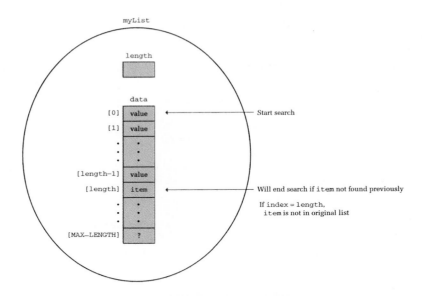

Then we can eliminate the condition that checks for the end of the list (index < length) (see Figure 13-2). Eliminating a condition saves the computer the time that would be required to test it. In this case, we save time during every iteration of the loop, so the savings add up quickly. Note, however, that we are gaining efficiency at the expense of space. We must declare the array size to be 1 larger than MAX_LENGTH to hold the sentinel value if the list becomes full. That is, we must change the private part of the class declaration as follows:

```
class List
{
    :
private:
    int       length;
    ItemType data[MAX_LENGTH+1];
};
```

Figure 13-2 reflects this change. The last array element shows an index of MAX_LENGTH rather than MAX_LENGTH−1, as in Figure 13-1.

The following function, IsPresent2, implements this new algorithm. After the search loop terminates, the function returns true if index is less than length; otherwise, it returns false.

```
bool List::IsPresent2( /* in */ ItemType item ) const

// Searches the list for item, reporting whether it was found

// Precondition:
//      item is assigned
```

```
// Postcondition:
//     data[0..length-1] are the same as at entry
//  && data[length] is overwritten to aid in the search
//  && Function value == true, if item is in data[0..length-1]
//                    == false, otherwise

{
    int index = 0;      // Index variable

    data[length] = item;           // Store item at position beyond
                                   //   end of list
    while (item != data[index])
        index++;

    return (index < length);
}
```

Note that the declaration of our `List` class in the file `list.h` includes the member function `IsPresent` but not `IsPresent2`. We have presented `IsPresent2` only to show you an alternative approach to implementing the search operation.

Sorting

Although we are implementing an unsorted list ADT, there are times when the user of the `List` class may want to rearrange the list components into a certain order just before calling the `Print` function. For example, the user might want to put a list of stock numbers into either ascending or descending order, or the user might want to put a list of words into alphabetical order. In software development, arranging list items into order is a very common operation and is known as **sorting.**

Sorting   Arranging the components of a list into order (for instance, words into alphabetical order or numbers into ascending or descending order).

If you were given a sheet of paper with a column of 20 numbers on it and were asked to write the numbers in ascending order, you would probably do the following:

1. Make a pass through the list, looking for the smallest number.
2. Write it on the paper in a second column.
3. Cross the number off the original list.
4. Repeat the process, always looking for the smallest number remaining in the original list.
5. Stop when all the numbers have been crossed off.

We can implement this algorithm directly in C++, but we need two arrays—one for the original list and a second for the sorted list. If the list is large, we might not have enough memory for two copies of it. Also, how do we "cross off" an array component? We could simulate crossing off a value by replacing it with some dummy value like INT_MAX. That is, we would set the value of the crossed-off variable to something that would not interfere with the processing of the rest of the components. However, a slight variation of our hand-done algorithm allows us to sort the components *in place*. We do not have to use a second array; we can put a value into its proper place in the list by having it swap places with the component currently in that position.

We can state the algorithm as follows. We search for the smallest value in the list and exchange it with the component in the first position in the list. We search for the next-smallest value in the list and exchange it with the component in the second position in the list. This process continues until all the components are in their proper places.

```
FOR count going from 0 through length-2
    Find minimum value in data[count . . length-1]
    Swap minimum value with data[count]
```

Figure 13-3 illustrates how this algorithm works.

Observe that we perform length-1 passes through the list because count runs from 0 through length-2. The loop does not need to be executed when count equals length-1 because the last value, data[length-1], is in its proper place after the preceding components have been sorted.

This sort, known as the *straight selection sort,* belongs to a class of sorts called selection sorts. There are many types of sorting algorithms. Selection sorts are characterized by finding the smallest (or largest) value left in the unsorted portion at each iteration and swapping it with the value indexed by the iteration counter. Swapping the contents of two variables requires a temporary variable so that no values are lost (see Figure 13-4).

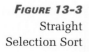

FIGURE 13-3
Straight
Selection Sort

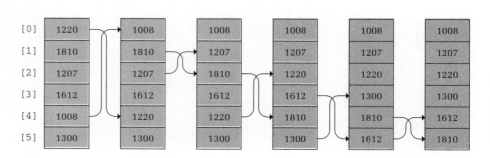

FIGURE 13-4
Swapping the
Contents of Two
Variables, x and y

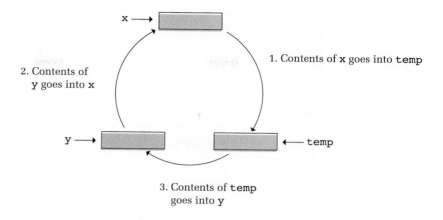

1. Contents of **x** goes into **temp**

2. Contents of
   y goes into **x**

3. Contents of **temp**
   goes into **y**

Here is the code for the sorting operation of the List class:

```
void List::SelSort()

// Sorts list into ascending order

// Postcondition:
//      data array contains the same values as data@entry, rearranged
//      into ascending order

{
    ItemType  temp;          // Temporary variable
    int       passCount;     // Loop control variable
    int       searchIndx;    // Loop control variable
    int       minIndx;       // Index of minimum so far

    for (passCount = 0; passCount < length - 1; passCount++)
    {
        minIndx = passCount;

        // Find the index of the smallest component
        // in data[passCount..length-1]

        for (searchIndx = passCount + 1; searchIndx < length;
                                              searchIndx++)
            if (data[searchIndx] < data[minIndx])
                minIndx = searchIndx;

        // Swap data[minIndx] and data[passCount]

        temp = data[minIndx];
        data[minIndx] = data[passCount];
        data[passCount] = temp;
    }
}
```

Note that with each pass through the outer loop, we are looking for the minimum value in the rest of the list (`data[passCount]` through `data[length-1]`). Therefore, `minIndx` is initialized to `passCount` and the inner loop runs from `searchIndx` equal to `passCount+1` through `length–1`. Upon exit from the inner loop, `minIndx` contains the position of the smallest value. (Note that the If statement is the only statement in the loop.)

Note also that we may swap a component with itself, which occurs if no value in the remaining list is smaller than `data[passCount]`. We could avoid this unnecessary swap by checking to see if `minIndx` is equal to `passCount`. Because this comparison would be made during each iteration of the outer loop, it is more efficient not to check for this possibility and just to swap something with itself occasionally. If the components we are sorting are much more complex than simple numbers, we might reconsider this decision.

This algorithm sorts the components into ascending order. To sort them into descending order, we would scan for the maximum value instead of the minimum value. To do so, we would simply change the relational operator in the inner loop from < to >. Of course, `minIndx` would no longer be an appropriate identifier and should be changed to `maxIndx`.

By providing the user of the `List` class with a sorting operation, we have not turned our unsorted list ADT into a sorted list ADT. The `Insert` and `Delete` algorithms we wrote do not preserve ordering by value. `Insert` places a new item at the end of the list, regardless of its value, and `Delete` moves the last item to a different position in the list. After `SelSort` has executed, the list items remain in sorted order only until the next insertion or deletion takes place. We now look at a sorted list ADT in which all the list operations cooperate to preserve the sorted order of the list components.

Sorted Lists

In the `List` class, the `IsPresent` and `IsPresent2` algorithms both assume that the list to be searched is unsorted. A drawback to searching an unsorted list is that we must scan the entire list to discover that the search item is not there. Think what it would be like if your city telephone book contained people's names in random rather than alphabetical order. To look up Mary Anthony's phone number, you would have to start with the first name in the phone book and scan sequentially, page after page, until you found it. In the worst case, you might have to examine tens of thousands of names only to find out that Mary's name is not in the book.

Of course, telephone books *are* alphabetized, and the alphabetical ordering makes searching easier. If Mary Anthony's name is not in the book, you discover this fact quickly by starting with the A's and stopping the search as soon as you have passed the place where her name should be.

Let's define a sorted list ADT in which the components always remain in order by value, no matter what operations are applied. Below is the slist.h file that contains the declaration of a SortedList class.

```
//******************************************************************
// SPECIFICATION FILE (slist.h)
// This file gives the specification of a sorted list abstract data
// type.  The list components are maintained in ascending order
// of value
//******************************************************************

const int MAX_LENGTH = 50;        // Maximum possible number of
                                  //   components needed
                                  // Requirement:
                                  //   MAX_LENGTH <= INT_MAX/2
typedef int ItemType;             // Type of each component
                                  //   (a simple type or string class)

class SortedList
{
public:
    bool IsEmpty() const;
        // Postcondition:
        //     Function value == true, if list is empty
        //                    == false, otherwise

    bool IsFull() const;
        // Postcondition:
        //     Function value == true, if list is full
        //                    == false, otherwise

    int Length() const;
        // Postcondition:
        //     Function value == length of list

    void Insert( /* in */ ItemType item );
        // Precondition:
        //     NOT IsFull()
        //  && item is assigned
        // Postcondition:
        //     item is in list
        //  && Length() == Length()@entry + 1
        //  && List components are in ascending order of value

    void Delete( /* in */ ItemType item );
        // Precondition:
        //     NOT IsEmpty()
```

```
    //   && item is assigned
    // Postcondition:
    //      IF item is in list at entry
    //          First occurrence of item is no longer in list
    //          && Length() == Length()@entry - 1
    //             && List components are in ascending order of value
    //      ELSE
    //             List is unchanged

bool IsPresent( /* in */ ItemType item ) const;
    // Precondition:
    //      item is assigned
    // Postcondition:
    //      Function value == true, if item is in list
    //                     == false, otherwise

void Print() const;
    // Postcondition:
    //      All components (if any) in list have been output

SortedList();
    // Constructor
    // Postcondition:
    //      Empty list is created
private:
    int       length;
    ItemType  data[MAX_LENGTH];
    void      BinSearch( ItemType, bool&, int& ) const;
};
```

How does the declaration of SortedList differ from the declaration of our original List class? Apart from a few changes in the documentation comments, there are only two differences:

1. The SortedList class does not supply a sorting operation to the client. Such an operation is needless, because the list components are assumed to be kept in sorted order at all times.
2. The SortedList class has an additional class member in the private part: a BinSearch function. This function is an auxiliary ("helper") function that is used only by other class member functions and is inaccessible to clients. We discuss its purpose when we examine the class implementation.

Let's look at what changes, if any, are required in the algorithms for the ADT operations, given that we are now working with a sorted list instead of an unsorted list.

Basic Operations

The algorithms for the class constructor, `IsEmpty`, `IsFull`, `Length`, and `Print` are identical to those in the `List` class. The constructor sets the private data member `length` to 0, `IsEmpty` reports whether `length` equals 0, `IsFull` reports whether `length` equals `MAX_LENGTH`, `Length` returns the value of `length`, and `Print` outputs the list items from first to last.

Insertion

To add a new value to an already sorted list, we could store the new value at `data[length]`, increment `length`, and sort the array again. However, such a solution is *not* an efficient way of solving the problem. Inserting five new items results in five separate sorting operations.

If we were to insert a value by hand into a sorted list, we would write the new value out to the side and draw a line showing where it belongs. To find this position, we start at the top and scan the list until we find a value greater than the one we are inserting. The new value goes in the list just before that point.

We can use a similar process in our `Insert` function. We find the proper place in the list using the by-hand algorithm. Instead of writing the value to the side, we shift all the values larger than the new one down one place to make room for it. The main algorithm is expressed as follows, where `item` is the value being inserted.

```
WHILE place not found AND more places to look
    IF item > current component in list
            Increment current position
    ELSE
            Place found
Shift remainder of list down
Insert item
Increment length
```

Assuming that `index` is the place where `item` is to be inserted, the algorithm for Shift List Down is

```
Set data[length]      =      data[length–1]
Set data[length–1]    =      data[length–2]
     ⋮                              ⋮
Set data[index+1]     =      data[index]
```

This algorithm is illustrated in Figure 13-5.

FIGURE 13-5

Inserting into a
Sorted List

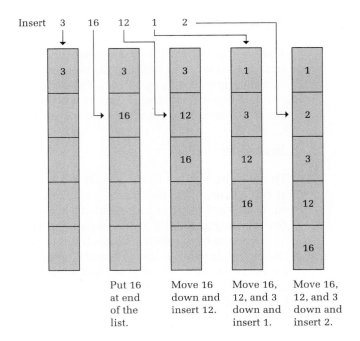

This algorithm is based on how we would accomplish the task by hand. Often, such an adaptation is the best way to solve a problem. However, in this case, further thought reveals a slightly better way. Notice that we search from the front of the list (people always do), and we shift down from the end of the list upward. We can combine the searching and shifting by beginning at the *end* of the list.

If `item` is the new item to be inserted, compare `item` to the value in `data[length-1]`. If `item` is *less*, put `data[length-1]` into `data[length]` and compare `item` to the value in `data[length-2]`. This process continues until you find the place where `item` is greater than or equal to the item in the list. Store `item` directly below it. Here is the algorithm:

```
Set index = length - 1
WHILE index ≥ 0 AND item < data[index]
    Set data[index + 1] = data[index]
    Decrement index
Set data[index + 1] = item
Increment length
```

What about duplicates? The algorithm continues until an item is found that is less than the one we are inserting. Therefore, the new item is inserted below a duplicate value (if one is there). Here is the code:

```
void SortedList::Insert( /* in */ ItemType item )

// Inserts item into the list

// Precondition:
//      length < MAX_LENGTH
//   && data[0..length-1] are in ascending order
//   && item is assigned
// Postcondition:
//      item is in the list
//   && length == length@entry + 1
//   && data[0..length-1] are in ascending order

{
    int index;      // Index and loop control variable

    index = length - 1;
    while (index >= 0 && item < data[index])
    {
        data[index+1] = data[index];
        index--;
    }
    data[index+1] = item;           // Insert item
    length++;
}
```

Notice that this algorithm works even if the list is empty. When the list is empty, `length` is 0 and the body of the While loop is not entered. So `item` is stored into `data[0]`, and `length` is incremented to 1. Does the algorithm work if `item` is the smallest? The largest? Let's see. If `item` is the smallest, the loop body is executed `length` times, and `index` is −1. Thus, `item` is stored into position 0, where it belongs. If `item` is the largest, the loop body is not entered. The value of `index` is still `length` − 1, so `item` is stored into `data[length]`, where it belongs.

Are you surprised that the general case also takes care of the special cases? This situation does not happen all the time, but it occurs often enough that it is good programming practice to start with the general case. If we begin with the special cases, we usually generate a correct solution, but we may not realize that we don't need to handle the special cases separately. So begin with the general case, then treat as special cases only those situations that the general case does not handle correctly.

This algorithm is the basis for another general-purpose sorting algorithm—an *insertion sort*. In an insertion sort, values are inserted one at a time into a list that was originally empty. An insertion sort is often used when input data must be sorted; each value is put into its proper place as it is read. We use this technique in the Problem-Solving Case Study at the end of this chapter.

Sequential Search

When we search for an item in an unsorted list, we won't discover that the item is missing until we reach the end of the list. If the list is already sorted, we know that an item is missing when we pass the place where it should be in the list. For example, if a list contains the values

```
  7
 11
 13
 76
 98
102
```

and we are looking for 12, we need only compare 12 with 7, 11, and 13 to know that 12 is not in the list.

If the search item is greater than the current list component, we move on to the next component. If the item is equal to the current component, we have found what we are looking for. If the item is less than the current component, then we know that it is not in the list. In either of the last two cases, we stop looking. We can restate this algorithmically with the following code, in which `found` is set to `true` if the search item was found.

```
// Sequential search in a sorted list

index = 0;
while (index < length && item > data[index])
    index++;

found = (index < length && item == data[index]);
```

On average, searching a sorted list in this way takes the same number of iterations to find an item as searching an unsorted list. The advantage of this new algorithm is that we find out sooner if an item is missing. Thus, it is slightly more efficient; however, it works only on a sorted list.

We do not use this algorithm to implement the `SortedList::IsPresent` function. There is a better algorithm, which we look at next.

Binary Search

There is a second search algorithm on a sorted list that is considerably faster both for finding an item and for discovering that an item is missing. This algorithm is called a *binary search*. A binary search is based on the principle of successive approximation. The algorithm divides the list in half (divides by 2—that's why it's called *binary* search) and decides which half to look in next. Division of the selected portion of the list is repeated until the item is found or it is determined that the item is not in the list.

This method is analogous to the way in which we look up a word in a dictionary. We open the dictionary in the middle and compare the word with one on the page that we turned to. If the word we're looking for comes before this word, we continue our search in the left-hand section of the dictionary. Otherwise, we continue in the right-hand section of the dictionary. We repeat this process until we find the word. If it is not there, we realize that either we have misspelled the word or our dictionary isn't complete.

The algorithm for a binary search is given below. The list of values is in the array data, and the value being looked for is item (see Figure 13-6).

1. Compare item to data[middle]. If item = data[middle], then we have found it. If item < data[middle], then look in the first half of data. If item > data[middle], then look in the second half of data.
2. Redefine data to be the half of data that we search next, and repeat step 1.
3. Stop when we have found item or know it is missing. We know it's missing when there is nowhere else to look and we still have not found it.

This algorithm should make sense. With each comparison, at best, we find the item for which we are searching; at worst, we eliminate half of the remaining list from consideration.

We need to keep track of the first possible place to look (first) and the last possible place to look (last). At any one time, we are looking only

FIGURE 13-6
Binary Search

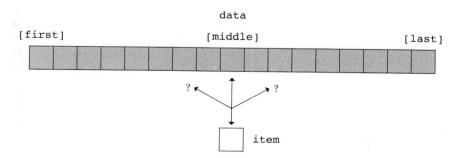

in data[first] through data[last]. When the function begins, first is set to 0 and last is set to length−1 to encompass the entire list.

Our three previous search algorithms have been Boolean observer operations. They just answer the question, Is this item in the list? Let's code the binary search as a void function that not only asks if the item is in the list but also asks which one it is (if it's there). To do so, we need to add two parameters to the parameter list: a Boolean flag found (to tell us whether the item is in the list) and an integer variable position (to tell us which item it is). If found is false, position is undefined.

```
void SortedList::BinSearch(
        /* in */   ItemType item,           // Item to be found
        /* out */ bool&     found,          // True if item is found
        /* out */ int&      position ) const // Location if found

// Searches list for item, returning the index
// of item if item was found.

// Precondition:
//     length <= INT_MAX / 2
//  && data[0..length-1] are in ascending order
//  && item is assigned
// Postcondition:
//     IF item is in the list
//         found == true  &&  data[position] contains item
//     ELSE
//         found == false  &&  position is undefined

{
    int first = 0;            // Lower bound on list
    int last = length - 1;    // Upper bound on list
    int middle;               // Middle index

    found = false;
    while (last >= first && !found)
    {
        middle = (first + last) / 2;
        if (item < data[middle])
            // Assert: item is not in data[middle..last]
            last = middle - 1;
        else if (item > data[middle])
            // Assert: item is not in data[first..middle]
            first = middle + 1;
        else
            // Assert: item == data[middle]
            found = true;
    }
    if (found)
        position = middle;
}
```

Should `BinSearch` be a public member of the `SortedList` class? No. The function returns the index of the array element where the item was found. An array index is useless to a client of `SortedList`. The array containing the list items is encapsulated within the private part of the class and is inaccessible to clients. If you review the `SortedList` class declaration, you'll see that `BinSearch` is a *private*, not public, class member. We intend to use it as a helper function when we implement the public operations `IsPresent` and `Delete`.

Let's do a code walk-through of the binary search algorithm. The value being searched for is 24. Figure 13-7a shows the values of `first`, `last`, and `middle` during the first iteration. In this iteration, 24 is compared with 103, the value in `data[middle]`. Because 24 is less than 103, `last` becomes `middle-1` and `first` stays the same. Figure 13-7b shows the situation during the second iteration. This time, 24 is compared with 72, the value in `data[middle]`. Because 24 is less than 72, `last` becomes `middle-1` and `first` again stays the same.

In the third iteration (Figure 13-7c), `middle` and `first` are both 0. The value 24 is compared with 12, the value in `data[middle]`. Because 24 is greater than 12, `first` becomes `middle+1`. In the fourth iteration (Figure 13-7d), `first`, `last`, and `middle` are all the same. Again, 24 is compared with the value in `data[middle]`. Because 24 is less than 64, `last` becomes `middle-1`. Now that `last` is less than `first`, the process stops; `found` is `false`.

The binary search is the most complex algorithm that we have examined so far. The following table shows `first`, `last`, `middle`, and `data[middle]` for searches of the values 106, 400, and 406, using the same data as in the previous example. Examine the results in this table carefully.

item	*first*	*last*	*middle*	*last[middle]*	*Termination of Loop*
106	0	10	5	103	
	6	10	8	200	
	6	7	6	106	found = true
400	0	10	5	103	
	6	10	8	200	
	9	10	9	300	
	10	10	10	400	found = true
406	0	10	5	103	
	6	10	8	200	
	9	10	9	300	
	10	10	10	400	
	11	10			last < first
					found = false

FIGURE 13-7
Code Walk-
Through of
`BinSearch`
Function (Search
Item Is 24)

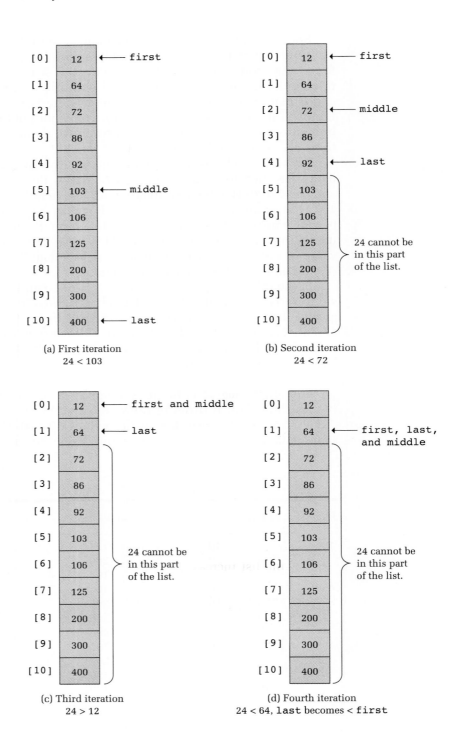

(a) First iteration
24 < 103

(b) Second iteration
24 < 72

(c) Third iteration
24 > 12

(d) Fourth iteration
24 < 64, `last` becomes < `first`

The calculation

```
middle = (first + last) / 2;
```

explains why the function precondition restricts the value of `length` to `INT_MAX/2`. If the item being searched for happens to reside in the last position of the list (for example, when `item` equals 400 in our sample list), then `first + last` equals `length + length`. If `length` is greater than `INT_MAX/2`, the sum `length + length` would produce an integer overflow.

Notice in the table that whether we searched for 106, 400, or 406, the loop never executed more than four times. It never executes more than four times in a list of 11 components because the list is being cut in half each time through the loop. The table below compares a sequential search and a binary search in terms of the average number of iterations needed to find an item.

	Average Number of Iterations	
Length of List	Sequential Search	Binary Search
10	5.5	2.9
100	50.5	5.8
1000	500.5	9.0
10,000	5000.5	12.4

If the binary search is so much faster, why not use it all the time? It certainly is faster in terms of the number of times through the loop, but more computations are performed within the binary search loop than in the other search algorithms. So if the number of components in the list is small (say, less than 20), the sequential search algorithms are faster because they perform less work at each iteration. As the number of components in the list increases, the binary search algorithm becomes relatively more efficient. Remember, however, that the binary search requires the list to be sorted, and sorting takes time. Keep three factors in mind when you are deciding which search algorithm to use:

1. The length of the list to be searched
2. Whether or not the list is already sorted
3. The number of times the list is to be searched

Given the `BinSearch` function (a private member of the `SortedList` class), it's easy to implement the `IsPresent` function (a public member of the class).

```
bool SortedList::IsPresent( /* in */ ItemType item ) const

// Searches the list for item, reporting whether it was found

// Precondition:
//     length <= INT_MAX / 2
//   && data[0..length-1] are in ascending order
//   && item is assigned
// Postcondition:
//     Function value == true, if item is in data[0..length-1]
//                    == false, otherwise

{
    bool found;        // True if item is found
    int position;      // Required (but unused) argument for
                       //   the call to BinSearch

    BinSearch(item, found, position);
    return found;
}
```

The body of IsPresent calls BinSearch, obtaining the result of the search in the variables found and position. Like the children's game of Pass It On, IsPresent receives the value of found from BinSearch and simply passes it on to the client (via the return statement). The body of IsPresent is not interested in where the item was found, so it ignores the value returned in the position argument. Why did we include this third argument when we designed BinSearch? The answer is that the Delete operation, which we look at next, calls BinSearch and *does* use the position argument.

Deletion

In the List::Delete function, we deleted an item by moving up the last component in the list to fill the deleted item's position. Although this algorithm is fine for unsorted lists, it won't work for sorted lists. Moving the last component to an arbitrary position in the list is almost certain to disturb the sorted order of the components. We need a new algorithm for sorted lists.

Let's call BinSearch to tell us the position of the item to be deleted. Then we can "squeeze out" the deleted item by shifting up all the remaining array elements by one position:

```
BinSearch(item, found, position)
IF found
    Shift remainder of list up
    Decrement length
```

The algorithm for Shift List Up is

```
Set data[position]     =     data[position+1]
Set data[position+1]   =     data[position+2]
       ⋮                            ⋮
Set data[length-2]     =     data[length-1]
```

Here is the coded version of this algorithm:

```cpp
void SortedList::Delete( /* in */ ItemType item )

// Deletes item from the list, if it is there

// Precondition:
//      0 < length <= INT_MAX/2
//   && data[0..length-1] are in ascending order
//   && item is assigned
// Postcondition:
//      IF item is in data array at entry
//          First occurrence of item is no longer in array
//       && length == length@entry - 1
//       && data[0..length-1] are in ascending order
//      ELSE
//          length and data array are unchanged

{
    bool found;       // True if item is found
    int position;     // Position of item, if found
    int index;        // Index and loop control variable

    BinSearch(item, found, position);
    if (found)
    {
        // Shift data[position..length-1] up one position

        for (index = position; index < length - 1; index++)
            data[index] = data[index+1];
        length--;
    }
}
```

THEORETICAL FOUNDATIONS

Complexity of Searching and Sorting

We introduced Big-O notation in Chapter 6 as a way of comparing the work done by different algorithms. Let's apply it to the algorithms that we've developed in this chapter and see how they compare with each other. In each algorithm, we start with a list containing some number of values, N.

In the worst case, our `List::IsPresent` function scans all N values to locate an item. Thus, it requires N steps to execute. On average, `List::IsPresent` takes roughly $N/2$ steps to find an item; however, recall that in Big-O notation, we ignore constant factors (as well as lower-order terms). Thus, function `List::IsPresent` is an order N—that is, an $O(N)$—algorithm.

`List::IsPresent2` is also an $O(N)$ algorithm because even though we saved a comparison on each loop iteration, the same number of iterations are performed. However, making the loop more efficient without changing the number of iterations decreases the constant (the number of steps) that N is multiplied by in the algorithm's work formula. Thus, function `List::IsPresent2` is said to be a constant factor faster than `List::IsPresent`.

What about the algorithm we presented for a sequential search in a sorted list? The number of iterations is decreased for the case in which the item is missing from the list. However, all we have done is take a case that would require N steps and reduce its time, on average, to $N/2$ steps. Therefore, this algorithm is also $O(N)$.

Now consider `BinSearch`. In the worst case, it eliminates half of the remaining list components on each iteration. Thus, the worst-case number of iterations is equal to the number of times N must be divided by 2 to eliminate all but one value. This number is computed by taking the logarithm, base 2, of N (written $\log_2 N$). Here are some examples of $\log_2 N$ for different values of N:

N	Log_2N
2	1
4	2
8	3
16	4
32	5
1024	10
32,768	15
1,048,576	20
33,554,432	25
1,073,741,824	30

As you can see, for a list of over 1 billion values, `BinSearch` takes only 30 iterations. It is definitely the best choice for searching large lists. Algorithms such as `BinSearch` are said to be of *logarithmic order*.

Now let's turn to sorting. Function `SelSort` contains nested For loops. The total number of iterations is the product of the iterations performed by the two loops. The outer loop executes $N - 1$ times. The inner loop also starts out executing $N - 1$ times, but steadily decreases until it performs just one iteration: The inner loop executes $N/2$ iterations. The total number of iterations is thus

$$\frac{(N - 1) \times N}{2}$$

Ignoring the constant factor and lower-order term, this is N^2 iterations, and `SelSort` is an $O(N^2)$ algorithm. Whereas `BinSearch` takes only 30 iterations to search a sorted array of 1 billion values, putting the array into order takes `SelSort` approximately 1 billion times 1 billion iterations!

We mentioned that the `SortedList::Insert` algorithm forms the basis for an insertion sort, in which values are inserted into a sorted list as they are input. On average, `SortedList::Insert` must shift down half of the values ($N/2$) in the list; thus, it is an $O(N)$ algorithm. If `SortedList::Insert` is called for each input value, we are executing an $O(N)$ algorithm N times; therefore, an insertion sort is an $O(N^2)$ algorithm.

Is every sorting algorithm $O(N^2)$? Most of the simpler ones are, but $O(N \times \log_2 N)$ sorting algorithms exist. Algorithms that are $O(N \times \log_2 N)$ are much closer in performance to $O(N)$ algorithms than are $O(N^2)$ algorithms. For example, if N is 1 million, then an $O(N^2)$ algorithm takes a million times a million (1 trillion) iterations, but an $O(N \times \log_2 N)$ algorithm takes only 20 million iterations—that is, it is 20 times slower than the $O(N)$ algorithm but 50,000 times faster than the $O(N^2)$ algorithm.

Now let's turn our attention to another example of array-based lists—a special kind of array that is useful when working with alphanumeric character data.

Understanding Character Strings

Ever since Chapter 2, we have been using the `string` class to store and manipulate character strings.

```
string name;

name = "James Smith";
len = name.length();
    ⋮
```

In some contexts, we think of a string as a single unit of data. In other contexts, we treat it as a group of individually accessible characters. In particular, we think of a string as a variable-length, linear collection of homogeneous components (of type char). Does this sound familiar? It should. As an abstraction, a string is a list of characters that, at any moment in time, has a length associated with it.

Thinking of a string as an ADT, how would we implement the ADT? There are many ways to implement strings. Programmers have specified and implemented their own string classes—the string class from the standard library, for instance. And the C++ language has its own built-in notion of a string: the **C string.** In C++, a string constant (or string literal, or literal string) is a sequence of characters enclosed by double quotes:

`"Hi"`

A string constant is stored as a char array with enough components to hold each specified character plus one more—the *null character.* The null character, which is the first character in both the ASCII and EBCDIC character sets, has internal representation 0. In C++, the escape sequence \0 stands for the null character. When the compiler encounters the string `"Hi"` in a program, it stores the three characters 'H', 'i', and '\0' into a three-element, anonymous (unnamed) char array as follows:

Unnamed array

[0]	'H'
[1]	'i'
[2]	'\0'

The C string is the only kind of C++ array for which there exists an aggregate constant—the string constant. Notice that in a C++ program, the symbols `'A'` denote a single character, whereas the symbols `"A"` denote two: the character 'A' and the null character.*

In addition to C string constants, we can create C string *variables.* To do so, we explicitly declare a char array and store into it whatever characters we want to, finishing with the null character. Here's an example:

---

* *C string* is not an official term used in C++ language manuals. Such manuals typically use the term *string.* However, we use *C string* to distinguish between the general concept of a string and the built-in array representation defined by the C and C++ languages.

```
char myStr[8];    // Room for 7 significant characters plus '\0'

myStr[0] = 'H';
myStr[1] = 'i';
myStr[2] = '\0';
```

C string In C and C++, a null-terminated sequence of characters stored in a `char` array.

In C++, all C strings (constants or variables) are assumed to be null-terminated. This convention is agreed upon by all C++ programmers and standard library functions. The null character serves as a sentinel value; it allows algorithms to locate the end of the string. For example, here is a function that determines the length of any C string, not counting the terminating null character:

```
int StrLength( /* in */ const char str[] )

// Precondition:
//      str holds a null-terminated string
// Postcondition:
//      Function value == number of characters in str (excluding '\0')

{
    int i = 0;    // Index variable

    while (str[i] != '\0')
        i++;
    return i;
}
```

The value of `i` is the correct value for this function to return. If the array being examined is

[0]	'B'
[1]	'y'
[2]	'\0'
[3]	
	.
	.
	.

then i equals 2 at loop exit. The string length is therefore 2.

The argument to the StrLength function can be a C string variable, as in the function call

```
cout << StrLength(myStr);
```

or it can be a string constant:

```
cout << StrLength("Hello");
```

In the first case, the base address of the myStr array is sent to the function, as we discussed in Chapter 12. In the second case, a base address is also sent to the function—the base address of the unnamed array that the compiler has set aside for the string constant.

There is one more thing we should say about our StrLength function. A C++ programmer would not actually write this function. The standard library supplies several string-processing functions, one of which is named strlen and does exactly what our StrLength function does. Later in the chapter, we look at strlen and other library functions.

Initializing C Strings

In Chapter 12, we showed how to initialize an array in its declaration by specifying a list of initial values within braces, like this:

```
int delta[5] = {25, -3, 7, 13, 4};
```

To initialize a C string variable in its declaration, you could use the same technique:

```
char message[8] = {'W', 'h', 'o', 'o', 'p', 's', '!', '\0'};
```

However, C++ allows a more convenient way to initialize a C string. You can simply initialize the array by using a string constant:

```
char message[8] = "Whoops!";
```

This shorthand notation is unique to C strings because there is no other kind of array for which there are aggregate constants.

We said in Chapter 12 that you can omit the size of an array when you initialize it in its declaration (in which case, the compiler determines its size). This feature is often used with C strings because it keeps you from having to count the number of characters. For example,

```
char promptMsg[] = "Enter a positive number:";   // Size is 25
char errMsg[] = "Value must be positive.";       // Size is 24
```

Be very careful about one thing: C++ treats initialization (in a declaration) and assignment (in an assignment statement) as two distinct operations. Different rules apply. Remember that array initialization is legal, but aggregate array assignment is not.

```
char myStr[20] = "Hello";    // OK
  ⋮
myStr = "Howdy";             // Not allowed
```

C String Input and Output

In Chapter 12, we emphasized that C++ does not provide aggregate operations on arrays. There is no aggregate assignment, aggregate comparison, or aggregate arithmetic on arrays. We also said that aggregate input/output of arrays is not possible, with one exception. C strings are that exception. Let's look first at output.

To output the contents of an array that is *not* a C string, you aren't allowed to do this:

```
int alpha[100];
  ⋮
cout << alpha;   // Not allowed
```

Instead, you must write a loop and print the array elements one at a time. However, aggregate output of a null-terminated `char` array (that is, a C string) is valid. The C string can be a constant (as we've been doing since Chapter 2):

```
cout << "Results are:";
```

or it can be a variable:

```
char msg[8] = "Welcome";
    ⋮
cout << msg;
```

In both cases, the insertion operator (<<) outputs each character in the array until the null character is found. It is up to you to double-check that the terminating null character is present in the array. If not, the << operator will march through the array and into the rest of memory, printing out bytes until—just by chance—it encounters a byte whose integer value is 0.

To input C strings, we have several options. The first is to use the extraction operator (>>), which behaves exactly the same as with `string` class objects. When reading input characters into a C string variable, the >> operator skips leading whitespace characters and then reads successive characters into the array, stopping at the first trailing whitespace character (which is not consumed, but remains as the first character waiting in the input stream). The >> operator also takes care of adding the null character to the end of the string. For example, assume we have the following code:

```
char firstName[31];    // Room for 30 characters plus '\0'
char lastName[31];

cin >> firstName >> lastName;
```

If the input stream initially looks like this (where ❏ denotes a blank):

❏❏John❏Smith❏❏❏25

then our input statement stores 'J', 'o', 'h', 'n', and '\0' into `firstName[0]` through `firstName[4]`; stores 'S', 'm', 'i', 't', 'h', and '\0' into `lastName[0]` through `lastName[5]`; and leaves the input stream as

❏❏❏25

The >> operator, however, has two potential drawbacks.

1. If the array isn't large enough to hold the sequence of input characters (and the '\0'), the >> operator will continue to store characters into memory past the end of the array.
2. The >> operator cannot be used to input a string that has blanks within it. (It stops reading as soon as it encounters the first whitespace character.)

To cope with these limitations, we can use a variation of the get function, a member of the istream class. We have used the get function to input a single character, even if it is a whitespace character:

```
cin.get(inputChar);
```

The get function also can be used to input C strings, in which case the function call requires two arguments. The first is the array name and the second is an int expression.

```
cin.get(myStr, charCount + 1);
```

The get function does not skip leading whitespace characters and continues until it either has read charCount characters or it reaches the newline character '\n', whichever comes first. It then appends the null character to the end of the string. With the statements

```
char oneLine[81];    // Room for 80 characters plus '\0'
   ⋮
cin.get(oneLine, 81);
```

the get function reads and stores an entire input line (to a maximum of 80 characters), embedded blanks and all. If the line has fewer than 80 characters, reading stops at '\n' but does not consume it. The newline character is now the first one waiting in the input stream. To read two consecutive lines worth of strings, it is necessary to consume the newline character:

```
char dummy;
   ⋮
cin.get(string1, 81);
cin.get(dummy);          // Eat newline before next "get"
cin.get(string2, 81);
```

The first function call reads characters up to, but not including, the '\n'. If the input of dummy were omitted, then the input of string2 would read *no* characters because '\n' would immediately be the first character waiting in the stream.

Finally, the ignore function—introduced in Chapter 4—can be useful in conjunction with the get function. Recall that the statement

```
cin.ignore(200, '\n');
```

says to skip at most 200 input characters but stop if a newline was read. (The newline character *is* consumed by this function.) If a program inputs a long string from the user but only wants to retain the first four characters of the response, here is a way to do it:

```
char response[5];        // Room for 4 characters plus '\0'

cin.get(response, 5);    // Input at most 4 characters
cin.ignore(100, '\n');   // Skip remaining chars up to and
                         //    including '\n'
```

The value 100 in the last statement is arbitrary. Any "large enough" number will do.

Here is a table that summarizes the differences between the >> operator and the get function when reading C strings:

Statement	Skips Leading Whitespace?	Stops Reading When?
cin >> inputStr;	Yes	At the first trailing whitespace character (which is *not* consumed)
cin.get(inputStr, 21);	No	When either 20 characters are read or '\n' is encountered (which is *not* consumed)

Finally, we revisit a topic that came up in Chapter 4. Certain library functions and member functions of system-supplied classes require C strings as arguments. An example is the ifstream class member function named open. To open a file, we pass the name of the file as a C string, either a constant or a variable:

```
ifstream file1;
ifstream file2;
char     fileName[51];   // Max. 50 characters plus '\0'

file1.open("students.dat");
cin.get(fileName, 51);          // Read at most 50 characters
cin.ignore(100, '\n');          // Skip rest of input line
file2.open(fileName);
```

As discussed in Chapter 4, if our file name is contained in a `string` class object, we still can use the `open` function, *provided* we use the `string` class member function named `c_str` to convert the string to a C string:

```
ifstream inFile;
string   fileName;

cin >> fileName;
inFile.open(fileName.c_str());
```

Comparing these two code segments, you can observe a major advantage of the `string` class over C strings: A string in a `string` class object has unbounded length, whereas the length of a C string is bounded by the array size, which is fixed at compile time.

C String Library Routines

Through the header file `cstring`, the C++ standard library provides a large assortment of C string operations. In this section, we discuss three of these library functions: `strlen`, which returns the length of a string; `strcmp`, which compares two strings using the relations less-than, equal, and greater-than; and `strcpy`, which copies one string to another. Here is a summary of `strlen`, `strcmp`, and `strcpy`:

Header File	Function	Function Value	Effect
`<cstring>`	`strlen(str)`	Integer length of `str` (excluding '\0')	Computes length of `str`
`<cstring>`	`strcmp(str1, str2)`	An integer < 0, if `str1` < `str2` The integer 0, if `str1` = `str2` An integer > 0, if `str1` > `str2`	Compares `str1` and `str2`
`<cstring>`	`strcpy(toStr, fromStr)`	Base address of `toStr` (usually ignored)	Copies `fromStr` (including '\0') to `toStr`, overwriting what was there; `toStr` must be large enough to hold the result

The strlen function is similar to the StrLength function we wrote earlier. It returns the number of characters in a C string prior to the terminating '\0'. Here's an example of a call to the function:

```
#include <cstring>
    ⋮
char subject[] = "Computer Science";

cout << strlen(subject);    // Prints 16
```

The strcpy routine is important because aggregate assignment with the = operator is not allowed on C strings. In the following code fragment, we show the wrong way and the right way to perform a string copy.

```
#include <cstring>
    ⋮
char myStr[100];
    ⋮
myStr = "Abracadabra";          // No
strcpy(myStr, "Abracadabra");   // Yes
```

In strcpy's argument list, the destination string is the one on the left, just as an assignment operation transfers data from right to left. It is the caller's responsibility to make sure that the destination array is large enough to hold the result.

The strcpy function is technically a value-returning function; it not only copies one C string to another, but also returns as a function value the base address of the destination array. The reason why the caller would want to use this function value is not at all obvious, and we don't discuss it here. Programmers nearly always ignore the function value and simply invoke strcpy as if it were a void function (as we did above). You may wish to review the Background Information box in Chapter 8 entitled "Ignoring a Function Value."

The strcmp function is used for comparing two strings. The function receives two C strings as parameters and compares them in *lexicographic* order (the order in which they would appear in a dictionary)—the same ordering used in comparing string class objects. Given the function call strcmp(str1, str2), the function returns one of the following int values: a negative integer, if str1 < str2 lexicographically; the value 0, if str1 = str2; or a positive integer, if str1 > str2. The precise values of the negative integer and the positive integer are unspecified. You simply test to see if the result is less than 0, 0, or greater than 0. Here is an example:

```
if (strcmp(str1, str2) < 0)    // If str1 is less than str2 ...
    ⋮
```

We have described only three of the string-handling routines provided by the standard library. These three are the most commonly needed, but there are many more. If you are designing or maintaining programs that use C strings extensively, you should read the documentation on strings for your C++ system.

String Class or C Strings?

When working with string data, should you use a class like `string`, or should you use C strings? From the standpoints of clarity, versatility, and ease of use, there is no contest. Use a string class. The standard library `string` class provides strings of unbounded length, aggregate assignment, aggregate comparison, concatenation with the + operator, and so forth.

However, it is still useful to be familiar with C strings. Among the thousands of software products currently in use that are written in C and C++, most (but a declining percentage) use C strings to represent string data. In your next place of employment, if you are asked to modify or upgrade such software, understanding C strings is essential. Additionally, *using* a string class is one thing; *implementing* it is another. Someone must implement the class using a concrete data representation. In your employment, that someone might be you, and the underlying data representation might very well be a C string!

PROBLEM-SOLVING CASE STUDY

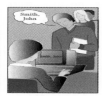

Exam Attendance

Problem: You are the grader for a U.S. government class of 200 students. The instructor has asked you to prepare two lists: students taking an exam and students who have missed it. The catch is that he wants the lists before the exam is over. You decide to write a program for your notebook computer that takes each student's name as the student enters the exam room and prints the lists of absentees and attendees for your instructor.

Input:
A list of last names of the students in the class (file `roster`), which was obtained from a master list in order of Social Security number
Each student's last name as he or she enters the room (standard input device)
(In this class, there are no duplicate last names.)

PROBLEM-SOLVING CASE STUDY _cont'd._

Output:
A list of those students taking the exam
A list of those students who are absent

Discussion: How would you take attendance by hand? You would stand at the door with a class roster. As each student came in, you would check off his or her name. When all the students had entered, you would go through the roster, making a list of those present. Then you would do the same for those who were absent.

This by-hand algorithm can serve as a model for your program. As each student enters the room, you enter his or her name at the keyboard. Your program scans the list of students for that name and marks that the student is present. When the last student has entered, you can enter a special sentinel name, perhaps "EndData," to signal the program to print the lists.

You can simulate "Mark that the student is present" by maintaining two lists: notCheckedIn, which initially contains all the student names, and thosePresent, which is initially empty. To mark a student present, delete his or her name from the notCheckedIn list and insert it into the thosePresent list. After all students have entered the exam room, the two lists contain the names of those absent and those present.

Your program must prepare the initial list of students in notCheckedIn from the class roster file, which is ordered by Social Security number. If you enter the names directly from the roster, they will not be in alphabetical order. Does that matter? Yes, in this case it does matter. The size of the class is 200, and the students need to enter the exam room with minimum delay (because most arrive just before the exam starts).

The length of the list and the speed required suggest that a binary search is appropriate. A binary search requires that the list be in sorted order. The names in the input file are not in alphabetical order, so your program must sort them. You can input all the names at once and then sort them using a function like SelSort, or you can use an insertion sort, inserting each name into its proper place as it is read. You decide to take the second approach because you can use the SortedList class of this chapter directly. This class provides such an Insert operation as well as a BinSearch operation.

Data Structures and Objects:
A SortedList object containing names of students not yet checked in
    (notCheckedIn)
A SortedList object containing names of students who have checked in
    (thosePresent)

PROBLEM-SOLVING CASE STUDY cont'd.

Main   Level 0

> Open roster file for input (and verify success)
> Get class roster
> Check in students
> Print lists

Get Class Roster (Inout: notCheckedIn, roster)   Level 1

> Read stuName from roster file
> WHILE NOT EOF on roster
>   notCheckedIn.Insert(stuName)
>   Read stuName from roster file

Check in Students (Inout: notCheckedIn, thosePresent)

> Print "Enter last name"
> Read stuName
> WHILE stuName isn't "EndData"
>   Process stuName
>   Print "Enter last name"
>   Read stuName

Process Name (In: stuName; Inout: notCheckedIn, thosePresent) Level 2

> IF notCheckedIn.IsPresent(stuName)
>   thosepresent.Insert(stuName)
>   notCheckedIn.Delete(stuName)
> ELSE
>   Print "Name not on roster."

PROBLEM-SOLVING CASE STUDY cont'd.

Print (In: notCheckedIn, thosePresent)   **Level 1**

> Print "The following students are taking the exam."
> thosePresent.Print()
> Print "The following students have missed the exam."
> notCheckedIn.Print()

The design is now ready to be coded.

Because our program uses the `SortedList` class, we need

```
#include "slist.h"
```

to insert the appropriate declarations into the program. But we must make sure that `MAX_LENGTH` and `ItemType` in the file `slist.h` are correct for our problem. Our lists should hold up to 200 student names, and the type of each list component is `string`. Thus, we edit `slist.h` as follows:

```
const int MAX_LENGTH = 200;
typedef string ItemType;
```

Then we recompile `slist.cpp` into `slist.obj`. To run our Exam program, we link its object code file with the object code file `slist.obj`.

Module Structure Chart:

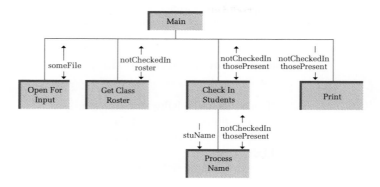

PROBLEM-SOLVING CASE STUDY *cont'd.*

(The following program is written in ISO/ANSI standard C++. If you are working with pre–standard C++, see the alternate version of the program in the PRE_STD directory of the program disk, available at the publisher's Web site, www.jbpub.com/disks.)

```cpp
//*****************************************************************
// Exam program
// This program compares students who come to take an exam against
// a class roster.  A list of students who took the exam and a list
// of students who missed the exam are printed.
// Assumption: Max. number of student names in roster file is
// MAX_LENGTH, which is defined in slist.h
//*****************************************************************
#include <iostream>
#include <fstream>      // For file I/O
#include <string>       // For string class
#include "slist.h"      // For SortedList class

const string END_DATA = "EndData";      // Sentinel value for
                                        //    student name

void CheckInStudents( SortedList&, SortedList& );
void GetClassRoster( SortedList&, ifstream& );
void OpenForInput( ifstream& );
void Print( SortedList, SortedList );
void ProcessName( string, SortedList&, SortedList& );

int main()
{
    SortedList notCheckedIn;  // List of students not yet checked in
    SortedList thosePresent;  // List of students present at exam
    ifstream roster;          // Input file to be analyzed

    OpenForInput(roster);
    if ( !roster )
        return 1;

    GetClassRoster(notCheckedIn, roster);
    CheckInStudents(notCheckedIn, thosePresent);
    Print(notCheckedIn, thosePresent);
    return 0;
}

//*****************************************************************
```

PROBLEM-SOLVING CASE STUDY cont'd.

```
void OpenForInput( /* inout */ ifstream& someFile )    // File to be
                                                       // opened
// Prompts the user for the name of an input file
// and attempts to open the file

{
    .
    .        (Same as in previous case studies)
    .
}

//*****************************************************************

void GetClassRoster(
        /* inout */ SortedList& notCheckedIn,    // List of students
        /* inout */ ifstream&    roster     )    // Roster data file

// Reads the class roster from the data file

// Precondition:
//     notCheckedIn is the empty list
// Precondition:
//     The roster file has been successfully opened for input
//  && The no. of student names in the file <= MAX_LENGTH (defined
//        in slist.h)
// Postcondition:
//     notCheckedIn contains the student names read from the file

{
    string stuName;       // An input student name

    roster >> stuName;
    while (roster)
    {
        notCheckedIn.Insert(stuName);
        roster >> stuName;
    }
}

//*****************************************************************

void CheckInStudents(
        /* inout */ SortedList& notCheckedIn,    // List of students
        /* inout */ SortedList& thosePresent )   // List of students

// Inputs student names from standard input,
// marking students present
```

PROBLEM-SOLVING CASE STUDY cont'd.

```
// Precondition:
//     notCheckedIn contains names of all students in class
//   && thosePresent is empty
// Postcondition:
//     The user has been repeatedly prompted to enter student names
//   && thosePresent contains all the valid input names
//   && notCheckedIn contains all student names except the valid
//       input names
//   && For all input names not found in the notCheckedIn list,
//       an error message has been printed

{
    string stuName;      // Name of student who is checking in

    cout << "Enter last name: ";
    cin >> stuName;
    while (stuName != END_DATA)
    {
        ProcessName(stuName, notCheckedIn, thosePresent);
        cout << "Enter last name: ";
        cin >> stuName;
    }
}


//******************************************************************

void ProcessName(
        /* in */     string         stuName,        // Input student name
        /* inout */  SortedList&    notCheckedIn,   // List of students
        /* inout */  SortedList&    thosePresent )  // List of students

// Searches for stuName in the notCheckedIn list.  If stuName
// is found, it is inserted into thosePresent and deleted from
// notCheckedIn.  Otherwise, an error message is printed.

// Precondition:
//     stuName is assigned
// Postcondition:
//     IF stuName is in notCheckedIn@entry
//         stuName is in thosePresent
//       && stuName is not in notCheckedIn
//     ELSE
//         An error message has been printed

{
    if (notCheckedIn.IsPresent(stuName))
    {
```

PROBLEM-SOLVING CASE STUDY *cont'd.*
_____

```
            thosePresent.Insert(stuName);
            notCheckedIn.Delete(stuName);
    }
    else
            cout << "Name not on roster." << endl;
}


//****************************************************************

void Print( /* in */ SortedList notCheckedIn,      // List of students
            /* in */ SortedList thosePresent )     // List of students

// Prints the names of those taking the exam, then the names
// of those who are absent

// Postcondition:
//      Contents of thosePresent and notCheckedIn have been printed

{
    cout << endl << "The following students are taking the exam."
        << endl;
    thosePresent.Print();

    cout << endl << "The following students have missed the exam."
        << endl;
    notCheckedIn.Print();
}
```

Testing: The list manipulation operations Insert, Delete, BinSearch, and Print must be tested with different sized lists: an empty list, a one-item list, a list of maximum length, and several sizes in between. The BinSearch routine must be tested by searching for items that are in the list, items that are not in the list, at least one item that compares less than the first item in the list, at least one item that compares greater than the last item in the list, the last item, and the first item.

In testing the overall logic of the program, names read from the keyboard must be spelled incorrectly as well as correctly. The following data represents a sample data set.

Roster File

Dale
MacDonald
Weems
Vitek
Westby
Smith

PROBLEM-SOLVING CASE STUDY cont'd.

```
Jamison
Jones
Kirshen
Gleason
Thompson
Ripley
Lilly
Headington
```

Copy of the Screen During the Run

```
Input file name: roster.dat
Enter last name: Weems
Enter last name: Dale
Enter last name: McDonald
Name not on roster.
Enter last name: MacDonald
Enter last name: Vitek
Enter last name: Westby
Enter last name: Gleason
Enter last name: EndData

The following students are taking the exam.
Dale
Gleason
MacDonald
Vitek
Weems
Westby

The following students have missed the exam.
Headington
Jamison
Jones
Kirshen
Lilly
Ripley
Smith
Thompson
```

By assuming that all students have unique last names, we have simplified the problem somewhat. Case Study Follow-Up Exercise 1 asks you to expand the program to account for duplicate last names.

Testing and Debugging

In this chapter, we have discussed, designed, and coded algorithms to construct and manipulate items in a list. In addition to the basic list operations `IsFull`, `IsEmpty`, `Length`, and `Print`, the algorithms included three sequential searches, a binary search, insertion into sorted and unsorted lists, deletion from sorted and unsorted lists, and a selection sort. We have already tested `SortedList::Insert`, `SortedList::Delete`, and `SortedList::BinSearch` in conjunction with the case study. Now we need to test the other searching algorithms and the functions `List::Insert`, `List::Delete`, and `List::SelSort`. We can use the same scheme that we used to test `BinSearch` to test the other search algorithms. We should test `List::Insert`, `List::Delete`, and `List::SelSort` with lists containing no components, one component, two components, MAX_LENGTH − 1 components, and MAX_LENGTH components.

When we wrote the precondition that the list was not full for operation `List::Insert`, we indicated that we could handle the problem another way—we could include an error flag in the function's parameter list. The function would call `IsFull` and set the error flag. The insertion would not take place if the error flag were set to `true`. Both options are acceptable ways of handling the problem. The important point is that we clearly state whether the calling code or the called function is to check for the error condition. However, it is the calling code that must decide what to do when an error condition occurs. In other words, if errors are handled by means of preconditions, then the user must write the code to guarantee the preconditions. If errors are handled by flags, then the user must write the code to monitor the error flags.

Testing and Debugging Hints

1. Review the Testing and Debugging Hints for Chapter 12. They apply to all one-dimensional arrays, including C strings.
2. Make sure that every C string is terminated with the null character. String constants are automatically null-terminated by the compiler. On input, the >> operator and the `get` function automatically add the null character. If you store characters into a C string individually or manipulate the array in any way, be sure to account for the null character.
3. Remember that C++ treats C string initialization (in a declaration) as different from C string assignment. Initialization is allowed, but assignment is not.
4. Aggregate input/output is allowed for C strings but not for other array types.

5. If you use the >> operator to input into a C string variable, be sure the array is large enough to hold the null character plus the longest sequence of (nonwhitespace) characters in the input stream.

6. With C string input, the >> operator stops at, *but does not consume,* the first trailing whitespace character. Likewise, if the get function stops reading early because it encounters a newline character, the newline character is not consumed.

7. When you use the strcpy library function, ensure that the destination array is at least as large as the array from which you are copying.

8. General-purpose functions (such as ADT operations) should be tested outside the context of a particular program, using a test driver.

9. Choose test data carefully so that you test all end conditions and some in the middle. End conditions are those that reach the limits of the structure used to store them. For example, in a list, there should be test data in which the number of components is 0, 1, and MAX_LENGTH, as well as between 1 and MAX_LENGTH.

Summary

This chapter has provided practice in working with lists stored in one-dimensional arrays. We have examined algorithms that insert, delete, search, and sort data stored in a list, and we have written functions to implement these algorithms. We can use these functions again and again in different contexts because they are members of general-purpose C++ classes (List and SortedList) that represent list ADTs.

C strings are a special case of char arrays in C++. The last significant character must be followed by a null character to mark the end of the string. C strings are less versatile than a string class. However, it pays to understand how they work because many existing programs in C and C++ use them, and string classes often use C strings as the underlying data representation.

Quick Check

1. The following code fragment implements the "Delete, if it's there" meaning for the Delete operation in an unsorted list. Change it so that the other meaning is implemented; that is, there is a precondition that the item *is* in the list. (pp. 751–752)

```
index = 0;
while (index < length && item != data[index])
    index++;
if (index < length)
{                                    // Remove item
    data[index] = data[length-1];
    length--;
}
```

2. In a sequential search of an unsorted array of 1000 values, what is the average number of loop iterations required to find a value? What is the maximum number of iterations? (pp. 772–773)

3. The following program fragment sorts list items into ascending order. Change it to sort into descending order. (pp. 755–758)

```
for (passCount = 0; passCount < length - 1; passCount++)
{
    minIndx = passCount;
    for (searchIndx = passCount + 1; searchIndx < length;
                                            searchIndx++)
        if (data[searchIndx] < data[minIndx])
            minIndx = searchIndx;
    temp = data[minIndx];                    // Swap
    data[minIndx] = data[passCount];
    data[passCount] = temp;
}
```

4. Describe how the `SortedList::Insert` operation can be used to build a sorted list from unsorted input data. (pp. 761–764)

5. Describe the basic principle behind the binary search algorithm. (pp. 765–769)

6. Using Typedef, define an array data type for a C string of up to 15 characters plus the null character. Declare an array variable of this type, initializing it to your first name. Then use a library function to replace the contents of the variable with your last name (up to 15 characters). (pp. 773–783)

Answers

1.
```
index = 0;
while (item != data[index])
    index++;
data[index] = data[length-1];
length--;
```

2. The average number is 500 iterations. The maximum is 1000 iterations. **3.** The only required change is to replace the < symbol in the inner loop with a >. As a matter of style, the name minIndx should be changed to maxIndx. **4.** The list initially has a length of 0. Each time a data value is read, insertion adds the value to the list in its correct position. When all the data values have been read, they are in the array in sorted order. **5.** The binary search takes advantage of sorted list values, looking at a component in the middle of the list and deciding whether the search value precedes or follows the midpoint. The search is then repeated on the appropriate half, quarter, eighth, and so on, of the list until the value is located.

6.
```
typedef char String15[16];

String15 name = "Anna";

strcpy(name, "Rodriguez");
```

Exam Preparation Exercises

1. What three factors should you consider when you are deciding which search algorithm to use on a list?

2. The following values are stored in an array in ascending order.

   28 45 97 103 107 162 196 202 257

   Applying function List::Search2 to this array, search for the following values and indicate how many comparisons are required to either find the number or find that it is not in the list.

   a. 28
   b. 32
   c. 196
   d. 194

3. Repeat Exercise 2, applying the algorithm for a sequential search in a sorted list (page 764).

4. The following values are stored in an array in ascending order.

   29 57 63 72 79 83 96 104 114 136

   Apply function SortedList::BinSearch with item = 114 to this list, and trace the values of first, last, and middle. Indicate any undefined values with a *U*.

5. A binary search is always better to use than a sequential search. (True or False?)

6. a. Using Typedef, define a data type NameType for a C string of at most 40 characters plus the null character.

   b. Declare a variable oneName to be of type NameType.

   c. Declare employeeName to be a 100-element array whose elements are C strings of type NameType.

7. Given the declarations

```
typedef char NameString[21];
typedef char WordString[11];

NameString firstName;
NameString lastName;
WordString word;
```

   mark the following statements valid or invalid. (Assume the header file cstring has been included.)

   a. `i = 0;`
```
      while (firstName[i] != '\0')
      {
          cout << firstName[i];
          i++;
      }
```
   b. `cout << lastName;`
   c. `if (firstName == lastName)`
```
          n = 1;
```
   d. `if (strcmp(firstName, lastName) == 0)`
```
          m = 8;
```
   e. `cin >> word;`

   f. `lastName = word;`
   g. `if (strcmp(NameString, "Hi") < 0)`
       `n = 3;`
   h. `if (firstName[2] == word[5])`
       `m = 4;`

8. Given the declarations

```
typedef char String20[21];
typedef char String30[31];

String20 rodent;
String30 mammal;
```

write code fragments for the following tasks. (If the task is not possible, say so.)
   a. Store the string "Moose" into `mammal`.
   b. Copy whatever string is in `rodent` into `mammal`.
   c. If the string in `mammal` is greater than "Opossum" lexicographically, increment a variable `count`.
   d. If the string in `mammal` is less than or equal to "Jackal", decrement a variable `count`.
   e. Store the string "Grey-tipped field shrew" into `rodent`.
   f. Print the length of the string in `rodent`.

9. Given the declarations

```
const int NUMBER_OF_BOOKS = 200;

typedef char BookName[31];
typedef char PersonName[21];

BookName     bookOut[NUMBER_OF_BOOKS];
PersonName borrower[NUMBER_OF_BOOKS];
BookName     bookIn;
PersonName name;
```

mark the following statements valid or invalid. (Assume the header file `cstring` has been included.)
   a. `cout << bookIn;`
   b. `cout << bookOut;`
   c. `for (i = 0; i < NUMBER_OF_BOOKS; i++)`
       `cout << bookOut[i] << endl;`
   d. `if (bookOut[3] > bookIn)`
       `cout << bookIn;`
   e. `for (i = 0; i < NUMBER_OF_BOOKS; i++)`
       `if (strcmp(bookIn, bookOut[i]) == 0)`
         `cout << bookIn << ' ' << borrower[i] << endl;`
   f. `bookIn = "Don Quixote";`
   g. `cout << name[2];`

10. Write code fragments to perform the following tasks, using the declarations given in Exercise 9. Assume that the books listed in `bookOut` have been borrowed by the person listed in the corresponding position of `borrower`.

a. Write a code fragment to print each book borrowed by name.

b. Write a code fragment to count the number of books borrowed by name.

c. Write a code fragment to count the number of copies of bookIn that have been borrowed.

d. Write a code fragment to count the number of copies of bookIn that have been borrowed by name.

Programming Warm-up Exercises

1. Write a C++ Boolean function named Exclusive that has three parameters: item (of type ItemType), list1, and list2 (both of type List as defined in this chapter). The function returns true if item is present in either list1 or list2 but not both.

2. To this chapter's List class, we wish to add a value-returning member function named Occurrences that receives a single parameter, item, and returns the number of times item occurs in the list. Write the function definition as it would appear in the implementation file.

3. Repeat Exercise 2 for the SortedList class.

4. To this chapter's List class, we wish to add a Boolean member function named GreaterFound that receives a single parameter, item, and searches the list for a value greater than item. If such a value is found, the function returns true; otherwise, it returns false. Write the function definition as it would appear in the implementation file.

5. Repeat Exercise 4 for the SortedList class.

6. The SortedList::Insert function inserts items into the list in ascending order. Rewrite it so that it inserts items in descending order.

7. Rewrite the SortedList::Delete function so that it removes all occurrences of item from the list.

8. Modify function SortedList::BinSearch so that position is where item should be inserted when found is false.

9. Rewrite function SortedList::Insert so that it implements the first insertion algorithm discussed for sorted lists. That is, the place where the item should be inserted is found by searching from the beginning of the list. When the place is found, all the items from the insertion point to the end of the list are shifted down one position. (Assume that BinSearch has been modified as in Exercise 8.) Write the function definition as it would appear in the implementation file.

10. To the SortedList class, we wish to add a member function named Component that returns a component of the list if a given position number (pos) is in the range 0 through length − 1. The function should also return a Boolean flag named valid that is false if pos is outside this range. Write the function definition as it would appear in the implementation file.

11. To the SortedList class, we wish to add a Boolean member function named Equal that has a single parameter named otherList, which is an object of type SortedList. This function compares two lists for equality: the one represented by otherList and the one represented by the class object for which the function is called. The function returns true if the two lists are of the same length and each element in one list equals the corresponding element in the other list. Here is an example of a call to the Equal function:

```
if (myList.Equal(yourList))
    ⋮
```

Assume the Component function of Exercise 10 has been added as a member of the SortedList class. Write the function definition as it would appear in the implementation file.

Programming Problems

1. A company wants to know the percentages of total sales and total expenses attributable to each salesperson. Each person has a pair of data lines. The first line contains his or her name, last name first. The second line contains his or her sales (int) and expenses (float). Write a program that produces a report with a header line containing the total sales and total expenses. Following this header should be a table with each salesperson's name, percentage of total sales, and percentage of total expenses, sorted by salesperson's name.

   Use one of the list classes developed in this chapter, modifying it as follows. ItemType should be a struct type that holds one salesperson's information. Therefore, the list is a list of structs. Some member functions of the list class must be modified to accommodate this ItemType. For example, comparisons involving list components must be changed to comparisons involving *members* of list components (which are structs). Also, include a Component member function in your list class (see Programming Warm-up Exercise 10) to allow the client code to access components of the list.

2. Only authorized shareholders are allowed to attend a stockholders' meeting. Write a program to read a person's name from the keyboard, check it against a list of shareholders, and print a message saying whether or not the person may attend the meeting. The list of shareholders is in a file inFile in the following format: first name, blank, last name. Use the end-of-file condition to stop reading the file. The maximum number of shareholders is 1000.

   The user should be prompted to enter his or her name in the same format as is used for the data in the file. If the name does not appear on the list, the program should repeat the instructions on how to enter the name and then tell the user to try again. A message saying that the person may not enter should be printed only after he or she has been given a second chance to enter the name. The prompt to the user should include the message that a *Q* should be entered to end the program.

3. Enhance the program in Problem 2 as follows:
   a. Print a report showing the number of stockholders at the time of the meeting, how many were present at the meeting, and how many people who tried to enter were denied permission to attend.
   b. Follow this summary report with a list of the names of the stockholders, with either *Present* or *Absent* after each name.

4. An advertising company wants to send a letter to all its clients announcing a new fee schedule. The clients' names are on several different lists in the company. The various lists are merged to form one file, clientNames, but obviously, the company does not want to send a letter twice to anyone.

Write a program that removes any names appearing on the list more than once. On each line of data, there is a four-digit code number, followed by a blank and then the client's name. For example, Amalgamated Steel is listed as

```
0231 Amalgamated Steel
```

Your program is to output each client's code and name, but no duplicates should be printed.

Use one of the list classes developed in this chapter, modifying it as follows. ItemType should be a struct type that holds one company's information. Therefore, the list is a list of structs. Some member functions of the list class must be modified to accommodate this ItemType. For example, comparisons involving list components must be changed to comparisons involving *members* of list components (which are structs).

Case Study Follow-Up

1. The Exam program assumes that the students have unique last names. Rewrite the program so that it accommodates duplicate last names. Assume now that each line in the roster file contains a student's first and last names, with last name first.
2. The Exam program uses an insertion sort, placing each student's name into its proper place in the list as it is input. How would you rewrite the program to input all the names at once and then sort them using SelSort?
3. The Exam program uses a binary search to search the student list. Assuming a list of 200 students, how many loop iterations are required to determine that a student is absent? How many iterations would be required if we had used the algorithm for a sequential search of a sorted list instead of BinSearch?
4. Write a test plan for the functions SortedList::Insert and SortedList::BinSearch, assuming ItemType is int.
5. Write a test driver to implement your test plan.

14

Object-Oriented Software Development

GOALS

- To be able to distinguish between structured (procedural) programming and object-oriented programming.
- To be able to define the characteristics of an object-oriented programming language.
- To be able to create a new C++ class from an existing class by using inheritance.
- To be able to create a new C++ class from an existing class by using composition.
- To be able to distinguish between static and dynamic binding of operations to objects.
- To be able to apply the object-oriented design methodology to solve a problem.
- To be able to take an object-oriented design and code it in C++.

In Chapter 11, we introduced the concept of data abstraction—the separation of the logical properties of a data type from the details of how it is implemented. We expanded on this concept by defining the notion of an abstract data type (ADT) and by using the C++ class mechanism to incorporate both data and operations into a single data type. In that chapter and Chapter 13, we saw how an object of a given class maintains its own private data and is manipulated by calling its public member functions.

In this chapter, we examine how classes and objects can be used to guide the entire software development process. Although the design phase precedes the implementation phase in the development of software, we reverse the order of presentation in this chapter. We begin with *object-oriented programming,* a topic that includes design but is more about implementation issues. We describe the basic principles, terminology, and programming language features associated with the object-oriented approach. After presenting these fundamental concepts, we look more closely at the design phase—*object-oriented design.*

Object-Oriented Programming

Until now, we have used functional decomposition (also called *structured design*), in which we decompose a problem into modules, where each module is a self-contained collection of steps that solves one part of the overall problem. The process of implementing a functional decomposition is often called **structured** (or **procedural**) **programming.** Some modules are translated directly into a few programming language instructions, whereas others are coded as functions with or without arguments. The end result is a program that is a collection of interacting functions (see Figure 14-1). Throughout structured design and structured programming, data is considered a passive quantity to be acted upon by control structures and functions.

Structured design is satisfactory for programming in the small (a concept we discussed in Chapter 4) but often does not "scale up" well for programming in the large. In building large software systems, structured design has two important limitations. First, the technique yields an inflexible structure. If the top-level algorithm requires modification, the changes may force many lower-level algorithms to be modified as well. Second, the technique does not lend itself easily to code reuse. By *code reuse* we mean the ability to use pieces of code—either as they are or adapted slightly—in other sections of the program or in other programs. It is rare to be able to take a complicated C++ function and reuse it easily in a different context.

A methodology that often works better for creating large software systems is object-oriented design (OOD), which we introduced briefly in Chapter 4. OOD decomposes a problem into objects—self-contained entities composed of data and operations on the data. The process of imple-

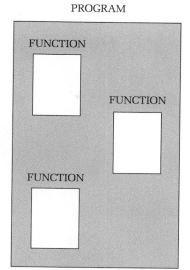

menting an object-oriented design is called **object-oriented programming (OOP).** The end result is a program that is a collection of interacting objects (see Figure 14-2). In OOD and OOP, data plays a leading role; the primary contribution of algorithms is to implement the operations on objects. In this chapter, we'll see why OOD tends to result in programs that are more flexible and conducive to code reuse than programs produced by structured design.

Several programming languages have been created specifically to support OOD and OOP: C++, Java, Smalltalk, Simula, CLOS, Objective-C, Eiffel, Actor, Object-Pascal, recent versions of Turbo Pascal, and others. These languages, called *object-oriented programming languages*, have facilities for

1. Data abstraction
2. Inheritance
3. Dynamic binding

You have already seen that C++ supports data abstraction through the class mechanism. Some non-OOP languages also have facilities for data abstraction. But only OOP languages support the other two concepts—*inheritance* and *dynamic binding*. Before we define these two concepts, we discuss some of the fundamental ideas and terminology of object-oriented programming.

FIGURE 14-2
Program Resulting
from Object-
Oriented
Programming

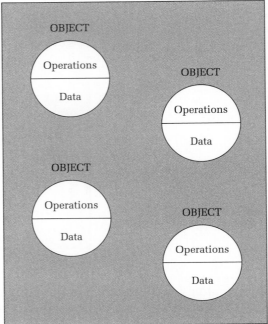

Structured (procedural) programming   The construction of programs that are collections of interacting functions or procedures.

Object-oriented programming (OOP)   The use of data abstraction, inheritance, and dynamic binding to construct programs that are collections of interacting objects.

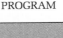 **Objects**

The major principles of OOP originated as far back as the mid-1960s with a language called Simula. However, much of the current terminology of OOP is due to Smalltalk, a language developed in the late 1970s at Xerox's Palo Alto Research Center. In OOP, the term *object* has a very specific meaning: It is a self-contained entity encapsulating data and operations on the data. In other words, an object represents an instance of an ADT. More specifically, an object has an internal *state* (the current values of its private data, called *instance variables*), and it has a set of *methods* (public operations). Methods are the only means by which an object's state can be inspected or modified by another object. An object-oriented program consists of a collection of objects, communicating with one another by *message passing*. If object A wants object B to perform some task, object A sends a message containing the name of the object (B, in this case) and the name of the particular method to execute. Object B responds by executing this method in its own way, possibly changing its state and sending messages to other objects as well.

As you can tell, an object is quite different from a traditional data structure. A C++ struct is a passive data structure that contains only data and is acted upon by a program. In contrast, an object is an active data structure; the data and the code that manipulates the data are bound together within the object. In OOP jargon, an object knows how to manipulate itself.

The vocabulary of Smalltalk has influenced the vocabulary of OOP. The literature of OOP is full of phrases such as "methods," "instance variables," and "sending a message to." Here are some OOP terms and their C++ equivalents:

OOP	C++
Object	Class object or class instance
Instance variable	Private data member
Method	Public member function
Message passing	Function call (to a public member function)

In C++, we define the properties and behavior of objects by using the class mechanism. Within a program, classes can be related to each other in various ways. The three most common relationships are as follows:

1. Two classes are independent of each other and have nothing in common.
2. Two classes are related by *inheritance*.
3. Two classes are related by *composition*.

The first relationship—none—is not very interesting. Let's look at the other two—inheritance and composition.

Inheritance

In the world at large, it is often possible to arrange concepts into an *inheritance hierarchy*—a hierarchy in which each concept inherits the properties of the concept immediately above it in the hierarchy. For example, we might classify different kinds of vehicles according to the inheritance hierarchy in Figure 14-3. Moving down the hierarchy, each kind of vehicle is more specialized than its *parent* (and all of its *ancestors*) and is more general than its *child* (and all of its *descendants*). A wheeled vehicle inherits properties common to all vehicles (it holds one or more people and carries them from place to place) but has an additional property that makes it more specialized (it has wheels). A car inherits properties common to all wheeled vehicles but also has additional, more specialized properties (four wheels, an engine, a body, and so forth).

The inheritance relationship can be viewed as an *is-a relationship*. Every two-door car is a car, every car is a wheeled vehicle, and every wheeled vehicle is a vehicle.

OOP languages provide a way of creating inheritance relationships among classes. In these languages, **inheritance** is the mechanism by which one class acquires the properties of another class. You can take an existing class A (called the **base class** or **superclass**) and create from it a new class B (called the **derived class** or **subclass**). The derived class B inherits all the properties of its base class A. In particular, the data and operations defined for A are now also defined for B. (Notice the is-a relationship—every B is also an A.) The idea, next, is to specialize class B, usually by adding specific properties to those already inherited from A. Let's look at an example in C++.

Inheritance   A mechanism by which one class acquires the properties—the data and operations—of another class.

Base class (superclass)   The class being inherited from.

Derived class (subclass)   The class that inherits.

FIGURE 14-3
Inheritance
Hierarchy

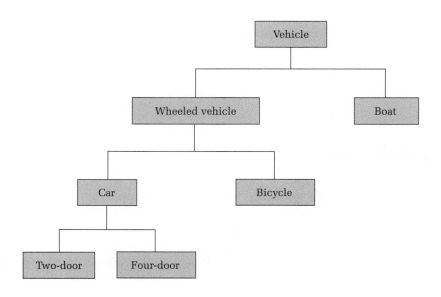

Deriving One Class from Another

Suppose that someone has already written a `Time` class with the following specification, abbreviated by omitting the preconditions and postconditions:

```
class Time
{
public:
    void Set( /* in */ int hours,
              /* in */ int minutes,
              /* in */ int seconds );
    void Increment();
    void Write() const;
    Time( /* in */ int initHrs,          // Constructor
          /* in */ int initMins,
          /* in */ int initSecs );
    Time();                              // Default constructor,
private:                                 //    setting time to 0:0:0
    int hrs;
    int mins;
    int secs;
};
```

This class is the same as our `TimeType` class of Chapter 11, simplified by omitting the `Equal` and `LessThan` member functions. Figure 14-4 displays a *class interface diagram* for the `Time` class. The public interface, shown as ovals in the side of the large circle, consists of the operations available to

FIGURE 14-4
Class Interface Diagram for `Time` Class

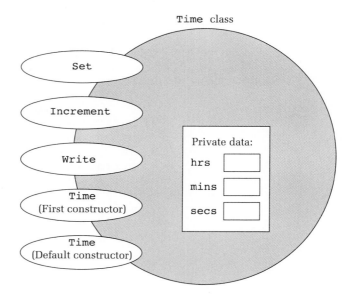

client code. The private data items shown in the interior are inaccessible to clients.

Suppose that we want to modify the Time class by adding, as private data, a variable of an enumeration type indicating the (American) time zone—EST for Eastern Standard Time, CST for Central Standard Time, MST for Mountain Standard Time, PST for Pacific Standard Time, EDT for Eastern Daylight Time, CDT for Central Daylight Time, MDT for Mountain Daylight Time, or PDT for Pacific Daylight Time. We'll need to modify the Set function and the class constructors to accommodate a time zone value. And the Write function should print the time in the form

```
12:34:10 CST
```

The Increment function, which advances the time by one second, does not need to be changed.

To add these time zone features to the Time class, the conventional approach would be to obtain the source code found in the time.cpp implementation file, analyze in detail how the class is implemented, then modify and recompile the source code. This process has several drawbacks. If Time is an off-the-shelf class on a system, the source code for the implementation is probably unavailable. Even if it is available, modifying it may introduce bugs into a previously debugged solution. Access to the source code also violates a principal benefit of abstraction: Users of an abstraction should not need to know how it is implemented.

In C++, as in other OOP languages, there is a far quicker and safer way in which to add time zone features: Use inheritance. Let's derive a new class from the Time class and then specialize it. This new, extended time class—call it ExtTime—inherits the members of its base class, Time. Here is the declaration of ExtTime:

```
enum ZoneType {EST, CST, MST, PST, EDT, CDT, MDT, PDT};

class ExtTime : public Time
{
public:
    void Set( /* in */ int       hours,
              /* in */ int       minutes,
              /* in */ int       seconds,
              /* in */ ZoneType timeZone );
    void Write() const;
    ExtTime( /* in */ int       initHrs,      // Constructor
             /* in */ int       initMins,
             /* in */ int       initSecs,
             /* in */ ZoneType initZone );
```

```
        ExtTime();                      // Default constructor,
                                        //   setting time to
private:                                //   0:0:0 EST
    ZoneType zone;
};
```

The opening line

```
class ExtTime : public Time
```

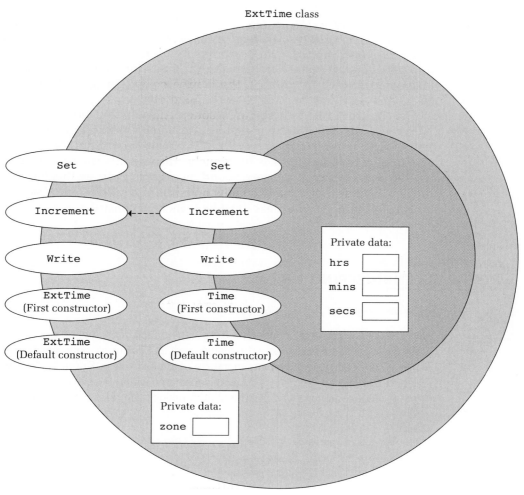

FIGURE 14-5
Class Interface Diagram for ExtTime Class

states that ExtTime is derived from Time. The reserved word public declares Time to be a *public base class* of ExtTime. This means that all public members of Time (except constructors) are also public members of ExtTime. In other words, Time's member functions Set, Increment, and Write can also be invoked for ExtTime objects.* However, the public part of ExtTime specializes the base class by reimplementing (redefining) the inherited functions Set and Write and by providing its own constructors.

The private part of ExtTime declares that a new private member is added: zone. The private members of ExtTime are therefore hrs, mins, secs (all inherited from Time), and zone. Figure 14-5 pictures the relationship between the ExtTime and Time classes.

This diagram shows that each ExtTime object has a Time object as a *subobject*. Every ExtTime is a Time, and more. C++ uses the terms *base class* and *derived class* instead of *superclass* and *subclass*. The terms *superclass* and *subclass* can be confusing because the prefix *sub-* usually implies something smaller than the original (for example, a subset of a mathematical set). In contrast, a subclass is often "bigger" than its superclass—that is, it has more data and/or functions.

In Figure 14-5, you see an arrow between the two ovals labeled Increment. Because Time is a public base class of ExtTime, and because Increment is not redefined by ExtTime, the Increment function available to clients of ExtTime is the same as the one inherited from Time. We use the arrow between the corresponding ovals to indicate this fact. (Notice in the diagram that Time's constructors are operations on Time, not on ExtTime. The ExtTime class must have its own constructors.)

SOFTWARE ENGINEERING TIP

Inheritance and Accessibility

With C++, it is important to understand that inheritance does not imply accessibility. Although a derived class inherits the members of its base class, both private and public, it cannot access the private members of the base class. Figure 14-5 shows the variables hrs, mins, and secs to be encapsulated within the Time class. Neither external client code nor ExtTime member functions can refer to these three vari-

---

* If a class declaration omits the word public and begins as

class DerivedClass : BaseClass

or if it explicitly uses the word private,

class DerivedClass : private BaseClass

then BaseClass is called a *private base class* of DerivedClass. Public members of BaseClass are *not* public members of DerivedClass. That is, clients of DerivedClass cannot invoke BaseClass operations on DerivedClass objects. We do not work with private base classes in this book.

ables directly. If a derived class were able to access the private members of its base class, any programmer could derive a class from another and then write code to directly inspect or modify the private data, defeating the benefits of encapsulation and information hiding.

Specification of the ExtTime Class

Below is the fully documented specification of the ExtTime class. Notice that the preprocessor directive

```
#include "time.h"
```

is necessary for the compiler to verify the consistency of the derived class with its base class.

```
//****************************************************************
// SPECIFICATION FILE (exttime.h)
// This file gives the specification of an ExtTime abstract data
// type.  The Time class is a public base class of ExtTime, so
// public operations of Time are also public operations of ExtTime.
//****************************************************************
#include "time.h"

enum ZoneType {EST, CST, MST, PST, EDT, CDT, MDT, PDT};

class ExtTime : public Time
{
public:
    void Set( /* in */ int       hours,
              /* in */ int       minutes,
              /* in */ int       seconds,
              /* in */ ZoneType timeZone );
        // Precondition:
        //     0 <= hours <= 23  &&  0 <= minutes <= 59
        //  && 0 <= seconds <= 59  &&  timeZone is assigned
        // Postcondition:
        //     Time is set according to the incoming parameters

    void Write() const;
        // Postcondition:
        //     Time has been output in the form HH:MM:SS ZZZ
        //     where ZZZ is the time zone

    ExtTime( /* in */ int       initHrs,
             /* in */ int       initMins,
             /* in */ int       initSecs,
             /* in */ ZoneType initZone );
```

```
                    // Precondition:
                    //    0 <= initHrs <= 23  &&  0 <= initMins <= 59
                    //  && 0 <= initSecs <= 59  &&  initZone is assigned
                    // Postcondition:
                    //     Class object is constructed
                    //  && Time is set according to the incoming parameters

                ExtTime();
                    // Postcondition:
                    //     Class object is constructed
                    //  && Time is 0:0:0 Eastern Standard Time
            private:
                ZoneType zone;
            };
```

With this new class, the programmer can set the time with a time zone (via a class constructor or the redefined `Set` function), output the time with its time zone (via the redefined `Write` function), and increment the time by one second (via the inherited `Increment` function):

```
// Client code:

#include "exttime.h"
  ⋮
ExtTime time1(8, 35, 0, PST);
ExtTime time2;                      // Default constructor called

time2.Write();                      // Outputs 0:0:0 EST
cout << endl;

time2.Set(16, 49, 23, CDT);
time2.Write();                      // Outputs 16:49:23 CDT
cout << endl;

time1.Increment();
time1.Increment();
time1.Write();                      // Outputs 08:35:02 PST
cout << endl;
  ⋮
```

Implementation of the `ExtTime` Class

The implementation of the `ExtTime` class needs to deal only with the new features that are different from `Time`. Specifically, we must write code to redefine the `Set` and `Write` functions and we must write the two constructors.

With derived classes, constructors are subject to special rules. At run time, the base class constructor is implicitly called first, before the body of the derived class's constructor executes. Additionally, if the base class constructor requires arguments, these arguments must be passed by the derived class's constructor. To see how these rules pertain, let's examine the implementation file exttime.cpp (see Figure 14-6).

FIGURE 14-6

ExtTime Implementation File

```
//****************************************************************
// IMPLEMENTATION FILE (exttime.cpp)
// This file implements the ExtTime member functions.
// The Time class is a public base class of ExtTime
//****************************************************************
#include "exttime.h"
#include <iostream>
#include <string>

using namespace std;

// Additional private members of class:
//     ZoneType zone;


//****************************************************************

ExtTime::ExtTime( /* in */ int      initHrs,
                  /* in */ int      initMins,
                  /* in */ int      initSecs,
                  /* in */ ZoneType initZone )


     : Time(initHrs, initMins, initSecs)

// Constructor

// Precondition:
//     0 <= initHrs <= 23  &&  0 <= initMins <= 59
//   && 0 <= initSecs <= 59  &&  initZone is assigned
// Postcondition:
//     Time is set according to initHrs, initMins, and initSecs
//     (via call to base class constructor)
//   && zone == initZone

{
    zone = initZone;
}


//****************************************************************

ExtTime::ExtTime()
```

Figure 14-6
ExtTime
Implementation
File
(continued)

```cpp
// Default constructor

// Postcondition:
//     Time is 0:0:0 (via implicit call to base class's
//     default constructor)
//   && zone == EST

{
    zone = EST;
}

//*******************************************************************

void ExtTime::Set( /* in */ int       hours,
                   /* in */ int       minutes,
                   /* in */ int       seconds,
                   /* in */ ZoneType timeZone )

// Precondition:
//     0 <= hours <= 23  &&  0 <= minutes <= 59
//   && 0 <= seconds <= 59  &&  timeZone is assigned
// Postcondition:
//     Time is set according to hours, minutes, and seconds
//   && zone == timeZone

{
    Time::Set(hours, minutes, seconds);
    zone = timeZone;
}

//*******************************************************************

void ExtTime::Write() const

// Postcondition:
//     Time has been output in the form HH:MM:SS ZZZ
//     where ZZZ is the time zone

{
    static string zoneString[8] =
    {
        "EST", "CST", "MST", "PST", "EDT", "CDT", "MDT", "PDT"
    };

    Time::Write();
    cout << ' ' << zoneString[zone];
}
```

In the first constructor in Figure 14-6, notice the syntax by which a constructor passes arguments to its base class constructor:

```
ExtTime::ExtTime( /* in */ int      initHrs,
                  /* in */ int      initMins,
                  /* in */ int      initSecs,
                  /* in */ ZoneType initZone )

    : Time(initHrs, initMins, initSecs)      ←      Constructor initializer

{
    zone = initZone;
}
```

After the parameter list to the ExtTime constructor (but before its body), you insert what is called a *constructor initializer*—a colon and then the name of the base class along with the arguments to *its* constructor. When an ExtTime object is created with a declaration such as

```
ExtTime time1(8, 35, 0, PST);
```

the ExtTime constructor receives four arguments. The first three are simply passed along to the Time class constructor by means of the constructor initializer. After the Time class constructor has executed (creating the base class subobject as shown in Figure 14-5), the body of the ExtTime constructor executes, setting zone equal to the fourth argument.

The second constructor in Figure 14-6 (the default constructor) does not need a constructor initializer; there are no arguments to pass to the base class's default constructor. When an ExtTime object is created with the declaration

```
ExtTime time2;
```

the ExtTime class's default constructor first implicitly calls Time's default constructor, after which its body executes, setting zone to EST.

Next, look at the Set function in Figure 14-6. This function reimplements the Set function inherited from the base class. Consequently, there are two distinct Set functions, one a public member of the Time class, the other a public member of the ExtTime class. Their full names are Time::Set and ExtTime::Set. In Figure 14-6, the ExtTime::Set function begins by "reaching up" into its base class and calling Time::Set to set the hours, minutes, and seconds. (Remember that a class derived from Time cannot access the private data hrs, mins, and secs directly; these variables are private to the Time class.) The function then finishes by assigning a value to ExtTime's private data, the zone variable.

The `Write` function in Figure 14-6 uses a similar strategy. It reaches up into its base class and invokes `Time::Write` to output the hours, minutes, and seconds. Then it outputs a string corresponding to the time zone. (Recall that a value of enumeration type cannot be output directly in C++. If we were to print the value of `zone` directly, the output would be an integer from 0 through 7—the internal representations of the `ZoneType` values.) The `Write` function establishes an array of eight strings and selects the correct string by using `zone` to index into the array. Why is `zoneString` declared to be `static`? Remember that by default, local variables in C++ are automatic variables—that is, memory is allocated for them when the function begins execution and is deallocated when the function returns. With `zoneString` declared as `static`, the array is allocated once only, when the program begins execution, and remains allocated until the program terminates. From function call to function call, the computer does not waste time creating and destroying the array.

Now we can compile the file `exttime.cpp` into an object code file, say, `exttime.obj`. After writing a test driver and compiling it into `test.obj`, we obtain an executable file by linking three object files:

1. `test.obj`
2. `exttime.obj`
3. `time.obj`

We can then test the resulting program.

The remarkable thing about derived classes and inheritance is that modification of the base class is unnecessary. The source code for the implementation of the `Time` class may be unavailable. Yet variations of this ADT can continue to be created without that source code, in ways the creator never even considered. Through classes and inheritance, OOP languages facilitate code reuse. A class such as `Time` can be used as-is in many different contexts, or it can be adapted to a particular context by using inheritance. Inheritance allows us to create *extensible* data abstractions—a derived class typically extends the base class by including additional private data or public operations or both.

Avoiding Multiple Inclusion of Header Files

We saw that the specification file `exttime.h` begins with an `#include` directive to insert the file `time.h`:

```
#include "time.h"

enum ZoneType {EST, CST, MST, PST, EDT, CDT, MDT, PDT};

class ExtTime : public Time
{
    ⋮
};
```

Now think about what happens if a programmer using the ExtTime class already has included time.h for other purposes, overlooking the fact that exttime.h also includes it:

```
#include "time.h"
#include "exttime.h"
```

The preprocessor inserts the file time.h, then exttime.h, and then time.h a second time (because exttime.h also includes time.h). The result is a compile-time error, because the Time class is defined twice.

The widely used solution to this problem is to write time.h this way:

```
#ifndef TIME_H
#define TIME_H
class Time
{
    ⋮
};
#endif
```

The lines beginning with "#" are directives to the preprocessor. TIME_H (or any identifier you wish to use) is a preprocessor identifier, not a C++ program identifier. In effect, these directives say:

If the preprocessor identifier TIME_H is not already defined, then

1. define TIME_H as an identifier known to the preprocessor,

and

2. let the declaration of the Time class pass through to the compiler.

If a subsequent #include "time.h" is encountered, the test #ifndef TIME_H will fail. The Time class declaration will not pass through to the compiler a second time.

Composition

Earlier we said that two classes typically exhibit one of the following relationships: They are independent of each other, they are related by inheritance, or they are related by **composition**. Composition (or **containment**) is the relationship in which the internal data of one class A includes an object of another class B. Stated another way, a B object is contained within an A object.

Composition (containment)   A mechanism by which the internal data (the state) of one class includes an object of another class.

C++ does not have (or need) any special language notation for composition. You simply declare an object of one class to be one of the data members of another class. Let's look at an example.

Design of a `TimeCard` Class

You are developing a program to manage a factory's payroll. Employees are issued time cards containing their ID numbers. When reporting for work, an employee "punches in" by inserting the card into a clock, which punches the current time onto the card. When leaving work, the employee takes a new card and "punches out" to record the departure time. For your program, you decide that you need a `TimeCard` ADT to represent an employee's time card. The abstract data consists of an ID number and a time. The abstract operations include Punch the Time, Print the Time Card Data, constructor operations, and others. To implement the ADT, you must choose a concrete data representation for the abstract data and you must implement the operations. Assuming an employee ID number is a large integer value, you choose the `long` data type to represent the ID number. To represent time, you remember that one of your friends has already written and debugged a `Time` class (we'll use the one from earlier in this chapter). At this point, you create a `TimeCard` class declaration as follows:

```
#include "time.h"
  ⋮
class TimeCard
{
public:
    void Punch( /* in */ int hours,
                /* in */ int minutes,
                /* in */ int seconds );
    void Print() const;
      ⋮
    TimeCard( /* in */ long idNum,
              /* in */ int  initHrs,
              /* in */ int  initMins,
              /* in */ int  initSecs );
    TimeCard();
private:
    long id;
    Time timeStamp;
};
```

FIGURE 14-7
Class Interface Diagram for TimeCard Class

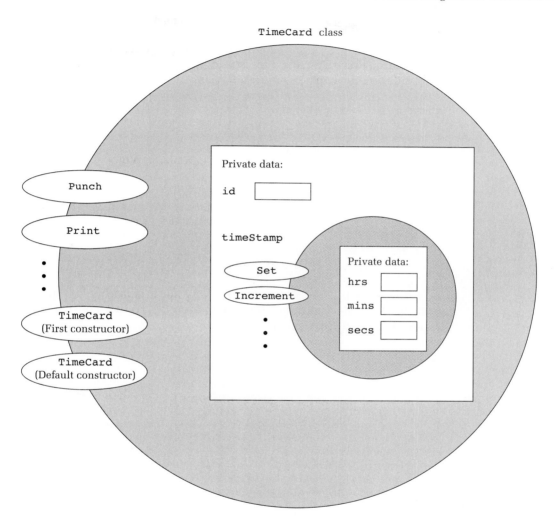

In designing the TimeCard class, you have used composition; a TimeCard object is composed of a Time object (and a long variable). Composition creates a *has-a relationship*—a TimeCard object *has a* Time object as a subobject (see Figure 14-7).

Implementation of the `TimeCard` Class

The private data of `TimeCard` consists of a `long` variable named `id` and a `Time` object named `timeStamp`. The `TimeCard` member functions can manipulate `id` by using ordinary built-in operations, but they must manipulate `timeStamp` through the member functions defined for the `Time` class. For example, you could implement the `Print` and `Punch` functions as follows:

```
void TimeCard::Print() const
{
    cout << "ID: "  << id << " Time: " ;
    timeStamp.Write();
}


void TimeCard::Punch( /* in */ int hours,
                      /* in */ int minutes,
                      /* in */ int seconds )
{
    timeStamp.Set(hours, minutes, seconds);
}
```

Implementing the class constructors is a bit more complicated to describe. Let's start with an implementation of the first constructor shown in the `TimeCard` class declaration:

```
TimeCard::TimeCard( /* in */ long idNum,
                    /* in */ int  initHrs,
                    /* in */ int  initMins,
                    /* in */ int  initSecs )

    : timeStamp(initHrs, initMins, initSecs)      ← Constructor initializer

{
    id = idNum;
}
```

This is the second time we've seen the unusual notation—the constructor initializer—inserted between the parameter list and the body of a constructor. The first time was when we implemented the parameterized `ExtTime` class constructor (Figure 14-6). There, we used the constructor initializer to pass some of the incoming arguments to the base class constructor. Here, we use a constructor initializer to pass some of the arguments to a member object's (`timeStamp`'s) constructor. Whether you are using inheritance or composition, the purpose of a constructor initializer is the same: to pass arguments to another constructor. The only difference is the following: With inheritance, you specify the name of the *base class* prior to the argument list, as follows.

```
ExtTime::ExtTime( /* in */ int      initHrs,
                  /* in */ int      initMins,
                  /* in */ int      initSecs,
                  /* in */ ZoneType initZone )

    : Time(initHrs, initMins, initSecs)
```

With composition, you specify the name of the *member object* prior to the argument list:

```
TimeCard::TimeCard( /* in */ long idNum,
                    /* in */ int  initHrs,
                    /* in */ int  initMins,
                    /* in */ int  initSecs )

    : timeStamp(initHrs, initMins, initSecs)
```

Furthermore, if a class has several members that are objects of classes with parameterized constructors, you form a list of constructor initializers separated by commas:

```
SomeClass::SomeClass( ... )

    : memberObject1(arg1, arg2), memberObject2(arg3)
```

Having discussed both inheritance and composition, we can give a complete description of the order in which constructors are executed:

Given a class X, if X is a derived class, its base class constructor is executed first. Next, constructors for member objects (if any) are executed. Finally, the body of X's constructor is executed.

When a `TimeCard` object is created, the constructor for its `timeStamp` member is first invoked. After the `timeStamp` object is constructed, the body of `TimeCard`'s constructor is executed, setting the `id` member equal to `idNum`.

The second constructor shown in the `TimeCard` class declaration—the default constructor—has no parameters and could be implemented as follows:

```
TimeCard::TimeCard()
{
    id = 0;
}
```

In this case, what happened to construction of the `timeStamp` member object? We didn't include a constructor initializer, so the `timeStamp` object is first constructed using the *default* constructor of the `Time` class, after which the body of the `TimeCard` constructor is executed. The result is a time card having a time stamp of 0:0:0 and an ID number of 0.

Dynamic Binding and Virtual Functions

Early in the chapter, we said that object-oriented programming languages provide language features that support three concepts: data abstraction, inheritance, and dynamic binding. The phrase *dynamic binding* means, more specifically, *dynamic binding of an operation to an object*. To explain this concept, let's begin with an example.

Given the `Time` and `ExtTime` classes of this chapter, the following code creates two class objects and outputs the time represented by each.

```
Time     startTime(8, 30, 0);
ExtTime endTime(10, 45, 0, CST);

startTime.Write();
cout << endl;
endTime.Write();
cout << endl;
```

This code fragment invokes two different `Write` functions, even though the functions appear to have the same name. The first function call invokes the `Write` function of the `Time` class, printing out three values: hours, minutes, and seconds. The second call invokes the `Write` function of the `ExtTime` class, printing out four values: hours, minutes, seconds, and time zone. In this code fragment, the compiler uses **static** (compile-time) **binding** of the operation (`Write`) to the appropriate object. The compiler can easily determine which `Write` function to call by checking the data type of the associated object.

Static binding   The compile-time determination of which function to call for a particular object.

In some situations, the compiler cannot determine the type of an object, and the binding of an operation to an object must occur at run time. One situation, which we look at now, involves passing class objects as arguments.

The basic C++ rule for passing class objects as arguments is that the argument and its corresponding parameter must be of identical type. With inheritance, though, C++ relaxes the rule. You may pass an object of a child class *C* to an object of its parent class *P*, but not the other way around—that is, you cannot pass an object of type *P* to an object of type *C*. More generally, you can pass an object of a descendant class to an object of any of its ancestor classes. This rule has a tremendous benefit—it allows us to write a single function that applies to any descendant class instead of writing a different function for each. For example, we could write a fancy Print function that takes as an argument an object of type Time or any class descended from Time:

```
void Print( /* in */ Time someTime )
{
    cout << "*************************" << endl;
    cout << "** The time is ";
    someTime.Write();
    cout << endl;
    cout << "*************************" << endl;
}
```

Given the code fragment

```
Time     startTime(8, 30, 0);
ExtTime endTime(10, 45, 0, CST);

Print(startTime);
Print(endTime);
```

the compiler lets us pass either a Time object or an ExtTime object to the Print function. Unfortunately, the output is not what we would like. When endTime is printed, the time zone CST is missing from the output. Let's see why.

The Slicing Problem

Our Print function uses passing by value for the parameter someTime. Passing by value sends a copy of the argument to the parameter. Whenever you pass an object of a child class to an object of its parent class using a pass by value, only the data members they have in common are copied. Remember that a child class is often "larger" than its parent—that is, it contains additional data members. For example, a Time object has three data members (hrs, mins, and secs), but an ExtTime object has four data members (hrs, mins, secs, and zone). When the larger class object is copied to the smaller parameter using a pass by value, the extra data members are discarded or "sliced off." This situation is called the *slicing problem* (see Figure 14-8).

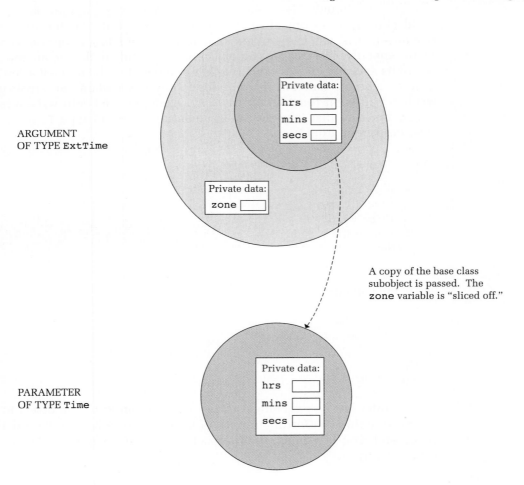

FIGURE 14-8
The Slicing Problem Resulting from Passing by Value

ARGUMENT
OF TYPE `ExtTime`

PARAMETER
OF TYPE `Time`

A copy of the base class
subobject is passed. The
`zone` variable is "sliced off."

(The slicing problem also occurs with assignment operations. In the statement

```
parentClassObject = childClassObject;
```

only the data members that the two objects have in common are copied. Additional data members contained in `childClassObject` are not copied.)

With passing by reference, the slicing problem does not occur because the *address* of the caller's argument is sent to the function. Let's change the heading of our `Print` function so that `someTime` is a reference parameter:

```
void Print( /* in */ Time& someTime )
```

Now when we pass endTime as the argument, its address is sent to the function. Its time zone member is not sliced off because no copying takes place. But to our dismay, the Print function *still* prints only three of endTime's data members—hours, minutes, and seconds.

Within the Print function, the difficulty is that static binding is used in the statement

```
someTime.Write();
```

The compiler must generate machine language code for the Print function at compile time, but the type of the actual argument (Time or ExtTime) isn't known until run time. How can the compiler know which Write function to use—Time::Write or ExtTime::Write? The compiler cannot know, so it uses Time::Write because the parameter someTime is of type Time. Therefore, the Print function always prints just three values—hours, minutes, and seconds—regardless of the type of the argument. Fortunately, C++ provides a very simple solution to our problem: *virtual functions.*

Virtual Functions

Suppose we make one small change to our Time class declaration: We begin the declaration of the Write function with the reserved word virtual.

```
class Time
{
public:
    ⋮
    virtual void Write() const;
    ⋮
private:
    ⋮
};
```

Declaring a member function to be virtual instructs the compiler to generate code that guarantees **dynamic** (run-time) **binding** of a function to an object. That is, the determination of which function to call is postponed until run time. (Note that to make Write a virtual function, the word virtual appears in one place only—the Time class declaration. It does not appear in the Write function definition that is located in the time.cpp file, nor does it appear in any descendant class—such as ExtTime—that redefines the Write function.)

Dynamic binding   The run-time determination of which function to call for a particular object.

Virtual functions work in the following way. If a class object is passed *by reference* to some function, and if the body of that function contains a statement

```
param.MemberFunc ( ... );
```

then

1. If `MemberFunc` is not a virtual function, the type of the *parameter* determines which function to call. (Static binding is used.)
2. If `MemberFunc` is a virtual function, the type of the *argument* determines which function to call. (Dynamic binding is used.)

With just one word—virtual—the difficulties we encountered with our `Print` function disappear entirely. If we declare `Write` to be a virtual function in the `Time` class, the function

```
void Print( /* in */ Time& someTime )
{
    ⋮
    someTime.Write();
    ⋮
}
```

works correctly for arguments either of type `Time` or of type `ExtTime`. The correct `Write` function (`Time::Write` or `ExtTime::Write`) is invoked because the argument carries the information necessary at run time to choose the appropriate function. Deriving a new and unanticipated class from `Time` presents no complications. If this new class redefines the `Write` function, then our `Print` function still works correctly. Dynamic binding ensures that each object knows how to print itself, and the appropriate version will be invoked. In OOP terminology, `Write` is a **polymorphic operation**—an operation that has multiple meanings depending on the type of the object that responds to it at run time.

Polymorphic operation   An operation that has multiple meanings depending on the type of the object to which it is bound at run time.

Here are some things to know about using virtual functions in C++:

1. To obtain dynamic binding, you must use passing by reference when passing a class object to a function. If you use passing by value, the compiler does not use the `virtual` mechanism; instead, member slicing and static binding occur.
2. In the declaration of a virtual function, the word `virtual` appears only in the base class, not in any derived class.
3. If a base class declares a virtual function, it *must* implement that function, even if the body is empty.
4. A derived class is not required to provide its own reimplementation of a virtual function. In this case, the base class's version is used by default.
5. A derived class cannot redefine the function return type of a virtual function.

Object-Oriented Design

We have looked at language features that let us implement an object-oriented design. Now let's turn to the phase that precedes implementation—OOD itself.

A computer program usually models some real-life activity or concept. A banking program models the real-life activities associated with a bank. A spreadsheet program models a real spreadsheet, a large paper form used by accountants and financial planners. A robotics program models human perception and human motion.

Nearly always, the aspect of the world that we are modeling (the *application domain* or *problem domain*) consists of objects—checking accounts, bank tellers, spreadsheet rows, spreadsheet columns, robot arms, robot legs. The computer program that solves the real-life problem also includes objects (the *solution domain*)—counters, lists, menus, windows, and so forth. OOD is based on the philosophy that programs are easier to write and understand if the major objects in a program correspond closely to the objects in the problem domain.

There are many ways in which to perform object-oriented design. Different authors advocate different techniques. Our purpose is not to choose one particular technique or to present a summary of all the techniques. Rather, our purpose is to describe a three-step process that captures the essence of OOD:

1. Identify the objects and operations.
2. Determine the relationships among objects.
3. Design the driver.

In this section, we do not show a complete example of an object-oriented design of a problem solution—we save that for the Problem-Solving Case Study at the end of the chapter. Instead, we describe the important issues involved in each of the three steps.

Step 1: Identify the Objects and Operations

Recall that structured design (functional decomposition) begins with identification of the major actions the program is to perform. In contrast, OOD begins by identifying the major objects and the associated operations on those objects. In both design methods, it is often difficult to see where to start.

To identify solution-domain objects, a good way to start is to look at the problem domain. More specifically, go to the problem definition and look for important nouns and verbs. The nouns (and noun phrases) may suggest objects; the verbs (and verb phrases) may suggest operations. For example, the problem definition for a banking program might include the following sentences:

... The program must handle a customer's savings account. The customer is allowed to deposit funds into the account and withdraw funds from the account, and the bank must pay interest on a quarterly basis. ...

In these sentences, the key nouns are

Savings account
Customer

and the key verb phrases are

Deposit funds
Withdraw funds
Pay interest

Although we are working with a very small portion of the entire problem definition, the list of nouns suggests two potential objects: savingsAccount and customer. The operations on a savingsAccount object are suggested by the list of verb phrases—namely, Deposit, Withdraw, and PayInterest. What are the operations on a customer object? We would need more information from the rest of the problem definition in order to answer this question. In fact, customer may not turn out to be a useful object at all. The nouns-and-verbs technique is only a starting point—it points us to *potential* objects and operations.

Determining which nouns and verbs are significant is one of the most difficult aspects of OOD. There are no cookbook formulas for doing so, and there probably never will be. Not all nouns become objects, and not all verbs become operations. The nouns-and-verbs technique is imperfect, but it does give us a first approximation to a solution.

The solution domain includes not only objects drawn from the problem domain but also *implementation-level* objects. These are objects that do not model the problem domain but are used in building the program itself. In systems with graphical user interfaces—Microsoft Windows or the Macintosh operating system, for example—a program may need several kinds of implementation-level objects: window objects, menu objects, objects that respond to mouse clicks, and so on. Objects such as these are often available in class libraries so that we don't need to design and implement them from scratch each time we need them in different programs.

Step 2: Determine the Relationships Among Objects

After selecting potential objects and operations, the next step is to examine the relationships among the objects. In particular, we want to see whether certain objects might be related either by inheritance or by composition. Inheritance and composition relationships not only pave the way for code reuse—as we emphasized in our discussion of OOP—but also simplify the design and allow us to model the problem domain more accurately. For example, the banking problem may require several kinds of savings accounts—one for general customers, another for preferred customers, and another for children under the age of 12. If these are all variations on a basic savings account, the is-a relationship (and, therefore, inheritance) is probably appropriate. Starting with a SavingsAccount class that provides operations common to any savings account, we could design each of the other accounts as a child class of SavingsAccount, concentrating our efforts only on the properties that make each one different from the parent class.

Sometimes the choice between inheritance and composition is not immediately clear. Earlier we wrote a TimeCard class to represent an employee's time card. Given an existing Time class, we used composition to relate TimeCard and Time—the private part of the TimeCard class was composed of a Time object (and an ID number). We could also have used inheritance. We could have derived class TimeCard from Time (inheriting the hours, minutes, and seconds members) and then specialized it by adding an extra data member (the ID number) and the extra operations of Punch, Print, and so forth. Both inheritance and composition give us four private data members: hours, minutes, seconds, and ID number. However, the use of inheritance means that all of the Time operations are also valid for TimeCard objects. A user of the TimeCard class could—either intentionally or accidentally—invoke operations such as Set and Increment, which are not appropriate operations on a time card. Furthermore, inheritance leads to a confused design in this example. It is not true that a TimeCard *is a* Time; rather, a TimeCard *has a* Time (and an ID number). In general, the best design strategy is to use inheritance for is-a relationships and composition for has-a relationships.

Step 3: Design the Driver

The final step is to design the driver—the top-level algorithm. In OOD, the driver is the glue that puts the objects (along with their operations) together. When implementing the design in C++, the driver becomes the main function.

Notice that structured design *begins* with the design of the top-level algorithm, whereas OOD *ends* with the top-level algorithm. In OOD, most of the control flow has already been designed in steps 1 and 2; the algorithms are located within the operations on objects. As a result, the driver often has very little to do but process user commands or input some data and then delegate tasks to various objects.

*S*OFTWARE ENGINEERING TIP

The Iterative Nature of Object-Oriented Design

Software developers, researchers, and authors have proposed many different strategies for performing OOD. Common to nearly all of these strategies are three fundamental steps:

1. Identify the objects and operations.
2. Determine the relationships among objects.
3. Design the driver.

Experience with large software projects has shown that these three steps are not necessarily sequential—step 1, step 2, step 3, then we are done. In practice, step 1 occurs first, but only as a first approximation. During steps 2 and 3, new objects or operations may be discovered, leading us back to step 1 again. It is realistic to think of steps 1 through 3 not as a sequence but as a loop.

Furthermore, each step is an iterative process within itself. Step 1 may entail working and reworking our view of the objects and operations. Similarly, steps 2 and 3 often involve experimentation and revision. In any step, we may conclude that a potential object is not useful after all. Or we might decide to add or eliminate operations on a particular object.

There is always more than one way to solve a problem. Iterating and reiterating through the design phase leads to insights that produce a better solution.

Implementing the Design

In OOD, when we first identify an object, it is an *abstract object.* We do not immediately choose an exact data representation for that object. Similarly, the operations on objects begin as *abstract operations,* because there is no initial attempt to provide algorithms for these operations.

Eventually, we have to implement the objects and operations. For each abstract object, we must

- Choose a suitable data representation.
- Create algorithms for the abstract operations.

To select a data representation for an object, the C++ programmer has three options:

1. Use a built-in data type.
2. Use an existing ADT.
3. Create a new ADT.

For a given object, a good rule of thumb is to consider these three options in the order listed. A built-in type is the most straightforward to use and understand, and operations on these types are already defined by the language. If a built-in type is not adequate to represent an object, you should survey available ADTs in a class library (either the system's or your own) to see if any are a good match for the abstract object. If no suitable ADT exists, you must design and implement a new ADT to represent the object.

Fortunately, even if you must resort to option 3, the mechanisms of inheritance and composition allow you to combine options 2 and 3. When we needed an `ExtTime` class earlier in the chapter, we used inheritance to build on an existing `Time` class. And when we created a `TimeCard` class, we used composition to include a `Time` object in the private data.

In addition to choosing a data representation for the abstract object, we must implement the abstract operations. With OOD, the algorithms that implement the abstract operations are often short and straightforward. We have seen numerous examples in this chapter and in Chapters 11 and 13 in which the code for ADT operations is only a few lines long. But this is not always the case. If an operation is extremely complex, it may be best to treat the operation as a new problem and use functional decomposition on the control flow. In this situation, it is appropriate to apply both functional decomposition and object-oriented methodologies together. Experienced programmers are familiar with both methodologies and use them either independently or in combination with each other. However, the software development community is becoming increasingly convinced that although functional decomposition is important for designing low-level algorithms and operations on ADTs, the future in developing huge software systems lies in OOD and OOP.

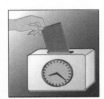

*P*ROBLEM-SOLVING CASE STUDY

Time Card Lookup

Problem: In this chapter, we talked about a factory that is computerizing its employee time card information. Work on the software has already begun, and you have been hired to join the effort. Each morning after the employees have punched in, the time card data (ID number and time stamp) for all employees is written to a file named `punchInFile`. Your task is to write a program that inputs the data from this file and allows the user to look up the time stamp (punch-in time) for any employee. The program should prompt the user for an ID number, look up that employee's time card information, and print it out. This interactive lookup process is repeated until the user types a negative number for the employee ID. The factory has, at most, 500 employees. If `punchInFile` contains more than 500 time cards, the excess time cards should be ignored and a warning message printed.

Input: Employee time card information (file stream `punchInFile`) and a sequence of employee ID numbers to be looked up (standard input device).
    Each line in `punchInFile` contains an employee's ID number (`long` integer) and the time he or she punched in (three integers—hours, minutes, and seconds):

```
246308 7 45 50
129336 8 15 29
```

The end-of-file condition signals the end of the input data.
    Interactive input from the user consists of employee ID numbers, entered one at a time in response to a prompt. A negative ID number signals the end of the interactive input.

PROBLEM-SOLVING CASE STUDY *cont'd.*

Output: For each employee ID that is input from the user, the corresponding time at which the employee punched in (or a message if the program cannot find a time card for the employee).

Below is a sample of the run-time dialogue. The user's input is highlighted.

```
Enter an employee ID (negative to quit): 129336
ID: 129336 Time: 08:15:29

Enter an employee ID (negative to quit): 222000
222000 has not punched in yet.

Enter an employee ID (negative to quit): -3
```

Discussion: Using structured design (functional decomposition), we would begin by thinking about the overall flow of control and the major actions to be performed. With object-oriented design, we consider the overall flow of control *last*.

We begin our design by identifying objects and their associated operations. The best place to start is by examining the problem domain. In object-oriented fashion, we search for important nouns and noun phrases in the problem definition. Here is a list of candidate objects (potential objects):

Factory
Employee
File `punchInFile`
ID number
Time card
Time stamp (punch-in time)
User

Reviewing this list, we conclude that the first two candidates—factory and employee—are probably not objects in the solution domain. In the problem we are to solve, a factory and an employee have no useful properties or interesting operations. Also, we can eliminate the last candidate listed—a user. *User* is merely a noun appearing in the problem definition; it has nothing to do with the problem domain. At this point, we can pare down our list of potential objects to the following:

File `punchInFile`
ID number
Time card
Time stamp

PROBLEM-SOLVING CASE STUDY cont'd.

To determine operations on these objects, we look for significant verb phrases in the problem definition. Here are some possibilities:

Punch a time card
Input data from the file
Look up time card information
Print out time card information
Input an employee ID

To associate these operations with the appropriate objects, let's make an *object table* as follows:

Object	Operation
File punchInFile	Input data from the file
ID number	Input an employee ID
Time card	Punch a time card
	Look up time card information
	Print out time card information
Time stamp	—

Analyzing the object table, we see that something is not quite right. For one thing, "Look up time card information" is not an operation on a single time card—it's more properly an operation that applies to a *collection* of time cards. What we're missing is an object that represents a list of time cards. That is, the program should read all the time cards from the data file and store them into a list. From this list, our program can look up the time card that matches a particular employee ID. Notice that this new object—the time card list—is an implementation-level object rather than a problem-domain object. This object is not readily apparent in the problem domain, yet we need it in order to design and implement the program.

Another thing we notice in the object table is the absence of any operations on the time stamp object. A little thought should convince us that this object simply represents the time of day. As with the Time class we discussed in this chapter, suitable operations might be to set the time and to print the time.

Here is a revised object table that includes the time card list object and refines the operations that might be suitable for each object:

PROBLEM-SOLVING CASE STUDY cont'd.

Object	Operation
File `punchInFile`	Open the file
	Input data from the file
ID number	Input an employee ID
	Print an employee ID
Time card	Set the ID number on a time card
	Inspect the ID number on a time card
	Punch the time stamp on a time card
	Inspect the time stamp on a time card
	Print the time card information
Time card list	Read all time cards into the list
	Look up time card information
Time stamp	Set the time of day
	Print the time

The second major step in OOD is to determine the relationships among the objects. Specifically, we're looking for inheritance and composition relationships. Our object table does not reveal any inheritance relationships. Using *is-a* as a guide, we cannot say that a time card is a kind of time stamp or vice versa, that a time card list is a kind of time card or vice versa, and so on. However, we find several composition relationships. Using *has-a* as a guide, we see that a time card has a time stamp as part of its state, a time card has an ID number as part of its state, and a time card list has several time cards as part of its state (see Figure 14-9). Discovery of these relationships helps us to further refine the design (and implementation) of the objects.

Now that we have determined a reasonable set of objects and operations, let's look at each object in detail. Keep in mind that the decisions we have made are not necessarily final. We may change our minds as we proceed, perhaps adding and deleting objects and operations as we focus in on a solution. Remember that OOD is an iterative process, characterized by experimentation and revision.

The `punchInFile` Object: This object represents an ordinary kind of input file with the ordinary operations of opening the file and reading from the file. No further design of this object is necessary. To implement the object, the obvious choice for a data representation is the `ifstream` class supplied by the C++ standard library. The `ifstream` class provides operations for opening and reading from a file, so we don't need to implement these operations ourselves.

The ID Number Object: This object merely represents an integer number (possibly large), and the only abstract operations we have identified are input and output. Therefore, the built-in `long` type is the most straightforward data representation. To implement the abstract operations of input and output we can simply use the `<<` and `>>` operators.

The Time Stamp Object: The time stamp object represents a time of day. There is no built-in type we can use as a data representation, but we can use an existing class—the `Time` class we worked with earlier in the chapter. The complete specification of the `Time` class appears below.

```
//********************************************************************
// SPECIFICATION FILE (time.h)
// This file gives the specification of a Time abstract data type
//********************************************************************
#ifndef TIME_H
#define TIME_H

class Time
{
public:
    void Set( /* in */ int hours,
              /* in */ int minutes,
              /* in */ int seconds );
        // Precondition:
        //     0 <= hours <= 23   &&   0 <= minutes <= 59
```

FIGURE 14-9
Composition
Relationships
Among Objects

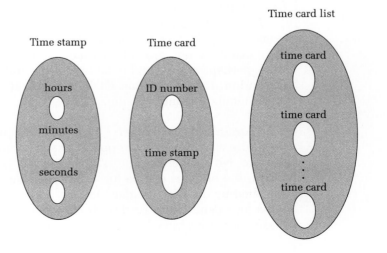

PROBLEM-SOLVING CASE STUDY cont'd.

```
                          //   && 0 <= seconds <= 59
                          // Postcondition:
                          //      Time is set according to the incoming parameters

                    void Increment();
                          // Postcondition:
                          //      Time has been advanced by one second, with
                          //      23:59:59 wrapping around to 0:0:0

                    void Write() const;
                          // Postcondition:
                          //      Time has been output in the form HH:MM:SS

                    Time( /* in */ int initHrs,
                          /* in */ int initMins,
                          /* in */ int initSecs );
                          // Precondition:
                          //      0 <= initHrs <= 23   &&  0 <= initMins <= 59
                          //   && 0 <= initSecs <= 59
                          // Postcondition:
                          //      Class object is constructed
                          //   && Time is set according to the incoming parameters

                    Time();
                          // Postcondition:
                          //      Class object is constructed  &&  Time is 0:0:0
              private:
                  int hrs;
                  int mins;
                  int secs;
              };
              #endif
```

(We surround the code with the preprocessor directives

```
#ifndef TIME_H
#define TIME_H
  ⋮
#endif
```

to prevent multiple inclusion of the Time class declaration in cases where a new class is created from Time by inheritance or composition. You may wish to review the section "Avoiding Multiple Inclusion of Header Files" in this chapter.)

You have already seen the implementations of the Time class member functions. They are the same as in the TimeType class of Chapter 11.

By declaring a time stamp object to be of type `Time`, we can simply implement our time stamp operations as calls to the `Time` class member functions:

```
Time timeStamp;

timeStamp.Set(hours, minutes, seconds);
timeStamp.Write();
```

Notice that the abstract operations we listed for a time stamp do not include an increment operation. Should we rewrite the `Time` class to eliminate the `Increment` function? No. Wherever possible, we want to reuse existing code. Let's use the `Time` class as it exists. The presence of the `Increment` function does no harm. We simply have no need to invoke it on behalf of a time stamp object.

Testing: Testing the `Time` class amounts to testing each of its member functions. In the Testing and Debugging section of Chapter 11, we described at length how to test a similar class, `TimeType`. `Time` is identical to `TimeType` except for the absence of two member functions, `Equal` and `LessThan`.

The Time Card Object: A time card object represents a pair of values: an employee ID number and a time stamp. The abstract operations are those we listed in our object table. There is no built-in type or existing C++ class that we can use directly to represent a time card, so we'll design a new class. (We sketched a `TimeCard` class earlier in the chapter, but it was not complete.)

Here is a possible specification of the class. Notice that we have added a new operation that did not appear in our object table: a class constructor.

```
//****************************************************************
// SPECIFICATION FILE (timecard.h)
// This file gives the specification of a TimeCard ADT
//****************************************************************
#ifndef TIMECARD_H
#define TIMECARD_H

#include "time.h"

class TimeCard
{
public:
    void Punch( /* in */ int hours,
```

```
                         /* in */ int minutes,
                         /* in */ int seconds );
              // Precondition:
              //      0 <= hours <= 23  &&  0 <= minutes <= 59
              //   && 0 <= seconds <= 59
              // Postcondition:
              //      Time is punched according to the incoming parameters

         void SetID( /* in */ long idNum );
              // Precondition:
              //      idNum is assigned
              // Postcondition:
              //      ID number on the time card is idNum

         long IDPart() const;
              // Postcondition:
              //      Function value == ID number on the time card

         Time TimePart() const;
              // Postcondition:
              //      Function value == time stamp on the time card

         void Print() const;
              // Postcondition:
              //      Time card has been output in the form
              //          ID: 235658 Time: 08:14:25

         TimeCard();
              // Postcondition:
              //      Class object is constructed with an ID number of 0
              //      and a time of 0:0:0
     private:
         long id;
         Time timeStamp;
     };
     #endif
```

The private part of this class declaration shows very clearly the composition relationship we proposed earlier—namely, that a time card object is composed of an ID number object and a time stamp object.

To implement the abstract operations on a time stamp, we must implement the `TimeCard` class member functions. Earlier in the chapter, we showed how to implement the constructor, `Punch`, and `Print` functions, so we do not repeat the discussion here. Now we must implement `SetID`, `IDPart`, and `TimePart`. These are easy. The body of `SetID` merely sets the private variable `id` equal to the incoming parameter, `idNum`:

```
id = idNum;
```

The body of IDPart needs only to return the current value of id, and the body of TimePart simply returns the current value of the private object timeStamp. Here is the implementation file containing the definitions of all the TimeCard member functions:

```
//**************************************************************
// IMPLEMENTATION FILE (timecard.cpp)
// This file implements the TimeCard class member functions
//**************************************************************
#include "timecard.h"
#include <iostream>

using namespace std;

// Private members of class:
//      long id;
//      Time timeStamp;

//**************************************************************

TimeCard::TimeCard()

// Default constructor

// Postcondition:
//      Time is 0:0:0 (via implicit call to timeStamp object's
//      default constructor)
//   && id == 0

{
    id = 0;
}

//**************************************************************

void TimeCard::Punch( /* in */ int hours,
                      /* in */ int minutes,
                      /* in */ int seconds )
```

PROBLEM-SOLVING CASE STUDY *cont'd.*

```
// Precondition:
//      0 <= hours <= 23  &&  0 <= minutes <= 59
//      && 0 <= seconds <= 59
// Postcondition:
//      Time is punched according to hours, minutes, and seconds

{
    timeStamp.Set(hours, minutes, seconds);
}

//****************************************************************

void TimeCard::SetID( /* in */ long idNum )

// Precondition:
//      idNum is assigned
// Postcondition:
//      id == idNum

{
    id = idNum;
}

//****************************************************************

long TimeCard::IDPart() const

// Postcondition:
//      Function value == id

{
    return id;
}

//****************************************************************

Time TimeCard::TimePart() const

// Postcondition:
//      Function value == timeStamp

{
    return timeStamp;
}

//****************************************************************
```

<u>PROBLEM-SOLVING CASE STUDY</u> *cont'd.*

```
void TimeCard::Print() const

// Postcondition:
//      Time card has been output in the form
//         ID: 235658 Time: 08:14:25

{
    cout << "ID: " << id << " Time: ";
    timeStamp.Write();
}
```

Testing: These functions are all very easy to test. Because the Time class has already been tested and debugged, the Punch function (which calls Time::Set) and the Print function (which calls Time::Write) should work correctly. Also, none of the TimeCard member functions use loops or branching, so it is sufficient to write a single test driver that calls each of the member functions, supplying argument values that satisfy the preconditions.

The Time Card List Object: This object represents a list of time cards. Once again, we'll write a new C++ class for this list because no built-in type or existing class will do.

In Chapter 13, we introduced the list as an ADT and examined typical list operations: insert an item into the list, delete an item, report whether the list is full, report whether the list is empty, search for a particular item, sort the list items into order, print the entire list, and so forth. Should we include all these operations when designing our list of time cards? Probably not. It's unlikely that a list of time cards would be considered general-purpose enough to warrant the effort. Let's stick to the operations we listed in the object table:

Read all time cards into the list
Look up time card information

To choose a data representation for the list, let's review the relationships among the objects in our program. We said that the time card list object is composed of time card objects. Therefore, we can use a 500-element array of TimeCard class objects to represent the list, along with an integer variable indicating the length of the list (the number of array elements that are actually in use).

Before we write the specification of the TimeCardList class, let's review the operations once more. The lookup operation must search the array for a particular time card. Because the array is potentially very large (500 elements), a binary search is better than a sequential search. However, a binary search requires the array elements to be in sorted order. We must

PROBLEM-SOLVING CASE STUDY *cont'd.*

either insert each time card into its proper place as it is read from the data file or sort the time cards after they have been read. Chapter 13's Exam Attendance case study used the former approach. For variety, let's take the latter approach and add another operation—a sorting operation. (We'll use the selection sort we developed in Chapter 13.) Finally, we need one more operation to initialize the private data: a class constructor. Here is the resulting class specification:

```cpp
//****************************************************************
// SPECIFICATION FILE (tclist.h)
// This file gives the specification of TimeCardList, an ADT for a
// list of TimeCard objects.
//****************************************************************
#ifndef TCLIST_H
#define TCLIST_H

#include "timecard.h"
#include <fstream>

using namespace std;

const int MAX_LENGTH = 500;    // Maximum number of time cards

class TimeCardList
{
public:
    void ReadAll( /* inout */ ifstream& inFile );
        // Precondition:
        //     inFile has been opened for input
        // Postcondition:
        //     List contains at most MAX_LENGTH employee time cards
        //     as read from inFile. (Excess time cards are ignored
        //     and a warning message is printed)

    void SelSort();
        // Postcondition:
        //     List components are in ascending order of employee ID

    void BinSearch( /* in */   long       idNum,
                    /* out */  bool&      found,
                    /* out */  TimeCard&  card  ) const;
        // Precondition:
        //     List components are in ascending order of employee ID
        //  && idNum is assigned
        // Postcondition:
        //     IF time card for employee idNum is in list
```

```
    //           found == true  &&  card == time card for idNum
    //      ELSE
    //           found == false  &&  value of card is undefined

TimeCardList();
    // Postcondition:
    //      Empty list created
private:
    int       length;
    TimeCard data[MAX_LENGTH];
};
#endif
```

The `BinSearch` function is a little different from the one we presented in Chapter 13. There, it was a private member function that returned the index of the array element where the item was found. Here, `BinSearch` is a public member function that returns the entire time card to the client.

Now we must implement the `TimeCardList` member functions. Let's begin with the class constructor. Remember that when a class X is composed of objects of other classes, the constructors for those objects are executed before the body of X's constructor is executed. When the `TimeCardList` constructor is called, all 500 `TimeCard` objects in the private `data` array are first constructed. These objects are constructed via implicit calls to the `TimeCard` class's default constructor. (Recall from Chapter 12 that an array of class objects is constructed using the class's default constructor, not a parameterized constructor.) After the `data` array elements are constructed, there is nothing left to do but to set the private variable `length` equal to 0:

```
TimeCardList::TimeCardList()

// Postcondition:
//      Each element of data array has an ID number of 0
//      and a time of 0:0:0 (via implicit call to each array
//      element's default constructor)
//   && length == 0

{
    length = 0;
}
```

To implement the `ReadAll` member function, we use a loop that reads each employee's data (ID number and hours, minutes, and seconds of the punch-in time) and stores the data into the next unused element of the data array. The loop terminates either when end-of-file occurs or when the length of the array reaches MAX_LENGTH. After exiting the loop, we are to print a warning message if more data exists in the file (that is, if end-of-file has not occurred).

ReadAll (Inout: inFile)

```
Read idNum, hours, minutes, seconds from inFile
WHILE NOT EOF on inFile AND length < MAX_LENGTH
        data[length].SetID(idNum)
        data[length].Punch(hours, minutes, seconds)
        Increment length by 1
        Read idNum, hours, minutes, seconds from inFile
IF NOT EOF on inFile
        Print warning that remaining time cards will be ignored
```

The implementation of the SelSort member function has to be slightly different from the one we developed in Chapter 13. Remember that SelSort finds the minimum value in the list and swaps it with the value in the first place in the list. Then the next-smallest value in the list is swapped with the value in the second place. This process continues until all the values are in order. The location in this algorithm that we must change is where the minimum value is determined. Instead of comparing two time cards in the list (which doesn't make any sense), we compare the *ID numbers* on the time cards. To inspect the ID number on a time card, we use the observer function IDPart provided by the TimeCard class. The statement that did the comparison in the original SelSort function must be changed from

```
if (data[searchIndx] < data[minIndx])
```

to

```
if (data[searchIndx].IDPart() < data[minIndx].IDPart())
```

We must make a similar change in the BinSearch function. The original version in Chapter 13 compared the search item with list components directly. Here, we cannot compare the search item (an ID number of type long) with a list component (an object of type TimeCard). Again, we must use the IDPart observer function to inspect the ID number on a time card.

PROBLEM-SOLVING CASE STUDY *cont'd.*

Below is the implementation file for the `TimeCardList` class.

```
//******************************************************************
// IMPLEMENTATION FILE (tclist.cpp)
// This file implements the TimeCardList class member functions.
// List representation: an array of TimeCard objects and an
// integer variable giving the current length of the list
//******************************************************************
#include "tclist.h"
#include <iostream>

using namespace std;

// Private members of class:
//    int       length;              Current length of list
//    TimeCard data[MAX_LENGTH];     Array of TimeCard objects


//******************************************************************

TimeCardList::TimeCardList()

// Default constructor

// Postcondition:
//     Each element of data array has an ID number of 0
//     and a time of 0:0:0 (via implicit call to each array
//     element's default constructor)
//  && length == 0

{
    length = 0;
}


//******************************************************************

void TimeCardList::ReadAll( /* inout */ ifstream& inFile )

// Precondition:
//     inFile has been opened for input
// Postcondition:
//     data[0..length-1] contain employee time cards as read
//     from inFile
//  && 0 <= length <= MAX_LENGTH
//  && IF inFile contains more than MAX_LENGTH time cards
//         Warning message has been printed and excess time cards
//         are ignored
```

PROBLEM-SOLVING CASE STUDY *cont'd.*

```
    {
        long idNum;      // Employee ID number
        int  hours;      // Employee punch-in time
        int  minutes;
        int  seconds;

        inFile >> idNum >> hours >> minutes >> seconds;
        while (inFile && length < MAX_LENGTH)
        {
            data[length].SetID(idNum);
            data[length].Punch(hours, minutes, seconds);
            length++;
            inFile >> idNum >> hours >> minutes >> seconds;
        }
        if (inFile)
            // Assert: inFile is not at end-of-file
            cout << "More than " << MAX_LENGTH << " time cards "
                 << "in input file.  Remainder are ignored." << endl;
    }


//*****************************************************************

void TimeCardList::SelSort()

// Postcondition:
//      data array contains the same values as data@entry, rearranged
//      into ascending order of employee ID

{
    TimeCard temp;       // Used for swapping
    int      passCount;  // Loop control variable
    int      searchIndx; // Loop control variable
    int      minIndx;    // Index of minimum so far

    for (passCount = 0; passCount < length - 1; passCount++)
    {
        minIndx = passCount;

        // Find the index of the smallest component
        // in data[passCount..length-1]

        for (searchIndx = passCount + 1; searchIndx < length;
                                                searchIndx++)
            if (data[searchIndx].IDPart() < data[minIndx].IDPart())
                minIndx = searchIndx;
```

PROBLEM-SOLVING CASE STUDY *cont'd.*

```
                    // Swap data[minIndx] and data[passCount]

            temp = data[minIndx];
            data[minIndx] = data[passCount];
            data[passCount] = temp;
        }
}


//******************************************************************

void TimeCardList::BinSearch( /* in */  long       idNum,
                              /* out */ bool&      found,
                              /* out */ TimeCard& card  ) const

// Precondition:
//      data[0..length-1] are in ascending order of employee ID
//   && idNum is assigned
// Postcondition:
//      IF time card for employee idNum is in list at position i
//          found == true  &&  card == data[i]
//      ELSE
//          found == false  &&  value of card is undefined

{
    int first = 0;          // Lower bound on list
    int last = length - 1;  // Upper bound on list
    int middle;             // Middle index

    found = false;
    while (last >= first && !found)
    {
        middle = (first + last) / 2;
        if (idNum < data[middle].IDPart())
            // Assert: idNum is not in data[middle..last]
            last = middle - 1;
        else if (idNum > data[middle].IDPart())
            // Assert: idNum is not in data[first..middle]
            first = middle + 1;
        else
            // Assert: idNum is in data[middle]
            found = true;
    }
    if (found)
        card = data[middle];
}
```

Testing: If we step back and think about it, we realize that if we write a test driver for the `TimeCardList` class, we will have written the main driver for the entire program! The big picture is that our program is to read in all the file data (function `ReadAll`), sort the time cards into order (function `SelSort`), and look up the time card information for various employees (function `BinSearch`). Therefore, we defer a discussion of testing until we have looked at the main driver.

The Driver: The final step in OOD is to design the driver—the top-level algorithm. As is usually the case in OOD, the driver has very little to do but coordinate the objects that have already been designed.

Main   **Level 0**

```
Create empty list of time cards named punchInList
Open punchInFile for input and verify success
punchInList.ReadAll(punchInFile)
punchInList.SelSort()

Get idNum from user
WHILE idNum ≥ 0
        punchInList.BinSearch(idNum, found, punchInCard)
        IF found
                punchInCard.Print()
        ELSE
                Print idNum, " has not punched in yet."
        Get idNum from user
```

Get ID (Out: idNum)   **Level 1**

```
Print blank line
Prompt user for an ID number
Read idNum
```

PROBLEM-SOLVING CASE STUDY *cont'd.*

Module Structure Chart:

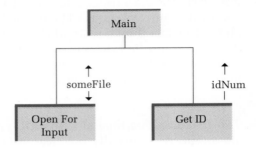

The PunchIn program showing the implementation of the driver follows. We use

```
#include "timecard.h"
```

to insert the TimeCard class declaration into the program, and we use

```
#include "tclist.h"
```

to insert the TimeCardList class declaration. (Recall that tclist.h also happens to #include the header file timecard.h. Thus, timecard.h gets inserted into our program twice. If we had not used the #ifndef directive at the beginning of timecard.h, we would now get a compile-time error for declaring the TimeCard class twice.)

To run the program, we link its object code file with the object code files tclist.obj, timecard.obj, and time.obj.

(The following program is written in ISO/ANSI standard C++. If you are working with pre–standard C++, see the alternate version of the program in the PRE_STD directory of the program disk, available at the publisher's Web site, www.jbpub.com/disks.)

```
//***************************************************************
// PunchIn program
// A data file contains time cards for employees who have punched
// in for work.  This program reads in the time cards from the
// input file, then reads employee ID numbers from the standard
// input.  For each ID number, the program looks up the employee's
// punch-in time and displays it to the user
//***************************************************************
#include <iostream>
#include <fstream>      // For file I/O
#include <string>       // For string class
```

PROBLEM-SOLVING CASE STUDY *cont'd.*

```cpp
#include "timecard.h"    // For TimeCard class
#include "tclist.h"      // For TimeCardList class

void GetID( long& );
void OpenForInput( ifstream& );

int main()
{
    ifstream      punchInFile;    // Input file of time cards
    TimeCardList  punchInList;    // List of time cards
    TimeCard      punchInCard;    // A single time card
    long          idNum;          // Employee ID number
    bool          found;          // True if idNum found in list

    OpenForInput(punchInFile);
    if ( !punchInFile )
        return 1;

    punchInList.ReadAll(punchInFile);
    punchInList.SelSort();

    GetID(idNum);
    while (idNum >= 0)
    {
        punchInList.BinSearch(idNum, found, punchInCard);
        if (found)
        {
            punchInCard.Print();
            cout << endl;
        }
        else
            cout << idNum << " has not punched in yet." << endl;
        GetID(idNum);
    }
    return 0;
}

//****************************************************************

void OpenForInput( /* inout */ ifstream& someFile )    // File to be
                                                       // opened

// Prompts the user for the name of an input file
// and attempts to open the file

// Postcondition:
//     The user has been prompted for a file name
//   && IF the file could not be opened
```

PROBLEM-SOLVING CASE STUDY *cont'd.*

```
//              An error message has been printed
// Note:
//     Upon return from this function, the caller must test
//     the stream state to see if the file was successfully opened

{
    •
    •    (Same as in previous case studies)
    •

}


//*****************************************************************

void GetID( /* out */ long& idNum )      // Employee ID number

// Prompts for and reads an employee ID number

// Postcondition:
//     idNum == value read from standard input

{
    cout << endl;
    cout << "Enter an employee ID (negative to quit): ";
    cin >> idNum;
}
```

Testing: To test this program, we begin by preparing an input file that contains time card information for, say, five employees. The data should be in random order of employee ID to verify that the sorting routine works properly. Using this input file, we run the program and supply the following interactive input: the ID numbers of all five employees in the data file (the program should print their punch-in times), a few ID numbers that are not in the data file (the program should print the message that these employees have not checked in yet), and a negative ID number (the program should quit). If the program tells us that one of the five employees in the data file has not checked in yet or prints a punch-in time for one of the employees not in the data file, the fault clearly lies with the punchInList object—the object responsible for reading the file, sorting, and searching. Using a hand trace, the system debugger, or debug output statements, we should check the TimeCardList member functions in the following order: ReadAll (to verify that the file data was read into the list correctly), SelSort (to confirm that the time card information ends up in ascending order of ID number), then BinSearch (to ensure that items in the list are indeed found and that items not in the list are reported as not there).

PROBLEM-SOLVING CASE STUDY cont'd.

One more thing needs to be tested. If the data file contains more than MAX_LENGTH time cards, the ReadAll function should print a warning message and ignore the excess time cards. To test this feature, we obviously don't want to create an input file with over 500 time cards. Instead, we go into tclist.h and change the const definition of MAX_LENGTH from 500 to a more manageable value—3, for example. We then recompile only tclist.cpp and relink all four object code files. When we run the program, it should read only the first three time cards from the file, print a warning message, and work with a list of only three time cards. Here is a sample run of the program using 3 as the value of MAX_LENGTH:

Input File

```
398405 7 45 04
290387 7 48 10
193847 7 53 20
938473 7 55 14
837485 8 00 00
385473 8 05 45
573920 8 12 13
483948 8 14 45
```

Copy of the Screen During the Run

```
Input file name: punchin.dat
More than 3 time cards in input file.  Remainder are ignored.

Enter an employee ID (negative to quit): 398405
ID: 398405 Time: 07:45:04

Enter an employee ID (negative to quit): 193847
ID: 193847 Time: 07:53:20

Enter an employee ID (negative to quit): 290387
ID: 290387 Time: 07:48:10

Enter an employee ID (negative to quit): 938473
938473 has not punched in yet.

Enter an employee ID (negative to quit): 111111
111111 has not punched in yet.

Enter an employee ID (negative to quit): -5
```

After testing this aspect of the program, we must not forget to change the value of MAX_LENGTH back to 500, recompile tclist.cpp, and relink the object code files.

Testing and Debugging

Testing and debugging an object-oriented program is largely a process of testing and debugging the C++ classes on which the program is built. The top-level driver also needs testing, but this testing is usually uncomplicated—OOD tends to result in a simple driver.

To review how to test a C++ class, you should refer back to the Testing and Debugging section of Chapter 11. There we walked through the process of testing each member function of a class. We made the observation that you could write a separate test driver for each member function or you could write just one test driver that tests all of the member functions. The latter approach is recommended only for classes that have a few simple member functions.

When an object-oriented program uses inheritance and composition, the order in which you test the classes is, in a sense, predetermined. If class X is derived from class Y or contains an object of class Y, you cannot test X until you have designed and implemented Y. Thus, it makes sense to test and debug the lower-level class (class Y) before testing class X. This chapter's Problem-Solving Case Study demonstrated this sequence of testing. We tested the lowest level class—the Time class—first. Next, we tested the TimeCard class, which contains a Time object. Finally, we tested the TimeCardList class, which contains an array of TimeCard objects. The general principle is that if class X is built on class Y (through inheritance or composition), the testing of X is simplified if Y is already tested and is known to behave correctly.

Testing and Debugging Hints

1. Review the Testing and Debugging Hints for Chapter 11. They apply to the design and testing of C++ classes, which are at the heart of OOP.
2. When using inheritance, don't forget to include the word public when declaring the derived class:

```
class DerivedClass : public BaseClass
{
      ⋮
};
```

The word public makes BaseClass a public base class of DerivedClass. That is, clients of DerivedClass can apply any public BaseClass operation (except constructors) to a DerivedClass object.

3. The header file containing the declaration of a derived class must #include the header file containing the declaration of the base class.

4. Although a derived class inherits the private and public members of its base class, it cannot directly access the inherited private members.

5. If a base class has a constructor, it is invoked before the body of the derived class's constructor is executed. If the base class constructor requires arguments, you must pass these arguments using a constructor initializer:

```
DerivedClass::DerivedClass( ... )
    : BaseClass(arg1, arg2)
{
    ⋮
}
```

If you do not include a constructor initializer, the base class's default constructor is invoked.

6. If a class has a member that is an object of another class and this member object's constructor requires arguments, you must pass these arguments using a constructor initializer:

```
SomeClass::SomeClass( ... )
    : memberObject(arg1, arg2)
{
    ⋮
}
```

If there is no constructor initializer, the member object's default constructor is invoked.

7. To obtain dynamic binding of an operation to an object when passing class objects as arguments, you must
   - Pass the object using passing by reference.
   - Declare the operation to be virtual in the class declaration.

8. If a base class declares a virtual function, it *must* implement that function even if the body is empty.

9. A derived class cannot redefine the function return type of a virtual function.

Summary

Object-oriented design (OOD) decomposes a problem into objects—self-contained entities in which data and operations are bound together. In OOD, data is treated as an active, rather than passive, quantity. Each object is responsible for one part of the solution, and the objects communicate by invoking each other's operations.

OOD begins by identifying potential objects and their operations. Examining objects in the problem domain is a good way to begin the process. The next step is to determine the relationships among the objects using inheritance (to express is-a relationships) and composition (to express has-a relationships). Finally, a driver algorithm is designed to coordinate the overall flow of control.

Object-oriented programming (OOP) is the process of implementing an object-oriented design by using language mechanisms for data abstraction, inheritance, and dynamic binding. Inheritance allows any programmer to take an existing class (the base class) and create a new class (the derived class) that inherits the data and operations of the base class. The derived class then specializes the base class by adding new private data, adding new operations, or reimplementing inherited operations—all without analyzing and modifying the implementation of the base class in any way. Dynamic binding of operations to objects allows objects of many different derived types to respond to a single function name, each in its own way. Together, inheritance and dynamic binding have been shown to reduce dramatically the time and effort required to customize existing ADTs. The result is truly reusable software components whose applications and lifetimes extend beyond those conceived of by the original creator.

Quick Check

1. Fill in the blanks: Structured (procedural) programming results in a program that is a collection of interacting _____, whereas OOP results in a program that is a collection of interacting _____. (pp. 802–805)
2. Name the three language features that characterize object-oriented programming languages. (pp. 802–805)
3. Given the class declaration

```
class Point
{
public:
    int X_Coord() const;        // Return the x-coordinate
    int Y_Coord() const;        // Return the y-coordinate
    Point( /* in */ int initX,  // Constructor
           /* in */ int initY );
private:
    int x;
    int y;
};
```

and the type declaration

```
enum StatusType {ON, OFF};
```

declare a class `Pixel` that inherits from class `Point`. Class `Pixel` has an additional data member of type `StatusType` named `status`; it has an additional member function `CurrentStatus` that returns the value of `status`; and it supplies its own constructor that receives three parameters. (pp. 805–812)

4. Write a client statement that creates a `Pixel` object named `onePixel` with an initial (*x*, *y*) position of (3, 8) and a status of `OFF`. (pp. 805–812)
5. Assuming `somePixel` is an object of type `Pixel`, write client code that prints out the current *x*- and *y*-coordinates and status of `somePixel`. (pp. 805–812)
6. Write the function definitions for the `Pixel` class constructor and the `CurrentStatus` function. (pp. 812–817)
7. Fill in the private part of the following class declaration, which uses composition to define a `Line` object in terms of two `Point` objects. (pp. 817–819)

```
class Line
{
public:
    Point StartingPoint() const;     // Return line's starting point
    Point EndingPoint() const;       // Return line's ending point
    float Length() const;            // Return length of the line
    Line( /* in */ int startX,       // Constructor
          /* in */ int startY,
          /* in */ int endX,
          /* in */ int endY   );
private:

};
```

8. Write the function definition for the `Line` class constructor. (pp. 820–822)
9. What is the difference between static and dynamic binding of an operation to an object? (pp. 822–827)
10. Although there are many specific techniques for performing OOD, this chapter uses a three-step process. What are these three steps? (pp. 827–830)
11. When selecting a data representation for an abstract object, what three choices does the C++ programmer have? (pp. 831–832)

Answers **1.** functions, objects **2** Data abstraction, inheritance, dynamic binding
3.
```
class Pixel : public Point
{
public:
    StatusType CurrentStatus() const;
    Pixel( /* in */ int     initX,
           /* in */ int     initY,
```

```
                    /* in */ StatusType initStatus );
    private:
        StatusType status;
    };
```

4. `Pixel onePixel(3, 8, OFF);`

5.
```
cout << "x-coordinate: " << somePixel.X_Coord() << endl;
cout << "y-coordinate: " << somePixel.Y_Coord() << endl;
if (somePixel.CurrentStatus() == ON)
    cout << "Status: on" << endl;
else
    cout << "Status: off" << endl;
```

6.
```
Pixel::Pixel( /* in */ int        initX,
              /* in */ int        initY,
              /* in */ StatusType initStatus )


    : Point(initX, initY)              // Constructor initializer
{
    status = initStatus;
}
```

7.
```
Point startPt;
Point endPt;
```

8.
```
Line::Line( /* in */ int startX,
            /* in */ int startY,
            /* in */ int endX,
            /* in */ int endY   )


    : startPt(startX, startY), endPt(endX, endY)
{
    // Empty body--nothing more to do
}
```

9. With static binding, the determination of which function to call for an object occurs at compile time. With dynamic binding, the determination of which function to call for an object occurs at run time. **10.** Identify the objects and operations, determine the relationships among the objects, and design the driver. **11.** Use a built-in data type, use an existing ADT, or create a new ADT.

Exam Preparation Exercises

1. Define the following terms:

structured design	method (of an object)
code reuse	is-a relationship
state (of an object)	has-a relationship
instance variable (of an object)	

2. In C++, inheritance allows a derived class to access directly all of the functions and data of its base class. (True or False?)

3. Given an existing class declaration

```
class Sigma
{
public:
    void Write() const;
        ⋮
private:
    int n;
};
```

a programmer derives a new class `Epsilon` as follows:

```
class Epsilon : Sigma
{
public:
    void Twist();
    Epsilon( /* in */ float initVal );
private:
    float x;
};
```

Then the following client code results in a compile-time error:

```
Epsilon someObject(4.8);

someObject.Write();    // Error
```

a. Why is the call to the `Write` function erroneous?
b. How would you fix the problem?

4. Consider the following two class declarations:

```
class Abc
{
public:
    void DoThis();
private:
    void DoThat();
    int   alpha;
    int   beta;
};

class Xyz : public Abc
{
public:
    void TryIt();
private:
    int gamma;
};
```

For *each* class, do the following:
a. List all private data members.
b. List all private data members that the class's member functions can reference directly.
c. List all functions that the class's member functions can invoke.
d. List all member functions that a client of the class may legally invoke.

5. A class X uses both inheritance and composition as follows. X is derived from class Y and has a member that is an object of class Z. When an object of class X is created, in what order are the constructors for classes X, Y, and Z executed?

6. With argument passing in C++, you can pass an object of an ancestor class to a parameter that is an object of a descendant class. (True or False?)

7. Consider the following two class declarations:

```
class A
{
public:
    virtual void Write() const;
    A( /* in */ char ch );
private:
    char c;
};


class B : public A
{
public:
    void Write() const;
    B( /* in */ char ch1,
       /* in */ char ch2 );
private:
    char d;
};
```

Let the implementations of the constructors and Write functions be as follows:

```
A::A( /* in */ char ch )
{
    c = ch;
}


void A::Write() const
{
    cout << c;
}
```

```
B::B( /* in */ char ch1,
      /* in */ char ch2 )

    : A(ch1)
{
    d = ch2;
}

void B::Write() const
{
    A::Write();
    cout << d;
}
```

Suppose that we declare two class objects, objectA and objectB:

```
A objectA('x');
B objectB('y', 'z');
```

a. If we write a global function PrintIt, defined as

```
void PrintIt( /* in */ A someObject )
{
    someObject.Write();
}
```

then what is printed by the following code segment?

```
PrintIt(objectA);
cout << endl;
PrintIt(objectB);
```

b. Repeat part (a), assuming that PrintIt uses passing by reference instead of passing by value:

```
void PrintIt( /* in */ A& someObject )
{
    someObject.Write();
}
```

c. Repeat part (b), assuming that Write is *not* a virtual function.

8. Define the following terms associated with object-oriented design:
problem domain
solution domain
implementation-level object

9. Mark each of the following statements as True or False.
   a. Every noun and noun phrase in a problem definition becomes an object in the solution domain.
   b. For a given problem, there are usually more objects in the solution domain than in the problem domain.
   c. In the three-step process for performing object-oriented design, all decisions made during each step are final.
10. For each of the following design methodologies, at what general time (beginning, middle, end) is the driver—the top-level algorithm—designed?
   a. Object-oriented design
   b. Structured design
11. Fill in each blank below with either *is-a* or *has-a*.
   In general, the best strategy in object-oriented design is to use inheritance for _____ relationships and composition for _____ relationships.

Programming Warm-up Exercises

1. For the Line class of Quick Check Question 7, implement the StartingPoint and EndingPoint member functions.
2. For the Line class of Quick Check Question 7, implement the Length member function. *Hint:* The distance between two points (x_1, y_1) and (x_2, y_2) is

$$\sqrt{(x_1 - x_2)^2 + (y_1 - y_2)^2}$$

3. The following class represents a person's mailing address in the United States.

```
class Address
{
public:
    void Write() const;
    Address( /* in */ string newStreet,
             /* in */ string newCity,
             /* in */ string newState,
             /* in */ string newZip    );
private:
    string street;
    string city;
    string state;
    string zipCode;
};
```

Using inheritance, we want to derive an international address class, InterAddress, from the Address class. For this exercise, an international address has all the attributes of a U.S. address plus a country code (a string indicating the name of the country). The public operations of InterAddress are Write (which reimplements the Write function inherited from Address) and a class constructor that receives five parameters (street, city, state, zip code, and country code). Write a class declaration for the InterAddress class.

4. Implement the InterAddress class constructor.

5. Implement the Write function of the InterAddress class.

6. Write a global function PrintAddress that takes a single parameter and uses dynamic binding to print either a U.S. address or an international address. Make the necessary change(s) in the declaration of the Address class so that PrintAddress executes correctly.

7. In Chapter 11, we developed a TimeType class (page 619) and a DateType class (page 625). Using composition, we want to create a TimeAndDay class that contains both a TimeType object and a DateType object. The public operations of the TimeAndDay class should be Set (with six parameters to set the time and day), Increment, Write, and a default constructor. Write a class declaration for the TimeAndDay class.

8. Implement the TimeAndDay default constructor.

9. Implement the Set function of the TimeAndDay class.

10. Implement the Increment function of the TimeAndDay class. (*Hint:* If the time part is incremented to midnight, increment the date part.)

11. Implement the Write function of the TimeAndDay class.

Programming Problems

1. Your parents are thinking of opening a video rental store. Because they are helping with your tuition, they ask you to write a program to handle their inventory.

   What are the major objects in a rental store? They are the items to be rented and the people who rent them. You begin with the abstraction of the items to be rented—video tapes. To determine the characteristics of a video object, you jot down a list of questions.

   - Should the object be one physical video tape, or should it be a title (to allow for multiple copies of a video)?
   - What information about each title should be kept?
   - Should the object contain a place for the card number of the person who has it rented?
   - If there are multiple copies, is it important to keep track of specific copies?
   - What operations should a video object be able to execute?

You decide that the basic object is the title, not an individual tape. The number of copies owned can be a data member of the object. Other data members should include the title, the movie stars, the producer, the director, and the production company. The system eventually must be able to track who has rented which videos, but this is not a property of the video object itself. You'll worry about how to represent the "has rented" object later. For now, who has which specific copy is not important.

The video object must have operations to initialize it and access the various data members. In addition, the object should adjust the number of copies (up or down), determine if a copy is available, check in a copy, and check out a copy. Because you will need to create a list of videos later, you decide to include operations that compare titles and print titles.

You decide to stop at this point, implement the video object, and test it before going on to the rest of the design.

2. Having completed the design and testing of the video object in Programming Problem 1, you are ready to continue with the original problem. Write a program to do the following tasks.
   a. Create a list of video objects.
   b. Search the list for a particular title.
   c. Determine if there are any copies of a particular video currently in the store.
   d. Print the list of video titles.

3. Now that the video inventory is under control, determine the characteristics of the customer and define a customer object. Write the operations and test them. Using this representation of a customer, write a program to do the following tasks.
   a. Create a list of customers.
   b. Search the list by customer name.
   c. Search the list by customer identification number.
   d. Print the list of customer names.

4. Combine the list of video objects and the list of customer objects into a program with the following capabilities.
   a. Check out a video.
   b. Check in a video.
   c. Determine how many videos a customer has (by customer identification number).
   d. Determine which customers have a certain video checked out (by title). (*Hint:* Create a `hasVideo` object that has a video title and a customer number.)

Case Study Follow-Up

1. Write a test plan for testing the `TimeCard` class.
2. Write a test driver to implement your test plan for the `TimeCard` class.

3. Object-oriented design makes code reuse easier and leads to flexible programs. See how easy it is to modify the case study's main driver so that it inputs *two* files (punchInFile and punchOutFile) and outputs not only the punch-in time but also the punch-out time for each employee whose ID is entered by the user. Make these modifications.

4. Revise the TimeCardList class by removing the SelSort function and modifying ReadAll so that it inserts each time card into its proper place in the list as it is read from the input file. Give both the specification and the implementation of the revised class.

15

Pointers, Dynamic Data, and Reference Types

GOALS

- To be able to declare variables of pointer types.
- To be able to take the addresses of variables and to access the variables through pointers.
- To be able to write an expression that selects a member of a class, struct, or union that is pointed to by a pointer.
- To be able to create and access dynamic data.
- To be able to destroy dynamic data.
- To be able to declare and initialize variables of reference types.
- To be able to access variables that are referenced by reference variables.
- To understand the difference between deep and shallow copy operations.
- To understand how C++ defines the term *initialization.*
- To be able to identify the four member functions needed by a C++ class that manipulates dynamic data.
- To be able to use pointers to improve program efficiency.

In the preceding chapters, we have looked at the simple types and structured types available in C++. There are only two built-in data types left to cover: **pointer** types and **reference** types (see Figure 15-1). These types are simple data types, yet in Figure 15-1 we list them separately from the other simple types because their purpose is so special. We refer to pointer types and reference types as *address types*. A variable of one of these types does not contain a data value; it contains the *memory address* of another variable or structure. Address types have two main purposes: They can make a program more efficient—either in terms of speed or in terms of memory usage—and they can be used to build complex data structures. In this chapter, we demonstrate how they make a program more efficient. Chapter 16 explains how to build complex structures using address types.

Pointers

In many ways, we've saved the best till last. Pointer types are the most interesting data types of all. Pointers are what their name implies: variables that tell where to find something else; that is, pointers contain the addresses or locations of other variables.

Pointer type   A simple data type consisting of an unbounded set of values, each of which addresses or otherwise indicates the location of a variable of a given type. Among the operations defined on pointer variables are assignment and testing for equality.

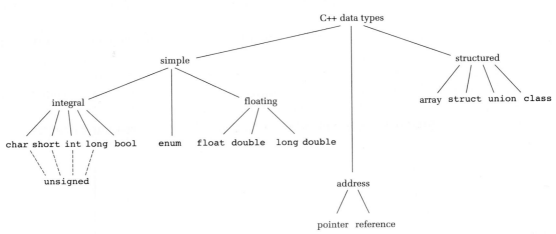

FIGURE 15-1
C++ Data Types

Let's begin this discussion by looking at how pointer variables are declared in C++.

Pointer Variables

Surprisingly, the word *pointer* isn't used in declaring pointer variables; the symbol * is used instead. The declaration

```
int* intPtr;
```

states that `intPtr` is a variable that can point to (that is, contain the address of) an `int` variable. Here is the syntax template for declaring pointer variables:

PointerVariableDeclaration

$$\left\{ \begin{array}{l} \text{DataType* Variable } ; \\ \text{DataType *Variable } , \text{*Variable} \dots ; \end{array} \right.$$

The syntax template shows two forms, one for declaring a single variable and the other for declaring several variables. In the first form, the compiler does not care where the asterisk is placed. Both of the following declarations are equivalent:

```
int* intPtr;
int *intPtr;
```

Although C++ programmers use both styles, we prefer the first. Attaching the asterisk to the data type name instead of the variable name readily suggests that `intPtr` is of type "pointer to `int`."

According to the syntax template, if you declare several variables in one statement you must precede each variable name with an asterisk. Otherwise, only the first variable is taken to be a pointer variable. The compiler interprets the statement

```
int* p, q;
```

as if it were written

```
int* p;
int  q;
```

To avoid unintended errors when declaring pointer variables, it is safest to declare each variable in a separate statement.

Given the declarations

```
int  beta;
int* intPtr;
```

we can make `intPtr` point to `beta` by using the unary `&` operator, which is called the *address-of* operator. At run time, the assignment statement

```
intPtr = &beta;
```

takes the memory address of `beta` and stores it into `intPtr`. Alternatively, we could initialize `intPtr` in its declaration as follows:

```
int  beta;
int* intPtr = &beta;
```

Suppose that `intPtr` and `beta` happen to be located at memory addresses 5000 and 5008, respectively. Then storing the address of `beta` into `intPtr` results in the relationship pictured in Figure 15-2.

Because actual numeric addresses are generally unknown to the C++ programmer, it is more common to display the relationship between a pointer and a pointed-to variable by using rectangles and arrows as in Figure 15-3.

To access a variable that a pointer points to, we use the unary `*` operator—the *dereference* or *indirection* operator. The expression

```
*intPtr
```

FIGURE 15-2

Machine-Level
View of a Pointer
Variable

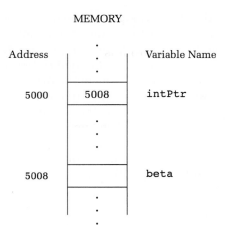

FIGURE 15-3
Abstract Diagram
of a Pointer
Variable

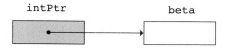

FIGURE 15-3
Abstract Diagram
of a Pointer
Variable

denotes the variable pointed to by `intPtr`. In our example, `intPtr` currently points to `beta`, so the statement

```
*intPtr = 28;
```

dereferences `intPtr` and stores the value 28 into `beta`. This statement represents **indirect addressing** of `beta`; the machine first accesses `intPtr`, then uses its contents to locate `beta`. In contrast, the statement

```
beta = 28;
```

represents **direct addressing** of `beta`. Direct addressing is like opening a post office box (P.O. Box 15, for instance) and finding a package, whereas indirect addressing is like opening P.O. Box 15 and finding a note that says your package is sitting in P.O. Box 23.

Direct addressing   Accessing a variable in one step by using the variable name.

Indirect addressing   Accessing a variable in two steps by first using a pointer that gives the location of the variable.

Continuing with our example, if we execute the statements

```
*intPtr = 28;
cout << intPtr << endl;
cout << *intPtr << endl;
```

then the output is

```
5008
28
```

The first output statement prints the contents of `intPtr` (5008); the second prints the contents of the variable pointed to by `intPtr` (28).

Let's look at a more involved example of declaring pointers, taking addresses, and dereferencing pointers. The following program fragment declares several types and variables. In this code, the `TimeType` class is the C++ class we developed in Chapter 11, with member functions `Set`, `Increment`, `Write`, `Equal`, and `LessThan`.

```
#include "timetype.h"    // For TimeType class
   ⋮
enum ColorType {RED, GREEN, BLUE};
struct PatientRec
{
    int idNum;
    int height;
    int weight;
};

int        alpha;
ColorType  color;
PatientRec patient;
TimeType   startTime(8, 30, 0);

int*        intPtr = &alpha;
ColorType*  colorPtr = &color;
PatientRec* patientPtr = &patient;
TimeType*   timePtr = &startTime;
```

The variables `intPtr`, `colorPtr`, `patientPtr`, and `timePtr` are all pointer variables. `intPtr` points to (contains the address of) a variable of type `int`, `colorPtr` points to a variable of type `Color`, `patientPtr` points to a struct variable of type `PatientRec`, and `timePtr` points to a class object of type `TimeType`.

The expression `*intPtr` denotes the variable pointed to by `intPtr`. The pointed-to variable can contain any `int` value. The expression `*colorPtr` denotes a variable of type `ColorType`. It can contain RED, GREEN, or BLUE. The expression `*patientPtr` denotes a struct variable of type `PatientRec`. Furthermore, the expressions `(*patientPtr).idNum`, `(*patientPtr).height`, and `(*patientPtr).weight` denote the idNum, height, and weight members of `*patientPtr`. Notice how the accessing expression is built.

`patientPtr`	A pointer variable of type "pointer to PatientRec."
`*patientPtr`	A struct variable of type `PatientRec`.
`(*patientPtr).weight`	The weight member of a struct variable of type `PatientRec`.

The expression `(*patientPtr).weight` is a mixture of pointer dereferencing and struct member selection. The parentheses are necessary because the dot operator has higher precedence than the dereference operator (see Appendix B for C++ operator precedence). Without the parentheses, the expression `*patientPtr.weight` would be interpreted wrongly as `*(patientPtr.weight)`.

When a pointer points to a struct (or a class or a union) variable, enclosing the pointer dereference within parentheses can become tedious.

In addition to the dot operator, C++ provides another member selection operator: ->. This *arrow operator* consists of two consecutive symbols: a hyphen and a greater-than symbol. By definition,

PointerExpression **->** MemberName

is equivalent to

(*PointerExpression).MemberName

Therefore, we can write (*patientPtr).weight as patientPtr->weight.

The general guideline for choosing between the two member selection operators (dot and arrow) is the following:

Use the dot operator if the first operand denotes a struct, class, or union variable; use the arrow operator if the first operand denotes a *pointer* to a struct, class, or union variable.

If we want to increment and print the TimeType class object pointed to by timePtr, we could use either the statements

```
(*timePtr).Increment();
(*timePtr).Write();
```

or the statements

```
timePtr->Increment();
timePtr->Write();
```

And if we had declared an array of pointers

```
PatientRec* patPtrArray[20];
```

and initialized the array elements, then we could access the idNum member of the fourth patient as follows:

```
patPtrArray[3]->idNum
```

Pointed-to variables can be used in the same way as any other variable. The following statements are all valid:

```
*intPtr = 250;
*colorPtr = RED;
patientPtr->idNum = 3245;
patientPtr->height = 64;
patientPtr->weight = 114;
patPtrArray[3]->idNum = 6356;
patPtrArray[3]->height = 73;
patPtrArray[3]->weight = 185;
```

Figure 15-4 shows the results of these assignments.

FIGURE 15-4

Results of
Assignment
Statements

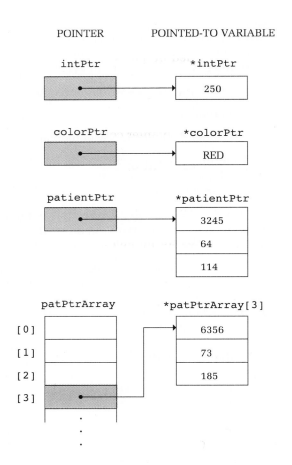

At this point, you may be wondering why we should use pointers at all. Instead of making `intPtr` point to `alpha` and storing 250 into `*intPtr`, why not just store 250 directly into `alpha`? The truth is that there is no good reason to program this way; on the contrary, the examples we have shown would make a program more roundabout and confusing. The major use of pointers in C++ is to manipulate *dynamic variables*—variables that come into existence at execution time only as they are needed. Later in the chapter, we show how to use pointers to create dynamic variables. In the meantime, let's continue with some of the basic aspects of pointers themselves.

Pointer Expressions

You learned in the early chapters that an arithmetic expression is made up of variables, constants, operator symbols, and parentheses. Similarly, pointer expressions are composed of pointer variables, pointer constants, certain allowable operators, and parentheses. We have already discussed pointer variables—variables that hold addresses of other variables. Let's look now at pointer constants.

In C++, there is only one literal pointer constant: the value 0. The pointer constant 0, called the *null pointer,* points to absolutely nothing. The statement

```
intPtr = 0;
```

stores the null pointer into `intPtr`. This statement does *not* cause `intPtr` to point to memory location zero; the null pointer is guaranteed to be distinct from any actual memory address. Because the null pointer does not point to anything, we diagram the null pointer as follows, instead of using an arrow to point somewhere:

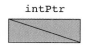

intPtr

Instead of using the constant 0, many programmers prefer to use the named constant NULL that is supplied by the standard header file `cstddef`:

```
#include <cstddef>
    ⋮
intPtr = NULL;
```

As with any named constant, the identifier NULL makes a program more self-documenting. Its use also reduces the chance of confusing the null pointer with the integer constant 0.

It is an error to dereference the null pointer, as it does not point to anything. The null pointer is used only as a special value that a program can test for:

```
if (intPtr == NULL)
    DoSomething();
```

We'll see examples of using the null pointer later in this chapter and in Chapter 16.

Although 0 is the only literal constant of pointer type, there is another pointer expression that is considered to be a constant pointer expression: an array name without any index brackets. The value of this expression is the base address (the address of the first element) of the array. Given the declarations

```
int   arr[100];
int* ptr;
```

the assignment statement

```
ptr = arr;
```

has exactly the same effect as

```
ptr = &arr[0];
```

Both of these statements store the base address of arr into ptr.

Although we did not explain it at the time, you have already used the fact that an array name without brackets is a pointer expression. Consider the following code, which calls a ZeroOut function to zero out an array whose size is given as the second argument:

```
int main()
{
    float velocity[30];
      ⋮
    ZeroOut(velocity, 30);
      ⋮
}
```

In the function call, the first argument—an array name without index brackets—is a pointer expression. The value of this expression is the base address of the velocity array. This base address is passed to the function. We can write the ZeroOut function in one of two ways. The first approach—one that you have seen many times—declares the first parameter to be an array of unspecified size.

```
void ZeroOut( /* out */ float arr[],
              /* in */  int   size  )
{
    int i;

    for (i = 0; i < size; i++)
        arr[i] = 0.0;
}
```

Alternatively, we can declare the parameter to be of type `float*`, because the parameter simply holds the address of a `float` variable (the address of the first array element).

```
void ZeroOut( /* out */ float* arr,
              /* in */  int    size )
{
    ⋮    // Function body is unchanged
}
```

Whether we declare the parameter as `float arr[]` or as `float* arr`, the result is exactly the same to the C++ compiler: Within the `ZeroOut` function, `arr` is a simple variable that points to the beginning of the caller's actual array (see Figure 15-5).

Even though `arr` is a pointer variable within the `ZeroOut` function, we are still allowed to attach an index expression to the name `arr`:

```
arr[i] = 0.0;
```

Indexing a pointer variable is made possible by the following rule in C++:

Indexing is valid for *any* pointer expression, not only an array name. (However, indexing a pointer makes sense only if the pointer points to an array.)

We have now seen four C++ operators that are valid for pointers: `=`, `*`, `->`, and `[]`. The following table lists the most common operations that may be applied to pointers.

FIGURE 15-5
A Parameter
Pointing to the
Caller's Argument

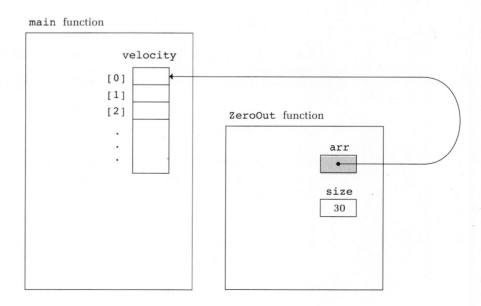

Operator	Meaning	Example	Remarks

=	Assignment	`ptr = &someVar;`
		`ptr1 = ptr2;`
		`ptr = 0;`
			Except for the null pointer, both operands must be of the same data type.

*	Dereference	`*ptr`	
==, !=, <, <=, >, and >=	Relational operators	`ptr1 == ptr2`	The two operands must be of the same data type.
!	Logical NOT	`!ptr`	The result is `true` if the operand is 0 (the null pointer), else the result is `false`.
[]	Index (or subscript)	`ptr[4]`	The indexed pointer should point to an array.
->	Member selection	`ptr->height`	Selects a member of the class, struct, or union variable that is pointed to.

Notice that the logical NOT operator can be used to test for the null pointer:

```
if ( !ptr )
    DoSomething();
```

Some people find this notation confusing because `ptr` is a pointer expression, not a Boolean expression. We prefer to phrase the test this way for clarity:

```
if (ptr == NULL)
    DoSomething();
```

When looking at the table, it is important to keep in mind that the operations listed are operations on pointers, *not* on the pointed-to variables. For example, if `intPtr1` and `intPtr2` are variables of type `int*`, the test

```
if (intPtr1 == intPtr2)
```

compares the pointers, not what they point to. In other words, we are comparing memory addresses, not `int`s. To compare the integers that `intPtr1` and `intPtr2` point to, we would need to write

```
if (*intPtr1 == *intPtr2)
```

In addition to the operators we have listed in the table, the following C++ operators may be applied to pointers: ++, --, +, -, +=, and -=. These operators perform arithmetic on pointers that point to arrays. For example, the expression ptr++ causes ptr to point to the next element of the array, regardless of the size in bytes of each array element. And the expression ptr + 5 accesses the array element that is five elements beyond the one currently pointed to by ptr. We'll say no more about these operators or about pointer arithmetic; the topic of pointer arithmetic is off the main track of what we want to emphasize in this chapter. Instead, we proceed now to explore one of the most important uses of pointers: the creation of dynamic data.

Dynamic Data

In Chapter 8, we described two categories of program data in C++: static data and automatic data. Any global variable is static, as is any local variable explicitly declared as static. The lifetime of a static variable is the lifetime of the entire program. In contrast, an automatic variable—a local variable not declared as static—is allocated (created) when control reaches its declaration and deallocated (destroyed) when control exits the block in which the variable is declared.

With the aid of pointers, C++ provides a third category of program data: **dynamic data.** Dynamic variables are not declared with ordinary variable declarations; they are explicitly allocated and deallocated at execution time by means of two special operators, new and delete. When a program requires an additional variable, it uses new to allocate the variable. When the program no longer needs the variable, it uses delete to deallocate it. The lifetime of a dynamic variable is therefore the time between the execution of new and the execution of delete. The advantage of being able to create new variables at execution time is that we don't have to create any more of them than we need.

Dynamic data   Variables created during execution of a program by means of special operations. In C++, these operations are new and delete.

The new operation has two forms, one for allocating a single variable and one for allocating an array. Here is the syntax template:

AllocationExpression

$$\left\{ \begin{array}{l} \textbf{new } \text{DataType} \\[1em] \textbf{new } \text{DataType } \textbf{[} \text{IntExpression } \textbf{]} \end{array} \right.$$

The first form is used for creating a single variable of type DataType. The second form creates an array whose elements are of type DataType; the desired number of array elements is given by IntExpression. Here is an example that demonstrates both forms of the new operation:

```
int*  intPtr;
char* nameStr;
```

`intPtr = new int;`	Creates a variable of type `int` and stores its address into `intPtr`.
`nameStr = new char[6];`	Creates a six-element `char` array and stores the base address of the array into `nameStr`.

Normally, the new operator does two things: It creates an uninitialized variable (or an array) of the designated type, and it returns a pointer to this variable (or the base address of an array). However, if the computer system has run out of space available for dynamic data, the program terminates with an error message.*

Variables created by new are said to be on the **free store** (or **heap**), a region of memory set aside for dynamic variables. The new operator obtains a chunk of memory from the free store, and, as we will see, the delete operator returns it to the free store.

Free store (heap)   A pool of memory locations reserved for allocation and deallocation of dynamic data.

A dynamic variable is unnamed and cannot be directly addressed. It must be indirectly addressed through the pointer returned by the new operator. Below is an example of creating dynamic data and then accessing the

---

* Technically, if the new operator finds that no more memory is available, it generates what is called a bad_alloc exception—a topic we do not discuss further. Unless we write additional program code to deal explicitly with this bad_alloc exception, the program simply terminates with a message such as "ABNORMAL PROGRAM TERMINATION."

In pre–standard C++, an entirely different approach was used. If new found no more memory available, it returned the null pointer rather than a pointer to a newly allocated object. The code invoking new could then test the returned pointer to see whether the allocation succeeded.

data through pointers. The code begins by initializing the pointer variables in their declarations.

```
#include <cstring>    // For strcpy()
    ⋮
int*  intPtr = new int;
char* nameStr = new char[6];

*intPtr = 357;
strcpy(nameStr, "Ben");
```

Recall from Chapter 13 that the `strcpy` library function requires two arguments, each being the base address of a `char` array. For the first argument, we are passing the base address of the dynamic array on the free store. For the second argument, the compiler passes the base address of the anonymous array where the C string "Ben" (including the terminating null character) is located. Figures 15-6a and 15-6b picture the effect of executing this code segment.

a. ```
int* intPtr = new int;
char* nameStr = new char[6];
```

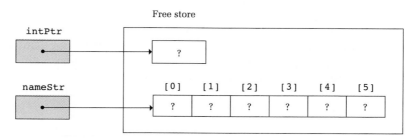

b. ```
*intPtr = 357;
strcpy(nameStr, "Ben");
```

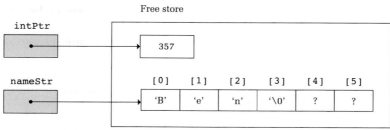

FIGURE 15-6

Allocating Dynamic Data on the Free Store

Dynamic data can be destroyed at any time during the execution of a program when it is no longer needed. The built-in operator `delete` is used to destroy a dynamic variable. The `delete` operation has two forms, one for deleting a single variable, the other for deleting an array:

DeallocationExpression

$$\left\{ \begin{array}{l} \textbf{delete} \text{ Pointer} \\[1em] \textbf{delete [ ]} \text{ Pointer} \end{array} \right.$$

Using the previous example, we can deallocate the dynamic data pointed to by `intPtr` and `nameStr` with the following statements.

`delete intPtr;`   Returns the variable pointed to by `intPtr` to the free store to be used again. The value of `intPtr` is then undefined.

`delete [] nameStr;`   Returns the array pointed to by `nameStr` to the free store to be used again. The value of `nameStr` is then undefined.*

After execution of these statements, the values of `intPtr` and `nameStr` are undefined; they may or may not still point to the deallocated data. Before using these pointers again, you must assign new values to them (that is, store new memory addresses into them).

Until you gain experience with the `new` and `delete` operators, it is important to pronounce the statement

`delete intPtr;`

accurately. Instead of saying "Delete `intPtr`," it is better to say "Delete the variable *pointed to* by `intPtr`." The `delete` operation does not delete the pointer; it deletes the pointed-to variable.

When using the `delete` operator, you should keep two rules in mind.

1. Applying `delete` to the null pointer does no harm; the operation simply has no effect.

---

* The syntax for deallocating an array, `delete [] nameStr`, may not be accepted by some prestandard compilers. Early versions of the C++ language required the array size to be included within the brackets: `delete [6] nameStr`. If your compiler complains about the empty brackets, include the array size.

2. Excepting rule 1, the `delete` operator must only be applied to a pointer value that was obtained previously from the `new` operator.

The second rule is important to remember. If you apply `delete` to an arbitrary memory address that is not in the free store, the result is undefined and could prove to be very unpleasant.

Finally, remember that a major reason for using dynamic data is to economize on memory space. The `new` operator lets you create variables only as they are needed. When you are finished using a dynamic variable, you should `delete` it. It is counterproductive to keep dynamic variables when they are no longer needed—a situation known as a **memory leak**. If this is done too often, you may run out of memory.

Memory leak   The loss of available memory space that occurs when dynamic data is allocated but never deallocated.

Let's look at another example of using dynamic data.

```
int* ptr1 = new int;     // Create a dynamic variable
int* ptr2 = new int;     // Create a dynamic variable

*ptr2 = 44;              // Assign a value to a dynamic variable
*ptr1 = *ptr2;          // Copy one dynamic variable to another
ptr1 = ptr2;            // Copy one pointer to another
delete ptr2;            // Destroy a dynamic variable
```

Here is a more detailed description of the effect of each statement:

`int* ptr1 = new int;`	Creates a pair of dynamic variables of type `int` and stores their locations into `ptr1` and `ptr2`.
`int* ptr2 = new int;`	The values of the dynamic variables are undefined even though the pointer variables now have values (see Figure 15-7a).
`*ptr2 = 44;`	Stores the value 44 into the dynamic variable pointed to by `ptr2` (see Figure 15-7b).
`*ptr1 = *ptr2;`	Copies the contents of the dynamic variable `*ptr2` to the dynamic variable `*ptr1` (see Figure 15-7c).
`ptr1 = ptr2;`	Copies the contents of the pointer variable `ptr2` to the pointer variable `ptr1` (see Figure 15-7d).

```
delete ptr2;
```
Returns the dynamic variable *ptr2 back to the free store to be used again. The value of ptr2 is undefined (see Figure 15-7e).

In Figure 15-7d, notice that the variable pointed to by ptr1 before the assignment statement is still there. It cannot be accessed, however, because no pointer is pointing to it. This isolated variable is called an **inaccessible object.** Leaving inaccessible objects on the free store should be considered a logic error and is a cause of memory leaks.

Notice also that in Figure 15-7e ptr1 is now pointing to a variable that, in principle, no longer exists. We call ptr1 a **dangling pointer.** If the program later dereferences ptr1, the result is unpredictable. The pointed-to value might still be the original one (44), or it might be a different value stored there as a result of reusing that space on the free store.

Inaccessible object   A dynamic variable on the free store without any pointer pointing to it.

Dangling pointer   A pointer that points to a variable that has been deallocated.

Both situations shown in Figure 15-7e—an inaccessible object and a dangling pointer—can be avoided by deallocating *ptr1 before assigning ptr2 to ptr1, and by setting ptr1 to NULL after deallocating *ptr2.

```
#include <cstddef>    // For NULL
   :
int* ptr1 = new int;
int* ptr2 = new int;

*ptr2 = 44;
*ptr1 = *ptr2;
delete ptr1;          // Avoid an inaccessible object
ptr1 = ptr2;
delete ptr2;
ptr1 = NULL;          // Avoid a dangling pointer
```

Figure 15-8 shows the results of executing this revised code segment.

Reference Types

According to Figure 15-1, there is only one built-in type remaining: the **reference type.** Like pointer variables, reference variables contain the addresses of other variables. The statement

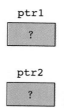

INITIAL CONDITIONS

a.
```
int* ptr1 = new int;
int* ptr2 = new int;
```

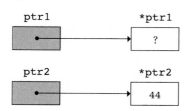

d. `ptr1 = ptr2;`

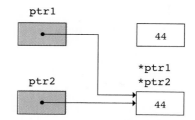

b. `*ptr2 = 44;`

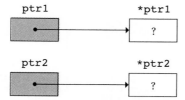

e. `delete ptr2;`

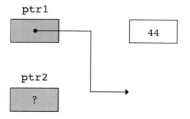

c. `*ptr1 = *ptr2;`

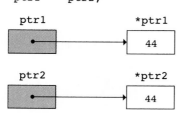

FIGURE 15-7
Results from Sample Code Segment

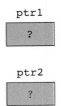

INITIAL CONDITIONS

a. `int* ptr1 = new int;`
   `int* ptr2 = new int;`

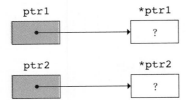

b. `*ptr2 = 44;`

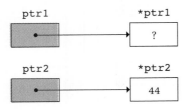

c. `*ptr1 = *ptr2;`

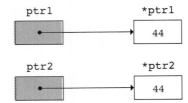

d. `delete ptr1;`

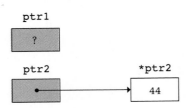

e. `ptr1 = ptr2;`

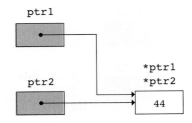

f. `delete ptr2;`

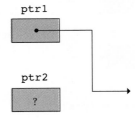

g. `ptr1 = NULL;`

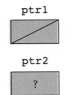

FIGURE 15-8
Results from Sample Code Segment After It Was Modified

```
int& intRef;
```

declares that `intRef` is a variable that can contain the address of an `int` variable. Here is the syntax template for declaring reference variables:

ReferenceVariableDeclaration

$$\begin{cases} \text{DataType\& Variable ;} \\ \text{DataType \&Variable , \&Variable \ldots ;} \end{cases}$$

Although reference variables and pointer variables both contain addresses of data objects, there are two fundamental differences. First, the dereferencing and address-of operators (`*` and `&`) are not used with reference variables. After a reference variable has been declared, the compiler *invisibly* dereferences every single appearance of that reference variable. This difference is illustrated below:

Using a Reference Variable	**Using a Pointer Variable**
`int  gamma = 26;`	`int  gamma = 26;`
`int& intRef = gamma;`	`int* intPtr = &gamma;`
`// Assert: intRef points`	`// Assert: intPtr points`
`//          to gamma`	`//          to gamma`
`intRef = 35;`	`*intPtr = 35;`
`// Assert: gamma == 35`	`// Assert: gamma == 35`
`intRef = intRef + 3;`	`*intPtr = *intPtr + 3;`
`// Assert: gamma == 38`	`// Assert: gamma == 38`

Some programmers like to think of a reference variable as an *alias* for another variable. In the preceding code, we can think of `intRef` as an alias for `gamma`. After `intRef` is initialized in its declaration, everything we do to `intRef` is actually happening to `gamma`.

The second difference between reference and pointer variables is that the compiler treats a reference variable as if it were a *constant* pointer. It cannot be reassigned after being initialized. In fact, absolutely no operations apply directly to a reference variable except initialization. (In this context, C++ defines initialization to mean (a) explicit initialization in a declaration, (b) implicit initialization by passing an argument to a parameter, or (c) implicit initialization by returning a function value.) For example, the statement

```
intRef++;
```

does not increment `intRef`; it increments the variable to which `intRef` points. Why? Because the compiler implicitly dereferences each appearance of the name `intRef`.

The principal advantage of reference variables, then, is notational convenience. Unlike pointer variables, reference variables do not require the programmer to continually prefix the variable with an asterisk in order to access the pointed-to variable.

Reference type   A simple data type consisting of an unbounded set of values, each of which is the address of a variable of a given type. The only operation defined on a reference variable is initialization, after which every appearance of the variable is implicitly dereferenced.

A common use of reference variables is to pass nonarray arguments by reference instead of by value (as we have been doing ever since Chapter 7). Suppose the programmer wants to exchange the contents of two `float` variables with the function call

```
Swap(alpha, beta);
```

Because C++ normally passes simple variables by value, the following code fails:

```
void Swap( float x, float y )
// Caution: This routine does not work
{
    float temp = x;

    x = y;
    y = temp;
}
```

By default, C++ passes the two arguments by value. That is, *copies* of `alpha`'s and `beta`'s values are sent to the function. The local contents of `x` and `y` are exchanged within the function, but the caller's arguments `alpha` and `beta` remain unchanged. To correct this situation, we have two options. The first is to send the addresses of `alpha` and `beta` explicitly by using the address-of operator (`&`):

```
Swap(&alpha, &beta);
```

The function must then declare the parameters to be pointer variables:

```
void Swap( float* px, float* py )
{
    float temp = *px;

    *px = *py;
    *py = temp;
}
```

This approach is necessary in the C language, which has pointer variables but not reference variables.

The other option is to use reference variables to eliminate the need for explicit dereferencing:

```
void Swap( float& x, float& y )
{
    float temp = x;

    x = y;
    y = temp;
}
```

In this case, the function call does not require the address-of operator (&) for the arguments:

```
Swap(alpha, beta);
```

The compiler implicitly generates code to pass the addresses, not the contents, of `alpha` and `beta`. This method of passing nonarray arguments by reference is the one that we have been using all along and continue to use throughout the book.

By now, you have probably noticed that the ampersand (&) has several meanings in the C++ language. To avoid errors, it pays to keep these meanings distinct from each other. Below is a table that summarizes the different uses of the ampersand. Note that a *prefix* operator is one that precedes its operand(s), an *infix* operator lies between its operands, and a *postfix* operator comes after its operand(s).

Position	Usage	Meaning
Prefix	&Variable	Address-of operation
Infix	Expression & Expression	Bitwise AND operation (mentioned, but not explored, in Chapter 10)
Infix	Expression && Expression	Logical AND operation
Postfix	DataType&	Data type (specifically, a reference type) *Exception*: To declare two variables of reference type, the & must be attached to each variable name: `int &var1, &var2;`

Classes and Dynamic Data

When programmers use C++ classes, it is often useful for class objects to create dynamic data on the free store. Let's consider writing a variation of the `DateType` class of Chapter 11. In addition to a month, day, and year, we want each class object to store a message string such as "My birthday" or "Meet Al." When a client program prints a date, this message string will be printed next to the date. The obvious thing to do is to use an object of class `string` to hold the message string. However, to demonstrate allocation and deallocation of dynamic data, let's use a C string to hold the message.

To keep the example simple, we supply only a bare minimum of public member functions. We begin with the class declaration for a `Date` class, abbreviated by leaving out the function preconditions and postconditions.

```
class Date
{
public:
    void Print() const;                      // Output operation
    Date( /* in */ int       initMo,         // Constructor
          /* in */ int       initDay,
          /* in */ int       initYr,
          /* in */ const char* msgStr );
private:
    int   mo;
    int   day;
    int   yr;
    char* msg;
};
```

In the class constructor's parameter list, we could just as well have declared msgStr as

```
const char[] msgStr
```

instead of

```
const char* msgStr
```

Remember that both of these declarations are equivalent as far as the C++ compiler is concerned. They both mean that the parameter being received is the base address of a C string.

As you can see in the private part of the class declaration, the private variable msg is a pointer, not a char array. If we declared msg to be an array of fixed size, say, 30, the array might be either too large or too small to hold the msgStr string that the client passes through the constructor's argument list. Instead, the class constructor will dynamically allocate a char array of just the right size on the free store and make msg point to this array. Here is the implementation of the class constructor as it would appear in the implementation file:

```
#include <cstring>     // For strcpy() and strlen()
    ⋮
Date::Date( /* in */ int           initMo,
            /* in */ int           initDay,
            /* in */ int           initYr,
            /* in */ const char* msgStr   )
{
    mo = initMo;
    day = initDay;
    yr = initYr;
    msg = new char[strlen(msgStr) + 1];
    // Assert:
    //      Storage for dynamic C string is now on free store
    //      and its base address is in msg
    strcpy(msg, msgStr);
    // Assert:
    //      Incoming string has been copied to free store
}
```

The constructor begins by copying the first three incoming parameters into the appropriate private variables. Next, we use the new operator to allocate a char array on the free store. (We add 1 to the length of the incoming string to leave room for the terminating '\0' character.) Finally, we use strcpy to copy all the characters from the msgStr array to the new dynamic array. If the client code declares two class objects with the statements

```
Date date1(4, 15, 2001, "My birthday");
Date date2(5, 12, 2001, "Meet Al");
    :
```

then the two class objects point to dynamic `char` arrays as shown in Figure 15-9.

Figure 15-9 illustrates an important concept: a `Date` class object does not encapsulate an array—it only encapsulates *access* to the array. The array itself is located externally (on the free store), not within the protective abstraction barrier of the class object. This arrangement does not violate the principle of information hiding, however. The only access to the array is through the pointer variable `msg`, which is a private class member and is therefore inaccessible to clients.

Notice that the `Date` class allocates dynamic data, but we have made no provision for deallocating the dynamic data. To deal adequately with class objects that point to dynamic data, we need more than just a class constructor. We need an entire group of class member functions: a class constructor, a *class destructor*, a *deep copy operation*, and a *class copy-constructor*. One by one, we will explain each of these new functions. But first, here is the overall picture of what our new class declaration looks like:

```
class Date
{
public:
    void Print() const;                      // Output operation
    void CopyFrom( /* in */ Date otherDate ); // Deep copy operation
    Date( /* in */ int        initMo,        // Constructor
          /* in */ int        initDay,
          /* in */ int        initYr,
          /* in */ const char* msgStr );
```

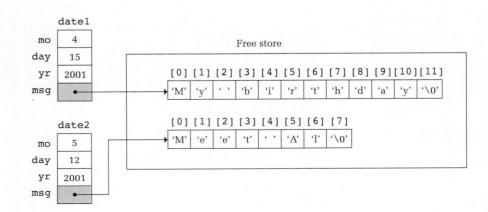

```
        Date( const Date& otherDate );          // Copy-constructor
        ~Date();                                 // Destructor
    private:
        int    mo;
        int    day;
        int    yr;
        char*  msg;
};
```

This class declaration includes function prototypes for all four of the member functions we said we are going to need: constructor, destructor, deep copy operation, and copy-constructor. Before proceeding, let's define more precisely the semantics of each member function by furnishing the function preconditions and postconditions. We have placed the complete specification of the Date class in its own figure—Figure 15-10—so that we can refer to it later.

FIGURE 15-10
Specification of
the Date Class

```
//*****************************************************************
// SPECIFICATION FILE (date.h)
// This file gives the specification of a Date abstract data
// type representing a date and an associated message
//*****************************************************************

class Date
{
public:
    void Print() const;
        // Postcondition:
        //      Date and message have been output in the form
        //          month day, year      message
        //      where the name of the month is printed as a string

    void CopyFrom( /* in */ Date otherDate );
        // Postcondition:
        //      This date is a copy of otherDate, including
        //      the message string

    Date( /* in */ int         initMo,
          /* in */ int         initDay,
          /* in */ int         initYr,
          /* in */ const char* msgStr   );
        // Constructor
        // Precondition:
        //      1 <= initMo <= 12
        //   && 1 <= initDay <= maximum number of days in initMo
        //   && 1582 < initYr
        //   && msgStr is assigned
        // Postcondition:
```

FIGURE 15-10
Specification of
the Date Class
(continued)

```
//      New class object is constructed with a date of
//      initMo, initDay, initYr and a message string msgStr

Date( const Date& otherDate );
    // Copy-constructor
    // Postcondition:
    //      New class object is constructed with date and
    //      message string the same as otherDate's
    // Note:
    //      This constructor is implicitly invoked whenever a
    //      Date object is passed by value, is returned as a
    //      function value, or is initialized by another
    //      Date object in a declaration

~Date();
    // Destructor
    // Postcondition:
    //      Message string is destroyed
private:
    int   mo;
    int   day;
    int   yr;
    char* msg;
};
```

Class Destructors

The Date class of Figure 15-10 provides a destructor function named ~Date. A class destructor, identified by a tilde (~) preceding the name of the class, can be thought of as the opposite of a constructor. Just as a constructor is implicitly invoked when control reaches the declaration of a class object, a destructor is implicitly invoked when the class object is destroyed. A class object is destroyed when it "goes out of scope." (An automatic object goes out of scope when control leaves the block in which it is declared. A static object goes out of scope when program execution terminates.) The following block—which might be a function body, for example—includes remarks at the locations where the constructor and destructor are invoked:

```
{
    Date conf(1, 30, 2002, "Conference");      ← Constructor is invoked
                                                 here
    ⋮
}            ← Destructor is invoked here because conf goes out of scope
```

In the implementation file `date.cpp`, the implementation of the class destructor is very simple:

```
Date::~Date()

// Destructor

// Postcondition:
//      Array pointed to by msg is no longer on the free store
{
    delete [] msg;
}
```

You cannot pass arguments to a destructor and, as with a class constructor, you must not declare the data type of the function.

Until now, we have not needed class destructors. In all previous examples of classes, the private data has been enclosed entirely within the abstraction barrier of the class. For example, in Chapter 11, a `TimeType` class object encapsulates all of its data:

startTime

hrs	8
mins	30
secs	20

When `startTime` goes out of scope, destruction of `startTime` implies destruction of all of its component data.

With the `Date` class, four data items are enclosed within the abstraction barrier, but the array is not (see Figure 15-9). Without the destructor function ~`Date`, destruction of a class object would deallocate the *pointer* to the dynamic array, but would not deallocate the array itself. The result would be a memory leak; the dynamic array would remain allocated but no longer accessible.

Shallow Versus Deep Copying

Next, let's look at the `CopyFrom` function of the `Date` class (see Figure 15-10). This function is designed to copy one class object to another, *including the dynamic message array*. With the built-in assignment operator (=), assignment of one class object to another copies only the class members; it does *not* copy any data pointed to by the class members. For example, given the `date1` and `date2` objects of Figure 15-9, the effect of the assignment statement

```
date1 = date2;
```

is shown in Figure 15-11. The result is called a **shallow copy** operation.
The pointer is copied, but the pointed-to data is not.

   Shallow copying is perfectly fine if none of the class members are
pointers. But if one or more members are pointers, then shallow copying
may be erroneous. In Figure 15-11, the dynamic array originally pointed to
by the date1 object has been left inaccessible.

   What we want is a **deep copy** operation—one that duplicates not only
the class members but also the pointed-to data. The CopyFrom function of
the Date class performs a deep copy. Here is the function implementation:

```
void Date::CopyFrom( /* in */ Date otherDate )

// Postcondition:
//      mo == otherDate.mo
//      && day == otherDate.day
//      && yr == otherDate.yr
//      && msg points to a duplicate of otherDate's message string
//         on the free store

{
    mo = otherDate.mo;
    day = otherDate.day;
    yr = otherDate.yr;
    delete [] msg;                                // Deallocate the
                                                  //    original array
    msg = new char[strlen(otherDate.msg) + 1];    // Allocate a new
                                                  //    array
    strcpy(msg, otherDate.msg);                   // Copy the chars
}
```

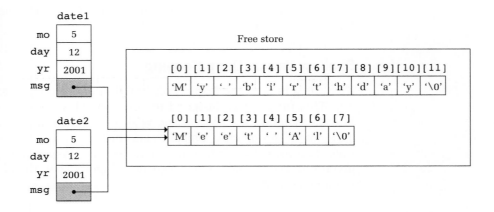

Figure 15-11
A Shallow Copy
Caused by the
Assignment
date1 = date2

First, the function copies the month, day, and year from the `otherDate` object into the current object. Next, the function deallocates the current object's dynamic array from the free store, allocates a new dynamic array, and copies all elements of `otherDate`'s array into the new array. The result is therefore a deep copy—two identical class objects pointing to two identical (but *separate*) dynamic arrays. Given our `date1` and `date2` objects of Figure 15-9, the statement

```
date1.CopyFrom(date2);
```

yields the result shown in Figure 15-12. Compare this figure with the shallow copy pictured in Figure 15-11.

Shallow copy   An operation that copies one class object to another without copying any pointed-to data.

Deep copy   An operation that not only copies one class object to another but also makes copies of any pointed-to data.

Class Copy-Constructors

As we have just discussed, the built-in assignment operator (=) leads to a shallow copy when class objects point to dynamic data. The issue of deep versus shallow copying can also appear in another context: initialization of one class object by another. C++ defines initialization to mean the following:

1. Initialization in a variable declaration

    ```
    Date date1 = date2;
    ```

2. Passing a copy of an argument to a parameter (that is, passing by value)

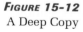

FIGURE 15-12

A Deep Copy

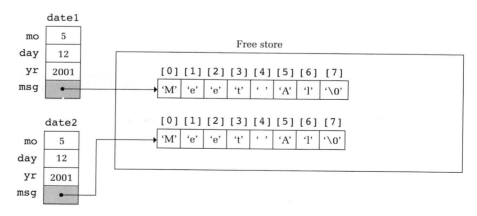

3. Returning an object as the value of a function

```
return someObject;
```

By default, C++ performs such initializations using shallow copy semantics. In other words, the newly created class object is initialized via a member-by-member copy of the old object without regard for any data to which the class members may point. For our `Date` class, the result would again be two class objects pointing to the same dynamic data.

To handle this situation, C++ has a special kind of constructor known as a *copy-constructor*. In a class declaration, its prototype has the following form:

```
class SomeClass
{
public:
    ⋮
    SomeClass( const SomeClass& someObject );    // Copy-constructor
    ⋮
};
```

Notice that the function prototype does not use any special words to suggest that this is a copy-constructor. You simply have to recognize the pattern of symbols: the class name followed by a parameter list, which contains a single parameter of type

```
const SomeClass&
```

For example, our `Date` class declaration in Figure 15-10 shows the prototype of the copy-constructor to be

```
Date( const Date& otherDate );
```

If a copy-constructor is present, the default method of initialization (member-by-member copying) is inhibited. Instead, the copy-constructor is implicitly invoked whenever one class object is initialized by another. The following implementation of the copy-constructor for the `Date` class shows the steps that are involved:

```
Date::Date( const Date& otherDate )

// Copy-constructor

// Postcondition:
//     mo == otherDate.mo
//  && day == otherDate.day
//  && yr == otherDate.yr
```

```
//   && msg points to a duplicate of otherDate's message string
//      on the free store

{
    mo = otherDate.mo;
    day = otherDate.day;
    yr = otherDate.yr;
    msg = new char[strlen(otherDate.msg) + 1];
    strcpy(msg, otherDate.msg);
}
```

The body of the copy-constructor function differs from the body of the `CopyFrom` function in only one line of code: The `CopyFrom` function executes

```
delete [] msg;
```

before allocating a new array. The difference between these two functions is that `CopyFrom` is copying to an *existing* class object (which is already pointing to a dynamic array that must be deallocated), whereas the copy-constructor is creating a new class object that doesn't already exist.

Notice the use of the reserved word `const` in the parameter list of the copy-constructor. The word `const` ensures that the function cannot alter `otherDate`, even though `otherDate` is passed by reference.

As with any nonarray variable in C++, a class object can be passed to a function either by value or by reference. Because C++ defines initialization to include passing by value, copy-constructors are vitally important when class objects point to dynamic data. Assume that we did not include a copy-constructor for the `Date` class, and assume that the following call to the `DoSomething` function uses a pass by value:

```
int main()
{
    Date quizDate(2, 18, 2002, "Geography quiz");
      ⋮
    DoSomething(quizDate);
      ⋮
```

Without a copy-constructor, `quizDate` would be copied to the `DoSomething` function's parameter using a shallow copy. A copy of `quizDate`'s dynamic array would *not* be created for use within `DoSomething`. Both `quizDate` and the parameter within `DoSomething` would point to the same dynamic array (see Figure 15-13). If the `DoSomething` function were to modify the dynamic array (thinking it is working on a *copy* of the original), then after the function returns, `quizDate` would point to a corrupted dynamic array.

FIGURE 15-13
Shallow Copy
Caused by a Pass
by Value without a
Copy-Constructor

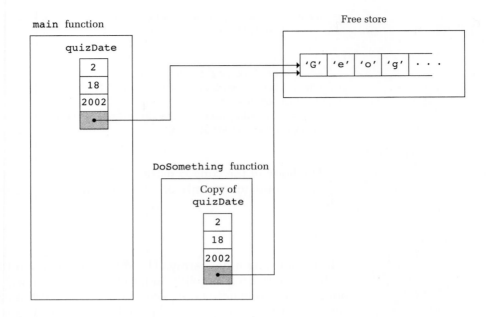

In summary, the default operations of assignment and initialization may be dangerous when class objects point to dynamic data on the free store. Member-by-member assignment and initialization cause only pointers to be copied, not the pointed-to data. If a class allocates and deallocates data on the free store, it almost certainly needs the following suite of member functions to ensure deep copying of dynamic data:

```
class SomeClass
{
public:
      ⋮
    void CopyFrom( SomeClass anotherObject );
        // A deep copy operation

    SomeClass( ... );
        // Constructor, to create data on the free store

    SomeClass( const SomeClass& anotherObject );
        // Copy-constructor, for deep copying in initializations

    ~SomeClass();
        // Destructor, to clean up the free store
```

```
private:
      ⋮
};
```

At the beginning of this chapter, we said that pointers are used for two reasons: to make a program more efficient—either in speed or in memory usage—and to create complex data structures (called *linked structures*). We give examples of the use of pointers to make a program more efficient in the case studies in this chapter. Linked structures are covered in Chapter 16.

*P*ROBLEM-SOLVING CASE STUDY

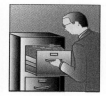

Personnel Records

Problem: We have a file of personnel records, and there is a great deal of data associated with each person. The task is to read in these records, sort them alphabetically by last name, and print out the sorted records.

Input: A file of personnel records (`masterFile`), in which each record corresponds to the data type `PersonnelData` in the declarations below.

```
struct AddressType
{
    string street;
    string city;
    string state;
};
struct PersonnelData
{
    string      lastName;
    string      firstName;
    AddressType address;
    string      workHistory;
    string      education;
    string      payrollData;
};
```

Each of the eight character strings (last name, first name, street address, city, state, work history, education, and payroll data) is on a separate line in `masterFile`, and each string may contain embedded blanks.

The number of records in the file is unknown. The maximum number of employees that the company has ever had is 1000.

Output: The contents of `masterFile` with the records in alphabetical order by last name.

Discussion: Using object-oriented design (OOD) to solve this problem, we begin by identifying potential objects and their operations. Recall that a good way to start is to examine the problem definition, looking for important nouns and noun phrases (to find objects) and important verbs and verb phrases (to find operations). Additionally, implementation-level objects usually are necessary in the solution. Here is an object table for this problem:

Object	Operation
File `masterFile`	Open the file
	Input data from the file
Personnel record	Read a record
	Print a record
Record list	Read all personnel records into the list
	Sort
	Print all records in the list

Notice that the record list object is an implementation-level object. This object is not readily apparent in the problem domain, yet we need it in order for the operation of sorting to make any sense. ("Sort" is not an operation on an individual personnel record; it is an operation on a *list* of records.)

The second major step in OOD is to determine if there are any inheritance or composition relationships among the objects. Using *is-a* as a guide, we do not find any inheritance relationships. However, the record list object and the personnel record object clearly are related by composition. That is, a record list *has a* personnel record within it (in fact, it probably contains many personnel records). Discovery of this relationship helps us as we proceed to design and implement each object.

The `masterFile` Object: For the concrete representation of this object, we can use the `ifstream` class supplied by the standard library. Then the abstract operations of opening a file and reading data are naturally implemented by using the operations already provided by the `ifstream` class.

PROBLEM-SOLVING CASE STUDY cont'd.

The Personnel Record Object: We could implement this object by using a C++ class, hiding the data members as private data and supplying public operations for reading and writing the members. (Also, we might need to provide observer and transformer operations that retrieve and store the values of individual members.) Instead, let's treat this particular object as passive data (in the form of a struct with all members public) rather than as an active object with associated operations. We'll use the struct declarations shown earlier (AddressType and PersonnelData), and we can implement the reading and writing operations by using the >> and << operators to input and output individual members of the struct.

The Record List Object: This object represents a list of personnel records. Thinking of a list as an ADT, we can use a C++ class to conceal the private data representation and provide public operations to read records into the list, sort the list, and print the list.

To choose a concrete data representation for the list, we remember the composition relationship we proposed—namely, that a record list is composed of one or more personnel record objects. Therefore, we could use a 1000-element array of PersonnelData structs, along with an integer variable to keep track of the length of the list. But there are two disadvantages to using an array of structs in this particular problem.

First, the PersonnelData structs are quite large (let's say 1000 bytes each). If we declare a 1000-element array of these structs, the compiler reserves 1,000,000 bytes of memory even though the input file may contain only a few records!

Second, the act of sorting an array of structs can take a lot of time. Consider the selection sort we introduced in Chapter 13. In the SelSort function, the contents of two variables are swapped during each iteration. Swapping two simple variables is a fast operation. If large structs are being sorted, however, swapping two of them can be time-consuming. The C++ code to swap two structs is the same, regardless of the size of the structs—ordinary assignment statements will do. But the length of time to make the swap varies greatly depending on the size of the structs. For example, it may take ten times as long to swap structs with 20 members as it does to swap structs with 2 members.

If we are dealing with large structs, we can make the sorting operation more efficient and save memory by making the structs dynamic variables and by sorting pointers to the structs rather than sorting the structs themselves. This way, only simple pointer variables are swapped on each iteration, rather than whole structs.

The SelSort function has to be modified somewhat to sort large structs rather than simple variables. The structs themselves are dynamically allocated, and a pointer to each is stored in an array. It is these pointers that are swapped when the algorithm calls for exchanging two values.

We have to declare an array `ptrList`, which holds pointers to the personnel records, to be the maximum size we might need. However, we create each `PersonnelData` variable only when we need it. Therefore, room for 1000 pointers is set aside in memory for the `ptrList` array, but at run time there are only as many `PersonnelData` variables in memory as there are records in the file (see Figure 15-14).

The `ptrList` array before and after sorting is shown in Figure 15-15. Note that when the algorithm wants to swap the contents of two structs, we swap the pointers instead.

Now that we have chosen a concrete data representation for the personnel record list, we should review the ADT operations once more. We identified three operations: read all the records into the list, sort the list, and print all the records in the list. Because our data representation uses dynamically allocated data, we must consider supplying additional operations: a class constructor, a class destructor, a class copy-constructor, and a deep copy operation. At a minimum, we need a constructor to initialize the private data and a destructor to deallocate all the `PersonnelData` variables from the free store. (Case Study Follow-Up Exercise 3 asks you to write the copy-constructor and deep copy operations.)

Below is the specification of the `RecordList` class. Notice that we use a Typedef statement to define the identifier `PersonPtr` as a synonym for the type `PersonnelData*`. Thereafter, we can declare the `ptrList` array as

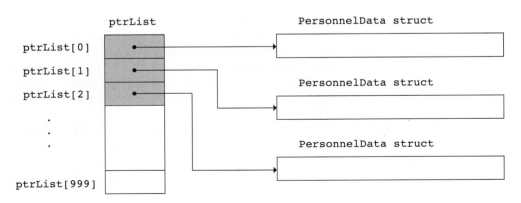

FIGURE 15-14

Array of Pointers to `PersonnelData` Structs

PROBLEM-SOLVING CASE STUDY *cont'd.*

```
PersonPtr ptrList[MAX_EMPL];
```

instead of

```
PersonnelData* ptrList[MAX_EMPL];
```

```cpp
//****************************************************************
// SPECIFICATION FILE (reclist.h)
// This file gives the specification of RecordList, an ADT for a
// list of personnel records.
//****************************************************************
#ifndef RECLIST_H
#define RECLIST_H

#include <fstream>    // For file I/O
#include <string>     // For string class

using namespace std;

const int MAX_EMPL = 1000;      // Maximum number of employees

struct AddressType
{
    string street;
    string city;
    string state;
};
struct PersonnelData
```

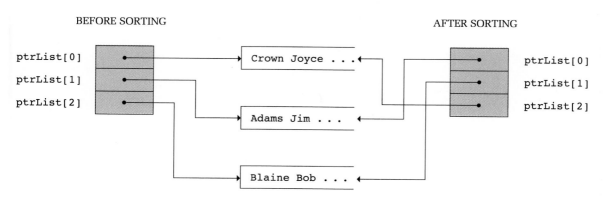

FIGURE 15-15
ptrList Array Before and After Sorting

PROBLEM-SOLVING CASE STUDY cont'd.

```
{
    string      lastName;
    string      firstName;
    AddressType address;
    string      workHistory;
    string      education;
    string      payrollData;
};

typedef PersonnelData* PersonPtr;

class RecordList
{
public:
    void ReadAll( /* inout */ ifstream& inFile );
        // Precondition:
        //     inFile has been opened for input
        //  && inFile contains at most MAX_EMPL records
        // Postcondition:
        //     List contains employee records as read from inFile

    void SelSort();
        // Postcondition:
        //     List is in ascending order of employee last name

    void PrintAll();
        // Postcondition:
        //     All employee records have been written to
        //     standard output

    RecordList();
        // Postcondition:
        //     Empty list created

    ~RecordList();
        // Postcondition:
        //     List destroyed
private:
    PersonPtr ptrList[MAX_EMPL];
    int       length;
};
#endif
```

Now we are ready to implement the `RecordList` member functions. We begin with the class constructor, whose sole task is to initialize the private variable `length` to 0.

The class constructor RecordList ( )

```
Set length = 0
```

To implement the `ReadAll` member function, we use a loop that repeatedly does the following: allocates a dynamic `PersonnelData` struct, reads an employee record into that struct, and stores the pointer to that struct into the next unused element of the `ptrList` array.

ReadAll (Inout: inFile)

```
Set aPerson = new PersonnelData              // Allocate a dynamic struct
Get a record from inFile into
     the struct pointed to by aPerson
WHILE NOT EOF on inFile
     Set ptrList[length] = aPerson           // Store pointer into array
     Increment length
     Set aPerson = new PersonnelData         // Allocate a dynamic struct
     Get a record from inFile into
          the struct pointed to by aPerson
```

The pseudocode step "Get a record from inFile ... " appears twice in `ReadAll`. This step breaks down into several substeps: read the last name, check for end-of-file, read the first name, and so on. To avoid physically writing down the substeps twice, let's write a separate "helper" function named `GetRecord`. In GetRecord's parameter list, `aPerson` is a pointer to a `PersonnelData` struct.

PROBLEM-SOLVING CASE STUDY *cont'd.*

GetRecord (Inout: inFile; In: aPerson)

```
Read aPerson->lastName from inFile
IF EOF on inFile
      Return
Read aPerson->firstName from inFile
Read aPerson->address.street from inFile
Read aPerson->address.city from inFile
Read aPerson->address.state from inFile
Read aPerson->workHistory from inFile
Read aPerson->education from inFile
Read aPerson->payrollData from inFile
```

The SelSort function is nearly the same as in Chapter 13. The original SelSort finds the minimum value in the list and swaps it with the value in the first place in the list. Then the next-smallest value in the list is swapped with the value in the second place. This process continues until all the values are in order. The location in this algorithm that we must change is where the minimum value is determined. Instead of comparing two components in the list, we compare the last-name members in the structs to which these components point. The statement that did the comparison in the original SelSort function must be changed from

```
if (data[searchIndx] < data[minIndx])
```

to

```
if (ptrList[searchIndx]->lastName
     < ptrList[minIndx]->lastName)
```

The remaining member functions—PrintAll and the class destructor—are straightforward to implement.

PROBLEM-SOLVING CASE STUDY *cont'd.*

PrintAll ( )

```
FOR index going from 0 through length - 1
     Print ptrList[index]->lastName, ", ", ptrList[index]->firstName
     Print ptrList[index]->address.street
     Print ptrList[index]->address.city, ", ", ptrList[index]->address.state
     Print ptrList[index]->workHistory
     Print ptrList[index]->education
     Print ptrList[index]->payrollData
```

The class destructor ~RecordList ( )

```
FOR index going from 0 through length - 1
     Deallocate the struct pointed to by ptrList[index]
```

Below is the implementation file for the RecordList class.

```cpp
//******************************************************************
// IMPLEMENTATION FILE (reclist.cpp)
// This file implements the RecordList class member functions.
// List representation: an array of pointers to PersonnelData
// structs and an integer variable giving the current length
// of the list
//******************************************************************
#include "reclist.h"
#include <iostream>
#include <cstddef>      // For NULL

using namespace std;

// Private members of class:
//     PersonPtr ptrList[MAX_EMPL];     Array of pointers
//     int       length;               Number of valid pointers
//                                        in ptrList

    void GetRecord( ifstream&, PersonPtr );    // Prototype for "helper"
                                               //    function
```

PROBLEM-SOLVING CASE STUDY cont'd.

```
//*****************************************************************

RecordList::RecordList()

// Default constructor

// Postcondition:
//     length == 0

{
    length = 0;
}

//*****************************************************************

RecordList::~RecordList()

// Destructor

// Postcondition:
//     Structs pointed to by ptrList[0..length-1]
//     are no longer on the free store

{
    int index;    // Loop control variable

    for (index = 0; index < length; index++)
        delete ptrList[index];
}

//*****************************************************************

void GetRecord( /* inout */ ifstream& inFile,
                /* in */     PersonPtr aPerson )

// Reads one record from file inFile

// Precondition:
//     inFile is open for input
//   && aPerson points to a valid PersonnelData struct
// Postcondition:
//     IF input of the lastName member failed due to end-of-file
//         The contents of *aPerson are undefined
//     ELSE
//         All members of *aPerson are filled with the values
//         for one person read from inFile
```

<u>PROBLEM-SOLVING CASE STUDY</u> *cont'd.*

```cpp
{
    getline(inFile, aPerson->lastName);
    if ( !inFile )
        return;
    getline(inFile, aPerson->firstName);
    getline(inFile, aPerson->address.street);
    getline(inFile, aPerson->address.city);
    getline(inFile, aPerson->address.state);
    getline(inFile, aPerson->workHistory);
    getline(inFile, aPerson->education);
    getline(inFile, aPerson->payrollData);
}


//******************************************************************

void RecordList::ReadAll( /* inout */ ifstream& inFile )

// Precondition:
//      inFile has been opened for input
//   && inFile contains at most MAX_EMPL records
// Postcondition:
//      ptrList[0..length-1] point to dynamic structs
//      containing values read from inFile

{
    PersonPtr aPerson;    // Pointer to newly input record

    aPerson = new PersonnelData;
    GetRecord(inFile, aPerson);
    while (inFile)
    {
        ptrList[length] = aPerson;        // Store pointer into array
        length++;
        aPerson = new PersonnelData;
        GetRecord(inFile, aPerson);
    }
}


//******************************************************************

void RecordList::SelSort()

// Sorts ptrList so that the pointed-to structs are in
// ascending order of last name

// Precondition:
//      ptrList[0..length-1] point to valid PersonnelData structs
```

PROBLEM-SOLVING CASE STUDY cont'd.

```
// Postcondition:
//      ptrList contains the same values as ptrList@entry, rearranged
//      so that consecutive elements of ptrList point to structs in
//      ascending order of last name

{
    PersonPtr  tempPtr;      // Used for swapping
    int        passCount;    // Loop control variable
    int        searchIndx;   // Loop control variable
    int        minIndx;      // Index of minimum so far

    for (passCount = 0; passCount < length - 1; passCount++)
    {
        minIndx = passCount;

        // Find the index of the pointer to the alphabetically first
        // last name remaining in ptrList[passCount..length-1]

        for (searchIndx = passCount + 1; searchIndx < length;
                                                  searchIndx++)
            if (ptrList[searchIndx]->lastName
                  < ptrList[minIndx]->lastName)
                minIndx = searchIndx;

        // Swap ptrList[minIndx] and ptrList[passCount]

        tempPtr = ptrList[minIndx];
        ptrList[minIndx] = ptrList[passCount];
        ptrList[passCount] = tempPtr;
    }
}

//******************************************************************

void RecordList::PrintAll()

// Precondition:
//      ptrList[0..length-1] point to valid PersonnelData structs
// Postcondition:
//      Contents of the structs pointed to by ptrList[0..length-1]
//      have been written to standard output

{
    int index;   // Loop control variable

    for (index = 0; index < length; index++)
    {
```

PROBLEM-SOLVING CASE STUDY cont'd.

```
        cout << ptrList[index]->lastName << ", "
             << ptrList[index]->firstName << endl;
        cout << ptrList[index]->address.street << endl;
        cout << ptrList[index]->address.city << ", "
             << ptrList[index]->address.state << endl;
        cout << ptrList[index]->workHistory << endl;
        cout << ptrList[index]->education << endl;
        cout << ptrList[index]->payrollData << endl << endl;
    }
}
```

Testing: As with any C++ class, testing RecordList amounts to testing each of its member functions. To test the ReadAll function, a test driver that invokes only ReadAll would not be useful; we would also need to invoke PrintAll to check the results. Likewise, a test driver cannot invoke only PrintAll without first putting something into the list (by invoking ReadAll). Thus, a minimal test driver must open a data file, call ReadAll, then call PrintAll. But now the test driver is almost identical to the main driver for the entire program, the only difference being that the main driver calls SelSort after calling ReadAll. Therefore, we postpone a detailed discussion of testing until we have written the main driver.

The Driver: The third step in OOD is to design the driver—the top-level algorithm. In this program, all the driver has to do is invoke the operations of the masterFile object and the record list object.

Main   **Level 0**

```
Create empty list of personnel records named list
Open masterFile for input and verify success
list.ReadAll(masterFile)
list.SelSort()
list.PrintAll()
```

Assumption: File masterFile contains no more than 1000 personnel records.

Module Structure Chart:

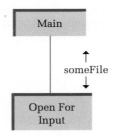

Below is the SortWithPointers program that implements our design. To run the program, we compile the source code files `reclist.cpp` and `sortwithpointers.cpp` into object code files `reclist.obj` and `sortwithpointers.obj`, then link the object code files to produce an executable file.

(The following program is written in ISO/ANSI standard C++. If you are working with pre–standard C++, see the alternate version of the program in the PRE_STD directory of the program disk, available at the publisher's Web site, `www.jbpub.com/disks`.)

```cpp
//****************************************************************
// SortWithPointers program
// This program reads personnel records from a data file,
// sorts the records alphabetically by last name,
// and writes them to the standard output device.
// Assumption: The input file contains at most 1000 records
//****************************************************************
#include <iostream>
#include <fstream>     // For file I/O
#include <string>      // For string class (for OpenForInput function)
#include "reclist.h"   // For RecordList class

using namespace std;

void OpenForInput( ifstream& );

int main()
{
    RecordList list;          // List of personnel records
    ifstream    masterFile;   // Input file of personnel records
```

PROBLEM-SOLVING CASE STUDY *cont'd.*

```
        OpenForInput(masterFile);
        if ( !masterFile )
            return 1;

        list.ReadAll(masterFile);
        list.SelSort();
        list.PrintAll();
        return 0;
    }


//****************************************************************

void OpenForInput( /* inout */ ifstream& someFile )      // File to be
                                                         // opened
// Prompts the user for the name of an input file
// and attempts to open the file

    {

        .
        .    (Same as in previous case studies)
        .

    }
```

Testing: To test this program, we begin by preparing an input file that contains personnel information for, say, ten employees. The data should be in random order by employee last name to make sure that the sorting routine works properly. Given this input data, we expect the program to output the personnel records in ascending order of last name.

File Data	**Expected Output**
Adams	Adams
:} Remainder of Adams's data	:} Remainder of Adams's data
Gordon	Cava
:} Remainder of Gordon's data	:} Remainder of Cava's data
Cava	Gleason
:	:
Sheehan	Gordon
:	:
McCorkle	Kirshen
:	:
Pinard	McCorkle
:	:
Ripley	Pinard
:	:

Kirshen	Ripley
⋮	⋮
Gleason	Sheehan
⋮	⋮
Thompson	Thompson

If we run the program and find too many or too few employee records printed out, or if the records are not in alphabetical order, the problem lies in the record list object—the object responsible for reading the file, sorting, and printing. Using a hand trace, the system debugger, or debug output statements, we should check the RecordList member functions in the following order: ReadAll (to verify that the file data was read into the list correctly), SelSort (to confirm that the records are ordered by employee last name), then PrintAll (to ensure that all records are output properly).

After the program works correctly for the file of test data, we should also run the program against the following files: a nonexistent file and an empty file. With a nonexistent file, the program should halt after the OpenForInput function prints its error message. With an empty file, the program should terminate successfully but produce no output at all. (Look at the loops in the ReadAll, SelSort, and PrintAll functions to see why.)

Are we required to test the program with a file of more than 1000 employee records? No. Clearly, the program would misbehave if the index into the ptrList array exceeded 999. However, our program correctly satisfies the problem definition, which states a precondition for the entire program—namely, that the input file contains at most 1000 records. The user of the program must be informed of this precondition and is expected to comply. If the problem definition were changed to eliminate this precondition, then, of course, we would have to modify the program to deal with an input file that is too long.

One final remark: For the SelSort function, what we have tested is that the program correctly sorts the data using pointers to dynamic variables of type PersonnelData. But the output may still be slightly wrong. Because SelSort compares the strings that make up the last names, it orders the names according to the machine's particular character set. As we mentioned earlier in the book, such comparisons can lead to problems when uppercase and lowercase characters are mixed. For example, in the ASCII set, Macartney would come *after* MacDonald. Case Study Follow-Up Exercise 1 asks you to modify SelSort so that it orders names regardless of the case of the individual characters.

PROBLEM-SOLVING CASE STUDY

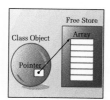

Dynamic Arrays

Problem: In Chapter 12, Programming Warm-up Exercise 9 described a "safe array" class (IntArray) that prevents array indexes from going out of bounds. The public member functions were as follows: a class constructor, to create an array of up to MAX_SIZE elements and initialize all elements to 0; a Store function, to store a value into a particular array element; and a ValueAt function, to retrieve the value of an array element. We want to enhance the IntArray class so that a client of the class can create an array of *any* size—a size that is not bounded by a constant MAX_SIZE. Furthermore, the client should be able to specify the array size at execution time rather than at compile time.

In this case study, we omit the Input and Output sections because we are developing only a C++ class, not a complete program. Instead, we include two sections entitled Specification of the Class and Implementation of the Class.

Discussion: In Chapter 12's IntArray class, the private part includes a fixed-size array of MAX_SIZE (which is 200) elements:

```
class IntArray
{
    ⋮
private:
    int arr[MAX_SIZE];
    int size;
};
```

Each class object contains an array of exactly 200 elements, whether the client needs that many or not. If the client requires fewer than 200 elements, then memory is wasted. If more than 200 elements are needed, the class cannot be used.

The disadvantage of any built-in array, such as arr in the IntArray class, is that its size must be known *statically* (at compile time). In this case study, we want to be able to specify the array size *dynamically* (at execution time). Therefore, we must design and implement a class (call it DynArray) that allocates dynamic data on the free store—specifically, an integer array of any size specified by the client code. The private part of our class will no longer include an entire array; rather, it will include a pointer to a dynamically allocated array:

```
class DynArray
{
```

```
     ⋮
private:
    int* arr;
    int  size;
};
```

Figure 15-9 depicted exactly the same strategy of keeping a pointer within a class object and letting it point to a dynamic array on the free store.

Specification of the Class: In choosing public operations for the DynArray class, we will retain the three operations from the IntArray class: ValueAt, Store, and a class constructor. The job of the constructor, when it receives a parameter arrSize, will be to allocate a dynamic array of exactly arrSize elements—no more and no less. Because DynArray class objects point to dynamic data on the free store, we also need a deep copy operation, a class copy-constructor, and a class destructor. Here is the specification of DynArray, complete with preconditions and postconditions for the member functions.

```
//****************************************************************
// SPECIFICATION FILE (dynarray.h)
// This file gives the specification of an integer array class
// that allows
//      1. Run-time specification of array size
//      2. Trapping of invalid array indexes
//      3. Aggregate copying of one array to another
//      4. Aggregate array initialization (for parameter passing by
//         value, function value return, and initialization in a
//         declaration)
//****************************************************************

class DynArray
{
public:
    int ValueAt( /* in */ int i ) const;
        // Precondition:
        //      i is assigned
        // Postcondition:
        //      IF i >= 0  &&  i < declared size of array
        //          Function value == value of array element
        //                                  at index i
        //      ELSE
        //          Program has halted with error message
```

PROBLEM-SOLVING CASE STUDY *cont'd.*

```
void Store( /* in */ int val,
            /* in */ int i   );
    // Precondition:
    //      val and i are assigned
    // Postcondition:
    //      IF i >= 0  &&  i < declared size of array
    //          val is stored in array element i
    //      ELSE
    //          Program has halted with error message

void CopyFrom( /* in */ DynArray array2 );
    // Postcondition:
    //      IF there is enough memory for a deep copy of array2
    //          This object is a copy of array2 (deep copy)
    //      ELSE
    //          Program has halted with error message

DynArray( /* in */ int arrSize );
    // Constructor
    // Precondition:
    //      arrSize is assigned
    // Postcondition:
    //      IF arrSize >= 1  &&  There is enough memory
    //          Array of size arrSize is created with all
    //          array elements == 0
    //      ELSE
    //          Program has halted with error message

DynArray( const DynArray& array2 );
    // Copy-constructor
    // Postcondition:
    //      IF there is enough memory
    //          New array is created with size and contents
    //          the same as array2 (deep copy)
    //      ELSE
    //          Program has halted with error message
    // Note:
    //      This constructor is implicitly invoked whenever a
    //      DynArray object is passed by value, is returned as
    //      a function value, or is initialized by another
    //      DynArray object in a declaration

~DynArray();
    // Destructor
    // Postcondition:
    //      Array is destroyed
```

```
private:
    int* arr;
    int  size;
};
```

Below is a simple client program that creates two class objects, x and y, stores the values 100, 101, 102, ... into x, copies object x to object y, and prints out the contents of y.

```
#include "dynarray.h"
#include <iostream>

using namespace std;

int main()
{
    int numElements;    // Array size
    int index;          // Array index

    cout << "Enter the array size: ";
    cin >> numElements;

    Dynarray x(numElements);
    Dynarray y(numElements);

    for (index = 0; index < numElements; index++)
        x.Store(index + 100, index);
    y.CopyFrom(x);
    for (index = 0; index < numElements; index++)
        cout << y.ValueAt(index);
    return 0;
}
```

If the input value for numElements is 20, the class constructor creates a 20-element array for x and initializes all elements to 0. Similarly, y is created with all 20 elements initialized to 0. After using the Store function to store 20 new values into x, the program does an aggregate copy of x to y using the CopyFrom operation. Then the program outputs the 20 elements of y, which should be the same as the values contained in x. Finally, both class objects go out of scope (because control exits the block in which they are declared), causing the class destructor to be executed for each object. Each call to the destructor deallocates a dynamic array from the free store, as we'll see when we look at the implementations of the class member functions.

Implementation of the Class: Next, we implement each class member function, placing the function definitions into a C++ implementation file `dynarray.cpp`. As we implement the member functions, we also discuss appropriate testing strategies.

The class constructor and destructor: According to the specification file, the class constructor should allocate an array of size `arrSize`, and the destructor should deallocate the array. The constructor must also verify that `arrSize` is at least 1. If this condition is met and allocation of the dynamic data succeeded, the constructor sets each array element to 0. (If the `new` operator fails to allocate the dynamic array, the program automatically terminates with an error message, thereby satisfying the stated postcondition.)

The class constructor DynArray (In: arrSize)

```
IF arrSize < 1
        Print error message
        Halt the program
Set size = arrSize
Set arr = new int[size]          // Allocate a dynamic array
FOR i going from 0 through size – 1
        Set arr[i] = 0
```

The class destructor ~DynArray ( )

```
Deallocate the array pointed to by arr
```

In the constructor, we allocate an integer array of `arrSize` elements and store its base address into the pointer variable `arr`. Remember that in C++ any pointer can be indexed by attaching an index expression in brackets. Therefore, the assignment statement

```
arr[i] = 0;
```

does exactly what we want it to do: it stores 0 into element `i` of the array pointed to by `arr`.

PROBLEM-SOLVING CASE STUDY cont'd.

Testing: Two things should be tested in the constructor: the If statement and the initialization loop. To test the If statement, we should try different values of the parameter `arrSize`: negative, 0, and positive. Negative and 0 values should cause the program to halt. To test the initialization loop, we can create a class object, use the `ValueAt` function to output the array elements, and verify that the elements are all 0:

```
DynArray testArr(50);

for (index = 0; index < 50; index++)
    cout << testArr.ValueAt(index) << endl;
```

Regarding the class destructor, there is nothing to test. The function simply deallocates the dynamic array from the free store.

The `ValueAt` and `Store` functions: The essence of each of these functions is simple: The `Store` function stores a value into the array, and `ValueAt` retrieves a value. Additionally, the function postconditions require each function to halt the program if the index is out of bounds.

ValueAt (In: i)

  Out: Function value

```
IF i < 0 OR i ≥ size
      Print error message
      Halt the program
Return arr[i]
```

Store (In: val, i)

```
IF i < 0 OR i ≥ size
      Print error message
      Halt the program
Set arr[i] = val
```

Testing: To test these functions, valid indexes (0 through `size`–1) as well as invalid indexes should be passed as arguments. Case Study Follow-Up Exercises 5 and 6 ask you to design test data for these finctions and to write drivers that do the testing.

PROBLEM-SOLVING CASE STUDY cont'd.

The class copy-constructor: This function is called whenever a new class object is created *and* initialized to be a copy of an existing class object.

The class copy-constructor DynArray (In: array2)

```
Set size = array2.size
Set arr = new int[size]          // Allocate a dynamic array
FOR i going from 0 through size – 1
    Set arr[i] = array2.arr[i]
```

Testing: A copy-constructor is implicitly invoked whenever a class object is passed by value as an argument, is returned as a function value, or is initialized by another class object in a declaration. To test the copy-constructor, you could write a function that receives a DynArray object by value, outputs the contents (to confirm that the values of the array elements are the same as in the caller's argument), and modifies some of the array elements. On return from the function, the calling code should print out the contents of the original array, which should be unchanged from the time before the function call. In other words, you want to verify that when the function modified some array elements, it was working on a *copy* of the argument, not on the argument itself.

The CopyFrom function: This function is nearly the same as the copy-constructor; it performs a deep copy of one class object to another. The important difference is that whereas the copy-constructor creates a *new* class object to copy to, the CopyFrom function is applied to an *existing* class object. The only difference in the two algorithms, then, is that CopyFrom must begin by deallocating the dynamic array that is currently being pointed to.

CopyFrom (In: array2)

```
Deallocate the dynamic array pointed to by arr
Set size = array2.size
Set arr = new int[size]          // Allocate a new dynamic array
FOR i going from 0 through size − 1
      Set arr[i] = array2.arr[i]
```

Testing: To test the CopyFrom function, we can use the client code we presented earlier:

```
for (index = 0; index < numElements; index++)
    x.Store(index + 100, index);
y.CopyFrom(x);
for (index = 0; index < numElements; index++)
    cout << y.ValueAt(index);
```

If the value of numElements is 20, the output should be the values 100 through 119, demonstrating that y is a copy of x.

Translating all of these pseudocode algorithms into C++, we obtain the following implementation file for the DynArray class.

```
//****************************************************************
// IMPLEMENTATION FILE (dynarray.cpp)
// This file implements the DynArray class member functions
//****************************************************************
#include "dynarray.h"
#include <iostream>
#include <cstddef>      // For NULL
#include <cstdlib>      // For exit()

using namespace std;

// Private members of class:
//     int* arr;             Pointer to array on free store
//     int  size;            Size of array


//****************************************************************

DynArray::DynArray( /* in */ int arrSize )

// Constructor
```

PROBLEM-SOLVING CASE STUDY *cont'd.*

```
// Precondition:
//      arrSize is assigned
// Postcondition:
//      IF arrSize >= 1  &&  There is room on free store
//            New array of size arrSize is created on free store
//         && arr == base address of new array
//         && size == arrSize
//         && arr[0..size-1] == 0
//      ELSE
//            Program has halted with error message

{
    int i;     // Array index

    if (arrSize < 1)
    {
        cout << "** In DynArray constructor, invalid size: "
            << arrSize << " **" << endl;
        exit(1);
    }
    size = arrSize;
    arr = new int[size];
    for (i = 0; i < size; i++)
        arr[i] = 0;
}


//****************************************************************

DynArray::DynArray( const DynArray& array2 )

// Copy-constructor

// Postcondition:
//      IF there is room on free store
//            New array of size array2.size is created on free store
//         && arr == base address of new array
//         && size == array2.size
//         && arr[0..size-1] == array2.arr[0..size-1]
//      ELSE
//            Program has halted with error message

{
    int i;     // Array index
```

PROBLEM-SOLVING CASE STUDY cont'd.

```
        size = array2.size;
        arr = new int[size];
        for (i = 0; i < size; i++)
            arr[i] = array2.arr[i];
}

//****************************************************************

DynArray::~DynArray()

// Destructor

// Postcondition:
//      Array pointed to by arr is no longer on the free store

{
    delete [] arr;
}

//****************************************************************

int DynArray::ValueAt( /* in */ int i ) const

// Precondition:
//      i is assigned
// Postcondition:
//      IF i >= 0  &&  i < size
//          Function value == arr[i]
//      ELSE
//          Program has halted with error message

{
    if (i < 0 || i >= size)
    {
        cout << "** In ValueAt function, invalid index: "
             << i << " **" << endl;
        exit(1);
    }
    return arr[i];
}

//****************************************************************

void DynArray::Store( /* in */ int val,
                      /* in */ int i   )
```

PROBLEM-SOLVING CASE STUDY cont'd.

```
// Precondition:
//      val and i are assigned
// Postcondition:
//      IF i >= 0  &&  i < size
//          arr[i] == val
//      ELSE
//          Program has halted with error message

{
    if (i < 0 || i >= size)
    {
        cout << "** In Store function, invalid index: "
            << i << " **" << endl;
        exit(1);
    }
    arr[i] = val;
}


//****************************************************************

void DynArray::CopyFrom( /* in */ DynArray array2 )

// Postcondition:
//      Array pointed to by arr@entry is no longer on free store
//   && IF free store has room for an array of size array2.size
//          New array of size array2.size is created on free store
//       && arr == base address of new array
//       && size == array2.size
//       && arr[0..size-1] == array2.arr[0..size-1]
//      ELSE
//          Program has halted with error message

{
    int i;     // Array index

    delete [] arr;
    size = array2.size;
    arr = new int[size];
    for (i = 0; i < size; i++)
        arr[i] = array2.arr[i];
}
```

Testing and Debugging

Programs that use pointers are more difficult to write and debug than programs without pointers. Indirect addressing never seems quite as "normal" as direct addressing when you want to get at the contents of a variable.

The most common errors associated with the use of pointer variables are as follows:

1. Confusing the pointer variable with the variable it points to
2. Trying to dereference the null pointer or an uninitialized pointer
3. Inaccessible objects
4. Dangling pointers

Let's look at each of these in turn.

If `ptr` is a pointer variable, care must be taken not to confuse the expressions `ptr` and `*ptr`. The expression

```
ptr
```

accesses the variable `ptr` (which contains a memory address). The expression

```
*ptr
```

accesses the variable that `ptr` points to.

`ptr1 = ptr2`	Copies the contents of `ptr2` into `ptr1`.
`*ptr1 = *ptr2`	Copies the contents of the variable pointed to by `ptr2` into the variable pointed to by `ptr1`.
`*ptr1 = ptr2`	Illegal—one is a pointer and one is a variable being pointed to.
`ptr1 = *ptr2`	Illegal—one is a pointer and one is a variable being pointed to.

The second common error is to dereference the null pointer or an uninitialized pointer. On some systems, an attempt to dereference the null pointer produces a run-time error message such as "NULL POINTER DEREFERENCE," followed immediately by termination of the program. When this event occurs, you have at least some notion of what went wrong with the program. The situation is worse, though, if your program dereferences an uninitialized pointer. In the code fragment

```
int   num;
int*  intPtr;

num = *intPtr;
```

the variable int Ptr has not been assigned any value before we dereference it. Initially, it contains some meaningless value such as 315988, but the computer does not know that it is meaningless. The machine simply accesses memory location 315988 and copies whatever it finds there into num. There is no way to test whether a pointer variable contains an undefined value. The only advice we can give is to check the code carefully to make sure that every pointer variable is assigned a value before being dereferenced.

The third error—leaving inaccessible objects on the free store—usually results from either a shallow copy operation or incorrect use of the new operator. In Figure 15-11, we showed how the built-in assignment operator causes a shallow copy; the dynamic data object originally pointed to by one pointer variable remains allocated but inaccessible. Misuse of the new operator also can leave dynamic data inaccessible. Execution of the code fragment

```
float* floatPtr;

floatPtr = new float;
*floatPtr = 38.5;
floatPtr = new float;
```

creates an inaccessible object: the dynamic variable containing 38.5. The problem is that we assigned a new value to floatPtr in the last statement without first deallocating the variable it pointed to. To guard against this kind of error, examine every use of the new operator in your code. If the associated variable currently points to data, delete the pointed-to data before executing the new operation.

Finally, dangling pointers are a source of errors and can be difficult to detect. One cause of dangling pointers is deallocating a dynamic data object that is pointed to by more than one pointer. Figures 15-7d and 15-7e pictured this situation. A second cause of dangling pointers is returning a pointer to an automatic variable from a function. The following function, which returns a function value of type int*, is erroneous.

```
int* Func()
{
    int n;
      ⋮
    return &n;
}
```

Remember that automatic variables are implicitly created at block entry and implicitly destroyed at block exit. The above function returns a pointer to the local variable n, but n disappears as soon as control exits the function. The caller of the function therefore receives a dangling pointer. Dangling pointers are hazardous for the same reason that uninitialized pointers are hazardous: When your program dereferences incorrect pointer values, it will access memory locations whose contents are unknown.

Testing and Debugging Hints

1. To declare two pointer variables in the same statement, you must use

   ```
   int *p, *q;
   ```

   You cannot use

   ```
   int* p, q;
   ```

   Similarly, you must use

   ```
   int &m, &n;
   ```

   to declare two reference variables in the same statement.
2. Do not confuse a pointer with the variable it points to.
3. Before dereferencing a pointer variable, be sure it has been assigned a meaningful value other than NULL.
4. Pointer variables must be of the same data type to be compared or assigned to one another.
5. In an expression, an array name without any index brackets is a pointer expression; its value is the base address of the array. The array name is considered a *constant* expression, so it cannot be assigned to. The following code shows correct and incorrect assignments.

   ```
   int   arrA[5] = {10, 20, 30, 40, 50};
   int   arrB[5] = {60, 70, 80, 90, 100};
   int*  ptr;

   ptr = arrB;    // OK--you can assign to a variable
   arrA = arrB;   // Wrong--you cannot assign to a constant
   ```
6. If ptr points to a struct, union, or class variable that has an int member named age, the expression

   ```
   *ptr.age
   ```

is incorrect. You must either enclose the dereference operation in parentheses:

```
(*ptr).age
```

or use the arrow operator:

```
ptr->age
```

7. The `delete` operator must be applied to a pointer whose value was previously returned by `new`. Also, the `delete` operation leaves the value of the pointer variable undefined; do not use the variable again until you have assigned it a new value.

8. A function must not return a pointer to automatic local data, or else a dangling pointer will result.

9. If `ptrA` and `ptrB` point to the same dynamic data object, the statement

```
delete ptrA;
```

makes `ptrB` a dangling pointer. You should now assign `ptrB` the value `NULL` rather than leave it dangling.

10. Deallocate dynamic data when it is no longer needed. Memory leaks can cause you to run out of memory space.

11. Inaccessible objects—another cause of memory leaks—are caused by
   a. shallow copying of pointers that point to dynamic data. When designing C++ classes whose objects point to dynamic data, be sure to provide a deep copy operation and a copy-constructor.
   b. using the `new` operation when the associated variable already points to dynamic data. Before executing `new`, use `delete` to deallocate the data that is currently pointed to.

Summary

Pointer types and reference types are simple data types for storing memory addresses. Variables of these types do not contain data; rather, they contain the addresses of other variables or data structures. Pointer variables require explicit dereferencing using the * operator. Reference variables are dereferenced implicitly and are commonly used to pass nonarray arguments by reference.

A powerful use of pointers is to create dynamic variables. The pointer is created at compile time, but the data to which the pointer points is created at run time. The built-in operator `new` creates a variable on the free store (heap) and returns a pointer to that variable. A dynamic variable is not given a name, but rather is accessed through a pointer variable.

The use of dynamic data saves memory space because a variable is created only when it is needed at run time. When a dynamic variable is no longer needed, it can be deallocated (using `delete`) and the memory space can be used again. The use of dynamic data can also save machine time when large structures are being sorted. The pointers to the large structures, rather than the large structures themselves, can be rearranged.

When C++ class objects point to data on the free store, it is important to distinguish between shallow and deep copy operations. A shallow copy of one class object to another copies only the pointers and results in two class objects pointing to the same dynamic variable. A deep copy results in two distinct copies of the pointed-to data. Therefore, classes that manipulate dynamic data usually require a complete collection of support routines: one or more constructors, a destructor (for cleaning up the free store), a deep copy operation, and a copy-constructor (for deep copying during initialization of one class object by another).

Quick Check

1. How would you declare each of the following pointer variables? (868–879)
   a. A variable `intPtr` that can point to a single `int` variable.
   b. A variable `arrPtr` that can point to a `float` array.
   c. A variable `recPtr` that can point to a structure of the following type.

   ```
   struct RecType
   {
       int    age;
       float height;
       float weight;
   };
   ```

2. Given the declarations

   ```
   int    someVal;
   float velocity[10];
   ```

   and the declarations in Question 1, answer the following.
   a. How would you make `intPtr` point to `someVal` and then use `intPtr` to store 25 into `someVal`?
   b. How would you make `arrPtr` point to `velocity` and then use `arrPtr` to store 6.43 into the third element of `velocity`? (pp. 868–879)

3. Given the declaration

   ```
   RecType oneRec;
   ```

   and the declarations in Question 1, answer the following.
   a. How would you make `recPtr` point to `oneRec`?
   b. What are two different expressions using `recPtr` that will store 120.5 into the `weight` member of `oneRec`? (pp. 868–879)

4. a. In a single statement, declare a pointer variable named `dblPtr` and initialize it to the address of a newly created dynamic variable of type `double`. Then, in a second statement, store 98.32586728 into the dynamic variable.

   b. In a single statement, declare a pointer variable named `list` and initialize it to the base address of a newly created dynamic array of 50 `int` elements. Then give a section of code that will zero out the array. (pp. 879–884)

5. Given the variables `dblPtr` and `list` of Question 4, show how to deallocate the dynamic data pointed to by `dblPtr` and `list`. (pp. 879–884)

6. Given the declaration and initialization

   ```
   float delta = -42.7;
   ```

   how would you declare a variable `gamma` to be of type "reference to `float`" and initialize it to contain the memory address of `delta`? (pp. 884–889)

7. Using the variable `gamma` of Question 6, how would you store the value 12.9 into `delta`? (pp. 884–889)

8. Which kind of copy operation—deep or shallow—copies one pointer to another without copying any pointed-to data? (pp. 890–897)

9. As defined by C++, assignment (using an assignment expression) and initialization are two different things. What are the three ways in which one C++ class object is initialized by another? (pp. 897–898)

10. In designing a C++ class whose class objects point to dynamic data, what are the four member functions you should provide? (pp. 900–901)

11. What are two ways in which pointers may be used to improve program efficiency? (p. 932)

Answers

1. ```
   int*     intPtr;
   float*   arrPtr;
   RecType* recPtr;
   ```
2. a. ```
      intPtr = &someVal;
      *intPtr = 25;
      ```
   b. ```
      arrPtr = velocity; (or arrPtr = &velocity[0];)
      arrPtr[2] = 6.43;
      ```
3. a. `recPtr = &oneRec;`
   b. ```
      (*recPtr).weight = 120.5;
      recPtr->weight = 120.5;
      ```
4. a. ```
      double* dblPtr = new double;
      *dblPtr = 98.32586728;
      ```
   b. ```
      int* list = new int[50];
      for (i = 0; i < 50; i++)
          list[i] = 0;
      ```
5. ```
   delete dblPtr;
   delete [] list;
   ```
6. `float& gamma = delta;` 7. `gamma = 12.9;` (Remember that once a reference variable is initialized, each appearance of the variable is *implicitly* dereferenced.) **8.** Shallow copying copies one pointer to another without copying any pointed-to data. **9.** a. Passing a class object as an argument using a pass by value. b. Initializing a class object in its declaration. c. Returning a class object as a function value. **10.** The class needs one or more constructors (to create the dynamic data), a destructor (to clean up the free store), a deep copy operation, and a copy-constructor (for deep copying during initializations). **11.** Pointers, when used with dynamic data, improve memory efficiency because we create only as many dynamic variables as are needed. With respect to time
   ```

efficiency, it is faster to move pointers than to move large data structures, as in the case of sorting large structs.

Exam Preparation Exercises

1. How does a variable of type `float*` differ from a variable of type `float`?
2. Show what is output by the following C++ code. If an unknown value gets printed, write a *U*.

```
int main()
{
    int   m;
    int   n;
    int*  p = &m;
    int*  q;

    *p = 27;
    cout << *p << ' ' << *q << endl;
    q = &n;
    n = 54;
    cout << *p << ' ' << *q << endl;
    p = &n;
    *p = 6;
    cout << *p << ' ' << n << endl;
    return 0;
}
```

3. Given the declarations

```
struct PersonType
{
    string lastName;
    char    firstInitial;
};
typedef PersonType* PtrType;

PersonType onePerson;
PtrType     ptr = &onePerson;
```

tell whether each statement below is valid or invalid.

a. `ptr.lastName = "Alvarez";`
b. `(*ptr).lastName = "Alvarez";`
c. `*ptr.lastName = "Alvarez";`
d. `ptr->lastName = "Alvarez";`
e. `*ptr->lastName = "Alvarez";`

4. What C++ built-in operation releases the space reserved for a dynamic variable back to the system?

5. Given the declarations

    ```
    int* ptrA;
    int* ptrB;
    ```

    tell whether each code segment below results in an inaccessible object, a dangling pointer, or neither.

    a.
    ```
    ptrA = new int;
    ptrB = new int;
    *ptrA = 345;
    ptrB = ptrA;
    ```

    d.
    ```
    ptrA = new int;
    ptrB = new int;
    *ptrA = 345;
    *ptrB = *ptrA;
    ```

    b.
    ```
    ptrA = new int;
    *ptrA = 345;
    ptrB = ptrA;
    delete ptrA;
    ```

    e.
    ```
    ptrA = new int;
    ptrB = new int;
    *ptrA = 345;
    ptrB = new int;
    *ptrB = *ptrA;
    ```

    c.
    ```
    ptrA = LocationOfAge();
    ```

    where function `LocationOfAge` is defined as

    ```
    int* LocationOfAge()
    {
        int age;

        cout << "Enter your age: ";
        cin >> age;
        return &age;
    }
    ```

6. The only operation that affects the contents of a reference variable is initialization. (True or False?)
7. Given the declarations

    ```
    int  n;
    int& r = n;
    ```

    what does the following statement do?

    ```
    r = 2 * r;
    ```

    a. It doubles the contents of n.
    b. It doubles the contents of r.
    c. It doubles the contents of the variable that n points to.
    d. It doubles the contents of both r and n.
    e. Nothing—it results in a compile-time error.

8. Define the following terms:
    deep copy
    shallow copy
    class destructor
    class copy-constructor
9. By default, C++ performs both assignment and initialization of class objects using shallow copying. (True or False?)

10. Given the class declaration

```
class TestClass
{
public:
    void Write();
    TestClass( /* in */ int initValue );
    ~TestClass();
private:
    int privateData;
};
```

suppose that the member functions are implemented as follows:

```
void TestClass::Write()
{
    cout << "Private data is " << privateData << endl;
}


TestClass::TestClass( /* in */ int initValue )
{
    privateData = initValue;
    cout << "Constructor executing" << endl;
}


TestClass::~TestClass()
{
    cout << "Destructor executing" << endl;
}
```

What is the output of the following program?

```
#include "testclass.h"
#include <iostream>

using namespace std;

int main()
{
    int         count;
    TestClass anObject(5);

    for (count = 1; count <= 3; count++)
        anObject.Write();
    return 0;
}
```

11. Given the TestClass class of Exercise 10, what is the output of the following program?

```
#include "testclass.h"
#include <iostream>
```

```
using namespace std;

int main()
{
    int count;

    for (count = 1; count <= 3; count++)
    {
        TestClass anObject(count);
        anObject.Write();
    }
    return 0;
}
```

12. Let x and y be class objects of the DynArray class developed in this chapter.

```
DynArray x(100);
DynArray y(100);
```

What is the output of each of the following code segments?

a. ```
x.Store(425, 10);
y.CopyFrom(x);
x.Store(250, 10);
cout << x.ValueAt(10) << endl;
cout << y.ValueAt(10) << endl;
```

b. ```
x.Store(425, 10);
y = x;
x.Store(250, 10);
cout << x.ValueAt(10) << endl;
cout << y.ValueAt(10) << endl;
```

13. Given a class named IntList, which of the following is the correct function prototype for the class copy-constructor?
a. void IntList(IntList otherList);
b. IntList(IntList& otherList);
c. IntList(const IntList otherList);
d. void IntList(const IntList& otherList);
e. IntList(const IntList& otherList);

14. How can the use of pointers make a program run faster?

Programming Warm-up Exercises

1. a. Declare a pointer variable p and initialize it to point to a char variable named ch.
   b. Declare a pointer variable q and initialize it to point to the first element of a long array named arr.
   c. Declare a pointer variable r and initialize it to point to a variable named box of type

```
struct BoxType
{
    int length;
    int width;
    int height;
};
```

2. Using the variables p, q, and r of Exercise 1, write code to do the following:
   a. Store '@' into the variable pointed to by p.
   b. Store 959263 into the first element of the array pointed to by q.
   c. Store a length, width, and height of 12, 14, and 5 into the variable pointed to by r.

3. Write a Boolean value-returning function that takes two pointer variables—ptr1 and ptr2—as parameters. Both variables point to float data. The function should return true if the two pointers point to the same variable, and false otherwise.

4. Write a Boolean value-returning function that takes two pointer variables—ptr1 and ptr2—as parameters. Both variables point to float data. The function should return true if the values in the pointed-to variables are identical, and false otherwise.

5. Given the code segment

```
struct GradeType
{
    int   score;
    char grade;
};
typedef GradeType* PtrType;

PtrType p1;
PtrType p2;
PtrType p3;
PtrType p4;
    :
p4 = PtrToMax(p1, p2, p3);
```

the PtrToMax function returns a pointer: the value of p1, p2, or p3, whichever points to the struct with the highest value of score. Implement the PtrToMax function.

6. Write an If statement that compares the two dynamic int variables pointed to by variables p and q, puts the smaller into an int variable named smaller, and destroys the original two dynamic variables.

7. Declare all variables used in Exercise 6.

8. Given the declarations

```
int    numLetters;  // No. of letters in user's last name
int    i;           // Index variable
char* list;         // Pointer to array of letters in
                    //   user's last name
```

write a section of code that prompts the user for the number of letters in his or her last name, dynamically creates a char array of exactly the right size to hold the letters, inputs the letters, prints out the letters in reverse order (last through first), and deallocates the array.

9. Pretend that C++ provides pointer types but not reference types. Rewrite the following function using pointer variables instead of reference variables.

```
void AddAndIncr( /* in */     int   int1,
                 /* inout */  int&  int2,
                 /* out */    int&  sum  )
{
    sum = int1 + int2;
    int2++;
}
```

10. For the function of Exercise 9, change the function call

```
AddAndIncr(m, n, theirSum);
```

so that it corresponds to the new version of the function.

Programming Problems

1. Given two arrays a and b, we can define the relation a < b to mean a[0] < b[0] *and* a[1] < b[1] *and* a[2] < b[2], and so forth. (If the two arrays are of different sizes, the relation is defined only through the size of the smaller array.) We can define the other relational operators likewise. Enhance this chapter's DynArray class by adding two Boolean member functions, LessThan and Equal.

These functions can be thought of as *deep comparison* operations because the dynamic arrays on the free store are to be compared element by element. In other words, the function call

```
arr1.LessThan(arr2)
```

returns true if arr1's array elements are pairwise less than arr2's elements.

Test your two new functions with suitable test drivers and comprehensive sets of test data.

2. Referring to Programming Problem 1, the client code can simulate the other four relational operators (!=, <=, >, and >=) using only the Equal and LessThan functions. However, you could make the class easier to use by supplying additional member functions NotEqual, LessOrEqual, GreaterThan, and GreaterOrEqual. Add these functions to the DynArray class in addition to Equal and LessThan. (*Hint:* Instead of writing each of the algorithms from scratch, simply have the function bodies invoke the existing functions Equal and LessThan. And remember: Class members can refer to each other directly without using dot notation.)

Test your new functions with suitable test drivers and comprehensive sets of test data.

3. The size of a built-in array is fixed statically (at compile time). The size of a dynamic array can be specified dynamically (at run time). In both cases, however, once memory has been allocated for the array, the array size cannot change while the program is executing. In this problem, you are to design and test a C++ class that represents an *expandable array*—one that can grow in size at run time.

Using this chapter's DynArray class as a starting point, create a class named ExpArray. This class has all of DynArray's member functions plus one more:

```
void ExpandBy( /* in */ int n );
    // Precondition:
    //     n > 0
    // Postcondition:
    //     Size of array has increased by n elements
    //  && All of the additional n elements equal zero
```

Here is an example of client code:

```
ExpArray myArray(100);
// Assert: Class object created with array size 100
   ⋮
myArray.ExpandBy(50);
// Assert: Array size is now 150
```

(*Hint:* To expand the array, you should allocate a new, larger dynamic array on the free store, copy the values from the old dynamic array to the new, and deallocate the old array.)

Test your class with a suitable test driver and a comprehensive set of test data. Note that your test driver should exercise the other class member functions to be sure they still work correctly.

Case Study Follow-Up

1. Rewrite the RecordList::SelSort function from the SortWithPointers program so that it correctly orders the structs regardless of whether characters in the last names are uppercase or lowercase. (*Hint:* Temporarily convert all the characters in both strings to uppercase before making the comparison.)
2. Rewrite the RecordList::SelSort function from the SortWithPointers program so that it orders the structs by last name, then first name (in case two or more people have the same last name).
3. We want to add two member functions to the RecordList class of the SortWithPointers program: a copy-constructor and a deep copy operation.
   a. Give the specification of the copy-constructor (as it would appear in the class declaration), then give the implementation of the function.
   b. Give the specification of a CopyFrom function (as it would appear in the class declaration), then give the implementation of the function.
4. In the Dynamic Arrays case study, suppose that the DynArray class had been written to store float rather than int values:

```
class DynArray
{
```

```
public:
    float ValueAt( /* in */ int i ) const;
    void Store( /* in */ float val,
                /* in */ int     i    );
    void CopyFrom( /* in */ DynArray array2 );
    DynArray( /* in */ int arrSize );
    DynArray( const DynArray& array2 );
    ~DynArray();
private:
    float* arr;
    int    size;
};
```

Indicate precisely how the implementation of each of the six member functions would differ from the code presented in the case study.

5. a. Design the data sets necessary to thoroughly test the ValueAt function of the DynArray class (pages 918–927).

    b. Write a driver and test the ValueAt function using your test data.

6. a. Design the data sets necessary to thoroughly test the Store function of the DynArray class (pages 918–927).

    b. Write a driver and test the Store function using your test data.

16

Linked Structures

GOALS

- To understand the concept of a linked data structure.
- To be able to declare the data types and variables needed for a dynamic linked list.
- To be able to print the contents of a linked list.
- To be able to insert new items into a linked list.
- To be able to delete items from a linked list.

In the last chapter, we saw that C++ has a mechanism for creating dynamic variables. These dynamic variables, which can be of any simple or structured type, can be created or destroyed at any time during execution of the program using the operators `new` and `delete`. A dynamic variable is referenced not by a name but through a pointer that contains its location (address). Every dynamic variable has an associated pointer by which it can be accessed. We used dynamic variables to save space and machine time. In this chapter, we see how to use them to build data structures that can grow and shrink as the program executes.

Sequential Versus Linked Structures

As we have pointed out in previous chapters, many problems in computing involve lists of items. A list is an abstract data type (ADT) with certain allowable operations: searching the list, sorting it, printing it, and so forth. The structure we have used as the concrete data representation of a list is the array, a sequential structure. By *sequential structure* we mean that successive components of the array are located next to each other in memory.

If the list we are implementing is a sorted list—one whose components must be kept in ascending or descending order—certain operations are efficiently carried out using an array representation. For example, searching a sorted list for a particular value is done quickly by using a binary search. However, inserting and deleting items from a sorted list are inefficient with an array representation. To insert a new item into its proper place in the list, we must shift array elements down to make room for the new item (see Figure 16-1). Similarly, deleting an item from the list requires that we shift up all the array elements following the one to be deleted.

FIGURE 16-1
Inserting into a Sequential Representation of a Sorted List

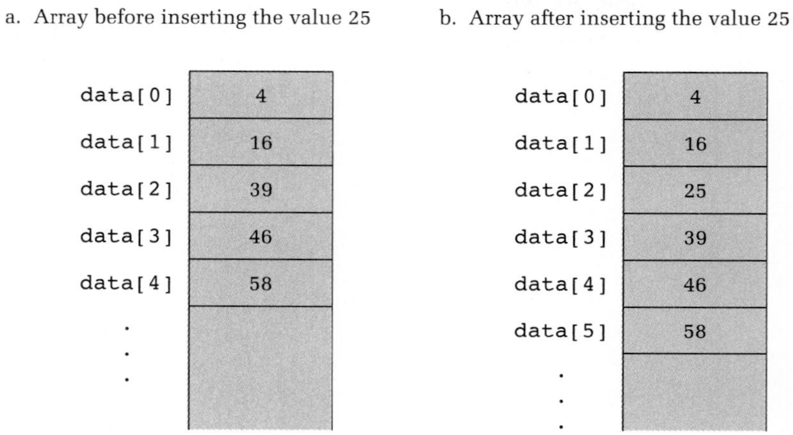

a. Array before inserting the value 25

data[0]	4
data[1]	16
data[2]	39
data[3]	46
data[4]	58
.	
.	
.	

b. Array after inserting the value 25

data[0]	4
data[1]	16
data[2]	25
data[3]	39
data[4]	46
data[5]	58
.	
.	
.	

When insertions and deletions are frequent, there is a better data representation for a list: the **linked list.** A linked list is a collection of items, called *nodes*, that can be scattered about in memory, not necessarily in consecutive memory locations. Each node, typically represented as a struct, consists of two members:

1. A component member, which contains one of the data values in the list
2. A link member, which gives the location of the next node in the list

Component	Link
(Data)	(Location of next node)

Figure 16-2 shows an abstract diagram of a linked list. An arrow is used in the link member of each node to indicate the location of the next node. The slash (/) in the link member of the last node signifies the end of the list. The separate variable `head` is not a node in the linked list; its purpose is to give the location of the first node.

Accessing the items in a linked list is a little like playing the children's game of treasure hunt—each child is given a clue to the hiding place of the next clue, and the chain of clues eventually leads to the treasure.

As you look at Figure 16-2, you should observe two things. First, we have deliberately arranged the nodes in random positions. We have done this to emphasize the fact that the items in a linked list are not necessarily in adjacent memory locations (as they are in the array representation of Figure 16-1). Second, you may already be thinking of pointers when you see the arrows in the figure because we drew pointer variables this way in Chapter 15. But so far, we have carefully avoided using the word *pointer;* we said only that the link member of a node gives the location of the next node. As we will see, there are two ways in which to implement a linked list. One way is to store it in an array of structs, a technique that does not use pointers at all. The second way is to use dynamic data and pointers. Let's begin with the first of these two techniques.

FIGURE 16-2
A Linked List

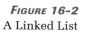

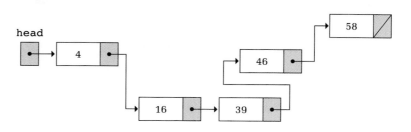

Linked list   A list in which the order of the components is determined by an explicit link member in each node, rather than by the sequential order of the components in memory.

Array Representation of a Linked List

A linked list can be represented as an array of structs. For a linked list of `int` components, we use the following declarations:

```
struct NodeType
{
    int component;
    int link;
};

NodeType node[1000];    // Max. 1000 nodes
int      head;
```

The nodes all reside in an array named `node`. Each node has two members: `component` (in this example, an `int` data value) and `link`, which contains the *array index* of the next node in the list. The last node in the list will have a `link` member of −1. Because −1 is not a valid array index in C++, it is suitable as a special "end-of-list" value. The variable `head` contains the

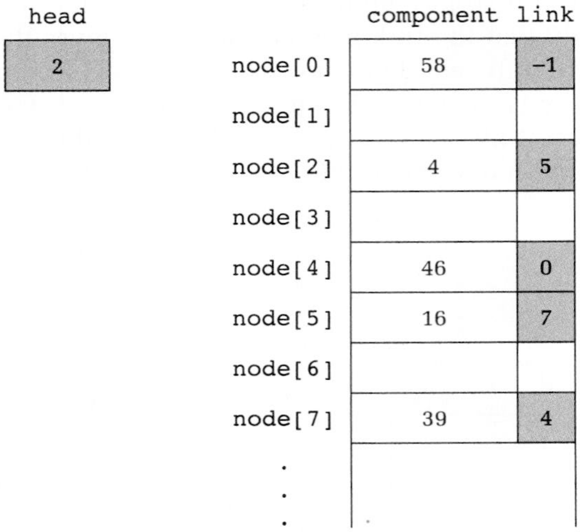

FIGURE 16-3

Array Representation of a Linked List

	head		component	link
	2	node[0]	58	−1
		node[1]		
		node[2]	4	5
		node[3]		
		node[4]	46	0
		node[5]	16	7
		node[6]		
		node[7]	39	4

array index of the first node in the list. Figure 16-3 illustrates an array representation of the linked list of Figure 16-2.

Compare Figures 16-1 and 16-3. Figure 16-1 shows a list represented directly as an array. Figure 16-3 shows a list represented as a linked list, which, in turn, is represented as an array (of structs). We said that when insertions and deletions occur frequently, it is better to use a linked list to represent a list than it is to use an array directly. Let's see why.

Figure 16-1 showed the effect of inserting 25 into the list; we had to shift array elements 2, 3, 4, ... down to insert the value 25 into element 2. If the list is long, we might have to move hundreds or thousands of numbers. In contrast, inserting the value 25 into the linked list of Figure 16-3 requires *no* movement of existing data. We simply find an unused slot in the array, store 25 into the component member, and adjust the link member of the node containing 16 (see Figure 16-4).

Before we introduce the second technique for implementing a linked list—the use of dynamic data and pointers—let's step back and look at the big picture. We are interested in the list as an ADT. Because it is an ADT, we must implement it using some existing data representation. One data representation is the built-in array, a sequential structure. Another data representation is the linked list, a linked structure. But a linked list is, itself, an ADT and requires a concrete data representation—an array of structs, for example. To help visualize all these relationships, we use an *implementation hierarchy diagram*, such as the one shown in Figure 16-5. In this diagram, each data type is implemented by using the data type(s) directly below it in the hierarchy.

FIGURE 16-4

Array Representation of Linked List After 25 Was Inserted

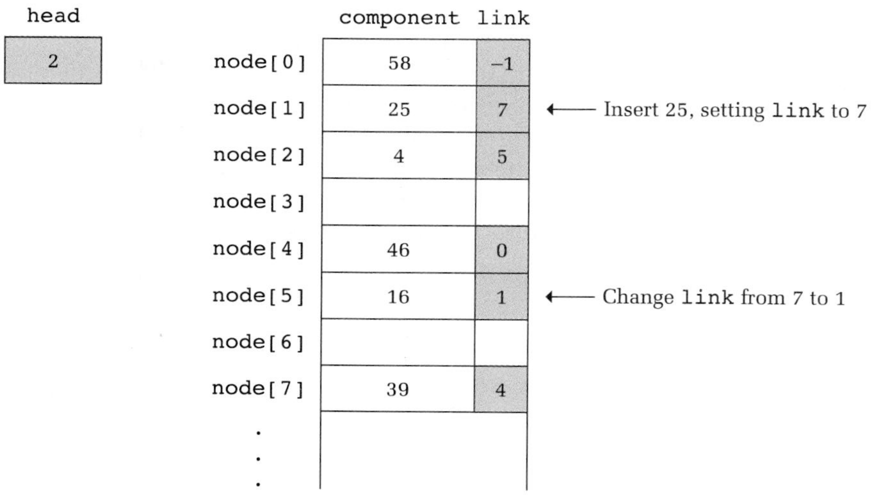

	component	link	
head			
2			
node[0]	58	−1	
node[1]	25	7	← Insert 25, setting link to 7
node[2]	4	5	
node[3]			
node[4]	46	0	
node[5]	16	1	← Change link from 7 to 1
node[6]			
node[7]	39	4	

FIGURE 16-5
Implementation
Hierarchy for a
List ADT

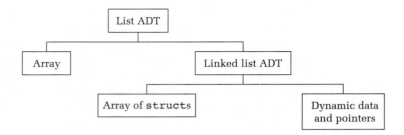

Dynamic Data Representation of a Linked List

Representing a list either as an array or as a linked list stored in an array of structs has a disadvantage: The size of the array is fixed and cannot change while the program is executing. Yet when we are working with lists, we often have no idea how many components we will have. The usual approach in this situation is to declare an array large enough to hold the maximum amount of data we can logically expect. Because we usually have less data than the maximum, memory space is wasted on the unused array elements.

There is an alternative technique in which the list components are dynamic variables that are created only as they are needed. We represent the list as a linked list whose nodes are dynamically allocated on the free store, and the link member of each node contains the memory address of the next dynamic node. In this data representation, called a **dynamic linked list,** the arrows in the diagram of Figure 16-2 really do represent pointers (and the slash in the last node is the null pointer). We access the list with a pointer variable that holds the address of the first node in the list. This pointer variable, named head in Figure 16-2, is called the **external pointer** or **head pointer.** Every node after the first node is accessed by using the link member in the node before it.

Such a list can expand or contract as the program executes. To insert a new item into the list, we allocate more space on the free store. To delete an item, we deallocate the memory assigned to it. We don't have to know in advance how long the list will be. The only limitation is the amount of available memory space. Data structures built using this technique are called **dynamic data structures.**

> **Dynamic data structure** A data structure that can expand and contract during execution.
>
> **Dynamic linked list** A linked list composed of dynamically allocated nodes that are linked together by pointers.
>
> **External (head) pointer** A pointer variable that points to the first node in a dynamic linked list.

To create a dynamic linked list, we begin by allocating the first node and saving the pointer to it in the external pointer. We then allocate a second node and store the pointer to it into the link member of the first node. We continue this process—allocating a new node and storing the pointer to it into the link member of the previous node—until we have finished adding nodes to the list.

Let's look at how we can use C++ pointer variables to create a dynamic linked list of float values. We begin with the declarations

```
typedef float ComponentType;

struct NodeType
{
    ComponentType component;
    NodeType*     link;
};
typedef NodeType* NodePtr;

NodePtr head;              // External pointer to list
NodePtr currPtr;           // Pointer to current node
NodePtr newNodePtr;        // Pointer to newest node
```

The order of these declarations is important. The Typedef for `NodePtr` refers to the identifier `NodeType`, so the declaration of `NodeType` must come first. (Remember that C++ requires every identifier to be declared before it is used.) Within the declaration of `NodeType`, we would like to declare `link` to be of type `NodePtr`, but we can't because the identifier `NodePtr` hasn't been declared yet. However, C++ allows *forward* (or *incomplete*) *declarations* of structs, classes, and unions:

```
typedef float ComponentType;

struct  NodeType;              // Forward (incomplete) declaration
typedef NodeType* NodePtr;

struct NodeType                // Complete declaration
{
    ComponentType component;
```

```
    NodePtr        link;
};
```

The advantage of using a forward declaration is that we can declare the type of `link` to be `NodePtr` just as we declare `head`, `currPtr`, and `newNodePtr` to be of type `NodePtr`.

Given the declarations above, the following code fragment creates a dynamic linked list with the values 12.8, 45.2, and 70.1 as the components in the list.

```
#include <cstddef>    // For NULL
    ⋮
head = new NodeType;
head->component = 12.8;
newNodePtr = new NodeType;
newNodePtr->component = 45.2;
head->link = newNodePtr;
currPtr = newNodePtr;
newNodePtr = new NodeType;
newNodePtr->component = 70.1;
currPtr->link = newNodePtr;
newNodePtr->link = NULL;
currPtr = newNodePtr;
```

Let's go through each of these statements, describing in words what is happening and showing the linked list as it appears after the execution of the statement.

head = new NodeType;   A dynamic variable of type `NodeType` is created. The pointer to this new node is stored into head. Variable head is the external pointer to the list we are building.

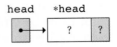

head->component = 12.8;   The value 12.8 is stored into the `component` member of the first node.

(see diagram next page)

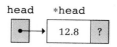

```
newNodePtr = new NodeType;
```

A dynamic variable of type `NodeType` is created. The pointer to this new node is stored into `newNodePtr`.

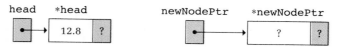

```
newNodePtr->component = 45.2;
```

The value 45.2 is stored into the `component` member of the new node.

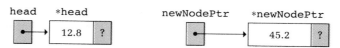

```
head->link = newNodePtr;
```

The pointer to the new node containing 45.2 in its `component` member is copied into the `link` member of `*head`. Variable `newNodePtr` still points to this new node. The node can be accessed either as `*newNodePtr` or as `*(head->link)`.

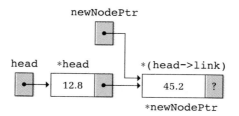

`currPtr = newNodePtr;`

The pointer to the new node is copied into `currPtr`. Now `currPtr`, `newNodePtr`, and `head->link` all point to the node containing 45.2 as its component.

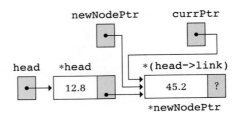

`newNodePtr = new NodeType;`

A dynamic variable of type `NodeType` is created. The pointer to this new node is stored into `newNodePtr`.

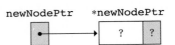

`newNodePtr->component = 70.1;`

The value 70.1 is stored into the component member of the new node.

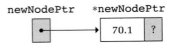

`currPtr->link = newNodePtr;`

The pointer to the new node containing 70.1 in the `component` member is copied into the `link` member of the node that contains 45.2.

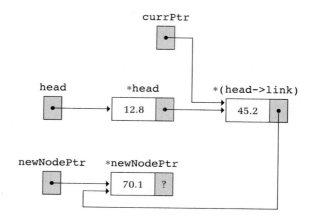

`newNodePtr->link = NULL;`

The special pointer constant NULL is stored into the `link` member of the last node in the list. When used in the `link` member of a node, NULL means the end of the list. NULL is shown in the diagram as a / in the `link` member.

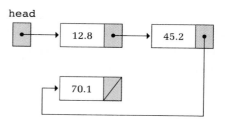

`currPtr = newNodePtr;`   `currPtr` is updated.

We would like to generalize this algorithm so that we can use a loop to create a dynamic linked list of any length. In the algorithm, we used three pointers:

1. `head`, which was used in creating the first node in the list and became the external pointer to the list.
2. `newNodePtr`, which was used in creating a new node when it was needed.
3. `currPtr`, which was updated to always point to the last node in the linked list.

When building any dynamic linked list by adding each new node to the end of the list, we always need three pointers to perform these functions. The algorithm that we used is generalized below to build a linked list of `int` numbers read from the standard input device. It is assumed that the user types in at least one number.

```
Set head = new NodeType
Read head->component
Set currPtr = head

Read inputVal
WHILE NOT EOF
      Set newNodePtr = new NodeType
      Set newNodePtr->component = inputVal
      Set currPtr->link = newNodePtr
      Set currPtr = newNodePtr
      Read inputVal
Set currPtr->link = NULL
```

The following code segment implements this algorithm. For variety, we define the component type to be `int` rather than `float`.

```
typedef int ComponentType;

struct  NodeType;               // Forward declaration
typedef NodeType* NodePtr;

struct NodeType
{
    ComponentType component;
    NodePtr       link;
};
```

```
NodePtr        head;              // External pointer to list
NodePtr        newNodePtr;        // Pointer to newest node
NodePtr        currPtr;           // Pointer to last node
ComponentType  inputVal;

head = new NodeType;
cin >> head->component;
currPtr = head;

cin >> inputVal;
while (cin)
{
    newNodePtr = new NodeType;              // Create new node
    newNodePtr->component = inputVal;       // Set its component value
    currPtr->link = newNodePtr;             // Link node into list
    currPtr = newNodePtr;                   // Set currPtr to last node
    cin >> inputVal;
}
currPtr->link = NULL;                       // Mark end of list
```

Let's do a code walk-through and see just how this algorithm works.

`head = new NodeType;`	A variable of type `NodeType` is created. The pointer is stored into `head`. Variable `head` will remain unchanged as the pointer to the first node (that is, `head` is the external pointer to the list).
`cin >> head->component;`	The first number is read into the `component` member of the first node in the list.
`currPtr = head;`	`currPtr` now points to the last node (the only node) in the list.
`cin >> inputVal;`	The next number (if there is one) is read into variable `inputVal`.
`while (cin)` `{`	An event-controlled loop is used to read input values until end-of-file occurs.
`newNodePtr = new NodeType;`	Another variable of type `NodeType` is created, with `newNodePtr` pointing to it.
`newNodePtr->component = inputVal;`	The current input value is stored into the `component` member of the newly created node.
`currPtr->link = newNodePtr;`	The pointer to the new node is stored into the `link` member of the last node in the list.

`currPtr = newNodePtr;`	`currPtr` is again pointing to the last node in the list.
`cin >> inputVal;`	The next input value (if there is one) is read in.
`}`	The loop body repeats again.
`currPtr->link = NULL;`	The `link` member of the last node is assigned the special end-of-list value `NULL`.

Following is the linked list that results when the program is run with the numbers 32, 78, 99, and 21 as data. The final values are shown for the auxiliary variables.

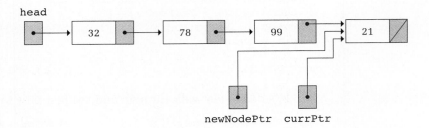

Algorithms on Dynamic Linked Lists

Now that we have looked at two examples of creating a dynamic linked list, let's look at algorithms that process nodes in a linked list. We need to be able to insert a node into a list, delete a node from a list, print the data values in a list, and so forth. For each of these operations, we make use of the fact that NULL is in the link member of the last node. NULL can be assigned to any pointer variable. It means that the pointer points to nothing. Its importance lies in the fact that we can compare the link member of each node to NULL to see when we have reached the end of the list.

As we develop these algorithms, we do so in the following context. We want to write a C++ class for a list (not linked list) ADT. As emphasized in Figure 16-5, a list ADT can be implemented in several ways. We choose a dynamic linked list as the data representation for a list, and we create the SortedList2 class whose specification is shown in Figure 16-6. (We use the name SortedList2 to distinguish this class from the SortedList class of Chapter 13.)

Figure 16-6
Specification of
the SortedList2
Class

```
//******************************************************************
// SPECIFICATION FILE (slist2.h)
// This file gives the specification of a sorted list abstract data
// type. The list components are maintained in ascending order of
// value
//******************************************************************

typedef int ComponentType;    // Type of each component
                              //    (a simple type or the string type)

struct NodeType;              // Forward declaration
                              //    (Complete declaration is
                              //    hidden in implementation file)
class SortedList2
{
public:
    bool IsEmpty() const;
        // Postcondition:
        //      Function value == true, if list is empty
        //                     == false, otherwise

    void Print() const;
        // Postcondition:
        //      All components (if any) in list have been output

    void InsertTop( /* in */ ComponentType item );
        // Precondition:
        //      item < first component in list
        // Postcondition:
        //      item is first component in list
        //   && List components are in ascending order

    void Insert( /* in */ ComponentType item );
        // Precondition:
        //      item is assigned
        // Postcondition:
        //      item is in list
        //   && List components are in ascending order

    void DeleteTop( /* out */ ComponentType& item );
        // Precondition:
        //      NOT IsEmpty()
        // Postcondition:
        //      item == first component in list at entry
        //   && item is no longer in list
        //   && List components are in ascending order

    void Delete( /* in */ ComponentType item );
        // Precondition:
```

FIGURE 16-6
Specification of
the SortedList2
Class
(continued)

```
//      item is somewhere in list
// Postcondition:
//      First occurrence of item is no longer in list
//      && List components are in ascending order

SortedList2();
    // Constructor
    // Postcondition:
    //      Empty list is created

SortedList2( const SortedList2& otherList );
    // Copy-constructor
    // Postcondition:
    //      List is created as a duplicate of otherList

~SortedList2();
    // Destructor
    // Postcondition:
    //      List is destroyed
private:
    NodeType* head;
};
```

In the class declaration, notice that the preconditions and postconditions of the member functions mention nothing about linked lists. The abstraction is a list, not a linked list. The user of the class is interested only in manipulating lists of items and does not care how we implement a list. If we change to a different implementation—an array, for example—the public interface remains valid.

The private data of the SortedList2 class consists of a single item: a pointer variable head. This variable is the external pointer to a dynamic linked list. As with any C++ class, different class objects have their own copies of the private data. For example, if the client code declares and manipulates two class objects like this:

```
SortedList2 list1;
SortedList2 list2;

list1.Insert(352);
list1.Insert(48);
list2.Insert(12);
    ⋮
if ( !list2.IsEmpty() )
    list2.DeleteTop(item);
```

then each of the two objects list1 and list2 has its own private head variable and maintains its own dynamic linked list on the free store.

In Figure 16-6, the specification file `slist2.h` declares a type `NodeType`, but only as a forward declaration. The only reason we need to declare the identifier `NodeType` in the specification file is so that the data type of the private variable `head` can be specified. In the spirit of information hiding, we place the complete declaration of `NodeType` into the implementation file `slist2.cpp`. The complete declaration is an implementation detail that the user does not need to know about. Here's how `slist2.cpp` starts out:

```
//***********************************************************************
// IMPLEMENTATION FILE (slist2.cpp)
// This file implements the SortedList2 class member functions
// List representation: a linked list of dynamic nodes
//***********************************************************************
#include "slist2.h"
#include <iostream>
#include <cstddef>        // For NULL

using namespace std;

typedef NodeType* NodePtr;
struct NodeType
{
    ComponentType component;
    NodePtr       link;
};

// Private members of class:
//      NodePtr head;              External pointer to linked list
    ⋮
```

To illustrate some commonly used algorithms on dynamic linked lists, let's look at the implementations of the `SortedList2` member functions. Creating an empty linked list is the easiest of the algorithms, so we begin there.

Creating an Empty Linked List   To create a linked list with no nodes, all that is necessary is to assign the external pointer the value `NULL`. For the `SortedList2` class, the appropriate place to do this is in the class constructor:

```
SortedList2::SortedList2()

// Constructor

// Postcondition:
//      head == NULL
```

```
{
    head = NULL;
}
```

As we discussed in Chapter 13, the implementation assertions (the preconditions and postconditions appearing in the implementation file) are often stated differently from the abstract assertions (those located in the specification file). Abstract assertions are written in terms that are meaningful to the user of the ADT; implementation details should not be mentioned. In contrast, implementation assertions can be made more precise by referring directly to variables and algorithms in the implementation code. In the case of the SortedList2 class constructor, the abstract postcondition is simply that an empty list (not a linked list) has been created. On the other hand, the implementation postcondition

```
// Postcondition:
//      head == NULL
```

is phrased in terms of our private data (head) and our particular list implementation (a dynamic linked list).

Testing for an Empty Linked List   The SortedList2 member function IsEmpty returns true if the list is empty and false if the list is not empty. Using a dynamic linked list representation, we return true if head contains the value NULL, and false otherwise:

```
bool SortedList2::IsEmpty() const

// Postcondition:
//      Function value == true, if head == NULL
//                     == false, otherwise

{
    return (head == NULL);
}
```

Printing a Linked List   To print the components of a linked list, we need to access the nodes one at a time. This requirement implies an event-controlled loop, where the event that stops the loop is reaching the end of the list. The loop control variable is a pointer that is initialized to the external pointer and is advanced from node to node by setting it equal to the link member of the current node. When the loop control pointer equals NULL, the last node has been accessed.

Print ( )

```
Set currPtr = head
WHILE currPtr doesn't equal NULL
     Print component member of *currPtr
     Set currPtr = link member of *currPtr
```

Note that this algorithm works correctly even if the list is empty (head equals NULL).

```
void SortedList2::Print() const

// Postcondition:
//      component members of all nodes (if any) in linked list
//      have been output

{
    NodePtr currPtr = head;       // Loop control pointer

    while (currPtr != NULL)
    {
        cout << currPtr->component << endl;
        currPtr = currPtr->link;
    }
}
```

Let's do a code walk-through using the following list.

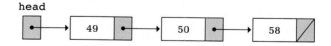

currPtr = head;   currPtr and head both point to
                                        the first node in the list.

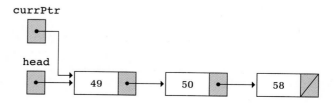

```
while (currPtr != NULL)
```
The loop body is entered because `currPtr` is not NULL.

```
cout << currPtr->component << endl;
currPtr = currPtr->link;
```
The number 49 is printed. `currPtr` now points to the second node in the list.

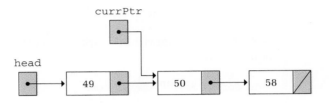

```
while (currPtr != NULL)
```
The loop body repeats because `currPtr` is not NULL.

```
cout << currPtr->component << endl;
currPtr = currPtr->link;
```
The number 50 is printed. `currPtr` now points to the third node in the list.

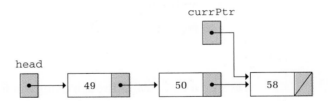

```
while (currPtr != NULL)
```
The loop body repeats because `currPtr` is not NULL.

```
cout << currPtr->component << endl;
currPtr = currPtr->link;
```
The number 58 is printed. `currPtr` is now NULL.

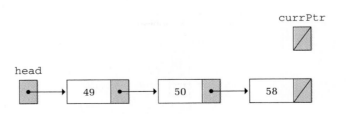

```
while (currPtr != NULL)
```
The loop body is not repeated because `currPtr` is NULL.

Inserting into a Linked List A function for inserting a component into a linked list must have an argument: the item to be inserted. The phrase *inserting into a linked list* could mean either inserting the component at the top of the list (as the first node) or inserting the component into its proper place according to some ordering (alphabetic or numeric). Let's examine these two situations separately.

Inserting a component at the top of a list is easy because we don't have to search the list to find where the item belongs.

InsertTop (In: item)

> Set newNodePtr = new NodeType
> Set component member of *newNodePtr = item
> Set link member of *newNodePtr = head
> Set head = newNodePtr

This algorithm is coded in the following function.

```
void SortedList2::InsertTop( /* in */ ComponentType item )

// Precondition:
//     component members of list nodes are in ascending order
//  && item < component member of first list node
// Postcondition:
//     New node containing item is at top of linked list
//  && component members of list nodes are in ascending order

{
    NodePtr newNodePtr = new NodeType;     // Temporary pointer

    newNodePtr->component = item;
    newNodePtr->link = head;
    head = newNodePtr;
}
```

The function precondition states that `item` must be smaller than the value in the first node. This precondition is not a requirement of linked lists in general. However, the `SortedList2` abstraction we are implementing is a sorted list. The precondition/postcondition contract states that *if* the client sends a value smaller than the first one in the list, then the func-

tion guarantees to preserve the ascending order. If the client violates the
precondition, the contract is broken.

The following code walk-through shows the steps in inserting a component with the value 20 as the first node in the linked list that was printed in the last section.

```
newNodePtr = new NodeType;
newNodePtr->component = item;
```
A new node is created.
The number 20 is stored into the component member of the new node.

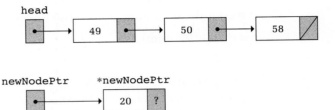

```
newNodePtr->link = head;
```
The link member of *newNodePtr now points to the first node in the list.

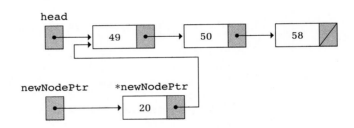

```
head = newNodePtr;
```
The external pointer to the list now points to the node containing the new component.

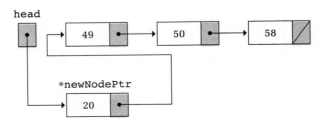

To insert a component into its proper place in a sorted list, we have to loop through the nodes until we find where the component belongs. Because the SortedList2 class keeps components in ascending order, we can recognize where a component belongs by finding the node that contains a value greater than the one being inserted. Our new node should be inserted directly before the node with that value; therefore, we must keep track of the node before the current one in order to insert our new node. We use a pointer prevPtr to point to this previous node. This method leads to the following algorithm:

Insert (In: item)

```
Set newNodePtr = new NodeType
Set component member of *newNodePtr = item
Set prevPtr = NULL
Set currPtr = head
WHILE item > component member of *currPtr
        Set prevPtr = currPtr
        Set currPtr = link member of *currPtr
Insert *newNodePtr between *prevPtr and *currPtr
```

This algorithm is basically sound, but there are problems with it in special cases. If the new component is larger than all other components in the list, the event that stops the loop (finding a node whose component is larger than the one being inserted) does not occur. When the end of the list is reached, the While condition tries to dereference currPtr, which now contains NULL. On some systems, the program will crash. We can take care of this case by using the following expression to control the While loop:

currPtr isn't NULL AND item > component member of *currPtr

This expression keeps us from dereferencing the null pointer because C++ uses short-circuit evaluation of logical expressions. If the first part evaluates to false—that is, if currPtr equals NULL—the second part of the expression, which dereferences currPtr, is not evaluated.

There is one more point to consider in our algorithm: the special case in which the list is empty or the new value is less than the first component in the list. The variable prevPtr remains NULL in this case, and *newNodePtr must be inserted at the top instead of between *prevPtr and *currPtr.

The following function implements our algorithm with these changes incorporated.

```
void SortedList2::Insert( /* in */ ComponentType item )

// Precondition:
//      component members of list nodes are in ascending order
//   && item is assigned
// Postcondition:
//      New node containing item is in its proper place
//         in linked list
//   && component members of list nodes are in ascending order

{
    NodePtr currPtr;        // Moving pointer
    NodePtr prevPtr;        // Pointer to node before *currPtr
    NodePtr newNodePtr;     // Pointer to new node

    // Set up node to be inserted

    newNodePtr = new NodeType;
    newNodePtr->component = item;

    // Find previous insertion point

    prevPtr = NULL;
    currPtr = head;
    while (currPtr != NULL && item > currPtr->component)
    {
        prevPtr = currPtr;
        currPtr = currPtr->link;
    }

    // Insert new node

    newNodePtr->link = currPtr;
    if (prevPtr == NULL)
        head = newNodePtr;
    else
        prevPtr->link = newNodePtr;
}
```

Let's go through this code for each of the three cases: inserting at the top (item is 20), inserting in the middle (item is 60), and inserting at the end (item is 100). Each insertion begins with the list below.

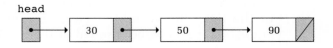

Insert(20)

```
newNodePtr = new NodeType;
newNodePtr->component = item;
prevPtr = NULL;
currPtr = head;
```

These four statements initialize the variables used in the searching process. The variables their contents are shown below.

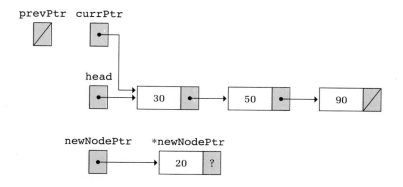

```
while (currPtr != NULL &&
    item > currPtr->component)

newNodePtr->link = currPtr;

if (prevPtr == NULL)
head = newNodePtr;
```

Because 20 is less than 30, the expression is `false` and the loop body is not entered.
`link` member of `*newNodePtr` now points to `*currPtr`.
Because `prevPtr` is `NULL`, the then-clause is executed and 20 is inserted at the top of the list.

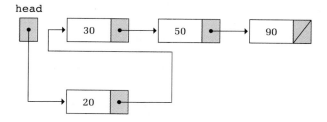

Insert(60)

```
newNodePtr = new NodeType;
newNodePtr->component = item;
prevPtr = NULL;
currPtr = head;
```

These four statements initialize the variables used in the searching process. The variables and their contents are shown below.

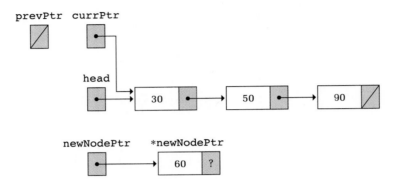

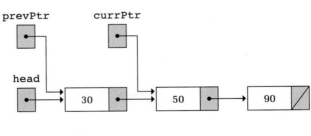

```
while (currPtr != NULL &&
    item > currPtr->component)

prevPtr = currPtr;
currPtr = currPtr->link;
```

Because 60 is greater than 30, this expression is true and the loop body is entered.
Pointer variables are advanced.

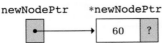

```
while (currPtr != NULL &&
    item > currPtr->component)

prevPtr = currPtr;
currPtr = currPtr->link;
```

Because 60 is greater than 50, this expression is `true` and the loop body is repeated.
Pointer variables are advanced.

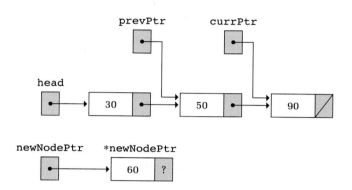

```
while (currPtr != NULL &&
    item > currPtr->component)

newNodePtr->link = currPtr;
```

Because 60 is not greater than 90, the expression is `false` and the loop body is not repeated.
`link` member of `*newNodePtr` now points to `*currPtr`.

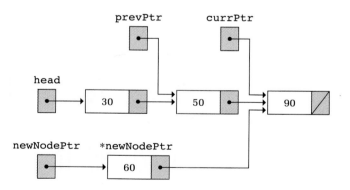

```
if (prevPtr == NULL)
prevPtr->link = newNodePtr;
```
Because `prevPtr` does not equal `NULL`, the else-clause is executed. The completed list is shown with the auxiliary variables removed.

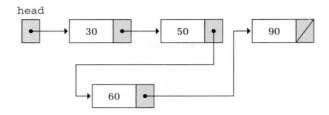

Insert(100)

We do not repeat the first part of the search, but pick up the walkthrough where `prevPtr` is pointing to the node whose component is 50, and `currPtr` is pointing to the node whose component is 90.

```
while (currPtr != NULL &&
    item > currPtr->component)

prevPtr = currPtr;
currPtr = currPtr->link;
```
Because 100 is greater than 90, this expression is `true` and the loop body is repeated. The pointer variables are advanced.

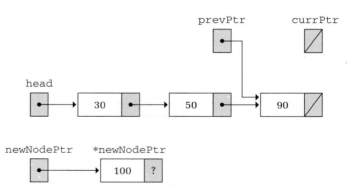

```
while (currPtr != NULL &&
    item > currPtr->component)

newNodePtr->link = currPtr;
```
Because `currPtr` equals `NULL`, the expression is `false` and the loop body is not repeated. `NULL` is copied into `link` member of `*newNodePtr`.

```
if (prevPtr == NULL)
prevPtr->link = newNodePtr;
```

Because `prevPtr` does not equal `NULL`, the else-clause is executed. Node `*newNodePtr` is inserted after `*prevPtr`. The list is shown with auxiliary variables removed.

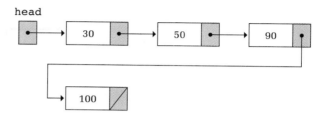

Deleting from a Linked List To delete an existing node from a linked list, we have to loop through the nodes until we find the node we want to delete. We look at the mirror image of our insertions: deleting the top node and deleting a node whose component is equal to an incoming parameter.

To delete the first node, we just change the external pointer to point to the second node (or to contain `NULL` if we are deleting the only node in a one-node list). The value in the node being deleted can be returned as an outgoing parameter. Notice the precondition for the following function: The client must not call the function if the list is empty.

```
void SortedList2::DeleteTop( /* out */ ComponentType& item )

// Precondition:
//      Linked list is not empty (head != NULL)
//   && component members of list nodes are in ascending order
// Postcondition:
//      item == component member of first list node at entry
//   && Node containing item is no longer in linked list
//   && component members of list nodes are in ascending order

{
    NodePtr tempPtr = head;     // Temporary pointer

    item = head->component;
    head = head->link;
    delete tempPtr;
}
```

We don't show a complete code walk-through because the code is so straightforward. Instead, we show the state of the data structure in two stages: after the first two statements and at the end. We use one of our previous lists. Following is the data structure after the execution of the first two statements in the function.

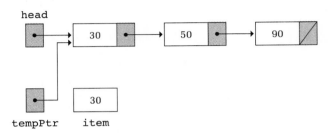

After the execution of the function, the structure is as follows:

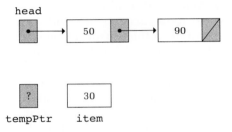

The function for deleting a node whose component contains a certain value is similar to the `Insert` function. The difference is that we are looking for a match, not a `component` member greater than our `item`. Because the function precondition states that the component we are looking for is definitely in the list, our loop control is simple. We don't have to worry about dereferencing the null pointer.

As in the `Insert` function, we need the node before the one that is to be deleted so we can change its `link` member. In the following function, we demonstrate another technique for keeping track of the previous node. Instead of comparing `item` with the `component` member of `*currPtr`, we compare it with the `component` member of the node pointed to by `currPtr->link`; that is, we compare `item` with `currPtr->link->component`. When `currPtr->link->component` is equal to `item`, `*currPtr` is the previous node.

```
void SortedList2::Delete( /* in */ ComponentType item )

// Precondition:
//      item == component member of some list node
//   && component members of list nodes are in ascending order
// Postcondition:
//      Node containing first occurrence of item is no longer in
//         linked list
//   && component members of list nodes are in ascending order

{
    NodePtr delPtr;      // Pointer to node to be deleted
    NodePtr currPtr;     // Loop control pointer

    // Check if item is in first node

    if (item == head->component)
    {
        // Delete first node

        delPtr = head;
        head = head->link;
    }
    else
    {
        // Search for node in rest of list

        currPtr = head;
        while (currPtr->link->component != item)
            currPtr = currPtr->link;

        // Delete *(currPtr->link)

        delPtr = currPtr->link;
        currPtr->link = currPtr->link->link;
    }
    delete delPtr;
}
```

Let's delete the node whose component is 90. The structure is shown below, with the nodes labeled as they are when the While statement is reached.

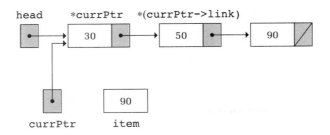

```
while (currPtr->link->component != item)   Because 50 is not equal
                                           to 90, the loop body is
                                           entered.
currPtr = currPtr->link;                   Pointer is advanced.
```

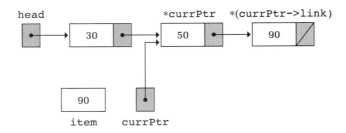

```
while (currPtr->link->component != item)   Because 90 is equal to
                                           90, the loop is exited.
delPtr = currPtr->link;
currPtr->link = currPtr->link->link;       The link member of the
                                           node whose compo-
                                           nent is 90 is copied
                                           into the link member
                                           of the node whose
                                           component is 50. The
                                           link member equals
                                           NULL in this case.
```

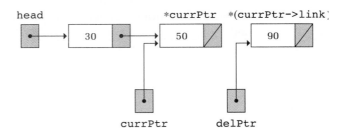

```
delete delPtr;
```

Memory allocated to `*delPtr` (the node that was deleted) is returned to the free store. The value of `delPtr` is undefined.

Note that NULL was stored into `currPtr->link` only because the node whose component is 90 was the last one in the list. If there had been more nodes beyond this one, a pointer to the next node would have been stored into `currPtr->link`.

Pointer Expressions

As you can see from the `SortedList2::Delete` function, pointer expressions can be quite complex. Let's look at some examples.

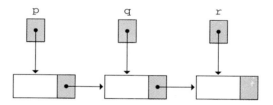

p, q, and r point to nodes in a dynamic linked list. The nodes themselves are `*p`, `*q`, and `*r`. Use the preceding diagram to convince yourself that the following are true.

```
p->link == q
```
`*(p->link)` is the same node as `*q`
```
p->link->link == r
```
`*(p->link->link)` is the same node as `*r`
```
q->link == r
```
`*(q->link)` is the same node as `*r`

And remember the semantics of assignment statements for pointers.

`p = q;`   Assigns the contents of pointer q to pointer p.

`*p = *q;`   Assigns the contents of the variable pointed to by q to the variable pointed to by p.

Classes and Dynamic Linked Lists

In Chapter 15, we said that classes whose objects manipulate dynamic data on the free store should provide not only a class constructor but also a destructor, a deep copy operation, and a copy-constructor. The SortedList2 class includes all of these except (to keep the example simpler) a deep copy operation. Let's look at the class destructor.

The purpose of the destructor is to deallocate the dynamic linked list when a SortedList2 class object is destroyed. Without a destructor, the linked list would be left behind on the free store, still allocated but inaccessible. The code for the destructor is easy to write. Using the existing member functions IsEmpty and DeleteTop, we simply march through the list and delete each node:

```
SortedList2::~SortedList2()

// Destructor

// Postcondition:
//     All linked list nodes have been deallocated from free store

{
    ComponentType temp;     // Temporary variable

    while ( !IsEmpty() )
        DeleteTop(temp);
}
```

The copy-constructor is harder to write. Before we look at it, we must stress the importance of providing a copy-constructor whenever we also provide a destructor. Pretend that SortedList2 doesn't have a copy-constructor, and suppose that a client passes a class object to a function using a pass by value. (Remember that passing an argument by value sends a *copy* of the value of the argument to the function.) Within the function, the parameter is initialized to be a copy of the caller's class object, including the caller's value of the private variable head. At this point, both the argument and the parameter are pointing to the same dynamic linked list. When the client function returns, the class destructor is invoked for the parameter, destroying the only copy of the linked list. Upon return from the function, the caller's linked list has disappeared!

By providing a copy-constructor, we ensure deep copying of an argument to a parameter whenever a pass by value occurs. The implementation of the copy-constructor, shown below, employs a commonly used algorithm for creating a new linked list as a copy of another.

```
SortedList2::SortedList2( const SortedList2& otherList )

// Copy-constructor

// Postcondition:
//      IF otherList.head == NULL   (i.e., the other list is empty)
//          head == NULL
//      ELSE
//          head points to a new linked list that is a copy of
//          the linked list pointed to by otherList.head

{
    NodePtr fromPtr;    // Pointer into list being copied from
    NodePtr toPtr;      // Pointer into new list being built

    if (otherList.head == NULL)
    {
        head = NULL;
        return;
    }

    // Copy first node

    fromPtr = otherList.head;
    head = new NodeType;
    head->component = fromPtr->component;

    // Copy remaining nodes

    toPtr = head;
    fromPtr = fromPtr->link;
    while (fromPtr != NULL)
    {
        toPtr->link = new NodeType;
        toPtr = toPtr->link;
        toPtr->component = fromPtr->component;
        fromPtr = fromPtr->link;
    }
    toPtr->link = NULL;
}
```

Choice of Data Representation

We have looked in detail at two ways of representing lists of components: one in which the components are physically next to each other (a direct array representation, as in Figure 16-1), and one in which the components are only logically next to each other (a linked list). Furthermore, a linked list is an abstraction that can be implemented either by using an array of structs or by using dynamically allocated structs and pointers (a dynamic linked list).

Let's compare the array representation with the dynamic linked list representation. (Throughout this discussion, we use *array* to mean a direct array representation, not an array of structs forming a linked list.) We look at common operations on lists and examine the advantages and disadvantages of each representation for each operation.

Common Operations

1. Read the components into an initially empty list.
2. Access all the components in the list in sequence.
3. Insert or delete the first component in a list.
4. Insert or delete the last component in a list.
5. Insert or delete the nth component in a list.
6. Access the nth component in a list.
7. Sort the components in a list.
8. Search the list for a specific component.

Reading components into a list is faster with an array representation than with a dynamic linked list because the new operation doesn't have to be executed for each component. Accessing the components in sequence takes approximately the same time with both structures.

Inserting or deleting the first component is much faster using a linked representation. Remember that with an array, all the other list items have to be shifted down (for an insertion) or up (for a deletion). Conversely, inserting or deleting the last component is much more efficient with an array; there is direct access to the last component, and no shifting is required. In a linked representation, the entire list must be searched to find the last component.

On average, the time spent inserting or deleting the nth component is about equal for the two types of lists. A linked representation would be better for small values of n, and an array representation would be better for values of n near the end of the list.

Accessing the nth element is *much* faster in an array representation. We can access it directly by using $n - 1$ as the index into the array. In a linked representation, we have to access the first $n - 1$ components sequentially to reach the nth one.

For many sorting algorithms, including the selection sort, the two representations are approximately equal in efficiency. However, there are some sophisticated, very fast sorting algorithms that rely on direct access to array elements by using array indexes. These algorithms are not suitable for a linked representation, which requires sequential access to the components.

In general, searching a sorted list for a specific component is much faster in an array representation because a binary search can be used. When the components in the list to be searched are not in sorted order, the two representations are about the same.

When you are trying to decide whether to use an array representation or a linked representation, determine which of these common operations are likely to be applied most frequently. Use your analysis to determine which structure would be better in the context of your particular problem.

There is one additional point to consider when deciding whether to use an array or a dynamic linked list. How accurately can you predict the maximum number of components in the list? Does the number of components in the list fluctuate widely? If you know the maximum and it remains fairly constant, an array representation is fine in terms of memory usage. Otherwise, it is better to choose a dynamic linked representation in order to use memory more efficiently.

*P*ROBLEM-SOLVING CASE STUDY

Simulated Playing Cards

Problem: As an avid card player, you plan to write a program to play solitaire once you have become thoroughly comfortable with dynamic data structures. As a prelude to that program, you decide to design a C++ class that models a pile of playing cards. The pile could be a discard pile, a pile of cards face up on the table, or even a full deck of unshuffled cards. The card pile will be structured as a dynamic linked list.

In this case study, we omit the Input and Output sections because we are developing only a C++ class, not a complete program. Instead, we include two sections entitled Specification of the Class and Implementation of the Class.

Discussion: Thinking of a card pile as an ADT, what kinds of operations would we like to perform on this ADT? You might come up with a different list, but here are some operations we have chosen:

Create an empty pile
Put a new card onto the pile
Take a card from the pile
Determine the current length of the pile
Inspect the *n*th card in the pile

We can base our design roughly on the `SortedList2` class of this chapter, but there are some differences. First, we should consider a card pile to be

PROBLEM-SOLVING CASE STUDY cont'd.

an unsorted list, not a sorted list, because the cards can be in random order in the pile. Second, the last two operations listed above were not present in SortedList2. These operations allow more flexibility in asking questions about the list. If we use a private variable to keep track of the current length of the list, we can ask at any time how many cards are in a pile. We also can simulate looking at a face-up pile of cards by using the last operation to inspect any card in the pile without removing it.

Before we write the class specification, we must decide how to represent an individual playing card. The suit of a card can be represented using an enumeration type. Rank can be represented using the numbers 1 through 13, with the ace as a 1 and the king as a 13. Each card is then represented as a struct with two members, suit and rank:

```
enum Suits {CLUB, DIAMOND, HEART, SPADE};

struct CardType
{
    Suits  suit;
    int    rank;        // Range 1 (ace) through 13 (king)
};
```

Below is the specification file cardpile.h, which provides the client with declarations for the CardType type and the CardPile class.

```
//******************************************************************
// SPECIFICATION FILE (cardpile.h)
// This file gives the specifications of
//   1. CardType--a data type representing an ordinary playing card
//   2. CardPile--an unsorted list ADT representing a pile
//      of playing cards
//******************************************************************
#ifndef CARDPILE_H
#define CARDPILE_H

enum Suits {CLUB, DIAMOND, HEART, SPADE};

struct CardType
{
    Suits  suit;
    int    rank;        // Range 1 (ace) through 13 (king)
};

struct NodeType;        // Forward declaration (Complete declaration
                        // is hidden in implementation file)
```

PROBLEM-SOLVING CASE STUDY *cont'd.*

```cpp
class CardPile
{
public:
    int Length() const;
        // Postcondition:
        //      Function value == number of cards in pile

    CardType CardAt( /* in */ int n ) const;
        // Precondition:
        //      n >= 1  &&  n <= Length()
        // Postcondition:
        //      Function value == card at position n in pile

    void InsertTop( /* in */ CardType newCard );
        // Precondition:
        //      newCard is assigned
        // Postcondition:
        //      newCard is at top of pile

    void RemoveTop( /* out */ CardType& topCard );
        // Precondition:
        //      Length() > 0
        // Postcondition:
        //      topCard == value of first component in pile at entry
        //   && topCard is no longer in pile

    CardPile();
        // Postcondition:
        //      Empty pile is created

    CardPile( const CardPile& otherPile );
        // Postcondition:
        //      Pile is created as a duplicate of otherPile

    ~CardPile();
        // Postcondition:
        //      Pile is destroyed
private:
    NodeType* head;
    int       listLength;
};

#endif
```

Implementation of the Class: For the data representation of a card pile, we use a linked list. Furthermore, we implement the linked list using dynamic data and pointers. Each node is of type NodeType, whose complete declaration (hidden in the implementation file) is as follows:

```
typedef NodeType* NodePtr;
struct NodeType
{
    CardType card;
    NodePtr  link;
};
```

The private variable head is the external pointer to the linked list, and the private variable listLength keeps track of the current length of the list.

The class constructor, copy-constructor, and destructor: These functions are essentially identical to those in the SortedList2 class. The only significant difference is in the constructor. In addition to setting head to NULL, the constructor must set listLength to 0.

The InsertTop and RemoveTop functions: These functions are the same as InsertTop and DeleteTop in the SortedList2 class, with the following differences. After inserting a new node, InsertTop must increment listLength; after deleting a node, RemoveTop must decrement listLength.

The Length function: Because the private variable listLength always indicates the current length of the list, no looping and counting are required. The function body is a single statement:

```
return listLength;
```

The CardAt function: To access the card at position *n* in the pile, we must start at the front of the list and sequence our way through the first *n* − 1 nodes. When we get to the desired node, we return the card member of the node as the function return value.

CardAt (In: n)

```
Set currPtr = head
FOR count going from 1 through n – 1
     Set currPtr = link member of *currPtr
Return card member of *currPtr
```

Here is the implementation file containing the definitions of the `CardPile` member functions:

```cpp
//****************************************************************
// IMPLEMENTATION FILE (cardpile.cpp)
// This file implements the CardPile class member functions
// List representation: a linked list of dynamic nodes
//****************************************************************
#include "cardpile.h"
#include <cstddef>        // For NULL

using namespace std;

typedef NodeType* NodePtr;
struct NodeType
{
    CardType card;
    NodePtr  link;
};

// Private members of class:
//      NodePtr head;              External pointer to linked list
//      int     listLength;        Current length of list

//****************************************************************

CardPile::CardPile()

// Constructor

// Postcondition:
//      head == NULL  &&  listLength == 0

{
    head = NULL;
    listLength = 0;
}
```

```
//*****************************************************************

CardPile::CardPile( const CardPile& otherPile )

// Copy-constructor

// Postcondition:
//      listLength == otherPile.listLength
//   && IF otherPile.head == NULL
//         head == NULL
//      ELSE
//         head points to a new linked list that is a copy of
//         the linked list pointed to by otherPile.head

{
    NodePtr toPtr;      // Pointer into new list being built
    NodePtr fromPtr;    // Pointer into list being copied from

    listLength = otherPile.listLength;
    if (otherPile.head == NULL)
    {
        head = NULL;
        return;
    }

    // Copy first node

    fromPtr = otherPile.head;
    head = new NodeType;
    head->card = fromPtr->card;

    // Copy remaining nodes

    toPtr = head;
    fromPtr = fromPtr->link;
    while (fromPtr != NULL)
    {
        toPtr->link = new NodeType;
        toPtr = toPtr->link;
        toPtr->card = fromPtr->card;
        fromPtr = fromPtr->link;
    }
    toPtr->link = NULL;
}


//*****************************************************************
```

PROBLEM-SOLVING CASE STUDY cont'd.

```
CardPile::~CardPile()

// Destructor

// Postcondition:
//      All linked list nodes have been deallocated from free store

{
    CardType temp;      // Temporary variable

    while (listLength > 0)
        RemoveTop(temp);
}

//*******************************************************************

int CardPile::Length() const

// Postcondition:
//      Function value == listLength

{
    return listLength;
}

//*******************************************************************

CardType CardPile::CardAt( /* in */ int n ) const

// Precondition:
//      1 <= n <= listLength
// Postcondition:
//      Function value == card member of list node at position n

{
    int     count;              // Loop control variable
    NodePtr currPtr = head;     // Moving pointer variable

    for (count = 1; count < n; count++)
        currPtr = currPtr->link;
    return currPtr->card;
}

//*******************************************************************

void CardPile::InsertTop( /* in */ CardType newCard )
```

```
// Precondition:
//      newCard is assigned
// Postcondition:
//      New node containing newCard is at top of linked list
//   && listLength == listLength@entry + 1

{
    NodePtr newNodePtr = new NodeType;     // Temporary pointer

    newNodePtr->card = newCard;
    newNodePtr->link = head;
    head = newNodePtr;
    listLength++;
}


//****************************************************************

void CardPile::RemoveTop( /* out */ CardType& topCard )

// Precondition:
//      listLength > 0
// Postcondition:
//      topCard == card member of first list node at entry
//   && Node containing topCard is no longer in linked list
//   && listLength == listLength@entry - 1

{
    NodePtr tempPtr = head;     // Temporary pointer

    topCard = head->card;
    head = head->link;
    delete tempPtr;
    listLength--;
}
```

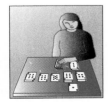

PROBLEM-SOLVING CASE STUDY

Solitaire Simulation

Problem: There is a solitaire game that is quite simple but seems difficult to win. Let's write a program to play the game, then run it a number of times to see if it really is that difficult to win or if we have just been unlucky.

PROBLEM-SOLVING CASE STUDY cont'd.

Although this card game is played with a regular poker or bridge deck, the rules deal with suits only; the face values (ranks) are ignored. The rules are listed below. Rules 1 and 2 are initialization.

1. Take a deck of playing cards and shuffle it.
2. Place four cards side by side, left to right, face up on the table.
3. If the four cards (or the rightmost four if there are more than four on the table) are of the same suit, move them to a discard pile. Otherwise, if the first one and the fourth one (of the rightmost four cards) are of the same suit, move the other two cards (second and third) to a discard pile. Repeat until no cards can be removed.
4. Take the next card from the shuffled deck and place it face up to the right of those already there. Repeat this step if there are fewer than four cards face up (assuming there are more cards in the deck).
5. Repeat steps 3 and 4 until there are no more cards in the deck. You win if all the cards are on the discard pile.

Figure 16-7 walks us through the beginning of a typical game to demonstrate how the rules operate. Remember that the game deals with suits only. There must be at least four cards face up on the table before the rules can be applied.

Input: The number of times the simulation is to be run (`numberOf-Games`), the number of times the deck is to be shuffled between games (`numberOfShuffles`), and an initial seed value for a random number generator (`seed`). We discuss the `seed` variable later.

Output: The number of games played and the number of games won.

Discussion: A program that plays a game is an example of a *simulation program*. The program simulates what a human does when playing the game. Programs that simulate games or real-world processes are very common in computing.

In developing a simulation, object-oriented design helps us decide how to represent the physical items being simulated. In a card game, the basic item is, of course, a card. A deck of cards becomes a list of 52 cards in the program. We can use a variation of the `CardPile` class developed in the previous case study to represent the deck.

Cards face up on the table and in the discard pile must also be simulated in this program. Putting a card face up on the table means that a card is being taken from the deck and put onto the table where the player can see it. The cards on the table can be represented by a `CardPile` class object. The rules that determine whether or not cards can be moved to the

<u>*PROBLEM-SOLVING CASE STUDY*</u> *cont'd.*

FIGURE 16-7
Solitaire Game

Initialize with the first 4 cards.

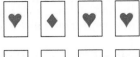

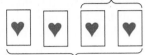

Remove the 2 inner cards.
Add 2 cards (need at least 4 cards to play).

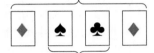

Remove all 4 cards.
Add 4 more cards.

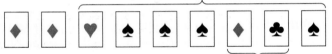

Remove the 2 inner cards.
Add 2 cards until another match.

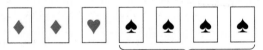

Remove the 2 inner cards from group of last 4.

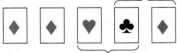

Remove the last 4 cards.
Add cards until another match.

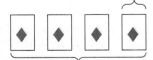

Remove the 2 inner cards from group of last 4.
Add cards until another match.

Remove all 4 cards.

.
.
.

discard pile are applied to the top four cards in this list—that is, the last four cards put into the list.

The discard pile is also a list of cards and can be represented as a `CardPile` class object. If no cards remain on the table (they are all on the discard pile) at the end of the game, then the player has won. If any cards remain on the table face up, the player has lost.

A linked list is a good choice for representing these three lists (the deck, the cards face up on the table, and the discard pile). The simulation requires a lot of deleting from one list and inserting into another list, and these operations are quite efficient with a linked list.

Using dynamic variables to represent our lists instead of a direct array representation saves memory space. If an array representation were used, three arrays of 52 components each would have to be created. In a dynamic linked representation, we use only 52 components in all, because a card can be in only one list at a time.

In our object-oriented design, we have now identified three objects: a card deck, an on-table pile, and a discard pile. A fourth object we'll use is a player object. This object can be thought of as a manager—it is responsible for coordinating the three card pile objects and playing the game according to the rules.

To determine the relationships among these four objects, we observe that the three card pile objects are independent of each other and are not related by inheritance or composition. However, the player object is composed of the other three objects—it *has a* deck, an on-table pile, and a discard pile as part or all of its internal data. This relationship is seen more clearly when we design and implement the player object.

The On-Table Pile and Discard Pile Objects: We can represent these objects directly using the `CardPile` class from the previous case study.

The Card Deck Object: We could represent this object using the `CardPile` class, but a full deck of cards is more specialized than an ordinary card pile. For example, the `CardPile` class constructor creates an empty pile, whereas we would like a new card deck to be created as a list of all 52 cards, arranged in order by suit and rank. Also, we would like to include two more operations that are appropriate for a card deck—one to shuffle the deck, the other to recreate the deck at the end of each game by gathering together all 52 cards from the on-table pile and the discard pile.

The easiest way to add these new operations to the `CardPile` class is to use inheritance. From the `CardPile` class we can derive a new `CardDeck` class that inherits the `CardPile` class members and adds the new functions. Inheritance is appropriate here because a card deck *is a* card pile (and more). Here is the class specification:

```
//*******************************************************************
// SPECIFICATION FILE (carddeck.h)
// This file gives the specification of a CardDeck class, derived
// from the CardPile class using inheritance
//*******************************************************************
#ifndef CARDDECK_H
#define CARDDECK_H

#include "cardpile.h"

const int DECK_SIZE = 52;

class CardDeck : public CardPile
{
public:
    void Shuffle( /* in */ int numberOfShuffles);
        // Precondition:
        //      Length of deck == DECK_SIZE
        //   && numberOfShuffles is assigned
        // Postcondition:
        //      The order of components in the deck has been
        //      rearranged numberOfShuffles times, randomly

    void Recreate( /* inout */ CardPile& pile1,
                   /* inout */ CardPile& pile2 );
        // Gathers cards from two piles and puts them back into deck
        // Precondition:
        //      Length of deck == 0
        //   && (Length of pile1 + length of pile2) == DECK_SIZE
        // Postcondition:
        //      Deck is the list consisting of all cards from
        //      pile1@entry followed by all cards from pile2@entry
        //   && Length of deck == DECK_SIZE
        //   && Length of pile1 == 0  &&  Length of pile2 == 0

    CardDeck();
        // Postcondition:
        //      List of DECK_SIZE components is created
        //      representing a standard deck of playing cards
        //   && Cards are in order by suit and by rank
private:
    void Merge( CardPile&, CardPile& );
};

#endif
```

PROBLEM-SOLVING CASE STUDY *cont'd.*

Notice in the CardDeck class declaration that the private part does not include any additional data members. The only private data is the data inherited from the CardPile class. However, the private part declares a member function named Merge. This function is not accessible to clients of CardDeck. As we see shortly, the Merge function is a "helper" function that is used by the Shuffle member function.

Now we implement the CardDeck member functions. We begin with the class constructor.

The class constructor CardDeck ( )

When a CardDeck class object is created, the constructor for its base class (CardPile) is implicitly executed first, creating an empty list. Starting with the empty list, we can generate the first card—the ace of clubs—and insert it into the list. The balance of the 52 cards can be generated in a loop. After every 13th card, we increment the suit and reset the rank to 1.

```
Set tempCard.suit = CLUB
Set tempCard.rank = 1
InsertTop(tempCard)                              // Insert into deck
FOR count going from 2 through 52
    Increment tempCard.rank
    IF tempCard.rank > 13
        Increment tempCard.suit
        Set tempCard.rank = 1
    InsertTop(tempCard)                          // Insert into deck
```

Although we don't use the rank of a card, we leave it there because we may want to print out the contents of the list during debugging. Also, the CardDeck class may be used in other simulations. The class should be tested with a complete representation of a deck of cards

Shuffle (In: numberOfShuffles)

When a human shuffles a deck of cards, he or she divides the deck into two nearly equal parts and then merges the two parts again. This process can be simulated directly (a simulation within a simulation). The list representing the deck can be divided into two lists, halfA and halfB. Then these two lists can be merged again. We use a random number generator to determine how many cards go into halfA. The rest go into halfB.

Through the header file cstdlib, the C++ standard library provides two functions for producing random numbers. The first, named rand, has the following prototype:

```
int rand();
```

Each time this function is called, it returns a random integer in the range 0 through RAND_MAX, a constant defined in cstdlib. (RAND_MAX is typically the same as INT_MAX.) Because we want our random number to be in the range 1 through 52, we use the conversion formula

Set sizeOfCut = rand( ) MOD 52 + 1

or, in C++,

```
sizeOfCut = rand() % 52 + 1;
```

Random number generators use an initial *seed* value from which to start the sequence of random numbers. The C++ library function srand lets you specify an initial seed before calling rand. The prototype for srand is

```
void srand( unsigned int );
```

If you do not call srand before the first call to rand, an initial seed of 1 is assumed. As you'll see in the initialization portion of our main function, we input an initial seed value from the user and pass it as an argument to srand.

PROBLEM-SOLVING CASE STUDY cont'd.

```
FOR count1 going from 1 through numberOfShuffles
        Create empty list halfA
        Create empty list halfB
        Set sizeOfCut = rand( ) MOD 52 + 1
        Move sizeOfCut cards from deck to halfA
        Move remaining 52–sizeOfCut cards from deck to halfB
        IF sizeOfCut <= 26
                Merge(halfA, halfB)
        ELSE
                Merge(halfB, halfA)
```

Merge (Inout: shorterList, longerList)

The merge algorithm takes a component alternately from each list without regard to the contents of the component. We call the `Merge` function with two arguments: the shorter list and the longer list.

```
WHILE more cards in shorterList
        shorterList.RemoveTop(tempCard)
        InsertTop(tempCard)                        // Insert into deck
        longerList.RemoveTop(tempCard)
        InsertTop(tempCard)
WHILE more cards in longerList
        longerList.RemoveTop(tempCard)
        InsertTop(tempCard)
```

Recreate (Inout: pile1, pile2)

The `Recreate` function takes an empty deck (an empty list) and gathers cards from two piles, putting them back into the deck.

PROBLEM-SOLVING CASE STUDY cont'd.

```
WHILE more cards in pile1
       pile1.RemoveTop(tempCard)
       InsertTop(tempCard)                      // Insert into deck
WHILE more cards in pile2
       pile2.RemoveTop(tempCard)
       InsertTop(tempCard)
```

Below is the implementation file for the `CardDeck` member functions.

```cpp
//*****************************************************************
// IMPLEMENTATION FILE (carddeck.cpp)
// This file implements the CardDeck class member functions.
// The CardPile class is a public base class of CardDeck
//*****************************************************************
#include "carddeck.h"
#include <cstdlib>       // For rand()

using namespace std;

const int HALF_DECK = 26;

// Additional private members of class (beyond those
// inherited from CardPile):
//     void Merge( CardPile&, CardPile& );        Used by the Shuffle
//                                                 function


//*****************************************************************

CardDeck::CardDeck()

// Constructor--creates a list of DECK_SIZE components representing
// a standard deck of playing cards

// Postcondition:
//     After empty linked list created (via implicit call to base
//     class constructor), all DECK_SIZE playing cards have been
//     inserted into deck in order by suit and by rank

{
    int        count;       // Loop counter
    CardType tempCard;      // Temporary card
```

PROBLEM-SOLVING CASE STUDY *cont'd.*

```
            tempCard.suit = CLUB;
            tempCard.rank = 1;
            InsertTop(tempCard);

            // Loop to create balance of deck

            for (count = 2; count <= DECK_SIZE; count++)
            {
                // Increment rank

                tempCard.rank++;

                // Test for change of suit

                if (tempCard.rank > 13)
                {
                    tempCard.suit = Suits(tempCard.suit + 1);
                    tempCard.rank = 1;
                }
                InsertTop(tempCard);
            }
        }


//******************************************************************

void CardDeck::Shuffle( /* in */ int numberOfShuffles)

// Rearranges the deck (the list of DECK_SIZE components) into a
// different order.  The list is divided into two parts, which are
// then merged.  The process is repeated numberOfShuffles times

// Precondition:
//      Length of deck == DECK_SIZE
//   && numberOfShuffles is assigned
// Postcondition:
//      The order of components in the deck has been rearranged
//      numberOfShuffles times, randomly

{
    CardType tempCard;    // Temporary card
    int      count1;      // Loop counter
    int      count2;      // Loop counter
    int      sizeOfCut;   // Size of simulated cut
```

PROBLEM-SOLVING CASE STUDY cont'd.

```
        for (count1 = 1; count1 <= numberOfShuffles; count1++)
        {
            CardPile halfA;     // Half of the list, initially empty
            CardPile halfB;     // Half of the list, initially empty

            sizeOfCut = rand() % DECK_SIZE + 1;

            // Divide deck into two parts

            for (count2 = 1; count2 <= sizeOfCut; count2++)
            {
                RemoveTop(tempCard);
                halfA.InsertTop(tempCard);
            }
            for (count2 = sizeOfCut+1; count2 <= DECK_SIZE; count2++)
            {
                RemoveTop(tempCard);
                halfB.InsertTop(tempCard);
            }
            if (sizeOfCut <= HALF_DECK)
                Merge(halfA, halfB);
            else
                Merge(halfB, halfA);
        }
    }


//*****************************************************************

void CardDeck::Merge( /* inout */ CardPile& shorterList,
                      /* inout */ CardPile& longerList  )

// Merges shorterList and longerList into deck

// Precondition:
//     Length of shorterList > 0  &&  Length of longerList > 0
//  && Length of deck == 0
// Postcondition:
//     Deck is the list of cards obtained by merging
//     shorterList@entry and longerList@entry into one list
//  && Length of shorterList == 0
//  && Length of longerList == 0

{
    CardType tempCard;    // Temporary card

    // Take one card from each list alternately
```

PROBLEM-SOLVING CASE STUDY *cont'd.*

```cpp
    while (shorterList.Length() > 0)
    {
        shorterList.RemoveTop(tempCard);
        InsertTop(tempCard);
        longerList.RemoveTop(tempCard);
        InsertTop(tempCard);
    }

    // Copy remainder of longer list to deck

    while (longerList.Length() > 0)
    {
        longerList.RemoveTop(tempCard);
        InsertTop(tempCard);
    }
}


//******************************************************************

void CardDeck::Recreate( /* inout */ CardPile& pile1,
                         /* inout */ CardPile& pile2 )

// Gathers cards from two piles and puts them back into deck

// Precondition:
//     Length of deck == 0
//  && (Length of pile1 + length of pile2) == DECK_SIZE
// Postcondition:
//     Deck is the list consisting of all cards from pile1@entry
//     followed by all cards from pile2@entry
//  && Length of deck == DECK_SIZE
//  && Length of pile1 == 0  &&  Length of pile2 == 0

{
    CardType tempCard;     // Temporary card

    while (pile1.Length() > 0)
    {
        pile1.RemoveTop(tempCard);
        InsertTop(tempCard);
    }
    while (pile2.Length() > 0)
    {
        pile2.RemoveTop(tempCard);
        InsertTop(tempCard);
    }
}
```

PROBLEM-SOLVING CASE STUDY cont'd.

The Player Object: This object manages the playing of the solitaire game. It encapsulates the card deck, on-table pile, and discard pile objects and is responsible for moving cards from one pile to another according to the rules of the game.

To represent the player object, we design a `Player` class with the following specification:

```
//**************************************************************
// SPECIFICATION FILE (player.h)
// This file gives the specification of a Player class that manages
// the playing of a solitaire game
//**************************************************************
#ifndef PLAYER_H
#define PLAYER_H

#include "cardpile.h"
#include "carddeck.h"

class Player
{
public:
    void PlayGame( /* in */  int    numberOfShuffles,
                   /* out */ bool& won                 );
        // Precondition:
        //     numberOfShuffles is assigned
        // Postcondition:
        //     After deck has been shuffled numberOfShuffles times,
        //     one game of solitaire has been played
        //  && won == true, if the game was won
        //          == false, otherwise
private:
    CardDeck deck;
    CardPile onTable;
    CardPile discardPile;

    void TryRemove();
    void MoveFour();
    void MoveTwo();
};

#endif
```

The `Player` class has one public operation, `PlayGame`, that plays one game of solitaire and reports whether the game was won or lost. The private part of the class consists of three class objects—`deck`, `onTable`, and `discardPile`—and three private member functions. These "helper" func-

PROBLEM-SOLVING CASE STUDY *cont'd.*

tions are used in the playing of the game and are not accessible to clients of the class.

PlayGame (In: numberOfShuffles; Out: won)

```
deck.Shuffle(numberOfShuffles)
WHILE more cards in deck
        // Turn up a card
        deck.RemoveTop(tempCard)
        onTable.InsertTop(tempCard)
        // Try to remove it
        TryRemove()
Set won = (onTable.Length( ) equals 0)
deck.Recreate(onTable, discardPile)
```

TryRemove ( )

To remove cards, we first need to check the first and fourth cards. If these do not match, we can't move any cards. If they do match, we check to see how many can be moved. This process continues until there are fewer than four cards face up on the table or until no move can be made.

```
Set moveMade = true
WHILE onTable.Length( ) >= 4 AND moveMade
      IF suit of onTable.CardAt(1) matches suit of onTable.CardAt(4)
              IF suit of onTable.CardAt(1) matches suit of onTable.CardAt(2) AND
                        suit of onTable.CardAt(1) matches suit of onTable.CardAt(3)
              Move four cards from onTable to discardPile
          ELSE
                        Move two cards—the second and third—from onTable to discardPile
      ELSE
              Set moveMade = false
```

PROBLEM-SOLVING CASE STUDY cont'd.

MoveFour ( )

```
FOR count going from 1 through 4
    onTable.RemoveTop(tempCard)
    discardPile.InsertTop(tempCard)
```

MoveTwo ( )

```
Save top card from onTable
Move top card from onTable to discardPile
Move top card from onTable to discardPile
Restore original top card to onTable
```

The implementations of the `Player` class member functions are shown in the `player.cpp` file below.

```cpp
//****************************************************************
// IMPLEMENTATION FILE (player.cpp)
// This file implements the Player class member functions
//****************************************************************
#include "player.h"

// Private members of class
//     CardDeck deck;              Deck of cards
//     CardPile onTable;           Cards face up on the table
//     CardPile discardPile;       Cards on discard pile
//
//     void TryRemove( CardPile&, CardPile& );
//     void MoveFour( CardPile&, CardPile& );
//     void MoveTwo( CardPile&, CardPile& );


//****************************************************************

void Player::PlayGame( /* in */  int    numberOfShuffles,
                       /* out */ bool&  won                )

// Places each card in the deck face up on the table
// and applies rules for moving
```

PROBLEM-SOLVING CASE STUDY *cont'd.*

```
// Precondition:
//      numberOfShuffles is assigned
// Postcondition:
//      After deck has been shuffled numberOfShuffles times,
//      all cards have been moved one at a time from deck to onTable
//   && Cards have (possibly) been moved from onTable to discardPile
//      according to the rules of the game
//   && won == true, if the game was won
//           == false, otherwise

{
    CardType tempCard;      // Temporary card

    deck.Shuffle(numberOfShuffles);
    while (deck.Length() > 0)
    {
        deck.RemoveTop(tempCard);
        onTable.InsertTop(tempCard);
        TryRemove();
    }
    won = (onTable.Length() == 0);
    deck.Recreate(onTable, discardPile);
}


//****************************************************************

void Player::TryRemove()

// If the first (top) four cards in onTable are the same suit,
// they are moved to discardPile.  If the first card and the fourth
// card are the same suit, the second and third card are moved from
// onTable to discardPile.  This process continues until no further
// moves can be made

// Precondition:
//      Length of onTable > 0
// Postcondition:
//      Cards have (possibly) been moved from onTable to discardPile
//      according to the above rules

{
    bool moveMade = true;      // True if a move has been made

    while (onTable.Length() >= 4 && moveMade)
        if (onTable.CardAt(1).suit == onTable.CardAt(4).suit)
```

```
                      // A move will be made

                      if (onTable.CardAt(1).suit == onTable.CardAt(2).suit &&
                          onTable.CardAt(1).suit == onTable.CardAt(3).suit)
                          MoveFour();   // Four alike
                      else
                          MoveTwo();    // 1st and 4th alike
                  else
                      moveMade = false;
        }


//****************************************************************

void Player::MoveFour()

// Moves the first four cards from onTable to discardPile

// Precondition:
//      Length of onTable >= 4
// Postcondition:
//      The first four cards have been removed from onTable and
//      placed at the front of discardPile

{
    CardType tempCard;     // Temporary card
    int      count;        // Loop counter

    for (count = 1; count <= 4; count++)
    {
        onTable.RemoveTop(tempCard);
        discardPile.InsertTop(tempCard);
    }
}


//****************************************************************

void Player::MoveTwo()

// Moves the second and third cards from onTable to discardPile

// Precondition:
//      Length of onTable >= 4
// Postcondition:
//      The second and third cards have been removed from onTable and
//      placed at the front of discardPile
//   && The first card in onTable at entry is still the first card
//      in onTable
```

PROBLEM-SOLVING CASE STUDY cont'd.

```
{
    CardType tempCard;      // Temporary card
    CardType firstCard;     // First card in onTable

    // Remove and save first card

    onTable.RemoveTop(firstCard);

    // Move second card

    onTable.RemoveTop(tempCard);
    discardPile.InsertTop(tempCard);

    // Move third card

    onTable.RemoveTop(tempCard);
    discardPile.InsertTop(tempCard);

    // Restore first card

    onTable.InsertTop(firstCard);
}
```

The Driver: We have now designed and implemented all the objects responsible for playing the solitaire game. All that remains is to write the top-level algorithm (the driver).

Main   **Level 0**

Create player—an object of type Player
Set gamesWon = 0
Prompt for and input numberOfGames
Prompt for and input numberOfShuffles
Prompt for and input seed
Use seed to initialize the random number generator

FOR gamesPlayed going from 1 through numberOfGames
     player.PlayGame(numberOfShuffles, won)
    IF won
        Increment gamesWon
Print numberOfGames
Print gamesWon

PROBLEM-SOLVING CASE STUDY *cont'd.*

Module Structure Chart:

```
┌─────────────┐
│    Main     │
└─────────────┘
```

(The following program is written in ISO/ANSI standard C++. If you are working with pre–standard C++, see the alternate version of the program in the PRE_STD directory of the program disk, available at the publisher's Web site, www.jbpub.com/disks.)

```cpp
//******************************************************************
// Solitaire program
// This program is a simulation of a card game.
// See text for rules of the game
//******************************************************************
#include "player.h"      // For Player class
#include <iostream>
#include <cstdlib>       // For srand()

using namespace std;

int main()
{
    Player player;              // Card-playing manager
    int     numberOfShuffles;   // Number of shuffles per game
    int     numberOfGames;      // Number of games to play
    int     gamesPlayed;        // Number of games played
    int     gamesWon;           // Number of games won
    int     seed;               // Used with random no. generator
    bool    won;                // True if a game has been won

    gamesWon = 0;
    cout << "Enter number of games to play: ";
    cin >> numberOfGames;
    cout << "Enter number of shuffles per game: ";
    cin >> numberOfShuffles;
    cout << "Enter integer seed for random no. generator: ";
    cin >> seed;
    srand(seed);                        // Seed the random no. generator

    for (gamesPlayed=1; gamesPlayed <= numberOfGames; gamesPlayed++)
    {
        player.PlayGame(numberOfShuffles, won);
        if (won)
            gamesWon++;
```

```
    }
    cout << endl;
    cout << "Number of games played: " << numberOfGames << endl;
    cout << "Number of games won: " << gamesWon << endl;
    return 0;
}
```

Testing: To test this program exhaustively, all possible configurations of a deck of 52 cards have to be generated. Although this is theoretically possible, it is not realistic. There are 52! (52 factorial) possible arrangements of a deck of cards, and 52! equals

$$52 \times 51 \times 50 \times ... 2 \times 1$$

This is a large number. Try multiplying it out.

Therefore, another method of testing is required. At a minimum, the questions to be examined are the following:

1. Does the program recognize a winning hand?
2. Does the program recognize a losing hand?

To answer these questions, we must examine at least one hand declared to be a winner and several hands declared to be losers. Specifying 20 as the number of games to play, we ran the program to see if there were any winning hands. There were none.

From past experience, we know this solitaire game is difficult. We let the simulation run, specifying 100 games and an initial seed of 3. There were two winning hands. Intermediate output statements were put in to examine the winning hands. They were correct. Several losing hands were also printed; they were indeed losing hands. Satisfied that the program was working correctly, we set up runs that varied in length, number of shuffles, and seed for the random number generator. The results are listed below. There is no strategy behind the particular choices of inputs; they are random.

Number of Games	Number of Shuffles	Seed	Games Won
100	1	3	2
100	2	4	0
500	3	4	3
1000	6	3	6
5000	10	327	11
10,000	4	4	40
10,000	4	3	45
10,000	4	120	44

Testing and Debugging

Testing and debugging a linked structure is complicated by the fact that each item in the structure contains not only a data portion but also a link to the next item. Algorithms must correctly account for both the data and the link.

When linked lists are implemented with dynamic data and pointers, the errors discussed in Chapter 15 can crop up: memory leaks, dangling pointers, and attempts to dereference a null pointer or an uninitialized pointer. Below are suggestions to help you locate such errors or avoid them in the first place.

Testing and Debugging Hints

1. Review the Testing and Debugging Hints for Chapter 15. They apply to the pointers and dynamic data that are used in dynamic linked lists.
2. Be sure that the link member in the last node of a dynamic linked list has been set to NULL.
3. When visiting the components in a dynamic linked list, be sure that you test for the end of the list in such a way that you don't try to dereference the null pointer. On many systems, dereferencing the null pointer causes a run-time error.
4. Be sure to initialize the external pointer to each dynamic data structure.
5. Do not use

   ```
   currPtr++;
   ```

   to make currPtr point to the next node in a dynamic linked list. The list nodes are not necessarily in consecutive memory locations on the free store.
6. Keep close track of pointers. Changing pointer values prematurely may cause problems when you try to get back to the pointed-to variable.
7. If a C++ class that points to dynamic data has a class destructor but not a copy-constructor, do not pass a class object to a function using a pass by value. A shallow copy occurs, and both the parameter and the argument point to the same dynamic data. When the function returns, the parameter's destructor is executed, destroying the argument's dynamic data.

Summary

Dynamic data structures grow and contract during run time. They are made up of nodes that contain two kinds of members: the component, and one or more pointers to nodes of the same type. The pointer to the first node is saved in a variable called the external pointer to the structure.

A linked list is a data structure in which the components are logically next to each other rather than physically next to each other as they are in an array. A linked list can be represented either as an array of structs or as a collection of dynamic nodes, linked together by pointers. The end of a dynamic linked list is indicated by the special pointer constant NULL. Common operations on linked lists include inserting a node, deleting a node, and traversing the list (visiting each node from first to last).

In this chapter, we used linked lists to implement lists. But linked lists are also used to implement many data structures other than lists. The study of data structures forms a major topic in computer science. Entire books and courses are developed to cover the subject. A solid understanding of the fundamentals of linked lists is a prerequisite to creating more complex structures.

Quick Check

1. What distinguishes a linked list from an array? (pp. 944–946)
2. Nodes in a linked list structure must contain a link member. (True or False?) (pp. 944–950)
3. The number of elements in a dynamic data structure must be determined before the program is compiled. (True or False?) (pp. 948–949)
4. When printing the contents of a dynamically allocated linked list, what operation advances the current node pointer to the next node? (pp. 960–963)
5. What is the difference between the operations of inserting a new item at the top of a linked list and inserting the new item into its proper position in a sorted list? (pp. 963–971)
6. In deleting an item from a linked list, why do we need to keep track of the previous node (the node before the one to be deleted)? (pp. 971–975)

Answers **1**. Arrays are data structures whose components are located next to each other in memory. Linked lists are data structures in which the locations of the components are defined by an explicit link member in each node. **2.** True; every node (except the first) is accessed by using the link member in the node before it. **3.** False; we do not have to know in advance how large it has to be. (In fact, we rarely know.) The only limitation is the amount of memory space available on the free store. **4.** The current node pointer is set equal to the link member of the current node. **5.** When inserting an item into position, the list must first be searched to find the proper place. We don't have to search the list when inserting at the top. **6.** Because we must set the link member of the previous node equal to the link member of the current node as part of the deletion operation.

Exam Preparation Exercises

1. Given the SortedList2 class of this chapter and a client's declaration

   ```
   SortedList2 myList;
   ```

   what is the output of each of the following code segments?

   a. myList.InsertTop(30);   b. myList.Insert(10);
       myList.InsertTop(20);   myList.Insert(20);
       myList.InsertTop(10);   myList.Insert(30);
       myList.Print();   myList.Print();

2. In a linked list, components are only logically next to each other, whereas in an array they are also physically next to each other. (True or False?)

3. Which of the following can be used to implement a list ADT?

   a. An array of the component type

   b. A linked list implemented using an array of structs

   c. A linked list implemented using dynamic structs and pointers

4. The following declarations for a node of a linked list are not acceptable to the C++ compiler:

   ```
   typedef T* P;
   struct T
   {
       float x;
       P      link;
   };
   ```

   Correct the problem by inserting another declaration before the Typedef statement.

5. What is the primary benefit of dynamic data structures?

6. This chapter's SortedList2 class represents a sorted list ADT. To make an *unsorted* list ADT, which of the following member functions could be removed: IsEmpty, Print, InsertTop, Insert, DeleteTop, and Delete?

7. Use the C++ code below to identify the values of the variables and Boolean comparisons that follow. The value may be undefined, or the expression may be invalid.

   ```
   struct NodeType;
   typedef NodeType* NodePtr;

   struct NodeType
   {
       int     number;
       char    character;
       NodePtr link;
   };

   NodePtr currPtr = NULL;
   NodePtr firstPtr = NULL;
   NodePtr lastPtr = NULL;

   currPtr = new NodeType;
   currPtr->number = 13;
   ```

```
currPtr->character = 'z';
currPtr->link = new NodeType;
lastPtr = currPtr->link;
lastPtr->number = 9;
firstPtr = new NodeType;
lastPtr->link = firstPtr;
firstPtr->number = 9;
firstPtr->character = 'h';
firstPtr->link = currPtr;
        ⋮
```

Expression	*Value*
a. `firstPtr->link->number`	_____
b. `firstPtr->link->link->character`	_____
c. `firstPtr->link == lastPtr`	_____
d. `currPtr->link->number`	_____
e. `currPtr->link == *lastPtr`	_____
f. `firstPtr == lastPtr->link`	_____
g. `firstPtr->number < firstPtr->link->number`	_____

8. Choose the best data structure (array or dynamic linked list) for each of the following situations. Assume unlimited memory but limited time.
   a. A list of the abbreviations for the 50 states
   b. A fixed list of 1000 to 4000 (usually 1500) elements that has elements printed according to position requests that are input to the program
   c. A list of an unknown number of elements that is read, then printed in reverse order

9. Choose the best data structure (array or dynamic linked list) for each of the following situations. Assume limited memory but unlimited time.
   a. A list of the abbreviations for the 50 states
   b. A fixed list of 1000 to 4000 (usually 1500) elements that has elements printed according to position requests that are input to the program
   c. A list of an unknown number of elements that is read, then printed in reverse order

10. What is the output of the following C++ code, given the input data 5, 6, 3, and 1?

```
struct PersonNode;
typedef PersonNode* PtrType;

struct PersonNode
{
    int     ssNum;
    PtrType next;
};

int     ssNumber;
PtrType ptr;
PtrType head = NULL;
```

```
cin >> ssNumber;
while (cin)
{
    ptr = new PersonNode;
    ptr->ssNum = ssNumber;
    ptr->next = head;
    head = ptr;
    cin >> ssNumber;
}
ptr = head;
while (ptr != NULL)
{
    cout << ptr->ssNum;
    ptr = ptr->next;
}
```

Programming Warm-up Exercises

1. To the SortedList2 class of this chapter, add a value-returning member function named Length that counts and returns the number of nodes in a list.
2. To the SortedList2 class, add a value-returning member function named Sum that returns the sum of all the data values in a list.
3. To the SortedList2 class, add a Boolean member function named IsPresent that searches a list for a particular value (passed as an argument) and returns true if the value is found.
4. To the SortedList2 class, add a Boolean member function named Equal that compares two class objects and returns true if the two lists they represent are identical.
5. The SortedList2 class provides a copy-constructor but not a deep copy operation. Add a CopyFrom function to the SortedList2 class that performs a deep copy of one class object to another.
6. To avoid special handling of empty linked lists for insertion and deletion routines, some programmers prefer to keep a dummy node permanently in the list. (The list is considered empty if it contains only the dummy node.) Rewrite the SortedList2 class to use a dummy node whose component value is equal to a constant named DUMMY. Do not keep any unnecessary code. (*Hint:* The first element of the list follows the dummy node.)
7. Given the declarations

```
struct NodeType;
typedef NodeType* NodePtr;

struct NodeType
{
    int     number;
    NodePtr link;
};
```

and the function prototype

```
void Exchange( /* in */ NodePtr head,
               /* in */ int     key );
```

implement the `Exchange` function. The function searches a linked list for the value given by key and exchanges it with the number preceding it in the list. If key is the first value in the list or if key is not found, then no exchange occurs.

8. Using the type declarations given in Exercise 7, write a function that reorganizes the items in a linked list so that the last item is first, the second to last is second, and so forth. (*Hint:* Use a temporary list.)

Programming Problems

1. In the Solitaire program in this chapter, all insertions into a linked list are made using the function `InsertTop`, and all the deletions are made using `RemoveTop`. In some cases, this is inefficient. For example, function `CardDeck::Recreate` takes the cards from onTable and moves them one by one to the deck. Then the cards on discardPile are moved one by one to the deck. It would be more efficient simply to concatenate (join) the deck list and the onTable list, then concatenate the resulting list and the discardPile list.

    To the `CardPile` class, add a member function whose specification is the following:

    ```
    void Concat( /* inout */ CardPile& otherList );
        // Postcondition:
        //      This list and otherList are concatenated (the front
        //      of otherList@entry is joined to the rear of this list)
        //   && otherList is empty
    ```

    Implement and test the `Concat` member function. Use it in the `CardDeck::Recreate` function of the Solitaire program to make the program more efficient.

2. In Chapter 11, the BirthdayCalls program uses a `DateType` class to process address book information found in a file friendFile. Entries in friendFile are in the form

    ```
    John Arbuthnot
    (493) 384-2938
    1/12/1970

    Mary Smith
    (123) 123-4567
    10/12/1960
    ```

    Write a program to read in the entries from friendFile and store them into a dynamic linked list ordered by birth date. The output should consist of a listing by month of the names and telephone numbers of the people who have birthdays each month.

3. In Chapter 15, the Personnel Records case study reads a file of personnel records, sorts the records alphabetically, and prints out the sorted records. Rewrite the program so that it reads each record and stores it into its proper position in a sorted list. Implement the list as a dynamic linked list using this chapter's SortedList2 class as a model. Note that the limit of 1000 employee records is no longer relevant because you are using a dynamic data structure.

4. This chapter's SortedList2 class implements a sorted list ADT by using a linked list. In turn, the linked list is implemented by using dynamic data and pointers. Reimplement the linked list using an array of structs. You will have to manage a "free store" within the array—the collection of currently unused array elements. To mimic the new and delete operations, your implementation will need two auxiliary functions that obtain and release space on the "free store."

Case Study Follow-Up

1. The CardDeck class is derived from the CardPile class using inheritance.
   a. List the names of all the public members of the CardDeck class.
   b. List the names of all the private members of the CardDeck class.
2. In the Shuffle function of the CardDeck class, why are the declarations of halfA and halfB located inside the body of the For loop? What would happen if the declarations were placed outside the loop at the top of the function?
3. Give the Player class more responsibility by making it prompt for and input the number of shuffles and the random number seed. Encapsulate the numberOfShuffles and seed variables within the Player class, and add two member functions named GetNumShuffles and GetSeed. Show the new class declaration and the implementations of the two new functions. Also, rewrite the main function, given these changes.

17

Recursion

G O A L S

- To be able to identify the base case(s) and the general case in a recursive definition.
- To be able to write a recursive algorithm for a problem involving only simple variables.
- To be able to write a recursive algorithm for a problem involving structured variables.
- To be able to write a recursive algorithm for a problem involving linked lists.

In C++, any function can call another function. A function can even call itself! When a function calls itself, it is making a **recursive call.** The word *recursive* means "having the characteristic of coming up again, or repeating." In this case, a function call is being repeated by the function itself. Recursion is a powerful technique that can be used in place of iteration (looping).

Recursive solutions are generally less efficient than iterative solutions to the same problem. However, some problems lend themselves to simple, elegant, recursive solutions and are exceedingly cumbersome to solve iteratively. Some programming languages, such as early versions of FOR-TRAN, BASIC, and COBOL, do not allow recursion. Other languages are especially oriented to recursive algorithms—LISP is one of these. C++ lets us take our choice: We can implement both iterative and recursive algorithms.

Our examples are broken into two groups: problems that use only simple variables and problems that use structured variables. If you are studying recursion before reading Chapter 11 on structured data types, then cover only the first set of examples and leave the rest until you have completed the chapters on structured data types.

What Is Recursion?

You may have seen a set of gaily painted Russian dolls that fit inside one another. Inside the first doll is a smaller doll, inside of which is an even smaller doll, inside of which is yet a smaller doll, and so on. A recursive algorithm is like such a set of Russian dolls. It reproduces itself with smaller and smaller examples of itself until a solution is found—that is, until there are no more dolls.The recursive algorithm is implemented by using a function that makes recursive calls to itself.

Recursive call A function call in which the function being called is the same as the one making the call.

In Chapter 8, we wrote a function named `Power` that calculates the result of raising an integer to a positive power. If X is an integer and N is a positive integer, the formula for X^N is

$$X^N = \underbrace{X \times X \times X \times X \times X \times \ldots \times X}_{N \text{ times}}$$

We could also write this formula as

$$X^N = X \times \underbrace{(X \times X \times ... \times X)}_{(N-1) \text{ times}}$$

or even as

$$X^N = X \times X \times \underbrace{(X \times X \times ... \times X)}_{(N-2) \text{ times}}$$

In fact, we can write the formula most concisely as

$$X^N = X \times X^{N-1}$$

This definition of X^N is a classic **recursive definition**—that is, a definition given in terms of a smaller version of itself.

Recursive definition   A definition in which something is defined in terms of smaller versions of itself.

X^N is defined in terms of multiplying X times X^{N-1}. How is X^{N-1} defined? Why, as $X \times X^{N-2}$, of course! And X^{N-2} is $X \times X^{N-3}$; X^{N-3} is $X \times X^{N-4}$; and so on. In this example, "in terms of smaller versions of itself" means that the exponent is decremented each time.

When does the process stop? When we have reached a case for which we know the answer without resorting to a recursive definition. In this example, it is the case where N equals 1: X^1 is X. The case (or cases) for which an answer is explicitly known is called the **base case**. The case for which the solution is expressed in terms of a smaller version of itself is called the **recursive** or **general case**. A **recursive algorithm** is an algorithm that expresses the solution in terms of a call to itself, a recursive call. A recursive algorithm must terminate; that is, it must have a base case.

Base case   The case for which the solution can be stated nonrecursively.

General case   The case for which the solution is expressed in terms of a smaller version of itself; also known as *recursive case*.

Recursive algorithm   A solution that is expressed in terms of (a) smaller instances of itself and (b) a base case.

Figure 17-1 shows a recursive version of the `Power` function with the base case and the recursive call marked. The function is embedded in a program that reads in a number and an exponent and prints the result.

FIGURE 17-1

Power Function

```
//*******************************************************************
// Exponentiation program
//*******************************************************************
#include <iostream>

using namespace std;

int Power( int, int );

int main()
{
    int number;             // Number that is being raised to power
    int exponent;           // Power the number is being raised to

    cin >> number >> exponent;
    cout << Power(number, exponent);  <——————— // Nonrecursive call
    return 0;
}


//*******************************************************************

int Power( /* in */ int x,    // Number that is being raised to power
           /* in */ int n )   // Power the number is being raised to

// Computes x to the n power by multiplying x times the result of
// computing x to the n - 1 power.

// Precondition:
//     x is assigned  &&  n > 0
// Postcondition:
//     Function value == x raised to the power n
// Note:
//     Large exponents may result in integer overflow

{
    if (n == 1)
        return x;  <——————————————————————— // Base case
    else
        return x * Power(x, n - 1);  <——————— // Recursive call
}
```

Each recursive call to Power can be thought of as creating a completely new copy of the function, each with its own copies of the parameters x and n. The value of x remains the same for each version of Power, but the value of n decreases by 1 for each call until it becomes 1.

Let's trace the execution of this recursive function, with number equal to 2 and exponent equal to 3. We use a new format to trace recursive routines: We number the calls and then discuss what is happening in paragraph form.

Call 1: Power is called by main, with number equal to 2 and exponent equal to 3. Within Power, the parameters x and n are initialized to 2 and 3, respectively. Because n is not equal to 1, Power is called recursively with x and n − 1 as arguments. Execution of Call 1 pauses until an answer is sent back from this recursive call.

Call 2: x is equal to 2 and n is equal to 2. Because n is not equal to 1, the function Power is called again, this time with x and n − 1 as arguments. Execution of Call 2 pauses until an answer is sent back from this recursive call.

Call 3: x is equal to 2 and n is equal to 1. Because n equals 1, the value of x is to be returned. This call to the function has finished executing, and the function return value (which is 2) is passed back to the place in the statement from which the call was made.

Call 2: This call to the function can now complete the statement that contained the recursive call because the recursive call has returned. Call 3's return value (which is 2) is multiplied by x. This call to the function has finished executing, and the function return value (which is 4) is passed back to the place in the statement from which the call was made.

Call 1: This call to the function can now complete the statement that contained the recursive call because the recursive call has returned. Call 2's return value (which is 4) is multiplied by x. This call to the function has finished executing, and the function return value (which is 8) is passed back to the place in the statement from which the call was made. Because the first call (the nonrecursive call in main) has now completed, this is the final value of the function Power.

This trace is summarized in Figure 17-2. Each box represents a call to the Power function. The values for the parameters for that call are shown in each box.

What happens if there is no base case? We have **infinite recursion,** the recursive equivalent of an infinite loop. For example, if the condition

```
if (n == 1)
```

were omitted, Power would be called over and over again. Infinite recursion also occurs if Power is called with n less than or equal to 0.

Infinite recursion   The situation in which a function calls itself over and over endlessly.

In actuality, recursive calls can't go on forever. Here's the reason. When a function is called, either recursively or nonrecursively, the computer system creates temporary storage for the parameters and the function's (automatic) local variables. This temporary storage is a region of memory called the *run-time stack.* When the function returns, its parame-

FIGURE 17-2
Execution of
`Power(2, 3)`

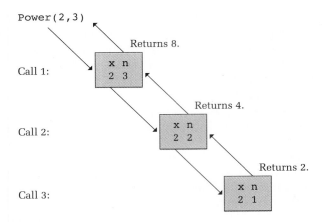

ters and local variables are released from the run-time stack. With infinite
recursion, the recursive function calls never return. Each time the function
calls itself, a little more of the run-time stack is used to store the new
copies of the variables. Eventually, all the memory space on the stack is
used. At that point, the program crashes with an error message such as
"RUN-TIME STACK OVERFLOW" (or the computer may simply hang).

Recursive Algorithms with Simple Variables

Let's look at another example: calculating a factorial. The factorial of a
number N (written $N!$) is N multiplied by $N - 1$, $N - 2$, $N - 3$, and so on.
Another way of expressing factorial is

$$N ! = N \times (N - 1)!$$

This expression looks like a recursive definition. $(N - 1)!$ is a smaller
instance of $N!$—that is, it takes one less multiplication to calculate $(N - 1)!$
than it does to calculate $N!$ If we can find a base case, we can write a
recursive algorithm. Fortunately, we don't have to look too far: 0! is
defined in mathematics to be 1.

Factorial (In: n)

```
IF n is 0
        Return 1
ELSE
        Return n * Factorial(n – 1)
```

This algorithm can be coded directly as follows.

```
int Factorial ( /* in */ int n )

// Precondition:
//      n >= 0
// Postcondition:
//      Function value == n!
// Note:
//      Large values of n may cause integer overflow

{
    if (n == 0)
        return 1;                       // Base case
    else
        return n * Factorial(n - 1);    // General case
}
```

Let's trace this function with an original n of 4.

Call 1: n is 4. Because n is not 0, the else branch is taken. The Return statement cannot be completed until the recursive call to Factorial with n − 1 as the argument has been completed.

Call 2: n is 3. Because n is not 0, the else branch is taken. The Return statement cannot be completed until the recursive call to Factorial with n − 1 as the argument has been completed.

Call 3: n is 2. Because n is not 0, the else branch is taken. The Return statement cannot be completed until the recursive call to Factorial with n − 1 as the argument has been completed.

Call 4: n is 1. Because n is not 0, the else branch is taken. The Return statement cannot be completed until the recursive call to Factorial with n − 1 as the argument has been completed.

Call 5: n is 0. Because n equals 0, this call to the function returns, sending back 1 as the result.

Call 4: The Return statement in this copy can now be completed. The value to be returned is n (which is 1) times 1. This call to the function returns, sending back 1 as the result.

Call 3: The Return statement in this copy can now be completed. The value to be returned is n (which is 2) times 1. This call to the function returns, sending back 2 as the result.

Call 2: The Return statement in this copy can now be completed. The value to be returned is n (which is 3) times 2. This call to the function returns, sending back 6 as the result.

Call 1: The Return statement in this copy can now be completed. The value to be returned is n (which is 4) times 6. This call to the function returns, sending back 24 as the result. Because this is the last of the calls to Factorial, the recursive process is over. The value 24 is returned as the

FIGURE 17-3

Execution of
Factorial(4)

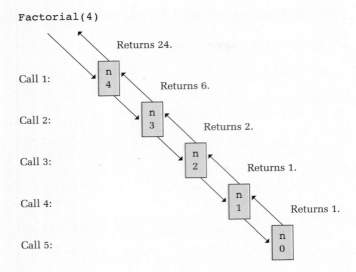

Factorial(4)

Returns 24.

Call 1: n 4

Returns 6.

Call 2: n 3

Returns 2.

Call 3: n 2

Returns 1.

Call 4: n 1

Returns 1.

Call 5: n 0

final value of the call to Factorial with an argument of 4. Figure 17-3 summarizes the execution of the Factorial function with an argument of 4.

Let's organize what we have done in these two solutions into an outline for writing recursive algorithms.

1. Understand the problem. (We threw this in for good measure; it is always the first step.)
2. Determine the base case(s).
3. Determine the recursive case(s).

We have used the factorial and the power algorithms to demonstrate recursion because they are easy to visualize. In practice, one would never want to calculate either of these functions using the recursive solution. In both cases, the iterative solutions are simpler and much more efficient because starting a new iteration of a loop is a faster operation than calling a function. Let's compare the code for the iterative and recursive versions of the factorial problem.

Iterative Solution

```
int Factorial ( /* in */ int n )
{
    int factor;
    int count;

    factor = 1;
    for (count = 2; count <= n; count++)
        factor = factor * count;
    return factor;
}
```

Recursive Solution

```
int Factorial ( /* in */ int n )
{
    if (n == 0)
        return 1;
    else
        return n * Factorial(n - 1);
}
```

The iterative version has two local variables, whereas the recursive version has none. There are usually fewer local variables in a recursive routine than in an iterative routine. Also, the iterative version always has a loop, whereas the recursive version always has a selection statement—either an If or a Switch. A branching structure is the main control structure in a recursive routine. A looping structure is the main control structure in an iterative routine.

In the next section, we examine a more complicated problem—one in which the recursive solution is not immediately apparent.

Towers of Hanoi

One of your first toys may have been three pegs with colored circles of different diameters. If so, you probably spent countless hours moving the circles from one peg to another. If we put some constraints on how the circles or discs can be moved, we have an adult game called the Towers of Hanoi. When the game begins, all the circles are on the first peg in order by size, with the smallest on the top. The object of the game is to move the circles, one at a time, to the third peg. The catch is that a circle cannot be placed on top of one that is smaller in diameter. The middle peg can be used as an auxiliary peg, but it must be empty at the beginning and at the end of the game.

To get a feel for how this might be done, let's look at some sketches of what the configuration must be at certain points if a solution is possible. We use four circles or discs. The beginning configuration is:

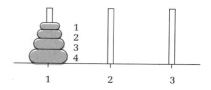

To move the largest circle (circle 4) to peg 3, we must move the three smaller circles to peg 2. Then circle 4 can be moved into its final place:

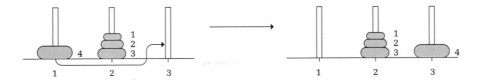

Let's assume we can do this. Now, to move the next largest circle (circle 3) into place, we must move the two circles on top of it onto an auxiliary peg (peg 1 in this case):

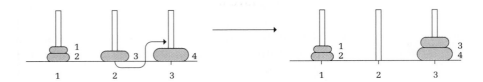

To get circle 2 into place, we must move circle 1 to another peg, freeing circle 2 to be moved to its place on peg 3:

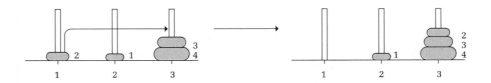

The last circle (circle 1) can now be moved into its final place, and we are finished:

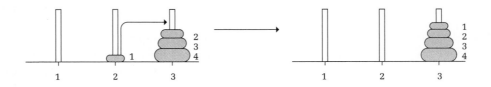

Notice that to free circle 4, we had to move three circles to another peg. To free circle 3, we had to move two circles to another peg. To free circle 2, we had to move one circle to another peg. This sounds like a recursive algorithm: To free the nth circle, we have to move $n - 1$ circles. Each stage can be thought of as beginning again with three pegs, but with one less circle each time. Let's see if we can summarize this process, using n instead of an actual number.

Get N Circles Moved from Peg 1 to Peg 3

Get n – 1 circles moved from peg 1 to peg 2
Move nth circle from peg 1 to peg 3
Get n – 1 circles moved from peg 2 to peg 3

This algorithm certainly sounds simple; surely there must be more. But this really is all there is to it.

Let's write a recursive function that implements this algorithm. We can't actually move discs, of course, but we can print out a message to do so. Notice that the beginning peg, the ending peg, and the auxiliary peg keep changing during the algorithm. To make the algorithm easier to follow, we call the pegs beginPeg, endPeg, and auxPeg. These three pegs, along with the number of circles on the beginning peg, are the parameters of the function.

We have the recursive or general case, but what about a base case? How do we know when to stop the recursive process? The clue is in the expression "Get *n* circles moved." If we don't have any circles to move, we don't have anything to do. We are finished with that stage. Therefore, when the number of circles equals 0, we do nothing (that is, we simply return).

```cpp
void DoTowers(
    /* in */ int circleCount,    // Number of circles to move
    /* in */ int beginPeg,       // Peg containing circles to move
    /* in */ int auxPeg,         // Peg holding circles temporarily
    /* in */ int endPeg      )   // Peg receiving circles being moved
{
    if (circleCount > 0)
    {
        // Move n - 1 circles from beginning peg to auxiliary peg

        DoTowers(circleCount - 1, beginPeg, endPeg, auxPeg);
        cout << "Move circle from peg " << beginPeg
             << " to peg " << endPeg << endl;

        // Move n - 1 circles from auxiliary peg to ending peg

        DoTowers(circleCount - 1, auxPeg, beginPeg, endPeg);
    }
}
```

It's hard to believe that such a simple algorithm actually works, but we'll prove it to you. Following is a driver program that calls the DoTowers function. Output statements have been added so you can see the values of the arguments with each recursive call. Because there are two recursive calls within the function, we have indicated which recursive statement issued the call.

```cpp
//******************************************************************
// TestTowers program
// This program, a test driver for the DoTowers function, reads in
// a value from standard input and passes this value to DoTowers
//******************************************************************
#include <iostream>
#include <iomanip>     // For setw()

using namespace std;

void DoTowers( int, int, int, int );

int main()
{
    int circleCount;     // Number of circles on starting peg

    cout << "Input number of circles: ";
    cin >> circleCount;
    cout << "OUTPUT WITH " << circleCount << " CIRCLES" << endl
         << endl;
    cout << "CALLED FROM  #CIRCLES" << setw(8) << "BEGIN"
         << setw(8) << "AUXIL." << setw(5) << "END"
         << "     INSTRUCTIONS" << endl
         << endl;
    cout << "Original   :";
    DoTowers(circleCount, 1, 2, 3);
    return 0;
}


//******************************************************************

void DoTowers(
    /* in */ int circleCount,     // Number of circles to move
    /* in */ int beginPeg,        // Peg containing circles to move
    /* in */ int auxPeg,          // Peg holding circles temporarily
    /* in */ int endPeg     )     // Peg receiving circles being moved

// This recursive function moves circleCount circles from beginPeg
// to endPeg.  All but one of the circles are moved from beginPeg
// to auxPeg, then the last circle is moved from beginPeg to endPeg,
// and then the circles are moved from auxPeg to endPeg.
// The subgoals of moving circles to and from auxPeg are what
// involve recursion
```

```
// Precondition:
//      All parameters are assigned  &&  circleCount >= 0
// Postcondition:
//      The values of all parameters have been printed
//   && IF circleCount > 0
//          circleCount circles have been moved from beginPeg to
//          endPeg in the manner detailed above
//      ELSE
//          No further actions have taken place

{
    cout << setw(6) << circleCount << setw(9) << beginPeg
        << setw(7) << auxPeg << setw(7) << endPeg << endl;
    if (circleCount > 0)
    {
        cout << "From  first:";
        DoTowers(circleCount - 1, beginPeg, endPeg, auxPeg);
        cout << setw(58) << "Move circle " << circleCount
            << " from " << beginPeg << " to " << endPeg << endl;
        cout << "From second:";
        DoTowers(circleCount - 1, auxPeg, beginPeg, endPeg);
    }
}
```

The output from a run with three circles follows. "Original" means that the parameters listed beside it are from the nonrecursive call, which is the first call to DoTowers. "From first" means that the parameters listed are for a call issued from the first recursive statement. "From second" means that the parameters listed are for a call issued from the second recursive statement. Notice that a call cannot be issued from the second recursive statement until the preceding call from the first recursive statement has completed execution.

OUTPUT WITH 3 CIRCLES

CALLED FROM	#CIRCLES	BEGIN	AUXIL.	END	INSTRUCTIONS
Original :	3	1	2	3	
From first:	2	1	3	2	
From first:	1	1	2	3	
From first:	0	1	3	2	
					Move circle 1 from 1 to 3
From second:	0	2	1	3	
					Move circle 2 from 1 to 2
From second:	1	3	1	2	
From first:	0	3	2	1	
					Move circle 1 from 3 to 2

From second:	0	1	3	2	
					Move circle 3 from 1 to 3
From second:	2	2	1	3	
From first:	1	2	3	1	
From first:	0	2	1	3	
					Move circle 1 from 2 to 1
From second:	0	3	2	1	
					Move circle 2 from 2 to 3
From second:	1	1	2	3	
From first:	0	1	3	2	
					Move circle 1 from 1 to 3
From second:	0	2	1	3	

▬ *Recursive Algorithms with Structured Variables*

In our definition of a recursive algorithm, we said there were two cases: the recursive or general case, and the base case for which an answer can be expressed nonrecursively. In the general case for all our algorithms so far, an argument was expressed in terms of a smaller value each time. When structured variables are used, the recursive case is often in terms of a smaller structure rather than a smaller value; the base case occurs when there are no values left to process in the structure.

We examine a recursive algorithm for printing the contents of a one-dimensional array of *n* elements to show what we mean.

Print Array

> IF more elements
>   Print the value of the first element
>   Print array of n – 1 elements

The recursive case is to print the values in an array that is one element "smaller"; that is, the size of the array decreases by 1 with each recursive call. The base case is when the size of the array becomes 0—that is, when there are no more elements to print.

Our arguments must include the index of the first element (the one to be printed). How do we know when there are no more elements to print (that is, when the size of the array to be printed is 0)? We know we have printed the last element in the array when the index of the next element to be printed is beyond the index of the last element in the array. Therefore, the index of the last array element must be passed as an argument. We call the indexes `first` and `last`. When `first` is greater than `last`, we are finished. The name of the array is `data`.

```
void Print( /* in */ const int data[],    // Array to be printed
            /* in */       int first,      // Index of first element
            /* in */       int last  )     // Index of last element
{
    if (first <= last)
    {                                                // Recursive case
        cout << data[first] << endl;
        Print(data, first + 1, last);
    }
    // Empty else-clause is the base case
}
```

Here is a code walk-through of the function call

```
Print(data, 0, 4);
```

using the pictured array.

    Call 1: `first` is 0 and `last` is 4. Because `first` is less than `last`, the value in `data[first]` (which is 23) is printed. Execution of this call pauses while the array from `first + 1` through `last` is printed.

    Call 2: `first` is 1 and `last` is 4. Because `first` is less than `last`, the value in `data[first]` (which is 44) is printed. Execution of this call pauses while the array from `first + 1` through `last` is printed.

    Call 3: `first` is 2 and `last` is 4. Because `first` is less than `last`, the value in `data[first]` (which is 52) is printed. Execution of this call pauses while the array from `first + 1` through `last` is printed.

    Call 4: `first` is 3 and `last` is 4. Because `first` is less than `last`, the value in `data[first]` (which is 61) is printed. Execution of this call pauses while the array from `first + 1` through `last` is printed.

    Call 5: `first` is 4 and `last` is 4. Because `first` is equal to `last`, the value in `data[first]` (which is 77) is printed. Execution of this call pauses while the array from `first + 1` through `last` is printed.

    Call 6: `first` is 5 and `last` is 4. Because `first` is greater than `last`, the execution of this call is complete. Control returns to the preceding call.

    Call 5: Execution of this call is complete. Control returns to the preceding call.

    Calls 4, 3, 2, and 1: Each execution is completed in turn, and control returns to the preceding call.

    Notice that once the deepest call (the call with the highest number) was reached, each of the calls before it returned without doing anything. When no statements are executed after the return from the recursive call to the function, the recursion is known as **tail recursion.** Tail recursion often indicates that the problem could be solved more easily using iteration. We used the array example because it made the recursive process easy to visualize; in practice, an array should be printed iteratively.

Tail recursion A recursive algorithm in which no statements are executed after the return from the recursive call.

Figure 17-4 shows the execution of the Print function with the values of the parameters for each call. Notice that the array gets smaller with each recursive call (data[first] through data[last]). If we want to print

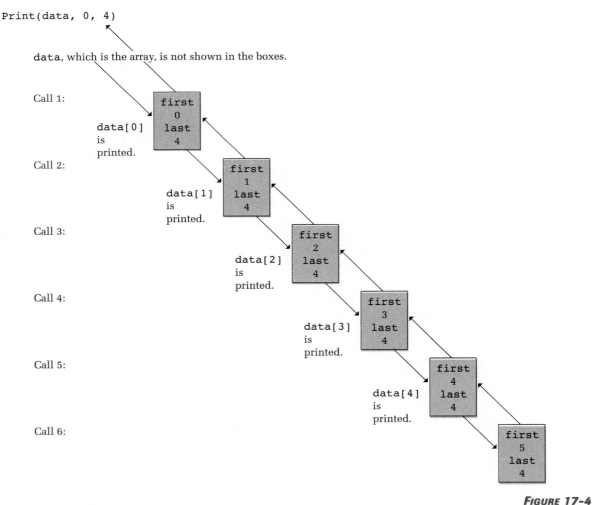

FIGURE 17-4
Execution of Print(data, 0, 4)

the array elements in reverse order recursively, all we have to do is interchange the two statements within the If statement.

Recursion Using Pointer Variables

The previous recursive algorithm using a one-dimensional array could have been done much more easily using iteration. Now we look at two algorithms that cannot be done more easily with iteration: printing a linked list in reverse order and creating a duplicate copy of a linked list.

Printing a Dynamic Linked List in Reverse Order

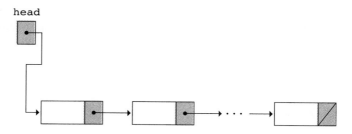

head

Printing a list in order from first to last is easy. We set a running pointer (ptr) equal to head and cycle through the list until ptr becomes NULL.

Print List (In: head)

```
Set ptr = head
WHILE ptr is not NULL
      Print ptr->component
      Set ptr = ptr->link
```

To print the list in reverse order, we must print the value in the last node first, then the value in the next-to-last node, and so on. Another way of expressing this is to say that we do not print a value until the values in all the nodes following it have been printed. We might visualize the process as the first node's turning to its neighbor and saying, "Tell me when you have printed your value. Then I'll print my value." The second node says to its neighbor, "Tell me when you have printed your value. Then I'll print mine." That node, in turn, says the same to its neighbor, and this continues until there is nothing to print.

Because the number of neighbors gets smaller and smaller, we seem to have the makings of a recursive solution. The end of the list is reached when the running pointer is NULL. When that happens, the last node can print its value and send the message back to the one before it. That node can then print its value and send the message back to the one before it, and so on.

RevPrint (In: head)

```
IF head is not NULL
        RevPrint rest of nodes in list
        Print current node in list
```

This algorithm can be coded directly as the following function:

```
void RevPrint( /* in */ NodePtr head )

// Precondition:
//      head points to a list node (or == NULL)
// Postcondition:
//      IF head != NULL
//          All nodes following *head have been output,
//          then *head has been output
//      ELSE
//          No action has taken place

{
    if (head != NULL)
    {
        RevPrint(head->link);                      // Recursive call
        cout << head->component << endl;
    }
    // Empty else-clause is the base case
}
```

This algorithm seems complex enough to warrant a code walk-through. We use the following list:

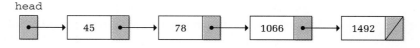

Call 1: head points to the node containing 45 and is not NULL. Execution of this call pauses until the recursive call with the argument head->link has been completed.

Call 2: head points to the node containing 78 and is not NULL. Execution of this call pauses until the recursive call with the argument head->link has been completed.

Call 3: head points to the node containing 1066 and is not NULL. Execution of this call pauses until the recursive call with the argument head->link has been completed.

Call 4: head points to the node containing 1492 and is not NULL. Execution of this call pauses until the recursive call with the argument head->link has been completed.

Call 5: head is NULL. Execution of this call is complete. Control returns to the preceding call.

Call 4: head->component (which is 1492) is printed. Execution of this call is complete. Control returns to the preceding call.

Call 3: head->component (which is 1066) is printed. Execution of this call is complete. Control returns to the preceding call.

Call 2: head->component (which is 78) is printed. Execution of this call is complete. Control returns to the preceding call.

Call 1: head->component (which is 45) is printed. Execution of this call is complete. Because this is the nonrecursive call, execution continues with the statement immediately following RevPrint(head).

Figure 17-5 shows the execution of the RevPrint function. The parameters are pointers (memory addresses), so we use → 45 to mean the pointer to the node whose component is 45.

FIGURE 17-5
Execution of
RevPrint(head)

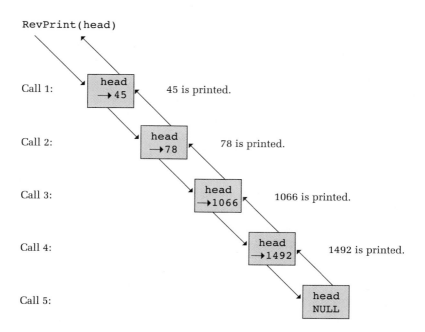

Copying a Dynamic Linked List

When working with linked lists, we sometimes need to create a duplicate copy (a *clone*) of a linked list. For example, in Chapter 16, we wrote a copy-constructor for the `SortedList2` class. This copy-constructor creates a new class object to be a clone of another class object, including its dynamic linked list.

Suppose that we want to write a value-returning function that receives the external pointer to a linked list (`head`), makes a clone of the linked list, and returns the external pointer to the new list as the function value. A typical call to the function would be the following:

```
NodePtr head;
NodePtr newListHead;
   ⋮
newListHead = PtrToClone(head);
```

Using iteration to copy a linked list is rather complicated. The following algorithm is essentially the same as the one used in the `SortedList2` copy-constructor.

PtrToClone (In: head)   // **Iterative algorithm**

  Out: Function value

```
IF head is NULL
        Return NULL

// Copy first node
Set fromPtr = head
Set cloneHead = new NodeType
Set cloneHead->component = fromPtr->component

// Copy remaining nodes
Set toPtr = cloneHead
Set fromPtr = fromPtr->link
WHILE fromPtr is not NULL
        Set toPtr->link = new NodeType
        Set toPtr = toPtr->link
        Set toPtr->component = fromPtr->component
        Set fromPtr = fromPtr->link
Set toPtr->link = NULL
Return cloneHead
```

A recursive solution to this problem is far simpler, but it requires us to think recursively. To clone the first node of the original list, we can allocate a new dynamic node and copy the component value from the original node into the new node. However, we cannot yet fill in the link member of the new node. We must wait until we have cloned the second node so that we can store its address into the link member of the first node. Likewise, the cloning of the second node cannot complete until we have finished cloning the third node. Eventually, we clone the last node of the original list and set the link member of the cloned node to NULL. At this point, the last node returns its own address to the next-to-last node, which stores the address into its link member. The next-to-last node returns its own address to the node before it, and so forth. The process completes when the first node returns its address to the first (nonrecursive) call, yielding an external pointer to the new linked list.

PtrToClone (In: fromPtr)   **// Recursive algorithm**

    Out: Function value

```
IF fromPtr is NULL
        Return NULL
ELSE
        Set toPtr = new NodeType
        Set toPtr->component = fromPtr->component
        Set toPtr->link = PtrToClone(fromPtr->link)
        Return toPtr
```

Like the solution to the Towers of Hanoi problem, this looks too simple; yet, it is the algorithm. Because the argument that is passed to each recursive call is fromPtr->link, the number of nodes left in the original list gets smaller with each call. The base case occurs when the pointer into the original list becomes NULL. Below is the C++ function that implements the algorithm.

```
NodePtr PtrToClone( /* in */ NodePtr fromPtr )

// Precondition:
//      fromPtr points to a list node (or == NULL)
// Postcondition:
//      IF fromPtr != NULL
//              A clone of the entire sublist starting with *fromPtr
//              is on the free store
//          && Function value == pointer to front of this sublist
//      ELSE
//              Function value == NULL
```

```
{
    NodePtr toPtr;       // Pointer to newly created node

    if (fromPtr == NULL)
        return NULL;                     // Base case
    else
    {                                    // Recursive case
        toPtr = new NodeType;
        toPtr->component = fromPtr->component;
        toPtr->link = PtrToClone(fromPtr->link);
        return toPtr;
    }
}
```

Let's perform a code walk-through of the function call

```
newListHead = PtrToClone(head);
```

using the following list:

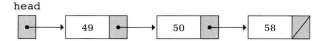

Call 1: fromPtr points to the node containing 49 and is not NULL. A new node is allocated and its component value is set to 49.

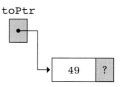

Execution of this call pauses until the recursive call with argument fromPtr->link has been completed.

Call 2: fromPtr points to the node containing 50 and is not NULL. A new node is allocated and its component value is set to 50.

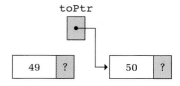

Execution of this call pauses until the recursive call with argument
fromPtr->link has been completed.

Call 3: fromPtr points to the node containing 58 and is not NULL. A
new node is allocated and its component value is set to 58.

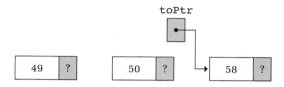

Execution of this call pauses until the recursive call with argument
fromPtr->link has been completed.

Call 4: fromPtr is NULL. The list is unchanged.

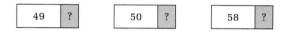

Execution of this call is complete. NULL is returned as the function value to
the preceding call.

Call 3: Execution of this call resumes by assigning the returned function value (NULL) to toPtr->link.

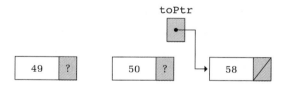

Execution of this call is complete. The value of toPtr is returned to the
preceding call.

Call 2: Execution of this call resumes by assigning the returned function value (the address of the third node) to toPtr->link.

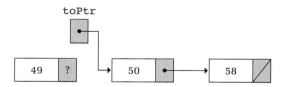

Execution of this call is complete. The value of toPtr is returned to the
preceding call.

Call 1: Execution of this call resumes by assigning the returned function value (the address of the second node) to toPtr->link.

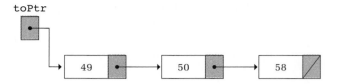

Execution of this call is complete. Because this is the nonrecursive call, the value of `toPtr` is returned to the assignment statement containing the original call. The variable `newListHead` now points to a clone of the original list.

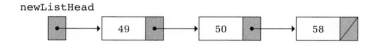

▁▁ *Recursion or Iteration?*

Recursion and iteration are alternative ways of expressing repetition in a program. When iterative control structures are used, processes are made to repeat by embedding code in a looping structure such as a While, For, or Do-While. In recursion, a process is made to repeat by having a function call itself. A selection statement is used to control the repeated calls.

Which is better to use—recursion or iteration? There is no simple answer to this question. The choice usually depends on two issues: efficiency and the nature of the problem being solved.

Historically, the quest for efficiency, in terms of both execution speed and memory usage, has favored iteration over recursion. Each time a recursive call is made, the system must allocate stack space for all parameters and (automatic) local variables. The overhead involved in any function call is time-consuming. On early, slow computers with limited memory capacity, recursive algorithms were visibly—sometimes painfully—slower than the iterative versions. However, studies have shown that on modern, fast computers, the overhead of recursion is often so small that the increase in computation time is almost unnoticeable to the user. Except in cases where efficiency is absolutely critical, then, the choice between recursion and iteration more often depends on the second issue—the nature of the problem being solved.

Consider the factorial and power algorithms we discussed earlier in the chapter. In both cases, iterative solutions were obvious and easy to devise. We imposed recursive solutions on these problems only to demonstrate how recursion works. As a rule of thumb, if an iterative solution is more obvious or easier to understand, use it; it will be more efficient. However, there are problems for which the recursive solution is more obvious or easier to devise, such as the Towers of Hanoi problem. (It turns out that the Towers of Hanoi problem is surprisingly difficult to solve using iteration.) Computer science students should be aware of the power of recursion. If the definition of a problem is inherently recursive, then a recursive solution should certainly be considered.

PROBLEM-SOLVING CASE STUDY

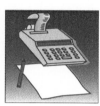

Converting Decimal Integers to Binary Integers

Problem: Convert a decimal (base-10) integer to a binary (base-2) integer.

Discussion: The algorithm for this conversion is as follows:

1.   Take the decimal number and divide it by 2.
2.   Make the remainder the rightmost digit in the answer.
3.   Replace the original dividend with the quotient.
4.   Repeat, placing each new remainder to the left of the previous one.
5.   Stop when the quotient is 0.

This is clearly an algorithm for a calculator and paper and pencil. Expressions such as "to the left of" certainly cannot be implemented in C++ as yet. Let's do an example—convert 42 from base 10 to base 2—to get a feel for the algorithm before we try to write a computer solution. Remember, the quotient in one step becomes the dividend in the next.

Step 1

$$
\begin{array}{r}
21 \quad \leftarrow \text{Quotient} \\
2\,\overline{)42} \\
\underline{4} \\
2 \\
\underline{2} \\
0 \quad \leftarrow \text{Remainder}
\end{array}
$$

Step 2

$$
\begin{array}{r}
10 \quad \leftarrow \text{Quotient} \\
2\,\overline{)21} \\
\underline{2} \\
1 \\
\underline{0} \\
1 \quad \leftarrow \text{Remainder}
\end{array}
$$

Step 3

$$
\begin{array}{r}
5 \quad \leftarrow \text{Quotient} \\
2\,\overline{)10} \\
\underline{10} \\
0 \quad \leftarrow \text{Remainder}
\end{array}
$$

Step 4

$$
\begin{array}{r}
2 \quad \leftarrow \text{Quotient} \\
2\,\overline{)5} \\
\underline{4} \\
1 \quad \leftarrow \text{Remainder}
\end{array}
$$

Step 5

$$
\begin{array}{r}
1 \quad \leftarrow \text{Quotient} \\
2\,\overline{)2} \\
\underline{2} \\
0 \quad \leftarrow \text{Remainder}
\end{array}
$$

Step 6

$$
\begin{array}{r}
0 \quad \leftarrow \text{Quotient} \\
2\,\overline{)1} \\
\underline{0} \\
1 \quad \leftarrow \text{Remainder}
\end{array}
$$

PROBLEM-SOLVING CASE STUDY cont'd.

The answer is the sequence of remainders from last to first. Therefore, the decimal number 42 is 101010 in binary.

It looks as though the problem can be implemented with a straightforward iterative algorithm. Each remainder is obtained from the MOD operation (% in C++), and each quotient is the result of the / operation.

```
WHILE number > 0
        Set remainder = number MOD 2
        Print remainder
        Set number = number / 2
```

Let's do a walk-through to test this algorithm.

Number	Remainder
42	0
21	1
10	0
5	1
2	0
1	1

Answer:	0	1	0	1	0	1
(remainder from step	1	2	3	4	5	6)

The answer is backwards! An iterative solution (using only simple variables) doesn't work. We need to print the last remainder first. The first remainder should be printed only after the rest of the remainders have been calculated and printed.

In our example, we should print 42 MOD 2 after (42 / 2) MOD 2 has been printed. But this, in turn, means that we should print (42 / 2) MOD 2 after ((42 / 2) / 2) MOD 2 has been printed. Now this begins to look like a recursive definition. We can summarize by saying that, for any given number, we should print number MOD 2 after (number / 2) MOD 2 has been printed. This becomes the following algorithm:

Convert (In: number)

```
IF number > 0
        Convert(number / 2)
        Print number MOD 2
```

PROBLEM-SOLVING CASE STUDY cont'd.

If number is 0, we have called Convert as many times as we need to and can begin printing the answer. The base case is simply when we stop making recursive calls. The recursive solution to this problem is encoded in the Convert function.

```
void Convert( /* in */ int number )    // Number being converted
                                        //   to binary
// Precondition:
//      number >= 0
// Postcondition:
//      IF number > 0
//          number has been printed in binary (base 2) form
//      ELSE
//          No action has taken place

{
    if (number > 0)
    {
        Convert(number / 2);                    // Recursive call
        cout << number % 2;
    }
    // Empty else-clause is the base case
}
```

Let's do a code walk-through of Convert(10). We pick up our original example at step 3, where the dividend is 10.

Call 1: Convert is called with an argument of 10. Because number is not equal to 0, the then-clause is executed. Execution pauses until the recursive call to Convert with an argument of (number / 2) has completed.

Call 2: number is 5. Because number is not equal to 0, execution of this call pauses until the recursive call with an argument of (number / 2) has completed.

Call 3: number is 2. Because number is not equal to 0, execution of this call pauses until the recursive call with an argument of (number / 2) has completed.

Call 4: number is 1. Because number is not equal to 0, execution of this call pauses until the recursive call with an argument of (number / 2) has completed.

Call 5: number is 0. Execution of this call to Convert is complete. Control returns to the preceding call.

Call 4: Execution of this call resumes with the statement following the recursive call to Convert. The value of number % 2 (which is 1) is printed. Execution of this call is complete.

Call 3: Execution of this call resumes with the statement following the recursive call to Convert. The value of number % 2 (which is 0) is printed. Execution of this call is complete.

Call 2: Execution of this call resumes with the statement following the recursive call to Convert. The value of number % 2 (which is 1) is printed. Execution of this call is complete.

Call 1: Execution of this call resumes with the statement following the recursive call to Convert. The value of number % 2 (which is 0) is printed. Execution of this call is complete. Because this is the nonrecursive call, execution resumes with the statement immediately following the original call.

Figure 17-6 shows the execution of the Convert function with the values of the parameters.

PROBLEM-SOLVING CASE STUDY

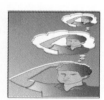

Minimum Value in an Integer Array

Problem: Find the minimum value in an integer array indexed from 0 through size − 1.

Discussion: This problem is easy to solve iteratively, but the objective here is to think recursively. The problem has to be stated in terms of a smaller case of itself. Because this is a problem using an array, a smaller case involves a smaller array. The minimum value in an array of size size is the smaller of data[size−1] and the smallest value in the array from data[0]...data[size−2].

Minimum (In: data, size)

```
Set minSoFar = Minimum(data, size − 1)
IF data[size−1] < minSoFar
        Return data[size−1]
ELSE
        Return minSoFar
```

PROBLEM-SOLVING CASE STUDY cont'd.

FIGURE 17-6
Execution of
Convert(10)

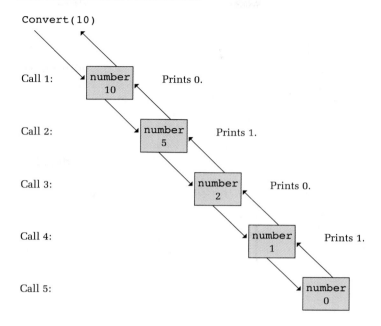

This algorithm looks reasonable. All we need is a base case. Because each recursive call reduces the size of the array by 1, our base case occurs when `size` is 1. We know the minimum value for this call: It is the only value in the array.

```
int Minimum(
        /* in */ const int data[],    // Array of integers to examine
        /* in */          int size  )  // One greater than index of
                                        //   last number in array
// Precondition:
//     data[0..size-1] are assigned
//   && size >= 1
// Postcondition:
//     Function value == smallest number in data[0..size-1]

{
    int minSoFar;        // Minimum returned from recursive call
```

FIGURE 17-7
Execution of
Minimum(data,5)

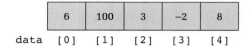

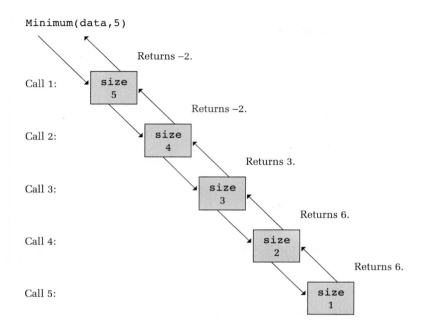

```
if (size == 1)
    return data[0];                         // Base case
else
{                                           // Recursive case
    minSoFar = Minimum(data, size-1);
    if (data[size-1] < minSoFar)
        return data[size-1];
    else
        return minSoFar;
}
}
```

We do not provide a code walk-through for this function. A diagram showing the parameters for each call appears in Figure 17-7.

Testing: To test this function, we need a driver program that reads values into an array, calls the function, and prints the result. The cases to be tested are the end cases (the minimum value is the first in the array, and the minimum value is the last in the array) and several cases between.

Testing and Debugging

Recursion is a powerful technique when used correctly. Improperly used, recursion can cause errors that are difficult to diagnose. The best way to debug a recursive algorithm is to construct it correctly in the first place. To be realistic, however, we give a few hints about where to look if an error occurs.

Testing and Debugging Hints

1. Be sure there is a base case. If there is no base case, the algorithm continues to issue recursive calls until all memory has been used. Each time the function is called, either recursively or nonrecursively, stack space is allocated for the parameters and automatic local variables. If there is no base case to end the recursive calls, the run-time stack eventually overflows. An error message such as "STACK OVERFLOW" indicates that the base case is missing.
2. Be sure you have not used a While structure. The basic structure in a recursive algorithm is the If statement. There must be at least two cases: the recursive case and the base case. If the base case does nothing, the else-clause is omitted. The selection structure, however, must be there. If a While statement is used in a recursive algorithm, the While statement usually should not contain a recursive call.
3. As with nonrecursive functions, do not reference global variables directly within a recursive function unless you have justification for doing so.
4. Parameters that relate to the size of the problem must be value parameters, not reference parameters. The arguments that relate to the size of the problem are usually expressions. Arbitrary expressions can be passed only to value parameters.
5. Use your system's debugger program (or use debug output statements) to trace a series of recursive calls. Inspecting the values of parameters and local variables often helps to locate errors in a recursive algorithm.

Summary

A recursive algorithm is expressed in terms of a smaller instance of itself. It must include a recursive case, for which the algorithm is expressed in terms of itself, and a base case, for which the algorithm is expressed in nonrecursive terms.

In many recursive problems, the smaller instance refers to a numeric argument that is being reduced with each call. In other problems, the smaller instance refers to the size of the data structure being manipulated.

The base case is the one in which the size of the problem (value or structure) reaches a point for which an explicit answer is known.

In the example for finding the minimum using recursion, the size of the problem was the size of the array being searched. When the array size became 1, the solution was known. If there is only one array element, it is clearly the minimum (as well as the maximum).

In the Towers of Hanoi game, the size of the problem was the number of discs to be moved. When there was only one left on the beginning peg, it could be moved to its final destination.

Quick Check

1. What distinguishes the base case from the recursive case in a recursive algorithm? (pp. 1014–1015)
2. What is the base case in the Towers of Hanoi algorithm? (pp. 1021–1025)
3. In working with simple variables, the recursive case is often stated in terms of a smaller value. What is typical of the recursive case in working with structured variables? (pp. 1026–1036)
4. In printing a linked list in reverse order recursively, what is the base case? (pp. 1029–1031)

Answers   **1.** The base case is the simplest case, the case for which the solution can be stated nonrecursively.   **2.** When there are no more circles left to move.   **3.** It is often stated in terms of a smaller structure.   **4.** When the value of the current node pointer is NULL.

Exam Preparation Exercises

1. Recursion is an example of
   a. selection
   b. a data structure
   c. repetition
   d. data-flow programming
2. A void function can be recursive, but a value-returning function cannot. (True or False?)
3. When a function is called recursively, the arguments and automatic local variables of the calling version are saved until its execution is resumed. (True or False?)
4. Given the recursive formula $F(N) = -F(N - 2)$, with base case $F(0) = 1$, what are the values of $F(4)$, $F(6)$, and $F(5)$? (If any of the values are undefined, say so.)
5. What algorithm error(s) leads to infinite recursion?
6. What control structure appears most commonly in a recursive function?
7. If you develop a recursive algorithm that employs tail recursion, what should you consider?
8. A recursive algorithm depends on making something smaller. When the algorithm works on a data structure, what may become smaller?
   a. Distance from a position in the structure.
   b. The data structure.
   c. The number of variables in the recursive function.

9. What is the name of the memory area used by the computer system to store a function's parameters and automatic local variables?

10. Given the following input data (where \n denotes the newline character):

    ABCDE\n

    what is the output of the following program?

```cpp
#include <iostream>

using namespace std;

void Rev();

int main()
{
    Rev();
    cout << endl;
    return 0;
}

//*************************************

void Rev()
{
    char ch;

    cin.get(ch);
    if (ch != '\n')
    {
        Rev();
        cout << ch;
    }
}
```

11. Repeat Exercise 10, replacing the Rev function with the following version:

```cpp
void Rev()
{
    char ch;

    cin.get(ch);
    if (ch != '\n')
    {
        cout << ch;
        Rev();
    }
}
```

12. Given the following input:

    15
    23

```
21
19
```

what is the output of the following program?

```
#include <iostream>

using namespace std;

void PrintNums();

int main()
{
    PrintNums();
    cout << endl;
    return 0;
}

//**************************************

void PrintNums()
{
    int n;

    cin >> n;
    if (cin)                    // If not EOF...
    {
        cout << n << ' ';
        PrintNums();
        cout << n << ' ';
    }
}
```

Programming Warm-up Exercises

1. Write a C++ value-returning function that implements the recursive formula $F(N) = F(N-1) + F(N-2)$ with base cases $F(0) = 1$ and $F(1) = 1$.

2. Add whatever is necessary to fix the following function so that Func(3) equals 10.

```
int Func( /* in */ int n )
{
    return Func(n - 1) + 3;
}
```

3. Rewrite the following DoubleSpace function without using recursion.

```
void DoubleSpace( /* inout */ ifstream& inFile )
{
    char ch;
```

```
        inFile.get(ch);
        if (inFile)                 // If not EOF...
        {
            cout << ch;
            if (ch == '\n')
                cout << endl;
            DoubleSpace();
        }
    }
```

4. Rewrite the following `PrintSquares` function using recursion.

```
void PrintSquares()
{
    int count;

    for (count = 1; count <= 10; count++)
        cout << count << ' ' << count * count;
}
```

5. Modify the `Factorial` function of this chapter to print its parameter and returned value indented two spaces for each level of call to the function. The call `Factorial(3)` should produce the following output:

```
3
  2
    1
      0
      1
    1
  2
6
```

6. Write a recursive value-returning function that sums the integers from 1 through *N*.

7. Rewrite the following function so that it is recursive.

```
void PrintSqRoots( /* in */ int n )
{
    int i;

    for (i = n; i > 0; i--)
        cout << i << ' ' << sqrt(double(i)) << endl;
}
```

8. The `RevPrint` function of this chapter prints the contents of a dynamic linked list in reverse order. Write a recursive function that prints the contents in forward order.

9. The `Print` function of this chapter prints the contents of an array from first element to last. Write a recursive function that prints from last element to first.

10. Given the following declarations:

```
struct NodeType;
typedef NodeType* PtrType;

struct NodeType
{
    int      info;
    PtrType link;
};

PtrType head;
int      key;
```

write a recursive value-returning function that searches a dynamic linked list for the integer value key. If the value is in the list, the function should return a pointer to the node where it was found. If the value is not in the list, the function should return NULL.

Programming Problems

1. Use recursion to solve the following problem.

    A *palindrome* is a string of characters that reads the same forward and backward. Write a program that reads in strings of characters and determines if each string is a palindrome. Each string is on a separate input line. Echo print each string, followed by "Is a palindrome" if the string is a palindrome or "Is not a palindrome" if the string is not a palindrome. For example, given the input string

    ```
    Able was I, ere I saw Elba.
    ```

    the program would print "Is a palindrome." In determining whether a string is a palindrome, consider uppercase and lowercase letters to be the same and ignore punctuation characters.

2. Write a program to place eight queens on a chessboard in such a way that no queen is attacking any other queen. This is a classic problem that lends itself to a recursive solution. The chessboard should be represented as an 8 × 8 Boolean array. If a square is occupied by a queen, the value is true; otherwise, the value is false. The status of the chessboard when all eight queens have been placed is the solution.

3. A maze is to be represented by a 10 × 10 array of an enumeration type composed of three values: PATH, HEDGE, and EXIT. There is one exit from the maze. Write a program to determine if it is possible to exit the maze from a given starting point. You may move vertically or horizontally in any direction that contains PATH; you may not move to a square that contains HEDGE. If you move into a square that contains EXIT, you have exited.

    The input data consists of two parts: the maze and a series of starting points. The maze is entered as ten lines of ten characters (P, H, and E). Each succeeding line contains a pair of integers that represents a starting point (that is, row and column numbers). Continue processing entry points until end-of-file occurs.

4. A group of soldiers is overwhelmed by an enemy force. Only one person can go for help because they have only one horse. To decide which soldier should go for help, they put their names in a helmet and put one slip of paper for each soldier with a number on it in another helmet. For example, if there are five soldiers, then the second helmet contains five pieces of paper with the numbers 1 through 5 each written on a separate slip.

    The soldiers arrange themselves in a circle and pull a name and a number from the helmets. Starting with the person whose name was pulled, they count off in a clockwise direction until they reach the number that was pulled. When the count stops, that soldier is eliminated from the circle. This continues until there is one soldier left, and that soldier rides for help.

    Implement this process in C++. The names are stored in a file, and the last name in the file is followed by the word STOP. Use a circular linked list to represent the soldiers (a circular linked list is one in which the link member of the last node points back to the first node instead of containing NULL). Use recursive functions to count around the circle and eliminate the soldiers. Output the total number of soldiers in the group, the names of the soldiers who were eliminated, and the name of the soldier who will go for help.

Case Study Follow-Up

1. What is the base case in the recursive Convert function?
2. In the recursive Minimum function, what is the first array index to be evaluated? Explain.
3. Rewrite the Minimum function, assuming the data structure is a dynamic linked list of integers instead of an array.

Appendix A   Reserved Words

The following identifiers are *reserved words*—identifiers with predefined meanings in the C++ language. The programmer cannot declare them for other uses (for example, variable names) in a C++ program.

and	double	not	this
and_eq	dynamic_cast	not_eq	throw
asm	else	operator	true
auto	enum	or	try
bitand	explicit	or_eq	typedef
bitor	export	private	typeid
bool	extern	protected	typename
break	false	public	union
case	float	register	unsigned
catch	for	reinterpret_cast	using
char	friend	return	virtual
class	goto	short	void
compl	if	signed	volatile
const	inline	sizeof	wchar_t
const_cast	int	static	while
continue	long	static_cast	xor
default	mutable	struct	xor_eq
delete	namespace	switch	
do	new	template	

Appendix B   Operator Precedence

The following table summarizes C++ operator precedence. Several operators are not discussed in this book (typeid, the comma operator, ->*, and .*, for instance). For information on these operators, see Stroustrup's *The C++ Programming Language,* Third Edition (Addison-Wesley, 1997).

In the table, the operators are grouped by precedence level (highest to lowest), and a horizontal line separates each precedence level from the next-lower level.

In general, the binary operators group from left to right; the unary operators, from right to left; and the ?: operator, from right to left. Exception: The assignment operators group from right to left.

Precedence (highest to lowest)

Operator	Associativity	Remarks
`::`	Left to right	Scope resolution (binary)
`::`	Right to left	Global access (unary)
`()`	Left to right	Function call and function-style cast
`[]` `->` `.`	Left to right	
`++` `--`	Right to left	++ and -- as postfix operators
`typeid` `dynamic_cast`	Right to left	
`static_cast` `const_cast`	Right to left	
`reinterpret_cast`	Right to left	
`++` `--` `!` Unary `+` Unary `-`	Right to left	++ and -- as prefix operators
`~` Unary `*` Unary `&`	Right to left	
`(cast)` `sizeof` `new` `delete`	Right to left	
`->*` `.*`	Left to right	
`*` `/` `%`	Left to right	
`+` `-`	Left to right	
`<<` `>>`	Left to right	
`<` `<=` `>` `>=`	Left to right	
`==` `!=`	Left to right	
`&`	Left to right	
`^`	Left to right	
`|`	Left to right	
`&&`	Left to right	
`||`	Left to right	
`?:`	Right to left	
`=` `+=` `-=` `*=` `/=` `%=`	Right to left	
`<<=` `>>=` `&=` `|=` `^=`	Right to left	
`throw`	Right to left	
`,`	Left to right	The sequencing operator, not the separator

Appendix C   A Selection of Standard Library Routines

The C++ standard library provides a wealth of data types, functions, and named constants. This appendix details only some of the more widely used library facilities. It is a good idea to consult the manual for your particular system to see what other types, functions, and constants the standard library provides.

This appendix is organized alphabetically according to the header file your program must #include before accessing the listed items. For example, to use a mathematics routine such as sqrt, you would #include the header file cmath as follows:

```
#include <cmath>
using namespace std;
  ⋮
y = sqrt(x);
```

Note that every identifier in the standard library is defined to be in the namespace std. Without the using directive above, you would write

```
y = std::sqrt(x);
```

C.1   The Header File cassert

assert(booleanExpr)
  Argument: A logical (Boolean) expression
  Effect: If the value of booleanExpr is true, execution of the program
                            simply continues. If the value of booleanExpr is false, execu-
                            tion terminates immediately with a message stating the Boolean
                            expression, the name of the file containing the source code, and
                            the line number in the source code.
  Function return value: None (a void function)
  Note: If the preprocessor directive #define NDEBUG is placed before
                            the directive #include <cassert>, all assert statements are
                            ignored.

C.2   The Header File cctype

isalnum(ch)
  Argument: A char value ch
  Function return value: An int value that is
                            - nonzero (true), if ch is a letter or a digit character ('A'–'Z',
                              'a'–'z', '0'–'9')
                            - 0 (false), otherwise

`isalpha(ch)`
Argument: A char value ch
Function return value: An int value that is
- nonzero (true), if ch is a letter ('A'–'Z', 'a'–'z')
- 0 (false), otherwise

`iscntrl(ch)`
Argument: A char value ch
Function return value: An int value that is
- nonzero (true), if ch is a control character (in ASCII, a character with the value 0–31 or 127)
- 0 (false), otherwise

`isdigit(ch)`
Argument: A char value ch
Function return value: An int value that is
- nonzero (true), if ch is a digit character ('0'–'9')
- 0 (false), otherwise

`isgraph(ch)`
Argument: A char value ch
Function return value: An int value that is
- nonzero (true), if ch is a nonblank printable character (in ASCII, '!' through '~')
- 0 (false), otherwise

`islower(ch)`
Argument: A char value ch
Function return value: An int value that is
- nonzero (true), if ch is a lowercase letter ('a'–'z')
- 0 (false), otherwise

`isprint(ch)`
Argument: A char value ch
Function return value: An int value that is
- nonzero (true), if ch is a printable character, including the blank (in ASCII, ' ' through '~')
- 0 (false), otherwise

`ispunct(ch)`
Argument: A char value ch
Function return value: An int value that is
- nonzero (true), if ch is a punctuation character (equivalent to isgraph(ch) && !isalnum(ch))
- 0 (false), otherwise

isspace(ch)
> *Argument:* A char value ch
> *Function return value:* An int value that is
> - nonzero (true), if ch is a whitespace character (blank, newline, tab, carriage return, form feed)
> - 0 (false), otherwise

isupper(ch)
> *Argument:* A char value ch
> *Function return value:* An int value that is
> - nonzero (true), if ch is an uppercase letter ('A'–'Z')
> - 0 (false), otherwise

isxdigit(ch)
> *Argument:* A char value ch
> *Function return value:* An int value that is
> - nonzero (true), if ch is a hexadecimal digit ('0'–'9', 'A'–'F', 'a'–'f')
> - 0 (false), otherwise

tolower(ch)
> *Argument:* A char value ch
> *Function return value:* A character that is
> - the lowercase equivalent of ch, if ch is an uppercase letter
> - ch, otherwise

toupper(ch)
> *Argument:* A char value ch
> *Function return value:* A character that is
> - the uppercase equivalent of ch, if ch is a lowercase letter
> - ch, otherwise

C.3 The Header File cfloat

This header file supplies named constants that define the characteristics of floating-point numbers on your particular machine. Among these constants are the following:

FLT_DIG	Approximate number of significant digits in a float value on your machine
FLT_MAX	Maximum positive float value on your machine
FLT_MIN	Minimum positive float value on your machine
DBL_DIG	Approximate number of significant digits in a double value on your machine
DBL_MAX	Maximum positive double value on your machine
DBL_MIN	Minimum positive double value on your machine
LDBL_DIG	Approximate number of significant digits in a long double value on your machine

LDBL_MAX	Maximum positive `long double` value on your machine
LDBL_MIN	Minimum positive `long double` value on your machine

C.4 The Header File `climits`

This header file supplies named constants that define the limits of integer values on your particular machine. Among these constants are the following:

CHAR_BITS	Number of bits in a byte on your machine (8, for example)
CHAR_MAX	Maximum `char` value on your machine
CHAR_MIN	Minimum `char` value on your machine
SHRT_MAX	Maximum `short` value on your machine
SHRT_MIN	Minimum `short` value on your machine
INT_MAX	Maximum `int` value on your machine
INT_MIN	Minimum `int` value on your machine
LONG_MAX	Maximum `long` value on your machine
LONG_MIN	Minimum `long` value on your machine
UCHAR_MAX	Maximum `unsigned char` value on your machine
USHRT_MAX	Maximum `unsigned short` value on your machine
UINT_MAX	Maximum `unsigned int` value on your machine
ULONG_MAX	Maximum `unsigned long` value on your machine

C.5 The Header File `cmath`

In the `math` routines listed below, the following notes apply.

1. Error handling for incalculable or out-of-range results is system dependent.
2. All arguments and function return values are technically of type `double` (double-precision floating-point). However, single-precision (`float`) values may be passed to the functions.

`acos(x)`
Argument: A floating-point expression x, where $-1.0 \le x \le 1.0$
Function return value: Arc cosine of x, in the range 0.0 through π

`asin(x)`
Argument: A floating-point expression x, where $-1.0 \le x \le 1.0$
Function return value: Arc sine of x, in the range $-\pi/2$ through $\pi/2$

`atan(x)`
Argument: A floating-point expression x
Function return value: Arc tangent of x, in the range $-\pi/2$ through $\pi/2$

`ceil(x)`
Argument: A floating-point expression x
Function return value: "Ceiling" of x (the smallest whole number $\ge$ x)

cos(angle)
Argument: A floating-point expression `angle`, measured in radians
Function return value: Trigonometric cosine of `angle`

cosh(x)
Argument: A floating-point expression x
Function return value: Hyperbolic cosine of x

exp(x)
Argument: A floating-point expression x
Function return value: The value e(2.718...) raised to the power x

fabs(x)
Argument: A floating-point expression x
Function return value: Absolute value of x

floor(x)
Argument: A floating-point expression x
Function return value: "Floor" of x (the largest whole number $\leq$ x)

log(x)
Argument: A floating-point expression x, where x > 0.0
Function return value: Natural logarithm (base e) of x

log10(x)
Argument: A floating-point expression x, where x > 0.0
Function return value: Common logarithm (base 10) of x

pow(x, y)
Arguments: Floating-point expressions x and y. If x = 0.0, y must be positive; if x $\leq$ 0.0, y must be a whole number
Function return value: x raised to the power y

sin(angle)
Argument: A floating-point expression `angle`, measured in radians
Function return value: Trigonometric sine of `angle`

sinh(x)
Argument: A floating-point expression x
Function return value: Hyperbolic sine of x

sqrt(x)
Argument: A floating-point expression x, where x $\geq$ 0.0
Function return value: Square root of x

```
tan(angle)
```
Argument: A floating-point expression `angle`, measured in radians
Function return value: Trigonometric tangent of `angle`

```
tanh(x)
```
Argument: A floating-point expression `x`
Function return value: Hyperbolic tangent of `x`

C.6 The Header File `cstddef`

This header file defines a few system-dependent constants and data types. From this header file, the only item we use in this book is the following symbolic constant:

`NULL`   The null pointer constant `0`

C.7 The Header File `cstdlib`

```
abs(i)
```
Argument: An `int` expression `i`
Function return value: An `int` value that is the absolute value of `i`

```
atof(str)
```
Argument: A C string (null-terminated `char` array) `str` representing a floating point number, possibly preceded by whitespace characters and a '+' or '−'
Function return value: A `double` value that is the floating-point equivalent of the characters in `str`
Note: Conversion stops at the first character in `str` that is inappropriate for a floating-point number. If no appropriate characters were found, the return value is system dependent.

```
atoi(str)
```
Argument: A C string (null-terminated `char` array) `str` representing an integer number, possibly preceded by whitespace characters and a '+' or '−'
Function return value: An `int` value that is the integer equivalent of the characters in `str`
Note: Conversion stops at the first character in `str` that is inappropriate for an integer number. If no appropriate characters were found, the return value is system dependent.

```
atol(str)
```
Argument: A C string (null-terminated `char` array) `str` representing a long integer, possibly preceded by whitespace characters and a '+' or '−'

Function return value:	A `long` value that is the long integer equivalent of the characters in `str`
Note:	Conversion stops at the first character in `str` that is inappropriate for a `long` integer number. If no appropriate characters were found, the return value is system dependent.

`exit(exitStatus)`

Argument:	An `int` expression `exitStatus`
Effect:	Program execution terminates immediately with all files properly closed
Function return value:	None (a void function)
Note:	By convention, `exitStatus` is 0 to indicate normal program completion and is nonzero to indicate an abnormal termination.

`labs(i)`

Argument:	A `long` expression `i`
Function return value:	A `long` value that is the absolute value of `i`

`rand()`

Argument:	None
Function return value:	A random `int` value in the range 0 through `RAND_MAX`, a constant defined in `cstdlib` (`RAND_MAX` is usually the same as `INT_MAX`)
Note:	See `srand` below.

`srand(seed)`

Argument:	An `int` expression `seed`, where `seed` $\geq$ 0
Effect:	Using `seed`, the random number generator is initialized in preparation for subsequent calls to the `rand` function.
Function return value:	None (a void function)
Note:	If `srand` is not called before the first call to `rand`, a `seed` value of 1 is assumed.

`system(str)`

Argument:	A C string (null-terminated `char` array) `str` representing an operating system command, exactly as it would be typed by a user on the operating system command line
Effect:	The operating system command represented by `str` is executed.
Function return value:	An `int` value that is system dependent
Note:	Programmers often ignore the function return value, using the syntax of a void function call rather than a value-returning function call.

C.8 The Header File `cstring`

The header file `cstring` (not to be confused with the header file named `string`) supports manipulation of C strings (null-terminated `char` arrays).

`strcat(toStr, fromStr)`

Arguments:	C strings (null-terminated `char` arrays) `toStr` and `fromStr`, where `toStr` must be large enough to hold the result
Effect:	`fromStr`, including the null character '\0', is concatenated (joined) to the end of `toStr`.
Function return value:	The base address of `toStr`
Note:	Programmers usually ignore the function return value, using the syntax of a void function call rather than a value-returning function call.

`strcmp(str1, str2)`

Arguments:	C strings (null-terminated `char` arrays) `str1` and `str2`
Function return value:	An `int` value < 0, if `str1` < `str2` lexicographically The `int` value 0, if `str1` = `str2` lexicographically An `int` value > 0, if `str1` > `str2` lexicographically

`strcpy(toStr, fromStr)`

Arguments:	`toStr` is a `char` array and `fromStr` is a C string (null-terminated `char` array), and `toStr` must be large enough to hold the result
Effect:	`fromStr`, including the null character '\0', is copied to `toStr`, overwriting what was there.
Function return value:	The base address of `toStr`
Note:	Programmers usually ignore the function return value, using the syntax of a void function call rather than a value-returning function call.

`strlen(str)`

Argument:	A C string (null-terminated `char` array) `str`
Function return value:	An `int` value ≥ 0 that is the length of `str` (excluding the '\0')

C.9 The Header File `string`

This header file supplies a programmer-defined data type (specifically, a *class*) named `string`. Associated with the `string` type are a data type `string::size_type` and a named constant `string::npos`, defined as follows:

`string::size_type`	An unsigned integer type related to the number of characters in a string
`string::npos`	The maximum value of type `string::size_type`

There are dozens of functions associated with the string type. Below are several of the most important ones. In the descriptions, s is assumed to be a variable (an *object*) of type string.

s.c_str()

    Arguments: None

    Function return value: The base address of a C string (null-terminated char array) corresponding to the characters stored in s

s.find(arg)

    Argument: An expression of type string or char, or a C string (such as a literal string)

    Function return value: A value of type string::size_type that gives the starting position in s where arg was found. If arg was not found, the return value is string::npos.

    Note: Positions of characters within a string are numbered starting at 0.

getline(inStream, s)

    Arguments: An input stream inStream (of type istream or ifstream) and a string object s

    Effect: Characters are input from inStream and stored into s until the newline character is encountered. (The newline character is consumed but not stored into s.)

    Function return value: Although the function technically returns a value (which we do not discuss here), programmers usually invoke the function as though it were a void function.

s.length()

    Arguments: None

    Function return value: A value of type string::size_type that gives the number of characters in the string

s.size()

    Arguments: None

    Function return value: The same as s.length()

s.substr(pos, len)

    Arguments: Two unsigned integers, pos and len, representing a position and a length. The value of pos must be less than s.length().

    Function return value: A temporary string object that holds a substring of at most len characters, starting at position pos of s. If len is too large, it means "to the end" of the string in s.

    Note: Positions of characters within a string are numbered starting at 0.

Appendix D   Using This Book with a Prestandard Version of C++

D.1   The string Type

Prior to the ISO/ANSI C++ language standard, the standard library did not provide a `string` data type. Compiler vendors often supplied their own programmer-defined types with names like `String`, `StringType`, and so on. The syntax and semantics of string operations often varied from vendor to vendor.

For readers with prestandard compilers, the authors of this book have created a data type named `StrType` that mimics a subset of the standard `string` type. The subset is sufficient to match the string operations displayed throughout this book.

The files related to `StrType` are available for download from the publisher's Web site (www.jbpub.com). Among the files is one called README.TXT, which explains how to compile the source code and link it with the programs you write. Another file is the header file `str-type.h`, which contains important declarations that define the `StrType` type. Programs that use `StrType` must #include this header file:

```
#include "strtype.h"
```

In the `#include` directive, you cannot place the file name in angle brackets (< >), which tell the preprocessor to look for the file in the standard include directory. Instead, you enclose the file name in double quotes (" "). The double quotes tell the preprocessor to look for the file in the programmer's current directory. Therefore, to use `StrType` in your program, you must (a) verify that the file `strtype.h` is in the directory in which you are currently working on your program, and (b) make sure your program uses the directive

```
#include "strtype.h"
```

Additional directions are given in README.TXT.

Throughout this book you can use `StrType` instead of the `string` data type as follows. First, in your variable declarations, substitute the word `StrType` for `string` as the name of the data type. Second, change the directive #include <string> to #include "strtype.h". For example, instead of

```
#include <string>
   ⋮
string lastName;
```

you would write

```
#include "strtype.h"
   ⋮
StrType lastName;
```

Finally, there is a restriction on performing input into `StrType` variables. Chapter 4 discusses the use of the >> operator and the `getline` function to input characters into a `string` variable. Using >> with StrType variables, at most 1023 characters can be read and stored into one variable. In practice, however, this isn't much of a restriction. It would be extremely rare for an input string to consist of that many characters. Input using getline is also restricted to 1023 characters. In the function call

```
getline(cin, myString);
```

in which myString is a StrType variable, the getline function does not skip leading white-space characters and continues until it either has read 1023 characters or it reaches the newline character '\n', whichever comes first. That is, getline reads and stores an entire input line (to a maximum of 1023 characters), embedded blanks and all. Note that for an input line of 1023 characters or less, the newline character *is* consumed (but is not stored into myString).

D.2   Standard Header Files and Namespaces

Historically, the standard header files in both C and C++ had file names ending in .h (meaning "header file"). Certain header files—for example, iostream.h, iomanip.h, and fstream.h—related specifically to C++. Others, such as math.h, stddef.h, stdlib.h, and string.h, were carried over from the C standard library and were available to both C and C++ programs. When you used an #include directive such as

```
#include <math.h>
```

near the beginning of your program, all identifiers declared in math.h were introduced into your program in global scope (as discussed in Chapter 8). With the advent of the *namespace* mechanism in ISO/ANSI standard C++ (see Chapter 2 and, in more detail, Chapter 8), all of the standard header files were modified so that identifiers are declared within a namespace called std. In standard C++, when you #include a standard header file, the identifiers therein are not automatically placed into global scope.

To preserve compatibility with older versions of C++ that still need the original files iostream.h, math.h, and so forth, the new standard header files are renamed as follows: The C++-related header files have the .h removed, and the header files from the C library have the .h removed *and* the letter *c* inserted at the beginning. Here is a list of the old and new names for some of the most commonly used header files.

Old Name	New Name
iostream.h	iostream
iomanip.h	iomanip
fstream.h	fstream
assert.h	cassert
ctype.h	cctype
float.h	cfloat
limits.h	climits
math.h	cmath
stddef.h	cstddef

```
stdlib.h        cstdlib
string.h        cstring
```

Be careful: The last entry in the list above refers to the C language concept of a string and is unrelated to the `string` type defined in the C++ standard library.

If you are working with a prestandard compiler that does not recognize the new header file names or namespaces, simply substitute the old header file names for the new ones as you encounter them in the book. For example, where we have written

```
#include <iostream>
using namespace std;
```

you would write

```
#include <iostream.h>
```

For compatibility, C++ systems are likely to retain both versions of the header files for some time to come.

D.3   The `fixed` and `showpoint` Manipulators

Chapter 3 introduces five manipulators for formatting the output: `endl`, `setw`, `fixed`, `showpoint`, and `setprecision`. If you are using a prestandard compiler with the header file `iostream.h`, the `fixed` and `showpoint` manipulators may not be available.

In place of the following code shown in Chapter 3,

```
#include <iostream>
using namespace std;
    ⋮
cout << fixed << showpoint;          // Set up floating-pt.
                                     //    output format
```

you can substitute the following code:

```
#include <iostream.h>
    ⋮
cout.setf(ios::fixed, ios::floatfield);
cout.setf(ios::showpoint);
```

These two statements employ some advanced C++ notation. Our advice is simply to use the statements just as you see them and not worry about the details. Here's the general idea. `setf` is a void function associated with the `cout` stream. (Note that the dot, or period, between `cout` and `setf` is required.) The first function call ensures that floating-point numbers are always printed in decimal form rather than scientific notation. The second function call specifies that the decimal point should always be printed, even for whole numbers. In other words, these two function calls accomplish the same effect as the `fixed` and `showpoint` manipulators.

Note: If your compiler complains about the syntax ios::fixed, ios::floatfield, or ios::showpoint, you may have to replace ios with ios_base as follows:

```
cout.setf(ios_base::fixed, ios_base::floatfield);
cout.setf(ios_base::showpoint);
```

D.4 The bool Type

Before the ISO/ANSI C++ language standard, C++ did not have a bool data type. Some pre-standard compilers implemented the bool type before the standard was approved, but others did not. If your compiler does not recognize the bool type, the following discussion will assist you in writing programs that are compatible with those in this book.

In versions of C++ without the bool type, the value 0 represents *false*, and any nonzero value represents *true*. It is customary in pre–standard C++ to use the int type to represent Boolean data:

```
int dataOK;
   ⋮
dataOK = 1;    // Store "true" into dataOK
   ⋮
dataOK = 0;    // Store "false" into dataOK
```

To make the code more self-documenting, many pre–standard C++ programmers define their own Boolean data type by using a *Typedef statement.* This statement allows you to introduce a new name for an existing data type:

```
typedef int bool;
```

All this statement does is tell the compiler to substitute the word int for every occurrence of the word bool in the rest of the program. Thus, when the compiler encounters a statement such as

```
bool dataOK;
```

it translates the statement into

```
int dataOK;
```

With the Typedef statement and declarations of two named constants, true and false, the code at the beginning of this discussion becomes the following:

```
typedef int bool;
const int true = 1;
const int false = 0;
   ⋮
```

```
bool dataOK;
   ⋮
dataOK = true;
   ⋮
dataOK = false;
```

Throughout the book, our programs use the words `bool`, `true`, and `false` when manipulating Boolean data. If your compiler recognizes `bool` as a built-in type, there is nothing you need to do. Otherwise, here are three steps you can take.

1. Use your system's editor to create a file containing the following lines:

    ```
    #ifndef BOOL_H
    #define BOOL_H
    typedef int bool;
    const int true = 1;
    const int false = 0;
    #endif
    ```

    Don't worry about the meaning of the first, second, and last lines. They are explained in Chapter 14. Simply type the lines as you see them above.
2. Save the file you created in step 1, giving it the name `bool.h`. Save this file into the same directory in which you work on your C++ programs.
3. Near the top of every program in which you need `bool` variables, type the line

    ```
    #include "bool.h"
    ```

    Be sure to surround the file name with double quotes, not angle brackets (< >). The quotes tell the preprocessor to look for `bool.h` in your current directory rather than the C++ system directory.

With `bool`, `true`, and `false` defined in this fashion, the programs in this book run correctly, and you can use `bool` in your own programs, even if it is not a built-in type.

Appendix E   Character Sets

The following charts show the ordering of characters in two widely used character sets: ASCII (American Standard Code for Information Interchange) and EBCDIC (Extended Binary Coded Decimal Interchange Code). The internal representation for each character is shown in decimal. For example, the letter *A* is represented internally as the integer 65 in ASCII and as 193 in EBCDIC. The space (blank) character is denoted by a "□".

Left Digit(s)	Right Digit → 0	1	2	3	4	5	6	7	8	9
	ASCII									
0	NUL	SOH	STX	ETX	EOT	ENQ	ACK	BEL	BS	HT
1	LF	VT	FF	CR	SO	SI	DLE	DC1	DC2	DC3
2	DC4	NAK	SYN	ETB	CAN	EM	SUB	ESC	FS	GS
3	RS	US	□	!	"	#	$	%	&	'
4	(	)	*	+	,	−	.	/	0	1
5	2	3	4	5	6	7	8	9	:	;
6	<	=	>	?	@	A	B	C	D	E
7	F	G	H	I	J	K	L	M	N	O
8	P	Q	R	S	T	U	V	W	X	Y
9	Z	[	\	]	^	_	`		a	b	c
10	d	e	f	g	h	i	j	k	l	m
11	n	o	p	q	r	s	t	u	v	w
12	x	y	z	{			}	~	DEL		

Codes 00–31 and 127 are the following nonprintable control characters:

NUL	Null character	VT	Vertical tab	SYN	Synchronous idle
SOH	Start of header	FF	Form feed	ETB	End of transmitted block
STX	Start of text	CR	Carriage return	CAN	Cancel
ETX	End of text	SO	Shift out	EM	End of medium
EOT	End of transmission	SI	Shift in	SUB	Substitute
ENQ	Enquiry	DLE	Data link escape	ESC	Escape
ACK	Acknowledge	DC1	Device control one	FS	File separator
BEL	Bell character (beep)	DC2	Device control two	GS	Group separator
BS	Back space	DC3	Device control three	RS	Record separator
HT	Horizontal tab	DC4	Device control four	US	Unit separator
LF	Line feed	NAK	Negative acknowledge	DEL	Delete

Left Digit(s)	Right Digit	EBCDIC									
		0	1	2	3	4	5	6	7	8	9
6						□					
7						¢	.	<	(	+		
8		&									
9		!	$	*	)	;	¬	−	/		
10								∧	,	%	_
11		>	?								
12			`	:	#	@	´	=	"		a
13		b	c	d	e	f	g	h	i		
14							j	k	l	m	n
15		o	p	q	r						
16			~	s	t	u	v	w	x	y	z
17									\	{	}
18		[	]								
19					A	B	C	D	E	F	G
20		H	I								J
21		K	L	M	N	O	P	Q	R		
22								S	T	U	V
23		W	X	Y	Z						
24		0	1	2	3	4	5	6	7	8	9

In the EBCDIC table, nonprintable control characters—codes 00–63, 250–255, and those for which empty spaces appear in the chart—are not shown.

Appendix F   Program Style, Formatting, and Documentation

Throughout this text, we encourage the use of good programming style and documentation. Although the programs you write for class assignments may not be looked at by anyone except the person grading your work, outside of class you will write programs that will be used by others.

Useful programs have very long lifetimes, during which they must be modified and updated. When maintenance work must be done, either you or another programmer will have to do it. Good style and documentation are essential if another programmer is to understand and work with your program. You will also discover that after not working with your own program for a few months, you'll be amazed at how many of the details you've forgotten.

F.1 General Guidelines

The style used in the programs and fragments throughout this text provides a good starting point for developing your own style. Our goals in creating this style were to make it simple, consistent, and easy to read.

Style is of benefit only for a human reader of your program—differences in style make no difference to the computer. Good style includes the use of meaningful variable names, comments, and indentation of control structures, all of which help others to understand and work with your program. Perhaps the most important aspect of program style is consistency. If the style within a program is not consistent, then it becomes misleading and confusing.

Sometimes, a particular style is specified for you by your instructor or by the company you work for. When you are modifying someone else's code, you should use his or her style in order to maintain consistency within the program. However, you will also develop your own, personal programming style based on what you've been taught, your own experience, and your personal taste.

F.2 Comments

Comments are extra information included to make a program easier to understand. You should include a comment anywhere the code is difficult to understand. However, don't overcomment. Too many comments in a program can obscure the code and be a source of distraction.

In our style, there are four basic types of comments: headers, declarations, in-line, and sidebar.

Header comments appear at the top of the program and should include your name, the date that the program was written, and its purpose. It is also useful to include sections describing input, output, and assumptions. Think of the header comments as the reader's introduction to your program. Here is an example:

```
// This program computes the sidereal time for a given date and
// solar time.
//
// Written By: Your Name
//
// Date Completed: 4/8/02
//
// Input: A date and time in the form MM DD YYYY HH MM SS
//
// Output: Sidereal time in the form HH MM SS
//
// Assumptions: Solar time is specified for a longitude of 0
//      degrees (GMT, UT, or Z time zone)
```

Header comments should also be included for all user-defined functions (see Chapters 7 and 8).

Declaration comments accompany the constant and variable declarations in the program. Anywhere that an identifier is declared, it is helpful to include a comment that explains its purpose. In programs in the text, declaration comments appear to the right of the identifier being declared. For example:

```
const float E = 2.71828;      // The base of the natural logarithms

float deltaX;                 // The difference in the x direction
float deltaY;                 // The difference in the y direction
```

Notice that aligning the comments gives the code a neater appearance and is less distracting.

In-line comments are used to break long sections of code into shorter, more comprehensible fragments. These are often the names of modules in your algorithm design, although you may occasionally choose to include other information. It is generally a good idea to surround in-line comments with blank lines to make them stand out. For example:

```
// Prepare file for reading

scoreFile.open("scores.dat");

// Get data

scoreFile >> test1 >> weight1;
scoreFile >> test2 >> weight2;
scoreFile >> test3 >> weight3;

// Print heading

cout << "Test Score   Weight" << endl;
```

Even if comments are not used, blank lines can be inserted wherever there is a logical break in the code that you would like to emphasize.

Sidebar comments appear to the right of executable statements and are used to shed light on the purpose of the statement. Sidebar comments are often just pseudocode statements from the lowest levels of your design. If a complicated C++ statement requires some explanation, the pseudocode statement should be written to the right of the C++ statement. For example:

```
while (file1 && file2)    // While neither file is empty...
{
    ⋮
```

In addition to the four main types of comments that we have discussed, there are some miscellaneous comments that we should mention. After the `main` function, we recommend using a row of asterisks (or dashes or equal signs or ...) in a comment before and after each function to help it to stand out. For example:

```
//********************************************************************

void PrintSecondHeading()
{
    ⋮
```

```
    }

    //*****************************************************************
```

In this text, we use C++'s alternative comment form

```
/* Some comment */
```

to document the flow of information for each parameter of a function:

```
void GetData( /* out */ int age,        // Patient's age
              /* out */ int weight )    // Patient's weight
{
    ⋮
}

void Print( /* in */     float val,     // Value to be printed
            /* inout */ int&  count )   // Number of lines printed
                                        //   so far
{
    ⋮
}
```

(Chapter 7 describes the purpose of labeling each parameter as /* in */, /* out */, or /* inout */.)

Programmers sometimes place a comment after the right brace of a block (compound statement) to indicate which control structure the block belongs to:

```
while (num >= 0)
{
    ⋮

    if (num == 25)
    {
        ⋮
    } // if
} // while
```

Attaching comments in this fashion can help to clarify the code and aid in debugging mismatched braces.

F.3 Identifiers

The most important consideration in choosing a name for a data item or function in a program is that the name convey as much information as possible about what the data item is or what the function does. The name should also be readable in the context in which it is used. For example, the following names convey the same information but one is more readable than the other:

```
datOfInvc        invoiceDate
```

Identifiers for types, constants, and variables should be nouns, whereas names of void functions (non-value-returning functions) should be imperative verbs or phrases containing imperative verbs. Because of the way that value-returning functions are invoked, their names should be nouns or occasionally adjectives. Here are some examples:

Variables	`address, price, radius, monthNumber`
Constants	`PI, TAX_RATE, STRING_LENGTH, ARRAY_SIZE`
Data types	`NameType, CarMakes, RoomLists, Hours`
Void functions	`GetData, ClearTable, PrintBarChart`
Value-returning functions	`CubeRoot, Greatest, Color, AreaOf, IsEmpty`

Although an identifier may be a series of words, very long identifiers can become quite tedious and can make the program difficult to read.

The best approach to designing an identifier is to try writing out different names until you reach an acceptable compromise—and then write an especially informative declaration comment next to the declaration.

Capitalization is another consideration when choosing an identifier. C++ is a case-sensitive language; that is, uppercase and lowercase letters are distinct. Different programmers use different conventions for capitalizing identifiers. In this text, we begin each variable name with a lowercase letter and capitalize the beginning of each successive English word. We begin each function name and data type name with a capital letter and, again, capitalize the beginning of each successive English word. For named constants, we capitalize the entire identifier, separating successive English words with underscore (_) characters. Keep in mind, however, that C++ reserved words such as `main`, `if`, and `while` are always lowercase letters, and the compiler will not recognize them if you capitalize them differently.

F.4 Formatting Lines and Expressions

C++ allows you to break a long statement in the middle and continue onto the next line. (However, you cannot split a line in the middle of an identifier, a literal constant, or a string.) When you must split a line, it's important to choose a breaking point that is logical and readable. Compare the readability of the following code fragments.

```
cout << "For a radius of " << radius << " the diameter of the cir"
    << "cle is " << diameter << endl;
```

```
cout << "For a radius of " << radius
        << " the diameter of the circle is " << diameter << endl;
```

When you must split an expression across multiple lines, try to end each line with an operator. Also, try to take advantage of any repeating patterns in the expression. For example,

```
meanOfMaxima = (Maximum(set1Value1, set1Value2, set1Value3) +
                Maximum(set2Value1, set2Value2, set2Value3) +
                Maximum(set3Value1, set3Value2, set3Value3)) / 3.0;
```

When writing expressions, also keep in mind that spaces improve readability. Usually you should include one space on either side of the = operator and most other operators. Occasionally, spaces are left out to emphasize the order in which operations are performed. Here are some examples:

```
if (x+y > y+z)
    maximum = x + y;
else
    maximum = y + z;
hypotenuse = sqrt(a*a + b*b);
```

F.5   Indentation

The purpose of indenting statements in a program is to provide visual cues to the reader and to make the program easier to debug. When a program is properly indented, the way the statements are grouped is immediately obvious. Compare the following two program fragments:

```
while (count <= 10)            while (count <= 10)
{                             {
cin >> num;                       cin >> num;
if (num == 0)                     if (num == 0)
{                                 {
count++;                              count++;
num = 1;                              num = 1;
}                                 }
cout << num << endl;              cout << num << endl;
cout << count << endl;           cout << count << endl;
}                             }
```

As a basic rule in this text, each nested or lower-level item is indented by four spaces. Exceptions to this rule are parameter declarations and statements that are split across two or more lines. Indenting by four spaces is a matter of personal preference. Some people prefer to indent by three, five, or even more than five spaces.

In this book, we indent the entire body of a function. Also, in general, any statement that is part of another statement is indented. For example, the If-Then-Else contains two parts, the then-clause and the else-clause. The statements within both clauses are indented four spaces beyond the beginning of the If-Then-Else statement. The If-Then statement is indented like the

If-Then-Else, except that there is no else-clause. Here are examples of the If-Then-Else and the If-Then:

```
if (sex == MALE)
{
    maleSalary = maleSalary + salary;
    maleCount++;
}
else
    femaleSalary = femaleSalary + salary;

if (count > 0)
    average = total / count;
```

For nested If-Then-Else statements that form a generalized multiway branch (the If-Then-Else-If, described in Chapter 5), a special style of indentation is used in the text. Here is an example:

```
if (month == JANUARY)
    monthNumber = 1;
else if (month == FEBRUARY)
    monthNumber = 2;
else if (month == MARCH)
    monthNumber = 3;
else if  nonth == APRIL)
    ⋮
else
    monthNumber = 12;
```

The remaining C++ statements all follow the basic indentation guideline mentioned previously. For reference purposes, here are examples of each.

```
while (count <= 10)
{
    cin >> value;
    sum = sum + value;
    count++;
}

do
{
    GetAnswer(letter);
    PutAnswer(letter);
} while (letter != 'N');

for (count = 1; count <= numSales; count++)
    cout << '*';
```

```
for (count = 10; count >= 1; count--)
{
    inFile >> dataItem;
    outFile << dataItem << ' ' << count << endl;
}

switch (color)
{
    RED    : cout << "Red";
             break;
    ORANGE : cout << "Orange";
             break;
    YELLOW : cout << "Yellow";
             break;
    GREEN  :
    BLUE   :
    INDIGO :
    VIOLET : cout << "Short visible wavelengths";
             break;
    WHITE  :
    BLACK  : cout << "Not valid colors";
             color = NONE;
}
```

Glossary

Abstract data type A data type whose properties (domain and operations) are specified independently of any particular implementation.

Abstract step A step for which some implementation details remain unspecified.

Abstraction barrier The invisible wall around a class object that encapsulates implementation details. The wall can be breached only through the public interface.

Aggregate operation An operation on a data structure as a whole, as opposed to an operation on an individual component of the data structure.

Algorithm A step-by-step procedure for solving a problem in a finite amount of time.

Anonymous type A type that does not have an associated type identifier.

Argument A variable or expression listed in a call to a function; also called *actual argument* or *actual parameter*.

Argument list A mechanism by which functions communicate with each other.

Arithmetic/logic unit (ALU) The component of the central processing unit that performs arithmetic and logical operations.

Array A collection of components, all of the same type, ordered on N dimensions ($N \geq 1$). Each component is accessed by N indexes, each of which represents the component's position within that dimension.

Assembler A program that translates an assembly language program into machine code.

Assembly language A low-level programming language in which a mnemonic is used to represent each of the machine language instructions for a particular computer.

Assignment expression A C++ expression with (1) a value and (2) the side effect of storing the expression value into a memory location.

Assignment statement A statement that stores the value of an expression into a variable.

Automatic variable A variable for which memory is allocated and deallocated when control enters and exits the block in which it is declared.

Auxiliary storage device A device that stores data in encoded form outside the computer's main memory.

Base address The memory address of the first element of an array.

Base case The case for which the solution can be stated nonrecursively.

Base class (superclass) The class being inherited from.

Binary operator An operator that has two operands.

Black box An electrical or mechanical device whose inner workings are hidden from view.

C string In C and C++, a null-terminated sequence of characters stored in a `char` array.

Central processing unit (CPU) The part of the computer that executes the instructions (program) stored in memory; made up of the arithmetic/logic unit and the control unit.

Class A structured type in a programming language that is used to represent an abstract data type.

Class member A component of a class. Class members may be either data or functions.

Class object (class instance) A variable of a `class` type.

Client Software that declares and manipulates objects of a particular class.

Communication complexity A measure of the quantity of data passing through a module's interface.

Compiler A program that translates a high-level language into machine code.

Complexity A measure of the effort expended by the computer in performing a computation, relative to the size of the computation.

Composition (containment) A mechanism by which the internal data (the state) of one class includes an object of another class.

Computer A programmable device that can store, retrieve, and process data.

Computer program A sequence of instructions to be performed by a computer.

Computer programming The process of planning a sequence of steps for a computer to follow.

Concrete step A step for which the implementation details are fully specified.

Constructor An operation that creates a new instance (variable) of an ADT.

Control abstraction The separation of the logical properties of an action from its implementation.

Control structure A statement used to alter the normally sequential flow of control.

Control unit The component of the central processing unit that controls the actions of the other components so that instructions (the program) are executed in the correct sequence.

Count-controlled loop A loop that executes a specified number of times.

Dangling pointer A pointer that points to a variable that has been deallocated.

Data Information in a form a computer can use.

Data abstraction The separation of a data type's logical properties from its implementation.

Data flow The flow of information from the calling code to a function and from the function back to the calling code.

Data representation The concrete form of data used to represent the abstract values of an abstract data type.

Data type A specific set of data values, along with a set of operations on those values.

Declaration A statement that associates an identifier with a data object, a function, or a data type so that the programmer can refer to that item by name.

Deep copy   An operation that not only copies one class object to another but also makes copies of any pointed-to data.

Demotion (narrowing)   The conversion of a value from a "higher" type to a "lower" type according to a programming language's precedence of data types. Demotion may cause loss of information.

Derived class (subclass)   The class that inherits.

Direct addressing   Accessing a variable in one step by using the variable name.

Documentation   The written text and comments that make a program easier for others to understand, use, and modify.

Driver   A simple `main` function that is used to call a function being tested. The use of a driver permits direct control of the testing process.

Dynamic binding   The run-time determination of which function to call for a particular object.

Dynamic data   Variables created during execution of a program by means of special operations. In C++, these operations are `new` and `delete`.

Dynamic data structure   A data structure that can expand and contract during execution.

Dynamic linked list   A linked list composed of dynamically allocated nodes that are linked together by pointers.

Editor   An interactive program used to create and modify source programs or data.

Encapsulation   Hiding a module implementation in a separate block with a formally specified interface.

Enumeration type   A user-defined data type whose domain is an ordered set of literal values expressed as identifiers.

Enumerator   One of the values in the domain of an enumeration type.

Evaluate   To compute a new value by performing a specified set of operations on given values.

Event counter   A variable that is incremented each time a particular event occurs.

Event-controlled loop   A loop that terminates when something happens inside the loop body to signal that the loop should be exited.

Expression   An arrangement of identifiers, literals, and operators that can be evaluated to compute a value of a given type.

Expression statement   A statement formed by appending a semicolon to an expression.

External (head) pointer   A pointer variable that points to the first node in a dynamic linked list.

External representation   The printable (character) form of a data value.

Field (member, in C++)   A component of a record.

File   A named area in secondary storage that is used to hold a collection of data; the collection of data itself.

Flow of control   The order in which the computer executes statements in a program.

Free store (heap) A pool of memory locations reserved for allocation and deallocation of dynamic data.

Function A subprogram in C++.

Function call (function invocation) The mechanism that transfers control to a function.

Function call (to a void function) A statement that transfers control to a void function. In C++, this statement is the name of the function, followed by a list of arguments.

Function definition A function declaration that includes the body of the function.

Function prototype A function declaration without the body of the function.

Function value type The data type of the result value returned by a function.

Functional cohesion A property of a module in which all concrete steps are directed toward solving just one problem, and any significant subproblems are written as abstract steps. Also, the principle that a module should perform exactly one abstract action.

Functional decomposition A technique for developing software in which the problem is divided into more easily handled subproblems, the solutions of which create a solution to the overall problem.

Functional equivalence A property of a module that performs exactly the same operation as the abstract step it defines. A pair of modules are also functionally equivalent to each other when they perform exactly the same operation.

General case The case for which the solution is expressed in terms of a smaller version of itself; also known as *recursive case*.

Hardware The physical components of a computer.

Hierarchical record A record in which at least one of the components is itself a record.

Identifier A name associated with a function or data object and used to refer to that function or data object.

Inaccessible object A dynamic variable on the free store without any pointer pointing to it.

Indirect addressing Accessing a variable in two steps by first using a pointer that gives the location of the variable.

Infinite recursion The situation in which a function calls itself over and over endlessly.

Information Any knowledge that can be communicated.

Information hiding The encapsulation and hiding of implementation details to keep the user of an abstraction from depending on or incorrectly manipulating these details.

Inheritance A mechanism by which one class acquires the properties—the data and operations—of another class.

Input/output (I/O) devices The parts of the computer that accept data to be processed (input) and present the results of that processing (output).

Interactive system A system that allows direct communication between user and computer.

Interface A connecting link at a shared boundary that permits independent systems to meet and act on or communicate with each other. Also, the formal description of the purpose of a subprogram and the mechanism for communicating with it.

Internal representation The form in which a data value is stored inside the memory unit.

Iteration An individual pass through, or repetition of, the body of a loop.

Iteration counter A counter variable that is incremented with each iteration of a loop.

Iterator An operation that allows us to process—one at a time—all the components in an instance of an ADT.

Length The number of values currently stored in a list.

Lifetime The period of time during program execution when an identifier has memory allocated to it.

Linked list A list in which the order of the components is determined by an explicit link member in each node, rather than by the sequential order of the components in memory.

List A variable-length, linear collection of homogeneous components.

Literal value Any constant value written in a program.

Local variable A variable declared within a block and not accessible outside of that block.

Loop A control structure that causes a statement or group of statements to be executed repeatedly.

Loop entry The point at which the flow of control reaches the first statement inside a loop.

Loop exit The point at which the repetition of the loop body ends and control passes to the first statement following the loop.

Loop test The point at which the While expression is evaluated and the decision is made either to begin a new iteration or skip to the statement immediately following the loop.

Machine language The language, made up of binary-coded instructions, that is used directly by the computer.

Member selector The expression used to access components of a struct or class variable. It is formed by using the struct or class variable name and the member name, separated by a dot (period).

Memory leak The loss of available memory space that occurs when dynamic data is allocated but never deallocated.

Memory unit Internal data storage in a computer.

Metalanguage A language that is used to write the syntax rules for another language.

Mixed type expression An expression that contains operands of different data types; also called *mixed mode expression*.

Module A self-contained collection of steps that solves a problem or subproblem; can contain both concrete and abstract steps.

Name precedence The precedence that a local identifier in a function has over a global identifier with the same name in any references that the function makes to that identifier; also called *name hiding.*

Named constant (symbolic constant) A location in memory, referenced by an identifier, that contains a data value that cannot be changed.

Named type A user-defined type whose declaration includes a type identifier that gives a name to the type.

Nonlocal identifier With respect to a given block, any identifier declared outside that block.

Object-oriented design (OOD) A technique for developing software in which the solution is expressed in terms of objects—self-contained entities composed of data and operations on that data.

Object-oriented programming (OOP) The use of data abstraction, inheritance, and dynamic binding to construct programs that are collections of interacting objects.

Object program The machine language version of a source program.

Observer An operation that allows us to observe the state of an instance of an ADT without changing it.

One-dimensional array A structured collection of components, all of the same type, that is given a single name. Each component (array element) is accessed by an index that indicates the component's position within the collection.

Operating system A set of programs that manages all of the computer's resources.

Out-of-bounds array index An index value that, in C++, is either less than 0 or greater than the array size minus 1.

Parameter A variable declared in a function heading; also called *formal argument* or *formal parameter.*

Peripheral device An input, output, or auxiliary storage device attached to a computer.

Pointer type A simple data type consisting of an unbounded set of values, each of which addresses or otherwise indicates the location of a variable of a given type. Among the operations defined on pointer variables are assignment and testing for equality.

Polymorphic operation An operation that has multiple meanings depending on the type of the object to which it is bound at run time.

Postcondition An assertion that should be true after a module has executed.

Precision The maximum number of significant digits.

Precondition An assertion that must be true before a module begins executing.

Programming Planning or scheduling the performance of a task or an event.

Programming language A set of rules, symbols, and special words used to construct a computer program.

Promotion (widening) The conversion of a value from a "lower" type to a "higher" type according to a programming language's precedence of data types.

Range of values The interval within which values of a numeric type must fall, specified in terms of the largest and smallest allowable values.

Record (structure, in C++) A structured data type with a fixed number of components that are accessed by name. The components may be heterogeneous (of different types).

Recursive algorithm A solution that is expressed in terms of (a) smaller instances of itself and (b) a base case.

Recursive call A function call in which the function being called is the same as the one making the call.

Recursive definition A definition in which something is defined in terms of smaller versions of itself.

Reference parameter A parameter that receives the location (memory address) of the caller's argument.

Reference type A simple data type consisting of an unbounded set of values, each of which is the address of a variable of a given type. The only operation defined on a reference variable is initialization, after which every appearance of the variable is implicitly dereferenced.

Representational error Arithmetic error that occurs when the precision of the true result of an arithmetic operation is greater than the precision of the machine.

Reserved word A word that has special meaning in C++; it cannot be used as a programmer-defined identifier.

Scope The region of program code where it is legal to reference (use) an identifier.

Scope rules The rules that determine where in the program an identifier may be accessed, given the point where that identifier is declared.

Self-documenting code Program code containing meaningful identifiers as well as judiciously used clarifying comments.

Semantics The set of rules that determines the meaning of instructions written in a programming language.

Shallow copy An operation that copies one class object to another without copying any pointed-to data.

Short-circuit (conditional) evaluation Evaluation of a logical expression in left-to-right order with evaluation stopping as soon as the final truth value can be determined.

Side effect Any effect of one function on another that is not a part of the explicitly defined interface between them.

Significant digits Those digits from the first nonzero digit on the left to the last nonzero digit on the right (plus any 0 digits that are exact).

Simple (atomic) data type A data type in which each value is atomic (indivisible).

Software   Computer programs; the set of all programs available on a computer.

Software engineering   The application of traditional engineering methodologies and techniques to the development of software.

Software piracy   The unauthorized copying of software for either personal use or use by others.

Sorting   Arranging the components of a list into order (for instance, words into alphabetical order or numbers into ascending or descending order).

Source program   A program written in a high-level programming language.

Static binding   The compile-time determination of which function to call for a particular object.

Static variable   A variable for which memory remains allocated throughout the execution of the entire program.

Structured data type   A data type in which each value is a collection of components and whose organization is characterized by the method used to access individual components. The allowable operations on a structured data type include the storage and retrieval of individual components.

Structured (procedural) programming   The construction of programs that are collections of interacting functions or procedures.

Stub   A dummy function that assists in testing part of a program. A stub has the same name and interface as a function that actually would be called by the part of the program being tested, but it is usually much simpler.

Switch expression   The expression whose value determines which switch label is selected. It cannot be a floating-point or string expression.

Syntax   The formal rules governing how valid instructions are written in a programming language.

Tail recursion   A recursive algorithm in which no statements are executed after the return from the recursive call.

Termination condition   The condition that causes a loop to be exited.

Test plan   A document that specifies how a program is to be tested.

Test plan implementation   Using the test cases specified in a test plan to verify that a program outputs the predicted results.

Testing the state of a stream   The act of using a C++ stream object in a logical expression as if it were a Boolean variable; the result is `true` if the last I/O operation on that stream succeeded, and `false` otherwise.

Transformer   An operation that builds a new value of the ADT, given one or more previous values of the type.

Two-dimensional array   A collection of components, all of the same type, structured in two dimensions. Each component is accessed by a pair of indexes that represent the component's position in each dimension.

Type casting   The explicit conversion of a value from one data type to another; also called type conversion.

Type coercion   The implicit (automatic) conversion of a value from one data type to another.

Unary operator   An operator that has just one operand.

Value parameter   A parameter that receives a copy of the value of the corresponding argument.

Value-returning function   A function that returns a single value to its caller and is invoked from within an expression.

Variable   A location in memory, referenced by an identifier, that contains a data value that can be changed.

Virus   A computer program that replicates itself, often with the goal of spreading to other computers without authorization, and possibly with the intent of doing harm.

Void function (procedure)   A function that does not return a function value to its caller and is invoked as a separate statement.

Answers to Selected Exercises

Chapter 1   Exam Preparation Exercises

2. Input: Source code file (program in a high-level language such as C++)
   Output: Object code file (machine language program). Some compilers also output a listing (a copy of the program with error messages and other information inserted).
4. The following are peripheral devices: disk drive, magnetic tape drive, printer, CD-ROM drive, auxiliary storage, LCD screen, and mouse. The arithmetic/logic unit, the memory, and the control unit are not peripherals.

Chapter 1   Case Study Follow-Up

1. There are many valid solutions to this question. Here is one way of dividing the problem:

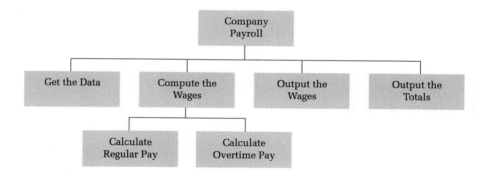

4. The remarks preceded by // are comments. The compiler ignores comments. They are included to help people (including the programmer) understand the program.

Chapter 2   Exam Preparation Exercises

1. a. invalid   b. valid   c. valid   d. invalid   e. valid   f. invalid   g. valid
   h. invalid
3. program—15; algorithm—14; compiler—3; identifier—1; compilation phase—12; execution phase—10; variable—11; constant—2; memory—13; syntax—6; semantics—8; block—7
4. a. reserved   b. programmer-defined   c. programmer-defined   d. reserved
   e. programmer-defined
7. a. `s1 = blues2 = bird`
   b. `Result:bluebird`
   c. `Result:   bluebird`
   d. `Result:   blue bird`

8. A rolling
   stone   ← One blank line

   gathers

                      ← Three blank lines

   nomoss
11. False
14. 1425B Elm St.
    Amaryllis, Iowa

Chapter 2   Programming Warm-up Exercises

2. ```
cout << "The moon" << endl;
cout << "is" << endl;
cout << "blue." << endl;
```
3. ```
string make;
string model;
string color;
string plateType;
char    classification;
```

Chapter 2   Case Study Follow-Up

1. In the line

   ```
cout << "beautiful Panhard, Texas! Now " << first << "I realize"
```

   replace Panhard, Texas with Wormwood, Massachusetts.
3. To insert blank lines in the form letter, you would use additional endl manipulators after the line

   ```
cout << "Argyle M. Sneeze" << endl << endl << endl << endl;
```

   For example, to add two more blank lines, the code would be

   ```
cout << "Argyle M. Sneeze" << endl << endl << endl << endl;
cout << endl << endl;
cout << "* Measured around the circumference of the packing"
```

Chapter 3   Exam Preparation Exercises

3. a. Floating point: 13.3333   b. Integer: 2   c. Integer: 5   d. Floating point: 13.75
   e. Integer: −4   f. Integer: 1   g. Illegal: 10.0 / 3.0 is a floating-point expression, but the % operator requires integer operands.
6. ```
Cost is
300
Price is 30Cost is 300
Grade A costs
300
```
9. a. iostream   b. cstdlib   c. cmath   d. iostream   e. iostream and iomanip
14. False
```

Chapter 3 Programming Warm-up Exercises

1. Only one line needs to be changed. In the following declaration, change 10 to 15:

   ```
   const int LBS = 10;
   ```

2. `sum = n * (n + 1) / 2;`
5. ```
   discriminant = sqrt(b * b - 4.0 * a * c);
   denominator = 2.0 * a;
   solution1 = (-b + discriminant) / denominator;
   solution2 = (-b - discriminant) / denominator;
   ```
9. The expression is `sentence.find("res")`. The first occurrence of the string "res" occurs at position 12.

Chapter 3 Case Study Follow-Up

1. The named constants make the program easier to read and understand. Also, to change one of the constants, you only need to change one line (the constant declaration) instead of changing every occurrence of the literal constant throughout the program.
2. Declare a constant ROUND_FACTOR (defined to be equal to the desired rounding factor, such as 100.0 for hundredths) and replace every occurrence of 10.0 with ROUND_FACTOR.

Chapter 4 Exam Preparation Exercises

2. a. `int1` contains 17, `int2` contains 13, and `int3` contains 7.
   b. The leftover values remain waiting in the input stream. These values will be read by subsequent input statements (or they will be ignored if no more input statements are executed).
6. True
8. `123 147`
13. Errors in the program are as follows:
    - The declaration of `outData` is missing:

      ```
      ofstream outData;
      ```

    - The opening of the input file is missing:

      ```
      inData.open("myfile.dat");
      ```

    - The statement

      ```
      cin >> n;
      ```

      does not read from the input file. Change `cin` to `inData`.
14. With the corrected version of the program in Exercise 13, file stream `inData` will still contain the value 144 after the program is executed. File stream `outData` will contain 144, followed by a newline character.
18. False. Class member functions are invoked by using dot notation.
      ```

Chapter 4   Programming Warm-up Exercises

1. `cin >> ch1 >> ch2 >> ch3;`
3. `cin >> length1 >> height1 >> length2 >> height2;`
4. In the following, the value 100 is arbitrary. Any value greater than 4 will work.

```
cin.get(chr1);
cin.ignore(100, '\n');
cin.get(chr2);
cin.ignore(100, '\n');
cin.get(chr3);
cin.ignore(100, '\n');
```

8.
```
#include <iostream>
#include <fstream>

using namespace std;

int main()
{
    int      val1;
    int      val2;
    int      val3;
    int      val4;
    ifstream dataIn;
    ofstream resultsOut;

    dataIn.open("myinput.dat");
    resultsOut.open("myoutput.dat");
    dataIn >> val1 >> val2 >> val3 >> val4;
    resultsOut << val1 << val2 << val3 << val4 << endl;
    return 0;
}
```

10. Note that the problem statement said nothing about getting into the car, adjusting seat-belts, checking the mirror, or driving away. Presumably those tasks, along with starting the car, are subtasks of a larger design such as "Go to the store." Here we are concerned only with starting the car itself.

Main Module

> Ensure car won't roll.
> Disengage gears.
> Attempt ignition.

Ensure Car Won't Roll

> Engage parking brake.
> Turn wheels into curb.

Disengage Gears

> Push in clutch with left foot.
> Move gearshift to neutral.
> Release clutch.

Attempt Ignition

Insert key into ignition slot.
Turn key to ON position.
Pump accelerator once.
Turn key to START position.
Release after engine catches or 5 seconds, whichever comes first.

Chapter 4 Case Study Follow-Up

1. Get Length and Width, Get Wood Cost, and Get Canvas Cost are input modules. Compute Dimensions and Costs is a computational module. Print Dimensions and Costs is an output module.

Chapter 5 Exam Preparation Exercises

2. a. No parentheses are needed.   b. No parentheses are needed.   c. No parentheses are needed.   d. ! (q && q)
6. a. 4   b. 2   c. 5   d. 3   e. 1
9. a. If-Then-Else   b. If-Then   c. If-Then   d. If-Then-Else
10. The error message is printed because there is a semicolon after the right brace of a block (compound statement).
13. Yes

Chapter 5 Programming Warm-up Exercises

2. In the following statement, the outer parentheses are not required but are included for readability.

```
available = (numberOrdered <= (numberOnHand - numberReserved));
```

4. In the following statement, the outer parentheses are not required but are included for readability.

```
leftPage = (pageNumber % 2 == 0);
```

6.
```
if (year % 4 == 0)
    cout << year << " is a leap year." << endl;
else
{
    year = year + 4 - year % 4;
    cout << year << " is the next leap year." << endl;
}
```

7.
```
if (age > 64)
    cout << "Senior voter";
else if (age < 18)
    cout << "Under age";
else
    cout << "Regular voter";
```

9.
```
// This is a nonsense program
if (a > 0)
    if (a < 20)
    {
        cout << "A is in range." << endl;
        b = 5;
    }
    else
    {
        cout << "A is too large." << endl;
        b = 3;
    }
else
    cout << "A is too small." << endl;
cout << "All done." << endl;
```

Chapter 5 Case Study Follow-Up

2. No. The data is only valid if each test score is nonnegative. Modifying the code to test whether the sum of the test scores is nonnegative will not catch the following invalid case: test1 = 100, test2 = 80, test3 = −20.

4. To input and compute the average of four scores, one control structure would need to be changed. The statement

```
if (test1 < 0 || test2 < 0 || test3 < 0)
    dataOK = false;
else
    dataOK = true;
```

would need to be replaced with

```
if (test1 < 0 || test2 < 0 || test3 < 0 || test4 < 0)
    dataOK = false;
else
    dataOK = true;
```

Note that the program would require other changes, but this is the only control structure that would need to be changed.

Chapter 6 Exam Preparation Exercises

3.
```
number = 1;
while (number < 11)
{
    cout << number << endl;
    number++;
}
```

4. Six iterations are performed.

9. Telephone numbers read in as integers have many different values that could be used as sentinels. In the United States, a standard telephone number is a positive seven-digit integer (ignoring area codes) and cannot start with 0, 1, 411, or 911. Therefore, a reasonable sentinel may be negative, greater than 9999999, or less than 2000000.

11. a. (1) Change < to <=. (2) Change 1 to 0. (3) Change 20 to 21.

    b. Changes (1) and (3) make count range from 1 through 21. Change (2) makes count range from 0 through 20.

Chapter 6 Programming Warm-up Exercises

1.
```
dangerous = false;
while ( !dangerous )
{
    cin >> pressure;
    if (pressure > 510.0)
        dangerous = true;
}
```

   or

```
dangerous = false;
while ( !dangerous )
{
    cin >> pressure;
    dangerous = (pressure > 510.0);
}
```

2.
```
count28 = 0;
loopCount = 1;
while (loopCount <= 100)
{
    inputFile >> number;
    if (number == 28)
        count28++;
    loopCount++;
}
```

5.
```
positives = 0;
negatives = 0;
cin >> number;
while (cin)        // While NOT EOF...
{
    if (number > 0)
        positives++;
    else if (number < 0)
        negatives++;
    cin >> number;
}
cout << "Number of positive numbers: " << positives << endl;
cout << "Number of negative numbers: " << negatives << endl;
```

6.
```
sum = 0;
evenInt = 16;
while (evenInt <= 26)
{
    sum = sum + evenInt;
    evenInt = evenInt + 2;
}
```

7.
```
hour = 1;
minute = 0;
am = true;
done = false;
while ( !done )
{
    cout << hour << ':';
    if (minute < 10)
        cout << '0';
    cout << minute;
    if (am)
        cout << " A.M." << endl;
    else
        cout << " P.M." << endl;

    minute++;
    if (minute > 59)
    {
        minute = 0;
        hour++;
        if (hour == 13)
            hour = 1;
        else if (hour == 12)
            am = !am;
    }
    if (hour == 1 && minute == 0 && am)
        done = true;
}
```

Chapter 6 Case Study Follow-Up

1. a. In the While loop, check for a negative income amount before processing it:

```
incFile >> sex >> amount;
femaleCount = 0;
femaleSum = 0.0;
maleCount = 0;
maleSum = 0.0;

while (incFile)
{
    cout << "Sex: " << sex << " Amount: " << amount << endl;
```

```
    if (amount < 0.0)                 // Check for invalid salary
        cout << "** Bad data--negative salary **" << endl;
    else
        if (sex == 'F')
        {
            femaleCount++;
            femaleSum = femaleSum + amount;
        }
        else
        {
            maleCount++;
            maleSum = maleSum + amount;
        }
    incFile >> sex >> amount;
}
```

2. Set 1:

    Empty file

    Set 2 (no males) :

    F 30000

    Set 3 (no females):

    M 30000

    Set 4 (invalid sex codes and income values):

    F 64000
    R 20000
    M 40000
    F -15000
    M 50000
    G 30000
    M -30000
    F 20000

Chapter 7   Exam Preparation Exercises

4. 5 3 13
   3 3 9
   9 12 30

7. For passing by value, parts (a) through (g) are all valid. For passing by reference, only parts (a) and (c) are valid.

8. 13571 (the memory address of the variable `widgets`).

10. The answers are 12 10 3

11. Variables in `main` just before `Change` is called: a = 10 and b = 7. Variables in `Change` at the moment control enters the function (before any statements are executed): x = 10, y = 7, and the value of b is undefined. Variables in `main` after return from `Change`: a = 10 (x in `Change` is a value parameter, so the argument a is not modified) and b = 17.

Chapter 7 Programming Warm-up Exercises

2.
```
void RocketSimulation( /* in */     float   thrust,
                       /* inout */ float& weight,
                       /* in */     int     timeStep,
                       /* in */     int     totalTime,
                       /* out */   float& velocity,
                       /* out */   bool&  outOfFuel )
```

5.
```
void Halve( /* inout */ int& firstNumber,
            /* inout */ int& secondNumber )

// Precondition:
//     firstNumber and secondNumber are assigned
// Postcondition:
//     firstNumber == firstNumber@entry / 2
//  && secondNumber == secondNumber@entry / 2

{
    ⋮
}
```

7. a. Function definition:

```
void ScanHeart( /* out */ bool& normal )

// Postcondition:
//     normal == true, if a normal heart rate (60-80) was input
//                      before EOF occurred
//            == false, otherwise
{
    int heartRate;

    cin >> heartRate;
    while ((heartRate < 60 || heartRate > 80) && cin)
        cin >> heartRate;

    // At loop exit, either (heartRate >= 60 && heartRate <= 80)
    // or EOF occurred

    normal = (heartRate >= 60 && heartRate <= 80);
}
```

b. Function invocation:

```
ScanHeart(normal);
```

8. a. Function definition:

```
void Rotate( /* inout */ int& firstValue,
             /* inout */ int& secondValue,
             /* inout */ int& thirdValue  )
```

```
// This function takes three parameters and returns their values
// in a shifted order

// Precondition:
//      firstValue, secondValue, and thirdValue are assigned
// Postcondition:
//      firstValue == secondValue@entry
//   && secondValue == thirdValue@entry
//   && thirdValue == firstValue@entry

{
    int temp;      // Temporary holding variable

    // Save value of first parameter

    temp = firstValue;

    // Shift values of next two parameters

    firstValue = secondValue;
    secondValue = thirdValue;

    // Replace value of final parameter with saved value

    thirdValue = temp;
}
```

b. Test program:

```
#include <iostream>

using namespace std;

void Rotate( int&, int&, int& );

int main()
{
    int int1;      // First input value
    int int2;      // Second input value
    int int3;      // Third input value

    cout << "Enter three values: ";
    cin >> int1 >> int2 >> int3;

    cout << "Before: " << int1 << ' ' << int2 << ' '
         << int3 << endl;
    Rotate(int1, int2, int3);
    cout << "After: " << int1 << ' ' << int2 << ' '
         << int3 << endl;
    return 0;
}
// The Rotate function, as above, goes here
```

Chapter 7 Case Study Follow-Up

2.  ```cpp
    void PrintData( /* in */ int    deptID,
                    /* in */ int    storeNum,
                    /* in */ float  deptSales )
    {
        string bar;    // Bar of asterisks

        cout << setw(12) << "Dept " << deptID << endl;
        cout << setw(3) << storeNum << "      ";
        bar = BarOfAsterisks(deptSales);
        cout << bar << endl;
    }
    ```

3. The `GetData` function would have the following statement added after the input statement that reads in numDays:

    ```cpp
    if (numDays < 0)
        cout << "** Data error--number of days for dept. " << deptId
             << " is negative **" << endl;
    ```

Chapter 8 Exam Preparation Exercises

1. True
5. 1 1
    1 2
    1 3
7. Yes
11. It is risky to use a reference parameter as a parameter of a value-returning function because it provides a mechanism for side effects to escape from the function. A value-returning function usually is designed to return a single result (the function value), which is then used in the expression that called the function. If a value-returning function declares a reference parameter and modifies the parameter (hence, the caller's argument), that function is returning more than one result, which is not obvious from the way the function is invoked. (However, an I/O stream variable *must* be declared as a reference parameter, even in a value-returning function.)

Chapter 8 Programming Warm-up Exercises

3.  ```cpp
    bool NearlyEqual( /* in */ float num1,
                      /* in */ float num2,
                      /* in */ float difference )
    ```

5.  ```cpp
    float CompassHeading( /* in */ float trueCourse,
                          /* in */ float windCorrAngle,
                          /* in */ float variance,
                          /* in */ float deviation     )


    // Precondition:
    //     All parameters are assigned
    // Postcondition:
    //     Function value == trueCourse + windCorrAngle +
    //                       variance + deviation
    ```
    ```

```
    {
        return trueCourse + windCorrAngle + variance + deviation;
    }
```

8. Function body for Hypotenuse function (assuming the header file cmath has been included in order to access the sqrt function):

```
    {
        return sqrt(side1*side1 + side2*side2);
    }
```

13. Below, the type of costPerOunce and the function return type are float so that the cost can be expressed in terms of dollars and cents (e.g., 1.23 means $1.23). These types could be int if the cost were expressed in terms of cents only (e.g., 123 means $1.23).

```
float Postage( /* in */ int    pounds,
               /* in */ int    ounces,
               /* in */ float  costPerOunce )

// Precondition:
//      pounds >= 0  &&  ounces >= 0  &&  costPerOunce >= 0.0
// Postcondition:
//      Function value == (pounds * 16 + ounces) * costPerOunce

    {
        return (pounds * 16 + ounces) * costPerOunce;
    }
```

Chapter 8   Case Study Follow-Up

3. Only the Get2Digits function needs to be modified. The test for whether the second character is a slash needs to be changed from

```
if (secondChar == '/')
```

to

```
if (secondChar == '/' || secondChar == '-')
```

4. Change the body of GetData so that it begins as follows:

```
    {
        bool badData;    // True if an input value is invalid

        badData = true;
        while (badData)
        {
            cout << "Enter the number of crew (1 or 2)." << endl;
            cin >> crew;
            badData = (crew < 1 || crew > 2);
            if (badData)
                cout << "Invalid number of crew members." << endl;
        }
```

```
          badData = true;
          while (badData)
          {
              cout << "Enter the number of passengers (0 through 8)."
                  << endl;
              cin >> passengers;
              badData = (passengers < 0 || passengers > 8);
              if (badData)
                  cout << "Invalid number of passengers." << endl;
          }
```

Continue in this manner to validate the closet weight (0–160 pounds), baggage weight (0–525 pounds), and amount of fuel loaded (10–565 gallons).

Chapter 9   Exam Preparation Exercises

2. False
4. False
6. MaryJoeAnneWhoops!
9. 1
13. False

Chapter 9   Programming Warm-up Exercises

```
1.  switch (grade)
    {
        case 'A' : sum = sum + 4;
                   break;
        case 'B' : sum = sum + 3;
                   break;
        case 'C' : sum = sum + 2;
                   break;
        case 'D' : sum++;
                   break;
        case 'F' : cout << "Student is on probation" << endl;
                   break;     // Not required
    }
2.  switch (grade)
    {
        case 'A' : sum = sum + 4;
                   break;
        case 'B' : sum = sum + 3;
                   break;
        case 'C' : sum = sum + 2;
                   break;
        case 'D' : sum++;
                   break;
        case 'F' : cout << "Student is on probation" << endl;
                   break;
```

```
                      break;      // Not required
      }
5.  do
    {
        cout << "Enter 1, 2, or 3: ";
        cin >> response;
    } while (response < 1 || response > 3);

6.  cin >> ch;
    while (cin)
    {
        cout << ch;
        cin >> ch;
    }
```

10. This solution returns proper results only if the precondition shown in the comments is true. Note that it returns the correct result for $base^0$, which is 1.

```
int Power( /* in */ int base,
           /* in */ int exponent )

// Precondition:
//      base is assigned  &&  exponent >= 0
//      && (base to the exponent power) <= INT_MAX
// Postcondition:
//      Function value == base to the exponent power

{
    int result = 1;      // Holds intermediate powers of base
    int count;           // Loop control variable

    for (count = 1; count <= exponent; count++)
        result = result * base;
    return result;
}
```

Chapter 9   Case Study Follow-Up

```
1.  void GetYesOrNo( /* out */ char& response )    // User response char
    {
        cin >> response;
        while (response != 'y' && response != 'n')
        {
            cout << "Please type y or n: ";
            cin >> response;
        }
    }
```

```
        void GetOneAmount( /* out */ float& amount )    // Rainfall amount
                                                        // for one month
        {
            cin >> amount;
            while (amount < 0.0)
            {
                cout << "Amount cannot be negative. Enter again: ";
                cin >> amount;
            }
        }
```

Chapter 10   Exam Preparation Exercises

3. a. `sumOfSquares += x * x;`
   b. `count--;`
      or
      `--count;`
   c. `k = (n > 8) ? 32 : 15 * n;`
5. Notice that
   the character \ is a backslash.
6. a. 1.4E+12 (to 10 digits)   b. 100.0 (to 10 digits)   c. 3.2E+5 (to 10 digits)
9. a. valid   b. invalid   c. invalid   d. valid
12. False. The angle brackets (< >) should be quotation marks.

Chapter 10   Programming Warm-up Exercises

2. `cout << "Hello\tThere\n\n\n\"Ace\"";`
6. `enum CourseType {CS101, CS200, CS210, CS350, CS375, CS441};`
8. `enum DayType {MONDAY, TUESDAY, WEDNESDAY, THURSDAY, FRIDAY};`
9.
```
    DayType CharToDay( /* in */ char ch1,
                       /* in */ char ch2 )

    // Precondition:
    //     ch1=='M' OR ch1=='W' OR ch1=='F' OR
    //     (ch1=='T' && ch2=='U') OR (ch1=='T' && ch2=='H')
    // Postcondition:
    //     Function value == MONDAY, if ch1=='M'
    //                    == TUESDAY, if (ch1=='T' && ch2=='U')
    //                    == WEDNESDAY, if ch1=='W'
    //                    == THURSDAY, if (ch1=='T' && ch2=='H')
    //                    == FRIDAY, if ch1=='F'

    {
        switch (ch1)
        {
            case 'M' : return MONDAY;
            case 'T' : if (ch2 == 'U')
                            return TUESDAY;
                       else
                            return THURSDAY;
```

```
                    case 'W' : return WEDNESDAY;
                    case 'F' : return FRIDAY;
                }
        }
```

Chapter 10 Case Study Follow-Up

5. The readability of the program is enhanced because we are using the actual values rather than char codes for the plays.

7. The data used in the book is a good data set. It tests each combination of 'R', 'P', and 'S' at least once and has an error in each data file. However, a comprehensive test plan must include data sets to test the following situations:
   - Player A wins.
   - Player B wins.
   - The game is a tie.
   - There is an error in both files at the same position.
   - fileA does not have enough plays.
   - fileB does not have enough plays.
   - Neither file has enough plays.

   Your test plan should include the data used for each case and the expected results.

Chapter 11 Exam Preparation Exercises

2.
```
struct RecType
{
    int    numDependents;
    float  salary;
    bool   hasMajorMed;
};
```

7. a. SomeClass and int b. Func1, Func2, Func3, and someInt c. object1 and object2 d. Func1, Func2, and Func3 e. Func1 and Func3 f. part (ii)

8. True

11. a. Only myprog.cpp must be recompiled. b. All of the object (.obj) files must be relinked. c. Only file2.cpp and file3.cpp must be recompiled. d. All of the object (.obj) files must be relinked.

Chapter 11 Programming Warm-up Exercises

1. a.
```
enum YearType {FRESHMAN, SOPHOMORE, JUNIOR, SENIOR};
enum SexType {M, F};

struct PersonType
{
    string    name;
    string    ssNumber;
    YearType  year;
    float     gpa;
    SexType   sex;
};
```

b.
```
PersonType person;
    ⋮
cout << person.name << endl;
cout << person.ssNumber << endl;
switch (person.year)
{
    FRESHMAN   : cout << "Freshman" << endl;
                 break;
    SOPHOMORE  : cout << "Sophomore" << endl;
                 break;
    JUNIOR     : cout << "Junior" << endl;
                 break;
    SENIOR     : cout << "Senior" << endl;
}
cout << person.gpa << endl;
if (person.sex == M)
    cout << "Male" << endl;
else
    cout << "Female" << endl;
```

3.
```
enum YearType {FRESHMAN, SOPHOMORE, JUNIOR, SENIOR};
struct DateType
{
    int month;
    int year;
};

struct StudentType
{
    string    name;
    long      studentID;
    int       hoursToDate;
    int       coursesToDate;
    DateType firstEnrolled;
    YearType year;
    float     gpa;
};
```

5. a.
```
if ( !time1.Equal(time2) )
    n = 1;
```
b.
```
if (time1.LessThan(time2) || time1.Equal(time2))
    n = 5;
```
c.
```
if (time2.LessThan(time1))
    n = 8;
```
d.
```
if ( !time1.LessThan(time2) )
    n = 5;
```
   or
```
if (time2.LessThan(time1) || time2.Equal(time1))
    n = 5;
```

7. Function specification (within the `TimeType` class declaration):

```
void WriteAmPm() const;
    // Postcondition:
    //      Time has been output in 12-hour form
    //          HH:MM:SS AM   or   HH:MM:SS PM
```

Function definition (omitting the postcondition to save space):

```
void TimeType::WriteAmPm() const
{
    bool am;          // True if AM should be printed
    int  tempHrs;     // Value of hours to be printed

    am = (hrs <= 11);
    if (hrs == 0)
        tempHrs = 12;
    else if (hrs >= 13)
        tempHrs = hrs - 12;
    else
        tempHrs = hrs;

    if (tempHrs < 10)
        cout << '0';
    cout << tempHrs << ':';
    if (mins < 10)
        cout << '0';
    cout << mins << ':';
    if (secs < 10)
        cout << '0';
    cout << secs;
    if (am)
        cout << " AM";
    else
        cout << " PM";
}
```

8. Function specification (within the `TimeType` class declaration):

```
long Minus( /* in */ TimeType time2 ) const;
    // Precondition:
    //      This time and time2 represent times in the same day
    // Postcondition:
    //      Function value == (this time) - time2, in seconds
```

Function definition (omitting the precondition and postcondition to save space):

```
long TimeType::Minus( /* in */ TimeType time2 ) const
{
    long thisTimeInSecs;   // This time in seconds since midnight
    long time2InSecs;      // time2 in seconds since midnight
```

```
                    // Using 3600 seconds per hour and 60 seconds per minute...

                    thisTimeInSecs = long(hrs)*3600 + long(mins)*60 + long(secs);
                    time2InSecs = long(time2.hrs)*3600 + long(time2.mins)*60 +
                                 long(time2.secs);
                    return thisTimeInSecs - time2InSecs;
                }
```

Chapter 11   Case Study Follow-Up

1. The class constructor `DateType()` is a constructor operation. `Set` and `Increment` are transformers. `Month`, `Day`, `Year`, `Print`, and `ComparedTo` are observers.

6. Assuming a variable `areaCode` is of type `int`, one solution is to print a leading zero if the area code is less than 100:

```
if (areaCode < 100)
    cout << '0';
cout << areaCode;
```

Another solution is to declare an area code to be a string rather than an `int`, thereby reading or printing exactly three characters each time I/O takes place.

Chapter 12   Exam Preparation Exercises

1. True

5. a. `enum BirdType {CARDINAL, BLUEJAY, HUMMINGBIRD, ROBIN};`
   b. `int sightings[4];`

7. 1 3 -2
   17 6 11
   4 2 2
   19 14 5
   11 15 -4

   52 40 12

9. `sample` [0] [1] [2] [3] [4] [5] [6] [7]

10	9	8	7	6	5	4	3

14. a. hierarchical record   b. record   c. record   d. array of records   e. array   f. array of hierarchical records   g. array of records

18. a. valid   b. valid   c. invalid   d. valid   e. invalid   f. invalid

20. a. True   b. False   c. True   d. True

Chapter 12   Programming Warm-up Exercises

1. `void Initialize( /* out */ bool failing[] )`

```
// Postcondition:
//      failing[0..NUM_STUDS-1] == false

{
```

```
        int index;    // Loop control and index variable

        for (index = 0; index < NUM_STUDS; index++)
            failing[index] = false;
    }
```

3.
```
   void SetPassing( /* inout */    bool passing[],
                    /* in */    const int  score[]    )

   // Precondition:
   //     score[0..NUM_STUDS-1] are assigned
   // Postcondition:
   //     For all i, where 0 <= i <= NUM_STUDS-1,
   //         IF score[i] >= 60, THEN passing[i] == true

   {
        int index;    // Loop control and index variable

        for (index = 0; index < NUM_STUDS; index++)
            if (score[index] >= 60)
                passing[index] = true;
   }
```

8. Below, assume the input will never exceed 500 parts.

```
   const int MAX_PARTS = 500;

   struct PartType
   {
        int    number;
        float  cost;
   };

   PartType part[MAX_PARTS];
   int      count = 0;

   cin >> part[count].number >> part[count].cost;
   while (cin)
   {
        count++;
        cin >> part[count].number >> part[count].cost;
   }
```

11.
```
    void Copy( /* in */   const TwoDimType data,
               /* out */        TwoDimType data2 )

    // Precondition:
    //     data[0..NUM_ROWS-1][0..NUM_COLS-1] are assigned
    // Postcondition:
    //     data2[0..NUM_ROWS-1][0..NUM_COLS-1] ==
    //         corresponding elements of array "data"
```

```
    {
        int row;        // Loop control and index variable
        int col;        // Loop control and index variable

        for (row = 0; row < NUM_ROWS; row++)
            for (col = 0; col < NUM_COLS; col++)
                data2[row][col] = data[row][col];
    }
```

16. Below, assume `ArrayType` is a two-dimensional integer array type with `NUM_ROWS` rows and `NUM_COLS` columns.

```
int RowSum( /* in */ const ArrayType arr,
            /* in */       int        whichRow,
            /* in */       int        colsFilled )

// Precondition:
//      colsFilled <= NUM_COLS  &&  whichRow < NUM_ROWS
//   && arr[whichRow][0..colsFilled-1] are assigned
// Postcondition:
//      Function value == arr[whichRow][0] + ...
//                        + arr[whichRow][colsFilled-1]

    {
        int col;        // Loop control and index variable
        int sum = 0;    // Accumulating sum

        for (col = 0; col < colsFilled; col++)
            sum = sum + arr[whichRow][col];
        return sum;
    }
```

Chapter 12   Case Study Follow-Up

1. No. If `firstList` were declared to be a `const` parameter, the compiler would not allow the function body to modify the array. Specifically, the statement

```
firstList[counter] = number;
```

would generate a compile-time error.

5. Only two lines in the program need to be changed—the constant declarations for `NUM_PRECINCTS` and `NUM_CANDIDATES`:

```
const int NUM_PRECINCTS = 12;
const int NUM_CANDIDATES = 3;
```

Chapter 13   Exam Preparation Exercises

6. a. `typedef char NameType[41];`
   b. `NameType oneName;`
   c. `NameType employeeName[100];`

7. a. valid b. valid c. invalid d. valid e. valid f. invalid g. invalid h. valid
9. a. valid b. invalid c. valid d. invalid e. valid f. invalid g. valid

Chapter 13 `Programming Warm-up Exercises

2.
```
int List::Occurrences( /* in */ ItemType item )

// Precondition:
//     item is assigned
// Postcondition:
//     Function value == number of occurrences of value "item"
//                        in data[0..length-1]

{
    int index;          // Loop control and index variable
    int counter = 0;    // Number of occurrences of item

    for (index = 0; index < length; index++)
        if (data[index] == item)
            counter++;
    return counter;
}
```

8. The `SortedList::BinSearch` function remains the same until the last If statement. This statement should be replaced with the following:

```
if (found)
    position = middle;
else
    position = first;
```

Also, the function postcondition should read as follows:

```
//     IF item is in list
//         found == true  &&  data[position] contains item
//     ELSE
//         found == false  &&  position is where item belongs
```

10.
```
void SortedList::Component(
        /* in */  int      pos,      // Desired position
        /* out */ ItemType& item,    // Item retrieved
        /* out */ bool&     valid )  // True if pos is valid

// Precondition:
//     pos is assigned
// Postcondition:
//     IF 0 <= pos < length
//         valid == true
//       && item == data[pos]
//     ELSE
//         valid == false
```

```
                    {
                        valid = (pos >= 0 && pos < length);
                        if (valid)
                            item = data[pos];
                    }
```

Chapter 13 Case Study Follow-Up

3. Using a binary search, the number of loop iterations for an unsuccessful search of 200 items is 8 (because $\log_2 128 = 7$ and $\log_2 256 = 8$). Using a sequential search of a sorted list, the worst-case number of loop iterations is 200, the best case is 1 iteration, and the average is 100.

Chapter 14 Exam Preparation Exercises

2. False
4. *Class Abc:*
   a. The private data members are alpha and beta.
   b. Functions DoThis and DoThat can reference alpha and beta directly.
   c. Functions DoThis and DoThat can invoke each other directly.
   d. Clients can invoke DoThis.
   Class Xyz:
   a. The private data members are alpha, beta, and gamma.
   b. Function TryIt can reference only gamma directly.
   c. Function TryIt can invoke the parent class's DoThis function directly. The syntax for the function call is Abc::DoThis().
   d. Clients can invoke DoThis and TryIt.
7. a. Member slicing occurs, and static binding is used. The output is

   x

   y

   b. Member slicing does not occur, and dynamic binding is used. The output is

   x

   yz

   c. Member slicing does not occur, but static binding is used. The output is

   x

   y

9. a. False   b. True   c. False

Chapter 14 Programming Warm-up Exercises

```
2.   #include <cmath>    // For sqrt()
        ⋮
     float Line::Length() const

     // Postcondition:
     //      Function value == length of this line
```

```
    {
        float diffX;    // Difference in x coordinates
        float diffY;    // Difference in y coordinates

        diffX = startPt.X_Coord() - endPt.X_Coord();
        diffY = startPt.Y_Coord() - endPt.Y_Coord();
        return sqrt(diffX*diffX + diffY*diffY);
    }
```

3.
```
    class InterAddress : public Address
    {
    public:
        void Write() const;
            // Postcondition:
            //      Address has been output

        InterAddress( /* in */ string newStreet,
                      /* in */ string newCity,
                      /* in */ string newState,
                      /* in */ string newZip,
                      /* in */ string newCountry );
            // Precondition:
            //      All parameters are assigned
            // Postcondition:
            //      Class object is constructed with private data
            //      initialized by the incoming parameters
    private:
        string country;
    };
```

7.
```
    class TimeAndDay
    {
    public:
        void Set( /* in */ int hours,
                  /* in */ int minutes,
                  /* in */ int seconds,
                  /* in */ int month,
                  /* in */ int day,
                  /* in */ int year     );
            // Precondition:
            //      0 <= hours <= 23   &&   0 <= minutes <= 59
            //   && 0 <= seconds <= 59  &&  1 <= month <= 12
            //   && 1 <= day <= maximum no. of days in month
            //   && year > 1582
            // Postcondition:
            //      Time and date are set according to the
            //      incoming parameters

        void Increment();
            // Postcondition:
```

```
//      Time has been advanced by one second, with
//      23:59:59 wrapping around to 0:0:0
//   && IF new time is 0:0:0
//           Date has been advanced to the next day

   void Write() const;
      // Postcondition:
      //      Time and date have been output in the form
      //          HH:MM:SS  month day, year

   TimeAndDay();
      // Postcondition:
      //      Class object is constructed with a time of 0:0:0
      //      and a date of January 1, 1583
private:
   TimeType time;
   DateType date;
};
```

Chapter 15   Exam Preparation Exercises

4. The delete operation releases the space reserved for a dynamic variable back to the system.
5. a. inaccessible object b. dangling pointer c. dangling pointer d. neither e. inaccessible object
7. The correct answer is (a).
11. Constructor executing
    Private data is 1
    Destructor executing
    Constructor executing
    Private data is 2
    Destructor executing
    Constructor executing
    Private data is 3
    Destructor executing
13. The correct answer is (e).

Chapter 15   Programming Warm-up Exercises

1. a. char* p = &ch;
   b. long* q = arr;
      or
      long* q = &arr[0];
   c. BoxType* r = &box;

2. a. *p = '@';
   b. *q = 959263;
   c. r->length = 12;   (*r).length = 12;
      r->width = 14;   *or* (*r).width = 14;
      r->height = 5;   (*r).height = 5;
```
```

6.  ```
    if (*p < *q)
        smaller = *p;
    else
        smaller = *q;
    delete p;
    delete q;
    ```

10. ```
    AddAndIncr(m, &n, &theirSum);
    ```

Chapter 15   Case Study Follow-Up

4. Change the function headings for `ValueAt` and `Store` so that the data types match those in the function prototypes. The bodies of `ValueAt`, `Store`, and the destructor do not need to be changed. Change the bodies of the constructor, copy-constructor, and `CopyFrom` functions by replacing

    ```
    arr = new int[size];
    ```

    with

    ```
    arr = new float[size];
    ```

Chapter 16   Exam Preparation Exercises

2. True
5. Dynamic data structures can expand and contract during program execution.
8. a. array   b. array   c. dynamic linked list

Chapter 16   Programming Warm-up Exercises

1. Function specification (within the `SortedList2` class declaration):

    ```
    int Length() const;
        // Postcondition:
        //      Function value == number of components in list
    ```

    Function definition:

    ```
    int SortedList2::Length() const
    {
        NodePtr currPtr = head;    // Loop control pointer
        int     count = 0;         // Number of nodes in list

        while (currPtr != NULL)
        {
            count++;
            currPtr = currPtr->link;
        }
        return count;
    }
    ```

5. The function heading is

    ```
    void SortedList2::CopyFrom( /* in */ SortedList2 otherList )
    ```

    (with a corresponding function prototype in the class declaration). The function body begins by deallocating the linked list pointed to by the current class object:

    ```
    ComponentType temp;    // Temporary variable

    while ( !IsEmpty() )
        DeleteTop(temp);
    ```

    After this deallocation, the rest of the body is identical to the body of the copy-constructor.

Chapter 16   Case Study Follow-Up

1. a. The functions Length, CardAt, InsertTop, RemoveTop, Shuffle, Recreate, and the class constructor are public members of the CardDeck class.
    b. The variables head and listLength and the function Merge are private members of the CardDeck class.

Chapter 17   Exam Preparation Exercises

2. False. Both void functions and value-returning functions can be recursive.
4. $F(4) = 1$, $F(6) = -1$, and $F(5)$ is undefined.
6. A selection control structure—either an If or a Switch statement
9. The run-time stack

Chapter 17   Programming Warm-up Exercises

1.  ```
    int F( /* in */ int n )
    {
        if (n == 0 || n == 1)
            return 1;
        else
            return F(n - 1) + F(n - 2);
    }
    ```

3.  ```
    void DoubleSpace( /* inout */ ifstream& inFile )
    {
        char ch;

        inFile.get(ch);
        while (inFile)              // While not EOF...
        {
            cout << ch;
            if (ch == '\n')
                cout << endl;
            inFile.get(ch);
        }
    }
    ```

8. In the If statement of the `RevPrint` function, change the sequence

    ```
    RevPrint(head->link);                        // Recursive call
    cout << head->component << endl;
    ```

    to

    ```
    cout << head->component << endl;
    RevPrint(head->link);                        // Recursive call
    ```

    and reword the function postcondition accordingly.

Chapter 17   Case Study Follow-Up

2. 0, the index of the first array element. The recursive algorithm starts at the fifth element but recursively calls itself until it reaches the first element, which is stored into `minSoFar`; then it compares `minSoFar` to the second element, and so on.